HUANG'S

Catheter Ablation of Cardiac Arrhythmias

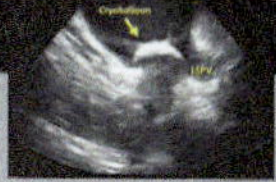
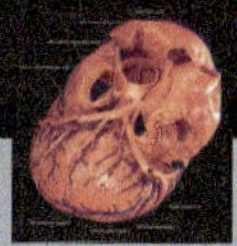
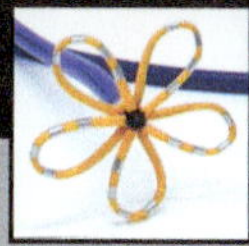
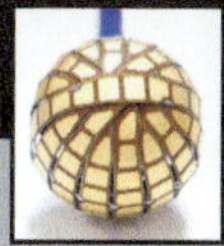
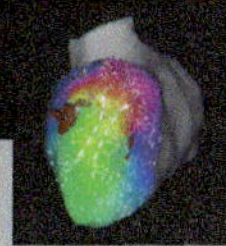

FIFTH EDITION

HUANG'S

Catheter Ablation of Cardiac Arrhythmias

Shoei K. Stephen Huang, MD, FHRS, FACC, FAHA

Professor Emeritus of Medicine and Former Director
Section of Cardiac Electrophysiology and Pacing
Texas A&M University Health Sciences Center
Temple, Texas

Jason S. Bradfield, MD, FHRS

Professor of Medicine
Associate Director
UCLA Cardiac Arrhythmia Center and EP Programs
Director
Specialized Program for Ventricular Tachycardia
UCLA Cardiac Arrhythmia Center
David Geffen School of Medicine at UCLA
Los Angeles, California

Kalyanam Shivkumar, MD, PhD

Professor of Medicine (Cardiology), Radiology and Bioengineering
Director
UCLA Cardiac Arrhythmia Center and EP Programs
Director and Chief
Cardiovascular and Interventional Programs
UCLA Health System
Editor-in-Chief
JACC: Clinical Electrophysiology
Los Angeles, California

ELSEVIER

Elsevier
1600 John F. Kennedy Blvd.
Ste 1800
Philadelphia, PA 19103-2899

HUANG'S CATHETER ABLATION OF CARDIAC ARRHYTHMIAS, FIFTH EDITION

ISBN: 978-0-323931106

Notice

Practitioners and researchers must always rely on their own experience and knowledge in evaluating and using any information, methods, compounds or experiments described herein. Because of rapid advances in the medical sciences, in particular, independent verification of diagnoses and drug dosages should be made. To the fullest extent of the law, no responsibility is assumed by Elsevier, authors, editors or contributors for any injury and/or damage to persons or property as a matter of products liability, negligence or otherwise, or from any use or operation of any methods, products, instructions, or ideas contained in the material herein.

Senior Content Strategist: Melanie Tucker
Senior Content Development Specialist: Vasowati Shome
Publishing Services Manager: Shereen Jameel
Senior Project Manager: Beula Christopher
Senior Designer: Renee Duenow

Printed in the United States of America by
Sheridan Kentucky, 100 US-60, Versailles, KY 40384
Last digit is the print number: 9 8 7 6 5 4 3

To my immediate family members,
including my dear wife, Su-Mei; my children, Priscilla, Melvin, and Jessica,
for all of their love, support, and sacrifice throughout my career;
to my beloved grandsons, Ethan, Titus, Miles, Philip, and Sammy;
and the first granddaughter, Lillian.

Additionally, I wish to dedicate this book to my unforgettable mentors,
Professors Pablo Denes, Robert Hauser, Gordon Ewy, Frank Marcus, and Joseph Alpert,
who have guided and inspired me throughout my training and career.

Shoei K. Stephen Huang, MD, FHRS, FACC, FAHA

To my wife Cindy, daughter Emersyn and son Hayden for being my inspiration
and to my parents, Laura and Robert (1926–2012) for their guidance.

Jason S. Bradfield, MD, FHRS

To the memory of my beloved parents, Ramanathan Kalyanam Iyer (1932–1992)
and Saraswathi Venkataraman Iyer (1934–2020). To my wife Preethi,
and our son Tejas, and my sister Nitya Kalyani.

Kalyanam Shivkumar, MD, PhD

CONTRIBUTORS

Amin Al-Ahmad, MD
Cardiac Electrophysiologist
Department of Cardiac Electrophysiology
Texas Cardiac Arrhythmia Institute
Austin, Texas

Jason G. Andrade, BSc, MD, FRCPC, FHRS
Associate Professor
Department of Medicine
University of British Columbia
Vancouver, British Columbia, Canada

Rishi Arora, MD
Professor of Medicine,
Director
Experimental Cardiac Electrophysiology,
Co-Director
Center for Arrhythmia Research
Feinberg Cardiovascular and Renal Research Institute
Northwestern University Feinberg School of Medicine
Chicago, Illinois

Arash Aryana, MD
Cardiac Electrophysiologist
Cardiac Arrhythmia Service
Mercy General Hospital and Dignity Health Heart and Vascular Institute
Sacramento, California

Nitish Badhwar, FACC, FHRS, FAHA
Director
Cardiac EP Training Program
Department of Medicine
Stanford University School of Medicine
Stanford, California

Mohamed Bassiouny, MD
Cardiac Electrophysiologist
Department of Cardiovascular Medicine, Electrophysiology Section
Texas Cardiac Arrhythmia
Austin, Texas

Shashank Behere, MD, CCDS
Assistant Professor
Section of Cardiology
Department of Pediatrics
Oklahoma University Health Sciences Center
Oklahoma City, Oklahoma

Aron Bender, MD
Cardiac Electrophysiologist
Department of Cardiology
University of California, Los Angeles
Los Angeles, California

Frank Bogun, MD
Professor of Medicine
Department of Internal Medicine
University of Michigan
Ann Arbor, Michigan

Stefano Bordignon, MD
Cardioangiologisches Centrum Bethanien (CCB)
Agaplesion Markus Hospital
Frankfurt, Germany

Jason S. Bradfield, MD, FHRS
Professor of Medicine,
Associate Director
UCLA Cardiac Arrhythmia Center and EP Programs;
Director
Specialized Program for Ventricular Tachycardia
UCLA Cardiac Arrhythmia Center
David Geffen School of Medicine at UCLA
Los Angeles, California

Eric Buch, MD
Professor of Medicine
Cardiac Arrhythmia Center
Division of Cardiology
University of California, Los Angeles
Los Angeles, California

J. David Burkhardt, MD
Director
Department of Electrophysiology
Texas Cardiac Arrhythmia
Austin, Texas

David J. Callans, MD
Associate Director of Electrophysiology
University of Pennsylvania Health System;
Professor of Medicine
Department of Medicine
University of Pennsylvania
Philadelphia, Pennsylvania

Jien-jiun Chen, MD
Attending Physician
Department of Internal Medicine
National Taiwan University Hospital, Yunliin Branch
DouLiu, Taiwan;
Clinical Assistant Professor of Medicine
College of Medicine
National Taiwan University
Taipei, Taiwan

Shaojie Chen, MD, PhD
Fellow
Department of Cardiology
Cardioangiologisches Centrum Bethanien (CCB)
Frankfurt am Main, Germany

Shih-Ann Chen, MD
Superintendent
Cardiovascular Center
Taichung Veterans General Hospital
Taichung, Taiwan;
Professor,
Faculty of Medicine
National Yang Ming Chiao Tung University;
Attending Physician
Department of Cardiology
Internal Medicine
Taipei Veterans General Hospital
Taipei, Taiwan;
Vice President
National Chung-Hsing University
Taichung, Taiwan

Christopher C. Cheung, MD, MPH, FRCPC
Assistant Professor
Department of Cardiology
University of Toronto
Toronto, Ontario, Canada

K.R. Julian Chun, MD
Head of Cardiology
Medizinische Klinik III
Cardioangiologisches Centrum (CCB)
Agaplesion Markus Hospital
Frankfurt, Germany

Wei-Hsin Chung, MD
UCLA Cardiac Arrhythmia Center
Ronald Reagan UCLA Medical Center
Los Angeles, California;
China Medical University Hospital
Taichung, Taiwan

Thomas Crawford, MD
Associate Professor of Medicine
Department of Internal Medicine
University of Michigan
Ann Arbor, Michigan

Robert D'Angelo, MD, MS
Fellow
Department of Cardiology
Beth Israel Deaconess Medical Center
Boston, Massachusetts

Andre d'Avila, MD, PhD
Director
Cardiac Arrhythmia Service
Beth Israel Deaconess Medical Center
Boston, Massachusetts

James P. Daubert, MD
Professor of Medicine
Department of Cardiology (Electrophysiology)
Duke University Medical Center
Durham, North Carolina

Mark J. Davies, MB, BChir, BSc (Hons), PhD
Consultant Cardiologist and Electrophysiologist
Department of Cardiology
Oxford University Hospitals NHS Foundation Trust
Oxford, United Kingdom

Luigi Di Biase, MD, PhD, FACC, FESC, FHRS
Section Head Electrophysiology
Professor of Medicine
Department of Cardiology
Albert Einstein College of Medicine at Montefiore Hospital
New York, New York;
Assistant Professor
Department of Biomedical Engineering
University of Texas
Austin, Texas

Juan Carlos Diaz, MD
Cardiologist and Electrophysiologist
Cardiac Arrhythmia and Electrophysiology Service
Clínica Las Vegas
Medellín, Colombia

Sanjay Dixit, MD
Professor
Department of Medicine
Hospital of The University of Pennsylvania
Philadelphia, Pennsylvania

Marc Dubuc, MD, FRCPC
Electrophysiologist
Electrophysiology Service
Department of Medicine
Montreal Heart Institute;
Associate Professor of Medicine
Department of Medicine
University of Montreal
Montreal, Quebec, Canada

Srinivas R. Dukkipati, MD
Co-Director
Cardiac Arrhythmia Service
Department of Cardiology
Icahn School of Medicine at Mount Sinai
New York, New York

Gregory K. Feld, MD
Professor of Medicine
Department of Cardiology
UCSD Health System
La Jolla, California

Lohit Garg, MD, FACC
Assistant Professor
Section of Electrophysiology
Division of Cardiology
University of Colorado School of Medicine
Aurora, Colorado

Alessio Gasperetti, MD, PhD
ARVC Post-Doctoral Fellow
Department of Cardiology,
Osler Housestaff
Department of Medicine
Johns Hopkins University
Baltimore, Maryland

Michael Ghannam, MD
Assistant Professor of Medicine
Department of Cardiovascular Medicine
University of Michigan
Ann Arbor, Michigan

Carola Gianni, MD, PhD
Texas Cardiac Arrhythmia Institute
St. David's Medical Center
Austin, Texas

Shana Greif, MD
Fellow Physician
Department of Electrophysiology
Stanford Health Care
Palo Alto, California

David E. Haines, MD
Professor
Department of Cardiovascular Medicine
Oakland University William Beaumont School of Medicine;
Director
Heart Rhythm Center
Department of Cardiovascular Medicine
William Beaumont University Hospital
Royal Oak, Michigan

Frederick T. Han, MD
Professor of Medicine
Department of Cardiovascular Medicine
University of California San Diego
La Jolla, California

Haris M. Haqqani, MBBS (Hons), PhD
Associate Professor
Faculty of Medicine
The University of Queensland;
Senior Electrophysiologist
Department of Cardiology
The Prince Charles Hospital
Brisbane, Australia

Justin Hayase, MD
Assistant Clinical Professor
Cardiac Arrhythmia Center
University of California Los Angeles
Los Angeles, California

Satoshi Higuchi, MD, PhD
Division of Cardiology
Section of Cardiac Electrophysiology
University of California San Francisco
San Francisco, California

Kurt S. Hoffmayer, MD, PharmD, FHRS
Division of Cardiology
Section of Cardiac Electrophysiology
University of California San Diego
San Diego, California

Rodney P. Horton, MD
Researcher
Department of Electrophysiology
Texas Cardiac Arrhythmia Institute
Austin, Texas

Henry H. Hsia, MD, FACC, FHRS
Professor of Medicine
Department of Electrophysiology, Cardiology
University of California San Francisco
San Francisco, California

Jonathan C. Hsu, MD, MAS
Professor
Department of Cardiac Electrophysiology
University of California San Diego
La Jolla, California

Weihow Hsue, DVM, DACVIM (Cardiology)
Assistant Professor
Department of Clinical Sciences
Cornell University College of Veterinary Medicine
Ithaca, New York

Shoei K. Stephen Huang, MD, FHRS, FACC, FAHA
Professor Emeritus of Medicine and Former Director
Section of Cardiac Electrophysiology and Pacing
Texas A&M University Health Sciences Center
Temple, Texas

Christopher Janson, MD
Assistant Professor
Department of Pediatrics
Perelman School of Medicine at the University of Pennsylvania
Philadelphia, Pennsylvania

Jonathan M. Kalman, MBBS, PhD
Director of Heart Rhythm Services
Department of Cardiology
Royal Melbourne Hospital;
Professor of Medicine
Department of Medicine
University of Melbourne
Melbourne, Australia

Mohamed H. Kanj, MD
Co-Director
Electrophysiology Laboratories
Robert and Suzanne Tomsich Department of Cardiovascular Medicine
Cleveland Clinic
Cleveland, Ohio

Rachel M. Kaplan, MD
Assistant Professor
Department of Cardiology
Medical University of South Carolina
Charleston, South Carolina

Iwanari Kawamura, MD
Assistant Professor
Department of Cardiology
Tokyo Medical and Dental University
Tokyo, Japan

Paul Khairy, MD, PhD
Professor of Medicine and André Chagnon Research Chair
Department of Cardiology
Montreal Heart Institute
Montreal, Quebec, Canada

Andy C. Kiser, MD, MBA
Physician-in-Chief
Cardiovascular Services
St. Clair Health;
Clinical Professor
Department of Cardiothoracic Surgery
University of Pittsburgh School of Medicine
Pittsburgh, Pennsylvania

Peter M. Kistler, PhD
Director of Electrophysiology
Department of Cardiology
Alfred Health
Melbourne, Australia

Bradley P. Knight, MD
Director of Electrophysiology
Department of Cardiology
Northwestern Medicine
Chicago, Illinois

Yuki Komatsu, MD, PhD
Associate Professor
Department of Cardiology
University of Tsukuba
Tsukuba, Japan

Jacob S. Koruth, MD
Assistant Professor of Medicine
Division of Cardiology
Mount Sinai Medical Center
New York, New York

Jamie L. Kowal, DO
Fellow
Department of Medicine
Division of Cardiovascular Medicine
Vanderbilt University Medical Center
Nashville, Tennessee

Bruce B. Lerman, MD
H. Altschul Master Professor of Medicine
Director
Greenberg Electrophysiology Institute;
Department of Medicine
Division of Cardiology
Cornell University Medical Center
New York Presbyterian Hospital
New York, New York

Jackson J. Liang, DO
Assistant Professor
Department of Cardiology
University of Michigan
Ann Arbor, Michigan

Lian-Yu Lin, MD, PhD
Professor
Division of Cardiology
Department of Internal Medicine
College of Medicine
National Taiwan University
Taipei, Taiwan

Ting-Tse Lin, MD, PhD
Attending Physician
Department of Internal Medicine
National Taiwan University Hospital
Taipei, Taiwan

Jeffrey C. Liu, MD, FHRS
Director
Cardiac electrophysiology
St. Clair Health
Pittsburgh, Pennsylvania

Li-Wei Lo, MD, PhD
Director
Heart Rhythm Center, Cardiovascular Center
Taipei Veterans General Hospital;
Professor
Faculty of Medicine
National Yang Ming Chiao Tung University
Taipei, Taiwan

Qing Lou, PhD
Principal Scientist
Cardiac Ablation Solution
Medtronic
Cleveland, Ohio

Varun Malik, MBBS (Hons), BMedSci (Hons), FRACP, PhD
Visiting Faculty
UCLA Cardiac Arrhythmia Center
University of California Los Angeles
Los Angeles, California;
Cardiologist and Cardiac Electrophysiologist
Centre for Heart Rhythm Disorders
University of Adelaide
Adelaide, Australia

Steven M. Markowitz, MD
Professor of Medicine
Department of Medicine
Weill Cornell Medical College
New York, New York

Nishaki K. Mehta, MD, FACC, FHRS, FAHA
Associate Professor
Department of Cardiovascular Medicine
Oakland University William Beaumont School of Medicine
Royal Oak, Michigan;
Adjunct Faculty
Department of Cardiovascular Medicine
University of Virginia
Charlottesville, Virginia

Gregory F. Michaud, MD
Director
Ventricular Tachycardia Ablation Program
Department of Cardiology
Massachusetts General Hospital
Boston, Massachusetts

John M. Miller, MD
Professor of Medicine
Department of Medicine
Indiana University School of Medicine;
Director
Cardiac Electrophysiology Services;
Department of Medicine
Indiana University Health
Indianapolis, Indiana

Jay A. Montgomery, MD
Associate Professor
Department of Medicine
Vanderbilt University Medical Center
Nashville, Tennessee

Jeremy P. Moore, MD, MS
Professor
Department of Pediatrics
Division of Pediatric Cardiology
University of California Los Angeles
Los Angeles, California

Shumpei Mori, MD, PhD
Department of Cardiology
Cardiac Arrhythmia Center
University of California Los Angeles
Los Angeles, California

Joshua D. Moss, MD
Professor of Clinical Medicine
Department of Cardiology-Electrophysiology
University of California San Francisco
San Francisco, California

Daniele Muser, MD
Adjunct Assistant Professor of Medicine
Division of Cardiac Electrophysiology
Department of Cardiovascular Medicine
Hospital of the University of Pennsylvania
Philadelphia, Pennsylvania;
Assistant Professor of Medicine
Department of Cardiac Electrophysiology
Humanitas University
Milan, Italy

Koonlawee Nademanee, MD
Professor of Medicine
Department of Medicine
Chulalongkorn University;
Director
Department of Cardiology
Heart Institute at Bumrungrad International Hospital
Bangkok, Thailand

Dustin Nash, MD
Cardiology Fellow
Department of Pediatrics
Children's Hospital of Philadelphia
Philadelphia, Pennsylvania

Andrea Natale, MD
Executive Medical Director
Texas Cardiac Arrhythmia Institute
St. David's Medical Center
Austin, Texas

Antoine Noel, MD, MSc
Fellow
Department of Electrophysiology
Montreal Heart Institute
Montreal, Quebec, Canada

Akihiko Nogami, MD, PhD
Professor
Department of Cardiology
University of Tsukuba, Tsukuba
Ibaraki, Japan;
President
Tokyo Heart Rhythm Hospital
Tokyo, Japan

Connor Oates, MD
Helmsley Center for Cardiac Electrophysiology
Icahn School of Medicine at Mount Sinai
New York, New York

Adam Oesterle, MD
Division of Cardiology
Department of Medicine
University of California San Francisco
Veterans Affairs Health Care System
San Francisco, California

Hakan Oral, MD
Professor of Internal Medicine
Department of Internal Medicine
Frederick G.L. Huetwell Professor of Cardiovascular Medicine
Department of Cardiovascular Medicine
Director
Cardiac Arrhythmia Service
University of Michigan
Ann Arbor, Michigan

Bhupesh Pathik, MBBS
Department of Cardiology
Royal Melbourne Hospital
Melbourne, Australia

Farshad Raissi, MD, MPH
Associate Professor
Department of Cardiovascular Medicine
University of California San Diego
La Jolla, California

Vivek Y. Reddy, MD
Helmsley Trust Professor of Medicine
Department of Cardiac Electrophysiology
Mount Sinai Medical Center
New York, New York

Melissa R. Robinson, MD
Clinical Associate Professor of Medicine
Department of Medicine
University of Washington
Seattle, Washington

Jorge E. Romero, MD, FACC, FHRS
Director
Arrhythmia and Electrophysiology Research;
Associate Director
Ventricular Arrhythmia Program
Department of Cardiac Electrophysiology
Brigham and Women's Hospital
Boston, Massachusetts

Javier E. Sanchez, MD
Texas Cardiac Arrhythmia Institute
St. David's Medical Center
Austin, Texas

Pasquale Santangeli, MD, PhD
Cardiac Electrophysiologist
Section of Electrophysiology
Division of Cardiovascular
Cleveland Clinic
Cleveland, Ohio

Melvin M. Scheinman, MD
Professor of Medicine
Department of Cardiology
University of California San Francisco
San Francisco, California

Boris Schmidt, MD, FHRS
Professor of Medicine
Agaplesion Markus Hospital
Cardioangiologisches Centrum Bethanien
Frankfurt, Germany

Maully Shah, MBBS
Director of Electrophysiology
Department of Pediatrics
Children's Hospital of Philadelphia
Philadelphia, Pennsylvania

Siddharth P. Shah, MD
Cardiac Electrophysiology Fellow
Department of Cardiovascular Medicine/Cardiac Electrophysiology
Indiana University School of Medicine
Indianapolis, Indiana

Kalyanam Shivkumar, MD, PhD
Professor of Medicine (Cardiology), Radiology and Bioengineering;
Director
UCLA Cardiac Arrhythmia Center and EP Programs;
Director and Chief
Cardiovascular and Interventional Programs
UCLA Health System;
Editor-in-Chief
JACC: Clinical Electrophysiology
Los Angeles, California

Konstantinos C. Siontis, MD
Assistant Professor
Department of Cardiovascular Medicine
Mayo Clinic
Rochester, Minnesota

Kyoko Soejima, MD
Professor of Medicine
Department of Cardiovascular Medicine
Kyorin University
Tokyo, Japan

Chandra Srinivasan, MD
Associate Professor
Department of Pediatrics
The Children's Hospital of Philadelphia, University of Pennsylvania
Philadelphia, Pennsylvania

Wilber Su, MD
Division of Cardiology
Banner - University, Medical Center Phoenix
University of Arizona
College of Medicine
Phoenix, Arizona

Takeki Suzuki, MD, MPH, PhD, MBA
Associate Professor
Department of Medicine
Indiana University
Indianapolis, Indiana

Hiroshi Tada, MD, PhD
Professor
Department of Cardiovascular Medicine Faculty of Medical Sciences
University of Fukui
Yoshida-gun, Japan

Tanyanan Tanawuttiwat, MD, MPH
Associate Professor
Department of Medicine
School of Medicine
Indiana University
Indianapolis, Indiana

Harikrishna Tandri, MD
Professor
Department of Medicine
Johns Hopkins University
Baltimore, Maryland

Patrick Tchou, MD
Cardiovascular Medicine
Heart and Vascular Institute
Cleveland Clinic
Cleveland, Ohio

Shota Tohoku, MD
Medical Doctor
Department of Cardiology
CCB Markus-Krankenhaus
Frankfurt, Germany

Cory M. Tschabrunn, PhD
Assistant Professor of Medicine
Division of Cardiovascular Medicine
University of Pennsylvania Perelman School of Medicine
Philadelphia, Pennsylvania

Roderick Tung, MD, FACC, FHRS
Professor of Medicine, Chief
Division of Cardiology;
Director
Banner Heart Institute;
Co-Director
Banner Health CV Service Line;
Director
Cardiovascular Clinical Research
The University of Arizona College of Medicine
Phoenix, Arizona

Wendy S. Tzou, MD, FACC, FHRS
Associate Professor of Medicine
Director of Cardiac Electrophysiology
Department of Medicine
Division of Cardiology
Electrophysiology Section
University of Colorado Anschutz Medical Campus
Aurora, Colorado

Akiko Ueda, MD, PhD
Associate Professor
Division of Advanced Arrhythmia Management
Department of Cardiovascular Medicine
Kyorin University Hospital
Mitaka-City, Japan

Jeremiah Wasserlauf, MD, MS
Cardiac Electrophysiologist
Department of Cardiology
North Shore University Health System
Evanston, Illinois

William Whang, MD, MS
Associate Professor
Department of Medicine
Icahn School of Medicine at Mount Sinai
New York, New York

PREFACE

(Shoei K. Stephen Huang)

On behalf of all the authors, I warmly welcome you to the fifth edition of *Huang's Catheter Ablation of Cardiac Arrhythmias*. This textbook represents the culmination of cutting-edge research, clinical expertise, and collective efforts by a dedicated team of healthcare professionals, cardiologists, and electrophysiologists. We aim to provide a comprehensive resource that probes into the intricacies of cardiac arrhythmias and their treatment through catheter ablation.

Albert Einstein rightly said, "The more I learn, the more I realize how much I don't know." We should also heed Abigail Adams' inspiring words, "Learning is not attained by chance; it must be sought for with ardor and diligence."

In the rapidly evolving field of cardiac electrophysiology, arrhythmia management has become increasingly complex and multidisciplinary. As such, our book will serve as a timely resource that imparts practical knowledge and fosters a holistic understanding of changing practices related to new mapping and ablation technologies. We have endeavored to create a clear road map for both newcomers and seasoned professionals to navigate the ever-expanding and shifting landscape of cardiac arrhythmia ablation.

Significant changes in this edition include the addition of several innovative chapters and insights from new authors, particularly regarding atrial fibrillation and ventricular tachycardias. We also removed obsolete content and updated every chapter to match the latest knowledge and application of ablation technologies.

Below are key features and topics covered in this textbook:

1. **Comprehensive Coverage:** We begin with the basics, covering the fundamental principles of cardiac electrophysiology, arrhythmia mechanisms, diagnosis, and the anatomy of the heart with numerous detailed topographic figures. The "key points" of each chapter, differential diagnosis, mapping, ablation techniques, targets for ablation, clinical outcomes, troubleshooting difficult cases, etc., are all systematically laid out to facilitate reading and maximize understanding.
2. **Biophysics of Contemporary Energy Sources for Catheter Ablation:** In addition to detailed descriptions of the biophysics of existing radiofrequency and cryothermal ablation energy, newer endoscopic laser and pulsed-field (electroporation) nonthermal ablations are also included to help understand the mechanisms of lesion formation, as well as the pros and cons of each of energy source.
3. **Ablation Techniques and Technologies:** Detailed discussions on catheter ablation techniques for each cardiac arrhythmia are woven throughout this textbook, including new strategies for atrial fibrillation ablation, ventricular tachycardia ablation, and more. A standalone chapter features a focused discussion on pulsed-field ablation and laser balloons for pulmonary vein isolation. We also explore the newest three-dimensional high-resolution mapping systems and imaging technologies.
4. **Patient Evaluation:** We delve into patient selection, preprocedural assessment, and perioperative care to help promote a holistic understanding of the ablation process.
5. **Clinical Insights:** Clinical pearls and expert insights are interspersed throughout the chapters. Some insightful procedural videos are included to illustrate key concepts and enhance your practical knowledge.
6. **Emerging Trends:** As the field of arrhythmia ablation continues to evolve, we highlight the latest advancements and future direction of catheter-based therapies.

We have crafted this textbook to cater to and reach a broad audience, from cardiology fellows and electrophysiology trainees to practicing clinicians and allied healthcare providers. Each chapter is designed to build upon the previous ones, offering a structured and intuitive learning experience. We believe this book will be an essential study tool in preparing for the exams of the Board of Clinical Cardiac Electrophysiology.

We have drawn deeply from our extensive and varied experiences and are pleased to offer this resource to inspire, educate, and empower healthcare professionals in the field of arrhythmia management for years to come. We trust this textbook will be a valuable companion in your journey to understanding and mastering the art and science of catheter ablation of cardiac arrhythmias.

With joy and thanks,
Shoei K. Stephen Huang, MD, FHRS, FACC, FAHA

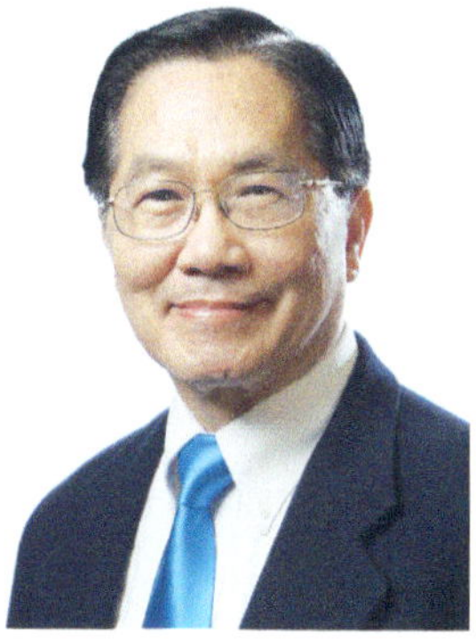

PREFACE

(Jason S. Bradfield and Kalyanam Shivkumar)

"The textbook" that cardiac electrophysiology fellows tend to read from cover to cover is *Huang's Catheter Ablation of Cardiac Arrhythmias*. This is indeed the book we have read and have recommended to our trainees for several years. It was therefore a great honor when Dr. Huang invited us to take over the role played by the previous coeditor and one of our beloved mentors and friends, Dr. John Miller.

We have structured the fifth edition of this book to include new content on cardiac anatomy and ablation technology while maintaining the incredibly well-written descriptions of the clinical and procedural evaluation of cardiac arrhythmias. Although the field of clinical cardiac electrophysiology and the associated technology continues to evolve rapidly, we believe that having a reliable and comprehensive reference is essential to those going through training or for physicians in practice dealing with complex clinical questions. Most importantly, that reference must provide the needed information in an understandable and accessible way, and we hope the readers, especially our younger colleagues, enjoy the fifth edition of this classic textbook.

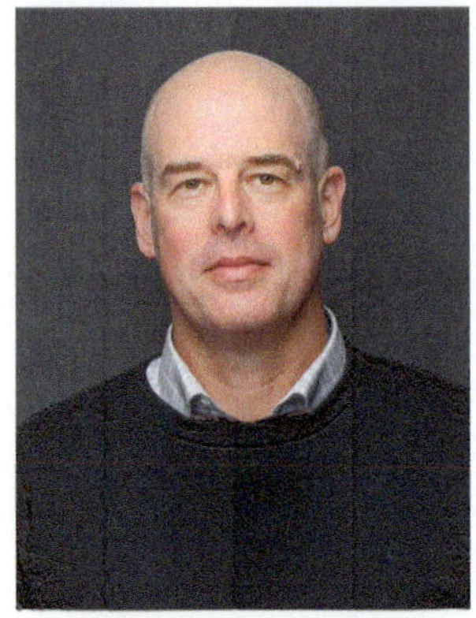

Jason S. Bradfield, MD, FHRS

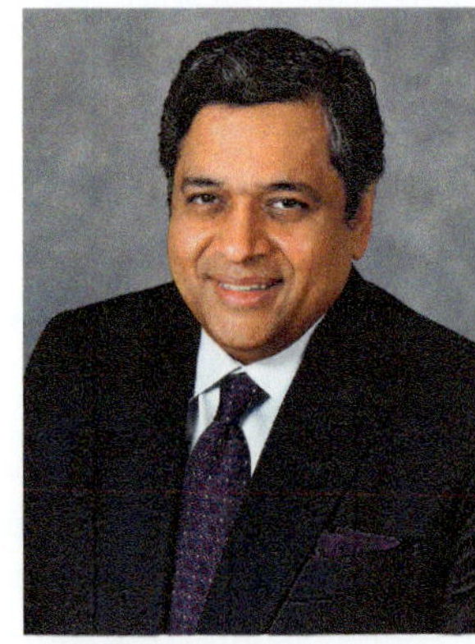

Kalyanam Shivkumar, MD, PhD

ACKNOWLEDGMENTS

I sincerely appreciate the extraordinary dedication of all the authors and contributors to this book. I particularly thank those new authors for their incredible efforts in making this updated edition possible.

Moreover, I am very grateful to Dr. Jason Bradfield for his hard work in assisting with the initial review/edit of many chapters of this textbook. I am also very much indebted to Dr. Kalyanam Shivkumar for his coordination of the authors and chapters.

Finally, special gratitude goes to Elsevier's wonderful staff – especially this book's publisher and Senior Content Strategist, Melanie Tucker; Senior Content Development Specialist, Vasowati Shome; and Senior Project Managers, Beula Christopher and Baljinder Kaur – all of whom exhibited the highest level of professionalism in shepherding this book to successful publication.

Shoei K. Stephen Huang, MD, FHRS, FACC, FAHA

CONTENTS

VIDEO CONTENTS

PART 1 Fundamental Concepts of Transcatheter Energy Delivery

1 Biophysics and Pathophysiology of Radiofrequency Lesion Formation

Video 1.1. Infrared thermal imaging of tissue heating during radiofrequency ablation with a closed irrigation catheter as seen from the surface of the tissue. Power is delivered at 30 W to blocks of porcine myocardium in a tissue bath. The surface of the tissue is just above the fluid level to permit thermal imaging of tissue and not the fluid. Temperature scale *(right)* and a millimeter scale *(top)* are shown in each panel.

Video 1.2. Infrared thermal imaging of tissue heating during radiofrequency ablation with a closed irrigation catheter as seen in cross section. Power is delivered at 30 W to blocks of porcine myocardium in a tissue bath. The surface of the tissue is just above the fluid level to permit thermal imaging of tissue and not the fluid. Temperature scale *(right)* and a millimeter scale *(top)* are shown in each panel.

2 Biophysics and Clinical Applications of Cryoablation

Video 2.1. Technical aspects of pulmonary vein isolation using Medtronic Arctic Front cryoballoon.

3 Biophysics and Clinical Applications of Laser Ablation

Video 3.1. Single-sweep pulmonary vein isolation with the X3 laser balloon. Graphic user interface of the endoscopic ablation system with a view at the RSPV ostium. There is complete circumferential balloon to tissue contact (no blood spilling). The shaft of the balloon catheter is located superior (10–1 o'clock). At first the laser generator is retracted to visualize the tissue exposure behind the shaft. Then the path of the laser beam is simulated by manually advancing the beam around the catheter shaft to ensure ablation in tissue rather than in blood. Finally, the application is started in RAPID model (e.g., the laser beam is continuously advanced in a clockwise fashion at a constant speed to deliver a full circular lesion set).

Video 3.2. Prerecorded live case of pulmonary vein isolation in a patient with symptomatic atrial fibrillation.

PART 2 Cardiac Mapping and Imaging

6 Cardiac Anatomy for Catheter Mapping and Ablation of Arrhythmias

Video 6.1. Progressive real dissection of the heart viewed from the right anterior oblique direction. Refer to Figs. 6.1 to 6.12.

Video 6.2. Progressive virtual dissection of the heart viewed from the left anterior oblique direction. Refer to Figs. 6.13 to 6.25.

Video 6.3. Rotational image of the three-dimensional virtual atrioventricular conduction system. Refer to Fig. 6.26.

Video 6.4. Consecutive histology slides of the sample involving the atrioventricular conduction axis. Refer to Figs. 6.27 and 6.28.

8 Fundamentals of Catheter Three-Dimensional Mapping Systems

Video 8.1. Ripple map of ventricular tachycardia (case shown in Fig. 8.5).

Video 8.2. Coherent map of ventricular tachycardia (case shown in Fig. 8.5).

Video 8.3. Activation map during left ventricular pacing (case shown in Fig. 8.6).

Video 8.4. Ventricular tachycardia activation map (case shown in Fig. 8.6).

10 Intracardiac Echocardiography, Computed Cardiac Tomography, and Magnetic Resonance Imaging for Guiding Mapping and Ablation

Video 10.1. Example of atrial ICE "survey." From the "home position" in mid-right atrium, clockwise rotation to the ICE catheter brings into sequential view: the anterior left atrium; the mitral valve and left atrial appendage (LAA); the left pulmonary veins (PVs); the posterior LA wall; and the right PVs.

Video 10.2. Example of direct visualization of left atrial structures with the ICE probe positioned within the left atrium. The ICE catheter can be advanced in the left atrium via a patent foramen ovale or within the same transseptal access used for mapping/ablation.

Video 10.3. ICE-guided LAA occlusion. Images are obtained with the ICE probe advanced to the left atrium. The delivery sheath is positioned coaxially to the LAA ostium and the device is deployed.

Video 10.4. Example of utilization of the CARTO Sound module to facilitate epicardial ablation of a VT substrate adjacent to the left phrenic nerve. An epicardial balloon is deployed in the pericardial space to mechanically displace the left phrenic nerve. The position of the ablation catheter on ICE is highlighted with a *green marker*, proving contact with the underlying epicardium and adequate separation with the parietal pericardium.

Video 10.5. Example of visualization of abnormal anteroseptal substrate with ICE and real-time monitoring of contact between the mapping multipolar grid catheter and the endocardium.

PART 3 Catheter Ablation of Atrial Tachycardias and Flutters

12 Ablation of Cavotricuspid Isthmus–Dependent Atrial Flutters

Video 12.1. Acutus map of typical AFL. RAO (*left panel*) and LAO caudal view (*right panel*) and LAO (*right panel*) views of the RA are shown during CCW typical atrial flutter. This is a noncontact map obtained with

Video 14.7. Atriotomy circuit in a patient undergoing pulmonary vein isolation for atrial fibrillation. Extrapulmonary vein substrates are often present in patients with congenital heart disease and should be targeted concurrently at procedures performed for atrial fibrillation.

Video 14.8. Example of counterclockwise cavotricuspid isthmus–dependent intra-atrial reentrant tachycardia in a patient after the Mustard operation. Following catheter ablation at the cavotricuspid isthmus on either side of the surgical baffle, a slower clockwise atriotomy circuit was induced and was also targeted for catheter ablation.

Video 14.9. Biatrial tachycardia after the Senning operation. A large macroreentrant circuit is shown traversing a posteroinferior isthmus below the expected location of the surgical counterincision and anastomosis that is part of this operative strategy.

Video 14.10. Catheter ablation for intra-atrial reentrant tachycardia after the atriopulmonary Fontan operation. The tachycardia circuit passes through a gap in a prior catheter ablation line where it was successfully interrupted with lesions placed to avoid the nearby phrenic nerve.

Video 14.11. Example of a commonly encountered tachycardia circuit after the lateral tunnel Fontan operation. The wavefront passes below scar at the free wall of the morphologic right atrium (within the lateral tunnel) where it was successfully targeted by catheter ablation. The pulmonary venous atrium was a bystander to the reentrant tachycardia.

Video 14.12. Example of intra-atrial reentry after the extracardiac Fontan operation. Although the tachycardia circuit is relatively straightforward, access to the pulmonary venous atrium can be challenging and requires congenital interventional experience.

Video 14.13. Example of biatrial reentry after the Bjork Fontan. The tachycardia wavefront can be seen passing to the morphologic left atrium through the coronary sinus and reentering the right atrium through the expected location of Bachmann bundle.

PART 4 Catheter Ablation of Atrial Fibrillation

15 Pulmonary Vein Isolation Using Radiofrequency Energy Ablation Technologies

Video 15.1. Intracardiac echocardiographic view showing a transseptal puncture.

Video 15.2. Intracardiac echocardiographic view of the left atrium, panning from the mitral valve to the right pulmonary veins.

Video 15.3. Small pericardial effusion as shown on intracardiac echocardiographic view (left ventricle and right ventricle).

16 Pulmonary Vein Isolation by Cryoballoon Catheter

Video 16.1. Complete cryoballoon ablation case from groin access to all pulmonary vein isolation with commentary using intracardiac echocardiogram and three-dimensional mapping system.

PART 5 Catheter Ablation of Atrioventricular Nodal Reentry Tachycardia and the Atrioventricular Junction

25 Ablation/Modification of Atrioventricular Junction for Heart Rate Control of Permanent Atrial Fibrillation

Video 25.1. Atrioventricular junction ablation by right-sided approach in a patient with drug-refractory atrial fibrillation. A VVIR pacemaker was implanted initially and was set to VOO mode. Distal bipole of ablation catheter recorded an atrial (A)–to–ventricular (V) electrogram ratio of 1:1.5 and a small His potential (H). The proximal bipole of ablation catheter recorded only A without V signal. An accelerated junctional rhythm followed by backup ventricular pacing at 40 per minute developed within 15 seconds after radiofrequency energy was delivered.

PART 6 Catheter Ablation of Accessory Atrioventricular Connections

26 Ablation of Free Wall Accessory Pathways

Video 26.1. Video in right anterior oblique and left anterior oblique views for ablation of a left free wall accessory pathway via the aortic left ventricular retrograde approach. After crossing the aortic valve, the catheter is turned counterclockwise to rotate the tip posteriorly toward the mitral valve annulus, which is identified approximately by the coronary sinus catheter. The catheter flexion is then opened on the annulus. The catheter can be turned to the proper position sitting on the annulus. To give a lesion, the catheter may be placed just under the annulus on the ventricular side. Once it is positioned under the mitral annulus, it is usually not freely movable.

Video 26.2. Video in right anterior oblique and left anterior oblique views for ablation of a left free wall accessory pathway via the transseptal approach. After crossing the interatrial septum, the catheter is kept curved as it maps along the mitral annulus, which is identified approximately by the coronary sinus catheter. The catheter can be turned anteriorly or posteriorly to position more on the ventricular or atrial side of the annulus. Catheter contact can be adjusted by opening and closing the flexion of the catheter and by moving the sheath up and down.

Video 26.3. Video in right anterior oblique and left anterior oblique views for ablation of a right free wall accessory pathway. The tricuspid annulus is marked approximately by a 20-electrode halo catheter. The ablation catheter is moved along the annulus using the sheath to keep it along the annulus. For posterior-lateral to lateral pathways an SR-1 or SR-2 sheath may be helpful.

Video 26.4. Map was produced using the 64-electrode Intellamap Orion catheter manufactured by Boston Scientific MA on the Rhythmia HD system.

PART 7 Catheter Ablation of Ventricular Tachycardias

32 Ablation of Idiopathic Left and Right Ventricular and Fascicular Tachycardias

Video 32.1. Propagation map during verapamil-sensitive left fascicular ventricular tachycardia (VT). Although the earliest myocardial activation site was observed at the inferoapical septum, diastolic potential could not be recorded in this patient. Because radiofrequency (RF) energy applications to the exit site and a linear RF lesion about 10 mm proximal to the VT exit were ineffective, more proximal linear lesion was applied.

Video 32.2. Propagation map during the nonreentrant fascicular ventricular tachycardia (VT) with right bundle branch block and left-axis deviation. Tags indicate the sites with the presystolic Purkinje potential during VT. The earliest Purkinje potential was recorded at the basal inferior wall, and radiofrequency current delivered to this site suppressed the VT.

33 Ablation of Ventricular Tachycardia in Coronary Artery Disease

Video 33.1. Intracardiac echocardiography (ICE) clip displaying the left ventricular long axis section as seen from the ICE catheter placed in the basal right ventricle. The HD Grid multipolar catheter is placed in basal inferoseptal left ventricle underneath the posteromedial papillary muscle, in close proximity to a false tendon. The catheter is in good contact with the left ventricular endocardium and was not causing any ectopy during mapping in this location.

37 Epicardial Approach to Catheter Ablation of Ventricular Tachycardia

Video 37.1. Pericardial tenting. Use of fluoroscopy and contrast to visualize tenting and puncture of pericardium with entry into the pericardial space.

Video 37.2. Pericardial wire. Importance of lateral anterior oblique view to confirm wire entry into the pericardial to the left lateral heart border, which excludes inadvertent right ventricular puncture.

41 Hybrid Approaches for Catheter Ablation of Ventricular Tachycardia

Video 41.1. Thoracotomy with epicardial mapping. View of the directly exposed anterolateral left ventricle (*left video*) and infarcted zone (*middle video*). Direct mapping with HD Grid (Abbott, Chicago, IL; *arrow*) on the surface of epicardium (*right video*).

Video 41.2. Epicardial mapping and termination of ventricular tachycardia. Demonstrates the propagation map during ventricular tachycardia with a slow conduction zone over the *light blue dot* area where diastolic potential was obtained. Ablation with cryothermal energy resulted in prolongation of the cycle length of tachycardia from 659 ms to 709 ms and termination of VT during ablation.

Video 41.3. CryoICE catheter (AtriCure). Shows that the catheter can be shaped using the provided tool or manually to optimize contact on the epicardial surface (*left video*). *Middle video* demonstrated the stability of CryoICE catheter during cryothermal ablation. The *right video* shows that the lesion was created immediately and 5 minutes after ablation.

PART 8 Miscellaneous Topics

43 Atrial Transseptal Catheterization

Video 43.1. The virtual fluoroscopic rotational image with shell-like reconstructions of the right atrium, left atrium, bronchi, and proximal aorta. (Refer to Fig. 43.7.)

Video 43.2. Phased-array intracardiac echocardiography image showing a large thrombus attached to the transseptal sheath during tenting of the fossa ovalis. (Refer to Fig. 43.11.)

Video 43.3. Fluoroscopic cine loops in the right anterior oblique and left anterior oblique projections demonstrating transseptal catheterization under fluoroscopic guidance. Contrast medium is injected through the Brockenbrough needle to demonstrate tenting of the interatrial septum. Contrast washout within the left atrium is shown after needle crossing. (Refer to Fig. 43.17.)

Video 43.4. Progressive virtual dissection of the heart viewed from the right anterior oblique direction. (Refer to Figs. 43.18, 43.19.)

Video 43.5. Progressive virtual dissection of the heart viewed from the left anterior oblique direction. (Refer to Figs. 43.18, 43.19.)

Video 43.6. Mechanical or radial intracardiac echocardiography clip taken during transseptal catheterization. Tenting of the fossa ovalis is seen. (Refer to Fig. 43.20.)

Video 43.7. A baseline survey of the atrial anatomy is routinely performed before transseptal catheterization. The phased-array intracardiac echocardiography catheter is rotated in a clockwise fashion from the initial mid right atrium (i.e., "home" view). (Refer to Fig. 43.21.)

Video 43.8. Sequential phased-array intracardiac echocardiography clips demonstrating different orientations of the transseptal apparatus. (Refer to Fig. 43.23.)

Video 43.9. Phased-array intracardiac echocardiography clip showing a patent foramen ovale. The corresponding color Doppler clip is shown in the *right panel.* (Refer to Fig. 43.24.)

Video 43.10. Phased-array intracardiac echocardiography clip demonstrating a large aneurysm of the interatrial septum. (Refer to Fig. 43.25.)

Video 43.11. A double interatrial septum imaged with phased-array intracardiac echocardiography. Note the echodense substance present within the lumen bounded by the two surfaces of the septum. (Refer to Fig. 43.26.)

Video 43.12. Phased-array intracardiac echocardiography clip from a patient with a prior transseptal catheterization for atrial fibrillation ablation. Note the heterogeneity in thickness of the fossa ovalis, which tapers significantly toward its inferior margin. (Refer to Fig. 43.28.)

Video 43.13. Phased-array intracardiac echocardiography clip taken from transseptal catheterization in a patient with a septal occlusion device. Note the region of intact fossa ovalis at the inferior margin of the device. Tenting of the transseptal sheath is seen in this region. (Refer to Fig. 43.29.)

Video 43.14. Fluoroscopy cine loops (right anterior oblique and left anterior oblique projections) taken during transseptal catheterization facilitated by the SafeSept transseptal guidewire (Pressure Products, San Pedro, CA). (Refer to Fig. 43.33.)

Video 43.15. Phased-array intracardiac echocardiography clip taken from transseptal catheterization facilitated by the NRG radiofrequency transseptal needle (Baylis Medical, Montreal, Canada). Note the characteristic echo artifact and microbubble formation during radiofrequency application. (Refer to Fig. 43.34.)

44 Special Considerations for Ablation in Pediatric Patients

Video 44.1. This video is the same geometry as Fig. 44.10 but with a propagation map using the CARTO 3 system (Biosense Webster Inc., Diamond Bar, CA). The *green* represents the wave propagation, with the wavefront on the atrial geometry. The wavefronts collide at the marked "collision." The His bundle and the CS are labeled. In this case, there was a good correlation between the area of wavefront collision and the low-voltage bridge where successful SP ablation was performed.

Video 44.2. The video depicts the same geometry as Fig. 44.15B. Open window propagation map of AVRT using the Ensite X system (Abbott Inc.) in the same patient is shown. The *white* represents the AVRT wave propagation via left cAP, with the wavefront on the purple atrial geometry, proceeding in the direction of the *arrows*. *cAP,* Concealed accessory pathway.

Video 44.3. The video depicts the same geometry as Fig. 44.15B. Open window SparkleMap (Ensite X system, Abbott Inc.) replays AVRT via left cAP with a representation of the activation proceeding in the direction of the arrows overlaying the voltage map on the three-dimensional geometry model. A full RF lesion set at the site of successful AP elimination is shown. *cAP,* Concealed accessory pathway.

Video 44.4. The video depicts the same geometry as Fig. 44.29B. Propagation map of right atrial appendage tachycardia generated with Advisor HD Grid using Ensite X Cardiac Mapping System and VoXel Mode (Abbott Inc.). The *white* represents the focal atrial tachycardia wave propagation from the tip of the atrial appendage on the *purple* atrial geometry.

Video 44.5. Vector SparkleMap (Ensite X, Abbott Inc.) shows the right AA tachycardia with a representation of the activation on the three-dimensional geometry model shown in Fig. 44.29B. Wavefront is shown proceeding in the direction of the *arrows*.

Video 44.6. Termination of right atrial appendage tachycardia with TactiCath irrigated-tip Contact Force Ablation Catheter, Sensor Enabled (Abbott Inc.) at 4 seconds. Termination occurred with power of 30 W, and catheter had contact force of 7*g*. Note change in P wave from negative to positive in lead V_1.

Video 44.7. Intracardiac echocardiography (CartoSound, Biosense Webster Inc.) used for anatomical visualization and catheter contact with right ventricular moderator band during ventricular tachycardia ablation in patient shown in Fig. 44.32.

PART 1

Fundamental Concepts of Transcatheter Energy Delivery

1

Biophysics and Pathophysiology of Radiofrequency Lesion Formation

Nishaki K. Mehta, David E. Haines

KEY POINTS

- Radiofrequency (RF) energy induces thermal lesion formation through resistive heating of myocardial tissue. Tissue temperatures of 50°C or higher are necessary for irreversible injury.
- Under controlled conditions, RF lesion size increases with increasing delivered power, electrode–tissue interface temperature, electrode diameter, and contact force.
- Power density declines with the square of distance from the source, and steady-state tissue temperature declines inversely with distance from the heat source.
- The ultimate RF lesion size is determined by the zone of acute necrosis as well as by the region of microvascular injury.
- Electrode cooling reduces the efficiency of tissue heating. For a fixed energy delivery, blood flow over the electrode–tissue interface reduces lesion width on the surface by convective tissue cooling. Ablation catheter irrigation increases lesion size by allowing the operator to increase the power that can be delivered before limiting electrode–tissue interface temperatures are achieved.
- Avoiding collateral injury while maintaining lesion transmurality when ablating thin-walled structures is challenging because present technology does not allow the operator to monitor lesion formation in real time. Use of high-power short-duration energy delivery and algorithms incorporating parameters such as power, duration, and contact force may improve predictability of lesion formation.
- New multielectrode catheters with balloon platforms may allow single-shot RF ablation of pulmonary veins.

When Huang and colleagues first introduced radiofrequency (RF) catheter ablation in 1985[1] as a potentially useful modality for the management of cardiac arrhythmias,[2] few would have predicted its meteoric rise. In the past three decades, it has become one of the most useful and widely used therapies in the field of cardiac electrophysiology. RF catheter ablation has enjoyed a high efficacy and safety profile, and indications for its use continue to expand. Improvements in catheter design have continued to enhance the operator's ability to target the arrhythmogenic substrate, and modifications in RF energy delivery and electrode design have resulted in more effective energy coupling to the tissue. It is likely that most operators view RF catheter ablation as a "black box" in that once the target is acquired, they need only to push the button on the RF generator. However, gaining insight into the biophysics of RF energy delivery and the mechanisms of tissue injury in response to this intervention will help the clinician optimize catheter ablation, which may ultimately enhance its efficacy and safety.

BIOPHYSICS OF RADIOFREQUENCY ENERGY TISSUE HEATING

Resistive Heating

The RF energy is a form of alternating electrical current that generates a lesion in the heart through electrical heating of the myocardium. A common form of RF ablation found in the medical environment is electrocautery, which is used for tissue cutting and coagulation during surgical procedures. The goals of catheter ablation with RF energy are to transform electromagnetic energy into thermal energy in the tissue and to destroy the arrhythmogenic tissues by heating them to a lethal temperature. The mode of direct tissue heating by RF energy is resistive (electrical) heating. As electrical current passes through a resistive medium, the voltage drops and heat is produced (similar to the heat that is created in an incandescent lightbulb). The RF electrical current is typically delivered in a unipolar fashion with completion of the circuit through an indifferent electrode placed on the skin. An oscillation frequency of 500–750 kHz is usual. Lower frequencies are more likely to stimulate cardiac muscle and nerves, resulting in arrhythmias and pain sensation. Much higher frequencies (in the microwave range) are less effective at transferring the electromagnetic energy to the tissue; therefore, complex and expensive catheter antenna designs must be used.[3]

Resistive heat production within the tissue is proportional to the RF power density, and that, in turn, is proportional to the square of the current density (Table 1.1). When RF energy is delivered in a unipolar fashion, the current distributes radially from the source. The current density decreases in proportion to the square of the distance from the RF electrode source. Thus, direct resistive heating of the tissue decreases rapidly with

TABLE 1.1 Equations Describing Biophysics of Radiofrequency Ablation

$V = I R$	Ohm's law V—voltage I—current R—resistance
$\text{Power} = V I (\cos \alpha)$	Cos α—phase shift between voltage (V) and current (I) in alternating current
$\text{Current density} = 1/4\pi r^2$	I—total electrode current r—distance from electrode center
$SAR = \lvert E\rvert^2\sigma/r = \lvert J\rvert^2\sigma\lvert r$	SAR—heat production per unit of volume of tissue σ tissue electrical conductivity r—tissue mass density E—electrical field strength J—electrical current density
$J = I\pi\lvert r^2$	I—current, r—distance of spherical boundary from electrode center in conductive medium
$\text{SAR at boundary} \propto I^2/r^4$	
$T(t) = T_{ss} + (T_{initial} - T_{ss})\ e^{-t}/\tau$	Monoexponential relationship between tissue temperature (T) and duration of radiofrequency energy delivery (t). $T_{initial}$—starting tissue temperature T_{ss}—tissue temperature at steady state τ—time constant
$r/r_i = (t_0 - T)/(t - T)$	Relationship between tissue temperature and distance from heat source in ideal system r—distance from center of heat source r_i—radius of heat source t_0—temperature at electrode–tissue interface T—basal tissue temperature t—temperature at radius r

increased distance from the electrode (Fig. 1.1). As a result, only a narrow band of tissue in close contact with the catheter electrode (2–3 mm) is heated directly. Heating of deeper tissue layers occurs passively through heat conduction.[4]

Thermal Conduction

Most of the tissue heating resulting in the formation of lesion during RF catheter ablation occurs as a result of thermal conduction from the direct resistive heat source. Transfer of heat through tissue follows basic thermodynamic principles and is represented by the bioheat transfer equation.[5] Change in tissue temperature with increasing distance from the heat source is called the *radial temperature gradient*. At the onset of RF energy delivery, the temperature is very high at the source of heating and falls off rapidly over a short distance (Fig. 1.1 and Videos 1.1 and 1.2). As time progresses, more thermal energy is transferred to deeper tissue layers by thermal conduction. The tissue temperature at any given distance from the heat source increases in a monoexponential fashion over time. Sites close to the heat source have a rapid rise in temperature (a short half-time of temperature rise), whereas sites remote from the source heat up more slowly.[6] Eventually, the entire electrode–tissue system reaches steady state, meaning that the amount of energy entering the tissue at the thermal source equals the amount of energy that is being dissipated at the tissue margins beyond the lesion border. At steady state, the radial temperature gradient becomes constant. If RF power delivery is interrupted before steady state is achieved, tissue temperature will continue to rise in deeper tissue planes as a result of thermal conduction from more superficial layers heated to higher temperatures. The temperatures at deeper sites may continue to rise several degrees over several seconds due to *thermal latency.* The important clinical implication is that active ablation, with its beneficial or adverse effects, will continue for a certain period despite cessation of RF current flow.[7]

The mechanism of tissue injury in response to RF ablation is thermal, and the isotherm of irreversible injury (the temperature at the border zone of the ablative lesion) is reproducible. Experimental studies predict this temperature with hyperthermic ablation to be approximately 50°C,[3] although alternative methods propose that this critical temperature may be higher.[8] One may predict the three-dimensional temperature gradients with thermodynamic modeling and finite-element analysis and by doing so can predict the anticipated lesion dimensions and geometry with the 50°C isotherm. In a steady-state theoretical model of thermal ablation, it is predicted that radial temperature gradient is inversely proportional to the distance from the heat source. The 50°C isotherm boundary (lesion radius) increases in distance from the source in direct proportion to the temperature at that source. In the absence of convective cooling, it has been demonstrated that the lesion depth and diameter are best predicted by the electrode–tissue interface temperature.[4] In the clinical setting, however, the opposing effects of convective cooling by circulating blood flow diminish the value of electrode-tip temperature monitoring to assess lesion size.

It has been predicted and demonstrated that the radius of the lesion is directly proportional to the radius of the heat source (Fig. 1.2).[9] When one considers the virtual heat source radius as the shell of direct resistive heating in tissue contiguous to the electrode, it is not surprising that larger electrode diameter, length, and contact area all result in a larger source radius and larger lesion size and that this may result in enhanced procedural success. Higher power delivery increases not only the source temperature but also the radius of directly heated tissue (i.e., the heat source), thereby increasing lesion size in two ways. This has been confirmed in the clinical setting with the use of large-tip catheters and cooled-tip catheters.[10–12]

Sudden Impedance Rise

While the peak tissue temperature increases during ablation, the temperature at greater tissue depths also increases. A very high source temperature, therefore, should theoretically yield a very deep 50°C isotherm temperature and, in turn, very large ablative lesions. Unfortunately, this process is prevented in the biological setting because of the formation of coagulum and char at the electrode–tissue interface when temperatures exceed 100°C. At 100°C, blood literally begins to boil with generation of showers

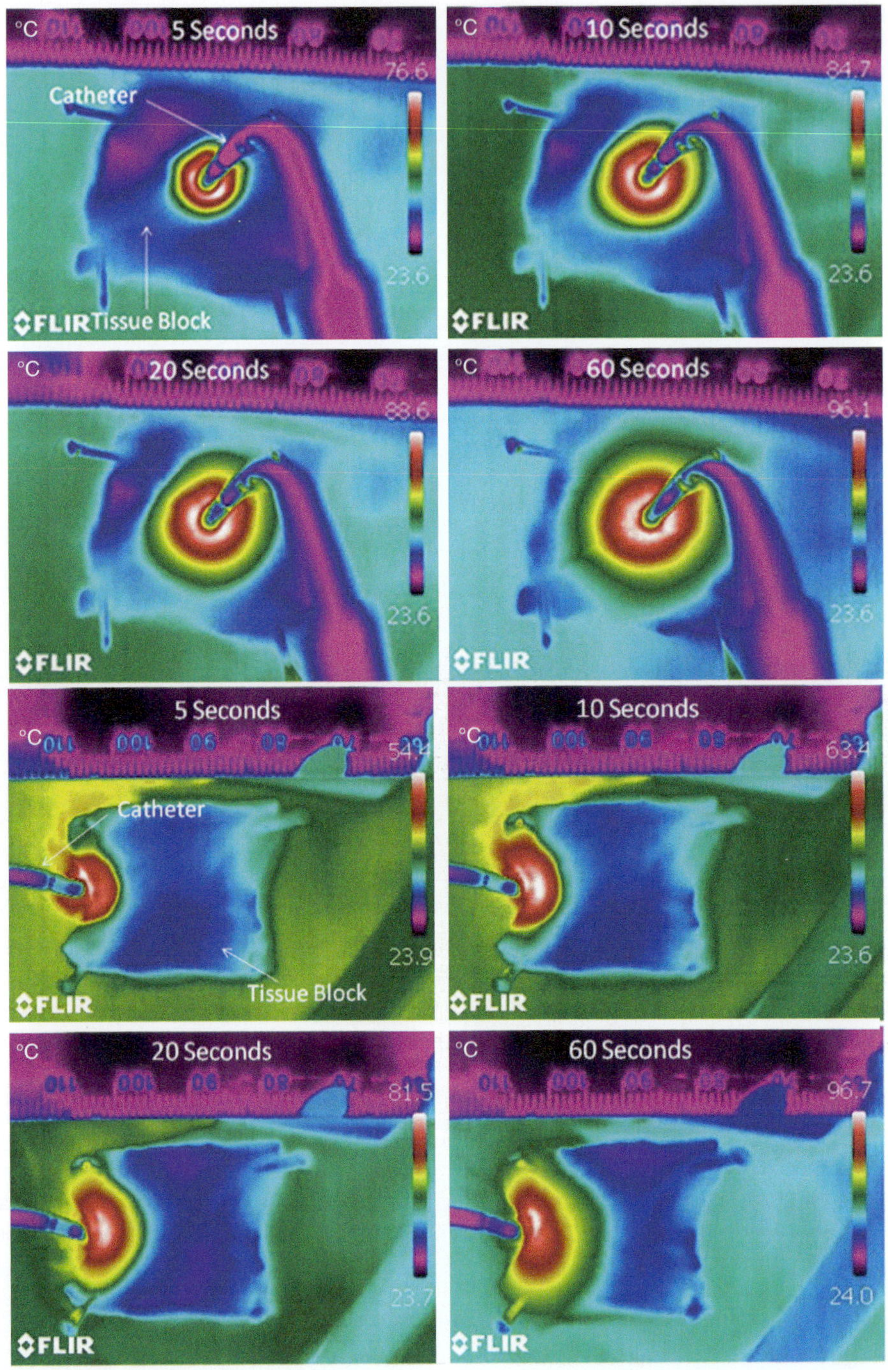

A

B

Fig. 1.1 Infrared thermal imaging of tissue heating during radiofrequency ablation with a closed irrigation catheter. Power is delivered at 30 W to blocks of porcine myocardium in a tissue bath. The surface of the tissue is just above the fluid level to permit thermal imaging of tissue and not the fluid. Temperature scale *(right)* and a millimeter scale *(top)* are shown in each panel. (A) When viewed from the surface, there is radial heating of the tissue from the electrode. (B) Tissue heating visualized in cross section. The electrode is partially submerged in the fluid bath and perpendicular to the upper edge of the tissue. In both cases, very high tissue temperatures (>96°C) are achieved at 60 seconds because of the absence of fluid flow over the tissue surface.

of microbubbles.[13] As the blood and tissue in contact with the electrode catheter desiccate, the residue of denatured proteins adheres to the electrode surface. These substances are electrically insulating and result in a smaller electrode surface area available for electrical conduction. In turn, the same magnitude of power is concentrated over a smaller surface area, and the power density increases. The electrode rapidly becomes encased in coagulum. In a study testing ablation with a 2-mm-tip electrode in vitro and in vivo, a measured temperature of at least 100°C correlated closely with a sudden rise in electrical impedance (Fig. 1.3).[14] All modern RF energy ablation systems have an automatic energy cutoff if a rapid rise in electrical impedance is

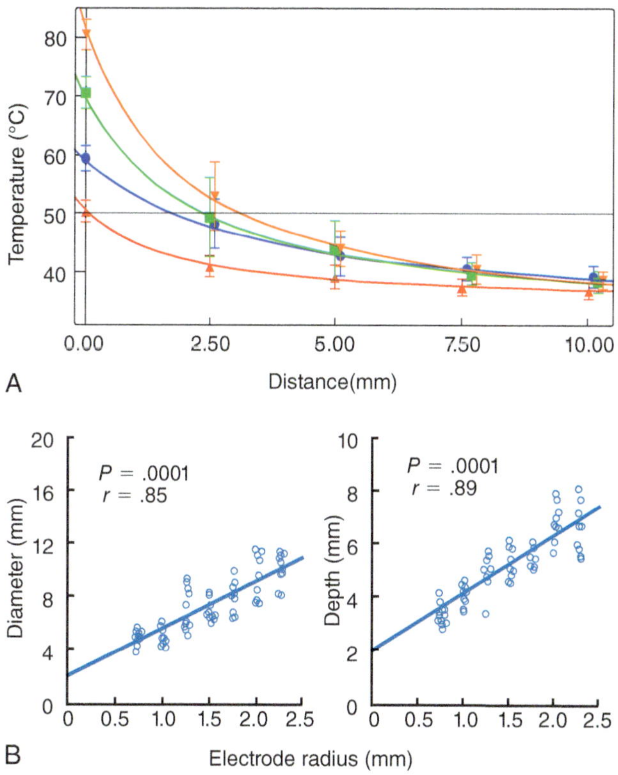

Fig. 1.2 (A) Radial temperature gradients measured during in vitro catheter ablation with source temperatures varying from 50°C to 80°C. The tissue temperature falls in an inverse proportion to distance. The *horizontal line* represents the 50°C isothermal line. The point at which the radial temperature gradient crosses the 50°C isotherm determines the boundary of the lesion. A higher source temperature results in a greater lesion depth. (B) Lesion depth and diameter are compared with the electrode radius in temperature-feedback power-controlled radiofrequency ablation. A larger-diameter ablation electrode results in higher power delivery and a proportional increase in lesion dimension.

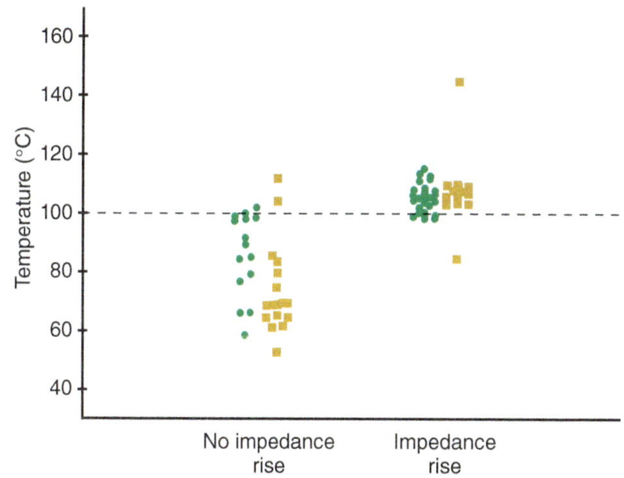

Fig. 1.3 The association of measured electrode-tip temperature and sudden rise in electrical impedance is shown in this study of radiofrequency catheter ablation with a 2-mm-tip ablation electrode in vitro *(blue circles)* and in vivo *(yellow squares)*. The peak temperature recorded at the electrode–tissue interface is shown. Almost all ablations without a sudden rise in electrical impedance had a peak temperature of 100°C or less, whereas all but one ablation manifesting a sudden rise in electrical impedance had peak temperatures of 100°C or more. (From Haines DE, Verow AF. Observations on electrode–tissue interface temperature and effect on electrical impedance during radiofrequency ablation of ventricular myocardium. *Circulation.* 1990;82:1034–1038.)

observed. When high temperatures and sudden rises in electrical impedance are observed, there is concern about the accumulation of char and coagulum, with the subsequent risk of char embolism. Reports of asymptomatic cerebral embolic lesions on diffusion weighted imaging–magnetic resonance (MR) images after atrial fibrillation ablation highlight the clinical significance of microembolism.[15,16] Anticoagulation and antiplatelet therapies have been proposed as preventative measures,[17] but meticulous sheath management avoidance of excessive heating at the electrode–tissue interface remains the best strategy to avoid this risk.[18]

Convective Cooling

The major thermodynamic factor opposing the transfer of thermal energy to tissue is convective cooling. Convection is the process in which heat is rapidly distributed through a medium by active mixing of that medium. In the case of RF catheter ablation, the heat is produced by resistive heating and transferred to deeper layers by thermal conduction. Simultaneously, the heat is conducted back into the circulating blood pool and metal electrode tip. Because the blood is moving rapidly past the electrode and over the endocardial surface, and because water (the main constituent of blood) has a high heat capacity, a large amount of the heat produced at the site of ablation can be carried away by the blood. Right bundle branch ablation under direct observation was performed in a Langendorff-perfused canine heart preparation. When pulsatile flow was streamed past the ablation electrode, the power requirements to cause block increased fourfold.[19] Convective cooling is such an important factor that it dominates the thermodynamics of catheter ablation.[20] Efficiency of energy coupling to the tissue can be as low as 10%, depending on electrode size, catheter stability, and position relative to intracavitary blood flow.[21] Unstable, sliding catheter contact results in significant tip cooling and decreased efficiency of tissue heating.[22] This is most often observed with ablation along the tricuspid or mitral valve annuli, or on the left pulmonary vein ridge.

Paradoxically, the convective cooling phenomenon has been used to increase lesion size. As previously noted, maximal power delivery during RF ablation is limited by boiling of blood and coagulum formation at the electrode tip. However, if the tip is cooled, a higher magnitude of power may be delivered without a sudden rise in electrical impedance. The higher magnitude of power increases the depth of direct resistive heating and, in turn, increases the radius of the effective heat source. In addition, higher temperatures are achieved 3–4 mm below the surface, and the entire radial temperature curve is shifted to a higher temperature over greater tissue depth. The result is a greater 50°C isotherm radius and a greater depth and diameter of the lesion. Nakagawa and coworkers demonstrated this phenomenon in a blood-superfused exposed thigh muscle preparation. In this study, intramural tissue temperatures 3.5 mm from the surface averaged 95°C with an irrigated-tip catheter despite a mean electrode–tissue interface

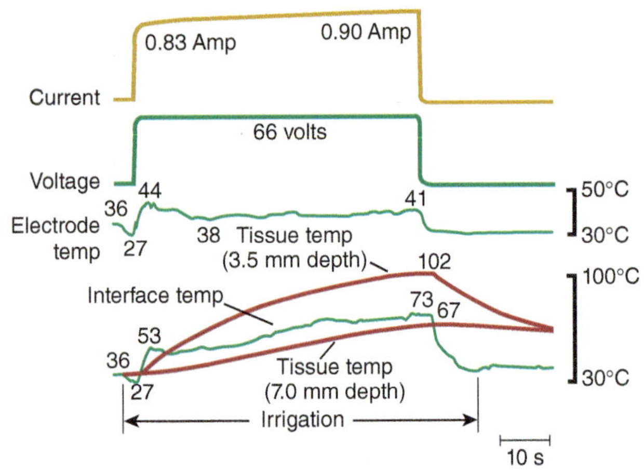

Fig. 1.4 Current, voltage, and temperatures measured during radiofrequency catheter ablation with a perfused-tip electrode catheter in a canine exposed thigh muscle preparation are shown. Temperatures were recorded within the electrode, at the electrode–tissue interface, and within the muscle below the ablation catheter at depths of 3.5 and 7 mm. Because the electrode–tissue interface is actively cooled, high current and high voltage levels can be used. This results in an increased depth of direct resistive heating and superheating of the tissue below the surface of ablation. The peak temperature in this example at a depth of 3.5 mm was 102°C, and at 7 mm was 67°C, indicating that the 50°C isotherm defining the lesion border was significantly deeper than 7 mm. (From Nakagawa H, Yamanashi WS, Pitha JV, et al. Comparison of in vivo tissue temperature profile and lesion geometry for radiofrequency ablation with a saline-irrigated electrode versus temperature control in a canine thigh muscle preparation. *Circulation.* 1995;91:2264–2273.)

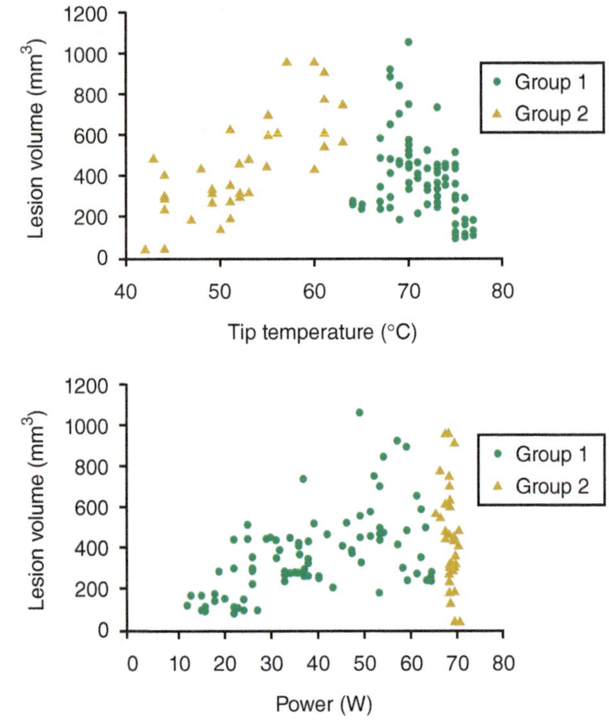

Fig. 1.5 Temperatures measured at the tip of the electrode during experimental radiofrequency ablation and power are compared with the resulting lesion volume in this study. A maximal power of 70 W was used. If lesion creation was not power limited *(group 1)*, the lesion volume was a function of the delivered power. However, if lesion production was limited by the 70-W available power maximum *(group 2)*, the temperature measured at the electrode tip correlated with lesion size. (From Petersen HH, Chen X, Pietersen A, et al. Lesion dimensions during temperature-controlled radiofrequency catheter ablation of left ventricular porcine myocardium: impact of ablation site, electrode size, and convective cooling. *Circulation.* 1999;99:319–325.)

temperature of 69°C. Lesion depths were 9.9 mm compared with 6.1 mm in a comparison group of temperature-feedback power control delivery with no electrode irrigation (Fig. 1.4). An important finding of this study was that 6 of 75 lesions had a sudden rise in electrical impedance associated with an audible pop. In these cases, the intramural temperature exceeded 100°C, resulting in sudden steam formation and a steam pop. The clinical concern about pop lesions is that sudden venting of steam to the endocardial or epicardial surface (or both) can potentially cause perforation and tamponade.[23] Monitoring intramyocardial steam formation with near-field ultrasound to terminate energy delivery before steam venting can occur has been proposed as a method of mitigating this risk.[24]

The observation of increasing lesion size with ablation-tip cooling holds true only when the ablation is not power limited. If the level of power used is insufficient to overcome the heat lost by convection, the resulting tissue heating may be inadequate. In this case, convective cooling will dissipate a greater proportion of energy with less tissue heating. The resulting lesion may be smaller than it would be if there was no convective cooling. As power is increased to a higher level, more energy will be converted into tissue heat, which results in larger lesions. If power is unlimited and temperature-feedback power control delivery is used, greater magnitudes of convective cooling will allow for higher power levels and very large lesions. Thus, paradoxically in this situation, lesion size may be inversely related to the electrode–tissue interface temperature if the ablation is not power limited.[25] However, if power level is fixed (most commercial RF generators limit power delivery to 50 W for use with standard catheters), lesion size increases in proportion to the electrode–tissue interface temperature even in the setting of significant convective cooling (Fig. 1.5).[26]

The magnitude of convective cooling that is achieved with irrigated catheters is relatively small compared to the circulating blood pool, but this cooling can occur in the highly localized region at the electrode–tissue interface. The main effect of irrigation is to prevent excessive surface heating, boiling, char formation, and impedance rise despite use of high-power amplitude. High versus low irrigation rates do not affect the ablation lesion depth if power is constant. However, high irrigation rates do result in smaller lesion diameter on the endocardial surface. Thus, if thin-walled tissues are being ablated (e.g., posterior left atrial wall), then using high irrigation flow rate will not alter risk of injury to collateral structures, but it will decrease ablation efficacy by reducing superficial lesion size.[27]

Electrode-tip cooling can be achieved passively or actively. Passive tip cooling occurs when the circulating blood flow cools the mass of the ablation electrode and cools the electrode–tissue interface. This can be enhanced by using a large ablation electrode[28] or by using an electrode material with high thermal conductivity, such as gold[29,30] or diamond.[31] Active tip cooling can be realized with a closed or open perfused-tip system. One design recirculates the saline through a return port, and the opposing design infuses the saline through weep holes in the electrode into the bloodstream. Both designs are effective and result in larger lesions and greater procedure efficacy than standard RF catheter ablation,[32,33] although open irrigation is preferred because operators observe less tendency for formation of thrombus compared to closed systems. Present-day electrode geometries vary considerably, tip irrigation is used routinely, and standard catheters embed their thermocouples within the mass of the electrode tip, thereby providing evidence of tip cooling with irrigation but no ability to detect tissue heating. A new generation of temperature-sensing catheters offers to improve this scenario. Six miniature thermocouple sensors have been positioned immediately below the electrode surface and distributed around the tip of a force-sensing catheter, significantly improving ability to predict catheter orientation and lesion depth.[34]

Because the peak tissue temperature is shifted from the endocardial surface to deeper intramyocardial layers, there is a risk of excessive intramural heating and pop lesions. The challenge for the clinician lies with the fact that with varying degrees of convective cooling, there is no reliable method for monitoring whether tissue heating is inadequate, optimal, or excessive. Cooling at the electrode–tissue interface limits the value of temperature monitoring to prevent excess power delivery and steam pops. New technologies such as MR thermography[35] or near-field ultrasound-guided ablation[36] may allow the operator to visualize lesion formation real time during energy delivery and more precisely adjust power and magnitude of convective cooling to optimize lesion formation. Catheter ablation in the pericardial space is a unique condition. Because there is no circulating blood, there is no convective cooling whatsoever. Ablations performed with conventional RF catheters yield very small lesions. Perfused-electrode catheters are usually used in this setting to provide some surface cooling and allow ablation at higher powers. In particular, linear ablation tools designed for surgical ablation of atrial fibrillation from the epicardial surface require cooling to achieve transmural atrial lesions.[37,38]

Catheter Contact Force and Orientation

It has long been appreciated that electrode–tissue contact force is an important factor in successful RF energy lesion formation. With increasing force, greater proportion of the electrode surface area is in contact with the tissue, and there is more efficient energy coupling. In addition with thin-walled tissues, the endocardial surface is slightly depressed with increasing contact force and the tissue is somewhat thinner at the contact point. This increases the likelihood that the RF lesion will be transmural. In recent years, force-sensing catheters have been developed that use either fiber-optic or piezoelectric components attached to a flexible catheter tip that can accurately measure the force applied to the tip electrode of the catheter. Lesions created with higher contact force (>20*g* force) were larger and required lower powers than lesions created with lower contact force.[39] Contact force catheters have also been used to determine that the average force needed for atrial perforation in a swine model was 175*g* force (range, 77–376*g* force).[40] Force-sensing catheters have been tested extensively in the clinical setting. Successful catheter ablation has been associated with higher contact forces, and higher forces that have been applied over longer durations (the force–time integral).[41,42] However, there is a concern that using greater contact force and longer durations during ablation of the posterior left atrial wall may have contributed to a higher risk of atrial-esophageal fistula.[43]

Catheter orientation will affect lesion size and geometry. Perpendicular catheter orientation results in less electrode surface area in contact with the tissue and more surface area in contact with the circulating blood pool. Parallel catheter orientation provides more electrode–tissue contact. With unrestricted power delivery, the parallel orientation should produce the larger lesion. In perfused-tip catheters, parallel orientation also results in more active tissue cooling and smaller lesion sizes than a perpendicular orientation.[44] The resultant interplay among active cooling, passive cooling, and power availability or limitation determines whether the lesions will be larger or smaller in these varying conditions. If perfused-tip catheters are positioned in a parallel orientation with greater tissue cooling, the lesions are smaller in vitro because of diminished efficiency of energy delivery. The effects of catheter orientation are less important with 4- or 5-mm-tip catheters but become more dominant when 8- or 10-mm tips are used.

Electrical Current Distribution

Catheter ablation depends on the passage of RF electrical current through tissues. As tissue contact improves, the impedance of the RF electrical circuit decreases since there is lower impedance at an electrode–tissue interface than at an electrode–blood interface.[45,46] A strong correlation is observed between effective lesion formation and rate of impedance fall during energy delivery because hotter tissue has a lower impedance than cooler tissue. Impedance monitoring as an indicator of effective tissue heating is further refined when measurements are taken between microelectrodes at the catheter tip and local impedance instead of system impedance is reported.[47] Impedance can be monitored to mitigate risk of sudden steam pops,[48] and if no impedance drop is observed, catheter repositioning is warranted.[49]

The magnitude of tissue heating is determined by the current density; in turn, the distribution of RF field around the electrodes in unipolar, bipolar, or phased RF energy delivery will determine the distribution of tissue heating. If energy is delivered in a unipolar fashion in an isotropic medium from a spherical electrode, current density around the electrode should be uniform. As geometries and tissue properties change, heating becomes nonuniform. Standard 4- or 5-mm electrode tips are small enough so that heating around the tip is fairly evenly distributed, even with varying tip contact angle to the tissue.[50]

With catheter irrigation, power distribution during RF ablation can be modulated by altering the tonicity of the irrigation solution. If more power is channeled through the tissue rather than into the blood pool and irrigation solution, the lesion size should be larger. This can be accomplished by using lower-tonicity saline with higher impedance as the irrigation liquid. Experimentally, this resulted in 60% larger lesion volumes.[51]

Fat is distributed widely on the epicardium of the heart and reduces both electrical and thermal conductivity. Epicardial ablation over fat will result in minimal ablation of the underlying myocardium. Conversely, ablation of tissue insulated by fat outside of the ablation target will produce an insulating effect, with higher temperatures for longer durations after cessation of energy delivery.[52] Fat dispersed within chronic ventricular scar may account for the difficulty in deep lesions during ablation of ventricular tachycardia.[53]

Bipolar ablation uses a second active ablation electrode rather than a dispersive electrode, and the current flows between the two electrodes with heating occurring at both electrodes. For symmetrical ablation at both active electrodes of the bipole, it is important that the electrodes are similar in size, because heating is proportional to power density, which is a function of both power and electrode surface area. With bipolar delivery, the electrical field is densest between the electrodes, so some additional volume heating may be achieved in the intervening tissues if the interelectrode spacing is close. It is possible to simultaneously deliver both unipolar RF energy to multiple poles and bipolar energy between poles by altering the phase of RF signal between the two electrodes or by using a duty cycle to alternate from unipolar to bipolar. The blended unipolar–bipolar RF lesion from contiguous electrodes will be deeper than a pure bipolar ablation but more continuous than a pure unipolar ablation.[54]

Dispersive Electrode

To complete the electrical circuit for unipolar RF delivery, a dispersive electrode (ground electrode) is applied to the patient's skin. Within the full circuit, the electrode–tissue interface is only one component of the system resistance, and only one site where energy is dissipated as heat. The other components of the system consume RF energy in proportion to the local impedance. Therefore, a lower impedance dispersive electrode–tissue interface will make more RF energy available to ablate the targeted tissue. (Fig. 1.6). Vigorous skin prep and using more than one dispersive electrode will both improve ablation and reduce risk of skin burns. Nath and associates reported that in the setting of system impedance higher than 100 Ω, adding a second dispersive electrode increased the peak electrode-tip temperature during clinical catheter ablation (Fig. 1.7).[55] The actual locations of the dispersive electrodes are less important because electrical field distribution is relatively uniform around the ablation electrode, but shorter path length from the ablation to dispersive electrode may increase lesion size.[56]

Edge Effect

Electrical field lines are not entirely uniform around the tip of a unipolar ablation electrode. The distribution of field lines from an electrode source is affected by changes in electrode geometry. At points of geometric transition, the field lines become more concentrated. This so-called edge effect can result in significant nonuniformity of heating around electrodes. The less symmetrical the electrode design (such as those found with long electrodes), the greater is the degree of nonuniform heating. McRury and coworkers tested ablation with 12.5-mm-long electrodes and found that a centrally placed temperature sensor significantly underestimated the peak electrode–tissue interface temperature.[57] Finite-element analysis demonstrated a concentration of electrical current at each edge of the electrode (Fig. 1.8). When dual thermocouples were placed on the edge of the electrode, the risk of coagulum formation and impedance rise was significantly reduced during ablation testing in vivo.

TISSUE PATHOLOGY AND PATHOPHYSIOLOGIC RESPONSE TO RADIOFREQUENCY ABLATION

Gross Pathology and Histopathology of the Ablative Lesion

The endocardial surface in contact with the ablation catheter shows pallor and sometimes a small depression caused by volume loss of the acute lesion. If excessive power has been applied, there may be visible coagulum or char adherent to the ablation site. On sectioning the acute lesion produced by RF energy, a central zone of pallor and tissue desiccation characterizes its gross appearance. There is volume loss, and the lesion frequently has a teardrop shape with a narrower lesion width immediately subendocardially and a wider width 2–3 mm below the endocardial surface. This is because of surface convective cooling by the endocardial blood flow. Immediately outside the pale central zone is a band of hemorrhagic tissue. Beyond that border, the tissue appears relatively normal. The acute lesion border, as assessed by vital staining, correlates with the border between the hemorrhagic and normal tissue (Fig. 1.9). The histologic appearance of the lesion is consistent with coagulation necrosis. There are contraction bands in the sarcomeres, nuclear pyknosis, and basophilic stippling consistent with intracellular calcium overload.[58]

The temperature at the border zone of an acute hyperthermic lesion assessed by vital staining with nitro blue tetrazolium was observed to be 52°C–55°C in one study[3] and 60°C in another.[59] However, it is likely that the actual isotherm of irreversible thermal injury occurs at a lower temperature boundary outside the lesion boundary and that it cannot be identified acutely. Coagulation necrosis is a manifestation of thermal inactivation of the contractile and cytoskeletal proteins in the cell. Changes in the appearance of vital stains are caused by loss of enzyme activity, as is the case with nitro blue tetrazolium or triphenyl tetrazolium chloride staining and dehydrogenase activity.[60] Therefore, the acute assessment of the lesion border represents the border of thermal inactivation of various proteins, but the ultimate viability of the cell may depend on the integrity of more thermally sensitive organelles such as the plasma membrane (see later discussion). In the clinical setting, recorded temperature does correlate with response to ablation. In patients with manifest Wolff-Parkinson-White syndrome, the reversible accessory pathway conduction block with a nonirrigated catheter was observed at a mean electrode temperature of 50°C ± 8°C,

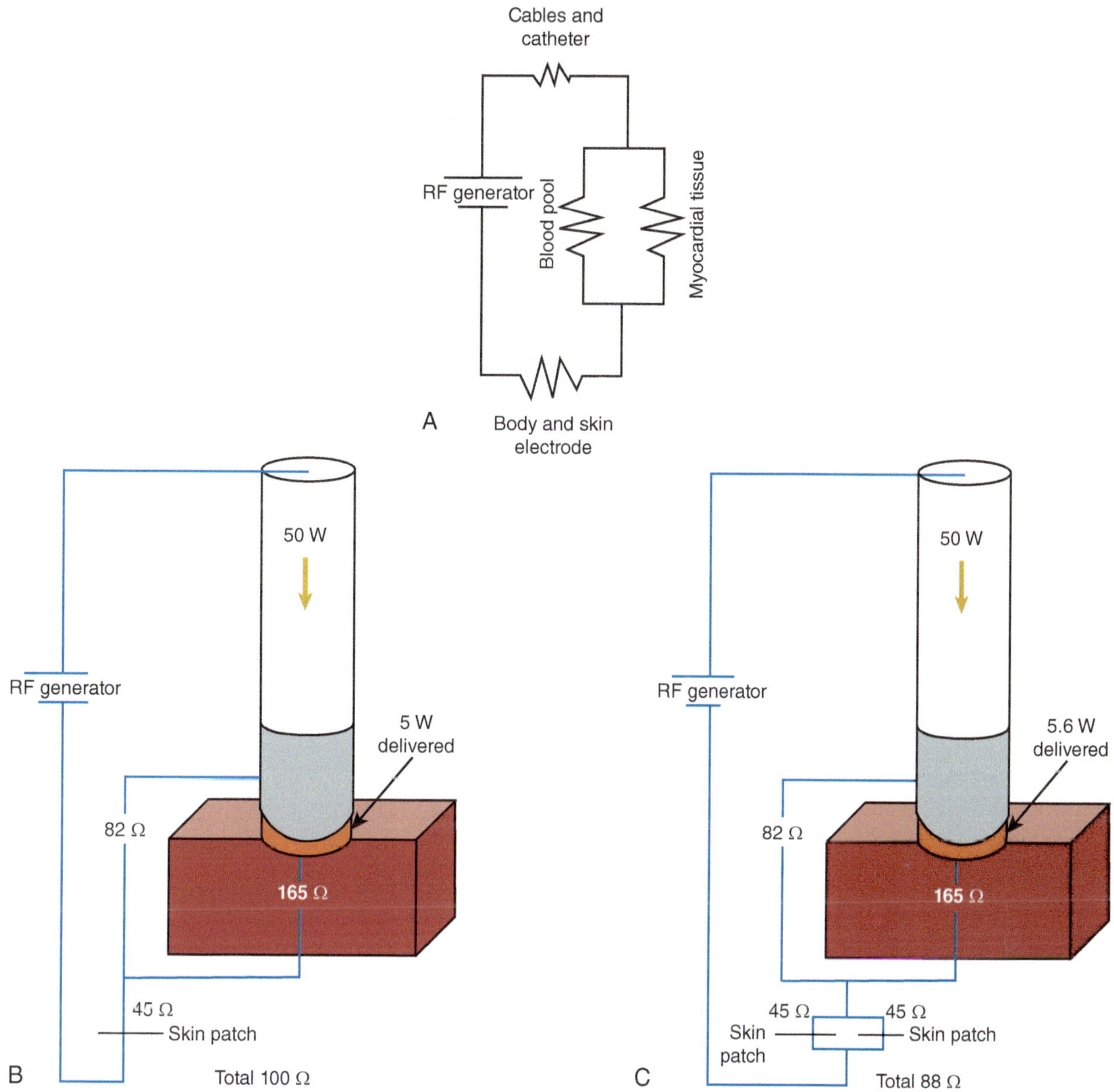

Fig. 1.6 Circuit diagrams for radiofrequency (RF) ablation. (A) From the RF generator, the cables and catheter present minimal resistance. The myocardial tissue and blood pool represent resistance circuits in parallel from the distal electrode. The return path from the ablation electrode to the generator comprises the patient's body and dispersive electrode in series. (B) Hypothetical resistances for RF ablation circuit path. The resistance of the blood pool is about half than that of the myocardial tissue. In this situation, for 50 W of energy delivered to the catheter, only 5 W is deposited in the myocardial tissue because of shunting of current through the lower resistance blood pool and power loss in the return path. (C) Effect of adding a second dispersive skin electrode to the circuit. Assuming that the impedance of each dispersive electrode is 45 Ω and the generator voltage is constant, the total ablation circuit impedance is decreased by 12%. This allows for greater current delivery through the circuit and a proportional increase in power delivered to the tissue.

whereas the permanent block occurred at a temperature of 62°C ± 15°C.[61] In a study of electrode-tip temperature monitoring during atrioventricular junctional ablation, an accelerated junctional rhythm was observed at a mean temperature of 51°C ± 4°C. Permanent complete heart block was observed at ablation temperatures of 60°C ± 7°C.[62] Because the targeted tissue was likely millimeters below the endocardial surface, the temperatures recorded by the catheter were expected to be higher than those achieved intramurally at the critical site of ablation.

The subacute pathology of the RF lesion is like what is observed with other types of injury. Although the appearance of typical coagulation necrosis persists, the lesion border becomes more sharply demarcated with infiltration of mononuclear inflammatory cells. A layer of fibrin adheres to the lesion surface, coating the area of endothelial injury. After 4–5 days, the transition zone at the lesion border is lost, and the border between the RF lesion and surrounding tissue becomes sharply demarcated. The changes in the transition zone within the first hours and days after ablation likely account for the phenomena of early arrhythmia recurrence (injury with recovery)[63] or delayed cure (progressive injury caused by the secondary inflammatory response).[64] The coagulation necrosis in the body of the lesion shows early evidence of fatty infiltration. By 8 weeks after the ablation procedure, the necrotic zone is replaced with fatty tissue, cartilage, and fibrosis and can be surrounded by chronic inflammation.[65] The chronic RF ablative lesion evolves into a uniform scar. Like any fibrotic scar, there is significant contraction of the scar with healing. Relatively large and wide acute linear lesions have the final gross appearance of narrow lines of glistening scar when examined 6 months after the ablation procedure.[66] The uniformity of the healed lesion accounts for the absence of any proarrhythmic effect of RF catheter ablation, unless multiple lesions with gaps are made. A group of patients who underwent pulmonary vein ablation and had clinical recurrence had full-thickness pulmonary vein antral biopsies at the time of a follow-up surgical maze procedure. Fifty percent of those specimens showed viable myocardium with or without scar on histopathologic analysis, explaining the reestablishment of pulmonary vein conduction after the acute catheter procedure.[59]

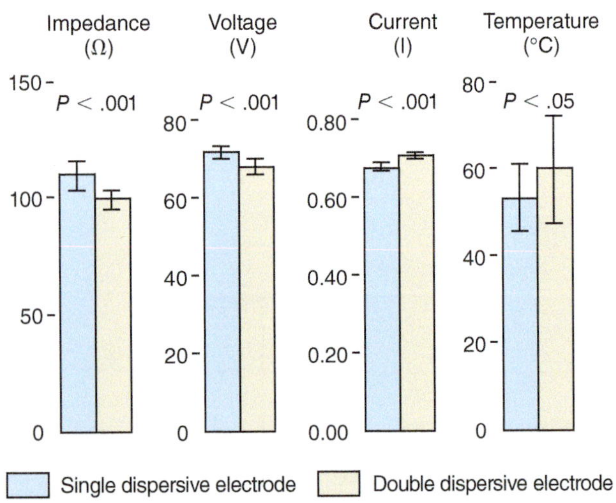

Fig. 1.7 Impedance, voltage, current, and catheter-tip temperature readings during radiofrequency catheter ablation in a subset of patients with a baseline system impedance of more than 100 Ω. Ablations using a single dispersive electrode were compared with those using a double dispersive electrode. A lower system impedance was observed with addition of the second dispersive patch. This resulted in a greater current delivery and higher temperatures measured at the electrode–tissue interface. (From Nath S, DiMarco JP, Gallop RG, et al. Effects of dispersive electrode position and surface area on electrical parameters and temperature during radiofrequency catheter ablation. *Am J Cardiol.* 1996;77:765–767.)

Radiofrequency Lesion Ultrastructure

The ultrastructural appearance of the acute RF lesion offers some insight into the mechanism of tissue injury at the lesion border zone. In cases of experimental RF ablation in vivo, ventricular myocardium was examined in a band 3 mm from the edge of the acute pathologic lesion as defined by vital staining (Fig. 1.10). It showed marked disruption in cellular architecture characterized by dissolution of lipid membranes and inactivation of structural proteins. The plasma membranes were severely disrupted or missing. There was extravasation of erythrocytes and complete absence of basement membrane. The mitochondria showed marked distortion of architecture with swollen and discontinuous cristae membranes. The sarcomeres were extended with loss of myofilament structure or were severely contracted.

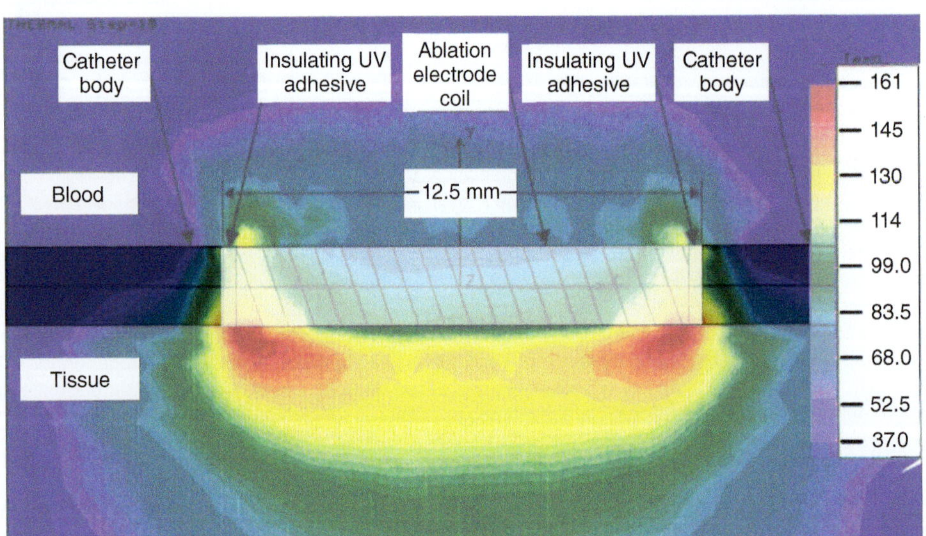

Fig. 1.8 Steady-state temperature distribution derived from a finite-element analysis of radiofrequency ablation with a 12-mm-long coil electrode. In this analysis, the electrode temperature at the center of the electrode was maintained at 71°C. The legend of temperatures is shown at the right of the graph and ranges from the physiologic normal (*violet* = 37°C) to the maximal tissue temperature (*red* = 161°C) located below the electrode edges. There is a significant gradient of heating between the peak temperatures at the electrode edges and the center of the electrode. *UV,* ultraviolet. (From McRury ID, Panescu D, Mitchell MA, Haines DE. Nonuniform heating during radiofrequency catheter ablation with long electrodes: monitoring the edge effect. *Circulation.* 1997;96:4057–4064.)

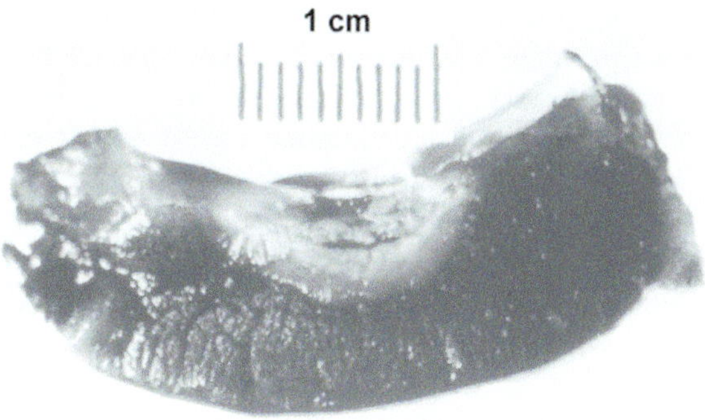

Fig. 1.9 Typical appearance of radiofrequency catheter ablation lesion. There is a small central depression with volume loss, surrounded by an area of pallor, then a hemorrhagic border zone. The specimen has been stained with nitro blue tetrazolium to differentiate viable from nonviable tissue.

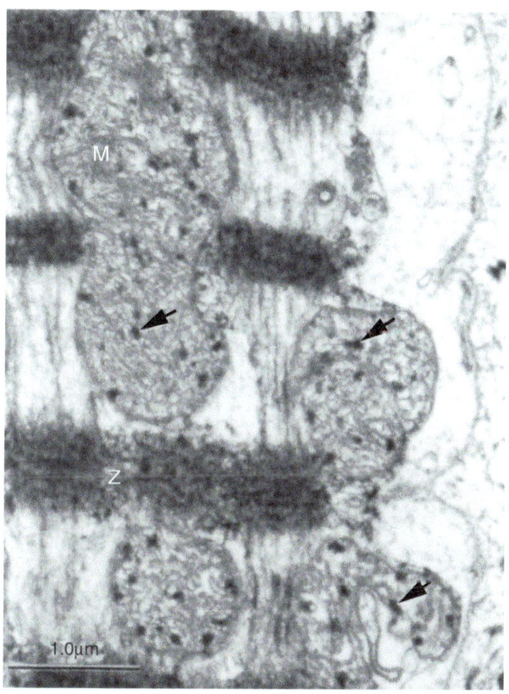

Fig. 1.10 Electron micrograph of a myocardial sample 3 mm outside of the border zone of acute injury created by radiofrequency catheter ablation. There is severe disruption of the sarcomere with contracted Z bands, disorganized mitochondria, and basophilic stippling *(arrows)*. Bar scale is 1.0 µm. *M*, mitochondria; *Z*, Z-bands. (From Nath S, Redick JA, Whayne JG, Haines DE. Ultrastructural observations in the myocardium beyond the region of acute coagulation necrosis following radiofrequency catheter ablation. *J Cardiovasc Electrophysiol.* 1994;5:838–845.)

The T tubules and sarcoplasmic reticulum were either absent or severely disrupted. Gap junctions were also either severely distorted or absent. Thus, even though the tissue examined was outside of the border of the acute pathologic lesion, the changes were profound enough to conclude that some progression of necrosis would occur within this border zone. The band of tissue 3–6 mm from the edge of the pathologic lesion was examined, and it showed significant ultrastructural abnormalities but not as severe as those described closer to the lesion core. Severe abnormalities of the plasma membrane were still present, but gap junctions and mitochondria were mainly intact. The sarcomeres were variable in appearance, with some being relatively normal and some partially contracted. Although ultrastructural disarray was observed in the 3- to 6-mm zone, the myocytes appeared to be viable and would likely recover from the injury.[67]

Radiofrequency Ablation and Arterial Perfusion

In addition to direct injury to the myocytes, RF-induced hyperthermia has an effect on the myocardial vasculature and the myocardial perfusion. Impairment of the microcirculation likely contributes to lesion formation by an ischemic mechanism. A previous study examined the effects of microvascular perfusion during acute RF lesion formation. In open-chest canine preparations, the left ventricle was imaged with ultrasound from the epicardial surface, and a myocardial echocardiographic contrast agent was injected into the left anterior descending artery during endocardial RF catheter ablation. After ablation, the center of the lesion showed no echo contrast, consistent with severe vascular injury and absence of blood flow to that region. In the border zone of the lesion, a halo effect of retained myocardial contrast was observed. This suggested marked slowing of contrast transit rate through these tissues. The measured contrast transit rate at the boundary of the gross pathologic lesion was 25% ± 12% of the transit rate in normal tissue. In the 3-mm band of myocardium outside of the lesion edge, the contrast transit was 48% ± 27% of normal, and in the band of myocardium 3–6 mm outside of the lesion edge, the transit rate was 82% ± 28% of normal ($P < .05$ for all comparisons). The ultrastructural appearance of the arterioles demonstrated marked disruption of the plasma membrane and basement membrane and extravasation of red blood cells in these regions of impaired myocardial perfusion. Although the relative contribution of microvascular injury and myocardial ischemia to ultimate lesion formation is unknown, it may play a role in lesion extension during the early phases after ablation.[68] Clinically, this phenomenon has been demonstrated with late gadolinium enhancement MR imaging (MRI). Regions of nonenhancement, indicating microvascular injury, on the MRI acquired immediately after ablation correlated best with scar observed on MRI 3 months later.[69]

The effect of RF heating on larger arteries is a function of the size of the artery, the arterial flow rate, and the proximity to the RF source. The heat-sink effect of coronary blood flow is protective of the vascular endothelium. With higher-power output of new ablation technologies, however, the convective cooling of the arterial flow may be overwhelmed, and there may be an increased risk of vascular injury. In one study, flow rate through a marginal artery (or intramural perfusion cannula) in an in vitro rabbit heart preparation was varied between 0 and 10 mL/minute. A pair of epicardial ablations was produced with epicardial RF energy applications. Even at low flow rates, there was substantial sparing of the artery and the surrounding tissue owing to the heat-sink effect of the arterial flow (Fig. 1.11). However, if 45 W of power was applied along with RF electrode-tip cooling, complete ablation of the tissue contiguous to the intramural perfusion cannula was achieved.[70] Although this may be a desirable effect in the setting of small perfusing arteries through a region of conduction critical for arrhythmia propagation,

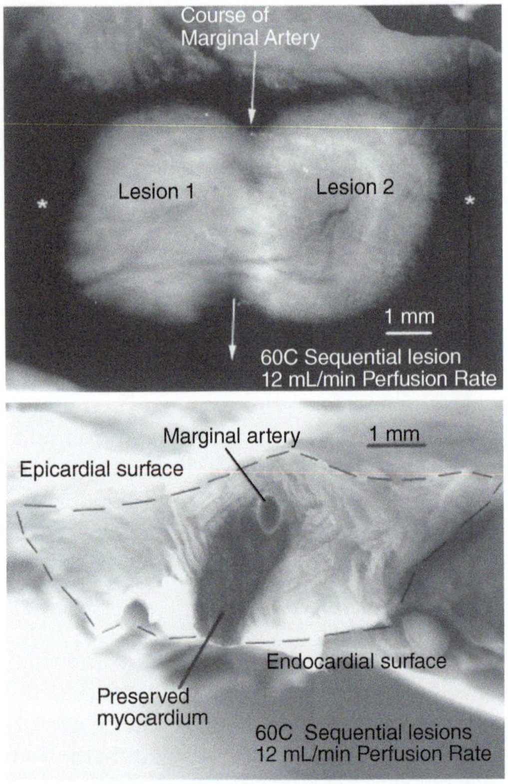

Fig. 1.11 *Top,* Epicardial view of two radiofrequency lesions created during perfusion of a penetrating marginal artery in a rabbit heart. The lesions show central pallor that is apparent after vital staining. The course of the artery is marked. The *asterisks* mark the line used for perpendicular sectioning of the lesion. *Bottom,* Cross-section through the middle of lesion perpendicular to marginal artery. The *broken lines* outline the lesion boundary. A region of myocardial sparing contiguous to the penetrating marginal artery (labeled) is apparent. Electrical conduction was present across this bridge of viable myocardium postablation. (From Fuller IA, Wood MA. Intramural coronary vasculature prevents transmural radiofrequency lesion formation: implications for linear ablation. *Circulation.* 2003;107:1797–1803.)

it is not desirable if the artery is a large epicardial artery that happens to be contiguous to an ablation site, as is sometimes the case with accessory pathway or slow atrioventricular nodal pathway ablation, ablation in the tricuspid–subeustachian isthmus for atrial flutter, or epicardial ablation.[71,72] Cases of arterial injury have been reported, particularly with the use of large-tip catheters or tip-cooling technologies that allow for application of high RF powers.[73,74] In particular, when high-power ablation is required within the coronary sinus or great cardiac vein, it is prudent to define the course of the arterial anatomy to avoid unwanted arterial thermal injury. Because greater destructive power is possible, the operators need to be aware of using only enough power that is required to achieve complete ablation of the targeted tissue to achieve the goal of arrhythmia ablation.

Collateral Injury from Ablation

The injury to targeted myocardium is usually achieved if an effort is made to optimize electrode–tissue contact. To ensure procedural success, particularly with ablation of more complex substrates such as those found with atrial fibrillation, operators have used several large-lesion RF technologies such as cooled-tip, perfused-tip, or large-tip catheters. However, with deep lesions sometimes comes unintended collateral injury to contiguous structures. Therefore, an understanding of the anatomic relationships and careful titration of RF energy delivery can avoid adverse consequences of ablation in most cases. A rare but dangerous complication of ablation of the posterior left atrium is esophageal injury, often leading to atrioesophageal fistula or esophageal perforation.[73] The esophagus is located immediately contiguous to the atrium in most patients, with a distance from atrial endocardium to esophagus as small as 1.6 mm.[74] Hyperthermic injury leads to damage to structural proteins resulting in significant reduction in tensile strength of the esophageal musculature.[75] This, coupled with esophageal mucosal injury and ulcer formation, likely leads to ultimate perforation with a high case-fatality rate. Other structures that can be damaged with pulmonary vein isolation procedures are vagal and phrenic nerves.[76,77] Although these nerves usually regenerate after several months, permanent palsy can occur. Avoiding injury to these structures while achieving reliable transmural ablation of the myocardium can be challenging.

The standard approach to minimizing heating of extracardiac structures has been to limit power amplitude and carefully monitor heating with multiple modalities (temperature, impedance drop, microbubbles on intracardiac echocardiogram imaging). However, longer durations of delivery that are required when lower powers are used promote heating of deeper tissue layers. Conversely, high power with short ablation duration exploits different rates of temperature rise between superficial and deep tissue layers. Whereas superficial tissues heat very rapidly, deeper tissues require heat conduction from the source of resistive heating and heating is delayed. Thus, short-duration RF delivery preferentially heats the superficial tissues, resulting in successful ablation of the thin-walled myocardium while avoiding excess heating of deeper structures. Reduction in catheter irrigation will also increase superficial lesion width and promote continuity and contiguity of adjacent lesions.[27]

A complication of ablation of atrial fibrillation that was prevalent when ablation was being performed within the vein was pulmonary vein stenosis.[78] If the temperature rise of the venous wall is excessive, irreversible changes in the collagen and elastin of the vein wall will occur. In vitro heating of pulmonary vein rings showed a 53% reduction in circumference and a loss of compliance with hyperthermic exposure at or above 70°C. After exposure to those temperatures, results of the histologic examination showed loss of the typical collagen structure, presumably caused by thermal denaturation of that protein.[79] For this reason, most pulmonary vein isolation is now performed outside the vein in the pulmonary vein antrum.

CELLULAR MECHANISMS OF THERMAL INJURY

The therapeutic effect of RF catheter ablation is caused by electrical heating of tissue and thermal injury. The field of hyperthermia is broad, and the effects of long-duration exposures to mild and moderate hyperthermia have been well characterized in the oncology literature. Thermal injury is dependent on both time and temperature. For example, when human bone marrow cells in culture are exposed to a temperature of 42°C, cell survival is 45% at 300 minutes. However, when those cells are heated to 45.5°C, survival at 20 minutes is only 1%.[80] Data regarding the effects of brief exposure of myocardium to higher temperatures, as is the case during catheter ablation, are more limited and are reviewed in this section. The central zone of the ablation lesion reaches high temperatures and is simply coagulated. Lower temperatures are reached during the ablation in the border zones of the lesion. The responses of the various cellular components to low and moderate hyperthermia determine the pathophysiologic response to ablation. The thermally sensitive elements that contribute to overall thermal injury to the myocyte are the plasma membrane with its integrated channel proteins, the nucleus, and the cytoskeleton. Changes in these structures that occur during hyperthermic exposure all contribute to the ultimate demise of the cell.

Plasma Membrane

The plasma membrane is very thermally sensitive. A pure phospholipid bilayer will undergo phase transitions from a relatively solid form to a semiliquid form as temperature rises. Addition of integral proteins and the varying composition of the phospholipids with regard to the saturation of the hydrocarbon side chains affect the degree of membrane fluidity in eukaryotic cells. In one study, cultured mammalian cell membranes were found to have a phase transition at 8°C and a second transition between 22°C and 36°C. No phase changes were seen in the 37°C–45°C temperature range, but studies have not been performed examining this phenomenon in sarcomeres or at temperatures above 45°C.[81] Regarding the function of integral plasma membrane proteins during exposure to heating, both inhibition and accentuation of protein activity have been observed. Stevenson and colleagues reported an increase in intracellular potassium (K^+) uptake in cultured Chinese hamster ovary cells upon heating up to 42°C. This was blocked by ouabain, indicating an increased activity of the sodium (Na^+),K^+–adenosine triphosphatase pump.[82] Nath and colleagues examined action potentials in vitro in a superfused guinea pig papillary muscle preparation. In the low hyperthermic range between 38°C and 45°C, there was an increase in the maximal dV/dt (rate of phase 0 depolarization) of the action potential, indicating enhanced Na^+ channel kinetics. In the moderate hyperthermia range from 45°C–50°C, the maximal dV/dt decreased below baseline values. The mechanism of this Na^+ channel inhibition was hypothesized to be either partial thermal inactivation of the Na^+ channel or, more likely, voltage-dependent Na^+ channel inactivation caused by thermally mediated cellular depolarization[83] (see later discussion).

Cytoskeleton

The cytoskeleton is composed of structural proteins that form microtubules, microfilaments, and intermediate filaments. The microfilaments coalesce into stress filaments. These include the proteins actin, actinin, and tropomyosin and form the framework to which the contractile elements of the myocyte attach. The cytoskeletal elements may have varying degrees of thermal sensitivity depending on the cell type. For example in human erythrocytes, the cytoskeleton is composed predominantly of the protein spectrin. Spectrin is thermally inactivated at 50°C. When erythrocytes are exposed to temperatures above 50°C, the erythrocytes rapidly lose their biconcave shape.[84] There is no scientific literature reporting the inactivation temperature of the cytoskeletal proteins in myocytes. However, electron micrographs of the border zone of RF lesions show significant disruption in the cellular architecture with loss of the myofilament structure.[67] In the central portion of the RF lesion, thermal inactivation of the cytoskeleton contributes to the typical appearance of coagulation necrosis.

Nucleus

The eukaryote nucleus shows evidence of thermal sensitivity in both structure and function. Nuclear membrane vesiculation, condensation of cytoplasmic elements in the perinuclear region, and a decrease in heterochromatin content have been described.[85,86] The nucleolus appears to be the most heat-sensitive component of the nucleus. Whether hyperthermia induces DNA strand breaks is controversial. One reproducible finding after hyperthermic exposure is the elaboration of nuclear proteins called *heat shock proteins* (HSPs). Although the function of HSPs has not been entirely elucidated, they appear to exert a protective effect on the cell. It is hypothesized that 70-kDa HSP facilitates the effective production and folding of proteins and assists their transit among organelles.[87]

Cellular Electrophysiology

Hyperthermia leads to dramatic changes on the electrophysiology of myocardium. The thermal sensitivity of myocytes has been tested in a variety of experimental systems, and the mechanisms of the electrophysiologic responses to catheter ablation have been elucidated. In one series of in vitro experiments, isolated superfused guinea pig papillary muscles were subjected to 60 seconds of exposure to hyperthermic superfusate at temperatures varying from 38°C to 55°C.[83] Action potentials were recorded continuously during and after the hyperthermic pulse. If resting membrane potential was not restored after return to normothermia, the muscle was discarded, and testing proceeded with a new tissue sample. The resting membrane potential was assessed in unpaced preparations, and the action potential amplitude, duration, dV/dt, and excitability were tested during pacing. The preparations maintained a normal resting membrane potential in the low hyperthermic range (<45°C). In the intermediate hyperthermic range (45°C–50°C), the myocytes showed a temperature-dependent depolarization that was reversible on return to normothermic superfusion. Finally, experiments in the high hyperthermic range (>50°C) typically resulted in irreversible depolarization, contracture, and death (Fig. 1.12). There was a temperature-dependent decrease in action potential amplitude between 37°C and 50°C as well as an inverse linear relationship between temperature and action potential duration. With increasing temperatures, the dV/dt increased, but above 46°C, this measurement began to decrease in preparations that had a greater magnitude of resting membrane potential depolarization.

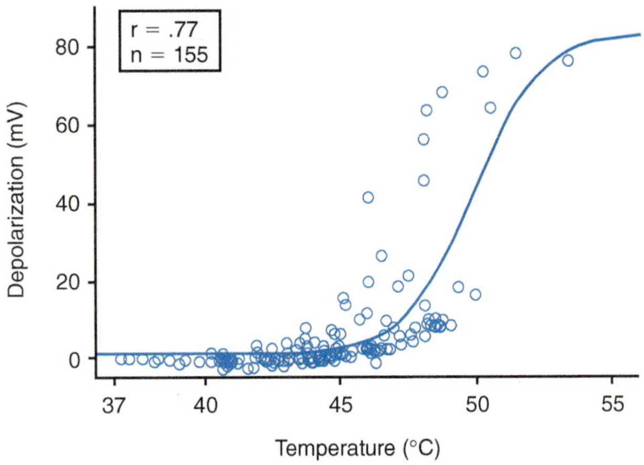

Fig. 1.12 The magnitude of depolarization of guinea pig papillary muscle cells exposed to 1-minute pulses of hyperthermic perfusate versus perfusate temperature. At temperatures below 45°C, little depolarization is seen. The cells have progressive depolarization between 45°C and 50°C. Above 50°C, few recordings are made because most cells have irreversible contracture and death. (From Nath S, Lynch C III, Whayne JG, Haines DE. Cellular electrophysiological effects of hyperthermia on isolated guinea pig papillary muscle: implications for catheter ablation. *Circulation*. 1993;88:1826–1831.)

Spontaneous automaticity was observed in both paced and unpaced preparations at a median temperature of 50°C, compared with a temperature of 44°C in preparations without automaticity.[83] The occurrence of automaticity in unpaced preparations in the setting of hyperthermia-induced depolarization suggested abnormal automaticity as the mechanism. Beginning at temperatures higher than 42°C, loss of excitability to external-field stimulation was seen in some paced preparations and was dependent on the resting membrane potential. Mean resting membrane potential observed with loss of excitability was −44 mV, compared with −82 mV for normal excitability. The superfusate temperature measured during reversible loss of excitability was 43°C–51°C, but irreversible loss of excitability (cell death) occurred only at temperatures of 50°C or higher. Thus, it appeared from these experiments that there was increased cationic entry into the hyperthermic cell and that the resultant depolarization led to loss of excitability and cell death.

Calcium Overload and Cellular Injury

In a preparation similar to that described previously, Everett and colleagues further elucidated the specific mechanisms for cellular depolarization and death in response to hyperthermia.[88] Isolated superfused guinea pig papillary muscles were attached to a force transducer to assess the pattern of contractility with varying hyperthermic exposure. Consistent with the observations of resting membrane potential changes during heating, there was a reversible increase in tonic resting muscle tension at temperatures between 45°C and 50°C. Above 50°C, the preparations showed evidence of irreversible contracture. This suggested that hyperthermia was causing calcium entry into the cell and ultimately calcium overload. This hypothesis was confirmed with calcium-sensitive fluo-3-acetoxymethyl (AM) dye. Hyperthermic increases in papillary muscle tension correlated well with fluo-3-AM luminescence. To elucidate the mechanism of calcium entry into the cell and its role in cellular injury, preparations were pretreated with either a calcium channel blocker (cadmium or verapamil) or an inhibitor of the sarcoplasmic reticulum calcium pump (thapsigargin). Preparations heated to 42°C–44°C showed no significant changes in tension at baseline or with drug treatment. Upon exposure to 48°C, treatment with calcium channel blockers did not reduce the increase in resting tension or fluo-3-AM fluorescence, suggesting that the increase in cytosolic calcium was not the consequence of channel-specific calcium entry into the cell. By contrast, thapsigargin treatment led to irreversible papillary muscle contracture at lower temperatures (45°C–50°C) than that observed without this agent. For preparations heated to 48°C, there was a greater increase in muscle tension and fluo-3-AM fluorescence in the thapsigargin group compared with controls (Fig. 1.13). The authors concluded that hyperthermia results in significant increases in intracellular calcium, probably because of nonspecific transmembrane transit through thermally induced sarcolemmal pores. With increased intracellular calcium entry, the sarcoplasmic reticulum acts as a protective buffer against calcium overload, unless this function is blocked with an agent like thapsigargin. In this case, cell contracture and death occur at lower temperatures than expected.[88]

Conduction Velocity

Simmers and coworkers have examined the effects of hyperthermia on impulse conduction in vitro in a preparation of superfused canine myocardium.[19] The average conduction velocity at baseline temperatures of 37°C was 0.35 m/second. When the superfusate temperature was raised, conduction velocity increased to supernormal values, reaching a maximum of 114% of baseline at 42.5°C. At temperatures above 45.4°C, conduction velocity slowed down. Transient conduction block was observed between 49.5°C and 51.5°C; above 51.7°C permanent block was observed (Fig. 1.14).[91] These findings are exactly concordant with the temperature-related changes in cellular electrophysiology described previously. In a related experiment, the authors assessed myocardial conduction across a surgically created isthmus during heating with RF energy. The temperatures recorded during transient conduction block (50.7°C ± 3.0°C) and permanent conduction block (58.0°C ± 3.4°C) were nearly identical to those temperature ranges recorded in the experiments performed with hyperthermic perfusate. The authors concluded that the sole effects of RF ablation on the electrophysiologic properties of the myocardium were hyperthermic and that there was no additional pathophysiologic response that could be attributed to direct effects of passage of electrical current through the tissue.[89] It is unknown whether these changes in conduction velocity are solely caused by changes in intracellular ionic concentrations or whether thermal injury to gap junctions may also be implicated.

DETERMINANTS OF EFFECTIVE LESION FORMATION

Targeting

The success of catheter ablation is dependent on several factors. The first and foremost factor is optimizing the targeting of

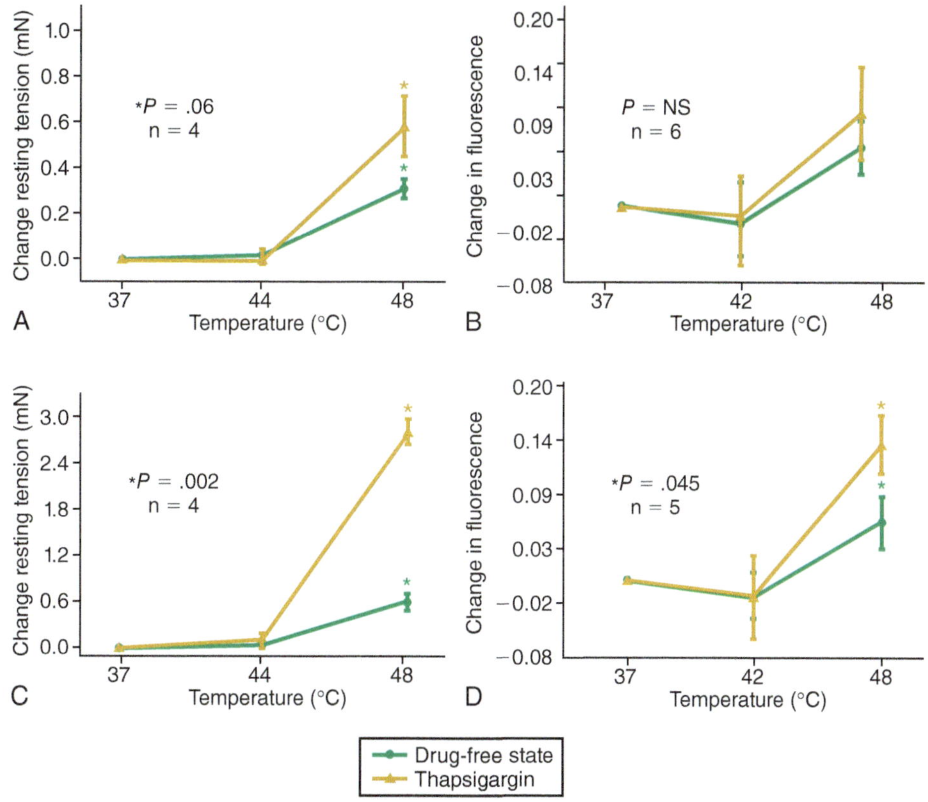

Fig. 1.13 The effects of hyperthermic exposure on calcium entry into cells were tested in isolated superfused guinea pig papillary muscles. A change in resting tension was used as a surrogate measure for cytosolic calcium concentration (A, C), and a change in fluo-3-acetoxymethyl (fluo-3-AM) fluorescence was used as a direct measure of free cytosolic calcium (B, D). With exposure to mild hyperthermia (42°C–44°C), little change in calcium levels was observed. With moderate hyperthermia (48°C), however muscle tension and fluo-3-AM fluorescence increased significantly. This increase was not channel specific because calcium-channel blockade with cadmium or verapamil did not alter this response (A, B). The response was accentuated by thapsigargin (C, D), an agent that blocks calcium reuptake by the sarcoplasmic reticulum. (From Everett TH, Nath S, Lynch C III, et al. Role of calcium in acute hyperthermic myocardial injury. *J Cardiovasc Electrophysiol.* 2001;12:563–569.)

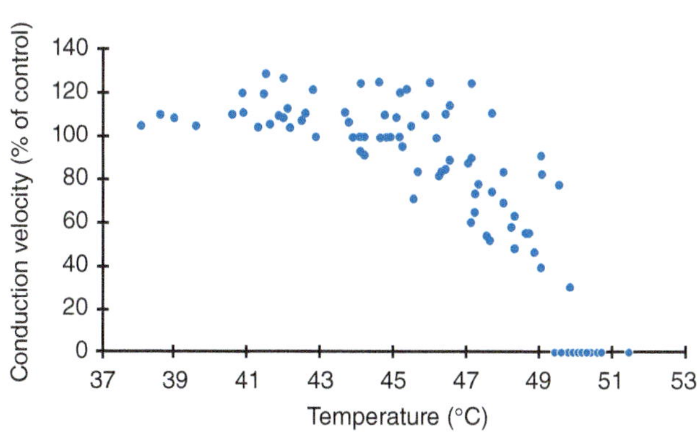

Fig. 1.14 Conduction velocity of myocardium in superfused canine myocardium in vitro versus the temperature of the superfusate. A mild augmentation of conduction velocity caused by an increase in dV/dt is observed at temperatures up to 45°C. Between 45°C and 50°C, conduction velocity falls, and above 50°C, conduction is blocked. (From Simmers TA, de Bakker JM, Wittkampf FH, Hauer RN. Effects of heating on impulse propagation in superfused canine myocardium. *J Am Coll Cardiol.* 1995;25:1457–1464.)

the arrhythmogenic substrate. It is intuitive that increasing the size and depth of an ablative lesion will not improve the ablation success if the site selected for ablation is poor. To optimize site selection, it is necessary to understand the physiology and the anatomy of the arrhythmia in its entirety. The proximity of the electrode to the target will be the most important factor for ablation success.

Tissue Composition

Lesion sizes are decreased in areas of dense scar. In addition an insulating layer of fat as thin as 2 mm overlying myocardial tissue (as in epicardial ablation) will prevent formation of a lesion with RF energy delivery.[90]

Power

Lesion size is proportional to power. Any method that will allow for greater power deposition into the tissue will result in more tissue heating and greater depth of thermal injury. In addition to power amplitude, efficiency of power coupling to the tissue (i.e., how much power is converted into tissue heat and how much is "wasted" with convective cooling) will affect ultimate lesion size.

Electrode Temperature

The electrode is passively heated by conduction of heat from the tissue during ablation. Lesion size increases directly with electrode temperature up until the point of coagulum formation and impedance rise. The relationship between lesion size and electrode temperature is confounded by the effects of convective cooling and catheter motion in vivo.

Peak Tissue Temperature

Because of convective cooling, electrode temperature underestimates peak tissue temperature—the real determinant of lesion size. Future sensors such as infrared, microwave, or ultrasound detectors may allow the operator to monitor actual lesion growth. Real-time MRI may guide ablation and provide real-time thermography or imaging of lesion formation.

Electrode Contact Force

Greater electrode–tissue contact force increases lesion size by improving electrical coupling with the tissue, increasing the electrode surface area in contact with the tissue, and reducing the shunting of current to the blood pool. In addition, greater contact force may prevent the electrode from sliding with cardiac motion. The optimal electrode contact force is believed to be 20–40*g* force.[6,39,41,42] Excessive contact that buries the electrode in the tissue, however, may prevent convective cooling of the electrode and reduce current delivery.

Convective Cooling

Ultimately, lesion size is a function of tissue heating, and tissue heating is a function of the magnitude of RF power that is converted into heat in the tissues. The greater the magnitude of power delivered to the tissue, the greater is the lesion size. Convective cooling at the electrode–tissue interface, either active or passive, will allow the operator to increase safely the power amplitude before impedance rises. However, if the ablation is power limited (i.e., the power amplitude is fixed throughout the ablation), greater degrees of convective cooling will draw heat from the tissue surface to create a smaller endocardial lesion diameter, especially at the endocardial surface, and smaller lesion volume. The two factors that affect passive cooling at the electrode–tissue interface are the magnitude of regional blood flow and the stability of the electrode catheter on the tissue surface. Catheter motion over the tissue greatly increases the loss of heat to the blood pool. Intramyocardial blood flow draws heat from the tissue and not from the electrode and therefore decreases lesion size.

Electrode Size

When the goal is to maximize lesion size, larger electrodes will always be better than smaller electrodes. Larger electrodes increase the surface area and allow the operator to deliver higher total power without excessive current density at the electrode–tissue interface. Thus, coagulum formation with a sudden rise in electrical impedance can be avoided despite high total power delivery. The higher power delivery to the tissue increases the depth of direct volume heating and in turn increases the size of the virtual heat source. This translates directly into a larger lesion. As is the case with cooled electrodes, a large electrode will result in larger lesion formation only if it is accompanied by higher power delivery. If a large electrode is used with lower power, a larger endocardial surface area may be ablated, but the lesion will not be as deep. The RF energy delivery to multiple electrodes may simultaneously produce a large lesion as well, but other issues such as catheter and target geometry may limit energy coupling to the tissue if the electrode–tissue contact is poor.

Duration of Energy Delivery

Tissue temperature follows a monoexponential rise during RF delivery (Table 1.2) until steady state is achieved. The half-time for lesion formation is 5–10 seconds for conventional ablation. Therefore, lesion formation is assumed to be nearly complete after 45–60 seconds (five half-lives). Large lesion technologies such as irrigated-tip catheters have a longer half-time of lesion growth, and in these cases continued energy application for 2 minutes or longer may result in some incremental gain in lesion depth. High-power short-duration (HPSD) energy delivery will maximize heating in the first 2–3 mm and lessen heating in deeper layers.[27]

Ablation Circuit Impedance

For RF ablation, reducing resistance within the cables and dispersive electrode current path will increase current delivery to the tissue. Using 0.45% saline as an irrigation solution may result in greater current density and heating within the tissue. Placing dispersive electrodes on the trunk rather than on the thigh and using two dispersive electrodes particularly when baseline impedance is high will maximize tissue heating.

Electrode Orientation

For nonirrigated electrodes with unrestricted power, an orientation parallel to the tissue generally results in larger lesions because of a larger electrode area in contact with the tissue and less current shunting to the blood pool. For irrigated electrodes delivering high-power outputs, the parallel electrode orientation may result in smaller lesion sizes because of a greater magnitude of tissue cooling.[44]

Electrode Geometry

Very long electrodes will provide greater surface area, allow higher power delivery, and usually yield larger lesions. If the electrode is too long, however, efficiency of electrode coupling to the tissue is lost, and lesion size is not increased.[26] In addition, power is concentrated at points of geometric transitions (the edge effect), resulting in the possibility of excess heating at the electrode edges and less heating in the middle of the electrode.[57]

Electrode Material

Electrode materials with high heat-transfer characteristics (such as gold and diamond) are more effectively cooled by passive blood flow and may allow for greater energy deliveries.[29,30]

TABLE 1.2 Factors Influencing Radiofrequency Lesion Size

Factor	Effect on Lesion Size
Targeting	Close proximity to the target improves likelihood of success even with a small lesion size
Tissue composition	Smaller lesion sizes in scar and fat
Power	Directly proportional to lesion size
Ablation electrode temperature	Underestimates peak tissue temperature because of convective cooling effects
Peak tissue temperature	Directly proportional to lesion size
Electrode–tissue contact force	Directly proportional to lesion size
Convective cooling – Electrode–tissue interface Active—perfused tip catheter Passive—large tip, sliding contact – Intramyocardial arterial flow	– With fixed energy delivery, reduces lesion size – With unlimited energy, increases lesion size
Electrode size	Directly proportional to lesion size provided unrestricted power
Duration energy delivery	Monoexponential relation to lesion size with half-time lesion formation of 5–10 seconds
Ablation circuit impedance	Lower body and dispersive (skin) patch resistance increases current delivery Shunting current through blood decreases impedance but can reduced lesion size
Electrode orientation	For nonirrigated electrode, parallel orientation increases lesion size For irrigated electrode, perpendicular orientation increases lesion size
Electrode geometry	Effects lesion size and shape by concentrating current density at electrode edges and asymmetries
Electrode material	Higher heat conductive materials increase lesion size by electrode cooling
RF characteristics	
– Pulsed	– May increase lesion size by allowing electrode cooling
– Phased	– Increases continuity of linear lesions formed with multi-electrode arrays
– Frequency	– Reduced heating efficiency at higher (MHz) frequencies

Characteristics of Radiofrequency Energy

Very high frequencies of alternating current lead to less efficient tissue heating, and lower frequencies may result in tissue stimulation causing pain and arrhythmias. Pulsed RF current may allow for more electrode cooling than unmodulated RF and therefore increase power delivery. With multielectrode ablation arrays, phased RF among the electrodes allows for more continuous linear lesions (Fig. 1.15).

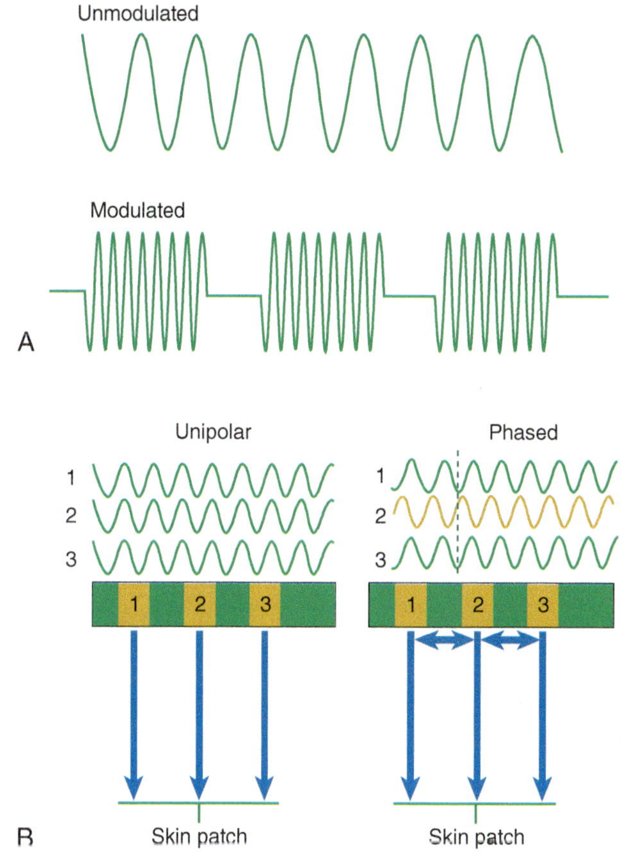

Fig. 1.15 (A) Unmodulated and modulated patterns of radiofrequency (RF) power. The modulated waveform is pulsed with periods of oscillating voltage separated by periods of quiescence. (B) Unipolar and phased RF deliveries from a multielectrode array. With the unipolar delivery, the oscillating voltages among the electrodes are all in phase, and therefore there is no electrical potential for current flow between electrodes. With phased RF, the oscillations in voltage among contiguous electrodes are out of phase, creating an electrical potential for current to flow between electrodes as well as to the dispersive skin electrode.

IMPROVING RADIOFREQUENCY ABLATION EFFECTIVENESS

High-Power Short-Duration

This is an umbrella term that encompasses combining high power (arbitrarily defined as 40–90 W) and short duration (15 seconds or less) for ablation instead of the traditional low-power long-duration (LPLD) RF ablation.[91,92] The premise of HPSD lies in the fact that the fastest change in lesion formation occurs within the first 10 seconds with greatly diminishing returns beyond 20 seconds of RF application. Therefore, beyond the constraints of time of RF application, power then becomes the main driver to augment lesion depth.[93] This modality creates a larger zone of direct resistive heating with less total energy deposition, limiting the extent of conductive heating. The lesions are generally wider with shallower depth but over all have similar volumes as traditional lesions. HPSD offers a theoretical advantage to reduce the risk of collateral injury, especially germane to esophageal damage during ablation in the posterior left atrium. Animal studies suggest that the standard ablation settings had endocardial preservation owing to the irrigation-induced endocardial cooling, which leads to incomplete lesion formation. HPSD abolishes this element of endocardial sparing.[91] Therefore, the resultant HPSD lesions are oval in cross section compared to the traditional tear drop morphology with standard application.

Unfortunately, increasing power increases risk of steam pops. The very HPSD (vHPSD) ablation catheter platform QDot (Biosense Webster, Diamond Bar, CA) attempts to address this risk and can deliver 90 W over 4 seconds. The algorithm can modulate power based on the thermocouple with the highest heating (65°C) and mitigate the risk of steam pop.[92] In vivo models have suggested more contiguous and transmural lesions with no evidence of collateral pulmonary parenchymal injury compared to 30 W at 30 s[94]; however, rates of esophageal injury by MRI are similar to those seen with standard ablation.[94] Single-center clinical studies have demonstrated reduction in ablation, fluoroscopy, and overall procedure times while maintaining excellent long-term outcomes.[92,95]

Indices of Successful Ablation

Proprietary indices that use algorithms with various input variables selected during ablation have been used to assist the operator in creating durable ablative lesions. The Ablation Index (AI) (Biosense Webster) is calculated using ablation time, energy, contact force, and catheter stability. Targeting AI >550 in the anterior wall and >400 over the posterior wall demonstrated 96% AF freedom off antiarrhythmic drugs at 6 months,[96] and a randomized clinical trial demonstrated shorter procedure time but no difference in long-term outcomes of AF ablation with AI-guided lesion delivery.[97] The Lesion Size Index (LSI) (Abbott Laboratories, Chicago, IL) also incorporates the AI parameters plus impedance drop. An LSI >5.5–6 led to 86% and 83% freedom at 1 year from AF in one single-center trial.[98] Other surrogate endpoints of value include unipolar electrogram modification, loss of pace capture, and fall in local or system impedance in response to RF energy delivery.

Advanced Radiofrequency Catheter Designs

While RF remains the workhorse for most ablations, the point-by-point application requires a certain degree of dexterity, learning curve, and time. Balloon RF technology aspires to rapid and easy single-shot isolation of the pulmonary veins. It provides an alternative to other balloon-based technologies like cryotherapy and laser energy delivery.

The Satake hot balloon system is approved in Japan and has shown comparable outcomes to rhythm control in paroxysmal AF population.[99] It is composed of a highly compliant polyurethane balloon that has an electrode within the balloon to directly heat the saline. Tissue is ablated by thermal conduction from the hot balloon surface. This technology does not prevent the infrequent complications of esophageal injury and pulmonary vein stenosis.[100]

The Luminize/Apama balloon (Boston Scientific, Marlborough, MA) platform has 12 proximal and 6 distal electrodes. It has the ability of pacing and sensing with microelectrodes and has LED lighting to provide real-time visualization of tissue contact. The AF-FICIENT 1 trial has demonstrated a high rate of acute isolation (98%) with 78% freedom from AF at 6 months.[101]

The Heliostar (Biosense Webster, Irvine, CA) incorporates 10 flexible, gold irrigated catheter electrodes. Similar to the Luminize platform, Heliostar has the ability to pace and sense but also permits integration with three-dimensional mapping system and fluoroscopic visualization. Its feasibility was demonstrated in the SHINE trial, where 85 patients with paroxysmal AF underwent PV isolation with a 72% freedom of atrial arrhythmias at 12 months.[102]

The Kardium Globe catheter is not balloon based but rather consists of a nonirrigated multielectrode array of 122 gold-plated electrodes mounted on 16 ribs, of which 24 electrodes can permit RF delivery at a time in a temperature-controlled mode. The electrodes can pace, sense, and deliver RF current. A temperature sensor map helps determine atrial tissue contact, and activation mapping shows wavefront propagation. The Global AF study showed 99% acute pulmonary vein isolation in 60 patients and 72% freedom from AF at 12 months.[103]

BIOPHYSICS OF PULSED-FIELD ABLATION COMPARED TO RADIOFREQUENCY ABLATION

Pulsed-field ablation (PFA) promises to be a dominant modality of catheter ablation going forward (see Chapter 4). Both RFA and PFA create ablative lesions with the passage of electrical current into tissue, but the mechanism of injury with PFA is electrical not thermal. The differences in the two energy forms are summarized in Table 1.3. The very high-voltage and very short-duration pulses cause electroporation and electropermeabilization of the cell membrane. In the lower range, the pores are very transitory, allowing passage of macromolecules intracellularly without killing the cells (reversible electroporation). Higher voltages lead to organelle

TABLE 1.3 Radiofrequency Ablation Versus Pulsed-Field Ablation

	Radiofrequency Ablation	Pulsed-Field Ablation
Electrical Parameters		
Voltage	10–100 V	500–3000 V
Waveform	Sinusoidal	Monophasic or biphasic DC
Frequency	500–750 kHz	300 kHz–10 MHz
Pulse duration	Continuous	10 ns–100 μs
Number of pulses	1	1–200
Biological Parameters		
Mode of injury	Thermal	Electrical, dielectric breakdown
Mechanism of death	Necrosis	Apoptosis, necroptosis, pyroptosis, necrosis
Main target of injury	Sarcolemmal membrane, plasma membrane	Organelles

damage, irreversible electropermeabilization and cell death. If even higher voltages are used, the thermal threshold is crossed, and targeted tissues begin to show desiccation and protein denaturation. Thermal effects are best avoided to minimize the risk of coagulum and other particulate material forming at the ablation site.

CONCLUSION

The RF catheter ablation has been the dominant modality for ablative therapy of arrhythmias. This technology is simple and has a high success rate and a low complication rate. An appreciation of the biophysics and pathophysiology of RF energy heating of myocardium during catheter ablation will help the operator make the proper adjustments to optimize ablation safety and success. A tissue temperature of 50°C needs to be reached to achieve irreversible tissue injury. This likely occurs because of sarcolemmal membrane injury and intracellular calcium overload. The 50°C isotherm determines the boundary of the lesion. Greater lesion size is achieved with higher power delivery and higher intramural tissue temperatures. Energy coupling to tissue is optimized by ensuring optimal catheter contact force into tissue. Monitoring surface temperature in noncooled catheters is useful in preventing boiling of blood with coagulum formation and a sudden increase in electrical impedance. Irrigated-tip catheters are effective at allowing the operator to increase power resulting in increased lesion depth. A full understanding of the biophysics of catheter ablation and the anatomy and physiology of the arrhythmogenic substrate will allow the operator to select the optimal ablation approach. The future will likely see widespread adoption of pulsed-field ablation, particularly for the ablation of atrial fibrillation, but RF ablation will certainly remain a mainstay in light of its long record of safety, efficacy, and predictability.

REFERENCES

Please refer to the e-book for a complete list of references.

2

Biophysics and Clinical Applications of Cryoablation

Antoine Noel, Jason G. Andrade, Paul Khairy, Marc Dubuc

KEY POINTS

- The biophysics and mechanisms of cryothermal injury comprise the following general phases: freeze–thaw, hemorrhage and inflammation, replacement fibrosis, and apoptosis.
- Cryoablation lesion size is determined by refrigerant flow rate, electrode size, electrode contact pressure, electrode orientation, duration of energy delivery, and electrode temperature.
- Advantages of cryoablation include the ability to titrate temperature/duration to produce reversible lesions before permanent tissue destruction (cryomapping), decreased risk of thromboembolism, superior catheter stability, and lesser risk of injury to vascular structures.
- Cryoablation has been applied clinically to a variety of arrhythmic substrates including atrioventricular (AV) nodal ablation, AV nodal reentrant tachycardia, mid- and paraseptal pathways, ventricular tachycardia, atrial flutter, and atrial fibrillation.

INTRODUCTION

The introduction of percutaneous direct-current ablation over 30 years ago launched an era of interventional cardiac electrophysiology that transformed the management of cardiac arrhythmias. Direct-current ablation was later supplanted by radiofrequency (RF) energy, which offered a more attractive safety and efficacy profile. Transcatheter RF ablation was broadly disseminated as the procedure of choice, with expanding indications that paralleled the growing global experience and knowledge base. Although the benefits of RF ablation became widely appreciated, limitations were noted, such as thromboembolization, inadvertent collateral damage to surrounding vascular and electrical structures, and the limited ability to assess electrophysiologic effects before permanent lesion creation.

The scientific community therefore persevered in its efforts to further improve patient safety and procedural outcomes by seeking alternative sources of energy and developing ablation systems capable of creating deeper, larger, and more contiguous lesions. It is within this context that cryothermal energy ablation emerged as an alternative treatment modality. With the first transcatheter procedure performed in humans at the Montreal Heart Institute in August 1998, the collective experience has increased exponentially over the past 25 years.[1] Potential advantages were recognized, including an impressive safety record with decreased thrombogenic potential, improved catheter stability during cryoapplications, lesser propensity to damage vascular structures, the ability to produce reversible electrophysiologic effects before permanent lesion creation, and decreased levels of pain perceived by patients.

The purpose of this chapter is to provide the clinical electrophysiologists, trainees, and cardiologists with a solid understanding of the field of cryoablation, beginning with a brief historical overview, discussion of biophysics, and depiction of the components of a transvenous catheter cryoenergy delivery system. Advantages and limitations of cryoablation are reviewed, and current clinical applications are discussed.

HISTORY OF CRYOTHERMAL ENERGY USE IN CARDIOVASCULAR MEDICINE

The use of cold temperatures to elicit a specific tissue response has a long history of effective medical use. The concept of cooling to treat medical disorders dates to the ancient Egyptians, who described the use of hypothermic therapy between 3000 and 1600 BC.[2,3] In the mid-1800s, iced saline was used for the treatment of carcinomas of the cervix and breast, followed by the topical use of liquid oxygen, nitrogen, and hydrogen for superficial carcinomas in the early 1900s. In 1948, Hass and coworkers first described predictable controlled myocardial lesions with cryoenergy using carbon dioxide as a refrigerant.[4,5] In 1964, Lister and coworkers described the application of cryoenergy to the cardiac conduction tissue by suturing a 4-mm U-shaped silver tube delivering cold energy near the bundle of His.[6] Thus although not novel as an energy modality, harnessing cryoenergy into a steerable transcatheter format represented a significant landmark in the history of arrhythmia therapy. Table 2.1 summarizes key historical landmarks in the development of a transvenous cryoablation system for cardiac arrhythmias.[3,4,6–11]

TABLE 2.1 Historical Landmarks in Cardiac Cryoablation

Year	Authors (Ref. No.)	Contribution
1948–1951	Hass and colleagues[4,5]	Cryothermal myocardial lesions
1963	Cooper and Lee[7]	Cryosurgical apparatus development
1964	Lister and coworkers[6]	Cryothermal energy used to retard conductive tissue with evidence of reversibility
1977	Harrison and coworkers[8]	Surgical application of cryothermal energy by handheld probe
1991	Gillette and coworkers[9]	Percutaneous application of cryothermal energy by transvenous catheter in animals
1998	Dubuc and coworkers[10]	Use of steerable cryocatheter system with pacing and recording electrodes
2001	Dubuc and coworkers[11]	Percutaneous transvenous catheter cryoablation in humans

From Khairy P, Dubuc M. Transcatheter cryoablation. In: Liem LB, Downar E, eds. *Progress in Catheter Ablation.* Dordrecht, The Netherlands; 2001:391.

The modern era of cryosurgery was initiated by Cooper and Lee when vacuum-insulated cryosurgical probes cooled by liquid nitrogen (−196°C) were introduced in the early 1960s.[12] Evolving from Cooper's apparatus, in which cooling was produced by a liquid-to-gas phase change in nitrogen, novel cryoprobes were developed using the Peltier effect (i.e., thermoelectric cooling by passing a direct current through dissimilar metal junctions) or cooling by the Joule–Thomson effect (i.e., cooling from the expansion of a highly compressed nonideal gas into a region of low pressure).

In the 1970s, the rigid handheld cryothermal ablation probes were adapted for cardiac surgical applications as an alternative to open surgical dissection for the treatment of refractory arrhythmic substrates.[8,13–15] In 1977, separate reports from Harrison and coworkers and Gallagher and coworkers demonstrated the efficacy of cryothermal ablation for supraventricular arrhythmic substrates.[13] Under cardiopulmonary bypass, Harrison and coworkers produced complete atrioventricular (AV) nodal block using a handheld bipolar electrode probe by cooling the His bundle in 20 dogs and achieved AV block in three patients with refractory supraventricular tachycardia.[8] Long term follow up on a larger series was later reported, with AV block successfully achieved in 17 of 22 patients. That same year, Gallagher and coworkers reported the first two cases of successful cryosurgical accessory pathway ablation.[13] Reports were also published on novel approaches obviating the need for extracorporeal bypass (i.e., ablation within the coronary sinus or right coronary fossa, or through the use of dual atriotomy incisions) and targeting selected patients with refractory ventricular arrhythmias (often as an adjunct to more extensive surgery including aneurysmectomy, subendocardial resection, encircling endocardial ventriculotomy, coronary artery bypass grafting, and valvular replacement).[15–27] Surgical cryoablation has also been described for less common arrhythmias including nodoventricular tachycardia,[28] sinoatrial reentrant tachycardia,[29] disabling ventricular bigeminy,[30] bundle branch reentry tachycardia,[31] and fetal malignant tachyarrhythmias.[32]

Gillette and coworkers reported the first animal study using a transvenous cryocatheter in 1991.[9] In five miniature swine, complete AV block was produced with an 11-F cryocatheter cooled by pressurized nitrous oxide with a limited success attributed to limited maneuverability as well as the lack of recording electrodes. Transcatheter cryoablation was revived several years later, ultimately leading to clinical use. In 1998, the first animal experiment using a steerable cryocatheter with integrated recording and pacing electrodes was reported.[10] This 9-F catheter system used halocarbon 502 (Freon) as a refrigerant. Chronic histology was later characterized, with sharply demarcated ultrastructurally intact lesions devoid of thrombus. These and other preclinical studies contributed importantly to the understanding of the impact of cooling rate and catheter-tip temperature on tissue effects.[10,23,24,33,34]

BIOPHYSICS AND MECHANISMS OF CRYOTHERMAL ENERGY TISSUE INJURY

The ultimate purpose of cryoablation is to freeze tissue in a discrete and focused fashion to destroy cells in a precisely targeted area. The application of cryothermal energy results in the formation of an ice ball. Cooling first occurs at the distal catheter tip in contact with endocardial tissue. Freezing then extends radially into the tissue, establishing a temperature gradient. The lowest temperature and fastest freezing rate are generated at the point of contact, with slower tissue cooling rates at the peripheral regions.[10,34–37] The mechanisms of tissue damage are complex and still debated but involve freezing and thawing, hemorrhage and inflammation, replacement fibrosis, and apoptosis (Fig. 2.1).[38]

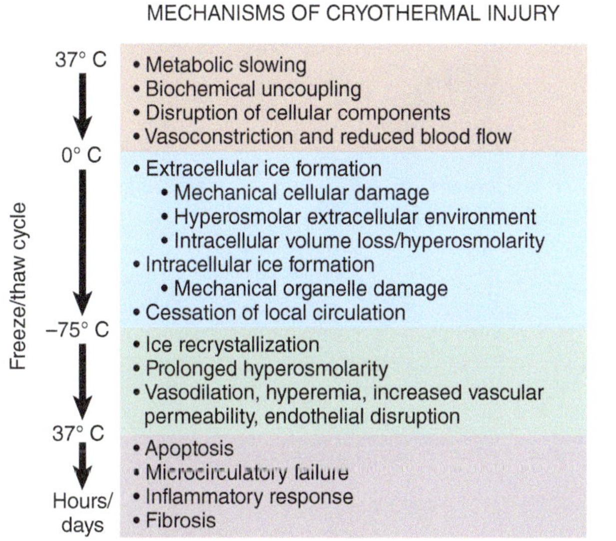

Fig. 2.1 Mechanisms of cryothermal injury during the freeze-thaw cycle of catheter cryoablation.

Tissue hypothermia causes cardiomyocytes to become less fluidic as metabolism slows, ion pumps to lose transport capabilities, and intracellular pH to become more acidic.[33] These effects may be transient, depending on the interplay between temperature and duration. The shorter the exposure to a hypothermic insult and/or the warmer the temperature, the faster the cells recover. As a clinical correlate, this characteristic feature of cryoenergy permits functional assessment of putative ablation sites (i.e., cryomapping) without cellular destruction.

By contrast, the hallmark of permanent tissue injury induced by hypothermia is the formation of ice crystals. As cells are rapidly cooled to freezing temperatures, ice crystals are first formed within the extracellular matrix and then intracellularly.[39] The size of ice crystals and their density are dependent on the combination of the following: proximity to the cryoenergy source, local tissue temperature achieved, and rate of freezing. Initially, ice crystals are formed exclusively in the extracellular space as the tissue temperature drops below −15°C. Progressive cooling to below −40°C results in the formation of intracellular ice crystals.[39] Although ice crystals are associated with mechanical cellular disruption, the predominant mechanism of cellular injury is biochemical.[40–42] The formation of extracellular ice crystals results in the extracellular space becoming relative hypertonic. To reestablish osmotic equilibrium, there is a compensatory egress of water from the intracellular to the extracellular space, with subsequent cellular shrinkage, resulting in intracellular desiccation.[42] Further, the newly established osmotic gradient precipitates a diffusion gradient between extracellular and intracellular spaces, resulting in the net movement of hydrogen ions (H^+) out of the cell and the migration of solute ions into the cell. A concomitant increase in the intracellular saline concentration with a reduction in intracellular pH results in cellular protein damage, enzyme system impairment, and adverse effects on lipoprotein components of the plasma membrane.[42,43] Of all the cytoplasmic components, the mitochondria are particularly sensitive and are the first structures to suffer irreversible damage.[44–46]

Upon completion of the freezing phase, the tissue passively returns to body temperature resulting in a thawing effect. This second phase induces cellular damage through a combination of two mechanisms. First, recrystallization and coalescence of intracellular and extracellular ice crystals increase the osmotic damage and generate shear forces, which further disrupt tissue architecture.[41,47] Second, restoration of microcirculatory function is associated with a hyperemic vascular response characterized by hemorrhage and inflammation (coagulation necrosis; Fig. 2.2A).[33,38–40] Specifically, blood vessel walls become porous, leading to increased capillary permeability, and subsequent interstitial edema. This vascular congestion, combined with endothelial injury, induces platelet aggregation and microthrombi formation and culminates in vascular obliteration and ischemic cellular necrosis. As such, although the central region subjected to the coldest freezing temperatures undergoes direct cellular damage, the surrounding microvascular injury results in the extension of tissue destruction.

The final phase of cryoinjury begins concurrent to thawing and is characterized by reactive inflammation, followed by tissue repair and replacement fibrosis. Over the subsequent weeks, these processes culminate in the generation of a mature lesion (see Fig. 2.2B), which has a distinct, well-circumscribed central region of dense fibrosis surrounded by a narrow border zone of variable cellular death (because of microvascular injury and apoptosis).[48]

CRYOABLATION TECHNICAL ASPECTS

Console and Catheters

Although insights gained from the extensive cryosurgical experience invaluably contributed to the conceptualization of the modern transvenous catheter cryoablation system, a significant number of engineering advances were required to achieve safe and effective delivery of cryorefrigerant to the tip of a steerable percutaneous catheter. The system has undergone various modifications since its conception in the early

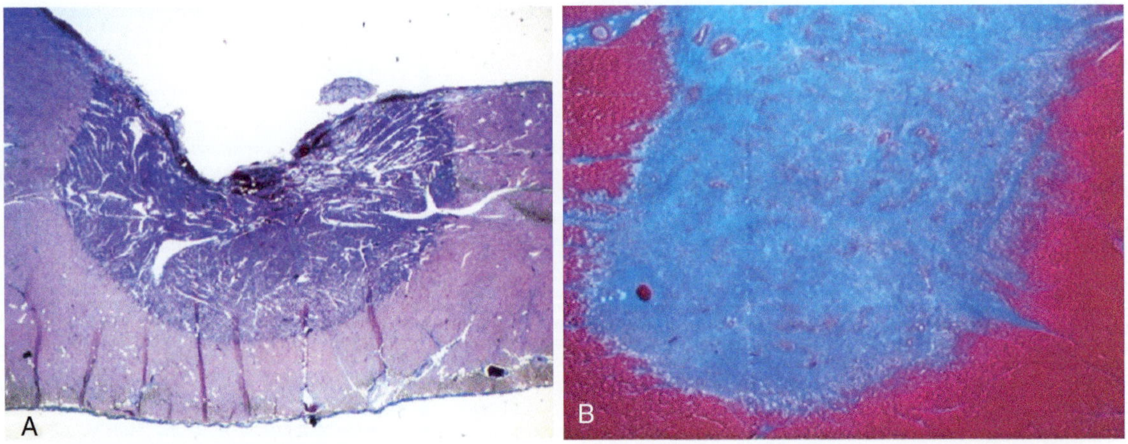

Fig. 2.2 (A) Low-power photomicrograph of a subacute cryothermal lesion; well-circumscribed borders of the lesion are seen. (B) Medium-power photomicrograph of a chronic cryothermal lesion with preserved tissue architecture. Both lesions were performed in the left ventricular myocardium of a mongrel dog with a 4-minute cryoapplication to −55°C.

1990s, but the basic design has remained constant. Specifically, the modern transvenous deflectable cryocatheter consists of a hollow shaft with a closed distal end containing a cooling electrode tip, integrated thermocouple device, and three proximal ring electrodes for recording and pacing (Fig. 2.3). A central CryoConsole (Medtronic CryoCath LP, Pointe-Claire, QC, Canada) contains the cryorefrigerant fluid (Fig. 2.4).[48] The cooling liquid travels through the inner delivery lumen to the catheter tip, where the cryorefrigerant is pressurized and released. This accelerated liquid-to-gas phase change results in rapid cooling of the distal tip. The gas is then conducted away from the catheter tip through a second coaxial return lumen maintained under vacuum and evacuated in the hospital medical gas disposal system.

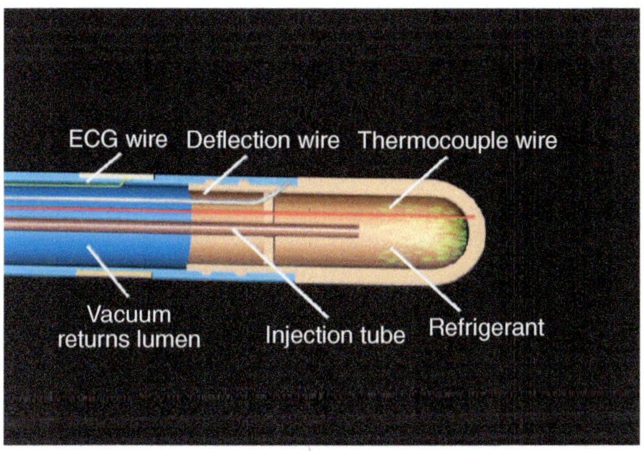

Fig. 2.3 Schematic diagram demonstrating the internal design of the CryoCath Freezor cryocatheter and its distal tip cooling by the Joule-Thomson effect. The electrocardiogram (ECG) wire, deflection wire, thermocouple wire, central injection tube, and vacuum return tip and lumen are shown. Refrigerant is injected from the central injection lumen into the distal tip, where it rapidly evaporates. The cooling of the tip causes formation of ice ball around the external portion of the distal tip with freezing of adjacent tissue. (Courtesy Medtronic CryoCath LP, Montreal, QC, Canada.)

The console allows the operator two different modes of operation. The first is the *cryomapping* mode in which the tip is cooled to a temperature not lower than −30°C for a maximum of 80 seconds, to prevent irreversible tissue damage. The second mode is *cryoablation,* which results in cooling of the catheter tip to at least −75°C for a programmable period (nominally 4 minutes), producing the permanent lesion. The cryomapping mode can be used for an indefinite number of times before cryoablation. Cryoablation may be initiated at any time during a cryomapping application or from the onset if the operator wishes to forego the cryomapping function.

Although the core tenets of its design have remained largely unchanged, the transvenous cryoablation catheter has undergone significant evolutionary advances over the years. The refrigerant has progressed from halocarbon 502 (Freon) to Genetron AZ-20 to the current nitrous oxide–generating lower catheter temperatures and faster freezing rates. Catheter diameter has been reduced from 9 F to 7 F, while larger electrode-tip sizes were introduced (4, 6, and 8 mm; Fig. 2.5). Steering mechanisms were developed and refined. Finally, with the introduction of innovative catheter configurations (focal, linear, circular, and balloon-based apparatuses), diverse clinical applications have been explored. Thus within a relatively brief time frame, the initial 9-F focal cryoablation catheter with slow cooling and a temperature limit of −50°C was transformed into the modern 7-F catheter with rapid cooling and achievable temperatures below 80°C.

In addition, expandable 23-mm (currently abandoned) and 28-mm diameter cryoballoon (CB) catheters (Arctic Front; Medtronic CryoCath LP) were specifically designed to isolate pulmonary veins (PVs) in patients with atrial fibrillation (AF; Fig. 2.6). The basic design and function of the CB catheter differ from the focal catheter in three major respects. First, instead of a rigid cooling electrode tip, the distal CB catheter consists of dual polyurethane and polyester balloons. Second, the CB is larger than the focal catheter (10.5-F outer diameter) and

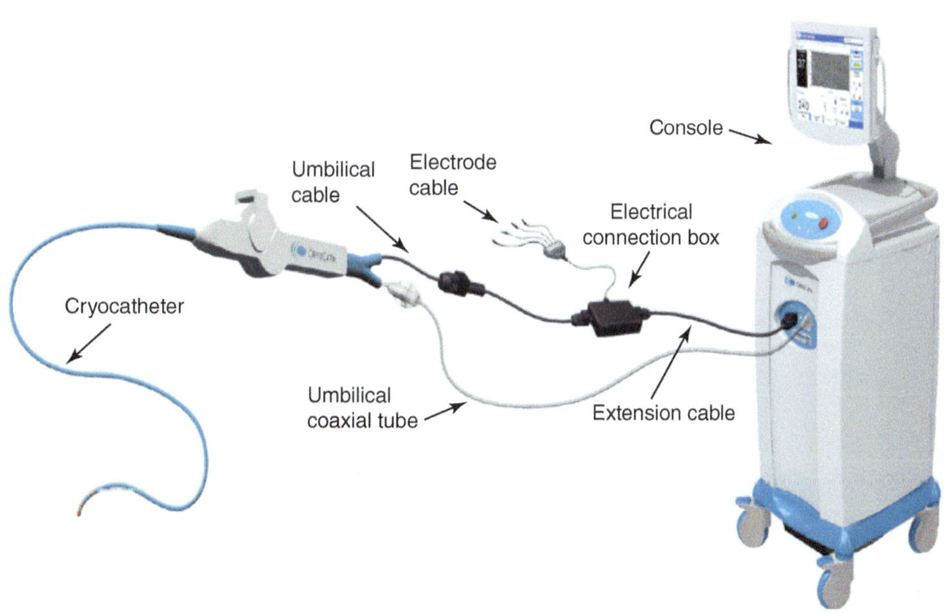

Fig. 2.4 Cryoablation console and connectors. (Courtesy Medtronic CryoCath LP, Montreal, QC, Canada.)

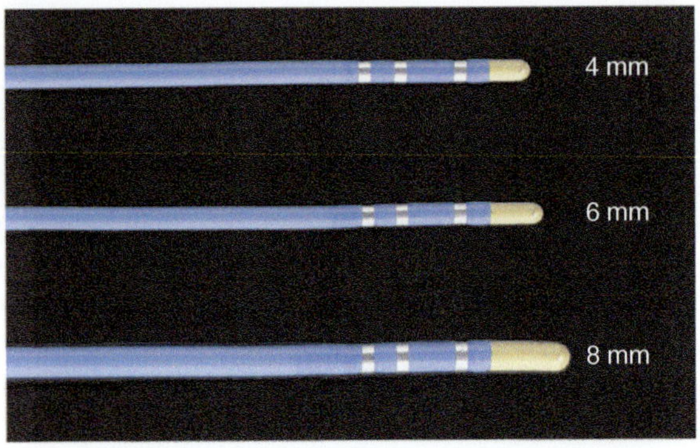

Fig. 2.5 Cryoablation catheters with 4-, 6-, and 8-mm distal electrode tips. (Courtesy Medtronic CryoCath LP, Montreal, QC, Canada.)

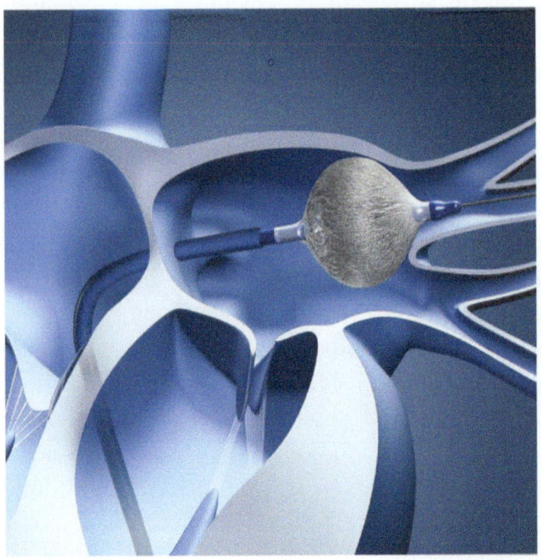

Fig. 2.6 Medtronic Arctic Front balloon cryoablation catheter. This catheter has a 10-F shaft with a lumen to permit over-the-wire placement at the ostium of the pulmonary veins and comes in balloon sizes of 23 and 28 mm. (Courtesy Medtronic CryoCath LP, Montreal, QC, Canada.)

requires the use of a 15-F (outer diameter) deflectable delivery sheath (FlexCath; Medtronic CryoCath LP). Third, the CB is deployed using an over-the-wire technique with a central lumen that permits a guidewire for positioning/support or a small-diameter circular diagnostic catheter for monitoring of PV potentials, as well as contrast injection to ensure adequate positioning. Moreover, the CB catheter underwent an evolutionary revision (Fig. 2.7). In the first-generation catheter, 6.2 L per minute of vapor was sprayed to the distal face of the balloon through four jets positioned at 90 degrees from one another, slightly distal to the CB equator. This resulted in a band of optimal cooling that was relatively equatorial and nonuniform between the two CB sizes. Specifically, given the identical refrigerant delivery mechanisms, the larger surface area associated with the 28-mm CB meant that the cryorefrigerant was delivered in a relatively less concentrated manner, resulting in heterogeneous cooling across the anterior aspect of the CB. The second-generation catheter refined the design by repositioning the jets more distally, increasing the number of jets to eight, and increasing the flow rate in the larger CB catheter to ensure more uniform ablative temperatures around the entirety of the distal surface of the CB.

Determinants of Cryoablation Lesion Size

During catheter cryoablation, tissue temperatures follow a monoexponential decline toward steady-state values about the ablation electrode (Fig. 2.8).[49] The size of catheter-based cryoablation lesions is dependent on many factors (Table 2.2).[49] Analogous to electrical current for RF ablation, the refrigerant is the mediator of thermal change in cryoablation systems. Higher flow rates of refrigerant can extract more heat from the tissue, and therefore lesion sizes are increased. The more abrupt and deep the temperature drop is, the more significant

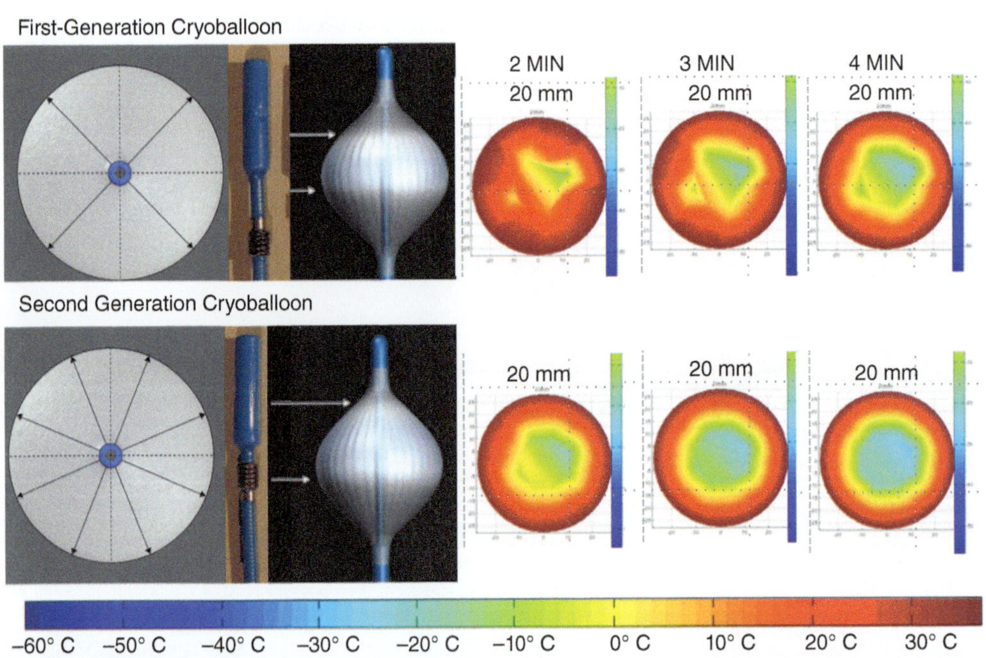

Fig. 2.7 Evolution of the cryoballoon from the first to the second generation (*left to right*). The combination of an increased number of jets (4–8) with a more distal positioning of the injection mechanism results in a wider band of more homogeneous cooling that is positioned slightly more toward the distal aspect of the balloon. (Courtesy Medtronic CryoCath LP, Montreal, QC, Canada.)

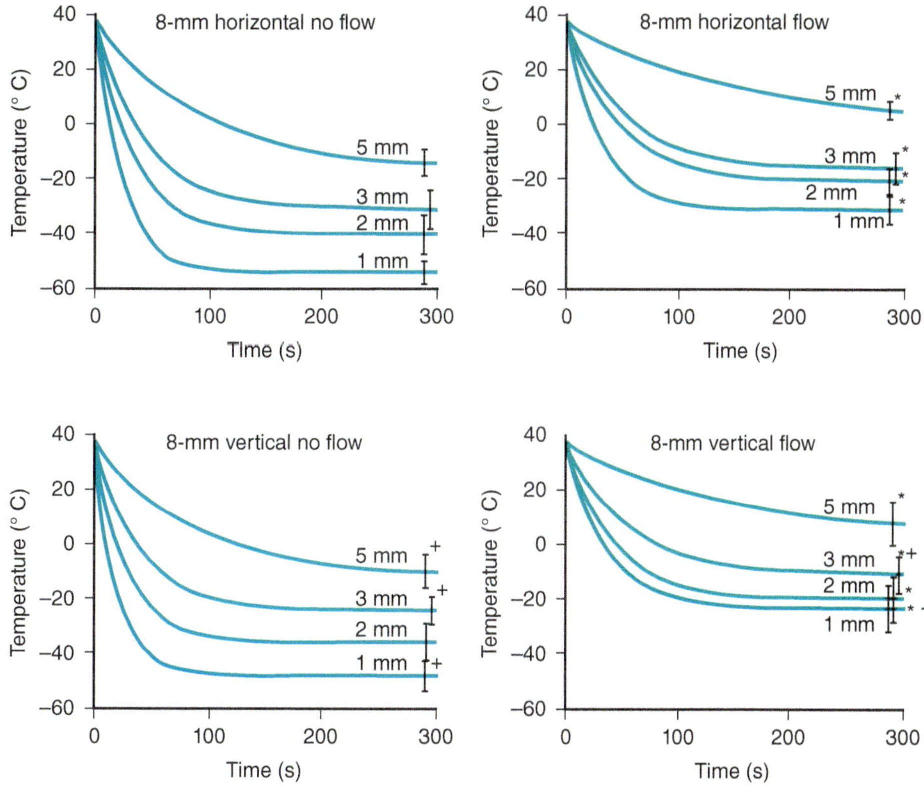

Fig. 2.8 Graphs of average tissue temperature versus time in isolated myocardial tissue undergoing catheter cryoablation. Temperature recordings are made at 1-, 2-, 3-, and 5-mm depths from an 8-mm-tip cryoablation catheter. The individual temperature curves each follow a monoexponential decrease over time. The vertical lines represent one standard deviation above and below the average temperature just before energy termination. The four graphs represent differing conditions of vertical (perpendicular) or horizontal (parallel) electrode orientation to the tissue and either the presence or absence of simulated blood flow over the electrode-tissue interface. Note the marked effect of convective warming on tissue temperatures. $*P < .05$ versus same condition except no flow, $+P < .05$ versus same condition except horizontal. (From Wood MA, Parvez B, Ellenbogen A, et al. Determinants of lesion sizes and tissue temperatures during catheter cryoablation. *PACE*. 2007;30:644-654.)

TABLE 2.2 Determinants of Lesion Size for Catheter Cryoablation

Factor	Effect On Lesion Size
Refrigerant flow rate	Increased flow increases lesion size
Electrode size	Increased electrode size allows greater refrigerant flow rates
Tissue contact	Increased contact pressure increases lesion size
Electrode orientation	Larger lesion sizes with horizontal (parallel) electrode orientation to tissue
Convective warming	Blood flow over electrode/tissue reduces lesion size
Electrode temperature	Colder temperature creates larger lesion[a]
Duration of energy application	Longer delivery produces larger lesion

Heat-extraction capacity of the refrigerant is important. A refrigerant with greater heat-extraction capacity may produce a larger lesion at a lower electrode temperature than a colder electrode using refrigerant with low heat-extraction capacity.
[a]See text.

the induced lesion is. In addition, refrigerants differ in their capacity to extract heat based on their physical properties and physical phase delivered to the electrode tip. For example, a colder gas phase of refrigerant may well produce a smaller lesion than a liquid refrigerant undergoing a phase change within the electrode at a warmer temperature. Larger electrode sizes appear tied to larger lesions by way of allowing greater refrigerant flow rates.[49] Lesion surface areas produced by 8-mm catheters are, on average, 92 mm^2 larger (177%) than by 4-mm catheters and 72 mm^2 larger (101%) than by 6-mm catheters.[50] The 8- and 6-mm catheters yield mean lesion volumes 253 mm^3 (248%) and 116 mm^3 (114%) larger than 4-mm catheters, respectively.[50] Lesion sizes also increase with greater electrode contact pressure and with greater electrode surface area in contact with the tissue to allow greater heat extraction from the tissue and less from the local blood pool.[49,50] Electrode orientations that are parallel with the tissue therefore produce larger lesions than perpendicular orientations because of greater thermal coupling with the tissue.[49-51] Convective warming of electrode and tissue by local blood flow has a detrimental effect on lesion formation.[52] In experimental preparations, simulated blood flow over cryoablation electrodes may reduce lesion volume by 75% compared with the absence of blood flow.[49] Even under strictly controlled experimental conditions, electrode temperature is an imperfect predictor of lesion size (Fig. 2.9). Because active cooling occurs

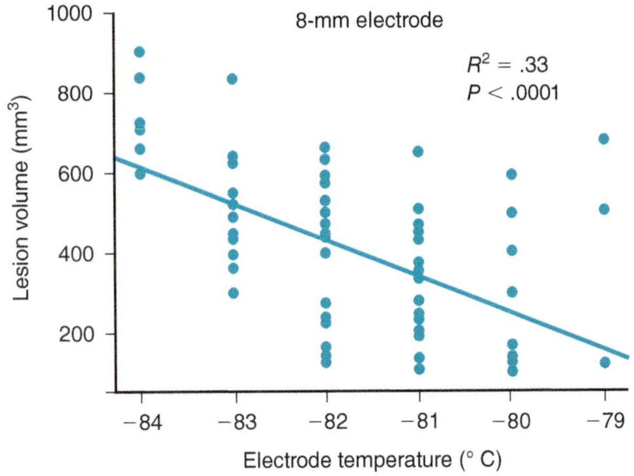

Fig. 2.9 Lesion volumes versus cryoablation electrode temperature in isolated ventricular myocardial tissue under controlled conditions of vertical or horizontal electrode orientation, tissue-contact pressure, and simulated blood flow over the electrode-tissue interface for an 8-mm-tip cryoablation catheter. Note the general trend toward larger lesions with colder electrode temperatures; however for any given electrode temperature, the resulting lesion size may vary by threefold to fourfold depending on conditions such as electrode orientation and convective warming from blood flow. (From Wood MA, Parvez B, Ellenbogen A, et al. Determinants of lesion sizes and tissue temperatures during catheter cryoablation. *PACE.* 2007;30:644-654.)

within the electrode and near the embedded thermocouple, electrode temperature is insensitive to other factors critical to lesion formation such as convective warming, contact pressure, and electrode orientation.[49] In addition, maximal electrode cooling may occur in the absence of any tissue contact. This differs from RF ablation in which the electrode is passively heated from contact with the tissue. In isolated tissue experiments, lesion dimensions were increased by prolonging energy delivery or by repeating the freeze–thaw cycle when compared with single 2.5-minute applications.[51]

Cryoablation Versus Radiofrequency Ablation

In comparison with RF catheter ablation, lesions associated with focal cryothermal ablation have a smaller surface area caused, in part, by cryoadhesion-induced loss of the brushing effect, with no difference in lesion depth.[48] Histologically, cryothermy results in a dense, homogeneous fibrosis that is clearly demarcated from normal myocardium (Fig. 2.10A, *right*).[3,37,47,48] By contrast, the hyperthermic injury induced by RF energy results in diffuse cellular destruction characterized by intralesional hemorrhage and ragged edges less clearly demarcated from normal myocardium (see Fig. 2.10A, *left*).[37] In addition, although devitalized, lesions produced by cryothermal ablation are associated with preservation of ultrastructural integrity, an observation that is attributed to the remarkable resilience of fibroblasts and collagen fibers to hypothermia.[53] Preservation of tissue ultrastructural integrity should theoretically result in a lower risk of myocardial perforation, esophageal injury, and aneurysmal dilation.[3,37,47,48,54] It may be speculated that lesions produced with cryoablation should be less arrhythmogenic (given that distinct border zones are less susceptible to spontaneous depolarization) and associated with a lower incidence of venous or arterial stenosis (given the minimal tissue contraction observed with lesion healing).[3,37,47,48,54] Thermal profiles for cryoablation and RF ablation lesions obtained by infrared thermography are shown in Fig. 2.10D.

Some factors influencing lesion size for catheter cryoablation are also critical to RF ablation, whereas others may have opposite effects for the two energy sources (Fig. 2.11).[55] Both modalities benefit from enhanced tissue-contact pressure and larger electrode sizes if the larger electrode allows greater refrigerant flow or electrical current to be delivered. Creation of larger lesions with cryoablation depends on conditions such as convective thermal effects and electrode orientation. For RF ablation, convective cooling of the electrode by local blood flow can enhance power delivery. For cryoablation, local blood flow can only be detrimental by warming the electrode and tissue.[49,55] For cryoablation and noncooled RF ablation, an electrode orientation parallel to the tissue enhances lesion size. For irrigated RF catheters, a parallel electrode orientation reduces lesion size.[55] Simultaneously applying standard RF and cryothermal energy through the same catheter may produce lesions of similar dimension to irrigated RF ablation.[56]

Cryomapping and Cryoablation Delivery

Standard ablation with the CryoCath system consists of advancing a steerable quadripolar catheter to the region of interest. The ablation target is identified with mapping techniques similar to RF ablation procedures. Once the target is identified, the operator may select between cryomapping and cryoablation modes. The cryomapping mode is typically used before cryoablation when the arrhythmia substrate is in the vicinity of the AV node/His–Purkinje conduction system. This mode consists of the use of milder freezing temperatures at the target lesion site to assess clinical effect (efficacy mapping) and ensure the absence of adverse clinical outcomes (safety mapping). The operator may choose to apply cryoablation directly if the region is deemed safe or at some distance from the conduction system. It is important to note that although safety and efficacy of mapping may be realized through the use of the cryomapping feature, a dynamic cryomapping process will naturally occur over the course of a cryoapplication as the hypothermic wavefront spreads centrifugally from the catheter tip to the surrounding tissue.[3,47,57] In effect, the cooling of cells with reversible electrophysiologic effects (e.g., cryoprobe temperature, 0°C to −30°C; tissue temperature, 0°C to −5°C) necessarily precedes irreversible tissue destruction (e.g., at temperatures of <−50°C to −60°C). Thus vigilance must be maintained throughout the cryoapplication when treating critical substrates (e.g., perinodal), because tissues not initially affected have the potential to undergo reversible suppression as the cryolesion continues to expand during cryoablation.

When temperatures reach −20°C, electrical noise appears on the distal electrode pair, with loss of the local electrogram signal because of the formation of the ice ball. This electrical

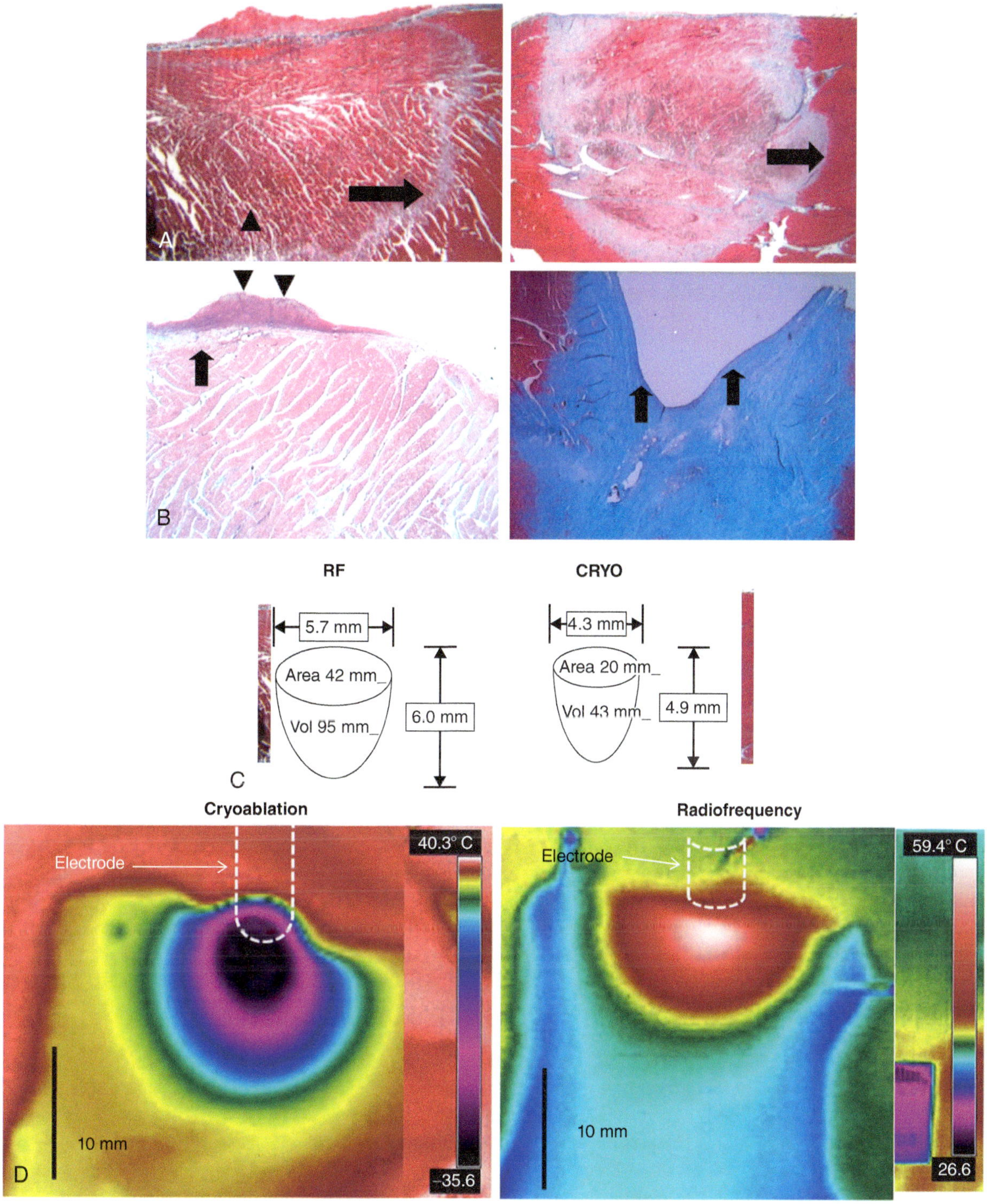

Fig. 2.10 (A) Photomicrographs of a chronic radiofrequency (RF) lesion (60 seconds at 70°C) (*left*) compared with a chronic cryothermal lesion (4 minutes at −75°C) (*right*). Note the hemispherical necrosis of the cryothermal lesion, as well as the discrete lesion demarcation (*right, arrow*) and preserved tissue architecture. By contrast, the RF lesion exhibits less discrete lesion demarcation (*left, arrow*) and less well-preserved architecture (*left, arrowhead*). (B) Photomicrographs of a chronic RF lesion (60 seconds at 70°C) (*left*) compared with a chronic cryothermal lesion (4 minutes at −75°C) (*right*). Note the well-preserved endothelium free of thrombus in the cryothermal lesion (*right, arrows*), compared with the disrupted endothelium (*left, arrow*) and associated thrombus (*left, arrowheads*) of the RF lesion. (C) Schematic diagram comparing lesion geometries between an RF lesion (*left*) and a cryoablation (CRYO) lesion (*right*). The RF lesion has similar depth but larger lesion volume and area. (D) Infrared thermal images of cryoablation lesion created with a 6-mm-tip electrode and RF lesion created with 4-mm internally irrigated electrode (25 W). The lesions are created in blocks of porcine ventricular myocardium in a warmed fluid path with the tissue surface exposed just above the fluid level. The outlines of the submerged electrode locations are shown. (A, *left*, from Khairy P, Chauvet P, Lehmann J, et al. Lower incidence of thrombus formation with cryoenergy versus radiofrequency catheter ablation. *Circulation*. 2003;107:2045–2050. C from Khairy P, Chauvet P, Lehmann J, et al. Lower incidence of thrombus formation with cryoenergy versus radiofrequency catheter ablation. *Circulation*. 2003;107:2045–2050.)

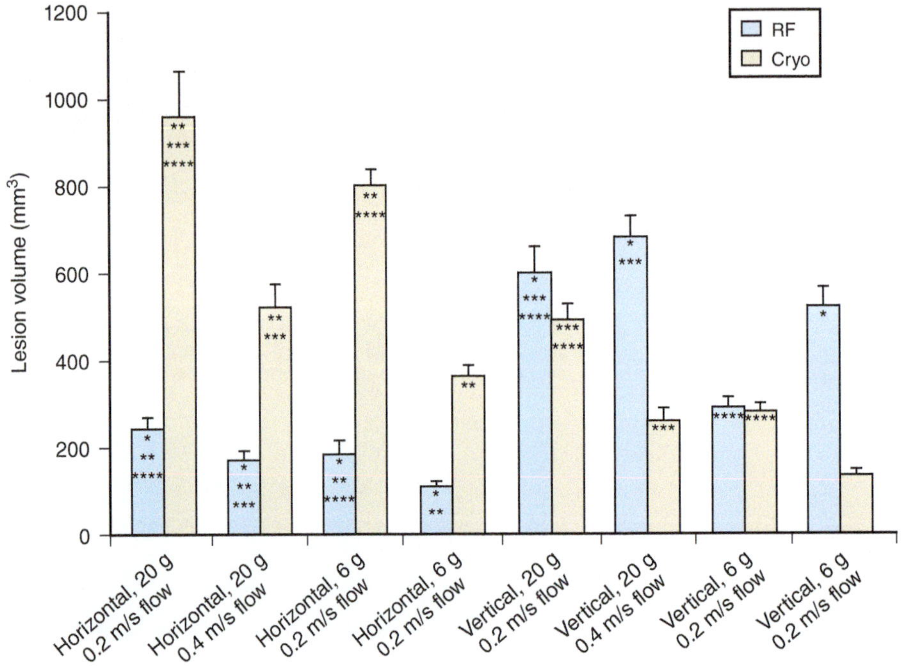

Fig. 2.11 Lesion volumes for irrigated radiofrequency (RF) ablation (*blue bars*) and cryoablation (*beige bars*) under various conditions of electrode orientation (vertical or horizontal), contact pressure (6 or 20 g), and simulated blood flow over the electrode-tissue interface (0.2 or 0.4 m/s). $*P < .05$ versus same conditions except cryoablation catheter, $**P < .05$ versus same conditions except vertical orientation, $***P < .05$ versus same conditions except 6-g pressure, $****P < .05$ versus same conditions except 0.4-m/s simulated blood flow. (From Parvez B, Pathak V, Schubert CM, Wood M. Comparison of lesion sizes produced by cryoablation and open irrigated radiofrequency ablation catheters. *J Cardiovasc Electrophysiol.* 2008;19:528–534.)

noise resolves once the temperature warms to over −20°C. During the time that temperatures remain colder than −20°C, the catheter adheres to the cardiac endocardial tissue and therefore allows the operator to perform programmed stimulation to confirm safety and/or efficacy without concern for catheter dislodgment. In the event of an undesirable effect, prompt termination of the application usually results in complete recovery within seconds after rewarming, with no permanent effect. If desired effects are confirmed, cryoablation is typically maintained for 4 minutes, largely because preclinical studies based on correlation between histopathologic analyses and visualization of ice ball formation demonstrated that the lesion increases in size during the first 2–3 minutes and reaches a plateau thereafter (Fig. 2.12A–C).[34] However chlorofluorocarbon agents have since been replaced by a more potent refrigerant, currently nitrous oxide (N_2O), which produces a faster drop in temperatures and lower absolute values. The standard 4-minute application has been questioned, with preclinical studies of focal cryocatheter[58] and CB[59] ablation suggesting that shorter application times (e.g., 2 minutes) suffice.

Although one application is typically sufficient to create permanent effects on conduction, double freeze–thaw cycles or multiple applications may be performed if desired or required to create more homogeneous necrosis.[34]

When performing PV isolation (PVI) for the treatment of AF with cryoenergy, the delivery tool is different and based on a balloon technology. The standard technique with the Arctic Front catheter consists of inserting a guidewire in a PV, advancing the catheter over the wire to the desired location, inflating the balloon, assessing tissue contact by injecting contrast through the catheter's central lumen demonstrating venous occlusion, in the absence of leaks, and applying 2–4 minutes of cryoablation.[59]

CLINICAL ADVANTAGES OF CRYOTHERMAL ENERGY FOR CATHETER ABLATION

Theoretical advantages of cryothermal over RF ablation are summarized in Table 2.3[3] and include reversibility, catheter stability, minimal risk of thromboembolism, safety near vascular structures, and decreased pain perception.

Reversible Effects

As previously discussed, one of the most exciting and truly remarkable characteristics of cryothermal energy is the ability to dynamically and prospectively assess the safety and efficacy of a potential ablation lesion site, because a period of reversible electrophysiologic tissue inhibition obligatorily precedes permanent tissue destruction (a process that can be dynamically manipulated by varying the temperature and/or time of application). Although extreme freezing (i.e., tissue temperatures colder than −50°C) results in near-instantaneous permanent tissue injury, a functional effect may be obtained at sublethal temperatures (i.e., −10°C to −25°C), with complete recovery of all electrophysiologic properties and

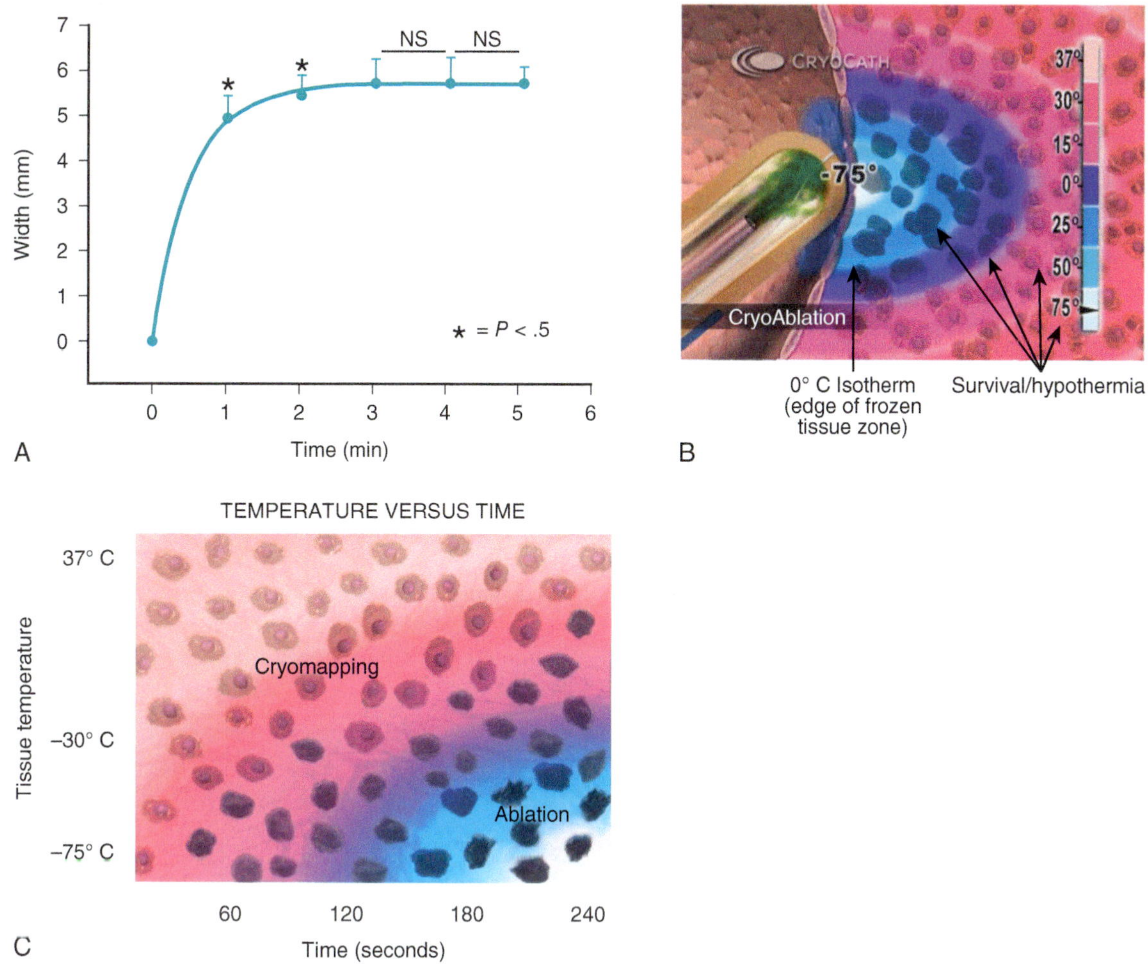

Fig. 2.12 (A) Plot of lesion width (mm) by time (min) of application demonstrating increase in lesion size during the first 3 minutes, with no substantial further increase thereafter. ∗$P < .5$ versus previous time. (B) Schematic diagram demonstrating that with freezing temperatures at the catheter tip, adjacent cardiac tissue is cooled, with formation of ice ball and outward expansion in a concentric fashion. The longer the catheter is cooled, the larger the formation of ice ball and the larger the lesion (until a plateau is reached). (C) Schematic plot of cryothermal energy delivery demonstrating the effect of temperature versus time. To create a permanent ablation lesion, the tissue adjacent to the catheter must reach a certain temperature, and this temperature must be applied for a given time. The colder the temperature, the shorter the duration of application required to achieve a permanent lesion. *NS*, Not significant. (A from Dubuc M, Roy D, Thibault B, et al. Transvenous catheter ice mapping and cryoablation of the atrioventricular node in dogs. *Pacing Clin Electrophysiol.* 1999;22:1488–1498. B and C, Courtesy Medtronic CryoCath LP, Montreal, QC, Canada.)

no histologically identifiable damage (Fig. 2.13*A–D*).[3,10,11,47] Not only is cryomapping theoretically possible, but the broad temperature/time window between reversible and irreversible effects renders this feature readily clinically applicable. Thus by identifying the desired substrate before definitive ablation, the appropriate catheter placement site may be confirmed to be efficacious (i.e., efficacy cryomapping) and/or safe (i.e., safety cryomapping). Reversible cryomapping may be of particular importance when ablating arrhythmogenic substrates located near critical sites such as the AV node, where a missed target lesion may have major consequences. Reversibility observed with cryothermal energy contrasts starkly with RF energy.[60] With RF ablation, hyperthermal tissue injury leading to reversible loss of excitability occurs at a median tissue temperature of 48°C, whereas irreversible tissue destruction occurs at tissue temperatures greater than 50°C.[60,61] The RF reversibility window is therefore too narrow for safe clinical applications.

Catheter Stability

With hypothermia generated at the distal cooling electrode, the cryocatheter adheres to tissue affording greater catheter stability.[62] Metaphorically, this has been likened to a wet tongue sticking to a frozen pole. The operator may let go of the catheter once it has adhered to the endocardial surface. Programmed electrical stimulation may be performed during cryoablation without concern for catheter dislodgment. Moreover, brushing effects that occur during beat-to-beat rocking heart motions and with respiratory variations are eliminated. This feature may be particularly advantageous if the arrhythmogenic substrate is located at a site where contact is difficult to maintain or ablation of nearby tissue is deemed hazardous (i.e., near the conduction

TABLE 2.3 Potential Advantages of Cryoablation Over Radiofrequency Ablation

Advantages	Clinical Implications
Catheter adhesiveness	Greater catheter stability Programmed stimulation may be performed during ablation Avoidance of brushing effects
Homogeneous sharply demarcated lesion	Less arrhythmogenic More controllable titration of lesion size
Preservation of ultrastructural integrity	Decreased risk of thrombus formation Absence of aneurysmal dilation or rupture
Reversible suppression of conduction tissue	Prediction of successful site Avoidance of unwanted lesions Ablation of high-risk substrates
Lesion limited by warming blood flow	Safety to nearby epicardial coronary arteries
Visualization by ultrasound	Real-time monitoring Confirmation of endocardial contact Defining optimal freezing parameters
Pain-free ablation	Discomfort minimized under conscious sedation

system, epicardial coronary arteries, or PVs).[10,11] It also permits ablation to be performed during tachycardia without the menace of catheter dislodgment upon abrupt arrhythmia termination. By contrast, catheter stability may be an issue during RF ablation. The catheter must be held in place by the operator to ensure adequate delivery of power and subsequent tissue heating, which may prove difficult in the beating heart. Such effects may be magnified during tachycardia, upon arrhythmia termination, and in patients with substantial valvular regurgitation. The lesser control and variable brushing effect may contribute to increasing the size, unpredictability, and imprecision of the lesion created.

Minimal Risk of Thromboembolism

To compare the propensity for RF and cryoenergy ablation to produce thrombus on the surface of the ablation lesion, a randomized preclinical study was conducted involving 197 ablation lesions in 22 dogs at right atrial, right ventricular, and left ventricular sites.[48] RF energy was five times more thrombogenic than cryoablation, as confirmed by results of histologic morphometric analyses 7 days after ablation. Moreover, thrombus

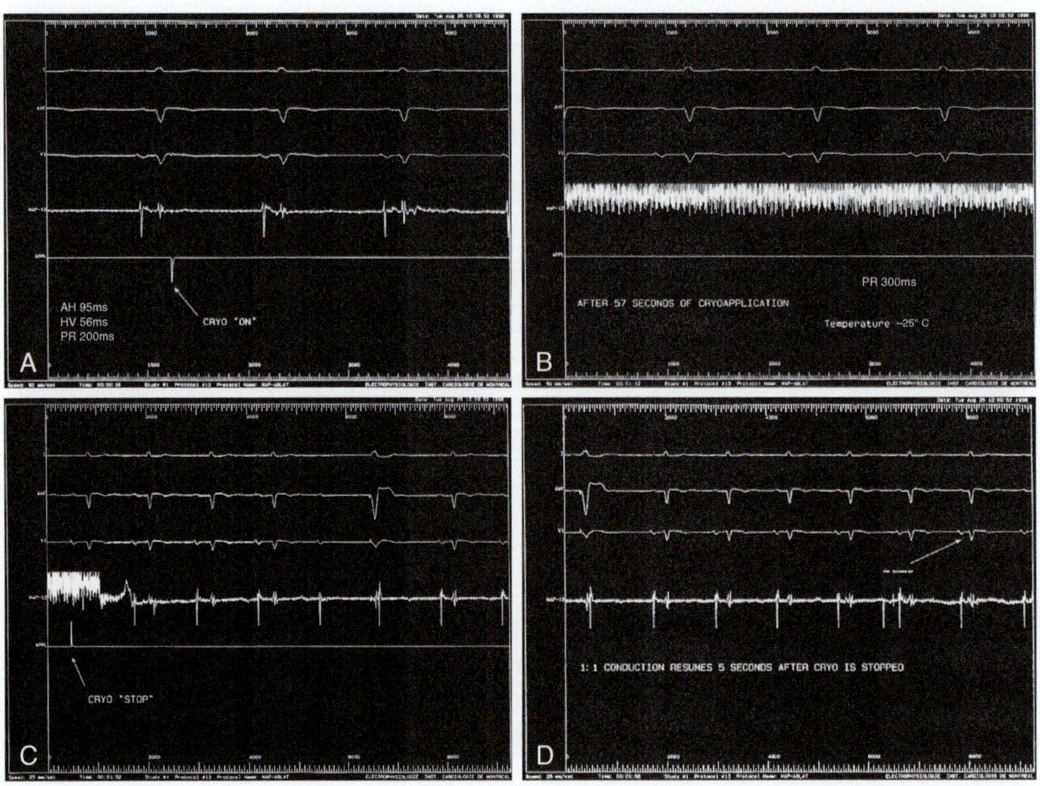

Fig. 2.13 Electrograms demonstrating the reversible effect of cryomapping on the AV node. For all panels, I, aV_F, and V_1 are surface electrocardiographic (ECG) recordings. (A) Normal baseline PR interval of 200 ms and AH interval of 95 ms before cryomapping application (paper speed = 50 mm/s). (B) After onset of cryomapping at a temperature of −25°C (evidenced by high-frequency signal on Map 1-2) for 57 seconds, the PR interval increased to 300 ms (paper speed = 50 mm/s). (C) At the end of the cryomapping application, a nonconducted atrial beat with a ventricular backup paced beat is shown. Upon rewarming, no further nonconducted atrial beats occurred (paper speed = 25 mm/s). (D) After 5 seconds of rewarming, normal 1:1 AV conduction resumed, and the PR interval returned to baseline (paper speed = 25 mm/s). *AH,* Atrium-to-His activation time; *AV,* atrioventricular; *HV,* His-to-ventricle activation time; *MAP 1-2,* signal from the distal electrode pair of the cryocatheter; *PR,* PR interval from the surface ECG. (From Dubuc M, Khairy P, Rodriguez-Santiago A, et al. Catheter cryoablation of the atrioventricular node in patients with atrial fibrillation: a novel technology for ablation of cardiac arrhythmias. *J Cardiovasc Electrophysiol.* 2001;12:439-444.)

volume was significantly greater with RF compared with cryoablation (see Fig. 2.10B, *left*). Interestingly, the extent of hyperthermic tissue injury was positively correlated with thrombus bulk. This was unlike cryoenergy, in which lesion dimensions were not predictive of thrombus size. It was conjectured that this disparity likely reflected the fact that intact tissue ultrastructure with endothelial cell preservation was maintained with cryoenergy. These results were later extended to larger-tip cryocatheters, further supporting the notion that the low risk of thrombosis is a feature of cryothermal energy, independent of lesion size.[50] Moreover, cryothermal ablation lesions are associated with a lesser degree of platelet and coagulation cascade activation when compared with RF ablation.[48,63,64] Although the true incidence of thromboembolism associated with RF ablation is likely underreported, especially for right-sided interventions, clinically important thrombi have been reported to occur in 1.8–2% of procedures in systemic cardiac chambers.[65,66]

Minimal Risk to Vascular Structures

Concerns have been raised regarding RF ablation adjacent to or within the coronary venous system or PVs.[62] Venous injury (including acute perforation and tamponade, and/or delayed fibrosis/stenosis), acute or subacute endoluminal venous thrombosis, and collateral damage to the esophagus and/or adjacent coronary arteries have been reported.[67] Perforation, tamponade, and coronary artery stenosis are potential complications. The circumflex and/or right coronary artery may course in close proximity to the arrhythmia substrate.[68–70] Moreover, the AV nodal artery passes near the mouth of the coronary sinus, and ablation may conceivably damage this small vessel.[71] Preclinical studies suggest a lower incidence of coronary artery stenosis following cryoablation compared with RF ablation. In an experimental study in swine submitted to cryoablation within the mid and distal coronary sinus, no angiographic coronary stenosis was observed and the medial and intimal layers of the coronary artery were preserved.[72] In a canine model, Aoyama and coworkers demonstrated that cryoablation in the coronary sinus within 2 mm of the left circumflex artery produced transmural myocardial lesions similar to RF energy but with a lesser risk of coronary artery stenosis.[73] Histologically, 50% of the animals randomized to RF energy had intimal coronary artery damage compared with none with cryoablation. These observations have been attributed to the resilience of fibroblasts and collagen fibers to hypothermic injury and to the protective heating effect of coronary arterial blood flow.[24,25] There is also growing evidence that cryoablation in close proximity to PVs is associated with a lesser risk of venous stenosis than RF energy.[74–76]

Painless

RF ablation may be painful to the patient under conscious sedation through direct stimulation of cardiac sensory nerves or pericardial or collateral visceral irritation, particularly when ablating near thin-walled or venous structures such as the posterior left atrium, coronary sinus, or posterior cavotricuspid isthmus. In contrast to RF catheter ablation, several studies have noted that pain perception, as assessed by standard Likert scales, is significantly less with cryoablation.[77–80] Thus, for select procedures associated with substantial patient discomfort, the use of cryoablation may theoretically result in lower anesthetic and analgesic requirements.[78–80] This is especially relevant for electrophysiology laboratories that do not use general anesthesia. However, it should be noted that in the case of AF ablation, a rare incidence of transient "ice cream headache" has been described during ablation.

Visualization by Ultrasound

In the 1990s, the ability to provide continuous real-time imaging of the freezing process was considered a major technologic advancement that sparked renewed interest in visceral cryosurgery.[33] Indeed, ultrasonographic monitoring of the freeze–thaw cycle and frozen tissue volume contributed to rapid improvements in hepatic and prostatic surgery. The ability to visualize formation of ice ball by ultrasonic means was likewise demonstrated in preclinical transcatheter cryoablation studies (Fig. 2.14A–C).[34] This feature of cryoablation has proved helpful in defining optimal freezing parameters.

CLINICAL APPLICATIONS

Since its inception, transcatheter cryoablation technology has substantially improved. The refrigerant was modified to allow lower temperatures and faster freezing rates, larger electrode-tip sizes emerged, and innovative catheters of differing configurations were manufactured. Diverse clinical applications have since been explored, as indications continue to be refined.[48,72,76,81–87]

Atrioventricular Nodal Ablation

Somewhat ironically, the first series of patients with transcatheter cryoablation underwent AV node ablation and pacemaker implantation as a rate-control strategy for permanent AF.[11] Although cryoablation is generally not advocated for this indication because of potentially lower long-term success rates, AV node ablation was deemed an appropriate substrate for the initial safety and feasibility studies. Indeed, in the very first study with the first-generation equipment (9-F catheter; suboptimal handling characteristics; minimum achievable temperature −55°C), AV node ablation was successful in 10 of 12 patients.[11]

Atrioventricular Nodal Reentrant Tachycardia

AVNRT is one of the most extensively studied arrhythmia substrates, as the unique properties of this arrhythmia are particularly well suited to cryoablation. Specifically, reversible tissue inhibition allows for the electrophysiologic evaluation of slow pathway conduction during mapping and/or ablation.[81] Catheter adherence minimizes the chance of inadvertent collateral damage and allows atrial extrastimulus testing to assess end points (such as disappearance of an A2-H2 jump, arrhythmia termination, and noninducibility) during the cryoapplication and without risk of catheter dislodgment.[81,88] Moreover, inadvertent permanent high-degree AV block is yet to be reported with cryoablation for AVNRT. In the ICY-AVNRT STUDY, 397 patients received cryoablation for AVNRT, 2 patients (0.005%)

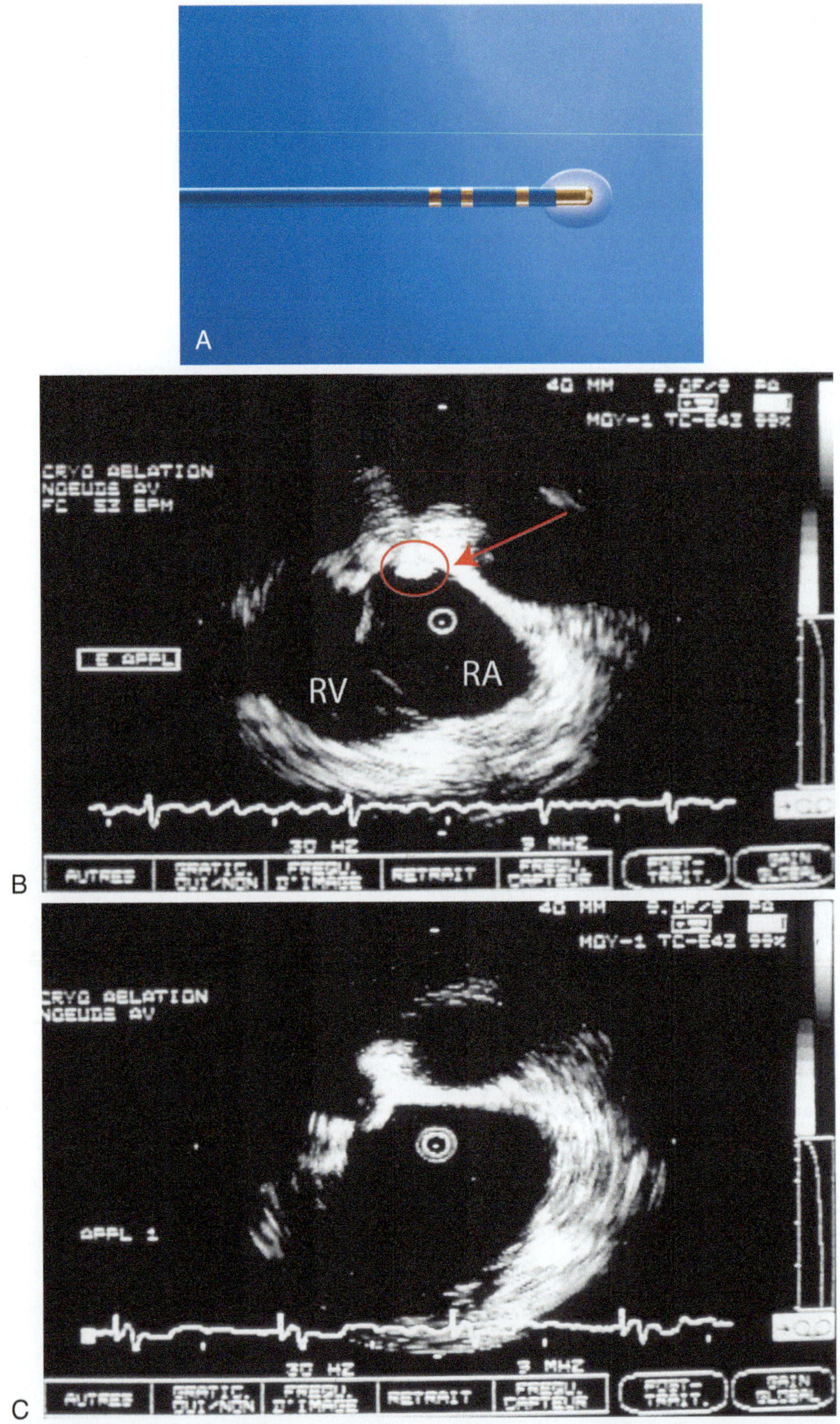

Fig. 2.14 (A) Ablation catheter adheres to adjacent cardiac tissue upon formation of an ice ball. (B) The catheter situated in the right atrium (RA) is indicated by the *arrow*. (C) After application of cryoenergy, the presence of an ice ball is seen as a hypoechoic zone bordered by a hyperechoic rim with posterior shadowing. *RV,* Right ventricle. (A courtesy Medtronic CryoCath LP, Montreal, QC, Canada. B, From Dubuc M, Khairy P, Rodriguez-Santiago A, et al. Catheter cryoablation of the atrioventricular node in patients with atrial fibrillation: a novel technology for ablation of cardiac arrhythmias. *J Cardiovasc Electrophysiol.* 2001;12:439-444.)

had a transient AV block, and no subject received a permanent pacemaker (in contrast to RF ablation, where the occurrence of complete AV block necessitating pacemaker implant remains significant at 0.8–2%).[89,90,92] Although preferences and practice patterns continue to vary, this superior safety profile has prompted some centers to adopt cryoablation as first-line therapy for the treatment of AVNRT.

In contrast to the well-established exceptional safety profile, some debate remains about long-term efficacy. In the first case series of 18 patients with cryoablation for AVNRT, cryomapping was demonstrated to be feasible, 17 patients underwent a successful ablation, and no recurrence was noted at 5 months of follow-up.[81] Important observations included the absence of an accelerated junctional rhythm during cryoablation, the ability to test for slow pathway conduction during the cryoapplication, and reversibility of AV block upon tissue rewarming.[79,82,91] In the prospective multicenter FROSTY cohort study, 103 patients with AVNRT had attempted cryoablation.[82] The acute procedural success rate was 91% using a 4-mm electrode-tip cryocatheter. At 6 months, arrhythmia-free survival in patients with acutely successful interventions was 94%. The more recent multicenter Intracardiac CrYoablation for AtrioVentricular Nodal Reentrant Tachycardia (ICY-AVNRT) study reported a 92.6% long-term success rate with a 6-mm electrode-tip cryocatheter.[92] Although these figures appear somewhat lower than historically reported success rates with RF ablation, large-scale direct and prospective comparisons to RF were not made.

In a small pilot study directly comparing acute and long-term success with cryoablation versus RF ablation for AVNRT, no statistically significant difference in acute success was noted (97% versus 98%).[93] However, long-term success rates favored RF. A separate study of 63 patients randomized to RF or cryoablation for AVNRT also noted equivalent acute procedural success rates.[94] The median number of cryothermal applications was significantly lower than the number of RF applications (two vs. seven). Fluoroscopy and procedural times were comparable. Long-term follow-up was later reported, suggesting no difference in outcomes.[95] In a systematic review that combined 22 published studies (2654 patients), cryothermal ablation had a high procedural success rate (95%; range 85–99%) that was comparable with RF catheter ablation (RFCA; 95–98%).[82,89,90,95–104] Long-term freedom from recurrent arrhythmia with cryoablation was reported to be 92.6% (range 89.5–94.8%), which was lower than historical observations with RF (93–97% freedom from recurrence).[92] Although historical comparisons between observational studies are fraught with potential biases, 11 comparative studies between cryothermy and RF catheter ablation for AVNRT (8 retrospective observational studies and 3 prospective randomized studies) reported comparable acute success rates.[95–104] In these studies, the procedure duration was globally similar, with a shorter fluoroscopy time with cryoablation. Although the long-term recurrence rate was statistically similar in 7 of the 11 studies, there was an overall trend that favored RF energy. It is important to note, however, that the lack of statistical significance is not synonymous with equivalency, which requires adequately powered studies.

Importantly, the risk of recurrence with cryoablation is sensitive to several modifiable factors, which are largely based on the fact that cryoablation for AVNRT differs from RF catheter ablation in several ways. For example (1) precise mapping is more critical than with RF because of the more focused nature of the cryolesion; (2) the ideal ablation site is generally more proximal (more atrial) and superior (higher up the septum; figure of Koch triangle and successful location of cryocatheter ablation)[92,105]; (3) the ability to test slow pathway conduction during ablation allows for an assessment of relative proximity of the catheter tip to the target tissue—an early time to effect is associated with a higher likelihood of delivering an efficacious lesion[81,88,105]; (4) repeated freeze–thaw cycles produce faster and more extensive tissue cooling, which extend the lethal effect of ablation to the outer limit of the frozen volume[106]; and (5) larger catheter-tip dimensions (6 and 8 mm) have been associated with increased procedural and long-term efficacy.[97,98,107,108] In a study of 289 patients with cryoablation using 4- or 6-mm electrode-tip catheters as a first-time procedure for AVNRT, a similar rate of acute procedural success was achieved.[107] However, recurrences were less common with 6-mm tips. Actuarial event-free survival rates at 1, 3, 6, and 12 months with 6- versus 4-mm electrode-tip catheters were 97%, 93%, 92%, and 89% versus 90%, 87%, 84%, and 77%, respectively, with no recurrence thereafter. Indeed, ablation with a 4-mm cryocatheter was associated with a 2.5-fold increased risk of recurrence. Hence, 4-mm electrode-tip cryocatheters were no longer used. (6) It remains debated whether the usual end points used with RF catheter ablation are applicable to cryoablation. Specifically, although persistent AV nodal physiology without more than a single echo beat on isoproterenol is an acceptable end point for RF catheter ablation after 30 minutes of observation, some studies suggest that a similar end point is appropriate for cryoablation, whereas others suggest that complete abolition of the slow pathway is preferable.[92,108–111] Long-term efficacy outcomes may continue to improve as operators gain experience, the procedure is further refined, and catheter designs evolve.

Septal and Para-Hisian Accessory Pathways

Most users of transcatheter cryoablation would probably agree that this technology permits them to tackle substrates that they would have otherwise refrained from ablating because of an unacceptably high risk of AV block using other energy modalities.[112,113] Midseptal and para-Hisian pathways are classic examples.[79,82,91] For septal pathways, including parahisian locations, AV block with RF ablation has ranged from 12.5% to 20%.[112,113] By contrast, in a study that included 11 anteroseptal and 8 midseptal accessory pathways undergoing cryoablation, transient atrium-to-His time prolongation was noted in 4 of 8 patients with midseptal pathways and not in any of the patients with anteroseptal pathways.[83] No permanent AV block occurred. Although the acute procedural success rate was reported at 100%, 20% recurred at 15 months of follow-up. The series was later extended to include a total of 39 patients with perinodal accessory pathways, 15 midseptal and 24 para-Hisian.[114] An acute success rate of 95% was achieved. Other series have reported similar acute successes.[79,115] As for AVNRT, permanent inadvertent AV block is yet to be reported with ablation of perinodal pathways, whereas right bundle branch block has occurred on occasion.

Atrial Flutter

The treatment of cavotricuspid isthmus–dependent atrial flutter by RF ablation has been associated with high success rates and improvements in quality of life. Although reported success rates are in the range of 80–100%, cavotricuspid isthmus ablation with RF may be painful during lesion delivery and is rarely complicated by AV block and/or injury to the circumflex or right coronary artery. Several studies assessed cryoablation for atrial flutter and reported comparable success and recurrence rates, with lower pain perception.[77,78,91,116,117]

In an observational study of 95 patients with attempted cavotricuspid isthmus ablation using 9-F 8-mm ($n = 52$) or 7-F 6-mm (n = 43) electrode-tip cryocatheters, a higher acute success rate was achieved with the larger catheters (100% vs. 88%).[118] Despite comparable outcomes, modest advantages favored the larger tip catheter with shorter fluoroscopy time and procedural duration and fewer applications. As an alternative technique, some investigators have advocated electrogram-guided hot spot focal ablation.[119] The authors placed an 8-mm electrode-tip cryocatheter at the isthmus, close to the mouth of the coronary sinus. The catheter is maneuvered laterally along the isthmus in search of electrograms with separated atrial and ventricular components and a local stimulus to onset time 70 ms or higher.[120] At these sites, cryoablation is performed at −75°C for 60 seconds. If conduction time across the cavotricuspid isthmus increases by 30–40 ms, an 8-minute cryoapplication is delivered. Although this approach was acutely successful, by 3 months of follow-up 44% no longer had bidirectional block on repeat testing.[119]

In comparison with conventional RF catheter ablation, similar freedom from recurrence (86% vs. 87% with RF ablation at 11.6 months of follow-up; $P = .84$) and fluoroscopy time (27.5 vs. 27.3 minutes with RF ablation; $P = .28$) have been reported with cryothermal ablation.[80] Although the procedural time has been reported to be significantly longer with cryothermal ablation (171.7 vs. 134.5 minutes with RF catheter ablation; $P < .001$), cryothermy results in a lesser degree of patient discomfort than RF energy.[77,78,80]

Atrial Fibrillation

Early attempts at PVI with cryoenergy were performed in a point-by-point manner similar to contemporary RF catheter ablation. Although the procedure was shown to be feasible and safe, it was associated with prohibitively long ablation and procedural durations (mean cryoablation time 65 ± 39 minutes per vein; mean total procedural time 7.5 ± 2 hours) and a disappointing long-term success rate (6% freedom from recurrent AF at 18 ± 9 months of follow-up).[75,76,121] In response to these limitations, a specialized curvilinear self-expanding 7 F Arctic Circle (Medtronic CryoCath LP) catheter was developed. Although acute isolation could be achieved in 91% of targeted PVs (4/45 PVs required focal RFCA for isolation), only 22% of patients (4/18) remained arrhythmia free after 14.8 ± 6.2 months of follow-up.[122]

Efforts to further refine the cryothermal energy delivery system for PVI spurred the designing of an expandable CB ablation catheter (Arctic Front; Medtronic CryoCath LP). To date, over 250,000 CB-based ablation (CBA) procedures have been performed worldwide. Video 2.1 shows a typical example of the technical aspects of pulmonary vein isolation using Medtronic Arctic Front cryoballoon. The first randomized trial comparing antiarrhythmic drug (AAD) therapy with CBA, the Sustained Treatment of Paroxysmal Atrial Fibrillation (STOP-AF) trial, enrolled 245 patients with paroxysmal AF and randomized them 2:1 to CBA (n = 163) or AAD therapy (n = 82).[123] Balloon-only PVI was realized in 90.8% of participants, with an overall procedural success rate (≥3 PVs isolated) of 98.2% when focal cryoablation touch-ups were added. Some 19% of patients required a repeat procedure within the 3-month blanking period. At 12 months of follow-up, 69.9% of the CB group versus 7.3% of the AAD group remained free of recurrent AF ($P < .001$) with a statistically significant improvement in symptoms and quality of life in the CBA group.

A meta-analysis examining the early experience with the first-generation CB catheter reported that CBA resulted in a high procedural success rate (>98% of patients achieving complete PVI) and 1-year freedom from recurrent AF (1-year single procedure off AADs success of 60%; 73% if a 3-month blacking period was included).[124] In comparison, long-term freedom from recurrent AF after RF catheter ablation has been reported to be 50–64% after a mean follow-up of 14 months in the meta-analysis by Calkins and coworkers, and 40% at 1 year in the prospective long-term cohort study by Weerasooriya and coworkers.[125,126]

As previously mentioned, the first generation of CBA catheters (Artic Front; 23 and 28 mm) included only four N_2O injectors. The cooling process was slower and less homogeneous than the second-generation CB (Artic Front Advance), built with eight injectors. Hence, procedural duration, time to isolation, and fluoroscopy times have since been significantly reduced.[127] Importantly, freedom from AF at 1 year was systematically improved, with reports indicating 80% event-free survival[127–131] The third-generation CB (Artic Front Advance Short Tip) facilitates analysis of PV potentials during cryoapplications[132] to obtain real-time recordings of time to isolation.

In 2016, a prospective randomized study on 762 patients demonstrated noninferiority of CBA versus RF ablation for paroxysmal AF. After a 1-year follow-up, the primary efficacy end point (supraventricular arrhythmia recurrence, AAD prescription, and/or repeated ablation) occurred in 138 patients in the CB group compared with 143 with RF ablation (34.6% and 35.9%, respectively; $P < .001$).[133] Likewise, the CIRCA-DOSE multicenter randomized clinical trial randomised 346 patients with drug-refractory paroxysmal AF to contact force-guided radiofrequency ablation (CF-RF), 4-minute (Cryo-4), or 2-minute (Cryo-2) cryoablation. All patients received an implantable loop recorder for AF recurrence detection. The primary outcome was documented recurrence of symptomatic or asymptomatic atrial arrhythmia (AF, atrial flutter, or atrial tachycardia) after the 3-month blanking period and within 1 year postprocedure or a repeat ablation procedure at any time. CF-RF and cryoballoon ablation resulted in no difference in 1-year efficacy (53.9%, 52.2% and 51.7% with CF-RF, Cryo-4, and Cryo-2, respectively, $P = .87$) and freedom from symptomatic atrial tachyarrhythmia (79.1%, 78.2%, and 73.3% with CF-RF, Cryo-4, and Cryo-2, respectively, $P = .26$). In a direct comparison to other contemporary AF ablation technologies, CBA is associated with procedures that are somewhat shorter than conventional irrigated RF ablation.[134–138,162]

However, fluoroscopy times remain longer with CBA because procedures are usually performed without electroanatomical mapping systems.[133] Despite these procedural differences, efficacy outcomes do not seem to differ between CBA and conventional irrigated RF catheter ablation, magnetic-guided RF, and duty-cycled multielectrode RF ablation.[134–139] Moreover, the rate of major complications with CBA is relatively low (<3–5%) in comparison with irrigated RF (5–6%).[125,140–142] With CBA, the reported rate of periprocedural stroke or transient ischemic attack (TIA) is 0.3, 0.6% for cardiac tamponade, and 1.8% for groin complications. Corresponding complication rates with RF ablation are 0.3–0.9% for stroke or TIA, 0.8–1.3% for cardiac tamponade, and 1–1.5% for groin complications.[124]

Although the global complication rate with CBA appears comparable to conventional irrigated RF ablation (10.2% vs. 12.8%, $P = .24$),[133] four types of complications merit further discussion. Phrenic nerve palsy (PNP) is the most frequently observed complication after CBA, with an estimated incidence of approximately 6% (range 3–11%), despite the interruption of ablation when impaired diaphragmatic excursion is detected by continuous abdominal palpation during continuous phrenic nerve pacing.[64,124,143] Although PNP has been observed with other ablation energy sources, it occurs more frequently with balloon-based technologies.[125,141,142] Fortunately, the majority of cases after CBA are transient, with <0.4% of PNPs persisting for >1 year.[124] Despite the rarity of its occurrence, the incidence of persistent PNP nevertheless appears to be approximately two times that reported with RF ablation (0.17%).[141] Although alternative monitoring techniques, such as continuous diaphragmatic visualization and/or auditory monitoring of diaphragmatic contraction, have been proposed, the use of diaphragmatic electromyography represents a potentially more sensitive technique.[143] During phrenic nerve pacing a reliable signal (the diaphragmatic compound motor action potential [CMAP]) can be easily recorded using surface electrodes. In preclinical studies it was demonstrated that it is technically possible to record high-quality diaphragmatic CMAP signals during CBA, and a 30% reduction in diaphragmatic CMAP amplitude reliably predicted impending hemidiaphragmatic paralysis (presaging diaphragmatic paralysis by abdominal palpation by a mean of 31 seconds). In a randomized preclinical study, the use of CMAP monitoring resulted in a significant reduction in the incidence of acute hemidiaphragmatic paralysis (50% vs. 100%; $P = .001$), persistent hemidiaphragmatic paralysis at 30 days (21% vs. 75%; multivariate odds ratio, 0.12; 95% confidence interval, 0.02–0.69; $P = .017$), and the histologic severity of phrenic nerve injury ($P = .001$) when compared with standard diaphragmatic palpation.[143,144]

Interestingly, the CMAP amplitude decreases more frequently during right superior PVI, as the phrenic nerve path courses along the right side of the heart.[145]

The second complication that warrants a more in-depth discussion is that of PV stenosis. Before the STOP-AF trial, multiple studies using systematic screening reported no PV stenosis (0/550 patients).[123,146–153] Conversely, the landmark STOP-AF trial reported a 3.07% (7/228 patients) incidence of radiographic PV stenosis. This incongruity likely reflects differences in criteria used to define the significance of PV stenosis. In the AF ablation literature, PV stenosis is most commonly defined on the basis of diameter measurements (typically as a reduction in PV diameter >70%).[154] By contrast, the STOP-AF trial defined PV stenosis as a >75% reduction in cross-sectional area from baseline, which corresponds to a 50% reduction in PV diameter.[123] As such, this more liberal definition may represent a relative overestimate of the rate of PV stenosis and limits direct comparisons with other studies. Even so, when the results of the STOP-AF trial were combined with other studies using systematic screening with noninvasive imaging, the incidence of radiographic PV stenosis was 0.90% (7/773 procedures), which is approximately half the rate observed in a large meta-analysis of conventional AF ablation with RF.[125,146–153] Reassuringly, the rate of symptomatic PV stenosis or PV stenosis requiring intervention was low (0.17%) and comparable with that observed with RF (0.1–0.3%).[125,141,142] In recent studies, the incidence of PV stenosis appeared to be negligible.[155]

The third is the possibility of esophageal injury after CBA. Four studies comprising 148 participants reported the results of systematic upper endoscopy after CBA.[149,156–158] Although two studies documented a 17% (6/35 patients) and 19% (6/32 patients) incidence of esophageal ulceration after CBA, two further studies failed to demonstrate thermal esophageal lesions in 38 and 43 patients who underwent systematic esophageal endoscopy. Similarly, although there were no cases of left atrial–esophageal fistula (0/1298 procedures) reported in the meta-analysis, subsequent case reports have emerged indicating that, although the possibility of atrial–esophageal fistula exists, the incidence is relatively rare (0.00018% with CBA vs. 0.018% with RF).

The last complication that warrants a more detailed discussion is that of systemic thromboembolism. Cerebral ischemic events are a recognized complication of percutaneous endocardial left atrial ablation. In the recent systematic review of CBA, the incidence of thromboembolic complications, including periprocedural stroke or TIA, was 0.32%, which compares favorably to conventional RF catheter ablation (0.3–0.94%).[125,141,142] Recognizing that not all embolic cerebral events lead to clinical symptoms, recent studies quantified microembolic signals (MESs) as a surrogate of subclinical disease. In a series of 30 patients, a significantly lower incidence of MES was noted in the middle cerebral arteries with CBA and irrigated RF catheters when compared with conventional nonirrigated RF.[159] Similarly, two studies comprising a total of 182 patients compared the incidence of silent cerebral ischemic lesions after PVI with duty-cycled multielectrode ablation, conventional irrigated-tip RFCA, and CBA. In both studies, the incidence of new silent cerebral ischemic lesions was found to be significantly higher with multielectrode ablation (37.5–38.9%) when compared with irrigated RF (7.4–8.3%) or CBA (4.3–5.6%).[160,161]

More recent studies have confirmed that CBA was effective and safe as the first-line therapy for paroxysmal AF. In the EARLY-AF trial, patients with symptomatic treatment-naïve paroxysmal AF were randomly assigned to cryoballoon ablation or antiarrhythmic drug therapy (AAD) for initial rhythm control. Patients received an implantable loop recorder for AF recurrence detection during a 12-month follow-up period. There was a significantly lower rate of AF recurrence with cryoballoon ablation than with AAD (42.9% versus 67.8% $p<0.001$) with a higher rate of serious adverse events in the AAD group (3.2% versus 4.0%).[163]

The STOP Persistent AF single-armed nonrandomized study found CBA to be safe and effective in treating patients with drug-refractory persistent AF characterized by continuous AF episodes <6 months. The primary efficacy endpoint was 12-month freedom from >30 seconds of AF, atrial flutter, or atrial tachycardia after a 90-day blanking period. At 12 months, the primary efficacy endpoint, as determined by noninvasive monitoring, was achieved in 54.8% of 165 ablated patients. Vascular pseudoaneurysm was the most serious safety outcomes of CBA PVI in this study (n = 2, 1.2%).[164]

In short, a single CBA procedure results in high acute and medium-term efficacy rates with a relatively low incidence of complications. The most frequent complication, PNP, is often transient and may be preventable. Moreover, rates of ischemic thromboembolic complications appear lower with CBA than other technologies, which may reflect maintenance of endocardial integrity and lower risk of thrombosis.

Ventricular Tachycardia

A few case series on cryoablation for ventricular tachycardia have been published.[162,163] Obel and coworkers reported three cases of left ventricular outflow tract tachycardia successfully ablated from the distal great cardiac vein.[164] In a larger series, cryoablation with an 8-mm-tip catheter was attempted in 14 patients with highly symptomatic frequent monomorphic ventricular premature beats or nonsustained ventricular tachycardia originating within the right ventricular outflow tract.[165] Cryoablation resulted in complete success in all but one patient. Three patients reported slight pain arising from local pressure of the catheter on the right ventricular outflow tract with no pain related to delivery of cryothermal energy. All patients with acutely successful procedures remained arrhythmia free at 3 months of follow-up.

Cryoablation in Children

Because of smaller anatomical structures and distressing consequences of inadvertent AV block, cryoablation has emerged as an attractive treatment option for several arrhythmia substrates in children. Fortunately, persistent AV block has not been reported with cryoablation in the young. In children with AVNRT, acute success rates are comparable to RF ablation. However, concerns persist over potentially higher recurrence rates.[166,167] Although these trends are not statistically significant and are influenced by learning curves and operator experience, the concerns are valid, particularly with 4-mm-tip cryocatheters. In addition, reported procedural times are longer with cryoenergy versus RF ablation (148 minutes vs. 112 minutes).[168]

Similar trends are noted with cryoablation of accessory pathways in children that are either close to the AV node or within the coronary venous system.[166,169] An acute success rate of 78% was noted in 35 young patients (mean age 15.6 years).[169] Permanent PR prolongation occurred in one patient and right bundle branch block in another. At median follow-up of 207 days, recurrences were noted in 45%. Younger patient age and midseptal pathways were associated with a higher likelihood of recurrence. Although acute success rates were comparable to RF ablation in a historical institutional control group, recurrences were significantly higher. The authors conjectured that safety benefits may nonetheless provide suitable compensation for higher recurrences. However, it is important to note that when applied to immature myocardium, the rate of expansion of cryoablation lesions is similar to RF catheter ablation.[170]

Reports of other substrates in children successfully cryoablated include ectopic atrial tachycardia,[166] junctional ectopic tachycardia,[166,167] and permanent junctional reciprocating tachycardia.[168]

Cryoablation in Congenital Heart Disease Patients

In patients with a congenital heart disease, particular indications may include presence of an intracardiac shunt to minimize thromboembolic risk[48] and anatomical displacement of the AV conduction system for cryomapping of the AV node and/or its inputs.[171] In several forms of congenital heart disease, the AV node and/or conduction system may be fragile or displaced. These include patients with AV septal defects, in whom the AV node is usually displaced inferiorly, anterior to the coronary sinus ostium, and congenitally corrected transposition of the great arteries (ccTGA) in whom the AV node is displaced anteriorly and laterally.[172,173] In other cases, location of the AV node may be uncertain and difficult to predict as a result of a distorted Koch triangle and reconstructed atrial anatomy. Iatrogenic damage to AV conduction in this subset of patients, particularly those with Fontan physiology, may be poorly tolerated, and pacemaker implantation, if required, may only be feasible surgically considering the lack of transvenous access to a ventricle. Avila et al.[174] reported that cryoablation was safe and feasible as a first-line therapy for treating perinodal arrhythmia substrates in adults with various forms of congenital heart disease associated with complex anatomies and/or displaced conduction systems.

NEW PERSPECTIVES

Recently, an ultra-low-temperature cryoablation system (UTLC, Adagio Medical, Inc, Laguna Hills, CA, USA) using nitrogen flow at a temperature of −196°C to cool an 11-cm ablation catheter was developed. Depending on anatomical targeting and ablation strategy, a single stylet-driven catheter can induce circular, linear, or focal lesions using exchangeable preshaped stylets. With a distal diagnostic segment and a proximal cryoablation element, this catheter is compatible with ≥8.5-F steerable sheaths and most mapping systems. PVI, left atrial posterior wall isolation, and a cavotricuspid isthmus flutter line can be performed with two consecutive freeze cycles of 60 seconds each. An oesophageal warming balloon catheter is used to maintain oesophageal temperature and prevent atrio-oesophageal fistulae during PVI. Ventricular lesions can be performed with longer duration (e.g., 240 seconds). Bourier et al. showed that ULTC created transmural, contiguous, and durable AV lesions in two large animal models. Local electrograms were eliminated after a single-shot application (92.5%

and 96.9% for atrial and ventricular lesions, respectively). For all other lesions, local electrograms were eliminated after the second ULTC application. Transmural lesions were confirmed using histology (1.96 ± 0.8 mm in atrial and 5.61 ± 2.2 mm in ventricular lesions) with well-delineated border zones and no evidence of injury to surrounding tissues. Coronary artery spasm with ST-elevation could be provoked with endocardial left ventricular lesions that was fully reversible and did not result in coronary injury.[175] Additional research is required to compare CBA to the newer energy modality, pulsed-field ablation, for which initial studies on PVI have reported promising results.[176]

REFERENCES

Please refer to the e-book for a complete list of references.

3

Biophysics and Clinical Applications of Laser Ablation

Boris Schmidt, Stefano Bordignon, Shaojie Chen, Shota Tohoku, K.R. Julian Chun

KEY POINTS

- Laser ablation represents a sound alternative energy source for catheter ablation of various cardiac arrhythmias.
- Laser produces well-defined transmural ablation lesions.
- Balloon-based laser ablation has become a well-established treatment option for patients with drug-refractory paroxysmal atrial fibrillation.
- Effective tissue exposure, however, is key to avoid coagulum formation and to ensure effective tissue ablation.

BIOPHYSICS OF LASER ABLATION

Laser is defined as "light amplification by stimulated emission of radiation." In other words, a lasing medium (e.g., a medium with identical molecules) housed in a chamber of reflecting surfaces is excited to a higher energy level and, after falling back into the baseline state, emits photons (i.e., electromagnetic radiation).[1] The emitted radiation consists of similar wavelengths and is spatiotemporally synchronized. As a consequence, laser is monochromatic (narrow spectrum), coherent (single phase), and collimated (parallel light waves).

This collimated light beam transports a high amount of energy. Depending on the lasing medium and the difference between the two energy states, laser is emitted at different wavelengths. In the ultraviolet and visible spectrum, argon and excimer lasers work at a wavelength of 300–700 nm. Argon, Nd:YAG (neodymium:yttrium-aluminum-garnet), and diode lasers are most commonly used for ablation of cardiac tissue.[2] The latter two lasers have a wavelength between 700 and 2000 nm (near infrared). Diode lasers have become increasingly popular for their technical features using semiconductors as a lasing medium.[3]

The biological effects depend on the absorption characteristics of the individual wavelength by the target tissue. The laser beam power decreases within the tissue due to scatter and absorption as well as the distance from the emitting source.[4] The primary absorption of the aforementioned diode laser with a wavelength of 980 nm occurs in water molecules, where the electromagnetic frequencies are converted into vibrational kinetic energy. As a consequence, water can be heated in a controlled fashion. Aside from direct heating, cellular lysis may also be achieved mechanically by shock waves.

Depending on the wavelength, maximum absorption occurs 2–4 mm below the endothelial level. Deeper lesion formation, however, can be reached by conductive heating. Given the precision of the collimated beam, laser lesions are well demarcated with narrow lines of margin.[5] Histologically, coagulation necrosis is observed similar to radiofrequency-induced lesion (Fig. 3.1). Transmurality can be achieved without charring at the endocardial surface if cooling is used.[6] This cooling can be achieved, for example, by a fluid-filled balloon on the endocardial surface. Preservation of the endothelial surface may be favorable in the clinical setting to avoid thrombus formation on the ablation lines. In preclinical studies with the 980-nm diode laser, only minimal endothelial disruption was observed and durable pulmonary vein isolation (PVI) was documented in 83% of all treated PVs.[7,8]

Laser energy may also be used for linear lesion creation. In canine studies, it was elegantly demonstrated that it was feasible to achieve 16- to 22-mm-long and 8- to 10-mm-wide transmural lesions using a 100-W Nd:YAG laser (Dornier Medical Systems, Kennesaw, GA) emitting continuous-wave radiation at a wavelength of 1.060 nm.[9] Most importantly, tissue temperatures were well controlled below 70°C, thus avoiding charring and vaporization, also referred to as steam pop.

Unlike other energy modalities, laser energy is absorbed by blood and, if delivered directly into blood, may lead to thermally induced coagulation as well as charring on the one side and insufficient energy delivery to tissue on the other side. In addition, perfused tissue exhibits different absorption characteristics; hence lesion size is altered.[10] However, when an unimpeded transmission of laser to tissue is achieved, there is hardly any loss of energy, which allows for optimal dosing and predictable lesions. Given the virtually absent loss of ablation energy to blood, much less energy is needed in comparison to radiofrequency current ablation (5.5–15 W versus 30–40 W for laser and radiofrequency current, respectively).

Different laser types exhibit different ablation characteristics. Argon laser, for example, is associated with a low scatter and a high absorption at the tissue surface. In order to avoid

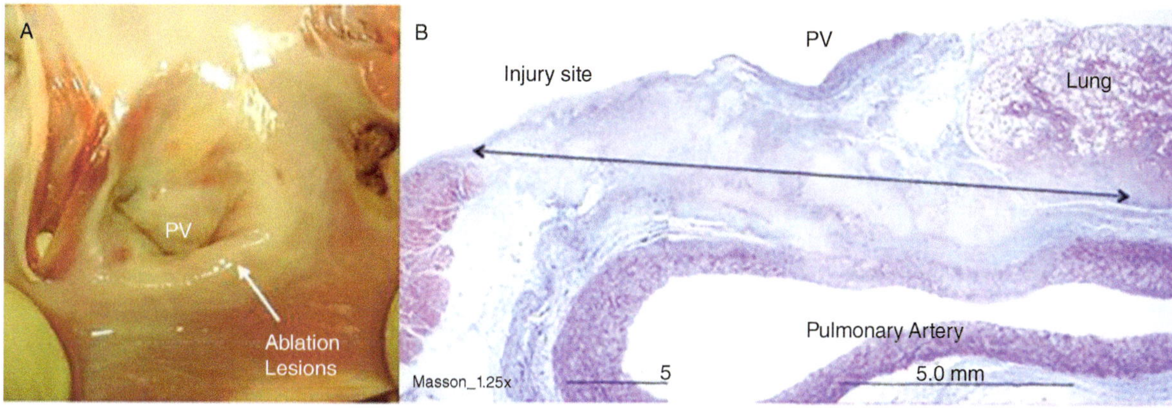

Fig. 3.1 Gross and histological assessment of chronic lesions. (A) Circumferential and contiguous lesions around the pulmonary vein (PV) of a pig are shown 4 weeks postablation. The lesions are paler and less intense than those seen acutely. (B) Histological section (Masson trichrome stain) showing a transmural lesion adjacent to the PV ostium is shown (*arrow*). The lesion extends into the adjacent lung and pulmonary artery. (From Dukkipati SR, Neuzil P, Skoda J, et al. Visual balloon-guided point-by-point ablation reliable, reproducible, and persistent pulmonary vein isolation. *Circ Arrhythmia Electrophysiol.* 2010;3:266–273.)

fiber-optic degradation, pulsed-laser beam application may be mandatory. In early feasibility studies, argon laser proved efficacious in ablating the conduction system in dogs.[11] However, ablation was associated with cardiac perforation in two of six animals. Histologically, tissue vaporization and thermal necrosis were found. In the clinical setting, argon laser was used for ablation of ventricular tachycardia during bloodless laser ventriculotomy and for atrioventricular accessory pathways.[12,13]

On the contrary, lasers with longer wavelengths, such as the Nd:YAG and diode lasers, have a higher scatter, and maximal absorption occurs below the tissue surface.[14] It appears that tissue vaporization is observed less commonly and intramyocardial coagulation necrosis can be created with endo- and epicardial sparing.[15] In several studies, large-volume lesions with up to 11-mm depth were created without evidence for perforation or endothelial damage, unlike lesions produced by radiofrequency current.[16] Another merit of diode lasers is customizing wavelength to the tissue properties targeted for ablation because absorption characteristics may vary.

Current technology (see below) uses a laser generator surrounded by a translucent balloon to occlude the pulmonary vein and to eliminate interjacent blood between the balloon surface and myocardium. Circulating fluid inside the balloon helps cool the tissue interface. The balloon design allows for circular ablation in a point-by-point manner. In preclinical studies, it was elegantly shown in chicken muscle preparations that lesion volume is determined by the total ablation energy delivered.[17] Moreover, contiguity of lesions was improved by a higher overlap ratio between spot lesions. In an attempt to continuously deliver laser energy to create contiguous and transmural circular lesions in a single sweep, a lesion formation computational model was created. The model accurately predicts lesion size and depth in human atrial myocardium by incorporating various variables such as scattering of light within target atrial tissue, absorption of light as a three-dimensional heat source, diffusion of the applied heat source within target tissue, heat removal by blood perfusion (per Pennes' classic bioheat),[18,19] metabolic tissue heating (per Pennes' classic bioheat), conduction of heat into adjoining tissue, convection of heat to/from balloon fill media and circulating blood, denaturing of tissue based on Arrhenius time–temperature integral, and coupling of tissue damage into previous processes' parameters. As a result, energy settings equivalent to manual spot lesions were developed. Mean lesion depths in the lesion formation model and in nonperfused fresh turkey thigh preparations differed by only 1.1–6.9% and were measured on average at 4.15–5.89 mm.

CLINICAL APPLICATIONS OF LASER ABLATION

Historically, laser ablation was evaluated for different cardiac arrhythmias (Table 3.1). In this chapter, studies for transvenous as well as surgical ablation are addressed.

TABLE 3.1 Overview of Clinical Indications for Ablation Using Laser Technology

Clinical Arrhythmia	Status Quo
Ventricular tachycardia	Epicardial ablation as well as endocardial during cardiac surgery Little to no experience for transvascular ablation
Atrial fibrillation	Proven noninferiority to standard technology for pulmonary vein isolation using the endoscopic ablation system
Supraventricular arrhythmias (Wolff-Parkinson-White, atrioventricular nodal reentrant tachycardia, inappropriate sinus tachycardias)	Subordinate role in clinical routine Historical experience during surgery for accessory pathways and smaller case series for transvascular ablation of inappropriate sinus tachycardia

SURGICAL ABLATION

Early clinical experience of surgical laser ablation was collected during mapping guided ablation of atrioventricular accessory pathways by using an argon laser.[13] The same argon laser was also used for ablation of malignant ventricular tachycardia originating from sites that were not amenable to surgical excision.[12] In the latter study, all ventricular tachycardias were rendered noninducible in four patients after bloodless ventriculotomy. Moreover, it was observed that higher laser energies are required to achieve similar lesion size in diseased as opposed to healthy ventricular myocardium.[20]

Consecutive studies also used the Nd:YAG laser for epicardial ablation of ventricular arrhythmias under cardiopulmonary bypass surgery.[21] Depending on baseline ejection fraction, procedural mortality ranged from 8% to 41%. With increasing experience and better patient selection, however, complication rates decreased and arrhythmia-free survival was reported to be as high as 78% during 17 months of follow-up.[22] In comparison to cryothermal ablation, the authors stressed the higher effectiveness in normothermic myocardium, the lack of temporary peripheral myocardial injury, and shorter ablation times.[23] For special indications such as Chagas disease, epicardial laser ablation may be the preferred choice.[24]

TRANSVENOUS ABLATION

Technical advancement was made to develop catheters with fiberoptics enabling an endocardial approach to ventricular substrates (Table. 3.2).[25] The key challenge was to design a fiberoptic that tolerates intracardiac manipulation, on the one hand, and that does not cause cardiac perforation, on the other hand.

Recently, a tripolar open irrigated electrode laser mapping and ablation catheter was developed.[26] This catheter is manipulated via a steerable delivery sheath and may deliver laser light at different wavelengths between 980 and 1470 nm while simultaneously mapping intracardiac electrograms. Clinical data exist for ablation of inappropriate sinus tachycardia as well as long-lasting persistent atrial fibrillation.[27,28] In the latter study, 48 patients were ablated with a 1064-nm continuous-wave Nd:Yag laser. Sites displaying high-rate electrical activity were targeted until sinus rhythm was achieved. As shown in Fig. 3.2, delivery of laser energy does not interfere with the recording of intracardiac electrograms.

More recently, a linear catheter was tested for its effectiveness to ablate the cavotricuspid isthmus in preclinical studies.[29] The 20-mm linear catheter may be introduced into the atrium via a steerable sheath and positioned at the cavotricuspid isthmus with intracardiac echo guidance (Fig. 3.3). Mean lesion length was 20.6 ± 1.65 mm. Transmurality of lesions was observed, and no evidence for charring or perforation was found.

The most commonly used laser ablation device for cardiac arrhythmias is the *endoscopic ablation system* (EAS), also referred to as the *laser balloon* (LB), for the treatment of drug-refractory paroxysmal atrial fibrillation. In the following, we provide a detailed description of the device.

TABLE 3.2 **Merits and Demerits of Laser as an Energy Source for Ablation of Cardiac Arrhythmias**

Merits	Demerits
Precise lesion delivery (depending on the device under visual guidance)	Complex catheter designs required (fiberoptics, balloons)
Hardly any energy loss into blood, thus predictable lesion volume with respective energy setting	Direct energy delivery into blood may lead to coagulum formation
Rare to no steam popping	Little to no experience for endocardial ventricular ablation
No noise on electrogram recordings during energy delivery	To date, no integration into three-dimensional mapping systems

The Endoscopic Ablation System (Laser Balloon)

The centerpiece of the EAS is a compliant balloon (Fig. 3.4). It is pear shaped and can vary in size from 7 to 42 mm by continuously flushing it with deuterium oxide (D_2O) mixed with contrast media. In the shaft of the balloon, there are several lumens for various purposes. Two lumens are used to continuously circulate the D_2O by a peristaltic pump. By varying the speed of the pump, the balloon can be inflated and deflated as needed in a seamless fashion. For this purpose, a controller is located at the proximal end of the catheter handle. Another lumen carries a glass fiber connected to a white light source. The laser generator is located in the central lumen. This 980-nm diode laser emits a beam perpendicular to the balloon surface. Because the diode laser beam is invisible, additional aiming beam lasers in green and red are used with the same optic fiber. While the red-green laser is nicely seen on tissue (light backgound), it disappears when targeting into blood. Therefore, a red aiming beam is added, which is clearly visible in blood. The laser beam covers approximately 30 degrees of an arc. In between energy deliveries, the operator advances the laser generator in a circular fashion via a steering wheel integrated in the catheter handle. To create a contiguous lesion set, it is advisable to overlap the individual lesions by 30–50%. The level of energy may be varied from 5.5 W to 12 W with predefined application times of 20–30 seconds per lesion.

In the latest EAS generation (X3), a motor drive was included into the catheter handle. The motor continuously advances the laser at a predefined speed of 2.2 degrees per second, thereby creating a circular lesion. This so-called RAPID mode may be used alternatively to the point-by-point ablation mode with manual adjustment of the laser application.

Ultimately, a 2F endoscope can be advanced to the distal end of the balloon to enable visual control of lesion delivery inside the beating heart.

Navigation of the balloon to the PVs is performed with the aid of a steerable sheath (12F inner diameter). To avoid cardiac perforation, the balloon is equipped with a flexible tip.

The catheter is connected to a specific workstation that houses a white light-source camera system and the laser generator. The graphical user interface is operative via a touch screen monitor and allows for selection of the ablation mode and power.

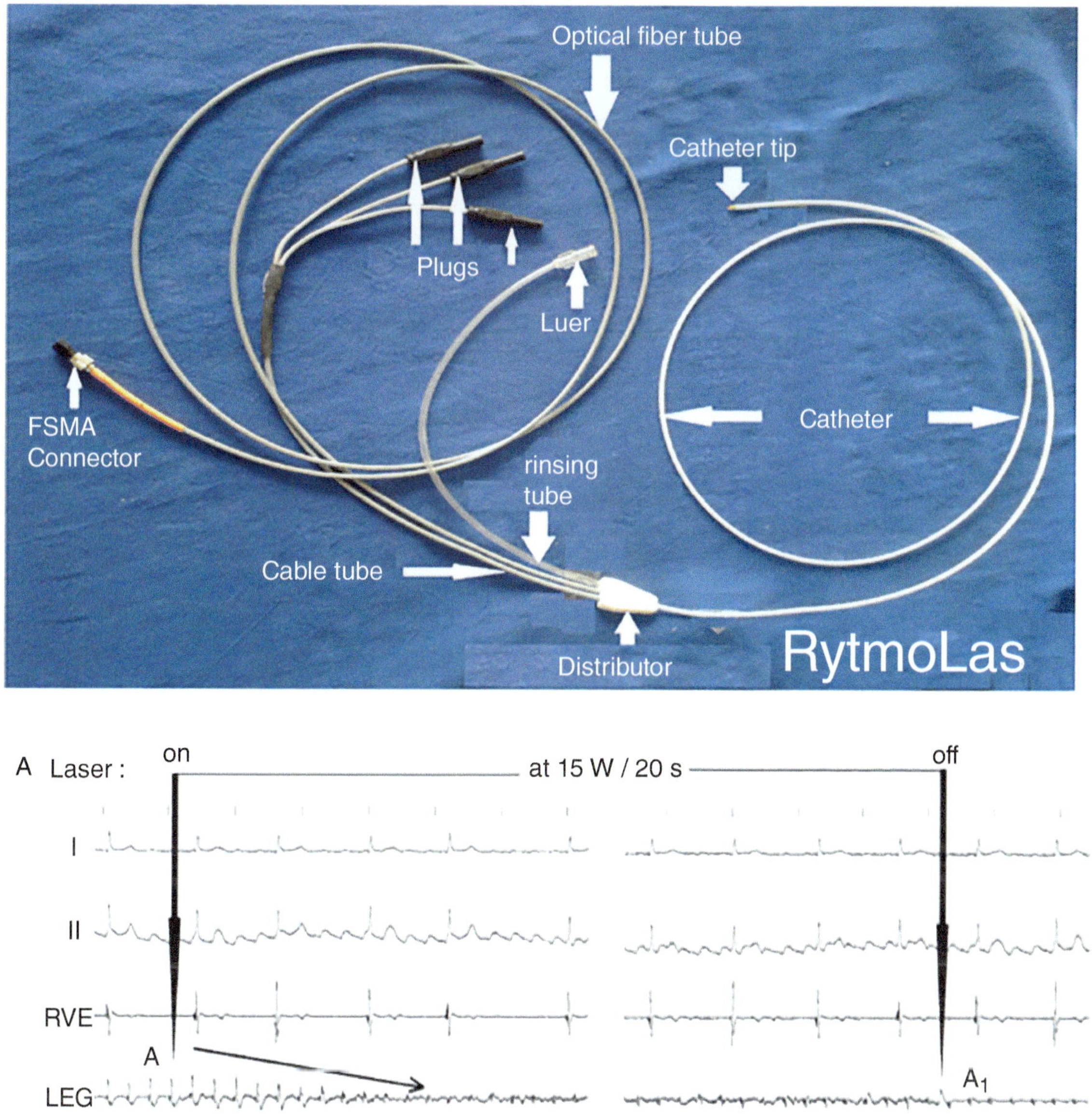

Fig. 3.2 Focal laser catheter for ablation and recording of intracardiac electrograms. *Lower panel,* Surface ECG (leads I and II) as well as intracardiac electrograms from the right ventricle (RVE) and the ablation site (LEG). While the local electrogram diminishes during ablation, no electrical noise is recorded, allowing for a precise interpretation of the local electrogram amplitude. (From Weber H, Sagerer-Gerhardt M, Heinze A. Laser catheter ablation of long-lasting persistent atrial fibrillation: longterm results. *J Atr Fibrillation.* 2017;10:1588. www.jafib.com.)

In addition, the endoscopic view is displayed to visually control the ablation. Aside from a live endoscopic view, in another panel the lesion set may be displayed by superimposed screenshot images of each energy application on top of the live image in order to facilitate a contiguous circular lesion. All ablation lesions may be tracked and reviewed at any time during the procedure using a designated software.

Pulmonary Vein Isolation With the EAS

While the EAS design allows for a wide-area circumferential PVI including both ipsilateral PVs into a figure-of-eight ablation lesion set, typically a sequential PVI approach is used with circular ablation at each individual PV.[30–32] The latter approach more reliably allows for gapless circular ablation and leads to a higher acute PVI rate as well as to better clinical outcome. Using the steerable sheath, the EAS balloon is navigated to the PV ostium and inflated until circumferential balloon-to-tissue contact is achieved without blood spilling in between the balloon surface and the antral tissue. In fact, the conformability of the balloon allows for ablation at virtually all PVs regardless of shape and size. Therefore, preprocedural 3D imaging may be performed but is not deemed a mandatory prerequisite.[33]

Under visual guidance, ablation lesions are deployed in a contiguous fashion. When the manual mode is applied, overlapping the individual lesions by 30–50% is recommended.[34] Energy is titrated from 5.5 to 12 W (20–30 seconds per each laser application time) according to the degree of tissue exposure. Usually, lesion deployment is started at one side of the

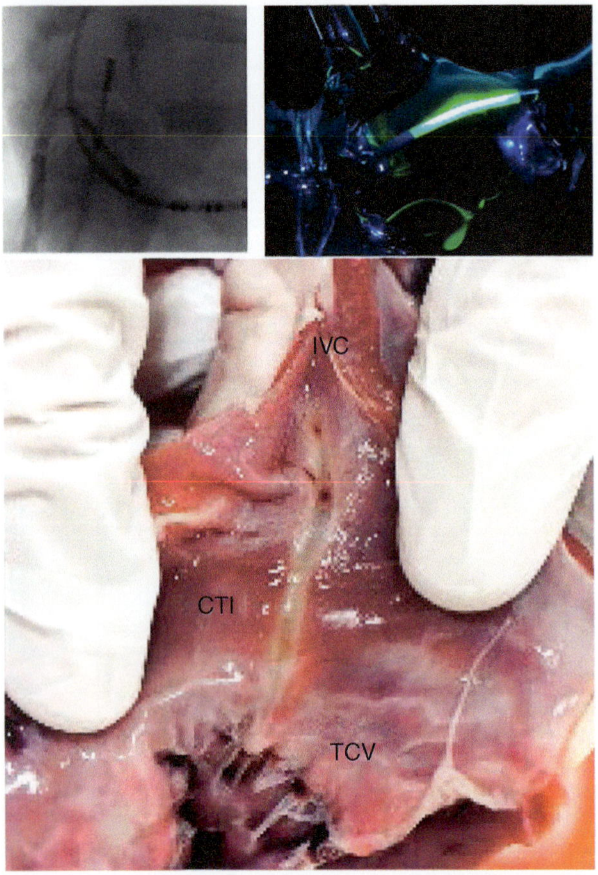

Fig. 3.3 Linear laser catheter for ablation of cavotricuspid atrial flutter. In the left upper panel, the 20-mm linear catheter is placed at the cavotricuspid isthmus (CTI) under fluoroscopy and intracardiac echo guidance. A diagnostic pacing catheter is placed in the coronary sinus. In the *right upper panel*, the linear laser catheter is shown. Please note, the laser active area visualized by a green low-energy diode laser. In the *lower panel*, a macroscopic view of the linear lesion is depicted. *IVC*, inferior vena cava; *TCV*, tricuspid valve. (From Krist D, Linz D, Schotten U, Zeemering S, Leenen D. A novel laser energy ablation catheter for endocardial cavo-tricuspid isthmus ablation and epicardial ventricular lesion formation: an in vivo proof-of-concept study. *Front Med Technol.* 2022;4:1–8.)

visible catheter shaft and continued until the other side was reached. In an attempt to expose the remaining part of antral PV tissue that lies behind the catheter shaft, a controlled rotation with the inflated balloon is performed. Next, the circular lesion set is completed.

The latest balloon generation now allows for RAPID mode ablation (e.g., a continuous laser energy delivery) while the beam is swept around the PV ostium at constant speed by an integrated motor drive (see Video 3.1). Initial studies showed that RAPID mode can be used in virtually all PVs.[35] Thereby, ablation and procedure times are dramatically reduced by 65% and 66%, respectively, at the same time maintaining efficacy of acute PVI with a single circular lesion set in 92% of PVs applied. Similar data were reported from a prospective registry.[36]

Theoretically, the use of RAPID mode turns the EAS into a single-sweep device (i.e., PVI with a single energy application). In a pilot study, the following technique was developed to achieve single-sweep PVI.[37] At first, the operator strived for optimal tissues exposure. After balloon positioning at the PV ostium, the laser generator was pulled back to obtain a circumferential view at the PV ostium. In case of 360-degree tissue exposure, the catheter shaft was positioned in the region with the broadest tissue corridor (usually posterior left atrial wall) to visualize the ablation path and subsequently allow for "blind spot" ablation behind the catheter shaft. Then, the ablation path was simulated by manually sweeping the aiming beam behind the shaft from one edge of the shaft to the other. If no or only minimal correction of the laser generator along the *z*-axis of the shaft was required to keep the beam on exposed tissue on both sides of the shaft, the individual PV is qualified for a RAPID ablation attempt. Using this approach, a total of 56% of all PVs in 100 consecutive patients were isolated by a single laser energy application. A prerecorded clinical case of EAS-guided PVI is available in Video 3.2.

It is of note that the catheter is not equipped with electrodes, thus precluding recording of electrophysiological signals. Hence, ablation is guided purely anatomically, and PV isolation has to be assessed with a diagnostic catheter thereafter. Direct lesion visualization, as demonstrated in animal experiments, is unreliable and limited to a subset of patients.

Safety Aspects and Precautions During PVI Using EAS

In general, balloon ablation technologies seem to have a favorable effect on procedural safety during PVI procedures with a significantly lower perforation rate.[38] Nonetheless, some strategies to mitigate the risk of ablation-associated complications are illustrated below.

Laser represents a thermal ablation modality. Thus, neighboring tissues are at potential risk for thermal injury during PVI procedures. Several clinical investigations have therefore focused on risk assessment as well as strategies to avoid these side effects.

Thermal Esophageal Injury

In order to prevent thermal esophageal injury, continuous esophageal temperature monitoring is recommended. In initial reports, a temperature cutoff of 39°C was recommended to cease energy applications at the posterior left atrial wall.[7] In later clinical investigations, gastroesophageal endoscopy was systematically performed to assess the incidence of thermal lesions.[39] This study confirmed the importance of temperature management showing that in 70% of all patients, the esophageal temperature rose above the preset cutoff of 38.5°C. In 82% of patients, no thermal injury was found. However, in 10% of cases, esophageal ulcerations were seen after the mean maximal temperature had reached >42°C. In a following study, it was demonstrated that esophageal temperature rather than ablation power determined the incidence of esophageal injury.[40]

Importantly, to date, no atrial-to-esophageal fistula has been reported after laser balloon ablation.[41] This underscores the effectiveness of esophageal temperature monitoring as a preventive measure in the setting of EAS ablation.

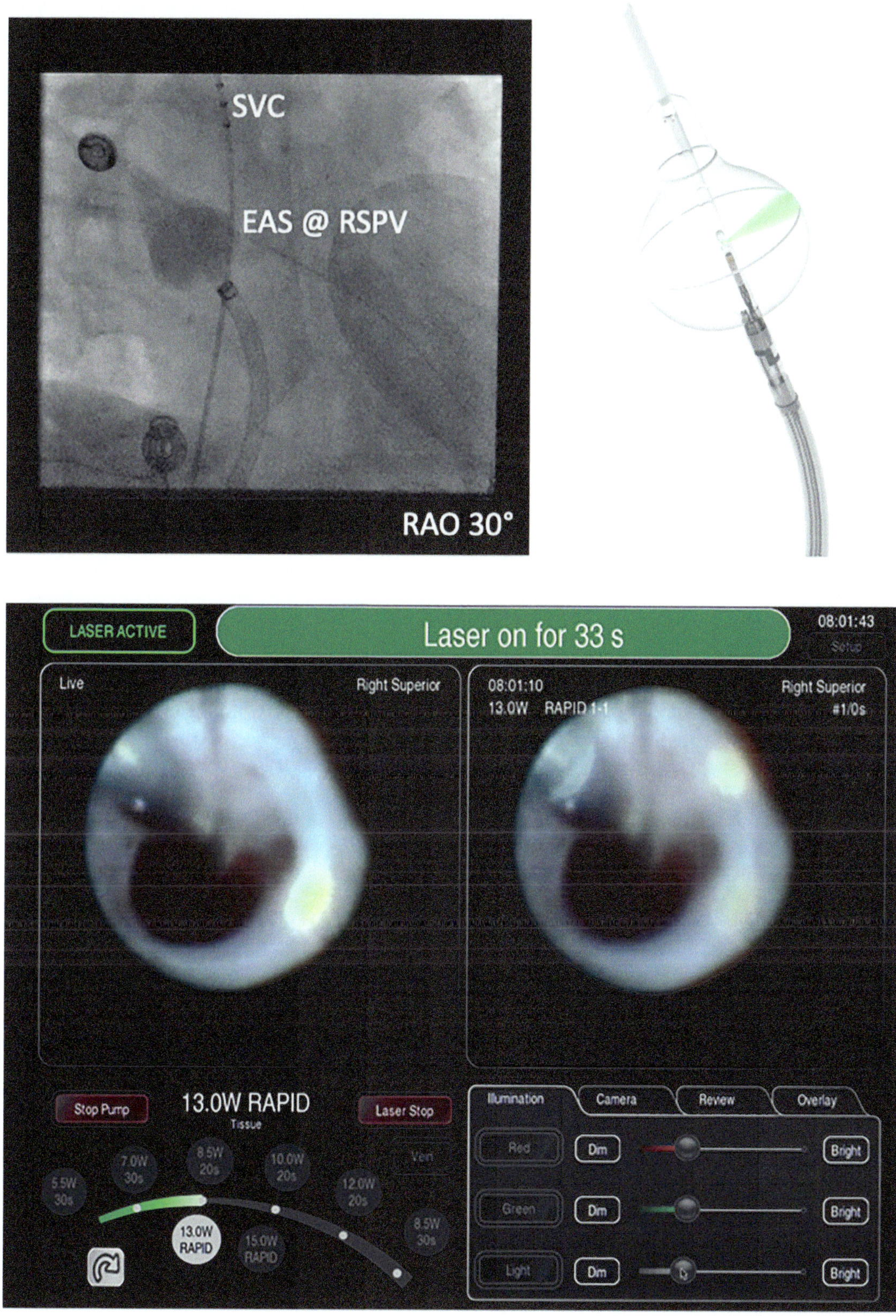

Fig. 3.4 Pulmonary vein isolation with the endoscopic ablation system (EAS). The balloon catheter is placed at the right superior pulmonary vein (RSPV) under fluoroscopic guidance (right anterior oblique [RAO] 30-degree view). *Lower panel,* Graphic user interface is depicted. It provides an endoscopic view at the completely occluded RSPV with a circumferential balloon to tissue contact (*left image,* live view). The *green point* reflects the aiming beam of the current diode laser position. It sweeps around the PV ostium in a continuous fashion. In the *lower part,* the various ablation settings (manual versus RAPID; 5.5–15 W) may be selected. The arrows serve to select the direction of the sweep. The right-sided endoscopic view is a live view and a superimposed screenshot of the first energy application. That allows the operator to determine the starting point of ablation in order to complete a circular lesion. The *top line* shows the elapsed application time.

Phrenic Nerve Injury

The phrenic nerve is at risk for thermal injury during ablation at the right-sided pulmonary veins. In a recently published meta-analysis, the risk for phrenic nerve injury (PNI) was estimated at 2.6% (1.4–3.9%).[41] Several strategies exist to mitigate the risk for PNI, including continuous high-output pacing from the superior vena cava, lowering of ablation energy at the anterior aspect of the PV ostium, andmaximum balloon inflation to increase the distance to the PN. The latter was identified to play a central role in avoiding PNI.[42] The use of recording the compound motor action potential remains controversial.[43] In comparison to the cryoballoon, the acute procedural risk for PNI seems to be lower (1.5% versus 4.2%); however, during follow-up beyond 3 months, persistence of diaphragmatic dysfunction is similar.[44]

Thromboembolic Complications and Silent Cerebral Lesions

In order to prevent cardioembolic stroke during EAS-guided PVI, the following precautions should be considered. First, it is advisable to keep the activated clotting time between 300 and 400 seconds. Second, energy delivery with power >5.5 W adjacent to or into blood must be avoided. Other than that, EAS-guided ablation has not been shown to be associated with an increased number of thromboembolic complications.

Moreover, clinical investigations have compared the silent cerebral embolic rate between laser balloon, irrigated radiofrequency, and cryoballoon ablation and did not find any significant differences.[45,46]

Clinical Outcomes

A sound number of clinical studies were performed to investigate the optimal use of the EAS as well as to compare it to other ablation technologies.

The largest prospective randomized study involving the EAS assessed the freedom from treatment failure during the first 12 months following ablation in comparison to irrigated radiofrequency-guided ablation in patients with drug-refractory paroxysmal AF.[47] A total of 353 patients were enrolled into the study. There was no statistically significant difference for the primary endpoint (61.1% versus 61.7% in the EAS and control groups, respectively). Moreover, no difference was found for the primary safety endpoint between the groups. As a conclusion, the authors stated that EAS-guided PVI proved noninferior to radiofrequency-guided ablation in patients with drug-refractory paroxysmal AF. Consequently, the device was approved for clinical use in the United States by the Food and Drug Administration in 2016.

When using continuous rhythm monitoring by implantable loop recorders, complete freedom from AF after a single EAS-guided ablation in an all-comer population (74% paroxysmal AF) was documented in 66.9% of all patients.[48]

Similarly, a randomized controlled multicenter study comparing EAS to irrigated radiofrequency-guided PVI was performed in patients with persistent AF. Again, freedom from atrial tachyarrhythmia recurrence was similar in both groups with 71.2% and 69.3% in the EAS and control groups, respectively ($P = .40$).[49]

Most recently, data were released from the first randomized study using two different balloon catheters.[50] In total, 200 patients with symptomatic AF were treated with either the EAS or the cryoballoon. After 12-month follow-up, no differences in rhythm control outcome were observed. However, procedural speed was in favor of the single-shot device.

Aside from the clinical arrhythmia recurrence rate, the performance of a particular ablation device should be evaluated (i.e., is durable PVI achieved after EAS guided ablation?).

Remapping studies of patients after EAS irrespective of their arrhythmia status revealed a durable PVI rate of 86%.[51] On a per-patient basis, 60% of remapped patients had complete durable PVI.

If patients undergo a second ablation procedure for symptomatic arrhythmia recurrences, the rate of durable PVI was found to be 61% using the second-generation EAS device as opposed to 82% using the X3 third-generation EAS.[52]

REFERENCES

Please refer to the e-book for a complete list of references.

4

Biophysics and Clinical Applications of Pulsed-Field Ablation

*Iwanari Kawamura, Connor Oates, Jacob S. Koruth**

KEY POINTS

- Pulsed-field ablation (PFA) is a nonthermal ablative modality that uses ultra-short high-voltage impulses. Above a certain threshold, irreversible permeability of the cell membrane occurs, as well as changes in the lipids and proteins embedded within the membrane. This increased permeability allows for inflow of otherwise membrane-impermeant molecules and outflow of critical molecules along with electrolyte balance that lead to cell death.
- Electrical field strengths that induce cell death can vary among cell types, and cardiomyocytes appear to be preferentially susceptible. The effect of PFA on the cell membrane can be reversible at lower field strengths.
- Catheter-based PFA has been explored as a novel energy source for cardiac ablation, with several reports demonstrating promise, especially for atrial ablation.
- Unlike thermal ablation, PFA offers the potential to spare collateral organs such as the phrenic nerve and the esophagus. Histologic changes after PFA include homogeneous fibrosis with absent risk of venous stenosis and evidence of nerve and vessel sparing.
- Our current knowledge of PFA is still in its early stages. Further research is needed to investigate its role in ventricular ablation as well as to better understand the risks of PFA, especially that of coronary artery spasm.

BIOPHYSICS OF LESION FORMATION

Pulsed-field ablation (PFA) is a nonthermal ablative energy modality that uses ultra-short high-voltage impulses and has unique tissue-selective ablative properties.[1–4] To understand PFA, one must view the targeted cell as a conductive component of tissue and pay particular attention to the dielectric phospholipid bilayer cell membrane that is responsible for the cell resting potential that exists across it. The mechanism of cell death from PFA has been traditionally ascribed to the theory of aqueous pore formation, widely referred to as electroporation. According to this concept, the electrical field induced by generating a high-voltage gradient created across a cell membrane reduces the energy required for spontaneous aqueous pore formation and facilitates the formation of pores that become increasingly more stable (Fig. 4.1A). These pores become permanent (i.e., irreversible electroporation occurs) when the electric field exceeds a critical threshold, which results in cell death due to increased membrane permeability.[5] It is important to appreciate that, at lower field strengths, pore formation remains transient, reversible electroporation occurs, and PFA does not lead to cell death. This reversible effect of pulsed fields is the basis for known therapies such as electrochemotherapy and other techniques used in cell biology.[6–8] As we describe later, the concept of reversible electroporation has potential applications in cardiac electrophysiology and their effects on cardiac function is an area of active investigation. More recently, the mechanism of PF on cell membranes has been broadened to include more than just pore formation, as chemical changes to the lipids and proteins have been found to occur as well (*electropermeabilization,* Fig. 4.1A).[9] The increased permeability that results after PFA allows for inflow of membrane-impermeant molecules and outflow of critical molecules from the cell's interior that then lead to cell death. One might think of the effects of electric fields on susceptible tissues, as manifesting in "zones" of reversible electroporation in the periphery with irreversible electroporation at the core of the field, and when the field exceeds a certain intensity, a zone of thermal effect may also be seen.

Pulsed electrical fields have demonstrated relative tissue-related specificity at doses used to ablate myocardium. Some bench experiments indicate that cardiomyocytes are more susceptible to ablation than esophageal smooth muscle, blood vessels, and nerves, although this differential sensitivity is not completely agreed upon, with other reports indicating similar sensitivity of cardiomyocytes and other tissues to PFA.[10,11] Tissue type, differences in cell size/orientation, and pulse design characteristics all affect the degree of irreversible electroporation/ablation that occurs with PFA.[12] Pulse characteristics include variables like voltage, monopolar versus bipolar, monophasic versus biphasic delivery, pulse duration, number of pulses, number of trains, and interphase intervals. Pulses delivered to

*Disclosure: Dr. Koruth serves as a consultant to Abbott/Acutus/Farapulse/Kardium. Dr. Koruth received research grants from Affera/Acutus/Cardiofocus/Kardium/LuxCath. Dr. Koruth holds stock options in Affera. Other authors have no conflicts to disclose.

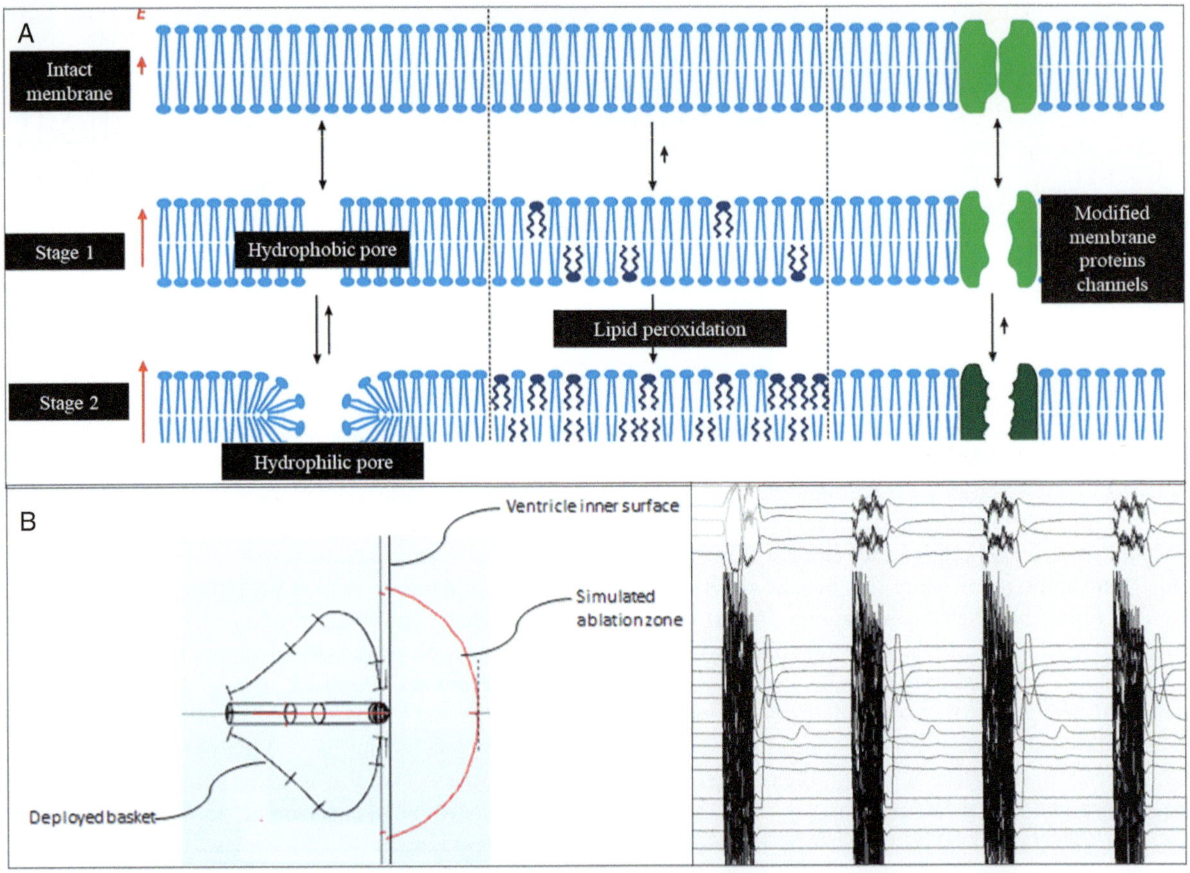

Fig. 4.1 Biophysics of pulsed-field ablation (PFA). (A) Conceptual scheme of molecular-level mechanisms of electropermeabilization, starting from an intact membrane (*top*). *Electroporation:* Electrically induced formation of aqueous pores in the lipid bilayer, shown here in two stages, with water molecules first penetrating the bilayer and thus forming an unstable hydrophobic pore (stage 1), and with adjacent lipids then reorienting with their polar headgroups toward these water molecules and thus forming a metastable hydrophilic pore (stage 2). Electrically induced chemical changes to membrane lipids, including peroxidation, which deforms their tails and increases the bilayer's permeability to water, ions, and small molecules and electrically induced modulation of membrane proteins' function, shown here for a voltage-gated channel. Arrow lengths for the electric field *(E, red)* correspond to its strength (i.e., amplitude of the electric pulse or pulses), while those for transitions between states of membrane permeability reflect the transition rate (*shorter arrow* = slower rate; not drawn to scale between the three mechanisms). (Adapted from Kotnik T, Rems L, Tarek M, et al. Membrane electroporation and electropermeabilization: mechanisms and models. *Annu Rev Biophys.* 2019;48:63-91.) (B) Figure diagram demonstrating the simulated ablation zone for a specific dose/electrode combination. (C) Joint pacing from coronary sinus and right ventricular catheters with QRS synchronized PFA pulses. (Adapted from Koruth JS, Kuroki K, Iwasawa J, et al. Endocardial ventricular pulsed field ablation: a proof-of-concept preclinical evaluation. *Europace.* 2020;22(3):434–439.)

the myocardium result in the saturation of multiple channels within the recording system (Fig. 4.1B, C). This characteristic signature of PFA is notably different from when radiofrequency (RF) current is applied in the electrophysiology laboratory. In general, monophasic PF configurations have largely been replaced by biphasic PFA for clinical cardiac ablation, given that monophasic delivery results in significant muscular and phrenic nerve stimulation requiring neuromuscular paralysis and general anesthesia. Modern biphasic PF pulses also elicit muscular and phrenic nerve activation but to lesser degrees, and certain waveforms have been optimized to allow for the ablation procedure to be completed with only deep sedation as opposed to general anesthesia and neuromuscular paralysis. The current required for myocardial PFA (often in the range of 1–2.5 kV for microsecond PFA) must be viewed as inherently stimulatory and explains why both myocardial, skeletal muscle, and phrenic never/diaphragm activation can occur during PFA delivery. The risk of ventricular activation during the vulnerable period, however, can result in ventricular arrhythmias (VAs) if PF is delivered in close proximity to the ventricles and can be avoided by synchronization of pulses to the R wave. Unsynchronized energy delivery to the left atrium appears safe thus far, and many clinical PFA systems currently do not gate their pulses during atrial ablation. High voltages, monopolar monophasic PF, and repeated applications are possible parameters to increase ablative effects.[13,14] In reality, PF pulse designs and effects are highly complex, and exceptions to these parameters exist. While a dose–response curve has been demonstrated for

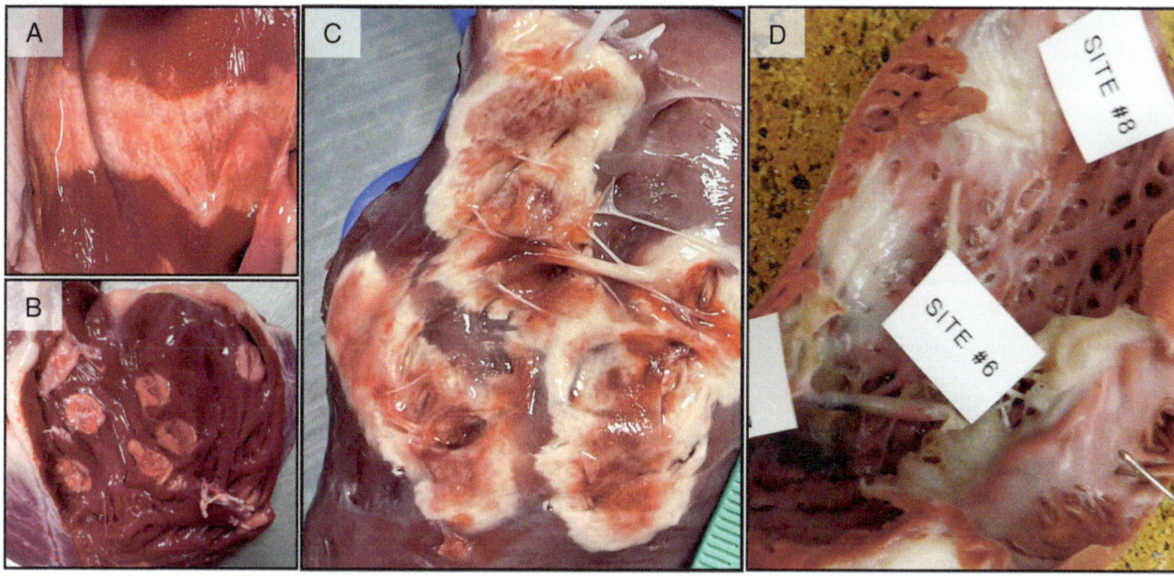

Fig. 4.2 Gross appearance of endocardial pulsed-field ablation (PFA) lesions. (A) Superior vena cava (opened along long axis) demonstrating well-demarcated wide acute homogeneous lesion (prefixation). (B) TTC-stained ventricle with discrete endocardial acute lesions demonstrating clear, oval, homogeneous PFA lesions. (Adapted from Koruth JS, Kuroki K, Kawamura I, et al. Focal pulsed field ablation for pulmonary vein isolation and linear atrial lesions: a preclinical assessment of safety and durability. *Circ Arrhythm Electrophysiol.* 2020;13:e008716.) (C) Appearance of linear acute lesion along the right ventricular endocardium where PFA lesions were applied using a focal PFA catheter. (Adapted from Kawamura I, Reddy VY, Santos-Gallego CG, et al. Electrophysiology, pathology, and imaging of pulsed field ablation of scarred and healthy ventricles in swine. *Circ Arrhythm Electrophysiol.* 2023;16(1):e011369.) (D) Well-demarcated chronic lesions with involvement of trabeculae and intracavitary structures such as the moderator band. (Adapted from Koruth JS, Kuroki K, Iwasawa J, et al. Endocardial ventricular pulsed field ablation: a proof-of-concept preclinical evaluation. *Europace.* 2020;22:434–439.)

cardiac ablation (i.e., increasing energy delivery results in bigger lesions), significant incremental energy also risks tissue heating, increased muscular contraction, electrical arcing, and barotrauma. The pursuit of a perfect dose that is sufficiently ablative yet retains myocardial selectivity and avoids thermal effects will be different for each technology. Careful technology specific modeling, animal experimentation, and detailed follow-up of initial clinical experience need to be performed.

BIOLOGICAL EFFECTS OF CARDIAC PULSED-FIELD ABLATION

PFA results in unique histologic features because of its nonthermal ablative mechanism—it irreversibly injures the myocardial cell membranes but with preservation of extracardiac tissue and the intervening connective tissue—thus uniquely sparing the structural integrity or scaffolding of the targeted tissue (myocardium). The mechanism of cell death from PFA is thought to include necrosis and apoptosis among several other potential mechanisms.[15] A detailed understanding of the time course and relative contributions of these and other mechanisms for contemporary waveforms used in cardiac ablation is still not well defined. Before we consider the effects of PFA on myocardium in detail, it is important to briefly understand the ablative effects of PFA on organs such as the liver, pancreas, kidneys, and prostate.[16-19] Clinical investigation of targeting these organs preceded cardiac PFA as an approach to treat parenchymal tumors and evaluation of its effects led to the unique appreciation of distinctive features of PFA, such as the preservation of nerves, blood vessels, and the underlying tissue architecture. This pattern of tissue selectivity is different from thermal energies, has been described to be consistent across various organs, and allows PFA to have a distinct advantage over the rather indiscriminate nature of thermal ablation.

Myocardial PF lesions were recently well characterized. While most reports are preclinical in nature and vary by catheter and pulse design, several features of myocardial PF lesions appear consistently. Myocardial lesions tend to have very discrete margins with narrow transition zones (unlike thermal lesions), and several reports demonstrate that best lesion visualization (on gross analysis) occurs a few hours after PF application (Fig. 4.2A, B). The lack of a clearly visible lesion immediately after a PFA application is consistent with its nonthermal mechanism. While some PFA technologies render a pale lesion with minimal intralesional hemorrhage, other technologies can result in central hemorrhagic changes (thought to be due to increased vascular permeability) and can give the lesions a central dark zone (Fig. 4.2C).[20] The shape of PFA lesions depends on the catheter footprint and does not propagate as duration of delivery is increased (unlike thermal ablation). It is useful to appreciate that the ablative zone for any PF catheter tip is a function of the electrical field that develops around the tip and that myocardial cells within the "ablative zone" of the electrical field are expected to be rendered nonfunctional. This concept of ablation is different from the dynamic thermal profile that is created over time around RF catheter tips.[21,22] Longer delivery times are needed with RF to achieve depths comparable to PFA, as RF lesion creation depends on both resistive and conductive heating. Understanding the "electrical field–based" ablation concept also allows one to appreciate the relevance of contact with tissue (a must for most thermal energies) in terms of both force exerted and coupling with tissue. In fact, detailed computational simulations suggest that, despite gaps of 2 mm between the PFA catheter tip and atrial tissue, adequate lesions can still be generated; if there is sufficient exposure of the tissue to a lethal electrical field, one can expect a lesion despite the lack of intimate contact.[12] This behavior also explains the striking, often homogeneous ablation of trabeculated tissue that is seen with PFA—an effect that is difficult to achieve with thermal ablation during which trabecular structures escape ablation due to poor contact over the duration of lesion (Fig. 4.2B). It should be noted that the energy delivered from a single point in a catheter during PFA decreases as a function of the square of the distance from the catheter. Since blood is generally more electrically conductive than cardiac tissue, there could be considerable loss of the electric current in areas of poor contact, thus limiting the depth of the lesion created. Nakagawa et al. showed that no detectable lesions were generated when the catheter was suspended 2 mm from the surface of the ventricular myocardium (using a 3.5-mm-tip catheter) and demonstrated that the treatment effect becomes markedly more pronounced with as little as 1g of force with lesion depth increasing as force was increased.[23] Verma et al. also demonstrated a linear relationship between lesion depth and tissue distance in their evaluation.[24] Therefore, one can conclude that electrode tissue proximity increases the likelihood of achieving desirable lesions by maximizing the electric field penetration into the target tissue, but, in general, PF may be more forgiving than thermal energies. One must also realize that the role of contact (force and/or stability) will also depend to an extent on the catheter size/design and the extent of the electrical field generated. Smaller catheter tips with poor coupling are more likely to create smaller lesions.

Another important feature of PFA lesions is the extent of acute electrical dysfunction that occurs immediately after PF delivery and the time course of recovery at different doses. We have indirect clinical and preclinical evidence that the area of immediate electrical stunning that occurs can exceed the dimension of the final lesion in some situations. This concept is supported by the near universal occurrence of acute PV isolation after PFA and the dramatic acute electrogram attenuation that occurs even when the applied dose does not result in chronic durability. This discordance between acute and chronic electrical effects is especially obvious with highly abbreviated PF pulses that result in reversible electroporation, and preclinical data have demonstrated the occurrence of unipolar changes that can extend beyond the actual site of ablation.[25–28] Surrogates of electrical dysfunction, such as electrogram amplitude reduction and increased pacing thresholds, have also been widely documented to occur immediately after pulse delivery. The ability of these metrics to predict durable lesions remains to be determined.

When PFA lesions are assessed at the chronic time point (>4 weeks) in preclinical studies, they are characterized by organized and homogeneous fibrotic replacement of the myocardium. PFA lesions often demonstrate a far more uniform appearance than typical thermal lesions (Fig. 4.2D) and characteristically exhibit a sharp, transitionless border between the lesion and adjacent myocardium. PFA lesions can also demonstrate tissue shrinkage, which becomes noticeable at the chronic time point (Fig. 4.2D, and Fig. 4.3B). The arteries, veins, and nerves within the myocardial lesions are mostly spared, which is an important differentiating feature of PFA compared to thermal energies (Fig. 4.3C, D). In contrast to PFA, RF lesions are characterized by a more heterogeneous healing pattern with regions of necrotic cardiomyocytes (coagulative necrosis) with surrounding fibrosis (Fig. 4.3A). A singularly distinctive feature of PFA when compared to thermal modalities is its ability to avoid the "heat sink effect." This property is often described to be one of the reasons why mitral isthmus block during left atrial ablation is difficult to achieve. Given its nonthermal ablative mechanism, PFA can avoid this effect. Preclinical evidence supports the occurrence of this phenomenon and shows that despite only endocardial PFA delivery at the mitral isthmus, evidence of ablation of the roof of coronary sinus can be seen (Fig. 4.4).

EFFECTS AND SAFETY OF PFA ON SPECIFIC TISSUE

The effects and safety of PFA on myocardium and neighboring structures comparing with other thermal modalities (RF ablation [RFA] and cryoablation) are summarized in Table 4.1.

Pulmonary Venous Tissue

The incidence of PV stenosis with RFA or cryoballoon ablation has been reported to range between 13% and 18%.[29,30] Although most PV stenosis is mild in severity, severe stenosis continues to occur, and fear of this adverse event sometimes limits the ability to deliver sufficient energy to ensure durable lesions. van Driel et al. compared the risk of PV stenosis between RFA and PFA (unipolar and monophasic).[31] In their study, PFA was associated with 11% decrease in the PV diameter immediately after ablation. However, by 3-month follow-up, the PV diameter had returned to normal with a 19% increase in size after PFA. In comparison, RFA was associated with a decrease in PV diameter both immediately postablation (a decrease of 23%) and at 3-month follow-up (−7%). More recently, similar results were observed with modern biphasic, bipolar PFA.[32] These preclinical findings are further supported by the clinical experience reported by Kuroki et al.[33] Investigators analyzed data from four clinical trials using either PFA or RFA in patients with paroxysmal atrial fibrillation (PAF). A total of 299 PVs were analyzed retrospectively from 80 patients who had undergone either PFA (n = 37) or RFA (n = 43), and an overall PV narrowing/stenosis (defined as >30%) was reported in 0% versus 12.0% of the PVs in patients who underwent PFA and RFA respectively. These data suggest that PFA even applied within the PV does not lead to narrowing of veins as seen with thermal energies. These early clinical findings need to be confirmed in the larger ongoing clinical trials; and while this stenosis-sparing

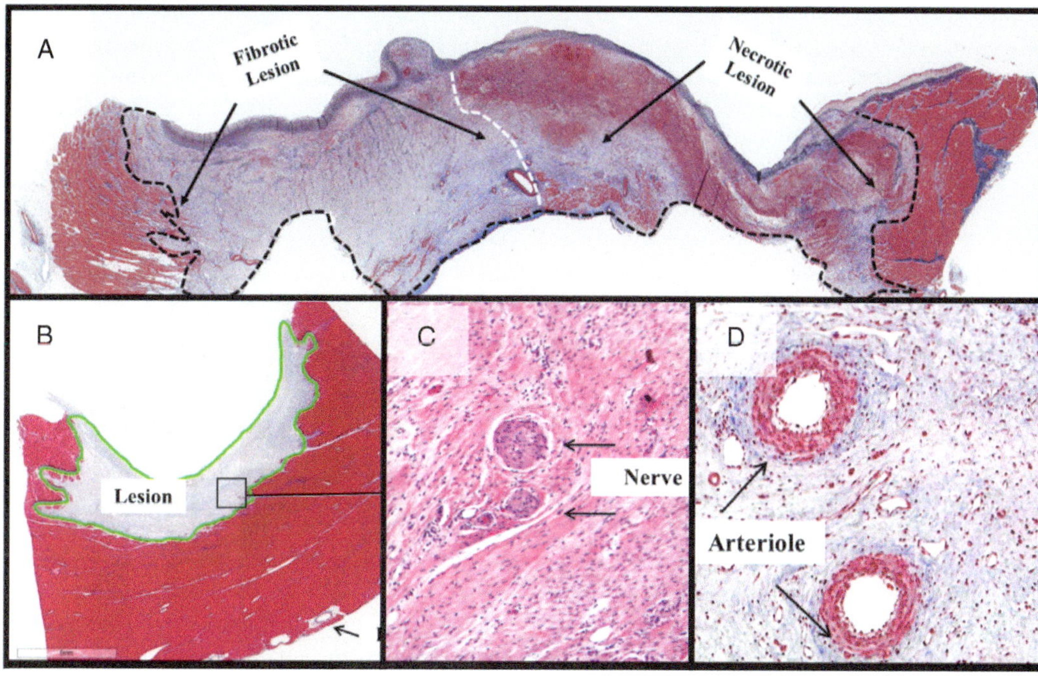

Fig. 4.3 Histology of pulsed-field ablation (PFA) lesions. (A) Section from left atrial roof demonstrating an area with homogeneous fibrosis on the left and a region with a necrotic lesion to the right, representing the histologic difference between PFA and radiofrequency ablation. (Adapted from Koruth JS, Kuroki K, Kawamura I, et al. Focal pulsed field ablation for pulmonary vein isolation and linear atrial lesions: a preclinical assessment of safety and durability. *Circ Arrhythm Electrophysiol.* 2020;13:e008716.) (B) Section demonstrating nontransmural lesions in the LV characterized by organized and homogeneous fibrotic replacement of the myocardium. (C) Two well preserved and viable nerve fascicles seen within fibrous tissue of PFA lesion. (D) Thickening of arteriolar walls (*black arrows*) with well-preserved endothelial lining and spared lumen as seen within the core of an ablation lesion (B, C, and D adapted from Koruth JS, Kuroki K, Iwasawa J, et al. Endocardial ventricular pulsed field ablation: a proof-of-concept preclinical evaluation. *Europace.* 2020;22:434–439.)

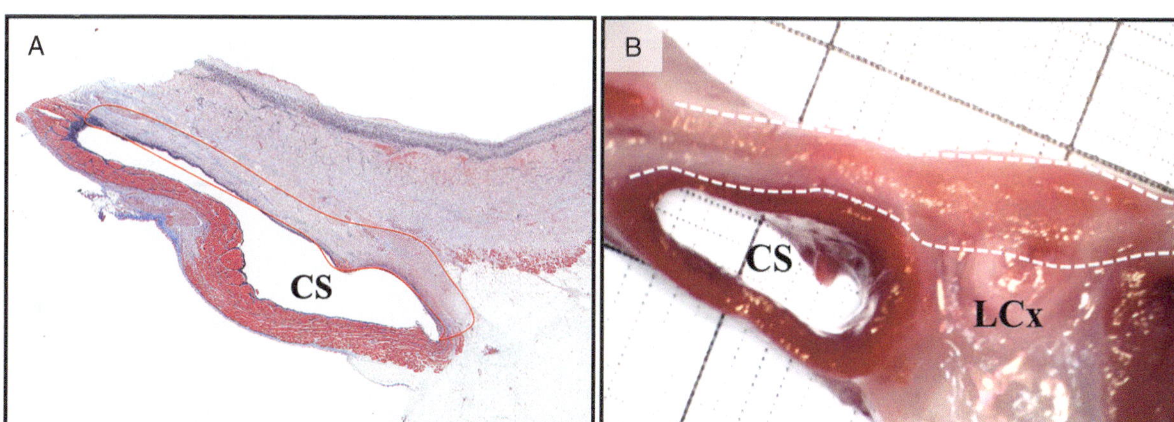

Fig. 4.4 Pulsed-field ablation (PFA) lesion on mitral isthmus. (A) Histology shows PFA lesions uniformly extended to roof of the coronary sinus (CS) despite only endocardial PFA delivery at the mitral isthmus. The CS musculature was replaced with homogeneous fibrosis, without distorting/occluding the lumen. The *red outlined circle* denotes the roof of the CS. (Adapted from Koruth JS, Kuroki K, Kawamura I, et al. Focal pulsed field ablation for pulmonary vein isolation and linear atrial lesions: a preclinical assessment of safety and durability. *Circ Arrhythm Electrophysiol.* 2020;13:e008716.) (B) Gross appearance of a mitral isthmus RF lesion with transmural ablation (*pale pink*, ablated) of the left atrium but with sparing of the roof of the coronary sinus (*bright red*, unablated). *LCx*, left circumflex coronary artery.

TABLE 4.1 Comparison of Efficacy and Safety Among Each Ablation Modality for Atrial Fibrillation

	PFA	RFA	Cryoablation
Procedure time for PVI	Significantly shortened	Can be short with HPSD	Can be short with TTI approach
PV durability	++	++	++
Esophageal safety	+++	+	++
Risk of PV stenosis	Very low	Low	Low
Risk of phrenic nerve palsy	Very low	Low	Occasional
Risk of cerebral embolism	Low	Low	Low
Risk of pericardial effusion	Low	Low	Low
Risk of coronary spasm	+++	+	Lower than RFA

HPSD, high-power short-duration; *PFA*, pulsed-field ablation; *PV*, pulmonary vein; *PVI*, pulmonary vein isolation; *RFA*, radiofrequency ablation; *TTI*, time to isolation.

effect appears to be a class effect across the PFA spectrum, a dedicated safety evaluation will be mandatory for different PFA technologies/doses.

Esophagus

Atrioesophageal fistula is a serious, life-threatening complication that can occur rarely with thermal ablation of the posterior left atrial wall.[34] One of the most attractive features of PFA is the early preclinical and clinical evidence indicating that PFA spares the esophagus despite creating durable left atrial lesions. We investigated the effect of PFA and RFA on esophagus in a porcine model in which we deflected the lower esophagus toward the inferior vena cava (IVC) to create a worst-case scenario of left atrial–esophageal proximity.[35] We delivered PFA from within the IVC at the sites of close esophageal contact to mimic delivery against the thin-walled left atrial posterior wall. Upon follow-up necropsy 1 month later, none of the animals in the PFA group demonstrated esophageal lesions on histopathologic exam. In contrast, injury was evident in all animals in the RFA group (Fig. 4.5). These findings confirm the findings of esophageal sparing that was demonstrated in a seminal, open-surgical preclinical assessment where PF was delivered directly atop the esophagus.[36] In that report, acute mucosal vesicle formation and minor chronic fibrotic changes in the muscularis layer were described, indicating that minor changes can occur with a worst case assessment of monophasic-monopolar delivery. In vitro reports using monolayers of cardiomyocytes, cortical neurons, and esophageal smooth muscles also demonstrated relative sparing of the esophagus, although such an assessment does not represent the anatomical complexities of the posterior left atrial–esophagus junction in humans.[10] While these findings are promising in that we may finally eradicate the dreaded risk of fistula, these preclinical insights are limited in terms of being technology and model specific. In fact, investigators have demonstrated that direct PF applications to the esophagus can generate transmural lesions, but this has not been shown with clinical PFA catheters.[37] Evidence of esophagus sparing has been also reported by using late gadolinium enhancement (LGE) MR imaging during the early clinical experience.[38] Cochet et al. described a cohort of 41 PAF patients undergoing PVI with PFA (n = 18) or thermal methods (n = 23, 16 RFA, 7 cryoballoon) where LGE MRI was performed before, acutely (<3 hours), and 3 months postablation. Acutely, thermal methods induced high rates of esophageal lesions (43%), whereas no lesions were observed with PFA, despite similar rates of direct contact between the esophagus and the ablation sites. Additional endoscopic evaluations performed after clinical case series have also demonstrated esophageal sparing and thus far the safety data are promising. However, data from larger trials are awaited to conclusively establish clinical safety.

Phrenic Nerve

Diaphragmatic paralysis due to phrenic nerve injury is another well-known complication of thermal energy ablation.[39,40] The effects of PF on the phrenic nerve has been explored by several investigators. Investigators demonstrated in swine that despite delivering 200 J PF (monophasic waveforms) within the SVC, the phrenic nerve could be reliably captured in 17 of 19 swine and in all 19 after a short waiting period.[41] We also demonstrated in a preclinical series that the phrenic nerve was spared despite ablation within the SVC with more modern PFA technologies.[42] More recently, investigators demonstrated a dose-dependent response for phrenic nerve function, highlighting the concept of reversible stunning that can occur. They demonstrated a correlation between the proximity of the catheter and phrenic nerve outcomes.[43] Even though the phrenic nerve was reversibly stunned postprocedure, gross and histopathologic evaluation yielded no injury in follow-up of their preclinical evaluation. This sparing of the phrenic nerve, despite closest delivery of PFA, is thought to occur due to the higher threshold for injury of the nerve compared to myocardial cells[10] and the poorly conductive myelin sheath that protects the nerve from the electrical field.[44,45] A recent largest multicenter survey of clinical PFA cases from Europe revealed no instances of phrenic nerve paralysis of the 1758 patients enrolled, although transient phrenic nerve injury was reported in 8 patients (0.46%).[46]

Microbubble Formation

Although symptomatic cerebral embolism after catheter ablation of AF is rare, the rate of asymptomatic cerebral embolism

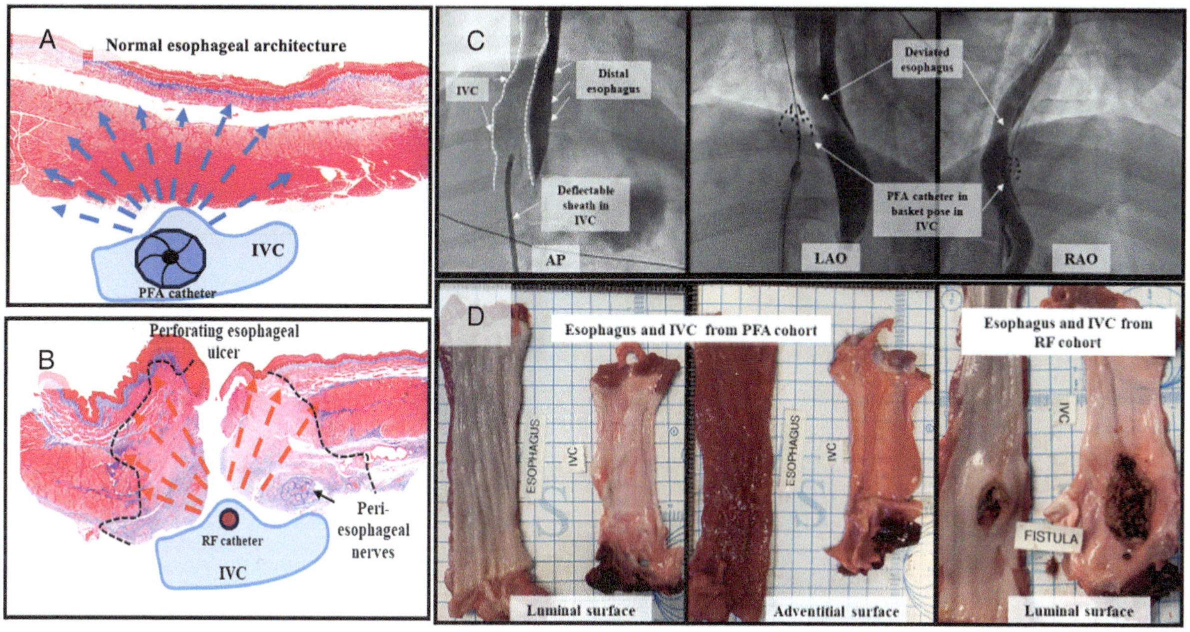

Fig. 4.5 Pulsed-field ablation (PFA) versus radiofrequency (RF) ablation on esophagus. (A) Shown are all four layers of the esophageal wall after PFA: tunica mucosa, tunica submucosa, tunica muscularis, and the outermost layer, tunica adventitia. These are all normal along the entire circumference of the esophagus. In particular, there is no evidence of ablation lesions in the outer layers of the tunica muscularis. (B) This section from RFA cohort depicts a perforating ulcer with disruption of the wall. (C) Fluoroscopic view of the esophageal injury model from PFA cohort. Contrast angiography was performed using a long deflectable sheath placed in the inferior vena cava (*IVC; outlined*). In the anteroposterior (AP) view, the IVC is seen rightward of the contrast-filled esophagus. Left and right anterior oblique (LAO and RAO) projections demonstrate the PFA catheter in basket pose forcefully pushed against the deviated esophagus. (D) Representative images demonstrating the normal luminal and adventitial surface of the esophagus after PFA on the left. Conversely, from the RF ablation cohort, a perforating ulcer is seen on the luminal aspect of the esophagus that was separated from a larger necrotic area opening into the inferior vena cava (*IVC*; esophagus-IVC fistula). (Adapted from Koruth JS, Kuroki K, Kawamura I, et al. Pulsed field ablation versus radiofrequency ablation: esophageal injury in a novel porcine model. *Circ Arrhythm Electrophysiol*. 2020;13:e008303.)

detected by MRI can be substantial.[47] A recent study evaluating the risk of cerebral embolism (DWI-FLAIR mismatch) after thermal energies used for PVI revealed an incidence of 39% (RFA 30%, cryoballoon 24%, hot balloon 34%, and laser balloon 39%).[48] PF delivered in the blood pool can generate microbubbles due to either hydrolysis or displacement of nitrogen gas. A preclinical report looked at the total volume and maximal diameter of bubbles produced from an investigational PFA system and compared this with RFA. Median bubble diameter was noted to be smaller for PFA than RFA (18 versus 30 μm, respectively).[49] Furthermore, PFA microbubbles were noted to be visible only during the few seconds of PF delivery, whereas RF bubbles persisted up to a minute after delivery. Microbubble formation can vary among PF technologies, with some resulting in easily visualized bubbles on intracardiac echocardiography and some technologies that create minimal bubble formation. The rate of cerebral embolism using PFA has not been well elucidated, but recent reports have described few incidents of cerebral infarction detected by MRI. These findings may represent embolic risks of left atrial ablation, and the data do not point to embolic risk from the microbubble formation itself.[50,51]

Ventricular Arrhythmias

The majority of recent PFA studies for atrial ablation have used ungated PF delivery given the arrhythmic safety demonstrated thus far (i.e., no VA have been reported clinically). Indeed, the electrical consequences of these pulses in the atrium (i.e., myocardial activation) have not been considered to be clinically relevant. However, PFA-related myocardial activation in the ventricle can be relevant and therefore likely more discernible and consequential. VAs have been reported during ventricular PFA in preclinical studies.[52] The mechanism of VA induction is likely related to rapid and repeated myocardial activation or activation during the vulnerable period, which is likely a class effect across PFA technologies. Further work is needed to better understand this interaction. It is unknown whether this risk of VA is particular to the animal models used (i.e., pigs are known to easily fibrillate during ventricular RFA) or if this will be a clinical concern in patients.[53] One solution for avoiding the risk of VA induction is to use QRS gating during PFA delivery, which, based on preclinical assessment, demonstrates reduced risk of VAs. Further dedicated evaluation of this phenomenon is needed, especially given the various technologies of specific pulse designs.

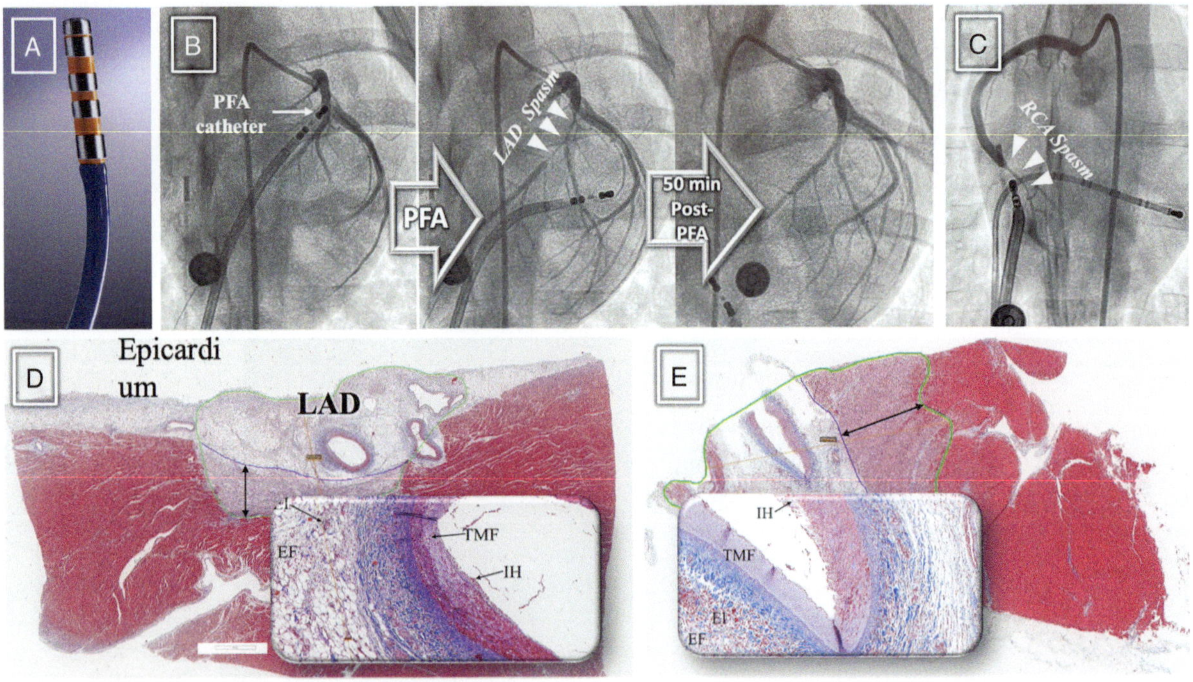

Fig. 4.6 Coronary artery spasms after pulsed-field ablation (PFA). (A) The focal PFA catheter. (B) Angiography before, spasm after, and resolution at 50 minutes. (C) Right coronary artery (RCA) spasm following endocardial PFA. (D) Histology at the site of the spasm reveals a preserved lumen and a shallow myocardial lesion (*double black arrow*). *Inset:* Left anterior descending artery (LAD) demonstrating tunica media fibrosis (TMF), intimal hyperplasia (IH), epicardial lymphocytic inflammation (EI), and epicardial fibrosis (EF). (E) Histology through the lateral right atrium: RCA is seen with preserved lumen, adjacent to the myocardial lesion. *Inset:* RCA demonstrates TMF, IH, EI, and EF. (Adapted from Koruth JS, Kawamura I, Buck E, et al. Coronary arterial spasm and pulsed field ablation: preclinical insights. *JACC Clin Electrophysiol.* In press.)

Coronary Spasm

Prior seminal preclinical reports using monophasic waveforms have shown the occurrence of transient coronary spasm in the setting of epicardial PFA.[54,55] More recently, this observation was reported to occur after endocardial delivery using a contemporary biphasic PFA waveform both in a patient and in preclinical reports with histologic changes of minimal intimal hyperplasia and medial fibrosis but with minimal to no loss of the lumen (Fig. 4.6).[56,57] The mechanism of spasm remains unknown; one potential mechanism could be activation of smooth muscle cells from the excitatory nature of PF and/or activation of autonomic input. Our observation of esophageal contraction during left atrial ablation,[58] as well as ventricular contraction during ventricular PFA,[52] gives the excitatory mechanism some support. Catheter design, contact force, pulse waveform, proximity, effect of arterial disease, susceptibility to spasm, and autonomic innervation/activation are all potential variables that may influence the risk of spasm. Further studies investigating safe "distance and dose" parameters as well as the effects of nitroglycerin to prevent or treat coronary spasm will be needed in addition to chronic histopathologic assessment of arteries that recover from coronary spasm. The relatively uncommon occurrence during atrial ablation reported thus far is reassuring, but this issue needs to be carefully evaluated and monitored as the clinical experience with PFA continues to grow.

Effects on the Conduction System

van Zyl et al. investigated the effect of PFA on the conduction system in a preclinical report and noted the occurrence of complete AV block, followed by recovery over time.[59] Infrahisian location of AV block was noted in some animals in that report, with persistence of bundle-branch block at follow-up in some instances. The investigators also indicated that the duration/degree of AV block appeared to be site and dose dependent, which is consistent with expected behavior of any ablative energy. The exact pathologic changes occurring with different doses within the conduction systems have not been described and need to be carefully explored. However, the data raise the provocative possibility that PFA, at certain doses, may be used to ablate myocardium while sparing the conduction system. Recent reports have also suggested this possibility.[60,61] A more detailed evaluation of this issue remains to be performed in order to provide definitive answers. This is especially important as selective ablation of the Purkinje fibers with PFA is being proposed.

ATRIAL PULSED-FIELD ABLATION

PFA can successfully create atrial lesions. This finding has been consistently demonstrated in several preclinical experiments with histologic evidence of consistent transmurality and contiguity (Fig. 4.2A and Fig. 4.3A).[42,62–64] Preclinical reports have also demonstrated that PFA can be used to durably isolate thoracic veins without risk of venous stenosis and phrenic nerve palsy.[42] These findings have led to the successful evaluation of PFA in the clinical setting with promising durability and safety thus far.

The first-in-human clinical trials (IMPULSE and PEFCAT) using a custom catheter were undertaken to assess the safety and efficacy of PFA in patients with PAF (see Chapter 17). They evaluated an over-the-wire 12-F catheter (Farawave, Farapulse, Inc., Menlo Park, CA) and a custom generator that delivers biphasic waveforms in a bipolar fashion (Farastar, Farapulse, Inc.).[26] The catheter consists of five splines, with four electrodes per spline and one electrode available for intracardiac electrogram recording, that can be deployed in either flower or basket configurations. The most recent updated results from this experience described findings from 121 patients (combined three trials: IMPULSE, PEFCAT, and PEFCAT II) and revealed that durable PVI (mandatory remapping was performed at 90 days) was achieved in 84.8% of PVs (64.5% of patients) and 96.0% of PVs (84.1% of patients), respectively, treated with the optimized biphasic energy PFA waveform.[65] In a subset of patients treated with the optimized PFA waveform freedom from AF and AFL or AT were 84.6% ± 6.0% and 84.5% ± 5.4% at 12 months, respectively. Additionally, a single-arm study of 25 patients with persistent AF (per AF) (PersAFOne: Pulsed Fields for Persistent Atrial Fibrillation) was performed to evaluate PFA using the above system for both PVI and posterior wall isolation.[66] In this report, a focal PFA catheter was also used for cavotricuspid isthmus (CTI) ablation and achieved block in 13 of 13 patients with a median time of 9 minutes. Invasive remapping at 3 months demonstrated durable isolation in 96% of PVs and 100% of the ablated posterior left atrial wall.

Several other technologies have since reported on their first-in-human evaluations. One such system uses a lattice-tip catheter (Sphere 9; Affera, Inc., Newton, MA) that can deliver both PF and RF using custom generators (HexaGen and HexaPulse, Affera, Inc.).[50] This 7.5F bidirectionally deflectable catheter has an expandable 9-mm-diameter lattice tip containing nine mini-electrodes/temperature sensors and location sensors allowing for three-dimensional localization within a custom mapping system. PFA is delivered in a monopolar fashion from the entire lattice tip (to a grounding electrode) using a proprietary biphasic waveform, and this technology can create focal lesions, allowing for lesion set flexibility. An initial report enrolled a total of 76 patients (55 with PAF and 21 with persistent AF) who underwent either RFA/PFA (n = 40) or PFA/PFA (n = 36). Regardless of the energy, electrical PVI was achieved in all 152 of 152 (100%) ipsilateral PV pairs with the lattice catheter alone. In addition, 13 of 14 mitral isthmus, 34 of 34 roof, and 44 of 44 CTI bidirectional block across the lines were successfully created. Similarly, another recent first-in-human experience (PULSED AF: Pulsed Field Ablation to Irreversibly Electroporate Tissue and Treat AF) evaluated the feasibility and efficacy of PVI using a circular multielectrode array catheter (PulseSelect; Medtronic, Inc, Minneapolis, MN).[67] Investigators reported the outcomes of the first 38 patients who underwent PVI for symptomatic PAF or persistent AF. Acute electrical isolation was achieved in 100% of pulmonary veins (n = 152). Several other PFA systems are currently undergoing clinical trials. While some of these catheters are by design created for pulmonary vein isolation, several other systems are capable of focal ablation and, thus, can in theory be used for several non–atrial fibrillation ablation procedures as well.

VENTRICULAR PULSED-FIELD ABLATION

Although well studied in both preclinical and clinical studies as a tool for atrial ablation, PFA's role in ventricular ablation is yet to be determined. The majority of the existing data describing the effects of PFA on ventricular myocardium are derived from preclinical reports that used a monophasic pulse delivered by an external defibrillator.[54,55,68–70] The authors of these landmark reports applied circular multielectrode or linear suction devices to the epicardial surface of swine ventricles and demonstrated that large PFA lesions can be created safely. These reports have cumulatively established that: (1) deep and wide ventricular lesions can be created, (2) this can be achieved with sparing of epicardial coronary arteries, and (3) there is a dose-dependent effect (i.e., lesion dimensions increase with the amount of energy delivered). However, energy delivery in these reports required either open surgical access or subxiphoid pericardial access. In theory, catheters designed to deliver focal PFA lesions have the potential to become an attractive alternative to currently available technologies for ventricular ablation, especially if they can deliver deep lesions consistently, rapidly, and safely. To address this issue, we performed preclinical evaluation of a focal PFA endocardial catheter in swine ventricles.[60] In this study, a prototype catheter delivered microsecond, bipolar- biphasic pulses to successfully create large (average depth of 6.5 ± 1.7 mm with maximum 9.4 mm) and homogeneous lesions in the ventricles with evidence of sparing of nerves and vessels on histology (Fig. 4.2D and Fig. 4.3B). It is important to note that with focal ablation, one is able to observe evidence of echocardiographic changes at the site of application over the course of the first 10 minutes that may reflect local tissue changes due to edema and other acute changes (Fig. 4.7). Other investigators as well as we have described the ability to create lesions with depths of up to 8.8 ± 0.7 mm using the lattice-tip catheter and have demonstrated that repeated applications promote lesion depth.[13] To further explore the effect of scar on PF lesion penetration, we created an "endocardium-only-homogeneous" scar model by using the large footprint of the lattice-tip catheter to create islands of PFA-induced scar. Four weeks later, PFA lesions were applied at multiple locations along the scar borders. This preclinical study demonstrated that acute PFA lesions extended beyond/deep to the scar in all examined sections (100%) with endocardial scar of a maximum depth of 4.2 mm. We also demonstrated the feasibility of epicardial PFA and demonstrated that these lesions were comparable to endocardial PFA lesions. This PFA-based scar assessment has obvious limitations: (1) ischemic and nonischemic cardiomyopathies often have patchy, heterogeneous scar that is often significantly thicker; and (2) clinical scars are, of course, more chronic in duration and may have other components such as calcification or intramural adipose tissue. However, this model

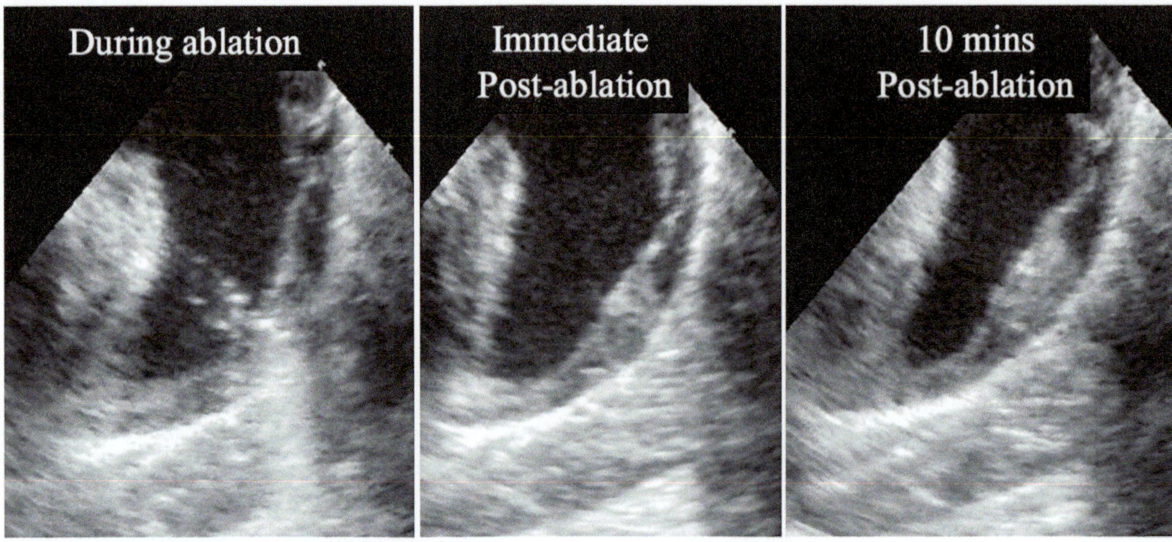

Fig. 4.7 PFA lesions on intracardiac echocardiography. The echocardiographic changes at application sites are not evident immediately after focal PFA using a prototype catheter, but regions of focal myocardial thickening with altered echogenicity at application sites can be observed over the course of the first 10 minutes.

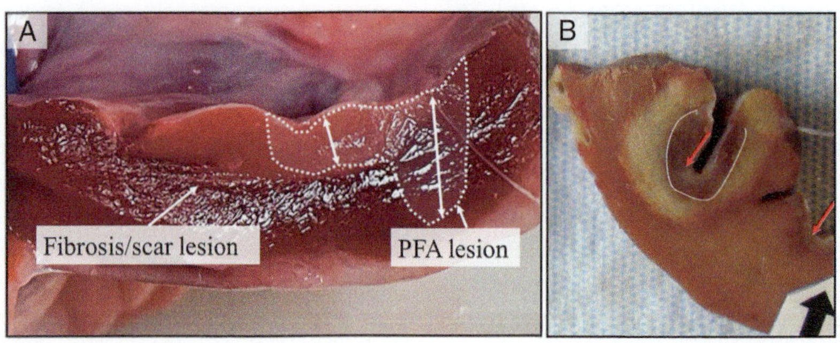

Fig. 4.8 Effect of pulsed-field ablation (PFA) on homogeneous chronic scar. (A) Concept illustration: Pale-pink region represents the outline of a chronic endocardial scar. Hypothesis: If PFA depth were to be affected by the presence of scar (*pale pink region*), then the acute lesion depth under endocardial scar would be diminished (left side, *white bidirectional arrow*) compared to what is achieved in nearby healthy adjacent myocardium (right side, *white bidirectional arrow*). The areas outlined by *white dotted lines* denotes presumptive PFA lesion if the chronic scar impede electrical field. (B) Gross specimen demonstrating a nontransmural acute lesion placed on a region of chronic scar in the left ventricle. The *white line* identifies the outer boundary of the chronic endocardial scar, which appears dark brown/red. Beyond this region is a circumscribed pale region that identified the acute PFA lesion that was placed over the chronic scar but is able to penetrate it. One can also appreciate that acute PFA (*pale area*) penetrates the chronic scar to the same depth, as is seen at the periphery of the chronic lesion. (A and B adapted from Kawamura I, Reddy VY, Wang BJ, et al. Pulsed field ablation of the porcine ventricle using a focal lattice-tip catheter. *Circ Arrhythm Electrophysiol.* 2022;15:e011120.)

allowed for a very controlled and easy-to-identify investigation of the impact of endocardial scarring on the penetrative capability of PFA in the setting of scar. By examining PFA applications placed on scar boundary regions, we were able to compare the PFA lesion extent directly beneath the endocardial scar to the healthy myocardial region (without scar) located at the boundary (Fig. 4.8). More recently, we demonstrated the ability of PF penetration of scar from myocardial infarction as well as from iatrogenic RF scar. This study showed PFA successfully penetrated scar without significant difference in lesion depth between lesions at the infarct border (5.9 ± 1.0 mm, $n = 41$) and healthy myocardium (5.7 ± 1.3 mm, $n = 26$). PFA penetration of both infarct and iatrogenic RF scar was observed in all examined sections (Fig. 4.9). These findings also confirm the finding of an important study that described the efficacy of PFA on infarcted and healthy myocardium.[71] In their study, the investigators described: (1) endocardial delivery of focal PFA in infarcted LV myocardium to be feasible, safe, and rapid, achieving depths from 4 to 8 mm; (2) lesions in infarcted myocardium were not significantly different in comparison to healthy myocardium; (3) a second multielectrode focal basket PFA catheter led to similar lesion depths, but with wider lengths compared with the linear focal catheter; and (4) in infarcted tissue, histologic lesion depths were greater with PFA compared with standard RFA (an important comparison). These findings have significant clinical relevance, since the inability to create deep lesions, especially in

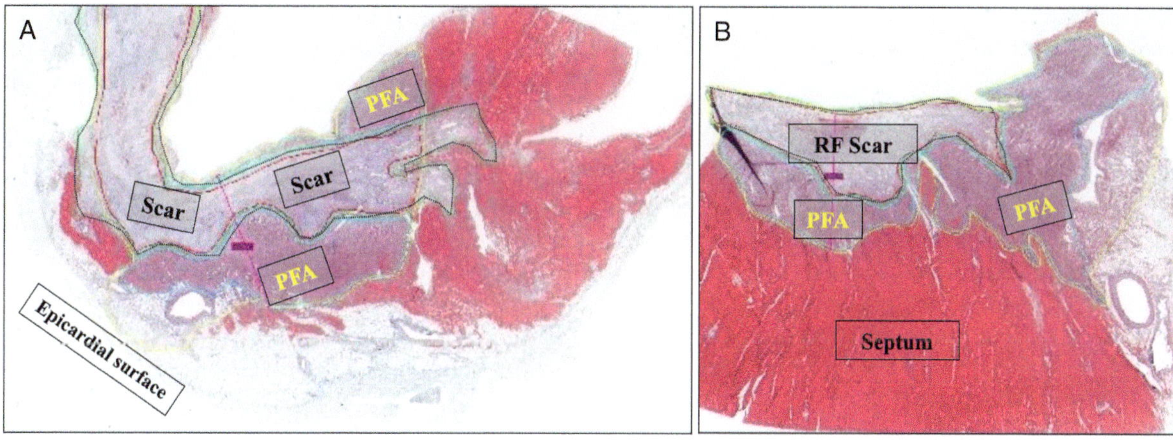

Fig. 4.9 Histology of pulsed-field ablation (PFA) lesions on ischemic and radiofrequency-induced chronic scar. Masson trichrome staining: chronic fibrotic scar is stained light blue, whereas the acute lesion is stained light purple with healthy myocardium staining red. (A) PFA lesion (enclosed in *yellow*) is demonstrated beyond chronic myocardial infarction scar (*black dotted line*). One can see subendocardial spared myocardium from the time of infarction that has been ablated as well. (B) PFA lesion (*yellow dotted line*) placed at the border of prior RF scar with demonstration of lesion below the RF scar (*black dotted line*). (Adapted from Kawamura I, Reddy V, Santos-Gallego CG, et al. Electrophysiology, pathology, and imaging of pulsed field ablation of scarred and healthy ventricles in swine. *Circ Arrhythm Electrophysiol.* 2022;15:e011120.)

the setting of scarred myocardium, has long been considered a limitation of current RF catheters. Although clinical data are lacking, PFA has certain characteristics that make it an attractive alternative/adjunct method for ablating VAs, and further work is needed to assess how effective this energy source will be. One must keep in mind that ventricular activation leading to arrhythmias, termination of VT from local capture, and local stunning related elimination of arrhythmias are potential challenges that may be experienced in the clinical setting and will need to be carefully explored.

"REVERSIBLE" ELECTROPORATION

Membrane pores that are created via pulsed fields can be either permanent, if the electric field is high enough, or temporary if the field is sublethal. In the latter case, pores have lifetimes ranging from milliseconds to minutes. In such instances, the pores can reseal once the electrical field is removed. Depending on pulse delivery settings, permeability of cells can be purposefully designed to be mostly or completely reversible (i.e., the cell will survive despite transient dysfunction because cell membrane integrity and electrical homeostasis remain preserved). Indeed, sublethal electric fields have long been used as a tool in cell biology, mostly as a technique to introduce biological material into cells.[6–8] In the myocardium, the same effect can be achieved, in theory, by using a tailored pulse that allows for reversible but not ablative effects (Fig. 4.10). This can be used as a diagnostic tool that temporarily disables electrical properties and then observing its effect on arrhythmia genesis and/or maintenance. Although the mechanism of stunning is not well defined, it likely results from a loss of cellular membrane selective permeability, altering transmembrane gradients that can lead to acute hyperpolarization of the membrane followed by a depression of excitability, reduction of amplitude of action potentials, and of the rate of rise of their upstroke (dV/dt).[72] The effect of such

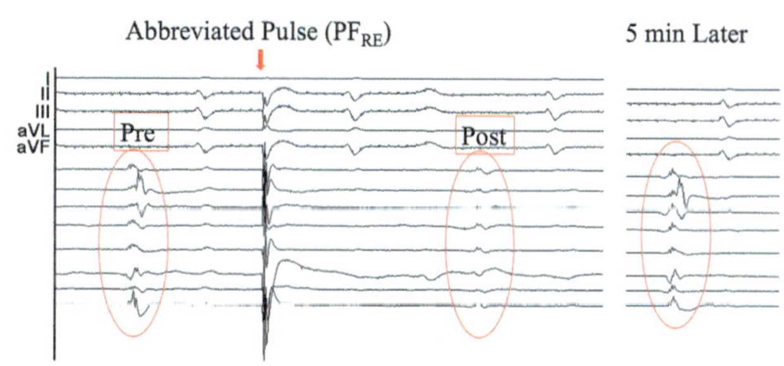

Fig. 4.10 Reversible pulsed-field ablation. Abbreviated pulsed electrical fields (PF_{RE}) (*red arrow*) resulting in diminished electrogram amplitude, which then recovers gradually with time. (Adapted from Koruth J, Kawamura I, Dukkipati S, et al. Dose-dependent transient AV nodal conduction block using reversible electroporation [Abstr]. *Heart Rhythm.* 2021;18:S4.)

abbreviated pulsed electrical fields (PF_{RE}) have been investigated in animal models. One such evaluation was performed by delivering PF_{RE} using a lattice-tip catheter to myocardial tissue in swine.[27] In this study, PF_{RE} was applied to left and right atrial sites in swine as well as to AV nodal tissue. In swine, post-PF_{RE} electrogram amplitudes demonstrated a mean reduction of 84% followed by recovery of up to 78% at 5 minutes. PF_{RE} over the AV node resulted in PR prolongation and complete AV block. There was complete recovery of the PR interval to baseline within seconds for the majority of applications. Other reports by van Zyl et al. have described transient acute damage to the Purkinje fibers evidenced by diminished Purkinje potentials but have noted preservation when examined chronically.[61] Further investigation is clearly needed to identify if these reversible effects come at a cost of some degree of cell death. Potential future applications include using these pulses to identify critical isthmuses in atrial flutters by slowing or terminating the tachycardia (inadvertent capture needs to be addressed if pulses are not synchronized), predicting the effect of ablation for accessory pathways and the impact of ablation at a putative driver site in persistent AF, etc.

SUMMARY

Pulsed fields and their effects on myocardium and neighboring structures are an evolving field that holds a lot of promise, especially in terms of efficacy and safety. While their role in PVI and posterior left atrial ablation progressively strengthens, its applicability elsewhere will require time and careful study. This chapter is by no means exhaustive, and we refer the readers to other summaries from colleagues who continue to expand this field with their investigations in the nearest future. As this exciting energy source evolves, we must demand and explore specific efficacy and safety concerns while keeping in mind that traditional energy sources that have matured over decades remain very useful and should not be simply forgotten.

REFERENCES

Please refer to the e-book for a complete list of references.

5

Contemporary Irrigated Radiofrequency Catheter Ablation

Robert D'Angelo, Arash Aryana, Andre d'Avila

KEY POINTS

- Irrigated ablation cools the tip of the ablation catheter to prevent excessive heating at the catheter–tissue interface, increasing lesion size through the delivery of increased power.
- Temperature monitoring is less reliable for cooled-tip radiofrequency (RF) ablation, and other parameters such as impedance, power, and contact force during RF ablation are used to guide ablation.
- Novel catheters, such as the QDOT Micro and Affera Sphere-9, integrate thermocouples into the catheter tip to allow for delivery of very high power (up to 90 W) with short lesion duration to reduce ablation time and minimize collateral tissue heating.
- High-power short-duration has supplanted low-power long-duration for the treatment of atrial fibrillation, with studies showing high procedural success rates, shorter procedures, and low complication rates.
- In ventricular tachycardia with intramyocardial origin, bipolar irrigated RF ablation or use of irrigate with lower ionic concentration (such as half-normal saline) can create larger and deeper lesions.
- Irrigated RF ablation from the coronary sinus can be used successfully to ablate accessory pathways and premature ventricular contractions/ventricular tachycardia in the left ventricular summit region.

INTRODUCTION

Radiofrequency (RF) ablation has become the standard energy source for the treatment of cardiac arrhythmias, including supraventricular tachycardia (SVT), atrial fibrillation (AF), and ventricular tachycardias (VTs).[1-5] RF was traditionally delivered using a nonirrigated 7F, 4-mm-tip electrode catheter, but energy delivery and resultant lesion size were limited by blood coagulum formation at the catheter–tissue interface.[6] Temperature control was later introduced to reduce excessive heating at the catheter-tissue interface and resultant coagulum formation, although lesion depth was limited to arrhythmogenic tissue within several millimeters of the ablation site.[7,8]

Cooling the ablation catheter helps prevent coagulum formation, permitting the delivery of higher power to create larger and deeper lesions.[6,9] Recently, ablation with high power (>50 W) short duration (HPSD) has shown promise in creating durable, transmural lesions for AF ablation. This chapter discusses the contemporary use of irrigated RF ablation for ablation of cardiac arrhythmias.

BIOPHYSICS OF IRRIGATED RADIOFREQUENCY ABLATION

For a given electrode size and tissue contact area, lesion size is a function of energy delivered to the tissue, with the relationship between power and duration as follows:

$$\text{Energy (Joules)} = \text{power (Watts)} \times \text{time (seconds)}$$

Energy is then converted to heat according to the specific heat capacity for myocardium and mass of the heated tissue according to the following formula[10,11]:

$$\Delta\,\text{Temperature} = \frac{\text{Energy}\,(J)}{\text{mass}\,(g) * \text{heat capacity}\,(J\,g^{-1}K^{-1})}$$

During application of RF energy, heating damages the myocardium due to a combination of resistive and conductive heating. There is a shell of resistive heating within a few millimeters of the catheter tip (Fig. 5.1), while thermal injury more than several millimeters away is due to conductive heating.[12,13] Resistive heating results when RF energy encounters an impedance at the catheter–tissue interface and within adjacent myocardium. The heating is rapid and associated with the direct application of RF energy. Conversely, conductive heating results from passive heat transferred from the core ablation lesion. If ablation is stopped before thermal equilibrium is reached (which can take up to 2 minutes), conductive heating continues.[10-12]

At higher power, lesion duration is often limited by impedance rise at the tissue–electrode interface as the tissue temperature reaches 100°C due to tissue desiccation and coagulum formulation. These impedance rises limit the duration of RF current delivery and total amount of energy delivered to the tissue, which limits lesion size. Please refer to Chapter 1 for details.

Temperature-controlled RF delivery minimizes impedance rise and coagulum formation but limits ability to deliver large

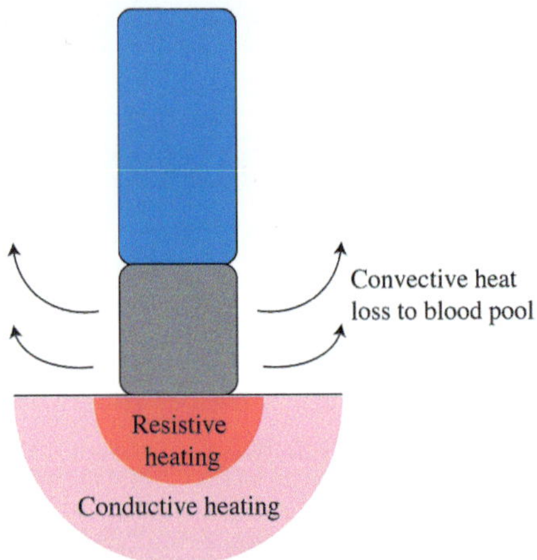

Fig. 5.1 Schematic drawing of radiofrequency catheter ablation on the endocardium demonstrating zones of resistive and conductive heating with convective heating loss into the blood pool and coronary arteries. Superficial tissue near the catheter is ablated by resistive heating, and deeper myocardium is heated by conductive heating.

lesions.[14–17] During temperature-controlled RF ablation, the tip temperature, tissue temperature, and lesion size are affected by electrode–tissue contact and cooling effects from blood flow. Additionally, lesion size is proportional to contact force. With improved contact, there is less cooling from the surrounding blood pool and the target temperature can be reached with lower power, resulting in relatively smaller lesions. With increased convective cooling from the blood pool, higher power settings are required to reach the target temperature, which can result in larger lesion size.

Cooling the electrode tip helps prevent impedance rises that limit power delivery, allowing for the creating of large lesions. Initially, larger ablation electrodes (8F, 8–10 mm in length) were used.[12,18,19] A larger electrode–tissue contact area leads to a greater volume of direct resistive heating and convective cooling of the electrode from ambient blood flow. This allows longer-duration lesions at a higher power, increasing lesion width and depth. However, a larger electrode introduces variability in tissue contact, reduces electrode temperature feedback, and may increase risk of coagulum formation.[12,13,15,20] These limitations led to the development of irrigated RF catheters.

Irrigated RF catheters use cool saline to decrease the temperature of the catheter tip, permitting creation of larger lesions (Fig. 5.2). Cool saline bathes the ablation electrode and dissipates heat generated during application of RF energy. Decreasing the electrode–myocardial interface temperature allows greater energy delivery prior to impedance rise or steam pop formation.[14,21,22] Additionally, irrigated catheters do not require convective cooling from the bloodstream, so RF power can be delivered at sites of low blood flow, such as the ventricular trabecular crevasse.[6]

There is still resistive heating at the electrode–myocardial interface during irrigated RF ablation, but the area of maximum temperature is located within the myocardium as opposed to at the electrode–myocardial interface. Nakagawa et al. demonstrated that the maximum temperature generated by irrigated RF application is several millimeters aways from the electrode–myocardial interface.[12,23] Irrigation does not increase the size of the lesion, but rather facilitates the delivery of increased power to the tissue without impedance rise or steam pop generation. This allows creation of a larger ablation lesion through delivery of increased power over a longer duration, thereby increasing total energy delivery to the tissue.

As the catheter tip is actively cooled, the temperature at the tip–tissue interface during irrigated ablation is often not reliable for determining the duration of RF application. The maximum temperature may be intramyocardial and surrounded by cooler areas of tissue. This can lead to intramyocardial steam and crater formation, possibly associated with dissection, perforation, and thrombus formation.[24] With the recent development of irrigated catheters with circumferential thermocouples, it is possible to use temperature control for guidance of irrigated RF ablation. In a study comparing temperature control versus power control using high power, temperature control was more effective in limiting steam pops, while maximizing lesion size.[25] Other irrigated catheter designs that have yet not been used commercially also use temperature control to reduce risk of tissue overheating.[26] These catheter designs incorporate thermocouple systems in the tip of the catheter that are robust to changes in catheter orientation. Small changes in tip temperature can then be extrapolated to tissue temperature to allow temperature-controlled irrigation RF ablation, limiting catheter tip temperature to 65°C.[27]

DESIGN OF IRRIGATED- AND COOL-TIP RADIOFREQUENCY CATHETERS

Cooling of the catheter tip during RF ablation is achieved by circulating saline through or around the tip of the ablation catheter while delivering RF current. Two different types of irrigation have been used to cool the catheter tip: closed-loop irrigation and open-irrigation (Fig. 5.3). With the closed-loop system, saline is circulated continuously within the electrode tip to cool the electrode. An open-irrigation catheter uses an internal thermocouple and multiple irrigation holes located around the electrode to cool the ablation catheter internally and externally as the catheter is continuously flushed with saline.

Closed-tip irrigation designs have been developed, such as the Boston Scientific Chilli Catheter (Boston Scientific Electrophysiology, San Jose, CA). This catheter circulates saline to the tip of the catheter during RF ablation and then returns it through a conduit in the catheter, avoiding infusion of saline into the body. This catheter has been used to ablate ventricular tachycardia from the epicardial space to avoid problems associated with fluid accumulation from open irrigation.[28] However, several experimental studies showed increased risk of thrombus formation and steam pops with a closed-tip irrigation compared to open-irrigated catheters.[29–31] While it may be possible to address some of these issues through alternate power settings and temperature control, open irrigation has become the standard of care.

Open irrigation catheters typically use a showerhead-type design (Biosense Webster, Diamond Bar, CA, and St. Jude

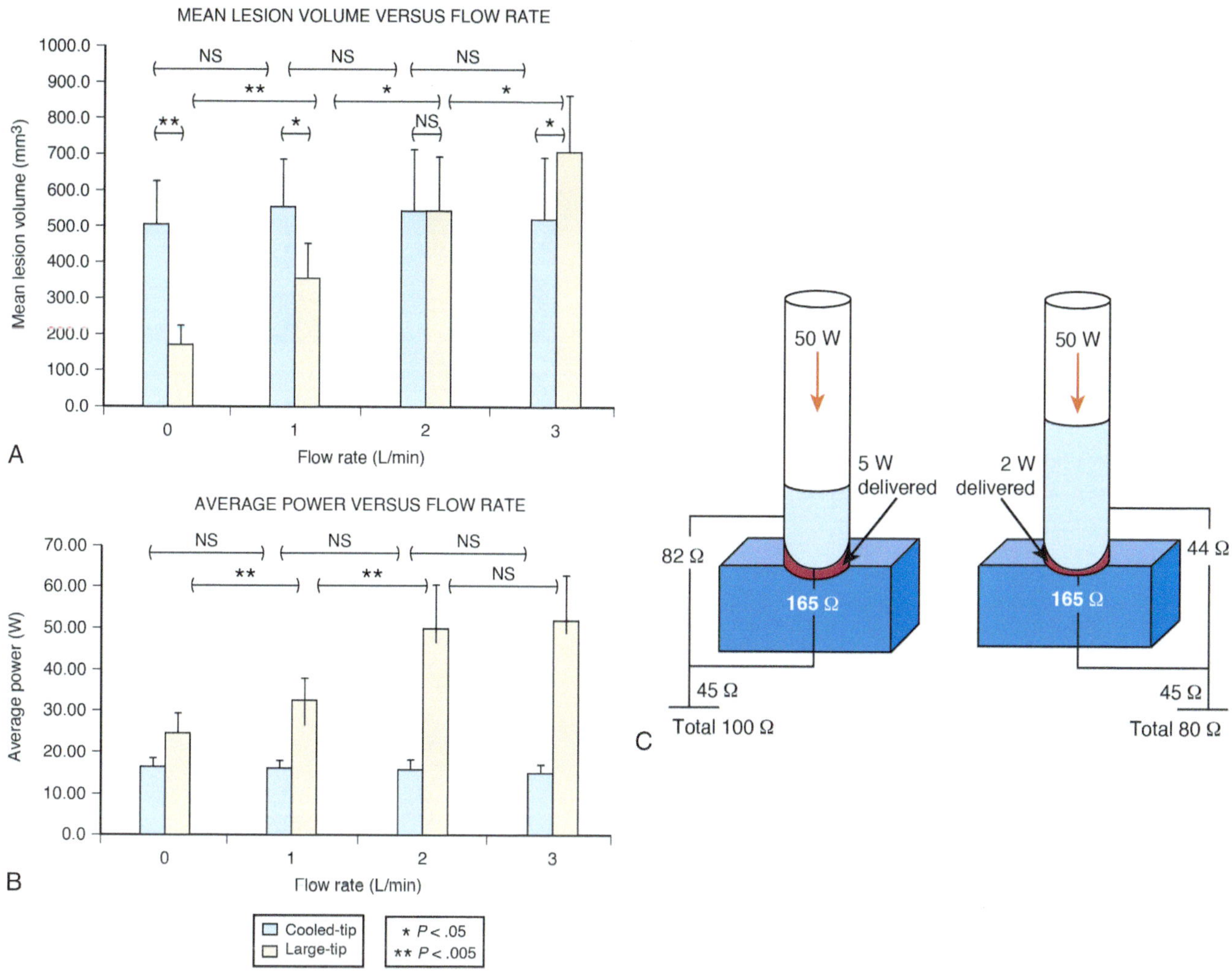

Fig. 5.2 (A) Relationship between lesion volume and superfusate flow rate with irrigated ablation catheter or large-tip (10 mm) electrodes in porcine ventricular tissue. Larger lesions could be produced with the large-tip catheter in temperature control mode (65–70°C) with increasing flow rate. Increased lesion size is due to delivery of increased power prior to reaching target electrode temperature (see B). There was no increase in lesion volume with irrigated electrode. (B) Average power delivered versus superfusate flow rate over the irrigated or large-tip electrodes. For the irrigated catheter, no further power could be delivered with increasing superfusate flow. For the large-tip electrode, increased superfusate flow allowed more power delivery through electrode cooling. This resulted in larger lesion size for the large-tip electrode. (C) Current shunting with large-tip ablation catheter. Theoretical ablations with 4-mm *(left)* and 8-mm *(right)* catheters are shown. The current path comprises the tissue resistance (165 Ω) and blood pool resistance in parallel and the resistance to the skin electrode in series; 50 W is delivered with each electrode. As the electrode diameter is the same for each catheter, the tissue resistances to each electrode are the same. The blood pool resistance is lower for the 8-mm electrode as greater surface area is in contact with the blood pool, shunting current away from the tissue (2 W versus 5 W delivered to the tissue) despite lower total resistance (80 W versus 100 W). This leads to a smaller lesion for the 8-mm electrode despite identical power deliveries. (A and B, from Pilcher TA, Sanford AL, Saul P, Dieter Haemmerich D. Convective cooling effect on cooled-tip catheter compared to large-tip catheter radiofrequency ablation. *Pacing Clin Electrophysiol.* 2006;29:1368–1374.)

Medical, St. Paul, MN). The ThermoCool SmartTouch Surround Flow (STSF) ablation catheter (Biosense Webster, Fig. 5.4) is approved by the U.S. Food and Drug Administration (FDA) for AF ablation. Cooling is achieved via six irrigation ports at the catheter tip with saline infusion at a rate of 17 or 35 mL/minute during RF application and 2 mL/minute at other times. A Nitinol spring-based contact sensor is integrated into the tip of the catheter, which converts spring displacement into force magnitude and direction. The Abbott Tacticath ablation catheter (Abbott Medical, Fig. 5.5) is also approved by the FDA for AF ablation. Cooling is achieved via six irrigation ports at the catheter tip with saline infusion rate of 17 or 30 mL/minute during RF application and 2 mL/minute at other times. In contrast to the Nitinol spring used in the ThermoCool, the Tacticath uses a triaxial optical force sensor.

Several designs for new irrigated-tip catheters are currently in testing (Fig. 5.6). The QDOT Micro catheter (Biosense Webster) uses an irrigation design similar to the SmartTouch STSF

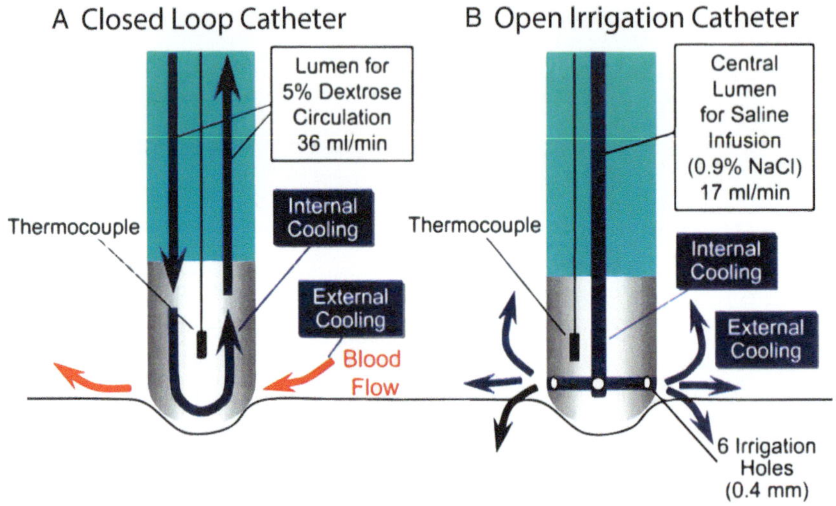

Fig. 5.3 Schematic representation of closed-loop and open-irrigation ablation catheters. (A) Closed-loop irrigation catheter circulates irrigant continuously through the tip electrode to cool the ablation electrode internally. (B) Open-irrigation catheter has irrigation holes that infuse normal saline at room temperature through the electrode and irrigation holes to provide internal and external electrode cooling. (Adapted from Yokoyama K, Nakagawa H, Wittkampf FHM, et al. Comparison of electrode cooling between internal and open irrigation in radiofrequency ablation lesion depth and incidence of thrombus and steam pop. *Circulation*. 2006;113(1):11–19.)

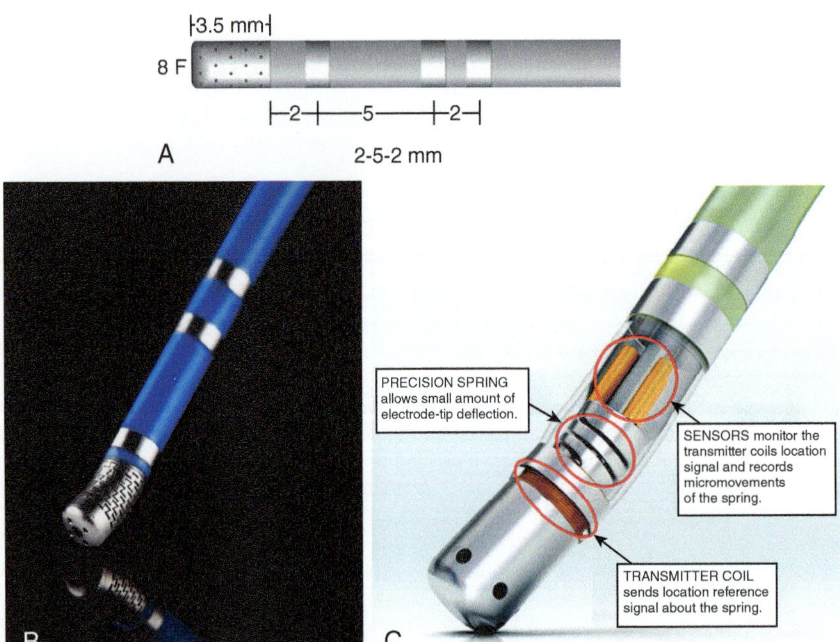

Fig. 5.4 (A) Biosense Webster ThermoCool SF ablation catheter with a porous tip and low flow rate; (B) St. Jude Therapy Cool Flex: unique laser cut catheter-tip electrode designed to provide an optimized irrigation flow distribution and better contact because of flexible tip. (C) Schematic illustration of catheter-force measurement technology through microdeformations of a precision spring connecting tip and shaft of the catheter (THERMOCOOLSMARTTOUCH; Biosense Webster, Diamond Bar, CA). This catheter is integrated into the Caro3 system (Biosense Webster). *SF*, Surround flow. (Reproduced with permission from Martinek M, Lemes C, Sigmund E, et al. Clinical impact of an open-irrigated radiofrequency catheter with direct force measurement on atrial fibrillation ablation. *PACE*. 2012;35:1312–1318.)

catheter, while integrating six thermocouples into the catheter tip for temperature sensing. This allows delivery of very HPSD lesions for AF ablation with temperature control.[32] Another design uses a 9-mm spherical lattice tip on an 8-F bidirectional irrigated catheter (Sphere-9, Affera Inc., Watertown, MA). Nine surface thermocouples are integrated into the catheter tip to allow for irrigated ablation with temperature control. The greater surface area of the lattice tip allows for lower current density, which enables delivery of increased power with lower risk of local tissue overheating.[26,33]

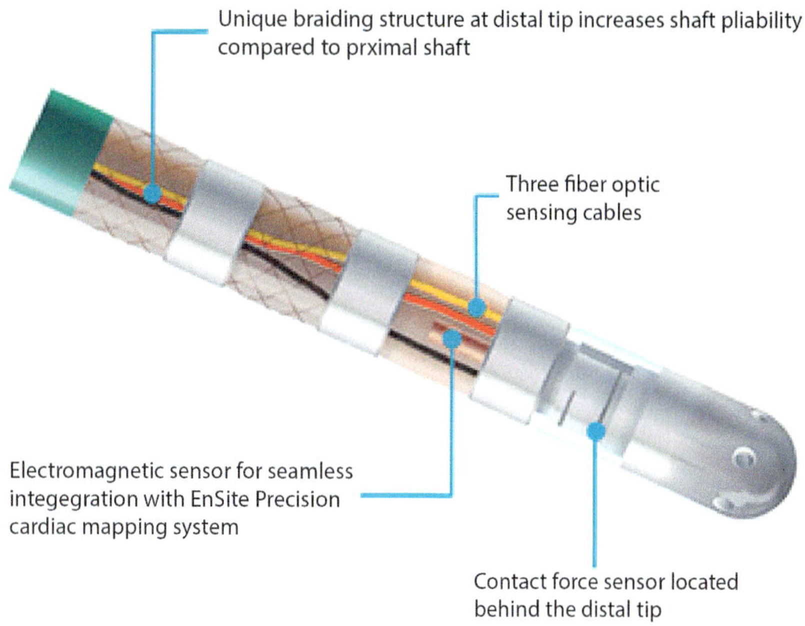

Fig. 5.5 Schematic drawing of open-irrigation Tacticath. This catheter has irrigation ports at the distal tip and integrates a trioptical force sensor to assess contact force. (Reproduced with permission of Abbott, © 2023. All rights reserved.)

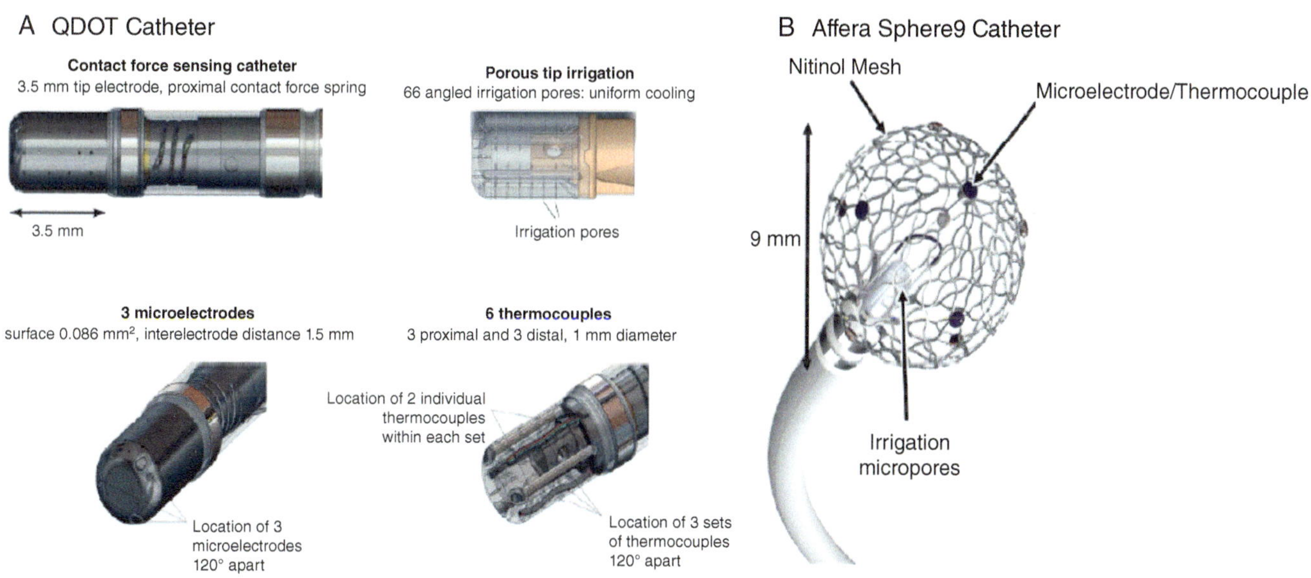

Fig. 5.6 (A, *left*), QDOT Micro Catheter uses an irrigation design similar to SmartTouch STSF, while integrating six thermocouples into the catheter tip for temperature sensing to allow for temperature-control in high power, short-duration lesion delivery. (B, *right*), Affera Sphere Catheter is a lattice-tip irrigated catheter with nine surface thermocouples to allow temperature-controlled ablation. Lower current density of the lattice-tip allows delivery of increased power without excessive local tissue heating. (Images used with permission from Medtronic, plc © 2023.)

TITRATING POWER AND DURATION DURING IRRIGATED RADIOFREQUENCY ABLATION

As with nonirrigated catheters, power has traditionally been set at the minimum required to destroy targeted tissue and reduce risk of complications. Electrode temperature is used to monitor tissue heating with nonirrigated catheters, but this is less reliable when using irrigation as the point of maximum heating is deep to the thermocouple. Consequently, other factors are useful to guide lesion characteristics, as outlined in Table 5.1.

The addition of contact force (CF)-sensing catheters adds a critical parameter to guide RF ablation. Low catheter–tissue CF is associated with ineffective lesion formation, whereas high contact force increases risk of steam pops and perforation.[34] CF affects lesion size at constant power and application duration, with greater contact force leading to larger lesions (Fig. 5.7).

TABLE 5.1 Evidence of Lesion Formation With Irrigated Radiofrequency Ablation Catheters

Reduction in local electrogram amplitude (>50%)
Impedance drop (5–10 Ω)
Emergence of double potentials, signifying local conduction block
Development of conduction block during pacing maneuvers
Tachycardia termination during ablation
Increase in local pacing threshold (>100%)

Force–time integral (FTI) has been studied as a parameter associated with transmural lesion formation in AF, with FTI >392 gram-seconds associated with transmural lesion formation.[34–36] FTI-targeted ablation improved results but was associated with high rates of recurrence of pulmonary vein potentials.[37]

Indices were created by manufacturers to predict ablation lesion quality by incorporating additional ablation parameters. Ablation Index (AI) is a proprietary formula (Biosense Webster) that incorporates power, CF, and time in a weighted formula to predict lesion depth[37] (see Chapter 1). The AI formula is shown below with constants replaced with letters.

$$\text{Ablation Index} = \left(K * \int_0^t CF^a(\tau) P^b(\tau) d\tau \right)^c$$

AI values of 550 for the anterior wall and 400 for the posterior wall of the left atrium were associated with higher rates of durable PV isolation in follow up (Fig. 5.8).[37,38] The Lesion Index (LSI) is another proprietary formula that includes contact force, ablation duration, and current (Abbott Medical, Chicago, IL). LSI >5 was associated with shorter procedure time, less RF, and fewer touch-up lesions.[39]

While power was traditionally titrated to the minimum required for ablation, recent studies have challenged use of a low-power, long-duration (LPLD) strategy for AF ablation. LPLD uses 25–35 W for 30–60 seconds per application, delivering up to 900 J. Approximately 10% of the total energy in each application is delivered to the myocardium, with the remainder dissipated within the blood pool.[12] HPSD is an alternative to LPLD that may help avoid collateral heating while delivering transmural lesions to the atrial myocardium. HPSD uses output of 50 W or greater for a shorter duration (typically 10–15 seconds), applying total energy of 500 J or less.[11,40,41] Most tissue damage is due to resistive heating, limiting conductive heating and potential damage to surrounding structures. Additional benefits include better lesion geometry, lesser influence of catheter stability on lesion formation, and better durability of electrical isolation.[10,11,27]

Studies have shown that lesion depth is related to total energy delivered rather than rate of energy delivery. In silico computer modeling showed similar lesion size between LPLD and HPSD groups with similar total energy delivery, although absolute tissue temperature is 5–8°C higher with HPSD (see Fig. 5.9).[41] Bhaskaran et al. compared lesion depth between 40 W/30 sec, 60 W/5 sec, and 80 W/5 sec and found all settings produced transmural lesions with similar lesion depth (2.1–2.2 mm) among groups. Steam pops incurred in 80-W and 40-W groups but not with intermediate power settings.[42] Bourier et al. showed similar lesion volume with LPLD and HPSD, although lesion width increased with higher power. Lesions were relatively shallower with higher power, although deep enough for transmurality (~3 mm) for AF ablation. There were diminishing returns with longer lesions, as the fastest increase in lesion size was within 10 seconds of RF delivery.[43] Wider lesions may occur due to the higher absolute temperature achieved with HPSD, whereas convective cooling may lead to shallower lesions. Additional experimental data

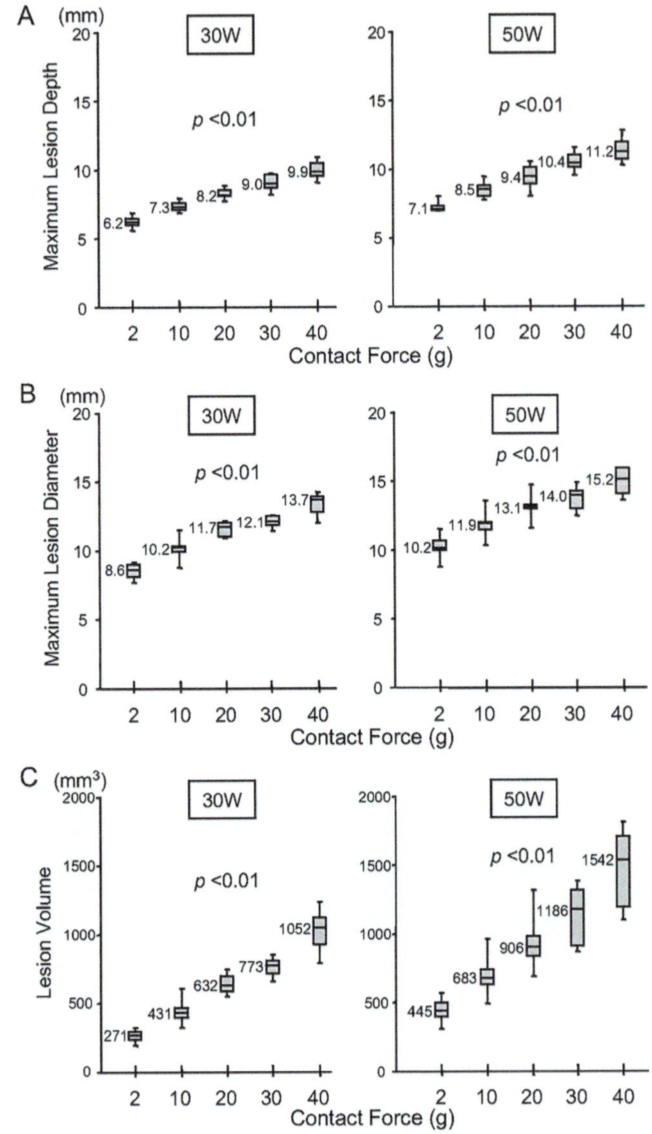

Fig. 5.7 Relationship between contact and radiofrequency (RF) lesion size in canine thigh muscle preparation. Lesion depth (A) and lesion volume (B) increased significantly with greater contact force for 30-W and 50-W RF applications. (Courtesy of Yokoyama K, Nakagawa H, Shah DC, et al. Novel contact force sensor incorporated in irrigated radiofrequency ablation catheter predicts lesion size and incidence of steam pop and thrombus. *Circ Arrhythm Electrophysiol.* 2008;1(5):354–362.)

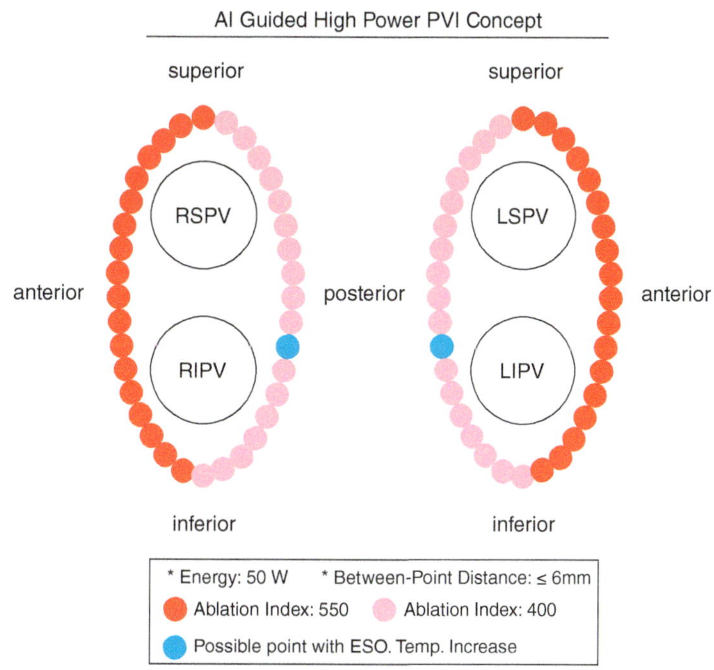

$$\text{Ablation Index} = \left(k * \int_0^t CF^{a}(\tau)\, P^{b}(\tau)\, d\tau \right)^c$$

Fig. 5.8 Ablation Index (AI) is a propriety formula created by Biosense Webster that incorporates power, time, and contact force. Chen et al. found that an AI-guided ablation strategy for pulmonary vein isolation was effective, targeting 550 for the anterior wall and 400 for the posterior wall using high power (50 W). (Courtesy of Chen S, Schmidt B, Bordignon S, et al. Ablation index-guided 50-W ablation for pulmonary vein isolation in patients with atrial fibrillation: procedural data, lesion analysis, and initial results from the FAFA AI High Power Study. *J Cardiovasc Electrophysiol.* 2019;30(12):2724–2731.)

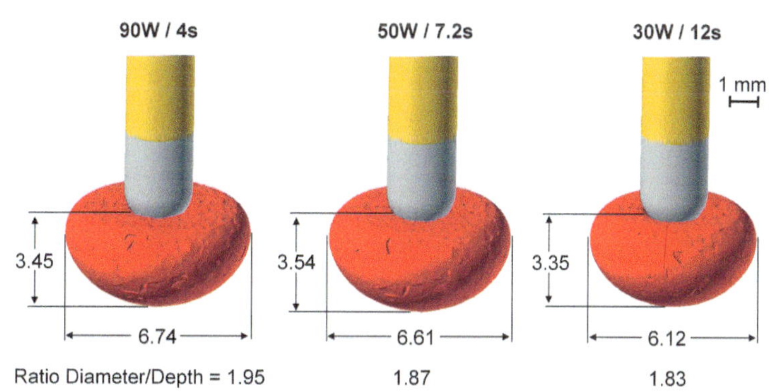

Fig. 5.9 In silico model showing similar lesion geometry for three power-duration settings (90 W/4 sec, 50 W/7.2 sec, 30 W/12 sec), each of which delivered 360 J. Lesion depth is similar among various power-duration settings, but lesions are relatively wider with higher power. (From Pérez JJ, D'Angelo R, González-Suárez A, et al. Low-energy (360 J) radiofrequency catheter ablation using moderate power–short duration: proof of concept based on in silico modeling. *J Interv Card Electrophysiol.* 2022;1–9.)

confirm these results, with greater ratio of endocardial heating to irrigation-mediated cooling in HPSD leading to less subendocardial sparing.[27]

HPSD is best suited for thin-walled structures (e.g., the atrium) and less well suited for thicker structures (e.g., left atrial appendage, lateral mitral annulus, ventricular myocardium), as maximum lesion depth is 3.5–4 mm using standard power and duration settings (Fig. 5.10).[27,40–43]

IRRIGATED RADIOFREQUENCY ABLATION OF ATRIAL FIBRILLATION

AF is the most common sustained cardiac rhythm disturbance, increasing in prevalence with age. Haissaguerre et al. first showed that potentials arising in or near the ostia of the pulmonary veins (PVs) can provoke atrial fibrillation, and elimination of these foci with catheter ablation can offer effective

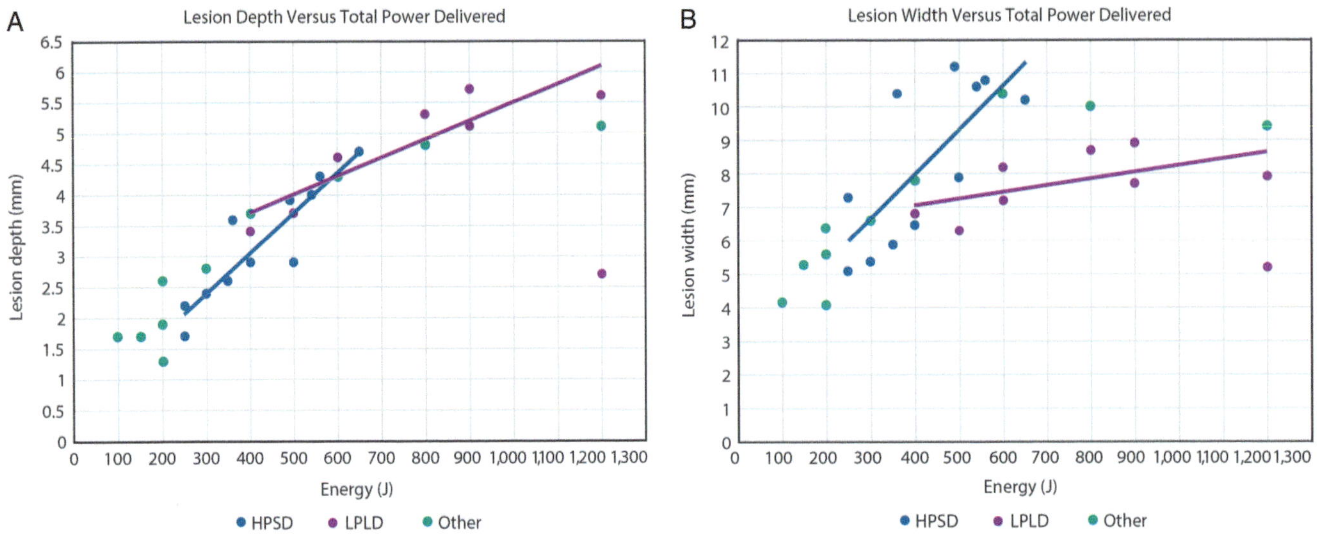

Fig. 5.10 Lesion geometry based on total energy delivered for high-power, short-duration (HPSD) and low-power, long-duration (LPLD) ablation strategies. (A) Lesion depth is similar for HPSD and LPLD within the range of energy typically delivered (400–900 J). (B) Lesions are wider with HPSD, likely as a consequence of higher absolute catheter–tissue temperature and reduced convective cooling. (From Kotadia ID, Williams SE, O'Neill M. High-power, short-duration radiofrequency ablation for the treatment of AF. *Arrhythm Electrophysiol Rev.* 2019;8(4):265–272.)

treatment.[44] The technique evolved from targeting individual foci within the veins to circumferential isolation of the entire PV musculature with an antral lesion set.

Successful ablation requires the creation of a long, contiguous, transmural lesion set to electrically isolate the pulmonary veins.[11,27,43] As described above, irrigated RF ablation with conventional settings typically uses 25–35 W for 30–60 seconds per lesion.[11,45] HPSD has recently supplanted LPLD for the treatment of atrial fibrillation as described above. Although few trials have directly compared HPSD and LPLD, there is a growing body of evidence that suggests advantages for treatment of AF.

Ablation with HPSD using 50 W was effective in achieving pulmonary vein isolation in several studies, with first-pass isolation rates up to 92%, when using contact force and ablation-index guided applications. Rates of complications were low, with only one patient having esophageal lesion on follow-up endoscopy without evidence of atrioesophageal fistula.[46–48] Another study using HPSD with 70-W lesions found similar efficacy without any significant periprocedural complications. Total procedure time was notably quicker compared to LPLD.[48]

Several recent studies have evaluated the safety and efficacy of a novel irrigated RF catheter that can deliver up to 90 W in a temperature-controlled mode (QDOT Micro Catheter, Biosense Webster). Delivery of 90 W over 4 seconds was effective in creating transmural lesions with similar safety profile in a swine model.[27] This preclinical model was validated in small clinical trials, demonstrating successful isolation with very high-power very short-duration ablation (vHPvSD, 90 W/4 sec) and no increase in complications.[32,49] One study evaluating the safety of vHPvSD ablation demonstrated very low risk of esophageal ulceration with an increase in asymptomatic cerebral events as detected by cerebral magnetic resonance imaging.[50] This complication was attributed to coagulum formation at the catheter tip and persisted with different iterations of the RF generator software.[51] This study also found low rates of first-pass isolation with vHPvSD (65% for left PVs; 38% for right PVs) compared to rates up to 92% using HPSD with 50 W. Low rates of first-pass isolation were attributed to difficulty in obtaining transmural lesions with short duration.[51] This may be attributable to difficulty in achieving stability with short lesion duration despite delivery of similar total energy with vHPvSD and HPSD.

IRRIGATED RADIOFREQUENCY ABLATION FOR ATRIAL FLUTTER

The most common type of atrial flutter is cavotricuspid isthmus (CTI) dependent, in which reentry is confined to the right atrium. The isthmus may have pouches, ridges, recesses, and trabeculations that make larger and deeper ablation lesions more advantageous for achieving block.

Jais and coworkers compared conventional and irrigated-tip catheter ablation of typical atrial flutter and showed that 100% of patients in the irrigated-tip group achieved successful creation of bidirectional isthmus block with significantly fewer RF applications and shorter procedure times as opposed to 85% of patients in the conventional RF group achieving bidirectional block.[52] Ilg and coworkers randomized 60 consecutive patients with typical atrial flutter to ablation with a 10-mm nonirrigated ablation catheter and an irrigated ablation catheter and found similar clinical efficacy, although with faster CTI block, with large-tip catheter. Notably, these trials were performed before introduction of contact force, and rates of successful CTI block were approximately 80% with large nonirrigated catheters.[53]

Another study assessed rates of CTI block using irrigated catheters with conventional power settings, 25–35 W over 15–35 seconds, finding first-pass success in 60% of cases with successful bidirectional block in 99% of cases. Although an AI target was not specified in this study, with AI of 500, there was a 93% first-pass rate without any complications.[54]

Golian et al. compared conventional ablation settings (30 W/30–40 sec) with HPSD (50 W/8–10 sec) for CTI ablation and found significantly shorter procedure times in the HPSD group along with lower rates of recurrence at 6-month follow-up (HPSD 0%; conventional 7%).[55]

IRRIGATED ABLATION FOR VENTRICULAR TACHYCARDIA

Subendocardial resection was introduced in the late 1970s as treatment for patients with ventricular tachycardia (VT) and ventricular aneurysms. This technique extended the excision for resection of the aneurysmal wall to the endocardial border zone. Preoperative and intraoperative endocardial and epicardial mapping suggested that these border zones served as critical sites for maintenance of VT. While subendocardial resection was effective, the procedure carried high operative mortality (5–15%), so techniques to target the endocardial substrate using catheter ablation were developed.[56] The first techniques for catheter ablation used 300-J direct current shocks from a 7F quadripolar catheter. RF ablation was later introduced to provide a more controlled and directed ablation, with irrigation allowing the creation of larger lesions.

Several trials have shown irrigated RF ablation to be effective in treating VT. Stevenson et al. enrolled 231 patients with infarct-associated recurrent VTs in the Multicenter Thermo-Cool VT Ablation Trial. Use of an irrigated-tip ablation catheter was successful in abolishing all inducible VTs in 49% of patients at 6-month duration, with a procedure mortality rate of 3% and a 1-year mortality rate of 18% (72.5% of deaths were attributable to ventricular arrhythmias).[57] A more recent study from Muser et al. that followed patients with nonischemic cardiomyopathy after irrigated catheter ablation found VT-free survival of 69% at 60 months and significant reduction in VT burden in patients who had recurrence.[58] Thirty-two percent of patients within this series required epicardial ablation. Open irrigation has been used in the epicardial space to avoid premature heating of the catheter tip. d'Avila et al. compared standard and irrigated ablation in the epicardial space and found that irrigated RF ablation created more effective lesions, particularly in areas with overlying epicardial adipose.[59] However, standard irrigation settings (13–30 mL/min) can result in significant intrapericardial fluid accumulation. Aryana et al. assessed the impact of irrigation flow rate (IFR) within the epicardial space and found that reduced IFRs (5–7 mL/min) yielded lesion sizes similar to high IFRs (>10 mL/min) without an increase in steam pop or tissue disruption. Additionally, presence of intrapericardial fluid significantly reduced lesion size (Fig. 5.11).[60]

VTs that originate from intramyocardial origins, including the interventricular septum, mid-myocardium, or papillary muscle, can be difficult to reach with standard irrigated ablation.

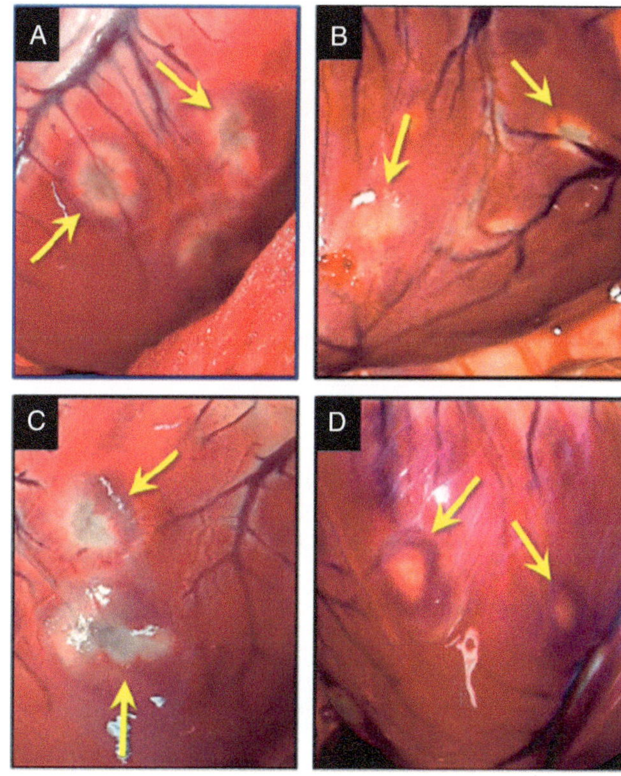

Fig. 5.11 Shown are gross analyses of in vivo epicardial lesions created with fixed power, contact force, and duration. (A) In the absence of intrapericardial fluid (IPF) with irrigation at 5 mL/minute. (B) In the presence of IPF with irrigation at 15 mL/minute. (C) In the absence of IPF with irrigation at 15 mL/minute. (D) In the presence of IPF with irrigation at 15 mL/minute. As seen, lesions generated in the absence of IPF (A and C) are significantly larger than those generated in the presence of IPF (B and D). Sizes of lesions created using 5 mL/min versus 15 mL/min do not appear to be significantly difference. (From Aryana A, O'Neill PG, Pujara DK, et al. Impact of irrigation flow rate and intrapericardial fluid on cooled-tip epicardial radiofrequency ablation. *Heart Rhythm.* 2016;13(8):1602–1611.)

In this situation, it is desirable to create a larger, deeper lesion. Two methods have been developed to deliver larger lesions: bipolar ablation and decreasing irrigant ionic concentration. In standard bipolar ablation, two open-irrigated catheters are used. One is placed at the endocardial site in the right or left ventricle, and the other is placed at the opposite epicardial, septal, or coronary sinus site. The catheter at the opposite site is designated as the grounding connection rather than the impedance patch. Ablation is performed with energy ranging from 30 W to 50 W. Several studies have assessed outcomes of bipolar ablation for treatment of refractory VT and found acute procedural success, although nearly half of patients had recurrence at 1 year. Procedural complications were more common, in part due to increased risk of steam pops.[61–63]

Another approach to creating larger lesions is altering the ionic concentration of the irrigant. Standard irrigated ablation is performed with normal saline (0.9% NaCl); however, irrigation with half normal saline (0.45% NaCl; HNS) can create larger and deeper lesions.[64,65] Nguyen at al. hypothesize that lower charge density of HNS facilitates RF current delivery to

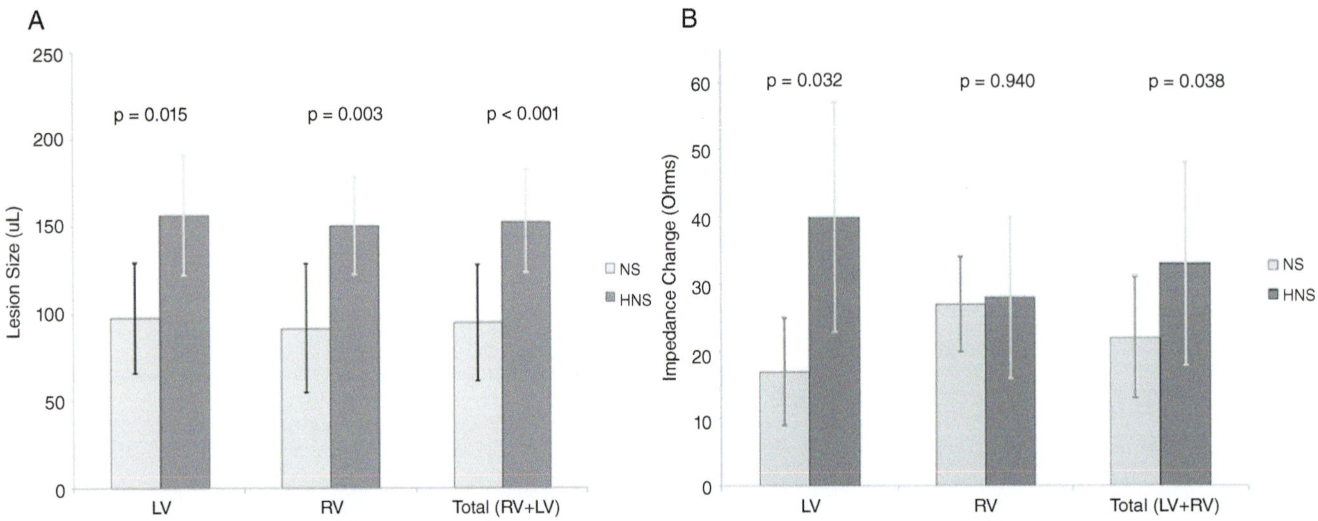

Fig. 5.12 (A) Comparison of lesion volumes after in vivo porcine ablation in the right ventricle (RV), left ventricle (LV), and combined LV and RV for half-normal saline (HNS) and normal saline (NS) irrigation. (B) Impedance changes after in vivo porcine ablation in the RV, LV, and RV and LV combined for HNS and NS. Overall, HNS resulted in deeper and larger lesions. Higher electrical impedance of HFS compared to NS leads to preferential flow of current to myocardium, which has relatively lower impedance. (From Nguyen DT, Gerstenfeld EP, Tzou WS, et al. Radiofrequency ablation using an open irrigated electrode cooled with half-normal saline. *JACC Clin Electrophysiol.* 2017;3(10):1103–1110.)

myocardium by decreasing loss to lower impedance environment around the catheter. They found that RF ablation with HNS created lesions that were 50% larger than standard applications (Fig. 5.12).[65] Larger lesion size may come with a tradeoff of increased risk of complications. Bennett et al. showed a higher risk steam pops with HNS or nonionic 5% dextrose in water (D5W), likely due to increased current delivery to the myocardium.[66]

IRRIGATED ABLATION FROM THE CORONARY SINUS FOR ACCESSORY PATHWAYS AND VENTRICULAR ARRHYTHMIAS

Between 5% and 17% of posteroseptal and left posterior accessory pathways are reportedly epicardial and can be ablated within a branch of the coronary sinus, on the floor of the coronary sinus, or within the coronary sinus diverticulum.[67] In the presence of a coronary sinus–ventricular accessory pathway, a nonirrigated catheter may occlude a branch of the coronary sinus and prevent cooling from ambient blood flow, leading to impedance rises. Irrigation permits delivery of increased power with less heating at the electrode–tissue interface.

A small percentage of left free-wall accessory pathways may also be epicardial, requiring ablation from within the coronary sinus. Other types of unusual accessory pathways that cannot be ablated with standard endocardial approach at the annulus have also been described.[68,69] These include accessory pathways that connect the right atrial appendage to the right ventricle that are successfully ablated using a transcutaneous pericardial approach and accessory pathways closely associated with the ligament of Marshall, ablated by targeting that ligament.[70–72] Several studies have shown that irrigated RF application can be useful for treatment of right posteroseptal accessory pathways resistant to nonirrgated catheter ablation, using temperature cutoff of 40–45°C.[73,74] Gulletta et al. prospectively followed 41 pediatric and adolescent patients who underwent RF ablation for Wolff-Parkinson-White syndrome using irrigated catheter with power titration from 15 W to 30 W in right-sided accessory pathways, 40 W in left-sided accessory pathways, and 20 W inside the coronary sinus with reported procedural success rate of 95.1% after the first procedure, with no complications or recurrence at 12 months.[75] Telishevska et al. showed a similar acute success rate between irrigated ablation with three-dimensional mapping (94.3%) versus nonirrigated ablation (94.2%) but significantly higher freedom from recurrence at 4 years (94% versus 81%) for right-sided accessory pathways.[76]

Ventricular arrhythmias arising from the left ventricular summit also remain a challenging target for ablation, although some can be ablated successfully from the coronary venous system (CVS). Mountantonakis et al. evaluated 47 patients who underwent ablation of non–scar-related ventricular arrhythmias from the CVS, with a success rate of 94% when ablated at the earliest CVS site. Ablation was performed using an irrigated catheter with starting power of 20 W, with lesion duration up to 60 seconds and maximum temperature of 45°C. The catheter was withdrawn to a proximal site if power delivery was limited due to wedging in a vein branch (Fig. 5.13).[77] In some cases, ablation from the CVS system is limited by ability to deliver adequate power resulting in sufficient lesion depth, which may be improved by using HNS or D5W as described above. Tung et al. successfully ablated a left ventricular summit ventricular

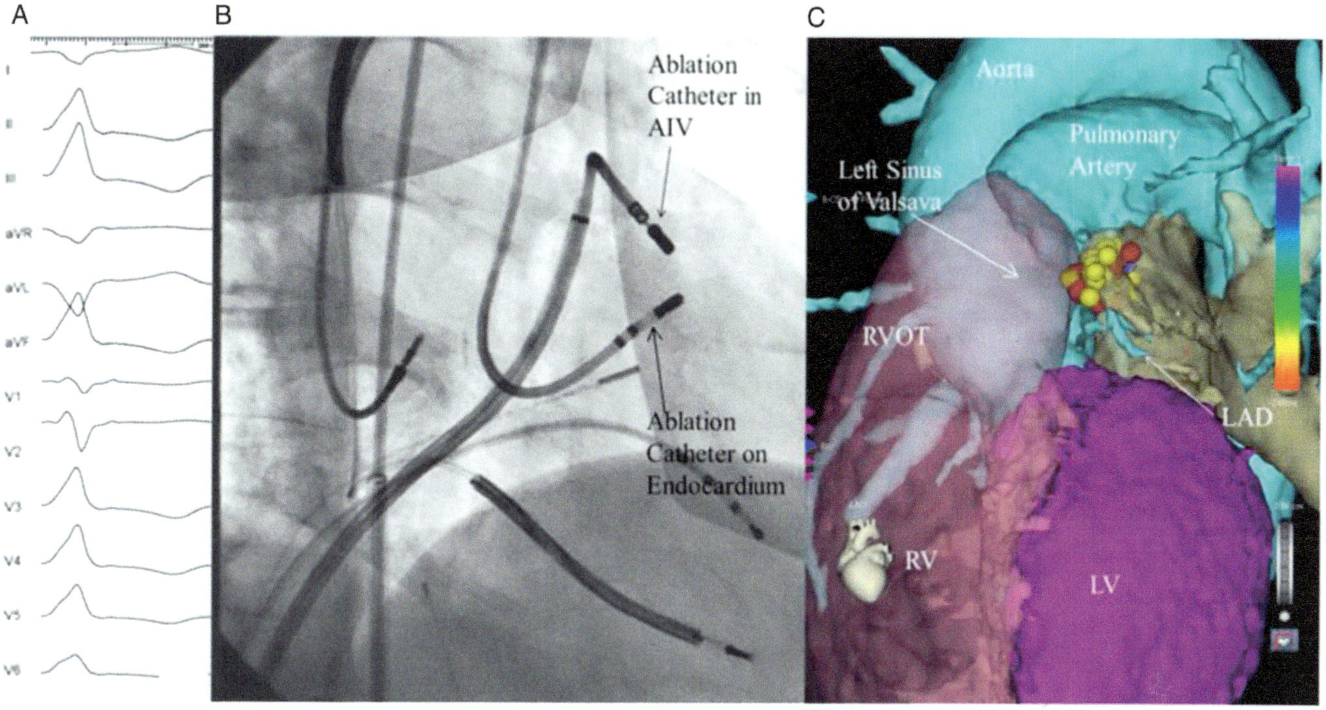

Fig. 5.13 Ventricular premature depolarization (VPD) originating from the anterior interventricular vein (AIV). (A) 12-lead ECG morphology of the clinical VPD, with left-bundle morphology with right inferior axis and precordial transition from negative to positive in lead V3. (B) Ablation catheter at site of earliest activation in AIV in RAO projection with additional catheter at endocardial site opposite successful ablation. (C) Merged image with electroanatomic map and computed tomographic scan. Course of AIV indicated by yellow points. Ablation was performed using an irrigated catheter, starting at 20 W and uptitrating to achieve 10- to 15-Ω drop with maximum temperature of 45°C for duration of 60 seconds. (From Mountantonakis SE, Frankel DS, Tschabrunn CM, et al. Ventricular arrhythmias from the coronary venous system: prevalence, mapping, and ablation. *Heart Rhythm.* 2015;12(6):1145–1153.)

tachycardia using an irrigated catheter within the distal great cardiac vein using nonionic irrigated RF ablation, after normal saline–irrigated ablation from the coronary sinus was unsuccessful.[78] High impedance within the CVS can limit lesion application, and therefore it is often necessary to increase the impedance cutoff to the maximum upper limit of the generator.

CONCLUSION

Research on irrigated ablation has been continuously evolving. Irrigated RF ablation allows for delivery of increased power to the myocardium, allowing formation of transmural lesions that lead to improved efficacy and lower recurrence rates. Irrigated RF ablation has been shown to be safe and effective for the treatment of several common arrhythmias including atrial flutter, atrial fibrillation, accessory pathways, and VT. Recently, new strategies for irrigated RF ablation have been developed, namely use of HPSD. This allows for delivery of equivalent total energy while favoring resistive heating over conductive heating to limit damage of adjacent structures. Newer irrigated electrode designs incorporate thermocouples and contact force sensors to enable temperature-controlled ablation with irrigated catheters that is safer and more efficacious. New designs that incorporate lattice-tip designs to lower-current density and enable greater power delivery to the myocardium are expected to revolutionize irrigated RF ablation.

REFERENCES

Please refer to the e-book for a complete list of references.

PART 2

Cardiac Mapping and Imaging

6

Cardiac Anatomy for Catheter Mapping and Ablation of Arrhythmias

Shumpei Mori, Jason S. Bradfield, Kalyanam Shivkumar

KEY POINTS

- Right and left anterior oblique directions remain fundamental for understanding cardiac anatomy for cardiac electrophysiologists.
- Serial progressive dissection of the entire heart will enhance comprehensive three-dimensional understanding of the cardiac anatomy.

INTRODUCTION

Precise understanding of cardiac anatomy is fundamental for cardiac electrophysiologists to secure procedural success and to avoid complications. The required anatomical knowledge is extensive. It involves the morphology and location of the heart within the thorax,[1] relationship between the heart and surrounding organs/tissues,[2,3] three-dimensional relationship among each chamber, anatomy of each intracardiac or extracardiac structures in association with cardiac silhouette and adjacent structures,[4–7] anatomy of the atrioventricular conduction system,[8–12] anatomy of the coronary arteries and veins,[2,13] anatomy of the pericardial space,[14,15] and anatomy of cardiac innervation.[16,17] Cardiac electrophysiologists are regularly required to focus on cardiac anatomy every time they perform invasive procedures. They also need to review cardiac anatomy when they encounter challenging cases. For the learning purpose, revisiting conventional dissection-based anatomy is an ideal option, as the real anatomy always provides the precise anatomical information with high spatial resolution. However, direct learning opportunity from the real dissection is significantly limited. Alternatively, numerous publications showing images from real dissection are currently available, in either analogue or digital fashion. However, if the structures are viewed from a nonclinical direction, they do not always provide clinically relevant information. Moreover, a two-dimensional single image is insufficient to show the three-dimensionality of the heart. Furthermore, to visualize the structures of interest, the heart is usually opened, which commonly cannot avoid significant distortion. This is even worse if the heart is fixed without pressure-perfusion fixation method, as it cannot prevent resultant collapse and distortion. In this chapter, therefore, the hearts are prepared using the pressure-perfusion fixation method.[2] This secures the heart to retain the physiological morphology during dissection. In addition to the real dissection, virtual dissection images[18] are used as an alternative approach to show the nuance of cardiac anatomy. Progressive dissection method, a serial stepwise approach to perform and record the dissection procedure that was preferentially used by Dr. Wallace A. McAlpine,[2] is applied to share three-dimensional features of the heart. To provide the best clinical relevance, all progressive dissection images are demonstrated from the right and left anterior oblique directions. Currently, it is a worldwide trend to reduce the fluoroscopy-guided procedure. However, these directions remain the gold standard for understanding cardiac anatomy, simply because they are appropriate directions to separate four chambers of the living heart within the chest.[3] Currently available learning sources showing progressive dissection viewed from these directions are surprisingly limited. Thus, serial comprehensive image sets prepared for this chapter will help in understanding the clinical anatomy of the heart. All directions are described using the attitudinally correct orientation.[2,3,19] As a rule, cranial, caudal, ventral, and dorsal orientations are described as superior, inferior, anterior, and posterior, respectively. The right and left orientations are described just as such. To clarify attitudinally correct orientation, substantial figures involve cross-shaped yellow direction indicators. To enhance the comprehensive and systematic visual learning, the atlas style[17] is used rather rather than the descriptive style.

PROGRESSIVE REAL DISSECTION OF THE HEART VIEWED FROM THE RIGHT ANTERIOR OBLIQUE DIRECTION

All the images were photographed using a digital single-lens reflex camera (Nikon D850, Nikon Corporation, Tokyo, Japan) at a dedicated photo studio established at the UCLA Cardiac Arrhythmia Center Anatomy Laboratory.[17] The heart was fixed with pressure-perfusion fixation method[2] and was placed on a special tripod with a rotational mount table.[2,17] Progressive real dissection was performed from the right heart side toward the left heart side. Images were recorded from the right anterior oblique direction (Figs. 6.1–6.12, Video 6.1).

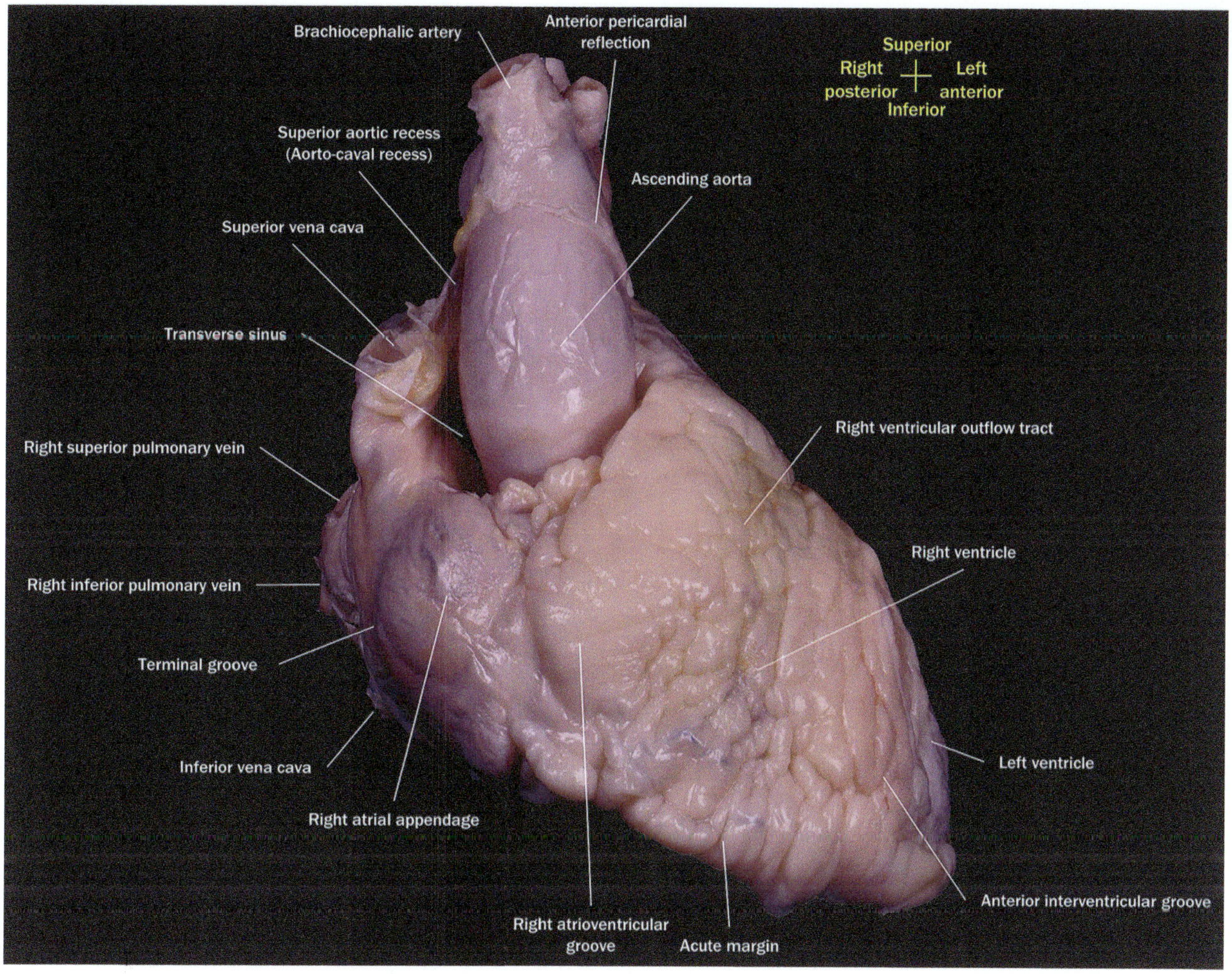

Fig. 6.1 The right atrium (*left*) and the right ventricle (*right*) divided by the right atrioventricular groove. Note the right atrial appendage is not covered by the epicardial fat. The right atrioventricular groove can be seen as the radiolucent band during the fluoroscopic procedure.[5] Generally, the radiolucent band tilts toward the left anteroinferior direction, which is the direction of the cardiac axis.[20] Thus, the radiolucent band works as the useful landmark to estimate the location of tricuspid annulus. This direction is not appropriate to separate the left heart from the right heart. The ascending aorta tilts toward the observer and also slightly tilts toward the right posterior direction.[21] On the contrary, the aortic arch runs away from the observer. The superior vena cava descends vertically behind the ascending aorta, whereas the orifice of the inferior vena cava opens toward right posteroinferior direction. The orifice of the right superior pulmonary vein is located behind the junction between the superior vena cava and the right atrial appendage, intervened by the posterior interatrial fold. The right phrenic nerve on the pericardium can descend very close to this fold between the right superior pulmonary vein and the superior vena cava at the level of the junction. The right-side entrance/exit of the transverse sinus is located between the ascending aorta and superior vena cava. The transverse sinus extends superiorly until it meets the pericardial reflection located near the orifice of the brachiocephalic artery. This allows the pericardial space termed the *superior aortic recess*, also referred to as the aortocaval recess.[2] As the transverse sinus is tight and bending, passing a catheter through it is not readily feasible.[14] The right-hand margin of the ventricular contour is consisted of the apical left ventricle.[22] The anterior interventricular groove is located vertically between the apical right and left ventricles. It contains the middle to distal part of the left anterior descending artery. The left anterior descending artery changes its course vertically along this groove, after skirting the right ventricular outflow tract and pulmonary root with its proximal horizontal segment.

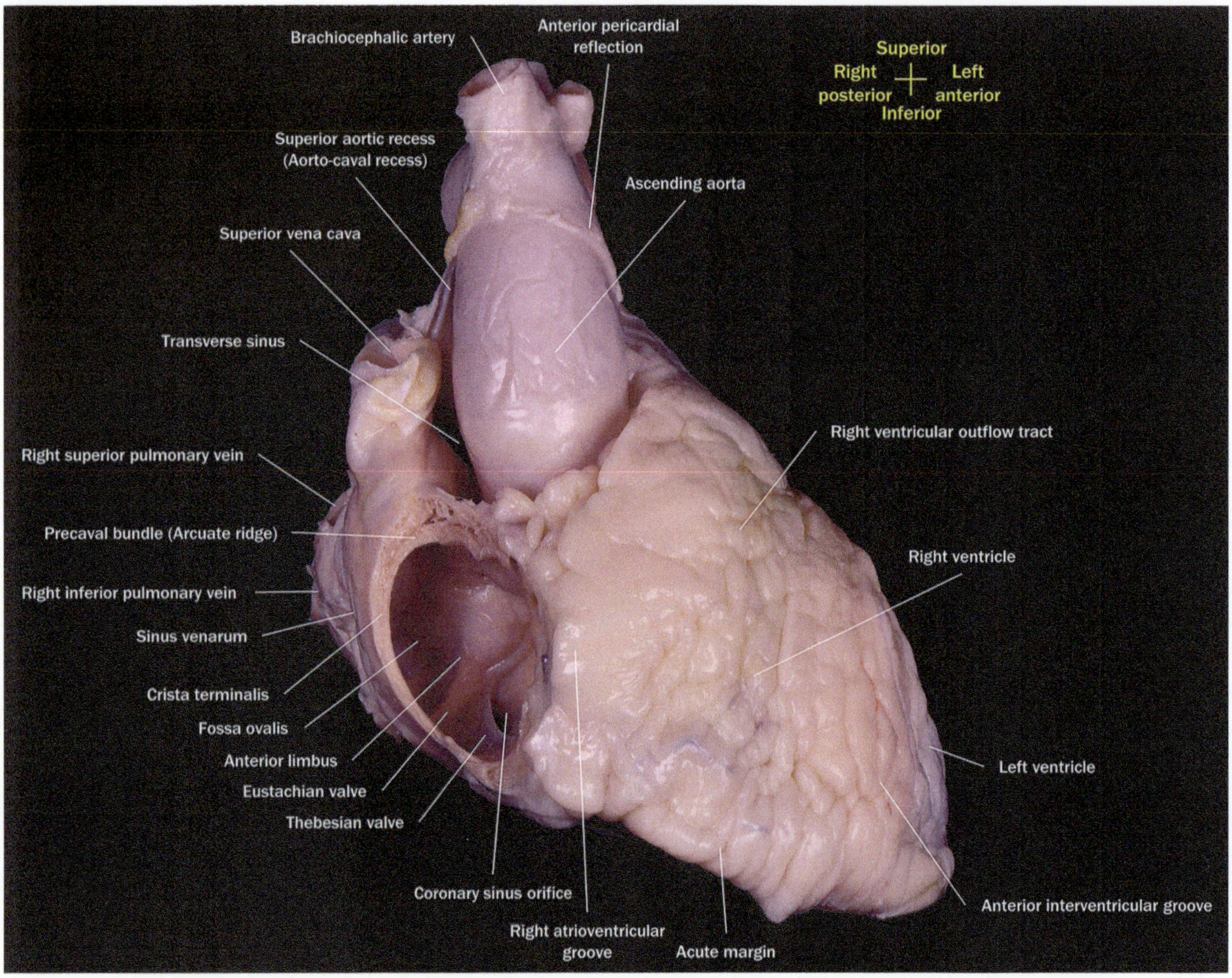

Fig. 6.2 Free wall of the right atrial appendage is removed. The right posterior incision is made along the crista terminalis running vertically between the sinus venarum and right atrial appendage. The crista terminalis continues to the precaval bundle, also referred to as the arcuate ridge, at the anterior part of junction between the superior vena cava and the right atrial appendage.[17] This precaval bundle is confluent with the Bachmann bundle behind the transverse sinus. The Eustachian valve is falciform valve guarding the medial and left anterior orifice of the inferior vena cava.[2] Its septal attachment is located on the anterior limbus of the fossa ovalis right posterior to the coronary sinus orifice. Notably, the height of this valve is higher in the medial part compared to the lateral part.[17] Thus, compared to the lateral side, ablation at the medial part of the cavotricuspid isthmus may risk insufficient contact of the tip, which requires U-turn approach.[17] The medial attachment of the Eustachian valve also corresponds to the location of the tendon of Todaro, the fibrous cord running within the right atrial wall, which cannot be seen without dissection.[2] However, as shown in this case, in some cases the endocardial fold created by the tendon of Todaro can be recognized in continuity with the medial attachment of the Eustachian valve. The tendon of Todaro merges with the central fibrous body beneath the noncoronary aortic sinus. The Thebesian valve is also falciform valve guarding inferior half of the coronary sinus orifice.[23] Thus to secure the smooth insertion of the catheters or electrodes into the coronary sinus orifice, approaching from the superior and medial side of the right atrium is important, rather than from the inferior and lateral side. The right posterior margin of the Thebesian valve is adjacent to the Eustachian valve. Both valves are orthogonal each other.[24] The extent of the Thebesian valve shows individual variation.[25] In some cases, it covers entire coronary sinus orifice with only slit-like opening at its superior corner, mimicking the coronary sinus atresia. The sinus venarum extends between the superior vena cava and inferior vena cava, medially to the crista terminalis.

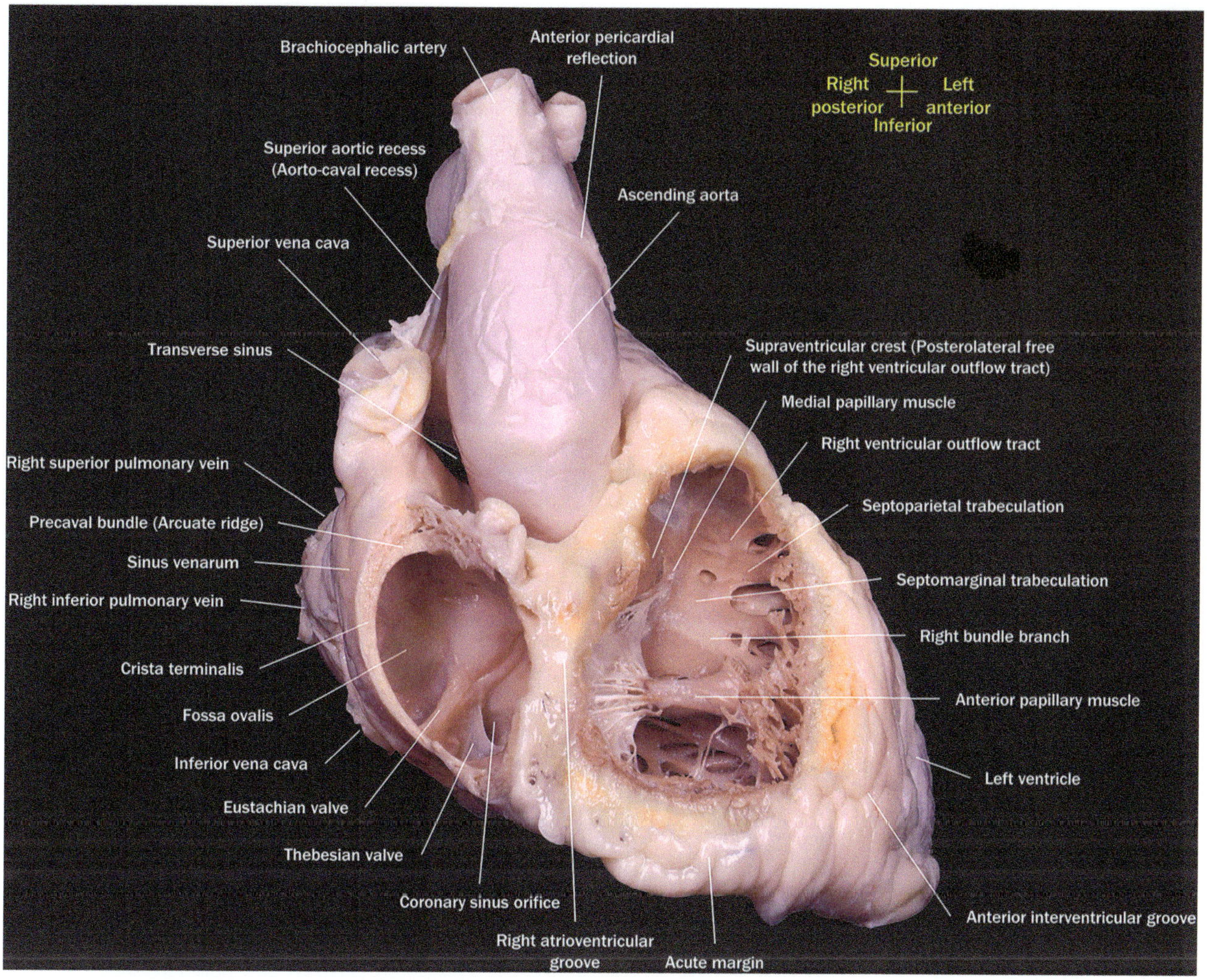

Fig. 6.3 Free wall of the right ventricle is partially removed. Note the anterior papillary muscle looks as if it floats horizontally within the right ventricle. On the septal surface of the right ventricle, thick muscular bundle is running between the right ventricular outflow and inflow is recognized. This is the septomarginal trabeculation, running almost horizontally or slightly inferiorly from the region left anterior to the aortic root toward the free wall. Whitish linear tissue observed on the septomarginal trabeculation involves the right bundle branch. The septomarginal trabeculation has Y-shaped limbs, superior and inferior ones. The superior limb directs toward the left adjacent pulmonary sinus, and the inferior limb directs toward the membranous septum. The medial papillary muscle is located at the Y-shaped bifurcation of the septomarginal trabeculation. It generally gives off the thick chorda tendineae supporting the anterosuperior tricuspid leaflet.[26] This tiny papillary muscle is located left anterior to the medial part of the supraventricular crest, which covers the right coronary aortic sinus anteriorly.[27] From the superior limb of the septomarginal trabeculation, several septoparietal trabeculations arise toward the left anterior free wall of the right ventricular outflow tract. Except for these trabeculations located at the medial and anterior free wall of the right ventricular outflow tract, the endocardial surface of the right ventricular outflow tract is relatively smooth. The septomarginal trabeculation, at the middle part of the right ventricle, gives off the moderator band. The base of the moderator band is located between the outflow, inflow, and apical trabeculation region. It traverses the right ventricle toward the free wall. Thickness and course of this peculiar bundle show individual variation,[28] and it can be even absent.[8] The moderator band connects at the base of the anterior papillary muscle. The medial papillary muscle, septomarginal trabeculation, and moderator band contain the right bundle branch, before it ramifies toward the right ventricular outflow tract, lateral free wall, apex, septum, and supraventricular crest from the base of the anterior papillary muscle.[8]

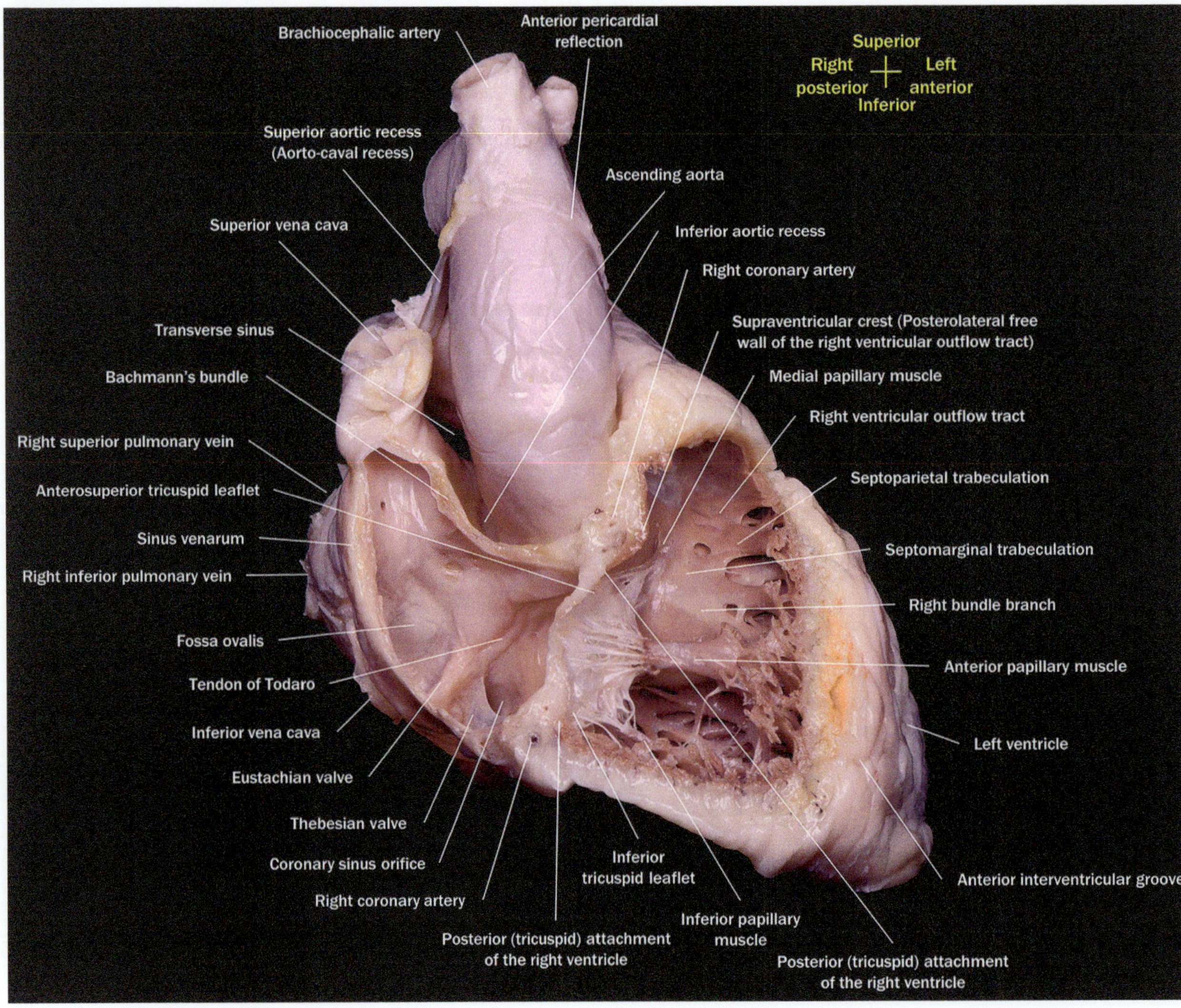

Fig. 6.4 Inferior and apical part of the free wall of the right ventricle is removed. Note the thinness of the right ventricular free wall. Also, the lateral part of the right atrioventricular groove is dissected to expose the lateral tricuspid annulus. Posterior (tricuspid) attachment of the right ventricle to the left ventricle corresponds to the atrioventricular junction of the right ventricular free wall.[2] Medial part of the right atrial appendage and sinus venarum is further opened. The medial papillary muscle gives off the chorda tendineae to the anterosuperior tricuspid leaflet. The chorda tendineae from the anterior papillary muscle supports the commissure between the anterosuperior and inferior tricuspid leaflets. The inferior papillary muscle gives off chorda tendineae to the inferior tricuspid leaflet. The sectional plane of the proximal and distal right coronary artery can be observed at the superior and inferior part of the right atrioventricular groove, respectively. The proximal right coronary artery is just behind the posterolateral free wall of the right ventricular outflow tract, also referred to as the supraventricular crest or ventriculoinfundibular fold. The distal right coronary artery lies inferior to the right atrial vestibule.[29] The close proximity of the right coronary artery to each right ventricular outflow tract and the right atrium indicates the potential risk of injury during catheter ablation.[30] On the medial wall of the right atrium, the fold created by the tendon of Todaro that directs from the Eustachian valve toward the central fibrous body is beautifully seen. The inferior extension of the transverse sinus behind the aortic root is referred to as the inferior aortic recess.[31] The space is located left anteriorly to the medial anterior wall of the right and left atria and reaching down to the level of the noncoronary aortic sinus. The precaval bundle is confluent with the Bachmann bundle at the level of the medial and anterior part of the junction between the superior vena cava and right atrial appendage.[2] The Bachmann bundle can be recognized as the focal thickening of the atrial wall facing the transverse sinus and ascending aorta.

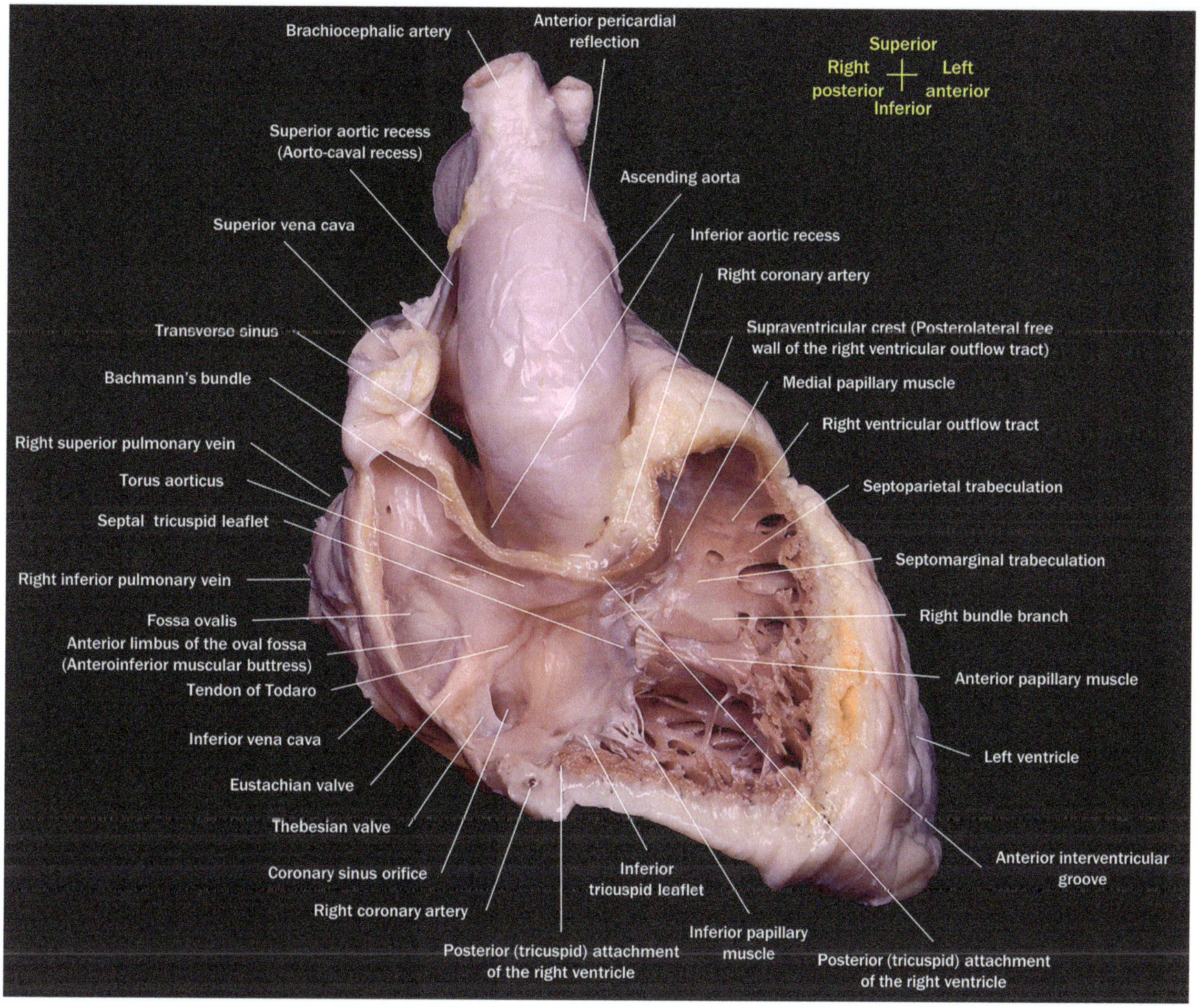

Fig. 6.5 Lateral part of the tricuspid leaflets is removed. The main body of the anterior papillary muscle is kept as is by cutting its chorda tendineae supporting the removed part of the leaflets. Entire septal tricuspid leaflet can be observed in its diastolic form. Note even in its diastolic form, the tip of the septal tricuspid leaflet does not reach to the vertical line placed at the level of the medial papillary muscle. Multiple small chorda tendineae originating directly from the ventricular septum anchor the leaflet. The color of the floor of the triangle of Koch, corresponding to the mid-paraseptal region, seems slightly yellowish, as it contains the adipose tissue of the inferior pyramidal space behind.[32] Anterior limbus of the fossa ovalis, corresponding to the anteroinferior muscular buttress between the fossa ovalis and triangle of Koch, is the muscular part of the atrial septum.[33,34] Superior to the triangle of Koch and left anterior to the fossa ovalis, the superior medial wall of the right atrium is facing the aortic root, intervened by the right-side transverse sinus.[1] At this region, anterior half of the noncoronary aortic sinus bulges toward the right atrium, which is referred to as the torus aorticus or right aortic mound. Any invasive procedures around this region have potential risks to injure the right atrium or aortic root, to create fistula between the aortic root and the right atrium, to induce the cardiac tamponade, and damage the fast pathway.[5,35]

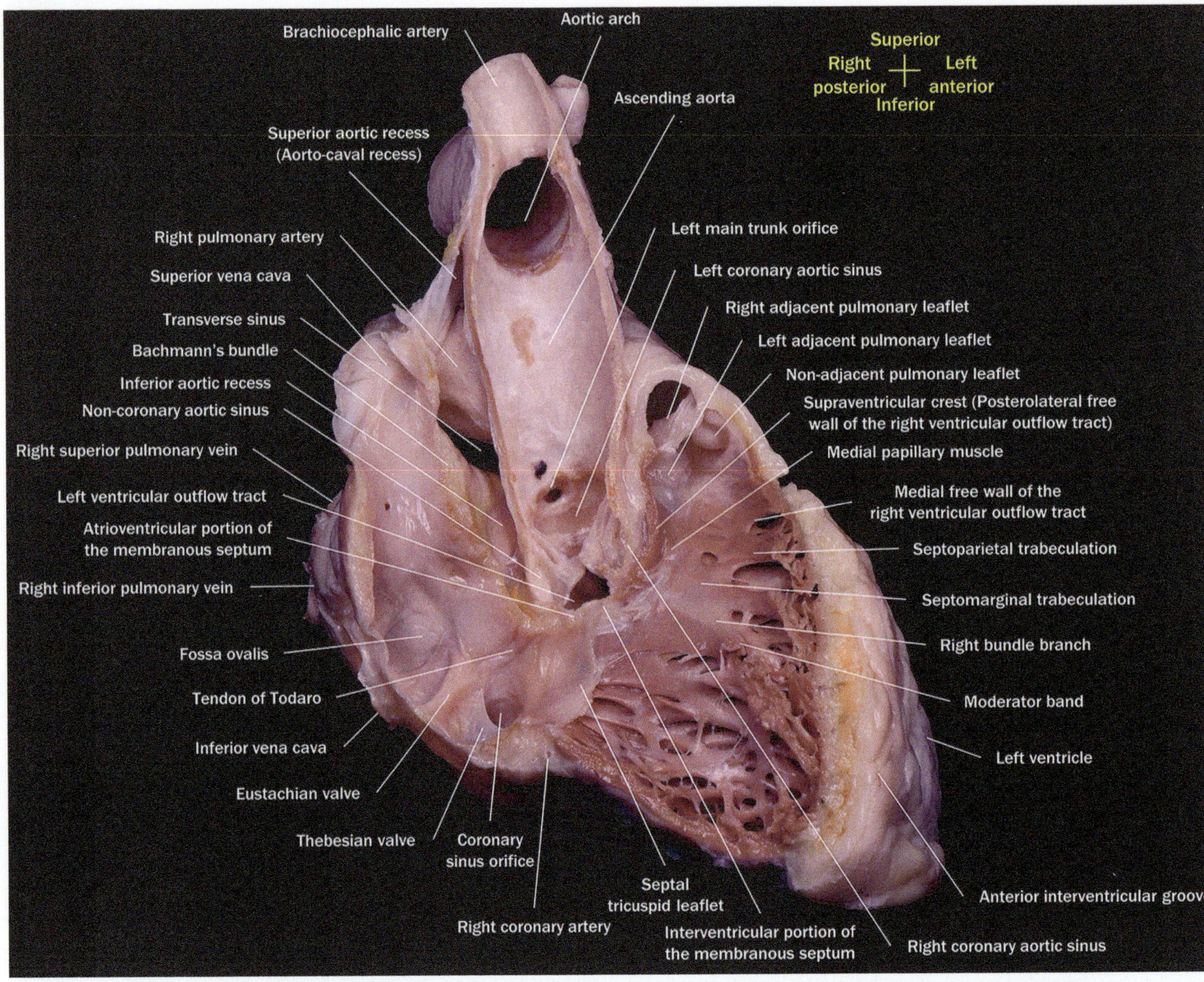

Fig. 6.6 The cutting plane is placed backward near the plane of the right-side ventricular septum. Note thinness of the membranous septum. Although the epicardial fat at the anterior interventricular groove is thick and apical trabeculations are prominent, note thinness of the free wall of the right ventricle. The aortic root and ascending aorta are opened to show the right and noncoronary aortic sinuses. Superior vena cava is also opened. The anterior papillary muscle is removed. The medial papillary muscle is located anterior to the right coronary aortic sinus. The ellipsoid shape of the sectioned moderator band is noted at the middle part of the right ventricle at the level of the apex of the triangle of Koch. The location of the origin of the moderator band defines the margin between the right ventricular outflow, right ventricular inflow, and apical trabeculation regions. The membranous septum is shown between the right and noncoronary aortic sinus. It is divided by the septal attachment of the septal tricuspid leaflet into atrioventricular and interventricular portions.[2,8,36] Behind the membranous septum, the left ventricular outflow tract is observed. The inferior aortic recess extends behind the noncoronary aortic sinus. The close proximity of the supraventricular crest, identical to the posterolateral free wall of the right ventricular outflow tract, and the right coronary aortic sinus is noted. The pulmonary artery is lifted up from the tricuspid valve by the right ventricular outflow tract and located left anterosuperior to the aortic root.[37] The right and left adjacent pulmonary sinuses are adjacent the aortic root or ascending aorta. Left adjacent leaflet, also referred to as the posterior pulmonary leaflet, is located most inferoposteriorly. Right and nonadjacent pulmonary leaflets are also referred to as the right anterior and left anterior pulmonary leaflets, respectively.[38] The part of the right ventricular outflow tract superior to the septomarginal trabeculation, which is located en face fashion to the observer, is the posterior and medial free wall.[2,17] This part is not the septal structure, but it is facing the anterior interventricular groove behind, suggesting the risk of free wall perforation.[39] The right pulmonary artery roofs the transverse sinus.

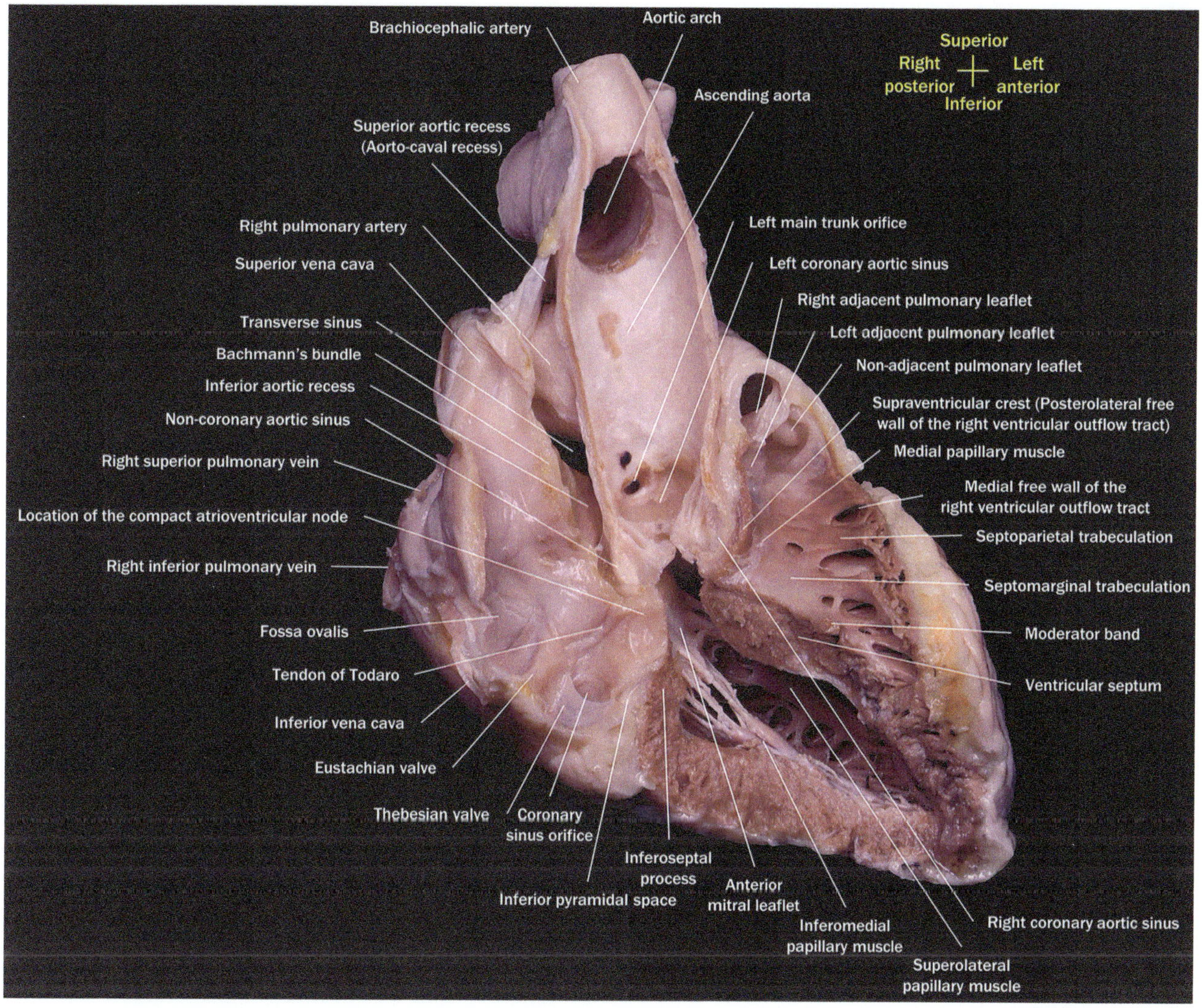

Fig. 6.7 Membranous septum and the part of the muscular ventricular septum is removed along the middle part of the septomarginal trabeculation. Note that in this section, the basal inferomedial part of the left ventricle shows process-like appearance directing toward the membranous septum. This part is not the ventricular septum but the inferomedial free wall facing the inferior pyramidal space. It is originally referred to as the posterosuperior process.[2] Attitudinally, however, the inferoseptal or inferomedial process should be appropriate.[40] The inferior pyramidal space is sandwiched between this process and the right atrium anterior to the coronary sinus orifice.[4] Thus, the septal isthmus between the tricuspid annulus and the coronary sinus orifice faces the process, intervened by the inferior pyramidal space. Therefore, ventricular arrhythmias originating from this process can be ablated from the left ventricle and right atrium.[40,41] Also, this part can be an alternative entrance to the left ventricle from the right atrium in the setting of double valve replacement.[42] The atrioventricular node is located between the tendon of Todaro and the membranous septum at the right posteroinferior margin of the atrioventricular portion of the membranous septum beneath the nadir of the noncoronary aortic sinus.[2,8,43] Both papillary muscles of the left ventricle are the free wall structure.[7] Superolateral papillary muscle, so-called anterolateral papillary muscle, is actually located left posterosuperior relative to the inferomedial papillary muscle, so-called posteromedial papillary muscle. The sectioned ventricular septum at the level of the outflow tract is seen tangentially, located inferior to the right ventricular outflow tract. It separates the right ventricular outflow tract from inferiorly located left ventricular outflow tract. This is because the right ventricular outflow tract overrides the left ventricular outflow tract in crisscross fashion.[3,6] Directional terminology of the ventricular outflow tract, however, remains controversial and confusing in the clinical settings. At least recognizing that the term *septal* cannot be applied in similar fashion as used for the ventricular inflow and apical regions is important.

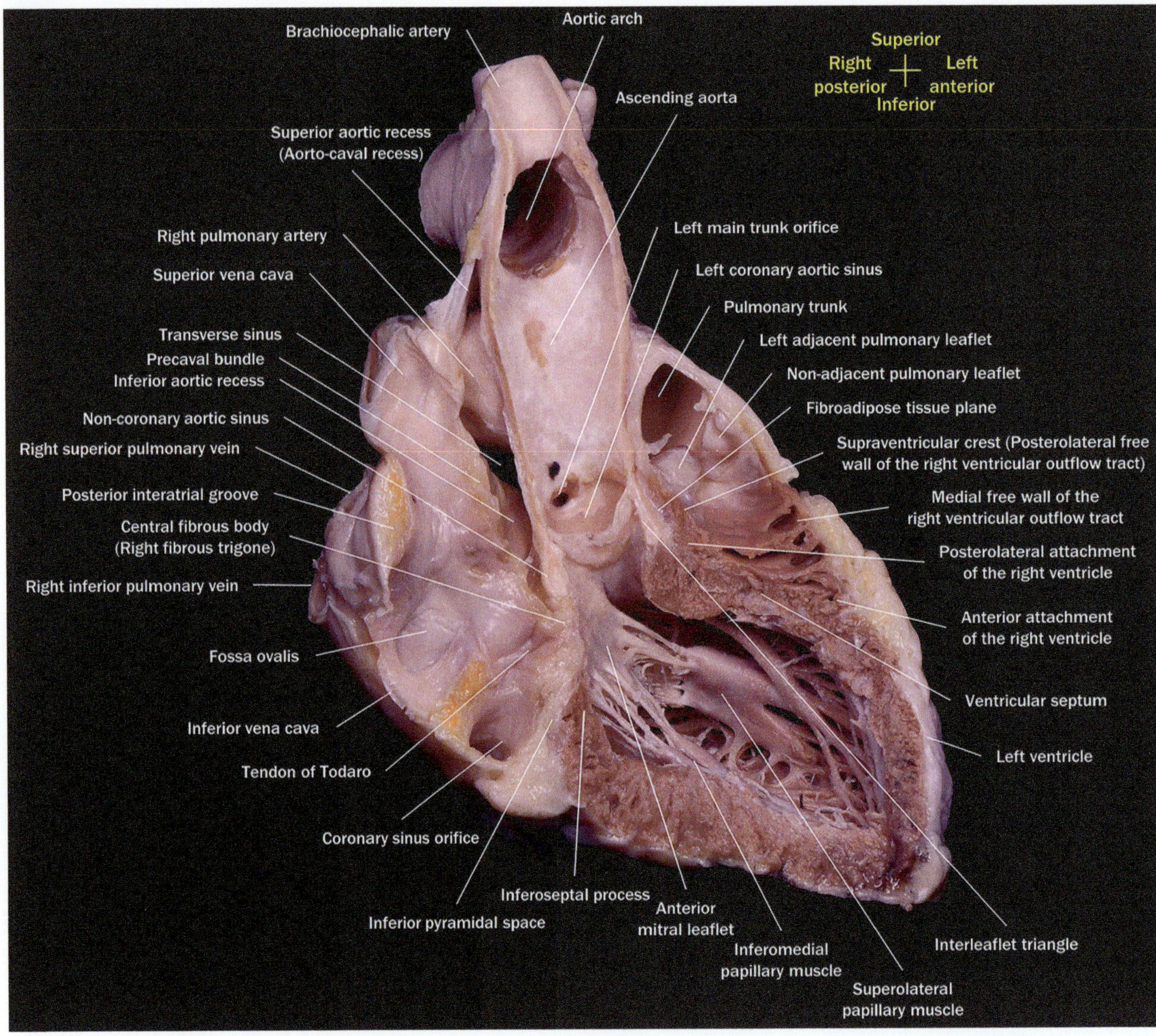

Fig. 6.8 The ventricular septum is removed along the superior margin of the septomarginal trabeculation. Orifice of the inferior vena cava is opened, and the Thebesian valve is removed. Note the close proximity of the right atrium and noncoronary aortic sinus. The anterior wall of the coronary sinus orifice faces the inferoseptal process intervened by the inferior pyramidal space. The ventricular septum at this superior level divides the right ventricular outflow tract from the inferiorly located left ventricle.[5] Posterolateral free wall of the right ventricular outflow tract faces the interleaflet triangle between the right and left coronary aortic sinuses, intervened by thin fibroadipose tissue plane.[6] Thus, at this region, the base of the interleaflet triangle is supported by the left ventricular free wall. The posterolateral free wall of the right ventricular outflow tract is located above the posterolateral attachment of the right ventricle to the left ventricle.[2,17] The medial free wall of the right ventricular outflow tract is located above the anterior attachment of the right ventricle to the left ventricle,[2,17] adjacent to the anterior interventricular groove. The right ventricular outflow tract wall located en face the observer is, therefore, not the septal structure but the posterior and medial free wall. Mitral valve is fixed in diastole shape. Only the anterior mitral leaflet can be recognized from this direction[7] as the posterior mitral leaflet is located behind. The plane cut also revealed adipose tissues at the base of the Eustachian valve and at the posterior interatrial groove, also referred to as the Waterston groove or the Sondergaard groove.[44] The latter groove is important for surgical approach to the left atrium and is related to the interatrial epicardial connection[45] using the interatrial muscular bridges.[46] The central fibrous body, also referred to as the right fibrous trigone,[2,47] is the central piece of the fibrous skeleton of the heart.[48] It carries the atrioventricular node on its right atrial side. It supports the bottom of the noncoronary aortic sinus, medial part of the anterior mitral leaflet, septal tricuspid leaflet, atrial septum, ventricular septum, and membranous septum.

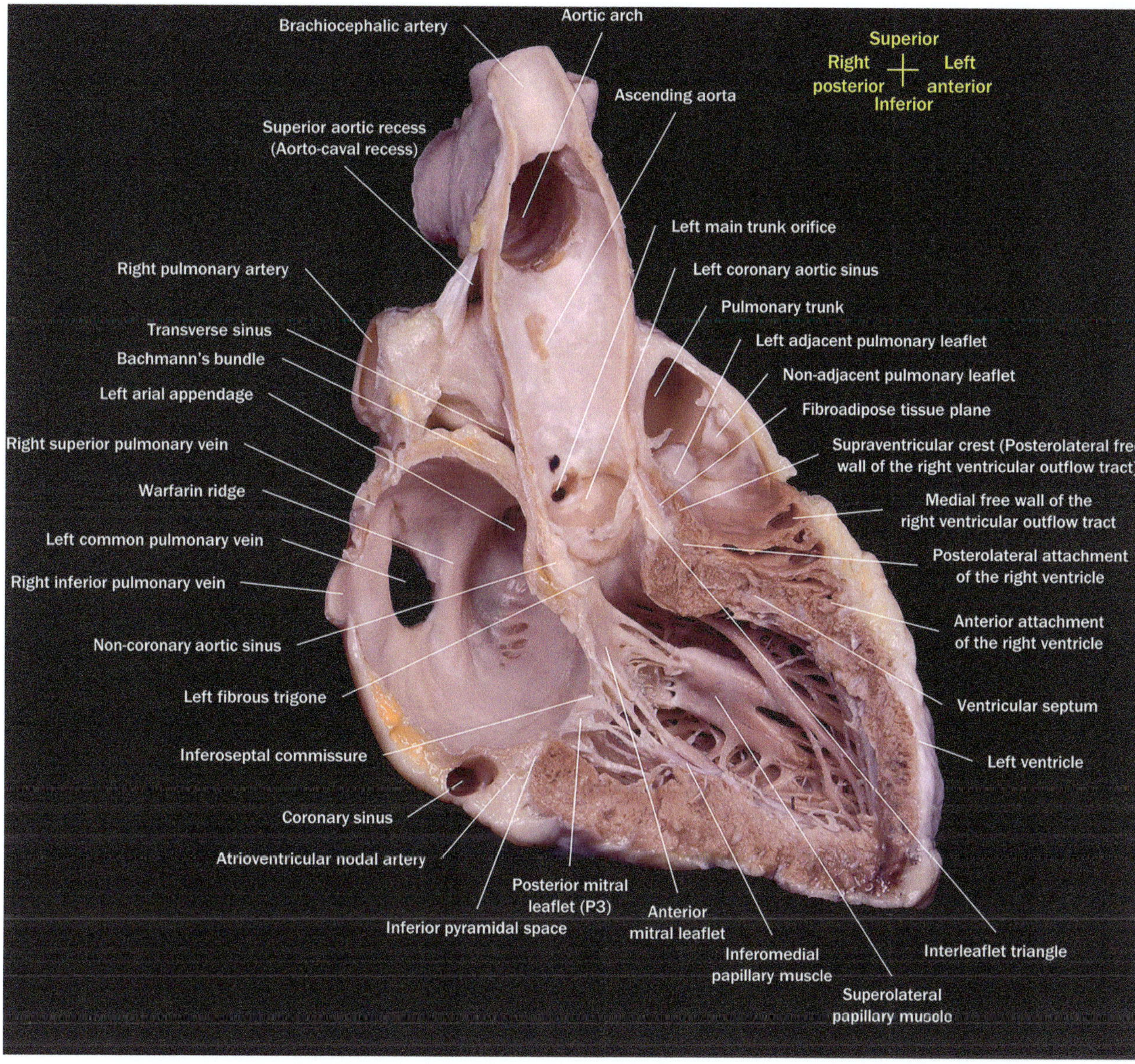

Fig. 6.9 The atrial septum and the inferoseptal process of the left ventricle are removed to show the anterior and posterior mitral leaflets. Note the close proximity of the left atrium and noncoronary aortic sinus. The chorda tendineae originating from the inferomedial papillary muscle supports the medial part of the mitral valve around the inferoseptal commissure. The chorda tendineae originating from the superolateral papillary muscle anchors the lateral part of the mitral valve around the superolateral commissure. The inferoseptal commissure is located at the inferior end of the right fibrous trigone. The coronary sinus is located inferior to the left atrium, embedded in the right posterior part of the inferior pyramidal space that continues to the left atrioventricular groove. The atrioventricular nodal artery originating from the left circumflex artery is noted. It ascends within this inferior pyramidal space toward the atrioventricular node, anterior to the coronary sinus orifice.[49] Orifices of the right pulmonary veins are on this plane. Orifice of the left common pulmonary vein is observed behind the orifice of the left atrial appendage, intervened by the Warfarin ridge. The right pulmonary artery lies on the roof/dome of the left atrium. The left fibrous trigone, supporting the lateral part of the anterior mitral leaflet, is related to the left coronary aortic sinus just posterior to its nadir. Anterior to this left fibrous trigone, free wall of the left ventricle supports the anterior half of the left coronary aortic sinus and interleaflet triangle between the right and left coronary aortic sinuses. Inferior end of the left fibrous trigone corresponds to the location of the superolateral commissure of the mitral valve.

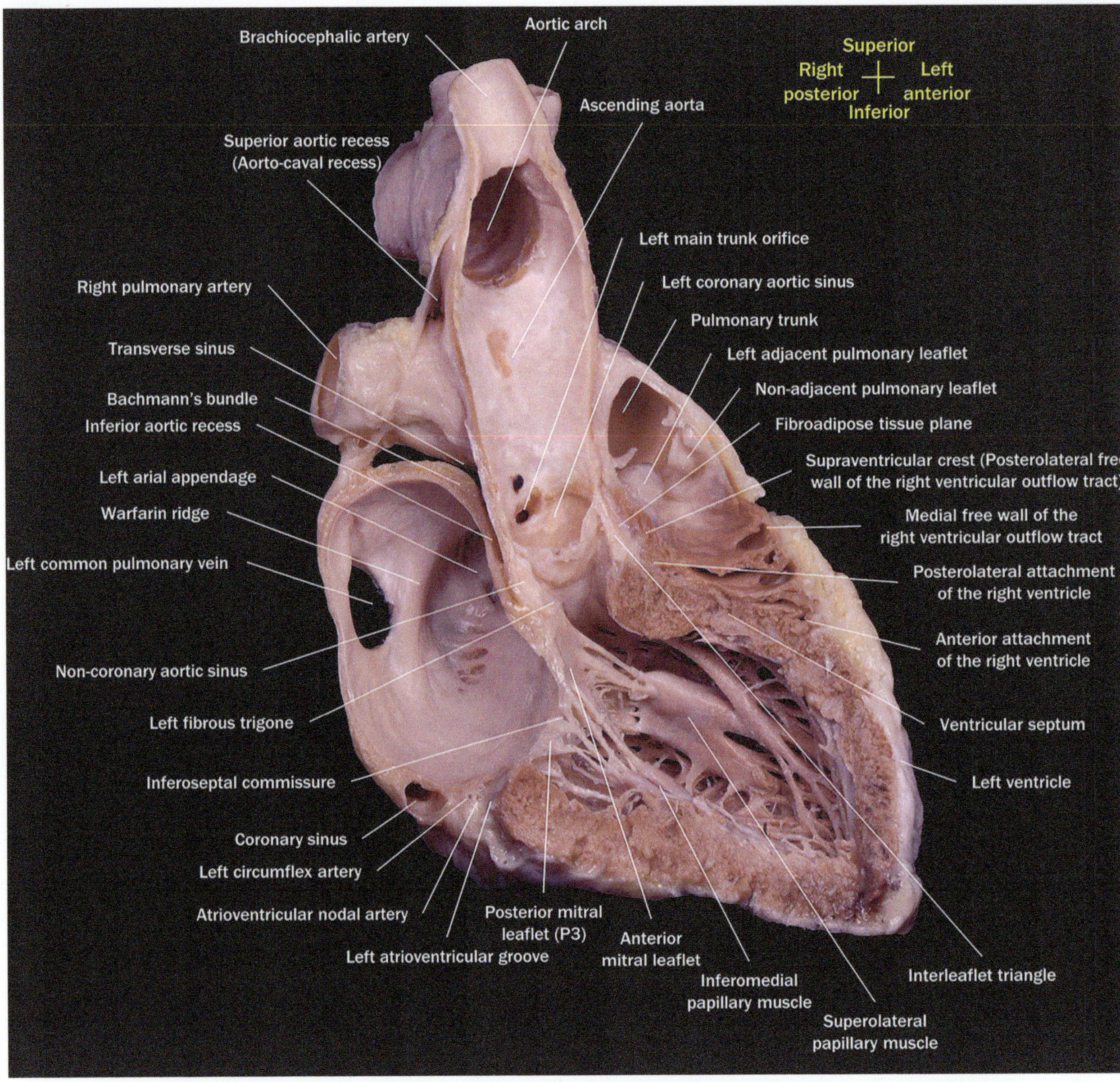

Fig. 6.10 The plane cut of the left atrium is placed backward at the level between the right and left pulmonary veins. Note the coronary sinus is located distant from the mitral annulus. The thickness of the left atrial wall shows variation.[50] The roof/dome and Bachmann bundle show relatively thick myocardium compared to the rest of the left atrium. Bachmann bundle is located at the superior part of the anterior wall of the left atrium and faces the ascending aorta intervened by the transverse sinus.[2,17] The atrioventricular nodal artery originates from the left circumflex artery. The coronary sinus is located behind the left circumflex artery and is exclusively related to the inferior left atrial vestibule. The transverse sinus extends posterior beneath the right pulmonary artery. The fibrous tissue connecting the left atrial roof and the right pulmonary artery is the location where the reflections of the oblique and transverse sinuses meet each other.[2,15,31]

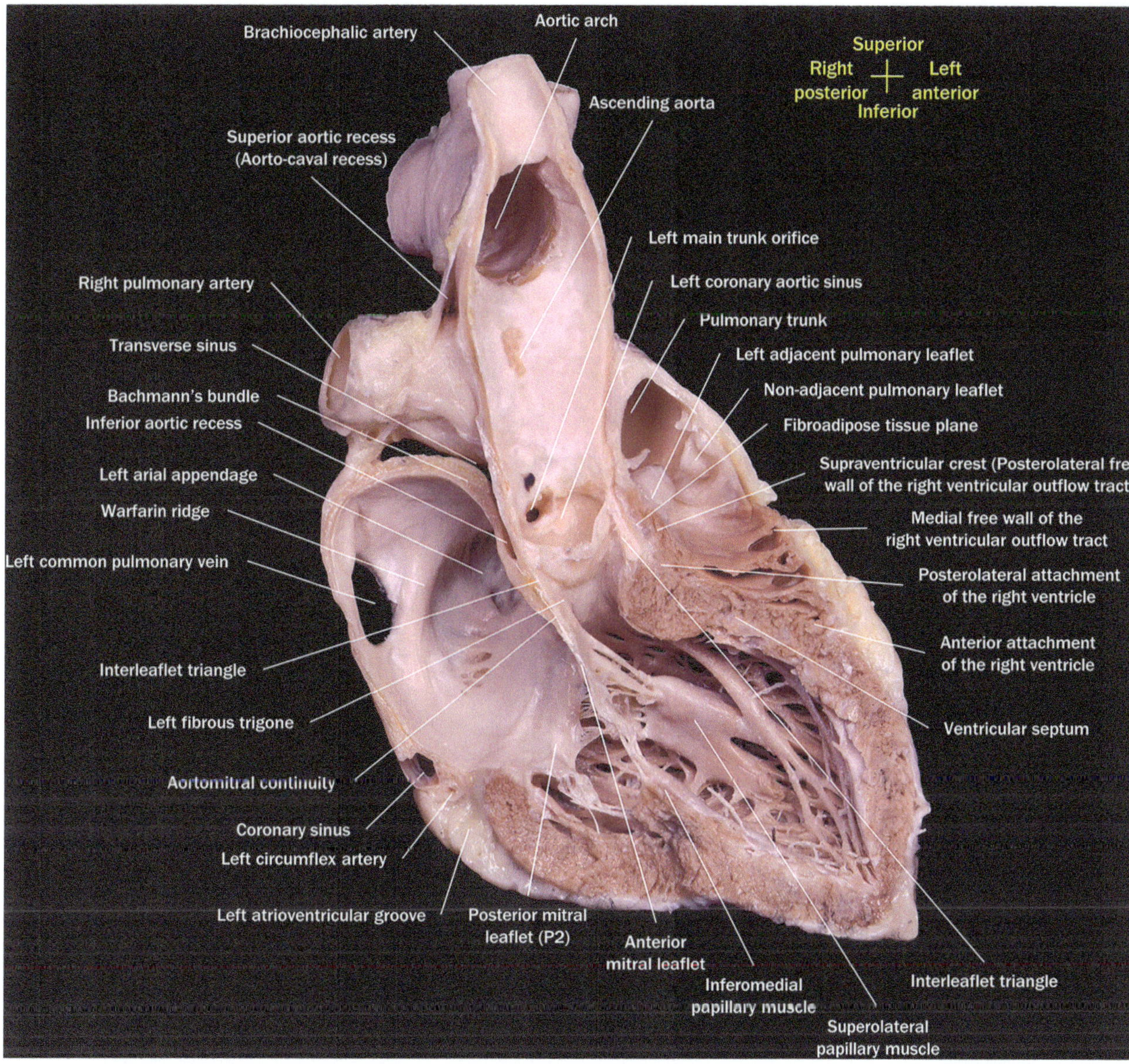

Fig. 6.11 Basal inferior left ventricular wall with medial scallop of the posterior mitral leaflet is removed to show the middle scallop of the posterior mitral leaflet (P2). Noncoronary aortic sinus is also removed to show the interleaflet triangle between the left and noncoronary aortic sinuses. Note the ventricular septum in this section separates the superiorly located right ventricular outflow tract from the inferiorly located left ventricle. The apex of the interleaflet triangle faces the anterior wall of the left atrium, intervened by the inferior aortic recess of the transverse sinus. The interleaflet triangle and anterior wall of the left atrium fuse together to create the aortomitral continuity at the base of the anterior mitral leaflet. The aortomitral continuity, also referred to as the aortomitral curtain[51] or intervalvular fibrosa/fibrous body,[52] generally lacks ventricular myocardium. In the field of electrophysiology, the left ventricular free wall at the left fibrous trigone, corresponding to the left ventricular summit, has been mistakenly deemed as the aortomitral continuity,[53] which is anatomically inaccurate and confusing. The left fibrous trigone supports the left side margin of the anterior mitral leaflet close to the nadir of the left coronary aortic sinus. Localized thinning of the cardiac apex can be noted. This is the normal finding that requires precaution during any invasive procedures within the left ventricle.[54] The median thickness and area of the left ventricular apical thinning are 0.9 mm and 5.6 mm^2, respectively. This area approximately equivalent to the cross-sectional areas of 8.0-F catheter.[54]

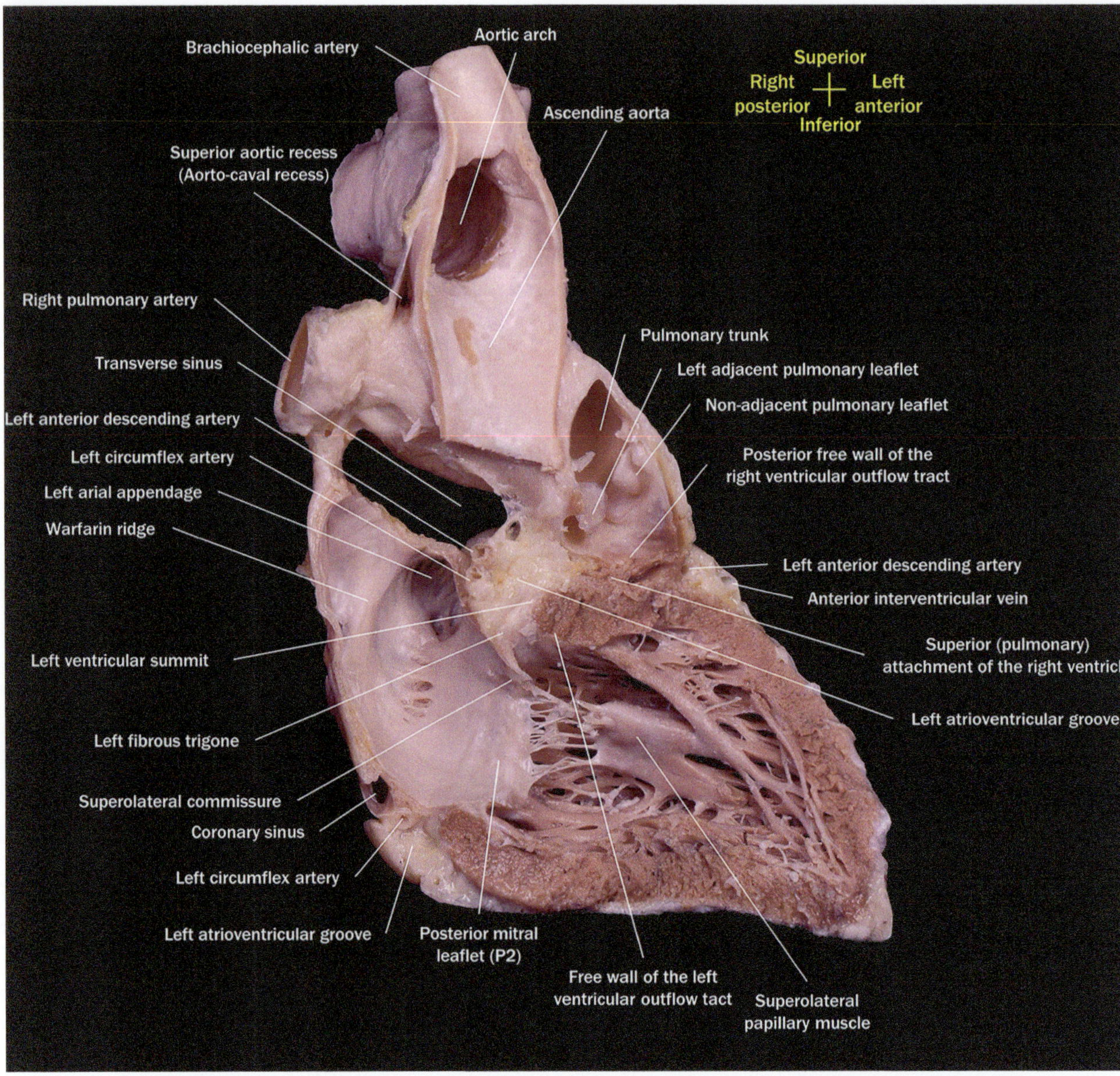

Fig. 6.12 The left coronary aortic sinus, proximal part of the ascending aorta, and posterolateral free wall of the right ventricular outflow are removed to show the structure behind the left coronary aortic sinus. Note the thin crest of the left ventricular summit beneath the thick left atrioventricular groove. The posterior free wall of the right ventricular outflow tract is located above the superior attachment of the right ventricle to the left ventricle[2,17] between the posterolateral and anterior attachments of the right ventricle. At this posterior free wall, the right ventricular outflow tract starts to detach from the basal left ventricle. This part is also referred to as the elevated infundibulum.[2] Posterior free wall of the right ventricular outflow tract faces the left ventricular summit, and its medial free wall is facing the proximal part of the anterior interventricular groove.[2,17] The left anterior descending artery skirts posterolateral to the elevated infundibulum before descending within the anterior interventricular groove accompanied by the anterior interventricular vein. Left-side entrance of the transverse sinus between the pulmonary trunk and left atrial appendage can be recognized. The left coronary aortic sinus faces thick adipose tissue of the proximal part of the left atrioventricular groove, which is located on the left ventricular summit. The proximal left atrioventricular groove contains the left anterior descending artery and left circumflex artery. This compartment, referred to as the left coronary fossa,[2] is surrounded by the left atrial anterior wall posteriorly, left atrial appendage laterally, pulmonary root and trunk anterosuperiorly, left fibrous trigone and left ventricular summit inferiorly, and left coronary aortic sinus medially. The anterior half of the left coronary aortic sinus and interleaflet triangle between the right and left coronary aortic sinuses are supported by the free wall of the left ventricular outflow tract.[3,55] The posterior half of the left coronary aortic sinus is supported by the left fibrous trigone, the firm fibrous tissue supporting the lateral part of the anterior mitral leaflet.[48]

PROGRESSIVE VIRTUAL DISSECTION OF THE HEART VIEWED FROM THE LEFT ANTERIOR OBLIQUE DIRECTION

We performed computed tomography of the heart fixed with pressure-perfusion fixation method using a commercially available 64-multidetector-row computed tomography scanner (SOMATOM Definition AS, Siemens Healthcare, Forchheim, Germany). All the images were reconstructed using a commercially available workstation (Ziostation2, version 2.9.8.4; AMIN Co., Ltd., Tokyo, Japan; Ziosoft Inc., Tokyo, Japan) with post-hoc modification using dedicated volume-rendering software (SARA-Engine, pita4 mobile LLC, San Francisco, CA). Progressive virtual dissection[18] was performed from the apical (ventricular) side toward the basal (atrial) side. Images were demonstrated from the left anterior oblique direction (Figs. 6.13–6.25, Video 6.2).

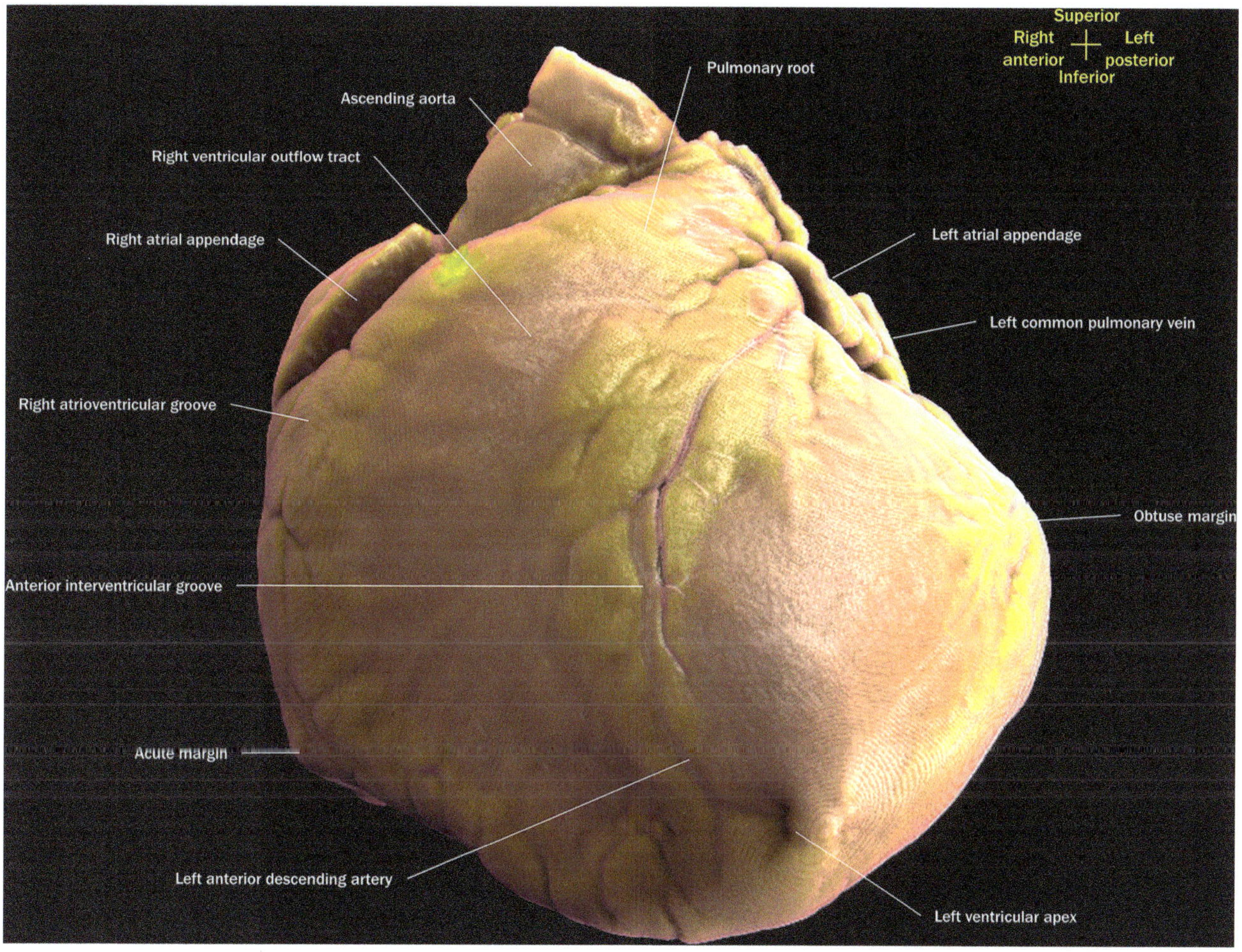

Fig. 6.13 The right heart except the outflow tract is seen on the left , and the left heart except the outflow tract is seen on the right divided by the anterior interventricular groove.[3] From this direction, the lateral wall of the chambers can be separated from the septal/medial wall of the chambers, except the outflow tract. The atria and ventricles cannot be separated from this direction. Nearly en face view of the atrioventricular valves is expected, if additional caudal angulation is applied against the cardiac axis.[3] The right ventricular outflow tract overrides the left ventricular outflow tract and the aortic root in crisscross fashion. Thus, the ventricular septum at the level of the outflow tract is located posteroinferior to the right ventricular outflow tract.[5] In contrast, at the level of the inflow tract and apical component, the ventricular septum is located medially relative to the bilateral free wall of both ventricles. The right atrial appendage covers the lateral side of the aortic root and is located on the right atrioventricular groove. In contrast, the left atrial appendage covers the lateral side of the pulmonary root and is located on the left atrioventricular groove. The left anterior descending artery is running within the anterior interventricular groove. Thus, apical segment of the left anterior descending artery is located medial to the left ventricular apex,[2] which commonly shows focal wall thinning[54] with vortex-shaped myocardial arrangement.[2] The acute margin of the heart is the margin between the right ventricular lateral free wall and right ventricular inferior free wall on the diaphragmatic surface. The obtuse margin of the heart corresponds to the lateral free wall of the left ventricle.[37]

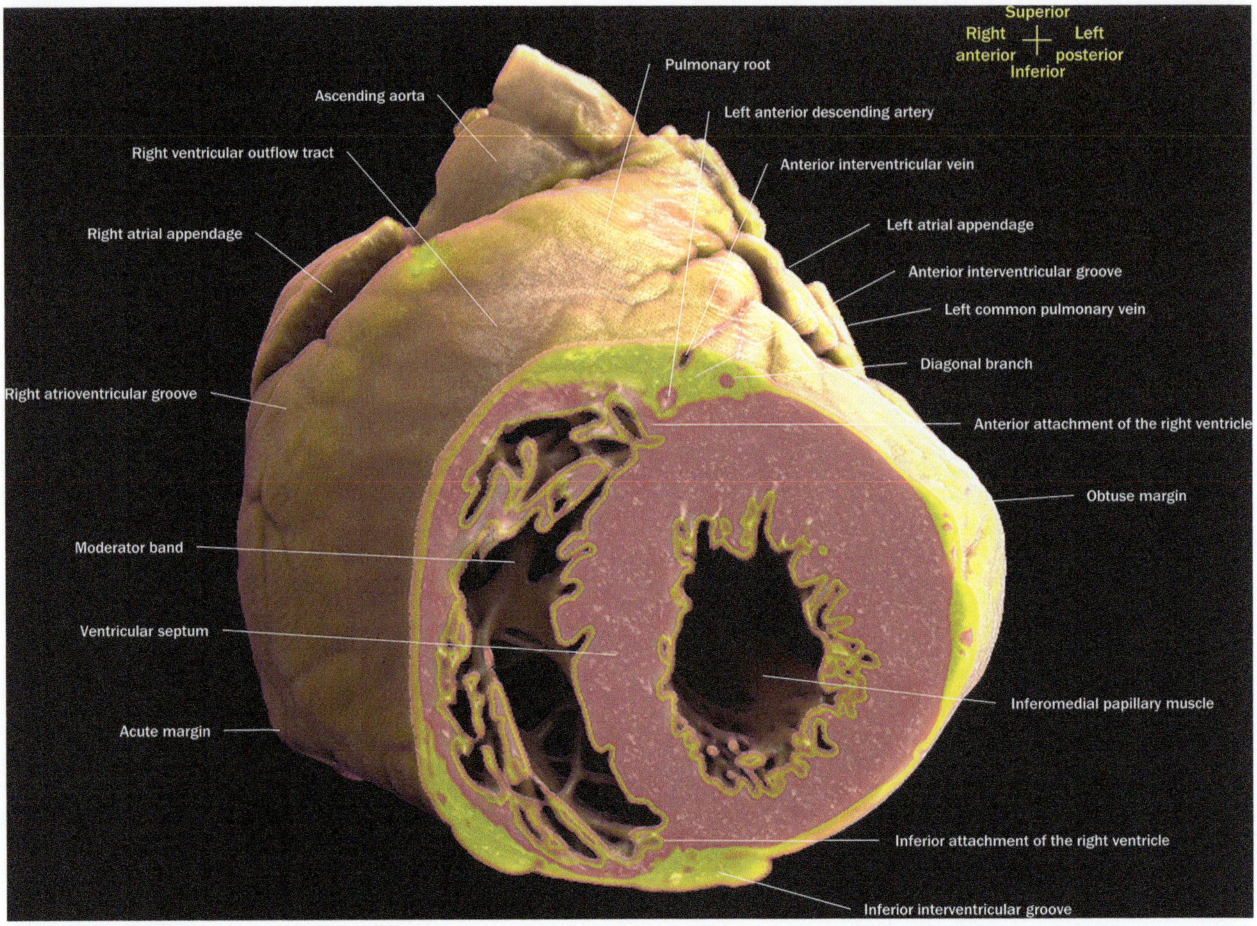

Fig. 6.14 Plane cut is performed at the level of the apical trabecular region. Note the thinness of the right ventricular free wall. The apical trabeculations in the left ventricle are fine. However, the apical trabeculations in the right ventricle are coarse.[56] The left anterior descending artery and anterior interventricular vein run within the anterior interventricular groove. The anterior attachment of the right ventricle[2,17] is adjacent to the anterior interventricular groove. Inferior attachment of the right ventricle[2,17] is located adjacent to the inferior interventricular groove. The diagonal branch is located on the anterior segment of the left ventricle.[17,57] The inferomedial papillary muscle is located at the margin between the inferior and inferolateral segments of the left ventricle.[7]

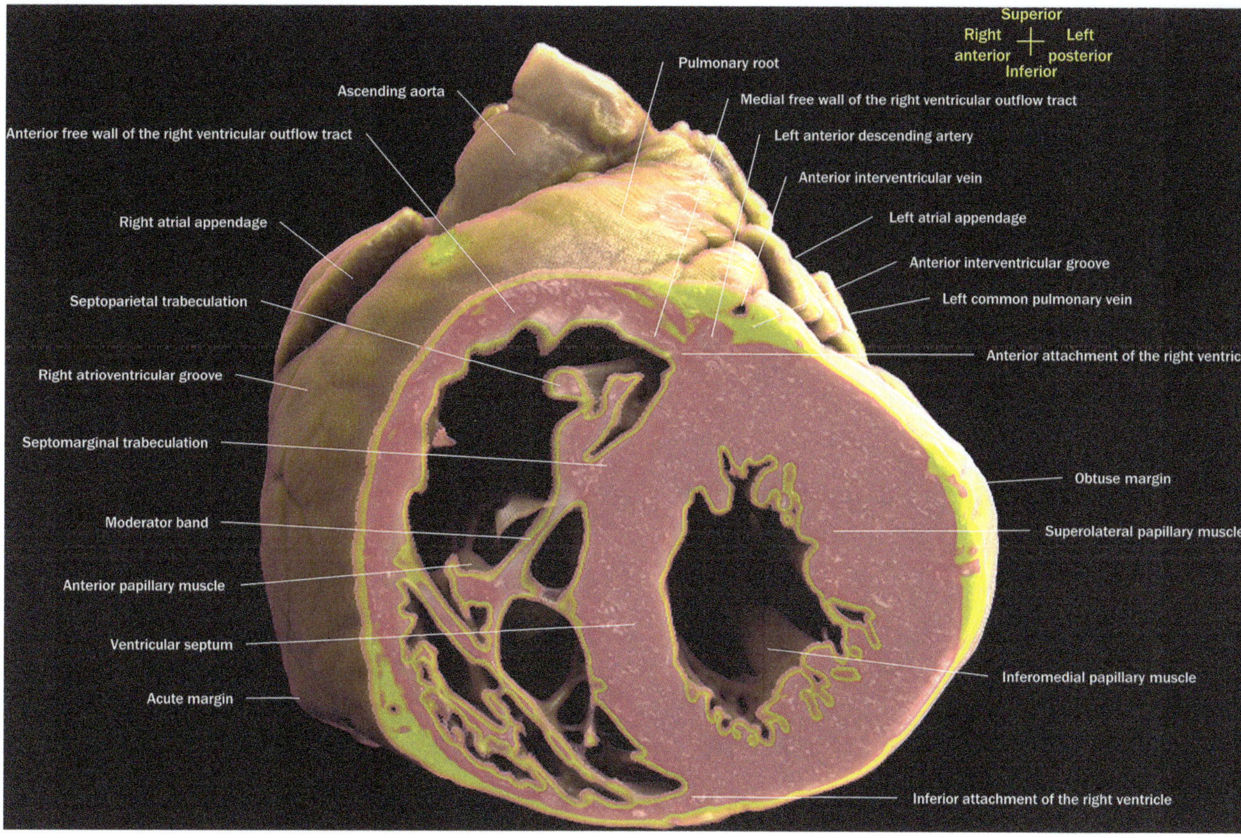

Fig. 6.15 Plane cut is made at the level of the moderator band. Note the trabeculations are less prominent in the right ventricular outflow tract except the septoparietal trabeculation. The moderator band arises from the septomarginal trabeculation. The moderator band continues to the base of the anterior papillary muscle after traversing the mid-right ventricle. All of these trabeculations contain the route of the right bundle branch, before it ramifies toward the right ventricular outflow tract, lateral free wall, apex, septum, and supraventricular crest.[2] The base of the anterior papillary muscle is supported by multiple apical trabeculations. Above the anterior attachment of the right ventricle, the medial free wall of the right ventricular outflow tract faces the anterior interventricular groove. This part, even if it is sometimes referred to as being "septal" viewed from the left anterior oblique direction, is actually not the septum but the free wall. This is the common site of right ventricular outflow tract perforation. On the left ventricular side, the superolateral papillary muscle is located at the anterolateral segment of the left ventricle.[7]

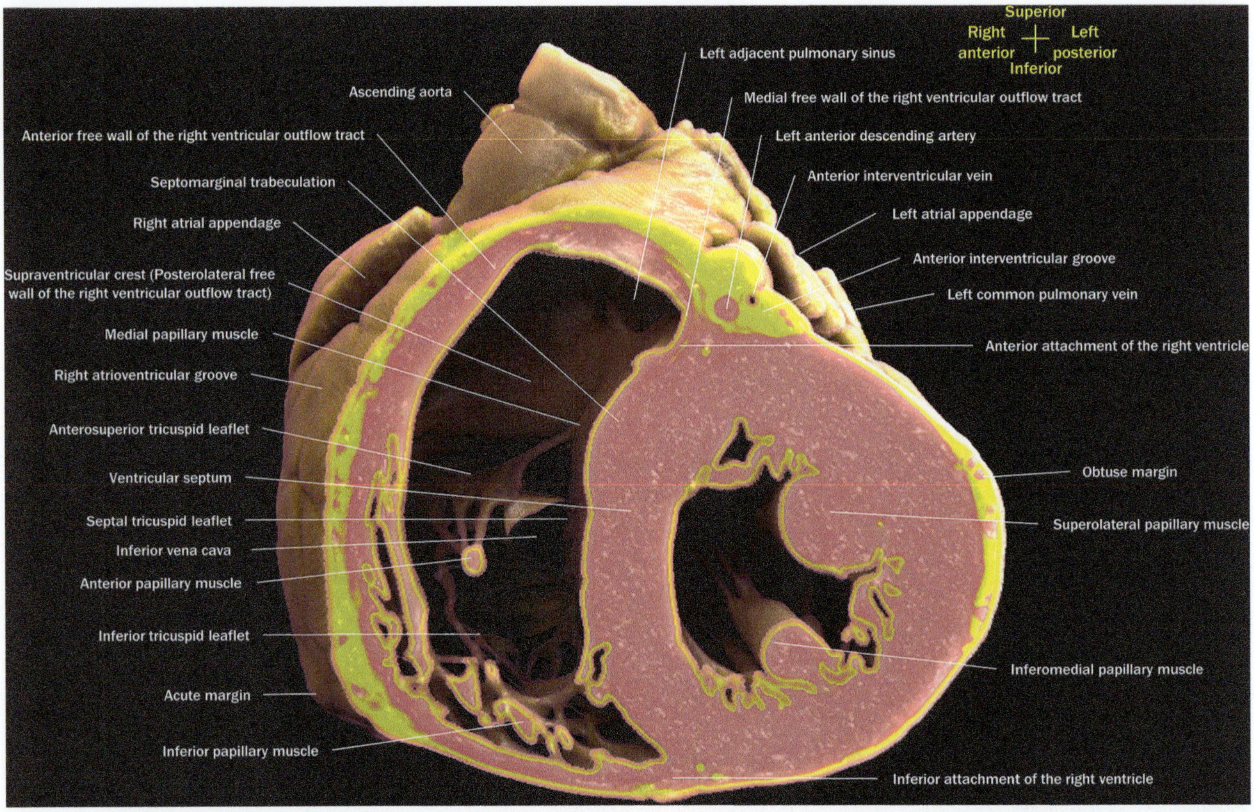

Fig. 6.16 The next plane cut is at the level of the left ventricular papillary muscle. Also, note the thinness of the medial free wall of the right ventricular outflow tract facing the anterior interventricular groove. In the right ventricle, the septomarginal trabeculation is observed as the focal rightward bulging of the ventricular septum at the anteroseptal segment of the left ventricle. At the base of this septomarginal trabeculation, small medial papillary muscle gives rise of the chorda tendinea to the medial part of the anterosuperior tricuspid leaflet. The chorda tendineae from the anterior papillary muscle anchors both anterosuperior and inferior tricuspid leaflets at their commissure.[26] The inferior tricuspid leaflet is also anchored by the inferior papillary muscle. The supraventricular crest traverse from the septal side to the lateral side at the posterolateral free wall of the right ventricular outflow tract between the tricuspid valve and pulmonary valve.[5] This structure is also referred to as the ventriculoinfundibular fold. In the left ventricle, the superolateral papillary muscle and inferomedial papillary muscle is almost aligned vertically on the free wall side.[7] The superolateral papillary muscle is located in the anterolateral segment of the left ventricle. The inferomedial papillary muscle is located at the margin between the inferior and inferolateral segments. The inferolateral segment between both papillary muscles is conventionally referred to as the posterior wall during the transthoracic echocardiography,[3] as the segment is visualized as the most distant region from the probe located in front of the right ventricular outflow tract during parasternal short-axis view. However, use of "posterior" for describing any part of the left ventricular segment has been deemed attitudinally inappropriate,[58] and it is no longer recommended by the guideline.[59] Rich trabeculations are observed on the free wall of the both ventricles, compared to smooth endocardial surface of the bilateral side of the ventricular septum and right ventricular outflow tract.

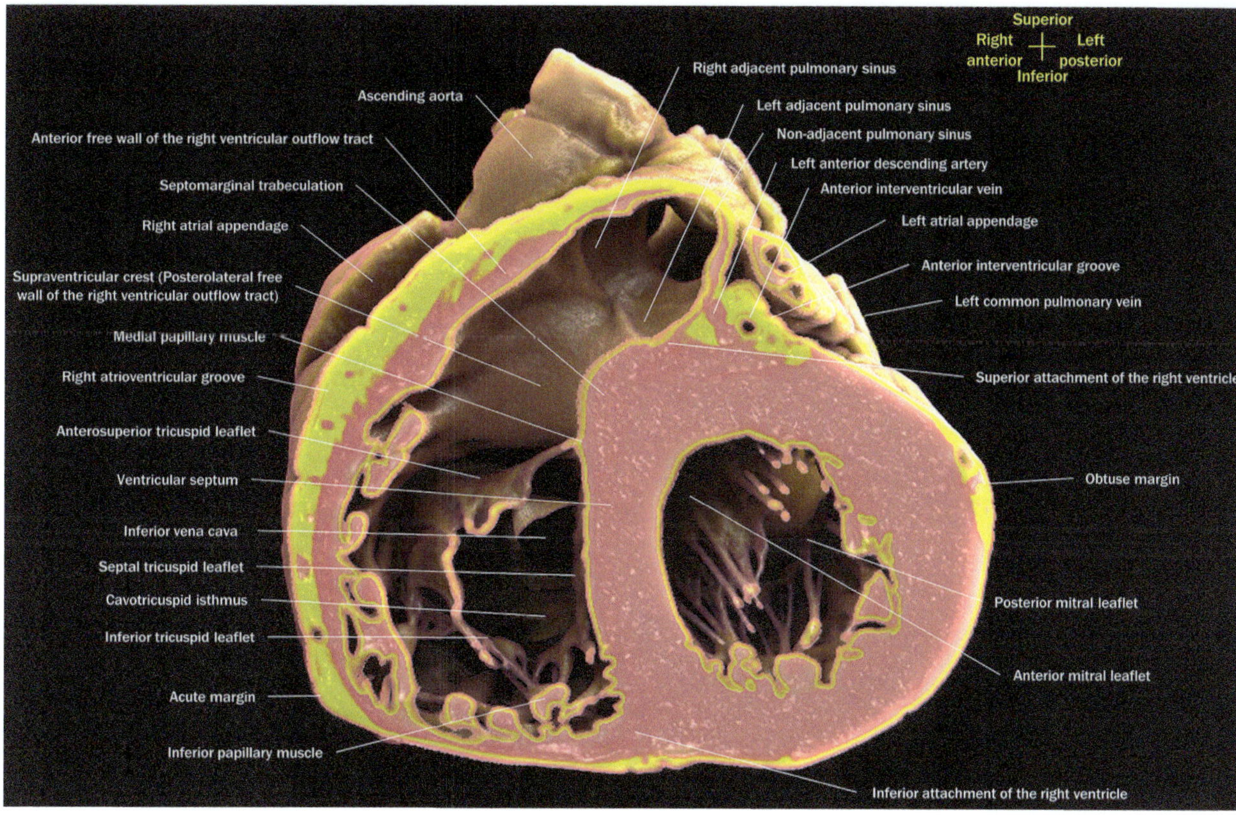

Fig. 6.17 The plane cut is then applied at the level of the medial papillary muscle located at the base of the septomarginal trabeculation located at the right-side basal anteroseptum. Note the smooth and less trabeculated right ventricular outflow tract and right-side ventricular septum, compared to the trabeculated free wall of the right ventricular inlet. The proximal right bundle branch runs near the base of the medial papillary muscle. At the level of the right ventricular outflow tract, ventricular septum, corresponding to the septomarginal trabeculation, is located left posteroinferior relative to the infundibulum, as the right ventricular outflow tract overrides the left ventricular outflow tract in crisscross fashion.[1,3,37] The right ventricular outflow is located left anterior to the aortic root. The tricuspid valve is separated from the pulmonary valve by the supraventricular crest. The supraventricular crest is orthogonal to the septomarginal trabeculation. Laterally, the supraventricular crest continues into multiple trabeculations on the free wall. The inferior papillary muscle gives multiple chorda tendineae at the commissure between the inferior and septal tricuspid leaflets. Behind the tricuspid valve, the inferior vena cava and cavotricuspid isthmus can be observed. The inferior vena cava is located medially within the right atrium along the atrial septum. In the left ventricle, the alignment of the anterior and posterior mitral leaflets is orthogonal to the alignment of the superolateral and inferomedial papillary muscles (Fig. 6.16). The superolateral and inferomedial papillary muscles give chorda tendinea to lateral and medial part of both anterior and posterior mitral leaflets, respectively. Thus, the inferoseptal commissure is anchored by the inferomedial papillary muscle, and the superolateral commissure is anchored by the superolateral papillary muscle.

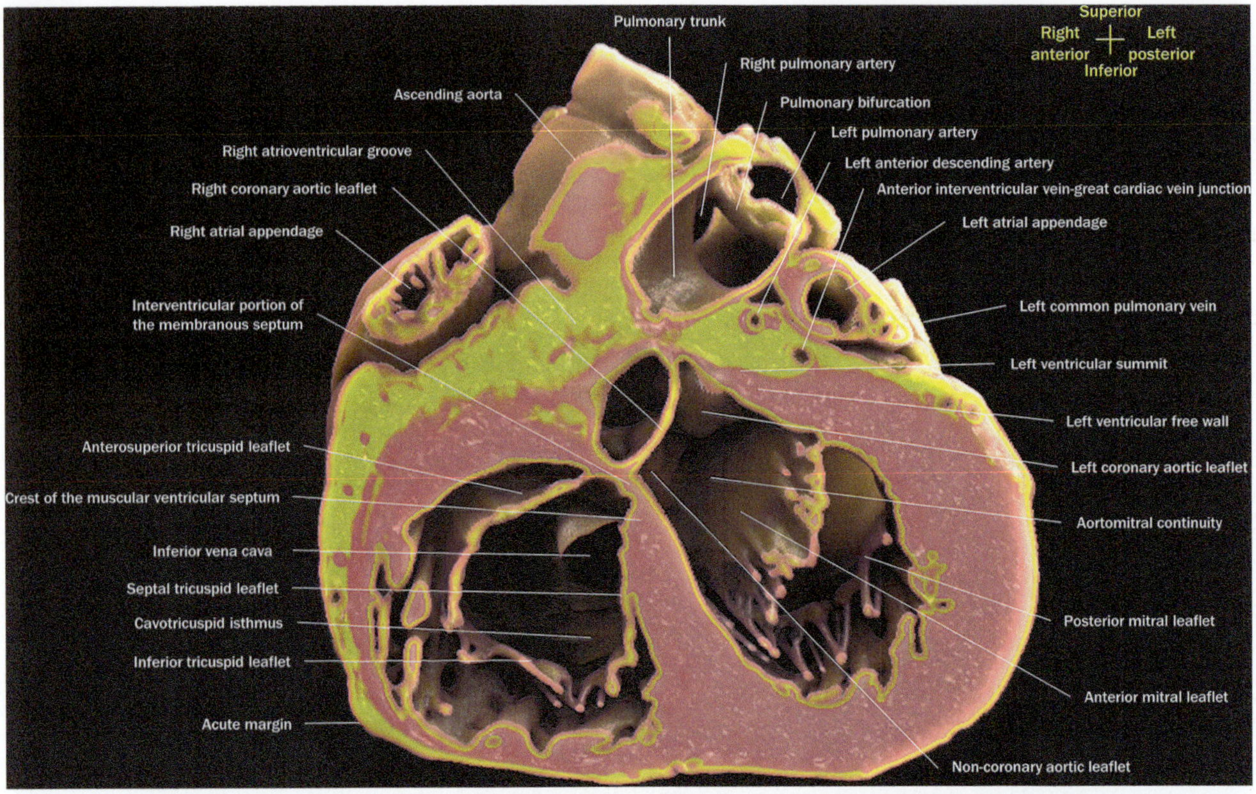

Fig. 6.18 Plane cut is made at the level of the right coronary aortic sinus. Note the centrally located right coronary aortic sinus at the base of both ventricles. Compared to Fig. 6.17, it is noted that the medial part of the supraventricular crest, where it meets the basal part of the septomarginal trabeculation, covers the right coronary aortic sinus. The interventricular portion of the membranous septum is located inferior to the right coronary aortic sinus. It is located at the commissure between the anterosuperior and septal tricuspid leaflets, superior to the crest of the muscular ventricular septum. The interventricular portion of the membranous septum divides the right ventricular inflow tract from the left ventricular outflow tract. The septal tricuspid leaflet, with its opening position, almost attaches to the right-side ventricular septum. Left ventricular sectional plane shows that the orifice of the mitral valve is not aligned horizontally, but it is quite oblique against the horizontal plane.[7] The left ventricular basal section shows reversed C-mark appearance. The opening segment of the reversed C-mark, corresponding to the left ventricular outflow tract, is located in the right anterosuperior position of the left ventricular section, behind the base of the septomarginal trabeculation (Fig. 6.17). The left ventricular free wall at the left ventricular summit supports the interleaflet triangle between the right and left coronary aortic sinuses. The aortic valve, specifically the non- and left coronary aortic leaflets, is in continuity with the anterior mitral leaflet through the aortomitral continuity. Free apices of the right and left atrial appendages are located on the thick right and left atrioventricular grooves, respectively, intervened by the pericardial space. These spaces work as the anterior entrance to the transverse sinus.[15]

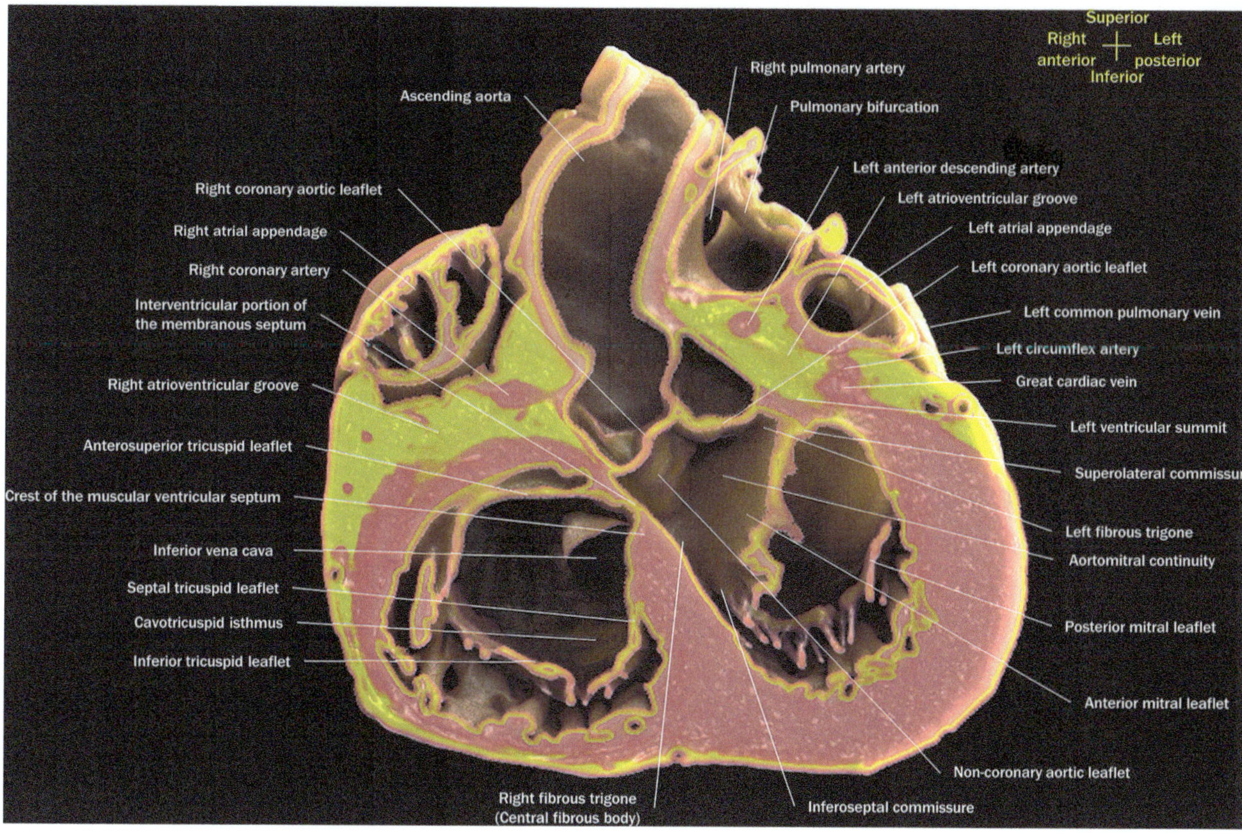

Fig. 6.19 The plane cut is advanced toward the level of the left coronary aortic sinus. Note the angulation created between the membranous septum and the crest of the ventricular septum, where the His-bundle electrode is usually fixed. The bundle of His, specifically the branching portion, is generally located on the crest of the ventricular septum at the inferior margin of the interventricular portion of the membranous septum.[2,8,43] The septal attachment of the septal tricuspid leaflet is located apically compared to the medial attachment of the medial scallop of the posterior mitral leaflet.[7] The right fibrous trigone, also referred to as the central fibrous body,[2,47] extends inferiorly from the nadir of the noncoronary aortic sinus. Its inferior end corresponds to the inferoseptal commissure of the mitral valve. The thin left ventricular free wall at the left ventricular summit supports the anterior half of the left coronary aortic sinus.[55] Behind this region, the left fibrous trigone extends from the nadir of the left coronary sinus. Its lateral end corresponds to the superolateral commissure of the mitral valve. The posterior halves of the non- and left coronary aortic sinuses continues to the aortomitral continuity at the base of the anterior mitral leaflet. The aortomitral continuity is the partition between the left ventricular outflow tract and the left atrium. It is in continuity with the interleaflet triangle between the non- and left coronary aortic sinuses. Both atrial appendages lie on the thick bilateral atrioventricular grooves intervened by the pericardial space. The medial part of the apex of the right atrial appendage is adjacent to the ascending aorta, whereas the medial part of the left atrial appendage is adjacent to the pulmonary trunk. The proximal left atrioventricular groove, which involves the left coronary artery and great cardiac vein, is surrounded by the left coronary aortic sinus medially, left ventricular summit inferiorly, pulmonary root anteriorly, pulmonary trunk superiorly, and left atrial appendage superolaterally.[2,60] From this view direction, the left atrial appendage, left ventricular summit, and superolateral commissure of the mitral valve are located on the vertical line corresponding to the 12 o'clock of the mitral annulus.

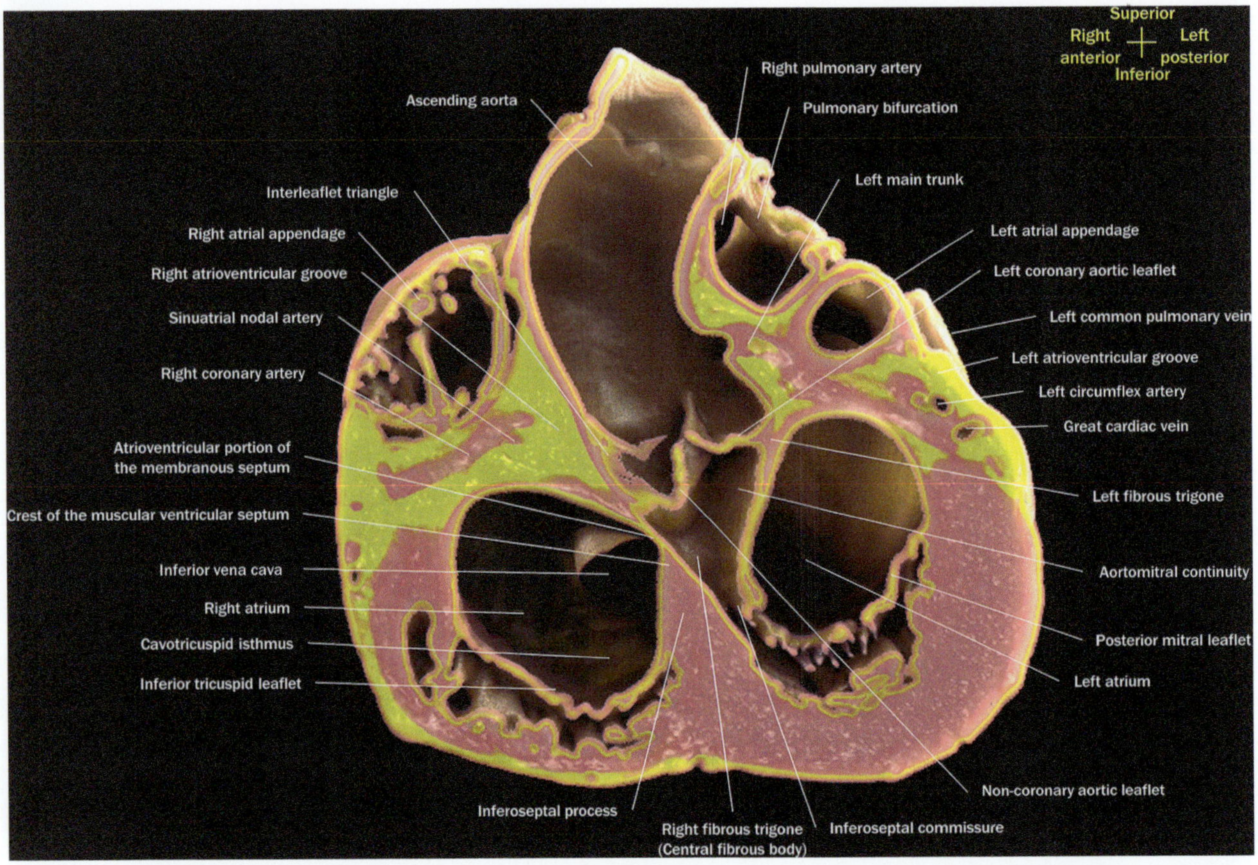

Fig. 6.20 The plane is advanced at the level of the atrioventricular portion of the membranous septum. Note the inferoseptal process divides the right atrium from the left ventricle. The interleaflet triangle between the right and noncoronary aortic sinuses faces the right atrioventricular groove,[6] intervened by the right-side transverse sinus. The atrioventricular portion of the membranous septum is located inferior to the interleaflet triangle. It divides the right atrium from the left ventricular outflow tract. Left laterally, it continues to the medial part of the right fibrous trigone. As indicated in Figs. 6.21, 6.26, and 6.28, the atrioventricular node is located at the right atrial side behind the central fibrous body.[8,61] Thus, the bundle of His, specifically the penetrating portion, penetrates this right fibrous trigone from the right posterior (basal) to left anterior (apical) directions toward the observer to appear on the crest of the ventricular septum at the inferior margin of the atrioventricular portion of the membranous septum.[8] The right atrial appendage is located superior to the right coronary artery. The pulmonary trunk is located superior to the left main trunk of the left coronary artery. The basal inferomedial left ventricular muscle facing the right atrium inferior to the membranous septum is referred to as the inferoseptal process.[40] At the left ventricular side, the inferior part of this inferoseptal process is related to the left ventricular inflow supporting the medial scallop of the posterior mitral leaflet. The superior part of this inferoseptal process is related to the left ventricular outflow medial to the aortomitral continuity. When viewed from this direction, the basal part of the left ventricular outflow tract shows a shape of a reversed pyramid, floored by the aortic valve superiorly, membranous septum and inferoseptal process medially, right fibrous trigone right posteriorly (basally), and aortomitral continuity laterally. The apex of the reversed pyramid corresponds to the inferoseptal commissure of the mitral valve. This apex continues to the subvalvular space of the posterior mitral leaflet,[2,48] also referred to as the mitral annular disjunction.[62,63] The left anterior surface of the pyramid has no wall structure and widely opens toward the middle part of the left ventricle as shown in Figs. 6.16 through 6.19.

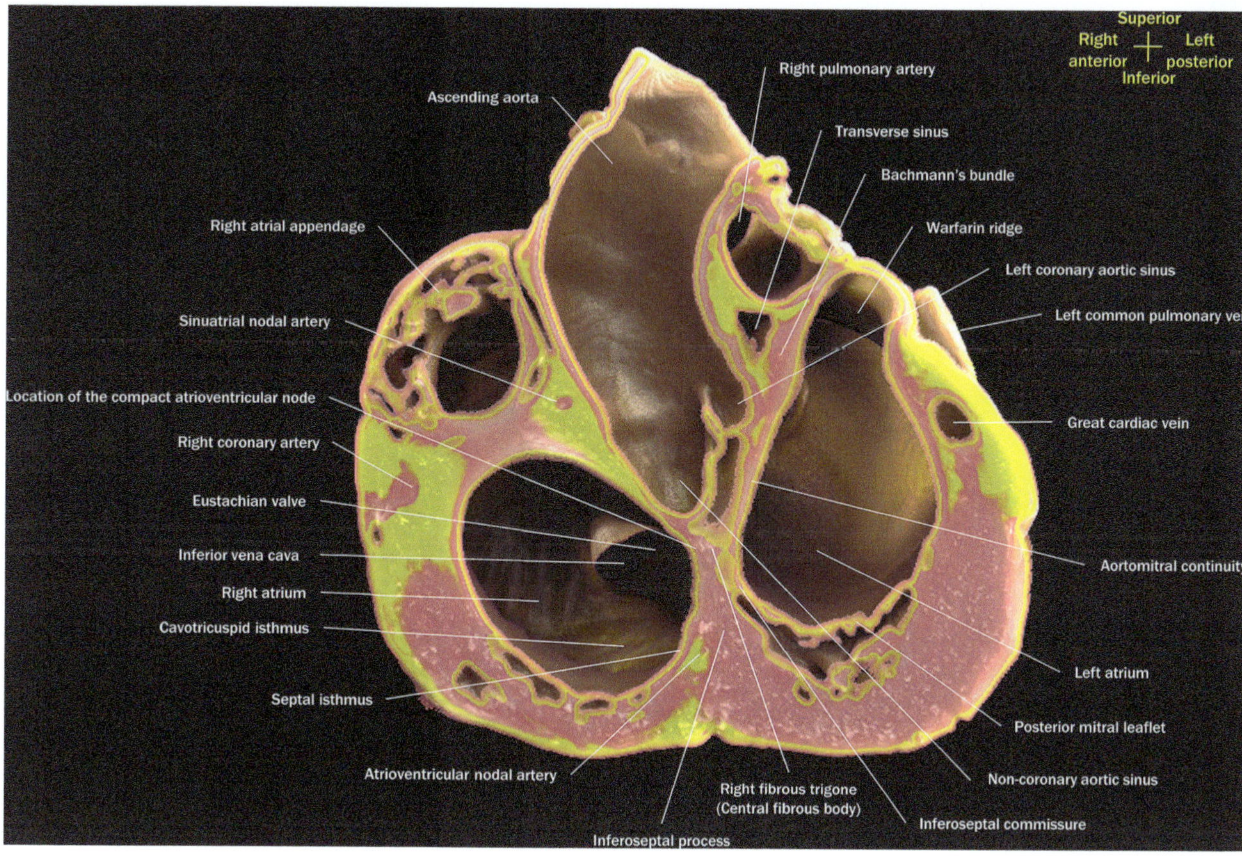

Fig. 6.21 The plane cut is advanced toward the nadir of the noncoronary aortic sinus. Note thin medial wall of the bilateral atria faces the noncoronary aortic sinus.[2,17,34] Thus, at these regions next to the noncoronary aortic sinus, they are the medial free wall of the atria but should not be deemed as the septal wall. The nadir of the noncoronary aortic sinus is supported by the central fibrous body, which is the firm fibrous tissue connecting the aortic root, atrial septum, ventricular septum, anterior mitral leaflet, septal tricuspid leaflet, and tendon of Todaro.[48] It is the central piece of the fibrous skeleton of the heart. The compact atrioventricular node lies on the right atrial side of this central fibrous body,[8,61] within the apex of the inferior pyramidal space wedging from the inferior crux of the heart.[4] The inferoseptal process, originally referred to as the posterosuperior process,[2] is the basal inferomedial left ventricle facing the right atrium.[40] However, it does not directly face the right atrium, but it is intervened by the inferior pyramidal space.[4] This inferior pyramidal space allows the atrioventricular nodal artery to ascend toward the atrioventricular node located between the left ventricle and right atrium.[32] The right atrium facing the inferoseptal process, corresponding the region between the septal tricuspid annulus and the coronary sinus orifice, is the septal isthmus. It is the common location to perform slow pathway modification. It should be noted that this septal isthmus is not seen tangentially from this direction, but rather facing the observer[32] along the funnel-shaped morphology of the septal isthmus continuing to the anterior wall of the coronary sinus (Fig. 6.22). The right sinuatrial nodal artery runs between the atrial appendage and the ascending aorta. The warfarin ridge, also referred to as the left atrial ridge or Coumadin ridge, is located between the orifice of the left atrial appendage and left pulmonary vein.[64] On its epicardial side, this ridge is the fold containing the vein/ligament of Marshall, persistent left superior vena cava if any, and left sinuatrial nodal artery taking the posterior course to the left atrial appendage.[2,65]

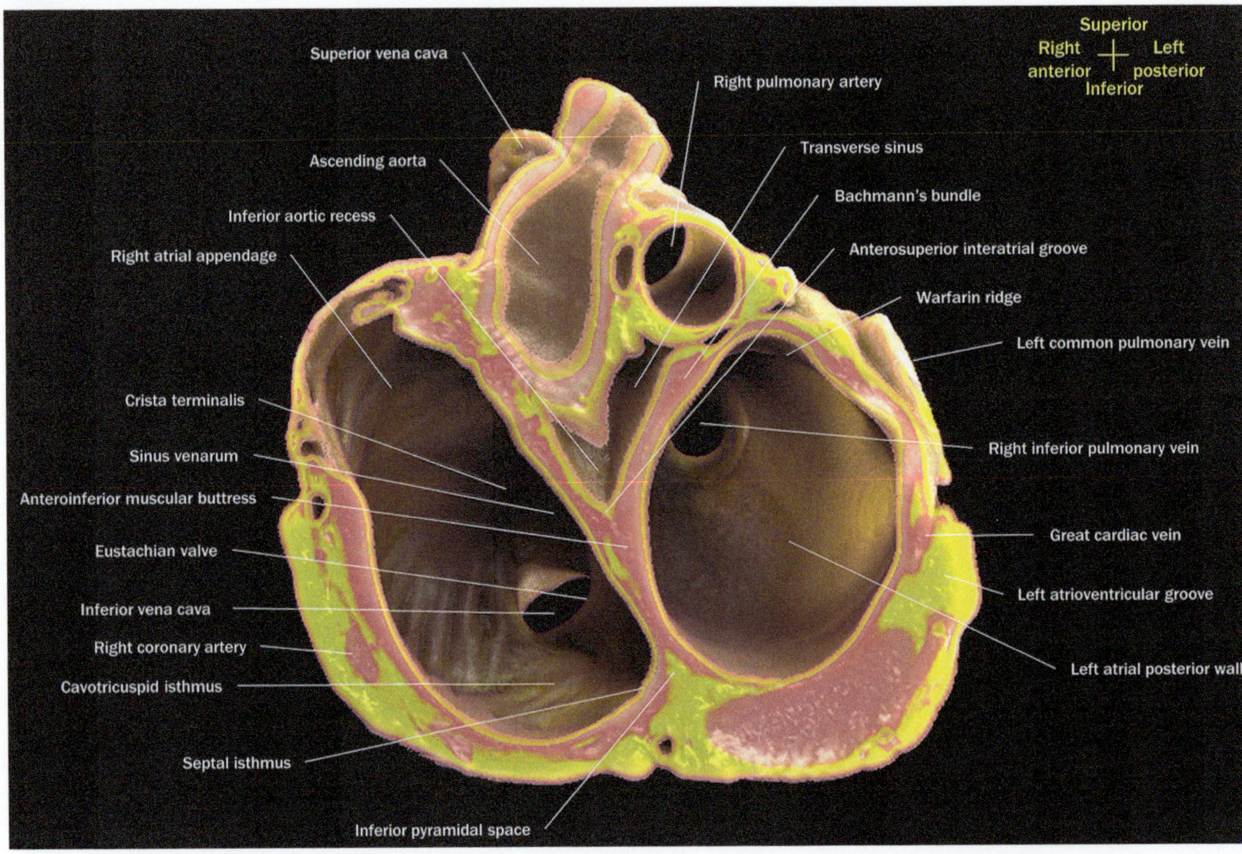

Fig. 6.22 The plane cut at the level of the transverse sinus shows bilateral atrium apical to the location of the fossa ovalis. Note the extensive pectinate muscles in the right atrial appendage compared to those confined within the left atrial appendage (Fig. 6.9). This section is also slightly apical to the coronary sinus orifice. The septal isthmus moved toward medial side compared to location indicated in Fig. 6.21. This indicates the funnel-shaped morphology of the septal isthmus continuing to the anterior wall of the coronary sinus ostium, rather than flat plane seen tangentially to the observer.[32] The right atrial appendage is large, showing extensive pectinate muscle surrounding the atrioventricular junction except the medial part.[66] On the other hand, the left atrial appendage is small, showing limited extension of the pectinate muscle relative to the atrioventricular junction (Fig. 6.19). Warfarin ridge is the epicardial fold containing the ligament of Marshall.[67] It gives off vestigial fold (Fig. 6.34), which is the original location of the left superior vena cava lateral to the left pulmonary artery.[2,15,31] The transverse sinus behind the ascending aorta and aortic root shows V-shaped morphology. The bottom of this V-shaped sinus corresponds to the inferior aortic recess behind the noncoronary aortic sinus.[14,31] It is the right pulmonary artery that is located on the left pulmonary roof/dome. The right pulmonary artery and the left atrial roof are intervened by the transverse sinus extending between them.

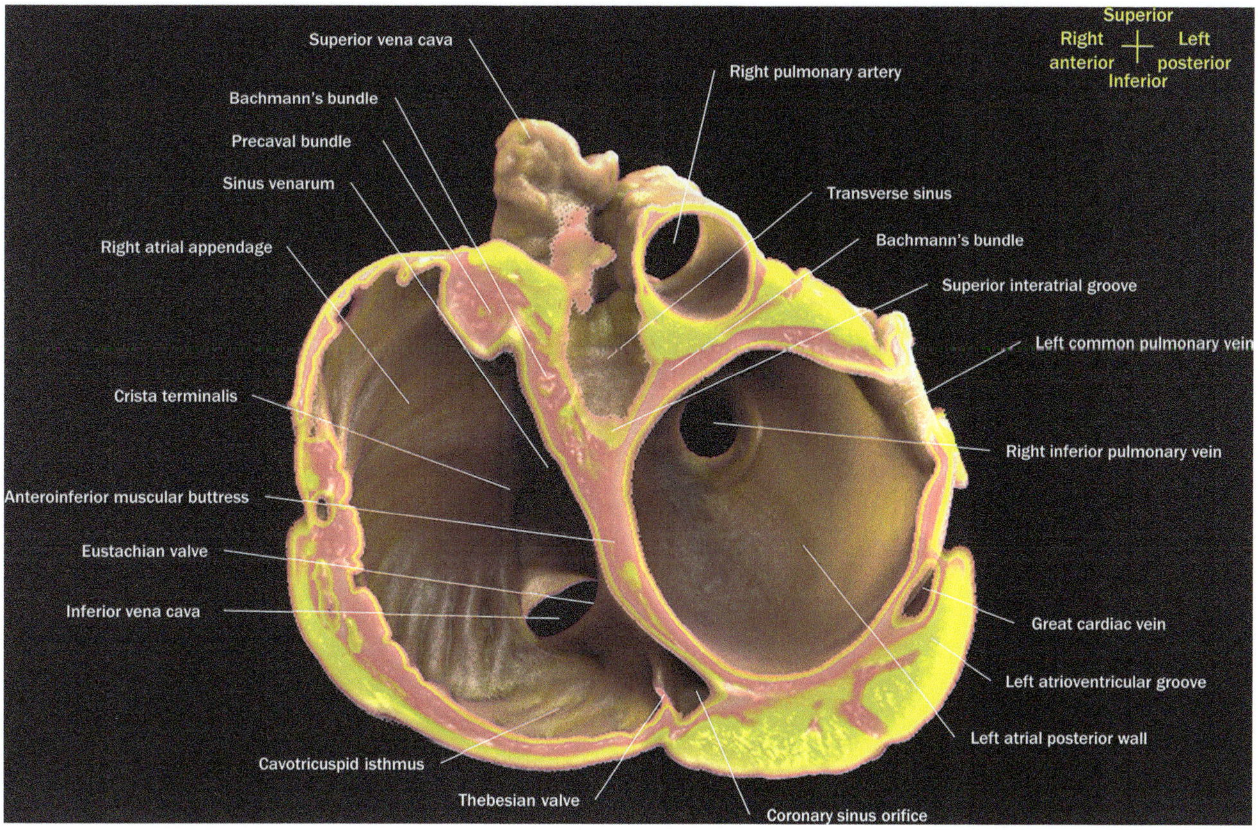

Fig. 6.23 The plane cut at the level of the coronary sinus orifice shows the Thebesian valve guarding the inferior half of the orifice of the coronary sinus.[23] Also, note the thickness of the anteroinferior muscular buttress compared to the primary septum at the floor of the fossa ovalis (Fig. 6.25). The anteroinferior muscular buttress is located between the fossa ovalis and triangle of Koch, and it is the muscular part of the atrial septum.[33,34] This section is still apical to the fossa ovalis. It is orthogonal to the Eustachian valve guarding the orifice of the inferior vena cava.[2,24] The height of the Eustachian valve is prominent in its medial part. Thus, appropriate contact of the ablation catheter during linear ablation along the cavotricuspid isthmus is expected to be more difficult in the medial part than the lateral part.[17] The crista terminalis is located medially relative to the lateral margin of the cardiac silhouette when viewed from this direction. It demarcates the margin between the right atrial appendage and the sinus venarum. The pectinate muscles run obliquely within the cavotricuspid isthmus. This structural anatomy shows wide individual variation and renders the cavotricuspid isthmus being a nonuniform structure.[44] The anteroinferior muscular buttress is the muscular thick part of the atrial septum that connects to the central fibrous body.[33,34] This corresponds to the anterior limbus of the fossa ovalis (Fig. 6.5).

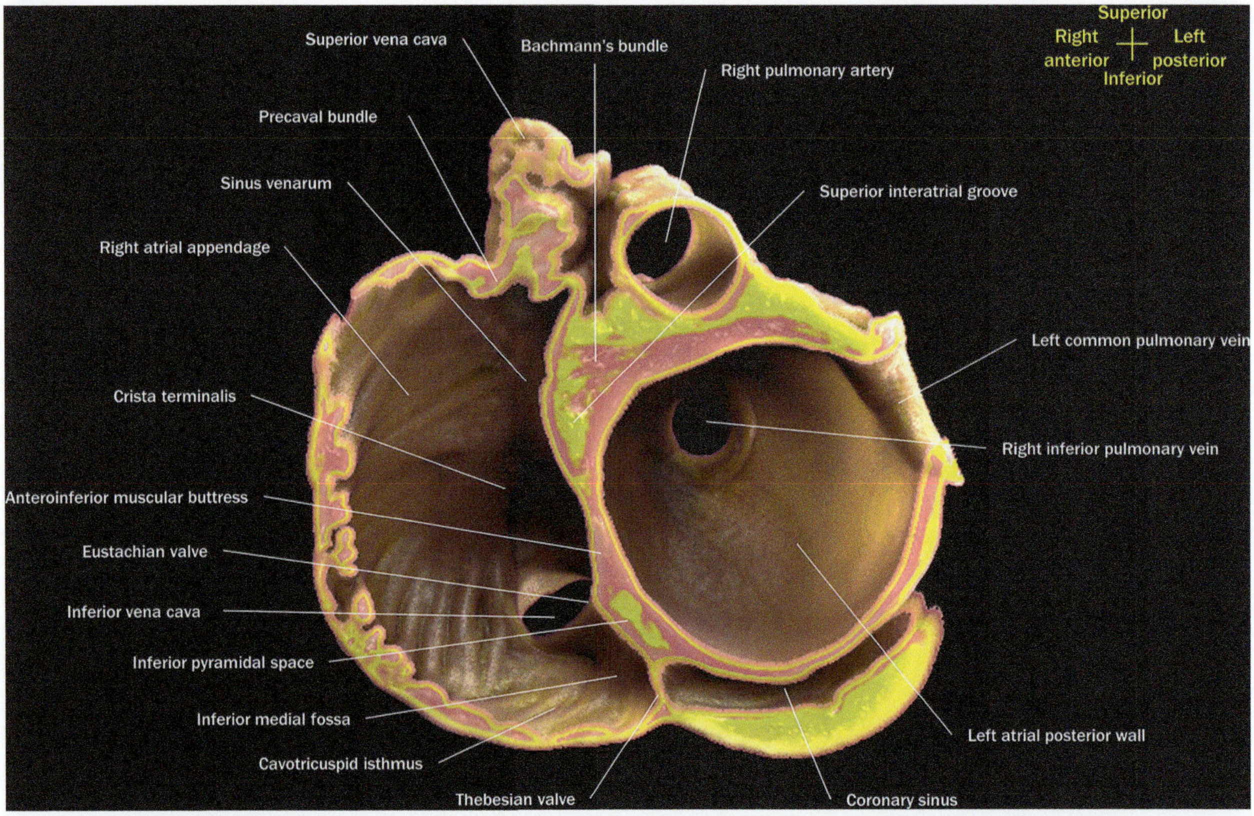

Fig. 6.24 The plane shows coronary sinus. Note the coronary sinus is related to the bottom of the left atrium, and the right pulmonary artery is related to the roof of the left atrium. This section is just at the anterior limbus of the fossa ovalis, corresponding to the anteroinferior muscular buttress.[33,34] In this view, the anteroinferior muscular buttress is sandwiched between the superior interatrial groove and inferior pyramidal space including the coronary sinus. These grooves between the atria, even if it is referred to as the secondary septum, is not the real septum but just the fold including the interatrial epicardial fibroadipose tissue. The Bachmann bundle bridges the superior interatrial fold behind the transverse sinus. It is originated from the precaval bundle, runs at the superior part of the anterior wall near the roof of the left atrium inferior to the right pulmonary artery, and ramifies toward both apical and basal side of the left atrial appendage.[2,17] The deep medial recess between the inferior vena cava and the coronary sinus orifice is referred to as the inferior medial fossa.[2] The bottom of the right atrium is located inferior than the bottom of the left atrium.

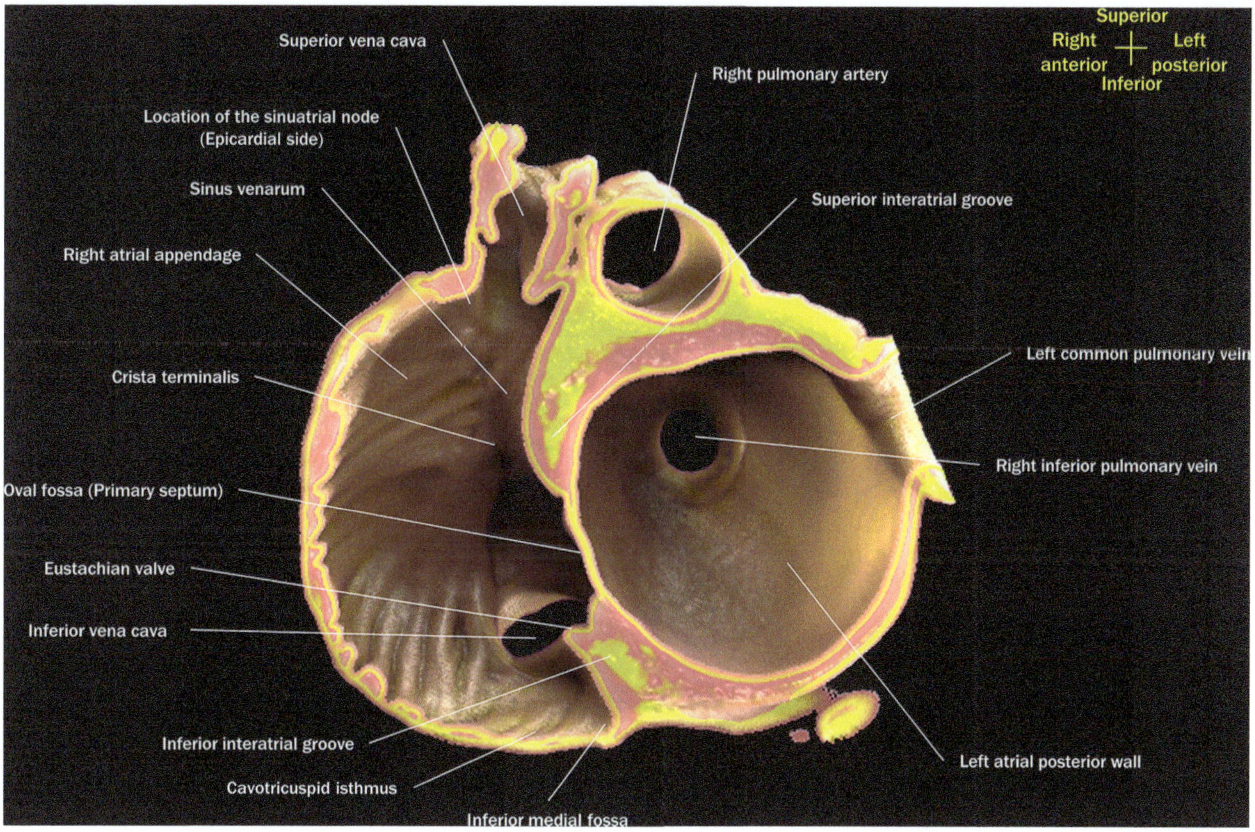

Fig. 6.25 The plane finally shows the primary septum at the floor of the fossa ovalis. Note the thinness and physiological tilting of the primary septum at the floor of the fossa ovalis. The primary septum is the true thin atrial septum surrounded by the superior and inferior interatrial groove. Both interatrial grooves are not the true anatomical septum but rather the folds protruding toward the fossa ovalis.[34] Thus, using the term *secondary septum* to indicate this fold is confusing.[34] Generally, the primary septum tilts toward the right anteroinferior direction along with the tilting of the proximal aorta.[5] The inferior medial fossa is facing the inferior interatrial groove. Thus, this region is also not the region cited as the "inferior interatrial septum."[68] In a case with elongated tortuous descending aorta, the aorta is potentially very close to this region.[5]

Anatomy of the conduction system.
See Figs. 6.26 through 6.28.

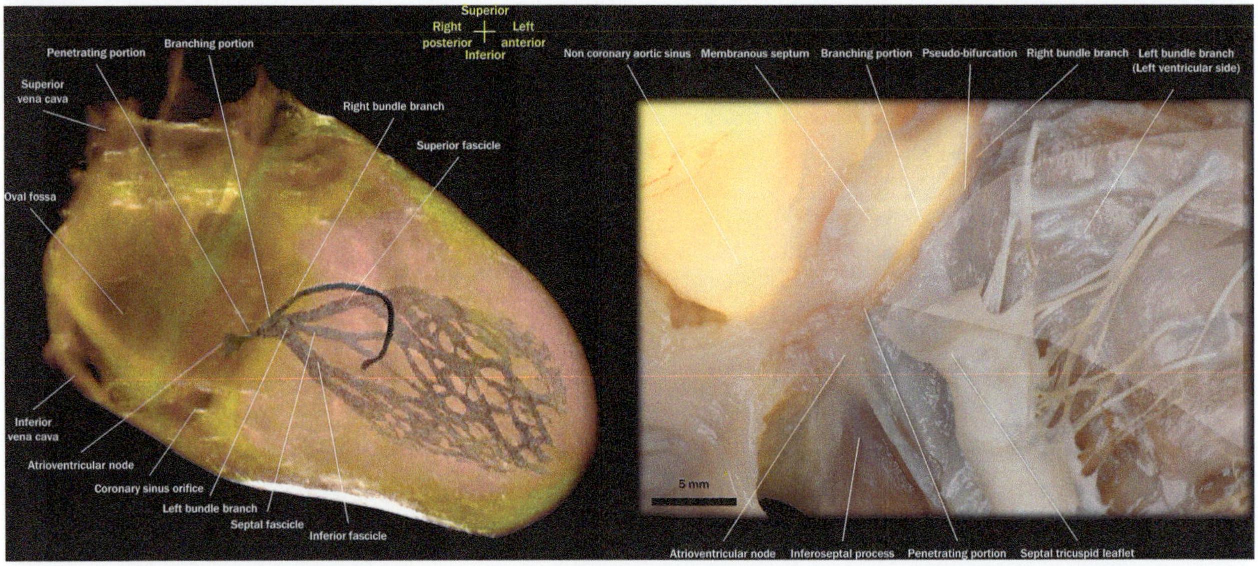

Fig. 6.26 *Left,* approximate location of the atrioventricular conduction system is illustrated and viewed from the right anterior oblique direction (Video 6.3). Note the size of each structure. The three-dimensional feature of the atrioventricular conduction axis can be appreciated within the context of cardiac contour. Attitudinally, so-called anterior and posterior fascicle is located superiorly and inferiorly, respectively.[1,69] This image is important for physiological pacing.[70,71] *Right,* the magnified image of the real dissection of the atrioventricular conduction axis viewed from the same direction. The atrioventricular node is located at the posteroinferior margin of the membranous septum, lying on the right atrial side of the central fibrous body inferior to the nadir of the noncoronary aortic sinus. After the short penetration of the central fibrous body, which is opened here, the atrioventricular conduction axis runs on the crest of the muscular ventricular septum at the inferior margin of the membranous septum. It gives off the left bundle branch[2,72] before giving off the right bundle branch. This part corresponds to the branching portion. Thus, although this part looks like a long single fiber from this direction, actually the thick proximal common left bundle branch is given off on the left ventricular subendocardium. The terminal bifurcation between the right and left bundle branches is referred to as the pseudo-bifurcation.[72] During the two-dimensional histologic evaluation, this pseudo-bifurcation is easily confused as the single point of branching. However, the branching starts more proximally soon after the penetration as discussed. If there is a longitudinal dissociation, therefore, the left bundle branch close to the pseudo-bifurcation should involve fibers going into the superior fascicle, and the left bundle branch close to the penetration portion should involve the fibers going into the inferior fascicle.[72] Injury around the pseudo-bifurcation will cause the right bundle branch block and left superior fascicle block as is common observation the clinical setting.

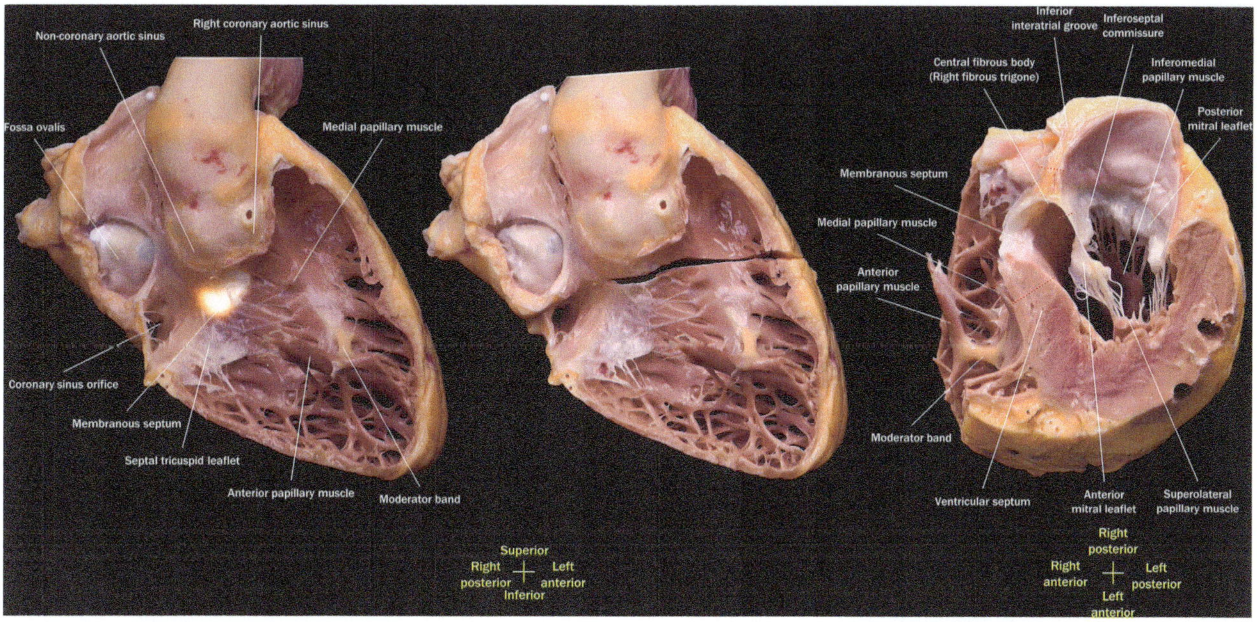

Fig. 6.27 This figure is created to appreciate the histologic images in Fig. 6.28. Note this sectional plane is not identical to the one to show the four-chamber image. Although it is generally neglected, understanding how the specimen is obtained in three-dimensional fashion is fundamental to appreciate the histology. Correlation between histology and gross anatomy is then appropriately recognized in the context of clinically relevant anatomy. *Left,* the right heart septal surface anatomy viewed from the right anterior oblique direction. Pressure-perfused fixed heart is prepared to retain the physiologic morphology. The membranous septum is transilluminated. *Middle,* the cutting plane. The cutting plane was nearly horizontal and is made along the middle part of the membranous septum, beneath the aortic root. The line is not exactly parallel to the inferior margin of the membranous septum, and it is not perpendicular to the tricuspid annular plane. On the atrial side, the plane goes through the anterior limbus of the fossa ovalis between the fossa ovalis and coronary sinus orifice. *Left,* sectioned plane viewed from the superior direction. Structures surrounding the membranous septum beneath the aortic root, including the ventricular septum, central fibrous body, interatrial groove, and anterior mitral leaflet, are observed. This orientation should be carefully appreciated to precisely correlate histologic findings with gross anatomy. The *red dotted lines* indicate the cutting edge to create the histologic sample for the staining as demonstrated in Fig. 6.28.

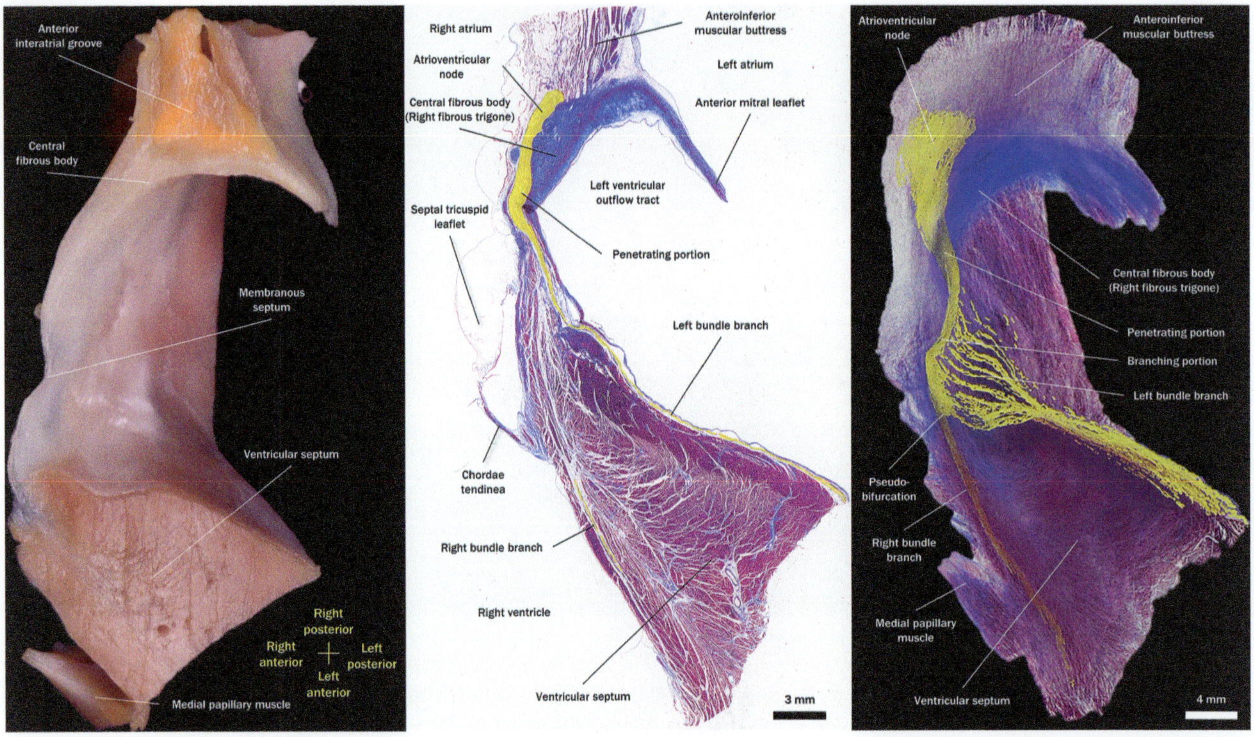

Fig. 6.28 *Left,* the gross image of the sample obtained in the way shown in Fig. 6.27. Note the topographic beauty of the atrioventricular bundle.[8] This sectional direction is almost identical to the one performed by Tawara.[8] *Middle,* the representative section at the level of the atrioventricular node with Masson trichrome stain. This deeper section corresponds to the posteroinferior margin of the membranous septum (27 of 46 slides from the surface). The conduction system is shown in *yellow.* In this particular section, the atrioventricular node, penetrating portion, and left bundle branch can be seen as the continuous structure. The course of the penetrating portion is from the right posterior to left anterior direction; in other words, it is basal to apical direction. On the right ventricular side, the right bundle branch can be traced within the shallow region within the right-side ventricular septum. At the atrial septum, working myocardium, corresponding to the anteroinferior muscular buttress, directly attaches to the central fibrous body. The right atrial side of this atrial septal muscle also connects with the atrioventricular node via transitional cells. *Right,* digital overlaying of whole 46 histology sections cut every 200 μm (Video 6.4). In this way, three-dimensional anatomy of the atrioventricular conduction system can be appreciated with its corresponding gross anatomy.[73]

Anatomy of the coronary arteries.
See Figs. 6.29 through 6.31.

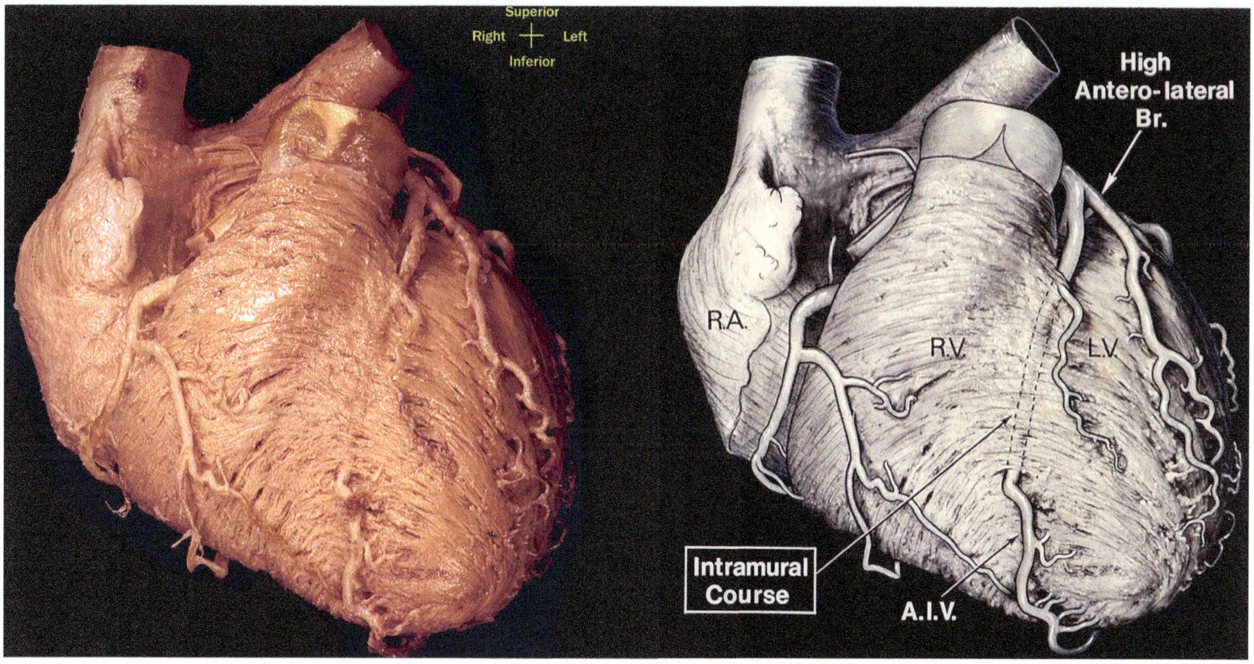

Fig. 6.29 All the epicardial fat is removed. The heart is viewed from the frontal direction. Note the myocardial bridge is found in the middle portion of the left anterior descending artery. The left anterior descending artery runs within the anterior interventricular groove between the right ventricle (R.V.) and left ventricle (L.V.). It is referred to as anterior interventricular branch (A.I.V.) by Dr. McAlpine (McAlpine WA. *Heart and Coronary Arteries: An Anatomical Atlas for Clinical Diagnosis, Radiological Investigation, and Surgical Treatment.* New York, NY: Springer-Verlag; 1975). The left ventricular apex is generally located lateral to the apical part of the left anterior descending artery. Intramural course of any branches of the epicardial coronary artery may risk inadvertent injury during endocardial ablation, ventricular pacing using active fixation leads,[74] and endomyocardial biopsy.[75] On the contrary, myocardial bridge, as well as thick epicardial fat, may have a protective role during epicardial ablation. *R.A.*, right atrium. (Illustration courtesy UCLA Cardiac Arrhythmia Center, Wallace A. McAlpine Collection [McAlpine WA. *Heart and Coronary Arteries: An Anatomical Atlas for Clinical Diagnosis, Radiological Investigation, and Surgical Treatment.* New York, NY: Springer-Verlag; 1975].)

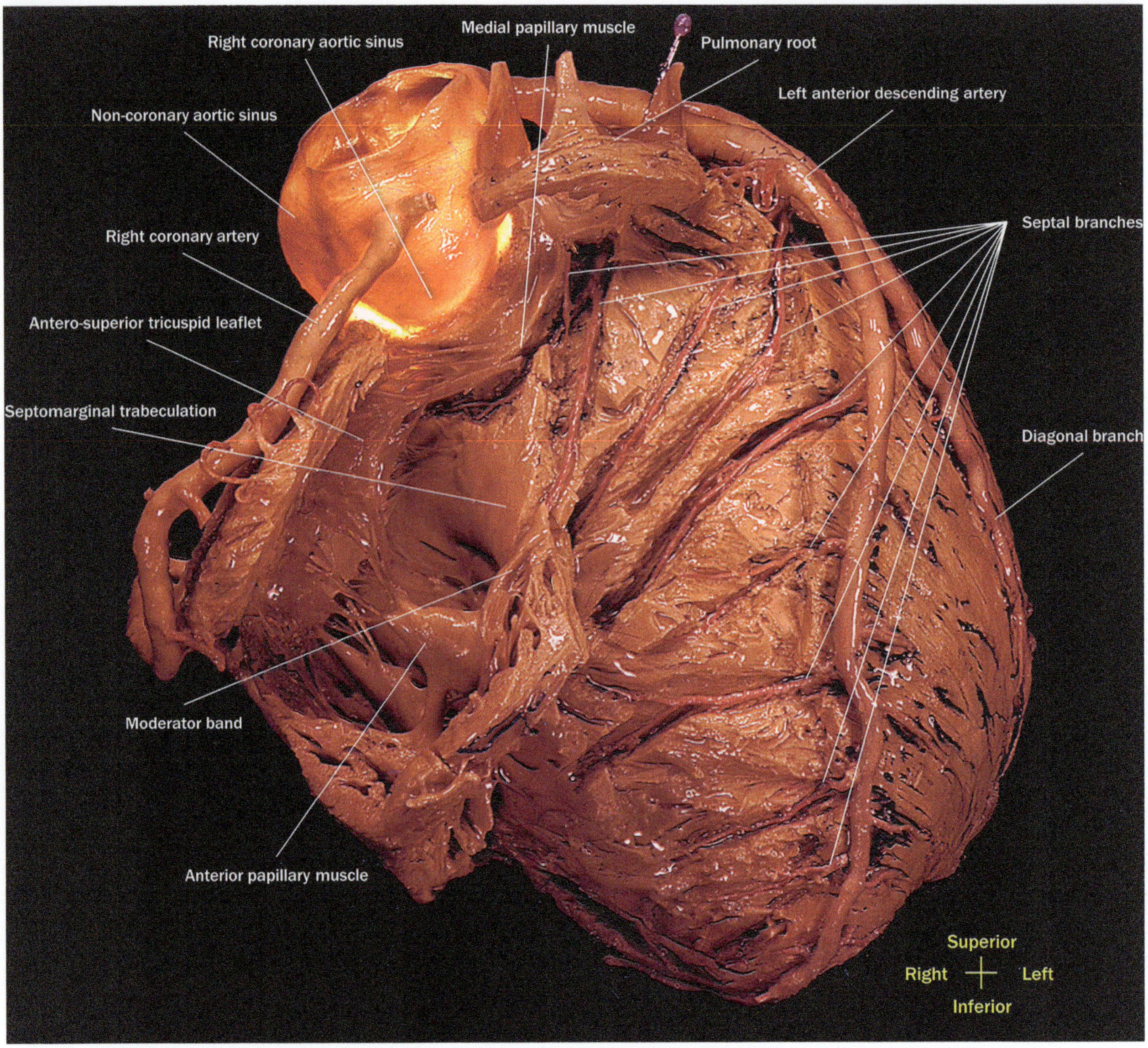

Fig. 6.30 All the epicardial fat is removed. Note multiple septal branches originating from the left anterior descending artery, which are beautifully exposed from the right-side ventricular septum. The heart is viewed from the frontal direction with a slightly cranial angulation. These septal branches perfuse superior two-thirds of the ventricular septum. The first and second septal branches, in this case, start to descend from the area behind the pulmonary root and distribute to the medial papillary muscle and septomarginal trabeculation at the base of the moderator band. As these structures involve the right bundle branch, infarction of these branches can cause right bundle branch block. Also, in the left ventricular side, these septal branches perfuse the left superior fascicle (Fig. 6.26), so-called anterior fascicle. Thus, infarction of these branches can also show left superior fascicular block. (Illustration courtesy UCLA Cardiac Arrhythmia Center, Wallace A. McAlpine Collection [McAlpine WA. *Heart and Coronary Arteries: An Anatomical Atlas for Clinical Diagnosis, Radiological Investigation, and Surgical Treatment.* New York, NY: Springer-Verlag; 1975].)

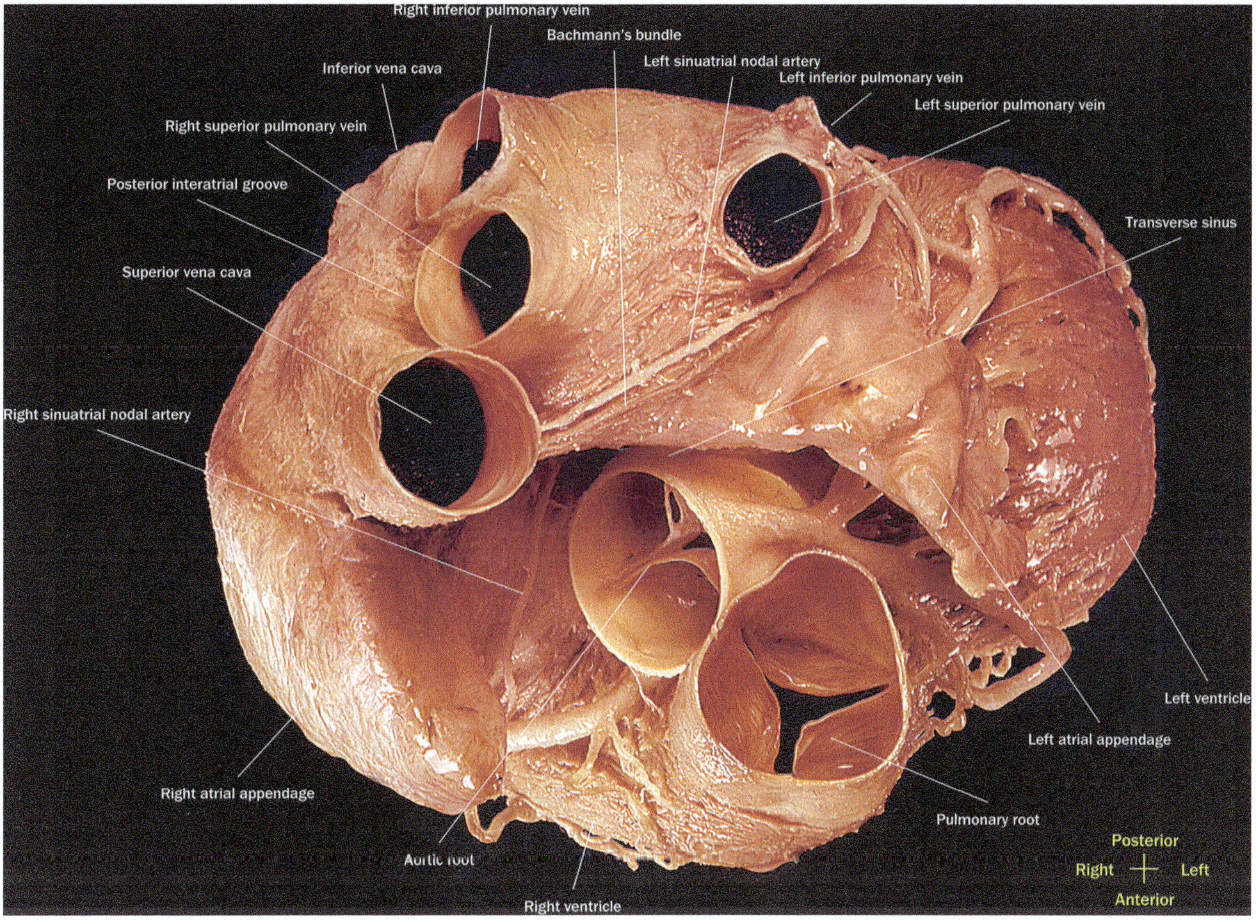

Fig. 6.31 All the epicardial fat is removed. The right and left sinuatrial nodal arteries are dissected. Note the topographic alignment of each structure viewed from the superior direction. The right sinuatrial nodal artery originates from the proximal right coronary artery and runs medial side of the right atrial appendage between the aortic root. Thus, an endocardial approach at the medial right atrial appendage near the proximal aorta may have a risk to injure this artery. The left sinuatrial nodal artery originates from the circumflex artery and runs posterior to the left atrial appendage. Then it runs within the fold between the left pulmonary veins and left atrial appendage before reaching on the Bachmann bundle located at the superior part of the left atrial anterior wall. These left sinuatrial nodal arteries, running either anterior or posterior to the left atrial appendage, are related to the Bachmann bundle[76] and often show intramural course. Thus, during endocardial ablation around the Bachmann bundle, including the linear ablation to create the anterior or roof lines preprocedural coronary angiography, may be indicated to evaluate anatomy of this left sinuatrial nodal artery. (Illustration courtesy UCLA Cardiac Arrhythmia Center, Wallace A. McAlpine Collection.[2])

Anatomy of the coronary veins.
See Figs. 6.32 and 6.33.

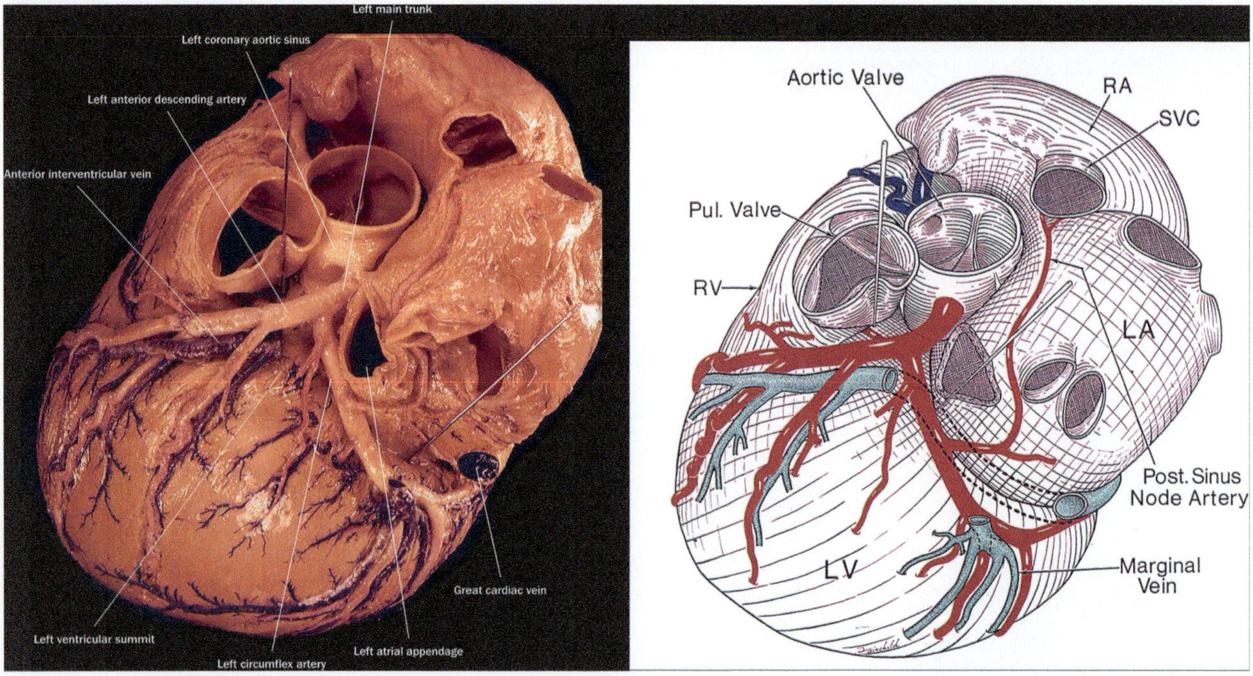

Fig. 6.32 The coronary venous system around the left ventricular summit is shown. Note this view provides the en face view of the left ventricular summit and best separates the left main trunk, proximal left anterior descending artery, and proximal left circumflex artery. The spatial relationship between coronary venous system, the pulmonary trunk, left coronary aortic sinus, left coronary artery, and left atrial appendage is illustrated. The anatomy of coronary venous system, including branching pattern of its tributaries, relationship with coronary arteries, distance from the left coronary aortic sinus, and distance from the left ventricular summit, are variable.[2,60] As demonstrated in this image, left anterior oblique and cranial direction is the optimal direction to obtain an en face view of the left ventricular summit, to evaluate the distance from the focus of arrhythmia to the coronary artery branches. *LA,* left atrium; *LV,* left ventricle; *RA,* right atrium; *RV,* right ventricle; *SVC,* superior vena cava. (Illustration courtesy UCLA Cardiac Arrhythmia Center, Wallace A. McAlpine Collection [McAlpine WA. *Heart and Coronary Arteries: An Anatomical Atlas for Clinical Diagnosis, Radiological Investigation, and Surgical Treatment.* New York, NY: Springer-Verlag; 1975].)

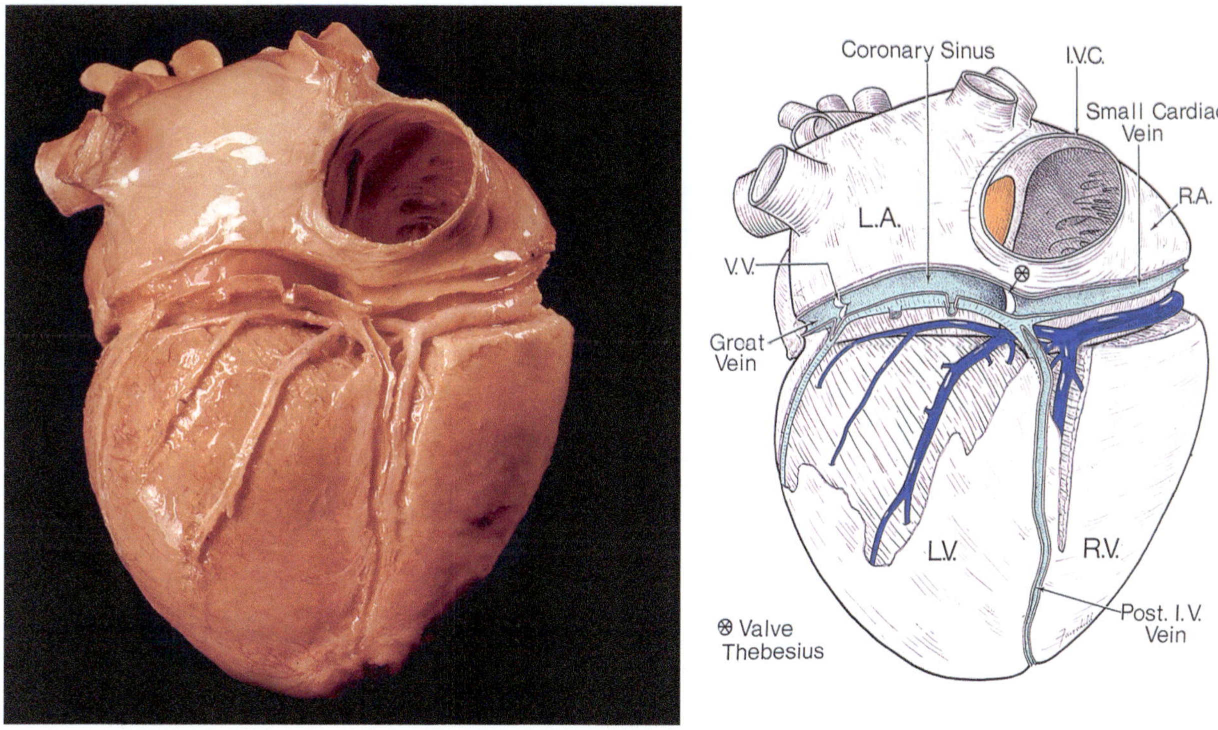

Fig. 6.33 All the epicardial fat is removed. Note the orifice of the inferior vena cava is paraseptal rather than lateral. The coronary sinus is opened and viewed from the inferior direction. The asterisk indicates the Thebesian valve. The Vieussens valve (V.V.) is shown between the coronary sinus and great cardiac vein. Middle cardiac vein is referred to as the posterior interventricular vein (Post.I.V. Vein) by Dr. McAlpine, even though he appreciated the importance of using attitudinally appropriate terminology. Thus, attitudinally, this middle cardiac vein can be better termed the *inferior interventricular vein*. The *orange area* seen via the orifice of inferior vena cava (I.V.C.) denotes the floor of the fossa ovalis, corresponding to the primary septum. *L.A.*, left atrium; *L.V.*, left ventricle; *R.A.*, right atrium; *R.V.*, right ventricle. (Illustration courtesy UCLA Cardiac Arrhythmia Center, Wallace A. McAlpine Collection [McAlpine WA. *Heart and Coronary Arteries: An Anatomical Atlas for Clinical Diagnosis, Radiological Investigation, and Surgical Treatment.* New York, NY: Springer-Verlag; 1975].)

Anatomy of the pericardial space.

See Fig. 6.34.

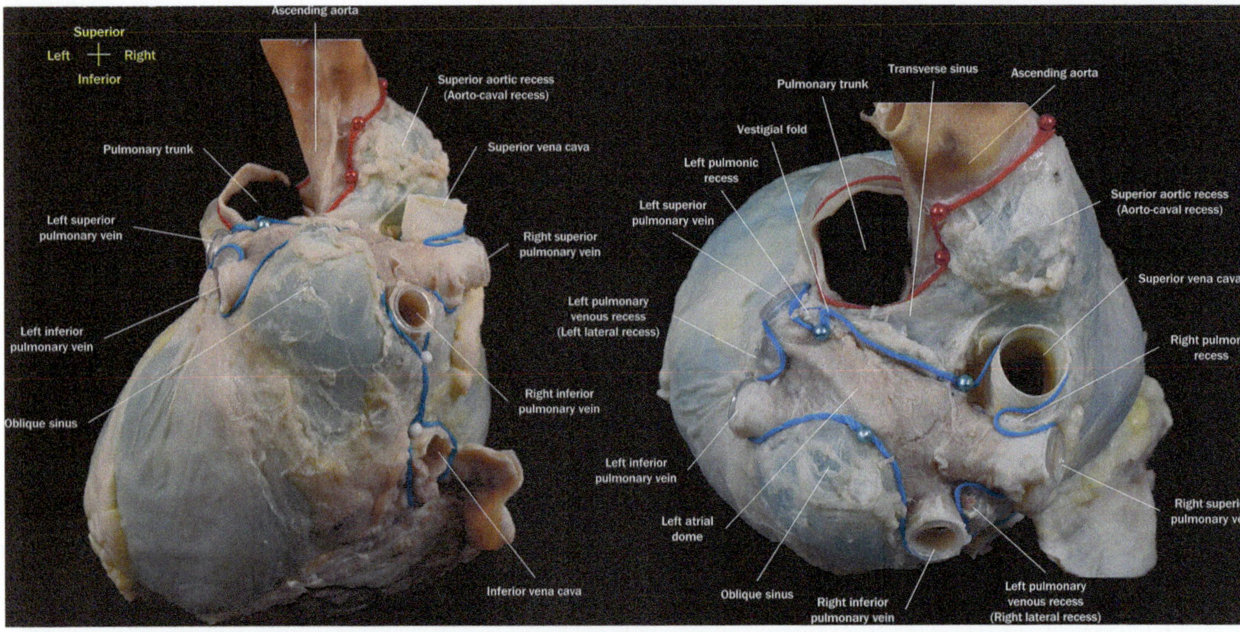

Fig. 6.34 Blue-colored agar is injected into the pericardial space. *Left,* Posterior view showing the oblique sinus between the right and left inferior pulmonary veins. Note the two areas surrounded by the red and blue strings. The red and blue strings demarcate the location of the pericardial reflections. Thus, the heart has two hila communicating with the mediastinum.[77] One is the superior hilum or arterial hilum (*red string*) surrounding the pulmonary trunk and ascending aorta. The other is the posterior hilum (*blue string*) or venous hilum surrounding the pulmonary veins, superior vena cava, and inferior vena cava. These two hila are the exclusive entrance or exit for any vessels and nerves to communicate with the heart within the pericardial space.[14,15] *Right,* The en face view of the posterior hilum viewed from the posterosuperior direction. It shows the bare roof/dome of the left atrium where it is not covered by the pericardial space. Thus, injury to this region cannot induce pericardial tamponade but creates mediastinal hematoma. Also, the inside area of the hilum is the region that cannot be approached via the epicardial approach. The transvers sinus is located between both hila of the heart.

Anatomy of the cardiac innervation.

See Figs. 6.35 and 6.36.

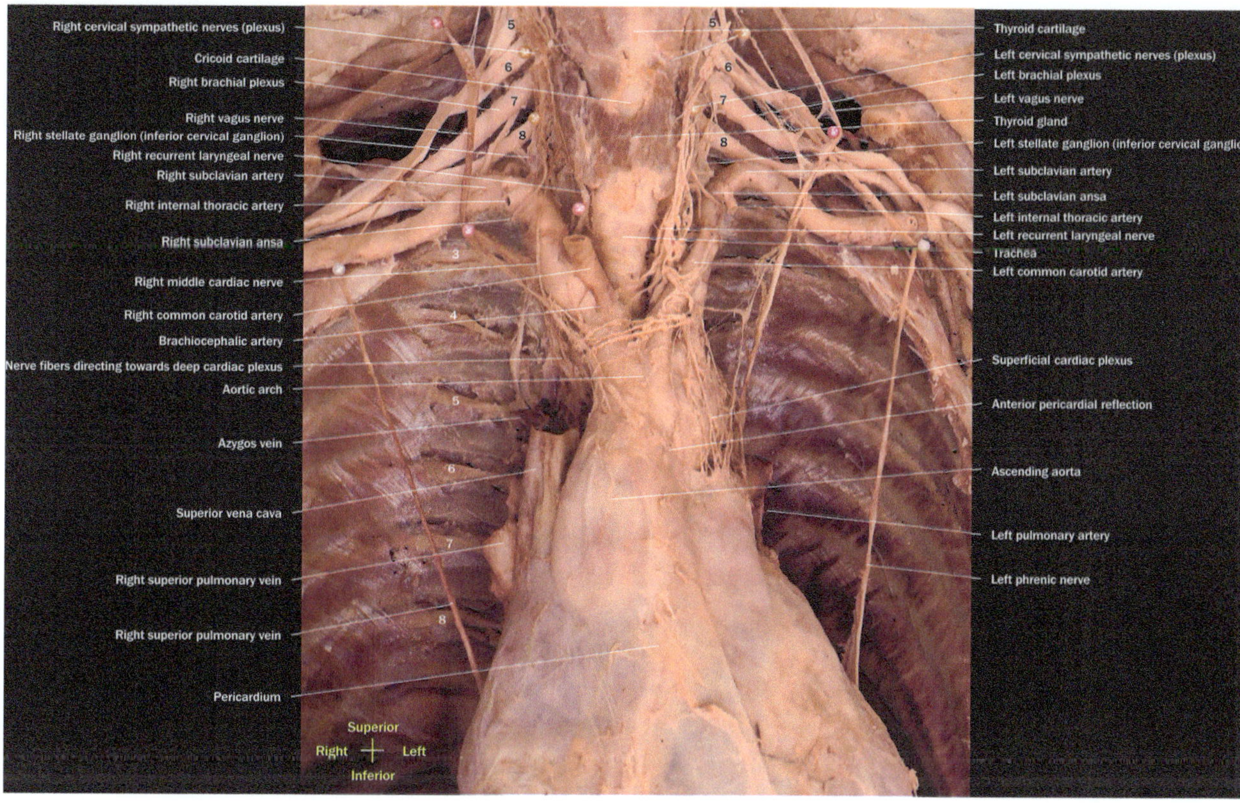

Fig. 6.35 Extracardiac nerve fibers communicating with the heart are dissected and viewed from the anterior direction.[17] The pericardium is left intact. Note the first through fourth intercostal nerves are located superior to the level of the aortic arch. Left anterior to the aortic arch, superior to the anterior pericardial refection, superficial cardiac plexus is demonstrated. The cervical sympathetic nerves are not a single tract but rather a plexus surrounding the common carotid artery. The left cervical sympathetic plexus gives off multiple cardiac nerves, mainly toward the superficial cardiac plexus. The superficial cardiac plexus also receives multiple cardiac nerves from the left vagus nerve. The left stellate ganglion with its subclavian ansa is seen behind the summit of the left subclavian artery. It also gives off multiple cardiac nerves joining both superficial and deep cardiac plexus. Right posterior to the aortic arch, behind the superior vena cava, the cardiac fibers originating from the right vagus nerve and right cervical sympathetic nerves create the plexus directing toward the deep cardiac plexus behind the pulmonary bifurcation anterior to the trachea. The right stellate ganglion behind the summit of the right subclavian artery also shows the subclavian ansa and gives off multiple cardiac nerves to the plexus. Multiple communication between those plexi is observed in front of the branches of the aortic arch. *Black numbers* indicate the cervical nerves of brachial plexi, and *white numbers* indicate the intercostal nerves.

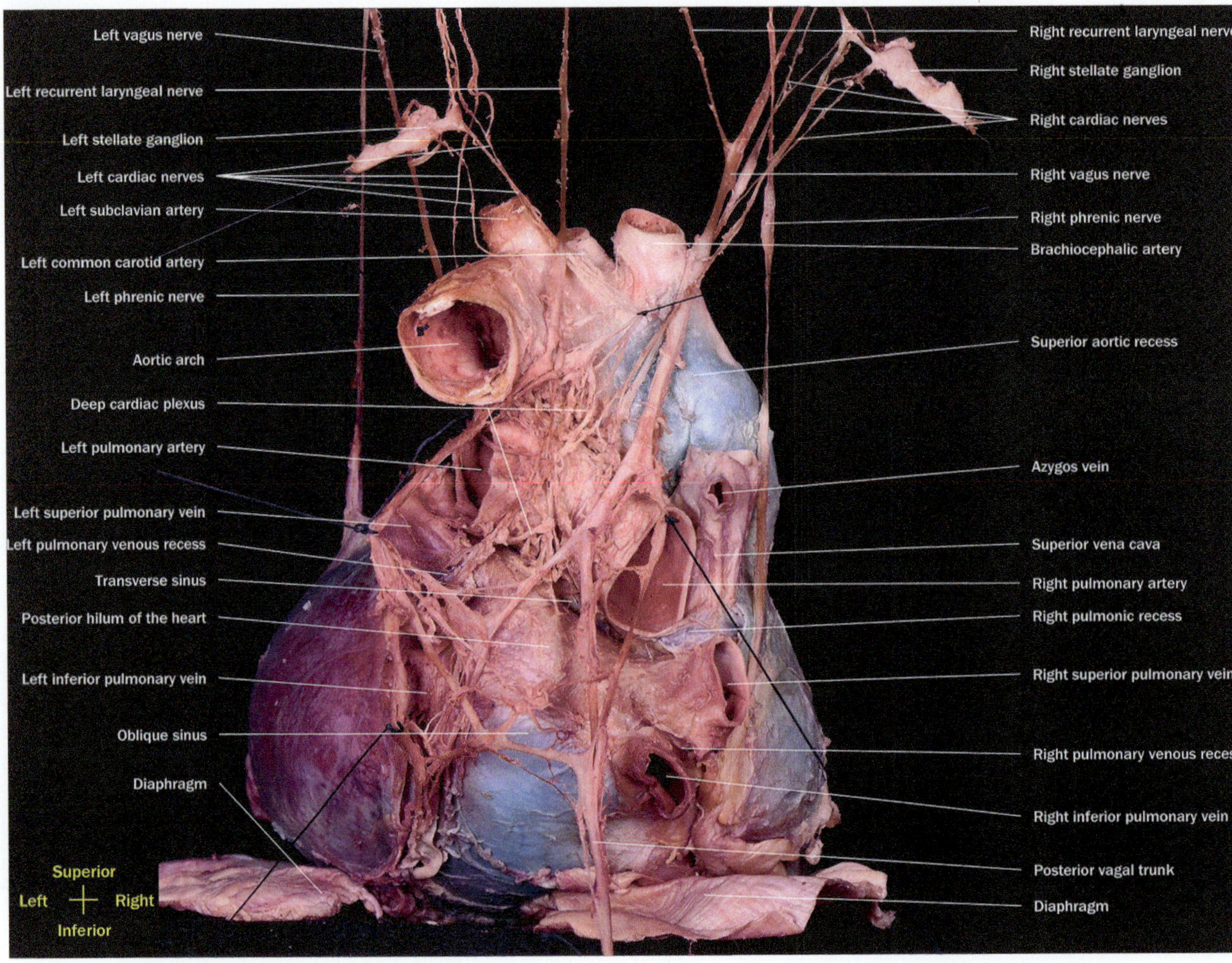

Fig. 6.36 The heart with intact pericardium is removed with the extracardiac nerve fibers communicating with the heart.[17] The heart is viewed from the posterior direction. The blue-colored agar is injected into the pericardial space. It shows the oblique sinus between the inferior pulmonary veins, transverse sinus beneath the pulmonary artery, and superior aortic recess inferoposterior to the orifice of the brachiocephalic artery. Note the roof/dome of the left atrium, corresponding to the pulmonary venous component,[78] is not covered by the pericardial space.[14,15] This region is referred to as the posterior hilum of the heart.[77] The deep cardiac plexus created from the multiple cardiac nerves coming from left recurrent laryngeal nerve, left stellate ganglion, right vagus nerve, and right stellate ganglion is observed behind the pulmonary bifurcation. Multiple fibers from this plexus can distribute to the heart via either superior (arterial) hilum of the heart or posterior (venous) hilum of the heart.[77]

CONCLUSION

Comprehensive progressive dissection images of the pressure-perfusion fixed hearts are demonstrated in an atlas style from the right and left anterior oblique directions. Additional real dissection images obtained from the Wallace A. McAlpine Collection or from the Anatomy Laboratory at the UCLA Cardiac Arrhythmia Center are prepared to cover the topics of the atrioventricular conduction system and epicardial or pericardial structures. Careful review of all of these serial images and supplementary videos will help in appreciation of three-dimensional and clinically relevant anatomy of the heart.

ACKNOWLEDGMENT

We thank individuals who have donated their bodies and tissues for the advancement of education and research. Special thanks to One Legacy Foundation and the NIH SPARC Program, which formed the basis for obtaining donor hearts for research and for funding this effort. We are also grateful to Prof. Warwick J. Peacock, Dr. Grace Chang, and Mr. Edwin Ng with the UCLA Surgical Sciences Laboratory and all the staff members of the UCLA Donated Body Program, Translational Research Imaging Center (Department of Radiology) at UCLA, and Translational Pathology Core Laboratory at UCLA for their support in dissection, image acquisition, and histological preparation. We would like to thank the family of Dr. Wallace A. McAlpine; his daughters, Ms. Laurel Flowers, Ms. Kim Renteria Clark, and Ms. Leigh McAlpine Whitten; and his son, Mr. Fraser McAlpine, for helping us locate his works. We thank Mr. Michael Papalucas, who expertly digitized the original slides made by Dr. McAlpine. We appreciate Mr. Kyle R. Adlaka with USC and Mr. Raj Bhatt with UCLA for their assistance in filming and modification of the images.

REFERENCES

Please refer to the e-book for a complete list of references.

7

Fundamentals of Intracardiac Mapping

Jeremiah Wasserlauf, Rishi Arora

KEY POINTS

- Intracardiac electrograms provide timing and morphologic information.
- Local tissue activation is best identified by the point of maximal downslope of unipolar electrograms and maximal amplitude of bipolar electrograms.
- The most common cardiac mapping techniques are substrate (voltage) mapping, activation mapping, pace mapping, and entrainment mapping.
- Atrial and ventricular pacing maneuvers performed in sinus rhythm and during tachycardia can be used to differentiate and diagnose cardiac arrhythmias.

This chapter discusses the fundamentals of intracardiac mapping as it relates to the mapping and ablation of cardiac arrhythmias. The initial sections are dedicated to the basis and methodology of intracardiac, extracellular recording techniques; this is followed by a description of intracardiac electrograms as recorded in the normal myocardium, and subsequently by a description of intracardiac signals in the abnormal heart. The remainder of the chapter is dedicated to the application of various endocardial mapping techniques, including activation, pace, and entrainment mapping, in the diagnosis and ablation of atrial and ventricular arrhythmias in both normal and diseased hearts. A focus on substrate mapping is provided in Chapters 8, 9, 19, and 36.

UNDERLYING BASIS FOR THE EXTRACELLULAR ELECTROGRAM

Cardiac electrical activity originates from activation of ion channels across cell membranes. The cardiac action potential is generated within individual cells and reflects cardiac electrical activation. Although some net charge flow occurs in the extracellular space, most cardiac electrical activity is generated within individual myocardial cells. Extracellular electrodes record potentials generated in the extracellular space and therefore differ markedly from action potentials recorded intracellularly. The differences are caused not only by differences in recording location (extracellular versus intracellular) but also by the inherent summation of electrical activity from multiple cells that occurs when an extracellular potential is generated.

The field of view of extracellularly recorded electrograms reflects the relative contribution of individual cells both near to and far from recording electrodes that generate extracellular potentials. Computer modeling studies have created simulated extracellular potentials using various assumptions regarding intracellular action potentials.[1] Factors that affect the field of view of recording electrodes are whether the recordings are unipolar or bipolar, interelectrode distance (for bipolar recordings), electrode size and composition, and inherent myocardial properties such as tissue resistivity and space constant. In view of the summation of intracellular potentials that occurs to generate extracellular potentials, some fundamental questions regarding cardiac mapping require further investigation. For example, when one asks the activation time determined from extracellular potentials, there may not be a single answer, because different cells within the field of view of an extracellular recording electrode may be activated at different times. Thus, uniform rules regarding interpretation of extracellular electrograms need to account for differences in underlying physiology, and different rules may be appropriate in different circumstances. For example, it has generally been accepted that the HV interval should be measured from the onset of the His-bundle electrogram. The basis for this approach is that regardless of the location of the recording electrode, one wishes to determine the onset of activation within the His bundle to best evaluate conduction time within the His–Purkinje system. By contrast, mapping of tachycardia origin uses techniques such as the baseline crossing in a bipolar electrogram that seeks to determine not the onset of activation but the occurrence of activation at a specific location and, in most cases, to predict the effects of ablation at that site. Thus, understanding the physiology that generates extracellularly recorded potentials and the purpose of a particular mapping technique is required to determine the best theoretical as well as practical techniques to use for intracardiac mapping.

ELECTROGRAM RECORDING: AMPLIFICATION, FILTERING, AND DIGITIZATION OF SIGNALS

Physiologic signals acquired through intracardiac electrodes are typically less than 10 mV in amplitude and therefore require

TABLE 7.1 Typical Filter Settings for Electrophysiology Laboratory Recordings

Recording	High Pass	Low Pass
Surface electrocardiogram	0.05–0.1 Hz	100 Hz
Bipolar intracardiac	30–50 Hz	300–500 Hz
Unipolar intracardiac	DC, 0.05 Hz	>500 Hz

DC, Direct current.

considerable amplification before they can be digitized, displayed, and stored. In most modern electrophysiology laboratories, the signal processor (filters and amplifiers), visualization screen, and recording apparatus are often incorporated as a computerized laboratory recording system. The amplifiers used for recording intracardiac electrograms must have functionality to modify gain as well as to alter both high-band-pass and low-band-pass filters to permit appropriate attenuation of the incoming signals.[2]

After amplification, signals are digitized and filtered by a computerized data-acquisition system and are written to a storage drive, while displaying signals in real time on a monitor. Digitization is a form of data reduction whereby an analog waveform is sampled at a constant rate (sampling rate) by an analog-to-digital (A/D) converter. The amplitude of the analog waveform is translated into a binary number (e.g., 8-, 10-, or 12-bit conversion resolution of the A/D converter), which represents the full dynamic input range of the A/D converter (typically ±2.5 or ±10 V). Sampling rates of 600 Hz or more allow for the recording of most of the data contained in the intracardiac electrogram waveforms, with most modern mapping systems sampling at or about 1000 Hz. The ideal system should be able to provide a variety of display configurations with a wide range of sweep speeds (most modern systems can display up to 400 mm/second) and should allow adjustment of the size and gain and other characteristics of the amplified electrogram.

Filtering is an important aspect of electrogram processing (Table 7.1). High-pass filters eliminate components below a given frequency (allowing signal content of higher frequency to pass without attenuation). In the surface electrocardiogram (ECG), components such as the T wave are of relatively low frequency, and high-pass filtering of 0.05–0.1 Hz is used to preserve these components while eliminating baseline drift. When examining bipolar intracardiac electrograms, high-frequency components are of the most interest, and high-pass filtering of 30–50 Hz is used to eliminate the low-frequency components. Unipolar electrograms usually go through a high-pass filter of 0.05 Hz, however, because the polarity of the signal (which reflects the direction of myocardial activation) and the signal morphology (and therefore low-frequency components) must be preserved. To eliminate noise at higher frequencies, low-pass filters are generally set to about 500 Hz for intracardiac signals (because there are essentially no intracardiac signals of interest much above 300 Hz).[3] Notch filters remove specific frequencies such as 60-Hz noise from power supplies. Fig. 7.1 shows the effect of different filter settings on intracardiac atrial, ventricular, and His–Purkinje signals.

UNIPOLAR AND BIPOLAR SIGNALS

The morphology and amplitude of the recorded electrograms depend on (1) the type of normal or abnormal depolarization responsible for the electrical potential and on local myocardial characteristics such as ischemia or infarction; (2) the orientation of the activation wavefront in relation to myocardial fiber orientation[4]; (3) the distance between the source of the potential and the recording electrode; (4) the size, configuration, and interpolar distance of the recording electrode[5]; (5) the orientation of the wavefront in relation to the poles of a bipolar electrode; (6) the conducting medium in which electrograms are recorded[6]; and (7) other factors.

The unipolar electrogram is recorded as the potential difference between a single electrode in direct contact with the heart (exploring electrode) and an indifferent electrode, which is placed at a distance from the heart[7] (such as in the inferior vena cava) or at the Wilson central terminal.[8] The recording is therefore not truly unipolar because all recordings depend on voltage differences between two poles; the unipolar designation signifies that one of the poles is distant from the heart. During cardiac activation, the approach of the dipole of an activation wavefront toward an exploring electrode gives a small positive deflection, and its passage gives a rapid deflection in the negative direction, with a final return to baseline.[9] The amplitude of the unipolar electrogram is proportional to the area of the dipole layer and the reciprocal value of the square of the distance between the dipole layer and the recording site.[10] Thus, the unipolar electrogram records a combination of local and distant electrical events, with the contribution of distant electrical events decreasing in proportion to the square of the distance from the exploring electrode.[11] As mentioned earlier, extracellular recordings are not synonymous with intracellular microelectrode recordings. Nonetheless, in normal myocardium with relatively homogeneous conduction and repolarization, several studies (as well as theoretical models) have shown conformity of activation times between intracellular microelectrode and extracellular recordings (Fig. 7.2), with the maximal downslope of the unipolar electrogram coinciding with the upstroke of the transmembrane potential.[12,13] Therefore, at least in normal hearts, there is agreement on using the maximal downslope of the unipolar electrogram for activation detection; there is significant controversy about the optimal value of the slope threshold. However, with recommended thresholds from different studies ranging from −0.2 to −2.5 mV/ms; the large range can be at least partially attributed to the fact that these studies were performed under a variety of different baseline conditions in normal, acutely ischemic as well as chronically infarcted hearts (animal and human).

The bipolar electrogram is recorded as the potential difference between two closely spaced electrodes in direct contact with the heart; it can be calculated as the difference between two unipolar electrograms at each of the two electrode sites[14] (Fig. 7.3). In the electrophysiology laboratory, this is typically done with analog amplifiers rather than with digital subtraction between unipolar signals. The amplitude of the bipolar electrogram is inversely proportional to the third power of the distance between recording site and dipole.[15]

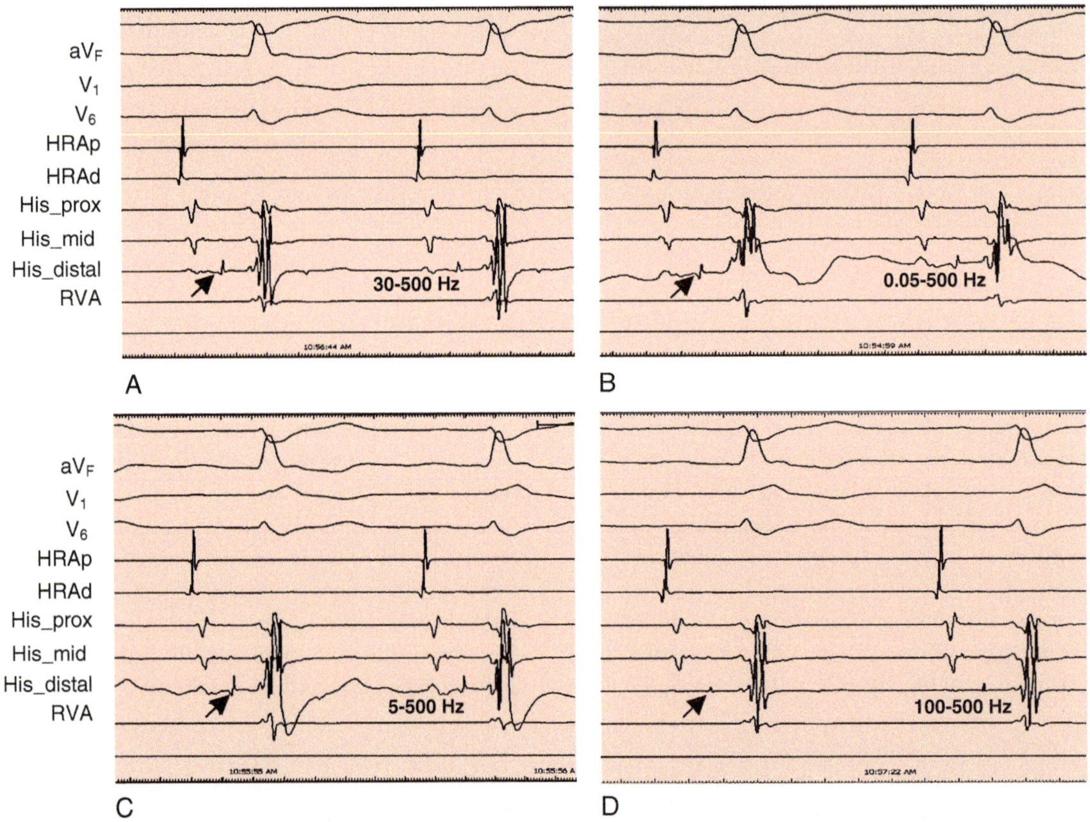

Fig. 7.1 Effects of various filtering frequencies on the morphologic appearance of intracardiac electrograms. (A–D) The tracings from *top* to *bottom* are electrocardiographic leads aVF, V1, V6, right atrial (HRAp, HRAd), three His bundle (His-prox, His-mid, His-distal) electrograms, and right ventricle (RVA). In each panel, both beats are of sinus origin. The top two His tracings (prox and mid), RA, and right ventricular (RV) tracings are filtered at 30–500 Hz (i.e., the usual filtering frequencies). The bottom His distal tracing shows the effect of various filtering frequencies on the appearance. The low-frequency signals are mostly eliminated at high–band-pass filter frequency settings > 10 Hz. Note that the high–band-pass setting reduces the overall magnitude of the electrogram, necessitating an increase in amplification. At all frequencies depicted, the His bundle deflection can be clearly identified. *His-distal*, distal His bundle; *His-mid*, middle His bundle; *His-prox*, proximal His bundle; *HRAd*, high right atrium distal; *HRAp*, high right atrium proximal. (From Akhtar M. Invasive cardiac electrophysiologic studies: an introduction. In Parmley WW, Chatterjee K [eds]: *Cardiology. Vol. 1. Physiology, Pharmacology, Diagnosis*. Philadelphia: Lippincott; 1991:1.)

The major advantage of bipolar recordings lies in the distinction between local and distant activity. A limitation of bipolar electrograms is their directional sensitivity; as a result, if the activation wavefront is parallel in relation to the electrode pair, the bipolar spike will be of maximal amplitude, whereas if it is perpendicular, both electrodes will record the same waveform at the same time, and no spike will result.[16] In addition, activation at the two poles of the bipolar electrogram is not simultaneous, making activation detection more difficult in bipolar electrograms. The following criteria have been suggested for activation detection in bipolar electrograms: (1) the maximal absolute value of the bipolar electrogram; (2) the first elevation of the electrogram of more than 45 degrees from the baseline (obviously subject to display gain); (3) the baseline crossing with the steepest slope; and (4) morphologic algorithms that search for symmetry in the bipolar waveform. Of these, the maximal amplitude of the bipolar electrogram is the most easily measured and has been shown to coincide closely with the maximal downslope of the unipolar electrogram (and the maximal upstroke of the monophasic action potential).[17]

The amplitude of voltage recordings is also influenced by characteristics of mapping catheters, consisting of electrode size, interelectrode spacing, and orientation relative to the myocardium. Contemporary high-density mapping catheters are designed with multiple electrodes with smaller electrode size and spacing as well as configurations for recording signals in multiple orientations.[18] This approach not only enables more rapid signal acquisition for annotation by electroanatomic mapping systems but also enhanced resolution to record near-field electrograms with sharp, high-voltage signals in areas of scar that would be obscured with traditional catheters (Fig 7.4). By additionally treating local propagation as a traveling wave with a single amplitude, speed, and direction across a multielectrode catheter, direction of activation can be displayed.[19]

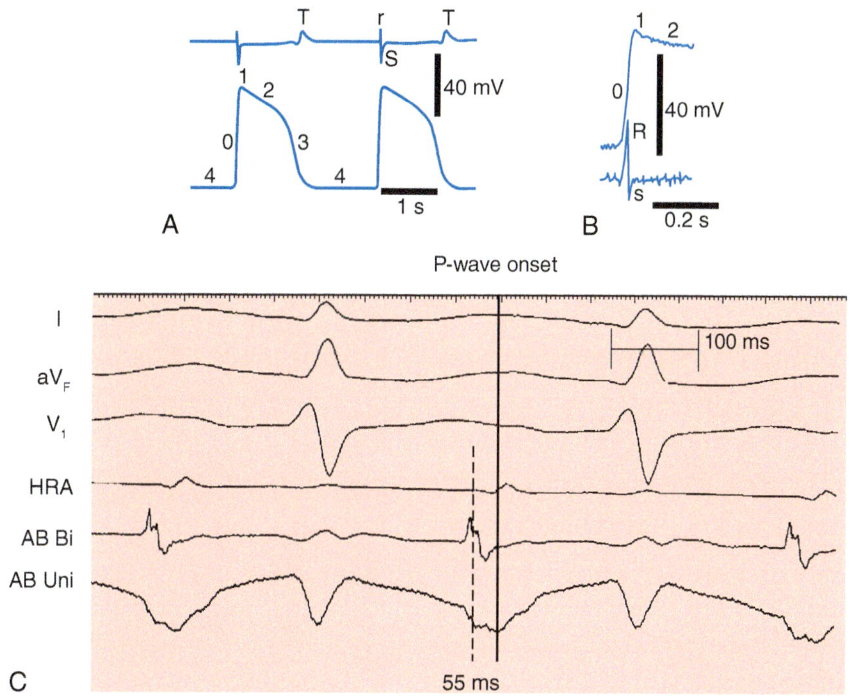

Fig. 7.2 Concordance between extracellular electrogram and intracellular action potential recordings. (A) Relationship between unipolar electrogram *(top trace)* and the transmembrane potential *(bottom trace)* recorded simultaneously from bullfrog ventricle. (B) Display of the initial part of the simultaneously recorded transmembrane action potential *(top trace)* and unipolar electrogram from a different frog *(bottom trace)*, showing concordance between the upstrokes of the two potentials. (C) Surface and intracardiac electrograms recorded during mapping of a right atrial tachycardia. The peak of the bipolar ablation electrogram (AB Bi) coincides with the maximal negative downslope of the distal ablation unipolar recording (AB Uni). These points reflect local activation time at the recording electrodes, and both precede P-wave onset by 55 ms. *HRA*, high right atrium. (A and B, Modified from Yoshida S. Simple techniques suitable for student use to record action potentials from the frog heart. *Adv Physiol Educ*. 2001;25:176–186, 2001.)

Recording Artifacts

The identification of artifactual electrograms is of crucial importance in any system of cardiac mapping and may have major influence on the final interpretation of an activation sequence, such as whether a fractionated electrogram represents a motion artifact or local activation in an assumed zone of slow conduction[20] (Table 7.2). Typical recording artifacts induced at the myocardium–electrode interface are (1) polarization of electrodes, which can cause slow shifts of the baseline of the signals; (2) local myocardial injury resulting from inappropriate pressure by recording electrodes[12]; (3) motion artifacts, which are often rhythmic and linked to cardiac events, therefore simulating fractionated electrograms, or which can be sudden shifts of potential that may be misinterpreted as activations by computer algorithms; (4) poor contact between electrode and myocardium, leading to heavier weighing of far-field effects and increased 50- or 60-Hz noise; (5) potentials produced by two electrodes from different catheters touching each other; and (6) repolarization signals masquerading as a mid-diastolic potential. Finally, intermittent recording of actual signals that do not repeat with every cycle (most typically signals that appear on alternate cycles during tachycardia) are problematic for computerized mapping algorithms. Ensuring good contact between the recording electrode and the underlying myocardium (to remove far-field effects), eliminating all possible sources of noise, including adequate grounding for 50–60 Hz (and if necessary, the use of notch filters), and locating preamplifiers and amplifiers as close as possible to the mapped heart may all help eliminate most of the artifacts that are seen in the clinical electrophysiology laboratory. Undue pressure by the recording catheter on the underlying myocardium can be reflected by the appearance of ST-segment elevation on the unipolar electrogram; slight catheter repositioning usually results in resolution of the ST segment to baseline. Motion artifact (from the patient or the surrounding environment) can be minimized by preventing contact between perfusion pumps and other equipment capable of generating cyclical noise with the patient table and mapping equipment.

CHARACTERISTICS OF INTRACARDIAC SIGNALS: NORMAL HEART

Unipolar endocardial electrograms obtained from experiments in normal canine hearts and from the human atrium and ventricle are characterized by a QS morphology with a rapid downstroke in the first part of the QRS complex (intrinsic deflection).[10,21] Bipolar endocardial electrograms in the normal human left ventricle from catheters with 10-mm interelectrode

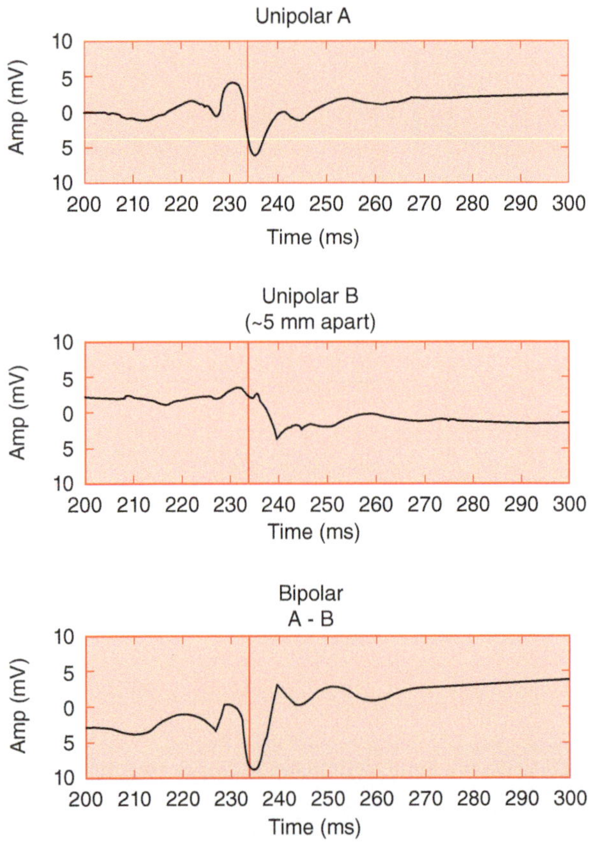

Fig. 7.3 Relationship between unipolar and bipolar electrograms. The bipolar electrogram represents the difference between two closely spaced unipolar electrodes that have the same reference. The result is that the far-field effects and noise that are present in both unipolar electrograms get canceled out. *Amp*, Amplitude.

distance have amplitudes greater than 3 mV and durations less than 70 ms, and no split, fractionated electrograms are found.[17] Unipolar and bipolar electrograms in diseased myocardium are typically characterized by slower upstrokes and fragmentation (see later discussion). Although slow conduction and fractionated, low-amplitude signals are not as widespread in the normal heart compared with the diseased atrium or ventricle; low-amplitude, high-frequency electrograms have been well described at the thoracic vein–atrium junction, within both the pulmonary veins and the vena cava,[22–24] as well as at other sites in the normal heart, such as the crista terminalis and coronary sinus.[25]

Electrical Abnormalities in the Absence of Structural Heart Disease

Electrograms need not be entirely normal even in the absence of overt fibrosis or fatty replacement. For example, low-amplitude, fractionated bipolar electrograms may be seen at the earliest activation sites of focal tachycardias, even in the presence of a normal looking unipolar electrogram. Fig. 7.5 shows the bipolar electrogram at the successful ablation site of two different focal tachycardias in the absence of any overt structural heart disease: a focal tachycardia originating from the coronary sinus ostium and a focal ventricular tachycardia (VT) arising from the inferolateral left ventricle. Late potentials

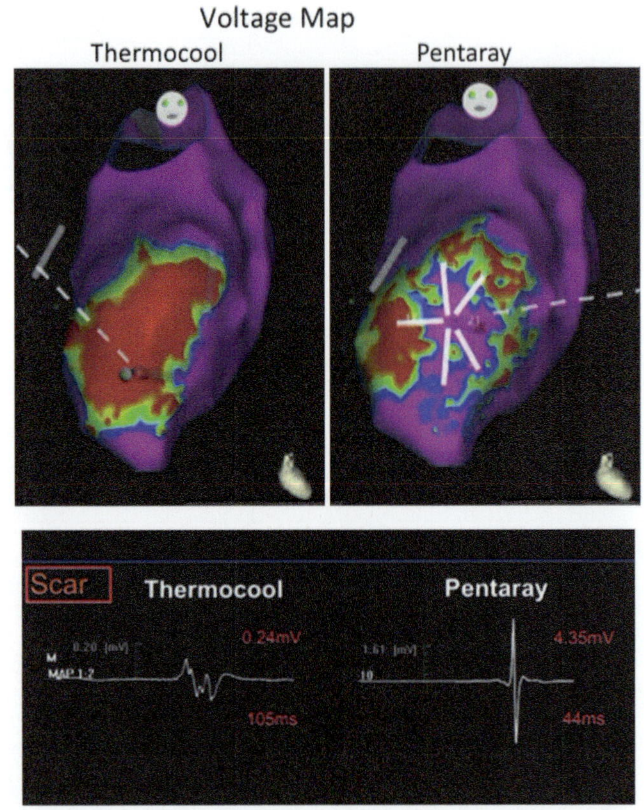

Fig. 7.4 Effect of electrode size and interelectrode spacing on electrograms. A voltage map generated by an ablation catheter (ThermoCool, *top left panel*; 3.5-mm tip and 1-mm ring) and multielectrode mapping catheter (Pentaray, *top right panel*; each electrode 0.8 mm^2) are shown. The red area is <0.5 mV. The bipolar signal recorded in the red area was 0.24 mV (*top left panel*) and was broad and fragmented. Recordings from the same site with a Pentaray show normal bipolar amplitude and width (*bottom panel*). (From Josephson ME, Anter E. Substrate mapping for ventricular tachycardia: assumptions and misconceptions. *JACC Clin Electrophysiol.* 2015;1(5):341–352.)

TABLE 7.2 Sources of Intracardiac Recording Artifacts

Cause	Manifestation
Electrode polarization	Electrogram drift
Excessive contact pressure	ST elevation
Catheter motion	Fractionation
Poor contact	Low amplitude
Contact with other catheters	High-frequency signals
Repolarization	Late or mid-diastolic potentials
Electromagnetic interference	High-frequency noise
Poor grounding	High-frequency noise

during sinus rhythm are also noted in hearts that are otherwise morphologically normal; Fig. 7.6 shows late potentials in the right ventricle of a patient who had exercise-induced left bundle branch block (LBBB) superior axis VT but with no evidence of scar or any other abnormality on ECG or cardiac magnetic resonance imaging (MRI).

The basis for these potentials is not entirely clear. In the absence of overt scar on sensitive imaging modalities such as

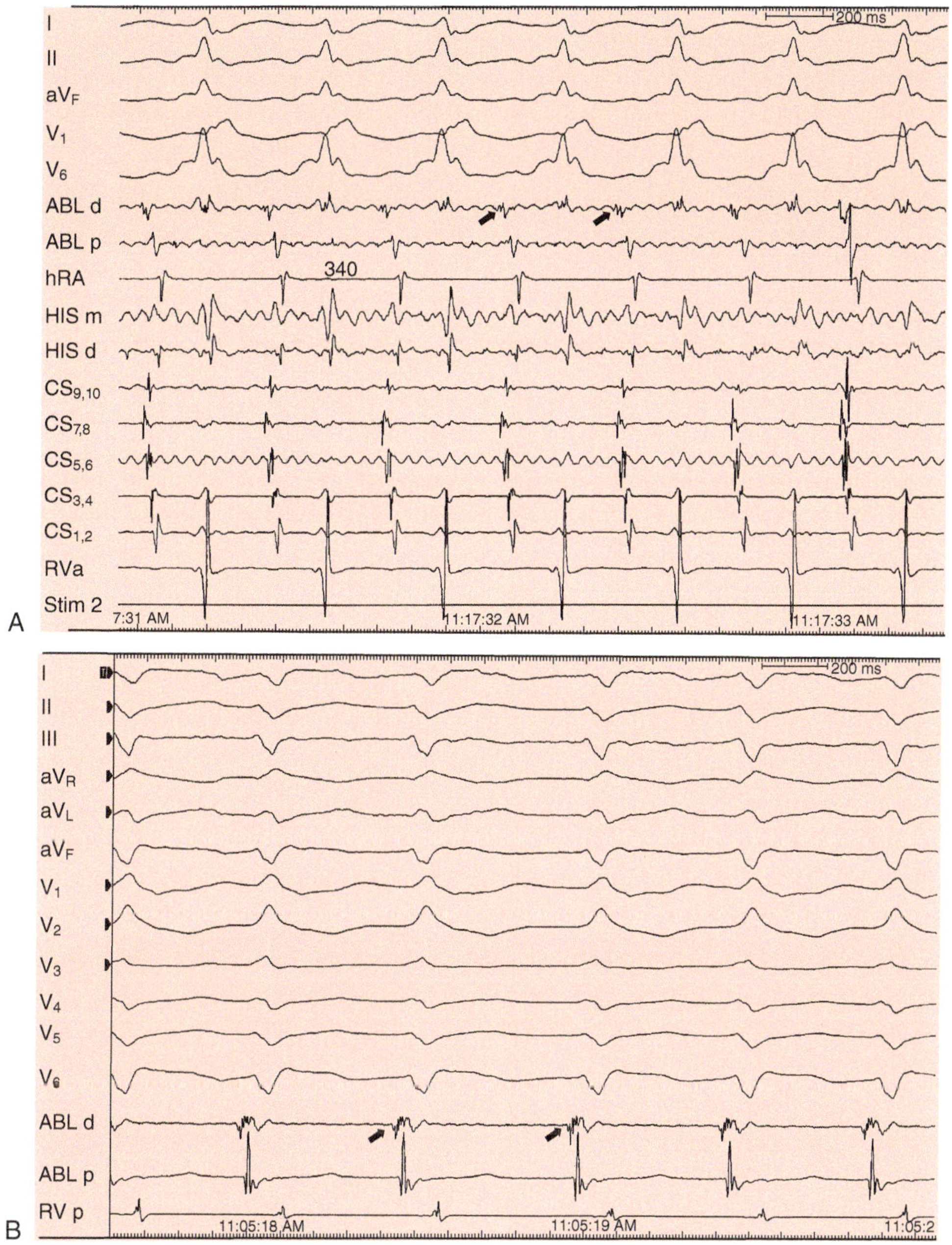

Fig. 7.5 Low-amplitude bipolar electrogram at successful ablation site of two focal tachycardias: a focal tachycardia originating from the ostium of the coronary sinus (A) and a focal ventricular tachycardia arising from the inferolateral left ventricle (B). In both instances, notice the lower amplitude and prolonged duration of the electrogram at the site of earliest activation (i.e., the ablation site) *(arrows)*. *ABL*, Ablation; *CS*, coronary sinus; *d*, distal; *HRA*, high right atrium; *m*, mid; *p*, proximal; *RV*, right ventricle.

MRI, it is tempting to speculate that at least some of the delay seen in these electrograms may be functional in nature. In fact, functional anisotropic conduction is well described in the normal heart (e.g., at the crista terminalis)[25] and may be responsible for the creation of macroreentrant circuits, such as isthmus-dependent atrial flutter. Anisotropic conduction has also been demonstrated within the pulmonary veins[26] and the superior vena cava. Fig. 7.7 shows that the conduction times into and out of the pulmonary vein can be very different, which is an example of anisotropic conduction.[27]

Conceivably, therefore, at least some of the focal tachycardias described in the normal heart may be microreentrant in origin. Other factors that have been postulated are poor intercellular coupling, such as that caused by decreased gap junctions at sites of origin of focal tachycardias, leading to decreased electrotonic inhibition of the focus by surrounding tissue.[28] In general, electrograms at successful ablation sites for focal tachycardias are less than 50 ms presystolic. However, pulmonary vein tachycardias are usually more than 50 ms presystolic, at least partially on account of the slow conduction noted in this area.

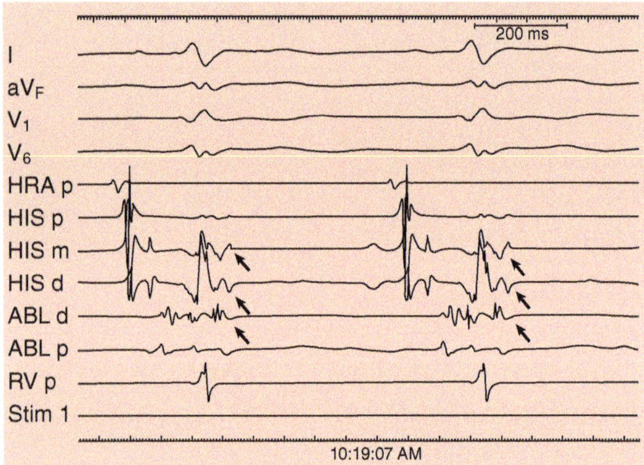

Fig. 7.6 Late systolic potentials in a heart with no known myocardial disease. The figure demonstrates late potentials that extend beyond the end of the QRS *(arrows)* at the septal right ventricle (base of the right ventricular outflow tract) of a patient who had exercise-induced left bundle superior axis ventricular tachycardia but no evidence of scar or any other abnormality on echocardiography or cardiac magnetic resonance imaging. *ABL*, Ablation; *d*, distal; *HRA*, high right atrium; *m*, mid; *p*, proximal; *RV*, right ventricle; *Stim*, stimulus.

Fractionated, bipolar electrograms (both during tachycardia and during sinus rhythm) have also been well described in idiopathic VT arising from the left ventricular septum. In fact, it is the presence of these Purkinje-like potentials some distance away from the septum that has led some to postulate a reentrant circuit of considerable size as the basis for this VT.[29] Split electrograms may sometimes be recorded in the normal heart, such as in the posteroseptal right atrium from conduction block across the Eustachian ridge.

Electrogram Abnormalities in the Presence of Structural Heart Disease

The signature of scar in the atrium or ventricle is a low-amplitude, high-frequency electrogram (during sinus rhythm or during tachycardia), with the duration and amplitude of the electrogram showing some correlation with the degree of slow conduction in and around the area of fibrosis.[30] Low-amplitude, fractionated electrograms may be recorded during or after the QRS complex and are typically less than 1 mV in amplitude; these can be recorded during sinus rhythm and VT. The characteristic unipolar electrogram in the setting of chronic myocardial scar, such as myocardial infarction, may show a single, rapid biphasic

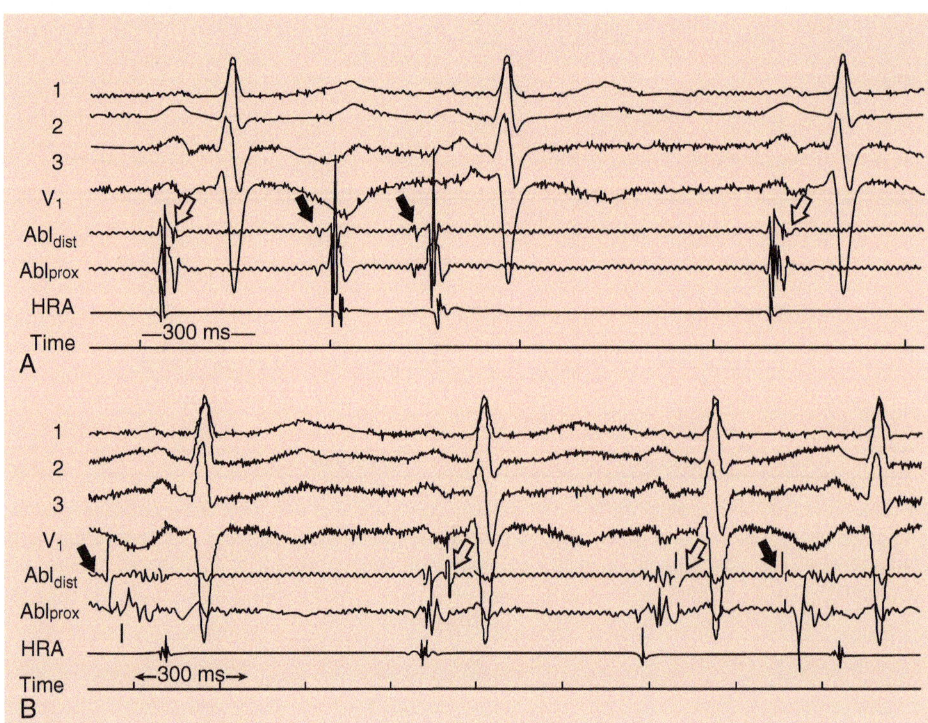

Fig. 7.7 Anisotropic conduction in the superior vena cava (SVC) and pulmonary vein. In both A and B, *open arrows* indicate atrial electrograms, and *solid arrows* indicate pulmonary vein potentials. (A) Sinus rhythm with conduction into the posterosuperior right atrium (close to its junction with the SVC). (B) The right superior pulmonary vein. In both A and B, the bipolar ablation electrogram shows an atrial signal followed by an SVC or a pulmonary vein myocardial signal. Atrial premature contractions (APCs) coming from the SVC or from pulmonary veins show the venous myocardial potential first, followed by the atrial myocardial signal. Note that conduction out of the SVC or pulmonary vein (APCs) is longer than conduction into the SVC or pulmonary vein during sinus rhythm. *ABL*, Ablation; *dist*, distal; *HRA*, high right atrium; *prox*, proximal. From Miller JM, Olgin JE, Das MK. Atrial fibrillation: what are the targets for intervention? *J Interv Card Electrophysiol.* 2003;9:249–257. With permission.

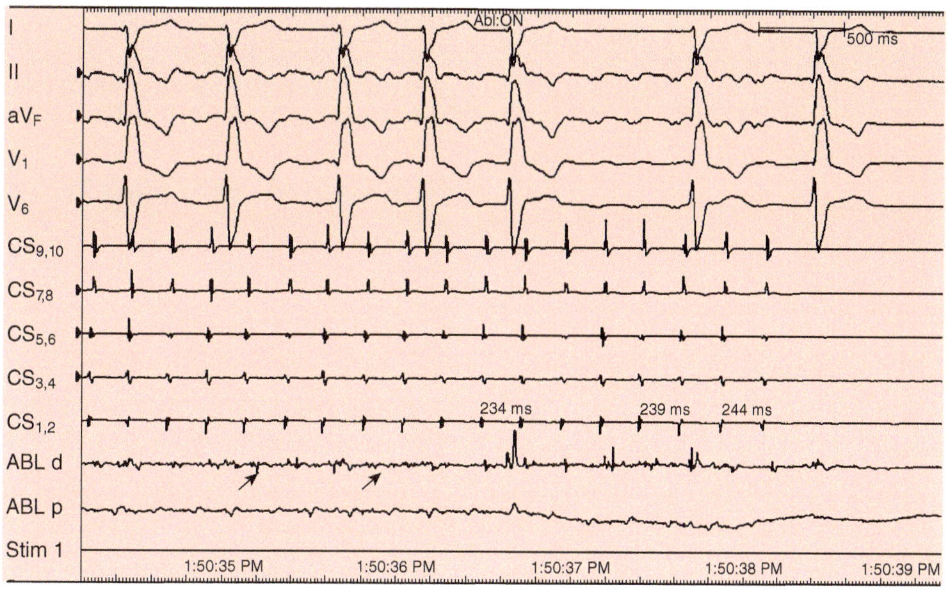

Fig. 7.8 Continuous, low-amplitude activity at the site of ablation in atrial flutter in the setting of D-transposition of the great arteries repair. In this patient, the atrial flutter was mapped to the subeustachian isthmus. The isthmus was first approached and ablated from the systemic or subaortic ventricle. However, the entire isthmus could not be ablated from the subaortic side (because of baffle and suture lines). Additional mapping and ablation were therefore performed through the baffle on the subpulmonic or left side. From the subpulmonic side, it was possible to reach a portion of the sub-Eustachian isthmus that had previously not been reached with a subaortic approach. Mapping along this portion of the sub-Eustachian isthmus (i.e., along the same line where ablation was performed from the right ventricle) revealed the continuous, low-amplitude activity shown by the *arrows*. Ablation here resulted in slowing and termination of the flutter. *ABL*, Ablation; *CS*, coronary sinus; *d*, distal; *p*, proximal; *Stim*, stimulus.

deflection of RS morphology following a wide QS potential, a double RS deflection, or fragmentation with multiple deflections.[31] Continuous, low-amplitude electrical activity, such as a fractionated electrogram spanning the entire tachycardia cycle length (TCL), can also be seen in the setting of myocardial scar or disease. Fig. 7.8 shows an example of low-amplitude continuous activity at a successful ablation site for a reentrant atrial tachycardia and flutter in a patient who had undergone Mustard repair for D-transposition of the great arteries.

Animal studies performed in the setting of experimental chronic myocardial infarction have examined the intracellular basis of the previously mentioned changes on the extracellularly recorded electrograms and have demonstrated that action potential amplitude and upstroke are similar to those of normal myocardium.[32,33] Despite the presence of normal action potentials, slow and discontinuous conduction is present, which may provide an electrophysiologic and anatomic basis for arrhythmias. One explanation of the low-amplitude, prolonged duration, and notched extracellular potentials in the infarcted areas is that the slow conduction represents activation of normal cells separated by areas of fibrous tissue producing discontinuities in conduction. Kadish and colleagues used vector mapping, a technique based on summing orthogonally bipolar electrograms, to determine the direction of activation in cardiac tissue and showed that although vector loops recorded from normal myocardial tissue were found to be smooth and pointing in a single direction, those recorded from areas of healed myocardial infarction were notched, irregular, and occasionally pointing in more than one direction.[34] Using the vector technique, the authors demonstrated complex activation patterns in areas where abnormal extracellular electrograms are recorded in which discrete activation times may be difficult to identify, such as in areas of fractionated electrograms where multiple peaks are present.[35]

Ischemic heart disease is by far the most common cause of scar in the ventricle, although less common conditions such as arrhythmogenic right ventricular (RV) dysplasia and cardiomyopathy may demonstrate similar electrophysiologic characteristics because of fibrofatty replacement in the right (and occasionally left) ventricle. Fibrosis has also been described in dilated cardiomyopathy but is seen less commonly than in ischemic heart disease. In the atrium, scar is commonly the result of surgery for congenital heart disease, with atrial septal defect repair, tricuspid atresia (Fontan repair), tetralogy of Fallot repair, and transposition of great arteries (Mustard–Senning repair) being the most common reasons for scar in the right atrium.[36] Left atrial surgery can create substrate for left or right atrial reentry,[37] the latter likely on account of cannulation sites during bypass. Similarly, extensive catheter ablation with multiple linear or multiple areas of focal lesions may also create substrate for subsequent development of left or right atrial tachyarrhythmias. Please see Chapters 13 and 14 for details.

As mentioned earlier, the low-amplitude electrograms during sinus rhythm are often noted late in systole; Fig. 7.9 shows an example of late systolic potentials in the right ventricle of a patient with arrhythmogenic RV dysplasia. Such low-amplitude,

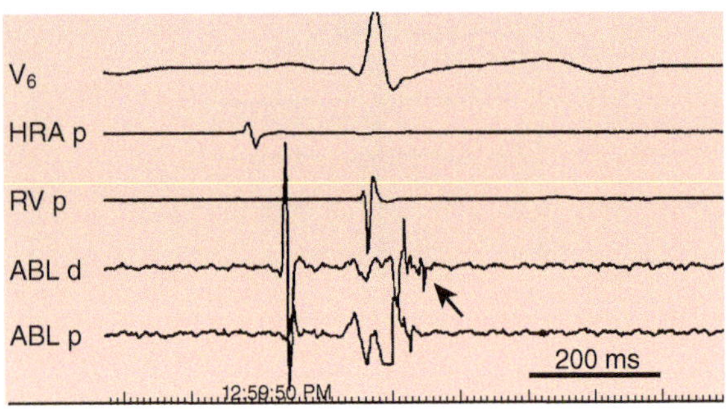

Fig. 7.9 Late potential mapping in the right ventricle. In a patient with arrhythmogenic right ventricular (RV) dysplasia, many of the electrograms were abnormal, especially at the RV inflow, the RV apex, and the RV outflow tract. The figure shows late potentials during sinus rhythm in the region of the RV apex on the ablation (ABL) catheter *(arrows)*. *d*, Distal; *HRA*, high right atrium; *p*, proximal.

high-frequency electrograms are thought to underlie the late potentials that are seen on a positive signal-averaged ECG.[38] Lately, there has been a renewed interest in local abnormal ventricular activities (LAVAs), some occurring before the end of QRS, in patients with structural heart disease. Jaïs and colleagues showed that a procedural end point of LAVA elimination was associated with mortality benefit and freedom from VT, compared with standard methods of VT mapping and ablation.[39] However, even though late potentials are typically seen in and around an area of scar or infarction and are frequently noted at or close to sites of successful ablation (of reentrant tachycardias), late potentials have not always been shown to be a clear predictor of ablation success.[40] They may lack specificity in that they may also be found at sites that are remote from a successful ablation site (indicating diseased myocardium in other areas). The presence of late potentials can also be dependent on the activation timing of the anatomic substrate, with LAVA seen more commonly in the epicardium rather than the endocardium and less frequently in the septum, which is activated early. The ability to distinguish late potentials (sometimes needing to decouple LAVA from the basic ventricular electrogram) is also dependent on conduction velocity in the diseased myocardium.[41]

A mapping strategy that focuses on slow conduction, distinct from late activation, has also been proposed to refine identification of ablation targets for ventricular tachycardia known as deceleration zones (DZs) when mapping in sinus rhythm. DZs can be displayed as isochronal late activation maps (ILAMs) acquired in sinus rhythm. Isochrones are segments of myocardial activation assigned a constant unit of time, meaning that the thickness of an isochrone illustrates the velocity (distance/time) of propagation. DZs are identified by crowding of multiple isochrones within a given radius of myocardium (Fig 7.10). Electrograms are annotated to the offset of the local bipolar electrogram, representing late activations, as opposed to the peak of the bipolar electrogram that is conventionally used. Aziz and colleagues demonstrated that targeted ablation of DZs (>3 isochrones within 1-cm radius) resulted in successful VT termination in 95% of cases in one series, supporting these zones as critical sites for VT that can be mapped in sinus rhythm and potentially reduce the need for more extensive voltage-guided substrate homogenization.[42]

A list of abnormal electrogram morphologies and the possible interpretations is given in Table 7.3.

ENDOCARDIAL MAPPING TECHNIQUES

Contact endocardial mapping can be performed during sinus rhythm as well as during tachycardia. Mapping techniques can be broadly categorized as follows: (1) activation sequence mapping, (2) fractionated local electrogram and voltage mapping, (3) pace mapping, (4) entrainment mapping, and (5) miscellaneous pacing maneuvers (performed during sinus rhythm or tachycardia). Although these techniques are usually used in combination, the relative utility of each depends on arrhythmia inducibility, hemodynamic and cycle length stability of the induced arrhythmia, underlying substrate (i.e., normal versus diseased heart), and arrhythmia mechanisms, among other factors. For example, entrainment can be used only in the setting of a sustained, rather regular reentrant arrhythmia. The previous two sections have described the electrogram and voltage characteristics in normal and diseased hearts. The following paragraphs describe the underlying basis for the remainder of the techniques and highlight their use (singly or in combination) in the diagnosis and ablation of atrial and ventricular arrhythmias.

Activation Sequence Mapping

The most commonly used method of identifying the optimal ablation site for a tachyarrhythmia is activation mapping to locate the site of earliest endocardial activation or to determine the activation sequence during the tachycardia. Focal arrhythmias are typically characterized by presystolic timings pre-P or pre-QRS less than 50 ms. By contrast, reentrant arrhythmias, both in the normal and in diseased hearts, typically demonstrate diastolic activity that is significantly earlier than 50 ms. In fact, for reentrant arrhythmias, intracardiac activity should be present at some point in the heart throughout the cardiac cycle. Electrograms are typically recorded through at least 70% of the TCL in macroreentrant arrhythmias. In the normal heart, such as in the setting of subeustachian isthmus–dependent typical atrial flutter, the macroreentrant circuit is of considerable size—bound by the two anatomic barriers of the crista terminalis and the tricuspid annulus—and need not demonstrate the low-amplitude, high-frequency electrograms that are typical of scar-related reentrant arrhythmias. In a reentrant VT in the setting of myocardial scar, a zone of slow conduction over a pathway of possibly quite complex geometry (e.g., nonlinear, nonhomogeneously anisotropic) provides the diastolic limb of the reentrant circuit. After emerging from the zone of slow conduction, the wavefront propagates rapidly throughout the ventricles to generate the QRS complex. Thus, early or presystolic activation occurs in close proximity to the exit region from the zone of slow conduction.

What is considered to be early activation and a suitable ablation site in a focal arrhythmia (30–50 ms presystolic) may not necessarily be early activation in a reentrant arrhythmia. Reentrant atrial tachycardias or VTs are typically characterized by

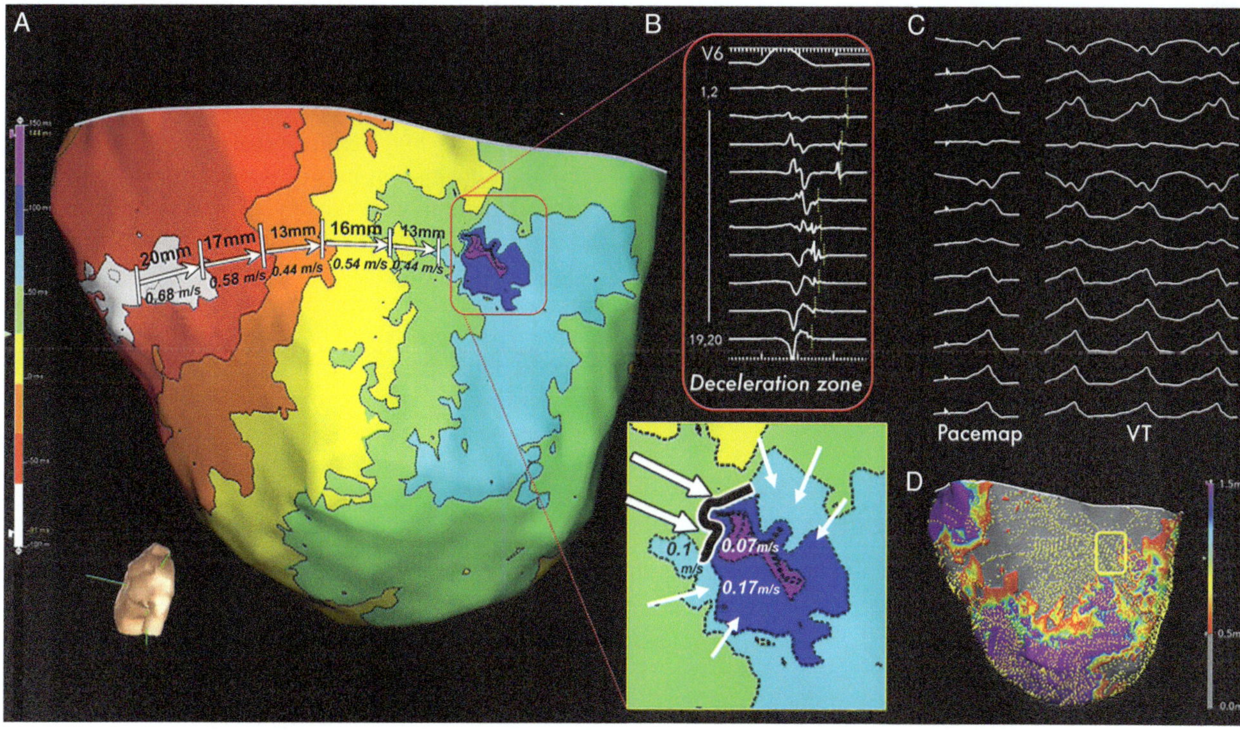

Fig. 7.10 Example of isochronal late activation mapping (ILAM) demonstrating single deceleration zone (DZ) due to localized line of conduction block. (A) Isochronal late activation map of left ventricular (LV) epicardium (left anterior oblique [LAO], cranial view) demonstrating activation of the left ventricle from anterior (white isochrone earliest) propagating posteriorly across the inferolateral wall (Ensite Precision, Abbott). The *white arrows* show the direction of wavefront activation with estimates of conduction velocity by distance over time. The entire window is divided evenly into eight colors of activation (see color bar for sequence) with the latest region of activation represented by the final purple isochrone. Uniform conduction with relatively even isochronal distribution is seen until the interface between the green and light blue isochrones. This discontinuity with isochronal crowding defines a deceleration zone, which is created by a small, localized line of epicardial conduction block (*black bold line with white outline* in the zoomed segment), which forces the activation around the line of block (*white arrows*). Slow conduction and late activation are spatially colocalized and conduction velocity estimates are between 0.07 and 0.17 m/s in this region. (B) Local electrograms are annotated to the offset of the latest component (*yellow dashed lines*) and discontinuous activation is evidenced by widely split electrograms on electrode pairs 1/2 to 7/8. (C) Pacing from the area activated distal to the line of block (multielectrode 7/8 with late potential) results in a perfect pace map match for the VT. D, Structural voltage map showing extensive nonspecific low-voltage area <1.5 mV and dense scar <0.5 mV. The mapping density is shown (*yellow dots*), and the *yellow box* outlines the deceleration zone. (From Aziz Z, Shatz D, Raiman M, et al. Targeted ablation of ventricular tachycardia guided by wavefront discontinuities during sinus rhythm. *Circulation*. 2019;140:1383–1397.)

TABLE 7.3 Abnormal Electrogram Morphologies

Morphology	Definition	Interpretations
Low amplitude	<0.5 mV in the atrium and <1.5 mV in the ventricle	Myocardial infarction, fibrosis, infiltrative process, poor contact, far-field
Fractionated	Prolonged (>70 ms), low-amplitude potential with multiple peaks or multiple baseline crossings	Peri-infarction, slow conduction, catheter motion, arborized myocardial connection
Split	>70 ms duration with two components separated by isoelectric interval	Local conduction block, surgical scar, slow conduction
Late component	Potential occurs after end of surface QRS or P wave	Delayed activation, line of block, slow conduction. Annotation to the offset of the local bipolar electrogram can be used to generate an isochronal late activation map (ILAM)
Continuous	Absence of isoelectric interval throughout diastole	Slow conduction, electromagnetic interference artifact
Mid-diastolic	Potential occurs in mid-diastole bounded by isoelectric intervals	Protected isthmus, bystander connection, repolarization, or motion artifact
Low frequency	Low depolarization velocity (*dV*/*dt*)	Far-field, artifact
Monophasic action potential	Injury current pattern	Excessive contact pressure, local tissue injury (unipolar)

earlier electrogram timing in diastole, with mid-diastolic (or even earlier) potentials (discussed later) having been correlated with successful ablation sites for these arrhythmias. Fig. 7.11 shows an example of atrial tachycardia that was induced in a patient with no known atrial disease; mapping with the ablation catheter revealed electrograms in and around the tricuspid annulus that were significantly more than 50 ms presystolic, thereby raising suspicion for a macroreentrant tachycardia; and a halo duodecapolar catheter was subsequently inserted into the right atrium and showed an activation sequence consistent with counterclockwise reentry around the tricuspid annulus (see Fig. 7.11B). Entrainment maneuvers confirmed the diagnosis and led to successful ablation of the arrhythmia at the cavotricuspid isthmus (CTI).

A related form of three-dimensional mapping, known as ripple (Carto3, Biosense Webster, Diamond Bar, CA), depicts electrograms in their entirety as vertical bars where the length of the bar, at a given time relative to a reference, is proportional to the amplitude of the electrogram at that time (Fig 7.12). The movement of adjacent bars illustrates the activation sequence of the arrhythmia and creates a ripple effect. Raw data provided by ripple mapping circumvent several limitations of traditional maps of local activation time: (1) a requirement for precise annotation of timing, and frequent need for manual adjustment due to errors, (2) interpolation of data between mapped points, which may be inaccurate, and (3) underrepresentation of important low-amplitude electrograms of long duration or double potentials, which can be highly important

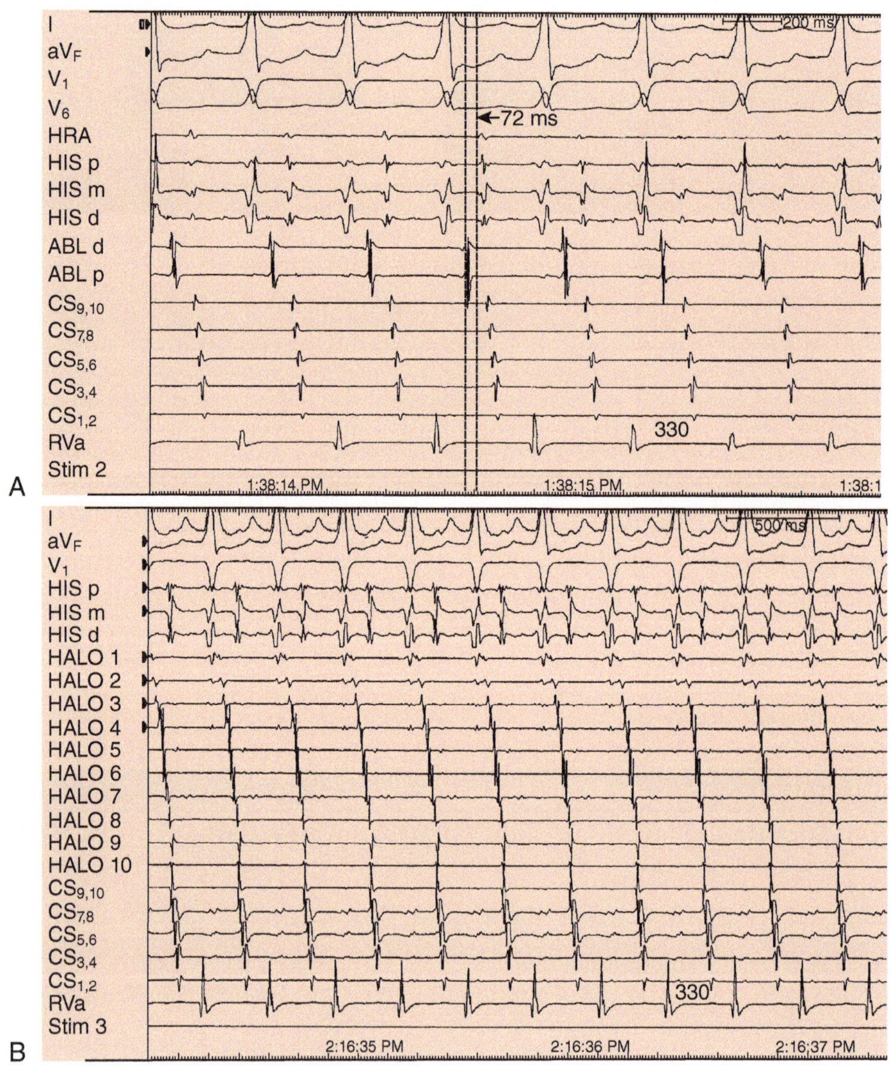

Fig. 7.11 Apparent atrial tachycardia with sites that had greater than 50 ms presystolic activation times in a patient with no known atrial disease. The P-wave morphology and cycle length suggested that atrial tachycardia rather than atrial flutter was present. However, the mid-diastolic activation times suggested reentry rather than focal tachycardia. (A) Mapping with the ablation catheter revealed electrograms in and around the tricuspid annulus that were >50 ms presystolic, thereby raising suspicion for a reentrant tachycardia. (B) A halo catheter inserted subsequently showed an activation sequence consistent with clockwise, isthmus-dependent atrial tachycardia and flutter. Entrainment maneuvers confirmed the diagnosis and led to successful ablation of the arrhythmia. *ABL*, Ablation; *CS*, coronary sinus; *d*, distal; *HRA*, high right atrium; *m*, mid; *p*, proximal; *Stim*, stimulus.

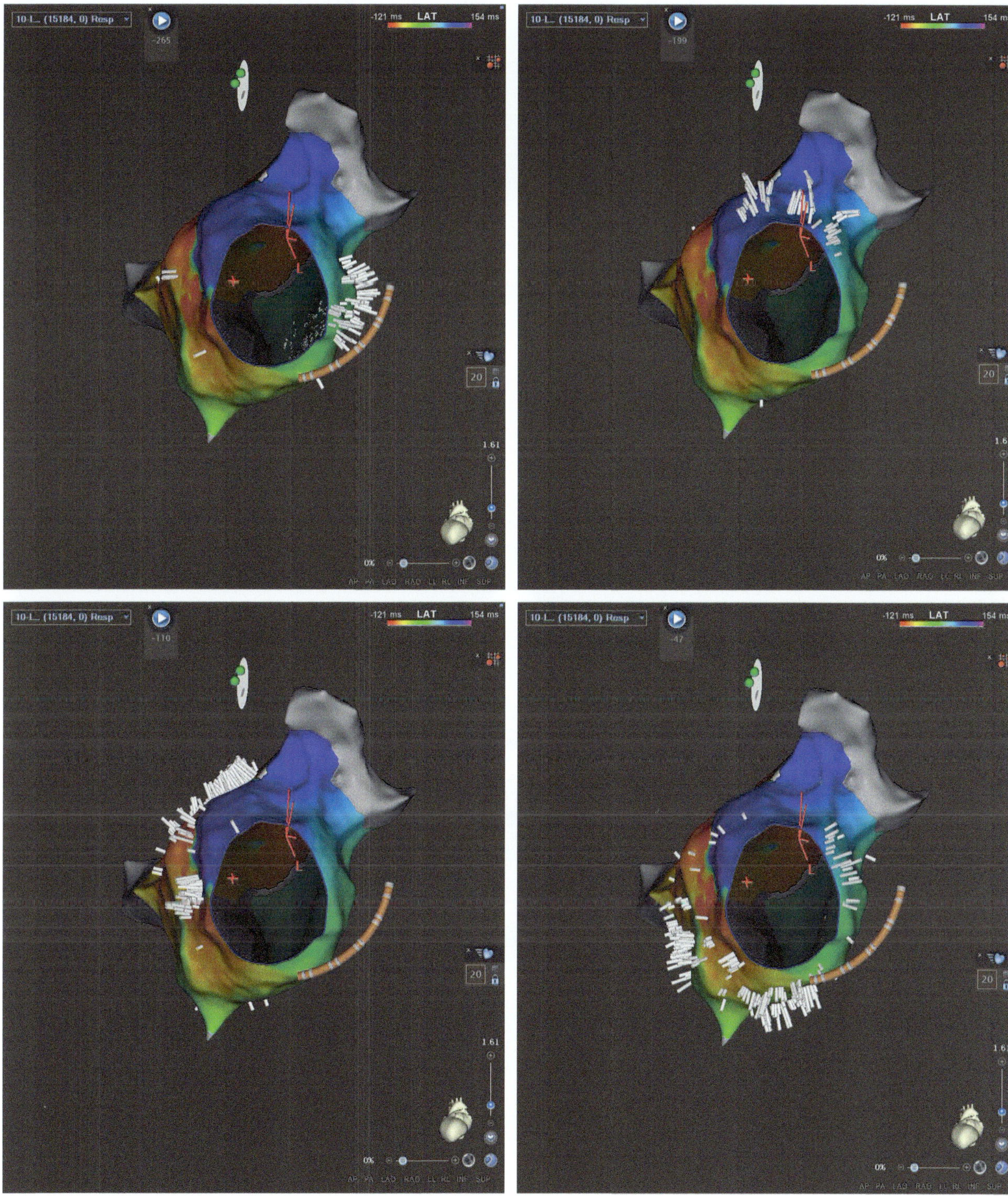

Fig 7.12 Ripple map of mitral annular flutter. *Panels 1 through 4* depict activation of the atrial flutter circuit with four sequential frames sampled from a live ripple map.

but omitted by methods that annotate only a single value of timing.[43,44]

Mid-Diastolic Potentials

If an intervening isoelectric segment exists between QRS complexes during VT, the prepotentials are called *mid-diastolic potentials* (Fig. 7.13); it has been suggested that they identify the region of slow conduction. These prepotentials may precede the major ventricular deflection by 10s to 100s of milliseconds.

It is important to demonstrate that during initiation and resetting of an arrhythmia, loss of the mid-diastolic potential is associated with termination of the arrhythmia.[29] Although there are some recent data to support the specificity of diastolic potentials during sinus rhythm as the potentially successful ablation

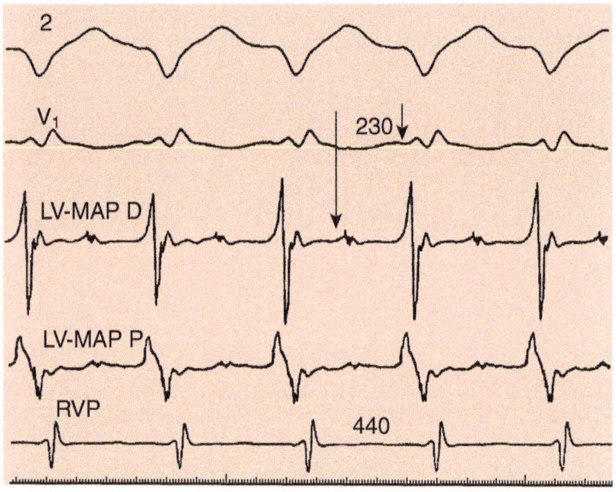

Fig. 7.13 Activation mapping in a diseased heart. The figure shows mid-diastolic potentials in the setting of infarct-related ventricular tachycardia (VT). Leads 2 and V1 are shown with distal (D) and proximal (P) bipolar signals recorded from a presumed protected isthmus of the VT circuit. An isolated mid-diastolic potential (*long arrow*) is recorded 230 ms before the QRS during VT (*short arrow*), with a cycle length of 440 ms. *LV,* Left ventricular; *MAP,* monophasic action potential. (From Josephson ME. *Clinical Cardiac Electrophysiology: Techniques and Interpretation,* 3rd ed. Philadelphia: Lippincott Williams & Wilkins; 2002.)

sites (i.e., critical isthmus sites during VT),[45] most studies have looked at diastolic potentials during sustained tachycardia as markers of a protected isthmus.

Mid-diastolic potentials that do not dynamically precede the QRS complex of the VT may represent blind-end alleys of late activation or motion artifact.[29,30] In one study, almost continuous electrical activity spanning the diastolic segment was frequently seen in patients with VT because of ischemic heart disease or arrhythmogenic RV dysplasia. However, in 85% of patients, the episodes of continuous electrical activity could be dissociated from the VT.[25] Such behavior is presumably caused by slow and stuttering conduction into areas of diseased myocardium not essential for ongoing tachycardia.

Unipolar Potential Mapping

Unipolar electrograms provide useful adjunctive mapping information to bipolar electrograms during mapping for focal atrial arrhythmias and VTs. Amerandral and associates noted that the presence of a QS complex was highly sensitive in identifying successful ablation sites.[46] However, nearly 70% of unsuccessful sites also manifested a QS unipolar complex, with QS complexes being recorded more than 1 cm away in 65% of patients.[47] The unipolar electrogram morphology with standard ablation electrodes is therefore a highly sensitive but nonspecific marker for target sites in patients with idiopathic RV and other VTs as well as atrial tachycardias. Unipolar electrograms are of limited use, however, in the setting of myocardial scar or fibrosis, because the criteria established for unipolar activation (i.e., peak depolarization velocity (dV/dt)) cannot be relied on in the presence of slow, disordered conduction, with the onset of unipolar recordings in this setting frequently showing a delayed initial deflection.

Much has been written about the use of the unipolar electrogram in localizing insertion and successful ablation sites for accessory pathways.[48] Note that most of these data are for anterograde mapping in the setting of overt preexcitation, although some investigators have demonstrated the use of unipolar mapping for retrogradely conducting accessory pathways.[49] Electrograms characteristic of the insertion sites of accessory pathways have been described in detail in Chapters 26–30 of this book.

Pace Mapping

Pace mapping involves manipulation of the mapping catheter to the region of origin of the tachycardia. Pacing at this site, using the same cycle length as the tachycardia, should generate P waves or QRS complexes resembling those during tachycardia. The greater the degree of concordance between the P-wave or QRS morphology during pacing and tachycardia, the closer the catheter is to the exit site of the tachycardia. In addition, a stimulus to QRS interval of more than 40–70 ms is an indication of slow conduction.

Pace mapping has advantages over activation mapping in that induction of arrhythmia is not required; as a result, it allows identification of the site of origin when the induced arrhythmia is poorly tolerated or when sustained tachycardia is not inducible by electrophysiologic techniques but when P-wave or QRS morphology from a 12-lead ECG is available. However, others have argued that pace mapping is not as sensitive or precise as activation mapping and may be more time consuming. Pace mapping has generally been more useful as a means of corroborating candidate ablation sites, with a combination of activation and pace mapping used to best identify the optimal target site of ablation. For generalized localization of an arrhythmia exit site, such as with substrate mapping of unstable ventricular arrhythmias, matching 10/12 leads may be sufficient. For precise arrhythmia localization, 12/12 leads should match the clinical tachycardia. Algorithms used in contemporary electroanatomic mapping systems can analyze the surface ECG morphology of paced complexes for correlation with a clinical arrhythmia and report the degree of correlation as a percentage match. A score in the range of 90% or higher is generally considered a high degree of correlation.[50]

Most investigators report successful ablation at sites with identical or nearly identical matches in all 12 surface leads.[51,52] Differences in QRS configuration between pacing and spontaneous tachycardia in a single lead may be critical. An example is shown in Fig. 7.14, in which ablation success was achieved (in the left coronary cusp) only at the site of a 12/12 or perfect pace map. Fig. 7.15 shows an example of premature ventricular complexes (PVCs) arising from the right coronary cusp. Unlike in Fig. 7.14A, in which there is a small R wave in the unipolar electrogram, the distal unipolar electrogram in Fig. 7.15A has a QS complex; pace mapping at this site also resulted in a nearly perfect pace map (see Fig. 7.15B). Ablation at this site resulted in elimination of all PVCs.

Pace mapping should be performed as close as possible to the cycle length of the spontaneous tachycardia to minimize rate-dependent aberration in paced P-wave or QRS configuration

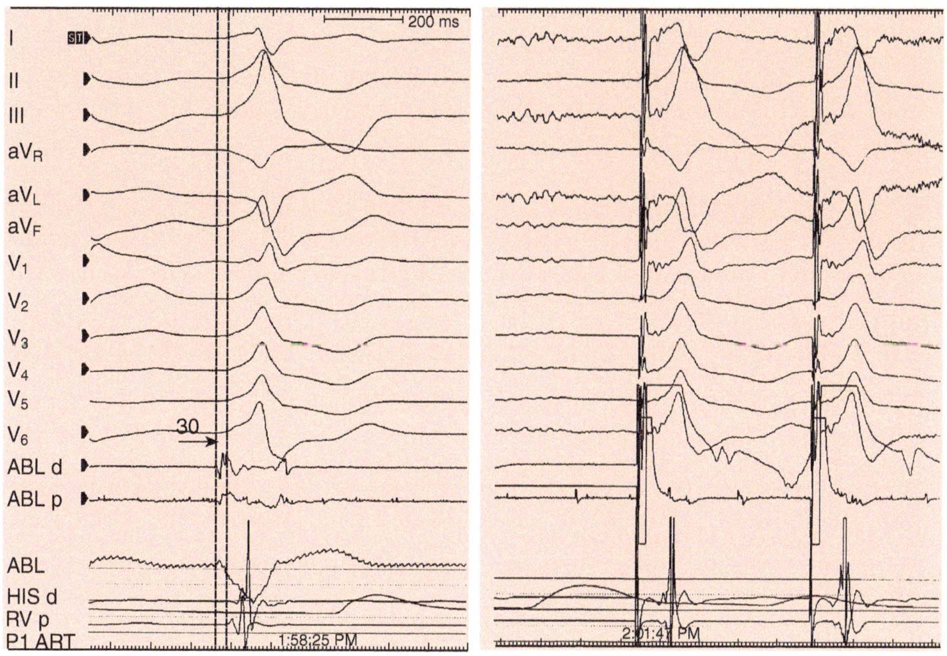

A B

Fig. 7.14 Excellent pace map in a patient with right bundle inferior axis premature ventricular contractions (PVCs). (A) Right bundle PVCs mapped to the left coronary cusp. The ablation catheter shows an activation time that was 30 ms presystolic. The distal unipolar electrogram coincides with the earliest bipolar electrogram. Note that the unipolar electrogram (ABL) has a small r wave before the inscription of the QS. (B) Pace mapping performed at the site shown in A revealed a 12/12 match with the PVC in A. It was decided to ablate at this site because activation sites with a QS pattern on the unipolar electrogram (i.e., no r wave) were <0.5 cm from the left main artery. Ablation resulted in termination of PVCs. *d*, Distal; *p*, proximal; *RV*, right ventricle.

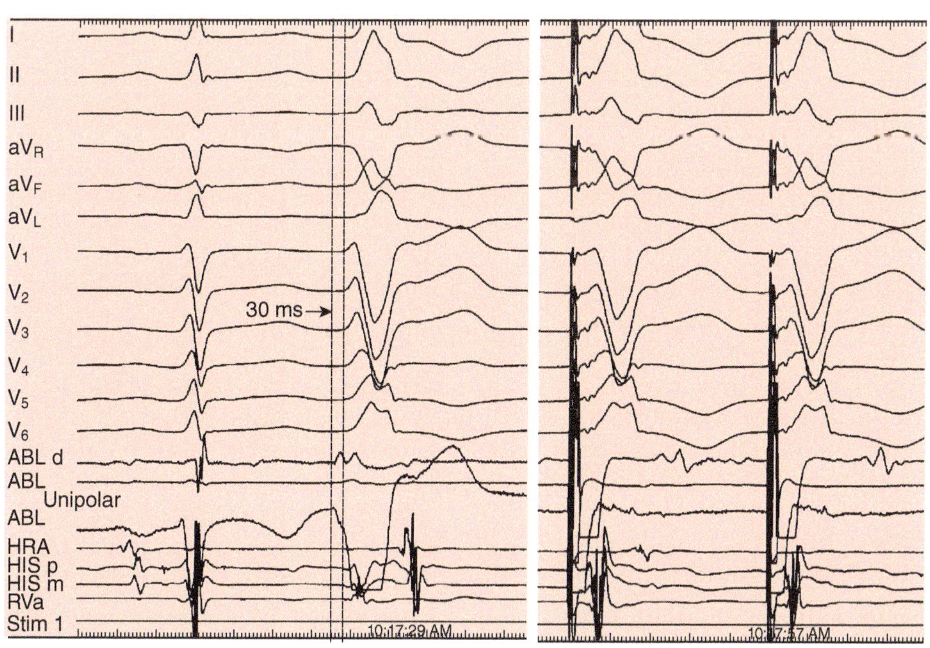

A B

Fig. 7.15 Excellent pace map in a patient with right coronary cusp premature ventricular contractions (PVCs). (A) Right bundle PVCs mapped to the right coronary cusp. The ablation catheter shows an activation time that was 30 ms presystolic. The distal unipolar electrogram coincides with the earliest bipolar electrogram and has a QS complex. (B) Pace mapping performed at the site shown in A revealed a 12/12 match with the PVC in A. Ablation at this site resulted in termination of PVC. *d*, Distal; *HRA*, high right atrium; *m*, mid; *p*, proximal; *Stim*, stimulus.

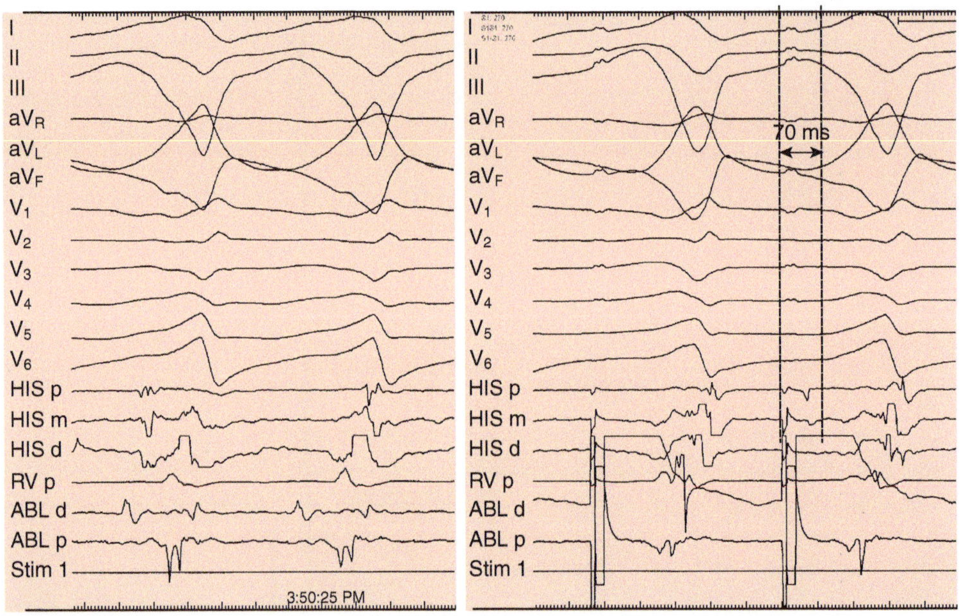

Fig. 7.16 Pace mapping in the setting of myocardial scar. (A) Ventricular tachycardia (cycle length, 260 ms). (B) Pace mapping in a region of scar (low-amplitude potentials) in the right ventricle of a patient with arrhythmogenic right ventricular dysplasia. Note the 12/12 leads pace map and the long, mid-diastolic stimulus-to-QRS interval (70 ms); the stimulus-to-QRS interval was suggestive of a location in the middle of a protected isthmus. The unusual morphology in lead V1 for a right ventricular origin may reflect surface lead placement. Ablation in this region rendered the ventricular tachycardia noninducible. *d*, Distal; *m*, mid; *p*, proximal; *Stim*, stimulus.

(owing to increasing degrees of incomplete repolarization and fusion with the preceding T wave during shorter cycle lengths).[53]

Pace mapping during sinus rhythm has been shown to be less sensitive in the setting of scarred myocardium, even when pacing is performed close to the tachycardia circuit. The activation wavefront may take the path of least resistance and, instead of mimicking the tachycardia wavefront (through the protected tachycardia isthmus), may activate normal myocardium first, thereby creating a very different pace map. In addition, the boundaries of a protected isthmus may be functional in nature, including in normal hearts, and therefore difficult to replicate with pacing during sinus rhythm. Several investigators have shown that pace mapping may be performed at the infarct border[54] with good sensitivity and specificity and can provide successful target sites for ablation based on the closeness of the pace map to the tachycardia and the stimulus-to-QRS interval (helping outline the critical isthmus from entrance to exit; Fig. 7.16).

Entrainment Mapping

Entrainment is one of the most powerful tools in the electrophysiologist's arsenal that serves the following purposes: (1) allows confirmation of reentry as the underlying mechanism of a sustained arrhythmia, (2) allows localization of an underlying reentrant circuit (e.g., to the right or left atrium in the setting of a reentrant atrial tachycardia), and (3) allows identification of myocardium that is critical to the reentrant circuit (i.e., critical isthmus). The critical isthmus may be narrow enough to be amenable to ablation, with resulting interruption of the tachycardia.[55] A full discussion of resetting curves, entrainment criteria, and the pitfalls of entrainment is beyond the scope of this chapter; the reader is referred to other authoritative texts for a more in-depth study of the principles of entrainment.[55–59]

Entrainment is continuous resetting of a reentrant circuit that has an excitable gap by a series of stimuli. The presence of entrainment is established when pacing at a rate slightly faster than the TCL accelerates all QRS complexes or P waves (or intracardiac electrograms) to the pacing rate and termination of pacing is followed by resumption of the same tachycardia with the presence of constant surface or intracardiac fusion during pacing (or progressive fusion during pacing at progressively faster cycle lengths). The four criteria for manifest entrainment are (1) constant fusion during overdrive pacing, except for the last captured beat, which is entrained but not fused; (2) progressive fusion during overdrive pacing at different cycle lengths; (3) localized conduction block to a site for one paced beat associated with interruption of the tachycardia, followed by activation of that site by the next paced beat from a different direction and with a shorter conduction time; and (4) a change in conduction time to and electrogram morphology at an electrode recording site when pacing at two different rates during a tachycardia (i.e., the intracardiac equivalent of criterion 2, because it may be difficult to visualize surface criteria in some cases, such as for atrial tachycardia).

Fig. 7.17 shows an example of manifest entrainment (based on intracardiac electrograms); activation around the tricuspid annulus is shown during overdrive pacing of what appeared to be typical, counterclockwise atrial flutter in a patient with a

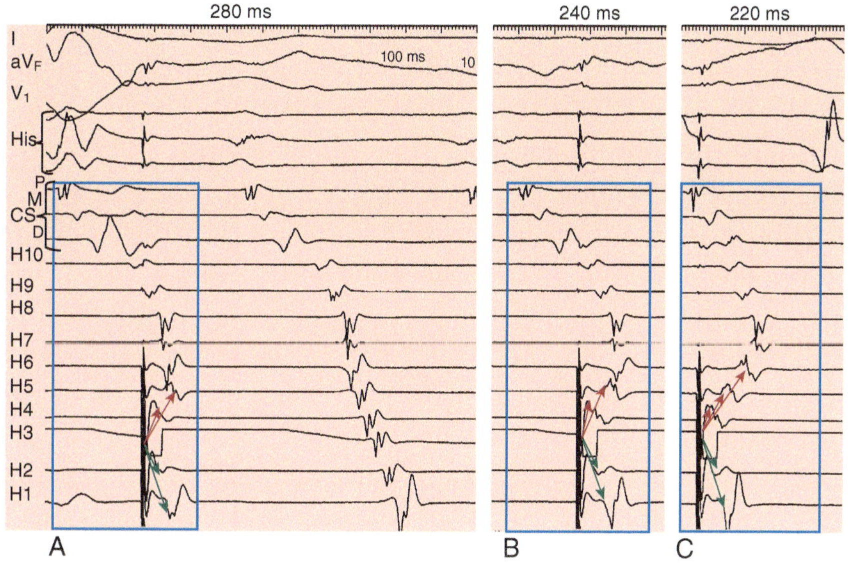

Fig. 7.17 Progressive fusion with demonstration of (manifest) entrainment. The figure shows activation around the tricuspid annulus during attempted entrainment of what appeared to be typical, counterclockwise atrial flutter in a patient with a normal heart. (A) Pacing from halo (H) 3 that is slightly faster than the tachycardia (entrainment) reveals fusion along the halo catheter; halo 5 is captured antidromically, but the rest of the halo is captured orthodromically (no change in activation sequence or polarity along the halo except in halo 7). (B) Pacing at 240 ms demonstrates progressive fusion: now halo 5 and halo 6 are captured antidromically (*red arrows*) show clear change in timing and morphology of halo 6 in B compared with A, thereby confirming entrainment (based on intracardiac fusion, the fourth entrainment criterion). (C) Pacing at 220 ms results in antidromic activation of halo 6 and halo 7. *CS*, Coronary sinus; *d*, distal; *m*, mid; *p*, proximal.

normal heart. Pacing at progressively faster rates demonstrates progressive fusion—one of the diagnostic criteria for entrainment and therefore reentry—which is best demonstrated by a change in activation (as well as timing) of the bipolar electrograms in the distal halo electrodes. In fact, even when changes in timing are subtle, electrogram morphology may provide important clues to a diagnosis.

After entrainment has been demonstrated (i.e., manifest entrainment), it can be used for mapping. Entrainment mapping is centered on obtaining a match between the entrained surface P wave or QRS complex or intracardiac electrograms and tachycardia morphology (concealed entrainment; discussed in a later section) and on obtaining a postpacing interval (PPI; described later) that is equal to the TCL. Although the demonstration of resetting with fusion (or manifest entrainment) confirms reentry, the presence of concealed entrainment allows the ablationist to hone in on a protected isthmus—a common site of ablation success. Concealed entrainment is characterized by a failure to demonstrate fusion (i.e., criteria 1, 2, and 4) during pacing from a protected isthmus within a tachycardia circuit (Fig. 7.18) and is associated with a PPI that is equal to the TCL. The PPI is the time between the last pacing stimulus that entrained the tachycardia and the next recorded electrogram at the pacing site. The PPI should be equal to the TCL within 20–30 ms if the pacing site is within a critical part of the reentrant circuit. If the pacing site is outside of the circuit, the PPI should be equal to the TCL plus the time required for the stimulus to propagate from the pacing site to the tachycardia circuit and back. Problems arise when the electrogram at the pacing site is distorted immediately after pacing. To overcome this shortcoming, alternative methods of estimating the PPI have been developed, such as the postpacing interval recorded at a remote electrode (PPIR) method and the N + 1 method. Both of these methods have been shown to be equivalent and comparable with the standard PPI (see Fig. 7.18D).[59]

Downstream Overdrive Pacing

More recently, the concepts involved with entrainment have been further expanded on, using downstream overdrive pacing (DOP) to rapidly detect fusion and diagnose macroreentrant atrial arrhythmias. Downstream overdrive pacing is an entrainment maneuver where atrial activation sequence can be used to differentiate macrorentrant from focal atrial tachycardias. The atrial tachycardia is overdrive paced with a multielectrode catheter at a site of activation downstream from the neighboring electrodes. This technique establishes the presence of fusion at a constant paced cycle minimally shorter than the tachycardia cycle length. Constant fusion is confirmed by measuring the time between the pacing stimulus (S) and the last upstream atrial electrogram (A_u) accelerated to the PCL (S-A_u). A short conduction time (S-A_u) would support a focal atrial tachycardia. A long conduction time (S-A_u) should be present only in macrorentrant atrial tachycardia unless a line of block or slow conduction is present (Fig. 7.19). Specifically, Barbhaiya and colleagues demonstrated that a macroreentrant circuit was confirmed with DOP when pacing near the circuit (PPI-TCL < 40 ms) and resulting in an S-A_u interval >75% of the TCL. In contrast, an S-A_u interval <25% of the TCL supported a focal AT or pacing at a site remote from a macroreentrant circuit.[60–61]

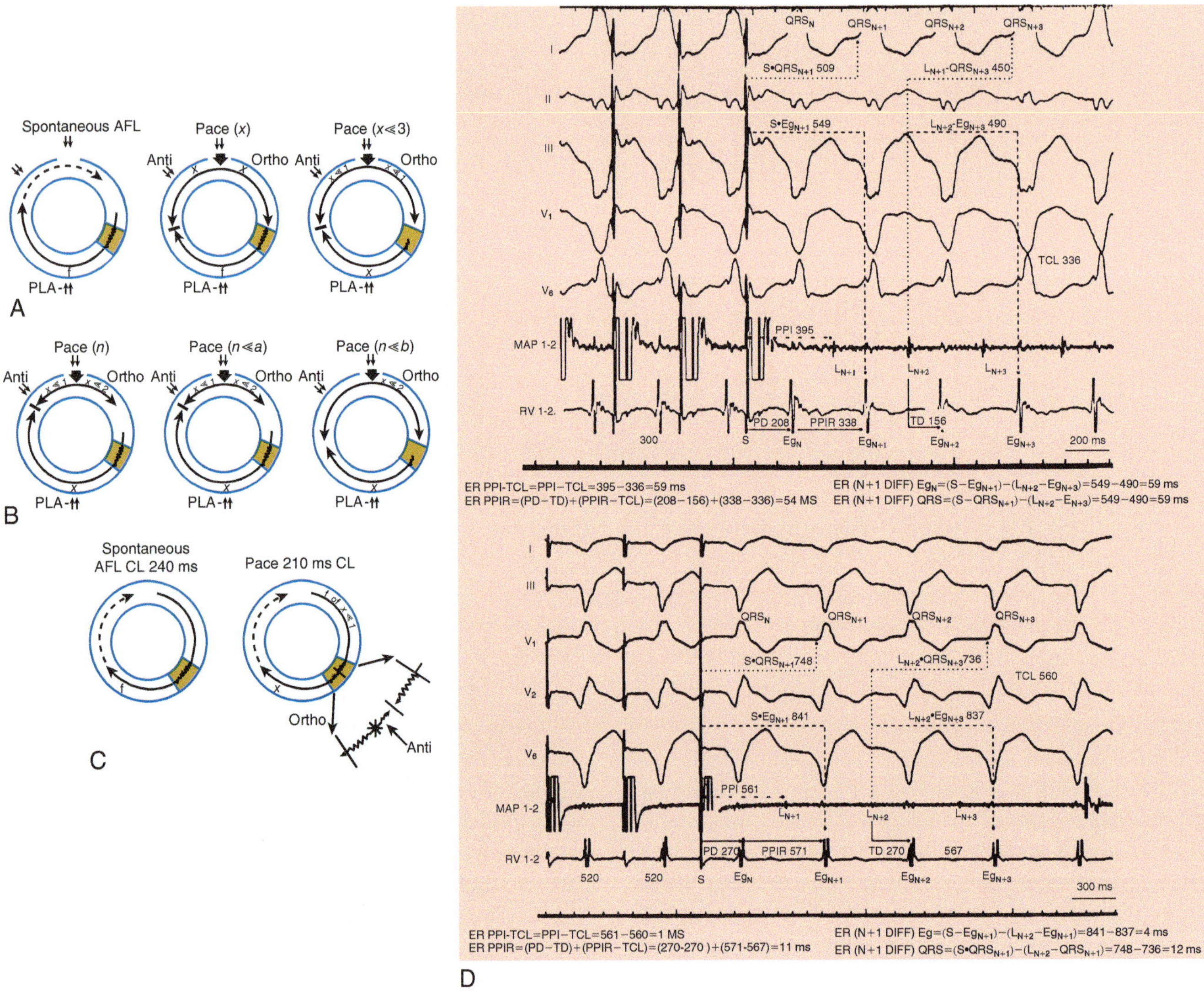

Fig. 7.18 Manifest and concealed entrainment of atrial flutter. The figure shows schematic diagrams of manifest and concealed entrainment, respectively. (A and B) Fixed and progressive fusion, respectively, with overdrive pacing during tachycardia; the contribution of the antidromic wavefront to the tachycardia morphology progressively increases. © Concealed fusion; that is, progressively faster pacing from a protected isthmus does not lead to manifest fusion because the antidromic wavefront does not contribute significantly to the morphology of the tachycardia beat. *Shaded areas* indicate protected isthmus. *AFL,* Atrial flutter; *anti,* antidromic; *CL,* cycle length; *n,* pacing cycle lengths with n > n + a > n + b; *ortho,* orthodromic; *PLA,* posteroinferior left atrium; *x,* pacing stimulus in a sequence of stimuli. (D) Alternative methods for estimating postpacing interval when the pacing electrogram is obscured. Comparison of conventional method and alternative methods for assessing entrainment response in ventricular tachycardia (VT) circuits. Surface electrocardiogram leads and intracardiac bipolar electrograms recorded from the mapping catheter (MAP 1–2) and from the reference catheter (RV 1–2) are shown. *Top panel:* Overdrive pacing from a bystander dead-end pathway entrains VT with concealed fusion. PPI is 395 ms, and TCL is 336 ms. PPI − TCL is 395 − 336 = 59 ms. Measurements for ER (*N* + 1 DIFF) using QRS complex as the reference point are as follows: S − QRS_{N+1} interval is 509 ms and L_{N+2} − QRS_{N+3} interval is 450 ms. ER (*N* + 1 $DIFF_{QRS}$) = (S − QRS_{N+1}) − (L_{N+2} − QRS_{N+3}) = 509 − 450 = 59 ms, and matches exactly measured PPI − TCL. Measurements using remote electrogram (RV 1–2) as the reference point are also presented: S − Eg_{N+1} interval is 549 ms and L_{N+2} − Eg_{N+3} interval is 490 ms and calculated ER (*N* + 1 $DIFF_{Eg}$) = (S − Eg_{N+1}) − (L_{N+2} − Eg_{N+3}) = 549 − 490 = 59 ms. Computations for the PPIR method are also: PD interval is 208 ms, TD interval is 156 ms, PPIR interval is 338 ms and almost matches TCL, which is 336 ms. Thus ER PPIR = (PD − TD) + (PPIR − TCL) = (208 − 156) + (338 − 336) = 52 + 2 = 54 ms. *Bottom panel,* VT entrained with concealed fusion during pacing from the isthmus of the VT circuit. PPI is 561 ms and TCL is 560 ms. PPI − TCL difference is 561 − 560 = 1 ms. Measurements for ER (*N* + 1 DIFF) using QRS complex as the reference point are as follows: S − QRS_{N+1} interval is 748 ms and L_{N+2} − QRS interval is 736 ms. Thus, ER (*N* + 1 $DIFF_{QRS}$) = (S − QRS_{N+1}) − (L_{N+2} − QRS_{N+3}) = 748 − 736 = 12 ms. Measurements using remote electrogram (RV 1–2) as the reference point are also presented. Eg − QRS_{N+1} interval is 841 ms and L_{N+2} − QRS interval is 837 ms and calculated. *AFL,* Atrial flutter; *anti,* antidromic; *CL,* cycle length; *ER,* entrainment response; *ERPPIR,* entrainment response (estimated PPI − TCL) by the PPI remote electrogram method; *MAP,* monophasic action potential; *n,* pacing cycle lengths with *n* > *n* + *a* > *n* + *b*; ortho, orthodromic; *PD,* pacing delay; *PLA,* posteroinferior left atrium; *PPI,* postpacing interval; *PPIR,* postpacing interval recorded at the remote electrode; *TCL,* tachycardia cycle length; *TD,* tachycardia delay; *x,* pacing stimulus in a sequence of stimuli. (A–C modified from Waldo AL. Atrial flutter: entrainment characteristics. *J Cardiovasc Electrophysiol.* 1997;8:337-352. D from Derejko P, Szumowski LJ, Sanders P, et al. Clinical validation and comparison of alternative methods for evaluation of entrainment mapping. *J Cardiovasc Electrophysiol.* 2009;20:741–748.)

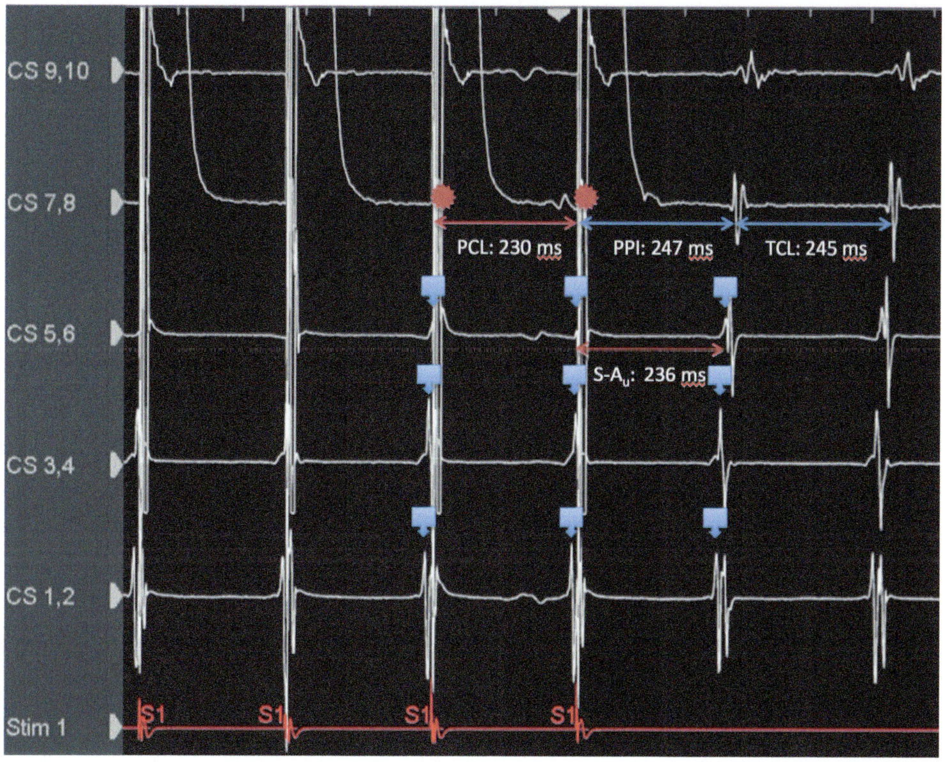

Fig 7.19 Downstream overdrive pacing (DOP) from the proximal coronary sinus in perimitral flutter. Pacing is performed from CS 7,8 (*brown star*) at a PCL of 230 ms. The PPI –TCL = 247 ms – 245 ms = 2 ms (<40 ms), which supports proximity to the circuit. The upstream electrodes are accelerated to the paced cycle length (*blue box arrows*). The S-Au time is 236 ms, which is 96% of the TCL (S-Au > 75%), suggesting fusion and supporting macroreentry as the mechanism of the tachycardia. *CS*, Coronary sinus; *Stim*, stimulus; PCL, paced cycle length; *PPI*, postpacing interval; *TCL*, tachycardia cycle length; *S-Au*, stimulus minus last upstream atrial electrogram.

Miscellaneous Pacing Maneuvers

Atrial or ventricular pacing during sinus rhythm or during tachycardia is a useful maneuver for determining the mechanism of a tachycardia and may also help in mapping a tachycardia (Table 7.4).

Response to Atrial or Ventricular Pacing

In the laboratory, overdrive ventricular pacing is performed to demonstrate entrainment in resetting a narrow-complex supraventricular tachycardia (SVT) with a concentric retrograde activation sequence, where ventricular pacing (entrainment) is performed as a diagnostic maneuver to differentiate between atrioventricular nodal reentrant tachycardia (AVNRT), atrioventricular reentrant tachycardia (AVRT), and atrial tachycardia. Pacing is set at 10–30 ms faster than the TCL for at least 8–10 beats to allow continuous resetting of the atrial rate to occur; the atrial activation sequence of the tachycardia must remain unchanged during orthodromic capture of an AVRT or reentrant atrial tachycardia circuit as well as during AVNRT. If the tachycardia resumes after pacing, a V-A-V versus a V-A-A-V response is evaluated on the return cycle,[62] with the latter indicating an atrial tachycardia. If a V-A-V response is noted, the stimulus-to-A (and His–atrial [HA], if a retrograde His is visible) interval is compared during pacing with the ventriculoatrial (VA; and HA) interval during tachycardia.[62–64] The PPI is also measured and compared with the TCL to differentiate between AVRT and AVNRT.[58] Fig. 7.20 shows examples of AVNRT and AVRT in response to ventricular entrainment.

Ventricular pacing can also be performed at the TCL during sinus rhythm, and the diagnostic criteria mentioned earlier (i.e., comparison of VA [>115 ms or <115 ms], stimulus to A [>85 ms or <85 ms], and HA [>−10 ms or <−10 ms] times during tachycardia and pacing) are used to differentiate between AVNRT and (septal) AVRT, respectively.[62–64] However, one should be aware of limitations to these maneuvers in a very slowly conducting septal accessory pathway (VA/TCL ≥ 40%).[65] One can also use these maneuvers (PPI-TCL and stimulus to A) when RV pacing results in induction of the SVT of interest.[66]

Even when an entrainment response does not occur, there are other helpful observations that can be gleaned at the onset of ventricular pacing during SVT. A typical scenario is termination of tachycardia during attempted ventricular entrainment as described earlier. A diagnosis of orthodromic reentrant tachycardia is likely if the atrial signal is reset during attempted RV pacing that results in fusion (similar to a His-refractory PVC response). AVNRT is more likely if atrial resetting, resulting in advanced fixed stimulus to A, required more than one fully paced RV beat.[67,68]

TABLE 7.4 Miscellaneous Pacing Maneuvers

	Diagnostic Purpose	Method	Requirements	Response to Pacing
Atrial Maneuver				
AOP	AVNRT versus AVRT versus AT	Entrainment of tachycardia: Atrial pacing at the TCL	1) Continuous resetting of atrial rate 2) Unchanged atrial activation sequence for orthodromic capture of AVRT, AVNRT, or reentrant atrial circuit	Compare AH intervals during A pacing compared with during tachycardia without pacing: 1) AT: Delta AH <20 ms 2) AVRT: Delta AH 20–40 ms 3) AVNRT: Delta AH >40 ms
AOP	JET versus AVNRT	Entrainment of tachycardia: Pace 10–30 ms faster than TCL for 8–10 beats in the ventricle	1) Continuous resetting of atrial rate 2) Unchanged atrial activation sequence for orthodromic capture of AVRT, AVNRT, or reentrant atrial circuit	1) JET; A-H-H-A response 2) AVNRT A-H-A response
AOP	Rule out AT	Entrainment of tachycardia: Atrial pacing at the TCL	1) Continuous resetting of atrial rate 2) Unchanged atrial activation sequence	VA linking: Consistent VA times postpacing
PACs	JET versus AVNRT	Input early-coupled PACs	Local electrogram from the PAC occurs before the immediate His activation	1) JET: Early-coupled PAC advances subsequent His 2) AVNRT: Early coupled PAC terminates tachycardia or delays next His
PACs	JET versus AVNRT	Input late-coupled PACS during His refractoriness	Local electrogram from the PAC occurs at or after the immediate His activation	1) JET: Late-coupled PAC fails to advance or delay subsequent His 2) AVNRT: Late-coupled PAC advances subsequent His, delays subsequent His, or terminates tachycardia
Ventricular Maneuver				
VOP	AVNRT versus AVRT versus AT	Entrainment of tachycardia: Pace 10–30 ms faster than TCL for 8–10 beats in the ventricle	1) Continuous resetting of atrial rate 2) Unchanged atrial activation sequence for orthodromic capture of AVRT, AVNRT, or reentrant atrial circuit 3) Tachycardia should resume after pacing	Assess response postpacing: 1) AT: V-A-A-V; 2) AVNRT or AVRT: V-A-V; 3) AVNRT: Stim A – VA > 85 ms or PPI-TCL > 115 ms
VOP	AVNRT versus AVRT	Entrainment of tachycardia: Pace 10–30 ms faster than TCL for 8–10 beats in the ventricle	1) Initially, ventricular capture with fusion 2) Then, full ventricular capture with resetting of atria	AVNRT > AVRT if more than 1 fully captured RV beat needed to advance the atrium
PVCs	1) Diagnose presence or absence of an accessory pathway 2) Diagnose possible participation of pathway in tachycardia	Input single PVCs during His refractoriness	Surface ECG fusion during PVC confirms His refractoriness	Presence of pathway: 1) Advance timing: of next atrial activation 2) Delay timing of next atrial activation* 3) Terminate tachycardia without atrial activation post fused PVC*

Table 7.4 illustrates atrial and ventricular pacing maneuvers to differentiate AVNRT, AVRT, AT, and JET.

A, Atrium; *AH*, atrial-His; *AOP*, atrial overdrive pacing; *AT*, atrial tachycardia; *AVRT*, atrioventricular reentrant tachycardia; *AVNRT*, atrioventricular nodal reentrant tachycardia; *ECG*, electrocardiogram; *H*, His; *JET*, junctional ectopic tachycardia; *PAC*, premature atrial contraction; *PPI*, postpacing interval; *PVC*, premature ventricular contraction; *TCL*, tachycardia cycle length; *V*, ventricle; *VA*, ventriculoatrial; *VOP*, ventricular overdrive pacing.

*Confirms the participation of the pathway as the retrograde limb of the tachycardia.

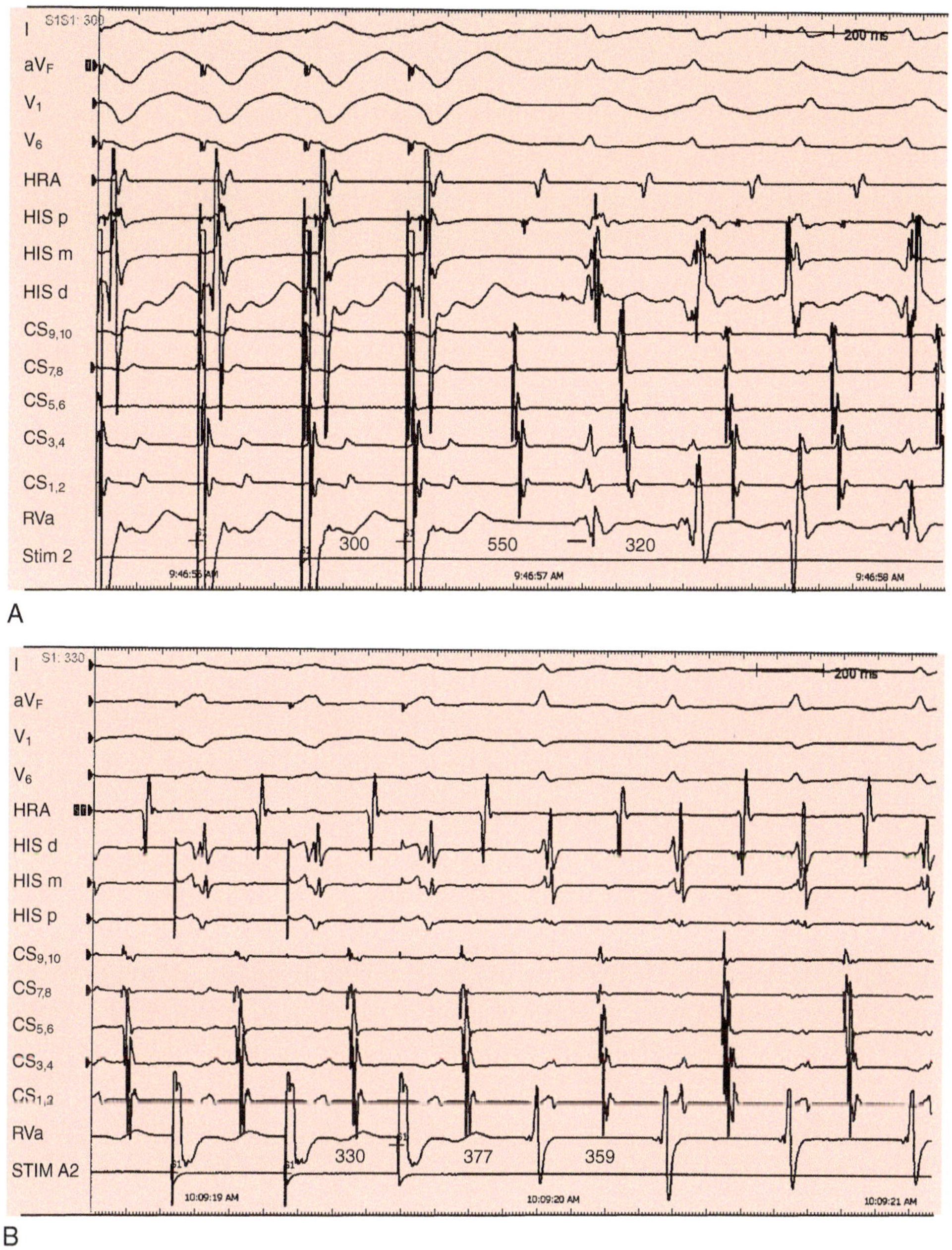

Fig. 7.20 Entrainment of supraventricular tachycardia. The figure demonstrates the response of atrioventricular nodal reentrant tachycardia (AVNRT) and atrioventricular reentrant tachycardia (AVRT; with concentric activation sequences) to entrainment from the ventricle. (A) Entrainment is consistent with AVNRT: the stimulus-to-A interval during ventricular pacing exceeds the VA interval during tachycardia by more than 85 ms. The postpacing interval (PPI) exceeds the tachycardia cycle length by more than 115 ms, also consistent with AVNRT. (B) Entrainment here is consistent with AVRT, with the difference between the stimulus-to-A interval (during pacing) and the VA interval (during tachycardia) being less than 85 ms and the PPI being about equal to the tachycardia cycle length. *CS*, Coronary sinus; *d*, distal; *HRA*, high right atrium; *m*, mid; *p*, proximal; *Stim*, stimulus.

Another maneuver that may be helpful in deciphering the mechanism of long RP SVTs is atrial pacing at the TCL; a comparison of AH times may allow differentiation among atrial tachycardia, AVNRT, and AVRT: AH intervals that occur during pacing are expected to be similar to those that occur during tachycardia ($\Delta AH \leq 20$ m) for atrial tachycardia but are longer during AVRT (ΔAH between 20 and 40 ms) and AVNRT ($\Delta AH \geq 40$ ms).[69] Similarly, atrial overdrive pacing can be helpful in excluding atrial tachycardia in the absence of VA linking.[62]

Atrial overdrive pacing can also help differentiate junctional ectopic tachycardia from AVNRT by documentation of an A-H-H-A response rather than an A-H-A response.[70]

Premature Ventricular Contractions During Narrow-Complex Tachycardia

It is almost a standard practice in most laboratories to deliver premature ventricular stimuli at the onset of a sustained, hemodynamically stable, and regular (i.e., no variability in cycle length)

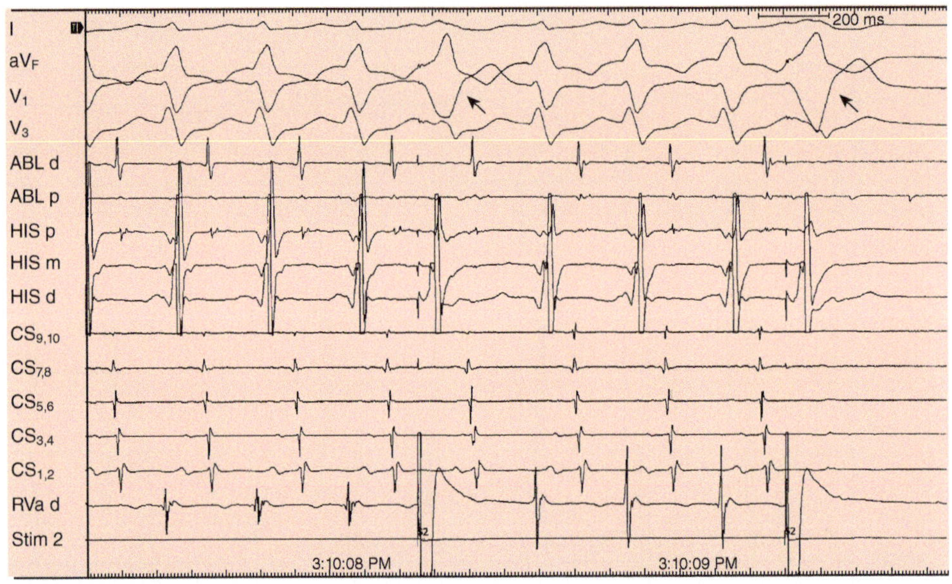

Fig. 7.21 Premature ventricular stimuli (PVCs) delivered during His refractoriness (during supraventricular tachycardia). Although no His depolarization is seen, the presence of electrocardiographic fusion during the first PVC, compared with the second PVC, which closely resembles a fully paced beat during sinus rhythm (not shown here), confirms anterograde His depolarization, thereby indicating His refractoriness during the first PVC. Termination of supraventricular tachycardia following the second PVC is not diagnostic since the stimulus appear to precede His refractoriness. *ABL*, Ablation; *CS*, coronary sinus; *d*, distal; *m*, mid; *p*, proximal; *Stim*, stimulus.

SVT. Exceptions to this rule are a regular tachycardia with changing VA times (indicating probable atrial tachycardia) and tachycardias lacking a 1:1 AV association (excluding AV reentry and making AVNRT unlikely). Single PVCs delivered during His refractoriness are of diagnostic utility if they advance or delay the timing of subsequent atrial activation or terminate the tachycardia without atrial activation. Each of these phenomena indicates the presence of a retrogradely conducting accessory pathway, with the latter two, if reproducible, confirming the participation of the pathway as the retrograde limb of the tachycardia. Although a PVC on His advancing the timing of atrial activation with the same activation sequence as the tachycardia is highly suggestive of a participating accessory pathway, it is by no means diagnostic, with an atrial tachycardia arising from close to the insertion of an accessory pathway being a remote possibility. Fig. 7.21 shows a PVC delivered during His refractoriness; although no His depolarization is seen, the presence of ECG fusion during the PVC confirms anterograde His depolarization, thereby indicating His refractoriness. More premature PVCs (more than 30 ms before the next expected His-bundle depolarization) delivered close to the site of earliest atrial activation can be considered diagnostic of the absence of an accessory pathway, if the atrium is not affected.[71] PVCs that reset the atrium can also help indicate the presence of an accessory pathway if they significantly change the VA time, such as during SVT with an eccentric retrograde atrial activation. An LBBB-type PVC (from the RV apex) that advances the atrium, along with an increase in the surface ECG VA interval, is diagnostic of a left-sided accessory pathway.

Premature Atrial Contractions During Narrow- and Wide-Complex Tachycardia

Delivery of premature atrial contractions (PACs) can also be useful during a narrow complex tachycardia. The most common application of this is during differentiation of AVNRT and junctional ectopic tachycardia. A late-coupled PAC would fail to perturb the His and TCL in junctional ectopic tachycardia, while perturbing (advancing or delaying) the subsequent His (or V with stable HV interval) deflection in AVNRT. An early-coupled PAC would be expected to advance the subsequent (n) His and V deflection in ectopic tachycardia while termination or delay ($n + 1$) would be seen in AVNRT.[72]

Late-coupled PACs can also be helpful in assessing participation of an antegradely conduction accessory pathway in the clinical tachycardia. A typical response can be advancement (85%) and, less often, delay of subsequent ventricular activation and resetting of TCL.[73] The utility of the PACs in the setting of wide-complex tachycardias is discussed in greater length in subsequent chapters of this book relating to specific AV connections.

Termination of Tachycardia During Pacing Maneuvers

If a narrow-complex tachycardia terminates during ventricular pacing without any change in the atrial cycle length (indicating no depolarization of the atrium by the ventricular stimuli), atrial tachycardia is excluded as a possible diagnosis (see the "Premature Ventricular Contractions During Narrow-Complex Tachycardia" section).

In certain cases, the mode of termination may provide valuable information about the location of a protected isthmus in the setting of a scar-related tachycardia. Fig. 7.22 shows left ventricle mapping during VT, with mid-diastolic recordings from a site on the anterior wall; pacing at this site showed that it was integral to the VT circuit. A single extrastimulus delivered at this site reproducibly terminated VT without local propagation or depolarization.[74] Moreover, a single extrastimulus delivered at this site during sinus rhythm–initiated VT. Radiofrequency

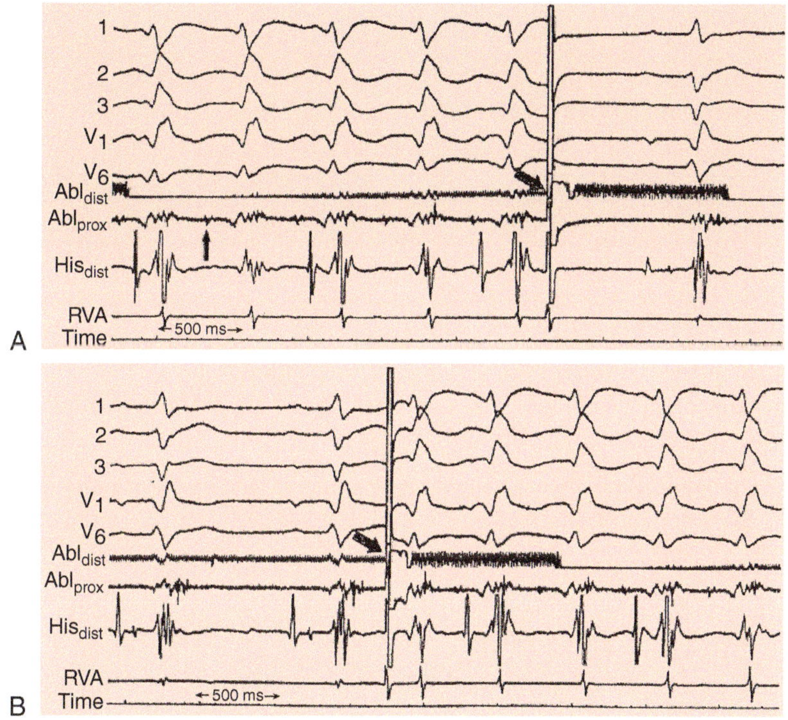

Fig. 7.22 Termination of ventricular tachycardia (VT) by a nonpropagated extrastimulus. (A) A single extrastimulus *(arrow)* terminated VT without local propagation. (B) A single extrastimulus delivered at this site during sinus rhythm initiated VT. See text for discussion. *ABL*, Ablation; *dist*, distal; *prox*, proximal. From Altemose GT, Miller JM. Termination of ventricular tachycardia by a nonpropagated extrastimulus. *J Cardiovasc Electrophysiol.* 2000;11:125, 2000. With permission.

energy delivered at this site terminated VT after one beat. This suggests that the ablation catheter tip was positioned in a critical portion of the circuit before tissues in the circuit immediately distal to this site had recovered excitability. The inference is that because the stimulus did not elicit a QRS complex, it affected cells that were in a protected area, such that (1) a single extrastimulus delivered at that site during sinus rhythm might have only one possible direction of propagation and could initiate VT and (2) this site would be an excellent ablation target site.

Electrogram Morphology in Response to Pacing

Close observation of electrogram morphology and polarity can also help differentiate between disparate activation pathways during electrophysiologic maneuvers performed in the absence of tachycardia. Bipolar electrogram morphology and polarity during atrial pacing, for example, can be helpful in targeting successful ablation sites in an otherwise normal, healthy heart in the setting of a reentrant tachycardia (e.g., during typical, CTI-dependent atrial flutter). Fig. 7.23 shows the local bipolar electrogram at a site where radiofrequency was applied with success; ablation had previously been performed along the CTI but without conduction block.

The ablation line was further explored for areas where conduction through the isthmus remained. At one site along the line of block, the electrogram shown in Fig. 7.23 was noted; although split, the electrograms were not as far apart as others along the ablation line. A single radiofrequency application at this site (applied during coronary sinus pacing) resulted in further separation of the electrograms (with a change in electrogram polarity for the second component of the split electrogram, indicating activation from the opposite direction) and evidence of conduction block on the halo catheter.

Bipolar electrograms have also been found to have use in mapping the pulmonary veins for ablation of atrial fibrillation. Sites where the bipolar electrogram changes direction or polarity—thought to indicate breakthroughs from the left atrium into the pulmonary vein—have been found to be predictive for ablation success of a myocardial sleeve (with resulting pulmonary vein isolation from the rest of the atrial myocardium; Fig. 7.24).[75]

Activation Sequence During Pacing Maneuvers

Close attention to atrial activation sequence and electrogram polarity during ventricular pacing (in sinus rhythm) can also provide important diagnostic clues to underlying accessory pathway and AV nodal physiology—clues that may be helpful to individualizing ablation strategies. Fig. 7.25 shows an example in which subtle changes in electrogram morphology are noted during ventricular pacing in the presence of a right lateral accessory pathway. Although a cursory look at the activation sequence suggests that fusion may be present in the first three beats (i.e., retrograde activation may progress up the accessory pathway and the AV node), because there is no significant change in timing of the high right atrial electrogram (i.e., the VA time between the first three complexes, which have a concentric retrograde activation sequence and the subsequent complexes, which have an eccentric retrograde sequence), the near reversal of polarity of the distal high right atrial electrogram in

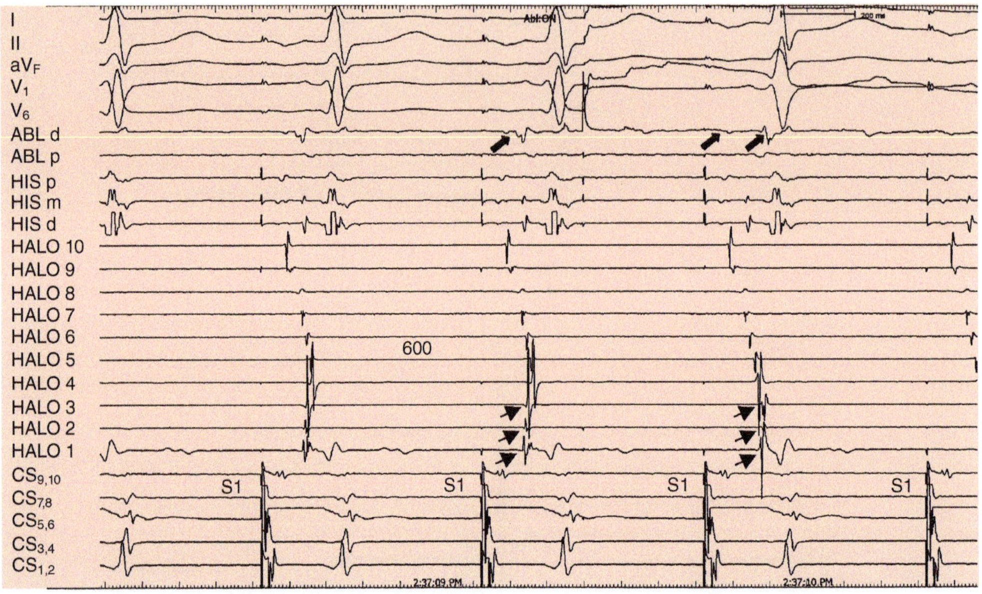

Fig. 7.23 Reversal of bipolar electrogram polarity with ablation. The figure shows right atrial electrograms from a patient undergoing ablation for typical, isthmus-dependent atrial flutter. Ablation had been performed along the isthmus but without resulting in conduction block. When the isthmus ablation line was further explored for nonablated areas, the electrograms shown here were recorded. The *first arrow* highlights the local bipolar electrogram at a 6-oclock position along the subeustachian isthmus, close to where radiofrequency had been applied previously. Although split, the electrograms were not as far apart here as at other sites along the ablation line. A single radiofrequency application at this site resulted in further separation of the electrograms *(double arrows)*, with a change in electrogram polarity for the second component of the split electrogram, indicating activation from the opposite direction, and evidence of conduction block on the halo catheter. *CS*, Coronary sinus; *dist*, distal; *m*, mid; *prox*, proximal.

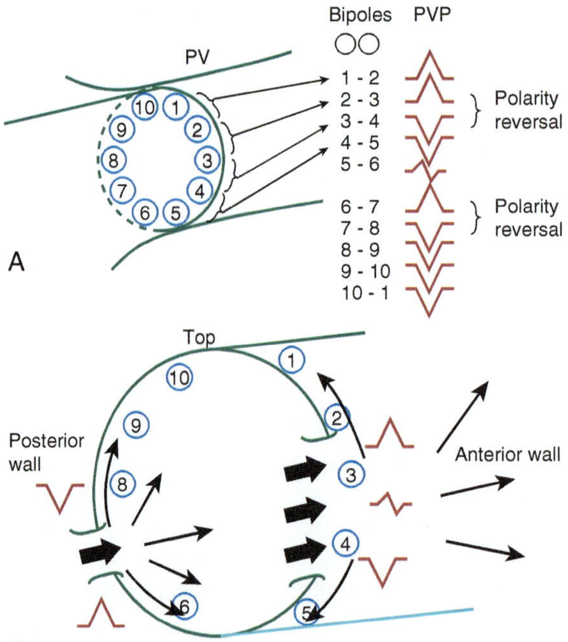

Fig. 7.24 Bipolar electrogram polarity reversal as an additional indicator of breakthroughs from the left atrium to the pulmonary veins. (A) Schematic representation of the circular mapping catheter with 10 electrodes. Pulmonary vein (PV) muscle potentials were recorded at the proximal PV in bipolar mode from 10 bipoles. Polarity reversal was defined as a sudden change of the main deflection of pulmonary vein potential (PVP) from positive to negative when analyzing adjacent bipoles in ascending order. (B) Schematic diagram of radial propagation of activation fronts from two different breakthroughs in the left superior PV. The numbers positioned at the ostium of the vein represent the 10 electrodes of the circular mapping catheter. There are two distinct breakthroughs, at both the anterior and posterior aspects of the vein. Radial propagation of the activation front through one breakthrough (posterior wall) is reflected by an electrogram polarity reversal across the adjacent two bipoles (6–7 and 7–8). In the case of wider breakthrough (anterior wall), an electrogram polarity reversal is observed across three consecutive bipoles (2–3, 3–4, and 4–5), with the intervening bipole (3–4) showing relatively isoelectric initial deflection. From Yamane T, Shah DC, Jais P, et al. Electrogram polarity reversal as an additional indicator of breakthroughs from the left atrium to the pulmonary veins. *J Am Coll Cardiol.* 2002;39:1337–1344. With permission.

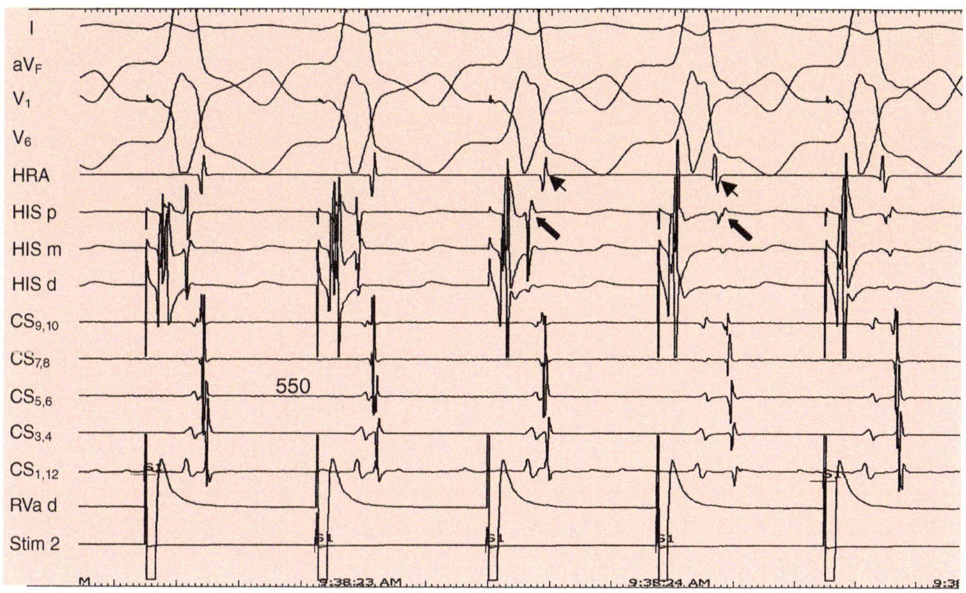

Fig. 7.25 Reversal of polarity in high right atrial (HRA) bipolar electrogram with a change in retrograde activation sequence during ventricular pacing. Subtle changes in electrogram morphology are noted during ventricular pacing (at 550 ms) in the presence of a right lateral accessory pathway. The first three beats suggest that activation is up the atrioventricular (AV) node, whereas the fourth and later beats show a change in activation sequence, with the HRA now being earliest, suggesting retrograde activation up a right-sided accessory pathway. Although the stimulus-to-atrium time in the HRA is about the same for both activation sequences, suggesting that fusion up the AV node and accessory pathway may be occurring during the first three beats, the polarity of the HRA electrogram changes with the second activation sequence. This suggests that retrograde activation for the first three beats is entirely up the AV node, whereas activation for the fourth and subsequent beats is entirely up the accessory pathway. *CS*, Coronary sinus; *dist*, distal; *m*, mid; *prox*, proximal; *Stim*, stimulus.

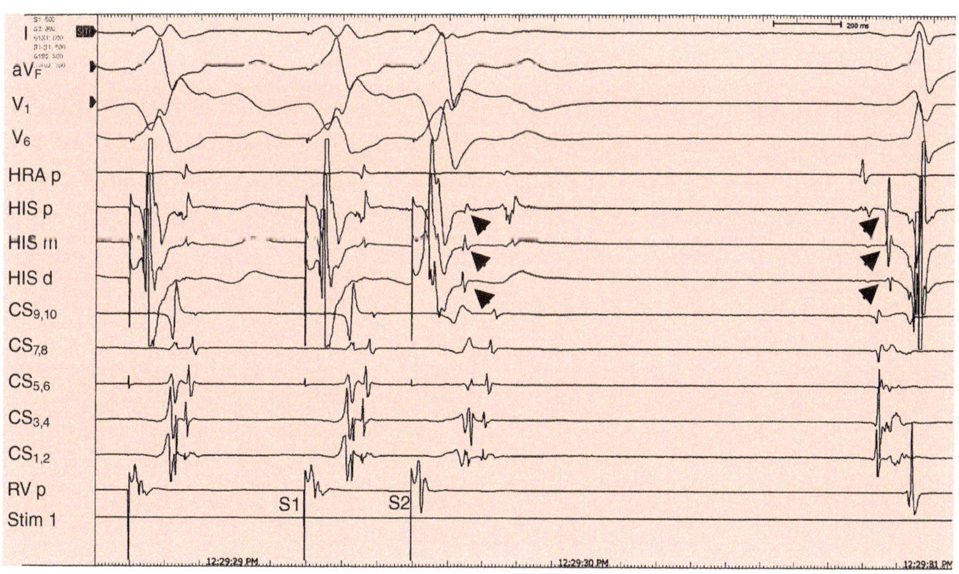

Fig. 7.26 Antegrade versus retrograde His bundle activation. An example of retrograde His bundle activation, as shown by the distal (d)–to–proximal (p) activation of the His bundle potential *(first set of arrows)* with a ventricular extrastimulus (seen clearly because of retrograde right bundle branch block with a prolonged VH time), as opposed to proximal-to-distal or antegrade activation during sinus rhythm *(second set of arrows)*. *CS*, Coronary sinus; *HRA*, high right atrial; *m*, mid; *RV*, right ventricle; *Stim*, stimulus.

the fourth and fifth complexes (compared with the first three complexes) suggests that retrograde activation for the first three complexes is solely up the AV node and solely up the accessory pathway for the fourth and fifth complexes. In fact, detailed assessment of atrial and AV accessory pathway activation direction using bipolar mapping has been performed by Damle and coworkers, who showed that vector mapping (performed by summing three orthogonally oriented bipolar electrograms) can help accurately localize accessory pathways insertion sites.[76]

Even if direct information is not present on a single bipolar electrogram (e.g., a high-frequency recording such as the His-bundle electrogram), analysis of the electrogram when performed in the presence of its neighboring electrograms may indicate direction of activation. Fig. 7.26 shows an example of

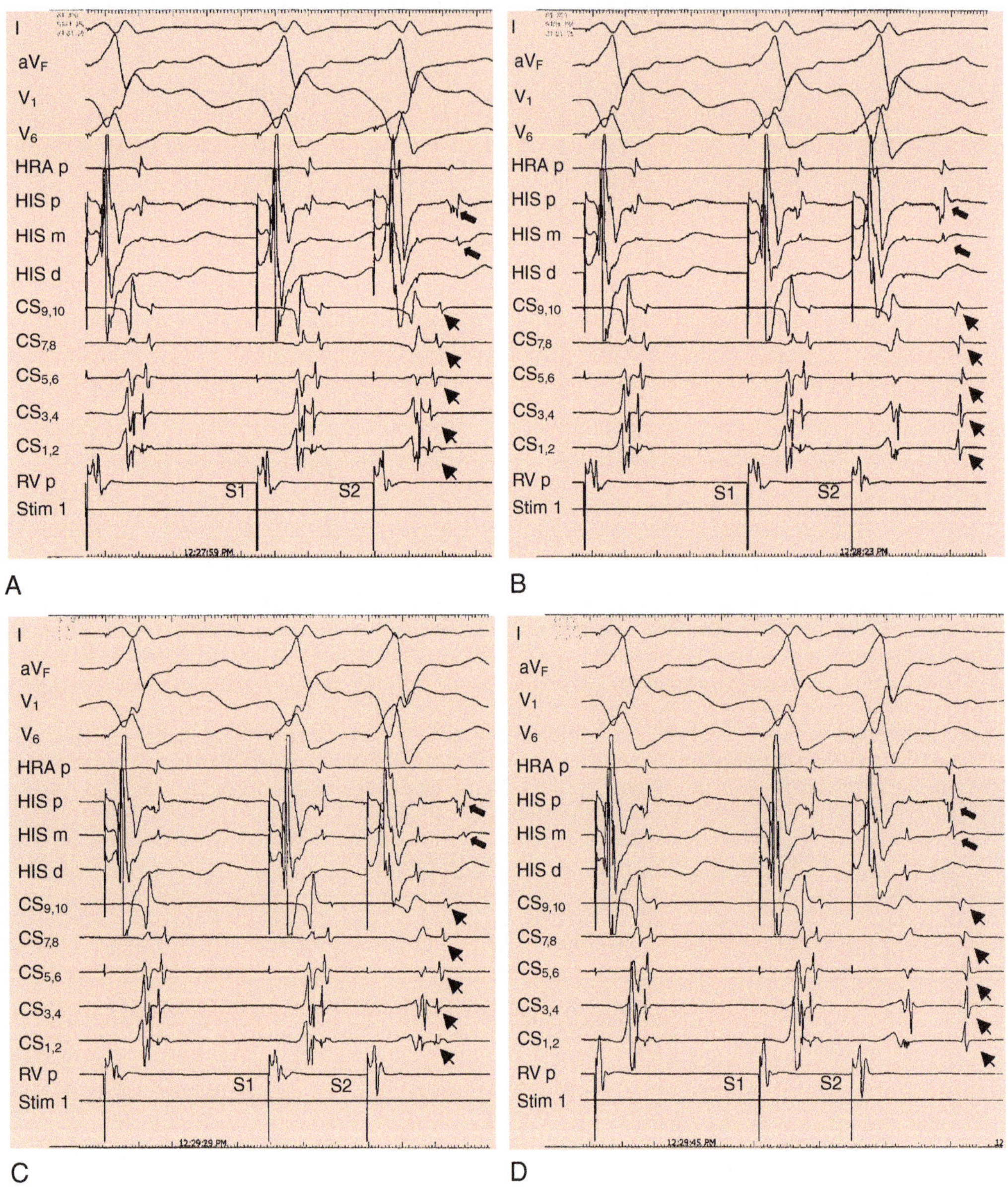

Fig. 7.27 Changes in retrograde activation sequence with ventricular pacing in a patient with a left lateral accessory pathway. Retrograde activation from the ventricular drive train appears to be fusion up the atrioventricular (AV) node and the accessory pathway. The VA time in the His bundle is shorter because the His is probably within the early portion of the QRS. Multiple activation sequences are detected by ventricular extrastimulus testing. In the same patient as in Fig. 7.17, disparate pathways of activation with single ventricular extrastimulus testing are shown. (A) Change in atrial activation in the His channel and in coronary sinus (CS) $_{9,10}$ (with a change in polarity in the latter) with the ventricular extrastimulus, with retrograde atrial activation appearing to go entirely up a left-sided accessory pathway. Note that a His deflection can be seen after the ventricular depolarization, suggesting retrograde right bundle branch block (caused by the premature extrastimulus) with activation up the left bundle branch. (B) With a more premature extrastimulus, the VH prolongs further; this is accompanied by a further increase in the VA time in the His recording channels, although the HA time remains unchanged. The atrial activation in the CS has now changed and is more concentric, suggesting activation up the AV node (i.e., block in the accessory pathway). (C) With a still more premature extrastimulus, there is conduction up the accessory pathway again (with a change in polarity in the CS electrograms); the timing and polarity of the His and HRA electrograms remains unchanged again, with the HA being constant. The retrograde activation represents fusion up the accessory pathway and the AV node. D, A further increase in prematurity of the extrastimulus results in block in the accessory pathway once again. There is a further increase in the VH time, with the VA time increasing accordingly (i.e., constant HA), indicating activation up the AV node. *d*, Distal; *HRA*, high right atrium; *m*, mid; *p*, proximal; *RV*, right ventricle; *Stim*, stimulus.

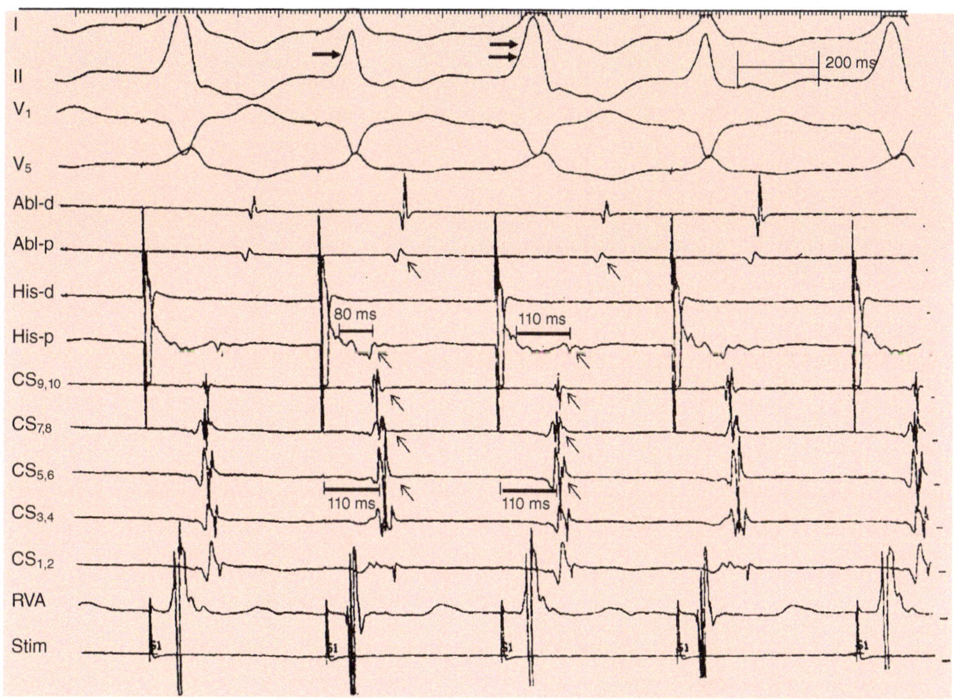

Fig. 7.28 Fusion up the AV node and an accessory pathway during para-Hisian pacing. Activation sequence is different between combined His and ventricular capture (narrow beat indicated by a *single, heavy arrow* in lead II) and ventricular capture (wider beat indicated by *two heavy arrows* in lead II). Closer inspection reveals that VA time is unchanged in $CS_{1,2}$ to $CS_{7,8}$ (110 ms in $CS_{5,6}$), indicating that atrial activation in these electrodes is through an accessory pathway. However, VA time during ventricular capture is longer in Abl (close to high right atrium), His-p (VA increases from 80–110 ms), and $CS_{9,10}$ compared with during para-Hisian capture, indicating that activation in these electrodes is up the AV node. *CS*, Coronary sinus; *d*, distal; *p*, proximal; *RVA*, right ventricular apex; *Stim*, stimulus.

retrograde His-bundle activation, as shown by the distal-to-proximal activation of the His-bundle potential with a ventricular extrastimulus (seen clearly owing to retrograde right bundle branch block with a prolonged VH time), as opposed to proximal-to-distal or antegrade activation during sinus rhythm (Fig. 7.27).

Para-Hisian Pacing

Para-Hisian pacing is of use in differentiating between a retrogradely conducting septal accessory pathway and the AV node. When direct His-bundle capture is obtained, retrograde conduction can occur rapidly over the AV node if retrograde septal conduction is present.[77] By contrast, if conduction is proceeding only up an accessory pathway, His-bundle capture will not alter the VA interval. Thus, the presence of a retrogradely conducting septal pathway can be identified by a fixed VA interval regardless of whether His capture occurs. Retrograde fusion complicates this finding. Shortening of the VA interval may occur if retrograde conduction is proceeding up both the AV node and an accessory pathway. In such a case, examination for closely spaced atrial recording sites can help identify a change in activation sequence that occurs when His bundle capture shortens the VA interval. An example of this is shown in Fig. 7.28; the activation sequence is different between para-Hisian capture (narrow beat indicated by a single, heavy arrow in lead II) and ventricular capture (wider beat indicated by two heavy arrows in lead II). Closer inspection reveals that VA time is unchanged in $CS_{1,2}$ to $CS_{7,8}$, indicating that atrial activation in these electrodes is through an accessory pathway. However, VA time during ventricular capture is longer in Abl (close to high right atrium), His, and $CS_{9,10}$ compared with during para-Hisian capture, indicating that activation in these electrodes is over the AV node. Fig. 7.29 shows a schematic outlining the use of para-Hisian pacing.

Fig. 7.30 shows another instance of a slowly conducting accessory pathway in which para-Hisian pacing may be fraught with error, with retrograde activation being different with ventricular compared with combined (ventricular and His bundle) capture; ventricular pacing alone causes a longer VA interval because conduction is over a posteroseptal pathway (although some AV nodal conduction, i.e., fusion, cannot be ruled out in the His-bundle recording) that conducts more slowly than the AV node. Combined His-bundle and ventricular capture causes conduction to proceed up the AV node but with a shorter VA time (and a different activation sequence than when retrograde conduction is over the accessory pathway).[78]

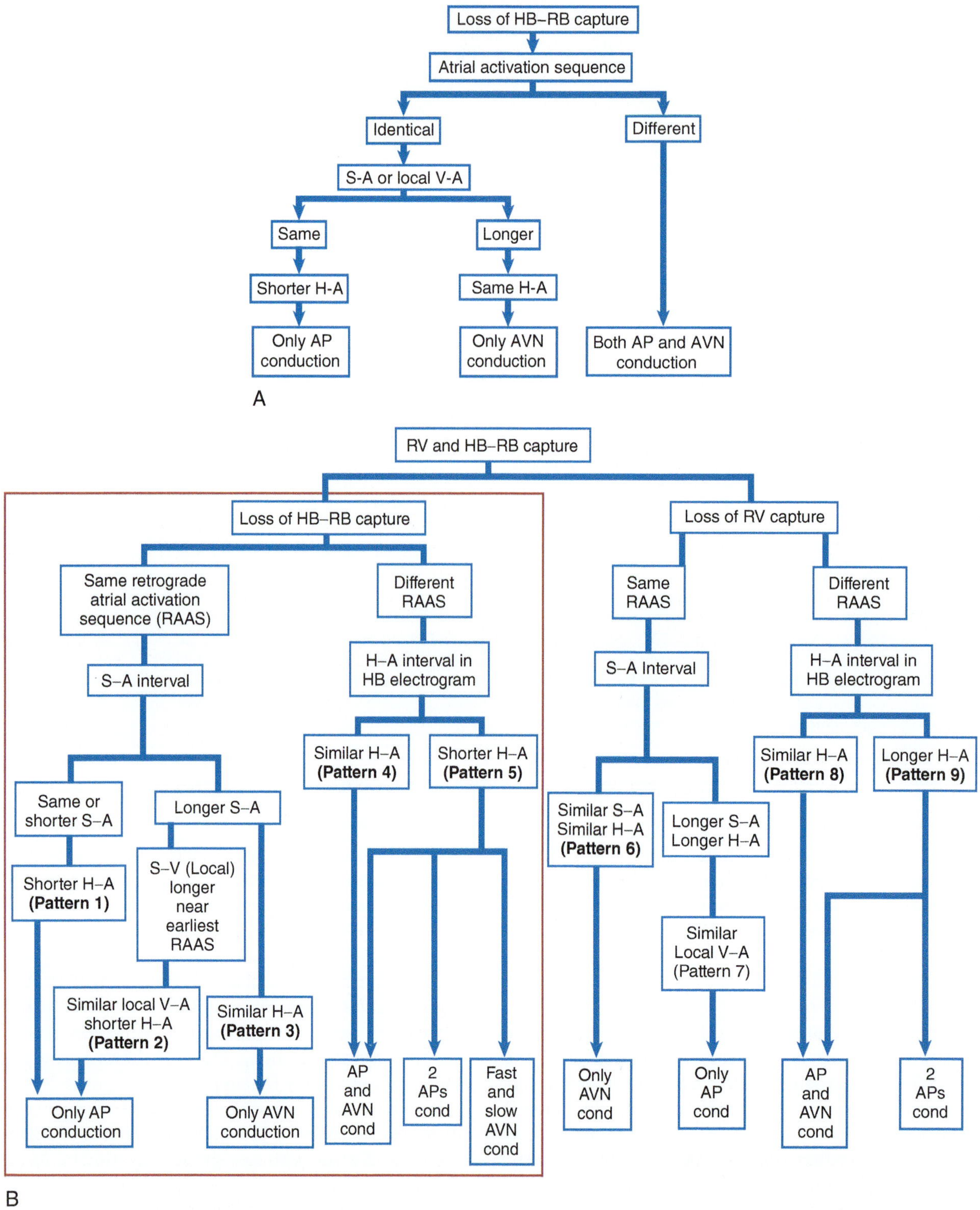

Fig. 7.29 (A) Abbreviated schematic for use in para-Hisian pacing to differentiate retrograde conduction over an accessory pathway from retrograde conduction over the atrioventricular (AV) node. (B) Complete schematic for para-Hisian pacing responses. The enclosed area corresponds to the three responses shown in panel A. *AP*, accessory pathway; *AVN*, atrioventricular node; *H-A*, interval from His bundle to atrial signal; *HB*, His bundle; *RAAS*, retrograde atrial activation sequence; *RB*, right bundle; *S-A*, interval from stimulus to atrial signal; *V-A*, interval from ventricular to atrial signal. In B, right, (Pattern 7) should be bold to be consistent with others. (A from Hirao K, Otomo K, Wang X, et al. Para-Hisian pacing: a new method for differentiating retrograde conduction over an accessory AV pathway from conduction over the AV node. *Circulation*. 1996;94:1027-1035. B from Nakagawa H, Jackman WM. Para-Hisian pacing. A useful clinical technique to differentiate retrograde conduction between accessory atrioventricular pathways and atrioventricular nodal pathways. *Heart Rhythm*. 2005;2:667–672.)

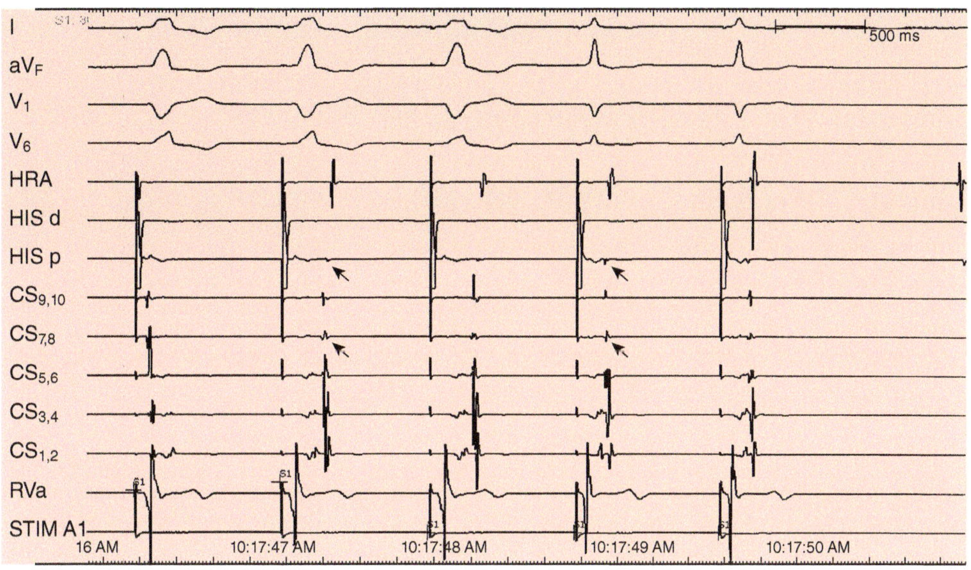

Fig. 7.30 Para-Hisian pacing is performed in a patient with a known posteroseptal pathway, with retrograde activation being different with ventricular compared with combined (i.e., ventricular and His bundle capture) pacing. The *first arrow* shows ventricular pacing (wider QRS) with a longer VA time, whereas the *second arrow* shows His bundle as well as ventricular capture (narrower QRS) with a shorter VA time. Note, however, that the retrograde activation sequence with the first beat is earliest in the proximal coronary sinus (CS), and with the second beat it is earliest at the AV junction. Conduction in the former instance is up a slowly conducting posteroseptal pathway, although some AV nodal conduction (i.e., fusion) cannot be ruled out in the His bundle recording; in the latter instance, conduction is up the AV node alone. See text for discussion. *CS*, Coronary sinus; *d*, distal; *HRA*, high right atrium; *p*, proximal; *Stim*, stimulus.

REFERENCES

Please refer to the e-book for a complete list of references.

8

Fundamentals of Catheter Three-Dimensional Mapping Systems

Akiko Ueda, Kyoko Soejima

KEY POINTS

- Currently, three commercial three-dimensional (3D) electroanatomical mapping systems are available.
- Each mapping system uses either magnetic or impedance-based technology for visualization.
- These systems obtain anatomical information by tracing catheter movement in the heart, creating a 3D reconstruction of the cardiac geometry.
- The systems simultaneously acquire and display electrical information pertaining to the geometry.
- The 3D mapping systems have greatly contributed to the reduction of radiation exposure during catheter ablation.
- Voltage maps have been used in substrate-based ablation strategies for scar-related ventricular tachycardia or atrial fibrillation.
- Activation maps obtained during sinus rhythm have recently been used as functional substrate maps to identify the critical isthmus.
- The type of mapping catheter, rhythm, and wavefront direction can affect both voltage and activation patterns.

INTRODUCTION

Three-dimensional (3D) electroanatomical mapping systems (EAMS) have been used clinically since the 1990s. Over the past 30 years, advancements in mapping systems have enormously contributed to a better appreciation of the mechanisms of complex arrhythmia, leading to an improvement in ablation outcomes and reduction of radiation exposure. A contemporary 3D mapping system is a critical tool for any type of ablation procedure.

Currently, three 3D mapping systems are commercially available: CARTO (Biosense Webster, Diamond Bar, California), EnSite (Abbott, St. Paul, Minnesota), and Rhythmia HDx (Boston Scientific, Marlborough, Massachusetts). The basic functions of these mapping systems are as follows: (1) simultaneous acquisition of anatomical and electrogram information, such as relative timing and voltage, by tracking catheter movement in the target heart chambers; (2) real-time display of the sensor-equipped catheters; (3) display of electrical information, such as voltage or wavefront activation on the integrated 3D geometry; and (4) tagging the area or point of interest on the reconstructed 3D geometry.

We discuss the characteristics of these mapping systems and dedicated mapping catheters and provide tips for appropriate mapping.

TECHNOLOGY USED IN 3D MAPPING SYSTEMS

To track and display catheters in real-time, 3D mapping systems use magnetic and/or impedance-based technologies. CARTO and Rhythmia HDx mainly adopt magnetic technology using sensor-equipped catheters for geometry reconstruction, but also display nonspecialized catheters without sensors using impedance-based technology. The most updated version of the EnSite system uses two mapping modes: a magnet-based mode named EnSite X and an impedance-based mode named EnSite NavX.

Magnetic Technology

In the CARTO system, a locator pad beneath the laboratory table contains nine coils that emit ultra-low-intensity magnetic fields (5×10^{-6} to 5×10^{-5} Tesla). The magnetic field strength from each coil is different and is detected by a location sensor embedded proximal to the tip of a specialized mapping catheter. The strength of each coil's magnetic field decays as a function of the distance from the coil. By integrating each coil's field strength and converting this measurement into a distance, the catheter-tip position is triangulated in space. The patient is positioned such that the heart is centrally positioned in the electromagnetic field. Six reference patch sensors placed on the patient's back and chest are used to monitor the patient's motion for correcting the reconstructed geometry. Once the dedicated mapping and ablation catheter is advanced into the chamber of interest, mapping points are acquired at the sites in contact with the surface. At each site, the local electrogram amplitude and electrical timing are recorded. In addition to catheter location, the orientation (roll, pitch, and yaw) of the catheter is determined. The accuracy of the system is <1 mm.[1,2] The most recent platform (CARTO-3) additionally uses current-based impedance catheter localization algorithms, allowing any type of catheter without sensors to be displayed on the map once the impedance data are collected by a sensor-equipped catheter.

The Rhythmia HDx with a proprietary 64-electrode mini-basket catheter (18-mm diameter) also uses magnetic technology for geometry reconstruction in conjunction with impedance-based technology for visualization of nondedicated catheters. The advantage of magnetic technology is the accuracy and stability of 3D geometry.

Impedance Technology

The EnSite NavX system uses impedance-based technology for catheter localization. An alternating current (8.136 kHz) is sequentially applied between three pairs of orthogonal (X, Y, and Z) surface electrode patches (Fig. 8.1). The magnitude of this current measured by the electrodes of any catheter within the field is proportional to the distance of the electrode from the surface electrode patches; therefore, the location of the catheter-tip is estimated and displayed in 3D space by triangulation. This is less accurate than magnetic location because of the nonhomogeneous impedance characteristics across the chest, and the introduction of additional fluid (e.g., saline irrigation) can cause dynamic changes in impedance during the procedure. However, a recent platform (EnSite Precision) improves the accuracy by using magnetic field scaling to correct the heterogeneous and variable distribution of impedance. The advantage of impedance technology is its "open platform," which allows the display of any type of catheter without a magnetic sensor.

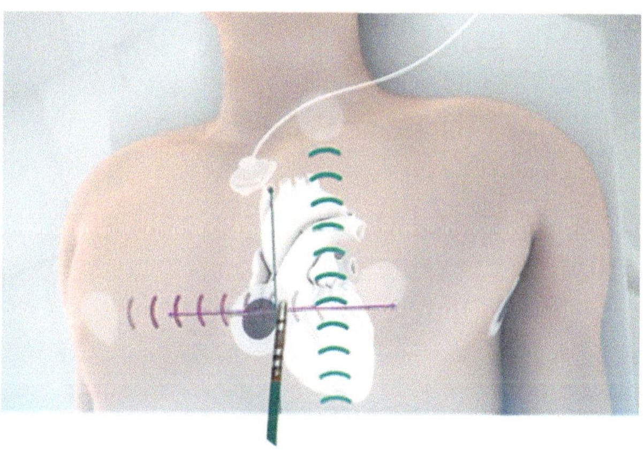

Fig. 8.1 EnSite NavX mapping system (impedance-based technology) (Abbott). Orthogonal surface patches are placed on the patient in the EnSite NavX system. A 5.68-kHz electrical signal is delivered alternately across each pair of patches, creating a voltage gradient along the axis between them. Once the gradient is established, any mapping, ablation, or diagnostic catheter can be placed in the field and act as a second receiver. The composite measurements represent the electrode positions of the catheters in three-dimensional virtual space. (Reproduced with permission of Abbott, © 2023. All rights reserved.)

Operators should understand the characteristics of each system and select a system suitable for the target tachycardia. Table 8.1 presents the characteristics of each mapping system.

FUNCTIONS (CAPABILITIES) OF 3D MAPPING SYSTEMS

Cardiac Geometry Reconstruction

Once the catheter is advanced into the chamber of interest, 3D geometry can be reconstructed by moving the catheter (sensor-equipped specialized catheter in a magnet-based mapping system/mode). An earlier 3D mapping system model displayed only the distal electrodes of the ablation catheter. Beat acceptance and annotation were conducted manually. Contemporary systems yield mapping with a multielectrode mapping catheter and automatic beat acceptance and annotation; therefore, detailed and accurate information can be obtained in a shorter time. Table 8.2 shows the lineups of the multielectrode catheters used for each mapping system. By imputing the electrode size and interelectrode space of a catheter, the system can accurately reconstruct and display the 3D position. Because most multielectrode mapping catheters are soft and flexible, the risk of cardiac perforation is minimized, and the catheters can be moved with limited use of fluoroscopy. Once the reconstruction of the chamber geometry is completed, the mapping and ablation catheters can be displayed in real time on the geometry at any arbitrary angle. The use of 3D mapping systems has significantly reduced the radiation exposure in various types of ablation procedures.[3–5] Through the development of mapping systems and catheters, fluoroscopy time and radiation dose in one center during atrial fibrillation (AF) ablation was reported to chronologically decrease from 61 minutes and 1365 mGy, respectively, in the early 2000s to 11 minutes and 200 mGy, respectively, in 2017.[6] Recently, near-zero fluoroscopic exposure ablation can be conducted under the guidance of 3D mapping systems and intracardiac echocardiography (ICE).[7,8]

TABLE 8.1 Specifications and Characteristics of Mapping Systems

Mapping System	Manufacturer	Technology for Point Acquisition	Dedicated Mapping Catheter	Ablation Catheter	Display Nonsensor Catheter	Image Integration
CARTO 3	Biosense Webster	Magnetic	Pentaray DecaNav	Smarttouch SF Smarttouch STSF	+ No data acquisition	+ CT/MRI/real-time ICE/fluoroscopy image
RHYTHMIA HDx	Boston Scientific	Magnetic	Intellamap Orion	Stable Point INTELLANAV MIFI OI	+ Data acquisition	+ CT/MRI
EnSite x	Abbott	Magnetic	Advisor HD grid Livewire	Tacti SE	+ No data acquisition	+ CT/MRI
EnSite Navx		Impedance	None (open platform)		+ data acquisition	

CT, computed tomography; *ICE*, intracardiac echocardiography; *MRI*, magnetic resonance imaging.

TABLE 8.2 Lineups of Dedicated Mapping Catheters

Multielectrode Catheter (Mapping System)	Number of Electrodes	Electrode Size (mm)	Edge-to-Edge Spacing (mm)	Center-to-Center Spacing (mm)
Pentaray (CARTO)	20	1	1-5-1	2-6-2
DecaNav (CARTO)	10	1	1-7-1	2-8-2
Lasso 2515 (CARTO)	20	1	1-5-1	2-6-2
Intellamap Orion (RHYTHMIA HDx)	64	0.9*0.45	1.6	2.5
Advisor HD grid HD wave solution (EnSite)	16	1	3	4
Livewire (EnSite)	20	1	2	3

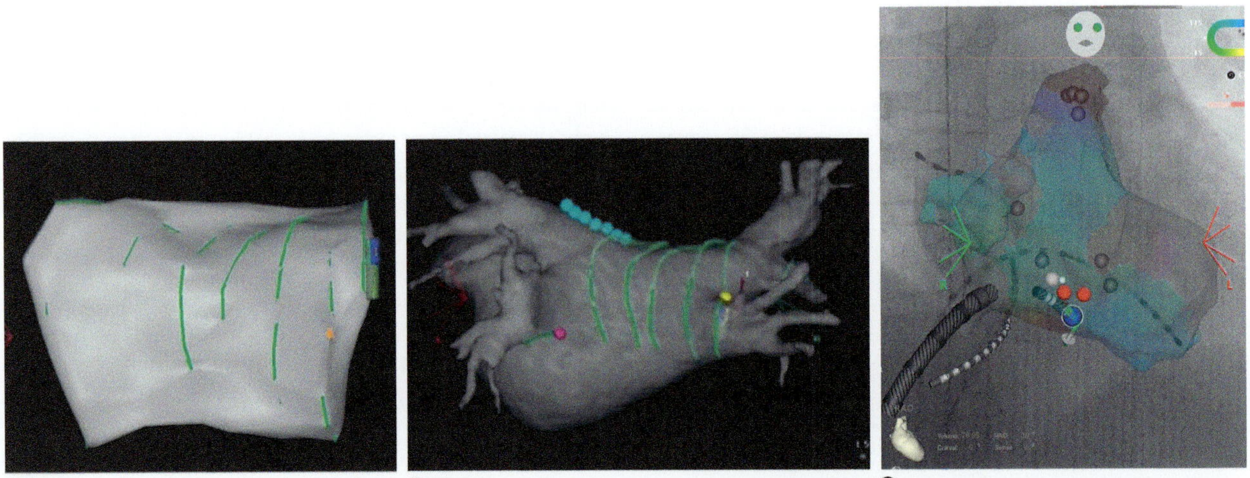

A B C

Fig. 8.2 Image integrations. (A) CARTOSOUND image of the left atrium with multiple planes of intracardiac echocardiography. (B) The computed tomography image merged with the geometry shown in A. (C) CARTOUNIVU image. Fluoroscopic images showing the positions of diagnostic catheters integrated with three-dimensional mapping.

Image Integration

The 3D mapping systems are equipped with image integration software that allows the superimposition of previously segmented computed tomography (CT) or magnetic resonance imaging (MRI) on the anatomical information acquired by mapping. This technique improves the accuracy of geometry creation, contributing to improved ablation outcomes and reduction of radiation exposure.[4,9] Preprocedural image data processing can provide information on the potential arrhythmogenic substrate in addition to anatomical information. For instance, delayed gadolinium enhancement on MRI is reportedly a useful guide for identifying critical isthmuses in scar-related ventricular tachycardias (VTs).[10]

Real-time anatomical information obtained from ICE can be integrated into the CARTO system. A 3D ultrasound image is acquired by a three-coil, electroanatomical mapping sensor and locator within the tip of the ICE catheter (SOUNDSTAR 3D catheter, Biosense Webster) and is displayed using the CARTOSOUND software.[11] The location and direction of the phased-array image fan, with characteristic pitch, yaw, and roll components of catheter-tip motion, are displayed within the *X*-, *Y*-, and *Z*-axes. Three-second segments of two-dimensional ICE images are acquired during electrocardiogram (ECG) gating. A single gated image is displayed on the ultrasound viewer, and the endocardial contour is manually or automatically traced (Fig. 8.2A, B). By repeating this process, a series of contours of the chamber is acquired and collated into a complete volume depicting point-to-point component interpolation. The advantage of this system is real-time appreciation of arrhythmic substrates, such as high-echogenic scars or thin aneurysms, as well as normal anatomy.[12,13] During ablation, monitoring the catheter contact and lesion formation can support effective and safe energy delivery.[14,15]

The CARTOUNIVU module can integrate fluoroscopic images into the 3D reconstructed map, enabling catheter manipulation of the acquired fluoroscopic images (Fig. 8.2C). Moreover, it provides information about the thorax, cardiac shadow, coronary angiography,[16] and esophagography, which were not previously available on the 3D mapping systems.[17]

Electrical Information

The 3D mapping systems collect electrical information, such as the amplitude of local unipolar and bipolar electrograms and activation timing during or after the completion of geometry reconstruction. Color-coded voltage and/or activation maps are displayed. The older systems could not display voltage and activation information simultaneously, but contemporary systems can display both types of information as an activation movie on the voltage map.

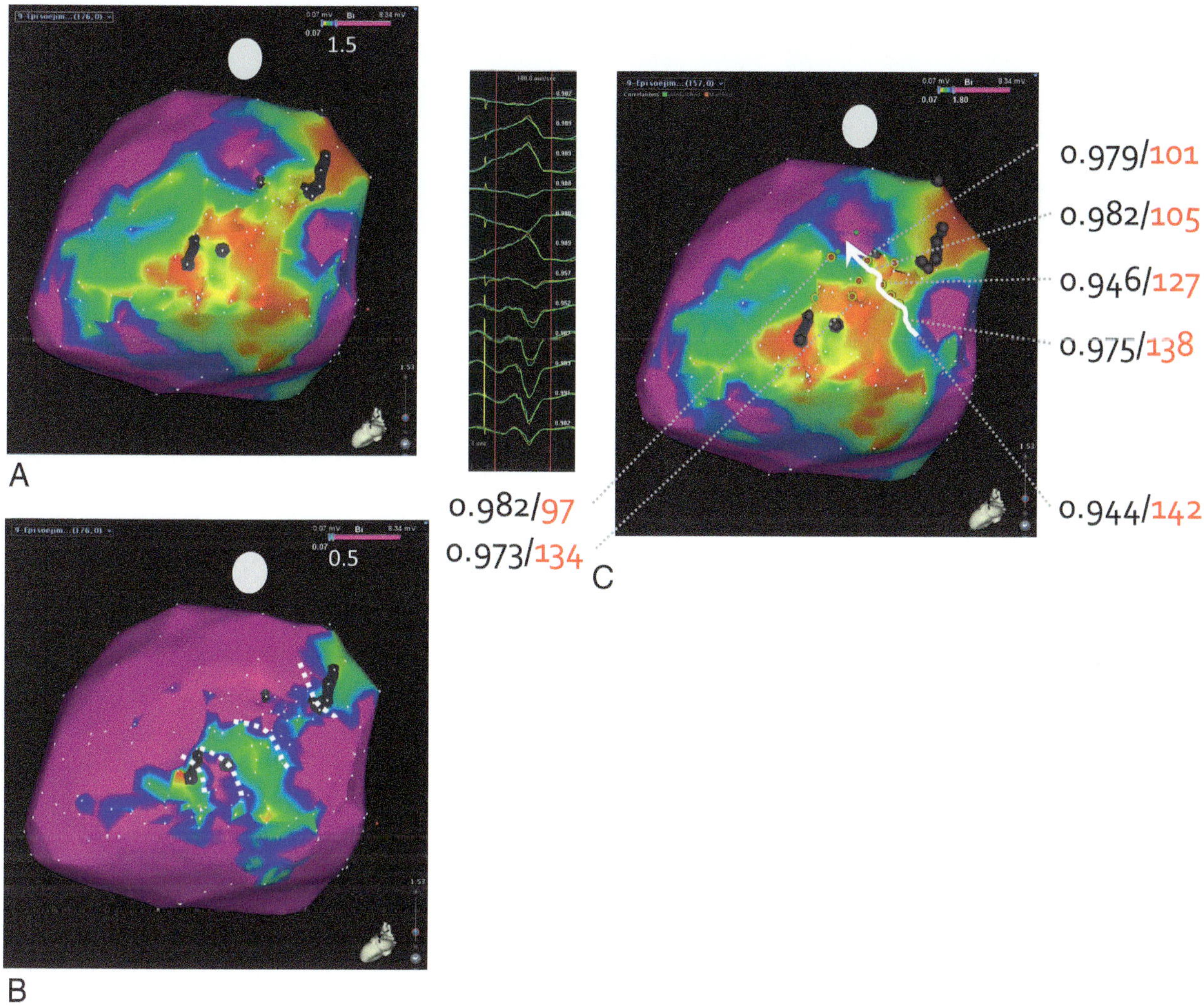

Fig. 8.3 Epicardial voltage maps. (A) Epicardial voltage map in a patient with dilated cardiomyopathy. A voltage of 1.5 mV or more is set as *purple*. Shown as an extensive low-voltage area in the posterior wall. (B) Epicardial voltage map in the same patient with an upper cutoff value of 0.5 mV, showing a relatively preserved voltage within an extensive low-voltage area (area marked by *dashed white lines*). (C) Pace mapping conducted in the corridor demonstrates excellent pace map–matching scores with various pacing latencies (shown as *red numbers*).

Voltage Map

The bipolar amplitude of the local electrogram correlates with histological information and demarcate infarct and border zone areas from healthy tissue.[12,18] Based on a validation study using the CARTO system, traditional bipolar amplitude cutoff values of 1.5 mV for normal ventricular tissue and 0.5 mV for dense scar have been used.[19] Dense scar is displayed as red and normal tissue as purple. Due to the increased field of view in unipolar recording, endocardial unipolar voltage < 8.3 mV in the left ventricle and 5.5 mV in the right ventricle are considered to reflect epicardial or midmyocardial scar tissue.[20,21] The unipolar information is often used to judge the necessity of mapping in the epicardium or opposite chamber.

Substrate ablation targeting low-voltage areas has become a cornerstone in VT ablation, and various strategies, such as linear ablation,[19] core isolation,[22] and scar homogenization,[23] have been reported. By adjusting the color range, a corridor of preserved myocardium in the low-voltage area can be revealed, aiding in the identification of the area of interest (Fig. 8.3).[24]

It should be noted that bipolar voltage can be affected by the catheter and wavefront direction. Bipolar recording obtained using smaller electrodes with narrower electrode spacing reflects more localized and detailed information about the area underneath the electrodes.[25] The low-voltage area can be enlarged by using a catheter with narrow interelectrode spacing and reduced via a wide interelectrode spacing.[26]

Catheter position relative to the wavefront direction can also affect voltage. When the bipolar pair of catheters is parallel to the wavefront direction, the amplitude of the bipolar electrogram—that is, the difference in each unipolar electrode amplitude—is maximized. When the bipolar pair of catheters is orthogonal to the wavefront direction, each unipolar electrode records the same amplitude simultaneously, resulting in a flat bipolar electrogram. Two maps created during pacing from two different sites revealed that more than half of the low-voltage

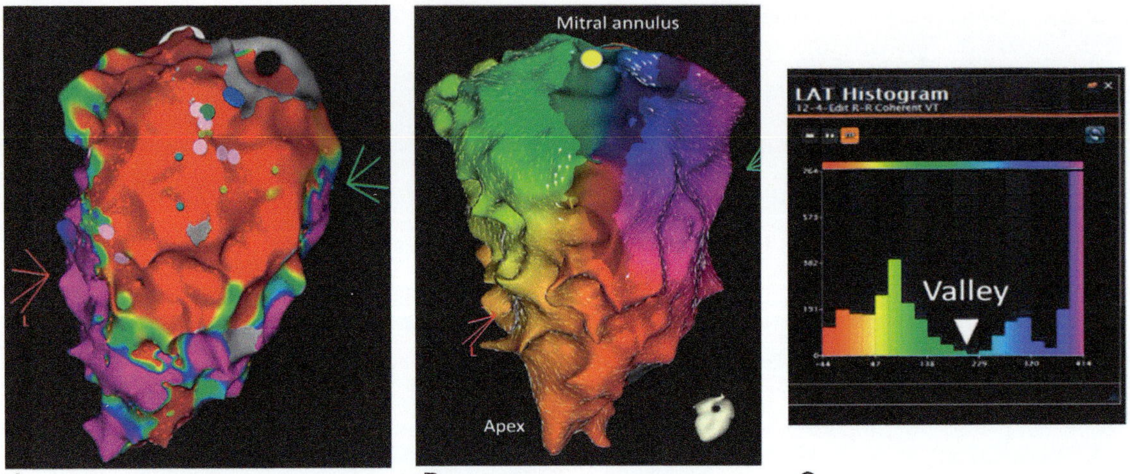

A B C

Fig. 8.4 Ventricular tachycardia mapping-1. (A) Voltage map in a patient with an old inferior myocardial infarction, showing extensive low-voltage areas in the inferior wall (color range: *purple* ≥1.5 mV, *red* < 0.5 mV). (B) Coherent map shows ventricular tachycardia circuit propagating around the low-voltage area. Thick arrows indicate slow conduction. (C) Histogram showing surface activation during the tachycardia cycle. The height of the bar indicates the activated area at a specific time; tall bar is the large area, and short bar is the small area activated (indicated as "valley"). The area activated in the "valley" corresponds to the *yellow tag* in Fig. 8.5B at the mitral annulus.

area did not overlap,[27] suggesting that wavefront direction can mask or unmask the low-voltage area.

Activation Map During Tachycardia

The system records the activation timing of each electrogram relative to the predefined timing reference. The difference in activation timings can be expressed by a color display function, and wavefront propagation can be visualized as a static image or a movie. Activation movies can be displayed on a voltage map. Activation mapping can be used for ablation targeting ectopic atrial or ventricular beats, and any regular tachycardia. The use of a multielectrode catheter reduces mapping time and can be accommodated in the mapping of VT in structural heart disease.

In the setting of mapping an ectopic beat or nonreentrant tachycardia, the activation map shows a focal, centrifugal pattern in which the activation starts from a small area and omnidirectionally spreads to the surrounding tissue. However, a focal activation pattern does not necessarily rule out a reentrant mechanism in the case of a microreentry or a single breakthrough site on the surface from the reentry circuit of the opposite surface or midmyocardium. When the activation timing covers the entire tachycardia cycle length, the tachycardia is likely to be a macroreentry in the mapped chamber. In cases with impaired myocardium or previous extensive ablation, prolonged conduction time in the chamber hinders the interpretation of the activation map. When the conduction time is equal to or exceeds the tachycardia cycle length, the activation map of a focal tachycardia may mimic macroreentry.[28] Additionally, inappropriately short or long window settings could result in misleading activation maps, which are discussed later in this chapter.

Tachycardia activation mapping is sometimes difficult to interpret in patients with previous ablations or severely diseased myocardium owing to inaccurate timing annotation of complex electrograms or passive diastolic activity. Coherent map technology (Biosense Webster) allows the automatic reannotation of the electrogram to the most reliable timing with appropriate coloring and shows the relative velocity and direction of the wavefront as vectors (Fig. 8.4, Videos 8.1 and 8.2). This can help delineate the complex tachycardia circuit.[29]

Activation Map During Sinus/Paced Rhythm

Late or delayed potentials recorded during sinus rhythm are considered important VT substrates. However, several recent studies showed that the critical site for VT is not the latest activation area but rather a more proximal site, where conduction often slows down.[30] Slow conduction in the diseased myocardium can lead to unidirectional conduction block, causing reentry.[31,32] Recently, various studies reported that the deceleration or steep activation gradient zones—that is, the conduction-slowing area—corresponded well to the VT isthmuses, and sinus/paced rhythm activation map using multielectrode catheters has gained interest as a functional substrate.[30,33–35] Such areas can be identified by the discontinuation or dense gathering of activation colors, "isochronal crowding." Because the functional substrate can dynamically change according to the wavefront direction or extrastimuli,[36] there is no definitive cutoff value for conduction velocity. In addition, when no clear functional substrate is identified in sinus rhythm activation mapping, changing the activation wavefront via pacing should be considered. Although the functional substrate is reported to have higher sensitivity and specificity for VT isthmuses than voltage maps or abnormal local electrograms,[37] additional techniques, including pace mapping, entrainment mapping, or limited VT activation mapping at the conduction slowing area, can elucidate the area of interest (Fig. 8.5, Videos 8.3 and 8.4).

Tagging Function

Sites with interesting electrograms, good responses to pacing, or ablation sites can be tagged on a 3D mapping system. Sequential tagging of ablation sites can guide a linear lesion set and help

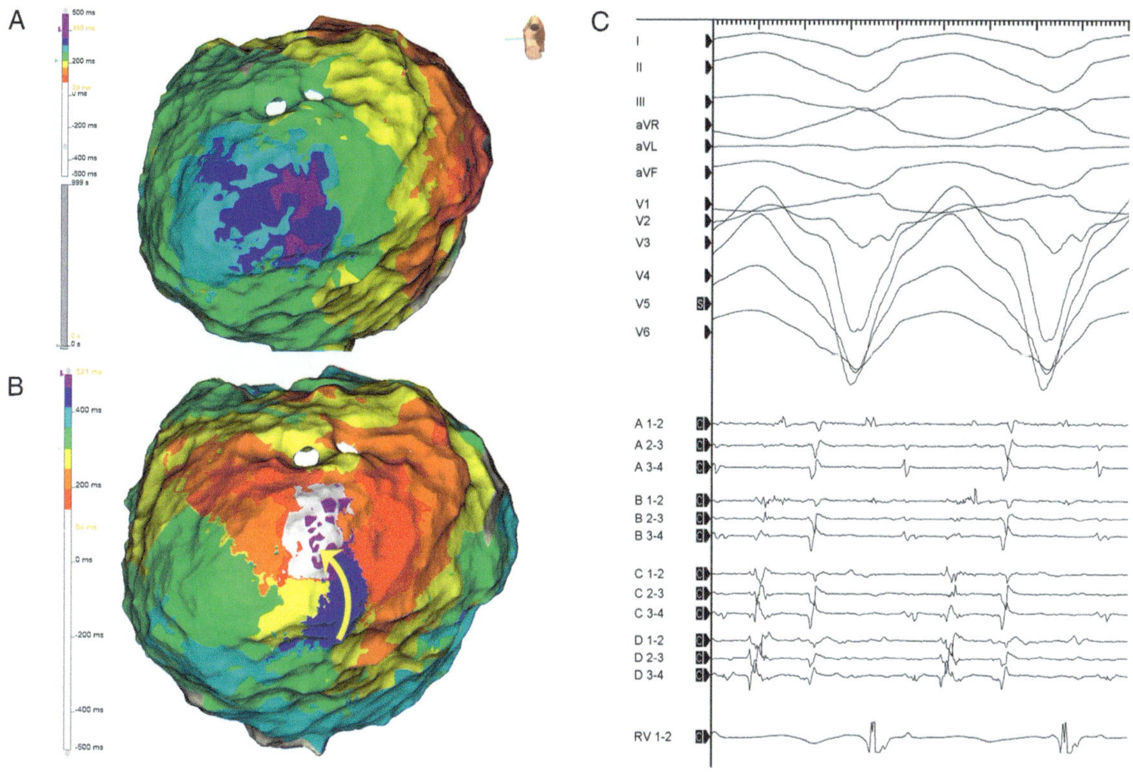

Fig. 8.5 Ventricular tachycardia mapping-2. (A) Isochronal map during left ventricular pacing in a patient with dilated cardiomyopathy. The apical area shows isochronal crowding, suggestive of conduction slowing. (B) Ventricular tachycardia activation map. The *white color* indicates the timing of QRS onset, and the *yellow arrow* indicates isthmus conduction, which corresponds well to the conduction slowing area during left ventricular pacing. (C) Diastolic electrograms recorded at the isthmus during ventricular tachycardia using an HD grid catheter. (Reproduced with permission of Abbott, © 2023. All rights reserved.)

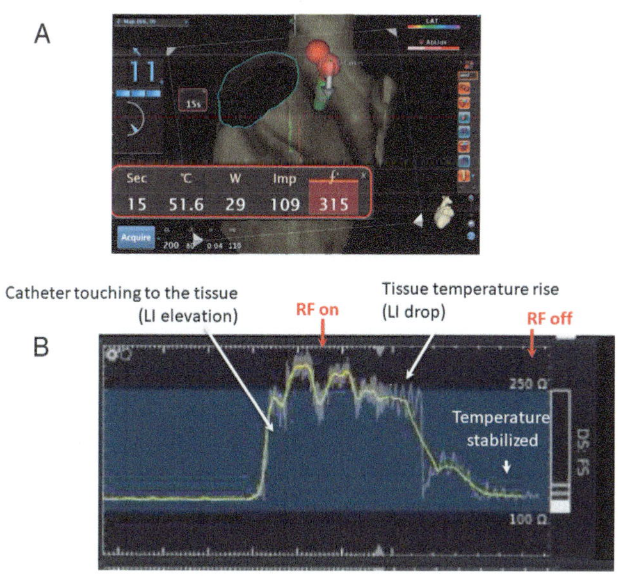

Fig. 8.6 Ablation lesion parameters. (A) Ablation tags in the CARTO mapping system. The ablation catheter is shown with an *arrow*, and the real-time contact force (11*g*) is shown on the *left*. *Lower left*, Parameters (duration, temperature, watt, impedance, and ablation index). (B) Changes in local impedance (LI) before, during, and after ablation.

identify gaps. Real-time contact-force monitoring of an ablation catheter with a sensor located at the tip has significantly improved the safety and efficacy of catheter ablation. In the CARTO and EnSite systems, the lesion dimension is expressed when using a dedicated ablation catheter for each system, as a parameter using the specialized formula combining radiofrequency (RF) power (W), RF duration (s), and contact force (*g*). When the value of the parameter increases and reaches a predefined level, a color-coded tag is displayed (Fig. 8.6A). The Stablepoint catheter, exclusive to the Rhythmia HDx system, has a unique profile for measuring the local impedance between the distal and proximal electrodes. With RF application, the local impedance drops by 20–35 Ω and plateaus. The Rhythmia system displays lesion formation based on this impedance drop (Fig. 8.6B).

STEP-BY-STEP GUIDE FOR MAPPING

Selecting Mapping Systems and Catheters

Each mapping system has unique features and adopts different parameters for ablation lesion formation, which is important for determining the best use of 3D EAMS. Mapping system and catheters should be selected based on the target tachycardia and mapping area. Multielectrode catheters are used for detailed mapping. A spherical catheter is unsuitable for epicardial mapping. For epicardial mapping via surgical pericardial access, impedance-based technology (EnSite NavX mode) should be avoided as the mapping area is exposed to air, resulting in distortion of the map.

Respiratory Acquisition

Respiratory heart motion of 1–2 cm must be considered. By acquiring the respiratory pattern before mapping (CARTO,

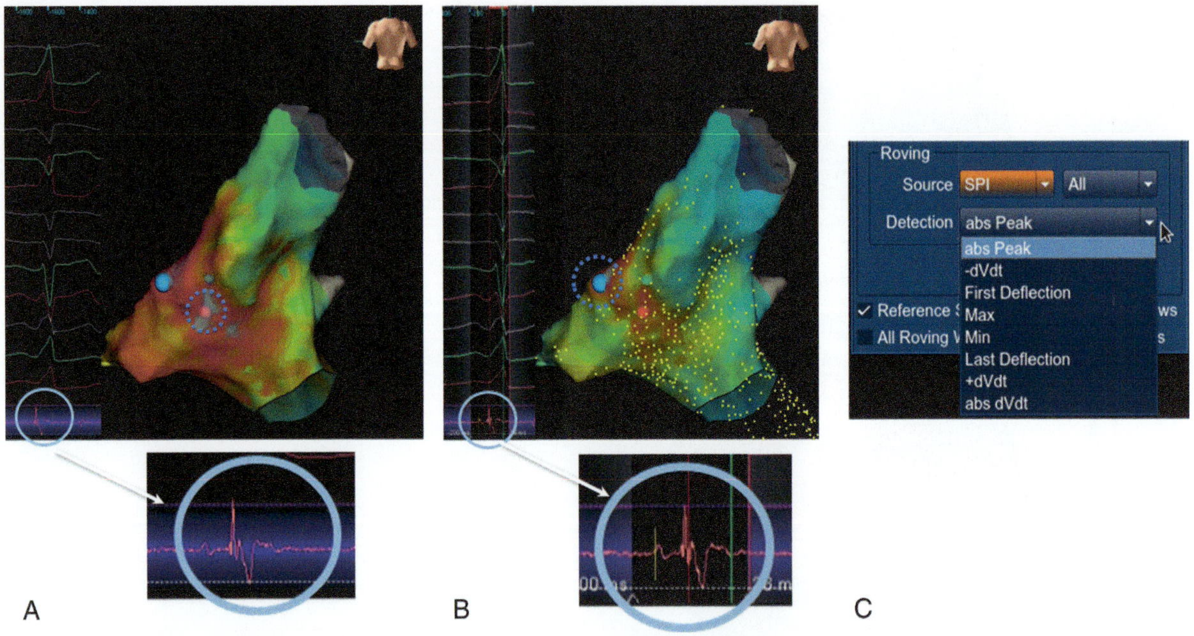

Fig. 8.7 Selection of local electrogram annotation timing in a patient with ventricular ectopy. (A) Right ventricular activation map, in which the annotation is set to –dV/dt. The system annotates the timing of the large signal but not at the small prepotential. (B) Reannotation at the first deflection changed the earliest activation site at *blue tag*. (C) EnSite system provides choice of annotation timing.

EnSite) or measuring the thoracic impedance from the body surface electrograms (Rhythmia HDx), the systems acquire mapping points exclusively during expiration. During the procedure, if the mode of respiration changes, such as with the use of continuous positive airway pressure, the respiratory pattern should be reacquired.

Timing Reference and Window of Interest

For atrial mapping, such as atrial tachycardia or targeting the atrial insertion site of the retrograde pathways, a stable atrial electrogram in the coronary sinus or right atrial appendage is often used as a timing reference. Surface electrocardiography is frequently used for ventricular mapping, such as premature ventricular complex (PVC), scar-related VTs, or ventricular insertion site of antegrade accessory pathways. Based on the characteristics of the selected electrogram or the surface ECG, the triggering criterion (reference annotation), including maximal or minimal deflection or maximal upslope (dV/dt), is selected so that electrogram data is acquired if the criteria are met. The nontargeted beat is screened out based on criteria such as cycle length, electrogram stability, and QRS morphology. Appropriate adjustment of the window of interest is important. For reentrant tachycardia mapping, the window is set to be equal to or slightly shorter than the tachycardia cycle length so that the whole activation can be obtained.

For ventricular substrate mapping during stable rhythm, the window after the QRS offset needs to be wide to obtain very late potentials.

Annotation Timing, Mapping Window

When recording a local bipolar electrogram obtained using a roving catheter, the activation timing relative to the reference is determined according to the predefined annotation setting. Annotation should be based on the local potential, often judged by the sharpest slope of dV/dt corresponding to the QS pattern of the unipolar electrogram. The detection of local timing is easy in normal tissues with simple electrograms. However, in abnormal tissues with fractionated multicomponent electrograms, it is difficult to determine the exact timing. Furthermore, a tiny prepotential followed by a larger electrogram is occasionally missed. Contemporary mapping systems automatically conduct all the processes of electrogram acquisition and annotation, but careful manual checks are required occasionally, especially for complex electrogram areas such as extensively delayed potentials. The EnSite system has a unique function in that the annotation timing, such as the first deflection, last deflection, and maximum positive or negative dV/dt, can be selected based on the operator's preference or clinical indication (Fig. 8.7).

ADDITIONAL FUNCTIONS

Pace Map–Matching

Pace mapping is often used to identify the site of origin of idiopathic ventricular ectopy and the distal isthmus of reentrant VTs. All EAMS install template-matching software that can compare the QRS morphologies of the target arrhythmia and paced beat. Using Pearson correlation analysis, the software compares each lead QRS morphology and calculates the matching score. The CARTO and EnSite systems can display a color-coded pace map–matching score map (PASO module, Biosense Webster; Score map, Abbott).

Annotation-Independent Activation Display

Ripple mapping in CARTO displays the activation wavefront as moving bars superimposed on a voltage map. The uniqueness

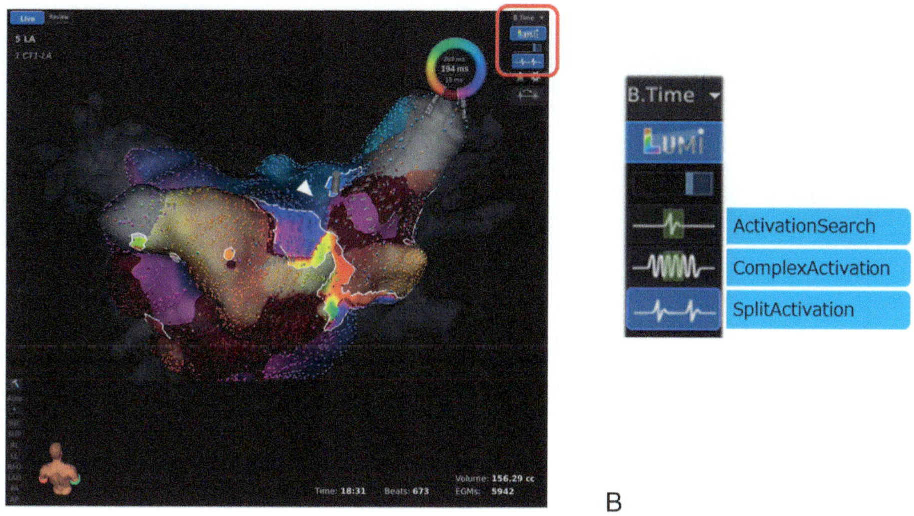

A B

Fig. 8.8 Functions in the Lumipoint software module. (A) Left atrial mapping during right atrial pacing after roof-line ablation. Areas with double potentials (split activation) were highlighted using the Lumipoint feature. By checking the area between the double potential recording areas, a gap in the line can be observed (shown with a *white arrow*). (B) Choice of functions in Lumipoint module (*red box*). ActivationSearch can highlight an area activated at a certain time. Complex activation can be used to highlight areas with fragmented electrograms. SplitActivation can highlight an area with split electrograms separated by >15 ms.

of this algorithm is that all the components of the bipolar electrogram at the corresponding cardiac surface are displayed as a dynamic bar. This is especially useful with a complex fractionated electrogram (CFAE), because identification of the local activation may be difficult. Ripple mapping during sinus rhythm can reportedly reveal a slow-conducting channel in the scar area, elucidating a potential VT isthmus.[37,38]

The Lumipoint software module, as a support tool in the Rhythmia HDx system, helps with quick analysis and interpretation of complex arrhythmias. For example, it can highlight an area harboring abnormal electrograms or an area activated at a certain time (Fig. 8.8). When focal tachycardia occurs, the site of origin may be a very limited area before spreading to the entire surface. When selecting the onset timing of the target P or QRS wave, the highlighted area corresponds to the origin of tachycardia. Some mapping systems can display a histogram that shows the activated surface area (*Y*-axis) in a certain phase of the mapping window (*X*-axis) (Fig. 8.4C). In focal tachycardia, the area highlighted at the onset of the *Y*-axis corresponds to the site of origin (Fig. 8.9). In macroreentrant tachycardia, the small value of the *Y*-axis implies that a very limited portion of the mapped surface is activated, suggesting activation through the narrow isthmus.

Local Activation Vector and Velocity Display

The most recent EnSite system can demonstrate a wavefront vector using omnipolar technology. Independent of global activation based on annotation timing, the activation direction is displayed as vectors of omnipolar electrograms, created from two bipolar electrogram pairs and three unipolar electrograms recorded using a grid catheter (Fig. 8.10A). The system also displays the relative velocity as a color-range algorithm (Fig. 8.10B).

Table 8.3 summarizes mapping information that can be displayed on the geometry.

USE IN VARIOUS ARRHYTHMIAS

Supraventricular Tachycardia

Although the use of the system in simple tachycardias, such as atrioventricular nodal reentrant tachycardia or atrioventricular reciprocating tachycardia, is not essential, displaying diagnostic catheters without specialized magnetic sensors in the His bundle region or coronary sinus may help reduce radiation exposure.

In atrial tachycardia following AF ablation or cardiac surgery, 3D mapping plays an important role by delineating previous ablation lines or cardiac incisions. A function that differentiates fragmented electrograms from double potentials helps identify the gap responsible for tachycardia. Occasionally, even a very detailed 3D activation map fails to define the tachycardia circuit, when basic electrophysiologic strategies such as entrainment pacing or a single extrastimulus can help identify the circuit.[39–41] In cases with multiple ablation procedures or atriotomy, appreciation of the sinus node location, intra-atrial conduction to the atrioventricular node, and conduction patterns in the left atrium are also important factors in designing ablation lines without interrupting atrial conduction.

Atrial Fibrillation

AF is the most commonly treated arrhythmia worldwide. Various supporting modules/software focusing on the AF substrate have been launched. CFAEs were the first reported AF substrate targets refractory to conventional pulmonary vein isolation.[42] All mapping systems now have a module that can record and highlight the CFAEs or fractionated electrograms based on algorithms with

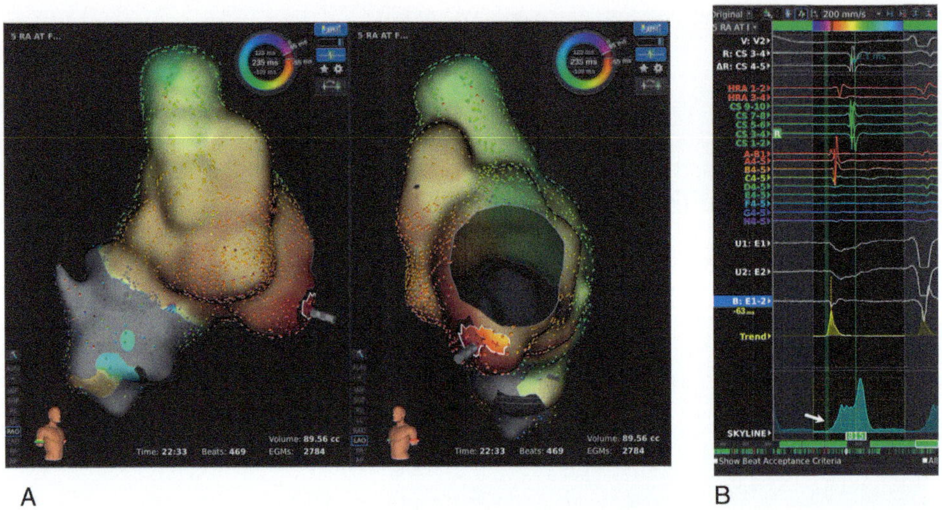

Fig. 8.9 Right atrial map during atrial tachycardia. (A) Right and left oblique views of the right atrium. The area of the earliest activation at the lower lateral tricuspid annulus is highlighted. (B) The *arrow* indicates the timing of atrial activation onset, which is highlighted. The area activated at this time corresponds to the area shown in A.

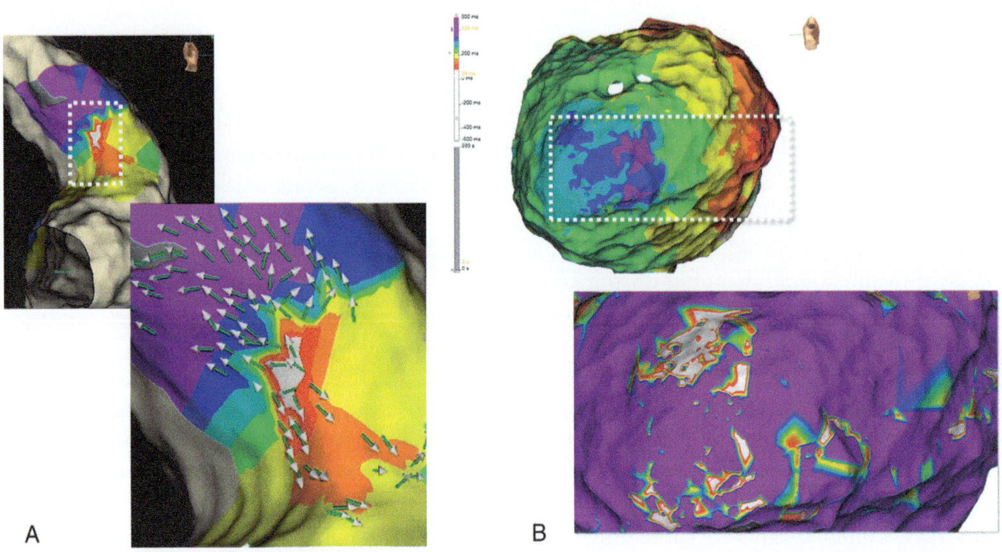

Fig. 8.10 Activation vector and wave speed map. (A) Activation map of the right ventricular ectopy using omnipolar electrograms. The magnified image of the marked area (dashed box) shows the activation vectors propagated from the earliest activation site. (B) Epicardial isochronal mapping during left ventricular pacing showing isochronal crowding in the apical area. Magnified image of the marked area (*dashed box*) with wave speed map demonstrates slow conduction shown in white (set as velocity <0.8 m/sec in this case).

cycle length, reproducibility, and average cycle lengths. CARTOFINDER is a module that detects rotational and focal activities during AF. Ablation targeting the non–pulmonary vein AF foci is another important strategy. The Lumipoint feature in Rhythmia HDx can highlight fractionated abnormal electrograms. Areas with fractionated electrograms in the atria during sinus or right atrial pacing can be the non–pulmonary vein AF foci.[43]

Premature Ventricular Complex/Idiopathic VT With Focal Mechanism

Activation mapping and pace mapping are used for PVC ablation. Once the QRS morphology of the target ventricular arrhythmia is recorded in the system, it can be used as a reference for activation mapping and template for pace mapping. The system acquires mapping information only when the QRS morphology matches the reference PVC to prevent nontargeted beat acquisition. The automatic annotation mode enables quick mapping, but careful screening to pick up a small prepotential is often needed (Fig. 8.8). The anatomy of the outflow tract, which is the most frequent source of idiopathic VAs, varies. The 3D mapping allows the acquisition of detailed anatomical and electrical information. Concomitant use of ICE or fluoroscopic image integration can help visualize the ostium of the coronary arteries in real time, which is useful for ablation of the coronary sinus of Valsalva.

TABLE 8.3 Information That Can Be Displayed on the Geometry

Map/Displayed Information	Description	Usage
Voltage map	Color-coded display of the local electrogram amplitude identification of abnormal low voltage area (scar)	Anatomical substrate map for scar-related VT, AF, AT
Activation map	Exhibiting the activation timing • Isochronal map by dividing total activation time into defined intervals • Movie (propagation map, sparkle map)	• Functional substrate map for scar-related VT (during sinus or paced rhythm) • Tachycardia map
Ripple map (CARTO)	Exhibiting the activation and amplitude of the electrogram as independent information on annotation timing • Can be replayed on voltage map	• Substrate map • Tachycardia map
Coherent map (CARTO)	Exhibiting the activation after reannotation of inadequate timing, with activation direction and relative velocity	• Substrate map • Tachycardia map
Lumipoint (Rhythmia HDx)	Exhibiting the arbitrary selected electrogram characteristics (double potentials, fragmentation) Highlighting the surface at selected activation phase independent on annotation timing	• Substrate map • Tachycardia map
Activation vector (EnSite)	Exhibiting wavefront vector as independent parameter on the global activation based on annotation timing activation based on annotation timing	• Substrate map • Tachycardia map
Wave speed (EnSite)	Exhibiting local wave speed using omnipolar technology	• Substrate map • Tachycardia map
CFAEs/fractionation	Exhibiting CFAEs or fractionation during atrial fibrillation based on the predefined definition	• AF

AF, atrial fibrillation; *CFAEs*, complex fractionated electrograms; *VT*, ventricular tachycardia.

Scar-Related VTs

The development of 3D mapping systems has affected the strategy of scar-related VT ablation. Detailed mapping with multielectrode catheters improves the identification of the critical isthmus. During sinus rhythm activation mapping, a strategy to annotate not at the –dV/dt but to the last deflection of the local electrogram has been reported.[30,33,44] Although it may cause far-field annotation, a sharp, spiky electrogram of a late timing recorded by a small electrode pair usually represents local delayed activation. The EnSite system allows annotation timing to the last deflection. When conducting VT activation mapping, quick electrogram acquisition that focuses on the timing and area of interest is important. VT activation mapping has been reported with the window setting restricted to the diastolic timing so that the isthmus can be detected efficiently without conducting whole activation mapping.[45] In this instance, the annotation timing is set to the first deflection in the EnSite system.

When targeting deep in the myocardium, sequential, simultaneous, or bipolar ablation are options. The use of a 3D mapping system facilitates positioning of the two ablation catheters with limited use of fluoroscopy.

REFERENCES

Please refer to the e-book for a complete list of references.

9

High-Resolution Three-Dimensional Mapping Systems

Weihow Hsue, Cory M. Tschabrunn

KEY POINTS

- The smaller electrode size and interelectrode distances of multielectrode catheters can record electrograms with higher bipolar voltage amplitude, shorter electrogram duration, and reduced fractionation, allowing more accurate annotation and improved visualization of heterogeneity within areas of low-voltage.
- Current multielectrode catheters include the Pentaray and Octaray with CARTO 3 (Biosense Webster), the Advisor HD Grid with Ensite X (Abbott), and the Intellamap Orion with Rhythmia HDx (Boston Scientific), each with their own advantages.
- Limitations of multielectrode catheters include inability to confirm adequate tissue contact, lack of specific bipolar voltage thresholds for each dedicated mapping catheter, possible need for extensive manual checks of electrogram annotation, and potential fibrillatory induction and physical entrapment of splines and baskets.

INTRODUCTION

The development of electroanatomical mapping technology during the 1990s transformed the field of cardiac electrophysiology. For the first time, it allowed direct visual localization of the mapping catheter and corresponding electrogram voltage and activation timing within a three-dimensional (3D) space.[1] Electroanatomical mapping technologies continue to evolve and are now routinely used for the guidance of catheter ablation procedures in patients with cardiac arrhythmias. The development and utilization of multielectrode mapping catheter technologies have provided further substantial insight into complex arrhythmia mechanisms and yielded significant clinical benefits for patients. To examine the current role of multielectrode mapping and detail our continued desire to achieve high-resolution mapping for a more comprehensive understanding of the mechanisms and pathophysiologic substrate underlying cardiac arrhythmias, this chapter will review (1) the advantages of multielectrode over point-by-point mapping, (2) types of multielectrode catheters, (3) limitations of high-resolution mapping, and (4) future perspectives.

POINT-BY-POINT VERSUS MULTIELECTRODE MAPPING

The ability to collect electrogram information accurately and efficiently is the cornerstone of electroanatomical mapping. However, electrogram voltage can be influenced by a variety of factors, including conduction velocity, fiber orientation and curvature, the relationship of fiber orientation to the propagating wavefront, tissue contact, fibrosis/fat, and, finally, characteristics of the recording catheter.[2–4] Conventional point-by-point mapping catheters typically have a large distal-tip electrode designed for radiofrequency energy delivery, but numerous studies indicate that smaller electrodes and closer center-to-center interelectrode spacing result in increased mapping resolution as each data point represents electrical activity from a smaller tissue size.[3,4]

The notion that electrode size and interelectrode spacing characteristics affect bipolar signal morphology and spatial resolution is not a new concept. Schaefer et al. demonstrated the mathematical relationship between electrode distance from the recording source (i.e., tissue) and the implications of unipolar and bipolar electrogram characteristics in 1951.[5] This initial work also introduced the concept that bipolar electrodes reduce far-field contamination, and this effect was maximized as interelectrode distance decreased. Durrer et al. validated this concept in 1957 in a canine left ventricle experimental model.[6] In more recent work, Stinnett-Donnelly et al. showed, using computational and in vitro models, that electrode spatial resolution is affected by electrode diameter, electrode length, interelectrode distance, and distance from the current source (tissue), and spatial resolution degrades with the increase of any of these four factors.[3] The angle of incidence (orientation of the catheter relative to the tissue) also has major implications that can impact the degree of signal cancellation and electrogram spatial resolution. Previous experimental studies have shown that electrograms in a nonparallel orientation (distal electrode in contact with tissue and proximal electrode not in contact) result in near-simultaneous activation of the distal and proximal unipolar electrograms.[7] This results in the bipolar summation that is subjected to significant cancellation, even in normal tissue. This is further complicated in the setting of tissue fibrosis due to nonuniform anisotropy and a significantly smaller degree of tissue mass being activated.

Consequently, conventional mapping catheters with a distal electrode that is > 3.5 mm, longer center-to-center interelectrode spacing, and predisposition to variable extremes in the angle of incidence inherently limit the spatial resolution of bipolar electrograms. As such, due to the presence of varying wavefronts in low-voltage scar areas, larger electrodes with greater far-field signaling are also more prone to document longer, more fractionated signals.[3,4] Conversely, because multielectrode catheters can record more data points with increased variability in the angle of incidence and the relationship to the vector of propagation, they are less susceptible to the cancellation effect of different bipolar vectors. By virtue of containing multiple electrodes, multielectrode catheters can also easily collect more electrograms over a shorter period of time.

Tung et al. performed one of the first preclinical studies comparing mapping resolution between contemporary linear and multielectrode mapping catheters. In a porcine model of infarction, they found that multipolar mapping achieves higher density in a shorter period of time and increases the detection of late potentials.[8] Similarly, Anter et al. directly compared voltage mapping between a linear catheter and a multielectrode catheter in 30 patients including 10 healthy volunteers and 20 patients with scar-related atrial tachycardia (AT).[9] In this study, a contemporary linear ablation catheter was used with a 3.5-mm distal electrode separated by 2 mm from a 2-mm proximal electrode, resulting in 4.75-mm center-to-center spacing (Thermocool, Biosense Webster). The multielectrode catheter was a 20-pole steerable catheter arranged in five soft radiating spines covering a diameter of 3.5 mm (Pentaray, Biosense Webster). It had 1-mm electrodes and recordings were performed with 2-mm interelectrode spacing and thus 3-mm center-to-center interelectrode spacing. Consistent with prior studies, multielectrode mapping resulted in significantly higher point density. Interestingly, patients with scar-related atrial arrhythmias had a smaller area of total low bipolar voltage area (defined as <0.5 mV) suggestive of the improved ability of the multielectrode catheter to detect areas of survived tissue. These differences remained significant after normalizing the maps for point density and interelectrode spacing, indicating that smaller-size electrodes are at least partially responsible for the improved resolution.

Similar results evaluating the same mapping catheters were demonstrated in a swine model consisting of 3 controls and 11 with chronic anterior wall infarction.[10] Within the infarcted group, the area of low bipolar voltage (<1.5 mV) was smaller (21.7 cm^2 versus 28.0 cm^2; $P = .003$) and had higher mean bipolar voltage amplitudes (0.99 ± 1.02 mV versus 0.57 ± 0.38 mV; $P = .001$) with multielectrode mapping compared to point-by-point mapping. In areas of very low bipolar areas (<0.5 mV), this difference was even more apparent in both size (7.1 cm^2 versus 15.2 cm^2; $P = .003$) and mean bipolar voltage amplitude (0.72 ± 0.81 mV versus 0.30 ± 0.12 mV; $P < .001$). Furthermore, electrograms recorded from multielectrode catheters were less fractionated (67% versus 95%; $P = .01$) and of shorter duration (73 ± 15 ms versus 97 ± 19 ms; $P = .001$), which enhances visualization of heterogeneity within the infarct zone and identification of voltage-preserved "channels"; cardiac magnetic resonance imaging and histology validated the presence of surviving myocardial bundles within these heterogeneous regions.

Findings from these initial studies have shown what has now become well accepted in the field: multielectrode catheters offer several advantages for mapping scar-related arrhythmias, including (1) smaller electrodes with closer interelectrode spacing that can record electrograms with higher bipolar voltage amplitude, shorter electrogram duration, and reduced fractionation, allowing more accurate annotation (which also applies to local activation time during activation mapping and interpretation of entrainment mapping) (Fig. 9.1); (2) larger footprints with the potential to record the entire circuit of reentrant tachycardias during a single beat and rapidly localize the circuit, which may be particularly beneficial in cases of poorly tolerated ventricular arrhythmias (Fig. 9.2); and (3) higher-mapping resolution that may identify heterogeneity within the area of low-voltage during sinus rhythm mapping, allowing localization of "channels" of surviving myocardial bundles that would otherwise be "contaminated" by surrounding fibrosis with the large distal electrode of a linear catheter (Fig. 9.3).

Nevertheless, large electrodes contribute to an extended "field of view" while smaller electrode catheters provide additional insight into the subendocardial surface. It is not that one is accurate and the other is inaccurate but rather that both recording modalities provide complementary information. This is well demonstrated in the examples shown in Fig. 9.4 and Fig. 9.5, which shows mapping from both a standard contact-force catheter and high-resolution catheter in two preclinical patients. In one subject (Fig. 9.4), a chronic, nonreperfused anterior infarction was created, resulting in transmural endocardial-to-epicardial LV scar. This transmural infarction is depicted with areas of low bipolar voltage (0.5–1.5 mV) and very low bipolar voltage (0.1–0.5 mV) recorded by both catheter types. In a different patient who underwent reperfusion myocardial infarction (Fig. 9.5), the more heterogenous subendocardial scar can be observed when mapping with the higher-resolution catheter. These examples also demonstrate the need for one to take care with the interpretation of these maps as the area of "normal" bipolar voltage (>1.5 mV) created with the high-resolution catheter does not necessarily indicate this entire area of tissue is normal, but rather there is survived subendocardial tissue bundles present. The area of larger, low bipolar voltage recorded with the conventional contact-force catheter in this same area is recording scar that is more midmyocardial and/or epicardial. This same principle is true when interpreting areas of low bipolar voltage with multielectrode catheters that are more prone to record "low-voltage" due to inadequate tissue contact and is why careful evaluation of electrogram characteristics is equally important during substrate mapping using non–contact-based catheters.

TYPES OF MULTIELECTRODE CATHETERS

Conventional point-by-point mapping catheters typically have a 3.5-mm electrode tip. Depending on the catheter, this distal tip electrode is separated by 0.5–2.5 mm from a proximal 1- to

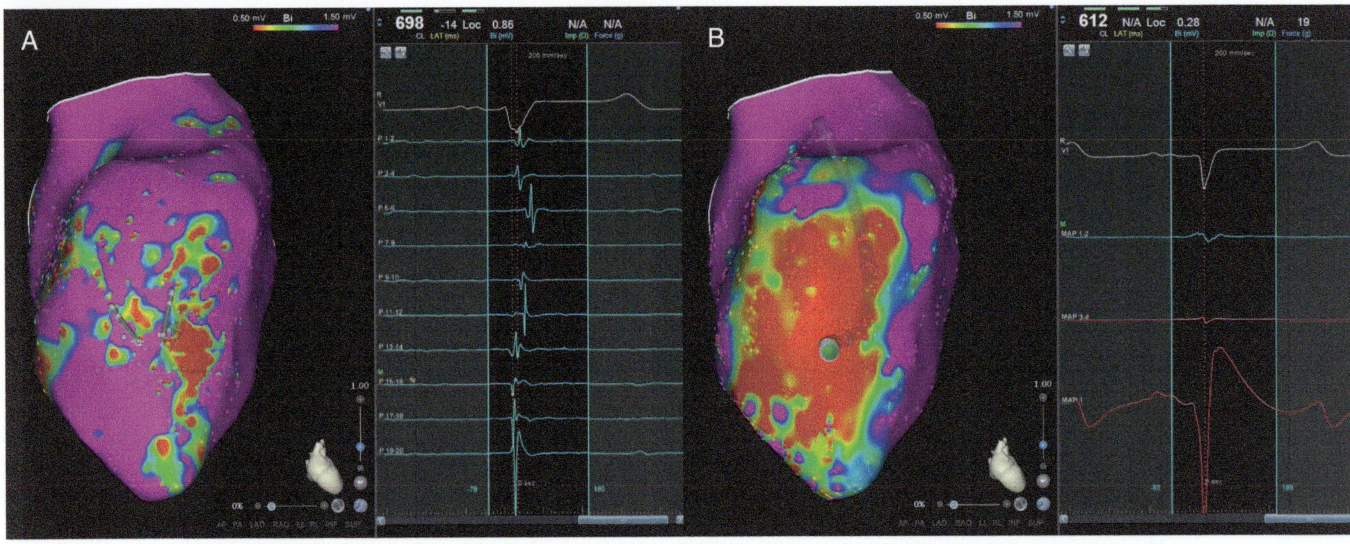

Fig 9.1 Electroanatomical maps (EAMs) of the left ventricle in an example of postinfarction swine using the CARTO 3 system. (A) High-resolution bipolar EAM made with the multielectrode 2–6–2 mm Pentaray catheter. (B) Standard bipolar EAM with a contact force ablation catheter. The maps are displayed in the anteroposterior view and with a bipolar voltage range of 0.5–1.5 mV. In this example of heterogeneous subendocardial scar, the mapping resolution within the area of low-voltage significantly diverged, whereas mapping with a linear catheter demonstrated homogeneous and confluent low-voltage area, mapping with a multielectrode catheter revealed channels of normal bipolar voltage amplitude and electrogram characteristics within the low-voltage zone.

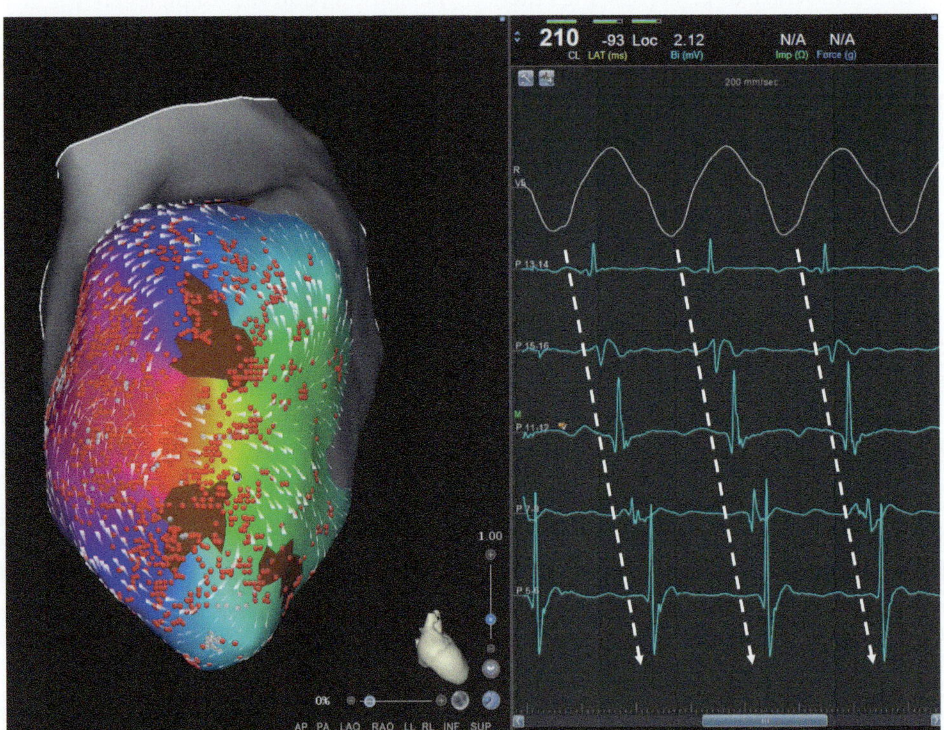

Fig 9.2 High-resolution left ventricular activation map 2–6–2 mm Pentaray catheter of monomorphic reentrant ventricular tachycardia in a postinfarction swine, obtained using the CARTO 3 system. Reentrant excitation recorded spanning the entire VT isthmus activation period is shown from a single recording site as depicted in the activation vectors shown. Near-field, sharp electrograms allow for accurate local activation time annotation and creation of high-resolution activation map of the VT.

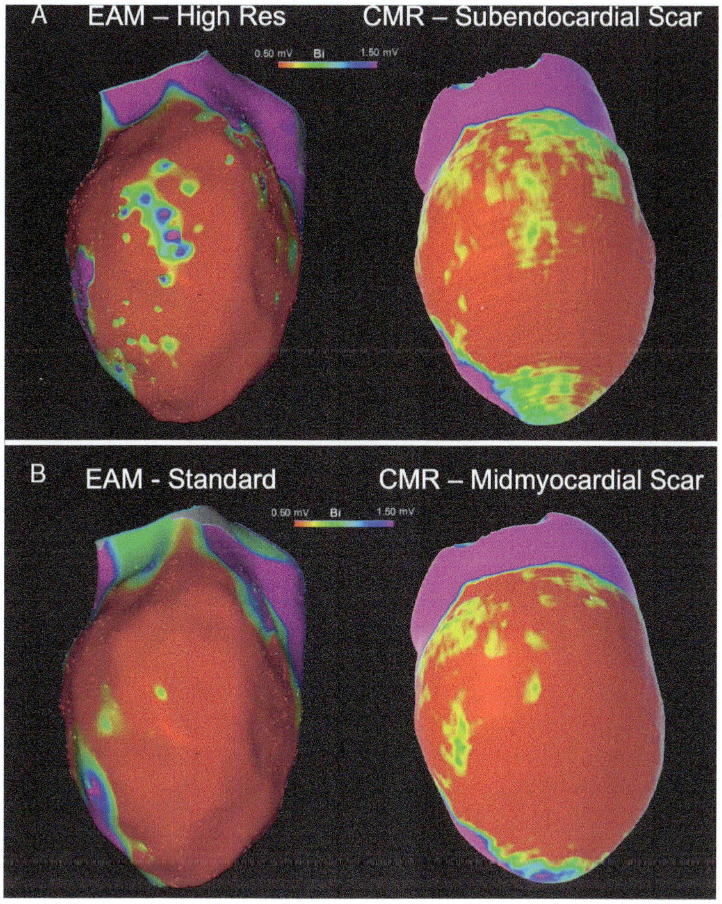

Fig 9.3 Additional example of electro-anatomical maps (EAMs) using the CARTO 3 system of the left ventricle in a chronic anterior infarct swine model. (A) High-resolution bipolar EAM made with the multielectrode 2–6–2 mm Pentaray catheter and cardiac magnetic resonance (CMR) imaging reconstruction of late-gadolinium (LGE) enhancement scar at the subendocardial surface (10% level of myocardium). (B) Standard bipolar EAM with a contact force ablation catheter and CMR image reconstruction of LGE at the midmyocardium (50%). The maps are displayed in the anteroposterior view and with a bipolar voltage range of 0.5–1.5 mV. In this example, there was only a small area of preserved voltage detected in the scar area consistent with the CMR LGE subendocardial reconstruction. The homogeneous scar pattern detected with the standard mapping catheter was consistent with the CMR LGE reconstruction of the midmyocardium, representative of the larger field of view present when recording with larger electrode sizes.

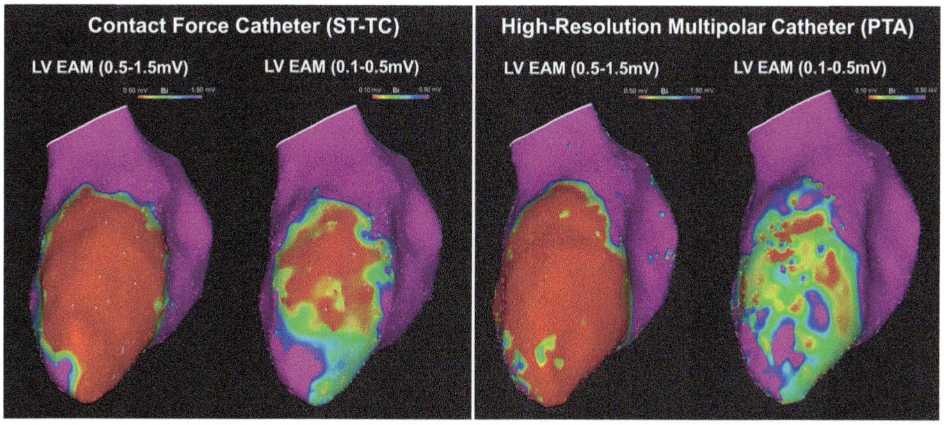

Fig 9.4 Electroanatomical maps (EAMs) of the left ventricle in a pre-clinical swine model of nonreperfusion myocardial infarction (MI) using the CARTO 3 system. *Left,* Left ventricular (LV) bipolar maps in the anterior-posterior view created with a standard contact-force catheter (Biosense Webster, Thermocool Smart-Touch). *Right,* LV bipolar maps generated with a high-resolution multipolar catheter (Biosense Webster, 2-6-2 mm Pentaray). Areas of low-voltage (0.5–1.5 mV) and very low-voltage (0.1–0.5 mV) are shown. Areas of consistent LV low and very low-voltage identified with both standard and high-resolution catheters is consistent with transmural infarction created in this nonreperfused model of MI.

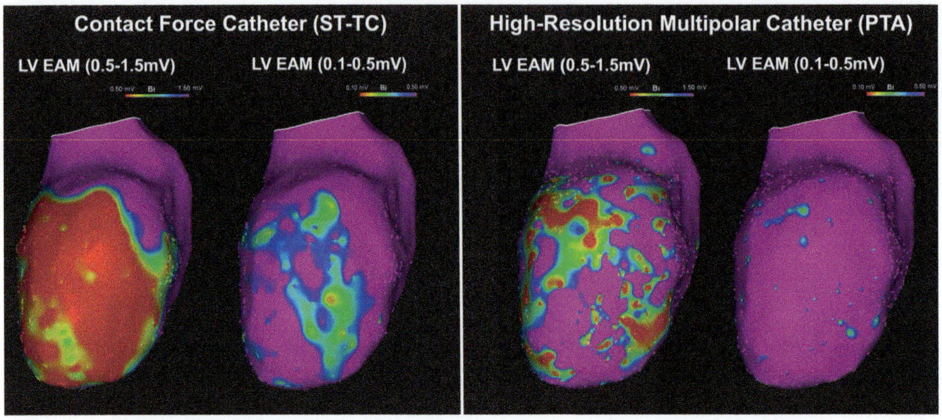

Fig 9.5 Electro-anatomical maps (EAMs) of the left ventricle in a preclinical swine model of reperfused myocardial infarction (MI) using the CARTO 3 system. *Left,* Left ventricular (LV) bipolar maps in the anteroposterior view created with a standard contact-force catheter (Biosense Webster, Thermocool Smart-Touch). *Right,* LV bipolar maps generated with a high-resolution multipolar catheter (Biosense Webster, 2-6-2 mm Pentaray). Areas of low-voltage (0.5–1.5 mV) and very low-voltage (0.1–0.5 mV) are shown. The heterogenous low-voltage areas seen with the high-resolution catheter is consistent with patchy, heterogeneous infarction with areas of survived subendocardial tissue bundles observed in this model of reperfused MI.

2-mm electrode, resulting in a center-to-center interelectrode spacing of ~2.50–5.0 mm (Table 9.1).[11] Many have a proximal 1-mm electrode, with a center-to-center interelectrode distance of ~3.25 mm. In contrast, multielectrode catheters often have 1-mm electrodes, 2-mm interelectrode spacing, and an overall 3-mm center-to-center interelectrode spacing. Currently, a variety of multielectrode catheters associated with the following commonly used 3D mapping systems are available: CARTO 3 (Johnson & Johnson, Biosense Webster), Ensite Precision and more recently Ensite X (Abbott), and Rhythmia (Boston Scientific). Table 9.1 provides a brief overview and a more comprehensive list of various catheter characteristics that are currently available for clinical use. (Please see Chapter 8 for more detailed descriptions of fundamental concepts of 3D mapping systems.)

Biosense Webster

The CARTO system consists of a location pad with three separate low-level magnetic field–emitting coils arranged as a triangle under the patient, six electrode patches positioned on the patient's back and chest, a data processing unit, and a graphic display unit to provide visualization of the electro-anatomical

TABLE 9.1 Electrode Configurations of Various Ablation and Multielectrode Mapping Catheters

Model	Manufacturer	Electrodes	Tip Electrode Size (mm)	Ring Electrode Size (mm)	Spacing (Edge to Edge)	Spacing (Center to Center)
Ablation Catheters						
QDOT Micro, CF	Biosense Webster	4 + 3ME	3.5	1	2-5-2	4.25
Thermacool ST, CF	Biosence Webster	4	3.5	1	1-6-2	3.25
Thermacool STSF, CF	Biosense Webster	4	3.5	1	2-5-2	4.25
FlexAbility	Abbott	4	4	1	1-4-1	3.5
Tacticath, CF	Abbott	4	3.5	1	2-5-2	4.25
MiFi	Boston Scientific	4		1	1.5	2.5
Intella MiFi	Boston Scientific	4 + 3ME	4	2	2.5-2.5-2.5	4.5
Multielectrode Catheters						
Decapolar	Biosense Webster	10	2.4	1	2-8-2	3
Pentaray	Biosense Webster	20		1	2-6-2 or 4-4-4	3
Octaray	Biosense Webster	48		0.5	1.5	2
Optrell	Biosense Webster	48		0.9 mm^2		2.4
LiveWire	Abbott	20	2	1	2-2-2	3
HD Grid	Abbott	16 or 32		1	3	4
IntellaMap Orion	Boston Scientific	64		0.9 × 0.45	1.6	2.5

CF, contact force; *ME*, mini- or micro-electrodes.

model being created. Three-dimensional localization is based on a hybrid of magnetic and current-based localization technologies with an accuracy of <1 mm. The Pentaray is the CARTO system's prototypical multielectrode catheter. It has 20 poles arranged in five flexible splines, with 1-mm electrodes separated by 4–4–4 or 2–6–2 spacing, that cover an area with a diameter of 3.5 cm when laid out flat. As discussed previously, many of the initial studies comparing multielectrode and point-by-point mapping used the Pentaray catheter as the representative multielectrode catheter. However, there are only a limited number of comparable studies investigating clinical outcomes. In the context of AT following atrial fibrillation (AF) termination, Bun et al. assessed multielectrode mapping using the Pentaray catheter against a historical group using conventional mapping.[12] Pentaray mapping acquired more points within a shorter period of time (449 ± 520 points within 14 ± 6 minutes versus 42 ± 18 points; $P < .0001$] within 33 ± 25 minutes ; $P = .05$), but more significantly all isthmuses were easily identified with Pentaray mapping than with conventional mapping (100% versus 87%; $P = .056$). This resulted in fewer recurrences in the Pentaray group during a mean follow-up of nearly 1 year (0 versus 23.5%; $P = .03$). For scar-related ventricular tachycardia (VT), Cano et al. evaluated the Pentaray catheter against a linear catheter in a clinical study involving 81 patients.[13] Again, the Pentaray catheter was associated with a significant shortening of the endocardial (38 ± 15 versus 56 ± 24 minutes; $P = .001$) and epicardial (28 ± 9 versus 41 ± 16 minutes; $P = .011$) mapping times, but with no differences in acute and long-term follow-up outcomes. Other studies found similar results, although some hint that patient outcomes may be improved.[14,15]

An advanced iteration of the Pentaray catheter, the Octaray, has since been evaluated.[16] The Octaray catheter extends the number of splines from five to eight and the total number of electrodes from 20 to 48 (each spline containing six electrodes); the size of each electrode is smaller in comparison with the Pentaray (0.9 versus 2.0 mm^2). The interelectrode spacing is 2 mm edge-to-edge and 2.5 mm center-to-center. Its uniform electrode spacing allows recording of overlapping electrograms (i.e., 1–2, 2–3, 3–4, etc.), such that the overall number of bipolar electrograms recorded at each beat is increased from 10–40. Fig. 9.6 demonstrates the electrode catheter configuration of both the Pentaray and Octaray catheters. The coverage area of the Octaray is similar to the Pentaray, although the mapping density is much higher (7 versus 2.5 electrodes/cm^2). Reflecting the ability of smaller electrode size and interelectrode distance to detect surviving myocardial tissue, the Octaray found higher voltage amplitudes (1.24 ± 1.12 mV versus 1.04 ± 1.27 mV; $P < .0001$) at sites of ablation gaps in experimental swine models, although ablation gaps were similarly identified by both catheters ($P = 1.0$).[16] This suggests that increased number of electrodes with smaller surface areas does not add significant value in identifying macroscopic ablation lines. Nevertheless, the same group found that the Octaray catheter identified a higher proportion of near-field local abnormal ventricular activities within the low-voltage area (53% ± 16% versus 34% ± 16%; $P = .03$) that were considered far-field electrograms by the Pentaray.[17] The Octoray was also advantageous for mapping hemodynamically unstable VTs due to is higher acquisition rate. Initial human experience with the Octaray was also positive, although rigorous clinical trials are needed for further assessment.[18]

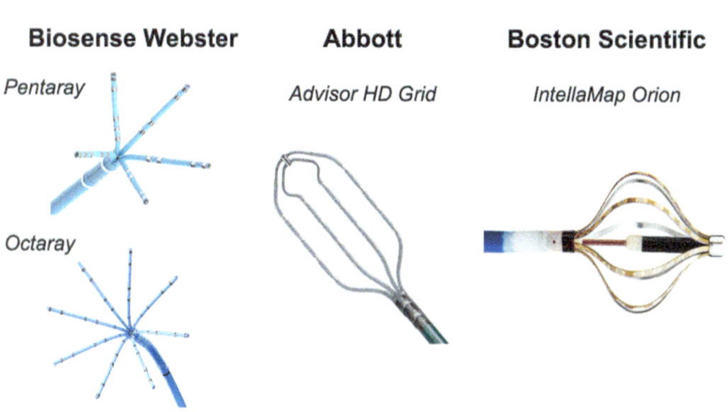

Fig 9.6 Images of contemporary multielectrode mapping catheters offered from the current three highest-volume vendors: Biosense Webster, Abbott Laboratories, and Boston Scientific.

Abbott

Set to replace the Ensite Precision, the Ensite X is the latest electroanatomical mapping system from Abbott that was approved by the FDA in 2022. The Ensite system consists of the Ensite amplifier that converts physiological signals from the patient to digital signals for the workstation, the field frame, the display workstation, and eight surface electrodes (three transthoracic pairs for three orthogonal axes and two patient reference sensors). Its representative multipolar catheter is the Advisor HD Grid. The Advisor HD Grid has four parallel splines forming a 1.3 × 1.3-cm^2 grid. Each spline has four electrodes that are 1 mm in size with 3–3–3 equidistant spacing. Electrodes on the same plane but different splines also have a 3-mm interelectrode spacing. Fig. 9.6 demonstrates the electrode catheter configuration of the Advisor HD grid. Direct comparison between multielectrode mapping and conventional point-by-point mapping for focal atrial and ventricular arrhythmias has been performed with this catheter in a case-matched cohort study encompassing 54 patients.[19] Mapping times (35 ± 24 versus 53 ± 31 minutes; $P = .03$) and procedural durations (126 ± 42 versus 153 ± 39 minutes; $P = .02$) were significantly shorter with grid catheter mapping. Although electrograms at successful ablation sites had earlier annotations with multielectrode mapping (39 ± 11 versus 33 ± 7 ms; $P = .02$), there were no differences in procedural success or arrhythmia recurrence.

Notably, the fixed-spacing grid conformation of the HD grid catheter allows for "omnipolar mapping." Bipolar electrograms exhibit variable morphology due to the interaction of the wavefront with the orientation of the electrode pair, which may lead to physiologically ambiguous characterization of the myocardium.[2] Consequently, bipolar voltage maps may display significant heterogeneity and compromised reproducibility. Introduced by Deno et al.[20] and validated by Massé et al.,[21] omnipolar electrogram methodology employs multiple electrodes and mathematical models of wave propagation to determine the direction of a traveling wave along the myocardial plane by interrogating its electric field. As such, all bipolar electrode orientations can be evaluated and the largest voltage value along the maximal bipole direction can be used. In preclinical studies involving swine models of myocardial infarctions,[22] omnipolar electrograms were 23–27% ($P < .05$) larger and had 38–47% ($P < .01$) less beat-by-beat variation than bipolar electrograms. Omnipolar-derived substrate maps were also closer in value with the surface area of endocardial infarction based on magnetic resonance late gadolinium enhancement. In human studies involving scar-related VT,[23–25] omnipolar mapping has also been associated with smaller scar areas and identification of greater number of conduction channels. Similarly, omnipolar technology may improve low-voltage–guided substrate ablation for AF.[26] In 36 patients undergoing ablation for AF, omnipolar mapping identified more PV sleeves and greater sleeve size ($P < .001$) than standard bipolar mapping using the same HD grid catheter.[27] This resulted in a change in ablation strategy in 64% of patient and increased number of ablation lesions for right (10.9 ± 1.55 versus 7.7 ± 1.13; $P = .005$) and left (8.56 ± 1.16 versus 6.62 ± 1.27; $P = .003$) veins, which may improve clinical outcomes.

Boston Scientific

The Rhythmia HDx mapping system uses a hybrid tracking technology with both magnetic and impedance-based localization features. For magnetic tracking, the system uses one sensor coil–embedded bac pack and a magnetic field generator. For impedance tracking, the impedance field is generated by applying current to the back patch, patches for the electrocardiographic limb leads, and the V_1, V_3, and V_6 chest leads. A 64-electrode mini-basket contact mapping array (Intellamap Orion) is available from Boston Scientific. The mini-basket catheter consists of eight splines, each containing eight electrodes. The surface area of each electrode is 0.4 mm^2, and the interelectrode spacing is 2.5 mm measured from center to center. The catheter is expandable to a nominal diameter of 18 mm and a maximal diameter of 22 when measured near its equator. The electrode catheter configuration of the Intellamap Orion catheter is shown in Fig. 9.6. To the authors' knowledge, no isolated analysis of the Orion catheter against point-by-point mapping has been performed for scar-related substrate, although it has been shown to record shorter durations of local sharp bipolar electrograms (54.95 ± 18.84 versus 71.22 ± 19.55 ms; $P = .001$) and increased incidence of late potentials (88% versus 60%; $P = .041$) in the voltage-transitional zone for idiopathic right ventricular outflow tract arrhythmias.[28] The low signal:noise ratio from the printed electrodes can be particularly beneficial in creating high-quality activation maps in complex disease substrate (Fig. 9.7). Comparative studies between different 3D electroanatomical mapping systems are lacking, but one study compared the Orion/Rhythmia system with the Pentaray/CARTO system in defining atrial low-voltage areas for AF ablation in 15 patients. The resulted showed comparable low-voltage areas between the two (Orion map = 4.3±6.4 cm^2, Pentaray map = 5.4±8.7 cm^2; $P = .69$), albeit the Orion map had a longer procedure time (23 ± 8 versus 12 ± 3 minutes; $P < .01$). However, the Orion documented low-voltage areas where the Pentaray recorded normal voltages (>0.5 mV) in 2 of 15 patients, although the results were not correlated to MRI findings and the Rhythmia system did not have a tissue proximity filter to avoid points with low tissue-electrode contact. Nevertheless, the Orion/Rhythmia system is associated with satisfactory procedural success for ventricular[29–31] and atrial[32,33] arrhythmias.

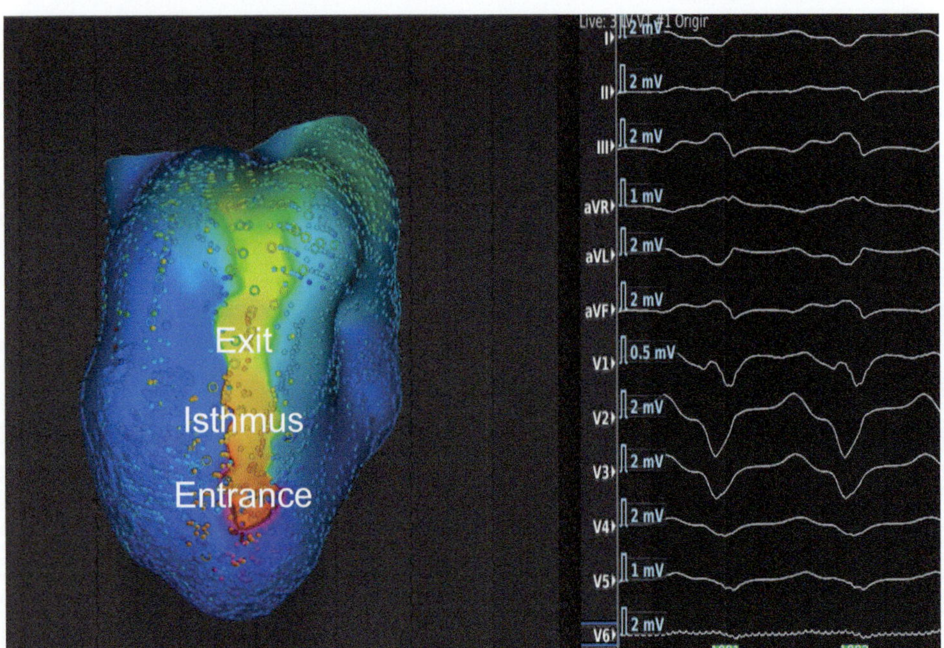

Fig 9.7 High-resolution map created using the IntellaMap Orion (Boston Scientific) and Rhythmia mapping system in a chronic anterior infarction porcine model demonstrating figure-of-eight reentrant VT. Entrance, isthmus, and exit of the VT is shown. (Adapted from Anter E, Tschabrunn CM, Buxton AE, Josephson ME. High-resolution mapping of postinfarction reentrant ventricular tachycardia: electrophysiological characterization of the circuit. *Circulation*. 2016;134(4):314–327.).

LIMITATIONS OF HIGH-RESOLUTION MAPPING

The signal amplitude, power spectrum, and fractionation of bipolar electrograms are commonly used to draw conclusions on underlying cardiac tissue characteristics. However, these features may be significantly affected by the distance and orientation of the mapping catheter bipole to the underlying tissue; adequate contact is thus considered determinant for credible characterization of the underlying arrhythmogenic substrate.[34] The most prevalent limitation of multielectrode catheters is the inability to ensure such adequate contact. Furthermore, even with perceived appropriate contact, contact force is unlikely to be uniform across all electrode pairs. In many instances, individual electrodes are intracavitary and completely devoid of contact with the myocardial surface. This is evident for basket catheters, where one hemisphere may not contact the myocardial surface due to its inherent geometric shape. In response to this limitation, 3D mapping systems have evolved to ascertain the relationship between the acquired point and the most outer aspects of the geometric chamber. Namely, points that are "internal" to the outer margin are not implemented into the working map display, so that the number of points that are used are a fraction of the total number of points sampled (e.g., the tissue proximity filter on the ConfiDENSE module on CARTO 3).[35]

Nevertheless, even among properly sampled signals, a rigid universal voltage threshold is unlikely to be consistent across the various electrode areas of commercially available catheters. Conventional scar and low bipolar voltage thresholds in the ventricular myocardium (0.5–1.5 mV) were based on mapping with a conventional electrode.[36] Based on the prior findings and comparison with MRI-derived substrate, an increasing linear relationship has been observed between optimal voltage thresholds for ventricular scar and wider bipole spacing.[37] In response, several authors have suggested specific bipolar voltage thresholds for each dedicated mapping catheter: 0.2–1 mV or 1.5 mV for the Pentaray and 0.1–1 mV for the Orion.[29,30] On the other hand, limited data exist for the atria. In a direct comparison between the Thermocool ablation catheter and the Pentaray multielectrode catheter, their respective mean bipolar electrogram amplitudes and the fifth percentile of the normal bipolar voltage distribution were similar. In this study, normal endocardial bipolar voltage amplitude was defined as ≥0.5 mV for both catheters.[9] Another small series found an excellent correlation between scar-distribution on CMR and high-density voltage mapping using the Orion multielectrode catheter during AT with a bipolar cut-off of 0.5 mV.[32] Clinical and experimental data all support the notion that larger electrodes with greater interelectrode spacing have a greater "antenna" than small electrode catheters with close interelectrode spacing (Fig. 9.3).

Although extremely rare, the conformation of individual catheters may have adverse effects that necessitate careful attention. In one study, two patients with inferior myocardial infarction experienced ventricular fibrillation during mapping when the Pentaray catheter was close to the posterior papillary muscle.[38] This suggests movement of splines may mechanically provoke premature beats when interacting with specific structures (e.g., papillary muscle, chordae tendineae, or left ventricular septum), with the potential of degenerating into ventricular fibrillation. In addition, there are isolated reports of entrapments within the Orion basket catheter. In one instance, a quadripolar diagnostic catheter was found to be entrapped within the splines of the basket catheter preventing retraction in the sheath.[39] In another instance, a remnant of a venous valve in the right internal iliac vein was entrapped between two splines of the basket catheter, and the tip of the catheter had to be surgically removed.[40] Particularly for mechanical valves, multielectrode catheters are at risk for entrapment and their use is considered off-label in these circumstances.[41,42]

FUTURE PERSPECTIVES OF HIGH-RESOLUTION MAPPING

With the advent of high-resolution mapping and the dramatic increases in the number of points that can be acquired, systemic manual checks of electrogram annotation can be cumbersome and paradoxically time consuming, especially if there are an overabundance of neighboring points around an inaccurate annotation. As such, accurate automatic annotation will become progressively more paramount. Recently, the Rhythmia system developed the first multiple criteria algorithm, where electrogram timing is derived from the combination of the maximum dV/dt from the unipolar electrogram and the maximum amplitude on the bipolar electrogram.[43] For fragmented or multiple potential electrograms, the system considers the timing in the surround area to select the potential to use for the timing annotation; if no statistical coherence is found between neighboring points, no color code is displayed. The window of interest is automatically set by the system at the cycle length value and centered on the main reference electrogram. Automatic electrogram acquisition occurs based on electrogram stability and respiration phase. In an experimental canine atrial linear lesion model, initial blinded examination of 73 activation maps accurately revealed the site of earliest atrial activation, the location and extent of the lines of conduction block, and the presence or absence of conduction through a gap.[43] Manual reannotation was only performed in 0.17% of the accepted electrograms for the purposes of presentation. Nevertheless, even with the most sophisticated automated mapping technology, it is likely that human input will always be warranted to correct for noise, artifacts, and near-field versus far-field determination.[44] Additionally, there is likely a limit to higher resolutions above which no appreciable differences in clinical outcomes are achieved. For example, it might be reasonable to hypothesize that increasing mapping density from 100 to 500 points may be clinically impactful, but adding another 1000 points to a 5000-point map may have diminishing returns. Furthermore, catheter ablation is typically targeted toward small, localized regions of interest, and high-resolution mapping is not indicated in locations remote from this site. As multielectrode catheters and automated mapping technology evolve, the value of mechanistic insights and clinical applicability must be considered.

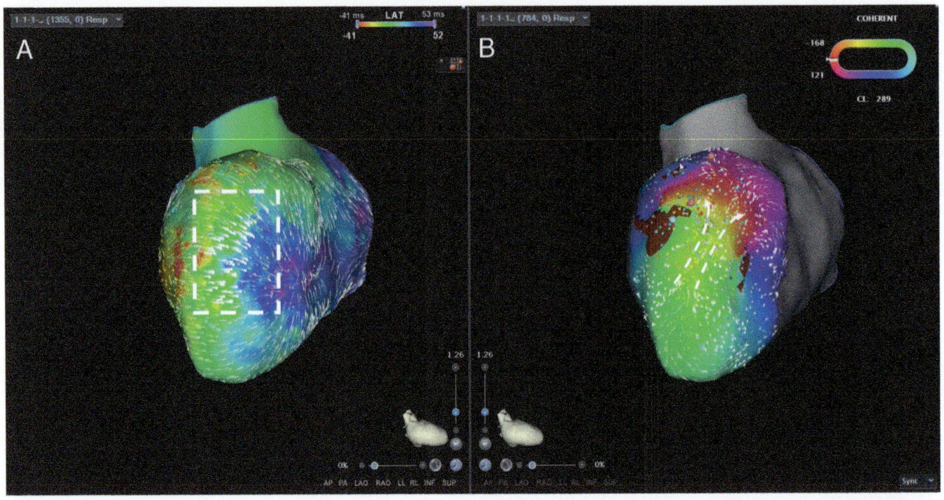

Fig 9.8 Identification of areas of slow conduction during substrate mapping using the CARTO 3 system. (A) High-resolution activation map during right ventricular (RV) pacing in a chronic anterior infarct swine model. Areas of slow conduction, represented by *bold arrows* in the vector map, are observed in the anterolateral aspect of the scar and highlighted in a *dotted line box*. (B) Detailed activation map of ventricular tachycardia (VT) in the same subject demonstrating co-localization of the area of slow conduction identified during RV pacing and the VT circuit.

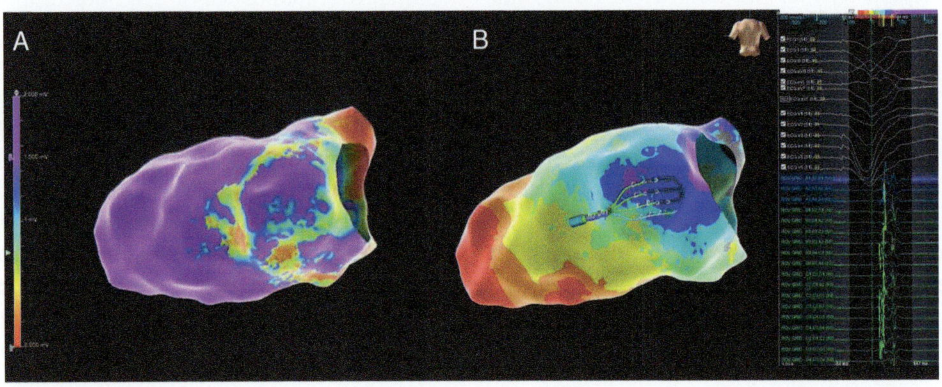

Fig 9.9 Identification of areas of slow conduction during substrate mapping using the Abbott Mapping system. (A) Endocardial left ventricular (LV) high-resolution bipolar voltage map (0.5–1.5 mV) generated using the Advisor HD Grid catheter in a patient with nonischemic cardiomyopathy. Areas of heterogenous basal lateral LV low-voltage demonstrated. (B) Activation map during right ventricular (RV) pacing reveals area of slow conduction within the area of patchy bipolar voltage scar. Fractionated and split recordings from this region of isochronal crowding indicative of deceleration during RV pacing are shown. Ablation in this region resulted in noninducibility of VT. (Case images courtesy of Dr. Timothy Markman.)

Notably, an emerging clinical application of high-resolution mapping for VT includes identifying areas of conduction slowing during sinus rhythm and/or pacing to identify regions within scar that may be particularly vulnerable to reentry. Because of the inherent hemodynamic instability resulting from VT, substrate modification has developed as an alternative to activation mapping, with a trend toward more extensive ablation strategies including substrate homogenization, core isolation, and complete elimination of local abnormal ventricular activity and late potentials.[45,46] However, these represent probabilistic strategies where greater extents of ablation translate to increased chances of disrupting a critical reentry site. Recently, functional substrate mapping incorporating deceleration zones and/or multiple wavefront analyses have been investigated, which promises to refine the approach and improve the sensitivity and specificity of mapping (Fig. 9.8 and Fig. 9.9).[47,48] Using high-resolution mapping (Ensite Precision with HD Grid), Aziz et al. created isochronal late activation maps annotated to the latest local electrogram deflection, and ablation was target at deceleration zones (three or more isochrones within 1-cm radius).[47] Anter et al. mapped the left ventricle from three directions (sinus rhythm or atrial pacing, right ventricular pacing, and left ventricular pacing), and ablation was applied to the cumulative area of slow activation (sum of all regions with activation times ≥40 ms per 10 mm).[48] The increased mapping speed and density bestowed by multielectrode mapping and automated mapping algorithms facilitate these opportunities to examine the substrate during electrophysiologic conditions, such as anisotropic conduction and varying coupling intervals, that more closely resemble VT (Fig. 9.10).

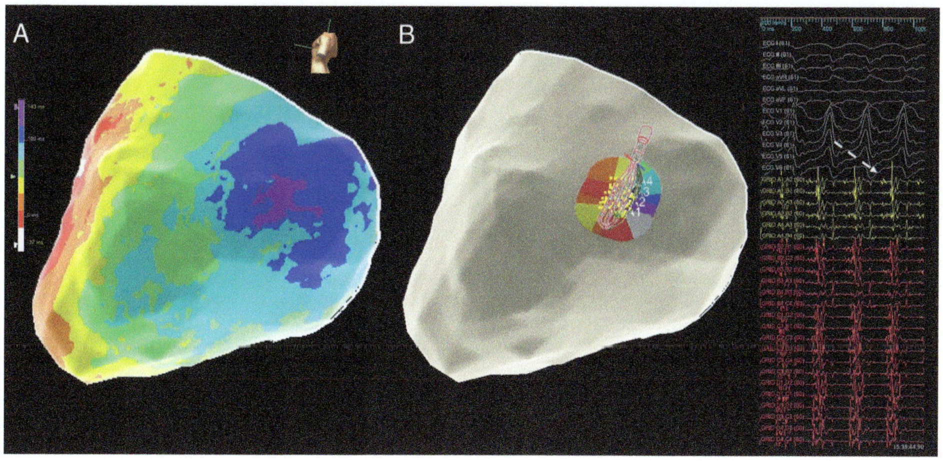

Fig 9.10 Identification of areas of slow conduction during substrate mapping and correlation with ventricular tachycardia (VT) circuit using the Abbott mapping system. (A) Epicardial high-resolution activation map during sinus rhythm generated using the Advisor HD Grid catheter in a patient with nonischemic cardiomyopathy and VT. Isochronal crowding is seen in the epicardial basal lateral left ventricle suggestive of slow conduction during sinus rhythm. (B) Limited activation map during unstable VT within the area of isochronal crowding shows reentrant excitation and mid-diastolic potentials. Ablation in this region resulted in VT noninducibility. (Case images courtesy of Dr. David Lin.)

CONCLUSION

Multielectrode and high-density mapping have clear benefits in delineating areas of arrhythmogenic substrate, improving accurate local activation time annotations, and decreasing mapping time. In addition to these clinical benefits, high-resolution mapping technologies have also provided important insights into disease pathology and complex arrhythmia mechanisms. Future engineering and computational technology developments to further improve accurate real-time signal annotation and better tissue contact algorithms are necessary and will further enhance the utility of high-resolution mapping during complex ablation procedures.

REFERENCES

Please refer to the e-book for a complete list of references.

10

Intracardiac Echocardiography, Computed Cardiac Tomography, and Magnetic Resonance Imaging for Guiding Mapping and Ablation

Daniele Muser, Pasquale Santangeli

KEY POINTS

- In the past two decades, different cardiovascular imaging modalities such as intracardiac echocardiography, cardiac magnetic resonance, and multidetector computed tomography have progressively achieved an established role in aiding catheter ablation procedures.
- Multimodality imaging is able to accurately define the arrhythmogenic substrate (i.e., presence and architecture of scar), and its integration with activation and voltage mapping data allows to identify ablation targets potentially improving procedural outcomes.
- Real-time imaging modalities such as intracardiac echocardiography allow for continuous monitoring of catheter position and early detection of complications.

INTRODUCTION

During the past few decades, catheter ablation has become an established treatment for a wide range of cardiac arrhythmias, offering the possibility of a lasting arrhythmia control for a substantial proportion of patients. The increasing procedural complexity has been paralleled by an increasing need for reliable imaging modalities to define the underlying arrhythmogenic substrate and plan the optimal procedural strategy, assist catheter manipulation for mapping and ablation, and monitoring of complications. Preprocedural imaging modalities such as multidetector cardiac computed tomography (MDCT) or cardiac magnetic resonance (CMR) have been extremely valuable to accurately characterize the cardiac anatomy and function and identify the underlying arrhythmogenic substrate with a substantial impact on the procedural approaches.[1–3] The findings from MDCT or CMR can be reconstructed in three-dimensional (3D) models and integrated with electroanatomical mapping systems to guide mapping and ablation.[1,3–5] Intracardiac echocardiography (ICE) is also an established role as intraprocedural imaging modality offering a variety of advantages such as assistance in positioning intracardiac catheters, confirmation of catheter contact, assessment of ablation lesion creation, visualization of the arrhythmia substrate and/or critical intracavitary structures, and detection and prevention of complications. This chapter provides an overview of the roles of ICE, MDCT, and CMR imaging to guide mapping and ablation of cardiac arrhythmias, with a particular focus on complex procedures such as ablation of atrial fibrillation (AF) and of ventricular tachycardia (VT).

INTRACARDIAC ECHOCARDIOGRAPHY

ICE Platforms

There are two commercially available types of ICE transducers: radial and phased-array systems. The radial ICE transducer, which currently is rarely used, is mounted on a 9-F nonsteerable catheter and emits an imaging beam at a 15-degree forward angle, perpendicular to the long axis of the catheter. The transducer is usually delivered through a curved or steerable introducer sheath into the chamber of interest. The transducer produces a 360-degree imaging plane perpendicular to the axis of the catheter. The radial ICE has a limited far-field resolution, necessitates imaging adjacent to the structure of interest, and it has been largely replaced by phased-array ICE catheters.

Two-dimensional phased-array ICE catheters contain 64-element transducers with variable frequency ranging from 4 to 10 MHz. The phased-array transducer is also capable of full spectral and color Doppler measurements, enhancing the physiologic data that can be obtained. The transducer is mounted on a multidirectional 8F–10F catheter. More recently, two novel phased-array 3D ICE catheters have received US Food and Drug Administration clearance and are available for clinical use: the 9-F VeriSight Pro (Philips, Eindhoven, Netherlands) and the 10-F NuVision (Nuvera, Los Gatos, CA) catheters (Fig. 10.1). These novel 3D ICE platforms have been designed with the intent of extending the capabilities of transesophageal echocardiography to ICE. Compared to regular 2D phased-array ICE catheters, 3D ICE platforms contain hundreds of element transducers, which allow the acquisition of volumes with a wider field of view, higher spatio-temporal resolution, and 90-degree volume imaging. Although 3D ICE may provide valuable

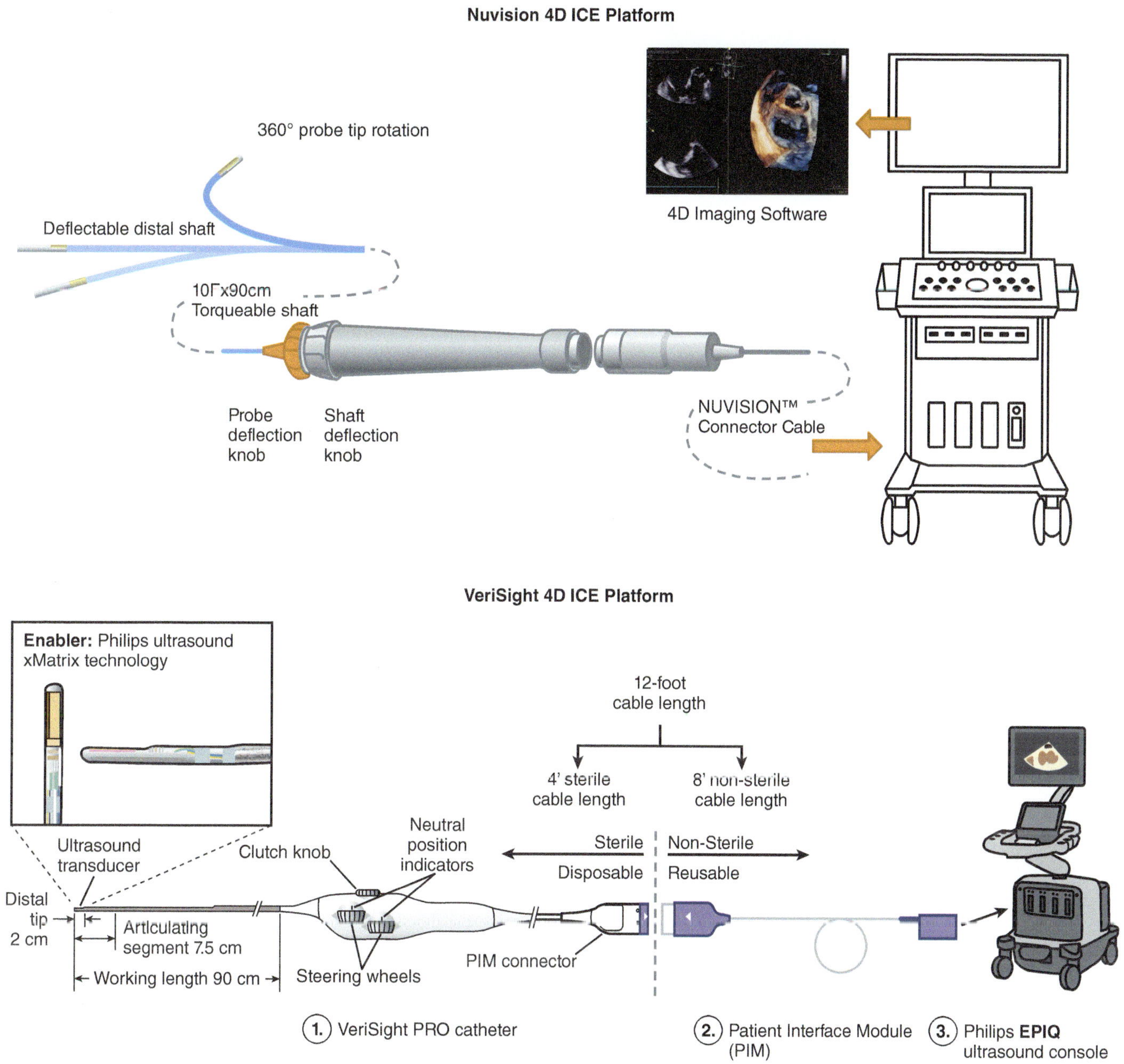

Fig. 10.1 Commercially available 4D ICE technologies. These novel ICE probes contain hundreds of element transducers, which allows us to acquire volumes with a wider field of view, higher spatiotemporal resolution, and 90 × 90-degree volume imaging.

additional information for cardiac structural procedures such as left atrial appendage closure or percutaneous valve interventions, the incremental value of 3D ICE imaging compared to regular 2D platforms for mapping and ablation procedures remains to be established.

ICE-Guided Transseptal Catheterization

ICE provides excellent real-time imaging to guide transseptal catheterization. The standard ICE views for transseptal access are obtained with the imaging transducer positioned in the mid right atrium (RA) and started from the "home view" with visualization of the tricuspid valve (TV) and the right ventricular (RV) inflow together with the noncoronary cusp and the aortic root region. Clockwise rotation to the ICE catheter brings into sequential view: the anterior left atrium; the mitral valve and left atrial appendage (LAA); the left pulmonary veins (PVs); the posterior LA wall; and the right PVs (Fig. 10.2 and Video 10.1). At variance with orthogonal fluoroscopy, the optimal site of the fossa ovalis to obtain access is easily determined with ICE imaging; for procedures that require catheter manipulation within the posterior LA, such as pulmonary vein isolation (PVI) for atrial fibrillation (AF), a more posterior transseptal access is typically performed, whereas for procedures that require catheter manipulation at the level of the mitral annulus (e.g., left ventricular [LV] access for VT ablation) or within the LAA, a more anterior approach is useful.

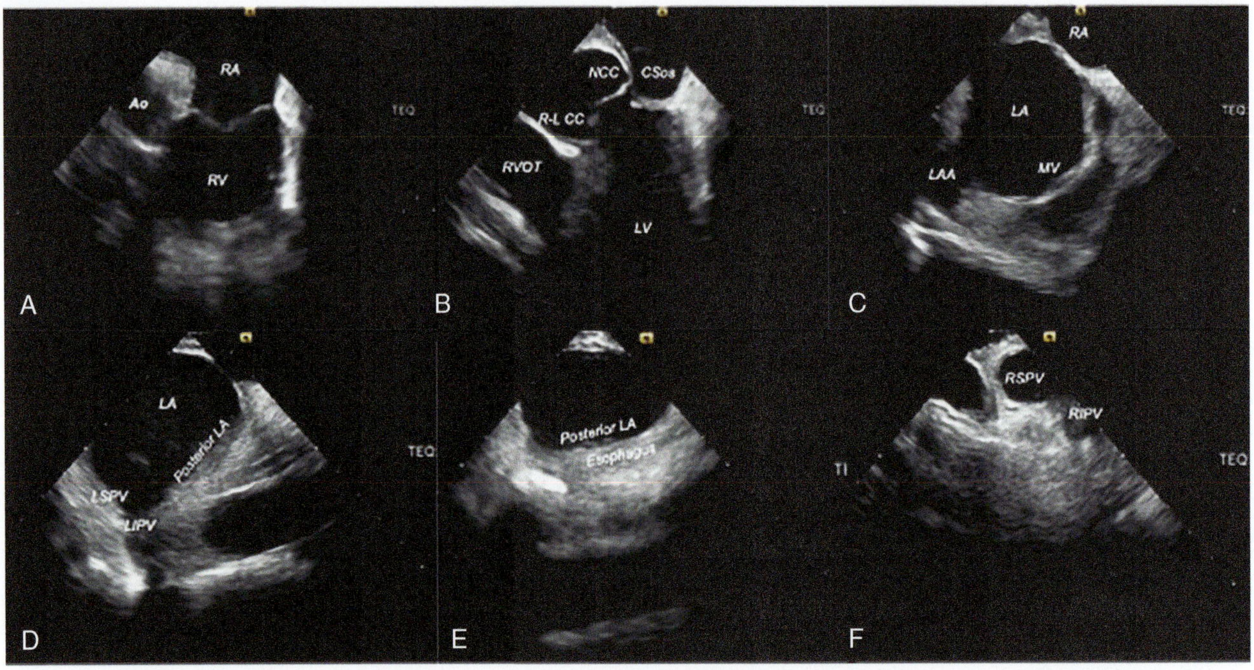

Fig. 10.2 Example of baseline ICE survey for AF ablation procedures. From the standard "home view" with the ICE in the mid right atrium (A) progressive clockwise rotation brings into view the anterior septum (B), the anterior fossa ovalis with far-field visualization of the LAA (C), the posterior fossa ovalis with far-field visualization of the left PVs (D), the posterior LA (E) and the right pulmonary veins (F).

Atrial Fibrillation Ablation

Pulmonary Vein Anatomy

Intraprocedural imaging with ICE allows for direct visualization of the PVs with an accurate definition of the anatomy and relationship with adjacent important structures like the LAA, the esophagus, and the interatrial septum. The left PVs can be visualized across the interatrial septum in the far-field view. Visualization of the right superior PVs may be challenging due to its septal location. However, in the large majority of cases, a good visualization of the right superior PV can be achieved with a slight anterior deflection of the ICE transducer toward the tricuspid annulus. In select cases, the ICE probe can be advanced in the LA via a patent foramen ovale or within the same transseptal access used for mapping/ablation. This maneuver significantly improves the visualization of the PV anatomy, esophagus, and LAA (Fig. 10.3 and Video 10.2). Visualization of the esophagus may allow for adjustment of the lesion set or of the ablation parameters. However, there is no evidence to date that direct esophageal visualization with ICE may reduce the incidence of thermal esophageal lesions or the risk of atrioesophageal fistula.

Left Atrial Appendage Visualization

In our institution, a detailed study of the LAA with ICE is routinely performed in addition or as an alternative to transesophageal echocardiogram in patients with inadequate preoperative anticoagulation and/or persistent AF. Although the gold standard for LAA imaging with ICE is obtained when the probe is deployed within the LA, several different LAA imaging planes can be obtained from adjacent cardiac chambers, including (1) from the RA across the atrial septum, (2) from the distal coronary sinus, or (3) from within the RV outflow tract and within the pulmonary artery (Fig. 10.4). The ICE-CHIP study has prospectively compared LAA imaging with transesophageal echo versus phased-array ICE; the study found incomplete LAA imaging with ICE in 15% of patients, as well as a lower sensitivity to detect LAA thrombus compared to TEE.[6] It is important to emphasize that the ICE-CHIP study only adopted LAA imaging from within the RA, which provides substantially less optimal imaging compared to the views that can be obtained from the RV outflow tract/pulmonary artery or from within the coronary sinus.[7,8] When the ICE probe is deployed within the LA, visualization of the LAA is optimal. This approach is routinely used to guide LAA occlusion procedures,[9] with optimal direct near-field visualization of the LAA ostium, LAA morphology, and depth in different lobes (Fig. 10.5 and Video 10.3).

Assessing Catheter Positioning and Contact

During LA ablation, ICE is useful when positioning the ablation and multipolar mapping catheters relative to the PV orifice. ICE imaging is also important to delineate the course of the esophagus along the LA posterior wall as well as the relationship between the esophagus and the PV antra. Direct imaging of the esophagus is crucial even when periprocedural esophageal temperature monitoring is performed because the size and location of the temperature probe sometimes grossly underestimate the dimension of the esophagus as directly visualized with ICE. Another important advantage of ICE imaging is the real-time assessment of tissue–catheter contact, which is particularly relevant when using catheters without

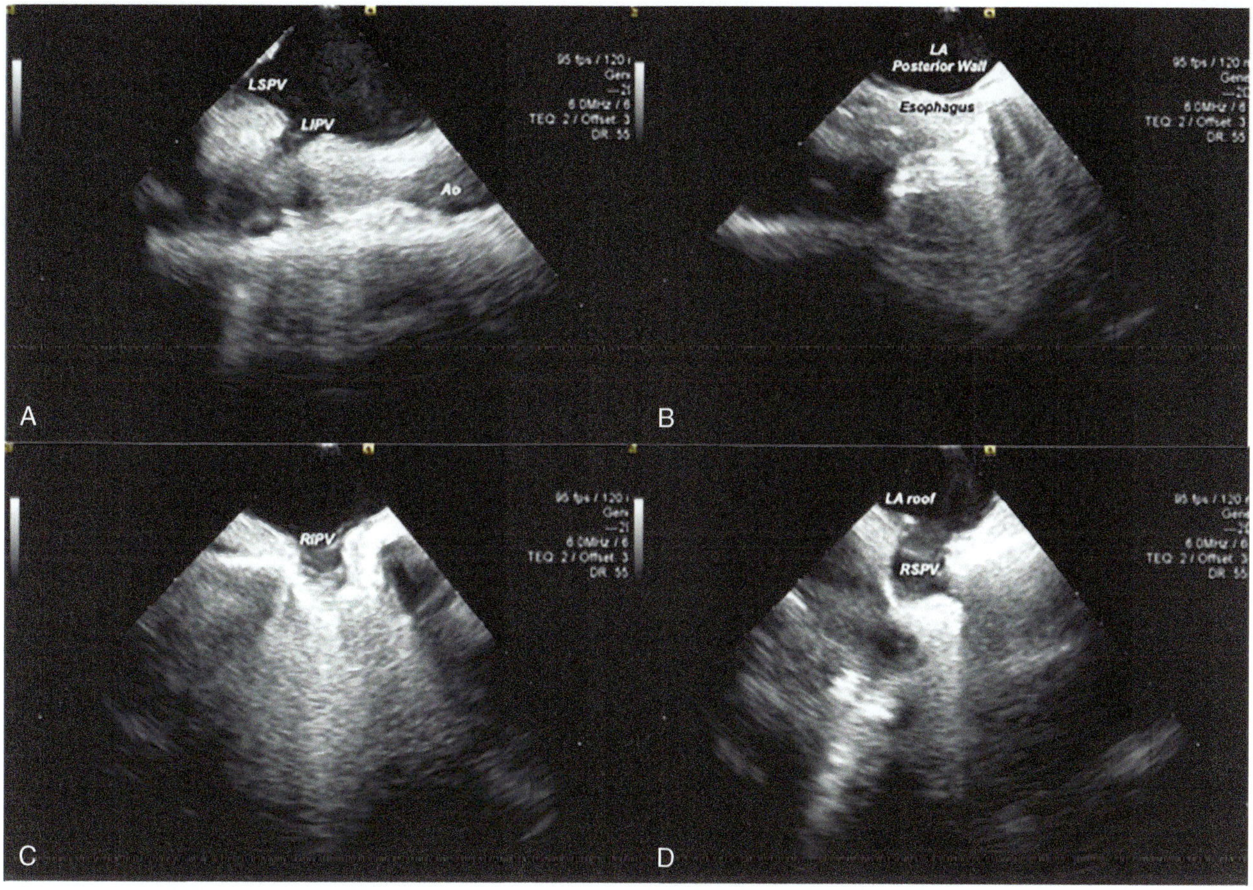

Fig. 10.3 Example of LA imaging with the ICE probe directly positioned within the LA via a transseptal approach. The quality of LA imaging is substantially improved with a better definition of the PV anatomy, posterior LA wall, and adjacent critical structures like the esophagus (A to D).

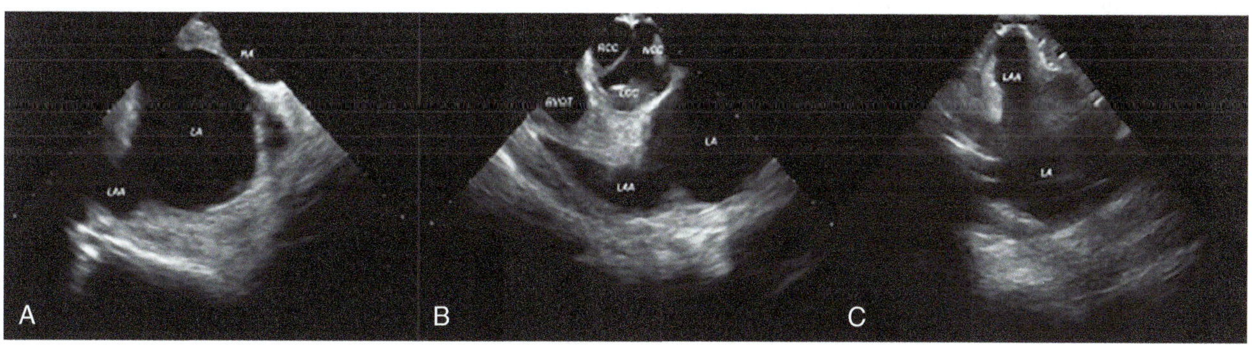

Fig. 10.4 Example of LAA imaging to define the anatomy and rule out thrombus. Three views are shown: a standard view from the mid RA with the LAA visualized in the far-field (A), a view from the RV outflow tract (B), and a view from the pulmonary artery (C).

direct contact force feedback (e.g., multipolar mapping catheters) but also relevant to integrate information obtained from catheters with direct catheter contact force measurement with intracardiac anatomical details. The CARTO Sound module facilitates this process by displaying the position of the ablation catheter (and of the anatomical sites mapped/ablated) in real-time on the 2D echo slice (Fig. 10.6 and Video 10.4). The development of probes capable of 3D imaging may provide even greater anatomical context, though with a concomitant reduction in spatial resolution.[10]

Ventricular Tachycardia Ablation

Outflow Tract Ventricular Arrhythmias

The complex three-dimensional anatomical relationships between different adjacent structures in the RV and LV outflow tracts poses substantial difficulties to mapping and ablation of VAs arising from this region.[11-13] Traditional RV and LV outflow tract mapping using a combination of fluoroscopy and intracardiac EGM characteristics is limited by the variable anatomy. The incorporation of ICE into these procedures has greatly improved the understanding of the anatomical relationships and common

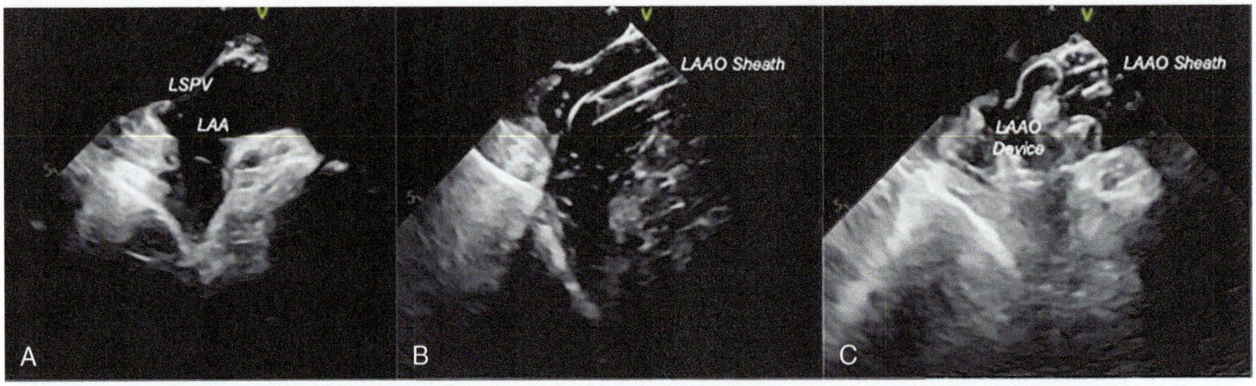

Fig. 10.5 Example of LAA imaging obtained with the ICE probe within the LA. In this case, the probe has been advanced to the left superior PV with excellent near-field visualization of the LAA (A). This approach is particularly helpful in guiding LAA occlusion procedures with optimal visualization of the deployment sheath (B) and LAA closure device (C).

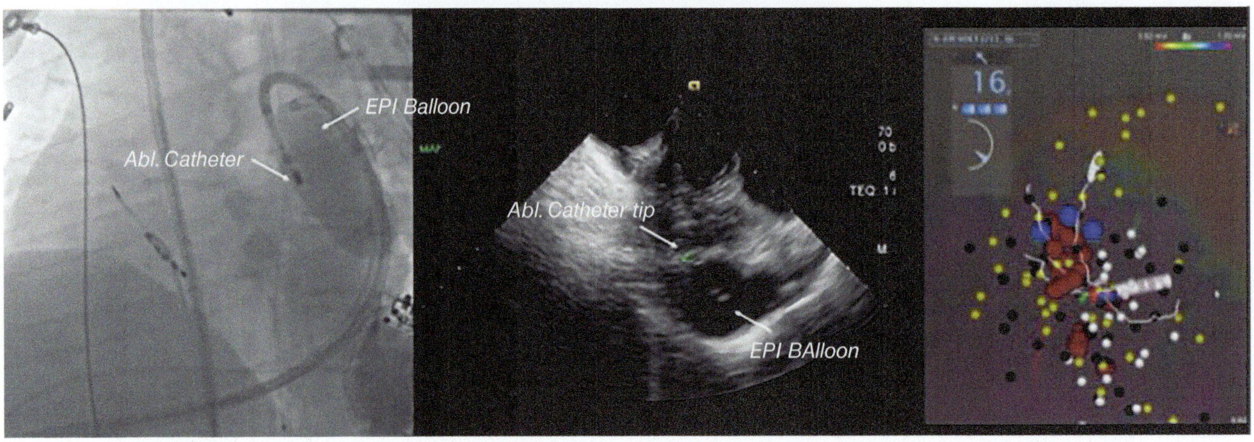

Fig. 10.6 Example of ICE integration with an electromagnetic mapping system during a case of epicardial catheter ablation of VT in a patient with nonischemic cardiomyopathy. In this case, the critical VT substrate was involving the epicardium adjacent to the left phrenic nerve and a pericardial balloon was used to dislodge the parietal pericardium (and adjacent left phrenic nerve). The correct position of the ablation catheter in between the epicardium and the pericardial balloon is visualized on ICE (*green tip*).

sites of origin. Imaging of the RV outflow tract is obtained by direct advancement of the ICE probe within the outflow tract region, which provides excellent near-field views (Fig. 10.7). From the "home view" by applying gentle anterior flexion of the ICE probe, the catheter can be easily passed through the tricuspid annulus into the RV. Clockwise torque brings into sequential view the RV septum, the LV cavity, and the outflow tract region. The RV outflow tract is usually imaged in the near field and in the long-axis view. From this view, the coronary cusp region can also be visualized in the short axis; the junction between the right and left coronary cusp defines the plane of the septum. The left pulmonic cusp is typically adjacent to the junction between the left and right pulmonic cusps and overlies the septal aspect of the left ventricular summit,[14] whereas the anterior pulmonic cusp is located at the most anterior aspect of the outflow tract region. A short-axis view of the pulmonic cusp is also obtainable from the RA free wall by applying anterior and leftward deflection to the probe.

The LV outflow tract can be visualized from the RA (clockwise rotation from the "home view") or from the RV (Fig. 10.8). When imaging from the RA, the aortic root is well seen in the long-axis view. This view provides adequate anatomical definition of the depth of the cusp (e.g., sinotubular junction, cusp nadir). The long-axis view also allows the operator to measure the vertical distance of the mapping catheter from the coronary arterial ostia and to define the degree of atherosclerosis/calcification in the ascending aorta. A similar long-axis view of the ascending aorta can be obtained by applying additional clockwise rotation to the ICE probe deployed within the RV outflow tract and once the standard short-axis view of the coronary cusp is obtained. Imaging the ascending aorta has important implications for the selection of the optimal access to the left ventricle (i.e., retrograde aortic vs. transseptal) in order to minimize risk of cerebral or systemic embolization.

Papillary Muscle Ablation

Traditional electroanatomical mapping of the RV and LV ventricle papillary muscles can be challenging due to their complex structure and intracavitary position. Furthermore, since ventricular arrhythmias originate from specific anatomical sites within the complex and variable anatomy of the individual

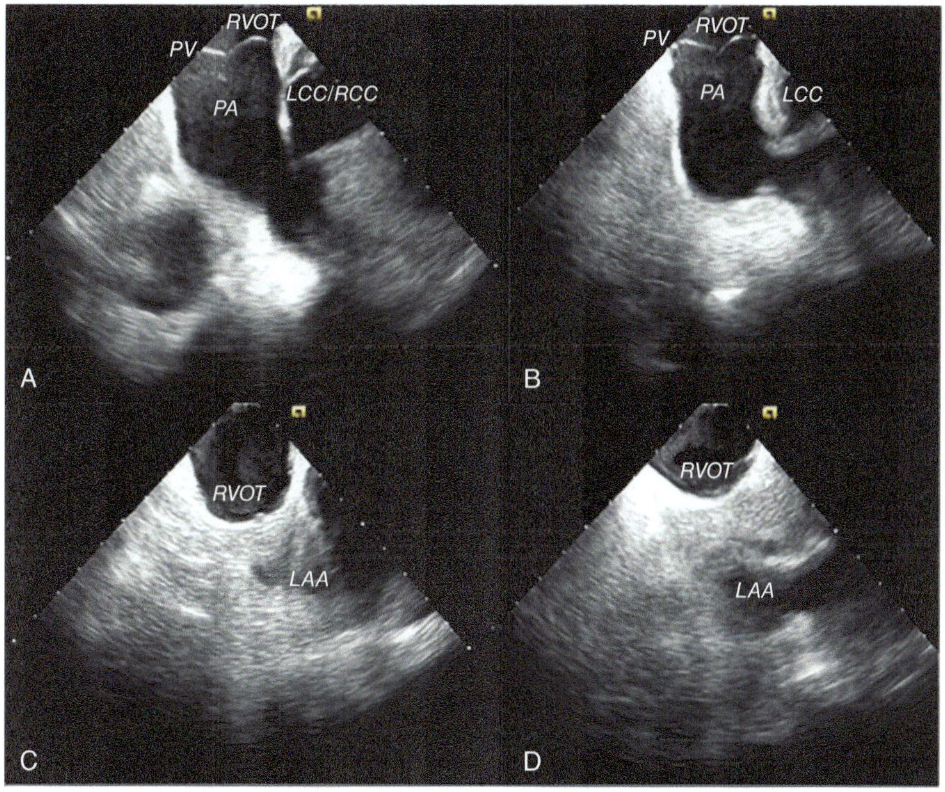

Fig. 10.7 ICE imaging of the right ventricular outflow tract showing "septal" views (A, B) and "free wall" views (C, D).

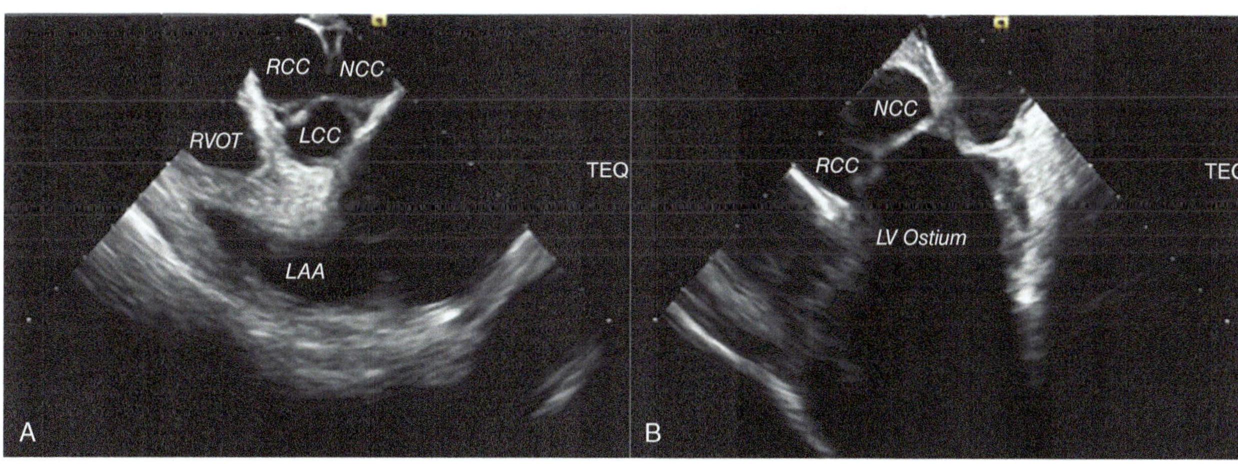

Fig. 10.8 ICE imaging of the right ventricular outflow tract. (A) A short-axis view showing the anatomy of the coronary cusps is obtained by advancing the ICE probe within the RV outflow tract. (B) A long-axis view can be obtained from the RA by clocking the ICE catheter from the "home view."

papillary muscles, precise positioning of the ablation catheter is required. Both the RV and LV papillary muscles can be anatomically well characterized by ICE. From the "home view," the RV inflow tract is imaged as well as the posterior RV papillary muscle. Advancement of the ICE catheter within the RV brings into view the moderator band and its continuation with the septal RV papillary muscle. Clockwise rotation of the transducer brings into view the insertion of the moderator band into the RV free wall. The septal RV papillary muscle(s) are often challenging to image given their small size and proximity to the interventricular septum and typically can be best imaged from the base of the RV outflow tract.

With clockwise rotation from the RV inflow, the LV posteromedial and anterolateral papillary muscles are sequentially imaged (Fig. 10.9).[15] Given the complex 3D structure of the RV and LV papillary muscles, intraprocedural imaging with ICE is crucial to guide mapping and ablation of these structures as conventional electroanatomical mapping systems are often insufficient to reproduce the papillary muscle anatomy, even when dedicated ICE integration softwares are implemented.

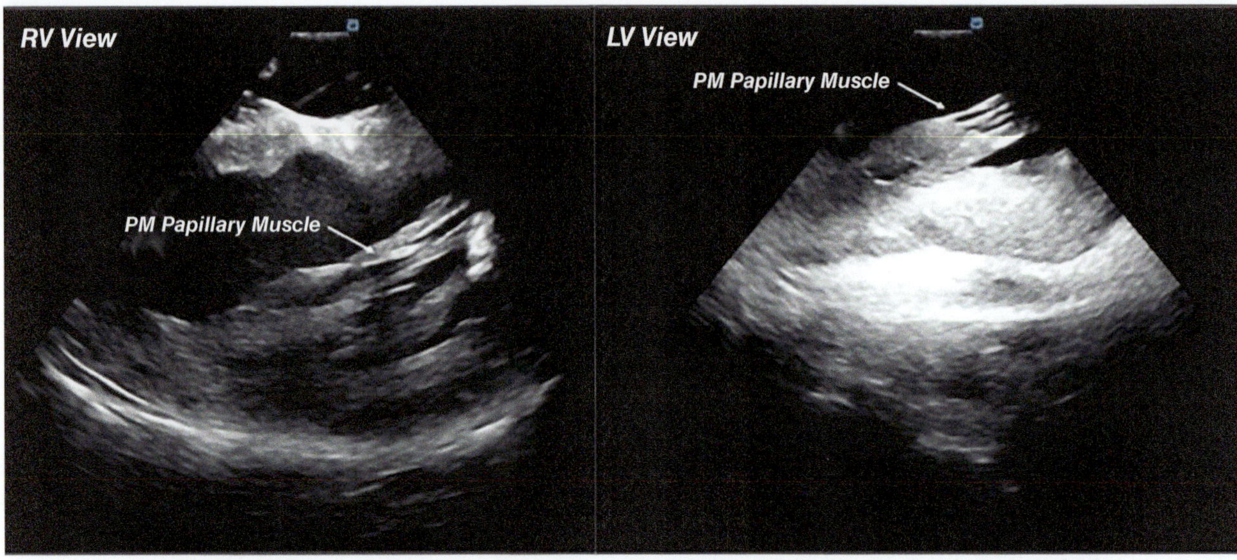

Fig. 10.9 Example of ICE imaging of LV papillary muscles. To enhance the definition of these intracavitary structures, advancement of the ICE probe within the LV (via an atrial transseptal puncture) may be needed.

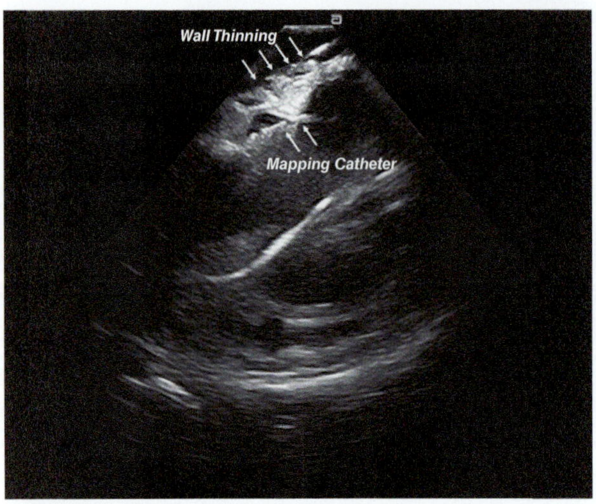

Fig. 10.10 Intraprocedural definition of abnormal LV substrate with ICE with evidence of focal hyperechoic areas with wall thinning.

Visualization of the Arrhythmia Substrate

In patients with scar-related VT, ICE provides an additional imaging tool for real-time visualization of the arrhythmia substrate. Typically, regions with abnormal substrate are characterized by segmental wall motion abnormalities and focal wall thinning/aneurysms (Fig. 10.10 and Video 10.5). Furthermore, since regions of fibrosis tend to be hyperechoic, it is possible to distinguish them from the surrounding healthy myocardium with ICE, particularly in the presence of larger and more confluent regions of fibrosis. Using the CARTO Sound system, diseased myocardial segments can be traced and transposed onto the 3D electroanatomical map.[16]

In select patients with nonischemic cardiomyopathy, ICE has also been shown able to detect confluent regions of intramural or epicardial fibrosis as an echo intense stripe surrounded by normal myocardium (Fig. 10.11).[17]

Detecting and Preventing Complications

The real-time imaging and excellent tissue resolution achieved with ICE provide optimal sensitivity to detect potential complications.

Intracardiac Thrombus

Occult thromboembolism represents an important source of morbidity from complex ablation procedures. The importance of adequate systemic anticoagulation during left-sided ablation procedures is paramount to decrease the risk of stroke and systemic thromboembolism. Sheath-associated thrombosis is occasionally seen despite aggressive anticoagulation, and if documented with ICE corrective measures may prevent systemic embolization. Furthermore, mobile thrombus has been documented with ICE in 30% of patients with implanted pacemaker and defibrillator leads and may also increase the risk of both acute and chronic embolic complications.[18]

Pericardial Effusion

The diagnosis of procedure-related pericardial effusion is often delayed until hemodynamic compromise occurs. The presence of intrapericardial fluid can be easily documented with the ICE catheter placed in the RV (Fig. 10.12). Also, from within the RA, views of the posterior LV can usually be obtained and allow for intraprocedural monitoring for effusion. It is our practice to screen for the presence of effusion periodically during the ablation procedure or with any change in hemodynamic parameters. In the absence of pericardial adhesions (e.g., from prior cardiac surgery), most patients have a circumferential fluid collection that is initially seen around the posterior LV (due to gravity). With early detection and prompt reversal of anticoagulation, some effusions will stabilize without the need for pericardiocentesis. If drainage is required, ICE may be used to guide the optimal location for pericardial puncture and document complete resolution.

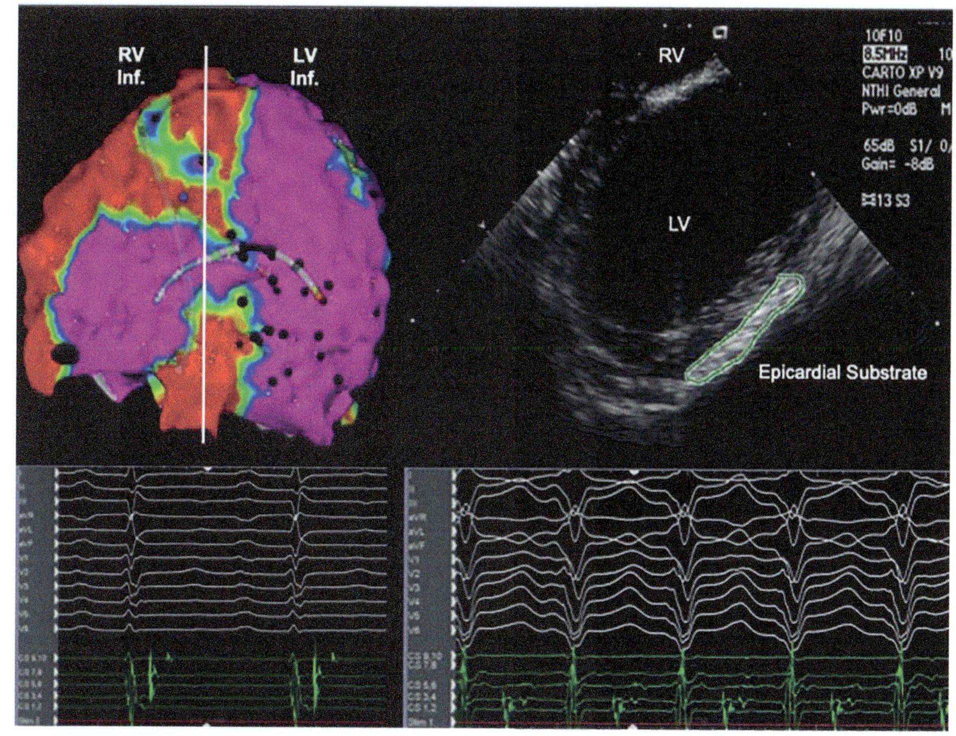

Fig. 10.11 Example of epicardial hyperechoic area in the LV inferior wall corresponding to critical abnormal substrate participating to VT.

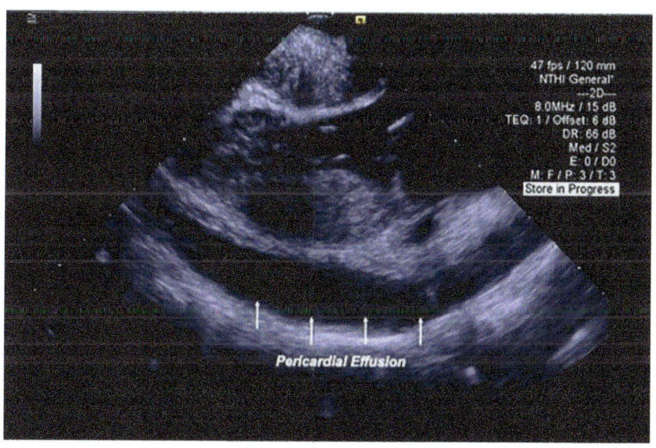

Fig. 10.12 Example of periprocedural pericardial effusion detected with ICE.

CARDIAC MAGNETIC RESONANCE

General principles and substrate characterization techniques

Among noninvasive cardiovascular imaging modalities, CMR has progressively acquired a central role, not only being able to accurately quantify cardiac chamber geometry and function with a high degree of reproducibility and avoiding exposure to ionizing radiation but also allowing myocardial tissue characterization, identifying the presence of structural abnormalities such as myocardial fatty replacement, myocardial edema, and necrosis/fibrosis that may be missed by other imaging modalities.[19,20] These characteristics make CMR particularly useful for the identification and characterization of the arrhythmogenic substrate. In particular, late gadolinium enhancement (LGE) imaging can detect replacement fibrosis as a potential substrate for reentrant arrhythmias.[21] The LGE imaging relies on the peculiar kinetic of gadolinium-chelated contrast agents (mainly gadolinium-diethylenetriamine pentaacetic acid [Gd-DTPA]). After bolus injection, Gd-DTPA transfers from the intravascular to the extracellular space (wash-in) while wash-out later occurs with renal clearance. The normal myocardium is characterized by fast wash-in/wash-out kinetics while scar tissue (due to extracellular volume expansion and poor venous drainage) has longer wash-out times determining a higher concentration of contrast agent several minutes after administration, thus rendering the area brighter (hyperenhanced) on T1-weighted images.[21]

After an electromagnetic pulse perturbates nuclear spins, magnetization returns to the equilibrium following an exponential process which has a time constant called relaxation time, representing the time to reach approximately 63% of magnetization recovery. Spin-lattice or T1 relaxation time is the time constant of recovery of longitudinal magnetization and primarily depends on the tissue composition itself including the presence of contrast agent. Differences in Gd-DTPA distribution are better appreciated ≥10 minutes after contrast injection, when equilibrium concentrations in the blood and myocardium have been reached resulting in shortening of the T1-relaxation time of scarred/fibrotic myocardium caused by the accumulation of the contrast agent, which translates into differences in signal intensity.[22]

Several signal intensity–based algorithms have been developed to further characterize the arrhythmogenic properties of myocardial scar being highly heterogeneous areas of scar, in which the coexistence of surviving myocardial fibers within scarred tissue (border zone), the ideal substrate for reentrant circuits as opposite to areas of dense scar (core).[23,24]

Ablation of Atrial Fibrillation

Even if the mechanisms behind AF genesis and maintenance are not completely understood, they typically involve the presence of triggers (pulmonary vein ectopies in most cases or non–pulmonary vein triggers from the LA posterior wall, coronary sinus, superior vena cava, and crista terminalis in 10–20% of cases) that initiates AF.[25] AF itself as well as comorbidities such as hypertension, dyslipidemia, chronic kidney disease, and diabetes and the presence of underlying structural heart disease lead to atrial remodeling characterized by progressive fibrosis deposition transforming paroxysmal AF into persistent and chronic forms.[26] There is evidence that atrial fibrosis can be visualized using LGE-CMR and used for management and treatment of arrhythmia, being a powerful predictor of outcomes of AF interventions.

Quantification of LA structure and function using CMR involves CMR angiography, which is acquired during continuous gadolinium injection and high-resolution respiratory navigated and ECG-gated, 3D LGE scans of the LA acquired in the same imaging session.[27] To minimize the effect of LA motion, imaging acquisition is performed during diastole.[27] Acquired images are then postprocessed and areas of fibrosis are identified on the basis of pixel signal intensity. Intensity thresholds in the range of 2–4 SDs from the mean are used to detect enhanced tissue. Fibrosis is generally quantified as volume or area percentage. In this regard, the group of the University of Utah has developed a staging system to describe atrial cardiomyopathy based on the LA wall enhancement as percentage of the total LA wall. In the Delayed Enhancement-MRI Determinant of Successful Catheter Ablation of Atrial Fibrillation (DECAAF) study, four stages were identified (stage I with <10%, stage II with ≥10% to <20%, stage III with ≥20% to <30%, and stage IV with ≥30% LGE).[2] The degree of atrial fibrosis has been correlated to outcomes after catheter ablation independently from AF type or associated comorbidities and to clinical outcomes such as stroke.[28,29] In the aforementioned DECAAF study enrolling patients with paroxysmal and persistent AF undergoing their first ablation procedure, the percentage of LA fibrosis was an independent predictor of AF recurrence even after adjustment for 10 demographic and clinical covariates with a 6% increase in 12-months AF recurrence rate every 1% increase in LGE extent (HR 1.06, 95% CI 1.03–1.09; $P < .001$).[2]

Integration of 3D-pixel intensity maps into electroanatomical mapping (EAM) systems has been tested to guide AF ablation and has been demonstrated to accurately localize gaps during redo PVI procedures, reducing procedural and radiofrequency time.[30] The use of areas of LGE-CMR as potential targets for ablation has also been proposed, but its utility in routine clinical practice is debated. A subanalysis of the DECAAF study suggested that residual fibrosis, defined as preexisting fibrosis not altered by the ablation procedure, was associated with higher incidence of recurrent AF.[31] On the other side, in the ALICIA trial in whom patients were randomized to PVI plus CMR-guided fibrosis ablation vs. PVI alone, no differences in terms of AF recurrence were detected at 12-month follow-up (recurrence rate 27.6% in the PVI-alone group vs. 27.8% in the CMR group).[32] The results of the DECAAF II trial, which enrolled 843 patients with persistent AF undergoing a first-time ablation procedure randomized in a 1:1 fashion to receive conventional PVI or PVI + fibrosis-guided ablation, showed no significant difference in the primary end point of AF recurrence between groups in the total study population. Recurrence of AF occurred in 175 (43%) patients in the intervention group and 188 (46.1%) patients in the control group ($P = .63$). In subgroup analyses, a trend was observed towards a lower rate of AF recurrence in the intervention group for patients with a Utah stage I or II fibrosis at baseline suggesting that PVI should remain the main ablation strategy in AF while targeting atrial fibrosis in AF patients with low levels of fibrotic disease (<20%) may help improve ablation outcomes.[33]

Ablation of Ventricular Tachycardia in Structural Heart Disease

Ventricular arrhythmias in patients with underlying structural heart disease (SHD) are typically sustained by scar-related reentry. The presence of surviving myocardial fibers within fibrous tissue leads to the formation of slow conduction pathways as well as to a dispersion of activation and refractoriness that constitute the milieu for reentrant circuits (Fig. 10.13).[34] The identification of such arrhythmogenic substrate by CMR tissue characterization techniques is of great value in aiding catheter ablation. The presence and distribution of LGE allow us to distinguish ischemic cardiomyopathy (ICM) from nonischemic cardiomyopathy (NICM). In ICM, LGE has a subendocardial distribution mirroring coronary artery territory, while in NICM, LGE has a mid-myocardial/subepicardial "patchy" distribution.[35]

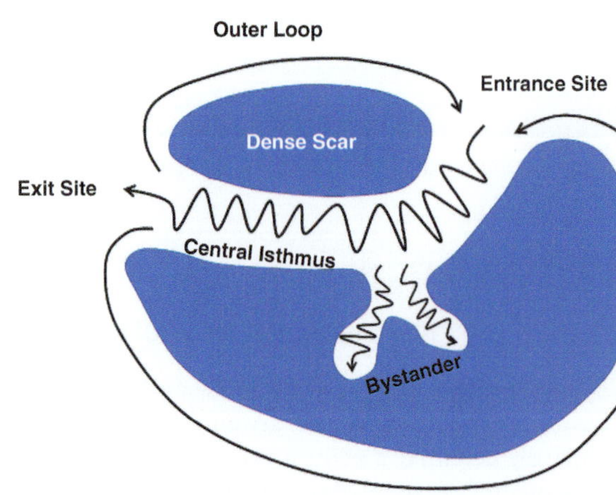

Fig. 10.13 Classic figure-of-eight reentry circuit as described by Stevenson et al. in 1993 (Stevenson WG, Khan H, Sager P, Saxon LA, Middlekauff HR, Natterson PD, Wiener I. Identification of reentry circuit sites during catheter mapping and radiofrequency ablation of ventricular tachycardia late after myocardial infarction. *Circulation.* 1993;88:1647-1670. doi:10.1161/01.cir.88.4.1647). *Blue regions* represent areas of dense scar. The activation wavefront propagates around two lines of conduction block sharing a central common isthmus. Bystander pathways represent areas of tissue activated by the wavefront but not playing an active role in the reentrant circuit.

The correlation between fibrosis detected by LGE and voltage abnormalities on EAM is well known in both ICM and NICM.[4,36–38] By merging LGE-CMR images with EAM voltage maps in postinfarction patients undergoing VT ablation, Desjardins et al. initially demonstrated a good correlation of both unipolar and bipolar low-voltage areas (LVAs) with the presence of CMR scar, with all critical sites of the VT circuit located within areas of LGE showing how noninvasive CMR scar characterization may facilitate VT mapping and ablation.[36] Similar findings have later been reported in NICM where areas of LGE present with two peculiar patterns: a predominant basal anteroseptal scar pattern, which can be found in about 40% of the patients, and a predominant inferolateral scar pattern, which can be found in about 50% of them.[4,38,39–41] The identification of scar and the distinction between those two patterns have important practical consequences in guiding the ablation strategy.[4] Patients with a predominant inferolateral scar distribution frequently have epicardial substrate (critical VT sites have been reported in the inferolateral epicardium in 63% of cases while only in 37% of them in the endocardial inferolateral LV), while those with a predominant anteroseptal scar pattern more often have intramural substrate (critical VT sites have been located in the aortic root and/or basal anteroseptal LV endocardium in 89% of such patients).[38] Although proximity to epicardial coronary vessels and phrenic nerve may preclude/limit ablation in up to half of patients with inferolateral scar, these patients still have a better VT-free survival (75% vs. 26% at 1.5 years follow-up; $P < .001$) and a lower need for redo procedures (7% vs. 59%; $P < .001$) compared to those with anteroseptal scar.[42] Besides location, scar transmurality has also been correlated with EGM characteristics such as amplitude, duration, and morphology (degree of fractionation) with highly fractionated EGM more likely to be found in regions with higher scar transmurality and most critical VT circuit sites located in regions with >25% scar transmurality.[39]

A CMR-based 3D reconstruction of cardiac anatomy and scar architecture allows the operator to plan the most appropriate ablation approach according to the location of the arrhythmogenic substrate and is particularly useful in cases of intramural or subepicardial scar. Use of this technology is especially useful after a previously failed endocardial catheter ablation procedure, allowing the operator to choose specific ablation tools (i.e., needle or bipolar ablation for intramural targets) and to avoid complication (i.e., detection of intracardiac thrombus).[43–45] An integrated imaging approach in which MDCT is used to precisely define cardiac anatomy including the course of coronary arteries and phrenic nerve as well as to identify pathological (i.e., due to previous myocardial infarction) regions of wall thinning (<5 mm) and LGE-CMR is used to identify areas of scar, have been recently proposed to guide VT ablation. Offline 3D reconstruction of a cardiac model including both MDCT and CMR data is merged by anatomical landmarks with EAM maps allowing for additional mapping focusing on the area of anatomical substrate (wall thinning on MDCT scan and LGE on CMR). Overall, 89% of critical VT sites and 85% of abnormal EGMs have been localized within the imaging-derived substrate. Moreover, image integration has been the reason for additional mapping and epicardial access in 57% and 33% of patients, respectively, leading to a tailored epicardial ablation strategy considering the course of the coronary vessels and the phrenic nerve.[3]

Other than influencing procedural strategy, image integration has been associated with higher VT-free survival over long-term follow-up.[46] A CMR-aided substrate catheter ablation approach targeting slow-conduction channels identified within the scar by LGE-CMR and then confirmed by electrophysiologic maneuvers has demonstrated to reduce procedural time and improve outcomes with up to 82% VT-free survival with CMR-aided catheter ablation compared to 56% of conventional ablation after a mean follow-up of 20 months (Fig. 10.14).[47] More recently, a CMR-only guided substrate catheter ablation approach in which targets were selected based only on the LGE-CMR information have been compared to a CMR-aided approach in which both LGE-CMR and EAM were used to select ablation targets and a classic approach based only on EAM without the use of CMR. This study showed that the CMR-guided approach is feasible, safe, and associated with shorter procedural, fluoroscopy, and radiofrequency times.[48] The CMR-guided approach was also associated with a significantly higher rate of VT noninducibility at the end of the procedure compared to both the CMR-aided and the no-CMR approach (18% vs. 32% and 46%; $P = .35$ and $P = .04$, respectively) and resulted in a lower 12-months VT recurrence rate compared to the no-CMR approach (4% vs. 25%; $P = .02$), while similar outcomes were found compared to the CMR-aided approach (4% vs. 7%; $P = .56$).[48] Tissue characterization by CMR has also been used to evaluate the efficacy of CA in terms of lesions depth showing that formation of irreversible radiofrequency lesions defined by areas of microvascular obstruction (MVO) surrounded by LGE are a reliable predictor of long-term VT-free survival regardless of acute procedural success.[49]

Future Perspectives

Even if the above results are promising, at the present time no randomized controlled clinical trials specifically designed to test the real incremental benefit of imaging integration compared to EAM alone are available. In this regard, a multicenter open-label randomized controlled trial (VOYAGE study) has recently been started and the preliminary results are expected to be released by August 2023.[50] Patients with scar-related VT and with an ICD or with ICD implantation expected within 1 month will be randomized to a CMR-aided/guided approach if suitable for CMR and MDCT or to a standard EAM-guided ablation approach if unsuitable for imaging or with image quality deemed not sufficient for postprocessing with a primary end point of 12-month VT recurrence, in order to test safety and efficacy of CMR-aided/guided catheter ablation.[50]

The presence of diffuse interstitial fibrosis undetectable by conventional LGE imaging, as not reaching the critical mass for detection, is well known, especially in the setting of NICM.[51] A mismatch between presence of LGE-CMR scar, LVA and critical VT sites on EAM have been reported.[52] In patients with NICM and VT, LVA on EAM in areas with absence of detectable LGE have been reported in about 36% of the cases with 34% of them having

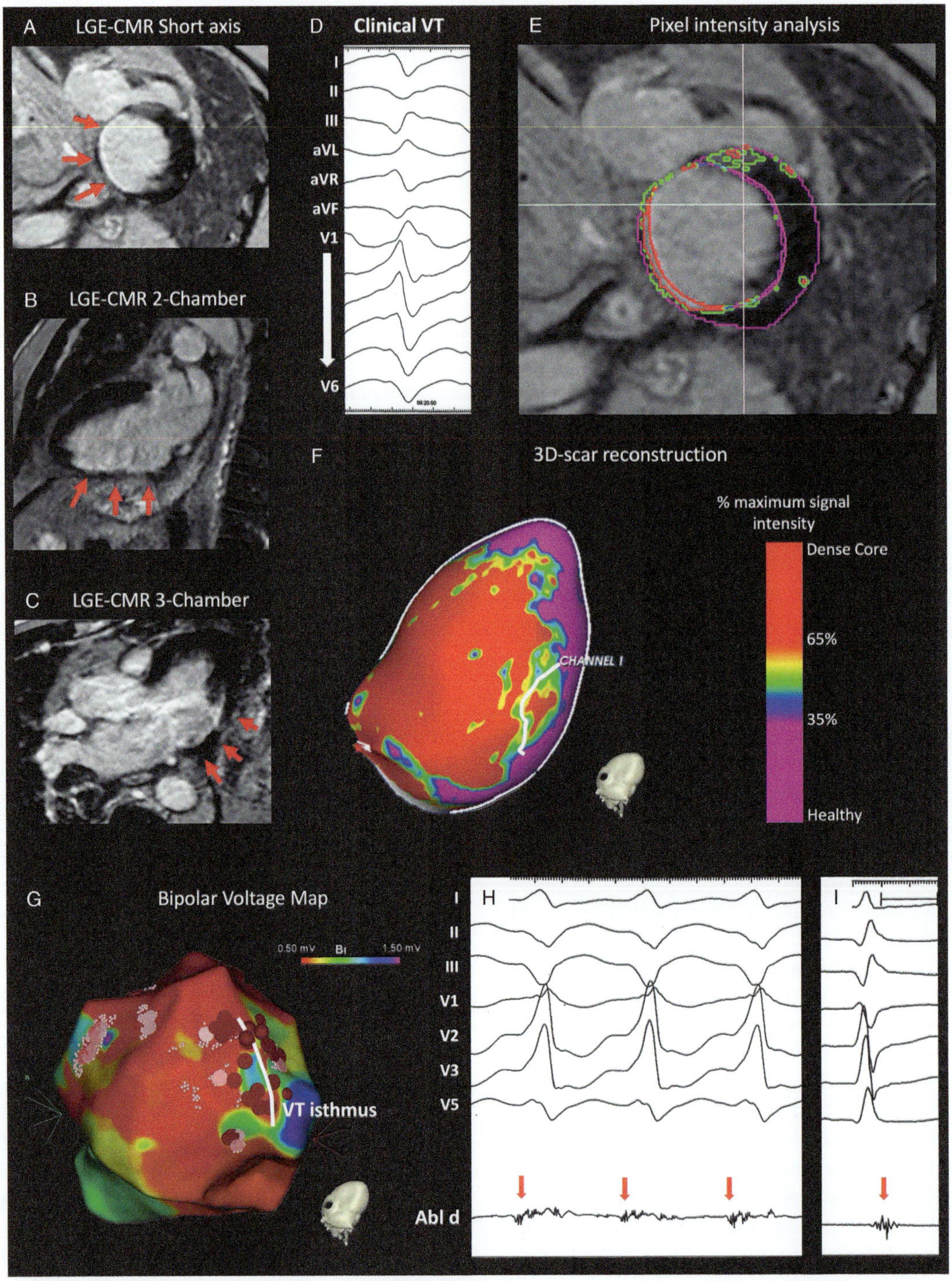

Fig. 10.14 Fifty-year-old man with previous inferolateral myocardial infarction showing a large area of transmural scar involving the inferior and inferolateral left ventricular walls on late gadolinium enhancement (LGE) cardiac magnetic resonance (A–C, *red arrows*) presenting with sustained VT (D). Pixel intensity analysis of CMR is performed with ADAS-VT (GalgoMedical, Barcelona, Spain) software (E) creating a three-dimensional reconstruction of the scar, which allows channels of viable myocardium to be identified within dense scar that may participate in the VT circuit (F, *white line*). Starting from the LGE short-axis stack (E), the software automatically calculates the signal intensity of each pixel of the image and projects it on a three-dimensional shell following color-coding (F). A signal intensity less than 35% of the maximum intensity is categorized as normal and represented by *purple color*. Scar areas are represented by a nonpurple range of colors, with the most abnormal signal (>65% of the maximum intensity) consistent with dense scar represented by *red color* (F). Bipolar voltage map (G) shows a low-voltage area (bipolar voltage <1.5 mV) consistent with the CMR-derived scar. A VT isthmus is identified by activation and entrainment mapping in the same location of the viable myocardium channel detected by CMR (G, *white line*) showing presystolic multicomponent fractionated activity during VT (H, *red arrows*) as well as late potentials during sinus rhythm (I, *red arrows*). Radiofrequency ablation (G, red dots) resulted in VT termination and noninducibility with programmed ventricular stimulation. (Reprinted from Muser D, Lavalle C, Guarracini F, Sassone B, Conte E, Magnani S, et al. Role of cardiac imaging in patients undergoing catheter ablation of ventricular tachycardia. *J Cardiovasc Med (Hagerstown)*. 2021;22:727–737. doi:10.2459/JCM.0000000000001121.)

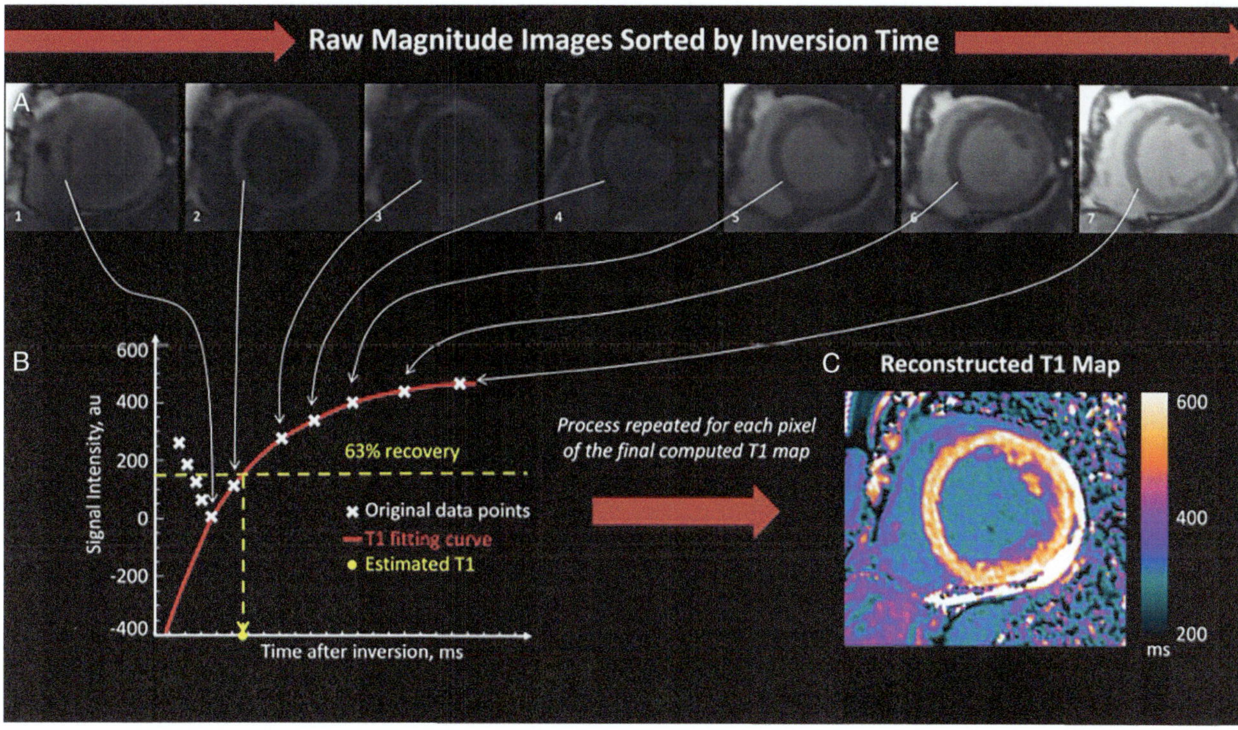

Fig. 10.15 Myocardial T1-mapping using the modified Look-Locker sequence with increasing inversion times (A). Multiple phases are acquired after an inversion pulse, then the software automatically determines pixel by pixel the signal intensity of each phase-image and subsequently plots it against the inversion time (B). Finally, the T1-time is automatically calculated by performing a curve fitting of the data points to an exponential recovery curve (B, *red curve*) representing the recovery of longitudinal magnetization. The T1-time is the constant of the exponential curve; it represents the time to reach approximately 63% of longitudinal magnetization recovery and it is used to generate a color-coded map (C). (Modified from Muser D, Nucifora G, Castro SA, Enriquez A, Chahal CAA, Magnani S, et al. Myocardial substrate characterization by CMR T1 mapping in patients with NICM and no LGE undergoing catheter ablation of VT. *JACC Clin Electrophysiol.* 2021;7:831–840. doi:10.1016/j.jacep.2020.10.002.)

at least one VT critical site localized within discordant areas.[52] In this setting, CMR T1-mapping allows the detection of areas with increased interstitial fibrosis as it influences the myocardial response to the magnetic field and, in particular, the T1-relaxation time (time required by tissue to reach approximately 63% of its longitudinal relaxation on a pixel-by-pixel basis (Fig. 10.15). Presence of interstitial fibrosis increases native T1-times by approximately 20%–30%. Areas of increased T1-time have been reported to be consistent with unipolar LVA on EAM and include VT critical sites in patients with NICM without detectable LGE potentially affecting postablation outcomes (Fig. 10.16).[53,54]

The possibility of CMR to provide a real-time imaging of ablation lesion formation is under investigation. Potential strategies include monitoring of tissue edema formation with T2-weighted imaging, documentation of MVO with T1-weighted imaging, and measurement of tissue temperature during radiofrequency energy delivery with T1-weighted thermometry. Such an approach may minimize x-ray exposure and enhance therapeutic efficacy by providing a direct correlation between lesions and ablation targets. Preliminary results mostly involving animal studies are promising, but performing catheter ablation procedures in a real-time CMR environment requires several technological improvements including CMR compatibility of electrophysiology catheters and mapping systems.[55,56]

Imaging-derived computational algorithms to noninvasively characterize VT circuits by translating imaging features into electrophysiological properties and simulate activation patterns are also under investigation and in the future could be used to predict ablation targets and guide ablation procedures without the need for VT induction and mapping.[57,58]

Recently, data on noninvasive ablation of VT using stereotactic radiotherapy have been reported suggesting a decrease in VT burden during follow-up.[59] However, invasive EAM was used to identify the ablation target. Future development of this approach may be a fully noninvasive procedure using imaging techniques combined with multielectrode body-surface ECG mapping to identify critical VT sites.[60]

MULTIDETECTOR COMPUTED TOMOGRAPHY

Ablation of Atrial Fibrillation

The main advantage of MDCT is its greater spatial resolution compared to other noninvasive imaging modalities such as CMR and transthoracic echocardiography. In the setting of supraventricular arrhythmias, MDCT can estimate atrial volumes without geometric assumptions providing a detailed geometric reconstruction, which is of great value in terms of preprocedural planning, especially for PVI by cryoablation, which is generally

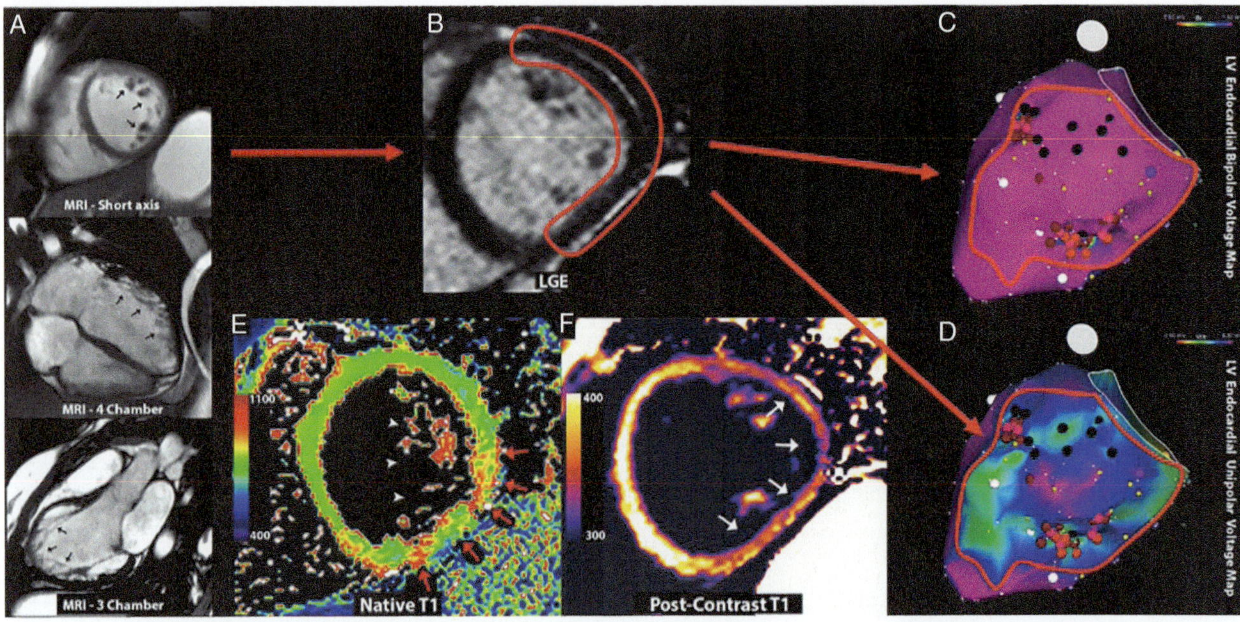

Fig. 10.16 Example of a patient with frequent premature ventricular contractions and left ventricular noncompaction studied with CMR (A, *black arrows*). The noncompacted walls do not show evidence of late gadolinium enhancement (B). Endocardial bipolar voltage map is normal (C), but the unipolar voltage map shows an area of low voltage in the inferior and lateral wall colocalizing with the noncompacted segments (D). Native T1 mapping revealed increased T1 relaxation time (E, *red color indicated by arrows*), and postcontrast T1 mapping revealed decreased T1 relaxation time (F, *white arrows*) consistent with interstitial fibrosis. This matches the region of unipolar voltage abnormality. (Reprinted from Muser D, Liang JJ, Witschey WR, Pathak RK, Castro S, Magnani S, et al. Ventricular arrhythmias associated with left ventricular noncompaction: electrophysiologic characteristics, mapping, and ablation. *Heart Rhythm.* 2017;14:166–175. doi:10.1016/j.hrthm.2016.11.014.)

performed without EAM reconstruction. In this regard, MDCT can accurately define the number and course of the pulmonary veins, the presence of common ostia, and the LAA location and morphology, as well as to screen for potential stenosis.[62] The thickness of LA walls can also be measured by MDCT, allowing for a more tailored radiofrequency energy delivery, taking into account sites of higher thickness.[63–65] Finally, MDCT allows the identification and estimation of extension of epicardial adipose tissue, which has been correlated with atrial remodeling and with the risk of recurrence after ablation.[66,67]

Ablation of Ventricular Tachycardia

Despite its widespread use, CMR applied to electrophysiology has several limitations in patients with cardiac implantable electronic devices, which are common, especially in patients presenting with VT. Both safety issues, such as local tissue heating, device software and hardware malfunction, and device chain-related artifacts, have been raised,[68,69] although there is mounting evidence that CMR can be performed safely in patients with cardiac implantable devices.[70] Even if the development of imaging techniques such as wideband CMR is progressively overcoming such limitations, the image quality may be suboptimal for detailed anatomical and substrate reconstruction and merging with EAM mapping systems.[71] In such scenarios, MDCT may represent an appropriate alternative. Compared to CMR, MDCT has a significantly higher spatial resolution (close to 0.5 mm on most systems compared to 1.4–2.0 mm) allowing for detailed 3D reconstruction of cardiac structures and making it the most effective imaging tool for detailed preprocedural definition of cardiac anatomy including coronary arterial and venous systems, valve apparatus, phrenic nerve, epicardial fat, and calcifications. Image integration of preacquired MDCT imaging into the EAM mapping system enables real-time visualization of chamber geometry, access route in case of epicardial approach, fat thickness, and epicardial coronary arteries during the procedure, thus improving the interpretation of bipolar electrograms and identification of ineffective or unsafe ablation sites and avoiding the need for repeated coronary angiography and phrenic pacing maneuvers.[5,72] In cases when epicardial access is needed, MDCT can be used to accurately assess the anatomical relationships between the pericardial space and neighboring structures in order to plan the optimal needle trajectory to minimize the risk of collateral damage of abdominal organs. Nonetheless, the identification of pericardial calcifications or thickening may suggest difficulties in catheter mobility within the pericardial space precluding epicardial mapping/ablation.[73]

Even if characterized by a lower contrast resolution (lower contrast-to-noise ratio) compared with LGE-CMR, MDCT can still be used for scar detection and characterization (Fig. 10.17).[74–76] Several MDCT image characteristics are used for scar definition, including wall thinning, hypoattenuation related to fatty metaplasia, decreased perfusion, and late hyperattenuation after contrast agent, with delayed hyperattenuation and wall thinning being the

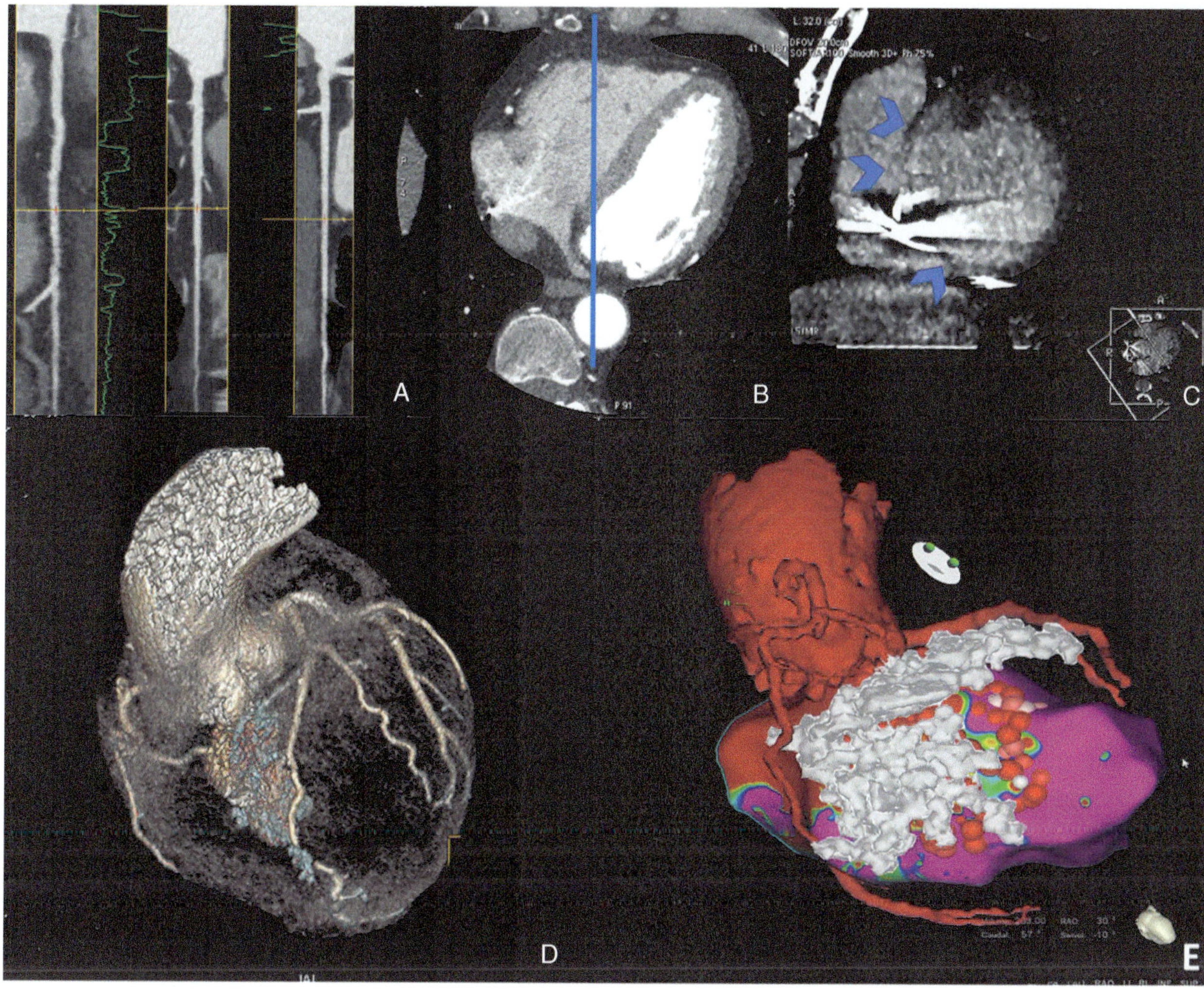

Fig. 10.17 A case of 67-year-old man with NICM and VT is shown. Standard MDCT acquisition on arterial phase enabled to exclude significative coronary artery disease (A) and provided important anatomical insight for possible epicardial approach (B). Late iodine CT scan (8 min after contrast medium administration) showed nonischemic myocardial scan with septal mid-wall distribution (*blue arrowhead* in C) as possible anatomical substrate of VT. Epicardial fat, coronary anatomy and myocardial scar information were exported in DICOM format and merged real time with electroanatomical evaluation (D and E). (Reproduced from Muser D, Lavalle C, Guarracini F, Sassone B, Conte E, Magnani S, et al. Role of cardiac imaging in patients undergoing catheter ablation of ventricular tachycardia. *J Cardiovasc Med (Hagerstown)*. 2021;22:727–737. doi:10.2459/JCM.0000000000001121.)

most used ones.[77,78] Of interest, a pilot study on 28 patients has described the possibility of evaluating diffuse myocardial fibrosis without contrast agents using dual-energy CT.[79] An overall good correlation between areas of wall thinning or areas of delayed attenuation on MDCT and LVA on EAM has been repeatedly reported, particularly in patients with ICM and transmural scar, whereas it is weaker in nontransmural scars or in patients with NICM.[77,78,80,81] More interestingly, areas of severe wall thinning (<2 mm) have been demonstrated to predict the presence of abnormal EGM with a specificity up to 100%, while areas with relatively preserved wall thickness (3–5 mm) crossing severely thinned areas have shown to identify channels of viable myocardium within dense scar colocalizing with critical sites of VT circuit.[82,83] Of note, 100% of VT isthmuses have been demonstrated to lay within CT channels, while about 50% of CT channels have been demonstrated to host critical VT isthmuses.[83] However, compared with LGE-CMR, the myocardial wall thickness assessment using MDCT fails to detect a significant proportion of LGE-CMR channels especially in presence of subendocardial or nontransmural scar.[84] Structural characteristics of the scar such as fatty metaplasia (identified as intramyocardial attenuation ≤30 HU) are also emerging as prognostically important, having been correlated with higher rates of VT recurrence and all-cause mortality.[85]

SUMMARY

Invasive and noninvasive imaging modalities are playing a growing role in all aspects of mapping and ablation of cardiac arrhythmias. Precise reconstruction of cardiac anatomy and its integration with electroanatomical mapping systems, identification of the arrhythmogenic substrate, planning of the optimal procedural strategy, assisting catheter manipulation, assessing lesion formation, and monitoring of complications are some of the main applications of imaging in the field of invasive electrophysiology. The main imaging modalities currently used are represented by CMR and CT, which have great contrast and spatial resolution and are of great value in reconstructing cardiac anatomy and characterizing the arrhythmogenic substrate, and by ICE, which has the main advantage of providing real-time information. The choice of the appropriate imaging modality should be tailored to patient characteristics and specific needs related to the procedure. In the future, advances in noninvasive imaging may also be able to provide specific ablation targets without the need for arrhythmia induction and mapping.

REFERENCES

Please refer to the e-book for a complete list of references.

PART 3

Catheter Ablation of Atrial Tachycardias and Flutter

11

Ablation of Focal Atrial Tachycardias

Jonathan M. Kalman, Bhupesh Pathik, Peter M. Kistler

KEY POINTS

Anatomy

- Atrial tachycardia (AT) foci exhibit a characteristic anatomical distribution in both atria.
- The right atrium is the most common location, with two-thirds of right-sided focal AT arising from the crista terminalis.

Pathophysiology

- Focal AT may be caused by microreentry, abnormal automaticity, or triggered activity.
- This mechanistic distinction is less relevant in the current era of radiofrequency ablation.

Arrhythmia Diagnosis

- Focal AT must be distinguished from other arrhythmias using both electrocardiographic clues and diagnostic approaches in the electrophysiology laboratory.
- Differential diagnoses include macroreentrant AT, atrioventricular nodal reentrant tachycardia, atrioventricular reentrant tachycardia, and inappropriate sinus tachycardia.

Mapping

- Initial evaluation of the P-wave morphology of the 12-lead electrocardiogram can indicate the likely region of origin of the focal AT.
- Detailed evaluation usually includes a three-dimensional mapping system looking for the earliest activity relative to P-wave onset.
- Anatomic sites in close proximity should be independently mapped.

Ablation

- Ablation endpoints include loss of all spontaneous AT activity and noninducibility.
- Ablation success rates in excess of 80–90% may be expected.

INTRODUCTION

Focal atrial tachycardia (AT) is the least common form of supraventricular tachycardia (SVT). It accounts for ~5–15% of SVT cases undergoing catheter ablation.[1,2] Focal AT is characterized by the presence of a discrete atrial focus with centrifugal spread of atrial activation away from that site.[3] Focal ATs are usually paroxysmal and self-limited, although, in some patients, focal AT may be incessant, which can lead to the development of tachycardia-mediated cardiomyopathy (TMC).[4] Focal AT may result in the initiation of other atrial arrhythmias such as atrial macroreentry or atrial fibrillation (AF) if the rate of focal firing is particularly rapid along with the development of secondary atrial remodeling.

Focal AT is frequently unresponsive to pharmacologic therapy. With the advent of catheter ablation, this type of tachycardia can be treated with high long-term success rates.[5-11] Importantly, mapping and ablation of focal AT are greatly facilitated by the characteristic anatomical distribution.[12] In addition, the use of sophisticated three-dimensional (3D) mapping technologies greatly facilitates accurate localization, but it is important to remember that P-wave analysis and conventional multipolar mapping techniques remain important adjunctive tools.[12]

Many different classic mechanisms of focal AT have been described, including abnormal automaticity, triggered activity, and microreentry.[13-18] However, the underlying mechanism seems less important in the ablation era because these diverse mechanisms manifest similarly on activation mapping.[3,19] We discuss the anatomical distribution, pathophysiology, mapping, and ablation techniques of this uncommon arrhythmia.

ANATOMY

AT foci do not originate in random locations throughout the atria but instead cluster in characteristic anatomical sites (Fig. 11.1 A, B).[20-28] The right atrium (RA) is the most common location with ~55–63% of foci originating in this chamber.[12,29] Within the RA, two-thirds of foci arise from along the crista terminalis (CT) with the superior and mid CT more common than the inferior CT.[23] Other common sites include the tricuspid annulus (TA),[27] the coronary sinus (CS) ostium,[26] the perinodal (para-Hisian) region, RA appendage (RAA),[28] and RA septum. In the left atrium (LA), the majority of foci originate from the pulmonary vein (PV) ostia[24] followed by the mitral annulus (MA),[25] left septum, LA appendage (LAA), and musculature within the CS body.[20] It is

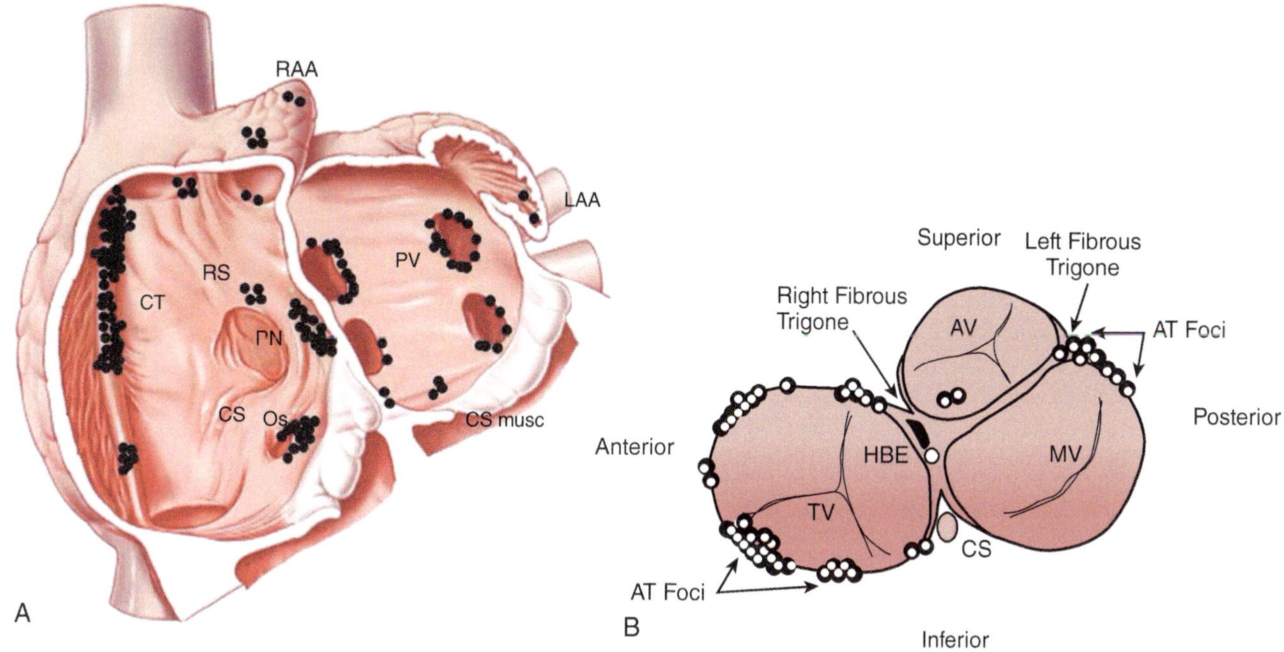

Fig. 11.1 (A) Schematic showing anatomic distribution of focal atrial tachycardias. (B) Distribution of tachycardia originating from the annular region and aortic cusp. *AT*, Atrial tachycardia; *AV*, atrioventricular; *CS*, coronary sinus, *CT*, crista terminalis, *HBE*, His bundle electrogram; *LA(A)* left atrial appendage; *MV*, mitral valve; *Os*, ostium; *PN*, perinodal; *PV*, pulmonary vein; *RA(A)* right atrial appendage; *RS*, right septum; *TV*, tricuspid valve.

important to be aware that despite this characteristic anatomical distribution, tachycardia foci may occur from unusual or previously undescribed sites.[30,31]

Crista Terminalis

In seminal work by Kalman et al. using intracardiac echocardiography, the CT was noted to be the location of two-thirds of focal AT arising from the RA.[22] The superior CT was the most common site, followed by the mid CT. Foci originating from the inferior CT were uncommonly observed. Focal AT from this site is more common in women, particularly above the age of 40 years, frequently has features to suggest microreentry (onset and termination with programmed stimulation), and may have multiple foci.[32] Although the reason for this characteristic distribution is unclear, there are certain electrophysiologic (EP) properties of the CT that may be important. The CT is a region of conduction anisotropy with poor transverse and rapid linear conduction,[33] potentially creating a substrate for microreentry in the context of atrial remodeling. Furthermore, the CT is the anatomical site along which the sinus pacemaker complex is distributed, and therefore is richly innervated with automatic tissue.[34]

In a discussion of tachycardias arising from the CT, it is worthwhile to consider whether sinus node reentry represents a distinct clinical entity. This tachycardia has been defined as an arrhythmia that can be induced and terminated with programmed stimulation with P-wave morphology (PWM) identical or similar to that of the sinus P wave. However, it is difficult to apply this definition strictly because of the variability in sinus PWM (e.g., sinus arrhythmia), and it can be argued that this arrhythmia is synonymous with an AT arising from the CT. As such, the use of this term should probably be discontinued.[19]

Tricuspid Annulus

In a series of consecutive patients with focal right atrial AT, 13% were reported to originate from the TA.[27] In this study, foci arose from either the superior TA or the inferoanterior TA with the latter being the most common site. An alternative series of patients with focal AT only observed foci arising from the superior TA.[35] Isolated case reports have reported focal AT originating from the inferolateral TA[36] and the anterolateral TA.[37] In two animal studies, McGuire et al. described the presence of cells with atrioventricular (AV) nodal–type characteristics around the entire TA.[38,39] These cells were histologically similar to the atrial cells but resembled nodal cells in their cellular electrophysiology, response to adenosine, and lack of connexin43. One may speculate that these cells serve as the substrate for AT originating from around the TA.

Coronary Sinus Ostium

Kistler et al. reported in ~7% of patients undergoing radiofrequency ablation (RFA) for focal AT, the AT focus originated from the CS ostium.[26] The CS ostium is characterized by the abrupt change in myocardial fiber orientation in the region of the Thebesian valve.[40] Most focal ATs originating from the CS ostium demonstrate properties suggestive of reentry. It is speculative whether this change in fiber orientation may provide the anisotropic conduction necessary to initiate reentry.

Midline Atrial Structures: Para-Hisian (Perinodal), Atrial Septal (Left or Right), and Noncoronary Cusp

There is considerable confusion about the origin and nomenclature of focal AT originating from the abovementioned anatomical regions.[21,22,41–48] The terms *para-Hisian* and *perinodal* have been used interchangeably. In addition, tachycardias described as arising from either the left or right side of the septum have also included tachycardias originating in the perinodal region. Furthermore, others have suggested that para-Hisian tachycardias are a subset of TA tachycardias because of their similar EP properties.[22] In addition, ATs originating from the noncoronary cusp have been viewed either as a distinct entity or, alternately, as an early exit region for a tachycardia that originates from the perinodal region or anterior septum.[22,47–49] In the latter of these hypotheses, the noncoronary cusp is thought to simply provide a safe approach to the ablation of an AT that actually originates from the perinodal area. It is the authors' opinion that tachycardias arising from each of the abovementioned regions should be viewed as a distinct clinical entity with careful mapping in each region. Rarely, AT has been described as arising from the left or right coronary cusps.[50,51]

Right Atrial Appendage

The hallmark of these uncommon tachycardias is that they are frequently incessant and therefore may be associated with TMC.[4] In a series of patients with RAA focal AT, Roberts-Thompson et al. observed that these arrhythmias arose from either the inferolateral base or the tip of the RAA.[28] The inferolateral base of the RAA was the most common location in this study. On the other hand, in a series by Freixa et al., the tip of the RAA was the most common site with 60% of foci arising from this location.[52] Both these studies noted that this tachycardia was more common in men.

Pulmonary Veins

The role of PV foci in the initiation of paroxysmal AF has been extensively documented.[53] These patients frequently demonstrate a spectrum of arrhythmias ranging from focal atrial ectopy and nonsustained AT to paroxysms of AF. In this patient population, there are multiple PV foci within each PV and from multiple PVs. As such, focal ablation is universally unsuccessful, and an approach that encompasses isolation is required. However, there is a group of patients with PV foci who demonstrate only focal AT as the clinical arrhythmia,[24,54,55] and in these patients the fundamental mechanism appears to be truly focal in the majority. Foci responsible for isolated AT tend to have longer cycle lengths and be ostially located rather than deep within the PV compared with foci associated with AF initiation. In addition, the foci arise more commonly from the superior PVs than the inferior PVs. AT originating from the PVs are virtually always spontaneous and rarely inducible with programmed stimulation, suggesting abnormal automaticity or triggered activity. In rare cases, PV AT has been induced by speech and deglutition[56–58] (Fig. 11.2). In some patients with PV AT, the arrhythmia may be incessant and result in TMC.[4] Although this appears to be fully reversible following catheter ablation, recent studies have suggested that subtle ventricular abnormalities may persist.[59] Given the focal nature of PV AT, these arrhythmias are curable in the long term with focal ablation. In a study by Teh et al. evaluating the long-term outcomes of patients with PV AT following catheter ablation, 96% were free from recurrence of AT off antiarrhythmic drugs at a mean follow-up of 7.2 ± 2.1 years.[55] None of the patients developed AF. In those patients with recurrences, in almost all instances this was from the original focus.[55]

Mitral Annulus

The MA is the second most common location of LA focal AT.[60] In a series of patients with LA focal AT by Hachiya et al., approximately one-third of foci originated from the MA. The superior region of the MA in close proximity to the aortomitral continuity (AMC) and the left fibrous trigone has been reported as the most common site of mitral annular focal AT.[25] Gonzalez et al. hypothesized using a murine model that embryologic remnants of specialized conducting tissue located in this region may provide the substrate for focal AT.[61] Furthermore, Wit et al. observed that muscle fibers of the anterior mitral valve leaflet were continuous with the LA myocardium.[62,63] These fibers exhibited AV nodal–type characteristics with both spontaneous automaticity and anisotropic conduction properties potentially providing the substrate for abnormal automaticity or microreentry.[62,63]

Left Atrial Appendage

LAA focal AT has been reported to most commonly arise from the base of the LAA. In a series by Yamada et al., all LAA foci arose from the base of the LAA, most commonly the medial side.[64] Rarely, LAA focal AT has been described as originating from the tip of the LAA[65] or the epicardium.[66]

Coronary Sinus Musculature

Badhwar et al. described an uncommon type of focal AT originating from within the CS musculature in ~3% of patients undergoing catheter ablation.[20] The mean distance from the CS ostium to the site of earliest endocardial activation recorded within the CS was 3.6 ± 0.5 cm. This site always preceded the earliest LA endocardial site during tachycardia. All patients were noted to have a sharp potential in the CS that preceded the CS atrial signal during tachycardia. In all patients, the tachycardia was successfully ablated within the CS.

PATHOPHYSIOLOGY

The pathophysiology leading to the development of focal AT remains unknown. When histologic examination has been possible in cases of focal AT, both normal and abnormal myocardia at the focal origin have been reported.[67–71] McGuire et al. reported four patients with abnormalities, two with extensive myocardial fibrosis and two with myocyte hypertrophy and endocardial fibrosis.[69] All had structural heart disease. Other reports have found mononuclear cell infiltration, mesenchymal cell proliferation, islets of fatty tissue, thinning, and blebs.[67,68,70] These may produce the substrate required for microreentry or abnormal automaticity.

Higa et al. demonstrated the existence of low-voltage zones suggesting the existence of localized atrial pathology in patients with focal AT.[72] The majority of focal ATs in this series originated within or on the border of a low-voltage zone. Many of

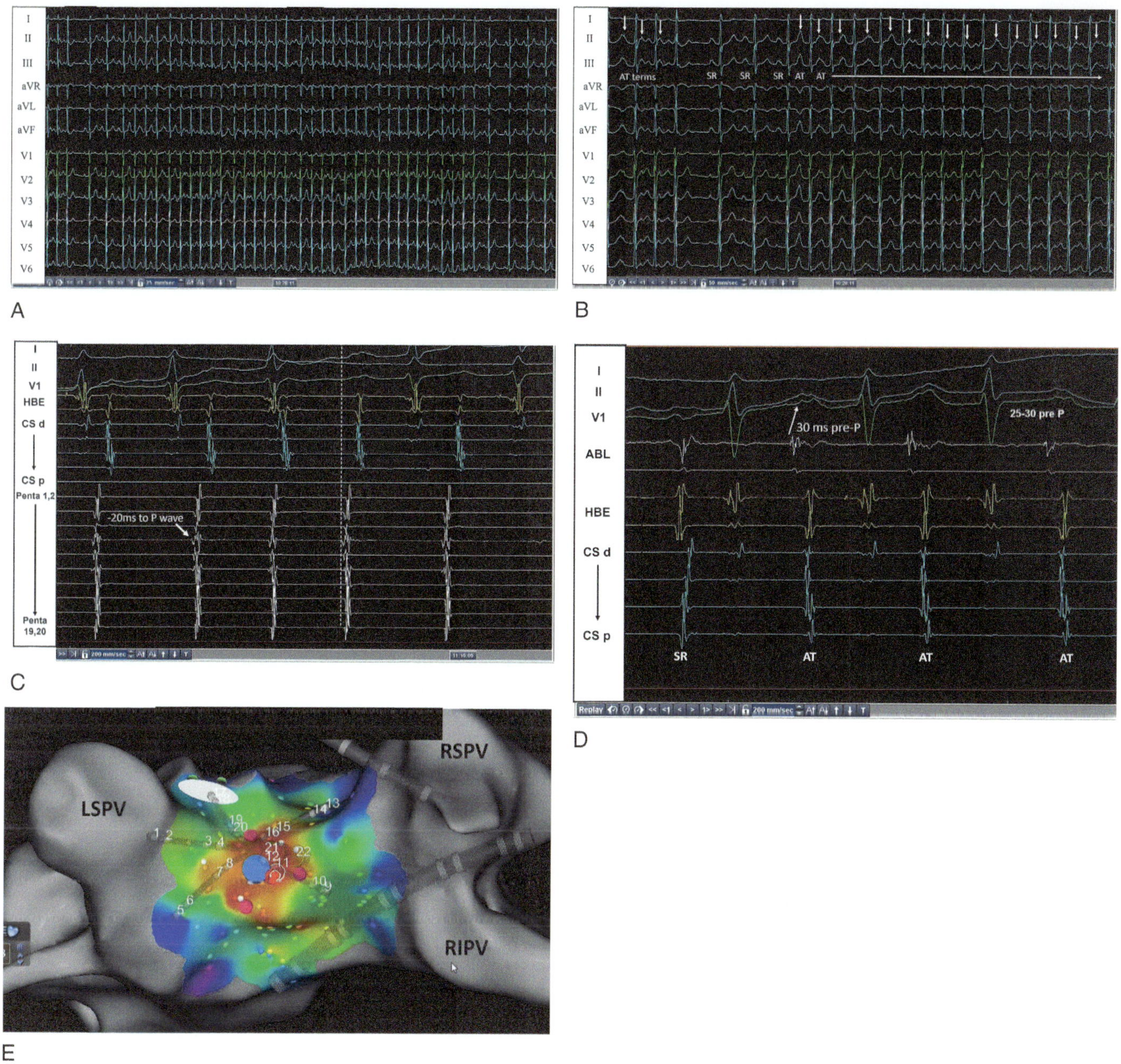

Fig 11.2 (A) A 68-year-old woman with talking-induced focal AT. This patient was referred for atrial fibrillation ablation. AT first appearance at 25-mm/s sweep speed; this continuous 12-lead rhythm trace resembles atrial fibrillation. (B) In this trace as 50-mm/sec sweep speed, it is apparent that there is organized activity throughout. On the left, a paroxysmal of AT terminates (*terms*) spontaneously, followed by three sinus beats and then reinitiation of the focal tachycardia. The P waves of the focal AT are arrowed in lead II. The varying degrees of P-wave fusion with the T wave and QRS create the impression of variability in P-wave morphology, but this is proved at mapping to be a single focal site of origin. The P-wave overlap with T wave and QRS also precludes a precise determination of the AT P-wave morphology, which would require analysis of a fully unencumbered AT P wave. (C) Mapping during ongoing tachycardia. Note that the CS is activated from distal to proximal, confirming a left atrial site of origin. However, the CS distal and the His A are almost "on time," indicating that the actual site of origin is distant from both of these widely separated recording sites. The PentaRay recordings with the catheter position in the LA roof between the superior PVs indicates earliest activation at PV 7, 8, 20 ms pre–P-wave onset. The local high density and high resolution (small electrodes with small interelectrode distance) provide very clear definition of the earliest site of AT origin even though all of the electrodes on the five PentaRay splines activate within 10–15 ms of each other. The resolution is much greater than a point-by-point map with a large bipole of an ablation catheter. (D) The ablation catheter (*ABL*) was subsequently positioned at the anatomical site of earliest activation defined by the PentaRay map. The fractionated signal is recorded 30 ms ahead of P-wave onset at the site of successful ablation. (E) Superior view looking down on the roof of the LA. The CARTO map indicates the PentaRay catheter position and the site of earliest activation in the roof of the LA (indicated by the *blue dot*) adjacent to bipole 7, 8. *AT*, Atrial tachycardia; *AV*, atrioventricular; *CS*, coronary sinus, *LA*, left atrium; *PV*, pulmonary vein.

these arose from the CT, which showed conduction anisotropy with rapid linear conduction and slowed transverse conduction.[33] It is possible that localized atrial myocardial abnormalities represent the substrate for focal AT. Consistent with these observations, several studies have found low-amplitude, fractionated electrograms at the site of successful ablation in patients with focal AT, representing slowed conduction and possibly atrial pathology.[23,73] Nevertheless, this has not been a universal finding and may be dependent on anatomical location such as the CT.

Whereas local structural abnormalities appear to most likely create the substrate for focal discharge or microreentry, focal AT may also exhibit EP characteristics suggestive of abnormal automaticity or triggered activity. Chen et al. performed a comprehensive evaluation of the mechanisms of AT in 36 patients using both pacing and pharmacologic maneuvers.[5] Automatic ATs were identified in seven patients by the following characteristics: (1) AT could be initiated only with isoproterenol; (2) programmed stimulation could not initiate or terminate AT; (3) AT could be transiently suppressed with overdrive pacing; (4) propranolol terminated all of the AT; (5) adenosine, dipyridamole, verapamil, Valsalva maneuver, carotid sinus massage, and edrophonium could not terminate the AT; and (6) monophasic action potential recordings did not find afterdepolarizations. AT related to triggered activity occurred in nine patients with the following features: (1) the initiation of AT was reproducible with atrial pacing and was dependent on achieving a critical range of atrial pacing cycle lengths; (2) just before the onset of AT, delayed afterdepolarizations were observed in the monophasic action potential recordings; (3) termination of AT was reproducible with programmed stimulation; (4) entrainment was not found, but overdrive suppression could be demonstrated; and (5) adenosine, dipyridamole, propranolol, verapamil, Valsalva maneuvers, carotid sinus massage, and edrophonium terminated the AT. AT arising from microreentry was identified in 20 patients. Their characteristics included the following: (1) AT could be reproducibly initiated and terminated with programmed stimulation; (2) fulfillment of the criteria for manifestation and concealed entrainment; (3) the interval between the initiating premature beat and the first beat of AT was inversely related to the premature coupling interval of atrial extrastimuli; and (4) adenosine, dipyridamole, and verapamil terminated the AT in most cases.

The limiting factor in the analysis of mechanisms is the significant overlap in EP characteristics. For example, programmed stimulation may initiate and terminate both triggered activity and microreentry. However, although triggered activity may be dependent on cycle length, abbreviation of pacing cycle lengths may also predispose to reentry.

The use of adenosine to differentiate between AT mechanisms has provided inconsistent results, which may in part reflect different definitions used in a range of studies. However, more recent studies using a strict differentiation between focal and macroreentrant AT have reported more consistent results.[16–18] Markowitz et al.[18] observed that focal automatic ATs could be transiently suppressed but not terminated with adenosine, and ATs with characteristics consistent with microreentry or triggered activity terminated with adenosine use. By contrast, macroreentrant ATs were insensitive to adenosine. Iwai et al. observed similar responses to adenosine and used 3D electroanatomical mapping to delineate the tachycardia circuit, ensuring a clear distinction between focal and macroreentry.[16]

In the era of catheter ablation, the relevance of tachycardia mechanism has been questioned. Chen et al. performed a literature search to determine whether mechanistic information altered ablation outcomes in patients with AT.[13] The ATs were categorized as either automatic or nonautomatic. This study found that the mechanism of AT did not predict successful ablation or recurrence of AT after the initial success.

Multiple Focal Atrial Tachycardia

This term must first be differentiated from the term *multifocal AT,* which refers to a continuously changing site of focal triggering most commonly observed in patients with advanced lung disease. Multiple focal ATs refer to the situation of having more than one sustained focal tachycardia. The second may be observed after ablation of the first, or rarely there may be competition between the two foci, with one triggering the other and vice versa. Hillock et al. described 10 patients in a series of 258 patients with AT who had more than one focus identified (4%).[32] The mean age of these patients was 54 years, and all were women. There were seven patients with two ATs each and three patients with three ATs each. The locations of AT were the CT, CS ostium, TA, MA, and PV ostium. Successful ablation was performed for 22/23 (96%) tachycardias, and there were no recurrences of AT in those patients with successful ablation during 2 years of follow-up.

Tachycardia-Mediated Cardiomyopathy and Focal Atrial Tachycardia

In a recent series of patients with focal AT, incessant AT occurred in 25% of patients and TCM was present in 10%.[4] TCM occurred in 37% of patients with incessant tachycardia. A comparison of the characteristics of patients with incessant AT who had TCM with those of patients who also had incessant AT but did not have TCM revealed no clear causative clinical differences, and it had been suggested that there may be an underlying genetic predisposition. Origin from atrial appendage sites was associated with a high incidence of incessant tachycardia (84%) and left ventricular (LV) dysfunction (42%). Origin from PV sites also carried a higher likelihood that the tachycardia would be incessant (59%). After successful ablation, LV function was restored in 97% of patients at a mean duration of 3 months. In long-term follow-up, LV function remained normal, but magnetic resonance imaging (MRI) revealed subtle abnormalities including minor LV dilatation, lower ejection fraction than the control group (while nevertheless in the normal range), and possible diffuse mild fibrosis on T_1 mapping.[59] There were no definite regions of delayed enhancement. The clinical relevance of these late findings remains unknown.

ARRHYTHMIA DIAGNOSIS AND DIFFERENTIAL DIAGNOSIS

Patients with focal AT may present with recurrent nonsustained bursts of narrow complex tachycardia or with sustained tachycardia, which at times can be difficult to differentiate from other SVT mechanisms or from atrial macroreentry.

Inappropriate Sinus Tachycardia Versus Focal Atrial Tachycardia

Differentiating AT from sinus tachycardia on the 12-lead electrocardiogram (ECG) can be difficult, particularly for tachycardias originating at the superior CT.[74] Although the P wave in AT usually has a different morphology to the sinus P wave, in AT from the superior CT, the P wave may be clinically indistinguishable. An abrupt onset and termination of the tachycardia, or warm up and cool down over three or four beats favors AT, whereas sinus tachycardia gradually increases and decreases in rate over ~30 seconds to several minutes. Inappropriate sinus tachycardia (IAST) invariably presents as a long RP tachycardia (RP > PR), whereas focal AT may be either long or short RP depending on the AT rate and AV nodal conduction properties. AT typically initiates with a tightly coupled P wave, which is not observed in IAST.

Patients with IAST have an abnormally fast resting heart rate with acceleration beyond that expected with minimal exercise. In one definition, the resting daytime heart rate exceeds 100 beats per minute and the average heart rate on 24-hour Holter monitor exceeds 90 beats per minute.[74] It is important to exclude secondary causes of sinus tachycardia before making this diagnosis. In general, EP testing is not indicated in these patients unless a focal AT is being considered. Some incessant ATs can have a persistently elevated 24-hour rate with blunted variability. In these cases, the P wave is often abnormal in morphology and the nocturnal rate remains elevated. However, even here there can be considerable variability. IAST should be distinguished from postural orthostatic tachycardia (POT) syndrome, which is characterized by a marked increase in rate (generally >30 beats per minute) during adoption of upright posture. This may represent an overlap syndrome.

In the EP laboratory, a typical feature of some forms of reentrant AT is that they are inducible with programmed stimulation. In the presence of isoproterenol, an automatic focal tachycardia will show sudden onset often with the initiating tachycardia P wave tightly coupled and located within the preceding T wave, and there is usually a sudden shift in the site of focal activation. In the case of IAST, there is a gradual increase in sinus rate with earliest activation at the superior CT.

To summarize, in comparison with IAST, focal AT (1) has sudden onset and termination; (2) frequently demonstrates tightly coupled activity with the P wave in the T wave at the time of onset (by contrast, IAST has gradual increase in rate); (3) has a fixed site of origin; acceleration may occur in response to isoproterenol, but the site of origin does not change (by contrast, in IAST, the site of activation shifts superiorly along the CT with isoproterenol); (4) demonstrates normal heart rate in between paroxysms of AT; and (5) frequently demonstrates a nonsinus PWM.

Atrial Tachycardia Versus Atrioventricular Nodal Reentrant Tachycardia/Atrioventricular Reentrant Tachycardia

Differentiation of AT from atrioventricular nodal reentrant tachycardia (AVNRT) or atrioventricular reentrant tachycardia (AVRT) on the 12-lead ECG can be difficult. Although most commonly associated with a long RP interval, AT can occur with either a short RP interval or a long RP interval depending on the tachycardia rate and the AV conduction interval at a given rate. It can therefore mimic either typical or atypical AVNRT and AVRT. If the ECG tracing shows persistent tachycardia with AV block or inconsistency (unhooking) of the ventriculoatrial (VA) relationship during ongoing tachycardia, then this suggests an AT. The observation of termination in which the last event is a nonpremature P wave generally excludes AT. Another clue to the diagnosis is the presence of an inferior P-wave axis. With some rare exceptions, this excludes AVRT or AVNRT as it suggests an origin high in the atrium. A superiorly directed P-wave vector may indicate AVRT or AVNRT or an AT focus originating from the CS ostium or annular structures. Automatic AT may also manifest with recurrent self-limiting bursts of tachycardia that can exhibit warm up and cool down phases, and this appearance is almost diagnostic of focal AT.

Several classical studies have proposed a variety of tachycardia features and pacing maneuvers to differentiate AT from AVNRT and AVRT in the EP laboratory.[75-80] Knight et al. investigated the diagnostic value of these features and pacing maneuvers in 196 patients with SVT, of whom 25 had AT.[79] Multiple baseline observations and tachycardia features were evaluated. Pacing maneuvers assessed were atrial pacing during SVT just below the tachycardia cycle length (TCL); atrial pacing during SVT at the longest cycle length that resulted in AV block; ventricular pacing during SVT just below the TCL; burst ventricular pacing for three to six beats at a cycle length of 200–250 ms; and scanning diastole with a premature ventricular extrastimulus. AT could not be consistently identified by any single feature or maneuver; however certain features were useful: AT required isoproterenol for induction more often than AVNRT or AVRT, although the predictive value was poor. Surprisingly, the presence of AV block with persistent tachycardia did not discriminate between AVNRT and AT. However, spontaneous termination of tachycardia with AV block excluded AT. This was seen in 28% of patients. Following ventricular pacing with atrial entrainment and an atrial activation sequence different from tachycardia, the presence of a V-A-A-V response was diagnostic of AT (Fig. 11.3). Inability to entrain the atrium during ongoing tachycardia caused by VA block had an 80% positive predictive value (PPV) for AT. Conversely, tachycardia termination during burst ventricular pacing that did not depolarize the atrium excluded the diagnosis of AT. AT was also excluded when a premature ventricular beat was introduced during the refractory period of the His bundle, and there was either advancement of atrial activation or tachycardia termination without atrial depolarization. The presence of a fixed VA interval on the first beat after atrial pacing (within

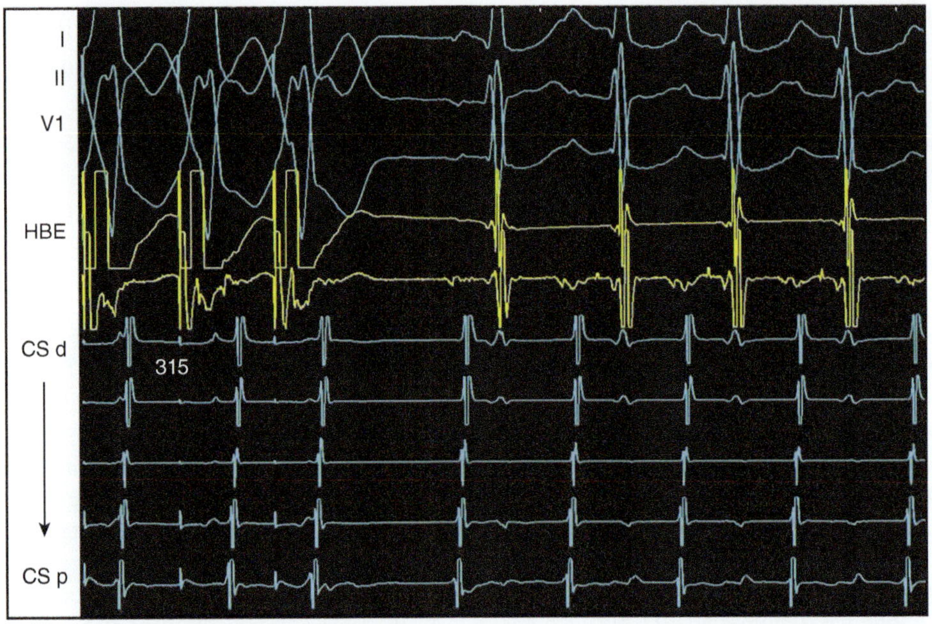

Fig. 11.3 Surface electrocardiography and intracardiac recordings at the initiation of an atrial tachycardia. Last two beats of a ventricular drive train followed by a ventricular extrastimulus *(left)*. The atrial activation follows the ventricular pacing. There is initiation of tachycardia with a V-A-A-V response indicating an atrial tachycardia. Note that this response applies equally on initiation as during entrainment. *CS*, Coronary sinus; *d*, distal; *HBE*, His bundle electrogram; *p*, proximal.

10 ms of the VA interval during tachycardia) had a high negative predictive value (NPV) for AT. However, this observation did not completely exclude AT, as apparent VA linking may occur because of coincidental events. Conversely, if the VA interval could be unhooked after the cessation of pacing, then AT is likely to be present. However, variable VA conduction can occur after pacing in AVNRT, and therefore this observation is not specific for AT.

Focal Atrial Tachycardia Versus Macroreentrant Atrial Tachycardia

In most cases of focal AT, it is possible to observe a discrete P wave with an intervening isoelectric interval (Table 11.1). However, when the atrial rate is very rapid and if atrial conduction slowing is present, there may be no isoelectric baseline and the appearance may mimic that of macroreentrant AT (see Chapter 13). Conversely, whereas macroreentrant AT frequently demonstrates a continuous undulation without an isoelectric period on the 12-lead ECG, patterns resembling focal AT (with an isoelectric period) have also been described particularly in the context of extensive atrial scarring and LA foci.[81,82] LA macroreentry in such patients can classically exhibit low-amplitude P waves and long isoelectric intervals. Ultimately, an EP study is required for a definitive diagnosis of focal AT.

In focal AT, the origin of atrial activation can be localized with endocardial mapping to a small area from which there is radial spread. Occasionally, the presence of anatomical or functional barriers conduction may result in regions of preferential conduction.[72] Nevertheless in focal AT, intracardiac recordings demonstrate large portions of the cycle length without activity, correlating with the isoelectric interval on the surface 12-lead ECG. Conversely, in macroreentrant AT, it is generally possible to record activity throughout the TCL. Furthermore, whereas focal AT caused by microreentry may be successfully entrained, the ability to entrain an AT with characteristics of being in the circuit (postpacing interval [PPI] minus the TCL of < 20 ms) from two sites greater than 2 cm apart is diagnostic of macroreentry.[2] It will be possible to entrain a reentrant focal AT, but the PPI-TCL will only indicate a site in the circuit in the immediate vicinity of the focus.[83]

The rate of the tachycardia does not help in discriminating between focal and macroreentrant AT, as the rate ranges of both focal AT and macroreentrant AT are too wide to be reliably used for determination of arrhythmia mechanism. The rate range of focal AT is usually between 130 and 250 beats per minute but may be as low as 100 beats per minute or as high as 300 beats per minute. Similarly, although macroreentrant AT usually has a rate between 240 and 310 beats per minute, conduction delays within the circuit either caused by atrial pathology or use of conduction slowing antiarrhythmic medications may slow the rate to less than 150 beats per minute.

With the advent of 3D mapping systems, small circuits with properties between those of microreentry and macroreentry have been described.[84,85] These reentrant circuits occur in a localized region with a diameter of 1–2 cm and have been described around a PV, in the anterior LA and in the septum (Fig. 11.4). Evidence of markedly slowed conduction is usually present, and many of these patients have had prior ablation procedures. These tachycardias often have a PMW consistent with a focal AT[84,85] (Box 11.1).

TABLE 11.1 Focal Atrial Tachycardia Versus Macroreentry or Small Circuit (Microreentry)

	Focal	Macroreentry	Microreentry
Most common SHD	None	SHD/CHD/AF RFA	AF RFA
ECG isoelectric interval	Yes	No	Yes
Record from >80% of CL	No	Yes	Yes
Entrain with PPI-TCL <20 ms	Yes	Yes	Yes
Entrain PPI-TCL < 20 ms, two sites > 2 cm apart	No	Yes	No
Activation pattern	Radial	Large loop	Radial
Ablation approach	Focal	Linear or focal	Focal

AF, atrial fibrillation; *AT,* atrial tachycardia; *CH(D)* coronary heart disease; *CL,* cycle length; *PPI,* postpacing interval; *RF(A),* radiofrequency ablation; *SH(D),* structural heart disease; *TCL,* tachycardia cycle length.

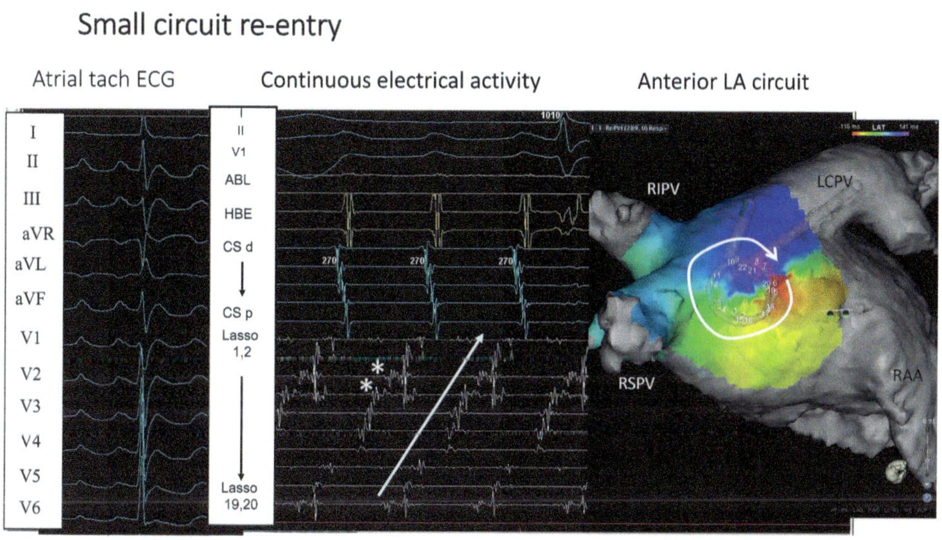

Fig. 11.4 Atrial tachycardia due to small circuit reentry in a patient with a history of persistent atrial fibrillation. Left panel, P-wave morphology, which is upright in V_1 (indicating a probable left atrial origin) and upright in inferior leads (indicating a probable superior origin). The signals in the middle panel recorded on a Lasso catheter in the anterior left atrium show activation spanning the entire cycle length. The asterisks indicate long fractionated multicomponent electrograms that span almost half the tachycardia cycle length and indicate a region of markedly slowed conduction necessary to maintain these small reentrant circuits. These signals reflect advanced atrial remodeling. The right panel shows an anatomical view of the left atrium viewed from superiorly. The Lasso catheter is shown in the anterior LA roof. The colour coding indicates the activation sequence from red through yellow, green, light blue, dark blue and purple. Where purple meets red is the "head meets tail" location of the reentrant circuit. The arrow indicates the activation sequence. This circuit was terminated by ablation at the site of the fractionated electrograms (asterisked).

MAPPING

One of the critical difficulties in mapping focal ATs is that in some patients, they may be quiescent while performing the EP procedure. Although some foci can be reliably initiated with programmed stimulation, those that cannot may be quiescent at the commencement of the procedure or become quiescent during the procedure, can prevent detailed mapping. The absence of frequent focal activity not only prevents mapping but also means that the procedural end point is uncertain. Although several pharmacologic approaches have been used to elicit focal firing (most commonly isoproterenol), the response is not consistent. Occasionally, patients are brought back for a further attempt at mapping and ablation at a time when the focus is active.

Mapping I: P-Wave Morphology

Although successful ablation will depend ultimately on detailed mapping, the PWM on the surface 12-lead ECG can provide important clues regarding the likely site of tachycardia origin, particularly given the classic anatomical localization of these foci. The PWM is determined by the site of origin and the pattern of atrial activation during AT. Several algorithms for localizing

BOX 11.1 Arrhythmia Diagnostic Criteria

Focal AT may be a long or short RP tachycardia. No single diagnostic maneuver for focal AT. Therefore, multiple approaches are used.

- ***Focal AT suggested in the following cases:***
  - Inferior P-wave axis
  - Multiple spontaneous bursts of tachycardia with warmup and cooldown
  - V-A-A-V response to ventricular overdrive pacing
  - Unhooking of the VA relationship (can occur in AVNRT)
- ***AT ruled out in the following cases:***
  - V-A-V response to ventricular overdrive pacing
  - Spontaneous termination with a nonpremature A as the last event
  - Advancement/delay or termination of the tachycardia with a ventricular extrastimulus when His bundle is refractory
  - Tachycardia termination with burst ventricular pacing that does not depolarize the atrium
  - Inability to entrain the atrium during ongoing tachycardia caused by VA block (can occur in AVNRT)
  - VA interval hooked on first return beat after atrial pacing (rarely can occur fortuitously)
- ***In comparison with IAST, focal AT***
  - Has sudden onset and termination or warms up and cools down within several beats
  - Frequently demonstrates tightly coupled activity with the P wave in the T wave at the time of onset. By contrast, IAST has gradual increase in rate
  - Has a fixed site of origin. Acceleration may occur in response to isoproterenol administration, but site of origin does not change. By contrast, in IAST the sites of activation shift superiorly along the crista with isoproterenol
  - Demonstrates normal heart rate in between paroxysms of atrial tachycardia
  - Frequently has a nonsinus P-wave morphology

AT, Atrial tachycardia; *AVNRT,* atrioventricular nodal reentrant tachycardia; *IAST,* inappropriate sinus tachycardia; *VA,* ventriculoatrial.

focal AT based on the PWM have been developed.[12,60,86,87] P waves are generally described as isoelectric, positive, negative, or biphasic (positive–negative or negative–positive), and a full description will include the presence of notching. Fig. 11.5A demonstrates an algorithm described by Kistler et al.,[12] and Fig. 11.5B,C shows examples of PWM for left and right focal ATs. Additional Fig. 11.6 provides an updated 2021 version of the P-wave algorithm.[88] In this updated version, focal AT arising from the CS os, right septum, perinodal region, left septum, noncoronary cusp, and superior mitral annular regions are grouped together as "para-septal" AT to reflect the inability of the P wave to adequately distinguish between these anatomically adjacent sites. In addition, the CS body was removed as this is an extremely rare site of origin.

There are several important caveats when interpreting the PWM. The first is that accurate localization depends on the absence of significant atrial structural abnormality or prior atrial surgery or ablation. Even PV isolation alone can markedly alter PWM caused by change in direction of activation.[89] Second, it is of critical importance to obtain a clear view of the P wave, particularly the initial vector direction, unencumbered by the preceding T-wave or QRS complex. This may be facilitated by vagal maneuvers, administration of adenosine or ventricular pacing. Third, the spatial resolution of the P wave for localizing foci in the atria may be as poor as 17 mm depending on the anatomical location.[86] The P wave alone cannot distinguish between closely spaced sites of origin as noted in the updated algorithm (Fig. 11.6).

Right or Left Atrial Site of Origin

Differentiating the atrium of origin before an ablation procedure has implications for planning whether LA access via transseptal puncture is necessary as well as in discussing the risks and success rates of RFA with the patient. In an important study by Kistler et al., these investigators developed an algorithm to localize focal AT based on the PWM.[12] The critical initial step in this algorithm was to focus on the PWM in V_1. This algorithm correctly identified the anatomical location of the focal AT in 93% of patients. In this algorithm, V_1 was most useful in differentiating between right and left ATs. A negative or biphasic (positive–negative) P wave in V_1 predicted a RA origin with 100% specificity, 100% PPV, 69% sensitivity, and 66% NPV. Conversely, a positive or negative–positive biphasic P wave in V_1 had 100% sensitivity, 81% specificity, 76% PPV, and 100% NPV for a LA origin. In this series, the PWM could not reliably distinguish between tachycardias located in close proximity to the septum (left versus right septal or perinodal).

P-Wave Morphology According to Anatomical Site of Origin: Crista Terminalis

The majority of these foci arise from the superior and mid CT and therefore may have similar PWM to sinus rhythm. Tada et al. found that a negative P wave in aVR predicted a CT origin compared with anterior RA foci with a sensitivity of 100% and specificity of 93%.[87] Kistler et al. found that a positive–negative P wave (or positive during both tachycardia and in sinus rhythm) in V_1, positive in lead I and II and negative in aVR predicted a CT origin with 93% sensitivity, 95% specificity, 84% PPV, and 98% NPV.[12] Although there may be overlap between the PWM of foci arising from the superior crista and right superior PV (RSPV) caused by the anatomical proximity of the two sites, these may be distinguishable on the basis of changes to the PWM in lead V_1 during tachycardia compared with sinus rhythm. In a RSPV focal AT, the P wave in V_1 will invariably be upright in V_1 in tachycardia and biphasic (positive–negative) in sinus rhythm. When a CT focal AT has an upright P wave in V_1 (~10%), it is invariably also upright during sinus rhythm.

Tricuspid Annulus and Right Atrial Appendage

Focal AT may arise from anywhere around the circumference of the TA. The PWM will vary markedly according to region on the TA in which the focus is located. Nevertheless a common feature of TA focal AT is the presence of an inverted P wave in V_1 and V_2 with late precordial transition to an upright appearance.[27] In general, the polarity of the P wave in leads II and III is deeply negative for an inferior location, and low amplitude positive or biphasic for a superior location. Other P-wave characteristics were positive in aVL and positive or isoelectric in lead I. Because of their close anatomical proximity, ATs arising from the RAA (especially from the lateral base of the appendage) are generally indistinguishable from superior TA foci (Fig. 11.7). In general, the P waves in V_1 and V_2 are negative (V_1 notching is frequently present) with variable precordial transition to positive in V6.[28,52] In the inferior leads, the P wave is characteristically low amplitude and positive.

Coronary Sinus Ostium

The PWM of CS ostium focal AT is highly characteristic with deeply inverted (negative) P waves in leads II, III, and aVF.[26] The P wave in V_1 is usually isoelectric–positive or negative–positive with variable precordial transition. The P waves are invariably positive in aVL and aVR.

Perinodal Region, Interatrial Septum

The PWM of perinodal and septal tachycardias is variable, and there is overlap between the left and right sides (Fig. 11.8). For right perinodal and right septal foci, an isoelectric P wave in V_1 is helpful if present (specificity and PPV of 100%) but is present in only 50% of cases.[12] Alternately the P wave in V_1 has been reported to be low-amplitude-negative, positive–negative biphasic, or in some instances negative–positive biphasic. Left septal and left perinodal foci may demonstrate either a biphasic negative–positive appearance or positive P wave in V_1.[45,90] In the inferior leads, the PWM is negative or negative–positive.[90] However, variable findings in the limb leads have been reported.[45] Some of the reported differences in PWM in this area may relate to how the septal region is defined. In some reports, this has

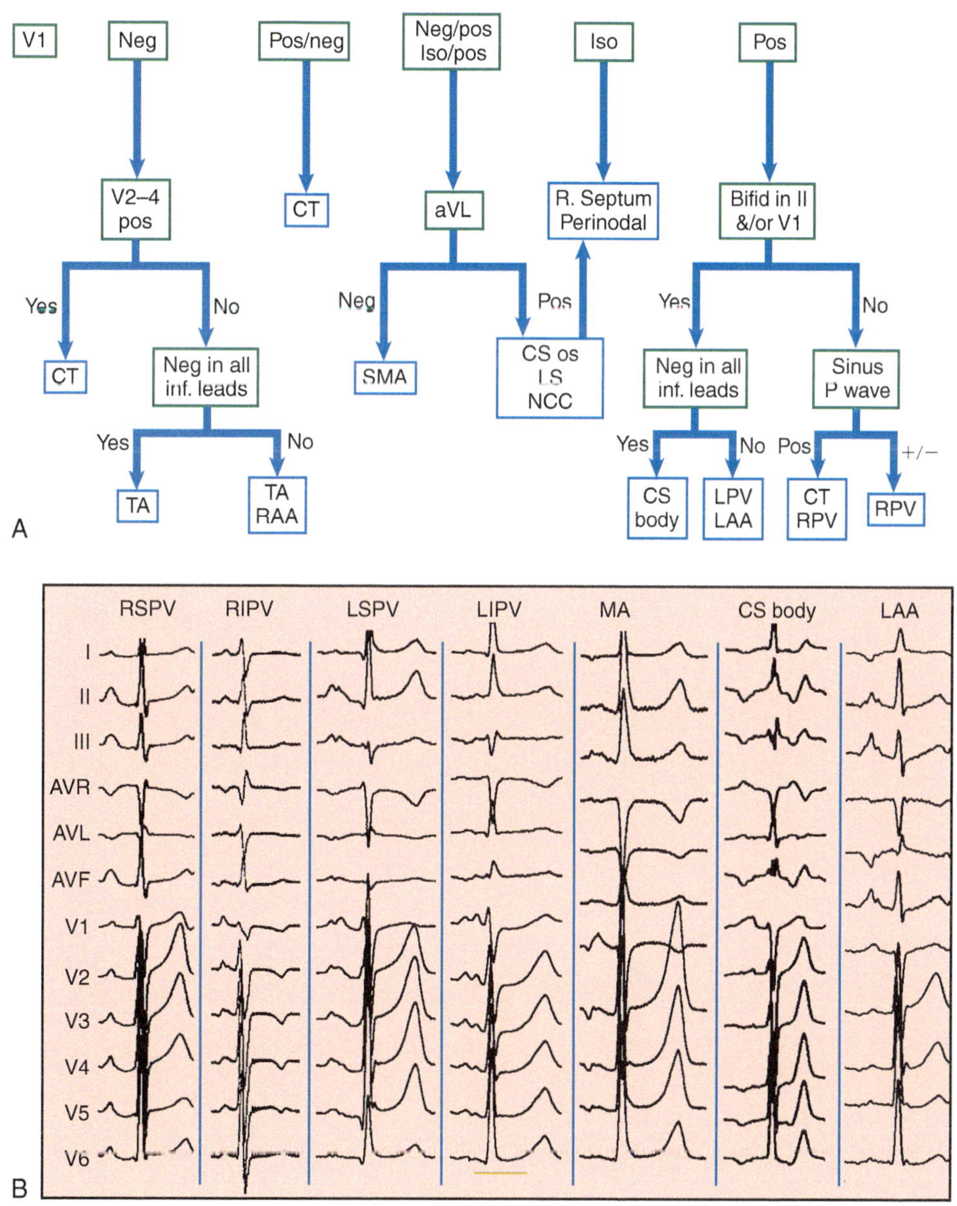

Fig. 11.5 (A) P-wave algorithm for identification of tachycardia origin. (B) Examples of P-wave morphology from typical left atrial origins.

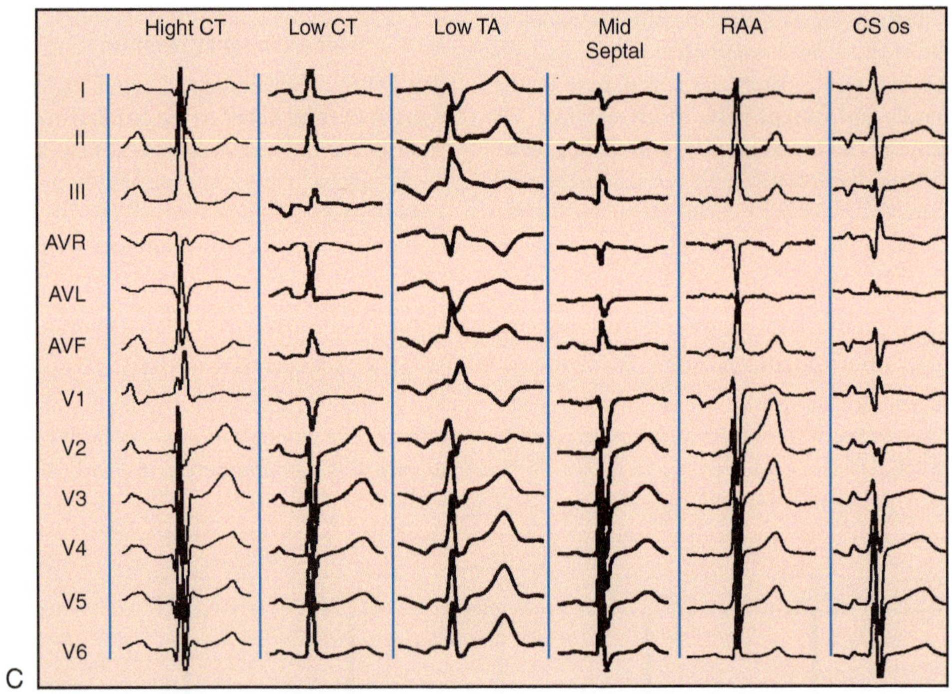

Fig. 11.5, cont'd (C) Examples of P-wave morphology from right atrial locations. *CS*, Coronary sinus, *CT*, crista terminalis, *HBE*, His bundle electrogram; *Iso*, isoelectric; *LA(A)* left atrial appendage; *LIPV*, left inferior pulmonary vein; *LPV*, left pulmonary vein; *LS*, lower septum; *LSPV*, left superior pulmonary vein; *M(A)* mitral annulus; *MV*, mitral valve; *NC(C) Neg*, negative; *Os*, ostium; *Pos*, positive; *PN*, perinodal; *PV*, pulmonary vein; *RA(A)* right atrial appendage; *RIPV*, right inferior pulmonary vein; *RPV*, right pulmonary vein; *RSPV*, right superior pulmonary vein; *SM(A)* superior mitral annulus; *T(A)* tricuspid annulus. (A, modified from Kistler PM, Roberts-Thomson K(C) Haqqani HM, et al. P-wave morphology in focal atrial tachycardia: development of an algorithm to predict the anatomic site of origin. *J Am Coll Cardiol.* 2006;48(5):1010–1017.)

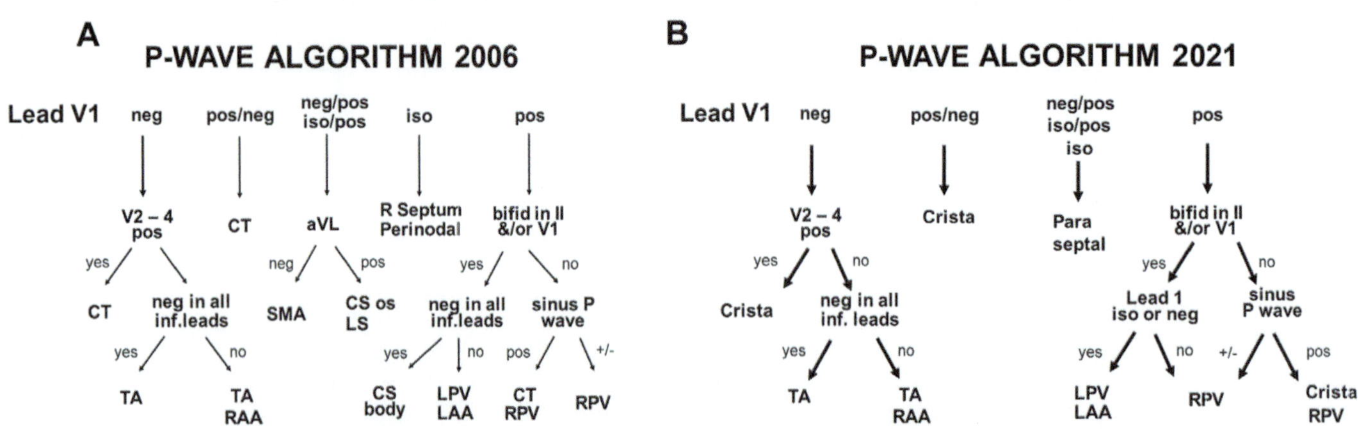

Fig. 11.6 Comparison of the original (A) and updated (B) P-wave algorithms.

included the fossa ovalis region and the septum primum and in others has referred to the region of Koch's triangle.[44] Recently the P-wave algorithm was updated to reflect the inability of the P wave to distinguish between closely spaced "para-septal" locations including the CS os, right septum, perinodal region, left septum, noncoronary cusp, and superior mitral annular regions[88] (Fig. 11.6).

Aorto-mitral Continuity and Noncoronary Cusp Focal Atrial Tachycardia

Although AT foci have been described from a range of MA sites, the majority cluster at the AMC adjacent to the left fibrous trigone (Fig. 11.9). ATs arising from this region characteristically have a biphasic negative–positive PWM in V_1 and an isoelectric or negative P wave in aVL (sensitivity of 88%, specificity 99%, PPV 88%, and NPV 99%).[25] The P wave in the inferior leads are usually low amplitude or isoelectric. Because of the close anatomical proximity, the P waves of focal AT originating from the noncoronary cusp of the aortic valve are very similar to those arising from the AMC. The P waves in leads V_1 and V_2 are also characteristically negative–aortomitral continuity positive as well as those in the inferior leads.[47] In this study, all nine patients had an upright P wave in leads I and aVL and this may serve as a distinguishing feature

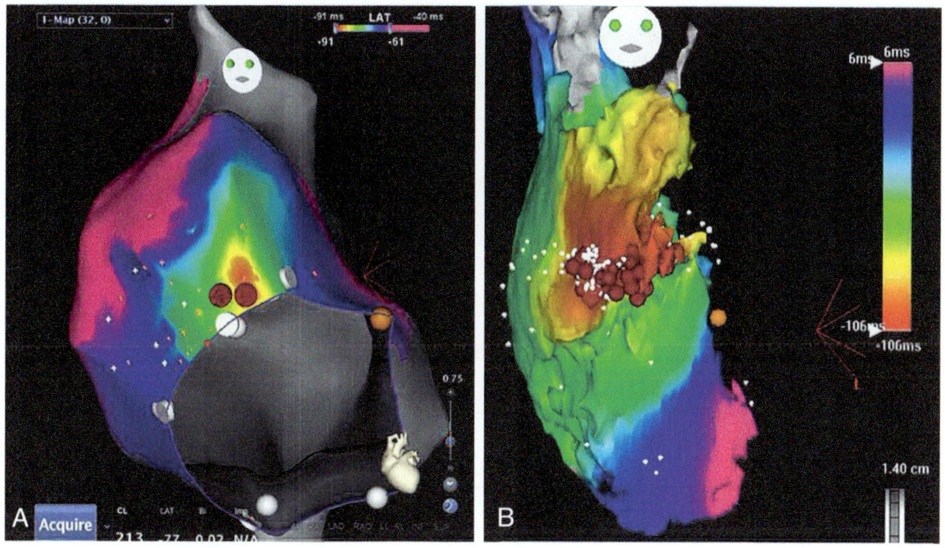

Fig. 11.7 (A) Left anterior oblique projection of the right atrial map of a superior tricuspid annular tachycardia. The geometry was created by the CARTO system, and the superimposed color map shows earliest activation at the superior tricuspid annulus (*TA*) at the site of successful ablation. (B) CARTO merge map from a patient with an incessant right atrial appendage tachycardia. Earliest colors in both maps are in *red* with radial spread away from this site. This focus was ablated at the lateral base of the right atrial appendage (*RAA*). The proximity of the superior TA to the RAA is highlighted by these examples.

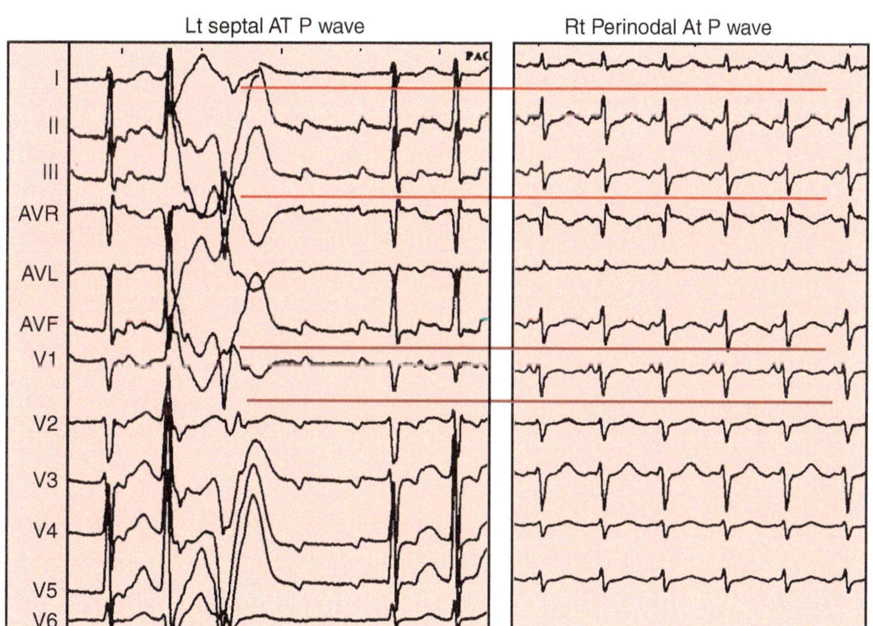

Fig. 11.8 Electrocardiography (ECG) from a left septal origin *(left)* and an ECG from a right perinodal location *(right)*. Note that both show the characteristic negative–positive V_1 morphology with similar morphology in inferior leads. This is a nonspecific pattern and can be observed from a variety of anatomical sites in this region (see text). *AT*, Atrial tachycardia.

from aortomitral focal AT. Nevertheless, there is considerable overlap of the PWM of noncoronary cusp AT with surrounding sites in close proximity (perinodal and septal regions) as described earlier.

Pulmonary Veins and Left Atrial Appendage

The posterior location of the PV ostia within the LA is reflected by the universal finding of a positive P wave in V_1 and across the precordial leads.[24] In almost all foci, the P wave is negative in aVR, and negative or isoelectric in aVL. Compared with the right-sided PVs, the left-sided PVs have a broader notched P wave in V_1 and in the inferior leads (Fig. 11.10). Right-sided PV foci usually have a positive P wave in lead I. The superior PVs invariably have a positive P wave in the inferior leads. The inferior PVs may have inverted, low-amplitude positive or isoelectric inferior P waves. Because

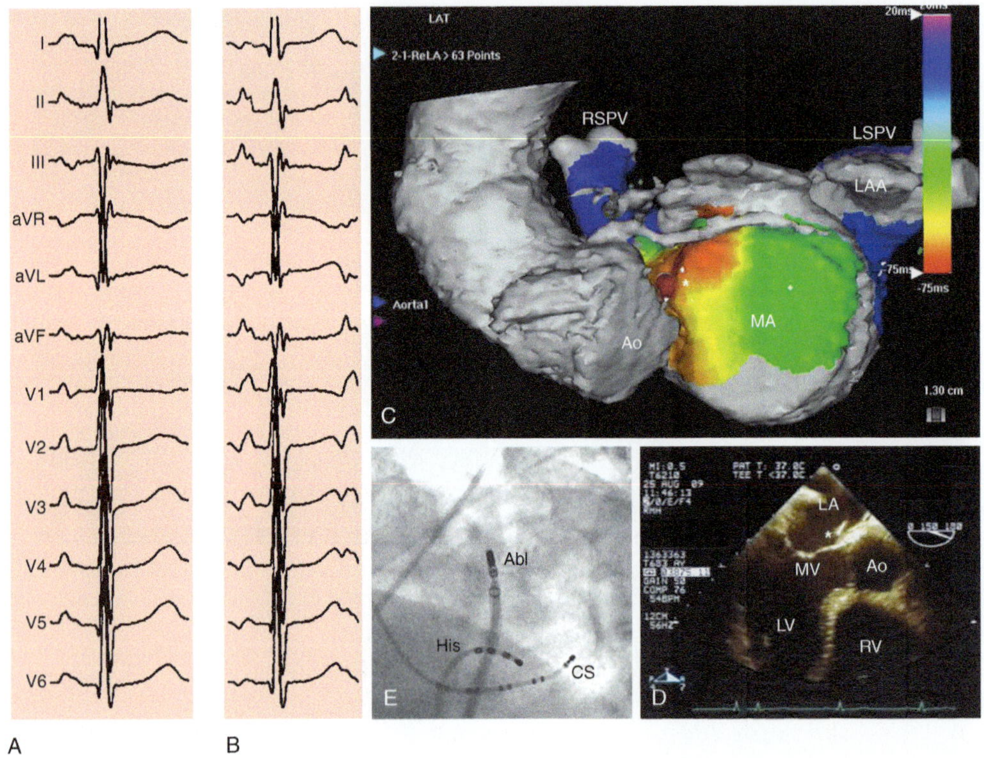

Fig. 11.9 Mitral annular tachycardia. (A) Sinus rhythm P wave. (B) Atrial tachycardia P wave showing negative–positive V_1 morphology and negative in a V_L. (C) The CARTO merge to computed tomography scan with earliest activation in *red* at the aortomitral continuity at the site of successful ablation *(red dot)*. (D) Transesophageal echocardiography image with the ablation catheter tip *(asterisk)* at the aortomitral continuity. (E) Left anterior oblique fluoroscopy projection at the same location. *Ao,* Aorta; *Cs,* coronary sinus; *L(A)* left atrium; *LA(A)* left atrial appendage; *LSPV,* left superior pulmonary vein; *LV,* left ventricle; *MA*; mitral annulus; *MV,* mitral valve; *RSPV,* right superior pulmonary vein; *RV,* right ventricle.

of the close proximity of the superior and inferior PVs and marked anatomical variation, distinguishing superior from inferior foci may be difficult.

The LAA is closely approximated with the left superior PV (LSPV) and as such has a similar PWM. A PWM that suggests an LSPV focus (broad upright and notched in V_1 and inferior leads) together with a deeply inverted P wave in lead I will most usually indicate a LAA focus (Fig. 11.11).[61] In recent studies, virtually all patients had negative P waves in leads I and aVL along with positive P waves in the inferior leads.[64,91] A negative P wave in leads I and aVL predicted a LAA focus with a sensitivity and specificity of 92% and 97%, respectively.

Coronary Sinus Midbody

Focal AT originating from several centimeters into the CS body characteristically demonstrate a PWM in V_1 that is broad and upright as the site of origin is leftward and posterior compared with the CS ostium.[20] The PWM in the inferior leads are deeply inverted and aVR is positive (see Fig. 11.5).

Mapping II: Endocardial Activation Mapping

Endocardial activation mapping is the most commonly used technique to identify the location of the AT focus. Mapping of focal AT will demonstrate atrial activation starting at a small area (focus) from which it spreads out centrifugally. It is very helpful to deploy standard mapping catheters that may provide a rapid guide to the anatomical region of interest (Fig. 11.12). Multipolar catheters will also give a rapid visual guide to when there is a change in tachycardia or in some cases when termination to sinus tachycardia occurs (see Fig. 11.12). Catheters will be placed as usual at the bundle of His area and within the CS to provide important mapping reference points. Other catheters may be deployed to provide higher-density mapping in the anatomical region of interest. These include multipolar catheters such as a CT catheter or a catheter deployed around the TA in the RA. Once the general location of the tachycardia has been identified a multi-electrode mapping catheter with high resolution (multiple bipoles with close spacing and small electrodes) should be deployed to precisely define the tachycardia origin. Such catheters include a circular mapping catheter, a PentaRay (BioSense Webster), a grid catheter (Abbott-St. Jude), or the Orion catheter (Boston Scientific) among others will provide the most rapid and precise localization of the focal site of tachycardia origin. For example, when a PV tachycardia is suspected, a circular catheter may help locate the focus or facilitate PV isolation. Alternately. for foci in the body of the atrium, a PentaRay, grid, or Orion catheter may be used. Once precise localization has been achieved, an ablation catheter can be easily moved to the anatomical location, activation timing confirmed, and successful ablation achieved. In general, activation times more than 20–30 ms before the P wave are observed at successful sites, but this is highly variable and dependent on

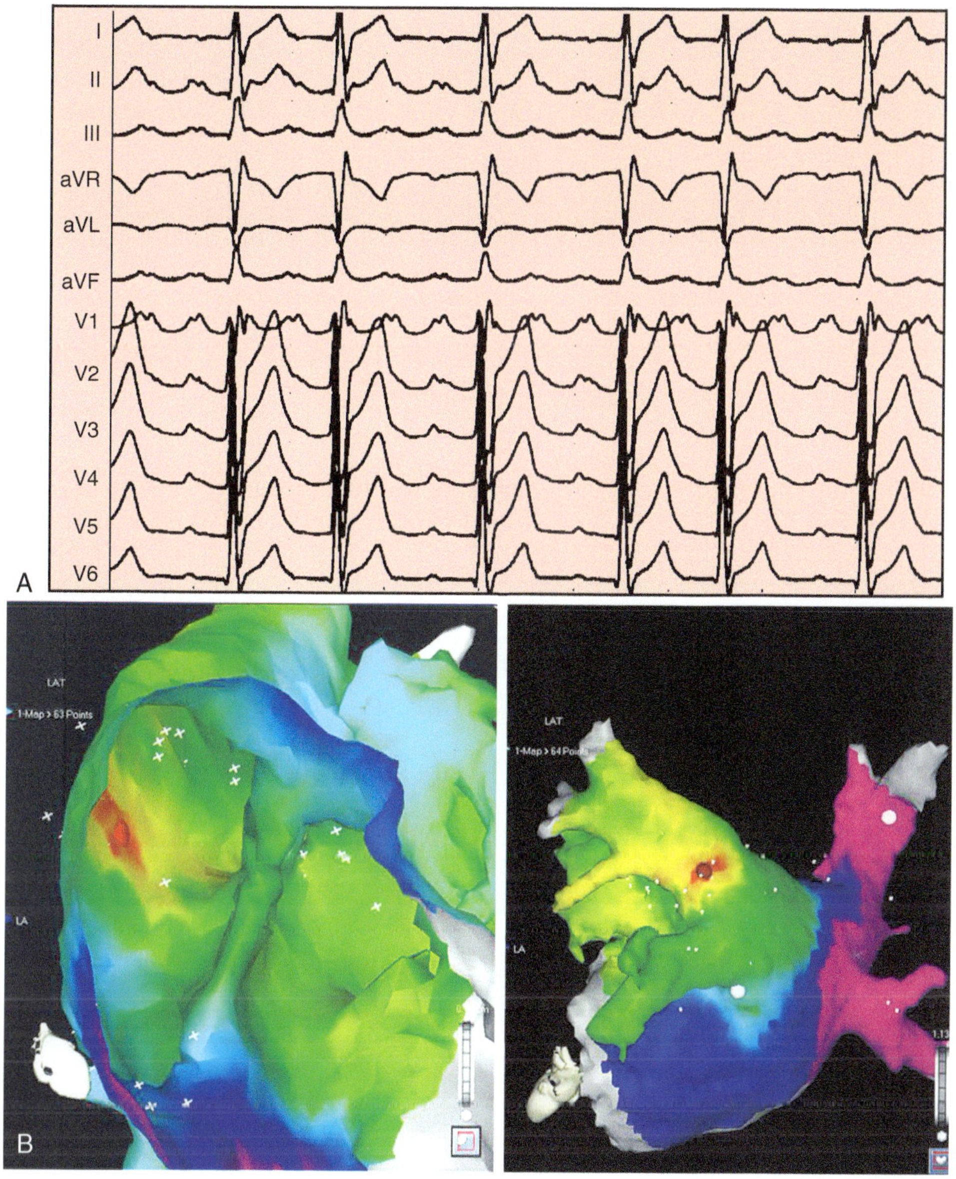

Fig. 11.10 (A) Electrocardiography from a 31-year-old male patient with an incessant atrial tachycardia arising from the left superior pulmonary vein. Note that the V_1 P wave is broad upright and notched as are the inferior P waves. The lead I P wave is isoelectric. (B) Demonstration of CARTO merge to the left atrial computed tomography scan with superimposed color map. Earliest activation and successful ablation were at the posterior inferior ostium of the left superior pulmonary vein. *Left panel,* endoluminal view; *right panel,* posterior view.

multiple factors such as clear observation of P-wave onset, and nature of local conduction. When the P-wave onset cannot be consistently observed, mapping can be performed with reference to a stable intracardiac fiducial point with a known relationship to P-wave onset.

Anatomical Relationships and Mapping Focal Atrial Tachycardia

The anatomical relationships described earlier under P-wave morphology are also important during catheter mapping. Some of the important relationships in this regard are as follows:

- Focal AT apparently originating from the superior CT or superior posterior RA should raise suspicion of a possible RSPV AT.
- Early activation at the CS ostium may suggest a CS ostium tachycardia but is also consistent with an origin from regions deep inside the CS, from the inferior TA, or from the perinodal region.
- Focal AT originating from the superior TA will have a very similar activation pattern to those from the base of the RAA.
- Focal AT arising apparently from the LSPV will need to be distinguished from those originating within the LAA.
- Finally, early activation in the perinodal region may indicate a focal AT originating from the TA in that region or alternately the LA or RA septum or aortic root or the aorto-mitral region. Knowledge about these critical anatomical relationships and the likely sites of AT origin will greatly facilitate mapping. A series of panels in Fig. 11.13 shows an example

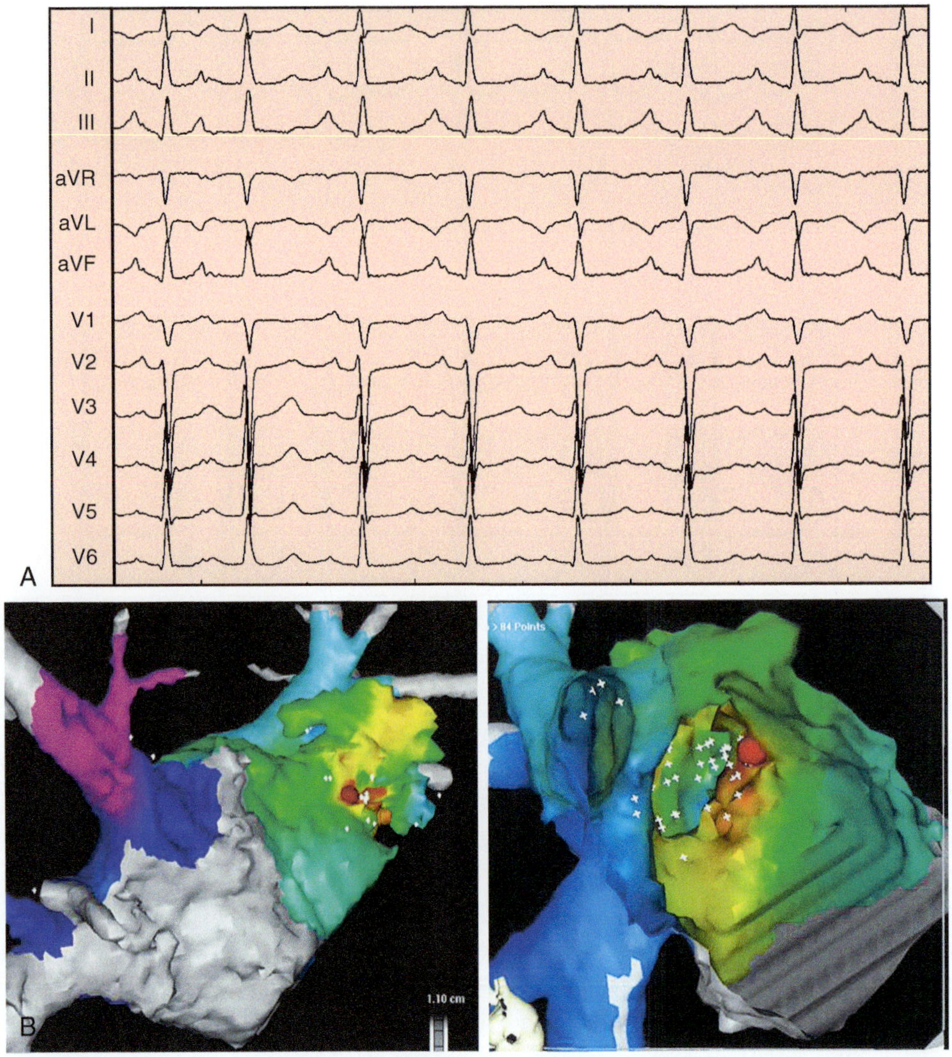

Fig. 11.11 (A) A 24-year-old female with incessant atrial tachycardia. P-wave morphology is broad, upright, and notched in V_1 and inferior leads, suggesting a left superior pulmonary vein origin. Deeply inverted P wave in lead I, however, suggests the adjacent left atrial appendage. (B) CARTO merge to computed tomography scan of segmented left atrium with superimposed color-coded activation map. *Left panel,* anterior view of the appendage; *right panel,* endoluminal view. Earliest activation in *red* is at the anterior base of the appendage with radial spread away from this position.

of a perinodal atrial tachycardia. The first two panels indicate the electrophysiology of the atrial tachycardia with variable VA time and ability to dissociate the ventricular activation from the ongoing tachycardia. Unmasking the otherwise undiscernible P wave following ventricular pacing allows us to determine that the His A is 30 ms pre–P indicating a site originating near to this location. A number of studies have indicated that many perinodal atrial tachycardias can be successfully ablated from the noncoronary cusp and mapping was performed in this anatomical location. Timing was similar to His A timing but attempted ablation at two different NCC sites was unsuccessful. Further mapping in the right perinodal region with breath hold under general anesthesia for catheter stability identified an activation time 90 ms pre–His A. Ablation here eliminated the tachycardia. Although the NCC can be a safe location to ablate some perinodal atrial tachycardias, this case demonstrates that this is not uniformly successful. The emphasis should always be on detailed mapping.

Right Atrium Versus Left Atrium: Endocardial Mapping

In addition to information from the PWM, the endocardial activation pattern can provide early clues to the need to perform transseptal puncture to map the LA. When CS activation is distal to proximal in sequence, this immediately denotes a LA site of origin. However, a proximal to distal sequence is also compatible with a LA origin, particularly for sites at the septum, AMC, or right-sided PVs. In general, for focal AT originating from the left atrium, there will be a large region on the right side of the septum and in the perinodal region with similar activation time. Furthermore, this is usually less than 15 ms pre–P wave. When earliest right-sided activation suggests a perinodal site of origin, it is important to map adjacent structures. In the RA, this will include the perinodal TA

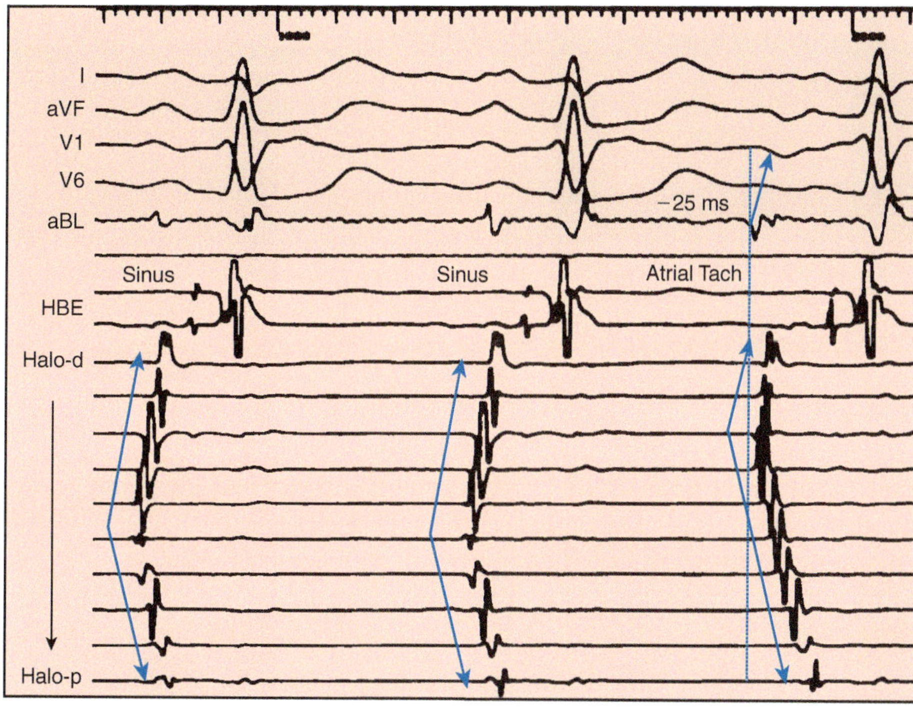

Fig. 11.12 Electrocardiography and intracardiac electrograms at spontaneous initiation of a tricuspid annular tachycardia. Note that a halo catheter around the tricuspid annulus shows a shift in the site of earliest activation, clearly indicating tachycardia onset. Note also that the general region of interest on the annulus is indicated by the catheter. Finally, the ablation electrogram shows an annular amplitude ratio (V > A) and is 25 ms pre–P at the site of successful ablation.

and adjacent RA septum. However, when earliest RA activity is perinodal, it is also important to map the left side of the septum and the aortic root for a noncoronary cusp origin. All these sites should be carefully mapped before commencing ablation.

Three-Dimensional Electroanatomical Mapping

The use of 3D mapping systems during mapping and ablation of focal AT is highly recommended. This technology registers the mapping information and provides a far greater anatomical resolution than that can be achieved with biplane fluoroscopy alone. A number of studies have demonstrated the ability of 3D electroanatomical mapping to provide a high-resolution map in the region of earliest activation and precisely locate the focus in relation to endocardial geometry.[92–95] The ability to import an MRI or cardiac computed tomography of the chamber of interest has further enhanced the appreciation of anatomical relationships and individual anatomical variations and as a result has further facilitated mapping.[93,94] It is now routine to use 3D mapping together with integrated multipolar catheters to precisely locate focal atrial tachycardias (Box 11.2).

Ablation

Characteristics of the Ablation Signal

Several criteria have been proposed to identify the signal at the AT focus. Fractionated electrograms are frequently found at the successful ablation site;[23,72,73] However, not all studies have reported this finding.[96] Unipolar recordings have also been used to successfully identify the site of tachycardia origin.[96,97] The presence of a negative deflection (QS pattern) with a rapid initial slope theoretically localizes the site of origin of the AT. Tang et al. analyzed the unipolar electrogram at both successful and unsuccessful ablation sites of focal AT. All the successful sites were characterized by the presence of the QS morphology.[98] An RS pattern was observed at unsuccessful sites. Furthermore, Poty et al. reported an acute success rate of 86% using unipolar recordings to identify the target site for ablation. [97]

Ablation Results

RFA has become the treatment of choice in symptomatic patients with focal AT. The focal AT ablation series have reported success rates from 69% to 100%.[5,6,13,20,23–27,37,47,73,97,99] Recurrence rates are generally low. In an analysis of 16 studies by Chen et al., the recurrence rate was 7%.[13] In that study, the authors analyzed predictors of success of RFA. An RA location was the only independent predictor of successful RFA. In other studies, it has been noted that patients who were male, had multiple foci, were older, and had coexisting cardiac disease had lower acute success rates.[13,100] In most series, ablation with RF has been used. However, others have reported successful use of cryoablation, particularly when the focus was in close proximity to the AV node.[101,102]

Although the approach in the majority of patients with focal AT is to map and ablate focally, there are some exceptions.

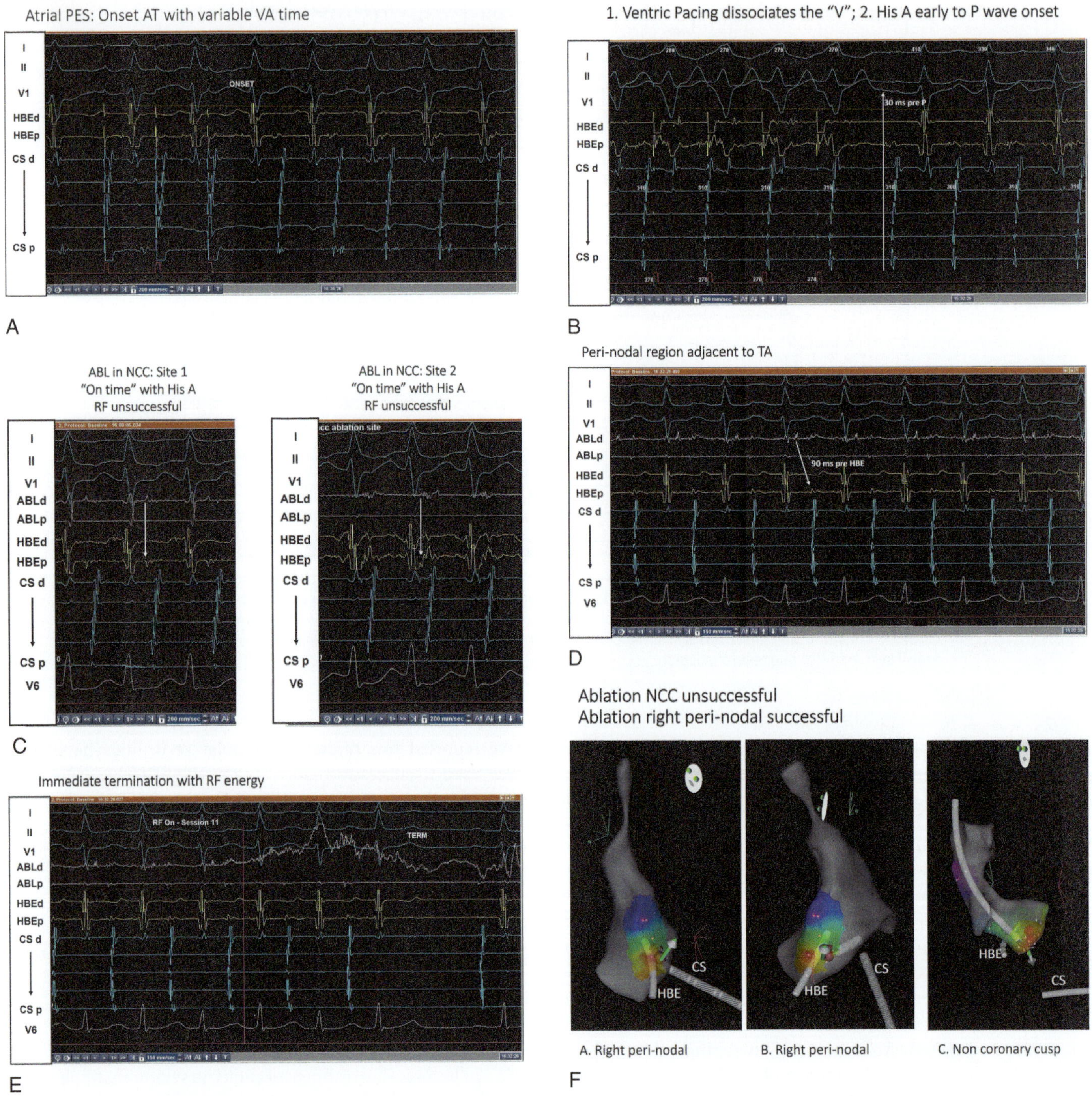

Fig. 11.13 (A) Atrial PES induces a sustained SVT. Note the variation in the VA time (progressive shortening) over the first four beats strongly suggestive of an atrial tachycardia. (B) Ventricular pacing at 270 ms is dissociated from the ongoing atrial tachycardia at 310 ms. This is highly suggestive of atrial tachycardia. Post ventricular pacing, there is a single visible P wave and timing is marked to the intracardiac electrograms. On this occasion, the His "A" is 30 ms pre–P-wave onset, suggesting a site of origin in this vicinity. (C) Mapping was undertaken in the noncoronary cusp with the ablation catheter at two sites within the cusp; both had identical timing to the His A (*arrows*). Ablation attempts within the cusp were unsuccessful. (D) With the ablation catheter repositioned to the perinodal region adjacent to the tricuspid annulus (note split A and AAV ratio of ~1), a very early atrial electrogram was recorded 90 ms ahead of the His A. Ablation at this site during breath hold (under GA) immediately terminated the tachycardia and rendered it noninducible. (E) Rapid termination of the atrial tachycardia within three beats of RF onset (marked by the *red line*). (F) A and B show two views of the ablation catheter on the perinodal tricuspid annulus at this site of successful ablation. C shows a view of the catheter in the noncoronary cusp at a site of unsuccessful ablation. The relationship to the His catheter and proximity to the successful ablation site on the *right* can be appreciated.

BOX 11.2 Target Sites

- Focus on anatomical sites (see Fig. 11.1).
- Detailed comparative mapping of sites in close anatomical proximity with early timing (electrograms):
  - Right atrial appendage and superior tricuspid annulus
  - Superior crista terminalis and right superior pulmonary vein
  - Left superior pulmonary vein and left atrial appendage
  - Perinodal (left and right), septal (left and right), near/on tricuspid, and mitral annuli, noncoronary cusp.
  - Coronary sinus ostium and tricuspid annulus
- Earliest activation time with regard to P-wave onset, usually > 15 ms but highly variable
- Unipolar QS
- Electrogram fractionation at successful site is neither sensitive nor specific

For PV foci, some have reported excellent results with circumferential isolation.[54] Although the preferred approach even in these cases is to ablate focally, in some instances if the focus is distally located or when focal activity becomes quiescent after the PV origin has been identified, then PV isolation may be needed. In cases of difficult to ablate appendage foci, there have been some reports of isolation of the appendage using a cryoballoon.[103] Others have reported successful epicardial ablation in refractory cases of LAA focal AT.[66,104] For refractory cases of LAA or RAA focal AT, others have described minimally invasive surgical approaches to ligate or excise the appendage with successful elimination of the tachycardia.[105–108]

TROUBLESHOOTING THE DIFFICULT CASE

A 25-year-old female was referred to our institution with recurrent palpitations. Symptoms had been present over many years, and episodes were triggered by coffee and exercise. A 12-lead ECG showed almost incessant AT with a ventricular rate of 110–120 beats per minute, alternating with several beats of sinus rhythm before reinitiation of tachycardia. A 24-hour ambulatory ECG monitor showed multiple episodes of AT with ventricular rates at times in excess of 200 beats per minute. A transthoracic echocardiogram revealed a structurally normal heart with normal LV systolic function. The patient had trialed flecainide, which was only partly effective and produced intolerable side effects. Finally, invasive cardiac EP study and RFA were initiated.

Procedure 1

On arrival in the EP laboratory, the patient was in sinus rhythm with runs of spontaneous AT, which became more persistent with isoproterenol infusion (Fig. 11.14). PWM was isoelectric–positive in V_1 and negative–positive in leads II, III, and aVF that was viewed as nonspecific but likely related to a midline structure. There were recurrent spontaneous bursts of AT with earliest activation in the distal CS bipole (Fig. 11.14B). Initial mapping within the RA, around the CS ostium, and the midseptal region showed earliest activation after the P-wave onset. CS diverticulum was not revealed by CS angiography. Transseptal access to the LA was achieved, and LA geometry was collected using an irrigated 3.5-mm ablation catheter and the CARTO electroanatomical mapping system (Biosense Webster, Diamond Bar, CA).

During tachycardia, the activation map demonstrated earliest atrial activity in the low posterior LA, immediately superior to the MA. When mapping with the ablation catheter, a relatively large area in the low posterior LA was activated within 10 ms, rendering the precise identification of the site of origin challenging. RFA was performed at putative sites of early activation in the low posterior LA (25 W irrigated caused by concern regarding esophageal proximity) and resulted in acceleration of the tachycardia but no termination. However, the tachycardia became progressively quiescent rendering mapping increasingly difficult. After the last RF application, no further tachycardia was observed even after provocation with isoproterenol. During a period of monitoring overnight, the patient had several short episodes of AT although the atrial rate was relatively slow. A 24-hour ambulatory ECG monitoring after discharge revealed AT recurrence, and therefore a further attempt at RFA was scheduled.

Procedure 2

On this occasion, a PentaRay NAV (Biosense Webster) multipolar mapping catheter with 1-mm electrode rings and 1-mm bipole spacing was used to facilitate greater mapping precision (Fig. 11.15). This identified early sharp signals at the low posterior LA ~20 ms pre–P-wave onset. The earliest signals were located ~1.5 cm above the mitral valve annulus. The ablation catheter was then positioned at this site using CARTO anatomical definition. The ablation catheter recorded a far less distinct early potential than that observed on the PentaRay (see Fig. 11.15B, C). The unipolar signal showed a QS pattern but was late with respect to the early potential. Ablation at this location (25 W irrigated) resulted in acceleration and termination of the tachycardia within 5 seconds. There was no recurrence of tachycardia over a 45-minute waiting period, which included isoproterenol provocation, or over the ensuing 6 months.

DISCUSSION

This case highlights the advantage of using a closely spaced 1-mm bipole with 1-mm electrodes for precise activation mapping compared with the recordings from the larger bipole of a 3.5-mm ablation tip electrode. The wider bipole summates regional activation, and details on critical activation time are lost. In a classical paper published almost 30 years ago, Ideker et al. described this as one of the key assumptions in activation mapping that may provide a misleading picture.[109] Ndrepepa et al. also demonstrated degradation in accuracy of activation timing with increasing bipolar spacing.[110] With

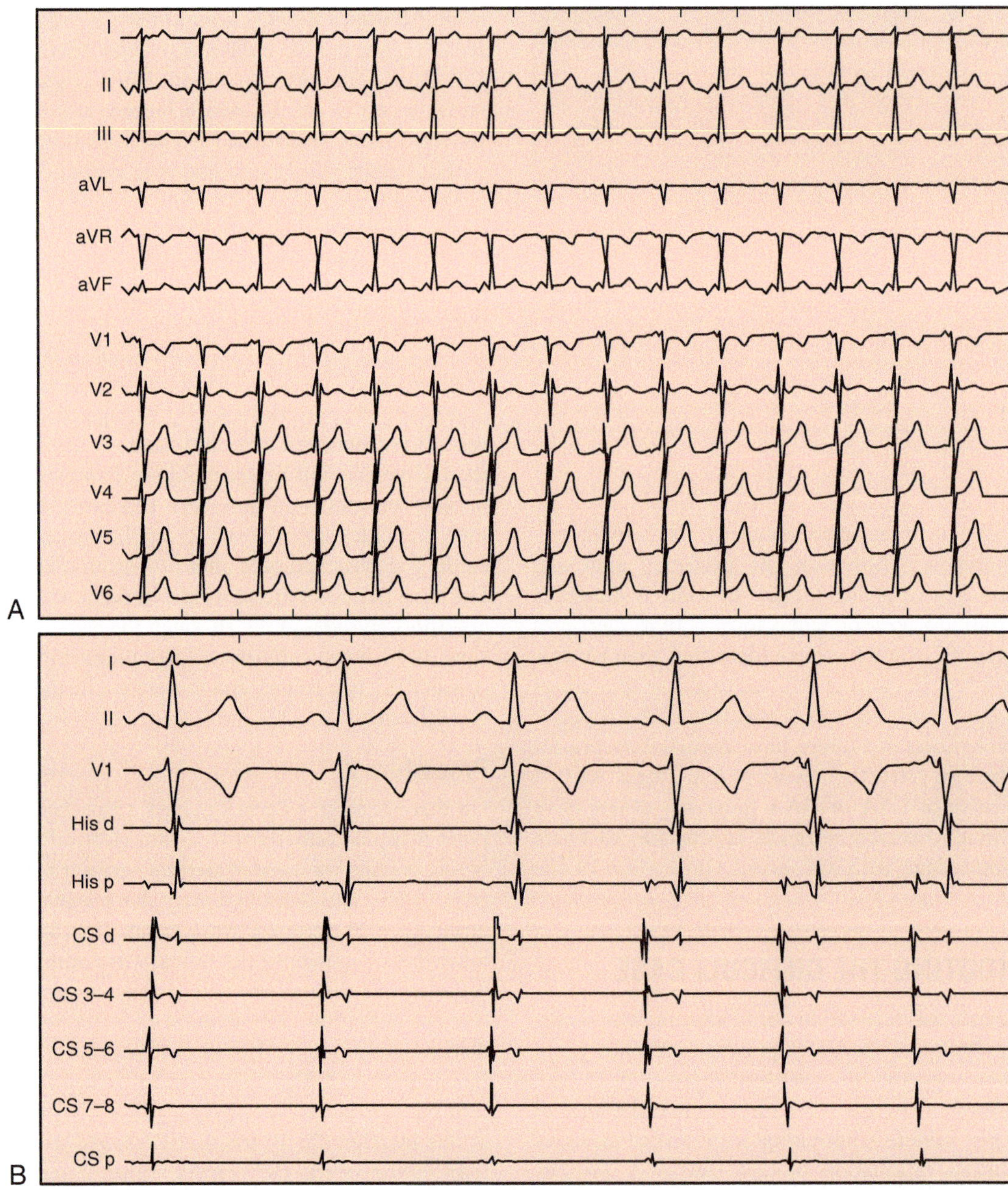

Fig. 11.14 (A) 12-lead electrocardiography (ECG) of atrial tachycardia. Note P-wave morphology: isoelectric-positive in V_1 and negative–positive in II, III, and aV_F. According to the algorithm, this pattern is suggestive of a *midline* location (noncoronary cusp, left or right septum, perinodal). (B) ECG and intracardiac electrograms at the spontaneous onset of tachycardia with earliest atrial activation noted in the distal coronary sinus (*CSd*) electrodes during atrial tachycardia in keeping with a left atrial focus. *L(A),* Left atrium; *LPV,* left pulmonary vein; *R(A)* right atrium.

the widespread use of the ablation catheter bipolar pair as the primary mapping approach for a range of arrhythmias, this important observation may be forgotten. This effect was amplified by the very rapid atrial conduction present in this young patient presumably caused by excellent cellular coupling. In this case, ablation electrode mapping resulted in a region in the posterior LA of almost 2 cm in diameter in which activation occurred within 10–15 ms. However, the 1-mm bipole of the PentaRay demonstrated a sharp early and localized potential at the site of tachycardia origin, which was much less obvious with the ablation catheter positioned at the same site (see Fig. 11.11C). In addition, the unipolar electrogram, although recording a QS pattern, did not reflect this earlier activity. This case provides a reminder of the importance of interelectrode distance in generating a precise activation map and highlights a potential pitfall when mapping is performed exclusively with the relatively wide bipole of an ablation catheter (Box 11.3).

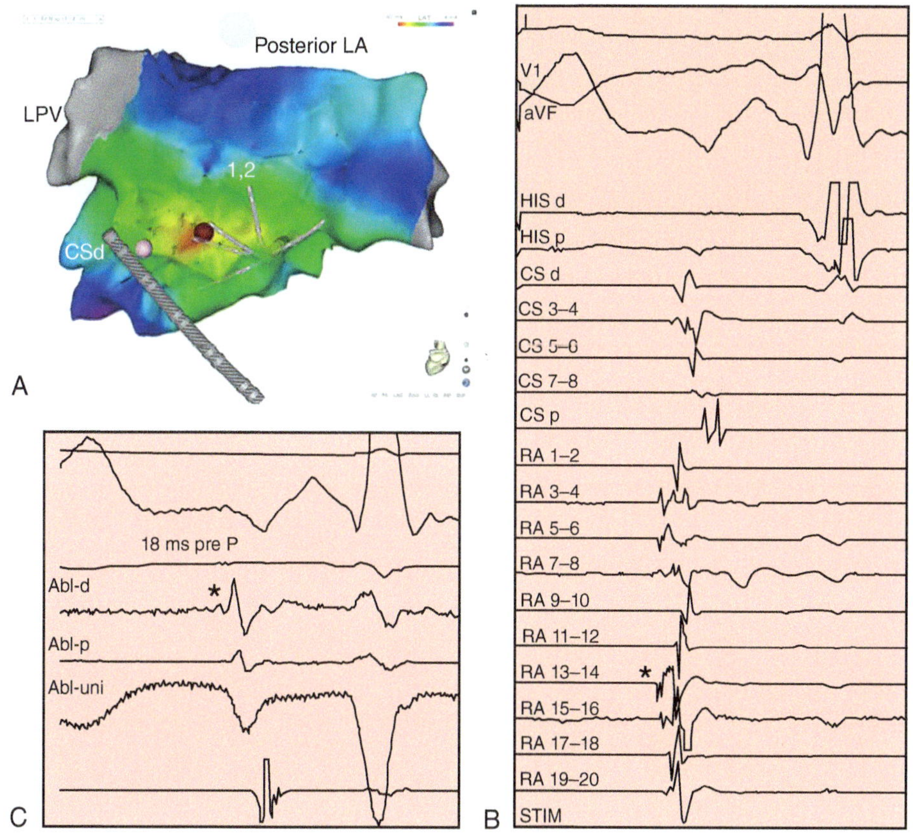

Fig. 11.15 (A) CARTO electroanatomical map of left atrial activation during atrial tachycardia. Earliest local activation time (*LAT*) indicated by *red*, with isochrones through the color spectrum to the latest activation delineated in *blue*. The PentaRay catheter can be seen positioned in the left atrium, and electrodes on the splines are labeled from distal to proximal in an anticlockwise direction. Electrodes 1 and 2 are labeled for orientation. Spline 4 is folded back such that it lies adjacent to spline 2, and earliest activity is on the distal bipole of this spline *(asterisk)*. Note the very sharp early signal. Earliest activation is evident in the low posterior left atrium (LA), and the *red sphere* denotes the position of successful ablation. (B) Intracardiac electrograms recorded by the PentaRay catheter during atrial tachycardia. Note earliest activation, 20 ms pre–P wave, at electrodes 5 and 6 and 13 and 14 (distal poles of spline 2 and 4, respectively). There is a low-amplitude high-frequency early potential at both sites. Note also that the remaining bipoles of the PentaRay catheter are rapidly activated within 10–15 ms. (C) Intracardiac electrograms recorded by the ablation catheter position at the site of earliest activation. The atrial electrogram on the ablation catheter is 18 ms pre–P wave and ablation at this site resulted in successful termination of the tachycardia. *Abl*, Ablation; *CS*, coronary sinus; *d*, distal; *LPV*, left pulmonary vein; *p*, proximal; *R(A)* right atrium; *STIM*, stimulus; *uni*, unipolar.

BOX 11.3 Troubleshooting the Difficult Case

- **Careful electrophysiologic confirmation of the diagnosis of focal AT.**
- **Reconfirm the diagnosis. Is this the same tachycardia or has it changed?**
  - A second focal atrial tachycardia
  - Atrioventricular nodal reentry or atrioventricular reentry
  - Sinus tachycardia while still on isoproterenol
  - Other approach: Repeat electrophysiologic diagnostic maneuvers. Reevaluate the P-wave morphology. Deploy multipolar catheters (rapid visual clue that tachycardia has changed). Remap.
- **Careful mapping of sites in close anatomical proximity.**
- **Improve mapping resolution with a closely spaced bipole.**
- **Avoid temptation to increase the RF power.**
  - More mapping rather than more power
  - The majority of atrial tachycardias can be successfully ablated with 30 W (irrigated tip)
  - Foci that require an epicardial approach are rare
- **If tachycardia is truly perinodal, (after conformation with mapping of left side and coronary cusp) consider use of cryoablation.**
  - In addition consider stopping the procedure to further discuss the risks.
  - Use of apnea under GA greatly enhances catheter stability, which is critical in this location

AT, Atrial tachycardia; *GA*, general anesthesia; *RF*, radiofrequency.

CONCLUSION

The majority of focal ATs originate from defined anatomical structures or sites within the atria. In patients without structural heart disease (or prior surgery or extensive ablation), wavefronts emanating from these sites produce a characteristic P-wave appearance that can facilitate targeted mapping. However, sites in close anatomical proximity will have overlap in P-wave appearance, and detailed mapping will be required. Endocardial activation mapping targeted to anatomical structures and facilitated by multipolar catheters can rapidly and simply identify critical regions of anatomical interest. The 3D mapping systems with imported computed tomography or MRI enhance mapping resolution and provide a precise appreciation of individualized anatomy.

REFERENCES

Please refer to the e-book for a complete list of references.

12

Ablation of Cavotricuspid Isthmus–Dependent Atrial Flutters

Gregory K. Feld, Jonathan C. Hsu, Kurt S. Hoffmayer, Frederick T. Han, Farshad Raissi

KEY POINTS

- The mechanism of most cavotricuspid isthmus (CTI)-dependent atrial flutter (AFL) is macroreentry around the tricuspid valve annulus (TVA).
- The diagnosis of CTI-dependent atrial flutter is made by demonstration of macroreentry around the TVA during entrainment at two or more sites around the tricuspid valve and demonstration of concealed entrainment from the CTI during AFL.
- The target for ablation of CTI-dependent AFL is the CTI, between the TVA and the inferior vena cava (IVC).
- Special equipment that may improve outcome or may be required to ablate the CTI includes a large-tip catheter (8- or 10-mm ablation electrode) with a high-power radiofrequency generator (up to 100 W) or an externally irrigated ablation catheter, a large-curve catheter, and a preformed or steerable sheath. An intracardiac echocardiographic (ICE) catheter, electroanatomical or noncontact three-dimensional mapping systems, or a multielectrode halo catheter may be useful but are not required.
- Sources of difficulty in ensuring long-term success may include complex anatomy (e.g., pouches, prominent Eustachian ridge) of the CTI, leading to failure to achieve bidirectional isthmus conduction block.
- Long-term success rates range from 90% to 95%, after achieving acute bidirectional CTI conduction block.

Cavotricuspid isthmus (CTI)-dependent atrial flutter (AFL) is a common atrial arrhythmia, often occurring in association with atrial fibrillation. It can cause significant symptoms because of a typically rapid ventricular rate and may cause embolic stroke and, rarely, a tachycardia-induced cardiomyopathy. The electrophysiologic substrate underlying CTI-dependent AFL has been shown to be macroreentry around the tricuspid valve annulus (TVA), with an area of concealed conduction in the CTI, anatomically bounded by the TVA anteriorly and the inferior vena cava (IVC) and Eustachian ridge posteriorly, with a line of conduction block along the crista terminalis. This electrophysiologic milieu produces a sufficiently long reentrant path length, relative to the average tissue wavelength around the TVA, to allow for sustained reentry. The triggers of AFL, commonly premature atrial contractions or nonsustained atrial fibrillation originating from the left atrium and pulmonary veins, most likely account for the fact that counterclockwise AFL (typical AFL) occurs most frequently clinically. AFL is also relatively resistant to pharmacologic suppression.

Because of the consistent and well-defined anatomical substrate and the typical pharmacologic resistance of CTI-dependent AFL, radiofrequency (RF) catheter ablation is established as a safe and effective first-line treatment. Although several approaches have been described for ablating CTI-dependent AFL, the most widely accepted technique is an anatomically guided approach targeting the entire CTI, resulting in a high efficacy rate for the cure of AFL, with minimal risk. This chapter reviews the electrophysiology of human CTI-dependent AFL and techniques currently used for its diagnosis, mapping, and ablation.

ATRIAL FLUTTER TERMINOLOGY

Because of the variety of terms used to describe AFL in humans in the past, including type 1 and type 2 AFL, typical and atypical AFL, counterclockwise (CCW) and clockwise (CW) AFL, and isthmus-dependent and non–isthmus-dependent AFL, the Working Group of Arrhythmias of the European Society of Cardiology and the North American Society of Pacing and Electrophysiology published a consensus document in 2001 in an attempt to develop a generally accepted standardized terminology for AFL.[1] The consensus was that the terminology "typical" and "type 1" AFL were most commonly used to describe CTI dependent, defined as macroreentrant right atrial tachycardia, and included both the CCW and CW variants rotating around the TVA. Therefore, the working group determined that CTI-dependent, right atrial macroreentrant tachycardia, rotating in the CCW direction around the TVA (when viewed from the right ventricle) would be termed typical AFL, and similar tachycardia rotating in the CW direction around the TVA would be termed reverse typical AFL.[1] For the purposes of this book, we will use the terms "typical" and "reverse typical AFL," or CTI-dependent AFL when being referred to jointly. Other rare isthmus-dependent AFL variants, including lower loop reentry and partial isthmus-dependent AFL, are also discussed in this chapter.

ANATOMY AND PATHOPHYSIOLOGY

The development of successful RF catheter ablation (RFCA) techniques for CTI-dependent AFL depended in part on the delineation of its electrophysiologic mechanism. Using advanced electrophysiologic techniques, including intraoperative and transcatheter activation mapping,[2-7] CTI-dependent AFL was shown to be caused by a macroreentrant circuit rotating in either a CCW (typical) or a CW (reverse typical) direction in the right atrium around the TVA, with an area of relatively slow conduction velocity in the low posterior right atrium (Figs. 12.1 and 12.2). The predominant area of slow conduction in the AFL reentry circuit has been shown to be in the CTI, through which conduction times may reach 80–100 ms, accounting for one-third to one-half of the AFL cycle length.[8-10]

The CTI is the target for ablation and warrants special attention. The CTI refers to right atrial myocardium between the TVA and IVC, which courses from the inferolateral to the posteromedial low right atrium and is anatomically bounded by the IVC and Eustachian ridge posteriorly and by the TVA anteriorly (see Figs. 12.1 and 12.2). These boundaries form lines of conduction block delineating a protected zone in the reentry circuit.[11-14] The presence of conduction block along the Eustachian ridge[11-14] has been confirmed by the demonstration of double potentials along its length during AFL (Fig. 12.3). The superomedial boundary of the CTI is the line between the septal insertion of the Eustachian ridge and the most inferior para-septal insertion of the tricuspid valve (TV) (i.e., the base of the triangle of Koch).[15,16] The inferolateral border of the CTI comprises the final ramifications of the pectinate muscles of the crista terminalis, but a precise lateral boundary is not well defined. In attitudinal orientation, the portion of the CTI adjacent to the tricuspid annulus is anterior and sometimes referred to as the vestibular portion of the CTI. The portion of the CTI that is adjacent to the IVC is attitudinally posterior and referred to as the membranous CTI. The middle portion of the CTI is referred to as the trabeculated CTI.[15]

The anatomy of the CTI can be assessed by computed tomography (CT) or magnetic resonance imaging (MRI) before ablation or by angiography, electroanatomical mapping, or echocardiography intraoperatively.[17-19] The CTI is typically 34 ± 5 mm in length when measured angiographically from the IVC to the TV. The CTI is usually subdivided into three sections: septal isthmus, central isthmus, and lateral isthmus (see Figs. 12.1 and 12.2).[15,19] In the electrophysiology laboratory, the septal isthmus is defined as that portion between 4 and 5 o'clock when visualized in the left anterior oblique (LAO) projection fluoroscopically. The central isthmus is that portion located at 6 o'clock, and the lateral isthmus is that starting at 7 o'clock.[15] The central isthmus (6 o'clock) marks the shortest distance between the IVC and tricuspid annulus (19 ± 4 mm, range 13–26 mm).[15] In addition, the central isthmus is the thinnest portion, ranging from an average of 3.5 mm near the TV to 0.8 mm in the middle portion.[15] The anterior (vestibular) portion of the CTI adjacent to the TV is entirely muscular, whereas the posterior (membranous) portion closest to the IVC is primarily fibrofatty tissue.[15] The muscle thickness is least in the central isthmus, greatest in the septal isthmus, and intermediate in the lateral isthmus.[15]

The anatomy of the CTI is highly variable but usually classified into three categories. A flat CTI shows 2 mm or less inferior concavity between the IVC and TV and is found in about 28% of patients.[18,19] A concave CTI with inferior concavity more than 2 mm in depth is found in about 20% of patients. In these, the average depth is 3.7 ± 0.8 mm.[19] In up to 83% of patients, the CTI shows a distinct inferior pouch (sub-Eustachian pouch or sinus of Keith) averaging 6.5 ± 2.2 mm in depth but up to 12.4 mm deep (see Figs. 12.1 and 12.2).[15-19] The pouch is separated from the TV by a smooth vestibular area (see Figs. 12.1 and 12.2).[19] The pouch itself may be symmetrical or asymmetrical, with extension toward the atrial septum. In anatomical studies, pouches are confined to the medial or septal CTI but are not seen in the lateral third of the CTI.[20] Other notable anatomical features influencing the success of CTI ablation are the presence of a prominent muscular Eustachian ridge in about 26% of patients and extension of pectinate muscles into the CTI in 70% of patients and even into the coronary sinus in 7%.[20] The thickness of the pectinate muscles is greatest laterally and diminishes toward the atrial septum. The presence of pectinate muscles in the CTI may be suggested by recording high-voltage electrograms (EGMs) from this area.[20] In autopsy specimens, CTI pectinate muscle extensions and CTI pouches tend to occur together.[20]

The crista terminalis forms another important boundary for CTI-dependent AFL. The crista terminalis leaves the superior right atrial septum and courses superiorly and anteriorly to the superior vena cava, and inferiorly along the posterolateral right atrial free wall to the IVC, where it then continues anteriorly and medially to form the Eustachian ridge. Double potentials have also been recorded along the crista terminalis,[11-14] suggesting that it too forms a line of block during AFL, separating the smooth septal right atrium from the trabeculated right atrial free wall (see Fig. 12.3). Such lines of block, which may be either functional or anatomical, are necessary for an adequate path length for reentry to be sustained, to prevent "short-circuiting" of the reentrant wavefront.[12-14,21]

Thus, during typical AFL, the activation wavefront traverses the CTI and exits medially, ascends the atrial septum, courses over the anterior right atrium, descends the right atrial lateral wall between the crista terminalis posteriorly and the TV anteriorly, and then enters the CTI laterally to complete the circuit.[12-14,21]

The medial and lateral CTI, which are contiguous, respectively, with the interatrial septum near the coronary sinus (CS) ostium and with the low lateral right atrium near the IVC (see Figs. 12.1 and 12.2), correspond to the exit and entrance to the CTI, depending on whether the direction of reentry is CCW or CW in the right atrium.[2-15] The presence of slow conduction in

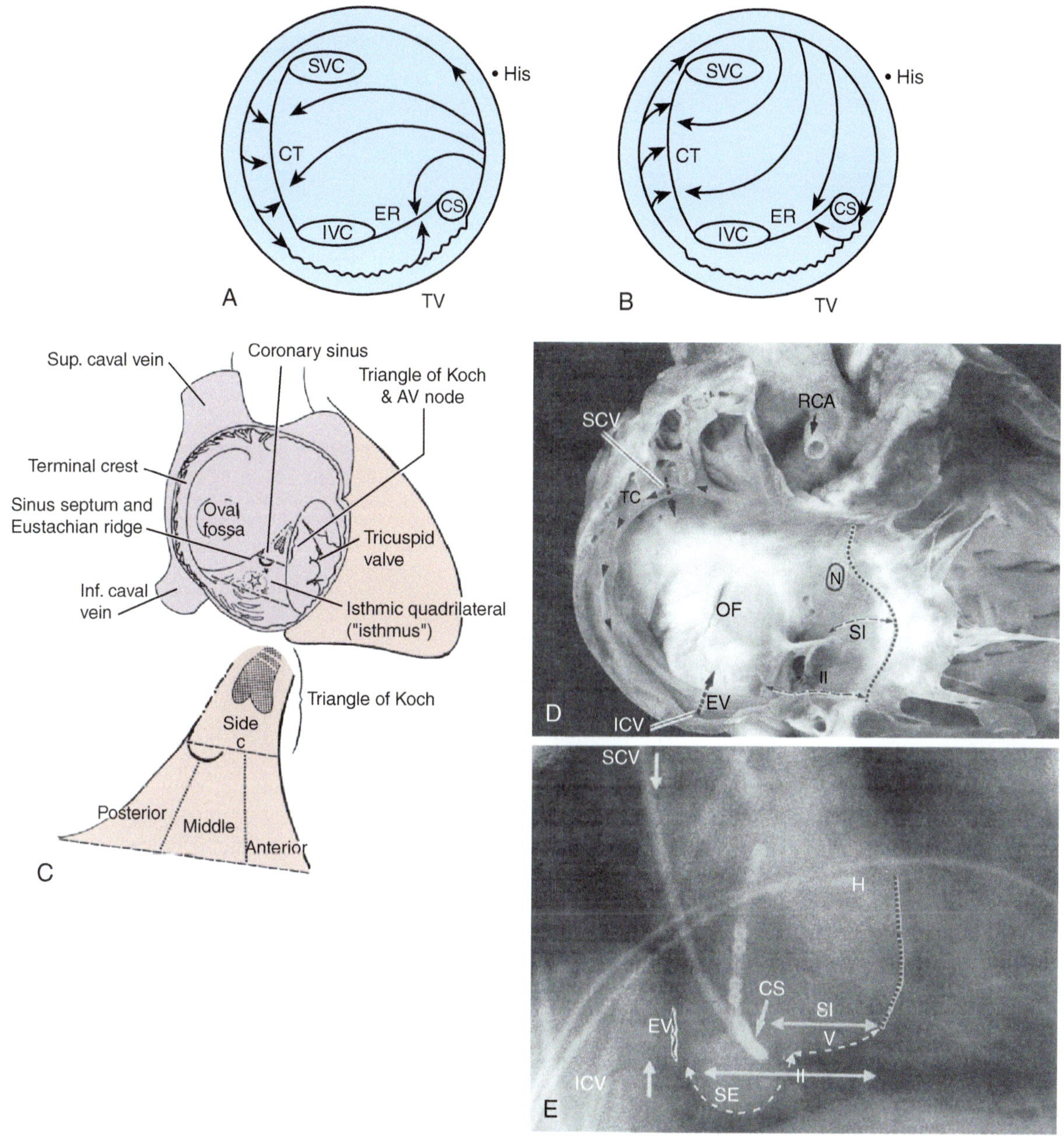

Fig. 12.1 Schematic diagrams showing the activation patterns of CTI-dependent AFL, as viewed from below the tricuspid valve (TV) annulus, looking up into the right atrium. In typical AFL (A), the reentrant wavefront rotates counterclockwise in the right atrium (RA), but in reverse typical AFL (B), reentry is clockwise. Note that the Eustachian ridge (ER) and crista terminalis (CT) form lines of block and that an area of slow conduction (wavy line) is present in the CTI (between the ER and TV annulus). *CS,* Coronary sinus ostium; *His,* His bundle; *SVC,* superior vena cava. (C–E) Anatomy of the CTI. A schematic diagram of the right atrium (C) shows the CTI (*expanded insert*), which is posterior and inferior to the triangle of Koch. Pathologic specimen (D) showing the heart in right anterior oblique (RAO) view. Note the complex anatomy of the cavotricuspid isthmus. The hinge of the TV is shown by the dotted line (E). *SI,* Septal isthmus; *II,* inferior isthmus; *EV,* Eustachian valve; *N,* AV nodal area; *OF,* foramen ovale; *SVC,* superior vena cava. € RAO angiogram of the CTI. A pouch-like sub-Eustachian sinus (SE) is seen adjacent to the vestibule region of the isthmus (V). *H,* His catheter. (From Cabrera JA, Sanchez-Quintana D, Ho SY, et al. The architecture of the atrial musculature between the orifice of the inferior caval vein and the tricuspid valve: the anatomy of the isthmus. *J Cardiovasc Electrophysiol.* 1998;9:1186–1195.)

the CTI, relative to the interatrial septum and right atrial free wall, may be caused in part by the anisotropic fiber orientation in the CTI.[7–10,22,23] This may also predispose to the development of unidirectional block during rapid atrial pacing, accounting for the observation that typical (CCW) AFL is more likely to be induced when pacing is performed from the CS ostium, and reverse typical (CW) AFL when pacing is from the low lateral right atrium.[24]

Lower-loop reentry is an isthmus-dependent flutter in which the caudal-to-cranial limb of the wavefront crosses over gaps

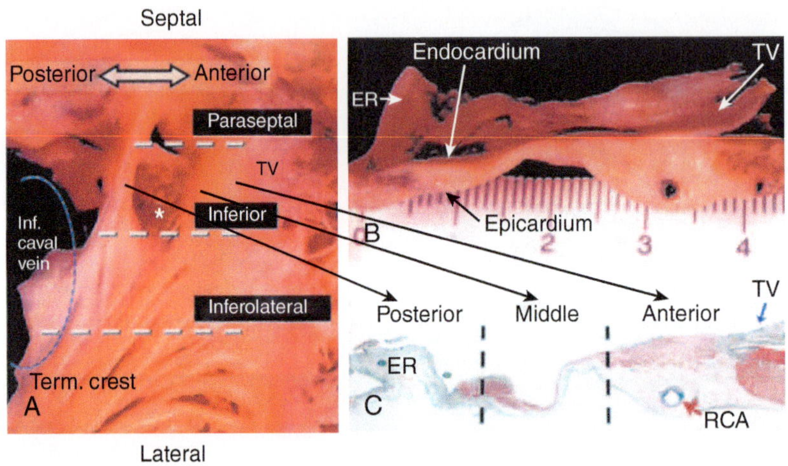

Fig. 12.2 (A) The endocardial surface of the right atrial cavotricuspid isthmus (CTI) is displayed to show the three levels. Note the pouch at the central isthmus and the distal ramifications of the terminal (Term.) crest that feed into the inferolateral CTI. (B and C) The CTI viewed in profile. The histologic section shows myocardium in *red* and fibrous tissue in *blue*. The anterior sector corresponds to the vestibule leading to the tricuspid valve (TV) and is related to the right coronary artery (RCA). The posterior sector is closest to the orifice of the inferior vena cava and contains the Eustachian valve or ridge (ER) (Masson trichrome stain). (From Cabrera JA. The inferior right atrial isthmus: further architectural insights for current and coming ablation technologies. *J Cardiovasc Electrophysiol*. 2005;16:402–408.)

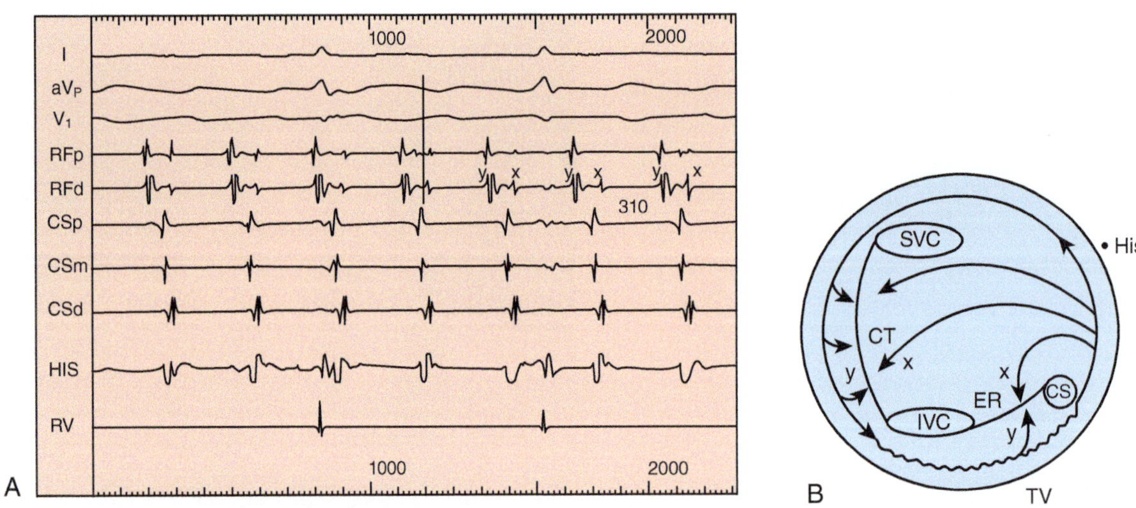

Fig. 12.3 (A) Surface electrocardiographic leads I, aVF, and V_1 and endocardial electrograms (EGMs) in a patient with typical atrial flutter (AFL) demonstrating double potentials (*x,y*) recorded along the Eustachian ridge (ER) by the ablation catheter (RFd and RFp). Note that the *x* and *y* potentials straddle the onset of the initial downstroke of the F wave in lead aVF (vertical line), indicating that the *x* potential is recorded immediately after the activation wavefront exits the sub-Eustachian isthmus and circulates around the coronary sinus above the ER. The *y* potential is recorded after the activation wavefront has rotated entirely around the atrium and is proceeding through the sub-Eustachian isthmus below the ER. Double potentials may similarly be recorded along the crista terminalis (CT). (B) Schematic diagram of the right atrium indicates where double potentials (*x,y*) may be recorded along the ER and CT during typical AFL. CSp, CSm, and CSd are electrograms recorded, respectively, from the proximal, middle, and distal electrode pairs on a quadripolar catheter in the coronary sinus (CS) with the proximal pair at the ostium. *His*, Electrogram from the His-bundle catheter; *IVC*, inferior vena cava; *RFp* and *RFd*, electrograms from the proximal and distal electrode pairs of the mapping and ablation catheter with the distal pair positioned on the ER; *RV*, right ventricle electrogram; *SVC*, superior vena cava; *TV*, tricuspid valve.

in the crista terminalis in the inferior to middle right atrium (Fig. 12.4A).[25,26] The circuit is essentially around the ostium of the IVC in the right atrium. The direction of rotation may be CW or CCW. This variant activation sequence may be sustained, or it may interconvert with other forms of AFL.

Partial isthmus flutter is another variant in which the CCW reentrant wavefront "short-circuits" through the Eustachian ridge barrier to pass between the IVC and the CS ostium (see Fig. 12.4B).[25] The wavefront then propagates in a CW direction through the medial end of the CTI to collide with the wavefront

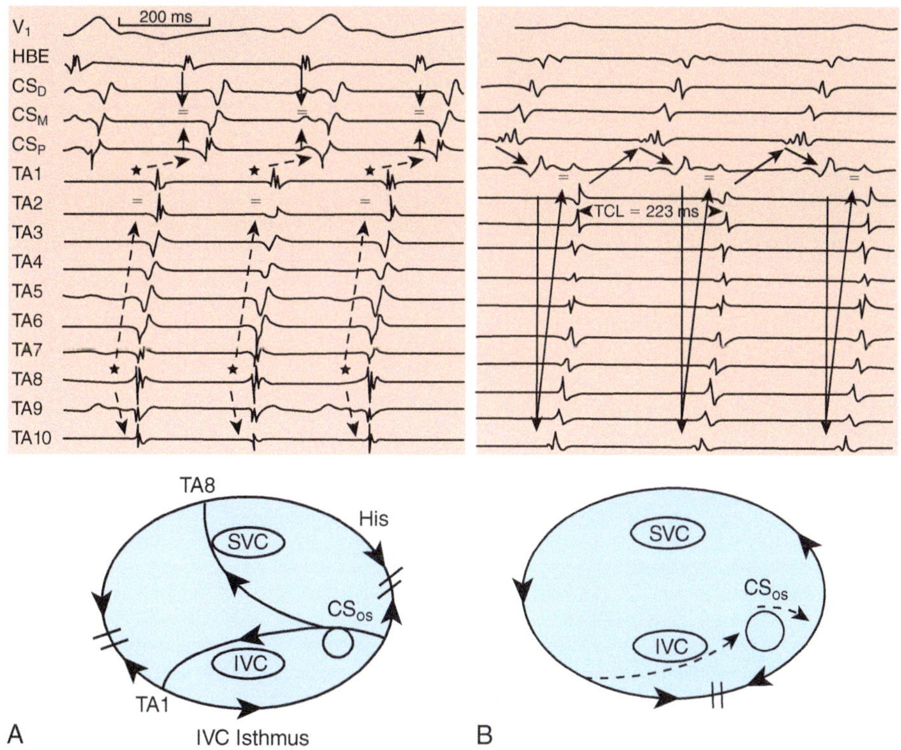

Fig. 12.4 Electrograms and schematic representation of atrial activation in lower-loop reentry and partial isthmus-dependent flutter. (A) During lower-loop reentry, the posterior right atrium is part of the reentry circuit around the inferior vena cava, and wavefronts collide in the lateral right atrium. The electrograms show multiple collisions at recording sites on the lateral right atrial wall TA1 and TA8 (*stars*). (B) During partial isthmus dependent flutter, the wavefront bypasses the anterior CTI near the TVA by passing through the Eustachian ridge posterior to the coronary sinus ostium (CSos). The coronary sinus ostium is activated prematurely, and the tachycardia is not entrained from the medial CTI itself. *IVC*, Inferior vena cava; *SVC*, superior vena cava; *TA1*, distal recording electrodes on halo catheter near lateral aspect of the CTI; *TA10*, proximal recording electrodes on halo catheter near upper septum. (From Yang Y, Cheng J, Bochoeyer A, et al. Atypical right atrial flutter patterns. *Circulation*. 2001;103:3092–3098.)

that is also conducting through the isthmus from its lateral aspect.

Intraisthmus reentry (IIR) is a microreentrant atrial flutter localized within the septal region of the CTI (Fig. 12.5). In a prospective series of patients with IIR reported by the Yang et al.,[27,28] around half of patients (57%) with intraisthmus had prior CTI ablation. IIR was often diagnosed in patients (21%) with recurrent atrial flutter after previous CTI ablation.

DIAGNOSIS

Surface Electrocardiography

The surface 12-lead electrocardiogram (ECG) is helpful in establishing a diagnosis of CTI-dependent AFL, particularly the typical form (Table 12.1). In typical AFL, an inverted sawtooth F-wave pattern is observed in the inferior ECG leads II, III, and aVF, with low-amplitude biphasic F waves in leads I and aVL, an upright F wave in precordial lead V_1, and an inverted F wave in lead V_6 (Fig. 12.6A). In contrast, in reverse typical AFL, the F-wave pattern on the 12-lead ECG is less specific and variable, often with a sine wave pattern in the inferior ECG leads (see Fig. 12.6B). The determinants of F-wave pattern on ECG are largely dependent on the activation sequence of the left atrium, resulting from reentry in the right atrium. Inverted F waves are inscribed in the inferior ECG leads in typical AFL, because of activation of the left atrium initially posteriorly near the CS, and upright F waves are inscribed in the inferior ECG leads in reverse typical AFL because of activation of the left atrium initially anteriorly, near Bachmann bundle.[29,30] However, because the typical and reverse typical forms of CTI-dependent AFL use the same reentry circuit, but in opposite directions, their rates are often similar. It has also been shown that the ECG presentation of typical AFL can be dramatically altered by ablation in the left atrium for atrial fibrillation.[31]

The ECG presentation of lower-loop reentry is highly variable, depending on the caudal-to-cranial level of wavefront breakthrough across the crista terminalis.[26] CCW lower-loop reentry may resemble typical AFL because of similar patterns of activation of the atrial septum and left atrium. A decrease in the late inferior forces may be evident in lower-loop reentry, because of wavefront collision in the lateral right atrium. With multiple or variable wavefront breaks in the lateral atrium, unusual and changing ECG patterns may be observed. Alternation of P-wave polarity from positive to negative in V_1 may occur.[26] CW lower-loop reentry typically demonstrates positive flutter waves in the inferior leads and negative flutter waves in V_1.

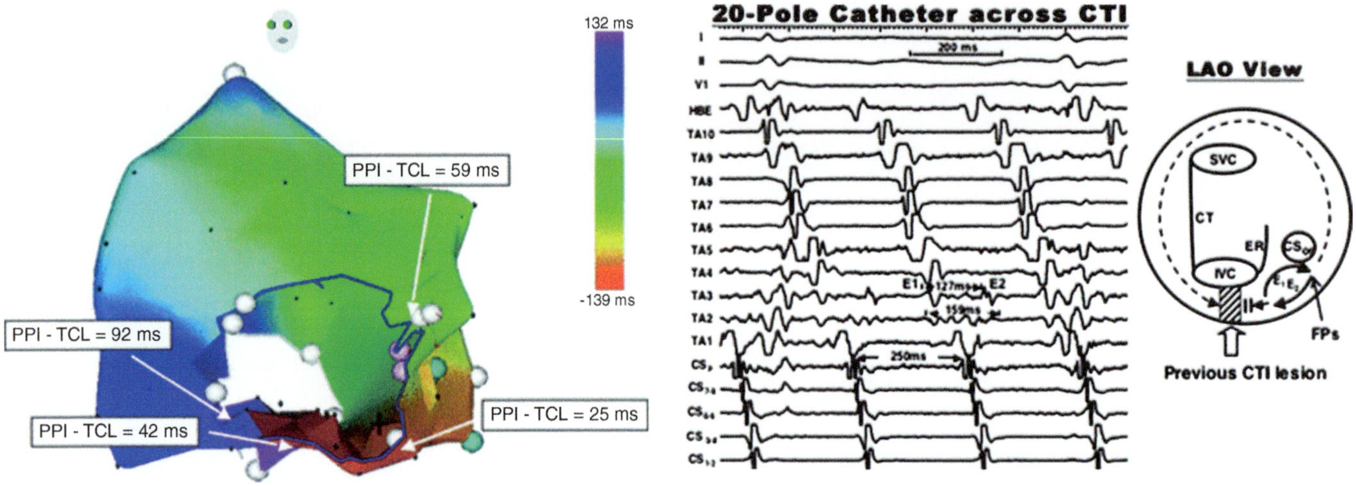

A B

Fig. 12.5 (A) CARTO map in a patient with intraisthmus reentry with a counterclockwise activation sequence around the tricuspid valve annulus (TVA). In the left anterior oblique (LAO) view, the earliest activation was at the septal cavotricuspid isthmus (CTI) and latest activation at the lateral CTI, resulting in an "early meets late" activation pattern at the CTI. The mapped cycle length spanned 99% of the tachycardia cycle length (TCL). However, the postpacing interval (PPI)-TCL interval, measured at different sites around the TVA, showed that only the septal CTI was in the circuit. (B) Simultaneous surface electrocardiogram recordings (leads I, II, and V_1), a His bundle (HBE), coronary sinus (CS), and duodecapolar catheter positioned around the TVA, with its distal electrode (TA1) across the CTI at CS ostium and proximal electrode (TA10) close to the high lateral TVA in a patient with typical AFL (cycle length 250 ms). The electrodes TA1–3 were located within the septal CTI (from the CS ostium to 6 o'clock on the TVA). Note the low-amplitude fractionated potentials (FPs) with a duration of 159 ms, recorded at TA2, which spanned 64% of the TCL, and the double potentials (DPs) with E1–2 interval of 127 ms recorded at TA3. A combination of the recordings from TA1 to TA3 (i.e., both FPs and DPs) spanned more than two-thirds of the TCL. In this patient, entrainment pacing from the septal CTI during the tachycardia showed a PPI–TCL ≤ 25 ms, whereas pacing from the lateral CTI showed a PPI–TCL greater than 25 ms. Radiofrequency catheter ablation at the septal CTI, where the FPs were recorded, terminated the AFL, and it was no longer inducible after ablation. The schematic diagram to the right of the figure shows the proposed reentrant circuit. (From Yang Y, Varma N, Badhwar N, et al. Prospective observations in the clinical and electrophysiologic characteristics of intra-isthmus reentry. *J Cardiovasc Electrophysiol.* 2010;21:1099–1106.)

TABLE 12.1 Diagnostic Criteria for Isthmus-Dependent Flutters

Type of Flutter	Criteria
Surface ECG	
Typical flutter	Sawtooth inverted F-wave pattern in the inferior ECG leads and in V_1
Reverse typical flutter	Sine-wave or upright F-wave pattern in the inferior ECG leads
Lower loop reentry	Variable; often resembles typical flutter if counterclockwise; clockwise rotation usually yields upright F waves inferiorly and inverted in V_1
Partial isthmus reentry	Poorly described; probably similar to typical flutter
EP Testing	
Isthmus-dependent flutters	Demonstration of entrainment criteria during pacing from the CTI, Including the following:
	First postpacing interval <30 ms longer than tachycardia cycle length
	Stimulus-to–F-wave interval equal to electrogram-to–F-wave interval on pacing catheter
	Identical paced F wave morphology and atrial activation sequence
	Macroreentrant RA activation by standard activation or electroanatomical mapping with entire tachycardia cycle length represented in right atrium
Typical flutter	Concealed entrainment from CTI and counterclockwise macroreentrant RA activation
Reverse typical flutter	Concealed entrainment from CTI and clockwise macroreentrant RA activation
Lower loop reentry	Concealed entrainment from both CTI and low posterior right atrium with clockwise or counterclockwise macroreentrant RA activation
Partial isthmus dependent	Concealed entrainment from lateral but not medial margin of CTI; early coronary sinus ostium activation during flutter; wavefront collision in CTI; counterclockwise macroreentrant RA activation

CTI, Cavotricuspid isthmus; *ECG*, electrocardiogram; *RA*, right atrial.

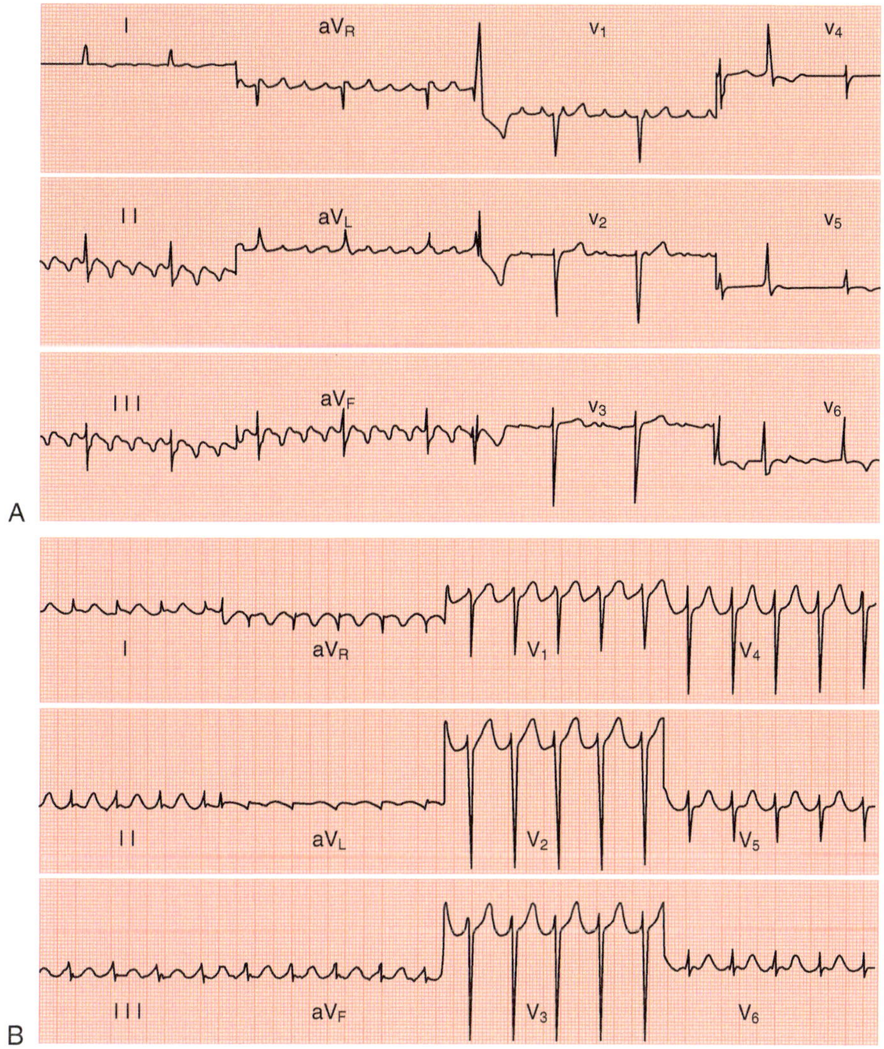

Fig. 12.6 (A) A 12-lead electrocardiogram recorded during typical atrial flutter (AFL). Note the sawtooth F-wave pattern in the inferior leads II, III, and aVF. Typical AFL is also characterized by flat to biphasic F waves in I and aVL, respectively; an upright F wave in V_1; and an inverted F wave in V_6. (B) 12-lead electrocardiogram from a patient with the reverse typical AFL. The F wave in reverse typical AFL has a less distinct, sine-wave pattern, in the inferior leads. In this case, the F waves are upright in the inferior leads II, III, and aVF; biphasic in leads I, aVL, and V_1; and upright in V_6.

The ECG description of partial isthmus-dependent flutter is incomplete, but it may be expected to resemble typical AFL, given their similar patterns of atrial activation.[25] The surface ECG pattern of IIR is variable, with 86% of cases resembling typical CCW AFL and 21% of cases exhibiting atypical AFL (positive F waves in inferior leads and V_1). In the majority of patients with IIR (79%), a distinct isoelectric period was observed between surface F waves, which were often low amplitude or flat.[27–29]

Electrophysiologic Study

Despite the use of the 12-lead ECG in making a presumptive diagnosis of typical AFL, an electrophysiologic study with mapping and entrainment should be performed to confirm the underlying mechanism if RFCA is to be successfully performed (see Table 12.1). This is particularly true in the cases of reverse typical AFL and CTI-dependent flutter following left atrial ablation, which are much more difficult to diagnose on 12-lead ECG.

For the electrophysiologic study of AFL, activation mapping may be performed using multielectrode catheters or three-dimensional (3D) electroanatomical computerized activation mapping systems. For standard multielectrode catheter mapping, catheters are positioned in the right atrium, His-bundle region, and CS. To most precisely elucidate the endocardial activation sequence, a duodecapolar catheter (e.g., halo 20-electrode mapping catheter) may be positioned in the right atrium around the TVA (Fig. 12.7). These catheters may extend to the lateral CTI or cross the entire CTI into the CS, depending on design. The latter obviates the need for a separate CS catheter. Recordings obtained during AFL from all electrodes are then analyzed to determine the right atrial activation sequence.

For patients who present to the laboratory in sinus rhythm, it is necessary to induce AFL to confirm its mechanism.

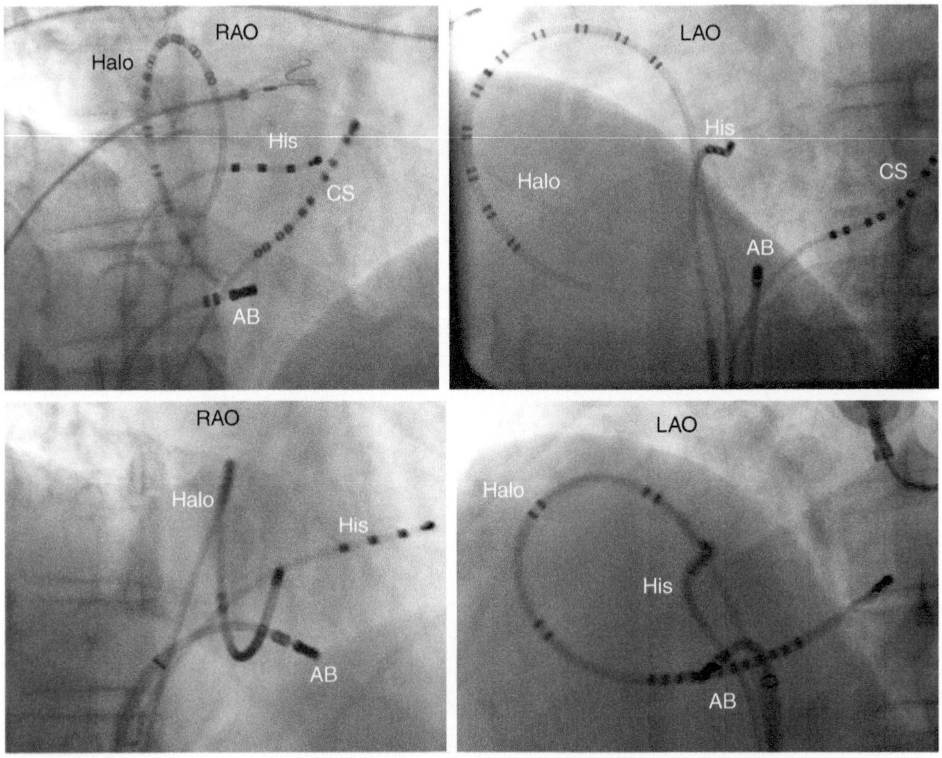

Fig. 12.7 Right anterior oblique (*left*) and left anterior oblique fluoroscopic (*right*) projections showing the intracardiac positions of the His bundle (His), coronary sinus (CS), halo (halo), and ablation catheters (AB). Two types of multielectrode mapping catheters are shown. This design (*top*) does not span the cavotricuspid isthmus (CTI). In this patient, the ablation catheter is septal and withdrawn to the posterior CTI near the inferior vena cava. This design (*bottom*) spans the CTI with closely spaced electrodes and continues into the coronary sinus. In this patient, the ablation catheter is over the central part of the CTI near the tricuspid valve annulus.

Induction of AFL is accomplished by atrial programmed stimulation or burst pacing, usually from the CS ostium or low lateral right atrium. The direction of AFL induced (e.g., CCW vs. CW) may depend in part on the pacing site. For burst pacing, cycle lengths between 180 and 240 ms are typically effective in producing unidirectional CTI block and inducing AFL. Induction of AFL typically occurs immediately after the onset of unidirectional CTI isthmus block or after a brief period of rapid atrial tachycardia or atrial fibrillation.[24] During electrophysiologic study, a diagnosis of either typical or reverse typical AFL is suggested by observing a CCW or CW activation pattern in the right atrium around the TVA, respectively. For example, as seen in Fig. 12.8A and Video 12.1 and Video 12.2, in a patient with typical AFL, the initial atrial activation is recorded at the CS ostium (i.e., CS os EGM), which is timed with the initial downstroke of the F wave in the inferior surface ECG leads, followed by caudal-to-cranial activation in the interatrial septum (i.e., His-bundle atrial EGM), then cranial-to-caudal activation in the right atrial free wall (i.e., proximal to distal EGMs on the duodecapolar catheter), and finally to the CTI (i.e., ablation catheter atrial EGM), demonstrating that the underlying mechanism is a CCW macroreentry circuit around the TVA encompassing the entire tachycardia cycle length. In a patient with reverse typical AFL, the mirror image of this activation pattern is seen (see Fig. 12.8B).

In addition, confirmation that the AFL reentry circuit uses the CTI, requires demonstration of classical criteria for entrainment, including concealed entrainment, during pacing from the CTI, and constant fusion from a site or sites outside the CTI (often the lateral right atrium).[5] Criteria for demonstrating concealed entrainment of AFL include acceleration of the tachycardia to the pacing cycle length without a change in the F-wave pattern on surface ECG or endocardial atrial activation pattern and EGM morphology, as well as immediate resumption of the tachycardia at the original cycle length on termination of pacing, including the first postpacing interval (i.e., the postpacing interval minus tachycardia cycle length, or PPI-TCL, should be less than 30 ms; Fig. 12.9). Concealed entrainment is further confirmed, during pacing from the CTI, if the stimulus-to–F-wave or stimulus-to-reference EGM interval during pacing, and the pacing electrode EGM-to–F-wave or pacing EGM-to-reference EGM interval during AFL are the same (see Fig. 12.9). Furthermore, during typical AFL, the stimulus-to–F-wave or stimulus-to-proximal CS EGM is shorter when the pacing site is medial, near the exit from the CTI (e.g., 30–50 ms), and longer when the pacing site is lateral, near the entrance to the CTI (e.g., 80–100 ms). The converse is true during reverse typical AFL. In contrast, pacing at sites outside the CTI results in manifest entrainment of AFL, with progressive fusion of the F postpacing interval wave pattern and endocardial atrial EGMs at progressively shorter cycle lengths faster than the AFL cycle length.

The diagnosis of lower loop reentrant AFL is confirmed by demonstration of concealed entrainment of the tachycardia from not only the CTI but also the inferoposterior right

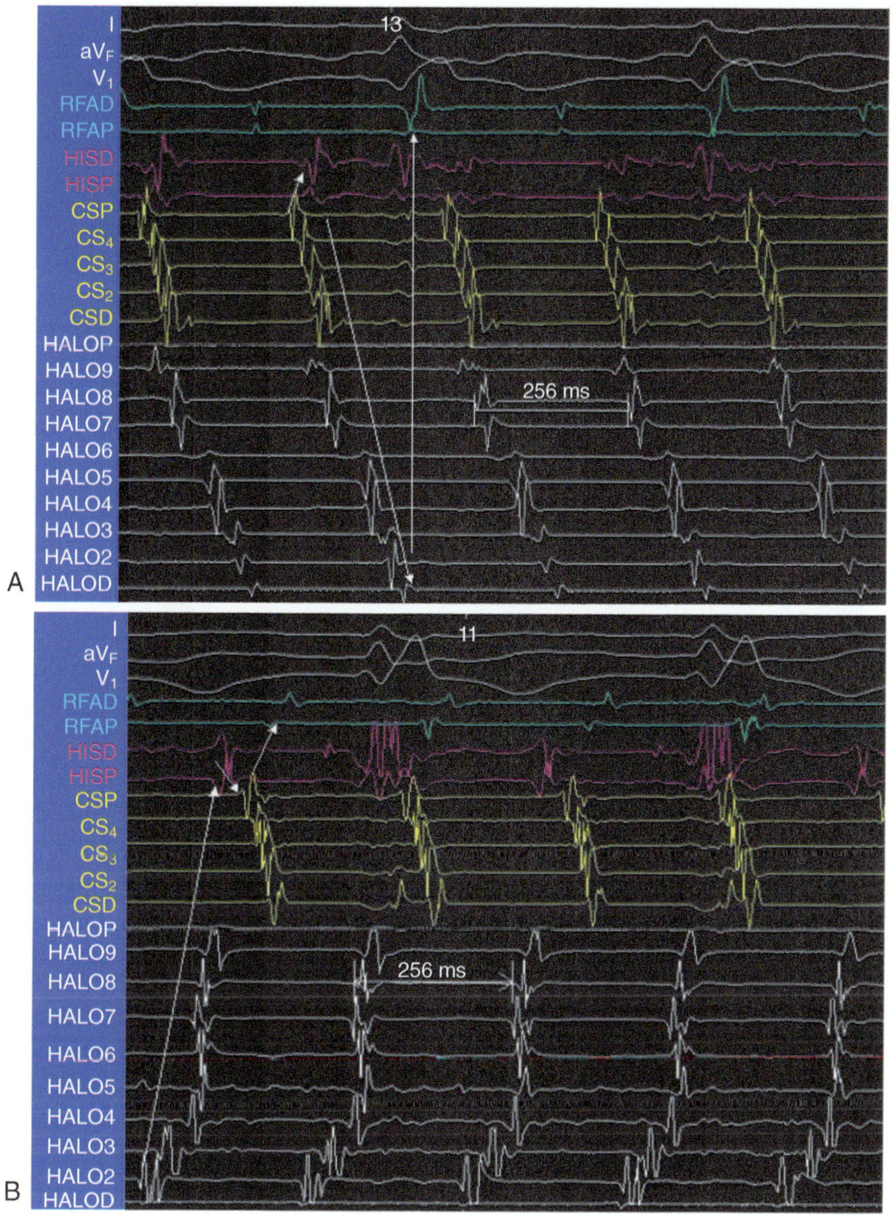

Fig. 12.8 Endocardial electrograms from the mapping and ablation, multielectrode halo, coronary sinus (CS), and His-bundle catheters and surface electrocardiogram leads I, aVF, and V_1, demonstrating a counterclockwise rotation of activation in the right atrium in a patient with typical atrial flutter (AFL) (A) and a clockwise rotation of activation in the right atrium in a patient with reverse typical AFL (B). The cycle length was 256 ms for both the typical and reverse-typical forms of AFL. *Arrows* demonstrate the activation sequence. The HALOD through HALOP tracings are 10 bipolar electrograms recorded from the distal (low lateral right atrium) to the proximal (high right atrium) poles of the 20-pole halo catheter positioned around the tricuspid valve annulus, with the proximal electrode pair at 1 o'clock and the distal electrode pair at 7 o'clock. CSP electrograms were recorded from the CS catheter proximal electrode pair positioned at the CS ostium, HISP electrograms from the proximal electrode pair of the His-bundle catheter, and RFAD electrograms from the mapping and ablation catheter positioned with the distal electrode pair in the cavotricuspid isthmus.

atrium.[25] Partial isthmus-dependent flutter is confirmed by the demonstration of concealed entrainment from the lateral margin of the CTI but not from the medial portion near the TVA. In addition, there is early activation of the CS ostium and evidence of wavefront collision within the medial CTI. Concealed entrainment should be demonstrable from the area of short-circuit between the Eustachian ridge and CS ostium.

The diagnosis of IIR is confirmed by demonstration of concealed entrainment only within the septal CTI near the CS ostium, while all other areas of the right atrium, left atrium, and CS are out of the circuit (PPI-TCL >25).[27,28] In addition, fractionated potentials and double potentials are often observed within the septal area of the CTI. In rare instances, concealed entrainment and fractionated potentials have also been observed at the

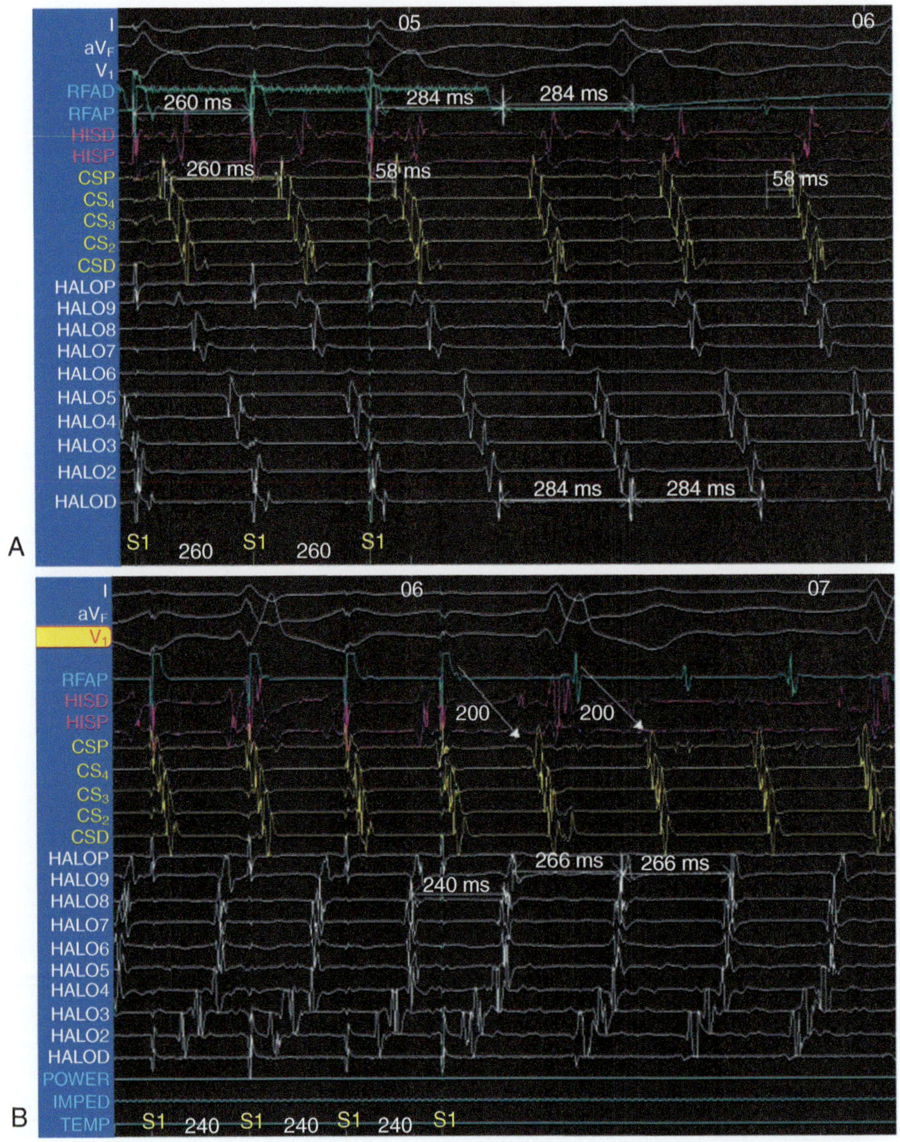

Fig. 12.9 Surface electrocardiogram (ECG) and endocardial electrogram (EGM) recordings during pacing entrainment from the cavotricuspid isthmus in patients with both typical atrial flutter (AFL) (A) and reverse-typical AFL (B). Note in both examples that the tachycardia is accelerated to the pacing cycle length and that the F-wave morphology on surface ECG and endocardial waveforms and the endocardial activation pattern are unchanged during pacing compared with AFL, indicating concealed entrainment. Furthermore, the stimulus-to–F-wave or local EGM intervals are comparable to the EGM-to–F-wave or local EGM intervals recorded on the mapping and ablation catheter (RFAD) during entrainment and AFL in both examples, indicating concealed entrainment. Halo catheter tracings are as described in Fig. 11.7. *CS*, Coronary sinus; *S1*, pacing stimulus artifact.

mid or anteroinferior CTI, indicating extension of the circuit more laterally.

Electroanatomical mapping may not have adequate resolution to identify this microreentrant circuit. It may demonstrate either a focal pattern with total mapped cycle length less than 60% of the tachycardia cycle length with earliest activation arising from the septal CTI near the CS ostium, or it may demonstrate a CCW reentrant pattern around the TVA, with the total mapped cycle length greater than 90% of the TCL, deceptively suggesting the presence of typical CTI-dependent AFL.

The differential diagnosis of AFL from other supraventricular arrhythmias is usually apparent given typical ECG manifestations and variable ventriculoatrial relationships. The most important distinction to be made is the exclusion of a focal atrial tachycardia. Rarely, focal atrial tachycardia in the low posteroseptal right atrium may be confused with AFL if unidirectional CTI conduction block (i.e., medial-to-lateral block) is present. Otherwise, the atrial tachycardia can be recognized by failure to entrain it from the CTI and by a radial activation pattern.

ABLATION

Techniques of Ablation

For ablation of CTI-dependent AFL, the most common approach is to create a line of bidirectional conduction block across the CTI, from the TVA to the IVC. For this purpose, a variety of mapping and ablation catheters, with different shapes and curve lengths, as well as RF generators, are available from several commercial manufacturers.[2–4,6,32–34] We prefer to use a standard-curve ablation catheter (Blazer 8-mm tip, mid-distal standard curve, Boston Scientific, Inc., Natick, MA) or an externally irrigated ablation catheter (Thermocool ST, Biosense Webster, Diamond Bar, CA; Tacticath, Abbott Laboratories, Chicago, IL) because it has been shown that the use of large-tip (8–10 mm) ablation catheters or irrigated ablation catheters reduces procedure durations and improves success rates compared with use of standard 4-mm RF electrodes.[35–37] The smaller electrode (3.5 mm) on irrigated catheter designs may provide better near-field EGM resolution than large-tip electrodes as well. Long, fixed-curve guide sheaths (e.g., SR0 or SL1, St. Jude, Inc., St. Paul, MN) or steerable deflectable sheaths (e.g., Agilis, St. Jude, Inc.) are also useful to improve catheter reach, stability, and tissue contact. There is also published evidence that large-tip ablation catheters are most useful for flat CTI anatomy, whereas irrigated designs may be more advantageous in the presence of CTI pouches.[38] When using fixed-curve or steerable sheaths, it is important that the curvatures of the sheath and catheter remain coaxial. Paradoxically, rotating the sheath to point into the septum may limit the septal motion of the catheter.

The target for CTI-dependent AFL ablation is the CTI (Table 12.2), which, when standard multipolar electrode catheters are used for mapping and ablation, is localized with a combined fluoroscopically and electrophysiologically guided approach.[2–4,6,32–42] The usual target for the ablation line is the central isthmus because the CTI is narrowest at this point (i.e., distance from TVA to IVC) and has the thinnest musculature.[15] This site is located at 6 o'clock in the LAO view (see Fig. 12.7). One drawback to ablation of the central isthmus is the frequent occurrence of pouches in this region. Pouches may be avoided by ablating the lateral isthmus (7 o'clock in LAO projection). However, there are thicker right atrial musculature and terminal pectinate muscles found here. The medial isthmus is devoid of pectinate musculature but contains the thickest atrial muscular layer and is nearest to the right coronary artery and AV nodal extensions. Typically, the ablation catheter is positioned using fluoroscopic guidance (see Fig. 12.7) or electroanatomical mapping, in the central CTI, with the distal ablation electrode on or near the TVA in the right anterior oblique (RAO) view, and midway between the septum and low right atrial free wall (6- or-7 o'clock position) in the LAO view. The distal ablation electrode position is then adjusted toward or away from the TVA, based on the ratio of atrial and ventricular EGM amplitudes (A/V ratio) recorded by the bipolar ablation electrode. An optimal ratio is 1:2 or 1:4 at the TVA, as seen in Fig. 12.8A on the ablation electrode. After the ablation catheter is positioned on or near the TVA, it is very slowly withdrawn during ablation toward the IVC while RF energy is applied continuously.

Alternatively, the ablation catheter can be withdrawn in a stepwise manner, a few millimeters at a time (usually less than or equal to the length of the distal ablation electrode), with 30- to 60-second pauses at each location, during a continuous or interrupted energy application. For irrigated electrodes, a maximal power of 35–50 W and a temperature of 40°C–45°C should be used.[35–38] In contrast, the large-tip (i.e., 8–10 mm) ablation catheters require a higher power, up to 100 W, to achieve target temperatures of 50°C–60°C, because of the greater energy-dispersive effects of the larger ablation electrode. Use of large-tip ablation catheters also requires the use of two grounding pads applied to the patient's skin to avoid skin burns.[38,40–42] Excessive impedance drops (i.e., >10–20 Ω from baseline) should be avoided, to prevent tissue overheating and steam pops. CTI ablation can be performed with standard 4-mm-tipped RF catheters (50 W, 50°C–65°C), although the use of these catheters is associated with longer procedure and ablation times, lower acute success rates, and much higher recurrence rates. EGM recordings may be used in addition to fluoroscopy to ensure that the ablation electrode is in contact with viable tissue in the CTI throughout each energy application. More recent studies have suggested that real-time contact force measuring catheters may help reduce total ablation time required to produce acute CTI conduction block, since standard surrogates of tissue contact (e.g., impedance, EGM amplitude) may not be adequate during CTI ablation.[43,44]

Ablation across the entire CTI (Fig. 12.10) may require several sequential 30- to 60-second energy applications during a stepwise catheter pullback, or a prolonged energy application of

TABLE 12.2 Targets for Ablation of Isthmus-Dependent Flutters

Type of Flutter	Targets
CTI dependent	CTI from TVA to IVC
	TVA to Eustachian ridge
	TVA to CS ostium to Eustachian ridge
	Maximal electrogram voltage recorded online
Partial isthmus dependent	CS ostium to IVC

CS, Coronary sinus; *CTI*, cavotricuspid isthmus; *IVC*, inferior vena cava; *TVA*, tricuspid valve annulus.

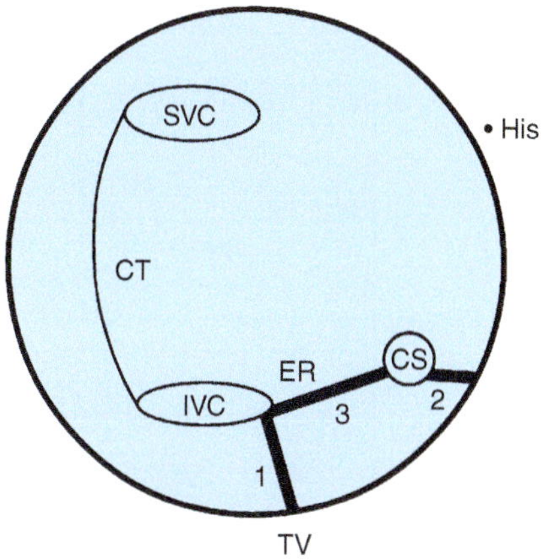

Fig. 12.10 Schematic diagram of the right atrium in the right anterior oblique view, showing the typical locations for linear ablation of the cavotricuspid isthmus (line 1), the tricuspid valve (TV)–coronary sinus (CS) isthmus (line 2), and the CS–inferior vena cava (IVC) isthmus (line 3). *CT*, Crista terminalis; *ER*, Eustachian ridge; *His*, His bundle; *SVC*, superior vena cava.

up to 120 seconds or longer during a continuous catheter pullback. The catheter should be gradually withdrawn until the distal ablation electrode no longer records an atrial EGM, indicating that it has reached the IVC, or until the ablation electrode is noted to abruptly slip off the Eustachian ridge. RF energy application should be immediately interrupted when the catheter has reached the IVC, because ablation in extracardiac venous structures is known to cause significant pain. Computerized 3D mapping systems are useful to document the anatomical placement of ablation lesions and decrease fluoroscopy use.[45] As the ablation catheter approaches the IVC, it is often useful to release the catheter curve slightly and withdraw the sheath and catheter as a unit to allow greater contact between the electrode and the CTI, before the catheter is withdrawn into the IVC.

Ablation of the TV-CS and CS-IVC isthmuses (see Fig. 12.10) may also be performed, using an approach similar to that used for CTI ablation.[46] However, for this approach to be successful, it may be necessary to ablate within the CS ostium, which may be associated with a higher risk of complications such as AV node block. It has also been reported that CTI-dependent AFL may be cured by ablating between the TVA and Eustachian ridge only, which is a narrower isthmus than the CTI.[47] During repeat ablation, it may be necessary to rotate the ablation catheter away from the initial line of energy application, either medially or laterally in the CTI, to create new or additional lines of block, or to use a higher power or higher ablation temperature, or both. In addition if ablation is initially attempted using a standard 4- to 5-mm-tip electrode and fails, repeat ablation with a large-tip electrode catheter or a cooled-tip ablation catheter may be successful.[35–42]

Ablation of partial isthmus-dependent flutter requires creation of a line of block from the CS ostium to the IVC, eliminating conduction across the Eustachian ridge. Completion of this line may convert the tachycardia to typical isthmus-dependent flutter, which then requires ablation of the entire CTI.[25]

In many cases, the CTI is composed of discrete muscle bundles embedded within connective tissue. Therefore, a continuous ablation line may be unnecessary to achieve conduction block. To reduce procedure times and unnecessary ablation, the maximal voltage-guided CTI technique has been introduced.[48,49] Bipolar EGMs are recorded from the ablation catheter in the central CTI during AFL or during CS pacing. As the catheter is withdrawn from the TVA to the IVC, the locations with the largest peak-to-peak bipolar voltage are marked. The ablation catheter is then returned to those sites of maximal voltage, and RF energy is delivered for 60 seconds or until there is greater than 50% reduction in the EGM voltage. The line is then remapped for the largest remaining EGM voltage and the procedure repeated until CTI block is confirmed. In randomized trials, the voltage-guided technique has been reported to reduce ablation time, number of lesions, and procedure and fluoroscopy times compared with the conventional anatomical approach.[48,49] However, whether such a limited approach will yield high long-term outcome results has not been studied.

After the termination of flutter, fewer than half of patients demonstrate bidirectional CTI block, and further ablation is often needed.[50] Persistent CTI conduction can be detected by pacing medial (i.e., proximal coronary sinus) or lateral (i.e., low lateral right atrium) to the ablation line and mapping the line for conduction gaps. The presence of split EGMs with less than 90 ms between EGM components is suggestive of a conductive gap in the line.[50] As the line is systematically mapped, the split EGM components draw closer together as the gap is approached. The gap itself is identified as a single or fractionated potential along the line bounded by split EGMs (Fig. 12.11).

Ablation of the CTI for AFL has also been performed using a linear microwave ablation catheter system (Medwaves, Inc., Rancho Bernardo, CA) with antenna lengths up to 4 cm.[51] These studies have shown the feasibility of linear microwave ablation of the CTI, which has the potential advantage of rapid ablation

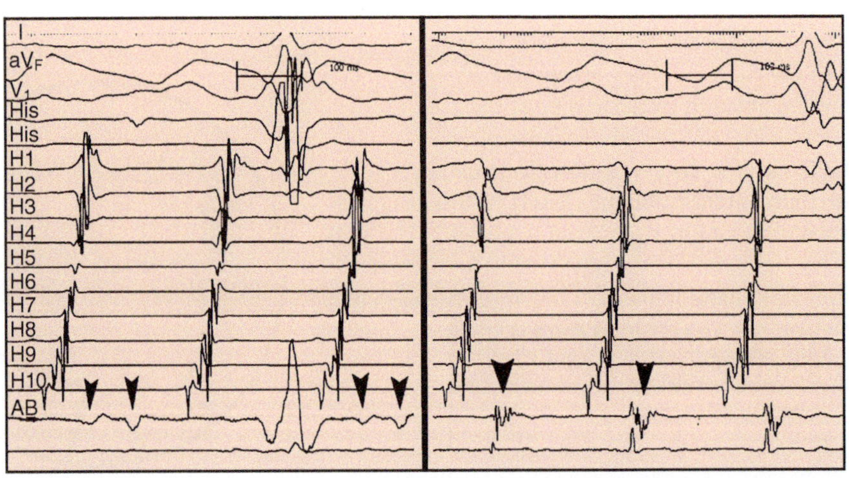

Fig. 12.11 Mapping for a gap in the ablation line in the cavotricuspid isthmus. In this patient, a previous attempt to terminate typical atrial flutter (AFL) had failed. *Left*, The ablation catheter (AB) records low-amplitude split electrograms (EGMs) (*arrowheads*) along the prior ablation line. The interval between EGM components was 70 ms during AFL. *Right*, With further interrogation of the ablation line, a site with a single-component, fractionated EGM (*arrowheads*) was identified. Ablation at this site terminated AFL in less than 2 seconds and created bidirectional block. Surface electrocardiogram leads I, aVF, and V_1 are shown. *His*, His channels; *H1 through H10*, halo catheter channels from distal to proximal.

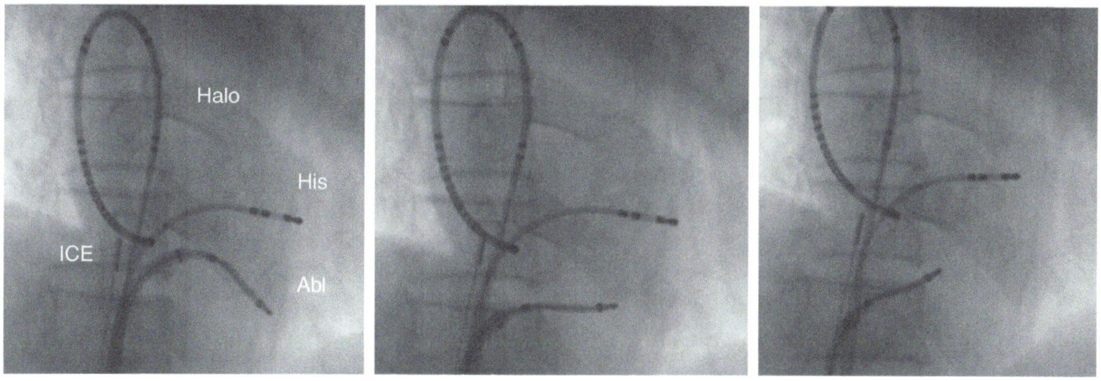

Fig. 12.12 Fluoroscopic right anterior oblique view of the Medwaves, Inc., microwave ablation (Abl) antenna positioned across the cavotricuspid isthmus (CTI). *Left,* Ablation antenna positioned near the tricuspid valve annulus (TVA). *Middle,* Ablation antenna at the middle CTI between the TVA and Eustachian ridge. *Right,* Ablation antenna withdrawn near the inferior vena cava. *Halo,* Halo catheter; *His,* His bundle; *ICE,* intracardiac echocardiography.

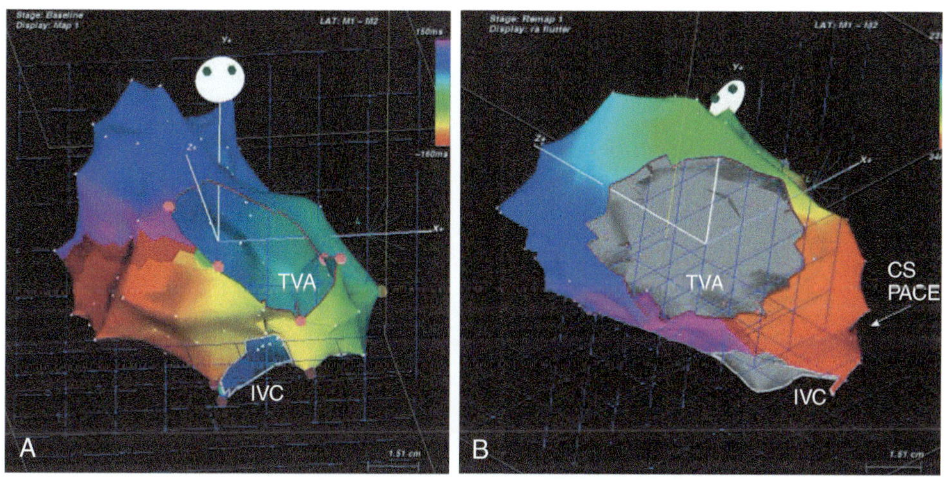

Fig. 12.13 Three-dimensional electroanatomical (CARTO system, Biosense Webster, Diamond Bar, CA) map of the right atrium in a patient with typical atrial flutter (AFL), before (A) and after (B) cavotricuspid isthmus (CTI) ablation. Note the counterclockwise activation pattern around the TVA during AFL (A, anteroposterior view), which is based on a color scheme indicating activation time from orange (early) to purple (late). After CTI ablation (B, left anterior oblique caudal view), during pacing from the coronary sinus (CS) ostium, there is evidence of medial-to-lateral CTI conduction block, as indicated by juxtaposition of orange and purple color in the CTI. *IVC,* Inferior vena cava; *TVA,* tricuspid valve annulus.

of the CTI with a single energy application over the entire length of the ablation electrode (Fig. 12.12). In addition, studies of catheter cryoablation (CCA) of the CTI have been done as well.[52,53] In a randomized trial of CCA using a 9-F catheter with an 8-mm tip compared to RFCA using an 8-F catheter with a 3.5-mm open irrigated tip, there was comparable acute and chronic efficacy (6 month) of CTI ablation, but longer procedure times with CCA.[52] This study also showed that CCA was perceived as less painful than RFCA.[52]

Computerized 3D mapping systems provide several advantages for CTI ablation but are not required for the procedure.[45] Electroanatomical mapping before ablation can demonstrate the reentry circuit, thus supporting the diagnosis (Fig. 12.13). In addition, 3D anatomical reconstruction may identify the presence of a CTI pouch, and high-voltage EGMs may indicate the presence of pectinate muscle extension into the CTI. During ablation, 3D mapping systems allow for documentation of each ablation lesion delivered, which may be helpful to complete an anatomically based ablation line and identify areas of anatomical gaps. Computerized mapping systems may therefore reduce fluoroscopy times by 50%, compared with conventional approaches.[45] After ablation, detailed electroanatomical mapping may be used to confirm the presence of CTI block or slow conduction as well.

Unlike typical AFL, reverse-typical AFL, lower-loop reentry, and partial isthmus flutter whose circuits all involve the lateral and central CTI, the ablation approach for IIR is slightly modified to interrupt the circuit located in the septal or medial CTI.[27,28] Successful ablation should be achieved by identifying and ablating the site with the longest fractionated potential associated with concealed entrainment and completing a septal CTI line from the tricuspid annulus to the IVC that includes this site.

Overcoming Difficult Cavotricuspid Isthmus Anatomy

The complex anatomy of the CTI may in some cases present difficulties for ablation. The most common problems encountered are the presence of a large CTI pouch, large pectinate muscles, and/or a prominent Eustachian ridge.[54] A pouch is a deep recess in the CTI, that may be skipped over by the ablation electrode during pullback (Fig. 12.14). The junction of the IVC and Eustachian ridge may form a "fulcrum" for the ablation catheter (see Fig. 12.14), preventing the distal ablation electrode from achieving adequate contact with the CTI, especially if there is a pouch in the CTI. The presence of a pouch may be identified by preprocedural CT or MRI, or more commonly by intracardiac echocardiography (ICE) or electroanatomical mapping, during the procedure. Right atrial angiography to identify CTI anatomy may also be performed by injecting 50 mL of contrast over 3–5 seconds through a 5-F pigtail catheter in the upper IVC or IVC–right atrial junction,[18] while imaging in the RAO view.

A CTI pouch may be avoided by a more lateral ablation line. Ablation within a CTI pouch may be accomplished by forming a 180-degree curvature on the ablation catheter (i.e., "knuckle maneuver") in the mid-tricuspid annulus and withdrawing the catheter to enter the pouch perpendicularly (Fig. 12.15). The curvature can be relaxed or tightened to reach the TVA and IVC ends of the pouch, respectively. Because of the restricted blood flow that may occur in a pouch, care should be taken to avoid excessive tissue heating and steam pops.

Large pectinate muscles should be suspected when recording high-voltage EGMs within the CTI during 3D electroanatomical mapping. These may potentially be avoided by ablation in the medial isthmus. Ablation of the high-voltage areas may require protracted (60–120 seconds) RF delivery. On the trabecular prominences, catheter contact may be unstable, whereas in the trabecular valleys, excessive electrode temperatures may result in steam pops (Fig. 12.16).[54] Preformed or deflectable sheaths may enhance tissue contact, and for irrigated ablation, lesion sizes are maximized with the electrode perpendicular to the tissue. And as noted earlier, a voltage-guided approach may limit unnecessary ablation.

A prominent Eustachian ridge can be detected by angiography or ICE (Fig. 12.17). The Eustachian ridge and adjacent tissue can be conductive and require ablation. Not only may the Eustachian ridge cause a fulcrum effect limiting distal ablation electrode contact with parts of the CTI as noted earlier; it may actually shield parts of the CTI entirely from ablation electrode contact (e.g., areas just anterior and below the Eustachian ridge). Again, by using the "knuckle maneuver," the electrode may be brought into contact with both the IVC and CTI sides of the Eustachian ridge for successful ablation (see Fig. 12.17).[54] This limitation may also be overcome by use of a preformed sheath

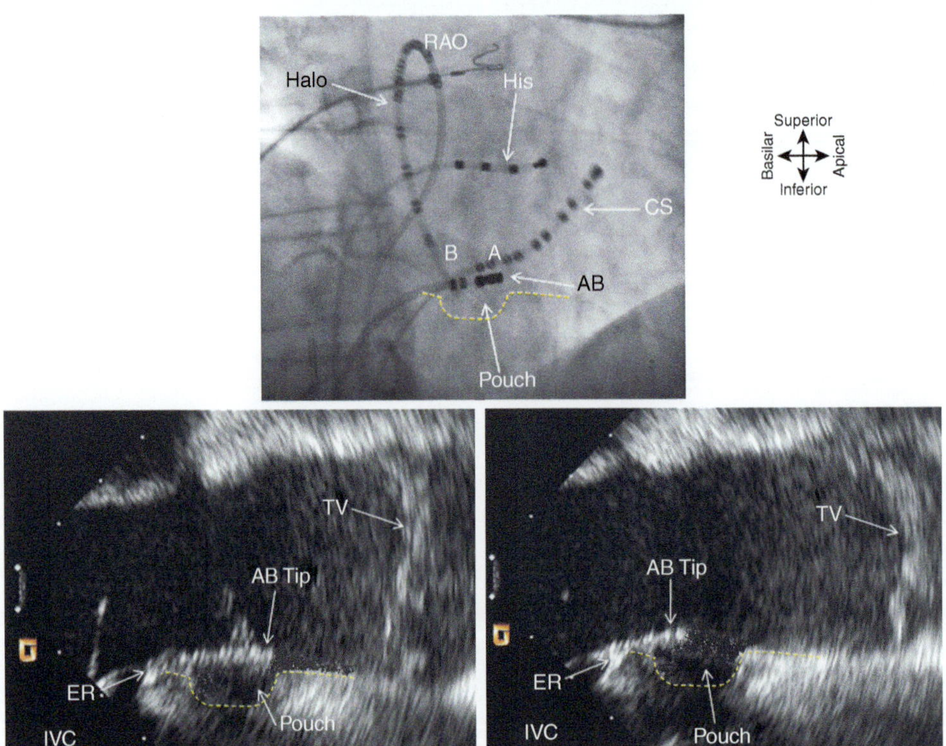

Fig. 12.14 A cavotricuspid isthmus (CTI) pouch. Right anterior oblique (RAO) fluoroscopic view of ablation catheters during CTI ablation (*top*). The *yellow dashed line* estimates the position of a large pouch visualized in this patient with intracardiac echocardiography (ICE) (*bottom*). As the ablation (AB) catheter is drawn toward the inferior vena cava (IVC) from point A to B, the tip of the catheter does not contact the floor of the pouch, and it is therefore not ablated. *Bottom left,* This ICE view demonstrates the pouch and ablation catheter skipping over the pouch in position A. The echo view is rotated to correspond to the fluoroscopic view. *Bottom right,* This ICE image corresponds to the ablation catheter at position B. The fulcrum created by the Eustachian ridge (ER) prevents the catheter from entering the pouch. *CS,* Coronary sinus catheter; *TV,* tricuspid valve.

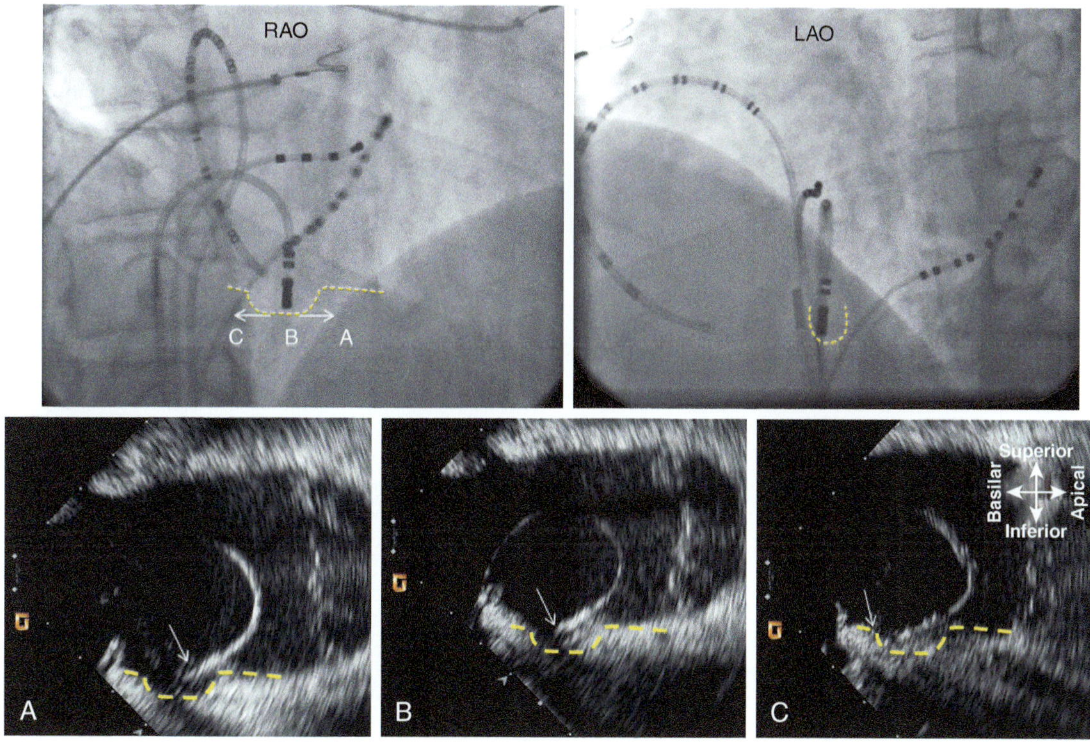

Fig. 12.15 Ablation within a cavotricuspid isthmus (CTI) pouch. *Top panels,* Right anterior oblique (RAO) and left anterior oblique (LAO) fluoroscopic views of the catheter positions. The *dashed yellow line* represents the estimated location of the pouch visualized on intracardiac echocardiography. With a 180-degree angle on the ablation catheter, the ablation electrode contacts the middle floor of the pouch (site B). By opening or closing the curve on the ablation catheter, the tricuspid valve annulus end (site A) and inferior vena cava end (site C) of the pouch can be reached, respectively. *Bottom panels,* Position of the ablation electrode at sites A, B, and C in the pouch. The *arrows* indicate the tip of the ablation catheter. The echo views are rotated to correspond to the RAO fluoroscopic image.

that directs the catheter anteriorly so that by placing a posterior curvature on the catheter body these areas can be reached (Fig. 12.18).

Occasionally, multielectrode catheters crossing the CTI map prevent contact between the ablation electrode and cardiac tissue (Fig. 12.19). When presented with this problem, the mapping catheter can be removed or the ablation catheter positioned beneath the halo (see Fig. 12.19).

End Points for Ablation

Ablation may be performed during sustained AFL or during sinus rhythm. If it is performed during AFL, the first end point is its termination during energy application (Fig. 12.20). However, even if AFL terminates, CTI conduction persists in more than half of patients.[50] Therefore, the entire CTI ablation should be completed before electrophysiologic testing to confirm bidirectional CTI conduction block. After completion of CTI ablation, as determined by fluoroscopic and electrophysiologic criteria described previously, testing can be performed immediately and repeated after at least 30 minutes to ensure that bidirectional CTI block has been achieved and is persistent (Table 12.3).[2–4,6,32–42,54–56] About 50% of patients demonstrate recurrent CTI conduction during the ablation procedure after CTI bidirectional block is initially documented.[53] Most reconnections occur within 10 minutes of initially "successful" CTI block, and multiple recurrences after repeat ablation within the same procedure are not uncommon. Both isoproterenol and adenosine infusion may unmask transient CTI block, but neither has been shown to predict late recurrence of CTI conduction or AFL.[57–58]

If AFL is not terminated during the first attempt at CTI ablation, the activation sequence and isthmus dependence of the AFL should be reconfirmed and ablation repeated. If AFL is terminated during ablation, pacing should be done at a cycle length faster than the intrinsic sinus cycle length (e.g., 700 or 600 ms) to confirm bidirectional conduction block in the CTI (Figs. 12.21–12.24). If ablation is done during sinus rhythm, pacing can also be done during energy application to monitor for the development of conduction block in the CTI (Fig. 12.25). The use of bidirectional conduction block as an end point for CTI ablation is associated with significantly lower recurrence rates of CTI-dependent AFL during long-term follow-up.[59–61]

Conduction in the CTI is typically evaluated after ablation by determining the right atrial activation sequence during pacing from the low lateral right atrium and CS ostium. It is important to pace at relatively slow rates, just above the sinus cycle length, during assessment for CTI block, because conduction block across the CTI may be functional or rate dependent in some cases. Conduction block across the crista terminalis may be functional in some patients as well, and at slow pacing rates

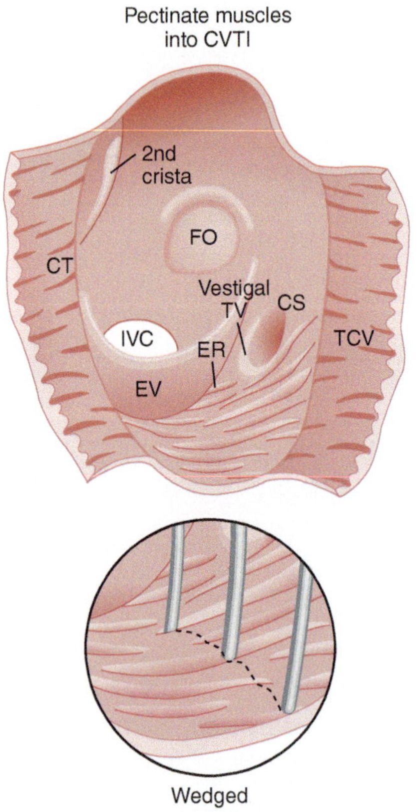

Fig. 12.16 This illustration demonstrated the potential difficulties in ablating the lateral cavotricuspid isthmus (CTI) in the presence of prominent pectinate muscles. On the tops of the muscle bundles, the catheter contact may be unstable. In the recesses between bundles, electrode overheating and low power delivery may result because of the absence of convective cooling. *CS*, Coronary sinus; *CT*, crista terminalis; *CVTI*, cavotricuspid isthmus; *ER*, Eustachian ridge; *EV*, Eustachian valve; *FO*, foramen ovale; *IVC*, inferior vena cava; *TCV*, tricuspid valve. (From Asirvatham S. Correlative anatomy and electrophysiology for the interventional electrophysiologist: right atrial flutter. *J Cardiovasc Electrophysiol*. 2009;20:113–122.)

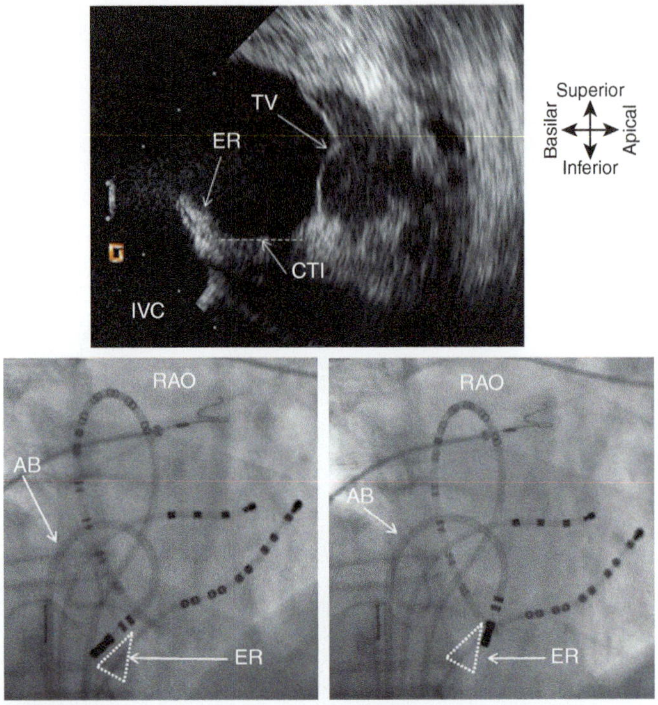

Fig. 12.17 Ablation of the Eustachian ridge (ER). *Top*, Prominent ER on intracardiac echocardiography. The echo views are rotated to correspond to the right anterior oblique (RAO) fluoroscopic image. *Bottom*, Estimated location of the ER and acute flexion of the ablation (AB) catheter to ablate both aspects of the ER facing the inferior vena cava (IVC) (*lower left*) and tricuspid valve (TV) (*lower right*).

conduction across the mid-crista region can result in uncertainty regarding the presence or absence of bidirectional conduction block after CTI ablation.[62–63]

Therefore, it may be necessary to pace not only from the proximal CS but also adjacent to the ablation line in the CTI, or in the posteroinferior right atrial septum, to confirm the presence of CTI conduction block.[64] Bidirectional conduction block after CTI ablation can be confirmed by demonstrating a cranial-to-caudal activation sequence over the lateral right atrium during pacing from the CS ostium or medial to the ablation line, and a cranial-to-caudal sequence over the right atrial septum during pacing from the lateral edge of the ablation line or the low lateral right atrium (see Figs. 12.21–12.24).[57–60] This sequence can be documented by multielectrode recordings or by electroanatomical 3D mapping. When using a multipolar electrode catheter to assess CTI block, it is important that the catheter be properly positioned near the TVA. Recordings are needed from immediately adjacent to the ablation line to assess for incomplete block or slow conduction through the ablation line. This can be performed using the multielectrode catheter crossing the ablation line or from the ablation catheter. A misleading activation sequence may be recorded if portions of the mapping catheter extend posterior to the crista terminalis or if the distal ablation electrode is posterior to the Eustachian ridge.[54] In addition during pacing medial to the ablation line, conduction posterior to the IVC can lead to the appearance of both pseudoconduction and pseudoblock through the CTI (Fig. 12.26).[54,65] In the case of pseudoblock, conduction from the medial pacing site (usually proximal coronary sinus) may conduct rapidly posterior to the IVC to activate the lateral CTI from lateral to medial, suggesting medial-to-lateral isthmus block despite persisting slow conduction through the isthmus. In this case, detailed mapping along the ablation line should identify gaps in the line. In the case of pseudoconduction, the posteriorly conducted wavefront activates the distal multielectrode mapping catheter in a CW pattern even when there is CTI block.

This is more likely to be seen if the distal electrodes on the multielectrode mapping catheter are displaced laterally and do not record from the immediate edge of the ablation line.[54] Pseudoconduction can be recognized by detailed mapping of sites spanning the ablation line. Theoretically, differential pacing maneuvers (see later) may also unmask these conduction patterns.

The creation of CTI conduction block is accompanied by prolongation of the activation time required for a pacing stimulus on one side of the ablation line to propagate to the opposite side of the line (trans-isthmus interval).[66] In this study, before ablation the trans-isthmus intervals averaged 100.3 ± 21 ms and

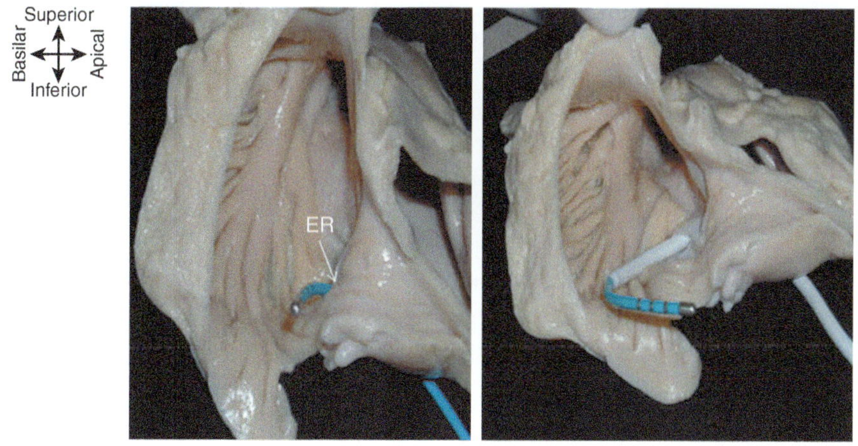

Fig. 12.18 In this autopsy heart specimen, the catheter excursion toward the septal cavotricuspid isthmus is restricted by the Eustachian ridge (ER) (*left*). A guiding sheath is used to direct the catheter anteriorly while curving the catheter posteriorly to reach around the ER (*right*). (From Asirvatham S. Correlative anatomy and electrophysiology for the interventional electrophysiologist: right atrial flutter. *J Cardiovasc Electrophysiol*. 2009; 20:113–122.)

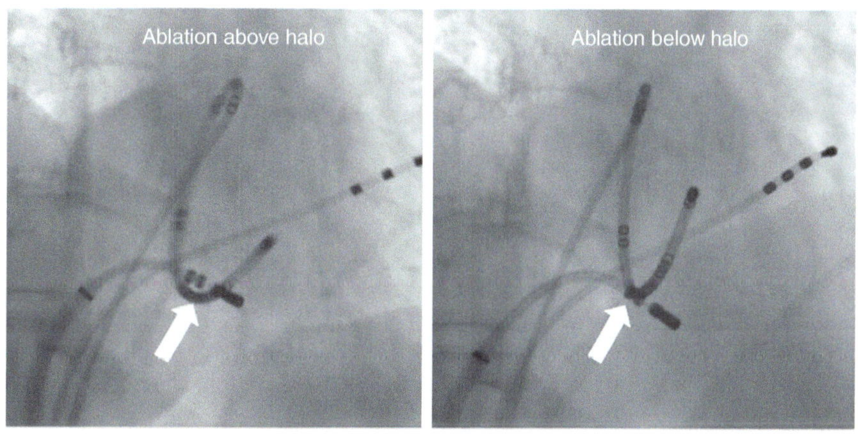

Fig. 12.19 Shielding of the cavotricuspid (CTI) by the halo catheter. In this patient, CTI conduction block could not be achieved after repeated ablation. The ablation catheter repeatedly coursed over the halo catheter that crosses the isthmus (*arrow, left*). By delivering lesions beneath the halo catheter (*arrow, right*), complete CTI block was achieved.

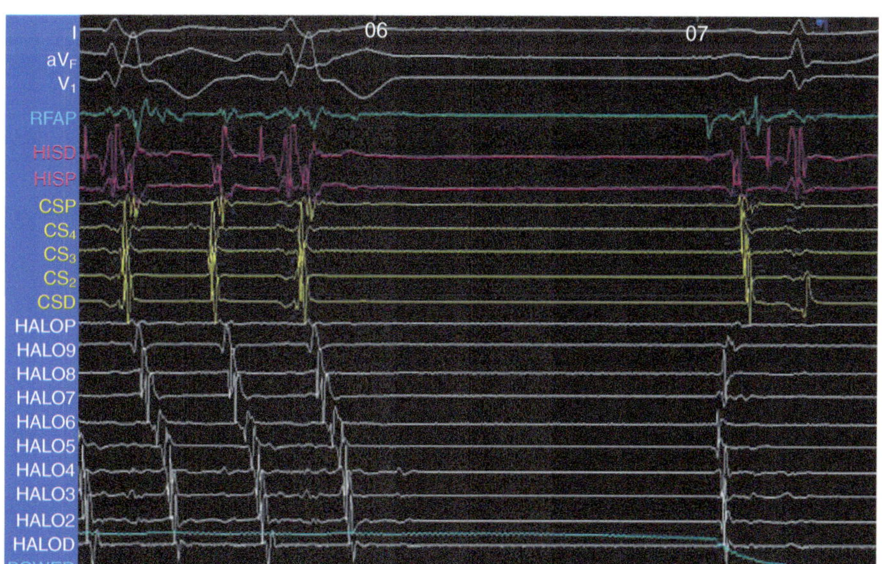

Fig. 12.20 Termination of typical atrial flutter (AFL) during radiofrequency catheter ablation using a slow drag technique across the cavotricuspid isthmus (CTI). AFL usually terminates just as the distal ablation electrode on the mapping and ablation catheter (RFAP) approaches the inferior vena cava. Conduction fails across the CTI, as indicated by block developing between the low lateral right atrium and coronary sinus typical AFL, or between the coronary sinus and the low lateral right atrium in the reverse typical AFL (not shown). The power readout from the radiofrequency energy generator is shown in the *bottom tracing*. *CS*, Coronary sinus.

TABLE 12.3 **Methods for Confirming Cavotricuspid Isthmus Block**

Method (Reference)	Criteria for CTI Block	SENS/ SPEC	PPV/ NPV	Comment
Atrial activation sequence	Cranial-to-caudal activation of right atrial inferolateral free wall with PCS pacing Cranial-to-caudal activation of right atrial septum with inferior lateral right atrial pacing			Requires careful mapping adjacent to ablation line on side contralateral to pacing to exclude slow conduction through the line.
Widely split electrograms (EGMs) along entire ablation line[68]	Interval between split atrial EGM components recorded along ablation line > 90 ms at all sites AND <15 ms maximal variation among all sites during pacing from PCS	100%/80%	86%/100%	Interval between electrogram recordings < 90 ms indicates gap in line. Recordings are from ablation catheter
Trans-isthmus interval[64]	CCW block: ≥50% increase in time interval between pacing stimulus from inferolateral TVA to the atrial EGM in the proximal CS CW block: >50% increase in time interval between pacing stimulus from PCS to the atrial EGM just lateral to ablation line	100%/80%	89%/100%	Minimal trans-isthmus interval associated with bidirectional CTI block approximately 140 ms
Differential pacing[66]	Shortening or no change in interval between pacing stimulus and latest component of split atrial EGM recorded over ablation line when pacing site moved from adjacent to line to 15 mm lateral to line When pacing close to the edge of ablation line, time to activation of contralateral side of ablation line shortens as pacing site moves away from ablation line	100%/75%	94%/100%	First pacing site should be immediately adjacent to ablation line Recording site should be immediately adjacent to ablation line
Electrogram polarity[69]	Loss of negative component of unipolar atrial EGM recorded just lateral to ablation line during PCS pacing or: Reversal of EGM polarity on 2 closely spaced bipoles just lateral to the ablation line during proximal CS pacing	89%/100%	100% (PPV)	Recording must be immediately adjacent to ablation line

CCW, Counterclockwise; *CS*, coronary sinus; *CTI*, cavotricuspid isthmus; *CW*, clockwise; *NPV*, negative predictive value; *PCS*, proximal coronary sinus; *PPV*, positive predictive value; *SENS*, sensitivity; *SPEC*, specificity, *TVA*, tricuspid valve annulus.

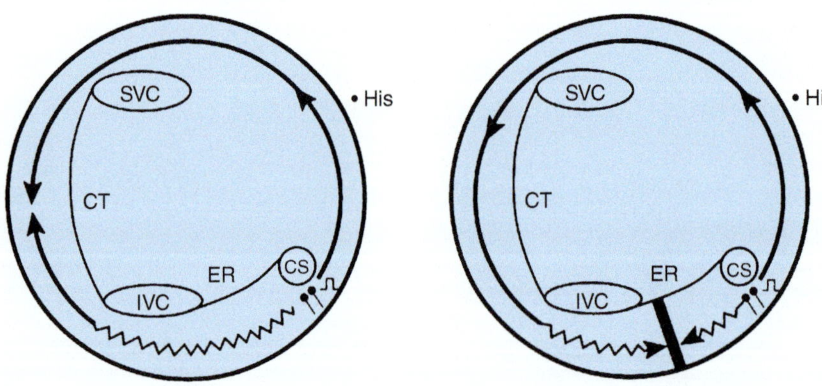

Fig. 12.21 Schematic diagrams of the expected right atrial activation sequence during pacing in sinus rhythm from the CS os before (*left*) and after (*right*) ablation of the cavotricuspid isthmus (CTI). Before ablation, the activation pattern during CS pacing is caudal to cranial in the interatrial septum and low right atrium, with collision of the septal and right atrial wavefronts in the mid-lateral right atrium. After ablation, the activation pattern during CS pacing is still caudal to cranial in the interatrial septum, but the lateral right atrium is now activated in a strictly cranial-to-caudal pattern (i.e., counterclockwise), indicating complete medial-to-lateral conduction block in the CTI. *CT*, Crista terminalis; *ER*, Eustachian ridge; *His*, His bundle; *IVC*, inferior vena cava; *SVC*, superior vena cava.

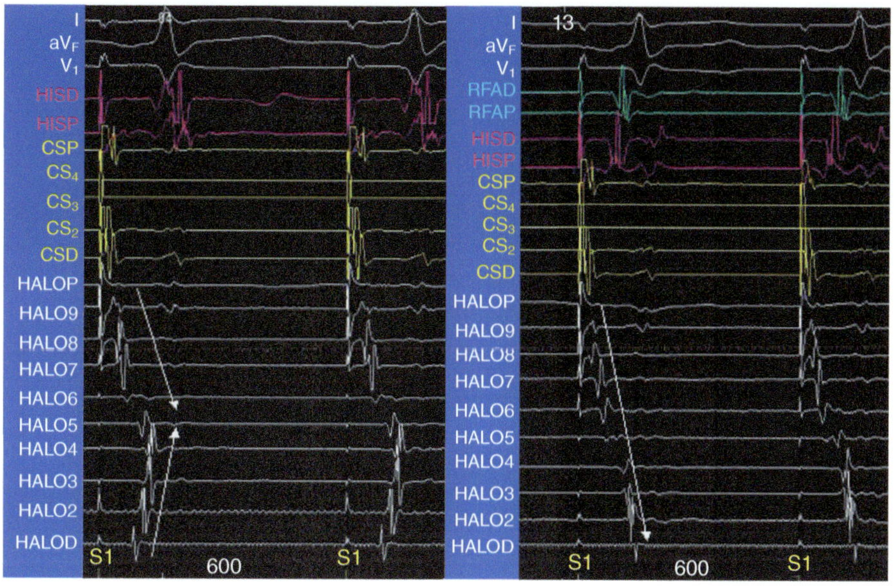

Fig. 12.22 Surface electrocardiogram (ECG) leads and right atrial endocardial electrograms recorded during pacing in sinus rhythm from the coronary sinus (CS) ostium before (*left*) and after (*right*) ablation of the cavotricuspid isthmus (CTI). Tracings include surface ECG leads I, aVF, and V_1 and endocardial electrograms from the proximal coronary sinus (CSP), His bundle (HIS), tricuspid valve annulus at 1 o'clock (HALOP) to 7 o'clock (HALOD), and high right atrium (RFA). Before ablation during CS pacing, there is collision of the cranial and caudal right atrial wavefronts in the mid-lateral right atrium (HALO5). After ablation, the lateral right atrium is activated in a strictly cranial-to-caudal pattern (i.e., counterclockwise), indicating complete medial-to-lateral conduction block in the CTI.

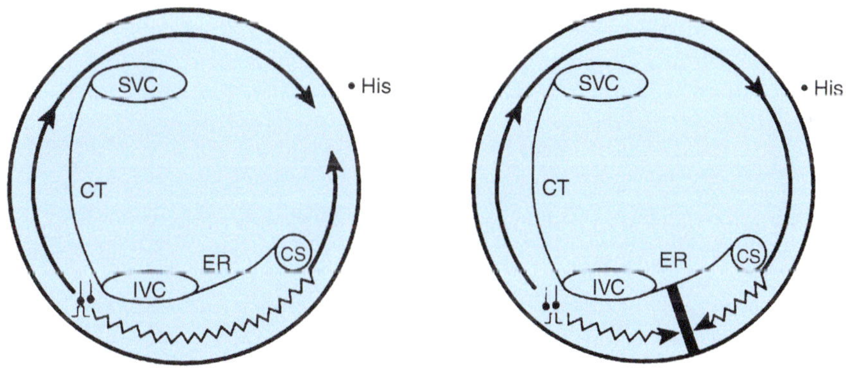

Fig. 12.23 Schematic diagrams of the expected right atrial activation sequence during pacing in sinus rhythm from the low lateral right atrium before (*left*) and after (*right*) ablation of the cavotricuspid isthmus (CTI). Before ablation, the activation pattern during coronary sinus (CS) pacing is caudal to cranial in the right atrial free wall, with collision of the cranial and caudal wavefronts (i.e., through the CTI) in the mid-septum; there is simultaneous activation at the His bundle (HISP) and proximal coronary sinus (CSP). After ablation, the activation pattern during low lateral right atrial sinus pacing is still caudal to cranial in the right atrial free wall, but the septum is now activated in a strictly cranial-to-caudal pattern (i.e., clockwise), indicating complete counterclockwise conduction block in the CTI. *CT*, Crista terminalis; *ER*, Eustachian ridge; *His*, His bundle; *SVC*, superior vena cava.

98.2 ± 25 ms in the CW and CCW directions, respectively (pacing at 500-ms cycle length). In the presence of bidirectional isthmus block, these times increased to 195.8 ± 30 ms and 185.7 ± 34 ms, respectively. Bidirectional CTI block never occurred with less than a 50% prolongation in the trans-isthmus interval. An increase in the trans-isthmus interval of 50% or greater provided 100% sensitivity, 80% specificity, 89% positive predictive value, and 100% negative predictive value in confirming CTI block.

The presence of bidirectional conduction block in the CTI is strongly supported by recording widely spaced double potentials along the entire ablation line, during pacing from the low lateral right atrium or CS ostium (see Fig. 12.25).[50,67] When pacing from the proximal CS, intervals of less than 90 ms between EGM components anywhere on the ablation line indicates persistent conduction through a gap (Fig. 12.27A).[50] When the interval between EGM components is more than 100 ms at all points along the ablation line and maximal variation in the interval is less than 15 ms among all points, it is highly likely that bidirectional CTI is present. When mapping an incomplete ablation line, additional lesions should be given to sites with intervals less than 100 ms between EGM components and at sites in which this interval is between 90 and 110 ms if the local

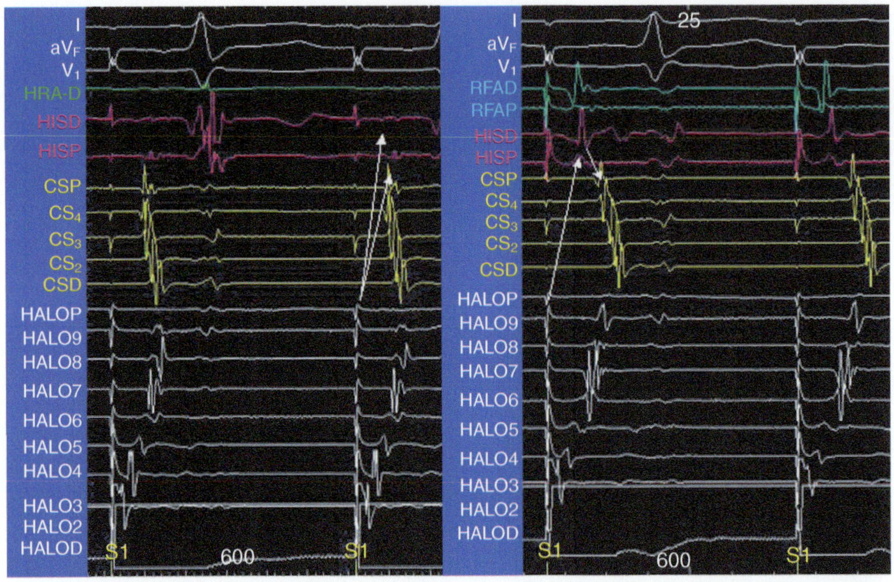

Fig. 12.24 Surface electrocardiogram (ECG) and right atrial endocardial electrograms during pacing in sinus rhythm from the low lateral right atrium before (*left*) and after (*right*) ablation of cavotricuspid isthmus. Tracings include surface ECG leads I, aVF, and V_1 and endocardial electrograms from the proximal coronary sinus (CSP), His bundle (HIS), tricuspid valve annulus at 1 o'clock (HALOP) to 7 o'clock (HALOD), and high right atrium (HRA or RFA). Before ablation, during low lateral right atrial pacing, there is collision of the cranial and caudal right atrial wavefronts in the mid-septum (HIS and CSP). After ablation, the septum is activated in a strictly cranial-to-caudal pattern (i.e., clockwise), indicating complete lateral-to-medial conduction block in the CTI.

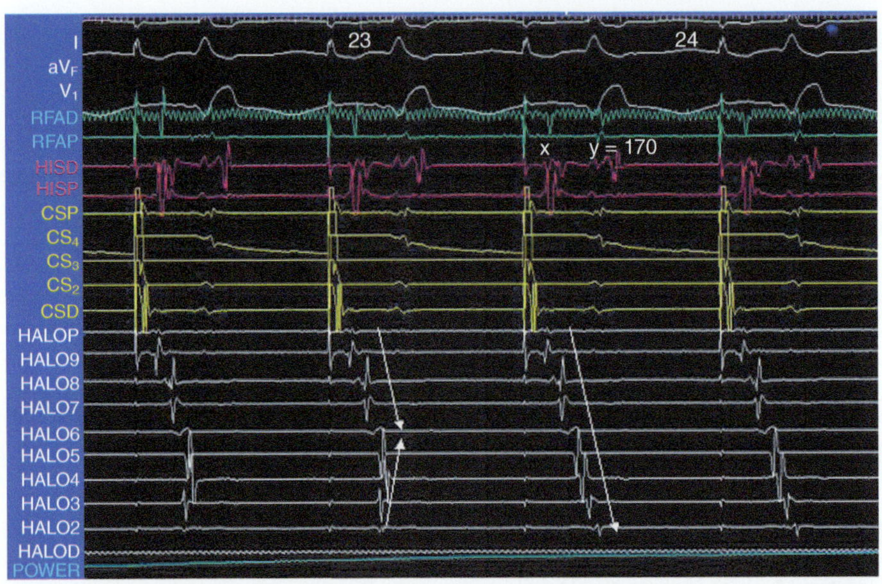

Fig. 12.25 Surface electrocardiogram leads I, aVF, and V_1, and endocardial electrograms from the coronary sinus (CS), His-bundle, halo, mapping and ablation (RF), and right ventricular catheters during radiofrequency catheter ablation of the cavotricuspid isthmus (CTI), while pacing from the CS ostium. Note the change in activation of the lateral right atrium on the halo catheter from a bidirectional to a unidirectional pattern, indicating the development of clockwise block in the CTI. This was associated with the development of widely spaced (170 ms) double potentials (*x,y*) on the ablation catheter in the CTI, further confirming medial-to-lateral conduction block. halo catheter and other tracings are as described in Fig. 11.7.

EGM characteristics suggest persistent conduction, including prolonged low-amplitude fractionated electrical activity in the interval between EGM components or if the second EGM component is positive in polarity. Points along the ablation line with intervals between EGM components of more than 110 ms rarely require further ablation at that site.

Differential pacing maneuvers can be used to further demonstrate functional linking of local EGMs to a single wavefront passing through the CTI in the presence of CTI conduction, or dissociation of the local EGMs in the case of conduction block.[68] In this technique, double potentials with an isoelectric interval (>30 ms) are recorded over the

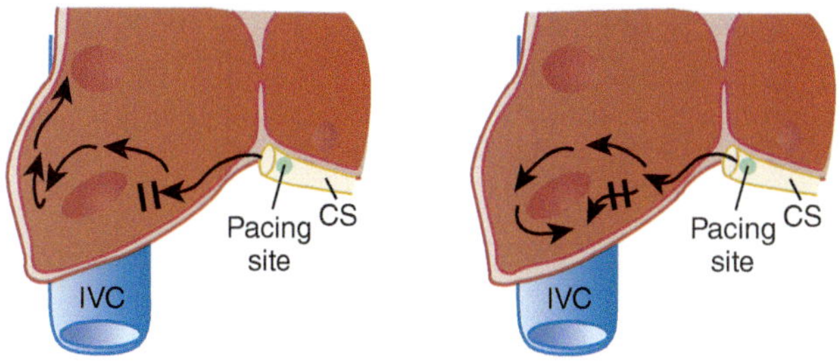

Fig. 12.26 Patterns of conduction in the low posterior right atrium to create pseudoconduction and pseudoblock after cavotricuspid isthmus ablation. See text for details. *CS*, Coronary sinus; *IVC*, inferior vena cava. (From Asirvatham S. Correlative anatomy and electrophysiology for the interventional electrophysiologist: right atrial flutter. *J Cardiovasc Electrophysiol.* 2009;20:113–122.)

ablation line during pacing from just lateral to the line (see Fig. 12.27B). The times from the stimulus to the initial and terminal components of the split EGMs are measured. The stimulus to first EGM component represents the time to activation of the ipsilateral side of the ablation line and should be 50 ms or less to demonstrate proximity. The pacing site is then moved 10–15 mm farther lateral (away from the ablation line) and pacing repeated. In the case of persistent CTI conduction, both components of the split EGM will be delayed or linked to the lateral to medial wavefront (see Fig. 12.27B). In the case of CTI block, however, the time to the first EGM component is delayed by 20 ± 9 ms, whereas the terminal component is advanced by 13 ± 8 ms, or unchanged in timing (see Fig. 12.27B). The delay in the terminal component indicates linking of this EGM, not to the lateral-to-medial wavefront but rather to that approaching the ablation line from the medial-to-lateral direction down the atrial septum. Using this method for detection of CTI block, the sensitivity has been shown to be 100%, specificity 75%, negative predictive value 94%, and positive predictive value 100%. For this technique to be reliable, it is important that the initial pacing site be as close as possible to the edge of the ablation line and that the more remote pacing sites be of limited distance from the first to maintain similar propagation wavefronts. For fractionated EGMs (more than three components) on the ablation line, the first and last components should be measured. This technique may clarify the origin of fractionated potentials as caused by a conduction gap or local activation inhomogeneities.

Variations on this and other pacing algorithms have been introduced over the past two decades to identify the occasional case where only conduction delay or incomplete conduction block (i.e., functional block) is suspected, especially when AFL is still inducible after initial ablation, in order to reduce risk of late recurrence of AFL (Fig. 12.28A, B).[69–71]

To expedite the assessment of bidirectional conduction block after CTI ablation and to obviate the need for multipolar electrode catheter recordings, algorithms based on reversal of EGM polarity near the ablation line and use of unipolar EGMs have also been used, with varying degrees of accuracy (Fig. 12.29).[72,73]

Simplified Approach to Ablation of Cavo-tricuspid Isthmus–Dependent Atrial Flutter

We have developed a simplified approach for CTI ablation in patients with isthmus-dependent AFL, using only two catheters. CTI ablation can be rapidly achieved with minimal fluoroscopy time using this approach. After percutaneous insertion via the right femoral vein, a steerable decapolar catheter is positioned in the CS with the proximal electrode pair at the ostium near the medial CTI, and an ablation catheter is flexed in the low lateral right atrium with the distal pair near the lateral CTI (Fig. 12.30A). Pacing from the proximal CS and the ablation catheter demonstrates bidirectional CTI conduction before, and block after, CTI ablation (see Fig. 12.30B,C). Using this simplified catheter approach, medial-to-lateral CTI conduction block is defined by both the presence of a high-to-low or descending (i.e., proximal to distal) activation sequence on the ablation catheter during pacing from the proximal CS, and bidirectional conduction block by demonstrating equal conduction times (i.e., >130 ms) from medial to lateral and from lateral to medial, during pacing from the proximal CS and low lateral RA, respectively. In addition, pacing from the proximal CS with the ablation catheter positioned on the ablation line will demonstrate widely spaced double potentials (Fig. 12.30D).

OUTCOMES AND COMPLICATIONS

Although early reports on RFCA for CTI-dependent AFL revealed high recurrence rates (i.e., 20–45%), increasing experience and advances in methodology and technology over time has resulted in acute and long-term success rates (defined as no recurrence of CTI-dependent AFL) as high as 85–95%.[1–6,32–44,61] For example, in a large meta-analysis comprising 10,719 patients, the long-term success rate for ablation with irrigated or large-tip RF catheters was 91% (95% confidence interval, 90–95%) (Table 12.4).[61] Contributing in large degree to these improved results has been the use of large-tip or irrigated ablation catheters, and the use of bidirectional CTI conduction block as a procedural end point.[32–44,61] Randomized comparisons of internally cooled, externally cooled, and large-tip ablation catheters also suggest a slightly better acute and chronic success rate with externally cooled ablation catheters.[35–38,44]

Despite the excellent acute and long-term results for AFL ablation, the development of atrial fibrillation after CTI ablation alone occurs at a high rate in this population (up to 67% over 5 years), especially if there is a history of atrial fibrillation or underlying heart disease before CTI ablation.[61,74,75] By meta-analysis, the occurrence rate of atrial fibrillation at 1- to 2-year follow-up was 23% in those without a history of atrial fibrillation before ablation and 53% in those with a prior history of atrial fibrillation.[61] At 5-year follow-up, the occurrence rate of atrial fibrillation was similar (i.e., 60%) regardless of atrial fibrillation history before ablation.[61]

Ablation of CTI-dependent AFL is relatively safe, with complication rates of 2.5–3.5%.[57] Most complications are caused by peripheral vascular injury (0.4% of patients), but serious complications can rarely occur, including heart block (0.2% of

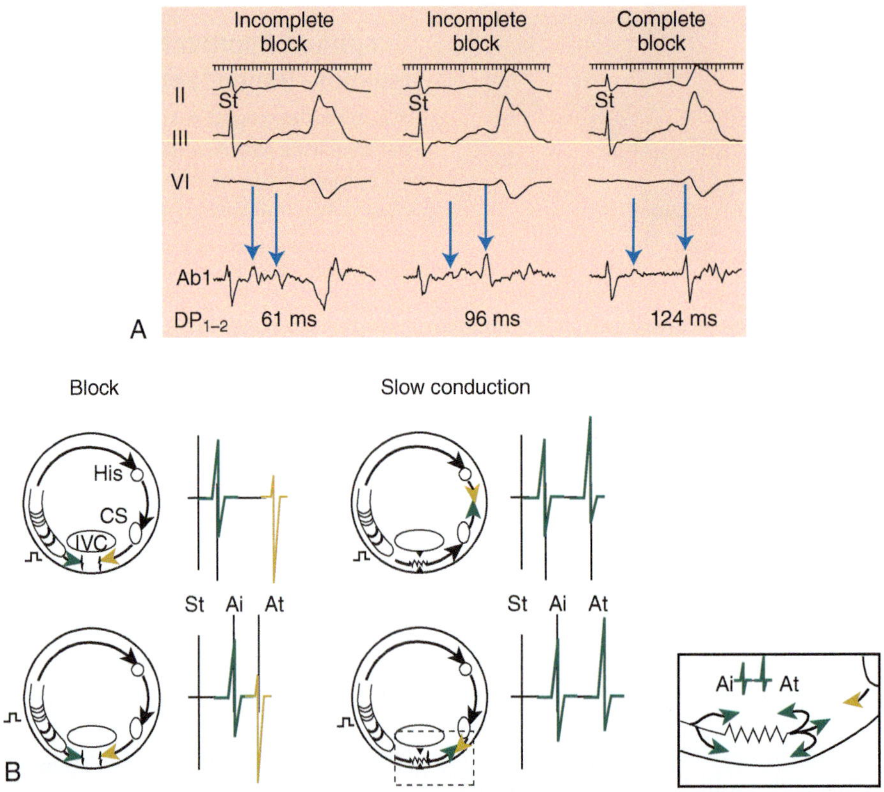

Fig. 12.27 Methods of determining bidirectional cavotricuspid isthmus (CTI) conduction block after ablation. (A) Recordings during coronary sinus (CS) pacing before (*left and middle*) and after (*right*) complete CTI block are shown. Displayed are leads II, III and V_1, electrograms recorded by the ablation catheter (Abl). The *arrows* in the electrograms recorded by the Abl point to the components of the double potentials (DPs). The Abl was positioned at exactly the same site in all three panels. *Left,* After several applications of radiofrequency energy along the ablation line, the interval separating the two components of DPs (DP1-2) is 61 ms, and there is incomplete block. *Middle,* After an additional application of radiofrequency energy, the DP1-2 interval increases to 96 ms, but isthmus block is still incomplete. *Right,* After a final application of radiofrequency energy, the DP1-2 interval lengthens to 124 ms, and now there is complete block. Note that when the DP1-2 interval was 96 ms, the segment separating the two components of the DP was not isoelectric, providing further evidence that there was a persistent gap in the ablation line. On the transition to complete block, the segment with the DP became isoelectric. *St,* Stimulus artifact. (From Tada H, Oral H, Sticherling C, et al. Double potentials along the ablation line as a guide to radiofrequency ablation of typical atrial flutter. *J Am Cardiol Coll.* 20001;38:750–755.) (B) Schematic representation of activation principles on which assessment is based. Right atrium and selected key structures [IVC, His bundle, coronary sinus ostium (Cs)] are shown in a cartoon format. A quadripolar catheter is shown and activation is pictured during distal bipole stimulation (*top row*) and proximal bipole stimulation (*bottom row*). Shown are activation patterns during complete isthmus block (*left*) and during persistent but slow isthmus conduction through a gap in the ablation line (*right*). During complete isthmus block, double potentials separated by an isoelectric interval are recorded on the ablation line as a result of two opposing fronts: a descending front (shown in *blue*) and another that detours around isthmus (in *brown*) give rise to double potentials Ai (initial potential) and At (terminal potential) (*blue* and *brown*, respectively). On changing to a proximal stimulation site, descending wavefront (in *blue*) has to travel a longer distance to reach line of block, whereas detouring wavefront (*brown*) has a shorter distance to travel; as a result, Ai (*blue*) is delayed, and At (*brown*) is advanced. During persistent isthmus conduction through a gap in the ablation line, double potentials are recorded as a result of delayed activation of downstream isthmus by the same blue front, and therefore both resulting potentials (Ai and At) are shown in *blue* (*inset, far right*). When stimulation is performed from a proximal site the activation pattern does not change, but the descending wavefront (*blue*) has a longer distance to travel to reach the isthmus line and as a result both blue potentials (Ai and At) are delayed. *St,* stimulus artifact. (From Shah D, Haissaguerre M, Takahashi A, et al. Differential pacing for distinguishing block from persistent conduction through an ablation line. *Circulation.* 2000;102:1517–1522.)

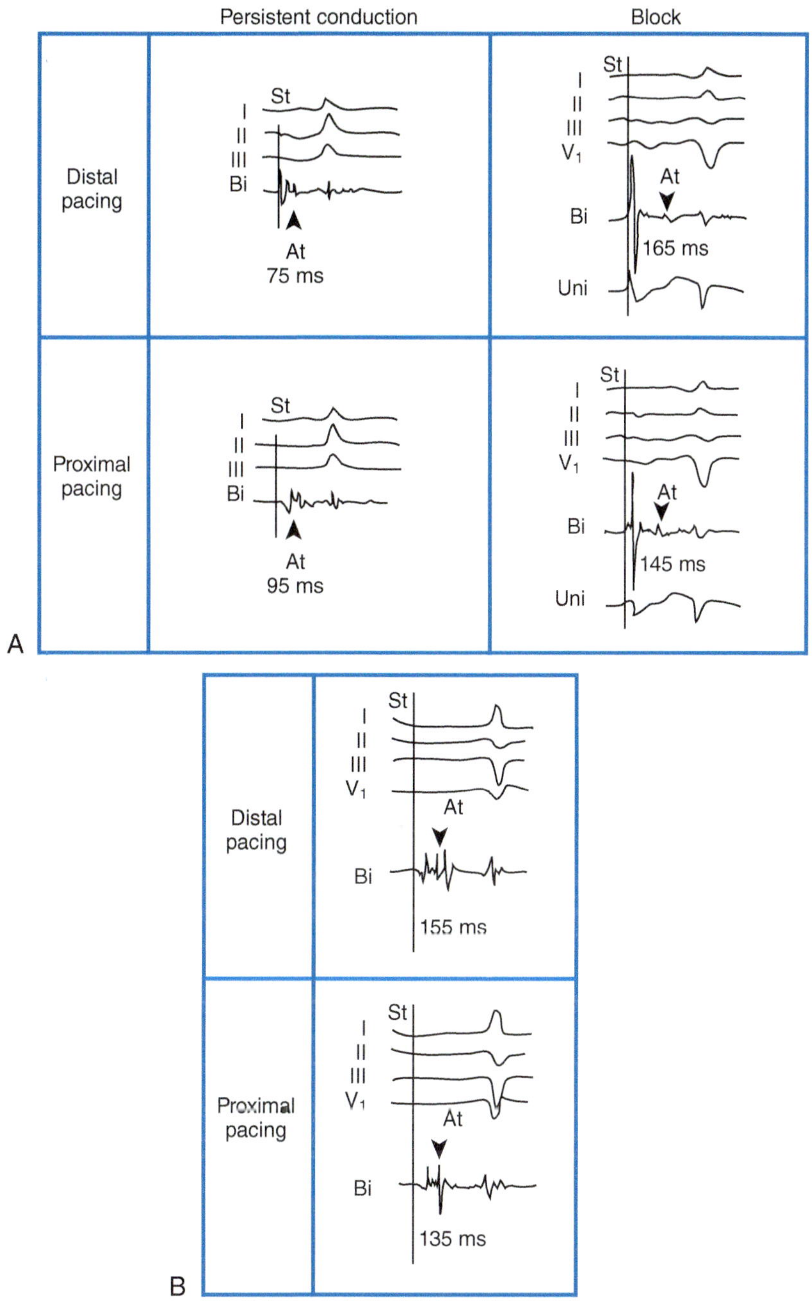

Fig. 12.28 Differential pacing to assess for cavotricuspid isthmus (CTI) conduction block. (A) Representative examples of assessment in different patients. *Top left,* Double potentials with a stimulus to second potential timing of 75 ms are recorded from isthmus during pacing from distal bipole. The stimulus to first potential timing is 20 ms. *Bottom left,* During pacing from the proximal bipole, both potentials are delayed by 20 ms so that second potential is now activated at 95 ms. This response indicates persistent conduction. Further ablation was performed in the CTI to produce complete conduction block. Surface electrocardiogram (ECG) leads shown are I, II, and III. *Right,* double potentials with a large first potential and a small second potential are recorded. During distal bipole pacing, as shown in the (*top*), first potential is activated at 15 ms, and second potential is activated at 165 ms after stimulus. During pacing from the proximal bipole (*middle*) the first potential is delayed by 20 ms and the second potential is advanced by 20 ms (145 ms). Note that morphology of both potentials remains unchanged, in bipolar as well as in unipolar electrograms (*bottom*). This response indicates complete isthmus block. Surface ECGs include leads I, II, III, and V_1. *Bi,* bipolar electrogram; *Uni,* unipolar electrogram. (B) Bystander slow conduction and complete block in the presence of a triple potential. A complex triple potential was recorded along the ablation line after documentation of complete CTI conduction block. Compared with the top tracing, which was recorded during stimulation from distal bipole, as shown on *bottom right,* which was recorded during proximal bipole stimulation, the first and second components are delayed identically without a change in their morphology by 25 ms, whereas the third and terminal component, which is also morphologically unchanged, is advanced by 20 ms (155–135 ms). This response indicates that complete conduction block exists between second and third components and that first two components are directly linked to each other by a single front of slow or circuitous conduction. (From Shah D, Haissaguerre M, Takahashi A, et al. Differential pacing for distinguishing block from persistent conduction through an ablation line. *Circulation.* 2000;102:1517–1522.)

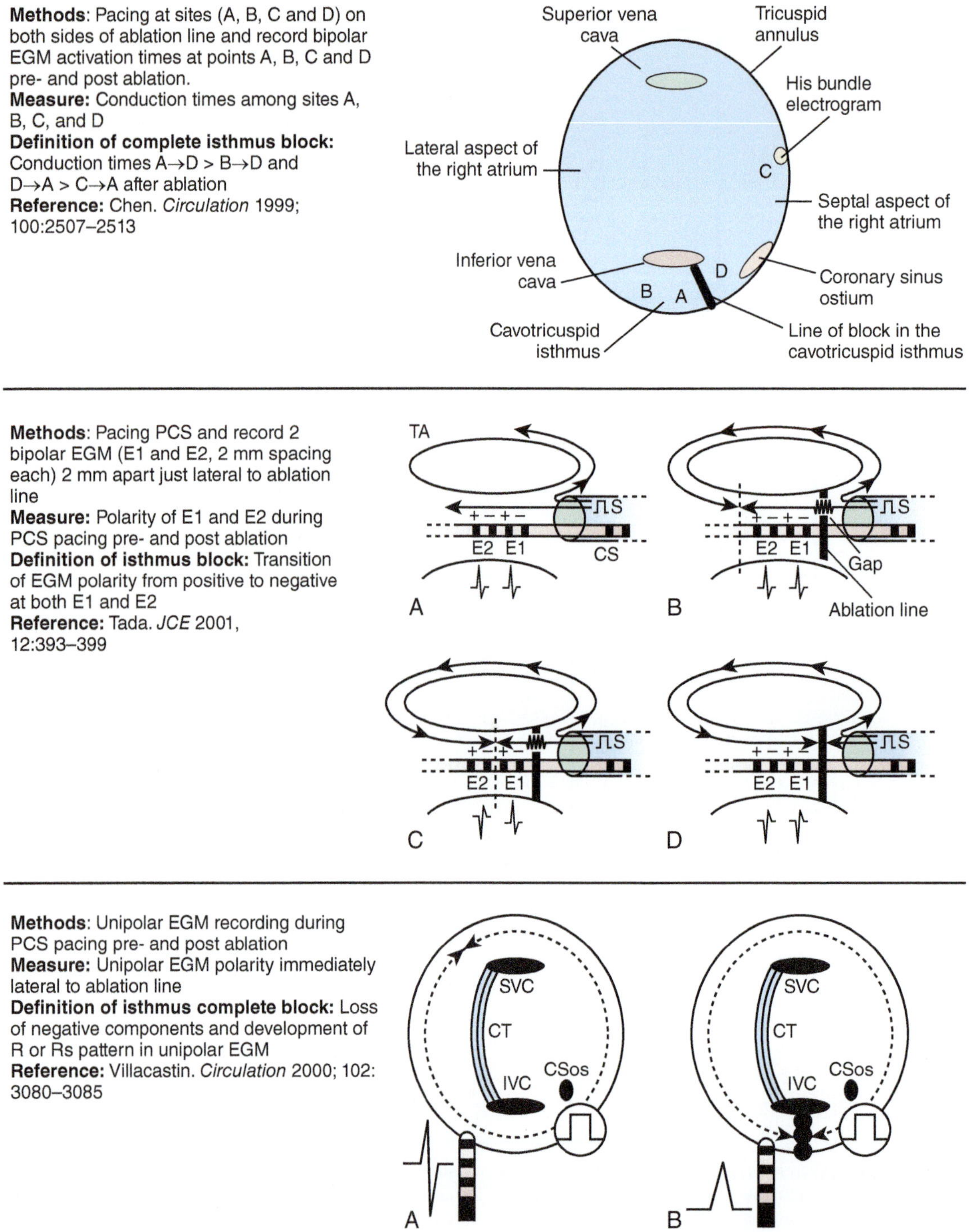

Fig. 12.29 Additional methods of defining cavotricuspid isthmus (CTI) conduction block. *Top,* Use of conduction times measured at line of block. In the presence of CTI block, moving the pacing site away from the ablation line shortens the distance to the contralateral side of the line and shortens the conduction time. In the presence of conduction through the line, the distance is prolonged, and the conduction times lengthen. *Middle,* Bipolar electrograms (EGMs) close to the edge of the ablation line reveal the direction of activation of each bipole. In the presence of CTI conduction block, both bipolar EGM pairs are activated by a wavefront propagating toward the ablation line. In the presence of CTI conduction block, one or both bipoles are activated by a wavefront propagating away from the ablation line. *Bottom,* In the presence of CTI conduction block, a unipolar EGM recorded immediately adjacent to the ablation line records only an activation wavefront approaching the electrode and no activation past the edge of the line. In this case, the EGM is entirely positive. *CS,* coronary sinus; *CSos,* coronary sinus ostium; *CT,* computed tomography; *IVC,* inferior vena cava; *PCS,* proximal coronary sinus; *SVC,* superior vena cava. (*Top panel* from Chen J, de Chilou C, Basiouny T, et al. Cavotricuspid isthmus mapping to assess bidirectional block during common atrial flutter radiofrequency ablation. *Circulation.* 1999;100:2507–2513; *middle panel* from Tada H, Oral H, Sticherling C, et al. EGM polarity and cavotricuspid isthmus block during ablation of typical atrial flutter. *J Cardiovasc Electrophysiol.* 2001;12:393–399; *bottom panel* from Villacastin J, Almendral J, Arenal A, et al. Usefulness of unipolar electrograms to detect isthmus block after radiofrequency ablation of typical atrial flutter. *Circulation,* 2000;102:3080–3085.)

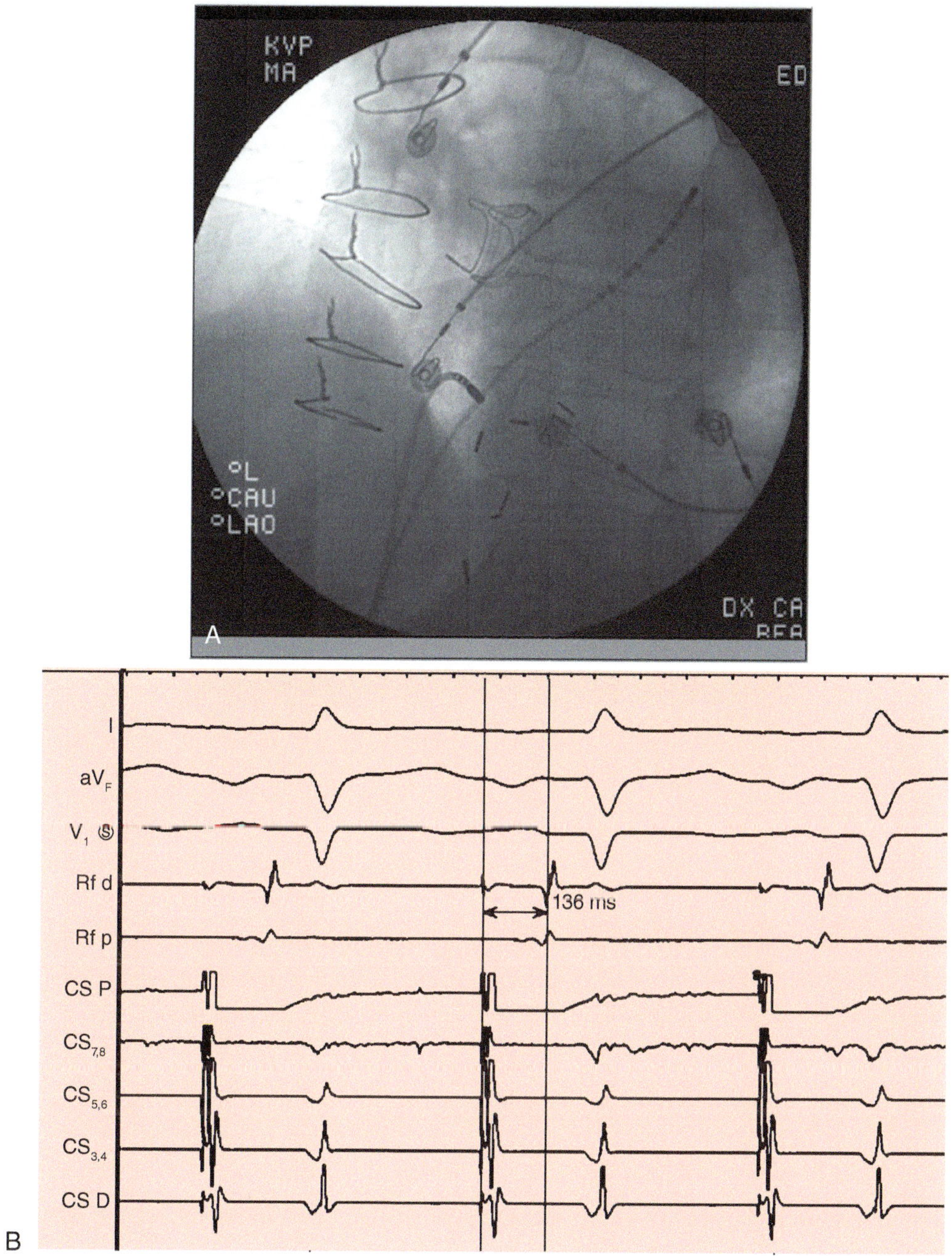

Fig. 12.30 (A) Left anterior oblique fluoroscopic projection showing the positions of the coronary sinus (CS) and ablation catheter after cavotricuspid isthmus (CTI) ablation to demonstrate conduction block. The proximal CS catheter electrode is positioned near the CS ostium, and the ablation catheter is positioned at the lateral CTI. (B) Surface electrocardiogram (ECG) and endocardial electrogram recordings during pacing from the proximal CS demonstrating a proximal to distal (high to low) activation sequence on the ablation catheter with a conduction time of 136 ms confirming medial to lateral CTI conduction block. *CSd-p*, Distal to proximal CS electrograms; *I*, *aVF*, and *V$_1$*, surface ECG leads; *RFd&p*, distal and proximal ablation catheter electrograms.

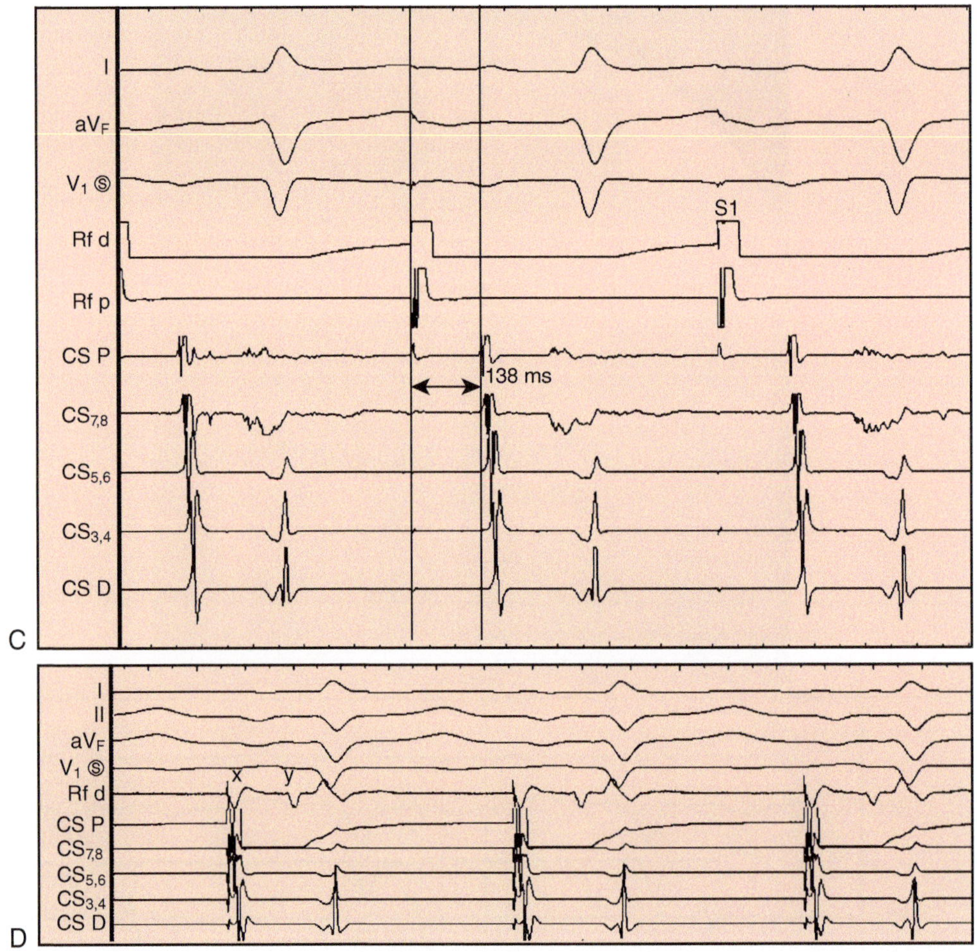

Fig. 12.30 cont'd (C) Surface ECG and endocardial electrogram recordings during pacing from the ablation catheter at the low lateral right atrium demonstrating a conduction time to the proximal CS of 138 ms, similar to the medial to lateral conduction time, confirming lateral to medial CTI conduction block. Abbreviations same as in 16B. (D) Surface ECG and endocardial electrogram recordings during pacing from the proximal CS demonstrating widely spaced (130 ms) double potentials (*X* and *Y*) at the ablation line, confirming medial to lateral conduction block. Abbreviations same as in previous figures. (From Sawhney NS, Wayne Whitwam W, Feld GK. Mapping of human atrial flutter and its variants. In: Shenasa M, Hindricks G, Borggrefe M, Briethardt G, eds. *Cardiac Mapping*, 4th ed. Hoboken, NJ: Wiley-Blackwell; 2012:191–212.)

TABLE 12.4 Meta-analysis of Ablation Outcomes Based on Catheter Technology

Catheter Type	Acute Success Number of Studies/Patients	Acute Success % (95% CI)	AFL Recurrence Number of Studies/Patients	AFL Recurrence % (95% CI)
4–6 mm RF	16/512	86 (78, 92)	17/529	18 (15, 21)
8–10 mm or irrigated RF	49/3098	94 (91, 95)	49/3052	7 (5, 8)

AFL, Atrial flutter; *RF* radiofrequency.

Data from Perez FJ, Schubert CM, Parvez B, et al. Long-term outcomes after catheter ablation of cavo-tricuspid isthmus dependent atrial flutter: a meta-analysis. *Circ Arrhythm Electrophysiol.* 2009;2:393–401..

patients), pericardial effusion and tamponade (0.1% of patients), myocardial infarction from right coronary artery injury, and thromboembolic events, including pulmonary embolism and stroke.[61]

Although conversion of AFL to sinus rhythm is less likely than atrial fibrillation to cause thromboembolic complications (e.g., stroke), there is still a significant risk, and oral anticoagulation before ablation must be considered in patients who have persistent CTI-dependent AFL.[76] This may be particularly important in those patients with depressed left ventricular function, mitral valve disease, or left atrial enlargement with spontaneous contrast (i.e., smoke) on echocardiography. As an alternative to oral anticoagulation, transesophageal echocardiography may be used to rule out left atrial clot immediately before CTI ablation, but subsequent to conversion of AFL to sinus rhythm during CTI ablation, oral anticoagulation must be continued for at least 30 days because of potential atrial stunning, similar to that seen following conversion of atrial fibrillation.[76]

TROUBLESHOOTING THE DIFFICULT CASE

Despite the high ablation success rates reported in recent studies, difficult AFL ablation cases may still be occasionally encountered. In these cases, several measures can be used to increase the likelihood of successful ablation (Fig. 12.31; Table 12.5). First, it is critically important to ensure that the mechanism of the spontaneous or induced AFL is CTI dependent. If multielectrode catheter mapping with pacing entrainment is not sufficient to confirm CTI dependence of the AFL, then 3D computerized activation mapping may be helpful for confirmation and to rule out other mechanisms. Once the CTI dependence of the AFL has been confirmed, if initial ablation attempts are unsuccessful, it is essential to ensure that the ablation catheter has reached the extreme borders of the CTI isthmus, including the TVA and Eustachian ridge or IVC. This may require the use of large-curve catheters or the use of preformed guiding sheaths, such as the Schwartz Left 1, Schwartz Right 0 (SL1, SR0), or ramp sheaths, to ensure catheter contact across the entire CTI. Careful mapping of the CTI with the mapping or ablation catheter may also help identify a gap in the ablation line (using criteria noted earlier), which, when ablated, may terminate AFL and produce bidirectional CTI conduction block (see Fig. 12.11). Persistent CTI conduction after initial failed ablation may sometimes be identified by 3D computerized activation mapping (Fig. 12.32), particularly if the use of standard multielectrode catheters has been unsuccessful.[77] Isthmus pouches are present in many patients and may not be ablated without specific catheter maneuvers. The presence of a pouch may be visualized by angiography, ICE, or electroanatomical mapping. The visualization of complex isthmus anatomy early in the case may facilitate a more rapid and successful conclusion.[78]

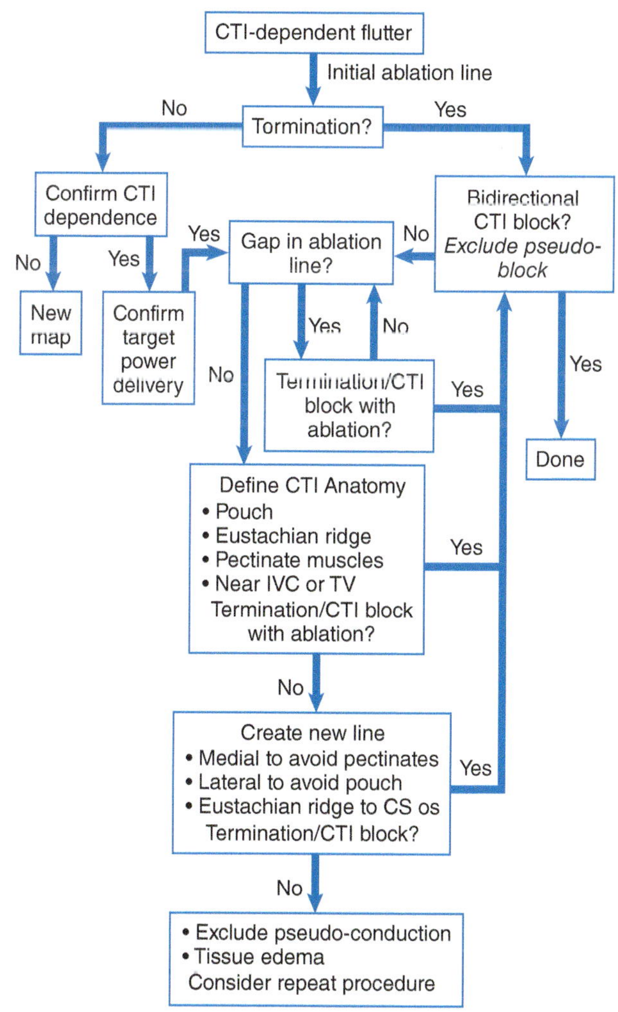

Fig. 12.31 Schematic diagram for sequence of events during cavotricuspid isthmus (CTI) ablation. *CS*, Coronary sinus; *IVC*, inferior vena cava; *TV*, tricuspid valve.

We recommend that ablation be performed in the 6 o'clock position on the TVA initially. If this is unsuccessful and CTI block cannot be achieved even after elimination of apparent gaps in the line, a new ablation line should be created more laterally, at the 7 or 8 o'clock position on the tricuspid annulus. Large right atrial trabeculae may enter the lateral CTI tangentially and require extensive ablation to achieve bidirectional conduction block. If this is also ineffective, an ablation line may then be created more medially, at the 5 o'clock position, but care must be taken in this position to monitor AV conduction because the risk for AV block is increased. It is important to give sufficient RF energy at each site. Marked tissue edema may occur after the initial energy delivery, thereby insulating the tissue from further ablation. If new lines fail, voltage-guided ablation of the CTI can be undertaken. Typically, an ablation temperature of 60°C is recommended for CTI ablation with a solid-tip nonirrigated ablation catheter, or a power of 40–45 W for irrigated catheters, but occasionally successful CTI ablation requires a temperature as high as 70°C for nonirrigated catheters or power as high as 50 W for irrigated catheters, respectively.[79] If standard ablation electrodes of 4 or 5 mm are used initially and ablation fails, the use of either a large-tip (8–10 mm) ablation catheter with a high-power generator or an irrigated-tip catheter is recommended. We prefer large-tip (8–10 mm) or cooled-tip catheters as the first-line approach for CTI ablation because they have been shown to have greater efficacy than standard catheters in most studies, or at least to produce CTI conduction block with fewer energy applications and shorter procedure times. The use of temperatures exceeding 70°C, with standard or large-tip ablation catheters, or energy exceeding 50 W with irrigated-tip catheters, in an attempt to improve success rates is not recommended because of the increased risk for steam pops, which can cause cardiac rupture.[79]

Various parameters measured during ablation, for example, contact force, impedance, and ablation duration, have been evaluated to determine if their use or any specific values can be correlated with improved acute and long-term outcomes after CTI ablation for atrial flutter. Monitoring these parameters may improve acute outcomes but not long-term

TABLE 12.5 Troubleshooting Difficult Cases

Problem	Cause	Solution
Lack of AFL termination	Non–CTI dependent AFL as original rhythm or change in circuit with ablation Incomplete ablation line because of poor tissue contact, low energy delivery, difficult anatomy Partial isthmus reentry	Repeat activation, entrainment mapping, map ablation line for gaps, use steerable or preformed sheath, use large tip or irrigated ablation catheter, angiography, ICE or EA mapping for pouch, large Eustachian ridge, pectinate muscles, confirm target energy delivery, deliver new line more lateral or medial, ablate under halo if crosses isthmus. Ablate between IVC and CS os.
Unable to achieve lasting bidirectional CTI	Incomplete ablation line because of poor tissue contact, low energy delivery, difficult anatomy Pseudo-conduction posterior to IVC Partial isthmus reentry Tissue edema after extensive ablation	Map ablation line for gaps, use steerable or preformed sheath, use large tip or irrigated ablation, angiography, ICE, EA mapping for pouch, large Eustachian ridge, pectinate muscles, deliver new line more lateral or medial, ablate under halo if crosses isthmus, confirm target energy delivery, detailed mapping with electrodes spanning ablation line, possibly differential pacing maneuvers. Ablate between Eustachian ridge and CS os. Create new ablation line, increase power delivery, schedule second procedure after tissue recovery.
Low RF energy delivery	Low blood flow caused by ablation in pouch, Eustachian ridge, or between pectinate muscles	Use irrigated catheter or cryoablation, create new line avoiding unfavorable anatomy
Poor catheter reach, stability, or unable to navigate to target sites	Enlarged right atrium/IVC, large Eustachian ridge (limits septal excursion), large pectinate muscles	Use preformed or steerable sheath to stabilize catheter, use longer reach and/or stiffer catheter, angle sheath anteriorly and catheter curvature posteriorly to reach around Eustachian ridge, ablation from superior vena cava approach.
Failure to attenuate/eliminate local electrograms	Low energy delivery Poor tissue contact Large pectinate muscles in CTI	See earlier. See earlier. Increase energy delivery, use sheaths, create new line medially.
Painful ablation	Electrical/thermal stimulation Deep sedation of cardiac nerves	Use deep sedation.
Changing atrial activation pattern during AFL	Figure-of-eight reentry in right atrium, intermittent crista terminalis breakthrough, intermittent lower loop-reentry	Remapping for sustained new activation patterns, use noncontact mapping, reassess after creating CTI block

AFL, Atrial flutter; *AV*, atrioventricular; *CS*, coronary sinus; *CTI*, cavotricuspid isthmus; *EA*, electroanatomical; *ICE*, intracardiac echocardiography; *IVC*, inferior vena cava; *os*, ostium; *RF*, radiofrequency energy.

outcomes.[80] In addition, computerized algorithms incorporating proportionately weighted composites of these various parameters, such as ablation index (AI), force-time integral (FTI), and lesion size index (LSI), have been introduced recently in the commonly used mapping systems that are currently available (e.g., Carto and Ensite systems). While utilization of these algorithms has been shown to reduce procedure and fluoroscopy times, overall number of ablation lesions required to achieve bidirectional CTI conduction block, and efficacy of achieving first-pass conduction block, they have not been shown to improve overall clinical outcomes and recurrence rates of atrial flutter, and this will require further study.[81–83] Thus we recommend that, when using a contact force measuring catheter, a contact force of at least 10*g* be achieved, and with any type of ablation catheter an impedance drop of at least 10 Ω be achieved (avoiding sudden impedance rises, which may portend a steam pop), and that ablation be performed at each location for a duration of at least 30 seconds, to help increase the likelihood of achieving first-pass conduction block.

Finally, if CTI conduction block cannot be achieved, and pseudoconduction is excluded, tissue edema may make further energy delivery futile and a second procedure may be necessary.

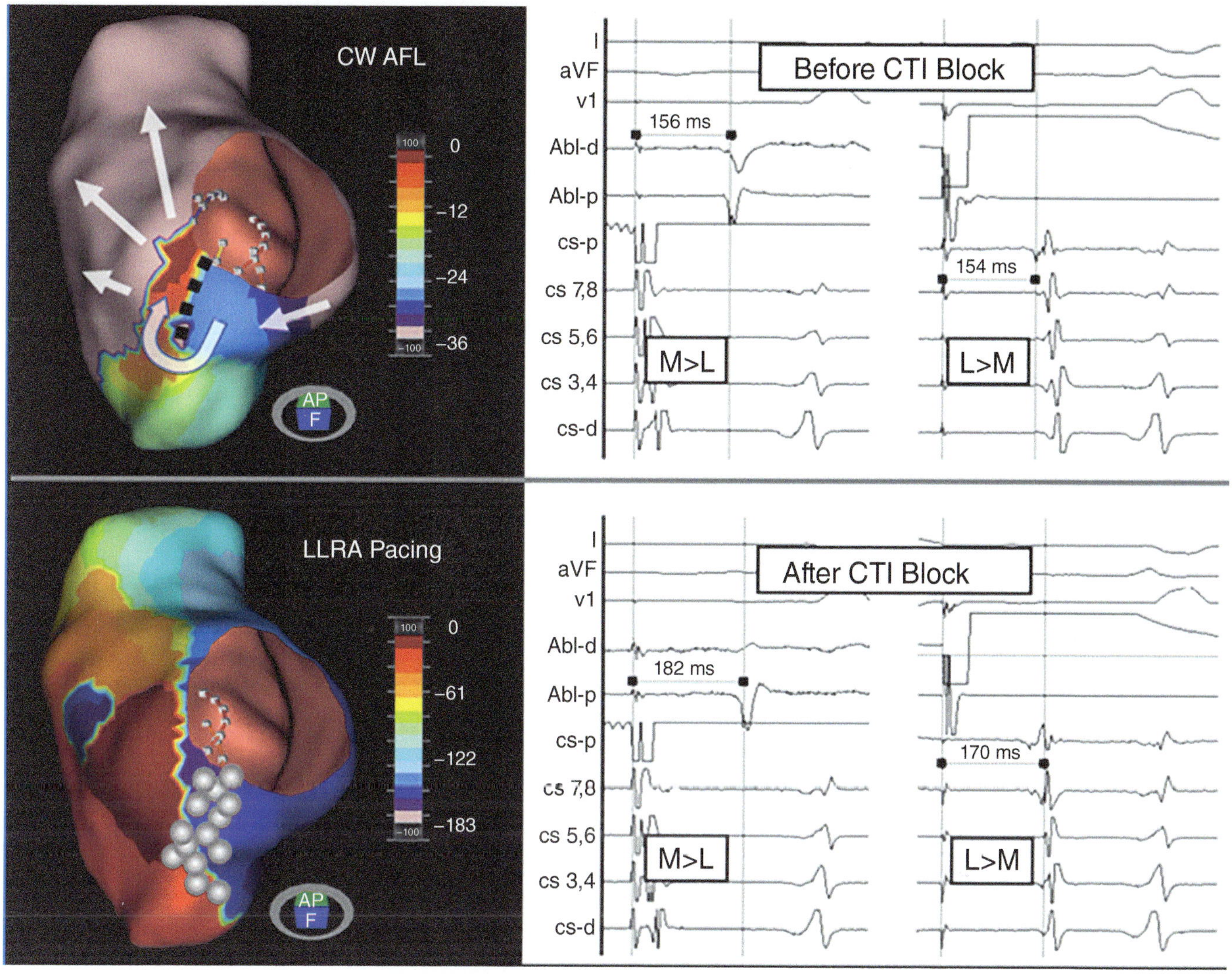

Fig. 12.32 Three-dimensional, high-density, noncontact (Acutus Medical, Inc. Carlsbad, CA) dipole density map of the right atrium during induced reverse typical AFL following initial CTI ablation attempt for typical AFL, demonstrating a conduction gap near the Eustachian ridge *(top left panel)*. Surface ECGs (leads I, aVF, and V1) and endocardial electrograms from the ablation and coronary sinus catheters during pacing from the proximal coronary sinus and low lateral right atrium *(top right)* showing trans-isthmus conduction times of 156 and 154 ms, respectively. Three-dimensional map following repeat ablation of the CTI near the Eustachian ridge demonstrating CTI conduction block *(bottom left)* and associated increase in trans-isthmus conduction times to 182 and 170 ms, respectively *(bottom right)*. AFL was no longer inducible after repeat ablation. *Abl-p and Abl-d*, proximal and distal electrograms from the ablation catheter; *CSp-CSd*, proximal through distal coronary sinus electrograms; *CTI*, cavotricuspid isthmus; *CW AFL*, Counterclockwise atrial flutter; *I, aVF, and V_1*, surface ECG leads; *LLRA* pacing, low lateral right atrial pacing; *M>L and L>M*, medial-to-lateral and lateral-to-medial trans-isthmus conduction.

REFERENCES

Please refer to the e-book for a complete list of references.

13

Ablation of Non–Isthmus-Dependent Flutters and Atrial Macroreentry

Steven M. Markowitz, Bruce B. Lerman

KEY POINTS

- Atypical or non–cavotricuspid isthmus–dependent atrial flutters require fixed or functional barriers and regions of slow conduction.
- Atypical flutters often occur after catheter ablation or surgical treatment of atrial fibrillation or after surgery that involves right or left atriotomies.
- Activation mapping is used to demonstrate reentrant circuits, mid-diastolic potentials, fractionated potentials, and double potentials.
- Entrainment distinguishes areas that participate in a tachycardia circuit from wavefronts that are passively activated.
- High-resolution mapping catheters and electroanatomical mapping systems are useful to map atypical flutters and identify critical isthmuses to target for ablation.
- Sources of difficulty include oscillations in atrial cycle length, conversion of atypical flutter to atrial fibrillation or other arrhythmias, interpretation and assignment of activation times to complex electrograms, achievement of transmural ablation with durable lines of conduction block, and recognition and ablation of epicardial connections.

INTRODUCTION

Atypical atrial flutters refer to a spectrum of arrhythmias that vary in location and circuit dimensions. Most atypical flutters encountered during electrophysiology procedures occur in patients who have had catheter ablation or surgical treatment for atrial fibrillation (AF), but these arrhythmias can also arise de novo in patients who have atrial myopathies. In this chapter, the term *atypical atrial flutter* will be used preferentially to refer reentrant circuits that are not dependent on the cavotricuspid isthmus (CTI). Atypical flutters may be classified based on their chamber of origin, size of the reentrant circuit, and site within a given atrium (Table 13.1).

ANATOMY

The specific configuration of a reentrant circuit depends on the local or global anatomy of the atrium, as well as the conduction and refractory properties of the atrial myocardium. As a general rule, reentry requires the presence of two limbs, which are anatomically and/or functionally contiguous but dissociated. These limbs are dependent on the presence of an inexcitable central barrier (i.e., atrioventricular annulus, venous ostium, or scar) or a functional line of block. In the right atrium (RA), natural barriers to conduction are the tricuspid annulus, inferior vena cava (IVC), superior vena cava (SVC), crista terminalis, Eustachian ridge, and fossa ovalis. In the left atrium (LA), the mitral annulus and pulmonary venous ostia serve as critical conduction barriers, along with electrically silent areas that may be found in myopathic atria or result from prior ablation or surgery.

PATHOPHYSIOLOGY

Atypical atrial flutters predominantly occur in patients with organic heart disease or after cardiac surgery or atrial fibrillation (AF) ablation. In patients with organic heart disease, the pathogenesis is thought to involve elevated atrial pressure, atrial distention, and activation of profibrotic signaling pathways, which cause interstitial fibrosis resulting in conduction slowing and block. Other important determinants are slowing of atrial conduction velocity, heterogeneity of atrial refractoriness, and initiating or triggering foci.

Fibrosis in the LA occurs in a variety of disease conditions, including systemic hypertension, rheumatic valve disease, hypertrophic cardiomyopathy, and other atrial myopathies. Areas of low voltage, consistent with diseased myocardium or scar, have been identified in various locations, such as the anterior, septal. or posterior walls of the LA and the lateral wall of the RA.[1–3] These areas of patchy scar create the substrate for macroreentry or localized reentry.

In response to premature stimuli or rapid atrial rates, arcs of functional block develop and—if of sufficient length—initiate and support reentry. Functional lines of block develop in structures such as the crista terminalis and the Eustachian ridge, both of which play a critical role in the formation of CTI-dependent atrial flutter.[4] Gaps in these functional lines of block,

TABLE 13.1 **Types of Nonisthmus-Dependent Atrial Flutters**

Circuit	Boundaries	Clinical Scenarios
RIGHT ATRIUM		
Upper loop reentry	SVC and crista terminalis	De novo or with CTI-dependent flutter
Right atrial free-wall reentry	Right atrial scar, lateral tricuspid annulus	Prior right atriotomy, atrial myopathy
Dual-loop reentry (combined lower loop, upper loop, free wall, and/or tricuspid valve)	Combinations of right atrial scar, SVC, tricuspid annulus, with or without CTI	Prior right atriotomy, atrial myopathy
LEFT ATRIUM		
Perimitral annular reentry	Mitral annulus, left atrial isthmus	Following left atrial ablation for AF, after maze surgery, de novo
Roof-dependent reentry	Wide-area antral isolation of pulmonary veins, possibly electrically active pulmonary vein tissue	Following left atrial ablation for atrial fibrillation with encircling lesions, after maze surgery, de novo
Anterior left atrial reentry	Scar in anterior or septal LA, mitral annulus	Following left atrial ablation for AF, atrial myopathy
Periseptal tachycardia	Right pulmonary veins and mitral annulus or fossa ovalis with right pulmonary veins or mitral annulus	Following atriotomy, left atrial ablation for atrial fibrillation, de novo
MISCELLANEOUS		
Lesional tachycardias	Surgical scars	Following left or right atriotomy, post maze surgery
Microreentry or localized reentry	Variable	Following left atrial ablation for AF, after maze surgery, atrial myopathy
Coronary sinus mediated reentry	Coronary sinus with left or right atrial myocardium	De novo

AF, Atrial fibrillation; *CTI,* cavotricuspid isthmus; *SV(C)* superior vena cava.

as in the crista terminalis, permit formation of atypical circuits. Functional lines of block may develop in many other locations, including variable sites in the LA. A combination of fixed and functional block has been demonstrated in animal models of lesional tachycardia, in which a line of functional block develops as an extension to a fixed anatomic lesion.[5] Functional lines of block have also been demonstrated clinically in flutter involving diseased myocardium in the anterior and septal LA.[6] In these cases, the anatomic lesions might not be large enough to support reentry, but the combined fixed and functional barriers provide critical path lengths needed to maintain reentry. Formation and breakdown of these arcs of block are responsible for interconversion of flutter circuits with each other and the transition to AF.

Atypical flutters are frequent after both catheter and surgical ablation. Discontinuities in ablation lines can result in unidirectional rate-dependent block or conduction slowing.[7] Commonly, endocardial gaps in linear ablation lines create the substrate for reentry. In other cases, failure to achieve transmural ablation results in epicardial connections with slow conduction and thus allow reentrant circuits to stabilize. Thus extensive ablation procedures for persistent AF, which may involve linear lesions and targeting of abnormal substrate, are associated with relatively high recurrence rates of ATs.[8] Furthermore, areas of excluded myocardium, such as those occurring with wide encircling pulmonary vein (PV) isolation, give rise to large central barriers that permit circus movement reentry. Many reentrant ATs are complex circuits that involve dual loops (figure-of-eight reentry) or, less commonly, triple loops.[9] In multiple loop tachycardias, conduction times are nearly equal around the individual loops, but sometimes a dominant circuit exists as a *driver,* which entrains other loops.

Small reentrant circuits, known as *localized reentry* or *microreentry*, can occur in a variety of clinical circumstances, such as catheter ablation of AF, surgical maze procedures, and surgical repair of congenital heart disease.[10,11] These small circuits can also occur de novo in diseased atria.[12] An arbitrary definition used in some studies to distinguish localized reentry from macroreentry is a circuit diameter <2–3 cm.[13] A unifying condition in cases of localized reentry is the presence of atrial fibrosis, as evidenced by their occurrence in areas of low voltage. Disruption of the myocardial architecture gives rise to markedly slow conduction, anisotropic differences in conduction velocity, and unidirectional block, which allow small circuits to develop and perpetuate. Evidence from high-resolution mapping shows that localized reentrant circuits consist of sequential corridors with very slow conduction.[13] Localized reentry has also been shown to occur adjacent to ablation lines or surgical incisions.

Cardiac surgery that involves atrial incisions is an important cause of atypical flutter. The location and extent of an incision, in addition to intrinsic disease of the atria, influence the likelihood of developing atypical flutter. Patients who have RA surgery are at risk of developing atypical flutter involving the surgical scar in the lateral RA, whereas those who have left atriotomies may develop atypical flutter in the LA.[14] In addition, patients who have right or left atriotomies are also prone to develop CTI-dependent flutter.

DIAGNOSIS

Macroreentrant Versus Focal AT

A fundamental consideration in evaluating atypical flutter is to establish if the arrhythmia is macroreentrant or focal in origin (Box 13.1), but the surface electrocardiogram (ECG) is usually not specific for the mechanism of an atypical flutter. In general, P-wave durations are shorter and surface isoelectric intervals are longer with focal tachycardias than with macroreentry.[15] A study of 75 patients with atypical flutters after AF ablation

BOX 13.1 Diagnostic Criteria

Macroreentrant Tachycardias

- Entrainment with fusion (with last beat entrained but not fused)
- Electroanatomic mapping of >90% of tachycardia cycle length with adjacent early and late areas of activation
- Insensitivity to adenosine (in dose sufficient to cause AV block)

Microreentrant Tachycardias or Localized Reentry

- Fragmented electrograms that encompass a large proportion of the tachycardia cycle length on single electrodes or multiple closely spaced electrodes
- Entrainment with progressively longer postpacing intervals at increasing distances from the apparent source
- Small circuit defined by electroanatomical mapping
- Insensitivity to adenosine (in dose sufficient to cause AV block)

Left Atrial Tachycardias

- Passive conduction in the RA, with early septal activation and fusion of wavefronts in the RA lateral wall
- Absence of RA activation during long segments of the cycle length (mapping <50% of tachycardia cycle length)
- Large variations in the RA cycle length with a relatively fixed cycle length in the LA
- Entrainment pacing at multiple sites in the RA yielding postpacing intervals >30 ms

AV, Atrioventricular; *LA,* left atrium; *RA,* right atrium.

found that a P-wave duration of <185 ms had a sensitivity of 85% and specificity of 97% in identifying a small reentrant circuit.[16] However, macroreentrant tachycardias may also have isoelectric intervals if part of the circuit consists of a slowly conducting isthmus generating little electric voltage.[17,18]

The electrocardiographic (ECG) morphology of atypical flutters is highly variable, and substantial overlaps exists between flutter morphologies arising from different anatomical circuits, so that localization of atrial flutters from the surface ECG has limited use. However, some broad generalizations can be made that distinguish CTI-dependent from non–CTI-dependent flutters, as well as right from left ATs.[19] CTI-dependent flutters often show characteristic morphologies, and recognizing deviation from these patterns allows one to conclude that a tachycardia might be atypical flutter. Typical counterclockwise CTI-dependent flutter usually has a superiorly directed flutter wave axis with a small terminal positive deflection in the inferior leads ("saw-tooth" pattern). Lead V_1 has an initial isoelectric or inverted component followed by a positive deflection, and the flutter wave transitions from positive to negative across the precordium. Clockwise CTI-dependent flutter is more variable, but it characteristically shows positive, notched flutter waves in the inferior leads and lead V_1 usually shows negative flutter waves. It should be emphasized that even CTI-dependent flutters can show variability in ECG morphology, and the "typical" patterns described above might also arise from non–CTI-dependent mechanisms, such as perimitral reentry. Typical CTI-dependent flutter that occurs after ablation for AF may lack the classic "saw-tooth" morphology,[20] although a transition from predominantly positive to negative P waves across the precordial leads is highly specific for peritricuspid reentry.[18]

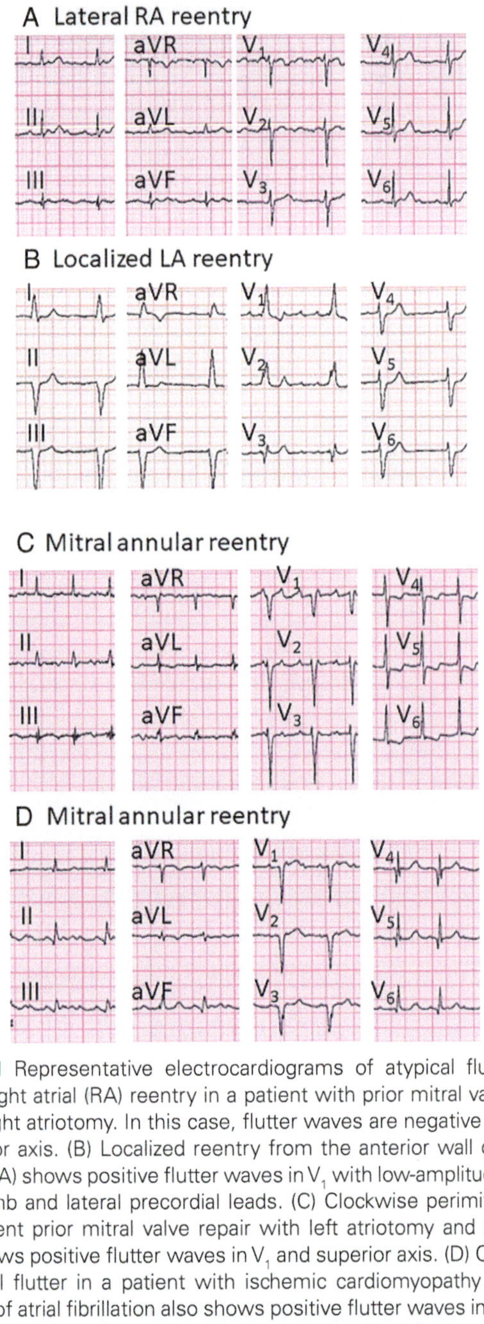

Fig. 13.1 Representative electrocardiograms of atypical flutters. (A) Lateral right atrial (RA) reentry in a patient with prior mitral valve repair with a right atriotomy. In this case, flutter waves are negative in V_1 with an inferior axis. (B) Localized reentry from the anterior wall of the left atrium (LA) shows positive flutter waves in V_1 with low-amplitude signals in the limb and lateral precordial leads. (C) Clockwise perimitral flutter in a patient prior mitral valve repair with left atriotomy and maze surgery shows positive flutter waves in V_1 and superior axis. (D) Clockwise, perimitral flutter in a patient with ischemic cardiomyopathy and prior ablation of atrial fibrillation also shows positive flutter waves in V_1, in this case with inferior axis, attributed to preexisting block in the cavotricuspid isthmus. Note the isoelectric intervals in perimitral flutter, illustrating that isoelectric intervals are not specific for focal tachycardia.

Generally, flutters that are predominately negative in V_1 arise from the RA, whereas those that show broad positive waves in V_1 (without isoelectric or negative initial components) usually arise from the LA (Fig. 13.1). Many LA flutters have low-amplitude deflections in the precordial leads and lateral limb leads, which reflect advanced atrial myopathy in these patients.[19,21] Detailed mapping studies of perimitral flutter permit some generalizations with regard to the flutter wave morphology and show that the frontal axis of the P wave in perimitral flutter is usually determined by RA activation.[22] Thus, counterclockwise perimitral flutters usually have inferior P-wave axes and clockwise atrial flutters have superior axes, as determined by wavefront propagation in the RA and septum. Exceptions occur when there is scar in the LA that interrupts interatrial conduction across Bachmann's bundle or prior ablation lesions such as block in the CTI. Isoelectric segments are usually present in perimitral flutter and correspond to activation of the diseased lateral LA. Despite these generalizations, localization of atypical flutters by ECG morphology is limited because the P waves are highly dependent on the extent and distribution of atrial fibrosis as well as prior interventions.

Evidence for a macroreentrant mechanism can be obtained through manifest entrainment, entrainment with concealed fusion (concealed entrainment), or electroanatomical mapping. Manifest entrainment is recognized as fixed fusion at any given paced cycle length and by progressive fusion with progressively rapid overdrive pacing.[23] Because the surface flutter wave may not be visible or may be obscured by ventricular depolarization or repolarization, intracardiac electrograms are used for identifying orthodromic and antidromic capture and the degree of fusion. Manifest entrainment with progressive fusion implies a dimensionality to the tachycardia circuit that includes separate entrance and exit sites, a condition that does not exist for focal tachycardia and is unlikely to be demonstrated for microreentry. "Downstream overdrive pacing" is a useful maneuver using multielectrode catheters that can confirm macroreentry.[24] If concealed fusion is identified when pacing from electrodes which are activated late compared to neighboring electrodes, then the tachycardia mechanism is very likely to be macroreentry (Fig. 13.2).

A pacing site is considered to be within a tachycardia circuit when the postpacing interval after entrainment is ≤30 ms greater than the tachycardia cycle length (Fig. 13.2). Entrainment from two opposite quadrants (such as septal and lateral LA, or anterior and posterior LA), each with return cycle lengths within 30 ms of the tachycardia cycle length, indicates the presence of a macroreentrant circuit.[25] Thus, *in-circuit* entrainment

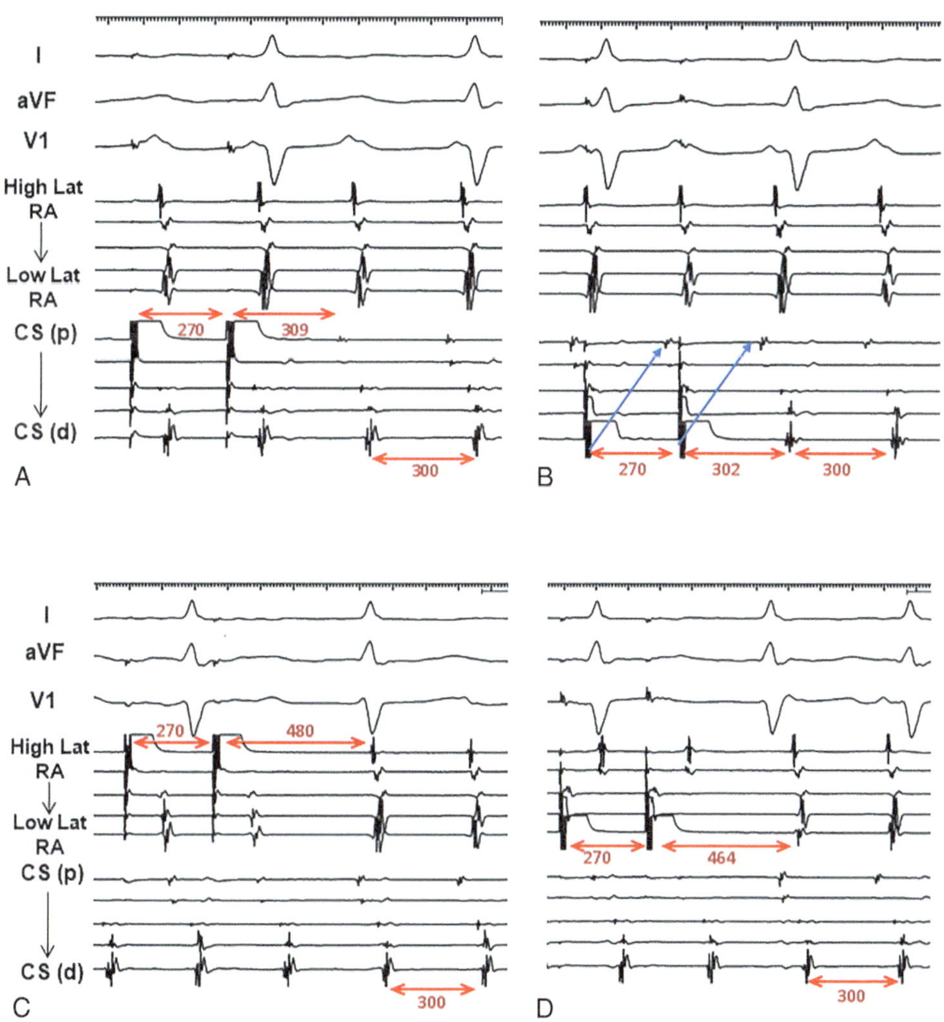

Fig. 13.2 Entrainment from multipolar catheters localizes a left atrial tachycardia. Activation of the coronary sinus (CS) is proximal to distal. Entrainment from the proximal and distal poles of the CS catheter (A and B) results in postpacing intervals nearly identical to the tachycardia cycle length. (B) Phenomenon of downstream overdrive pacing. Entrainment from the distal electrode of the CS catheters (downstream from the proximal electrodes) results in orthodromic capture of the proximal poles after conduction delay. (C and D) Entrainment from the high and low right atrium (RA), respectively, both of which show long postpacing intervals (as well as fusion of intracardiac electrograms during pacing), indicating that they are remote from the tachycardia circuit. These responses are consistent with a left atrial tachycardia, which was per-mitral reentry.

from the septal and lateral LA often indicates perimitral reentry; *in-circuit* entrainment from the anterior and posterior LA is consistent with a roof-dependent LA flutter. Entrainment may also give indirect information about the distance of a pacing site from the reentrant circuit, with shorter postpacing intervals indicating closer proximity to the circuit.

Entrainment is often needed to confirm if particular regions participate in the tachycardia, particularly if the electroanatomical map is ambiguous and it is difficult to distinguish critical components from bystander regions.[26–28] On occasion, localized reentrant arrhythmias occur on one side of a linear lesion and the electroanatomical map will give the inaccurate impression of macroreentry. In this case, entrainment would clarify that tissue on the opposite side of the line if passively activated.

Combining activation and entrainment mapping can rapidly identify a mechanism of atypical flutter.[25] Opposite activation sequences in the superior and inferior mitral annulus (e.g., lateral-to-septal activation along the superior annulus and septal-to-lateral activation along the inferior annuli) identify perimitral reentry. By contrast, similar directions of activation (e.g., lateral-to-septal) in both the superior and inferior annuli exclude perimitral reentry. Opposite activation along the anterior and posterior walls is seen with roof-dependent reentry.

Ultra-high-resolution mapping is indispensable for defining complex atypical circuits and identifying appropriate sites for ablation.[29–31] Mapping systems that display histograms of activation time and identify fractionated electrograms can help distinguish reentry from focal tachycardias and identify the timing and locations of critical isthmuses (Fig. 13.10). Recent iterations in mapping software display vectors of wavefront activation and conduction velocity, based on computational models derived from the unipolar electrograms or through the use of omnipolar electrogram analysis.[32,33]

The response to adenosine is useful in distinguishing reentrant from focal ATs, in that it exerts mechanistic-specific effects on atrial arrhythmias.[34] With rare exceptions, adenosine does not terminate the vast majority of reentrant atrial arrhythmias, whereas it either terminates focal ATs due to triggered activity and transiently suppresses focal AT due to enhanced automaticity (Fig. 13.3). Adenosine-insensitive ATs with apparently focal activation patterns show characteristics of localized reentrant circuits, including low-amplitude, long-duration fractionated electrograms, and can be entrained.[12] This direct tool provides a reliable means for establishing a tachycardia mechanism before mapping (Fig. 13.4).

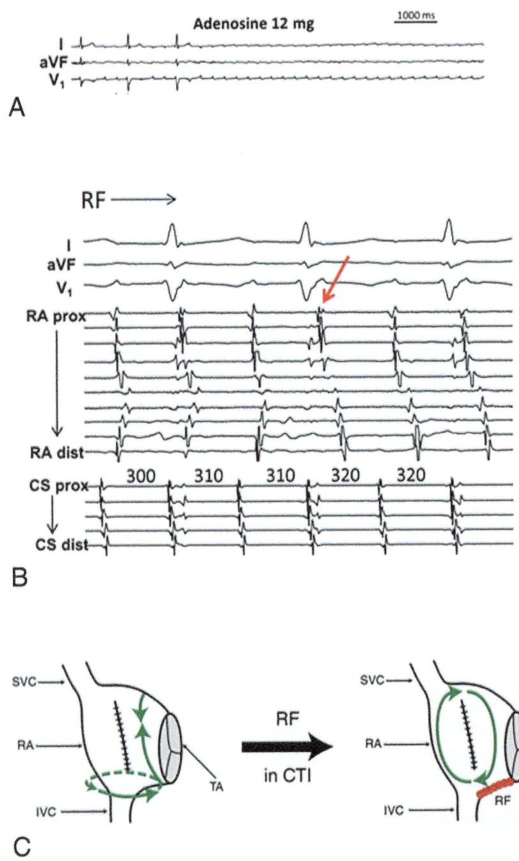

Fig. 13.3 Reentrant atrial tachycardia in a patient with a prior lateral right atriotomy. (A) The tachycardia is insensitive to adenosine, which is consistent with a reentrant mechanism. (B) A duodecapolar catheter in the lateral right atrium (RA) demonstrates fusion of wavefronts in the lateral wall. This pattern is consistent with lower loop reentry, with a circuit around the inferior vena cava (IVC). During ablation in the cavotricuspid isthmus, the tachycardia cycle length prolongs and activation in the lateral right atrium changes *(arrow)*, which is explained by interruption of lower loop reentry and the existence of a second circuit involving the lateral right atriotomy. (C) The change in the tachycardia circuit is illustrated graphically. *CS*, Coronary sinus; *CTI*, cavotricuspid isthmus; *RF*, radiofrequency; *SV(C)* superior vena cava; *T(A)* tricuspid annulus.

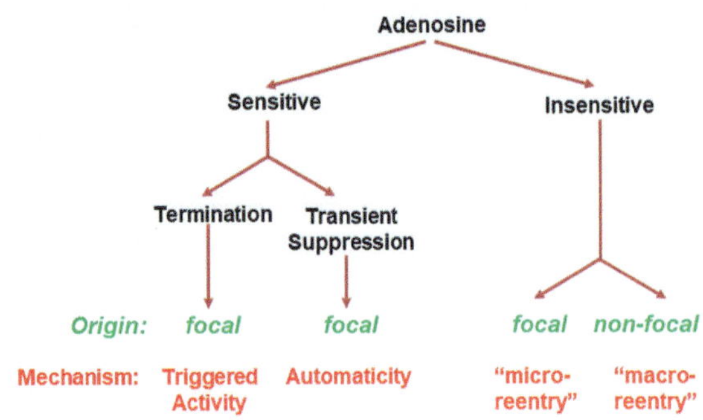

	Triggered Activity	Automaticity	"micro-reentry"	"macro-reentry"
Induction by PES	+	-	+	+
Termination by PES	+	-	+	+
Entrainment	-	-	+	+
Electrogram duration	N	N	L	N/L
Catecholamine facilitation	+	+	+/-	+/-

Fig. 13.4 Differentiating mechanisms of atrial tachycardia using adenosine and electrophysiological characteristics. Adenosine-sensitive atrial tachycardia is typically focal in origin and due to triggered activity or, far less commonly, automaticity. Adenosine-insensitive atrial tachycardia is either macroreentrant or microreentrant, depending on circuit size and the resolution of the mapping system. Entrainment with the postpacing interval (PPI) nearly equal to the atrial tachycardia cycle length (ATCL) is typical for "macro" or "micro" reentrant tachycardias. Markedly prolonged electrogram durations may be recorded at early sites in microreentrant tachycardias but are not typical at the origin of triggered and automatic rhythms. Electrogram durations at sites around a macroreentrant circuit might vary depending on local conduction characteristics. *L*, Long electrogram duration; *N*, normal duration; *PES*,programmed electrical stimulation. (Adapted with permission from Markowitz SM, Nemirovksy D, Stein KM, et al. Adenosine-insensitive focal atrial tachycardia: evidence for de novo micro-re-entry in the human atrium. *J Am Coll Cardiol*. 2007;49:1324–1333.)

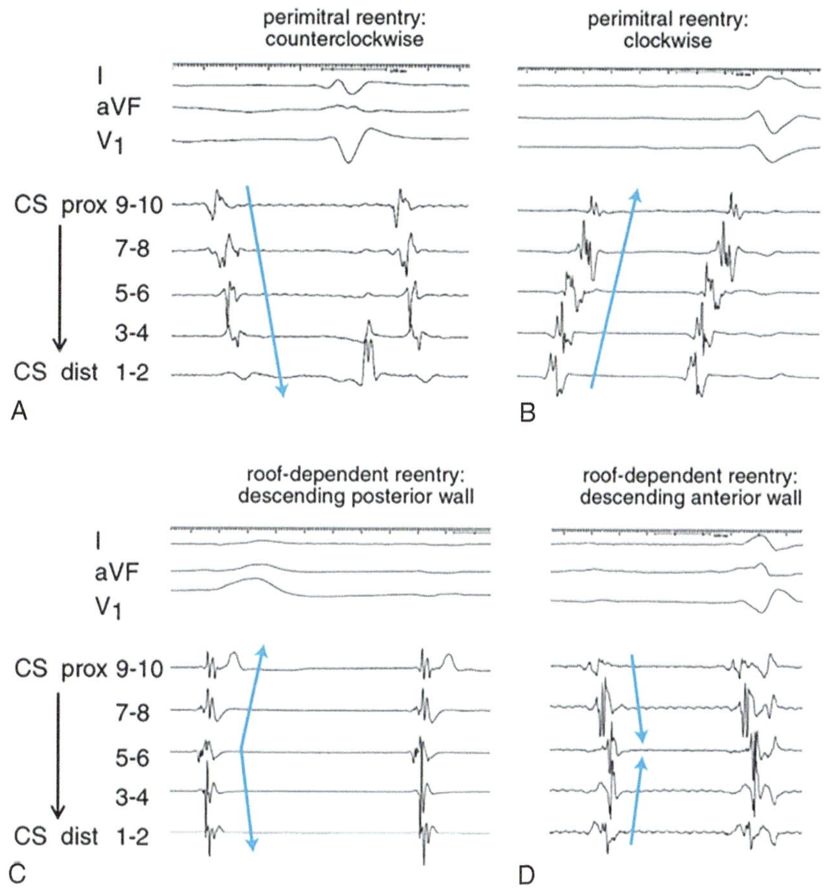

Fig. 13.5 Activation sequences of the coronary sinus (CS) in various forms of macroreentrant left atrial tachycardia. (A) Counterclockwise perimitral reentry gives rise to proximal-to-distal CS activation. (B) Clockwise perimitral reentry produces distal-to-proximal CS activation. (C) Roof-dependent atrial tachycardia with a descending wavefront in the posterior wall causes early activation in the mid CS, after which the impulse propagates both proximally and distally along the mitral annulus (*chevron pattern*). (D) Roof-dependent atrial tachycardia with a descending wavefront in the anterior wall causes fusion of wavefronts in the posterior mitral annulus (by the coronary sinus) because the impulse first activates the anterior mitral annulus and then bifurcates to activate the lateral and septal walls before fusing in the posterior annulus (*reverse chevron pattern*). Localized reentrant and focal tachycardias can also give rise to these patterns of activation depending on the location.

Localization of Reentry to the Right or Left Atrium

The activation pattern of the coronary sinus (CS) is useful in localizing ATs.[35,36] RA tachycardias typically exhibit proximal-to-distal activation in the CS, unless activation proceeds predominantly over Bachmann's bundle (or the catheter is positioned very distally in the CS), in which case the distal CS may be activated earlier. LA tachycardias show a variety of activation patterns depending on the particular reentrant circuit (Fig. 13.5). Some LA tachycardias, such as clockwise perimitral annular reentry and tachycardias originating near the lateral LA (by the left PVs or appendage), exhibit distal-to-proximal CS activation. However, a proximal-to-distal sequence does not necessarily localize the arrhythmia to the RA and may be seen with counterclockwise perimitral reentry or tachycardias involving the septum or right PVs. *Chevron* and *reverse chevron* activation patterns occur with roof-dependent LA macroreentry. The chevron pattern occurs when a wavefront descends the posterior wall and activates the mid-posterior mitral annulus and then propagates in both septal and lateral directions along the inferior LA. The reverse chevron pattern occurs when a wavefront descends the anterior LA wall and then fuses in the posterior mitral annulus. The location of a CS catheter will affect the likelihood of identifying these patterns; specifically, the chevron sequences would not necessarily be recognized if the CS catheter is positioned very distally in the great cardiac vein. A nearly simultaneous CS activation pattern distinguishes roof-dependent reentry from perimitral reentry with relatively high accuracy. The measurement of mitral annular activation time (earliest to latest activation times on a decapolar CS catheter) can distinguish peri-mitral flutter from roof-dependent LA flutter.[36,37] A mitral annular activation time of <40–45 ms with nonsequential activation identifies roof-dependent flutter with high sensitivity and specificity.

It is possible to establish a diagnosis of LA tachycardia during mapping in the RA and thus identify the need for transseptal catheterization and LA mapping. Criteria for identifying an LA origin through intracardiac mapping include the following:

1. Passive conduction into the RA, which may be demonstrated as fused wavefronts in the lateral wall of the RA.
2. Earliest RA activation in the septum, typically in the region of Bachmann's bundle or the CS ostium, especially if areas of early activation encompass a large area.[38]
3. Large variations in the RA cycle length with a relatively fixed cycle length in the LA, implying LA/RA dissociation or conduction block.
4. Entrainment pacing at multiple sites in the RA (including the CTI and the RA free wall) yielding postpacing intervals > 30 ms.

While fusion of wavefronts in the lateral wall of the RA is common during LA tachycardias, it is possible to record a single wavefront mimicking counterclockwise or clockwise atrial flutter. This situation depends on (1) the location of the multipolar catheter in the lateral wall, (2) the location of conduction breakthrough from the LA (i.e., preferential conduction over Bachmann's bundle or the CS), and (3) the presence of conduction block in the CTI. Typically, activation time in the RA is substantially less than the tachycardia cycle length. Exceptions occur when the tachycardia cycle length is short or if conduction is substantially slowed in the RA, incorrectly implying the presence of an RA tachycardia.

ABLATION

The guiding principle in ablating atypical flutters is to target a critical isthmus or component that participates in the tachycardia circuit (Box 13.2). The critical isthmus may be a narrow channel or a relatively broad region. In the case of dual-loop tachycardias, it is helpful to identify the common isthmus or corridor. Ablation can be performed by targeting the common isthmus or each loop separately. The technique of ablation involves the creation of a linear lesion between two electrically silent boundaries to transect the isthmus. Occasionally, a single radiofrequency (RF) application is enough to interrupt a narrow isthmus or localized reentry.

Most ablation for atypical flutters is performed with force-sensing, irrigated RF catheters. An impedance drop of ≥10 Ω during ablation is a specific indicator of effective RF lesion formation.[39] Other criteria for effective lesion creation include reduction in bipolar electrogram amplitude, a change in unipolar electrogram morphology (loss of S wave), failure to capture local tissue with high output pacing, and ablation indices that integrate power, force, and time.[40,41] Local impedance measured between microelectrodes on the tip of an ablation catheter provide reliable information about tissue heating. Optimal cut-off values for local impedance drop in predicting conduction block were found to be 16 Ω for the LA anterior wall or roof and 12 Ω for the posterior or inferior LA.[42]

In cases of linear lesions, bidirectional conduction block should be verified after ablation by pacing from either side of the ablation line and recording from the contralateral side. The detour of wavefronts around completed ablation lines can be displayed graphically with a reconstructed electroanatomical map during pacing or sinus rhythm (Fig. 13.6, Video 13.1). Widely spaced double potentials along an ablation line, while pacing from one side, provide supporting evidence for conduction block after ablation. The techniques of differential pacing can be used to support the presence of conduction block. This is based on the principle that pacing and recording close to a line of block result in longer conduction times than pacing or recording farther away from the line. Noninducibility of AT is another important end point of ablation. In cases of extreme conduction delay or epicardial bridges, criteria for conduction block across a line might be fulfilled, but a slower variant of the ablated AT could still be inducible (Table 13.2).

Pulsed-field ablation holds promise to create durable transmural lesions even in the presence of preexisting scar. While

BOX 13.2 Target Sites for Ablation

General Principles

- Critical isthmus identified by electroanatomical mapping bounded by two conduction barriers
- Entrainment demonstrates orthodromic capture of most of atrium (*concealed entrainment* is present) and postpacing interval minus tachycardia cycle length ≤30 ms

Ablation Strategies for Specific Arrhythmias

Upper Loop Reentry

- Gap in crista terminalis
- Linear ablation from SVC to scar or tricuspid annulus or intercaval line

RA Free-Wall Reentry

- Linear ablation from conduction barrier to IVC
- Linear ablation from conduction barrier to tricuspid annulus
- Linear ablation from conduction barrier to SVC

Perimitral Reentry

- Linear ablation from lateral mitral annulus to left inferior PV, with or without coronary sinus ablation
- Linear ablation from anterior mitral annulus to roof line or PV
- Linear ablation from septal mitral annulus to right PVs

LA Roof-Dependent Reentry

- Linear ablation between left and right superior PVs (roof line)
- Linear ablation between left and right inferior PVs (posterior wall)

LA Anterior Reentry

- Linear ablation in channel: from scar to mitral annulus, to PV, or neighboring scar

Left Septal Reentry

- Linear ablation from septum to mitral annulus
- Linear ablation from septum to right pulmonary

Lesional Tachycardia

- Linear ablation from scar boundary to anatomical barrier
- Gap within incomplete incisional lines

Localized Reentry

- Site with highly fragmented electrograms encompassing large percentage of tachycardia cycle length

IVC, Inferior vena cava; *LA*, left atrium; *RA*, right atrium; *SVC*, superior vena cava.

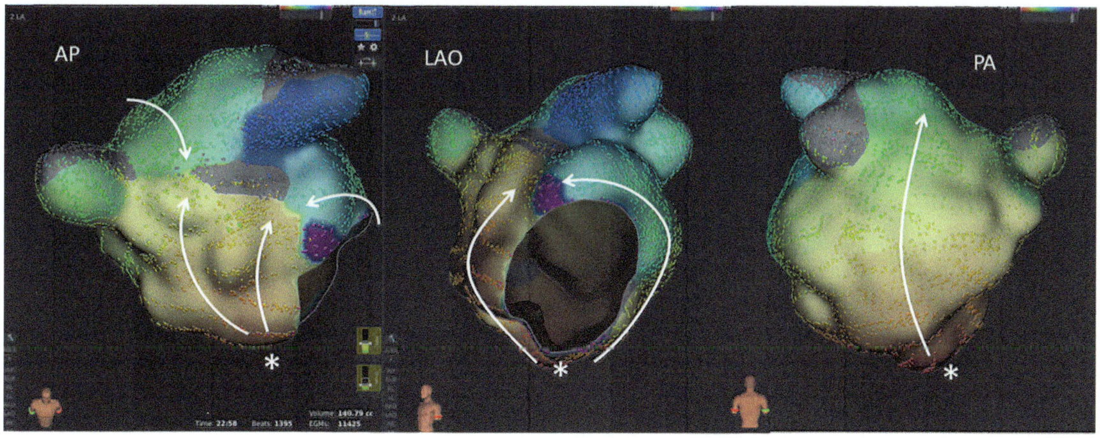

Fig. 13.6 Demonstrating line of block with electroanatomical mapping (Rhythmia) after ablation along the septal left atrium in the patient with roof dependent flutter depicted in Fig. 13.10. Pacing from the proximal coronary sinus *(asterisk)* results in wavefronts ascending the posterior wall and septum and counterclockwise around the mitral annulus, with collision in the superior septum. Projections are shown in modified anteroposterior (AP), left anterior oblique (LAO), and posteroanterior (AP). See Video 13.1.

TABLE 13.2 Troubleshooting Difficult Cases

Problem	Cause	Solution
Unstable rhythm interconverting with AF or other forms of atypical flutter	Instability of lines of block	• Limit atrial pacing and entrainment mapping • Consider noncontact electroanatomic mapping • Consider long linear lesions and/or ablation of atrial fibrillation • Identify and treat channels of slowly conducting tissue • Low-dose Class IC or III drug to stabilize reentry
Uninterpretable electroanatomical map	Incomplete map, failure to identify lines of block and areas of scar	• Use ultra-high-density mapping • Review voltage map to identify areas of scar and low-voltage, fragmented electrograms • Review annotation of electrograms • Use entrainment to identify critical components of tachycardia • Review previous surgery and ablation attempts
Failure to achieve conduction block in mitral isthmus	Persistent epicardial conduction	• Use irrigated radiofrequency catheter • Ablate within coronary sinus • Ethanol ablation in vein of Marshall • Alternative linear lesion
Failure to terminate tachycardia despite complete ablation line	Dual-loop reentry, epicardial connections, inaccurate mapping of critical isthmus	• Reevaluate cycle length, surface ECG, and activation sequence • Reevaluate map or re-map • Consider ablating epicardial connection
Unstable catheter during linear ablation	Large left atrium, limited catheter mobility	• Use adjustable or telescoping sheath system, change catheters, linear ablation array, robotic navigation

AF, Atrial fibrillation; *ECG,* electrocardiography.

initial applications of pulsed-field energy have centered on ablation of AF, the technology has been demonstrated to be effective in isolating the posterior LA and ablation in the roof and lateral mitral isthmus.[43,44] Catheters used with pulsed-field ablation include multielectrode arrays, and pulsed wave forms; generators are also being investigated for use with conventional RF ablation catheters.

Ablation Outcomes

Acute and long-term clinical outcomes depend on the specific arrhythmia targeted for ablation and the atrial substrate. Most studies show acute success rates of >85% for ablating atypical flutters in patients with or without prior ablation or surgery. However recurrences of atrial arrhythmias are common after ablation of atypical flutter (25–50% over 12–20 months), although subsequent arrhythmias may arise from different circuits or mechanisms.[10,45–47] Similarly high recurrence rates are seen in patients with atypical flutter after surgery for valve disease, particularly if patients also have documented AF.[48]

High-density mapping has been shown to result in better acute outcomes and fewer recurrences compared to lower-resolution catheter and mapping systems. One study compared a high-density grid catheter with circular mapping catheters in 82 patients with 142 atypical flutters.[49] Acute ablation success was highest in those with the grid catheter, particularly when used with the latest generation mapping system. This group also had fewer "unmappable" rhythms and better flutter-free survival. These results were replicated in another study of 87 patients, in whom higher acute and long-term success were obtained in those mapped with a high-density grid catheter.[50]

SPECIFIC FORMS OF ATYPICAL FLUTTER (SEE TABLE 13.1)

Upper Loop Reentry

This macroreentrant circuit involves reentry around the SVC and an area of fixed or functional conduction block adjacent to the SVC. Upper loop reentry may occur in patients who also have isthmus-dependent flutter but it also occurs in isolation or in those with a prior right atriotomy (Fig. 13.7; Video 13.2). The ECG in upper loop reentry mimics the morphology of clockwise CTI-dependent flutter, with an inferior flutter wave axis.[21] Electrograms may show a descending wavefront in the lateral RA, but if scar or conduction block extends inferior to the SVC, the pattern of activation may be more complex. Concealed entrainment may be demonstrated in the septum between the fossa ovalis and the SVC and in the high lateral RA. The most effective strategy is to identify a gap between nonconductive barriers, such as between adjacent regions of scar or between the SVC and scar.

Right Atrial Free-Wall Macroreentry

Macroreentry may occur in the free wall of the RA in patients with an atriotomy, but also has been reported in patients without prior cardiac surgery.[1,51,52] The pathophysiology of this arrhythmia is reentry around a line of block in the lateral RA, defined by an electrically silent area or a line of double potentials. Lateral right atriotomies are utilized for repair of congenital heart disease (such as atrial septal defects and more complex congenital disease), mitral and tricuspid valve surgery, and removal of atrial myxomas. In patients without an atriotomy, free wall reentry arises because of fixed scar in the lateral RA or rate-related functional block in the crista terminalis.

Mapping with conventional multipolar catheters reveals a line of double potentials in the lateral wall, which are widely split in the middle of the line and progressively narrow toward the end of the line where the wavefront pivots. Often, a fractionated potential is recorded at the inferior end of the line, reflecting the lower pivot point (Fig. 13.8). Entrainment from both sides of the central line of block results in postpacing intervals within 30 ms of the tachycardia cycle length, indicating that both limbs participate in the tachycardia circuit. The location of the upper pivot point may be in the upper free wall of the RA or involve the SVC. Other variants of RA free wall reentry show figure-of-eight patterns in the lateral wall. Catheter ablation may be performed by making a line of RF lesions between the lateral RA (the area of double potentials) and the IVC. Alternatively, ablation may be performed in the corridor between the line of block in the lateral wall and the tricuspid annulus or the crista terminalis. It is important to confirm line of block after interrupting lateral wall reentry. When ablation is performed from the lateral wall to the IVC, line of block can be demonstrated

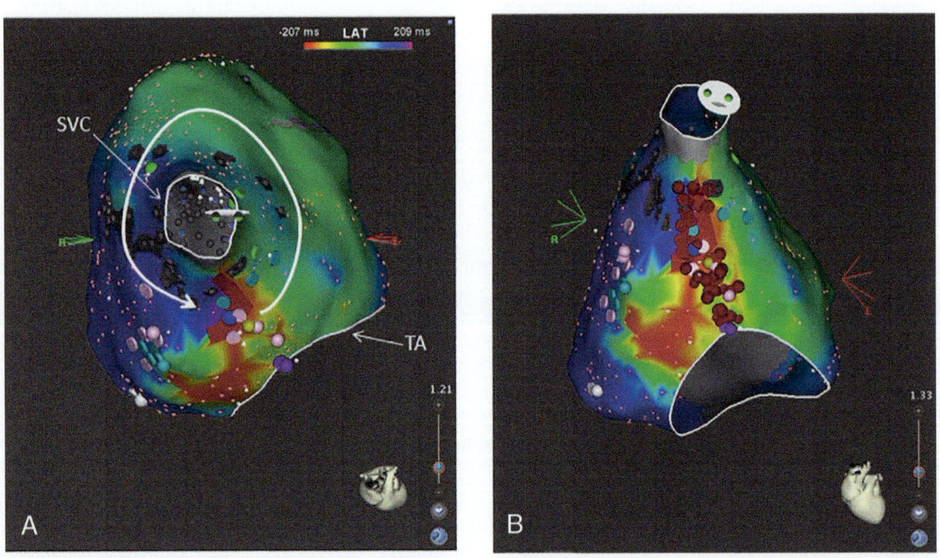

Fig. 13.7 Upper loop reentry in patient with prior mitral valve and maze surgery. (A) Superior projection of the electroanatomical map shows reentry around the superior vena cava (SVC). *Green tags* indicate sites where entrainment was consistent with participation in the tachycardia circuit. *Pink tags* indicate fractionated electrograms. (B) An ablation line between the SVC and anterior tricuspid annulus (TA) terminated the tachycardia.

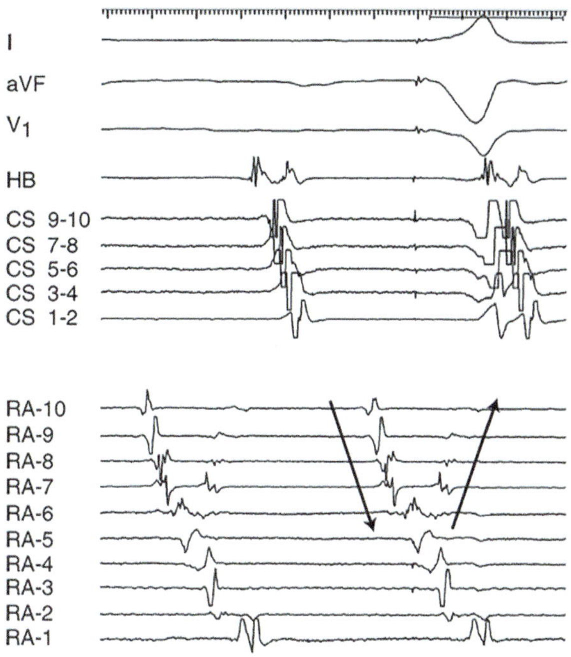

Fig. 13.8 Right atrial (RA) free-wall reentry. Double potentials in the lateral wall reflect descending and ascending wavefronts, with narrowing of the intervals between double potentials down the lateral wall and a fragmented electrogram reflecting a *pivot point* in pole RA-6 (RA-1, low lateral RA; RA-10, high lateral RA). *CS,* Coronary sinus.

by pacing and recording both anterior and posterior to the line (Fig. 13.9). Activation should proceed in a cranio-caudal direction on the side opposite the pacing site.[53,54]

Dual-Loop Right Atrial Macroreentry

Dual-loop reentry may occur in the RA in which two atypical circuits described earlier coexist or when one of the atypical circuits combine with rotation around the tricuspid annulus. Entrainment and electroanatomic mapping have been used to identify various combinations of reentry around the IVC (lower loop reentry), the tricuspid annulus, the SVC, and a conduction barrier in the lateral RA (Fig. 13.3). Ablation of one component usually transforms the tachycardia to another circuit. Dual-loop reentry is common in patients who have prior right atriotomies.[55] One example is reentry around the atriotomy scar that coexists with peritricuspid reentry. The flutter wave morphology may resemble typical flutter, and activation mapping may indicate reentry around the tricuspid annulus, which is confirmed with entrainment mapping in the CTI. If mapping in the lateral RA is not performed, the second component of this circuit might not be identified. A multipolar catheter is useful for demonstrating ascending and descending wavefronts on either side of a lateral atriotomy. Ablation in the CTI modifies but does not terminate the tachycardia, as evidenced by a change in activation pattern and/or cycle length (Fig. 13.3). This form of dual-loop reentry can be treated by creating two linear lesions to interrupt each reentrant loop (one in the CTI and another from the lateral atriotomy to the IVC or SVC) or ablating the common isthmus (e.g., between the lateral tricuspid annulus and the lateral atriotomy). Because catheter stability may be challenging in the lateral tricuspid annulus, many operators favor CTI and inferior RA lesions. As with single loop lateral wall reentry, it is important to verify line of block with pacing maneuvers in addition to noninducibility (Fig. 13.9). Some dual-loop tachycardias share a narrow common isthmus in the lateral wall that can be targeted for focal ablation (Video 13.3).

Ablation Outcomes for Atypical Right Atrial Flutters

The acute success rate of ablating lateral wall reentry generally exceeds 85%, but late recurrences of atrial arrhythmias are common. After ablation of macroreentrant AT in patients with right atriotomies, 55–75% of patients remain free of arrhythmias during intermediate-term follow-up, but there are high rates of AF (up to 30%) during long-term follow-up.[56–58] Improvements in mapping and ablation technologies may improve long-term outcomes with regard to recurrences of the targeted arrhythmias, with acute success rates exceeding 90% and freedom from recurrences of 72–86%.[55,59] As with other arrhythmia substrates, higher long-term success is achievable with repeat ablations.[60] The issue of late AF is of particular importance in patients with arrhythmogenic atrial substrate because patients may require anticoagulation and additional medical or ablative therapy during follow-up.

Perimitral Reentry

In typical forms of perimitral reentry, the entire tachycardia cycle length is accounted for around the mitral annulus. Variations of perimitral reentry occur in which the circuit involves only segments of the mitral annulus and the impulse detours around areas of scar (Fig. 13.10). A circuit around the mitral annulus may also coexist with a second loop, such as reentry around a set of PVs (*roof-dependent reentry*) or around scar in the anterior LA (Fig. 13.11). In cases of prior ablation, particularly if linear lesions were performed, the reentrant circuit may involve epicardial structures, such as the ligament of Marshall (LOM), muscu lar bundles connecting the LA to the sleeve that envelopes the CS and proximal great cardiac vein, or Bachmann's bundle. The presence of an epicardial bridge can be surmised when an electroanatomical maps does not encompass the complete tachycardia cycle length and there are apparent areas of "breakthrough" activation on the endocardial surface (Fig. 13.12; Video 13.4). In these situations, entrainment can confirm if macroreentry is present and what regions participate in the tachycardia.

Perimitral reentry is treated by creating a line of RF lesions between the mitral annulus and another electrical barrier. This barrier can be an electrically isolated PV or a line of block in the LA roof (Fig. 13.13). A common approach is to create a linear lesion from the lateral mitral annulus to the left inferior PV (*lateral mitral isthmus*). Completion of the ablation line in the *lateral mitral isthmus* may be difficult to achieve because of a CS muscular sleeve, and incomplete ablation can result in slow conduction and thus promote recurrent perimitral flutter. Achieving a line of block often requires ablation within the CS with an irrigated-tip catheter.[61] Ablation within the CS is performed at power settings of 20–30 W with irrigation rates of 17–60 mL/min, depending on the type of ablation catheter. Verification of a line of block along the *mitral isthmus* can be demonstrated

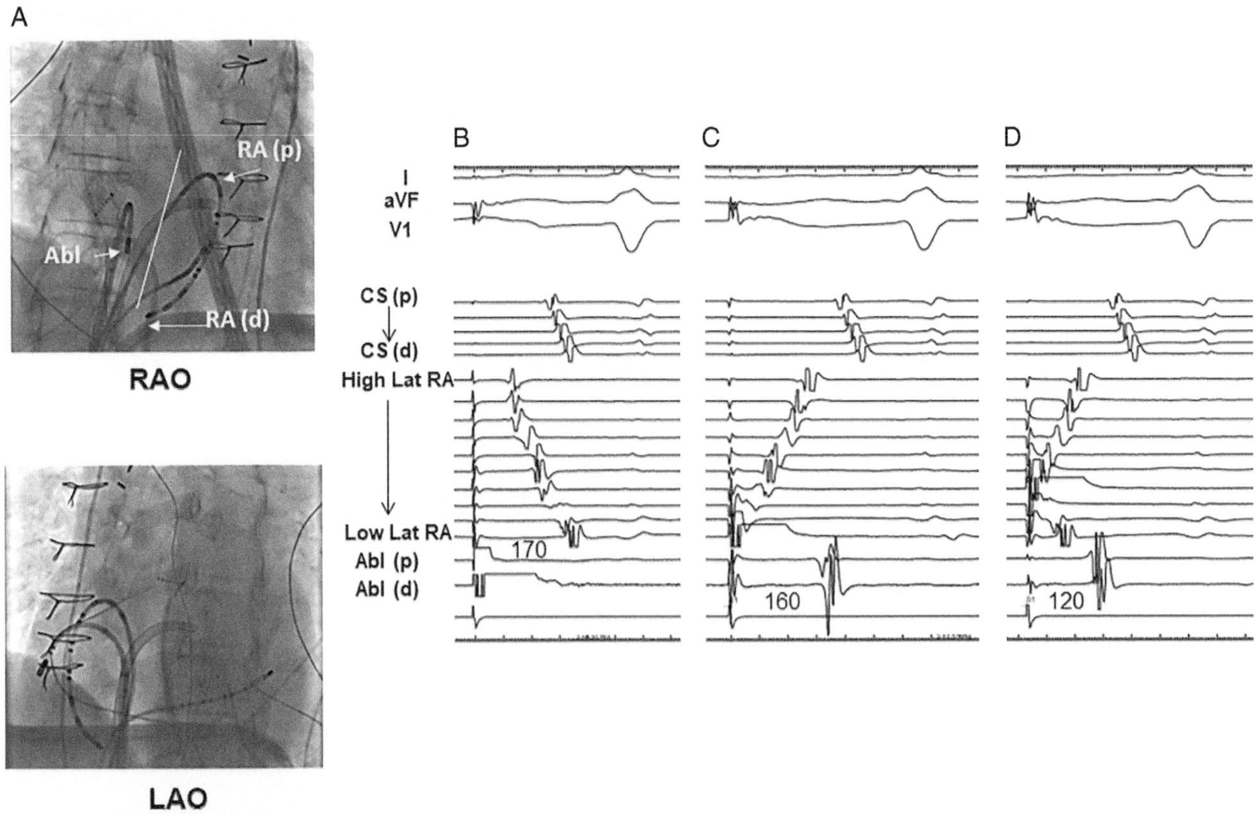

Fig. 13.9 Demonstration of bidirectional line of block in lateral wall of the right atrium (RA). The patient had incisional reentry around scar in the lateral RA. Ablation was performed between the scar in the lateral RA to the inferior vena cava. (A) Fluoroscopic images in right and left anterior oblique show a multipolar catheter in the RA anterior to a line of block; an ablation catheter (Abl) in the lateral RA positioned posterior to the line of block, and a coronary sinus catheter (CS). (B) During pacing from the ablation catheter, there is delay to the low right atrium (170 ms) with a descending wavefront on the multipolar catheter, consistent with propagation around the superior end of the line and down the anterolateral wall. (C) During pacing from the low lateral RA (RA 1-2) anterior to the line, there is similar delay to the ablation catheter on the other side of the line (160 ms). (D) Pacing higher on the anterolateral wall at RA 7-8 results in a shorter interval to the ablation catheter positioned posterior to the line (120 ms), since it is closer to the superior margin of the ablation line. *(d)*, Distal; *(p)*, proximal; *lat*, lateral; *LAO*, left anterior oblique; *RAO*, right anterior oblique.

by pacing on either side of the ablation line; the CS catheter is useful for assessing activation lateral to the line or it may cover both sides of the line of block (Fig. 13.14). If line of block is achieved, there should be proximal-to-distal CS activation during LA appendage pacing, and similar delay should occur to the appendage during distal CS pacing. In addition, the presence of double potentials along the line supports the existence of conduction block.

Epicardial connections involving the LOM and muscular bundles to the CS or great cardiac vein may remain after endocardial ablation in the lateral mitral isthmus ablation.[62–64] In fact, if conduction exists through epicardial connections, criteria for conduction block in the lateral isthmus might seem to be achieved ("pseudoblock"; see Table 13.2). In this case, pacing the LAA results in apparent focal activation of the posterolateral LA where the epicardial connection is located and conduction propagates toward the lateral ablation line. Further ablation along the Marshall bundle in the ridge between the PVs and appendage, at sites with long fragmented electrograms, might be needed to achieve true conduction block. Also, identifying connection sites in the great cardiac vein, along the atrial or free wall side of the vein, can facilitate complete conduction block.[64] Careful analysis of electrograms may show distinct local and far-field components, which reflect activation of the CS and the endocardial LA.[35] Analogously, "pseudoblock" can exist with an anteroseptal line if epicardial conduction exists over Bachmann's bundle or septal myocardium or if extremely slow conduction persists through a remaining endocardial channel (Fig. 13.15).[65]

Ethanol infusion in the vein of Marshall has been shown to improve success of lateral mitral isthmus ablation, facilitate isolation of the left PVs, and also reduce recurrences after ablation of persistent AF (Fig. 13.16, Video 13.5).[66–68] The vein of Marshall is located proximal to the valve of Vieussens and can be identified by venography extending posteriorly and superiorly from the CS toward the LA. The technique involves advancing an over-the-wire angioplasty balloon (1.5–2.5 mm × 6–8 mm) and occluding the vein with low-pressure inflation. Contrast injections verify occlusion of the vein and the specific venous anatomy. Ethanol (98–99%, 1–3 mL) is injected and repeated up to total

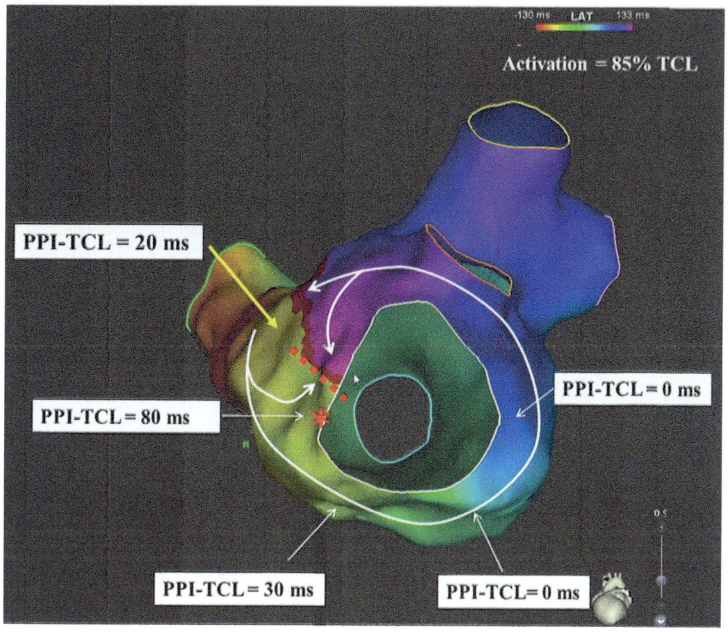

Fig. 13.10 Counterclockwise perimitral reentry treated with linear ablation with anteroseptal line between mitral annulus and right superior pulmonary vein (RSPV). During ablation, coronary sinus activation changed. Repeat entrainment mapping showed a long PPI-TCL in anteroseptal annulus *(asterisk)* but short PPI-TCL at gap by RSPV *(yellow arrow)*, indicating a gap by the RSPV and detour around an incomplete line of block *(dashed red line)*.

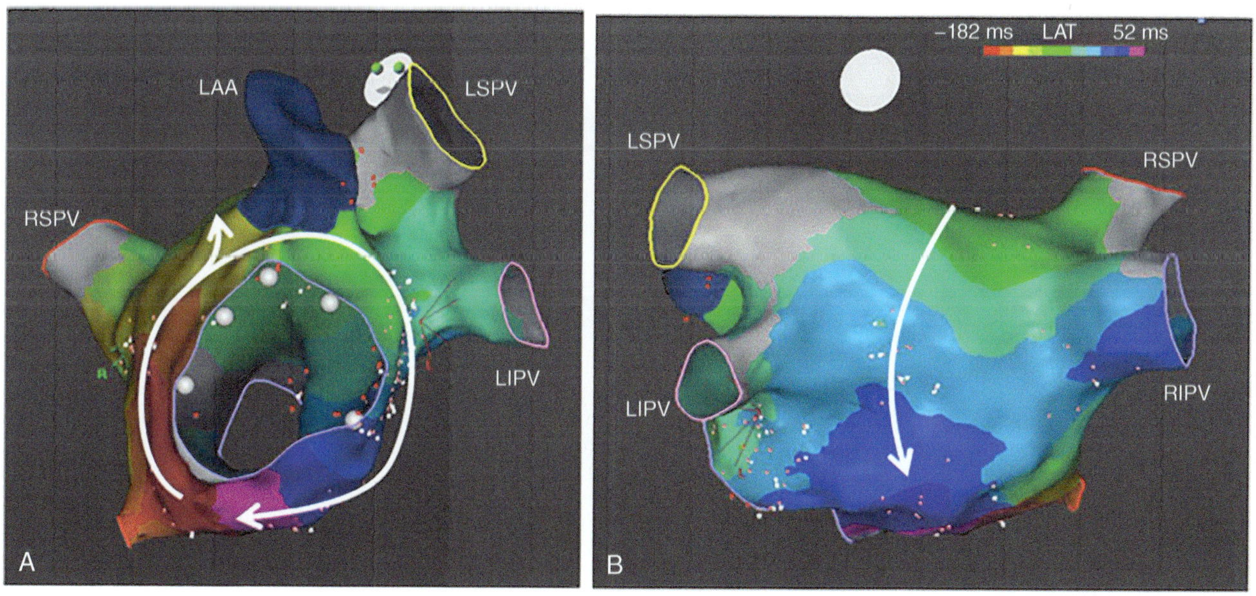

Fig. 13.11 Electroanatomical map (Carto) of a left atrial tachycardia with isochronal steps of 20 ms. The map demonstrates a dual-loop tachycardia, with one clockwise loop around the mitral annulus (A) and a second roof-dependent circuit around the right pulmonary veins with descending activation of the posterior wall (B). *LA(A),* Left atrial appendage; *LIPV,* left inferior pulmonary vein; *LSPV,* left superior pulmonary vein; *RIPV,* right inferior pulmonary vein; *RSPV,* right superior pulmonary vein.

dose of ~10 mL. Contrast staining of the atrial myocardium indicates endothelial disruption and effective ethanol ablation. After ethanol ablation, voltage mapping should reveal an expansion of low-voltage zone anterior and inferior to the left inferior PV. To achieve complete block in the lateral mitral isthmus, adjunctive ablation in the great coronary vein is needed about 50% of the time to target residual LA connections.[64] Complications of ethanol LOM ablation include venous rupture, tamponade, and delayed pericarditis.

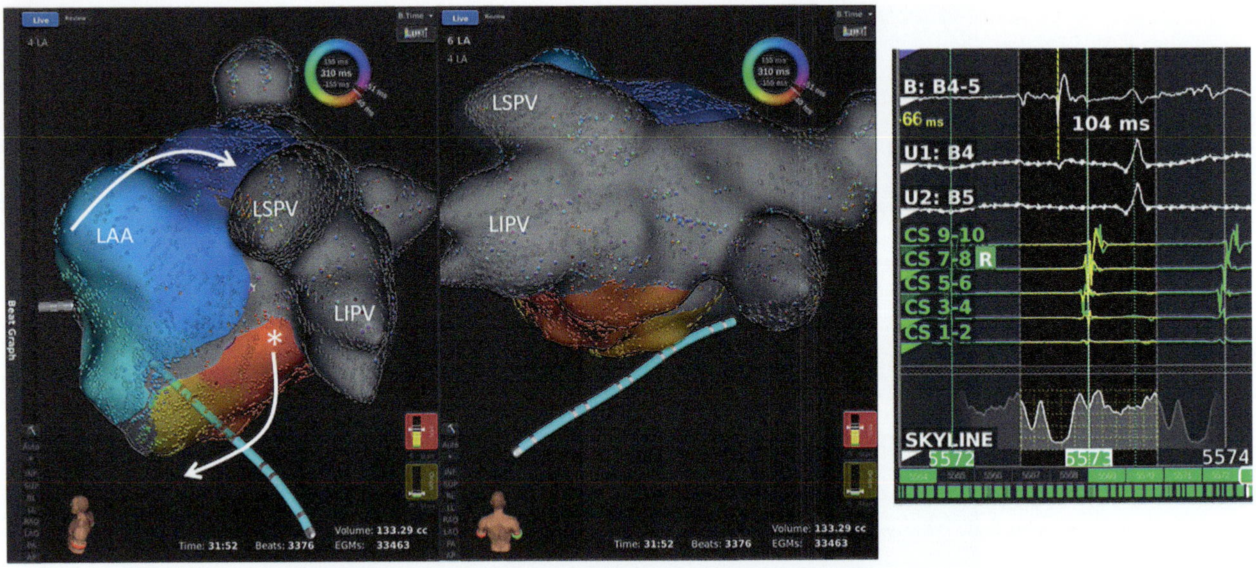

Fig. 13.12 Perimitral reentry with epicardial gap along ligament of Marshall mapped with Rhythmia. The patient underwent prior pulmonary vein isolation and posterior wall isolation and ablation along the lateral mitral isthmus between the annulus and left inferior pulmonary vein (LIPV). No discernable voltage is recorded along the mitral isthmus. The impulse propagates to the roof adjacent to the left superior pulmonary veins (LSPV) and then reappears anterior to the LIPV (*). Ablation along the ridge between the appendage and LSPV terminated the flutter. See Video 13.4.

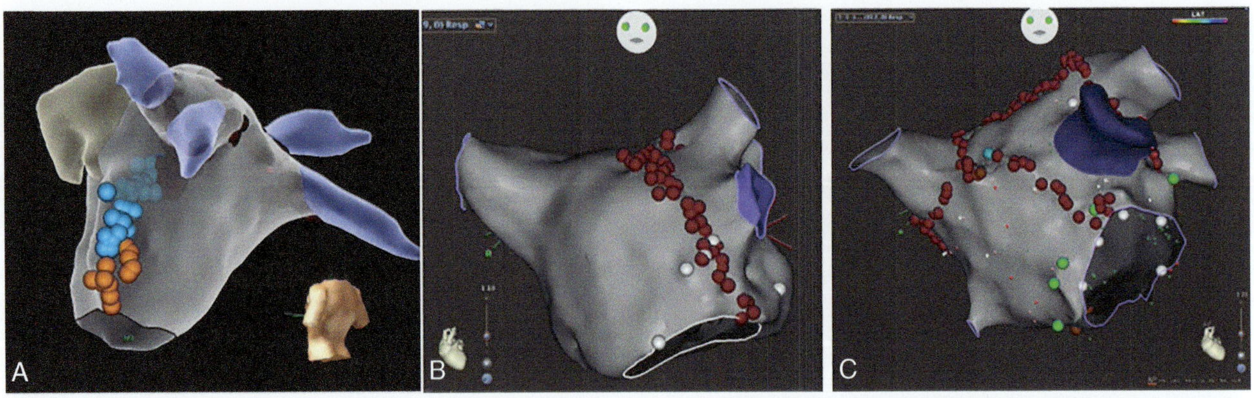

Fig. 13.13 Ablation lines for perimitral flutter. (A) Lateral mitral isthmus: Ablation is performed from the lateral mitral annulus to an electrically isolated left inferior pulmonary vein. This lesion set is created lateral to the appendage. Ablation in the coronary sinus is often required to achieve line of block. In this case, *blue tags* represent endocardial ablation lesions and the *orange tags* represent an ablation in the coronary sinus, which was required to achieve block in the lateral isthmus. (B) Anterior mitral line: Ablation is performed from the anterior mitral annulus to a roof line or an isolated left superior pulmonary vein. This lesions set is created medial to the appendage (*shaded in blue*). (C) Septal mitral line: Ablation is performed from the anterior or septal mitral annulus to an isolated right superior pulmonary vein.

Perimitral reentry can be also interrupted by creating a line of block in the anterior LA between the mitral annulus and the LA roof or the right PVs.[69,70] Conduction block can be verified by the demonstration of double potentials along the line during pacing adjacent to the line. To distinguish slow conduction from complete block, the technique of *differential pacing* may be used, which involves measuring conduction times between two catheters positioned just across the ablation line and then moving a catheter farther away from the line (Fig. 13.17). Pitfalls of creating an anterior mitral line include nontransmural lesions due to the thickness of Bachmann's bundle and delayed activation of the LA appendage. In the case of incomplete anterior mitral lines, complex biatrial tachycardia may result.

Left Atrial Roof-Dependent Reentry

Roof-dependent flutter refers to reentry around one or both sets of PVs, sometimes with corridors between areas of scar on the anterior or posterior walls (Fig. 13.18). This atypical flutter is usually treated with linear ablation between the left and right PVs. Transmural conduction block is more easily achieved by ablating along the posterior wall between the PVs compared to

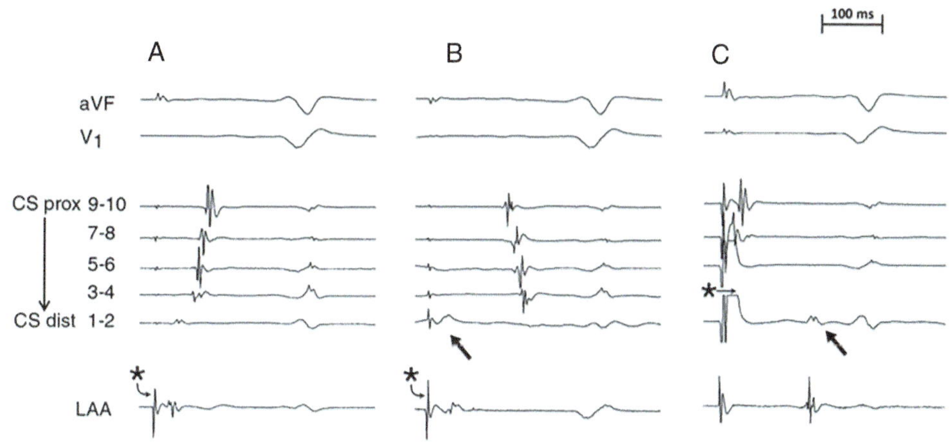

Fig. 13.14 Conduction block in the lateral mitral isthmus. (A) Pacing *(asterisk)* is performed from the left atrial appendage (LAA) before the ablation line was made between CS 1-2 and CS 3-4. Pacing from the appendage activates the coronary sinus (CS) from distal to proximal. (B) After the line is completed, conduction block is demonstrated by proximal to distal CS activation from CS 9-10 to 3-4. CS 1-2 is on the opposite (or anterior) side of the line *(arrow)*. (C) To assess conduction in the opposite direction, pacing is performed from the distal CS, in this case poles 3-4. After the line is completed, there is late activation of the adjacent distal pole (CS 1-2, *arrow*) and the appendage.

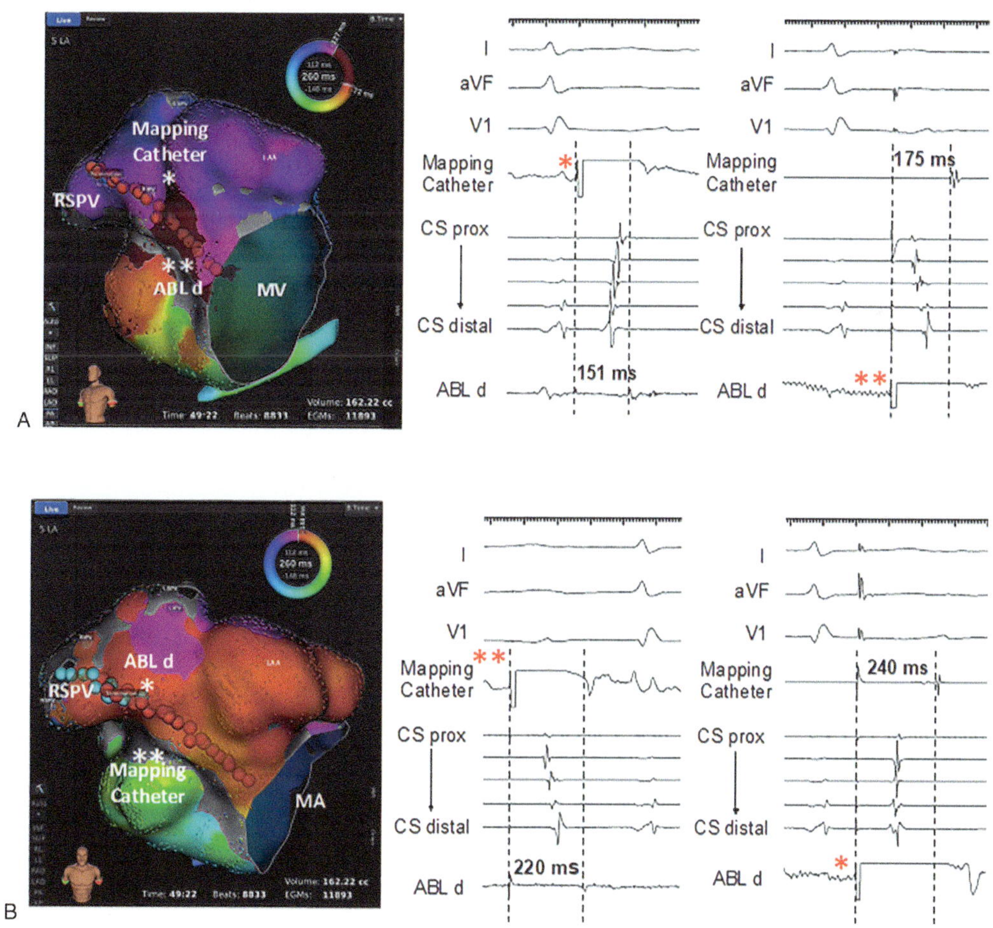

Fig. 13.15 Pseudoblock after initial anteromedial ablation lesion set from mitral annulus to right superior pulmonary vein (RSPV). (A) Pacing on opposite sides of the ablation line shows prolonged conduction times. Shown are electrograms from the coronary sinus (CS), distal electrodes from the ablation catheter (ABL d) and a selective recording from an ultra-high-density multielectrode mapping catheter. *Site of pacing from the mapping catheter; **site of pacing from the distal ablation catheter. (B) After additional ablation at a localized gap near the RSPV, complete line of block is demonstrated with further prolongation of conduction times, suggesting that previous apparent block was actually pseudoblock. *Aqua dots* represent additional ablation lesions after the initial anteromedial line was made. *Site of pacing from the distal ablation catheter; **site of pacing from the mapping catheter. (Modified from Goyal R, Markowitz SM, Cheung JW, Lerman BB. Diagnosing pseudo-conduction block across an anteromedial mitral ablation line: limitations of bidirectional and differential pacing. *Heart Rhythm Case Rep*. 2020;6:29-33. doi:10.1016/j.hrcr.2019.10.009.)

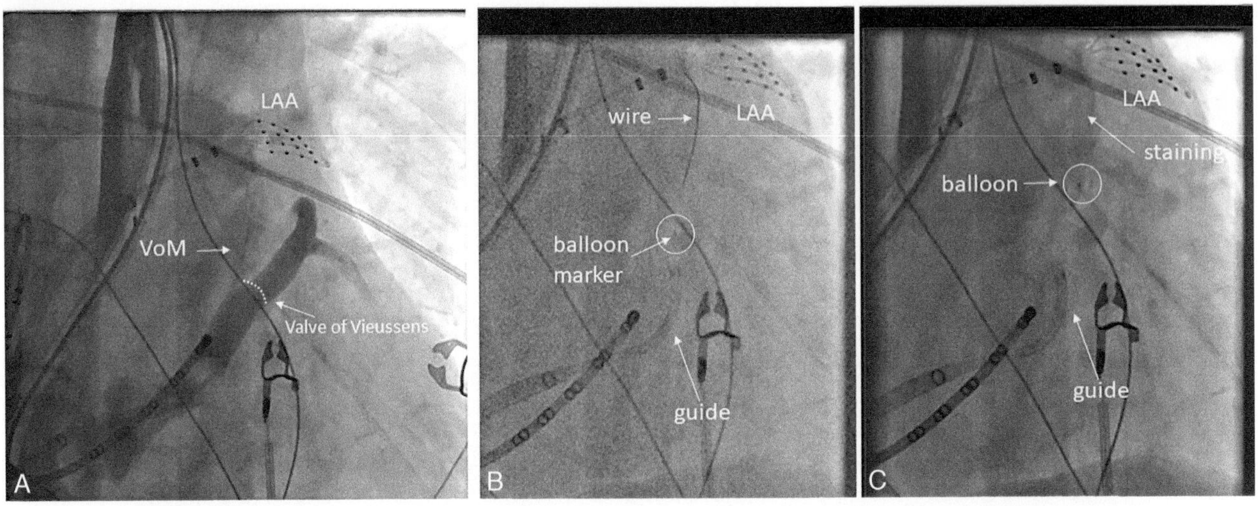

Fig. 13.16 Ethanol infusion in the vein of Marshall (VoM). (A) Coronary sinus venogram in right anterior oblique view shows the VoM takeoff proximal to the valve of Vieussens and coursing posterior and superior toward the orifice of the left atrial appendage (LAA), which is identified by the Pentaray catheter. (B) An 0.014" wire preloaded in an angioplasty balloon and advanced through a guide into the VoM. (C) The balloon is inflated, and contrast medium is injected through the balloon to confirm placement and occlusion of the vein, after which ethanol is infused. After ethanol infusion, contrast staining is visualized in the lateral LA in the left anterior oblique projection.

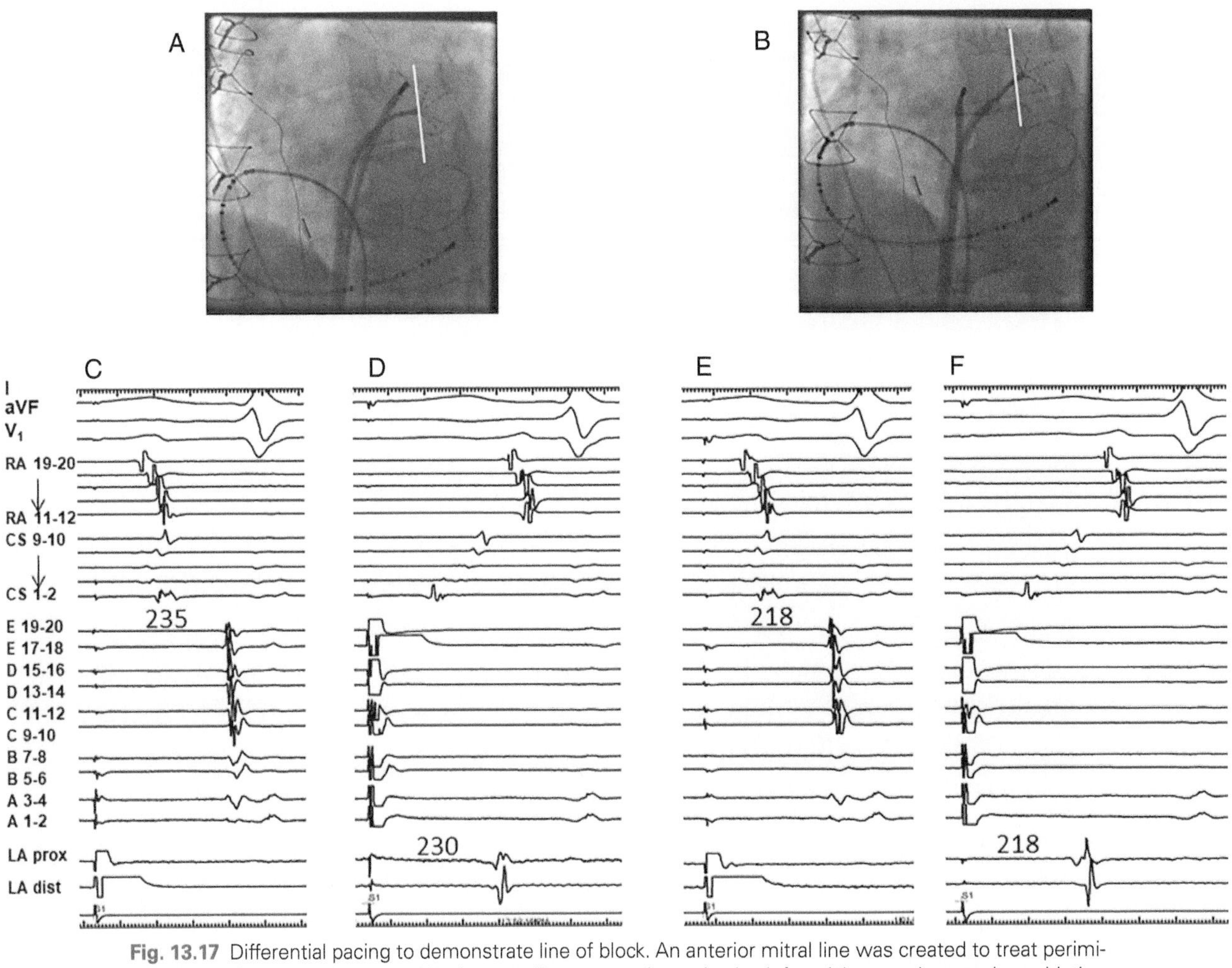

Fig. 13.17 Differential pacing to demonstrate line of block. An anterior mitral line was created to treat perimitral flutter. Fluoroscopic image (A) shows a Pentaray catheter in the left atrial appendage and an ablation catheter just medial to the ablation lesions, denoted by a white line. Pacing from the ablation catheter results in a delay of 235 ms to the appendage (C) and pacing from the appendage results in a similar delay of 230 ms of the ablation catheter on the medial side (D). When the ablation catheter is moved more medially and away from the line (B), there are shorter conduction times between the ablator and the appendage in both directions (E and F).

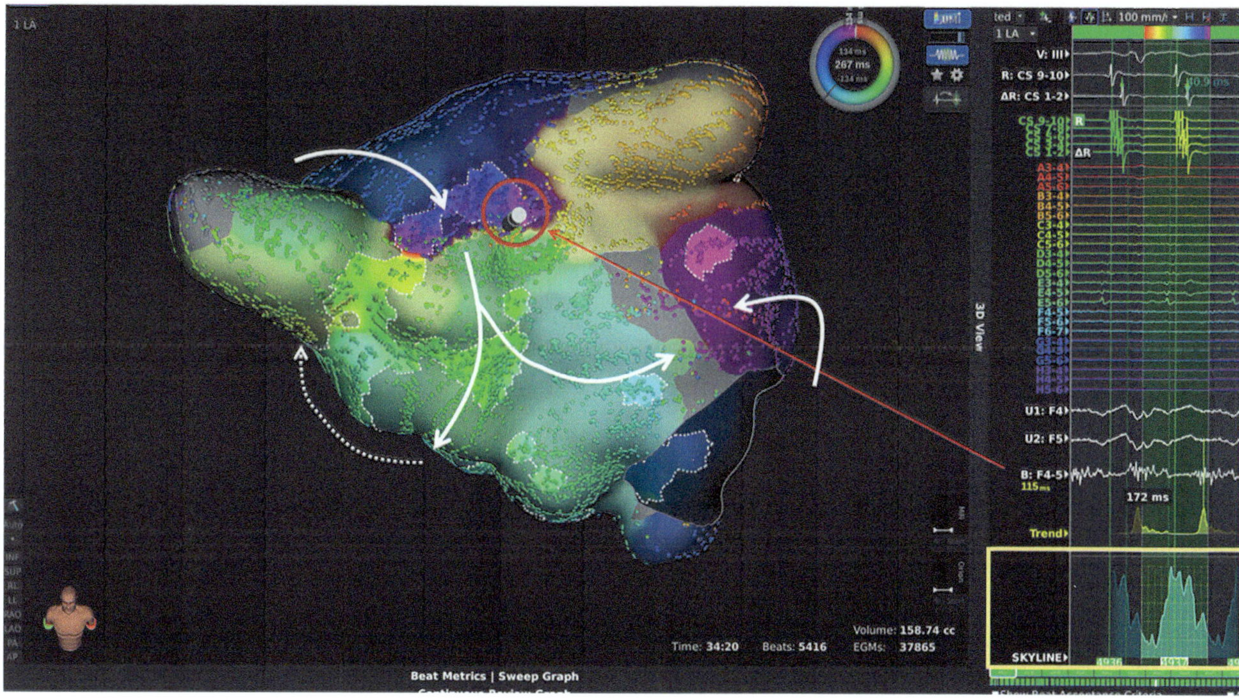

Fig. 13.18 Ultra-high-resolution map of roof-dependent flutter in a patient who had prior ablation of persistent atrial fibrillation. Reentry is present around the right pulmonary veins. Conduction block is present in the anterior LA. Rhythmia Lumipoint module highlights areas of fragmented electrograms, including the site indicated by red circle and displayed at right (*red arrow*). Histogram of electrograms displayed by activation time (Skyline, *orange box*) shows a valley that corresponds to the zone of slow conduction at the roof adjacent to the right superior pulmonary vein.

the LA roof because of the septopulmonary bundle that is found on the epicardial aspect of the LA dome and may be separated from endocardial fibers by adipose tissue.[71] In choosing posterior wall ablation with thermal energy, the operator must balance the risk of esophageal injury. Completeness of the line can be demonstrated by recording widely spaced double potentials along the ablation line during pacing from one side of the line.[72] The LA appendage may also be selected as a stable pacing site in the anterior segment of the LA. Activation of the posterior wall during appendage pacing should proceed from an inferior to superior direction, as the impulse diverts around the PVs to engage the posterior wall (Fig. 13.19). Analogously, pacing from the posterior wall should result in late activation of the anterior segment, including the appendage.

In cases of myopathy or prior ablation, a practical isthmus with slow conduction and fragmented electrograms may be identified by electroanatomic mapping and is the most suitable site for ablation (Fig. 13.18).

Anterior Left Atrial Reentry

Atypical flutters that arise de novo in the LA involve regions of patchy scar, which are identified as electrically silent or low-voltage areas that often involve the anterior or anteroseptal walls.[6,30,52] These ATs may take the form of reentry around an electrically silent patch in the anterior LA, with or without a second circuit such as perimitral reentry (Fig. 13.20, Video 13.6). There may be multiple zones of slow conduction along the reentrant path. Functional conduction block may contribute to stabilization of the reentrant circuit. Scar in the anterior LA is also implicated in complex perimitral circuits that deviate from the annulus and detour around areas of localized conduction block.[73] The ablation strategy for anterior wall reentry is to transect a critical isthmus, which may involve ablation from the scar to the mitral annulus or another anchoring site such as an isolated PV.

Septal Flutter

Reentry confined to the interatrial septum may occur in patients with prior atrial surgery or catheter ablation[74,75] and uncommonly in the absence of prior interventions among AF patients treated with antiarrhythmic drugs.[21,76] Typically, patients have low voltage in the interatrial septum with abnormal electrograms. Electroanatomical maps demonstrate centrifugal activation of both atria from the septum. Entrainment can identify participation of the circuit on either the left or right sides or on both opposing sides. Mapping and entrainment characteristics suggest that the circuits may occur within the septal tissue. In cases of atrial surgery, the reentrant circuits may be bounded by the right PVs posteriorly and the mitral annulus anteriorly, with double potentials defining a line of conduction block. Elimination of intraseptal flutters may be difficult owing to the thickness of the septum at the superior limbus, and effective ablation may involve treating both sides of the interatrial septum.

Biatrial Flutter

Biatrial flutter is found primarily among patients who have had extensive prior catheter ablations involving the anterior LA or septum.[77] In these cases, nontransmural ablation results in bridges, typically involving Bachmann's bundle, that permit

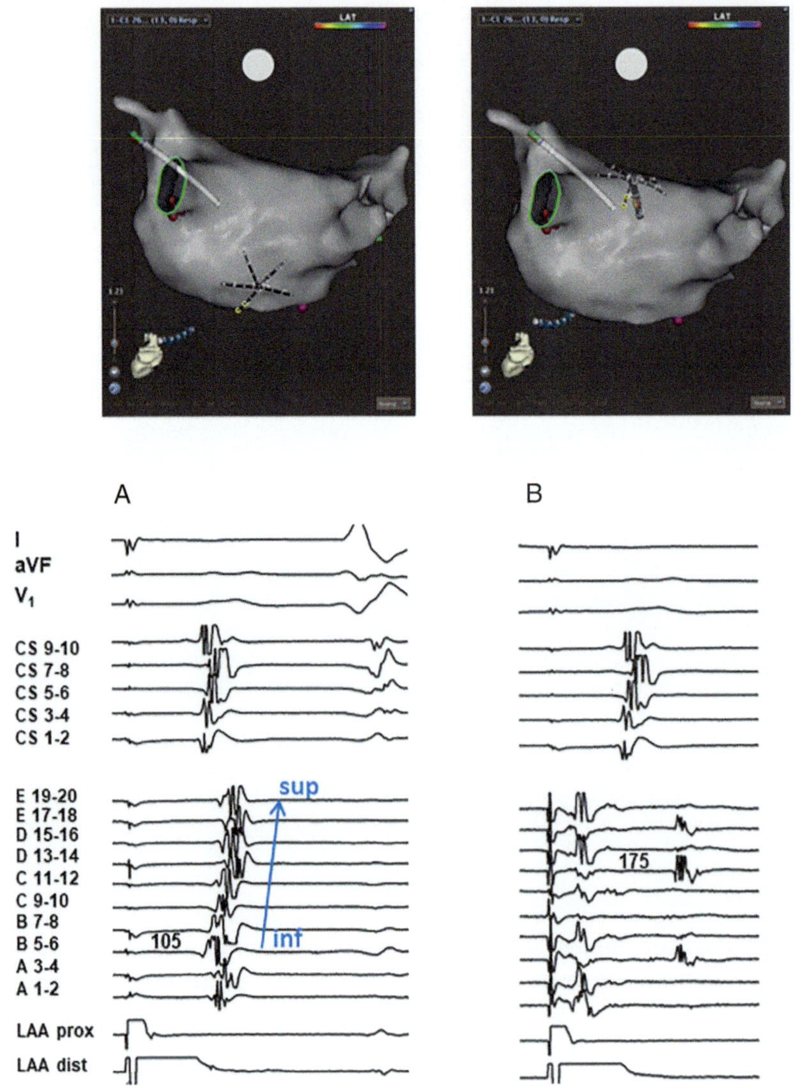

Fig. 13.19 Demonstrating line of block in the left atrial roof. (A) Pacing is performed from the ablation catheter, which is positioned in the left atrial appendage (LAA). A PentaRay catheter positioned in the low posterior left atrium demonstrates earliest activation in the most inferior electrodes (inf) and propagation to the superior electrodes (sup). (B) When the PentaRay is positioned in the anterior roof along the ablation line, straddling the roof ablation line, double potentials are demonstrated, with the second component activated later than any recording lower on the posterior wall as recorded on the coronary sinus (CS) catheter. *dist,* Distal; *prox,* proximal.

conduction between the anterior LA and the RA. These flutters should be suspected in patients who had extensive prior ablation when mapping of one chamber fails to delineate the complete tachycardia circuit. Some components of the circuit might not be accounted for if long epicardial bridges are involved, and there may be no discernible endocardial electrograms along the anterior or anteroseptal LA because of prior ablation. Entrainment from both atria will confirm biatrial participation.

Variants of biatrial flutter include reentry involving both the mitral and tricuspid annuli; the mitral annulus and atrial septum; and macroreentry involving both sides of the septum.[77] Ablation targets vary depending on the characteristics of the biatiral circuits and the locations of critical isthmuses. Sites of ablation have included the CTI, corridors in the LA, and connection sites in the RA.

Localized Reentrant ATs

Small reentrant circuits can occur in myopathic RA or LA after catheter or surgical ablation of AF but also in patients without prior interventions. A characteristic feature of *localized reentry* or *microreentry* is the presence of low-amplitude, long-duration, fractionated electrograms that occupy a small region of the atrium (Fig. 13.21).[16] Multielectrode catheters with closely spaced electrodes are useful for localizing the arrhythmia and identifying abnormal electrograms, which might not be identified with large-tip ablation catheters. Activation of the atria proceeds from this highly fractionated location. Electroanatomical maps will usually demonstrate a centrifugal activation pattern, but it may be difficult to assign activation times for highly fractionated points, which can make electroanatomic map difficult to interpret. Ultra-high-resolution mapping with automated

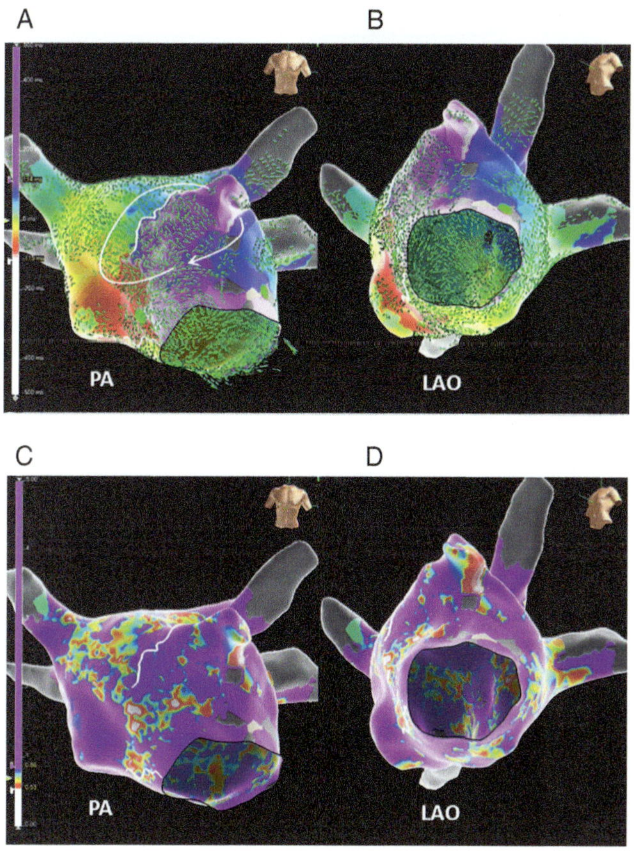

Fig. 13.20 Left atrial anterior wall reentry in a man without prior atrial intervention. (A and B) Activation map with Ensite X shows reentry around a line of block in the anterior LA. Vectors computed from omnipolar electrograms confirm the directions of activation and collision at the central line of block. Wavefronts also propagate around the mitral annulus in a counterclockwise direction. (C and D) Wavefront velocity is coded in this case with white <0.53 m/sec and blue >0.86 m/sec. Several areas of slow conduction are demonstrated around the reentrant path. Ablation was performed between the central line of block and the anterior mitral annulus. AP indicates anteroposterior; LAO, left anterior oblique.

annotation has proved useful in delineating complex circuits with long-duration electrograms (Fig. 13.22, Video 13.7).[29-31] Activation mapping can be supplemented with entrainment to localize these small circuits. Entrainment at or near the location of the small circuit will yield a postpacing interval within 30 ms compared to the tachycardia cycle length, whereas entrainment at increasing distance from the circuit results in a gradient of increasing postpacing intervals. Another characteristic of these arrhythmias is insensitivity to adenosine, which supports a reentrant mechanism rather than triggered activity or automaticity.[12] Focal ablation at sites with complex electrograms is often effective in terminating these arrhythmias.

Atypical Flutter After Catheter Ablation for AF

ATs may present as a late complication in <5–40% of patients who undergo catheter ablation for AF.[78] This complication is less common after segmental PV isolation, cryoballoon ablation, and multielectrode phased-RF ablation compared to wide encircling antral ablation using unipolar RF catheters. Even higher rates of AT occur after procedures that add additional substrate modification techniques, such as linear ablation in the LA, ablation of complex fractionated electrograms, and targeting of rotational activity. The majority of ATs that occur after catheter ablation are macroreentrant (~55–75%), with localized reentry accounting for a sizeable minority and true focal mechanisms occurring less frequently.[18,79] Gaps or inhomogeneities in ablation lines create the substrate for macroreentrant ATs, of which perimitral and roof-dependent reentry are the most common, although more complex variants are also encountered after extensive ablation. A specific type of reentry involves reconnected PVs, in which two gaps occur in a single PV or ipsilateral PVs; these can give rise to circuits with entrance and exit sites involving the PVs or more complex circuits also revolving around the contralateral PVs.[80,81] Localized reentry can occur near previous ablation lines, in areas of myopathic atria remote from prior ablation, and also in the LoM.[82] Gaps in prior ablation lines and localized circuits typically demonstrate low-amplitude, long-duration electrograms that are best identified with high-density mapping electrodes.[31]

In patients who have undergone previous PV isolation, a deductive stepwise approach using activation and entrainment mapping can be used to determine the mechanism of the AT and its general location.[25] Basic activation and entrainment mapping are used to rapidly identify or exclude perimetral, roof-dependent circuits, as well as CTI-dependent flutter. PV isolation should be confirmed and reisolation performed if necessary. Cycle length variation ≥15% should prompt a search for focal tachycardia. High-resolution mapping then identifies the specific pattern of activation and the practical isthmus for ablation.

For ATs that occur after catheter ablation of AF, freedom from recurrent atrial arrhythmias during follow-up is approximately 75% after one procedure,[78] and higher long-term success rates are attainable if patients have repeat procedures for recurrent arrhythmias.

Atypical Flutter After Maze Surgery

ATs that occur late after maze surgery demonstrate features similar to those that occur after catheter ablation of AF, but the locations of reentrant circuits are influenced by the surgical approach. Although most flutters after maze surgery are left-sided, typical RA flutter is not infrequent. RA reentrant circuits can also occur related to cannula locations or gaps in the RA ablation lines. In the LA, gaps in the posterior wall lesions and in connecting lesions to the mitral annulus have been described, resulting in roof-dependent and perimitral reentry (Fig. 13.23, Videos 13.8 and 13.9).[83-87] Reconnection of the PVs also account for recurrences after surgical ablation of AF, particularly if surgery involved the use of unipolar RF energy.[85] Focal ATs account for a minority of post-maze arrhythmias and arise from reconnected PVs or other sites in both atria. It is not clear whether gap-related flutters occur more commonly with a particular surgical modality (e.g., conventional incisions, bipolar RF, cryoablation, or microwave energy). Although some evidence suggests that gaps are less likely to occur across "cut-and-sew" lesions, reentrant arrhythmias due to incomplete lines of block

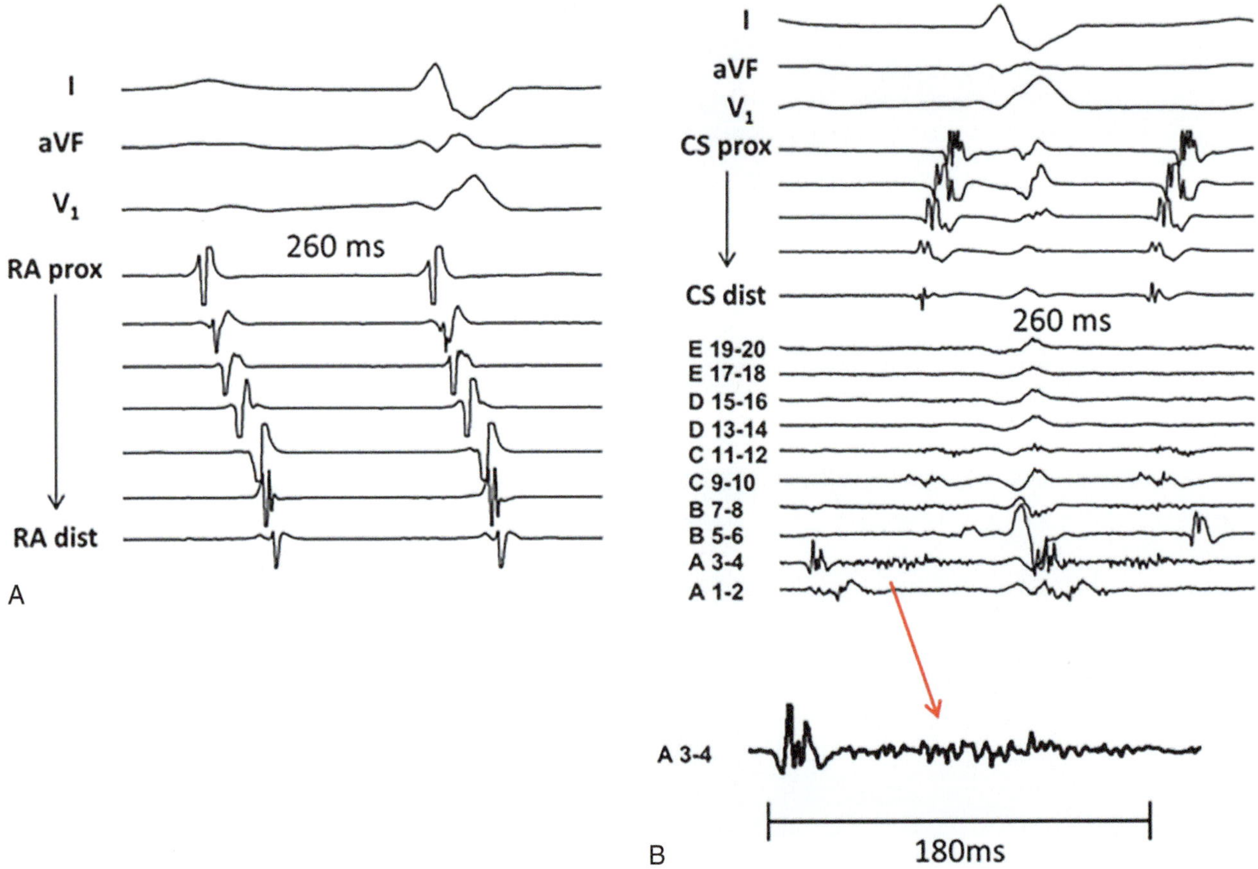

Fig. 13.21 Left atrial microreentrant tachycardia after catheter ablation of atrial fibrillation. (A) The right atrial (RA) activation sequence demonstrates a descending wavefront in the lateral wall because of prior ablation in the cavotricuspid isthmus. (B) A PentaRay catheter positioned anterior to the left inferior pulmonary vein shows a highly fractionated, low-amplitude electrogram (0.12–0.24 mV) on spline electrode A 3–4, which spans most of the tachycardia cycle length. *CS*, Coronary sinus.

have been documented after this approach. Catheter ablation of gap-related atrial flutter after maze surgery is feasible, using the same mapping techniques for other complex atrial reentrant circuits.

Atypical Flutter After Mitral Valve Surgery

Atypical flutters occur in both the RA and LA after mitral valve surgery.[1,14,54,88] The substrate for these arrhythmias involves atriotomy incisions as well as intrinsically diseased myocardium, giving rise to anatomic and functional regions of block as well as slowed conduction. It is helpful to ascertain the surgical approach used in a given patient, which informs the likely locations of atypical flutter and the approach to mapping (Fig. 13.24). Macroreentry is the predominant mechanism, and circuits often localize to the RA, including typical CTI-dependent flutter.[88] Reentry in the RA may be attributed to several factors, including surgical approaches to the mitral valve that involve RA incisions (such as the transseptal or superior septal approaches), cannula insertion in the RA, and underlying myocardial disease. Tachycardias in the RA are single- and dual-loop circuits that involve the RA free wall. Reentry involving scar in the RA side of the septum has also been reported after transseptal access of the mitral valve.[89] In these cases, ablation can be accomplished by creating lesions between the septal scar and the tricuspid annulus.

In the LA, areas of low voltage are often identified anterior to the right PVs, which correspond to LA incisions. Roof-dependent AT may be present with reentry around the right PVs (involving this zone of low voltage), but other circuits may involve a posterior scar or the mitral annulus. LA flutters are more common if mitral valve surgery is combined with a maze procedure.[88]

In a systematic review of 14 studies comprising 227 patients, ablation of ATs in patients with prior mitral valve surgery was acutely successful in 95% of patients, but maintenance of sinus rhythm after multiple procedures was 71% at midterm follow-up and 47% during long-term follow-up due to a high burden of late AF.[90]

Atypical Flutters After Orthotopic Cardiac Transplantation

The late development of AT after cardiac transplantation may be a sign of acute rejection, but such arrhythmias also occur

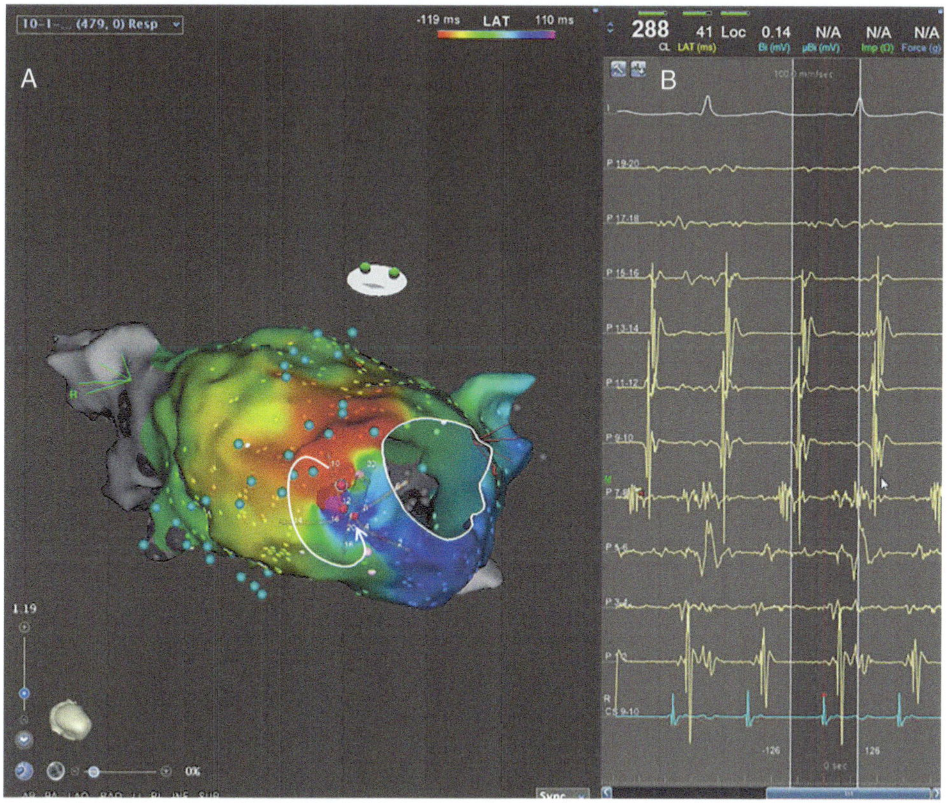

Fig. 13.22 Localized reentry in the left atrium in a man with a prior catheter ablation of long-standing persistent atrial fibrillation. (A) Carto activation map demonstrates a small circuit adjacent to the inferoseptal mitral annulus. There is an apparent circuit clockwise around the mitral annulus, but entrainment revealed the lateral LA did not participate in the tachycardia, illustrating the phenomenon of apparent or "pseudo"-reentry. (B) A Pentaray catheter in the inferior septum recorded electrograms spanning 85% for the tachycardia cycle length.

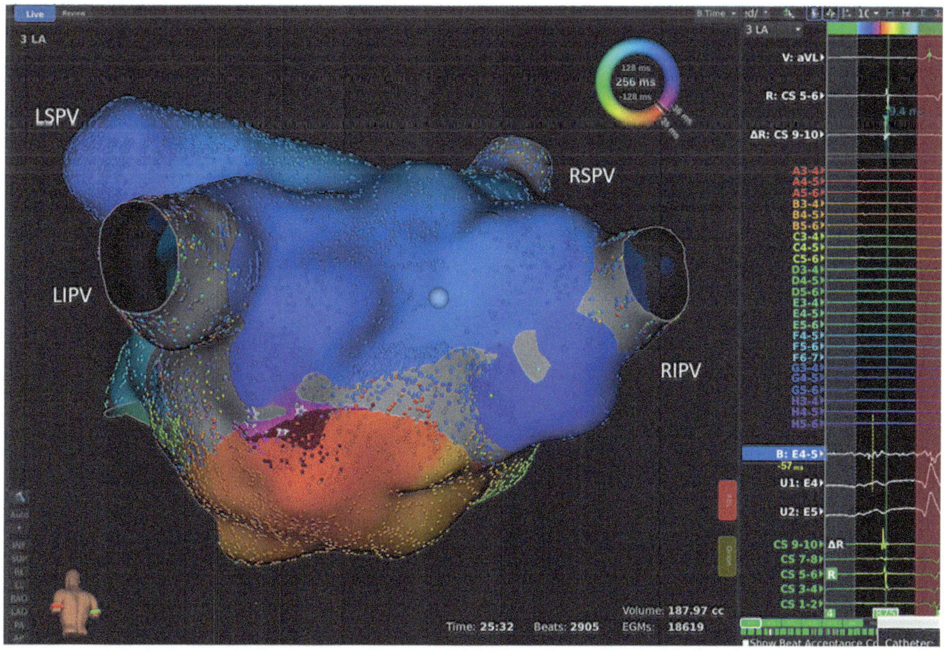

Fig. 13.23 Macroreentry in left atrium in patient with prior mitral valve repair and maze surgery. Rhythmia map with Orion catheter shows scar between the inferior pulmonary veins (PV) with a gap near the left inferior PV after adjusting the voltage mask to the noise level of the system. The impulse propagated through the gap, which demonstrated the fragmented electrogram at E4-5, and around the right PVs because of preexisting block in the lateral mitral isthmus. Focal ablation in this gap terminated with tachycardia and established line of block across the posterior wall. *LIPV,* Left inferior PV; *LSPV,* left superior PV; *P(A),* posteroanterior; *RIPV,* right inferior PV; *RSPV,* right superior PV. See Video 13.9.

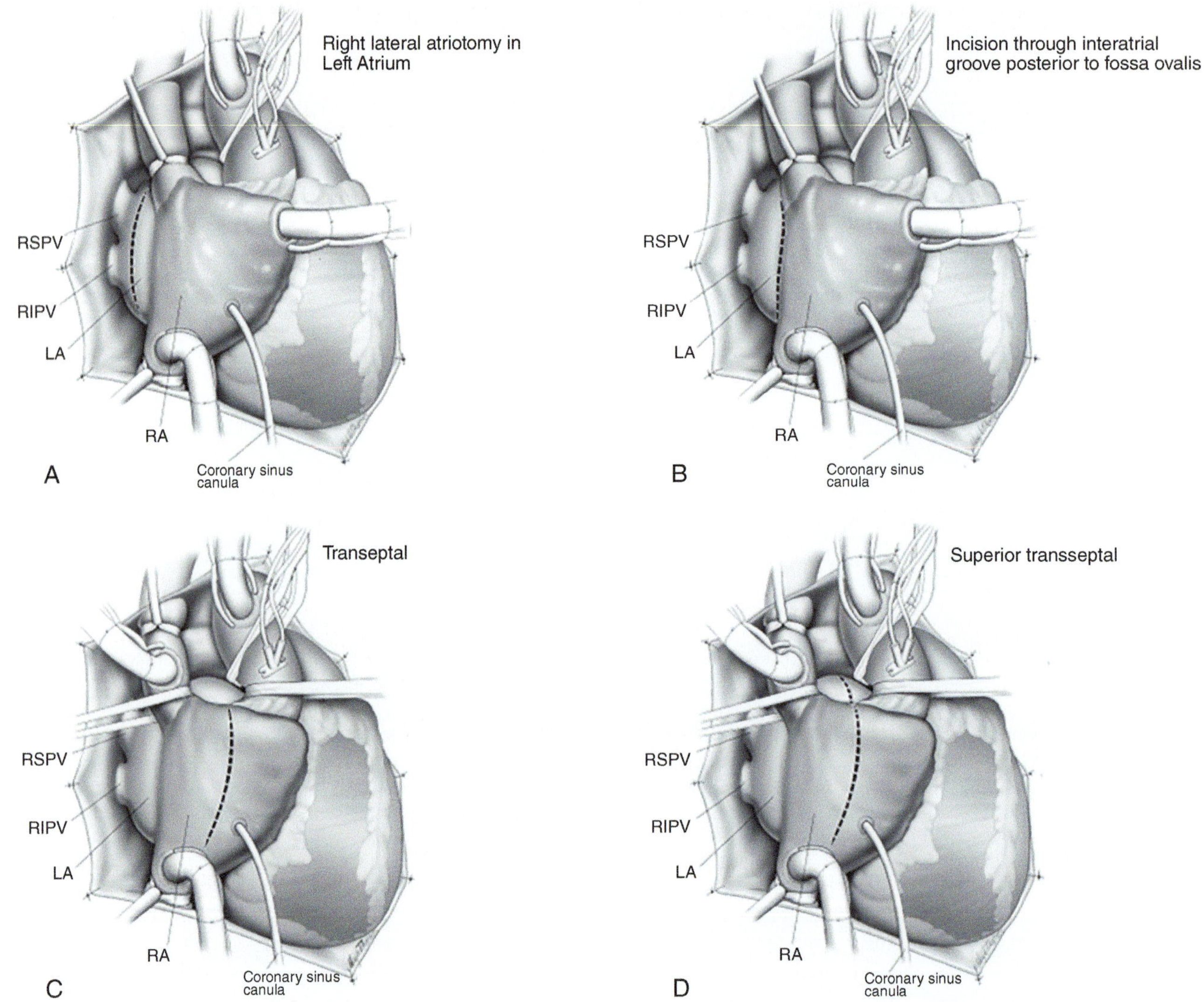

Fig. 13.24 Surgical approaches to the mitral valve. (A) Left atriotomy anterior to the right pulmonary veins. (B) Dissection in interatrial groove and incision posterior to fossa ovalis. (C) Transseptal approach with incision in the lateral right atrium (RA), followed by incision through the interatrial septum. (D) Superior transseptal approach with incision in the lateral RA which is carried over the superior aspect of the RA and through the interatrial septum and may involve the dome of the left atrium. (Modified from Markowitz SM, Brodman RF, Stein KM, Mittal S, Slotwiner DJ, Iwai S, Das MK, Lerman BB. Lesional tachycardias related to mitral valve surgery. *J Am Coll Cardiol.* 2002;39:1973–1983.)

in <5% of stable patients.[91,92] The most common atrial arrhythmias presenting late after transplant are macroreentrant ATs, but focal arrhythmias are also documented.[93] CTI-dependent flutter accounts for the majority of these arrhythmias in most series. The flutter morphology of CTI-dependent tachycardias posttransplantation is usually atypical. A variety of other atypical focal and macroreentrant circuits can occur in these patients and many involve scar or suture lines for the atrial anastomoses. A unique form of arrhythmia in transplant patients is related to conduction from recipient to donor atria across the atrial anastomoses. In cases of biatrial anastomoses, recipient-to-donor conduction can potentially occur in either the RA or LA. In cases of bicaval anastomoses, no recipient atrial myocardium exists in the RA, but the recipient LA can develop a connection to the donor LA, with tachycardia conducting from the recipient to the donor atria. These tachycardias can be targeted by identifying the breakthrough site in the donor atrium. Ablation at this site can dissociate the recipient and donor atria and prevent tachycardia in the donor heart. Macroreentrant circuits can also occur that involve isthmuses created by the anastomotic suture lines and other conduction barriers, such as the mitral annulus. Overall, organized ATs appear to arise more commonly from the RA than the LA of transplanted hearts. Catheter ablation of atrial tachyarrhythmias in this population is acutely successful in >90% of cases, although recurrent atrial arrhythmias occur in up to 20% over several years.[93,94]

REFERENCES

Please refer to the e-book for a complete list of references.

14

Ablation of Atrial Flutter/Tachycardia in Congenital Heart Disease

Jeremy P. Moore

KEY POINTS

- Atrial tachycardia in congenital heart disease is predominantly related to "intra-atrial reentrant" (IART) tachycardia (less commonly, focal atrial tachycardia), in the setting of adverse hemodynamic sequelae or iatrogenic, surgical scar.
- Classic electrophysiologic techniques supplemented with contemporary three-dimensional mapping tools both improve understanding of IART circuits and facilitate catheter ablation procedures for congenital heart disease.
- Atrial fibrillation is increasingly observed among the aging congenital heart disease population at a younger age than in acquired heart disease, and is believed to be caused by both conventional pulmonary vein and extrapulmonary vein triggers.
- Detailed understanding of congenital anatomy and the corresponding operative strategies are imperative for successful catheter ablation regardless of the catheter ablation target and assist the operator in avoiding collateral damage and procedural complications.
- Catheter ablation is increasingly successful and often serves as definitive therapy for atrial tachycardia; however, arrhythmia recurrence and atrial fibrillation still represent formidable challenges for the growing field of congenital electrophysiology.

INTRODUCTION

Supraventricular arrhythmia is a leading cause of both morbidity and mortality for patients with congenital heart disease (CHD).[1,2] It is the most frequent reason for CHD hospital admission and is associated with adverse events such as stroke and heart failure as well as a greater need for interventional procedures.[2–4] Supraventricular arrhythmia disproportionately affects CHD after cardiac repair, affecting more than 50% of adult patients during their lifespan, especially after right-sided congenital cardiac operations.[3,5] As the CHD population continues to grow, the burden of supraventricular arrhythmia will undoubtedly increase. Supraventricular arrhythmia has been identified as a clinical priority in the field of congenital cardiology and is a growing public health concern.

Of the supraventricular arrhythmias, atrial tachycardia is the most common subtype among CHD, and of these, intra-atrial reentrant tachycardia (IART) dominates the clinical spectrum. IART tends to be progressive and increasingly difficult to manage over time, often resulting in escalation of medical therapy.[6] Other than arrhythmia surgery, catheter ablation represents the only form of definitive therapy for IART. Catheter ablation has been shown to be superior to antiarrhythmic drugs for control of IART in CHD and results in substantial clinical improvement for the majority of patients.[7,8] Consensus guidelines recommend catheter ablation as a Class I indication for patients with CHD and symptomatic atrial tachycardia.[9]

GENERAL PRINCIPLES OF CATHETER ABLATION FOR CONGENITAL HEART DISEASE

Observations that IART circuits depend on wavefront propagation through relatively narrow and vulnerable conduction isthmuses ultimately resulted in the introduction of catheter ablation as the principal therapy for CHD. Historically, conduction isthmuses were identified by recognizing electrophysiologic surrogates of slow conduction, including fractionated signals and large changes in electrogram timing with small catheter movements through anatomically constrained regions bordering two nonconducting barriers.[10–12] Such barriers generally correspond to (1) anatomical structures such as the AV annulus, vena cava, or pulmonary veins, (2) inert material, such as surgical baffles or patch material, or (3) permanent or functional lines of conduction block such as atriotomy incisions, dense scarring, or the crista terminalis. Practically speaking, dense scar (i.e., inert surgical material or fibrotic myocardium) is defined by a bipolar tissue voltage <0.05 mV and an inability to capture the region with high-output pacing, whereas low-voltage but viable myocardial areas are defined by amplitudes between 0.05 and 0.5 mV. Similarly, discrete lines of conduction block during tachycardia are recognized by widely disparate (>50 ms separation) electrograms on the recording electrodes that demonstrate their greatest separation at the midpoint and converge at the end (Fig. 14.1).[12–15]

Entrainment techniques were used beginning with the first description of catheter ablation for CHD and were borrowed from early work used to understand the mechanism of

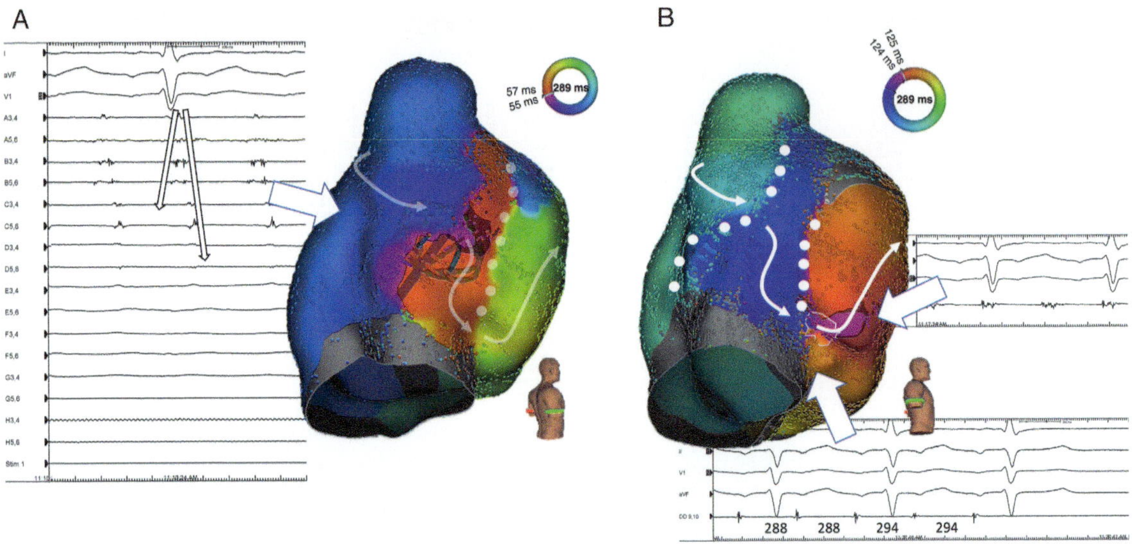

Fig. 14.1 Example of split potentials recorded on a multipolar basket electrode in a patient with tetralogy of Fallot and intra-atrial reentrant tachycardia within the right atrium. Incomplete conduction block corresponds to the expected course of the crista terminalis and intercaval scar. (A) With basket catheter placed against a zone of conduction block bordering a critical isthmus, progressively wider split potentials are observed as the dipoles extend inferiorly away from a conduction gap. (B) Application of radiofrequency energy at a critical isthmus where a continuous and fractionated electrogram is encountered, results in slowing and termination of the tachycardia without ectopic beats.

postinfarction reentrant ventricular tachycardia.[16,17] Accordingly, early mapping strategies relied on the surface p wave to define local atrial activation timing within the circuit, and the response to entrainment was used to clarify the functional properties of targeted site(s).[10,11,18,19] Further studies clarified the proper use of entrainment and have established its limitations.[20] From a practical standpoint, entrainment at a rate slightly faster than the underlying tachycardia that results in a postpacing interval of no more than 30 ms greater than the tachycardia cycle length and that is characterized by concealed fusion of the intracardiac wavefront is generally accepted as corresponding to a critical isthmus (Fig. 14.2). Among CHD patients, extensive surgical sequelae, scarring, and low-voltage regions may dispose to multiple competing wavefronts that can defy complete resolution even with the most sophisticated mapping tools.[21] Even with the introduction of fully automated mapping systems, tachycardia entrainment remains a major tool for the complete evaluation of IART.

With the introduction of three-dimensional (3D) electroanatomical mapping, greater understanding of critical isthmus sites in relation to their surrounding anatomy has become possible.[22] Lines of block and inert material are now routinely annotated on 3D mapping software and anatomical structures are defined for future reference.[14] The use of mapping technology improves the outcomes of catheter ablation for CHD[8] and given its value for mapping complex IARTs, the routine use of such systems is now recommended as a Class I indication for these procedures.[9] Recently, high-density and ultra-high-density mapping catheters and systems have enabled near instantaneous acquisition of large numbers of electrograms with the use of proprietary automated algorithms. These systems permit rapid, yet comprehensive chamber mapping that can facilitate complete delineation of the entire spatial course of wavefront propagation. The accompanying catheters are designed with closely spaced electrodes that optimize near-field electrogram discrimination and better characterize the tachycardia substrate. Novel mapping tools may also assist with the identification of critical isthmuses through informative visual displays of underlying electrophysiologic phenomena (Fig. 14.3).[23,24] Accordingly, a greater understanding of tachycardia circuits in CHD has been accompanied by newly described tachycardia mechanisms.[24–26] Nevertheless, it is necessary to remain cognizant of fundamental principles when using such systems as manual reannotation of complex signals may still be necessary.[27]

Although the mechanism of atrial tachycardia in CHD is chiefly related to macroreentry, focal AT (FAT) is implicated in up to 5–22% of cases.[28–35] FAT is almost always nonautomatic in its behavior but cannot be reliably differentiated further using conventional catheter-based techniques (though microreentry is widely considered to be the major electrophysiologic mechanism). FAT generally originates from the right atrium in CHD with a strong predilection for scar border zones (Fig. 14.4).[21,36] Sites of origin are characterized by low-amplitude, fractionated electrograms,[37] suggestive of nonuniform anisotropic conduction and poor cell-to-cell coupling from damaged myocardium.[38] Atrial activation conventionally constitutes <40% of the total cycle length for FAT, but the ratio increases with the degree of atrial myopathy (represented by low bipolar voltage) and slow transit through the atrial chamber.[21] Although FAT in CHD tends to be slower than macroreentrant AT, there is considerable overlap. In general, distinction by surface electrocardiography is unreliable and cannot be used to predict tachycardia mechanisms.[36]

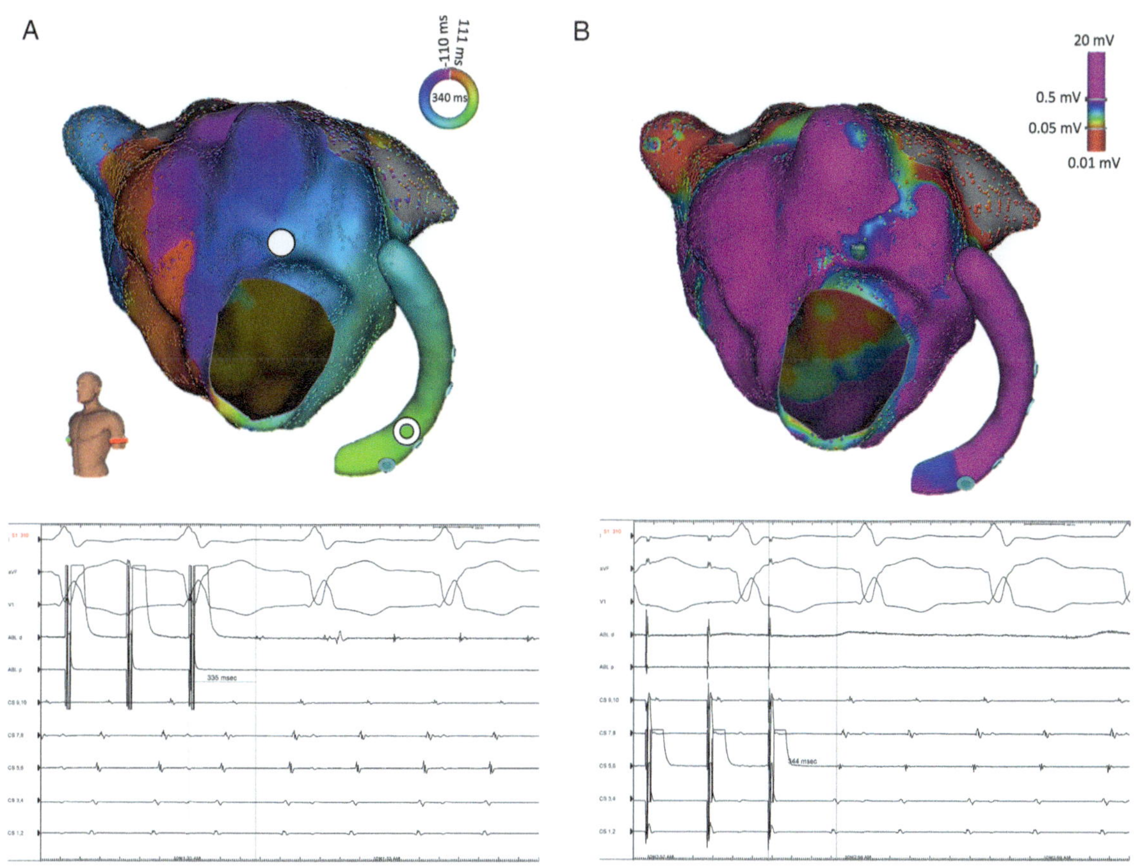

Fig. 14.2 Example of entrainment of a perimitral intra-atrial reentrant tachycardia in a patient with Ebstein anomaly after biatrial maze operation. (A and B) Activation and voltage maps created during tachycardia, respectively. There was a gap in an anterior mitral line where entrainment (*solid circle*) results in concealed fusion of the intracardiac electrograms and a postpacing interval equal to the tachycardia cycle length (*lower left*). Entrainment of tachycardia from the posterior coronary sinus electrode (*open circle*) results in manifest fusion but equivalent postpacing interval and tachycardia cycle length, consistent with an outer loop site (*lower right*).

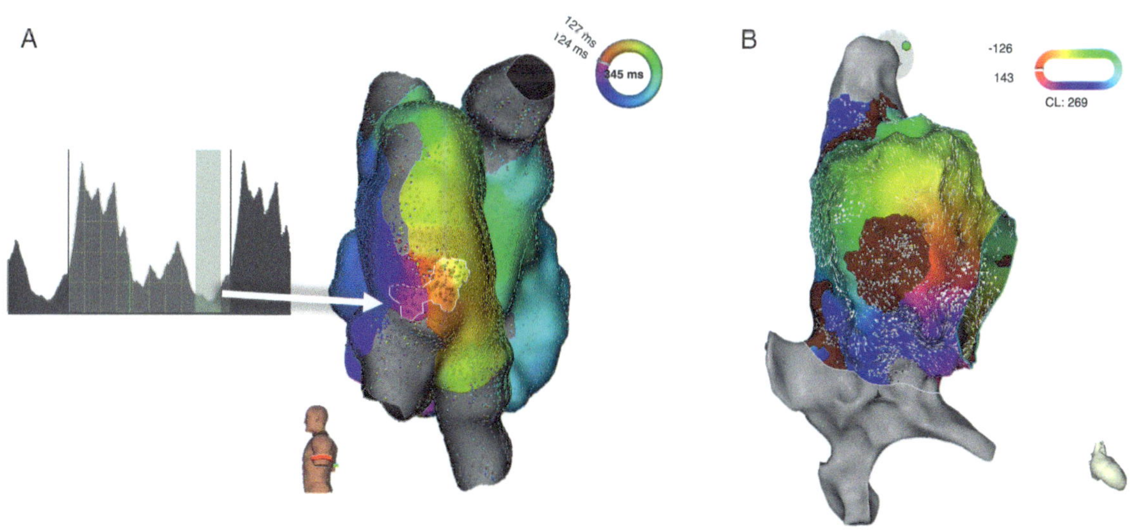

Fig. 14.3 Mapping tools to assist with intra-atrial reentrant tachycardia critical isthmus localization. (A) A trough in the global activation histogram is highlighted on the three-dimensional map. The histogram displays the proportion of activated surface area relative to the maximum instantaneous activated surface area throughout the tachycardia cycle. Critical isthmuses are typically characterized by limited activation through anatomically constrained areas. (B) A vector-based display of wavefront propagation shows both velocity and direction of local wavefront propagation. *Wider and shorter arrows* indicate slow conduction zones that are associated with critical isthmus sites.

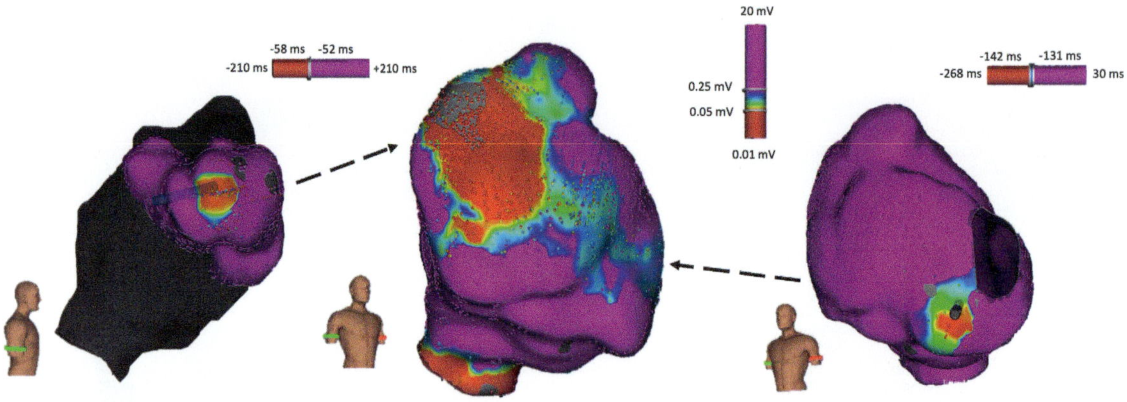

Fig. 14.4 Example of focal atrial tachycardias developing along scar border zones for congenital heart disease. This patient with pulmonary atresia with intact ventricular septum and Glenn anastomosis developed multiple episodes of supraventricular tachycardia and was found to have two separate focal atrial tachycardias near scarring in the right atrial free wall.

INTRA-ATRIAL REENTRANT TACHYCARDIA CIRCUIT CHARACTERISTICS IN CONGENITAL HEART DISEASE

IART circuits in CHD are often conceptualized by revolution of an activation wavefront around a fixed, identifiable central obstacle. In turn, central obstacles usually serve as the basis upon which these arrhythmias are described (Table 14.1). Early studies of postoperative IART demonstrated the importance of central obstacles arising from a variety of anatomical structures, surgical lesions, or acquired pathology.[22] More recent studies of conduction velocity have suggested that intrinsic differences exist between central obstacle categories in CHD. For example, standard anatomical obstacles (such as valve annuli) tend to be associated with faster and larger circuits, whereas obstacles resulting from acquired sequelae of prior cardiac operations are associated with slower and smaller circuits. For the latter, critical isthmus conduction velocity is often very slow (<0.15 m/s), with narrow channels of conduction that can be interrupted by limited catheter ablation (Fig. 14.5).[34,39] Diffusely low tissue voltage (<0.5 mV) is associated with this isthmus type.[40]

With rare exceptions, the most common IART isthmus encountered among patients with CHD (regardless of anatomy or operative strategy) is the anatomical equivalent of the cavotricuspid isthmus.[35,41,42] The central obstacle for this form of reentry is generally the AV valve annulus related to the inferior vena cava (tricuspid or mitral depending on the congenital lesion). In many cases, IART circuits are exceedingly complex yet still depend on the CTI or its equivalent.[41] A related variant that is frequently observed among CHD is lower loop reentry. This circuit is commonly observed among congenital lesions associated with severe right atrial enlargement, where the dilated inferior vena cava serves as a large, central obstacle yet the CTI remains the critical isthmus. Similar circuits can also be seen in other unrelated settings (Fig. 14.6, Video 14.1).[43] For patients with conventional morphologic right atrial anatomy, catheter ablation targeting CTI-dependent IART can proceed normally, with the operator remaining cognizant of tissue thickness, proximity to the coronary arteries, and the possibility of displaced AV nodal tissue (discussed in subsequent sections).

Another commonly observed central obstacle among CHD is the atriotomy, owing to the nearly ubiquitous presence of this surgical incision in the morphologic right atrial free wall (Figs. 14.3, 14.5, 14.7, and 14.8). Atriotomy scars can be distinguished from the nearby crista terminalis by their more anterior location and discrete boundaries, although the exact locations of the incisions themselves are highly variable and dependent

TABLE 14.1 Commonly Observed Reentrant Obstacles Among Congenital Heart Disease

Central Obstacle	Biventricular	DTGA S/M	AP Fontan	LT Fontan	EC Fontan
AV valve annulus	+++	+++	+	+	+
Atriotomy	+++	+	++	++	++
Crista terminalis	+	–	+	–	–
Septal patch	+	–	+	++	–
SVC (+ adjacent scar)	+	–	+	–	–
IVC	+/–	+/–	++	–	–
Morphologic RA scar	+	+/–	++	++	–

Abbreviations: *AP,* atriopulmonary; *AV,* atrioventricular; *DTGA-S/M,* D-transposition of the great arteries after Senning or Mustard operation; *EC,* extracardiac; *IVC,* inferior vena cava; *LT,* lateral tunnel; *RA,* right atrial; *SVC,* superior vena cava.

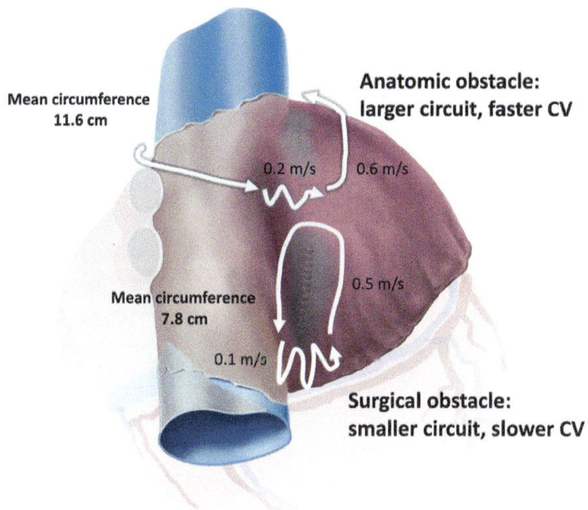

Fig. 14.5 Schematic of the posterolateral morphologic right atrium summarizing conduction velocity characteristics after congenital heart disease operations. Postoperative central obstacles (a surgical atriotomy is depicted in the lower portion of the figure) tend to be smaller and associated with slower conduction velocity as compared to the larger anatomical obstacles. *CV*, conduction velocity. (Adapted from Khale AK, et al. *JAHA*. 2019.)

on the prior surgical approach. The presence and participation of an atriotomy should be evaluated for all CHD undergoing catheter ablation, as atriotomy circuits may either operate independently or concurrently with other arrhythmias (e.g., dual loop reentry). Both more extensive atriotomy incisions (>5.1 cm) and those located adjacent to the tricuspid annulus are most likely to support reentry.[44] In other situations, atriotomy incision may serve to extend adjacent obstacles, increasing their effective size. This is particularly common for circuits related to the superior vena cava, often termed "upper loop reentry" (Figs. 14.5 and 14.7). These latter circuits tend to be large and their ablation targets variable. Ultimately, all forms of intra-atrial reentry can be associated with nearly any type of congenital heart defect and their relative frequency is likely underappreciated in the absence of comprehensive 3D mapping.

Other complex IART forms, often coexisting with the previously described circuits, have been identified in CHD. Among these, dual loop reentry has been implicated in 25–58% of IARTs in CHD.[45,46] Here, separate circuits propagate simultaneously around central obstacles that share a common anatomical isthmus. Most commonly, the tricuspid valve annulus serves as one central obstacle while a right atrial free wall atriotomy serves as another, especially when the latter is extensive (Fig. 14.7).[44,45] Often one loop is associated with a shorter cycle length and serves as the dominant loop. If faster loop is targeted first, the tachycardia will slow but will not terminate, despite successive ablation lesions. Conversely, if the slower tachycardia is first targeted, no change in cycle length is observed despite successful interruption of the related isthmus (Fig. 14.8, Videos 14.2 and 14.3).[45] In this situation, a change in p-wave morphology and coronary sinus activation may be the only indication of successful catheter ablation of the initial loop.[45,47]

A final IART mechanism, biatrial reentrant tachycardia, has recently been described among patients with CHD and highlights the successive advances in understanding the interatrial myoarchitecture and its relevance to IART.[26] Biatrial tachycardia is likely underdiagnosed in CHD, and its recognition has been shown to correlate with successive improvements in mapping technology. Such tachycardias are commonly observed in Fontan patients, including those with Bjork modification, as well as after the Senning operation. As catheter ablation of atrial fibrillation (AF) increases and IART is more frequently targeted within the left atrium, it is likely that this tachycardia will increasingly be seen among patients with biventricular congenital heart disease as well (Fig. 14.9, Video 14.4).

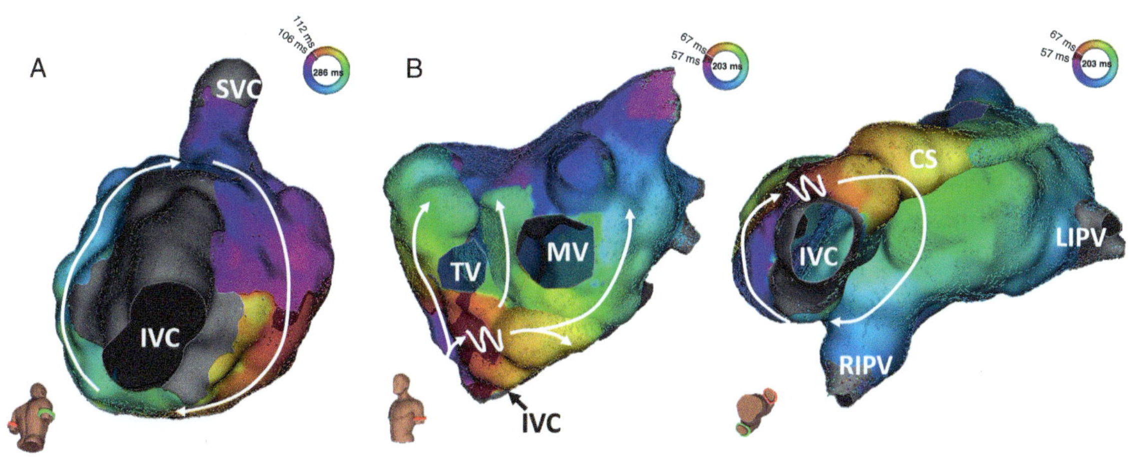

Fig. 14.6 Examples of lower loop reentry utilizing the cavotricuspid isthmus in congenital heart disease. (A) Clockwise reentry around the IVC in a patient with Ebstein anomaly and a severely dilated morphologic right atrium and IVC. (B) Lower loop reentry in a patient with mitral stenosis. Initial mapping appeared to demonstrate a focal tachycardia from the low right atrium, but on further inspection, a macroreentrant circuit was apparent around the IVC, using the coronary sinus and the septal aspect of the morphologic left atrium for the circuit. *CS*, coronary sinus; *IVC*, inferior vena cava; *LIPV*, left inferior pulmonary vein; *MV*, mitral valve; *SVC*, superior vena cava; *TV*, tricuspid valve.

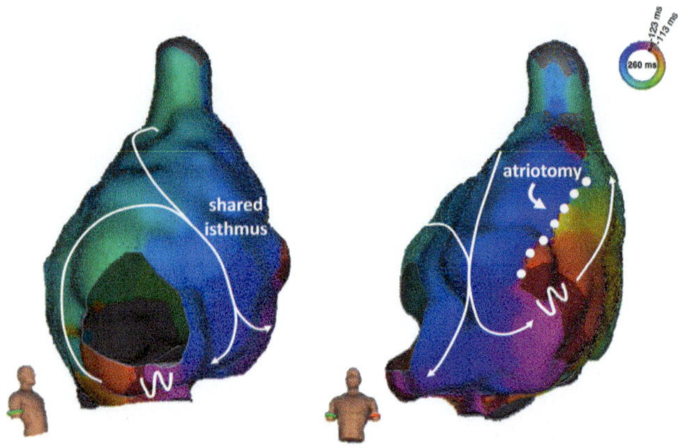

Fig. 14.7 Dual loop reentry in a patient with situs inversus and d-transposition of the great arteries following the Rastelli operation. There is clockwise rotation around the tricuspid annulus and counterclockwise rotation around the combined atriotomy incision and superior vena cava. A shared isthmus is present between the atriotomy incision and tricuspid annulus.

APPROACH TO CATHETER ABLATION

Due to anatomical and physiologic complexity, the American Heart Association/American College of Cardiology recommend that catheter ablation be performed by electrophysiologists with expertise in the management of adult CHD (Table 14.2).[48] Catheter ablation should be performed in dedicated electrophysiology laboratories where advanced mapping equipment and cardiac anesthesia is available. Procedures are generally performed with general anesthesia and endotracheal intubation. For patients who present to the catheterization laboratory in atrial tachycardia, uninterrupted anticoagulation is usually pursued, and transesophageal echocardiography is often performed to exclude left atrial thrombus.[49] Meticulous rate control and anesthetic management is vital for such patients to avoid the occasionally catastrophic consequence of 1:1 conduction that can result in marked hemodynamic compromise or even complete circulatory collapse for some congenital anomalies.

After vascular access is obtained, a multipolar diagnostic catheter is used as a fiduciary reference and is placed in the coronary sinus or the morphologic right atrium for patients with conventional anatomy. After the total cavopulmonary connection operation, diagnostic catheters are usually placed in the pulmonary artery where recording of nearby pulmonary venous atrial myocardium is possible. For patients after the Senning or Mustard operation, diagnostic catheters are typically placed either along the septal patch or within the morphologic left atrial appendage. A simplified approach using two catheters in CHD has been advocated by some and may decrease the amount of time required for the procedure and accelerate the postrocedure recovery.[46] Limitations of the latter approach include a reduced ability to discern subtle changes in the tachycardia circuit, followed by improper annotation of activation timing. For CHD in general, but especially when limited intracardiac diagnostic catheters are used, it is imperative to meticulously monitor the intracardiac activation sequence and cycle length as well as the surface electrocardiographic appearance for abrupt changes that suggest conversion to an alternate tachycardia to avoid contamination of the 3D map.[50]

Comprehensive mapping of the entire relevant chamber(s) is recommended in CHD given the common existence of atypical IART or dual loop circuits, even for patients with relatively simple anatomies (Fig. 14.10, Video 14.5). Review of the activation map will usually suggest a constrained region or "critical isthmus" at which the reentrant circuit can be targeted. It is generally advisable to target isthmuses associated with the lowest voltage and slowest conduction velocity in order to increase the probability of acute and long-term success.[46,51] In some cases, however, a greater likelihood of collateral damage demands that catheter ablation energy be delivered at an alternative area associated with less favorable conduction properties.[24,52] Careful selection of the most appropriate

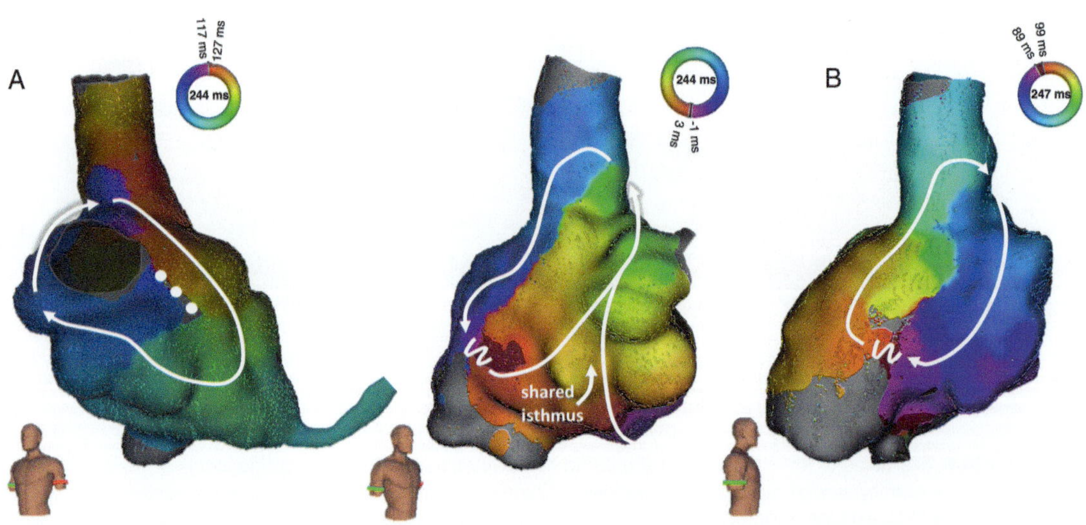

Fig. 14.8 Dual loop reentry after the Bjork operation for tricuspid atresia. (A) Catheter ablation was initially performed between the Bjork anastomosis and the inferior vena cava, but the cycle length was not affected despite documentation of complete conduction block. A second loop was evident at the right atrial free wall. (B) The alternate loop was mapped a second time in the opposite direction and ablated successfully at a gap near the inferior vena cava. *White circles* represent intra-atrial conduction block.

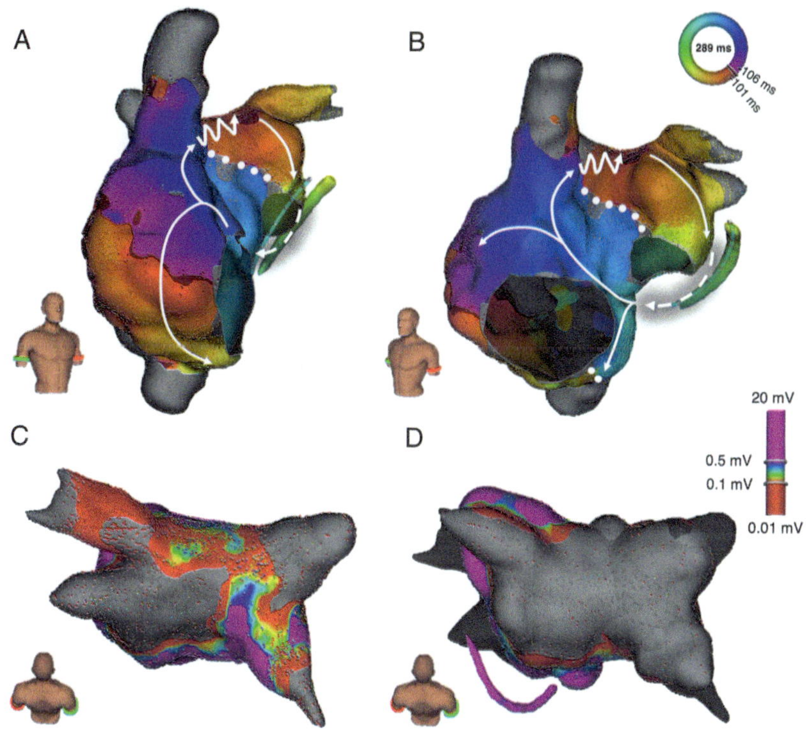

Fig. 14.9 Biatrial reentry in a patient with bicuspid aortic valve after the Ross operation. The patient had undergone cryoballoon pulmonary vein and LA posterior wall isolation with anterior mitral and cavotricuspid isthmus lines for persistent atrial fibrillation (*white circles* represent intra-atrial conduction block at the site of prior catheter ablation). (A and B) The patient developed postprocedural intra-atrial reentrant tachycardia, and a biatrial circuit utilizing the septopulmonary/Bachmann bundle (right → left) and coronary sinus connections (left → right) was diagnosed. (C) Reconnection of the left atrial posterior wall and right inferior pulmonary vein was evident at baseline. (D) With catheter ablation of epicardial connections at the septal left atrial roof, tachycardia was eliminated, and complete isolation of the left atrial posterior wall and pulmonary veins was observed.

TABLE 14.2 Challenges and Potential Solutions for Mapping and Catheter Ablation of Atrial Tachycardia in Congenital Heart Disease

Mapping	Potential Solutions
Multiple competing atrial arrhythmias	Multiple reference electrodes/multielectrode mapping/substrate ablation
Non sustained atrial tachycardia	Multielectrode mapping/substrate ablation
Limited reference electrodes	Esophageal/pulmonary artery electrodes*
Atypical mechanism (dual loop/biatrial reentry)	Comprehensive full chamber/biatrial mapping
Dissociated atrial myocardium	Meticulous exclusion of extraneous data
Pseudoreentry related to intra-atrial block	Ultra-high-density mapping/entrainment mapping
Identification of critical isthmus	Entrainment mapping/proprietary software algorithms
Presence of conduits/baffles	Preprocedural imaging/interventional expertise/RMN
Absence of femoral venous access	Hepatic access/remote magnetic navigation
Hypertrophied myocardium	Irrigated ablation/judicious selection of ablation targets
Protected atrial myocardium	Needle perforation/bipolar ablation/RMN
Catheter stability	Steerable sheath/intracardiac echocardiography/RMN
Latent substrates	Strict induction protocol/isoproterenol administration

Abbreviation: *RMN*, remote magnetic navigation.
*Select anatomies (e.g., extracardiac Fontan operation).

isthmus target is imperative to provide optimal catheter ablation outcomes.

After identification of the targeted isthmus, catheter ablation is nearly always performed with the use of irrigated radiofrequency energy.[9] Linear catheter ablation lesions are used to connect two nonconducting barriers to interrupt the tachycardia circuit. When targeting a critical IART isthmus, the tachycardia cycle length will most often progressively lengthen prior to termination (Fig. 14.1). The combination of tachycardia cycle length prolongation and termination without ectopic beats

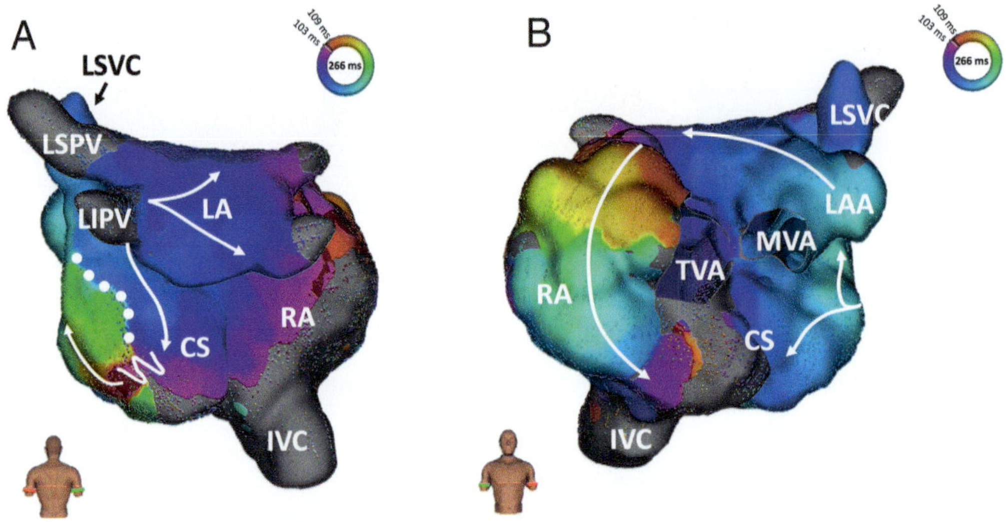

Fig. 14.10 Atypical intra-atrial reentrant tachycardia circuit after operative repair of atrioventricular septal defect with left superior vena cava to the coronary sinus. The coronary sinus had become massively enlarged over time and had formed a supernumerary atrial chamber. A left atrial appendage tachycardia was suspected after mapping of the left atrium at another hospital and catheter ablation was deferred. At repeat electrophysiology study with complete mapping of the atrial chambers, a reentrant circuit within the CS was diagnosed and successfully targeted by catheter ablation. *CS*, coronary sinus; *IVC*, inferior vena cava; *LAA*, left atrial appendage; *LIPV*, left inferior pulmonary vein; *LSPV*, left superior pulmonary vein; *MVA*, mitral valve annulus; *RA*, right atrium; *SVC*, superior vena cava; *TVA*, tricuspid valve annulus.

is taken as a favorable response to catheter ablation and confirms the critical nature of the targeted isthmus.[19] In general, split potentials are observed at the line of conduction block during effective isthmus interruption.[53] For some congenital heart defects, transmural isthmus interruption may be challenging due to signficiant atrial myocardial hypertrophy. This is particularly common for patients after an older-style Fontan operation where long-standing atrial hypertension can lead to atrial wall thickness that approaches the limits of radiofrequency energy delivery. In the modern era, irrigated radiofrequency energy is recommended for most CHD procedures to improve transmural ablation and has been shown to be effective when standard nonirrigated catheter ablation fails.[54,55]

After cardiac operations for repair of CHD, it is not uncommon for various types of intra-atrial block to occur, related to prior atriotomy incisions, baffle placement, maze lesions, or prior catheter ablation. Discontinuities in intra-atrial conduction can manifest as localized 2:1 block or even complete dissociation during tachycardia or sinus rhythm (Fig. 14.11), which can frustrate attempts at 3D mapping.[16] It is critical to recognize regions with dissociated atrial activity without delay to avoid erroneous incorporation into the activation map. Operationally, if a region of myocardium is not concordant with the rhythm of interest, it can be considered irrelevant to the tachycardia circuit and ignored. A useful technique is to label dissociated areas as dense scar on the activation map so that the aberrant timing is not included.

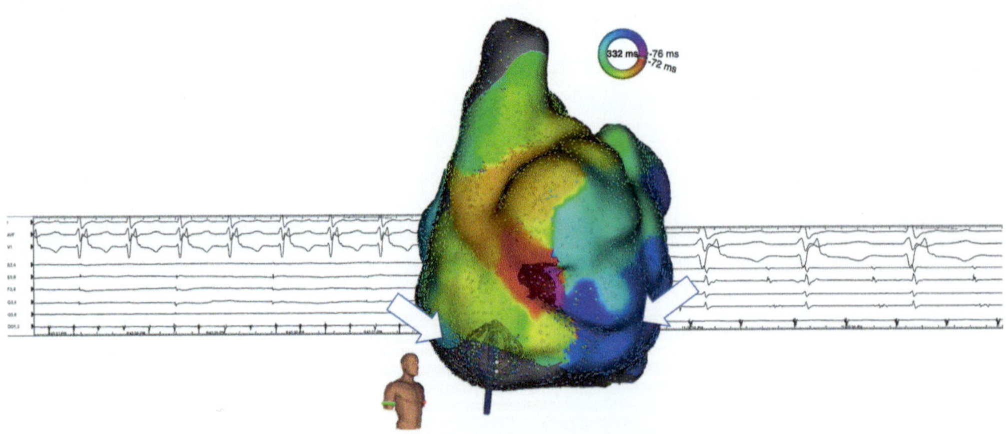

Fig. 14.11 Regions in the right atrium with dissociated electrograms during mapping of intra-atrial reentrant tachycardia after surgical repair of tetralogy of Fallot. Leftward panel (electrograms E–G recorded from the basket catheter) demonstrate a slow atrial rhythm unrelated to the tachycardia of interest, whereas the rightward panel shows electrograms recorded in a region associated with 2:1 entrance block. Failure to recognize dissociated rhythms and inadvertent incorporation into the electroanatomical map can confound circuit characterization during congenital heart disease procedures.

Following catheter ablation, bidirectional block across the newly formed lesion set is recommended.[56] This can be achieved through differential pacing maneuvers or formal 3D mapping. After targeting the CTI, demonstration of conduction block is usually straightforward but can be challenging for atypical circuits, especially those that are located within the pulmonary venous atrium. Here, multipolar electrode-based catheters can be useful. Repeat testing following catheter ablation is necessary to evaluate for additional, latent atrial tachycardias, which are quite common in CHD and represent a major mechanism for tachycardia recurrence.[32] There is no standardized protocol for repeat testing of IART in CHD patients; however, delivery of triple atrial extrastimuli along with incremental atrial pacing to a minimum cycle length of 200 ms is reasonable for the evaluation of latent substrates.[34] Isoproterenol should also be considered during repeat testing.[6,34] Finally, most series of catheter ablation for IART suggest additional arrhythmia subtypes are present (e.g. AVNRT, AVRT, twin AVRT) in 4–7% of cases,[34,57] such that comprehensive electrophysiologic evaluation is required regardless of the clinical indication.

Catheter Ablation of Atrial Fibrillation

AF has emerged as an important contributor to supraventricular tachycardia among patients with CHD. Its prevalence increases with age and surpasses IART by the age of 50 years.[58] Although classically related to pulmonary venous triggers, AF appears to represent a more diverse disease in CHD. There is emerging evidence to implicate morphologic right atrial substrates as AF drivers in many cases. For instance, fibrillatory conduction of rapid right atrial AT has been described. Conversely, substrate-based catheter ablation within the morphologic right atrium after atriopulmonary Fontan operation can eliminate AF without the need for PVI.[38,59,60] Accordingly, it has been unclear whether pulmonary vein isolation for the treatment of AF in CHD will yield equivalent results compared to the general population. To date, there is emerging evidence that pulmonary vein isolation in addition to catheter ablation targeting extrapulmonary vein triggers may yield good outcomes for CHD, but further study is required to firmly establish optimal catheter ablation strategies.[61]

POTENTIAL COMPLICATIONS AND COLLATERAL DAMAGE

CHD patients are at elevated risk of collateral injury during catheter ablation (Table 14.3). Anatomical variations in the location of the compact AV node and proximal His bundle represent a chief concern for select anatomies and require careful consideration to avoid unintended AV block. Cryoablation has been shown to be safe and effective for patients in whom the location of the AV node is either uncertain or is in known proximity to the location of planned catheter ablation.[62] As most arrhythmia substrates involve the morphologic right atrium, pacing for capture and subsequent delineation of the course of the right phrenic nerve is prudent whenever lesions are placed at the posterior-to-lateral morphologic right atrial wall (Fig. 14.12).[6] For some forms of CHD, one or more coronary arteries may

TABLE 14.3 Potential Complications and Steps That Can Be Taken to Avoid Them During Catheter Ablation in Congenital Heart Disease

Complication	Steps to Avoid
AV block	Preprocedural knowledge of congenital diagnosis and conduction system anatomy
Sinus node injury	Baseline mapping of sinus rhythm or subsidiary pacemaker
Coronary artery stenosis	Judicious ablation/intracardiac echocardiography/coronary angiography
Prolonged radiation	3D mapping/intracardiac echocardiography
Hemodynamic instability	Preprocedural rhythm control/inpatient optimization/congenital anesthesia expertise AV nodal agents/mechanical support
Phrenic nerve injury	Endocardial mapping of phrenic nerve course at posterolateral RA
Pericardial/intrathoracic hemorrhage	Preoperative advanced imaging/ echocardiographic guidance/interventional expertise
Systemic/pulmonary thromboembolism	Exclusion of right and left thrombus by transesophageal echocardiography/ heparinization

Abbreviations: *AV*, atrioventricular; *RA*, right atrium; *TEE*, transesophageal echocardiogram.

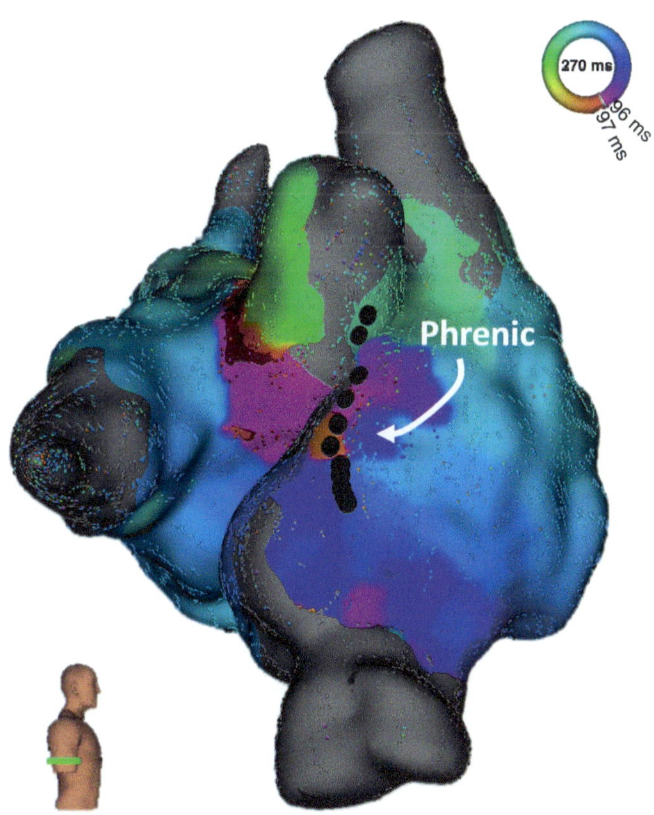

Fig. 14.12 Typical course of the phrenic nerve after Warden operation for sinus venosus defect with anomalous right superior pulmonary vein. The phrenic nerve was located near a potential ablation target requiring a modified strategy. *Black circles* represent locations that were associated with phrenic nerve capture during endocardial pacing.

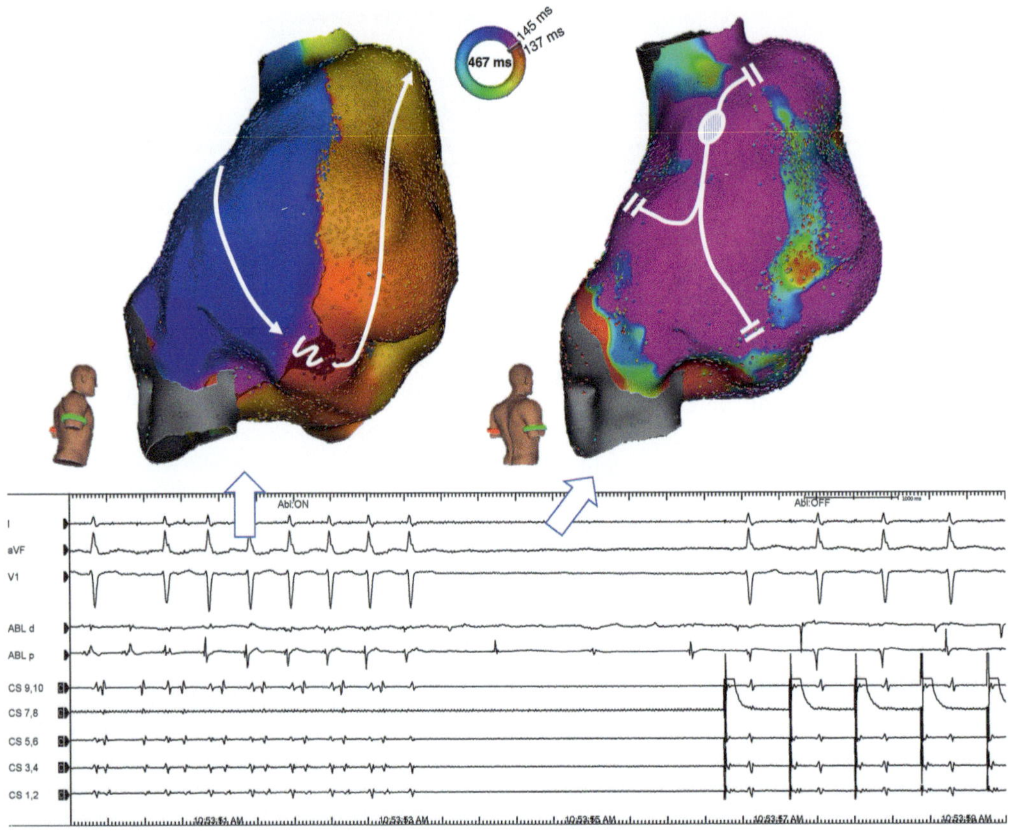

Fig. 14.13 Example of intra-atrial atrioventricular block developing during catheter ablation of an atriotomy circuit. Although wavefront propagation traversed the atrial septum during intra-atrial reentrant tachycardia, dissociation of the lateral right atrial wall from the left atrium developed during catheter ablation at a critical isthmus below the atriotomy (intact atrioventricular conduction during coronary sinus pacing is noted on the *right* of the recording). Intra-atrial conduction later resumed, and no further lesions were placed.

also lie close to the endocardium and pose a risk for stenosis and even myocardial infarction at the time of catheter ablation.[63] Catheter ablation for CHD may also occasionally require prolonged fluoroscopy or protracted procedural duration which carry risks of radiation-induced injury as well as volume overload and hemodynamic deterioration, especially for the more fragile postoperative physiologies. Judicious use of fluoroscopy during 3D mapping, supplemented with intracardiac echocardiography can limit radiation exposure for CHD.[64] Safe and effective catheter ablation also requires an in-depth knowledge of the embryology, anatomy, and electrophysiology that are all unique to these patients.

A rare complication, AV block can ensue in situations where multiple regions of intra-atrial block are preexisting, and when additional catheter ablation isolates a portion of the atrium containing the sinus node (Fig. 14.13). Careful evaluation of sinus activation is required to avoid this problem and may require baseline mapping in sinus rhythm.

CATHETER ABLATION FOR SPECIFIC FORMS OF CONGENITAL HEART DISEASE

Although general principles may apply, the technical approach to catheter ablation varies widely according to the underlying congenital anatomy and the type of operative repair. Not only are arrhythmia circuits closely associated to the underlying surgical anatomy, but the urgency of catheter-based therapy, the hemodynamic consequences of the arrhythmia, routes of catheter access to the underlying substrate, and likelihood of acute success all vary according to the anatomical and physiologic status of the patient. The fundamentals of catheter ablation for specific postoperative anatomies are discussed in the following sections. Although it is not possible to illustrate or describe all variations of arrhythmia circuits observed in CHD, representative examples of some of the most common forms are included.

Atrial Septal Defects

Atrial septal defects are highly prevalent CHD substrates and are strongly associated with both atrial flutter in younger, and AF in older, age groups. Although both CTI-dependent and atriotomy-related IART circuits are observed after operative repair, multiple variations are possible. For instance, dual loop tachycardia involving a combination of the cavotricuspid isthmus and atriotomy is common after ASD repair, in accord with the original description of this mechanism in a series of postoperative ASD patients.[65,66] In general, post-ASD atriotomy isthmuses tend to be relatively narrow, requiring a small number of lesions for transection.[39] A less commonly described tachycardia following operative or transcatheter ASD closure involves reentry around the defect itself (Fig. 14.14, Video 14.6).[12,16,47,66,67]

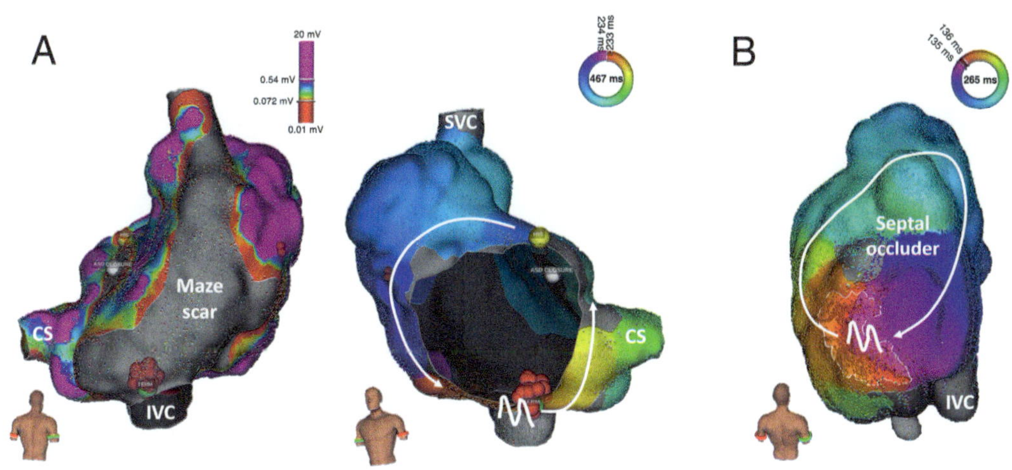

Fig. 14.14 Examples of intra-atrial reentrant tachycardia after ASD repair. (A) Despite prior right atrial maze operation, intra-atrial reentrant tachycardia used the cavotricuspid isthmus with a gap in the lateral tricuspid isthmus lesion. (B) Intra-atrial reentrant tachycardia using a transcatheter device that had been used to close an ASD was targeted with lesions between the device and the IVC. *CS*, coronary sinus; *IVC*, inferior vena cava; *SVC*, superior vena cava.

It is necessary for the operator to target all inducible tachycardia circuits to establish durable success. This is often best accomplished by full chamber mapping with complete delineation of single or multiple loops prior to attempted catheter interruption. Importantly, for older patients after surgical maze operation, atrial tachycardias are still observed in approximately 15% of patients. Remarkably, IART using the CTI is often observed despite biatrial maze operations, in part because the modified right atrial maze does not typically include direct transection of this isthmus (Fig. 14.14).[68]

Atrioventricular Septal Defect

Atrioventricular septal defects (AVSDs) develop when the cardiac endocardial cushions fail to fuse during embryologic development. Defects range from partial, transitional to complete and are associated with variable morphologic AV valve subtypes. A shared feature for all subtypes is inferior displacement of the AV node toward the crux of the heart where the atrial and ventricular septae are more closely aligned. For AVSDs, the surgical landmark to the location of the AV node is no longer the apex of the triangle of Koch but at a triangle delimited by the tendinous rim of the primum ASD, the inferior bridging leaflet of the atrioventricular valve and the ostium of the coronary sinus.[69] In the early era of operative repair, the septal patch was often placed to encircle this entire triangle, leaving the coronary sinus drainage to the morphologic left atrium. In these cases, the atrial septal remnant and coronary sinus are no longer easily accessible for catheter ablation (Fig. 14.15). Regardless of the operative approach, conduction system landmarks are often obscured so that catheter ablation at the posteroseptum should proceed cautiously to avoid unintended AV block.

Owing to the presence of an embryologic septal commissure ("cleft") between the anterior and posterior bridging leaflets, residual left-sided AV valve regurgitation or stenosis can be seen following operative repair. It has been demonstrated that AF arising after AVSD repair is related to the degree of residual left-sided AV valve regurgitation.[70] AF is increasingly recognized in this population and can develop irrespective of the surgical approach.[70] Catheter ablation must be directed toward both the AF and concomitant IART circuits that are frequent in this group (Fig. 14.16, Video 14.7).

Ebstein Anomaly

Ebstein anomaly is a rare congenital heart malformation characterized by apical displacement of the septal leaflet of the tricuspid valve. The ensuing tricuspid regurgitation and "atrialization" of the basal portions of the right ventricle promote right atrial enlargement and a propensity for atrial tachycardia. Although the most common arrhythmia substrate for patients with Ebstein anomaly is atrioventricular reentrant tachycardia related to the congenital presence of accessory pathways, atrial tachycardias are increasingly observed with age.[71] Prior to operative repair, the cavotricuspid isthmus is the most commonly implicated conduction isthmus. Catheter ablation procedures for Ebstein anomaly can be challenging due to massive enlargement of the right atrium and can be encumbered by multiple arrhythmia substrates (Fig. 14.17). Following tricuspid valve repair, IART circuits are typically more complex, especially when a maze procedure has been performed. Notably, CTI-dependent IART remains a prominent tachycardia mechanism despite prior right atrial maze operation, depending on the location of operative cryolesions.[68] When only tricuspid valve repair is necessary, postoperative catheter ablation targeting the CTI is generally feasible and associated with a favorable outcome.[72]

For patients with Ebstein anomaly in whom a tricuspid valve ring or replacement has been placed, catheter ablation procedures targeting the cavotricuspid isthmus are more challenging as atrial tissue can be excluded by the surgical prosthesis.[72] Usually the CTI can be transected with lesions placed at both the atrial and ventricular aspects of the isthmus.[72,73] When this is unsuccessful, however, unique approaches to obtain access to restricted tissues below the bioprosthetic ring or valve have been

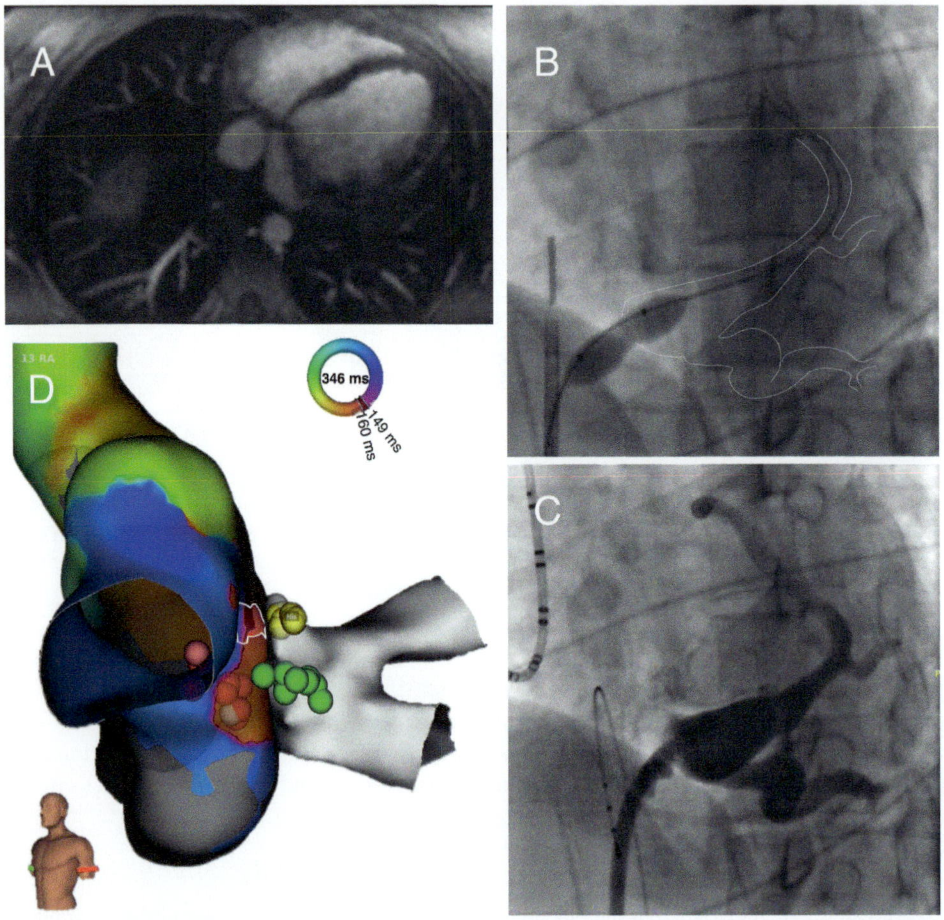

Fig. 14.15 Exclusion of the coronary sinus and septal right atrial remnant after atrioventricular septal defect operation. (A) Preoperative MRI shows discontinuity between the coronary sinus and the morphologic right atrium. (B and C) Access to the coronary sinus was achieved by radiofrequency wire perforation under intracardiac echocardiography guidance followed by serial balloon dilatations. (D) Although slow pathway modification was unsuccessful from the right atrial side, successful catheter ablation could be achieved after entry into the excluded chamber.

described, including subvalvular puncture or catheter ablation through the small cardiac vein.[73,74] Due to the difficulties that can arise after placement of surgical bioprosthetic material, preemptive catheter ablation or intraoperative cryoablation of the cavotricuspid isthmus has been proposed to prevent formidable challenges associated with postoperative catheter ablation.[72]

Owing to unique anatomy, catheter ablation of Ebstein anomaly is associated with unique risks compared to other forms of CHD. Anatomical proximity of the right coronary artery to the endocardium is a known feature and likely explains case reports describing coronary arterial injury.[75,76] Other potential complications of catheter ablation for Ebstein anomaly include AV block related to anatomically displaced conduction system, systemic thromboembolism through residual atrial level shunts, iatrogenic ventricular pseudoaneurysm, and ventricular fibrillation, among others.

Tetralogy of Fallot and Related Variants

Tetralogy of Fallot is the most common form of cyanotic CHD and is prevalent among catheter ablation series.[34] Patients with surgically repaired tetralogy of Fallot may develop increased right atrial filling pressure related to residual pulmonary valve dysfunction and right ventricular dilation. The emergence of atrial arrhythmia for the patient with tetralogy of Fallot may suggest a deterioration in right ventricular hemodynamics and is often a motivating factor to pursue reintervention on the pulmonary valve.[9] Independent risk factors for the development of both atrial tachycardia and AF for patients with TOF include right atrial enlargement, systemic hypertension and greater number of prior cardiac surgeries.[77]

Atrial tachycardias arising after operated tetralogy of Fallot are most often IARTs related to the cavotricuspid isthmus or right atrial free wall, where atriotomy and the crista terminalis circuits play a significant role (Fig. 14.2 and 14.11).[42,78] Dual loop reentry appears to be particularly common in this group of patients, often using the tricuspid annulus and atriotomy incisions or right atrial free wall scar (Fig. 14.18). Thorough evaluation of all inducible substrates is important to limit the risk for recurrent atrial tachycardia.

AF has also emerged as an important contributor to arrhythmia burden among patients with tetralogy of Fallot.[78] For these patients, the prevalence of AF exceeds that

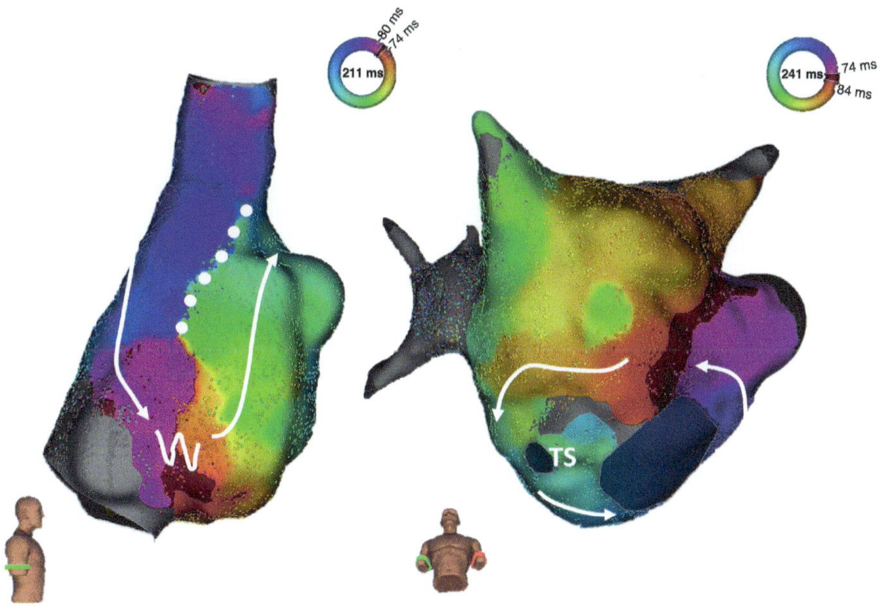

Fig. 14.16 Catheter ablation of multiple substrates after AV septal defect repair. The patient presented with both atrial fibrillation and atrial flutter and was referred for catheter ablation. At the procedure, both perimitral (*right figure*) and right atrial intra-atrial reentrant tachycardia (*left figure*) were observed and were targeted for catheter ablation along with pulmonary vein isolation. *White circles* represent intra-atrial conduction block along the crista terminalis. *TS*, transseptal puncture.

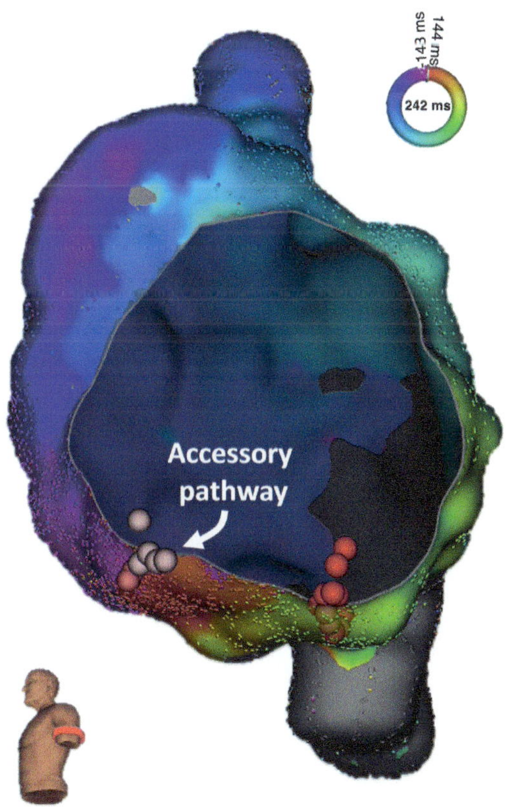

Fig. 14.17 Catheter ablation in unoperated Ebstein anomaly with considerable right atrial enlargement. Although intra-atrial reentrant tachycardia using the cavotricuspid isthmus was the targeted arrhythmia, a coexisting concealed accessory pathway was noted following catheter ablation. Comprehensive electrophysiologic evaluation is recommended for patients with Ebstein anomaly given a strong association with additional arrhythmia substrates.

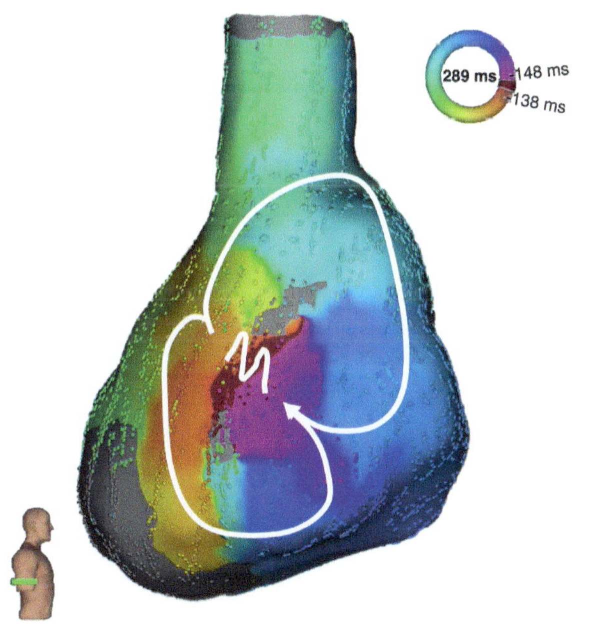

Fig. 14.18 Example of localized dual loop reentry in a patient with tetralogy of Fallot. There is a region of uneven scar at the right atrial free wall, likely related to prior atriotomy incision. Two reentrant loops are shown with a common isthmus between segments of scar where lesion delivery successfully eliminated tachycardia.

of atrial tachycardia by the age of 55 years and is more common among those with left ventricular dysfunction, left atrial enlargement, and older age.[77] Like many other forms of CHD, concomitant catheter ablation of both pulmonary vein triggers and IART circuits are often required in order to achieve long-term rhythm control.

Mustard and Senning Operation

The Mustard and Senning operations for D-transposition of the great arteries were profound innovations for patients with previously inoperable CHD. Although the two surgical techniques are highly distinct, both redirect systemic and pulmonary venous return to the contralateral ventricle and establish a physiology that is compatible with survival. Atrial tachycardias affect patients after the Mustard and Senning operation at an increased frequency compared to other forms of CHD, with 20% to 30% developing SVT after 10 years. Importantly, rapid conduction of atrial flutter in this group is associated with sudden cardiac death, so timely therapy is considered paramount.

Atrial tachycardia after the Mustard and Senning operation is usually related to IART within the morphologic right atrium, which is described postoperatively as the pulmonary venous atrium.[10] Circuits tend to use the cavotricuspid isthmus that are facilitated by a series of both permanent and functional boundaries posterior to a dilated tricuspid annulus, that include the septal patch, crista terminalis, and inferior vena cava.[35,79–82] Catheter ablation targeting the CTI is curative for this form of IART but is uniquely challenging, as the isthmus is often bisected by prior baffle material, Catheter ablation therefore usually requires access to both systemic and pulmonary venous chambers for isthmus transection (Fig. 14.19, Video 14.8).[83]

Other IART circuits may be found within the pulmonary venous atrium and include reentry related to the right-sided pulmonary veins and nearby surgical anastomosis in cases after the Senning or baffle operation.[81,84] Localized reentry in this region has been observed.[79] Circuits may use patches or incisions in the lateral wall of the pulmonary venous atrium after the Mustard operation and, rarely, lower loop reentry after both forms of operative repair.[79,81,85] Recently, a novel biatrial tachycardia has been described for the Senning operation that traverses the posterior surgical anastomosis with epicardial connections between morphologic right and left atria (Fig. 14.19, Video 14.9).[26] Finally, focal atrial tachycardias are frequently encountered, often arising from scar border zones, and are particularly common along the length of the septal patch (Fig. 14.20).[82]

Access to the pulmonary venous atrium is commonly achieved by trans-baffle puncture so that detailed mapping and catheter ablation can proceed via a direct approach. As opposed to other transseptal punctures, needle orientation after the Mustard or Senning operation is often directed rightward and superior given the unique orientation of the systemic and pulmonary venous baffles (Fig. 14.21). Supplemental imaging with contrast venography and transesophageal or intracardiac echocardiography are recommended. The presence of femoral venous occlusion may add to procedural complexity, given that many patients have undergone atrial septostomy as a palliative maneuver in the neonatal period.

As an alternative to the prograde approach, retrograde placement of the mapping and ablation catheter through both aortic and tricuspid valves has been used, primarily in a historical context.[10,18] Catheter manipulation is technically demanding from this approach, given multiple angulations required to reach the pulmonary venous atrium. Remote magnetic navigation has also more recently been reported to be useful in this scenario and has been applied with success.[28,86,87] Potential limitations include the inability to use high-density mapping or force-sensing catheters.

Atriopulmonary Fontan Operation

The earliest iteration of the Fontan operation involved a direct connection from the right atrium (typically the atrial appendage) to the pulmonary artery to provide passive venous flow to the pulmonary arterial circulation. This operation allowed the functionally single ventricle to act as a systemic pump, effectively separating two circulations into a series so that long-term survival could be achieved. The morphologic right atrial chamber inevitably, and gradually, dilates after this operation, which serves as the basis for multiple potential IART circuits. Pathologic changes observed after atriopulmonary Fontan operation

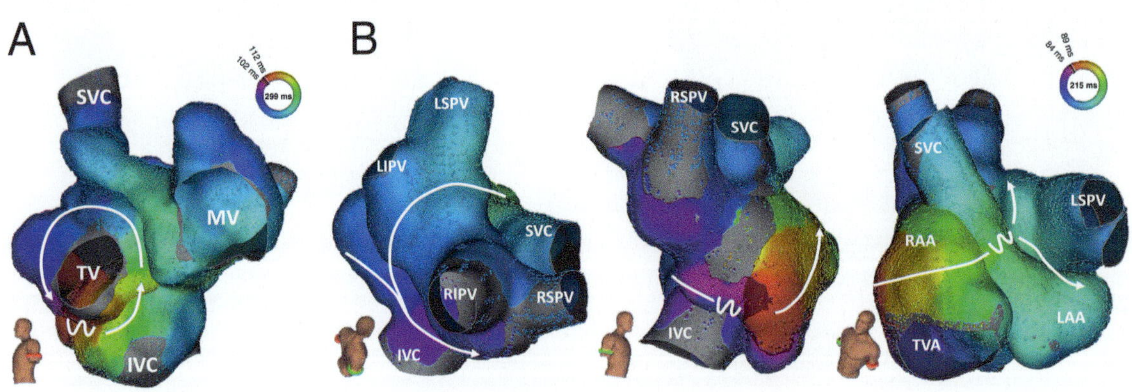

Fig. 14.19 Examples of intra-atrial reentrant tachycardia developing after the Mustard or Senning operation. (A) Intra-atrial reentrant tachycardia using the cavotricuspid isthmus after the Mustard operation. The targeted isthmus is located between the tricuspid annulus and the inferior vena cava that has been partitioned by a surgical baffle. (B) Biatrial tachycardia in a patient with prior Senning operation. A large circuit is present that uses both morphologic atria. An isthmus between the pulmonary venous anastomosis and the IVC was targeted successfully for catheter ablation. *IVC*, inferior vena cava; *LAA*, left atrial appendage; *LIPV*, left inferior pulmonary vein; *LSPV*, left superior pulmonary vein; *MV*, mitral valve; *RAA*, right atrial appendage; *RIPV*, right inferior pulmonary vein; *RSPV*, right superior pulmonary vein; *SVC*, superior vena cava; *TVA*, tricuspid valve annulus.

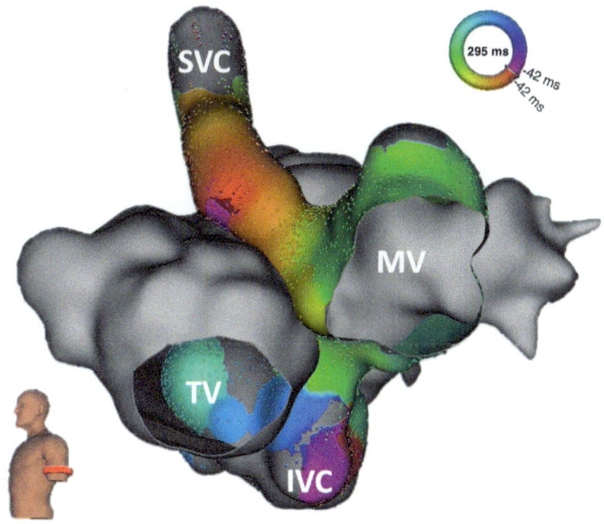

Fig. 14.20 Focal atrial tachycardia after the Mustard operation for D-transposition of the great arteries. Earliest atrial activation arises from the septal aspect of the superior venous baffle adjacent to dense scar corresponding to surgical patch material. The pulmonary venous atrium is shown without activation in grey. Notice that total atrial activation time represents a large proportion of the tachycardia cycle length for this patient with complex congenital heart disease.[21] *IVC*, inferior vena cava; *MV*, mitral valve; *SVC*, superior vena cava; *TV*, tricuspid valve.

include morphologic right atrial enlargement, mural thickening, and interstitial fibrosis, which are initially modest but increase progressively with time.[88] The development of IART after early iterations of the Fontan operation was quite common, with roughly 50% having from supraventricular arrhythmia within 10 years.[89] Importantly, low-voltage areas are associated with increased morphologic right atrial size and correlate with reduced acute and long-term catheter ablation success after the Fontan operation.[90] As opposed to other forms of CHD, free wall circuits appear to be the most common substrate.[18,57] Other reported mechanisms include those involving the right-sided AV valve to IVC,[91] septal patch, lower loop reentry, and reentry involving the atriopulmonary anastomosis (Fig. 14.22, Video 14.10).[43,57]

After the atriopulmonary Fontan operation, prior baffle placement may cover critical portions of the right atrial remnant that can support IART. In particular, the right-sided AV valve may be protected by patch material yet serve as the central obstacle for reentry. In most cases, conventional trans-baffle puncture into the morphologic left atrium can performed with deflection of the catheter through an atrial septal defect back toward this supra-annular chamber; however, an atrial septal defect is not always present (Fig. 14.23). In these cases, access to the remnant chamber can be quite challenging. An alternative option (when available) is remote magnetic navigation, which may permit retrograde access for these substrates.

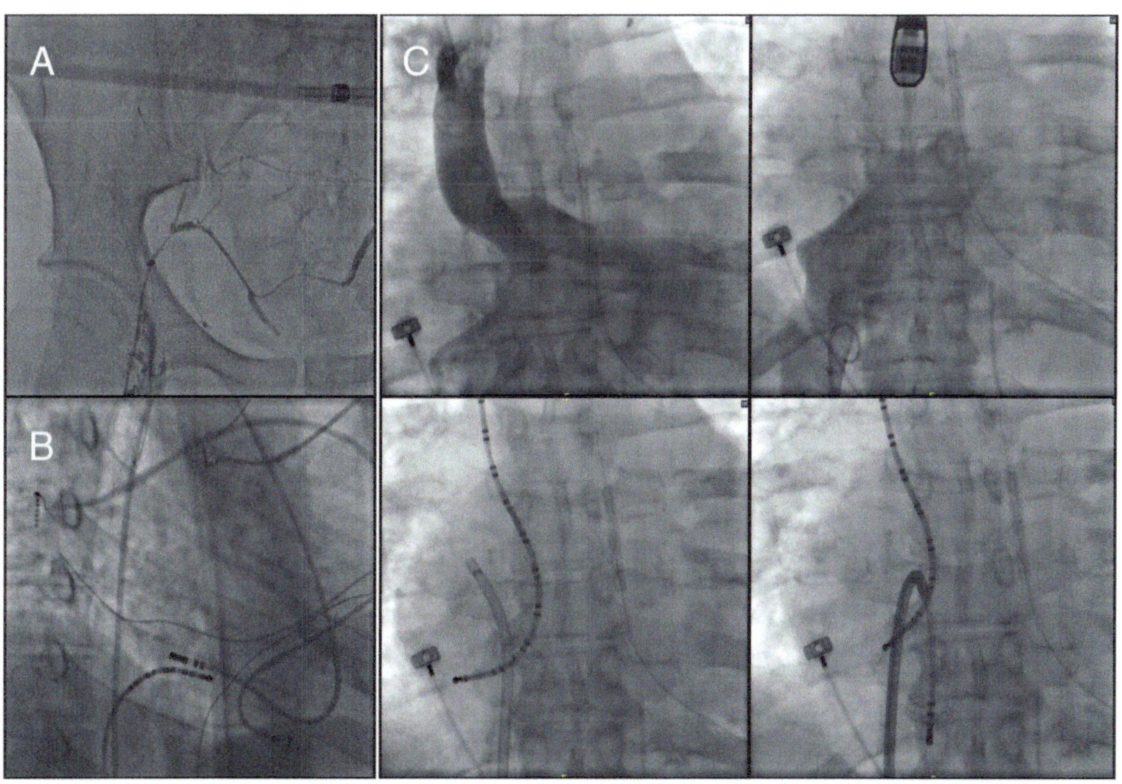

Fig. 14.21 Fluoroscopic views for the Mustard or Senning operation. (A) Right femoral venous occlusion after neonatal intervention. (B) Retrograde aortic access to the pulmonary venous atrium for ablation of the cavotricuspid isthmus. (C) Sequential venous angiography (superior and inferior) and trans-baffle sheath and catheter placement after the Senning operation. A multipolar electrode catheter has been placed inferiorly along the systemic venous baffle. The sheath has been advanced from below through an anterior and rightward baffle puncture, after which the catheter has been deflected downward to the cavotricuspid isthmus.

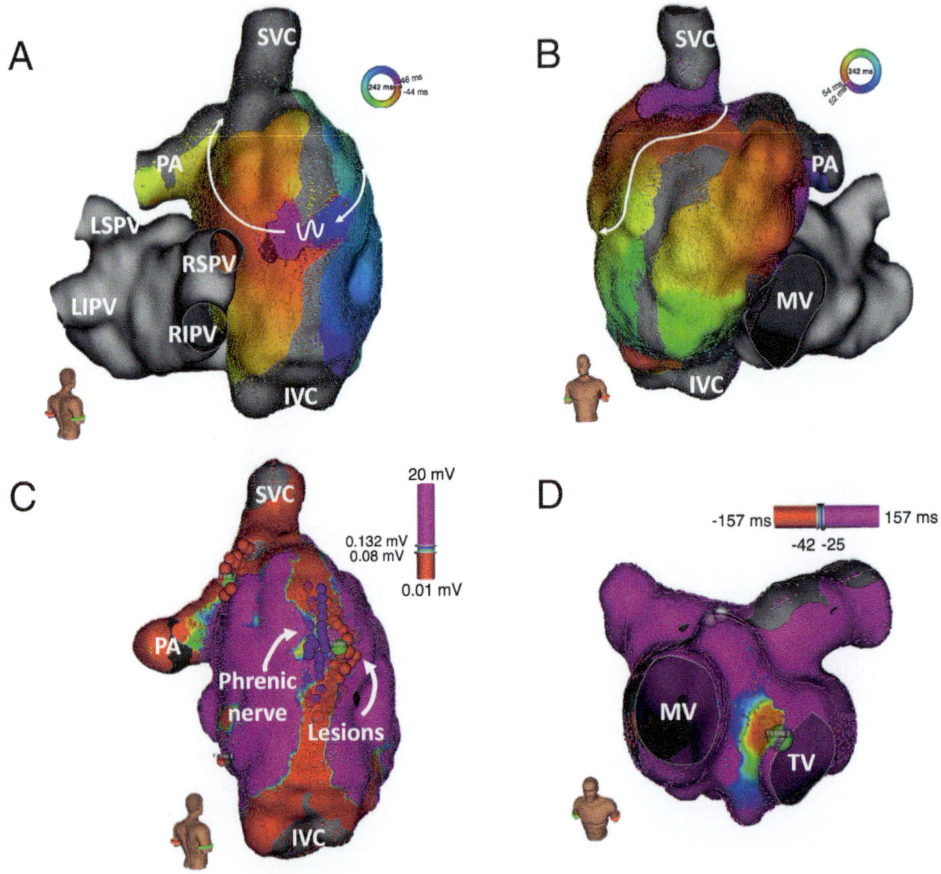

Fig. 14.22 Catheter ablation after atriopulmonary Fontan operation in a patient with congenitally corrected transposition and hypoplastic right ventricle. (A) A large reentrant circuit passes through a gap in a prior ablation line that had been cautiously placed as there was proximity to the phrenic nerve. The wavefront then passed through an isthmus between the SVC and atriopulmonary anastomosis. (B) The prior anterior ablation line was intact but had failed to interrupt the new circuit. (C) The course of the phrenic nerve is shown in relation to ablation lesions. (D) A focal atrial tachycardia from the tricuspid annulus was induced on isoproterenol and ablated following catheter ablation of the intra-atrial reentrant tachycardia in the same patient. *IVC*, inferior vena cava; *LIPV*, left inferior pulmonary vein; *LSPV*, left superior pulmonary vein; *PA*, pulmonary artery; *MV*, mitral valve; *RIPV*, right inferior pulmonary vein; *RSPV*, right superior pulmonary vein; *SVC*, superior vena cava; *TV*, tricuspid annulus.

Lateral Tunnel Fontan Operation

The lateral tunnel (LT) Fontan operation was initially proposed as a surgical solution to the suboptimal hemodynamics associated with the atriopulmonary Fontan. The operation involves the creation of an intracardiac atrial tunnel that connects the inferior and superior vena cava through the posterolateral morphologic right atrium. The approach favorably effects pulmonary hemodynamics and has been shown to delay the onset of atrial arrhythmia compared to prior iterations.

Tachycardia mechanisms following the LT Fontan are most often related to the isthmus between the right-sided AV valve annulus and the IVC, analogous to the CTI.[91,92] Early animal experiments suggested that the LT suture lines predispose to this mechanism by acting as an effective posterior boundary, creating a corridor between the baffle and the AV valve annulus.[93] This mechanism should be suspected for LT patients presenting with atrial tachycardia. Access to the pulmonary venous atrium is required for successful catheter ablation and can be accomplished via residual fenestration, baffle puncture, or retrograde approach.[91,92] Equally common are circuits related to the baffle suture line within the lateral tunnel itself (Fig. 14.24, Video 14.11). Concomitant arrhythmia mechanisms including twin AV nodal tachycardia and other typical forms of supraventricular tachycardia are also often jointly observed, as noted in published catheter ablation series.[92]

Extracardiac Fontan Operation

The most recent iteration of the Fontan operation involves the placement of an extracardiac conduit from the inferior vena cava to the pulmonary artery to reroute systemic venous return to the pulmonary circulation. Although associated with the lowest burden of supraventricular tachycardia developments compared to either the atriopulmonary or lateral tunnel Fontan,[94] after the extracardiac Fontan patients remain at risk for various forms of supraventricular tachycardia, including IART. As opposed to prior iterations, however, direct access to the pulmonary venous chamber is much more

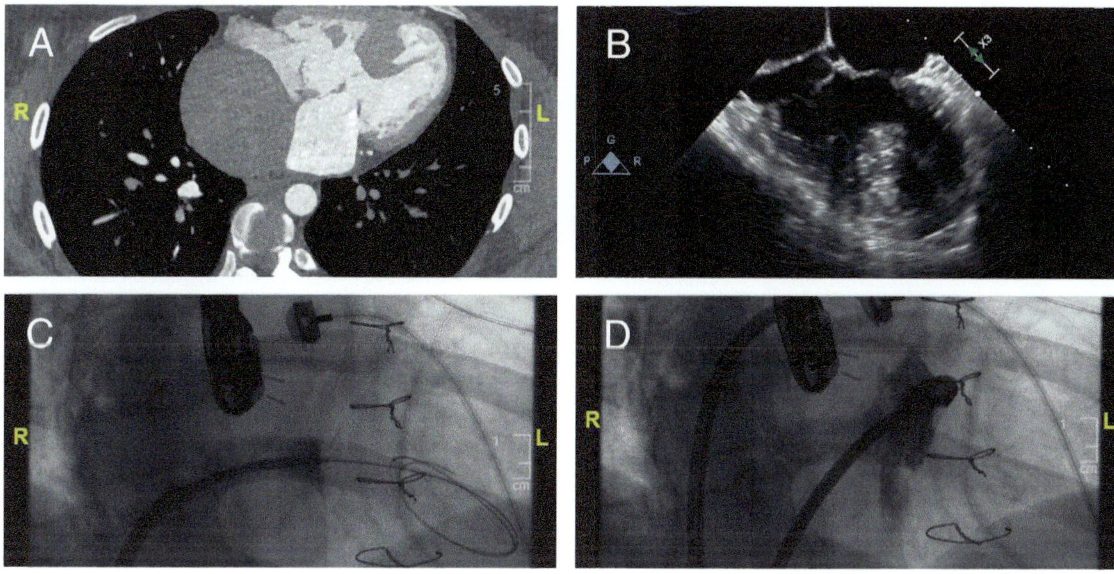

Fig. 14.23 Periannular intra-atrial reentrant tachycardia circuit in a patient with unbalanced atrioventricular septal defect after the atriopulmonary Fontan operation. (A) Preoperative computed tomography demonstrates an enlarged morphologic right atrial Fontan chamber with a patch that excludes the atrial remnant and cavotricuspid isthmus. (B) Transesophageal echocardiographic view of the remnant chamber used to guide the transbaffle puncture (note the intact atrial septum). (C and D) A radiofrequency wire has been used to perforate the baffle, after which the sheath has been advanced and contrast venography performed to opacify the chamber before catheter ablation.

challenging and various approaches to the substrate have been proposed.[95,96]

IART circuits are commonly related to the systemic AV valve and the oversewn remnant of the IVC, analogous to the CTI in the normal heart (Fig. 14.25, Video 14.12) however atriotomy circuits are also described.[95] Not uncommonly, patients with extracardiac Fontan have undergone a prior Fontan conversion operation with attendant atrial myocardial resection and intraoperative cryolesions. For these latter patients, IART circuits can be quite complex and more challenging to target. Not surprisingly, tachycardia recurrence despite successful catheter ablation is more common for this subgroup.[95]

Atypical circuits may also depend on the underlying congenital anatomy. For instance, intra-atrial reentry in the setting of tricuspid atresia often involves a region near the "dimple" at the floor of the atretic tricuspid valve. This structure along with the central fibrous body may serve as a central obstacle analogous to the tricuspid annulus in the normal heart.[50]

Other Types of Fontan Operation

Other iterations of the Fontan operation for palliation of the single ventricle exist and tachycardia circuits may vary according to the postoperative anatomy. For instance, IART after the Bjork operation has been shown to be associated with biatrial

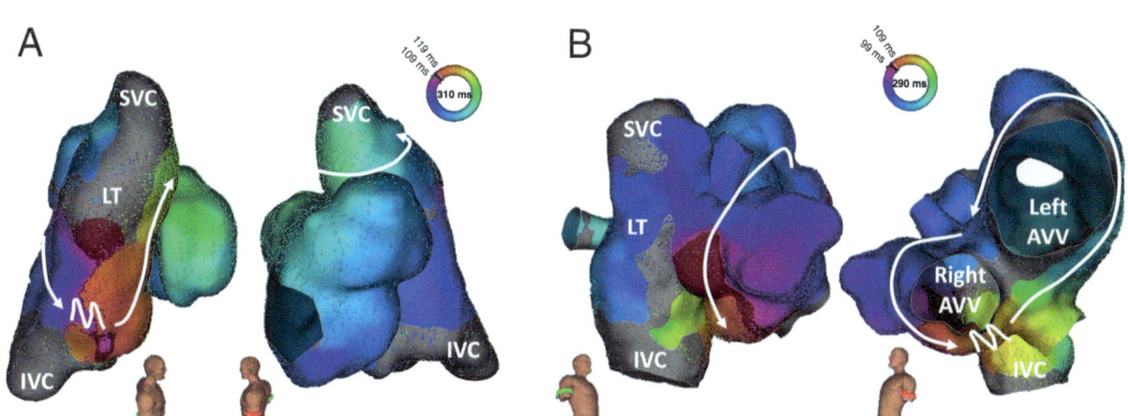

Fig. 14.24 Example of intra-atrial reentrant tachycardia circuits developing after the LT Fontan operation. (A) A free wall circuit uses a gap between the free wall baffle and the inferior vena cava and (B) intra-atrial reentrant tachycardia circuit within the pulmonary venous atrium. The latter used both atrioventricular valves as the central obstacle (biatrial circuit) and could be ablated by connecting the right AVV and the IVC. *AVV*, atrioventricular valve; *IVC*, inferior vena cava; *SVC*, superior vena cava; *LT*, lateral tunnel.

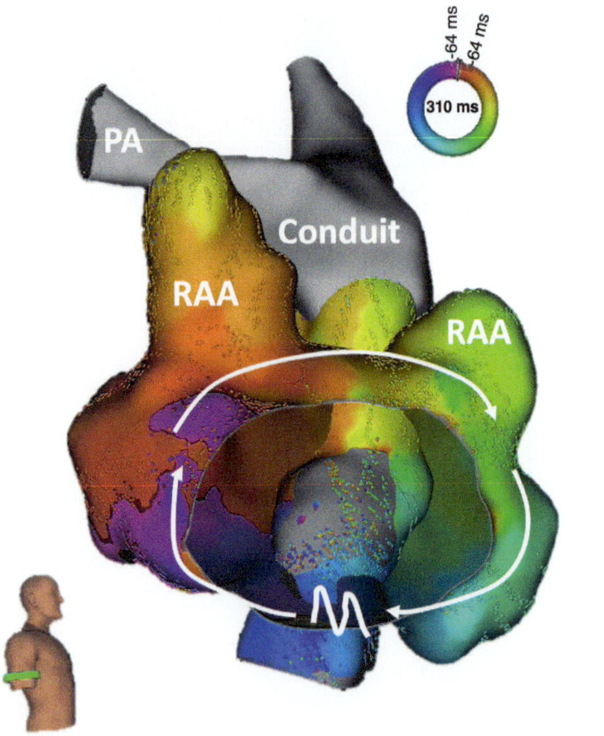

Fig. 14.25 Periannular intra-atrial reentrant tachycardia circuit in a patient with heterotaxy syndrome and unbalanced AV septal defect after the extracardiac Fontan operation. A large clockwise circuit is present, located entirely within the pulmonary venous atrium. Note that the inferior vena cava and conduit are leftward of the atrial chamber. *PA*, pulmonary artery; *RAA*, right atrial appendage.

reentry (Fig. 14.26, Video 14.13) as well as reentry in the right atrial free wall or the Bjork anastomosis itself (Fig. 14.8).[24,26] Other iterations of the total cavopulmonary connection, such as intra-atrial conduit, the extracardiac pericardial tunnel variations, and others exist and may be associated with unique technical and electrophysiologic challenges.

OUTCOMES OF CATHETER ABLATION IN CONGENITAL HEART DISEASE

Reported outcomes of catheter ablation for CHD vary widely in part due to differences in the definitions of success, inclusion criteria and procedural era. Notwithstanding these limitations, acutely successful elimination of all inducible tachycardias at the index procedure appears to be possible within the range of 75–93%[33,34,97,98] in the modern era with at least partial success in almost all procedures.[34] Although historically more complex anatomy (e.g., Mustard or Senning operation or postoperative Fontan status) had predicted procedural failure, this has not been observed in more recent studies.[34,99] For patients with moderate to complex forms of CHD, excellent catheter ablation outcomes are noted at dedicated CHD centers in the modern era.[100]

Similar to definitions of acutely successful catheter ablation, classification of recurrence has also varied between studies without a clear consensus as to the duration of episodes that meet the threshold for reporting, clinical significance of the recurrence arrhythmia, or type of rhythm (e.g., AF) included. The majority of recurrences appear to occur within 1 year following successful catheter ablation.[6,97] Despite this, it has been clearly demonstrated that among patients with CHD and atrial tachycardia, clinically oriented composite scores are improved despite tachycardia recurrence.[92] Multivariate predictors of tachycardia recurrence have included greater lesion complexity,[28,29] history of AF[34,98] or AF induction,[98] electrocardiographic evidence of intra-atrial delay,[98] catheter ablation targeting a non–CTI-dependent IART,[98] prior maze operation,[33] incomplete success,[34] and pulmonary venous atrial substrate.[34] Similarly, studies evaluating the mechanisms of tachycardia recurrences have been mixed. Whereas some studies have suggested recurrence of the same tachycardia circuit,[97,98] most studies suggest that recurrences represent tachycardias

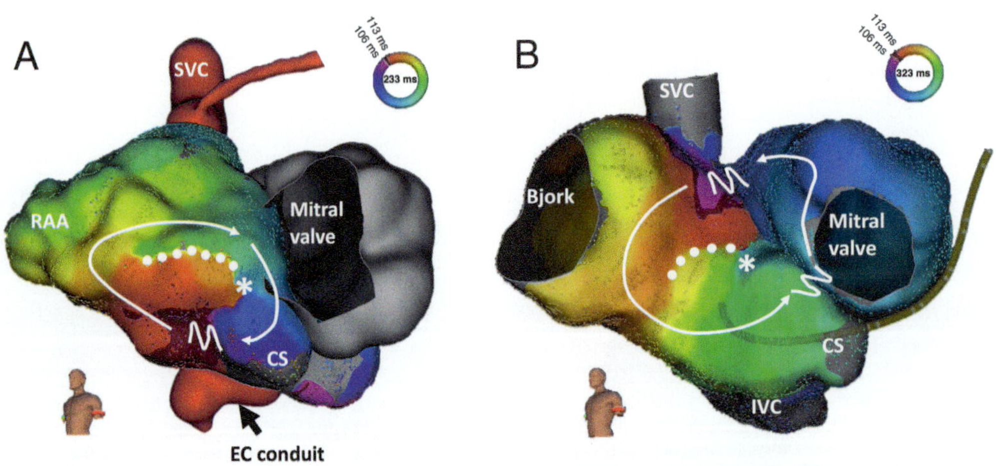

Fig. 14.26 Ultra-high-density maps for two patients with tricuspid atresia are shown. (A) After extracardiac Fontan operation, clockwise reentry around the atretic tricuspid valve is observed. The asterisk marks the expected location of the compact atrioventricular node near the ostium of the coronary sinus. Split potentials (*solid white circles*) are encountered along the expected location of the tendon of Todaro, which retains its normal anatomical positioning for this congenital anomaly. (B) Biatrial reentry is shown for a patient after the Bjork modification of the Fontan operation. Here, a larger circuit rotates around the same central obstacles as in panel A but also includes the atrial septal defect that was surgically closed. *CS*, coronary sinus; *EC*, extracardiac; *IVC*, inferior vena cava; *RAA*, right atrial appendage; *SVC*, superior vena cava.

unobserved at the index procedure.[33,34,101] Importantly, AF represents an increasing proportion of tachycardia recurrence in CHD.[34,98] It is expected that with further understanding of pathophysiologic substrates in conjunction with improving mapping and ablation technologies, outcomes will continue to improve for the CHD patient.

CONCLUSION

Beginning with the earliest observations among postoperative CHD, the complex interplay between anatomical lesions, surgical sequelae, and their vast manifestations have continued to fascinate the congenital electrophysiology community. Great strides in the understanding of IART mechanisms and the optimal strategies for catheter ablation have both improved acute procedural outcomes and reduced the probability of recurrence. A growing familiarity with complex anatomical and electrophysiologic substrates has permitted the development of reginal centers of excellence, further optimizing catheter-based outcomes. Despite these many advances, CHD catheter ablation remains one of the most challenging procedures for the practicing electrophysiologist, demanding a unique awareness of congenital anatomy, postoperative sequelae, and the overarching electrophysiology.

REFERENCES

Please refer to the e-book for a complete list of references.

PART 4

Catheter Ablation of Atrial Fibrillation

15

Pulmonary Vein Isolation Using Radiofrequency Energy Ablation Technologies

Carola Gianni, Pasquale Santangeli, Amin Al-Ahmad, J. David Burkhardt, Rodney P. Horton, Javier E. Sanchez, Andrea Natale

KEY POINTS

- Pulmonary vein isolation (PVI) is the cornerstone of current ablation techniques for the treatment of atrial fibrillation (AF).
- Confirmation of electrical isolation with a circular mapping catheter is crucial to improve the short- and long-term outcomes of this procedure.
- Wide antral PVI improves the long-term arrhythmia-free survival compared with ostial PVI.
- PV reconnection is a major contributor to AF recurrences after PVI, especially in patients with paroxysmal AF.
- Despite proven PVI, a subset of patients still experiences recurrent arrhythmia, mostly because of a higher prevalence of non-PV triggers.
- PVI is associated with worse arrhythmia-free survival in patients with nonparoxysmal AF than those with paroxysmal AF.

Pulmonary vein isolation (PVI) represents the cornerstone of current catheter ablation techniques for the treatment of atrial fibrillation (AF), with significantly improved efficacy compared with antiarrhythmic drug therapy as demonstrated in multiple randomized clinical trials.[1–3] After the pivotal demonstration by Haïssaguerre and coworkers that focal discharges from the pulmonary veins (PVs) are implicated in the initiation of AF, empirical PVI has been performed with the highest procedural success in patients with paroxysmal AF, in whom spontaneous PV firing is frequently the only trigger for AF paroxysms.[4] Over the years, PVI techniques have undergone a profound evolution, from initial attempts consisting of focal PV ablation of documented AF triggers within the PV to the current standard of care, that is empirical ablation targeting the junction between the PVs and the left atrium (LA), the PV antrum. To achieve PV antrum isolation, multiple approaches with different ablation strategies have been described; the technique currently endorsed by the HRS/EHRA/ECAS expert consensus statement on catheter and surgical ablation of AF consists of antral PVI confirmed by a circular mapping catheter (CMC).[5] In this chapter, the techniques and outcomes for different PVI techniques employing radiofrequency energy will be reviewed.

PREPROCEDURAL CONSIDERATIONS

Patient Selection

Current guidelines for the management of AF give a class I indication with the highest level of evidence to PVI in patients with symptomatic paroxysmal AF, who have failed treatment with at least one Class I or III antiarrhythmic drug (second-line treatment).[5–7] Based on the results of randomized trials,[3,8,9] PVI as first-line treatment in patients with no or minimal structural heart disease can be considered when performed in expert centers, where outcomes are comparable with antiarrhythmic drug (AAD) treatment, without an increase in complication rates.[1,10,11] To date, there is no indication for PVI to reduce cardiovascular morbidity/mortality or hospitalization.

Preprocedural Imaging

A baseline standard transthoracic echocardiogram is useful to assess LA dimensions, interatrial septum morphology, left ventricular ejection fraction, and other gross abnormalities in all patients before they undergo PVI. If INR is subtherapeutic or nonadherence to direct oral anticoagulants (DOACs) is suspected, a transesophageal echocardiography (TEE) is performed to rule out LAA thrombosis the day of the procedure.

Computed tomography (CT) or magnetic resonance imaging (MRI) can also be performed for a better definition of LA anatomy, which can be integrated with the mapping system at the time of the ablation procedure.

Antiarrhythmic Drugs

Patients undergoing PVI should have their AADs discontinued for at least 5 half-lives before the ablation procedure to facilitate the identification of AF triggers, especially those outside the PVs that are not empirically targeted. In this regard, although adequate drug washout can be achieved in reasonable time before the procedure for most AADs, patients receiving chronic treatment with amiodarone represent a unique challenge because of the long half-life of the drug, and thus require longer elimination time. There might be an incremental benefit of adequate preprocedural amiodarone washout, suggesting that discontinuation of the drug 4–6 months before the procedure increases the chance of disclosing latent non-PV trigger sites, resulting in better long-term arrhythmia-free survival.[12]

Anticoagulation Status

A proper anticoagulation status is crucial to minimize the risk of periprocedural thromboembolism and bleeding. In recent times, a substantial body of evidence has been built on the benefit of performing PVI under uninterrupted anticoagulation with both warfarin and the direct oral anticoagulants; this reduces the risk of stroke without increasing the risk of bleeding.[13–16] Of note, among the direct oral anticoagulants, our experience with uninterrupted dabigatran has been disappointing, with an increase in the risk of bleeding or thromboembolic complications compared with uninterrupted warfarin; therefore, we usually prefer to use warfarin or factor Xa inhibitors in the periablation setting.[17] Another important strategy to minimize the risk of periprocedural stroke is to administer an intravenous heparin bolus (usually 80 U/kg up to 10,000 U with warfarin, or 12,000–16,000 U with factor Xa inhibitors, based on the patient's weight and baseline INR) when vascular access is obtained. The goal is to achieve full anticoagulation (goal activated clotting time [ACT] between 350 and 500 seconds) before transseptal access, thus reducing the chance of thrombus formation when sheaths and catheters are in the LA.

PROCEDURAL CONSIDERATIONS

Anesthesia Protocol

The anesthesia protocol adopted during PVI can also affect the procedural results. Although moderate to deep sedation/anesthesia can be used, general anesthesia, with or without high-frequency jet ventilation, has the important advantage of controlling respiration by eliminating deep breathing. This improves catheter stability, leading to more effective RF energy delivery, thus reducing procedural times and improving long-term outcomes compared with conscious sedation.[8,9]

Vascular and Left Atrial Access

To reduce vascular complications, central venous access should be obtained with real-time ultrasound guidance; this reduces the number of attempts, time to access, and risk of arterial puncture.[18] Moreover, an arterial line for hemodynamic monitoring should not be placed routinely, given the higher risk of hematomas in anticoagulated patients. Noninvasive intermittent blood pressure monitoring every 2–5 minutes is generally sufficient. For LA access, two separate transseptal punctures are performed (one for the ablation catheter, the other for the CMC) under intracardiac echocardiography (ICE) guidance. The goal is to cross into the LA along the mid-posterior interatrial septum, such that the left-sided PVs are in clear view (Fig. 15.1, Video 15.1). To advance the transseptal needle, manual pressure can be used; to facilitate access, radiofrequency (RF) is frequently used, using either an electrocautery pen (cut at 20–40 W) and applied externally near the metal hub or

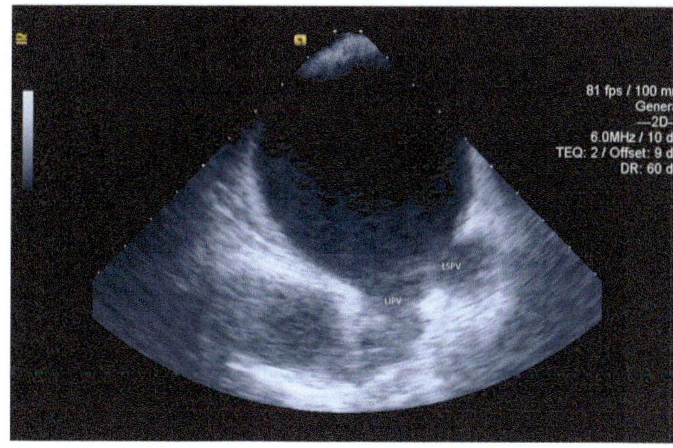

Fig. 15.1 Intracardiac echocardiographic image of the left pulmonary veins. *LSPV,* Left superior pulmonary vein; *LIPV,* left inferior pulmonary vein.

using a dedicated RF-powered transseptal needle (i.e., Baylis NRG). Although a second transseptal sheath can be introduced via wire exchange, a separate transseptal puncture minimizes sheath-to-sheath interaction.

LA access can be obtained using a variety of transseptal sheaths. In our center, we prefer sheaths with a moderate primary fixed curve and no secondary curve (50 degrees for the ablation catheter and 90 degrees for the CMC), which allow easier catheter maneuverability in the posterior aspect of the LA.

Techniques and Results of Pulmonary Vein Isolation

Triggers from the PVs represent the dominant mechanism of initiation of AF. The initial description of PV trigger ablation consisted of focal ablation within the PVs. This approach had minimal long-term benefit and was associated with a significant risk of PV stenosis.[4,19,20] Subsequent evolution of the procedure involved segmental ablation at the anatomic ostium of the PVs, as defined by angiography or ICE, to isolate muscle sleeve connections between the PV and LA electrically, an approach commonly referred to as segmental ostial PVI.[21] In addition to ostial PVI, initial attempts targeted only the PVs with evidence of arrhythmogenic activity. However, it was rapidly realized that empirical isolation of all PVs was necessary to increase the procedural success, as the majority of patients presented multiple arrhythmogenic PVs. In addition, symptomatic PV stenosis remained an important risk with ostial PVI, and AF triggers localized in the more proximal antral region were not addressed with such strategy. The technique further evolved targeting the LA tissue more proximal to the PV ostium, in a region defined as the PV antrum.[22–24]

To achieve antral PVI, multiple approaches have been described. The approach currently adopted in our institution is a wide PV antrum isolation (encompassing the LA posterior wall between the PVs) guided by a CMC and ICE (Fig. 15.2).[25] The importance of a wider antral isolation is the empirical elimination of triggers arising from the LA posterior wall, which should be considered as an extension of the PVs from an embryologic, anatomical, and electrophysiologic standpoint.[26] Compared with ostial PVI, wide antral PVI is associated with a significantly lower rate of arrhythmia recurrence, driven by a reduced rate of AF at follow-up without increasing the rate of periprocedural

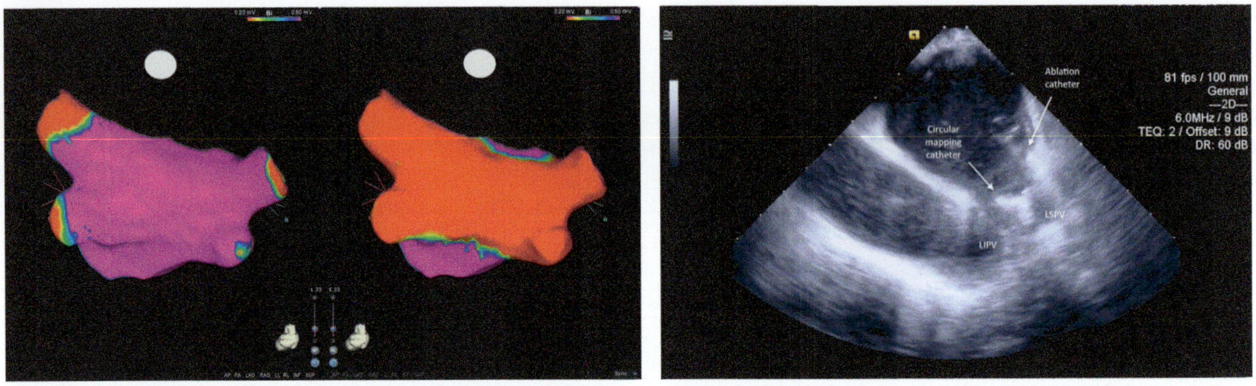

Fig. 15.2 Antral pulmonary vein isolation (PVI) with posterior wall isolation; *right*, intracardiac echocardiographic image of the circular mapping catheter and ablation catheter at the level of the left superior pulmonary vein antrum; *left*, posterior view of the left atrium showing voltage before and after antral PVI.

complications.[27,28] This approach has been demonstrated to be superior to other ablation techniques in studies of direct comparison, and is one of the most reproducible and standardized techniques to achieve PVI.[23,29–31] Circumferential PV ablation without confirmation of electrical isolation with a CMC has been demonstrated to be ineffective in achieving long-term arrhythmia control.[22,29,32] Moreover, adopting a CMC-guided approach also offers the potential advantages of shortening the procedural time, limiting the delivery of RF energy to discrete areas showing the earliest potentials (segmental approach).[23,33] By contrast, in a circumferential PV ablation approach, contiguous lesions are created without necessarily achieving complete conduction block, and postincisional reentrant atrial tachycardias are not uncommon.

Although not necessary, the use of a 3-dimensional electroanatomic mapping system, such as EnSite (Abbott, St. Jude Medical, St. Paul, MN), Carto 3 (Johnson & Johnson, Biosense Webster, Diamond Bar, CA), or Rhythmia (Boston Scientific, Malborough, MA), can facilitate PVI significantly, allowing efficient registration of ablation sites and documentation of the extent of antral ablation (Fig. 15.3). Mapping systems allow real-time display of any cardiac catheter during ablation; most importantly, their ability to display the CMC allows for very rapid creation of an LA volume map and facilitates the direction of the ablation catheter toward the desired poles. While maneuvering the CMC, care should be taken not to displace it anteriorly, as this can result in its entrapment in the mitral valve apparatus. Particular attention should be paid in the presence of a mechanical mitral valve, where even noncircular multipolar catheters can be entrapped as when they are maneuvered in the vicinity of the prothesis. The use of ICE during mapping facilitates locating the four PVs (Video 15.2). The left-sided PVs can be seen with clockwise rotation of the ICE catheter a few degrees past the left atrial appendage (LAA) and the mitral valve annulus, whereas to image the right PVs, the ICE catheter is advanced slightly and further rotated clockwise. Moreover, ICE has been shown to reduce PV stenosis, compared with PV angiography.[34] The LAA can be recognized by a high amplitude signal on the superior-anterior aspect of the LA.

The CMC is used as a roving catheter for mapping and directing the ablation catheter throughout the procedure (Fig. 15.4). It should be small enough to move within the chamber easily

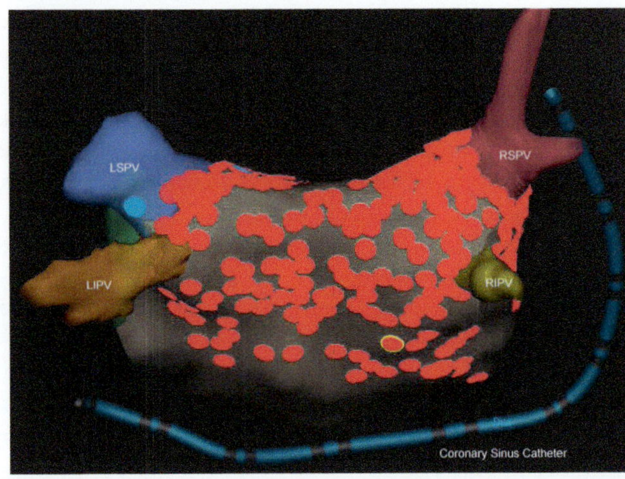

Fig. 15.3 Ablation lesions delivered to obtain antral pulmonary vein isolation. *LIPV*, Left inferior pulmonary vein; *LSPV*, left superior pulmonary vein; *RIPV*, right inferior pulmonary vein; *RSPV*, right superior pulmonary vein.

but of a large enough diameter that it does not readily fall deep inside the PVs. In most adults, a 20-mm, 10-pole CMC provides a balance between maneuverability and size. RF energy delivery with open-irrigation catheters is the standard of care in performing PVI. Open-irrigation catheters allow the use of greater power without a significant increase in temperature and clot formation, enabling more efficient and predictable energy delivery, resulting in larger ablation lesion sets. The main disadvantage of using open irrigation catheters is a higher risk of steam pops: there is a high discrepancy between the recorded tip temperature and the actual tissue temperature, so steam pops might occur even with "normal" tip temperature. These can be minimized with appropriate titration of energy delivery, as guided by monitoring any abrupt change in tip temperature, impedance, and if available, contact force. Our catheter of choice is a unidirectional open-irrigated 3.5-mm tip with an F curve. A smaller curve may be considered in the minority of patients with a very small LA (rare), whereas a J curve is necessary for patients with a larger LAs (more frequent in nonparoxysmal AF patients).

Using an irrigation-tip catheter, a power of 40 W (the temperature cut-off varies according to the type of ablation

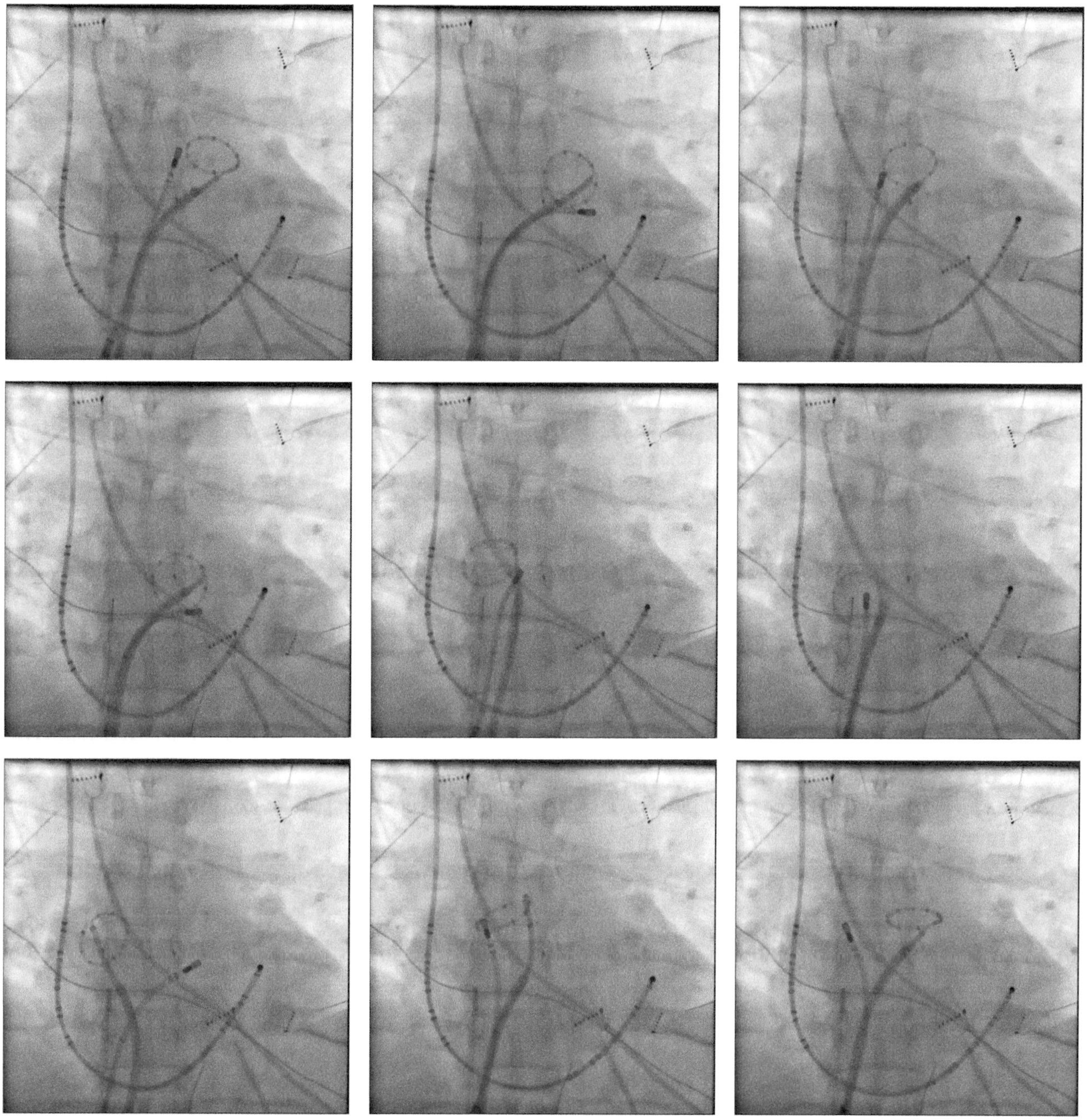

Fig. 15.4 Circular mapping catheter (CMC)-guided antral pulmonary vein isolation; the roving CMC is sequentially placed along the pulmonary vein antra and posterior wall.

catheter) is typically used. Occasionally, on the anterior aspect of the PVs (e.g., a thick ridge), a higher power is needed to achieve potential abatement, but with currently available irrigated-tip catheters, we generally do not exceed 45 W. In our practice, we mostly employ open-irrigation catheters with contact force feedback, which contain sensors that provide real-time information on the catheter–tissue contact, an important determinant of RF lesion size. To date, there are two commercially available contact force ablation catheters: TactiCath Quartz (Abbott-St. Jude Medical) and ThermoCool SmartTouch (Biosense Webster), using fiber-optic and spring microdeformation technology, respectively (Fig. 15.5). Achieving optimal contact force results in effective RF energy delivery and lesion formation; thus it is not surprising that contact force sensing ablation catheters have been shown to increase the efficacy of PVI in multiple randomized and nonrandomized studies.[35–40] With contact force sensing ablation catheters, when delivering 40 W of RF energy, our target contact force lies between 7 g and 15 g). RF energy is delivered for approximately 10–20 seconds per lesion site or until the electrical signals have diminished. In areas near the esophagus, energy delivery should be limited to up to 5 seconds per lesion site and the catheter should be constantly moved to distant areas during ablation to prevent esophageal heating. It is very important to monitor the esophageal temperature closely, frequently readjusting the esophageal probe so that it is close to

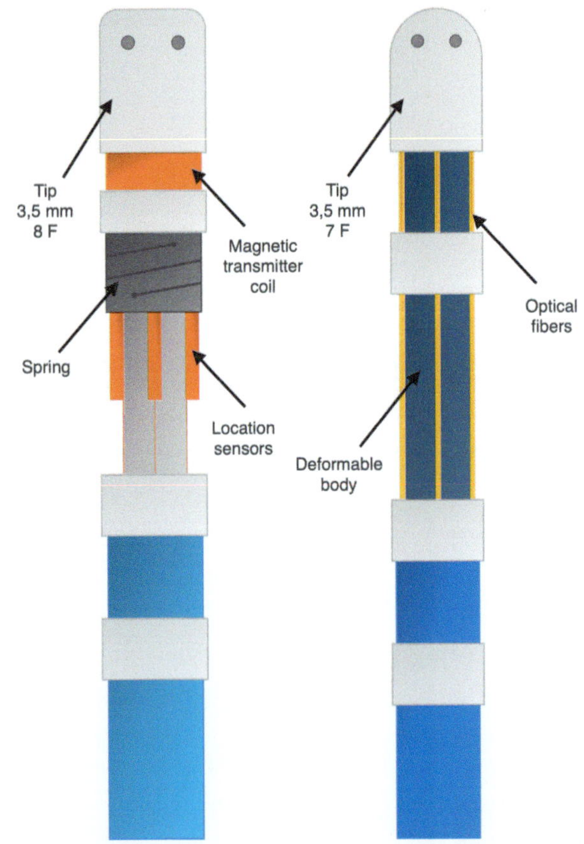

Fig. 15.5 Schematics of the two types of commercially available contact force catheters: *left*, electromagnetic (SmartTouch); *right*, fiber-optic (TactiCath Quartz). (From Bourier F, Gianni C, Dare M, et al. Fiberoptic contact-force sensing electrophysiological catheters: how precise is the technology? *J Cardiovasc Electrophysiol.* 2017;28:109–115.)

the ablation area. A rapid rise in temperature is often noted, and when this happens, the ablation catheter should be moved away or RF delivery stopped, independently of the absolute value of esophageal temperature recorded, which is a function of the temperature probe used[41] (i.e., presence and thickness of insulation) and patient's anatomy (i.e., distance between the LA and esophagus, esophageal width). Despite movement of the catheter, a delayed rise in esophageal temperatures is often observed. Generally, esophageal temperatures greater than 38°C–39°C should be avoided to minimize the risk of deep tissue injury. It is also important to note that the esophagus is wider than the temperature probe (Fig. 15.6); therefore, sometimes no or minimal temperature change is recorded, despite ablating over the esophagus, as assessed by ICE (Fig. 15.7). If ICE is not available, it is important to move quickly whenever ablating in the posterior wall regardless of the location of the esophageal probe.

We usually begin with ablation of the electrical potentials surrounding each PV. The end point of PVI is complete PV electrical isolation, as confirmed by entrance and exit block (Table 15.1). Entrance block is confirmed by the absence of electrical signals where these signals had been previously observed. Occasionally, dissociated PV potentials can be recorded (Fig. 15.8) to confirm exit block. In addition pacing from within the PV can be performed to confirm exit block, although this is

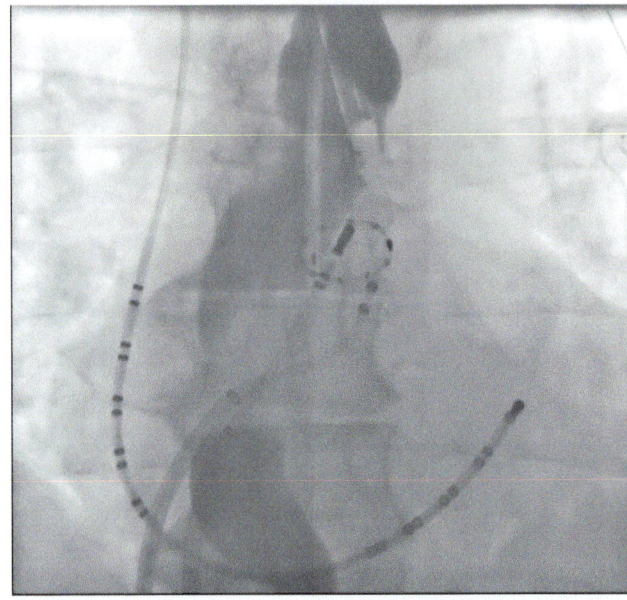

Fig. 15.6 Relationship between the esophageal probe and esophagus.

not necessary. Once PVI is achieved, we focus on the remaining antral areas. The CMC is particularly useful for identifying additional electrical potentials along the posterior wall and roof of the LA (see Fig. 15.4). The procedural endpoint is to eliminate all electrical activity in the antrum and roof of the LA (see Figs. 15.2 & 15.9). After PV antral isolation, with patients in sinus rhythm, 20–30 μg/kg/min of isoproterenol is infused to assess for PV reconnection and elicit non-PV triggers. If consistent (repetitive premature atrial contractions [PACs], PACs triggering atrial flutter/AF, and focal atrial tachycardia), their sites of origin are further targeted with ablation. We do not routinely use adenosine to test for acute PVI.[42]

As mentioned, most of the studies investigating the role of PVI for the long-term maintenance of sinus rhythm have predominantly enrolled patients with paroxysmal AF; thus far, the role of PV triggers in patients with nonparoxysmal AF has not been investigated in a systematic fashion. In addition, few data support the benefit of PVI in paroxysmal patients, also at the very long-term follow-up. However, the authors' experience suggests that some of the patients will develop non-PV triggers over times that are responsible for arrhythmia recurrence at long term. The clinical experience with PVI in patients with nonparoxysmal AF has consistently shown worse results compared

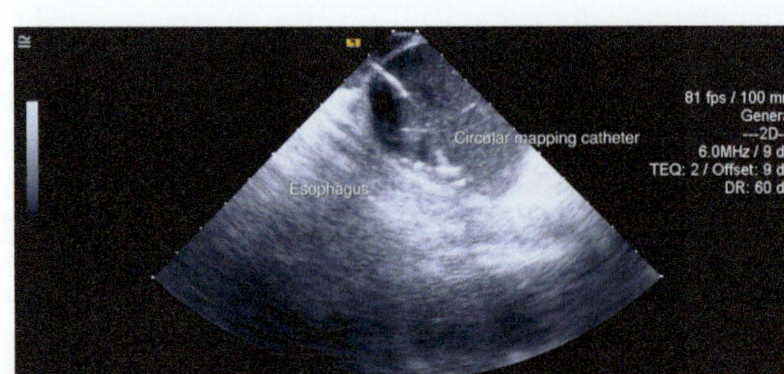

Fig. 15.7 Intracardiac echocardiographic image of the esophagus behind the left atrial posterior wall.

TABLE 15.1 End Points of Pulmonary Vein Isolation

	Definition	Pros	Cons
Entrance block	Elimination of all the potentials within the PV antrum, as assessed by a circular mapping catheter	Tested in multiple clinical studies	Rare cases of unidirectional entrance block have been described
Exit block	Failure to conduct from within the PV antrum to the atrium	Identifies bidirectional conduction block across the PV antrum	Not validated in large studies
Voltage reduction	Reduction of local voltages after circumferential PV ablation	—	Not equivalent to PVI, which has to be confirmed with a circular mapping catheter. Multiple randomized trials have demonstrated the ineffectiveness of this end point
Termination of AF	Restoration of sinus rhythm (or conversion to intermediate AT) during ablation	When achieved in the process of PVI (when the isolated PV remains in AF), proves the critical participation of the PV as a trigger for AF	Contradictory clinical data do not support the use of this end point during AF ablation

AF, Atrial fibrillation; *AT*, atrial tachycardia; *PV*, pulmonary vein; *PVI*, pulmonary vein isolation.

with paroxysmal patients, and PVI alone is largely insufficient to achieve satisfactory long-term arrhythmia-free survival in this cohort.[43,44] Thus far, the approach of most institutions is to provide extensive ablation targeting the LA substrate and areas demonstrating non-PV triggers, either spontaneously or after induction with drug challenges (e.g., isoproterenol) or pacing. However, the amount of additional ablation necessary in these patients to increase the procedural success is still a matter of controversy and goes beyond the scope of this chapter.

COMPLICATIONS OF PULMONARY VEIN ISOLATION

Because patients are anticoagulated, the most common complications are *vascular* (hematomas, pseudoaneurysm, and arteriovenous fistulas). These can be easily prevented using real-time ultrasound when obtaining central venous access.

Hemodynamic and temperature monitoring during the ablation procedure allows early detection and avoidance of the most serious complications of PVI: cardiac tamponade and atrial-esophageal fistula. Blood pressure drops, both sudden and gradual, should be evaluated carefully. A vagal response to ablation near the ganglionic plexi may result in transient sudden hypotension, usually associated with bradycardia (sinus arrest or atrioventricular block). If there is no immediate recovery, cardiac tamponade should be assumed until proven otherwise. Suspicion should be higher after a difficult transseptal puncture, a steam pop, or inadvertent application of excess pressure in the LAA or the roof of the LA. To determine early diagnosis of cardiac tamponade, it is important not to delay pericardiocentesis. A quick assessment to check for the presence of pericardial effusion can be easily and accurately performed with ICE (Video 15.3). If this is not available, fluoroscopy usually demonstrates a reduction in the excursion of the cardiac silhouette, better appreciated in the LAO view. Of note, especially after extensive ablation, it is not uncommon to detect mild pericardial effusion without hemodynamic compromise following the procedure. Most of these asymptomatic effusions can be managed conservatively.

PVI involves extensive burning near the esophagus, and atrial-esophageal fistulas can present in the weeks following ablation. Although exceedingly rare, they are frequently fatal; therefore, prevention and early diagnosis/treatment (surgical repair) are important to reduce mortality. During ablation, temperature monitoring and limitation of the duration of energy delivery when ablating in the posterior aspect of the LA (down to the CS) are vital to avoid excessive heating of the esophagus. A short course of prophylactic proton pump inhibitors and sucralfate can be prescribed. During follow-up, patient and physician awareness is the key. Patients should be instructed to immediately contact the electrophysiology service if fever, chest pain, neurologic symptoms, dysphagia, hematemesis, or melena occur.

Thermal injury can also result in phrenic nerve (PN) injury. This can be right sided when ablating in the right superior PV or performing isolation of the superior vena cava (SVC) or left sided when ablating inside the LAA. To prevent PN injury, it is important to avoid ablation inside the PVs or LAA, and to perform PN mapping when isolating the SVC. Patients with PN paralysis are usually asymptomatic, but they can present with dyspnea on exertion. There is no treatment, but the condition is usually transient, so observation is all that is needed. Dyspnea, with or without cough or hemoptysis, is also a presenting symptom of severe PV stenosis, which is a rare occurrence after true PVI, because RF energy is not delivered ostial or inside the PVs. PV stenosis is diagnosed with CT imaging, and if severe or symptomatic might require intervention (venoplasty and stenting).

To reduce periprocedural thromboembolic events, the procedure should be performed under uninterrupted oral anticoagulation and heparin administered transseptal access with goal ACT of 350 seconds or longer. To prevent air embolism, transseptal sheaths should be continuously flushed with 2–4 mL/mine of heparinized-saline using pressure bags set at 300–400 mmHg.

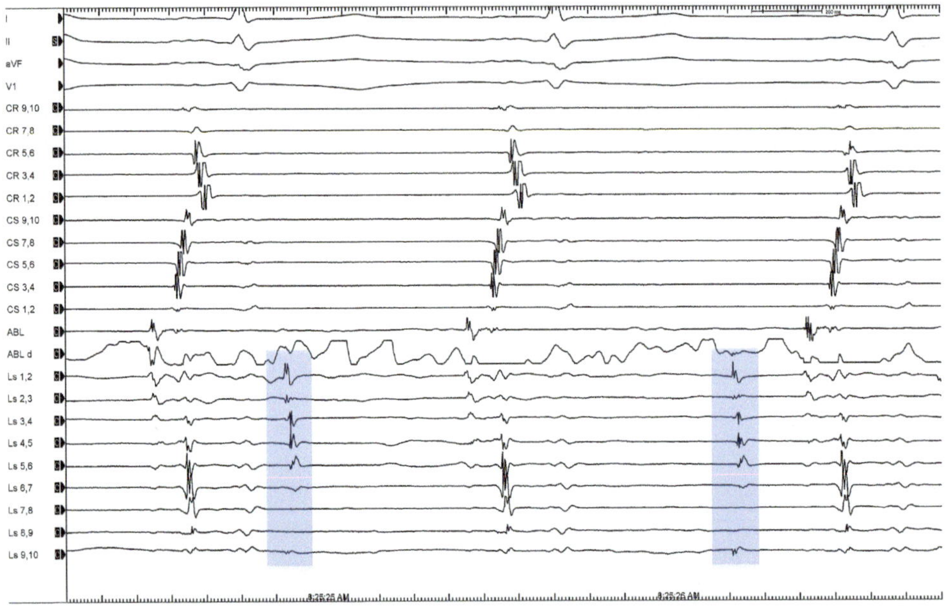

Fig. 15.8 Dissociated firing in the left superior pulmonary vein.

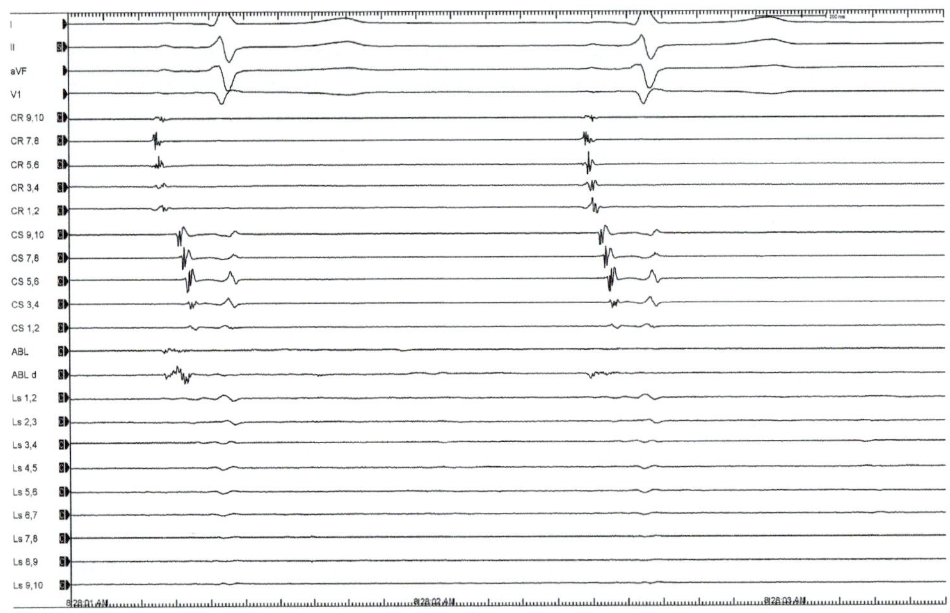

Fig. 15.9 Electrical silence in the left atrial posterior wall.

DIFFICULT CASES

Sometimes it is challenging to confirm entrance block for the presence of far-field electrograms caused by adjacent structures, such as the right atrium (RA) and LA for the right pulmonary veins, the SVC for the right superior pulmonary vein, the LA for the left pulmonary veins, or the LAA for the left superior pulmonary vein.[45] In these instances, pacing from the structure believed to be the origin of the far-field potential is useful to distinguish a local pulmonary vein potential and avoid unnecessary ablation. For example when LAA far-field is suspected (Fig. 15.10, top panel), it is important to compare the electrograms recorded by the CMC in sinus rhythm with those during pacing from the LAA. In sinus rhythm, there is simultaneous activation of the LAA and pulmonary veins, with signal overlap. With pacing within the LAA, the local electrograms are advanced and merge with the pacing artifact (Fig. 15.10, middle panel), whereas if pulmonary vein potentials are present, they are relatively delayed because of decremental conduction at the left atrial-pulmonary vein junction (Fig. 15.11, bottom panel). Other common problems encountered during PVI and their solutions are listed in Table 15.2.

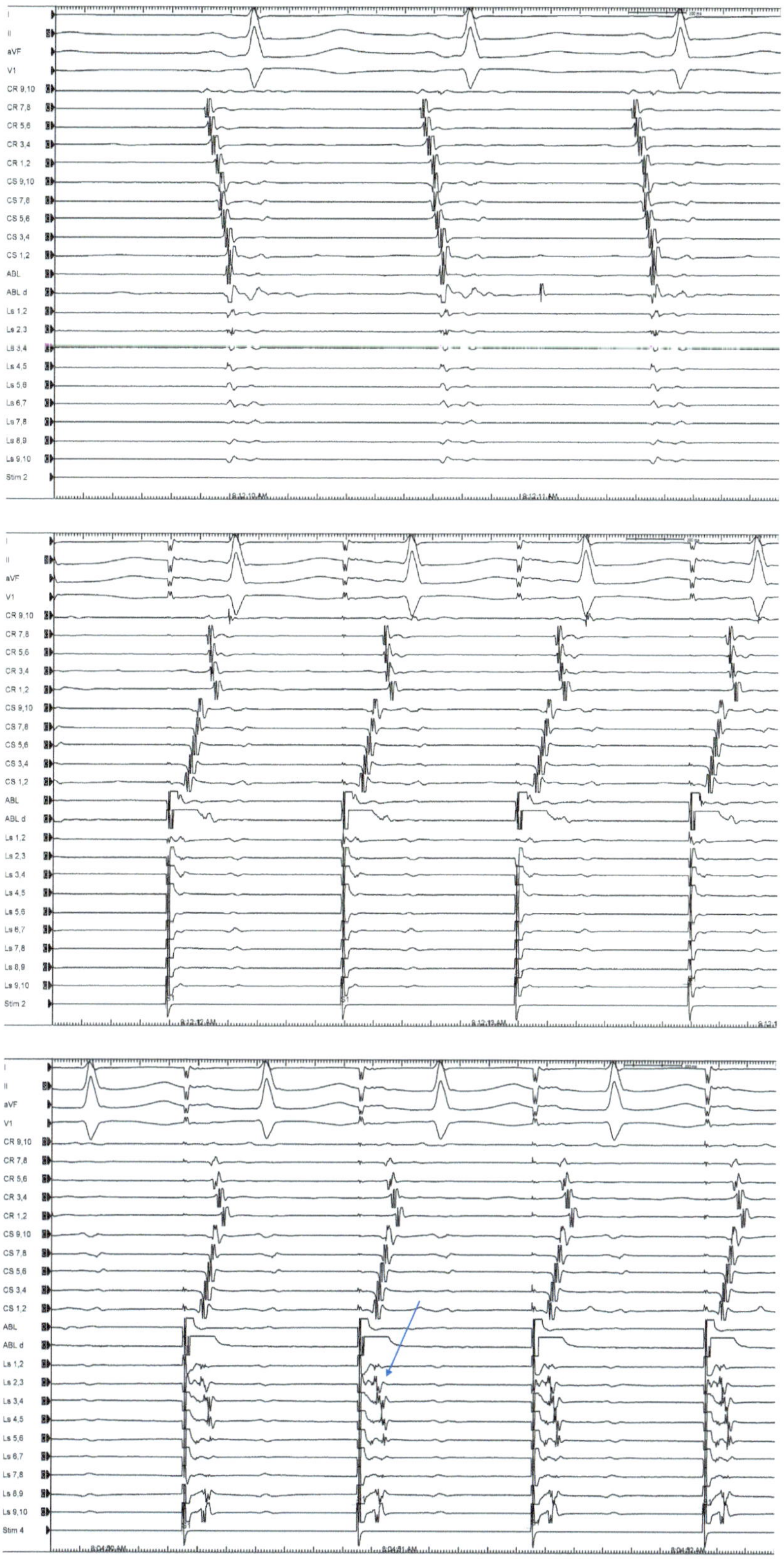

Fig. 15.10 How to distinguish far-field from the left atrial appendage (LAA); pacing from the LAA. See text for explanation. Blue arrow points to the captured LAA local electrogram.

POSTPROCEDURAL CONSIDERATIONS

Mechanisms of Arrhythmia Recurrence After Pulmonary Vein Isolation

Reconnection of the PVs represents the dominant mechanism of arrhythmia recurrence after PVI. Observational studies reporting the findings at repeat procedures in patients who already had PVI showed a prevalence of PV reconnection ranging from 80% to 100%.[46] The mechanisms underlying PV reconnection have not been fully elucidated; however, the delivery of nonpermanent lesions at the time of the index procedure with subsequent recovery of conduction after a transient phase of

TABLE 15.2 Troubleshooting the Difficult Cases of Pulmonary Vein Isolation

	Problem	Cause	Solution
Central venous access	Difficult access; vascular complications	Inability to obtain venous access; inadvertent arterial or lung puncture Arterial line for continuous systemic pressure monitoring	Real-time US-guided access ICE/US to monitor for intracardiac and vascular complications
CS cannulation	Difficult CS cannulation from the femoral vein; failure to achieve catheter stability/sufficient depth	Prominent eustachian valve; tortuous/ steep CS course	Superior access (right internal jugular vein > left axillary/antecubital vein); real-time imaging of the CS os with ICE deflectable catheter
Transseptal access	Cardiac tamponade; aortic root puncture; inability to obtain transseptal access	Inadvertent puncture posterior/anterior to the fossa ovalis Inadvertent puncture of the LA posterior/ lateral wall because of an aneurysmal interatrial septum; inability to obtain transseptal access because of a thick septum (e.g., status post cardiac surgery, ASD repair, lipomatous hypertrophy)	Real-time ICE-guided transseptal access Radiofrequency transseptal needle
Catheter manipulation	Difficult catheter manipulation, inadequate contact in the posterior aspect of the PVs/PW	Anterior transseptal puncture; single transseptal puncture	Double posterior transseptal puncture (i.e., obtain access while visualizing the PVs on ICE)
PVI	Inability to obtain PVI	Low power; inadequate contact Esophageal heating Electrical break through difficult to identify Misclassification of far-field activity	High power (40–45 W); contact force sensing ablation catheter; real-time visualization of the ablation catheter-tissue contact with ICE; general anesthesia steerable transseptal sheath; Short-lived (5–10 s), high-power (40 W), medium contact (5–10 g) lesions Cardioversion (if patient in AF); pacing from the CS (for the left-sided PVs) Differential pacing

ASD, atrial septal defect; *CS*, coronary sinus; *ICE*, intracardiac echocardiography; *LA*, left atrium; *PV*, pulmonary veins; *PVI*, pulmonary vein isolation; *PW*, left atrial posterior wall; *US*, ultrasound.

reversible tissue injury, along with inflammation and edema, has been claimed as the dominant mechanism underlying PV reconnection.[47]

Despite persistent PVI, a subset of patients still continues to experience recurrent arrhythmia.[48] The reasons underlying such a lack of sustained response to PVI are still unclear, although the occurrence of triggers outside the PV region has been shown to play an important role in numerous observational studies.[49] Of note, non-PV triggers are more prevalent in patients with nonparoxysmal AF, female gender, obesity, sleep apnea, older age, low left ventricular ejection fraction, severe left atrial scarring, hypertrophic cardiomyopathy, and mechanical mitral valve (Table 15.3). In these patients, we target non-PV triggers at the time of the first procedure.[48,50–58] Typically, non-PV triggers cluster in specific regions such as other thoracic veins (SVC, coronary sinus [CS], vein of Marshall), the LA posterior wall, crista terminalis, interatrial septum, and the LAA. In our center, we use high-dose isoproterenol infusion (20–30 μg/min for 10–15 minutes) to induce latent non-PV triggers. Mapping non-PV triggers is guided by multiple catheters positioned along both the RA and LA (Fig. 15.11): a 10-pole CMC in the left superior PV recording the far-field LAA activity, the ablation catheter in the right superior PV that records the far-field interatrial septum, and a 20-pole catheter with electrodes spanning from the SVC, RA/crista terminalis to the CS. With this simple catheter setup, when focal ectopic atrial activity is observed (a single ectopic beat is enough), their activation sequence is compared with that of sinus rhythm, allowing quick identification of their area of origin:

TABLE 15.3 Subset of Patients With Higher Prevalence of Nonpulmonary Vein Triggers

NON-PV TRIGGERS	
Nonparoxysmal AF	Low LVEF
Female gender	Severe LA scarring
Older age	Hypertrophic cardiomyopathy
Obesity	Mechanical mitral valve
Sleep apnea	

AF, atrial fibrillation; *LA*, left atrium; *LVEF*, left ventricular ejection fraction; *PV*, pulmonary vein.

- beats originating from the RA: earliest activation in the proximal duo-decapolar catheter; the specific activation sequence varies depending on the site of origin, resembling that of sinus rhythm for ectopies originating from the SVC (Fig. 15.12)
- beats originating from the interatrial septum area: both the CS and proximal duo-decapolar catheter are early, usually

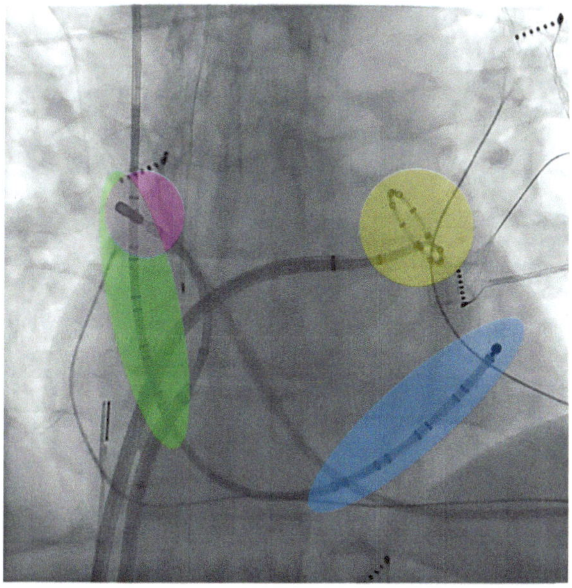

Fig. 15.11 Catheter setup to assess the origin of atrial ectopic activity during isoproterenol challenge: *green*, proximal duo-decapolar catheter (crista terminalis); *blue*, distal duo-decapolar catheter; *pink*, ablation catheter (right superior pulmonary vein > far-field interatrial septum); *yellow*, circular mapping catheter (left superior pulmonary vein > far-field left atrial appendage).

preceded by the far-field atrial activity recorded with the ablation catheter (Fig. 15.13)

- beats originating from the CS: earliest activation in the distal duo-decapolar catheter (Fig. 15.14)
- beats originating from the LAA: far-field activity in the CMC is early, preceding that recorded in the distal CS (Fig. 15.15)

For significant non-PV triggers (repetitive isolated beats, focal atrial tachycardias, or beats triggering AF/atrial flutter), a more detailed activation mapping is performed in the area of origin. A detailed description of the ablation strategy for non-PV triggers goes beyond the scope of this chapter, but briefly, significant non-PV triggers are targeted with focal ablation, exceptions being the triggers originating from the SVC, LAA, or CS, in which case complete isolation of these structures is the ablation strategy of choice.

Postprocedural Care and Follow-Up

A proper postprocedural management and follow-up is crucial for all patients undergoing PVI. In our institution all patients undergo strict monitoring for outcome and complications during overnight hospital stay. Ideally, patients should be given an event recorder for 3 months up to 1 year and asked to transmit their rhythm regularly, both at the time of symptoms and at least once a week if asymptomatic.[59] Moreover, all patients present for follow-up 3–4 months after the ablation, and 7-day Holter are obtained every 3 months for 1 year. We typically do not change the patient's antiarrhythmic regimen during the first 2–3 months, with the decision to discontinue, continue, or change antiarrhythmic drugs depending on the arrhythmia burden thereafter. Anticoagulation is continued in all patients for at least 3 months, whereas the decision to discontinue oral anticoagulation thereafter is taken on an individual basis, and it depends the patient's thromboembolic and bleeding risk as well as the success of the procedure (assessed with intense ECG monitoring). Patients with low thromboembolic risk (CHA_2DS_2-VASc/$CHADS_2$ score = 0) can be comfortably taken off oral anticoagulation after 3 months. The long-term stroke risk of patients with a higher thromboembolic risk following PVI ablation is not well studied, but those with lower risk and without recurrence of AF may be considered for discontinuation. In our center, we follow a standard, uniform, and validated protocol.[60] In brief, oral anticoagulation is discontinued,

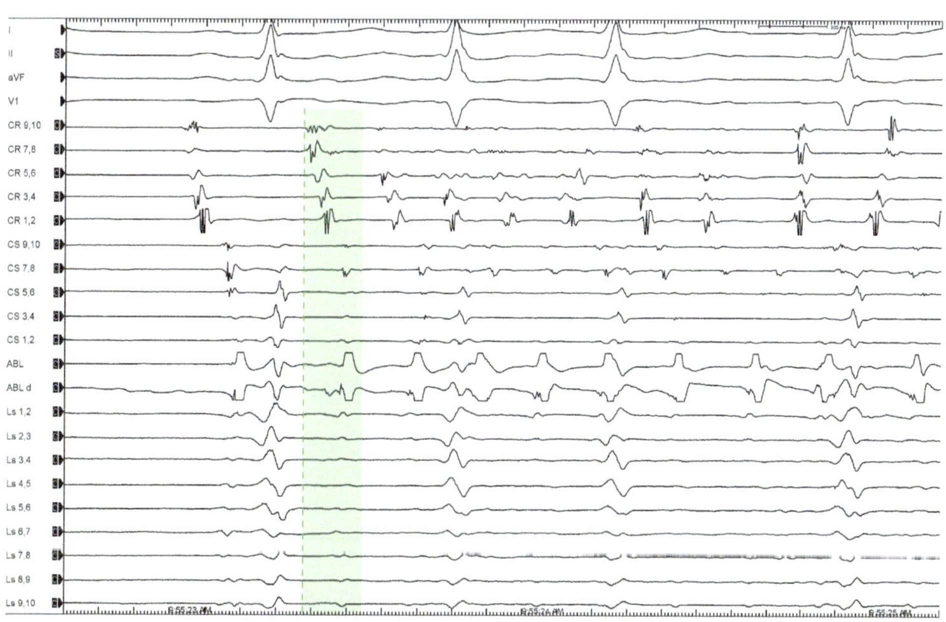

Fig. 15.12 Premature atrial beat (green shade) from the superior vena cava triggering atrial fibrillation. *ABL*, Ablation catheter; *CR*, crista; *CS*, coronary sinus; *Ls*, circular mapping catheter.

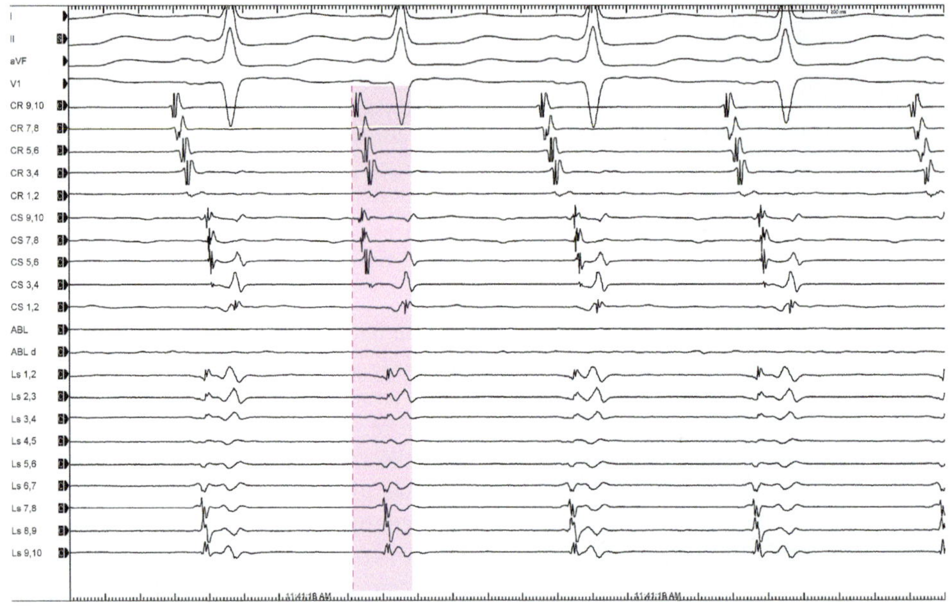

Fig. 15.13 Premature atrial beat (purple shade) from the interatrial septum. *ABL*, Ablation catheter; *CR*, crista; *CS*, coronary sinus; *Ls*, circular mapping catheter.

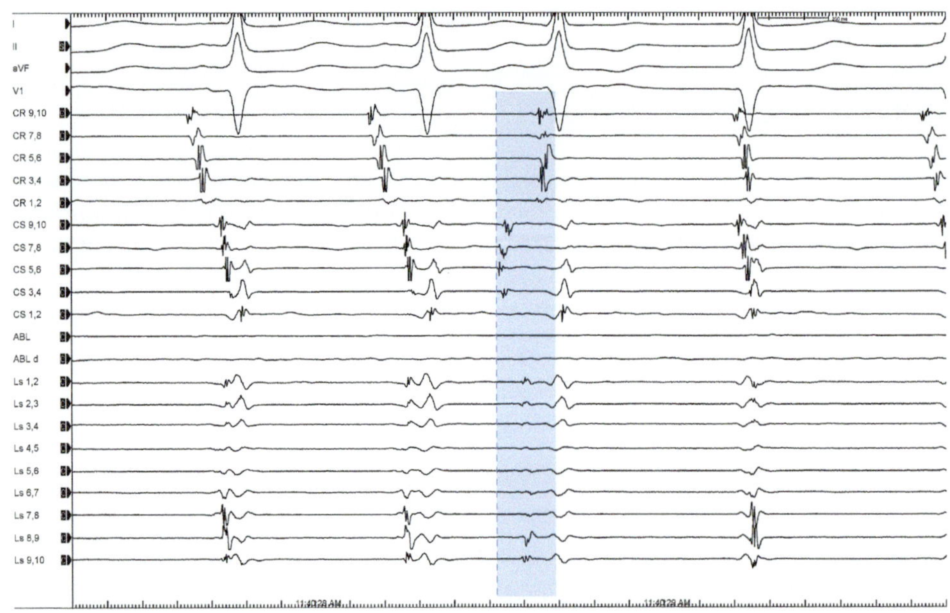

Fig. 15.14 Premature atrial beat (blue shade) from the mid-coronary sinus. *ABL*, Ablation catheter; *CR*, crista; *CS*, coronary sinus; *Ls*, circular mapping catheter.

regardless of the thromboembolic risk, if patients do not experience any recurrence of atrial tachyarrhythmias, severe PV stenosis (PV narrowing >70%), or severe LA mechanical dysfunction, as assessed by transthoracic echocardiography. Patients with a $CHADS_2$ score 1 or higher experiencing early recurrence of AF are maintained on oral anticoagulation for at least 6 months. In these patients, warfarin is discontinued if there is no AF recurrence without antiarrhythmic drugs. In case of new AF recurrence in patients with a $CHADS_2$ score 1 or higher, oral anticoagulation is restarted.

RADIOFREQUENCY-BALLOON ABLATION FOR PVI

Balloon-based ablation technologies have been developed with the aim of achieving PVI in shorter time (single-shot, relatively ostial PV isolation) and minimizing the operator dependency on manual procedures. Owing to the overall dismal results with PVI only in nonparoxysmal patients, balloon-based technologies should be recommended mostly in patients with paroxysmal AF.

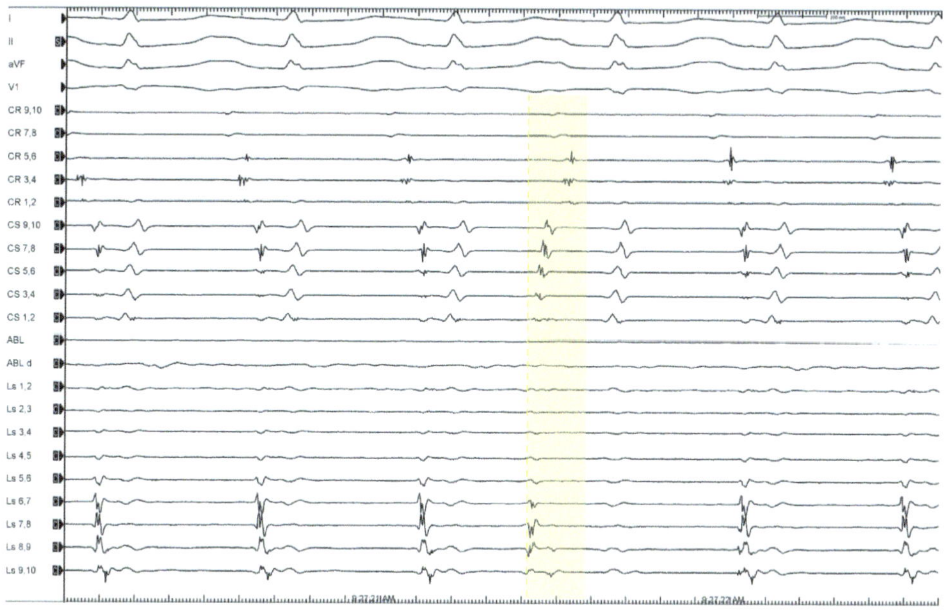

Fig. 15.15 Premature atrial beat (yellow shade) from the left atrial appendage. *ABL*, Ablation catheter; *CR*, crista; *CS*, coronary sinus; *Ls*, circular mapping catheter.

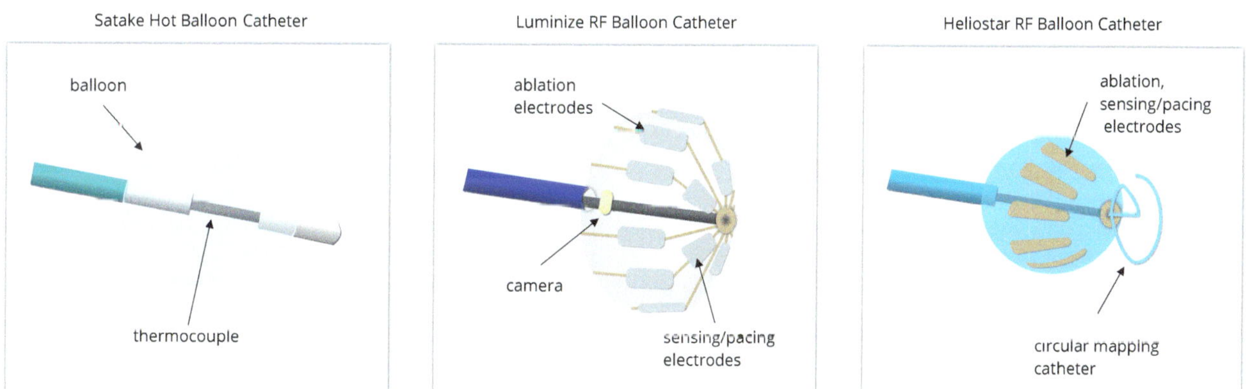

Fig. 15.16 Illustration of the three types of available radiofrequency balloon-based ablation devices: *left*, Satake Hot Balloon; *middle*, Luminize; *right*, Heliostar.

In addition to cryoenergy and laser, there are three available balloon-based devices that uses RF to obtain permanent lesions (Fig. 15.16; Table 15.4).[61] The Satake HotBalloon catheter[62–63] (Toray Industries, Tokyo, Japan) uses a compliant balloon (20–35 mm inflation diameter) filled with a saline/contrast solution to adapt to different PV anatomies. After positioning the balloon at the level of the PV ostium with the aid of a stiff wire, the balloon is inflated to occlude the PV and a central coil electrode delivers RF energy heating the solution. Power (up to 150 W) is delivered in a temperature-controlled fashion, to reach a target solution temperature of 65°C–75°C. The balloon surface heats the PV wall circumferentially through direct conductive heating, resulting in permanent, homogeneous, circumferential lesions. The Luminize RF balloon catheter[64] (Boston Scientific, Marlborough, MA; formerly, Apama Medical) is a 28-mm compliant balloon with 12 equatorial and 6 forward-facing, irrigated, flat electrodes wrapped on its extremity. In addition to these ablation electrodes, there are separate sense/pace electrodes, thus eliminating the need for a separate diagnostic catheter. The catheter also incorporates built-in cameras with LED lightning to provide real-time visualization of tissue–electrode contact. RF energy is delivered through the irrigated equatorial electrodes in a multipolar or unipolar fashion, which allows for quick circumferential as well as focal ablation, as needed. In clinical studies, Luminize has only been used in a multipolar ablation mode, in which 8–10 W of RF energy are delivered from each irrigated electrode for up to 60 seconds, according to the amount of impedance drop (>20% is indicative of adequate lesion formation) and time to PV isolation. The Heliostar RF balloon catheter[65] (Biosense Webster, Irvine, CA, USA) is a 28-mm compliant balloon is a with 10 irrigated, flexible, gold-plated electrodes that encompass the distal end of the balloon. Each electrode is equipped with an integrated thermistor to

TABLE 15.4 Comparison of Radiofrequency Balloon Ablation Technologies

	Balloon Compliance	Over the Wire	Built-in Camera	Contrast Injection	Pacing	Sensing	EAM System Integration	RF Delivery	Non-PV Ablation
Satake Hot Balloon	+++	Yes	No	Yes	No	Planned	No	RF to heat saline	Yes, with manipulation
Luminize	+	Yes	Yes	No	Yes	Yes	Planned	Unipolar or bipolar	Yes, with dedicated electrodes
Heliostar	++	Yes (CMC/ wire)	No	Yes	Yes	Yes	Yes	Unipolar	Yes, with manipulation

CMC, circular mapping catheter; *EAM*, electroanatomical mapping; *PV*, pulmonary vein; *RF*, radiofrequency.

monitor the tissue temperature and with sensors to allow their (magnet-based) visualization on the Carto 3 mapping system. All electrodes can ablate, sense and pace, but a separate small-sized (3-F) CMC is also provided to accurately detect time to PV isolation and manipulate the balloon within the LA. RF energy is delivered through each electrode independently in a unipolar fashion in temperature-controlled mode (maximum power 15 W, maximum temperature 55°C) for a maximum of 60 seconds per site. This allows for quick, single-shot circumferential (all electrodes) as well as segmental (selected electrode/s) ablation.

RF-balloon ablation technology has been used to successfully treat patients with paroxysmal AF, with the main reported complications mirroring those of standard RF catheter ablation, that is, PV stenosis, PN, and esophageal injury.[62–66] Of note, with Luminize and Heliostar, RF energy delivery can be selectively limited in the electrodes facing the esophagus, thus reducing the risk of esophageal injury.

CONCLUSION

PVI remains the cornerstone of catheter-based therapies for AF. Over the years, the PVI technique has undergone profound evolution; multiple clinical studies have been designed and conducted to evaluate the best ablation approach. Current guidelines recommend a wide antral PVI with confirmation of electrical isolation with a CMC. This approach has been demonstrated to optimize clinical success and minimize the risk of procedure-related complications. Available ablation tools for PVI are imperfect, and PV reconnection following a single PVI procedure still represents a major mechanism of recurrent arrhythmia after ablation. Ongoing research is evaluating novel ablation tools with the aim of reducing the operator dependency of PVI procedures, minimizing complications, and increasing the rate of permanent PVI.

REFERENCES

Please refer to the e-book for a complete list of references.

16

Pulmonary Vein Isolation Using the Cryoballoon Catheter

Justin Hayase, Aron Bender, Wilber Su, Eric Buch

KEY POINTS

Mapping

- The proximal-seal method is the best approach for antral pulmonary vein positioning of the cryoballon
- Pulmonary vein potentials should be recorded with a circular mapping catheter for mesaurement of time-to-isolation
- Creation of a post-ablation voltage map aids in cofirmation of wide antral isolation

Ablation Targets

- Cryoballoon lesions target isolation of the pulmonary veins and pulmonary vein antra

Special Equipment

- Cryoballoon ablation system: Flexcath sheath, cryoballoon
- Circular Achieve mapping catheter
- Optional: intracardiac echocardiography for transseptal catheterization

Sources of Difficulty

- Common pulmonary vein ostium or ovoid antrum will often require segmental ablation
- Phrenic nerve and esophageal proximity
- Cryoballoon dosing with time-to-effect monitoring requires real-time assessment of local pulmonary vein potentials

INTRODUCTION

Electrical isolation of the pulmonary veins (PVs) via antral isolation remains the foundation of catheter-based treatment for both paroxysmal and persistent atrial fibrillation (AF).[1] Focal ablation via radiofrequency (RF) energy delivery used to isolate the PVs can be technically demanding since it requires maintenance of stable, point-by-point catheter–tissue contact, is associated with a prolonged learning curve, and requires many contiguous, durable, transmural RF energy applications to isolate the PVs.[2] Unlike focal ablation for pulmonary vein isolation, cryoballoon ablation is a single-shot ablation tool that can achieve antral PV isolation with a predictable, homogeneous, and wide band of ablated myocardial tissue. Cryoballoon ablation has been demonstrated to be effective and reproducible among a vast group of operators, with randomized data showing similar efficacy and safety to RF ablation.[3,4] The unique histologic pattern of the lesion created by the cryoballoon has also been demonstrated to be advantageous; evidence suggests it preserves tissue architecture and may reduce the incidence of complications such as thromboembolic phenomena.[5,6]

Low rates of complications such as pulmonary vein stenosis, phrenic nerve injury, atrioesophageal (AE) fistula, stroke, and death have been reported based on worldwide experience.[7–9] The complications associated with cryoballoon ablation are dependent on dosing and technical factors. Availability of progressive generations of the cryoballoon and mapping tools along with refined technique and dosing norms have improved success, procedural duration, and complication rates of cryoballoon ablation.[4,10,11]

RANDOMIZED CONTROLLED TRIAL DATA

The EAST-AFNET 4 trial, which enrolled 2789 patients with AF diagnosed less than a year prior to enrollment, showed a benefit of a rhythm control strategy with a hazard ratio of 0.79 (96% confidence interval [CI], 0.66–0.94; $P = .005$) for a primary composite outcome of death from cardiovascular causes, stroke, or hospitalization with worsening of heart failure or acute coronary syndrome.[12] This study was followed by several large, randomized clinical trials comparing cryoballoon ablation with antiarrhythmic therapy for initial treatment of AF, particularly early in patients with paroxysmal AF.[7–9]

The STOP-AF trial randomized 203 patients with paroxysmal atrial fibrillation who had never previously received rhythm control treatment to either cryoballoon ablation or class I or III antiarrhythmic medications.[7] At 12 months, freedom from atrial arrhythmias was 74.6% in the ablation arm versus 45% in the antiarrhythmic drug arm ($P < .001$). EARLY-AF enrolled symptomatic patients with a diagnosis of paroxysmal atrial fibrillation within the last two years and randomized to either an initial strategy of cryoballoon ablation or antiarrhythmic medications, demonstrating a hazard ratio of 0.48 (95% CI 0.35–0.66) for atrial arrhythmia recurrence at one year (43% recurrence on loop recorder in the ablation group, 68% in the antiarrhythmic group).[8] In the Cryo-FIRST trial, 218 treatment-naïve patients with atrial fibrillation were randomized to cryoballoon catheter ablation versus antiarrhythmic medications and then followed for 12 months.[9] Freedom from atrial arrhythmias was 82% in the ablation arm versus 67.6% in the antiarrhythmic medication arm ($P < .001$). The EARLY-AF, STOP-AF, and Cryo-FIRST randomized controlled trials, taken together, significantly bolster the evidence supporting the use of cryoballoon catheter ablation for patients with symptomatic, paroxysmal atrial fibrillation, particularly early in the course of the arrhythmia.

PREPROCEDURAL CONSIDERATIONS

There are a number of preprocedural considerations for patients undergoing cryoballoon ablation for AF. Anticoagulation management is determined on a patient-by-patient basis to balance the risks and benefits to each individual. In general, uninterrupted oral anticoagulation should be considered for most patients presenting for ablation, typically for at least 30 days before the procedure. Preprocedural transesophageal echocardiogram to rule out left atrial thrombus is prudent in some AF patients with undergoing catheter ablation, especially those with inadequate preprocedural anticoagulation or very high stroke risk. The use of intracardiac echocardiography may be considered as an alternative, with results suggesting equivalence to TEE when used properly.[13] Additionally, use of cardiac computed tomography (CT) with intravenous contrast may also be used with a high negative predictive value.[14,15] Cardiac magnetic resonance imaging (MRI) may also be considered to rule out left atrial appendage thrombus, though with perhaps a lower sensitivity than alternative imaging modalities.[16]

Preprocedure cardiac MRI or CT scan imaging of the left atrium can be performed for fusion with the electroanatomical mapping system; however, cryoballoon is amenable to variable PV anatomies and can be successfully used without preprocedural imaging. The need for focal touch-up ablation following cryoballoon ablation has been minimal since the introduction of the second-generation cryoballoon, Arctic Front Advance (Medtronic, Minneapolis, MN).[6,17]

CRYOBALLOON ABLATION PROCEDURE

The availability of cryoballoon ablation tools should be reviewed by supportive staff before each case. Required and commonly used tools are listed (Table 16.1, Video 16.1).

Sedation and Anesthesia Considerations

The minimally invasive nature of cryoablation allows for modest procedure-related patient discomfort. The procedure can be performed under general anesthesia or conscious sedation. Patients without deep or general anesthesia are more likely to exhibit a vasovagal response during left superior PV ablation or thawing.[18,19] Because three-dimensional mapping is optional during cryoballoon procedures, potential patient motion that could compromise positional references is less of a concern. Further, Foley catheterization is not necessary because of the relatively short procedure time and lack of saline irrigation. If general anesthesia is used, it is critical to note that paralytics should be avoided after anesthesia induction to allow for effective phrenic nerve pacing during right-sided PV ablation.

TABLE 16.1 Cryoballoon Ablation Tools

Arctic Front Advance 28-mm cryoballoon (23-mm cryoballoon if all PV <15 mm)
Flexcath Advance deflectable sheath
Achieve mapping catheter 20 mm (15-mm Achieve if PV <15 mm)
Contrast agent and injection manifold
Pacing catheter for right phrenic nerve and right ventricle
Optional: 14 F dilator for femoral access, intracardiac echocardiogram

PV, Pulmonary vein.

Vascular Access

Cryoballoon access through the right femoral vein is preferred because of its proximity to the operator. Cryoballoon access is typically obtained via the Flexcath Advance deflectable, which has a 12-F inner diameter and a 14.5-F outer diameter. There is a step-up between the dilator and the sheath caused by the reinforced sheath tip, which allows balloon retraction without deformation. This may present difficulty in introducing the balloon through the femoral access site and crossing the interatrial septum. Dilation at the femoral access site with a short 14-F dilator aids smooth passage of the Flexcath. At least one additional venous access is necessary for phrenic nerve monitoring with pacing in the superior vena cava. Access for intracardiac ultrasound is optional but can aid in precisely locating the transseptal puncture site and reducing dependence on fluoroscopy during ablation. Therapeutic anticoagulation is recommended after femoral vein access and prior to transseptal access via intravenous heparin bolus with a target activated clotting time of at least 300 seconds, or according to the operator's convention, usually similar to left atrial RF ablation.

Transseptal Access

Careful placement of the transseptal access point maximizes the mechanical advantage of the catheter. A low and anterior transseptal puncture at the lower limbus of the septum is optimal (Fig. 16.1). In addition to the mechanical advantage, the tissue of the interatrial septum is more fibrous at the thinner portion

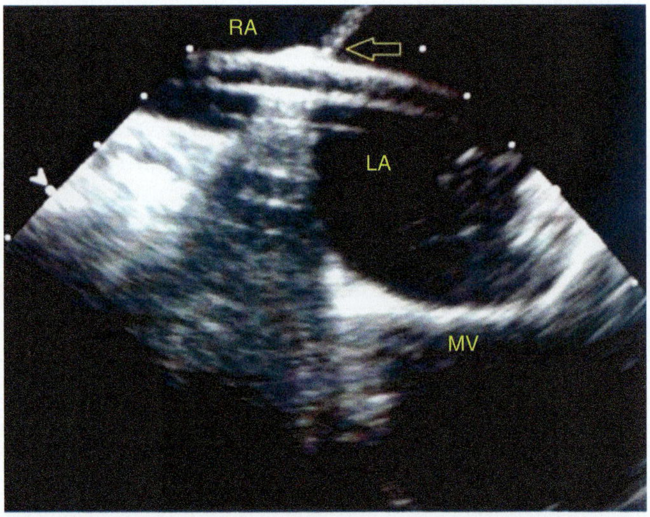

Fig. 16.1 Intracardiac echocardiogram view of the transseptal puncture at a more anterior and inferior site of the atrial septum. Here the Flexcath Advance is introduced through the inferior limbus *(arrow)* to reduce the possibility of iatrogenic atrial septal defect. *LA*, Left atrium; *MV*, mitral valve; *RA*, right atrium.

versus the limbus region, which is more muscular. This difference in tissue architecture eases the ability to puncture through the septum even though it is slightly thicker.[19,20] Initial transseptal access can typically be obtained with SL1 or similarly shaped sheath, including powered needle or wire transseptal access systems such as Versacross (Baylis Medical, Montreal, Quebec, Canada)[21] (see Chapter 43).

Exchange of the Flexcath Advance is accomplished with a guidewire of the operators' choice, preferably positioned at the left superior PV, or with an atraumatic pigtail wire. However, if a significant amount of resistance is encountered during the passage of the Flexcath, repositioning the guidewire with a deflection of the sheath toward the right superior PV may allow for a straighter passage; this maneuver is useful for more difficult septal punctures caused by a thick, fibrotic, or previously accessed septum. Predilatation of the septum using just the dilator from the Flexcath Advance may reduce resistance during the initial passage of the sheath. In addition, twisting or rotational motion may aid in the passage of the step-up portion between the dilator and the sheath. After insertion of the Flexcath Advance sheath, the dilator should be removed slowly. The sheath is aspirated by opening the side-arm while covering the valve with the left thumb. The sheath is typically flushed continuously with heparinized saline for the duration of left atrial dwell time.

The cryoballoon is prepared per the manufacturer's recommendation, immersing the balloon folds underwater and sliding the introducer over the balloon folds to remove air. As the cryoballoon is advanced into the sheath, care should be taken to avoid the introduction of air and bending of the cryoballoon. The Achieve should lead the advancement of the cryoballoon in the left atrium. To aid in localization, the end of the sheath is indicated by an initial white marker-band on the cryoballoon catheter. Exposure of the second white marker-band denotes full cryoballoon extension beyond the sheath.

Cryoballoon Maneuvers

Cryoballoon techniques are aimed at maximizing patient safety and procedural success. This section discusses maneuvers generally and is followed by cryoballoon dosing recommendations to minimize procedural complications. It should be noted that the cryoballoon is noncompliant and comes in both 23-mm and 28-mm diameter sizes. Most operators will find that the 28-mm cryoballoon works well for nearly all patients. In most PVs, the cryoballoon makes circumferential tissue contact for full occlusion, and because the balloon is substantially larger than the PV ostium, a wide area of PV antrum can be modified at once. However, because of the noncompliant nature of the cryoballoon and the ovoid shape of some PV antra, a mismatch of contact area is possible. Some PVs are simply unable to be engaged in such a way as to attain circumferential contact. Indeed, the more ovoid a PV ostium, the more likely that it will be necessary to perform segmental isolation by selectively making contact along the superior arc of the PV and, subsequently, the inferior arc, as shown in Fig. 16.2. The resulting antral modification closely resembles the typically intended wide area circumferential ablation around each of the PVs.

In general, cryoballoon ablation differs from that of radiofrequency catheter ablation in that most of the maneuvers depend on the sheath to define the angle of engagement rather than the cryoballoon itself. The maneuvers required to access each individual pulmonary vein are divided into steps, not always performed in this order: (1) Access the PV using Achieve (ideally the lower branch inferior PVs). (2) Inflate the cryoballoon within the left atrium to avoid PV injury. (3) Engage the PV and attempt to maximize cryoballoon-antrum contact. Sheath angulation and direction should be optimized to allow coaxial mechanical support. Orthogonal fluoroscopy views can aid in the assessment of sheath coaxial alignment. (4) Reposition the Achieve catheter to ensure PV signal monitoring to optimize dosing and to predict ablation success. (5) Use contrast injection, pressure wave monitoring, or intracardiac echocardiogram (ICE)[22] evaluation to minimize leak/optimize cryoballoon-PV engagement (Fig. 16.3). It is important to note that not all PVs can be occluded. (6) If the PV is completely occluded, relax forward motion and pull back the cryoballoon until contrast leak is seen around the true antrum. This step is critical and will ensure the cryoballoon is not deeply seated inside the PV (Fig. 16.4). (7) Initiate ablation for approximately 3 seconds to allow the cryoballoon to enlarge and increase in pressure before advancing the balloon toward the antrum for optimal ostial engagement. (8) Some operators may find it useful to check for leaks again during this final engagement with ICE or additional contrast injection within the first 10 seconds of ablation before the lumen is frozen. (9) Pacing of the phrenic nerve superior to the cryoballoon position should be performed during ablation of both right-sided PVs. Most operators start phrenic nerve pacing 30–60 seconds after the start of cryoablation of the right-sided PVs. To improve sensitivity, phrenic pacing output can be adjusted to just above the phrenic capture threshold. The right phrenic nerve is reliably located at the junction of the superior vena cava and the right subclavian vein. The general techniques for the cryoballoon maneuvers are summarized in Table 16.2.

Although inflation of the cryoballoon within the PV is not recommended, the inflation pressure without ablation is low and is unlikely to cause injury. However, ablation within the PV should never be performed; cryoballoon ablation within the PV is the most likely cause of PV stenosis with mechanical trauma and increases risk of collateral tissue damage such as lung and phrenic injury. Avoidance of deep seating the cryoballoon is particularly important in the right superior PV because of proximity to the phrenic nerve. Risk of phrenic nerve injury can be reduced by diligent placement of the cryoballoon at the antrum of the PVs with the maneuvers described earlier.[19]

Maneuvering the cryoballoon after ablation initiation should be avoided to prevent tissue injury. It is important to understand the limitations of maneuvers such as the "pull-down" method. In this method, the superior part of the cryoballoon is allowed to freeze for the first 60 seconds, which is followed by pulling down the cryoballoon to engage or seal off the inferior part of the PV. Although this maneuver often seems successful, one must understand the inherent risk of mechanical trauma to the PV. Further, in this method a layer of ice forms on the surface of the cryoballoon and acts as an insulator when the cryoballoon

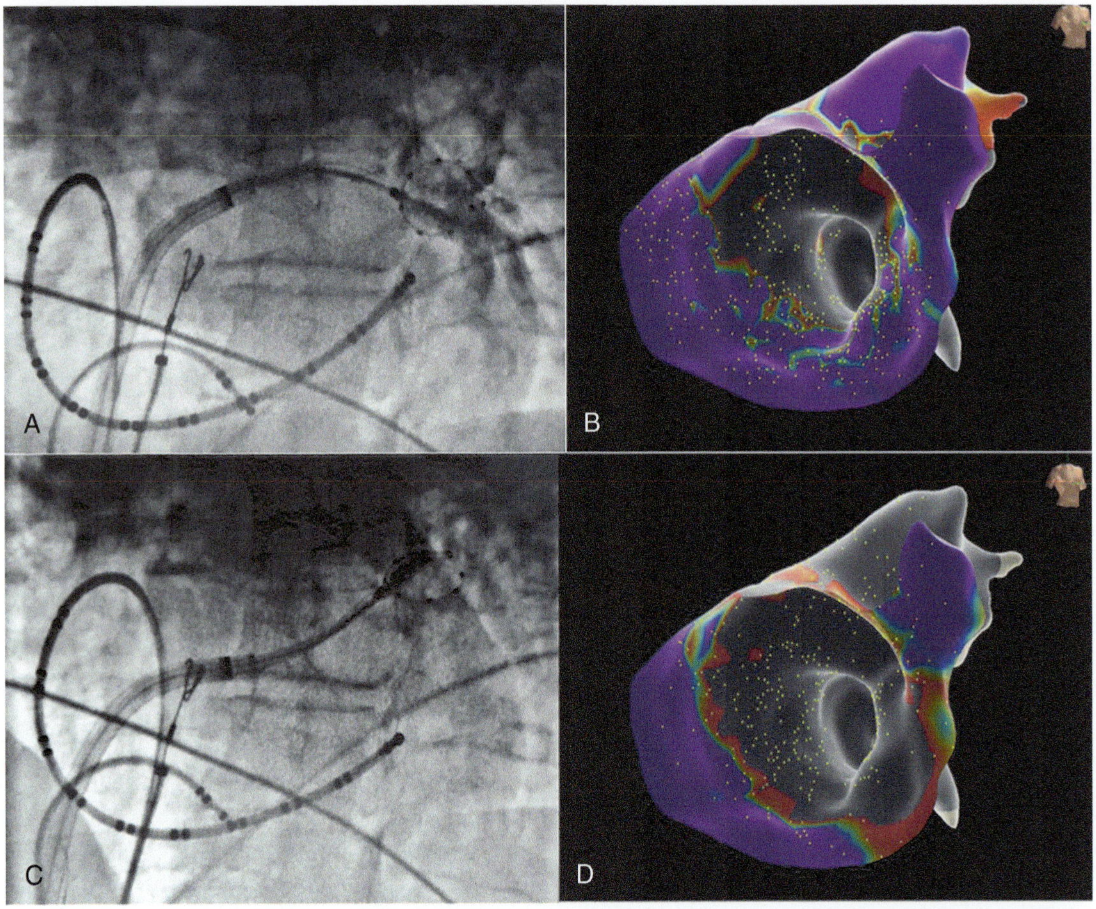

Fig. 16.2 Segmental isolation of a more ovoid pulmonary vein (PV) to achieve circumferential PV isolation with wide-area antral modification. (A) Cryoballoon with upper tilt and engagement in left anterior oblique (LAO) view and venogram. (B) resultant voltage map of upper tilt engagement. (C) Cryoballoon with lower tilt and engagement in LAO view. (D) Voltage map after the addition of the lower cryoballoon engagement to create a wide area circumferential lesion.

is pulled down, preventing effective ablation along the inferior PV. The inferior portion of the PV ablated during the pull-down may be acutely isolated, but it is often noted to recover upon follow-up. The appropriate way to ablate a PV antrum without a complete seal is to perform segmental ablation with the cryoballoon at two different angles: a superiorly directed ablation followed by an inferiorly directed ablation. The segmental approach is described in more detail in a later section. After cryoablation, the thawing process can be slow. The operator should not move the balloon catheter until the catheter temperature reading is close to body temperature to avoid tissue trauma due to residually frozen tissue.

Phrenic Nerve Preservation

Persistent right phrenic nerve injury is the most commonly reported serious complication in cryoballoon ablation, and it is caused by either ablation near the phrenic nerve deeper inside the PV or not monitoring the status of the phrenic nerve diligently during ablation of the right-sided PVs.[3,19] Most experienced operators have reported significantly lower incidence of phrenic nerve injury when using the proximal-seal method described earlier. However, because of the proximity of the phrenic nerve, monitoring diligently is required regardless of the balloon position.[19] Immediate termination of the cryoablation and immediate deflation of the balloon when a reduction in diaphragm motion is detected will minimize the likelihood of persistent phrenic nerve injury.

Various methods of phrenic monitoring have been studied. All rely on pacing the right phrenic nerve during ablation of all right-sided PVs. If paralytic was administered during the anesthesia induction, sufficient time is needed to allow the recovery of the phrenic nerve before the ablation of right-sided PV for adequate monitoring. Sugammadex (a neuromuscular relaxant drug) can be given to reverse residual paralysis if necessary. Consistent and stable phrenic capture for pacing is often found near the junction of the superior vena cava and right subclavian vein. Pacing cycle length of 1000–2000 ms is recommended. Direct palpation by placing a hand on the patient's abdomen can detect cyclical changes in the strength of the phrenic capture. Typically, phrenic nerve paralysis progresses rapidly during cryoballoon ablation, and rapid detection of the decrement in diaphragm contraction is critical for immediate return of phrenic nerve function.[19,23]

Other methods of phrenic nerve monitoring have been described, from intracardiac echocardiogram to monitor hepatic/diaphragmatic contraction, to fetal ultrasound for an audible warning.[24] One of the methods used to increase the sensitivity of early phrenic nerve injury detection is the use of compound motor action potential, and use of this technique has been reported to decrease the incidence of phrenic nerve injury to less than 1.5%.[25–27]

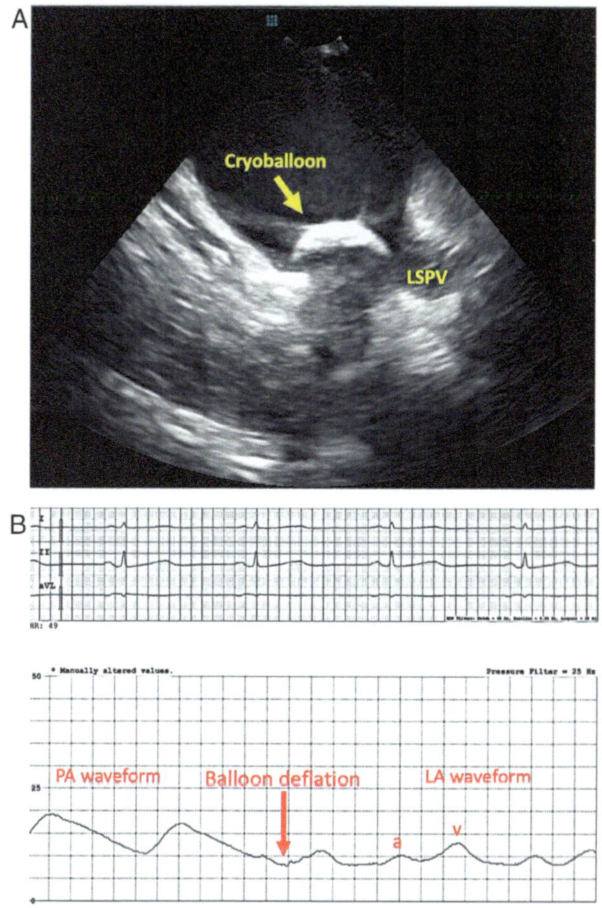

Fig. 16.3 Intracardiac echocardiography and pressure wave monitoring to guide cryoballoon occlusion. (A) Intracardiac echocardiographic image of the left atrium demonstrating the cryoballoon (*arrow*) in occlusive position within the left inferior pulmonary vein. The adjacent left superior pulmonary vein (LSPV) can also be visualized. (B) Pressure waveform during sinus rhythm showing pulmonary artery (PA) waveform at the start of the tracing with transition to a left atrial (LA) waveform following balloon deflation with distinct "a" and "v" waves.

TABLE 16.2 Cryoballoon Technique Key Points

Steps in pulmonary vein isolation using cryoballoon
1. Transseptal access at an anterior and inferior location
2. Select and access pulmonary vein with Achieve mapping catheter
3. Cryoballoon inflation in the left atrium
4. Engagement of cryoballoon with the pulmonary vein antrum
5. Contrast injection to assess occlusion using "proximal-seal method"
6. Adjust Achieve mapping catheter to record pulmonary vein electrogram
7. Begin cryoablation, record time-to-isolation
8. Dose cryoballoon appropriately, monitor for collateral injury with phrenic nerve in right-sided pulmonary vein. Esophageal temperature monitoring
9. Segmental isolation of the pulmonary vein antrum may be necessary for anatomically challenged antrum
10. Assessment of pulmonary vein isolation and antral modification postablation

When phrenic nerve injury is suspected, immediate termination of the ablation should be performed. Delivery of cryoenergy can be rapidly terminated by using a "double stop" technique for immediate cryoballoon deflation. This technique is considered safe without reported adverse events.[23] Reevaluation of the cryoballoon position should be done to ensure that a proximal-seal technique is performed to increase the distance between the balloon and the phrenic nerve at repeat ablation. If phrenic nerve recovery is not seen, repeat ablation should not be performed. Postprocedure inspiratory and expiratory chest radiography or ultrasound sniff test should be performed to establish the baseline of the phrenic nerve injury.[19] A summary of difficulties that may be encountered during the procedure and possible solutions is listed in Table 16.3.

CRYOBALLOON DOSING

Dosing: Background of First- Versus Second-Generation Cryoballoon

Cryoballoon dosing has evolved significantly since the introduction of the cryoballoon; it is directly related to procedural

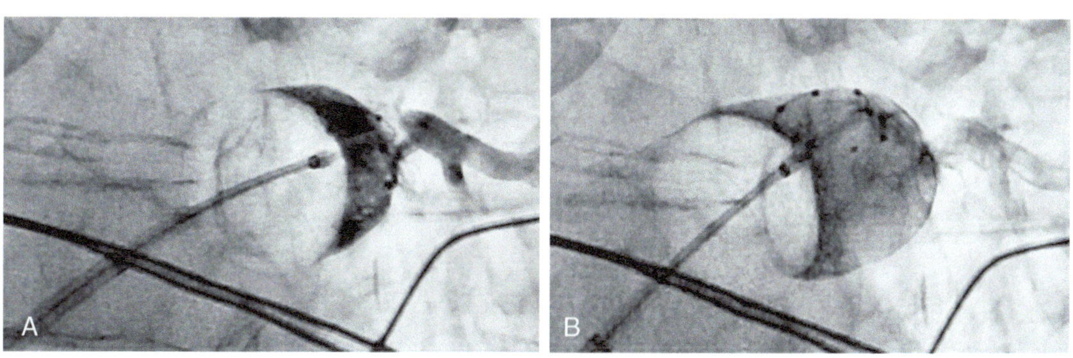

Fig. 16.4 Pull-back method to assess the location of pulmonary vein antrum. (A) Contrast venogram revealing good cryoballoon occlusion of the pulmonary vein. However, ablation at this point will yield a deeper lesion than intended. (B) Cryoballoon is pulled back to observe contrast leak on intracardiac ultrasound to identify the pulmonary vein antrum. Ablation should then be initiated for 2 to 3 seconds to increase the cryoballoon pressure before reengaging the balloon at the antrum at the ostium.

TABLE 16.3 Troubleshooting Difficult Cases

Problem	Causes	Solution
Inability to record TTI	Achieve mapping catheter deep inside the PV	Manipulation and pull-back of the Achieve Mapping toward front of the balloon or repositioning of the cryoballoon to allow the Achieve recording catheter
Inability to occlude PV	Mismatch of ovoid antrum to the round cryoballoon	Segmental isolation of the PV antrum instead of single freeze isolation
Long TTI	Poor or partial cryoballoon-PV contact	Assess area of poorer contact and perform segmental approach ablation to cover circumferentially
Recurrent AF	Extra PV triggers	Need for repeat mapping and ablation of extra-PV AF causes

AF, Atrial fibrillation; *PV*, pulmonary vein; *TTI*, time-to-isolation.

success and importantly, collateral injury and complications. Therefore this is perhaps the most important section of the chapter and will be discussed in detail.

Cryothermal ablation to cause myocardial cell death depends on a rapid rate of tissue temperature reduction, sufficiently low tissue temperature for an adequate duration, and can be enhanced with repeated freeze-refreeze cycling.[28] The cryoballoon is designed to provide a continuous, circumferential PV lesion via refrigerant delivery at the distal hemisphere of the cryoballoon. The first-generation cryoballoon (Arctic Front, Medtronic Inc., Minneapolis, MN) was introduced in 2006 with recommended dosing of 240 seconds, which was derived from experience with the 4-mm focal ablation catheter to create a permanent lesion. Using this dosing scheme, the STOP AF trial (NCT00523978) was designed to allow the use of 23- and/or 28-mm cryoballoon along with 8-mm focal cryoablation for possible touch-up for the treatment of paroxysmal AF, and the study reported a 12-month clinical rhythm control success of 69.9% versus 7.3% with antiarrhythmic drug use.[3]

Although the first-generation cryoballoon created adequate lesions at the four coldest points along the cryoballoon equator, uncontacted areas could leave gaps in the PV isolation. Due to this limitation, PV anatomical variations were often challenging. In response, some operators increased ablation time to try to compensate for the areas that were not adequately frozen. There were reports of ablation durations up to 300 seconds or more, and multiple applications at each PV were performed. Two reports of AE fistulas were potentially associated with increased dosing time beyond the original recommendation. Improvements in the second-generation cryoballoon (Arctic Front Advance, Medtronic Inc.) included increased refrigerant spray from four to eight ports that covered the entire front hemisphere of the cryoballoon, resulting in a more reliable circumferential lesion.[17] Initially, dosing recommendations remained at 240 seconds with repeated ablation, similar to that of the first-generation cryoballoon.[29] A comparative analysis between the first- and second-generation device has corroborated enhanced circumferential lesion with the second-generation cryoballoon in a canine model.[17] An improved rate of temperature drop, nadir temperature, prolonged thaw, and the ability to isolate PVs even with off-center engagement using the second-generation cryoballoon were immediately observed. However, an increase in collateral damage accompanied these improvements including lung injury, which manifested as coughing and hemoptysis and, importantly, reports of AE fistula.[30–33] Because of the increase in collateral injuries, an early consensus of experienced users recommended a reduction of ablation time from 240 to 180 seconds while maintaining consistent circumferential pulmonary vein isolation (PVI).[19]

Controllable factors that influence dosing of the cryoballoon include (1) cryoballoon-PV location and contact, (2) ablation time, and (3) repeat ablation time and location. Feedback obtained during the ablation is also used to determine dosing, which includes (1) time-to-isolation, (2) nadir temperature of the return gas, and (3) effects on phrenic nerve function and esophageal temperature. All of the aforementioned are important considerations of cryoballoon dosing to achieve the optimal balance between procedural success and avoiding complications.[19,34] The following sections will detail each of the individual feedback parameters observed during cryoballoon ablation to improve the user's understanding on its impact on safety and outcome.

Dosing: Cryoballoon–Pulmonary Vein Contact

Cryoballoon thermal transfer is largely dependent on the contact of the cryoballoon with the PV antrum. The cryoballoon central lumen accommodates a guidewire or the Achieve circular mapping catheter and allows contrast injection to assess cryoballoon-PV engagement.[19] The "proximal-seal method" should always be used to engage the PV-antrum (previously described in the technique section [see Fig. 16.4]) to ensure an antral location of the cryoballoon, which minimizes collateral injury to the lung as well as the phrenic nerve during right-sided PV ablation.

Cryoballoon-PV contact is certainly an important component of energy transfer to create a permanent lesion. When incomplete contact is observed with contrast leak, an incomplete lesion is expected. It is critical to note that although complete occlusion can render a single cryoballoon application effective, anatomical variability makes it difficult to achieve perfect contact with every PV. The cross-section of the noncompliant cryoballoon is circular, whereas PV antra are often ovoid; therefore, a single-freeze only approach to achieve complete, circumferential lesion at every PV is not currently feasible. When the cryoballoon-PV antrum engagement is axial, a nearly perfect wide area circumferential lesion can be created (Fig. 16.5A). However, when the PV antrum is ovoid, the cryoballoon-PV antrum engagement is off-axis and a more "tear-drop"–like lesion is created (see Fig. 16.5B). Although both lesions may create acute

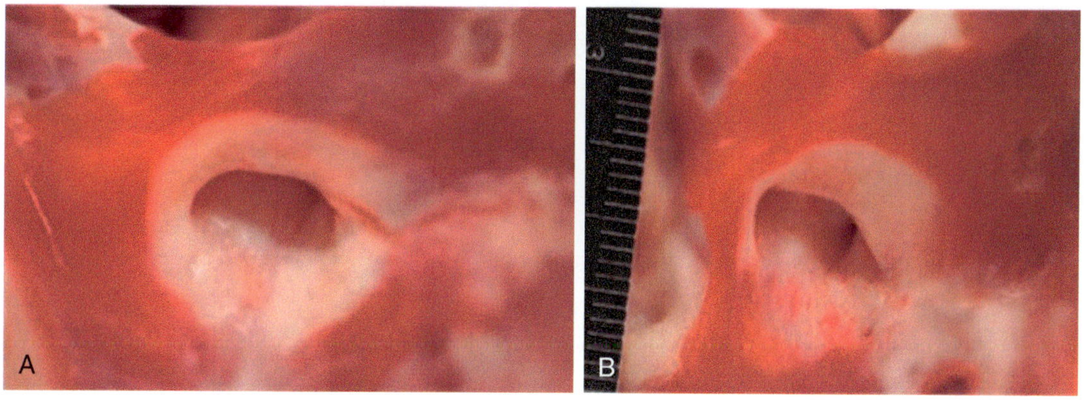

Fig. 16.5 (A) Canine pathology study demonstrating circumferential lesion with circumferential contact. (B) Canine pathology study demonstrating less circumferential lesion with a portion of the pulmonary vein with poorer contact (6 to 9 o'clock portion).

PVI, antral modification (which may be an important part of substrate modification and a more permanent PVI) may be improved with segmental ablation with a second cryoballoon lesion placed in the opposite direction of PV engagement (see Fig. 16.2).[19]

Dosing: Ablation Duration

Studies initially examined the reduction of dosing from 240 seconds with a 240-second refreeze ("bonus freeze" or "freeze-thaw-freeze") to a single freeze with the 28-mm second-generation cryoballoon and reported that a single freeze acutely isolated over 99% (176 of 177 PV) of the PVs investigated with 82% (36/44) of patients free from AF.[35] At the time of repeat ablation, 5 of 11 PVs (45%) that were initially ablated using single-freeze strategy were reconnected compared with no reconnected PVs in the bonus-freeze–treated group. Another study investigated a single 240-second ablation in 59 patients compared with 139 patients who received a bonus freeze and reported that 4 of 188 PVs (2%) in the single-freeze cohort had dormant conduction.[36] No clinically significant differences in terms of procedural differences or freedom from AF were identified between the two groups. Notably, time to isolation (TTI) was not tracked in these studies to evaluate PVI physiology, nor was a single-freeze technique expected to result in 100% PVI in anatomically challenged PV antrum that prevents perfect contact with the cryoballoon; it is expected that a segmental approach using the cryoballoon for complete PVI would have resulted in better efficacy in ovoid PV antra. A routine bonus freeze may not produce additive benefit if the cryoballoon positioning is identical in the two freezes; however, there may be benefits to a bonus freeze if the cryoballoon is repositioned to alter cryoballoon-PV antrum contact on the second freeze.

The duration of ablation required to produce a transmural lesion has been reported in limited clinical trials. The use of 180 seconds instead of the previously recommended 240 seconds with the second-generation cryoballoon did not reveal any significant clinical outcome differences.[37,38] Studies investigating a single, 180-second ablation have reported acute PVI in 94% of patients with 80% of patients free from AF at 1 year.[39] These findings were corroborated by Miyazaki et al., who delivered a 180-second, single ablation in 54 patients and assessed 217 PVs. They reported 1.3 ablations were needed per PV except for common PVs and ultimately 82% of patients were free from AF.[40] The STOP-AF First randomized trial used two 180-second duration freezes per pulmonary vein,[7] as did the EARLY AF randomized trial.[41]

As clinical evidence accumulated, dosing duration evolved from 240 seconds with a bonus freeze to 180 seconds with an optional bonus freeze.[35–38,40] Adequate lesion formation at the cryoballoon-PV interface is typically reliable, and additional assessment of other feedback parameters discussed will together ensure reliable PVI.

Dosing: Time-to-Isolation (TTI)

Use of the Achieve mapping catheter (Medtronic Inc., Minneapolis, MN) to assess real-time, acute physiology of PVI is a powerful predictor of permanent isolation of the PVs.[19] TTI is the only direct physiologic indication of the extent of circumferential tissue ablation; knowledge of TTI during a 180-second ablation will help differentiate whether additional ablation is necessary or whether that PV is at risk for reconnection. TTI gives the operator insight into when the tissue temperature likely has reached the target of less than −30°C for about 30 seconds, to achieve permanent irreversible tissue ablation (Fig. 16.6). Live monitoring of TTI can help differentiate near versus far-field signals; *near-field signals usually appear sharper and higher frequency, whereas far field signals usually appear more rounded and lower frequency*. The caveat is that signals from adjacent structures, such as the left atrial appendage from the left superior pulmonary vein, or the SVC from the right superior pulmonary vein, can have the appearance of near-field potentials. If operators mistake this as residual PV conduction and perform unnecessary additional ablation, there is an increased risk of collateral injury. Pacing in either the vein or the adjacent structure can help differentiate. But the most useful observation is progressive delay then disappearance of the local PV potentials during cryoablation, which would not be seen for far-field signals from adjacent structures.

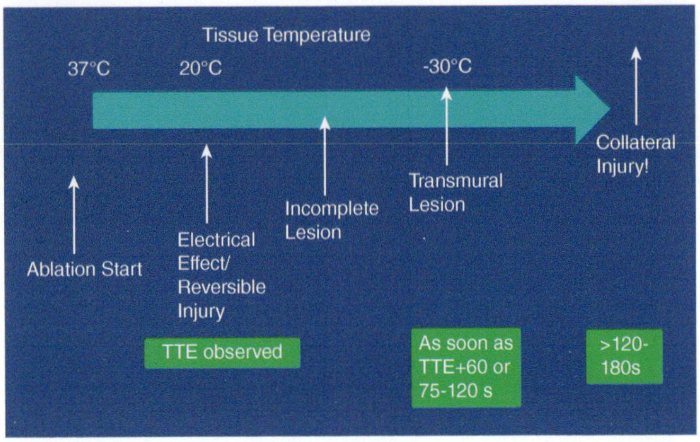

Fig. 16.6 Cryoballoon dosing, correlating observation of time-to-isolation/time-to-effect (TTE) to tissue temperature and permanence of lesion creation.

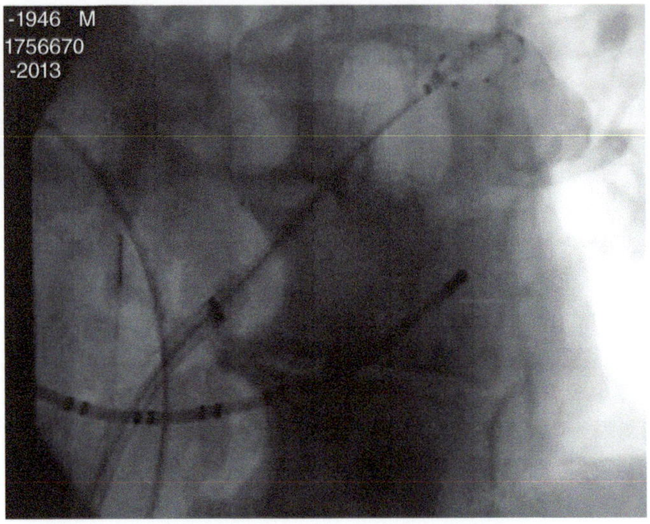

Fig. 16.7 Optimal Achieve position is demonstrated in Fig. 16.4. Note that the Achieve mapping catheter is reflected back toward the cryoballoon to record pulmonary vein isolation time-to-isolation.

From preclinical dosing studies to human procedural experiences, evidence supports that the shorter the TTI, the better the outcome and durability of PVI.[29,38,39,42] Techniques to measure TTI are important, and TTI has been recorded in in as many as 90% of PVs during ablation in experienced centers. The Achieve catheter has also been used as an anchoring wire by operators who feel it is important for stability; however many physicians suggest that the stability of the cryoballoon is more dependent on the position, angle, and stability of the sheath. The Achieve often records TTI effectively when retroflexed toward the surface of the cryoballoon (Fig. 16.7).

Human clinical data supports the use of TTI to assess permanence of PVI; a TTI greater than 60 seconds has been correlated to poorer long-term PVI.[38,39,42] Cinconte et al. examined the permanence of PVI in 212 patients, of which 41 patients experienced AF recurrence. Of the patients who experienced AF recurrence, 29/41 underwent a repeat ablation, which revealed 1.25 PV reconnections per patient. A TTI greater than 60 seconds was an independent predictor of PV reconnection in this cohort. Further, TTI was longer in reconnected PVs versus PVs that remained isolated (71.4 ± 18.8 vs. 42.3 ± 27.2 seconds, respectively; $P < .001$).[39] A TTI ≤60 seconds predicted long-term PVI with 86.7% sensitivity and 86.2% specificity.[39] Aryana et al. examined 71 patients with 111 PVs reconnected (1.56 PV per patient) and reported that reconnected PVs had a longer TTI compared with isolated PVs (67.6 ± 19.7 vs. 39.1 ± 11.7 seconds, respectively; $P < .001$). Multivariate analysis demonstrated that a TTI ≤60 seconds predicted durable PVI (83.3% sensitivity and 83.2% specificity; $P < .001$).[42] Ciconte et al. also examined 143 consecutive patients treated with cryoballoon ablation with a mean follow-up of 12.1 ± 4.4 months and reported that 80.4% of patients were AF free. In this study, TTI was also found to be a predictor of arrhythmia recurrences ($P = .02$), and that a TTI ≤40 seconds trended toward no recurrence (90% sensitivity and 81% specificity).[38] Consistent with what is reported in other studies, longer TTI predicted AF recurrence; every additional 10 seconds required for PVI increased the risk of recurrence by 1.3 times (95% confidence interval [CI], 1.21–1.34; $P < .01$).[38]

Titration of ablation time based on TTI versus standard 240 seconds freeze-thaw-freeze was tested in the ICE-T trial, where 100 patients were randomized 1:1 using a TTI dosing protocol.[43] TTI was observed in 79% of the total PVIs, and a TTI cut off of ≤75 seconds was used to define where a repeated freeze was not administered. A single freeze was administered in 88% of the treated PVs. Therefore fewer ablation applications were reported in the TTI-guided group compared with the control group (5 ± 1 vs. 8 ± 1; $P < .001$). Despite the reduced number of cryo applications, there was no difference in recurrence at 12 months (18% in control group vs. 12% in TTI-guided group, Log-rank $P = .804$).[43] Multivariate statistical analysis determined that TTI predicted AF recurrence ($P = .011$) and that a mean TTI ≥43 seconds predicted recurrent arrhythmias with 77% sensitivity and 74% specificity. There were no differences in complication rates between the two groups ($P = .06$).[43]

A prospective study using TTI as a guide to shorten ablation times and guide bonus freeze applications enrolled 355 patients in the TTI group compared with 400 control patients who underwent cryoablation using a conventional, nonstandardized approach.[44] This study reported that the TTI dosing protocol was associated with shorter (149 ± 34 vs. 226 ± 46 seconds; $P < .001$) and fewer (1.7 ± 0.8 vs. 2.9 ± 0.8 applications; $P < .001$) ablations, as well as reduced total ablation time (16 ± 5 vs. 40 ±14 minutes; $P < 0.001$), fluoroscopy time (13 ± 6 vs. 29 ± 13 minutes; $P < .001$), left atrial dwell time (51 ± 14 vs. 118 ± 25 minutes; $P < .001$), and total procedure time (84 ± 23 vs. 145 ± 49 minutes; $P < .001$). Not surprisingly, the nadir balloon temperature (−47 ± 8 vs. −48 ± 6°C; $P = .41$) and thaw times (43 ± 27 vs. 45 ± 19 seconds; $P = .09$) were not significantly different between the TTI-guided versus standard approach. Complications such as persistent phrenic nerve injury (0.6% vs. 1.2%; $P = .33$) and overall adverse events remained similar as did the 12-month freedom from all atrial arrhythmia recurrence between the TTI-guided versus control group, respectively (83% vs. 78%; $P = .14$). At the time of repeat ablation procedure for recurrent arrhythmias, there were significantly fewer PV reconnections in the TTI-guided group (5% vs. 19%; $P < .001$).

It is also important to again emphasize that the cryoballoon is noncompliant and circular. Anatomical variations of the PVs will not allow 100% PV occlusion with the cryoballoon, and a segmental ablation approach may be necessary. If the initial ablation did not achieve 100% occlusion and a short TTI was not observed, the initial ablation may be continued to treat the PV antrum in contact with the balloon and additional ablation should be performed to segmentally isolate the PV. In these circumstances, the initial ablation will likely create a PV delay, and the second ablation with different cryoballoon-PV engagement will complete the PVI. The cryoballoon can be directed toward the segment of the PV with residual conduction in order to complete PVI. Short TTI is likely still predictive of permanent PVI.

Dosing: Ablation Temperature

The cryoablation-console displays temperature during ablation that can be used to predict a successful ablation by depicting significant freezing/energy transfer. It is essential to understand that the temperature displayed on the console is not the temperature of the surface of the balloon or the tissue. Rather, the displayed temperature is the temperature of the return gas via a thermocouple located at the back of the cryoballoon. As the refrigerant exits the nozzle it sprays directly to the front hemisphere of the cryoballoon at about −80°C as it evaporates. After the gas is warmed by contact with the target tissue, the temperature of the return gas is displayed by the console and typically has a nadir reading between −30°C to −60°C during ablation. Multiple variables influence the temperature displayed, including collateral warming from the ipsilateral vein, area in contact with the antrum, angulation of the sensor inside the cryoballoon, and tissue heat sink. Therefore a temperature reading that is low is likely reflects low tissue temperature. However, a temperature reading that is higher does not necessarily indicate a poor ablation; a short TTI can be observed with a warmer temperature. The creation of irreversible cryothermal injury requires a sustained temperature below −30°C, as indicated by short TTE.[28] Data regarding nadir temperature as a predictor of durability of PVI are somewhat contradictory.[39,42,45–48] Compared with that of aforementioned TTI, temperature should not be used in isolation to inform dosing except to inform the decision to terminate the ablation if the nadir temperature reaches below −55°C.[19]

Dosing: Post-Ablation Rewarming

A prolonged post-ablation rewarming time is also predictive of a durable PVI.[28,42,45] However, it is also important to understand that the converse, a shorter rewarming time, may not always indicate a poor PVI. Several factors, including collateral warming, play a role in the rewarming time. Some studies have reported that the absence of a prolonged thaw time from −30°C to 15°C is predictive of AF recurrence, and further that thaw time ≤25 seconds predicted AF recurrence with 70% sensitivity and 69% specificity.[45] By contrast, a thaw time ≥67 seconds was associated with a durable PVI.[45] Similarly, a separate study recorded thaw time from the nadir to 0°C in 71/112 patients in whom 111/435 PVs were reconnected. In this study, they report that the thaw time was significantly longer in PVs that remained isolated (14.8 ± 10.9 vs. 7.1 ± 2.0 seconds; $P < .001$).[42] Further it was observed that TTI ≤60 seconds and a thaw time to 0°C ≥ 10 seconds were the sole predictors of durable PVI. When both short TTI and long thaw time were seen, there was a <1% risk of long-term PV reconnection (vs 75% risk with long TTI and short thaw time).[42] Therefore consideration of a prolonged thaw time can be useful when TTI cannot be observed, and it may inform the operator to avoid an immediate, consecutive ablation when thaw time is prolonged.

Dosing: Safety Considerations

The most important considerations of a dosing strategy are to minimize collateral injury and maximize patient safety. Safety considerations and best practices involve cryoballoon positioning, patient anatomy, temperature, dosing, and proximity to collateral structures. AE fistula is a rare complication of AF ablation,[30–32] and cryoablation can produce deep enough lesions to injure the esophagus if it is not properly monitored.[43,44] AE fistula has been the most devastating complication of ablation and with proper technique should be avoidable.

Luminal esophageal temperature (LET) monitoring is the primary method to prevent AE fistula, but it is not foolproof. If the thermocouple is not positioned near the coldest part of the esophagus, the extent of esophageal cooling will be underestimated. Despite the shortcomings, when the LET is observed to be low, a true-positive reading is important. Several studies have reported acceptable LETs by luminal esophageal probe and together have recommended a cut off temperature range of no lower than 10–15°C to minimize esophageal injury.[49–52]

Esophageal erosion and the relationship to LET during cryoballoon ablation was examined by Fürnkranz et al. in 32 patients who were treated with a 28-mm second-generation cryoballoon using two consecutive 240 second ablations. In this cohort, ablation was only terminated because of phrenic nerve injury or an LET less than 5°C. The investigators found no significant correlation between balloon nadir temperature and esophageal nadir temperature.[49] A subsequent esophageal scope was performed after the procedure (mean = 2 ± 1 days), and esophageal lesions were observed in 19% (6/32) of patients. Esophageal lesions were found in patients with LETs during ablation that were significantly lower than patients without lesions (0.3°C ± 8.9°C versus 22.3°C ± 8.3°C, respectively). Therefore LET below 12°C predicted an esophageal lesion with 100% sensitivity and 92% specificity (negative predictive value = 100% and positive predictive value = 71%). Metzner et al. also evaluated 50 patients during use of a 28-mm second-generation balloon with bonus freeze protocol, and LETs lower than 0°C were observed in six separate cryoapplications in five patients (range −1.5°C to −14.0°C) during ablation of the left inferior PV.[50] Esophageal examination performed after the procedure (mean = 2 ± 1 days) identified a thermal lesion (N = 1) or ulcerations (N = 5) in 12% (6/50) of patients. All patients that experienced esophageal thermal injury had a luminal LET below 2.9°C in at least one cryoapplication (range = −2.9°C to −14.0°C)[4] No esophageal thermal injury was detected if all LETs were ≥ 3.0°C. It is important to note that the LET often did not decrease significantly until after 180 seconds of ablation, or earlier with repeat freezing as esophageal and surrounding soft-tissue rewarming is slower than that of the atrial tissue. This supports the recommendation to not perform consecutive lesions when the PV is in close proximity to the esophagus or when a reduction of LET is observed.

Dosing: Conclusion

Dosing techniques to reduce complications while maximizing outcome include (1) optimizing cryoballoon-PV antral contact while using the proximal-seal method; (2) observing TTI to deliver the minimum effective duration and number of ablations; (3) avoiding consecutive ablation in the same location to allow collateral tissue rewarming; and (4) performing segmental PVI when necessary. Ablation should be terminated when the return gas temperature reading drops to below −55°C, and a reduction of the ablation time can be considered when the TTI is less than 30 seconds. In addition careful monitoring for collateral tissue injury to the phrenic nerve and esophagus along with the above-mentioned dosing practices should be implemented to take full advantage of the biophysics of cryoablation while maximizing safety.

POSTPROCEDURE CARE

Recovery

Postprocedural care varies depending on the sedation used and postprocedure team standard of care. In general, most physicians administer protamine to reverse heparin before venous sheaths are removed, and manual compression is applied. Many centers have used a "figure of 8 stitch" either with a surgical tie or with a three-way stopcock technique with good success.[53,54] Alternatively, use of commercially available vascular access closure devices may improve the time needed to achieve hemostasis and safely reduce time to ambulation following ablation.[55,56] Overall complications from femoral access are no greater than that of the prior radiofrequency experiences, despite the larger sheath used in cryoballoon.[4] Patients are advised to lie flat for at least 3–4 hours after sheath removal. Should hemostasis be maintained after 4 hours, resumption of oral anticoagulation is recommended. Patients are typically observed for 6 hours, or overnight for observation and discharged. Some investigators reinitiate antiarrhythmic agents that were discontinued before the procedure, with a plan to stop all antiarrhythmic agents after 1–3 months if the patient remains free from AF. A proton pump inhibitor is recommended for 30 days to reduce the risk of gastric acid contributing to esophageal injury.

Postprocedural Complications

Vascular access, procedural, and collateral injury such as to the phrenic nerve or esophagus comprise the majority of possible complications to monitor. The complication rates described are otherwise similar to conventional AF ablation, including complications at sites of vascular access such as groin hematoma and arterial pseudoaneurysm.[4] Atrial-esophageal fistulas have been described in patients undergoing cryoablation, but since the reduction of dosing below 180 seconds, incidence has been less than 1 in 10,000. Avoidance of consecutive lesions and early termination of ablation using TTI or nadir temperature has minimized the incidence of AE fistula. However, if this complication does occur, early recognition is critical to saving a patient's life, as early surgical intervention appears to be the only effective remedy. Low incidence of cerebrovascular events was reported in large studies such as the Fire and Ice Trial, where two patients had stroke or transient ischemic events in both the cryoablation arm and the radiofrequency ablation arm out of 374 and 376 patients, respectively. In this trial, whereas ten patients had phrenic nerve injury at discharge, only two and one patients had phrenic nerve injury at 3 and 12 months, respectively.[4] Injury to the right phrenic nerve can be minimized by exclusive use of the 28-mm cryoballoon and most importantly, use of the proximal-seal method. Phrenic nerve palsy often does not require supportive care, as patients are rarely highly symptomatic at rest. All cases of right phrenic nerve palsy in several trials resolved spontaneously, and it has been rare for phrenic nerve palsy to persist after the procedure when cryoablation is terminated early. The list of potential complications is summarized in Table 16.4; they can be minimized with proper cryoballoon techniques and dosing considerations.

TABLE 16.4 List of Potential Complications

Potential Complications	Incidence
Groin access complication: hematoma/arterial-venous fistula	1–3%
Phrenic nerve paralysis (transient vs. persistent)	1–8% vs. <1%
Pulmonary vein stenosis	<1%
Hemoptysis or bronchial complication	<1%
Gastroparesis	<1%
Stroke/transient ischemic attack	<1%
Cardiac tamponade or pericardial effusion	<1%
Atrioesophageal fistula	<0.003%

Follow-Up

Routine follow-up is carried out per operator preferences or Heart Rhythm Society recommendations. Clinic visits with repeated 24-hour or 7-day ambulatory rhythm monitoring document procedural outcomes. In most research studies, recurrence is defined as any documented episode of atrial tachyarrhythmia (either symptomatic or asymptomatic) lasting for more than 30 seconds. Current guidelines indicate that patients with CHADSVASC2 scores of 2 or higher should be maintained on anticoagulation, regardless of the apparent success or failure of the ablation procedure.

Repeat Ablation

Cryoballoon ablation has improved clinical outcomes and the quality of the life for patients suffering from AF.[4] Different challenges and considerations for a repeat ablation after the index cryoballoon ablation need to be weighed carefully, as most of the PV antrum is likely isolated during an index procedure that followed appropriate dosing and cryoballoon technique. Therefore the repeat ablation toolset should not include cryoballoon, but rather preferentially use irrigated radiofrequency ablation for extra-PV sites and lines for the treatment of mappable arrhythmias, although the optimal ablation approach for recurrence despite isolated veins has not been established.

CONCLUSION

Cryoballoon ablation is a safe and predictable toolset to generate a reliable large-area PV antral isolation for the treatment of AF. Its reproducibility amongst a wide range of operators have made it an easier technology to adopt with a shorter learning curve and consistent outcomes. Understanding of the science of cryoballoon technology has been an ongoing discovery process since its launch, and best practices continue to be improved. To improve outcomes and to minimize potential complications, technical and dosing recommendations were discussed in detail—access technique, transseptal cryoballoon maneuvers, dosing, and avoidance of complications. The use of cryoballoon beyond paroxysmal and early-persistent AF has also been recognized, and some limited data for use in long-standing persistent AF and its use to modify extra-PV targets have had initial success. Future design improvements in cryoballoon, including modifications of size, compliance, cryothermal transfer, and improved balloon PV antrum contact, are already underway to improve the safety and reliability of the procedure.

REFERENCES

Please refer to the e-book for a complete list of references.

17

Pulmonary Vein Isolation Using Pulsed-Field Ablation or Laser Balloon

Jacob S. Koruth, Iwanari Kawamura, Vivek Y. Reddy

KEY POINTS

- Pulsed-field ablation can achieve pulmonary vein isolation either via a one-shot device or by focal catheter with excellent durability and fast procedural time. Beyond pulmonary vein isolation, lesions such as left posterior wall isolation, mitral isthmus line, roof line, and cavotricuspid line can be also achieved.
- With a nonthermal modality, pulsed-field ablation can create cardiac lesions with limited collateral tissue injuries, but the incidence of coronary spasm should be carefully considered.
- There remain certain unknowns with PFA, such as the impact of lack of effective autonomic modulation resulting from the sparing of ganglionated plexi. This has the potential to limit its efficacy on atrial fibrillation control despite an increase in PVI durability; ongoing studies are needed to provide better insight.
- Laser balloon ablation, in its more recent iteration, achieves rapid antral isolation that is enabled by the motorized movement of the laser arc and a conformable balloon that allows for better antral fit and wider antral lesions.

PULSED-FIELD ABLATION FOR PULMONARY VEIN ISOLATION

Basic Principle

Various technologies using different energy sources are now widely used for pulmonary vein isolation (PVI).[1] Although these have proven to be largely safe and effective, there continue to be reports of severe complications such as pulmonary vein (PV) stenosis, phrenic nerve palsy, and atrioesophageal fistulas, the latter often culminating in death.[2–5] Common to many of the currently used thermal energy sources is that these can ablate all exposed and proximate tissues indiscriminately. Pulsed-field ablation (PFA), on the other hand, is a nonthermal ablative modality in which ultra-short high-voltage impulses are applied to target tissue. This destabilizes cell membranes by forming irreversible aqueous pores and changing the lipids and proteins embedded in the membrane, culminating in cell death. Most importantly, various tissues have specific threshold electrical field strengths that induce cell death, and cardiomyocytes appear to be preferentially susceptible. That is, PFA can create irreversible cardiac lesions by sparing the adjacent tissue such as the phrenic nerve or esophagus. It is in this clinical setting that PFA or irreversible electroporation is poised to become an important energy source (also see Chapter 4).

The beginnings of present-day PFA can be traced to direct current (DC) catheter ablation, a technique used to perform

Disclosure: Vivek Reddy's disclosures with medical companies (unrelated to this manuscript) include: Abbott (Consultant), Ablacon (Consultant, Equity), Acutus Medical (Consultant, Equity), Affera (Consultant, Equity), (Apama Medical-Boston Scientific (Consultant, Equity), APN Health (Consultant, Equity), Aquaheart (Consultant, Equity), Atacor (Consultant, Equity), AtiAN (Consultant), Autonomix (Consultant, Equity), Axon Therapies (Consultant, Equity), Backbeat (Consultant, Equity), BioSig (Consultant, Equity), Biosense-Webster (Consultant), BioTel Heart (Consultant), Biotronik (Consultant), Boston Scientific (Consultant), Cardiac Implants (Consultant, Equity), CardiaCare (Consultant, Equity), Cardiofocus (Consultant), Cardionomic (Consultant), CardioNXT / AFTx (Consultant, Equity), Circa Scientific (Consultant, Equity), CoreMap (Consultant), CoRISMA (Consultant, Equity), Corvia Medical (Consultant, Equity), Dinova-Hangzhou Nuomao Medtech (Consultant, Equity), East End Medical .(Consultant, Equity), EBR (Consultant), EPD-Philips (Consultant, Equity), EP Frontiers (Consultant, Equity), Epix Therapeutics (Consultant, Equity), EpiEP (Consultant, Equity), Eximo (Consultant, Equity), Farapulse-Boston Scientific (Consultant, Equity), Fire1 (Consultant), Gore & Associates (Consultant), HRT (Consultant, Equity), Impulse Dynamics (Consultant), Intershunt (Consultant, Equity), Javelin (Consultant, Equity), Kardium (Consultant, Equity), Keystone Heart (Consultant, Equity), LuxMed (Consultant, Equity), Manual Surgical Sciences (Equity), Medlumics (Consultant, Equity), Medtronic (Consultant), Middlepeak (Consultant, Equity), Neutrace (Consultant, Equity), Newpace (Equity), Nuvera-Biosense Webster (Consultant, Equity), Philips (Consultant), Pulse Biosciences (Consultant), Restore Medical (Consultant, Equity), Sirona Medical (Consultant, Equity), Surecor (Equity), Valcare (Consultant, Equity) and Vizaramed (Equity).

Jacob Koruth's disclosures: Consultant–Abbott, Farapulse, Pulse Biosciences, Cardiofocus, Affera and Grant Support–Farapulse, Pulse Biosciences, Cardiofocus, Affera, Equity: Affera cardiac ablation in the 1980s.[6–8] During the early years of catheter ablation, DC ablation was largely used for ablation of the bundle of His for refractory supraventricular arrhythmias and for ventricular tachycardia. Despite its efficacy, it was ultimately abandoned in favor of radiofrequency (RF) ablation due to the risk of serious complications such as barotrauma, cardiac rupture, and skeletal muscle stimulation (requiring general anesthesia and neuromuscular paralysis).[9–11] To reduce the incidence of barotrauma, which is the result of a high-pressure shock wave–like phenomenon (caused by arcing through an electrically isolating gas bubble around the ablation electrode), low-energy DC ablation was subsequently developed.[12–16] Early reports of ablation lesions created with this approach have similarities to current PFA lesions. However, this favorable modification did not gain sufficient traction and was quickly replaced by an easier-to-titrate and -deliver energy source: RF.

Among the early descriptions of PFA, Wittkampf et al. were among the first to demonstrate the feasibility of using electroporation as an approach to cardiac ablation (ventricular and PV ablation) in a series of preclinical experiments.[17] One of the early reports described a chronic swine series, where they administered up to four 200-J monophasic shocks per PV, delivered between a circular multielectrode catheter and a return patch (monopolar). After 3 weeks, they demonstrated reduced PV electrogram amplitudes and increased pacing thresholds, with histologic lesions as deep as 3.5 mm. More recent focused preclinical experiments on atrial ablation have demonstrated the feasibility and safety of PFA for both PV and left atrial (LA) ablation. These reports have also demonstrated durable PV isolation and use of more modern endocardial catheters with custom generators/waveforms.[18,19]

Pulmonary Vein Isolation with Single-Shot PFA Devices

An initial evaluation of endocardial and epicardial PFA for patients with paroxysmal AF, enrolling a total of 22 patients across two centers, in an open-label, nonrandomized study.[20] The endocardial PFA system used in this report consisted of a custom-built generator that was capable of delivering programmed bipolar waveforms (900–1000 V) and an endocardial PFA catheter designed for delivering energy at a PV antrum delivered via a 13-F steerable sheath (Iowa Approach Inc., Menlo Park, CA). For epicardial ablation, a linear ablation catheter was designed to deliver PFA (2100–2400 V) in a box format around the PVs. The study demonstrated that endocardial PFA was acutely successful in all 57 PVs in 15 patients (100%) with the average number of ablation lesions needed being 3.3 ± 0.5/PV. The total time for PFA delivery was noted to be less than 60 seconds per patient, translating to a catheter dwell time of 26 ± 4.3 minutes and an overall procedural time of 67 ± 10.5 minutes. Epicardial ablation with PFA was performed in a subset of six patients who were undergoing cardiac surgery for mitral (n = 3) or aortic valve (n = 3) or coronary artery bypass grafting (n = 1). Both the PVs and posterior LA were electrically isolated after two consecutive applications in six patients: the system failed to deliver appropriately in one patient due to technical problems. There were no adverse events in any of the patients at the 1-month follow-up. These promising acute results led to the subsequent first-in-human clinical trials (IMPULSE and PEFCAT), which by design required protocol-driven invasive second procedures to assess PV durability at the 3-month time point in follow-up, an important step given that it was a new energy source.[21]

These two clinical trials, IMPULSE and PEFCAT, evaluated the safety and effectiveness of catheter-based PFA in patients with paroxysmal AF using a subsequent-generation over-the-wire 12-F catheter (Farawave, Farapulse-Abbott, Inc., Menlo Park, CA; Fig. 17.1) and its custom generator that could deliver either biphasic or monophasic waveforms in a bipolar fashion (Farastar, Farapulse-Abbott, Inc.). The catheter has five splines, each containing four electrodes, and can be deployed in either a basket or flower petal configurations. The ablative energy was delivered from all electrodes with the third electrode on each spline being able to record electrograms as well. The catheter was also rotated between applications to ensure circumferential coverage. The ablation protocol underwent consecutive evolutionary modifications: from monophasic to biphasic pulses, and then stepwise optimization of the biphasic waveform, pulse sequence, and deployment strategies. Finally, a total of 81 patients underwent PVI and had their PV isolated acutely by monophasic (n = 15) or biphasic (n = 66) PFA with ~3 minutes of delivery/patient, skin-to-skin procedure time of 92.2 ± 27.4 minutes, and fluoroscopy time of 13.1 ± 7.6 minutes (Fig. 17.1). With successive waveform refinement, durability at 3 months continue to improve, and beyond a single procedure-related pericardial tamponade, there were no additional primary adverse events over the 120-day median follow-up, inclusive of stroke, phrenic nerve injury, PV stenosis, and esophageal injury.

Recently this experience was updated and the authors reported on a total of 121 patients with 1-year outcomes (a combination of three trials: IMPULSE, PEFCAT, and PEFCAT II).[22] Acute PVI was again achieved in 100% of PVs with PFA alone. There was no evidence of (1) waveform discontinuities suggestive of "arcing," (2) ventricular tachyarrhythmias, or (3) significant repolarization abnormalities on 12-lead electrocardiography. Monophasic and biphasic PFA waveforms were used in the first 15 and subsequent 106 patients (57 patients with the early biphasic waveforms or other delivery protocols and 49 subsequent patients with the optimized biphasic waveforms), respectively. All monophasic and the first biphasic PFA were performed under general anesthesia; the remaining 105 biphasic procedures used conscious sedation. Biphasic deliveries were well tolerated; mild degrees of muscle activation and transient cough were noted, but with adequate sedation, this did not result in disruption of energy delivery. PV remapping was performed in 110 patients at 93.0 ± 30.1 days and demonstrated durable PVI in 84.8% of PVs (64.5% of patients) for the entire cohort, and in 96.0% of PVs (84.1% of patients) who were treated with the optimized biphasic energy PFA waveform. In addition, this study also suggested that the use of intracardiac echocardiography likely led to improved PVI durability (from 91.8% to 98.2% [$P = .022$]) in the optimized waveform

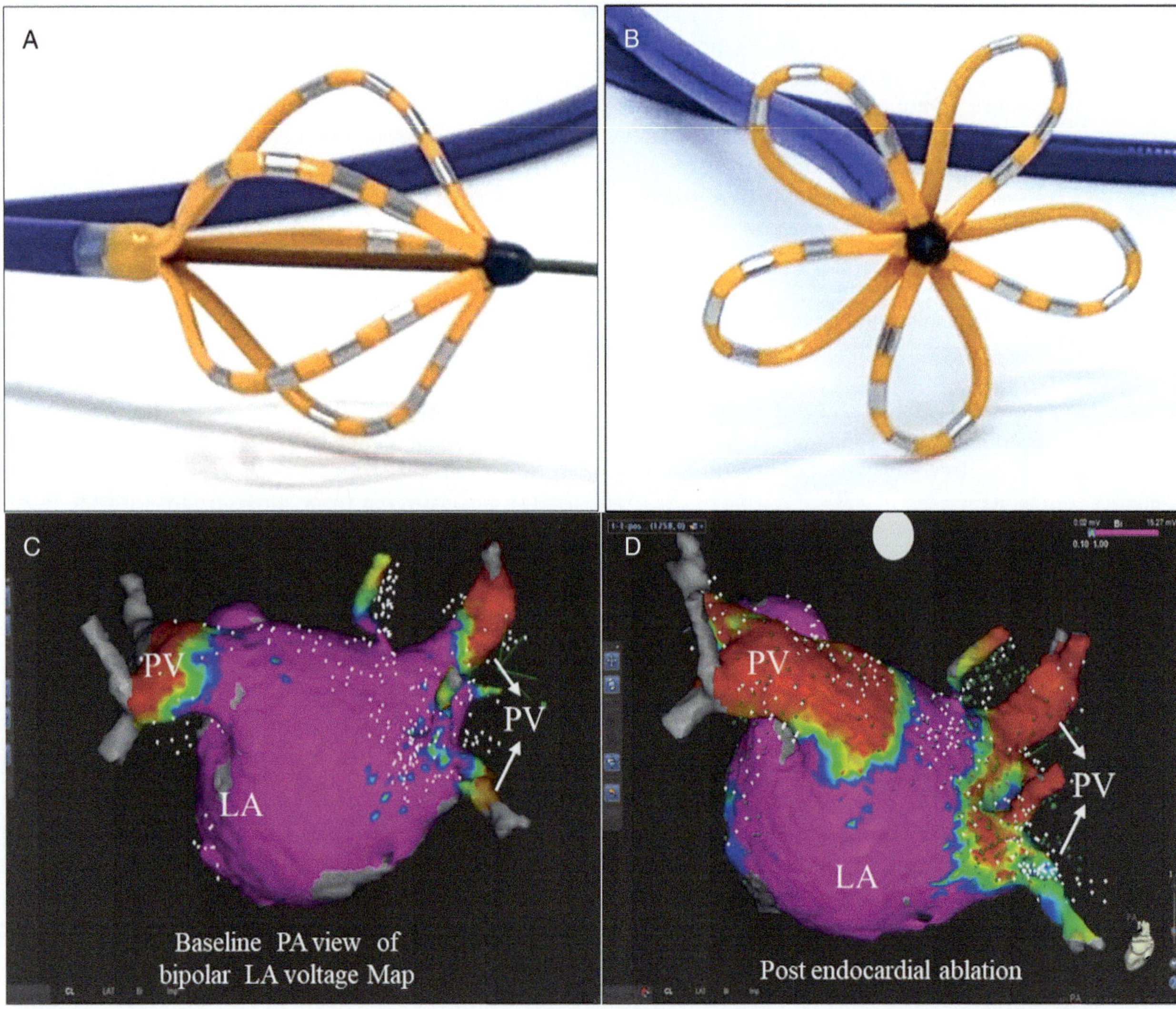

Fig. 17.1 The PFA catheter is shown over a guidewire with its splines in either the basket deployment pose (A) or the flower petal deployment pose (B). Posterior LA views of baseline voltage map (C) and post-ablation map (D). At baseline, the electrical activity was noted at the PV ostia; the low voltage observed distally in the PVs is normal. After endocardial ablation (D), the voltage amplitudes are diminished in the PVs. (Adapted from Reddy VY, Koruth J, Jais P, et al. Ablation of atrial fibrillation with pulsed electric fields: an ultra-rapid, tissue-selective modality for cardiac ablation. *JACC Clin Electrophysiol*. 2018;4(8):987–995.)

cohort. Primary adverse events occurred in 2.5% of patients (two pericardial effusions or tamponade, one hematoma); in addition, there was one transient ischemic attack. Importantly, there were no cases of atrioesophageal fistula, stroke, PV stenosis >70%, or phrenic nerve injury. Delayed enhancement magnetic resonance imaging revealed that the esophagus was unaffected.[23]

The 1-year Kaplan-Meier estimates for freedom from any atrial arrhythmia for the entire cohort and for the optimized biphasic energy PFA waveform cohort were 78.5 ± 3.8% and 84.5 ± 5.4%, respectively. The data beyond 1-year follow-up were available for 112 of 121 patients, with follow-up of 1049 ± 205 days.[24] Patients had no long-term ablation-related adverse events, including no deaths (1 patient had a brain tumor treated with radiation). Long-term efficacy data was available for 81 of 121 patients, with follow-up of up to 1116 ± 193 days. Repeat catheter ablation after the 1-year time point was performed on 10 of 78 (12.8%) patients. The mean time to reablation was 934 ± 269 days. Of these 10 patients, 3 had initially received the optimized PFA waveform at the index procedure—all PVs had remained isolated at both the protocol-mandated remapping procedure and at the late reablation procedure. The remaining seven patients had initially received their index PVI procedures with earlier versions of the PFA waveforms. Data at reablation was available for six of the seven patients: one patient had two PVs reconnected, three patients had one PV reconnected, and two patients had a durable PVI.

Adjunctive ablation beyond PVI using this single-shot device has also been performed: an issue relevant for the non–PV-based substrate that has been implicated in persistent AF. A single-arm study of 25 patients with persistent AF (PersAFOne: Pulsed Fields for Persistent Atrial Fibrillation) was performed to evaluate PFA using the above system for both PVI and left atrial posterior wall (LAPW) isolation.[25] In this report, acute

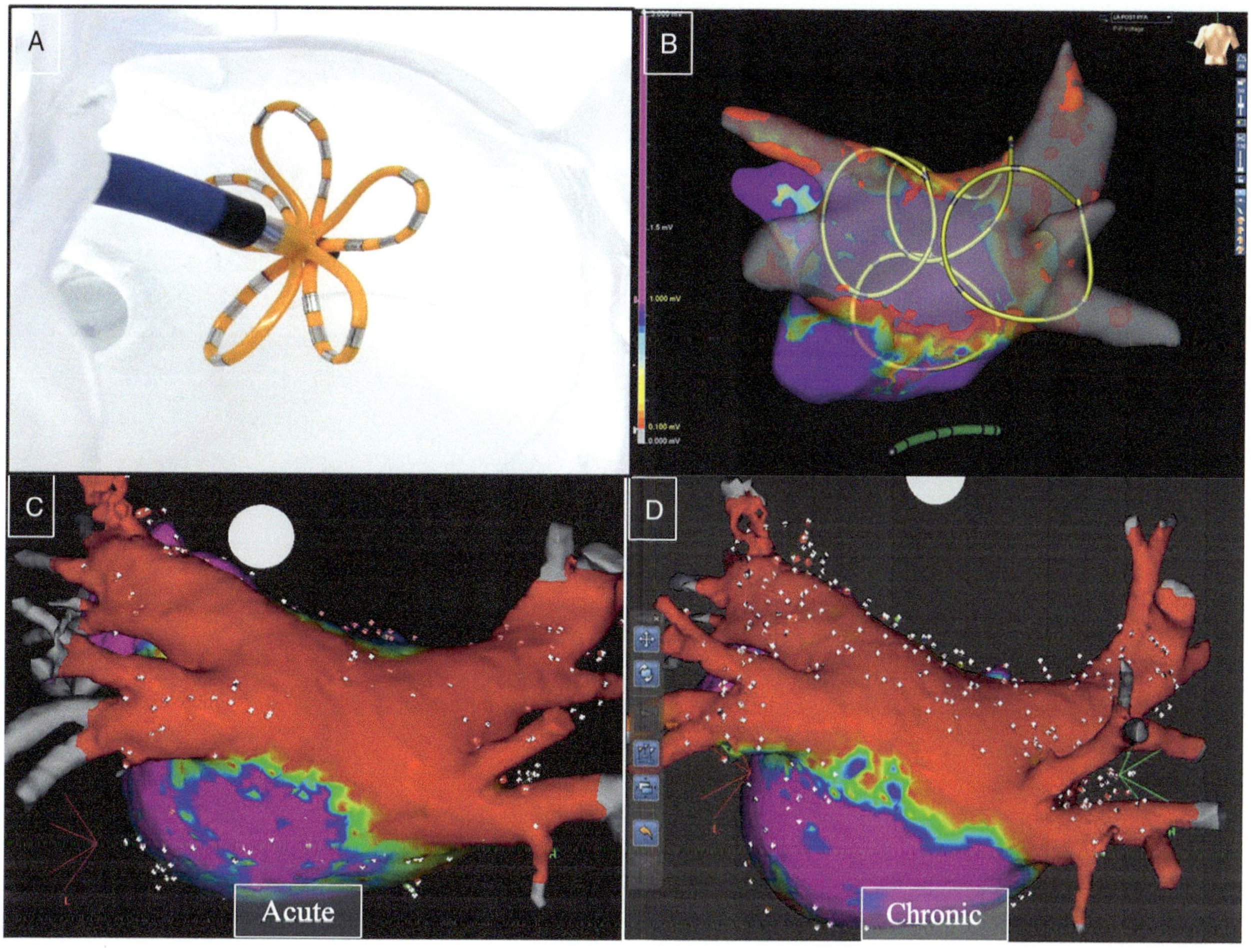

Fig. 17.2 (A) Demonstrative image shows the configuration of PFA catheter when it attaches the left atrial posterior wall. (B) Electroanatomical mapping demonstrates the 4 PVs and the left atrial posterior wall after PFA (gray indicates low voltage, <0.1 mV; purple indicates preserved voltage, >0.5 mV). Four circular renditions of the catheter catalog four discrete, overlapping positions of the PFA catheter in the flower pose during left atrial posterior wall isolation. Electroanatomical maps of immediately postablation (C) and follow-up (D) in the same patient, created by CARTO mapping system. The low-voltage area of follow-up is nearly identical to baseline. (Adapted from Reddy VY, Anic A, Koruth J, et al. Pulsed field ablation in patients with persistent atrial fibrillation. *J Am Coll Cardiol.* 2020;76(9):1068–1080.)

PVI (96 of 96 PVs) and LAPW ablation (24 of 24 patients) was acutely successful in all cases. The median time for PVI and LAPW isolation was 22 minutes and 10 minutes, respectively. In addition, a focal PFA catheter (Faraflex, Farapulse, Inc.) was also used for cavotricuspid isthmus (CTI) ablation and was able to achieve block in 13 of 13 patients with a median time of 9 minutes. Postprocedure esophagogastroduodenoscopy and repeat cardiac computed tomography revealed no mucosal lesions or PV narrowing, respectively. Invasive remapping demonstrated durable isolation (defined by entrance block) in 82 of 85 PVs (96%) and 21 of 21 LAPWs (100%) treated with the pentaspline catheter (Fig. 17.2). In three patients, there was localized scar regression of the LAPW ablation, albeit without conduction breakthrough. This study has extended the potential role of PFA to non-PV structures by showing rapid and efficient LAPW isolation.

Since its approval in Europe in March 2021, several single-center studies investigating its safety, and short-term outcomes have been published.[26–29] MANIFEST-PF was conducted to survey the performance of this system in an unselected patient population in routine clinical practice in Europe.[30] This retrospective survey included all 24 clinical centers using the pentaspline PFA catheter after its regulatory approval, including all patients treated at those centers since approval. With an average of 73 patients treated per center (range 7–291), the full cohort included 1758 patients: mean age was 61.6 years (range 19–92), and 34.2% were female. This was the first ablation procedure for 93.5% of patients. The type of AF treated was paroxysmal (57.5%), persistent (35.2%), or long-standing persistent (3.9%) with a subset of patients classified as repeat AF ablation or other LA flutters (2.9%). Most procedures were successful in 99.9% (range 98.9–100%). The mean procedure time was 65 minutes (range 38–215). There were no esophageal complications, symptomatic PV stenosis, or phrenic nerve injuries persisting past hospital discharge. Major complications (1.6%) were pericardial tamponade (0.97%) and stroke (0.4%); one stroke resulted in death (0.06%). Minor complications (3.9%) were primarily vascular (3.3%) but also included transient phrenic nerve paresis

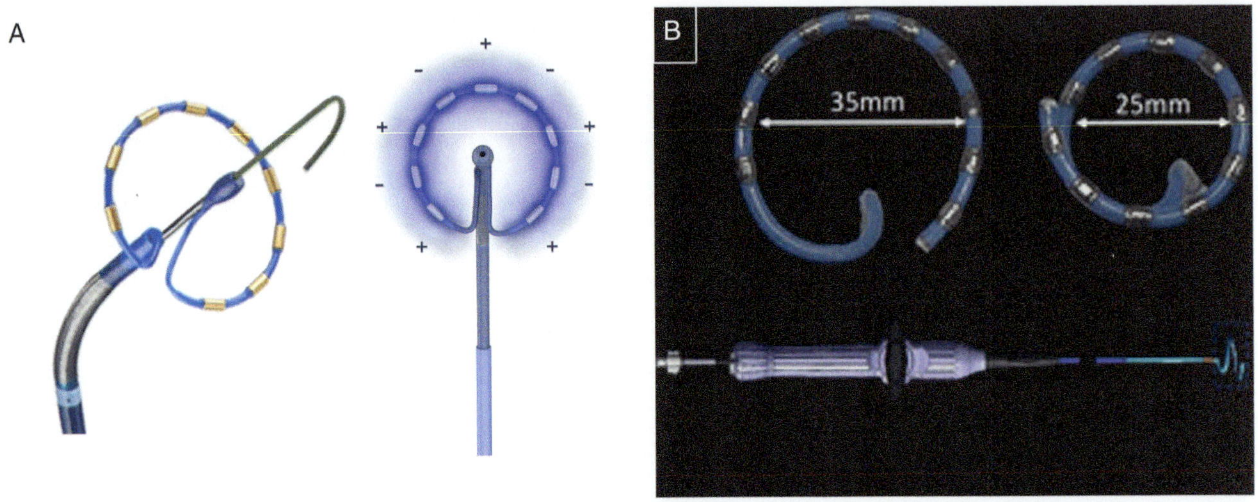

Fig. 17.3 (A) PFA catheter with an array of nine gold circular electrodes (electrode length, 3 mm; 20° forward-tilted array with diameter of 25 mm; 9F shaft). (B) A circular multielectrode catheter with variable expansion ranging from 25 to 35 mm. It includes 10 electrodes capable of PFA in bipolar configuration. A magnetic sensor allows visualization by the electroanatomical mapping system. (Adapted from Verma A, Boersma L, Haines DE, et al. First-in-human experience and acute procedural outcomes using a novel pulsed field ablation system: the PULSED AF Pilot Trial. *Circ Arrhythm Electrophysiol.* 2022;15(1):e010168, and Yavin H, Brem E, Zilberman I, et al. Circular multielectrode pulsed field ablation catheter lasso pulsed field ablation: lesion characteristics, durability, and effect on neighboring structures. *Circ Arrhythm Electrophysiol.* 2021;14(2):e009229.)

(0.46%) and TIA (0.11%). Rare complications included coronary artery spasm, hemoptysis, and dry cough persistent for 6 weeks (n = 1; 0.06% each).

There are currently two undergoing randomized controlled trials (ADVENT and BEAT-AF) in the US and Europe, respectively, that will further assess the safety and efficacy of PFA using this system and will be very important reports whose results will confirm or refute what has been reported on this technology thus far.

Several other single-shot PFA technologies are in development and evaluation. We briefly describe a few such catheters for which clinical data have been reported recently. PULSED AF (Pulsed Field Ablation to Irreversibly Electroporate Tissue and Treat AF) was a nonrandomized, prospective, multicenter, global, premarket clinical study that evaluated the feasibility and efficacy of PVI using a circular multielectrode array catheter (PulseSelect; Medtronic, Inc.; Fig. 17.3).[31] The PF generator delivers a biphasic, bipolar waveform (500–1500 V) through a 25-mm, 20° forward tilted array that mounts nine gold electrodes (9-F shaft and 25-mm diameter). Each electrode is 3 mm in length and capable of recording as well as pacing. Investigators described that acute electrical isolation was achieved in 100% of PVs (n = 152) in the 38 patients with a skin-to-skin procedure time of 160 ± 91 minutes, LA dwell time of 82 ± 35 minutes, and fluoroscopy time of 28 ± 9 minutes. An average of 8.2 ± 4.2 energy applications were delivered around each of the PVs. No serious adverse events related to the PFA system were observed in any patients out to 30 days postprocedure, but there were no specific assessments performed (esophageal, PV, or brain MRI imaging/assessment).

Another technology that is currently being evaluated is a 7.5-F bidirectional, variable circular catheter (Biosense Webster, Diamond Bar, CA; Fig. 17.3) that is capable of mapping as well as ablation. A clinical study (INSPIRE, Treatment of Paroxysmal Atrial Fibrillation by Pulsed Field Ablation System with Irreversible Electroporation [IRE]) is currently evaluating this catheter as well as its multichannel generator that delivers bipolar and biphasic PFA. The catheter is positioned at the venous ostia/antral regions and prescriptive pulsing regimens are followed.

Another combined mapping and PF ablation catheter presently undergoing evaluation is a multielectrode spherical array that consists of 16 flat ribs with 122 gold-plated electrodes (Globe, Kardium Inc, Burnaby, BC, Canada; Fig. 17.4). Its electrodes have multiple functions; in addition to ablation, each electrode can record electrograms and pace and measure current, temperature, and tissue contact. Electrograms and maps of measured voltage, temperature, and tissue contact can be reviewed in real time during a procedure and are stored to enable full procedure replay. Each electrode is capable of delivering PF energy in bipolar, biphasic fashion using up to 64 electrodes simultaneously. A dual-generator design allows for switching between PF and RF (temperature-controlled) energies without having to remove the catheter/switch cables, thereby allowing utilization of a single electroanatomical map. The array's electrodes are located on flexible electronic circuits that are laminated onto thin, rounded stainless steel ribs. The catheter is 16 F and advanced through a custom deflectable sheath into the LA. The coiled ribs are fanned open, forming a spherical array with a diameter of 30 mm. First-in-man feasibility and safety assessments have been completed and larger studies are being planned.

Pulmonary Vein Isolation With Focal PFA Catheters

Although single-shot designs have simpler workflow approaches to achieving PVI, focal catheters capable of delivering PFA may

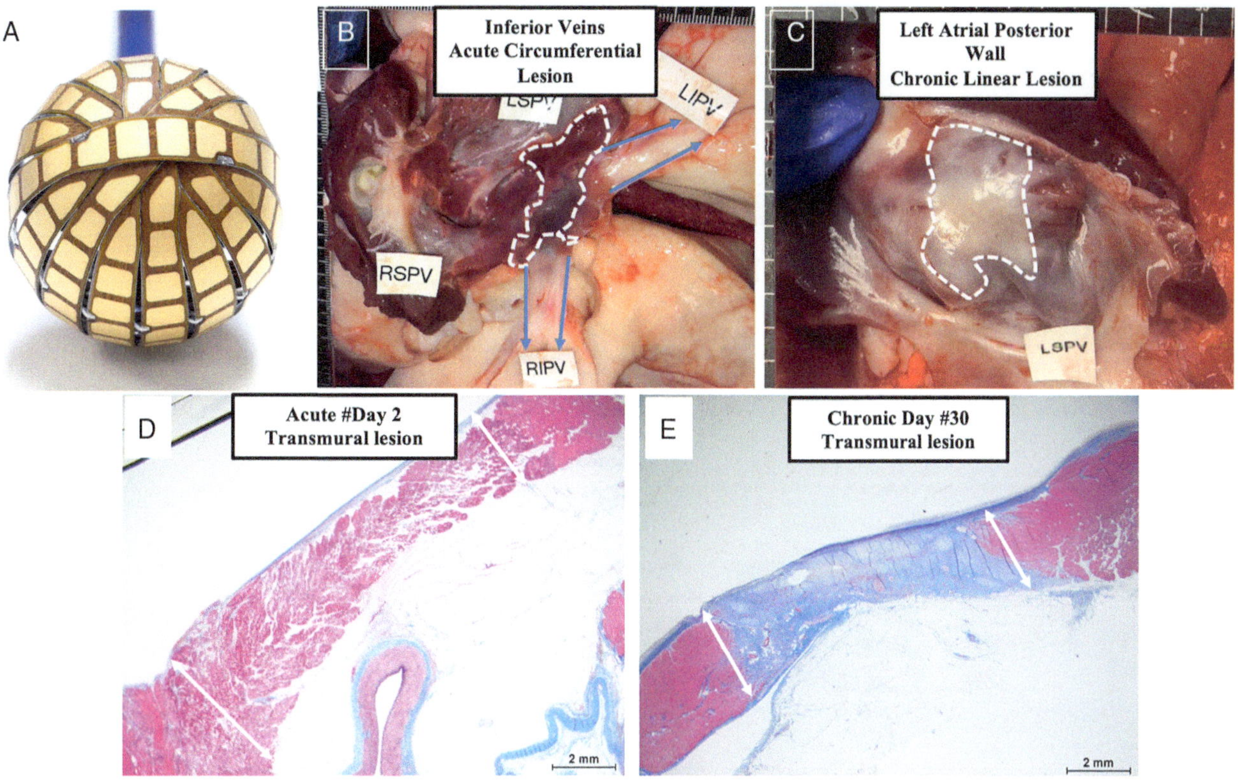

Fig 17.4 (A) Multielectrode array with 122 gold-plated electrodes. (B) Inferior veins subacute circumferential lesion with wide confluent band. (C) Appearance of PF lesion at the left atrial posterior wall in chronic phase. (D) Transmural PF lesion at 2 days with cardiomyocytes at varying stages of necrosis, edema, and variable degree of hemorrhage. (E) Transmural PF lesion at 30 days replaced with fibrous connective tissue.

be advantageous given their flexibility in delivering diverse lesion sets. In addition, focal catheters can be used for several non-PV ablation procedures in both the atrium and ventricles. Recently, a 7.5-F catheter with a compressible spheroid-shaped 9-mm-diameter lattice tip with nine minielectrodes and surface thermocouples was introduced (Sphere-9; Affera, Inc., Newton, MA). This catheter can deliver either PF or RF using custom generators (HexaGen and HexaPulse, Affera, Inc.) and is linked to an electroanatomical mapping system (Hexamap, Affera, Inc.) using a magnetic sensor within the lattice tip (Fig. 17.5). Catheter–tissue contact is assessed by continuously evaluating the impedance between each minielectrode and center electrode. Voltage and activation maps can be created simultaneously with anatomy acquisition. Each minielectrode incorporates a temperature sensor for temperature-controlled saline-irrigated RFA from the entire conductive lattice tip (the typical setting is 3–7 seconds with a target surface temperature of 73–75°C). PFA is delivered in a monopolar fashion from the entire lattice tip (to a grounding electrode) using a biphasic waveform that consisted of a train of microsecond-scale pulses delivered over 3–5 seconds, with total current delivery between 24 and 32 amperes.

In a three-center, single-arm, first-in-human trial, the safety and feasibility of this focal RF and PF system were assessed.[32] Toggling between energy sources, point-by-point PV encirclement was performed using biphasic PFA posteriorly and either temperature-controlled irrigated RFA (RF/PF strategy) or PFA anteriorly (PF/PF strategy) (Fig. 17.6). The 76-patient cohort included 55 paroxysmal and 21 persistent AF patients undergoing either RF/PF (n = 40) or PF/PF (n = 36). Acute electrical PVI was achieved in all 152 of 152 ipsilateral PV pairs. The therapy duration time (transpiring from first to last lesion) was 22.6 ± 8.3 min/patient with a mean of 50.1 RF/PF lesions/patient. Linear lesions were also created using either PFA or RFA across 14 mitral (4 RF only/2 combined with RF and PF/8 PF only), 34 left atrium roof (12 RF only/22 PF only), and 44 cavotricuspid isthmus (36 RF only/8 PF only) lines, with therapy duration times of 5.1 ± 3.5, 1.8 ± 2.3, and 2.4 ± 2.1 min/patient, respectively. Acute bidirectional block across the lines was obtained in 13/14 mitral isthmus, 34/34 roof, and 44/44 cavotricuspid isthmus lines successfully with the lattice tip catheter alone. Overall, the system successfully alternated between PF and RF during the procedure; there were no perceptible differences in electrogram reduction and catheter/ map behavior between modalities.

There were no instances of pericardial tamponade, phrenic nerve paralysis, PV stenosis, stroke, atrioesophageal fistula, or death. Postprocedure esophagogastroduodenoscopy (in 60 patients at 1.6 ± 1.1 days) revealed no esophageal injury in the PF/PF cases (0 of 24; 0%) and only minor mucosal thermal injury in 2 of 36 (5.6%) RF/PF cases, thought to be due to inadvertent posterior delivery of RF energy. Postprocedure brain MRIs were performed in 51 of 76 (67%) patients at 1.2 ± 0.6 days, revealing silent cerebral events (DWI-positive/FLAIR-negative) and silent cerebral lesions (DWI-positive/FLAIR-positive) in 5 (9.8%) and 3 (5.9%) of 51 patients, respectively. An

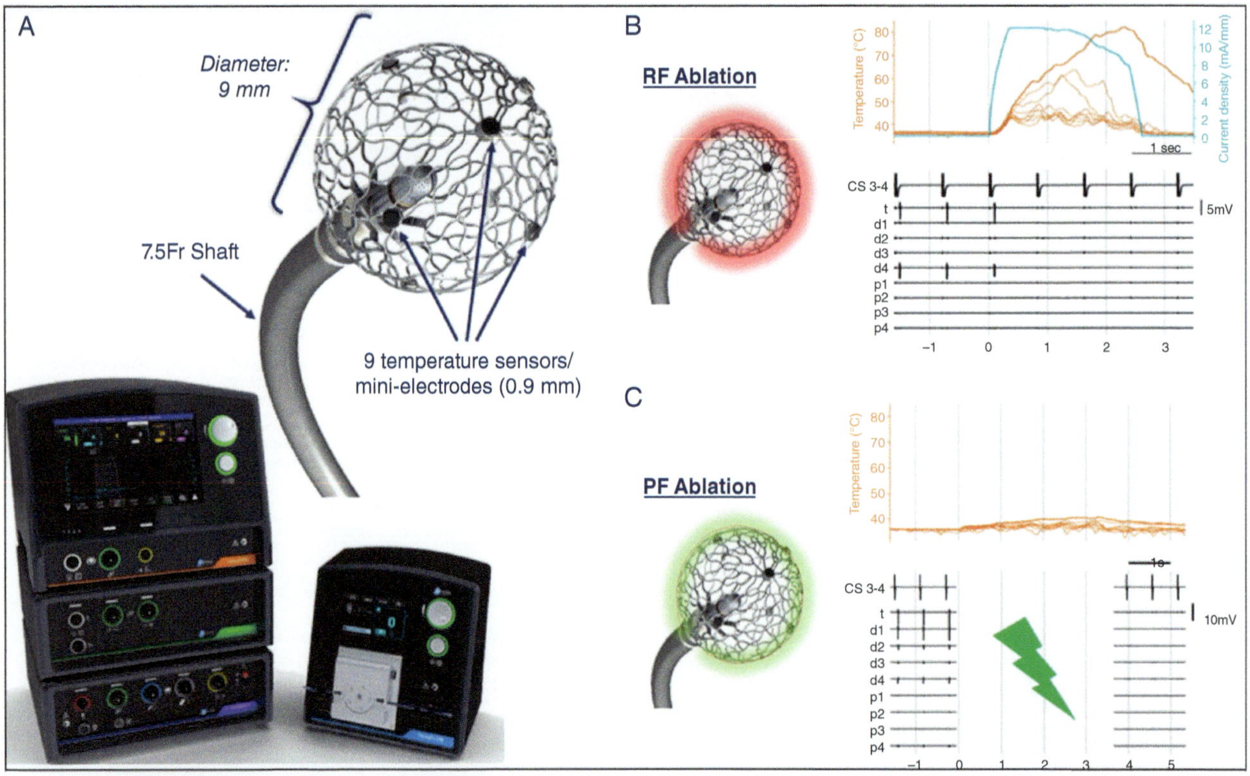

Fig. 17.5 (A) The lattice catheter and radiofrequency/pulsed field (RF/PF) ablation system. The system includes the lattice-tip catheter, an integrated mapping system, high-current RF and PF generators, and an irrigation pump. The expanded lattice electrode (diameter 9 mm) contains nine minielectrodes with embedded thermocouples. (B) RF energy emanates from the entire lattice framework to create a uniform current cloud, and the generator uses a temperature-controlled mode to modulate current output based on the hottest thermocouple. (C) Alternatively, the system can toggle to deliver PF energy instead. During PFA, lasting 3–5 seconds, there is minimal temperature elevation observed on the thermocouples. (Adapted from Reddy VY, Anter E, Rackauskas G, et al. Lattice-tip focal ablation catheter that toggles between radiofrequency and pulsed field energy to treat atrial fibrillation: a first-in-human trial. *Circ Arrhythm Electrophysiol.* 2020;13(6):e008718.)

ongoing randomized study evaluating this catheter against RF ablation should provide additional insights into the efficacy and safety of this approach.

PFA and Their Effect on Ganglionated Plexi

The GPs are part of the intrinsic cardiac autonomic nervous system (ANS) and are located primarily in the epicardium of the heart, particularly in the atria.[33] Given the importance of their contribution to both initiation and maintenance of AF, ablative modification of the GPs has been long considered as an approach to improve outcomes of AF ablation.[34–36] Compared to the standard thermal ablation, PFA appears to less effectively ablate GPs, possibly due to its tissue selectivity despite the frequent occurrence of GP stimulation during the pulse train. To determine whether PFA has a different effect than thermal ablation on resting heart rates after ablation, patients presenting in sinus rhythm after either (1) PFA (n = 20) using a pentaspline PFA catheter, (2) RFA (n = 20) using an irrigated RF balloon catheter, or (3) cryoballoon ablation were compared in recent report.[37] Given that heart rate (HR) and HR variability have been reported as indicators of autonomical remodeling after GP ablation, preablation and 3-month ECGs were also collected to assess the HR.[38] In contrast to RFA or cryoablation, PFA did not demonstrate an increase in HR at 3-month follow-up. Similarly, another report by Stojadinović et al. described less reduction of parasympathetic innervation after PFA compared to RFA by using extracardiac high-frequency stimulation.[39] They enrolled 31 AF patients who underwent PVI either using a lattice-tip PF catheter (n = 18) or a standard RF irrigation catheter (n = 13) to compare their impacts on the vagal innervation of the sinoatrial node and AV node. They demonstrated that PF-treated patients had less reduction of responsiveness of both sinus and AV nodes to vagal stimulation compared to RF-treated patients.

A separate study evaluating the acute effect of epicardial PFA on the GPs by measuring atrial effective refractory period (AERP) has also been recently reported.[40] Atrial GPs were ablated in 19 patients undergoing elective open-chest CABG surgery, using a monopolar, monophasic PFA system (AtriAN Medical LLC). An average AERP extension of 21% was obtained from 13 valid pre- and post-ablation datasets (changed from 233 ± 51 ms to 260 ± 55 ms; $P < .01$) after ablating GPs in the oblique, right superior, transverse, left superior, and ligament of Marshall. Extension of AERP as shown in this report can potentially reduce AF recurrences and further longer-term studies are needed.

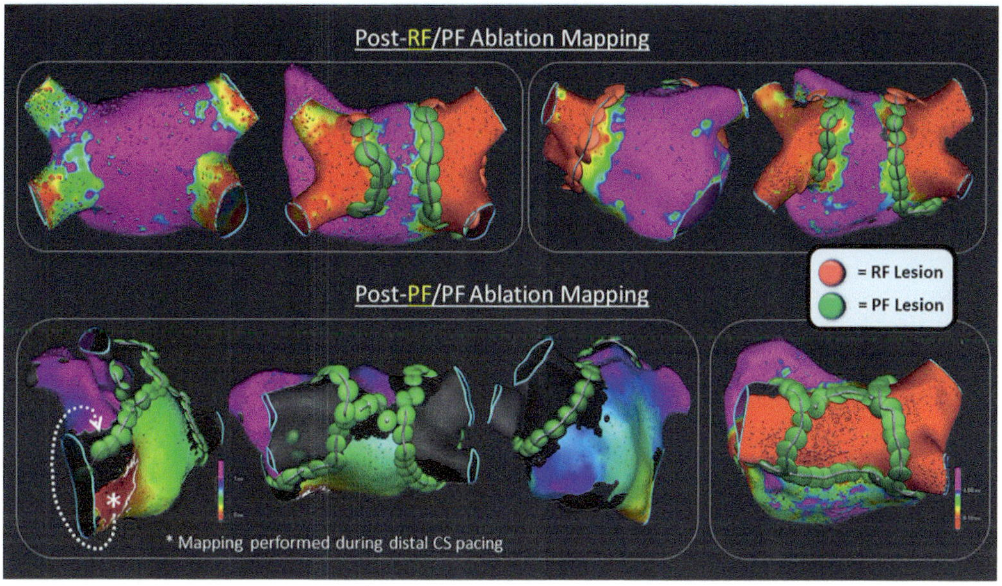

Fig. 17.6 Atrial fibrillation ablation using a radiofrequency/pulsed field (RF/PF) or PF/PF strategy. Shown are various examples of AF ablation using either an RF/PF (*above*) or a purely PF/PF (*below*) strategy. In addition to extraostial PVI, the *bottom-left* images also depict completed mitral isthmus and left atrial roof lines, whereas the *bottom-right* image shows a left atrial posterior box lesion set. *CS,* Coronary sinus. (Adapted from Reddy VY, Anter E, Rackauskas G, et al. Lattice-tip focal ablation catheter that toggles between radiofrequency and pulsed field energy to treat atrial fibrillation: a first-in-human trial. *Circ Arrhythm Electrophysiol.* 2020;13(6):e008718.)

Level of Pulmonary Vein Isolation with Single-Shot PFA Catheters

In contrast to thermal energy approaches for AF ablation, PFA appears to be less dependent on forceful tissue contact although electrode tissue proximity is known to be important for deep lesions.[41] This unique characteristic of PFA allows for easier isolation of PVs even when anatomical variants exist.[25] Since wide-area PV antral ablation is thought to result in improved AF ablation outcomes, circumferential PVI typically involves substantial antral ablation.[42] Balloon ablation catheters can create antral lesions but are highly reliant on tissue contactof left atrial and PV anatomy.[43,44] Focal RFA catheters can target any level of isolation as per the operator's desire, but are frustrated by the time required and the challenge of making multiple contiguous lesions.[45] To assess the level of isolation after PFA, we compared the level of electrical isolation after PFA (n = 20, pentaspline catheter, Farapulse) versus thermal ablation (n=39: 29 RFA, 6 cryoballoon, and 4 visually guided laser balloons), for patients with durable PVI.[46] This study demonstrated that there was no significant difference between the PFA and thermal ablation cohorts for both veins and the nonablated posterior wall. Another interesting finding from this study was that notch-like normal voltage areas were seen at the posterior aspect of the carina in the cryo and laser balloon subcohort, but not in the PFA and RFA cohorts (Fig. 17.7). Those notch-like normal voltage areas appeared to reflect the design of the balloon technologies. Gunawardene et al. also evaluated the extent of lesions immediately after PVI performed with the Farapulse system with ultra-high-density mapping and reported similar findings.[47]

While the goal of PFA is irreversible injury, depending on the device design and pulse parameters used by a given system, cell permeability with PFA also has the potential to be reversible.[48] That is, cells may survive because of the reestablishment of cell membrane integrity and electrical homeostasis. Thus, beyond each PFA lesion's zone of irreversible electroporation and cell death, there may be a surrounding zone of reversible electroporation with acute cell injury that recovers with time. Accordingly, using a pentaspline PF catheter, the level of electrical PVI that is observed acutely after PFA was assessed acutely and chronically to establish if it regressed over time.[49] This study revealed there was no significant difference in either left- and right-sided PV antral isolation areas or nonablated posterior wall area when comparing immediately post-PFA and ~3 months later. However, this analysis should be performed with each PFA technology and waveform, as this lack of regression may not be true for all.

PULMONARY VEIN ISOLATION WITH LASER BALLOON

Basic Principles

The ability of laser energy to be highly focused permits high-power density to be administered to the target tissue. Diode lasers use semiconductors and emit wavelengths between 700 and 1500 nm (near-infrared) whereas solid lasers are neodymium-doped yttrium–aluminum–garnet (Nd–YAG) and holmium and emit energy in the infrared spectrum of 1064–2000 nm.[50–54] Tissue ablation is thermal in nature, and this effect is a function of the laser power density in tissue. During tissue irradiation, light is scattered and absorbed to an extent that depends on beam diameter and the optical properties of the tissue. The energy is selectively absorbed by tissue to a depth of several

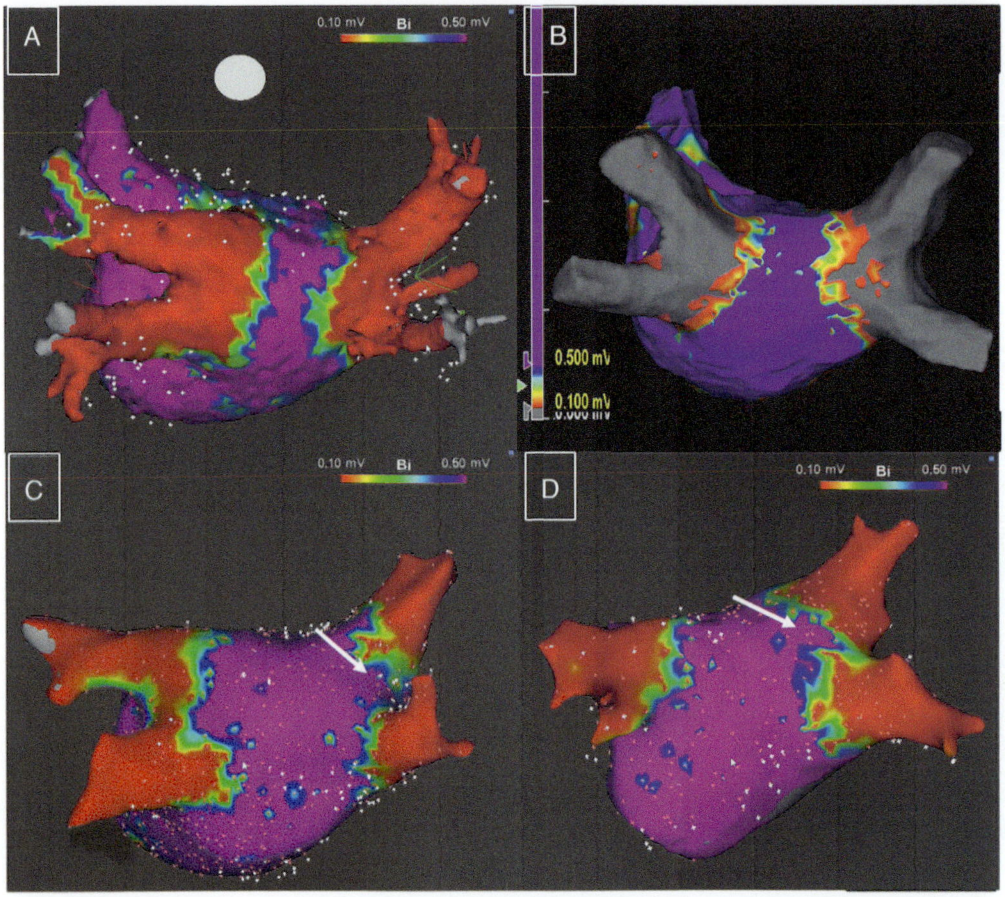

Fig. 17.7 Representative voltage maps of chronic post pulmonary vein isolation with different modalities. (A) Pulsed field ablation. (B) Radiofrequency ablation. (C) Cryoballoon ablation. (D) Visually guided laser balloon. In the balloon subcohorts, there were notch-like areas of normal voltage at the carinal areas (*white arrows*). (Adapted from Kawamura I, Neuzil P, Shivamurthy P, et al. How does the level of pulmonary venous isolation compare between pulsed field ablation and thermal energy ablation (radiofrequency, cryo, or laser)? *Europace*. 2021;23(11):1757–1766.)

millimeters and produces heating of a volume of tissue.[55] Tissue heating produces focal myocardial tissue ablation by vaporization and coagulation necrosis. The volume of coagulated tissue can vary depending on laser energy absorption (transfer ratio) in the irradiated tissue.[56] Tissue temperatures in excess of 100°C typically cause tissue vaporization, whereas those in the range of 42°C–65°C cause tissue damage from protein denaturation.[57,58] The power of the laser decreases with distance within the tissue in an exponential manner. The rate of decay is multifactorial and involves laser beam absorption, scatter, as well as the distance from the laser source.[59] Tissue injury may progress beyond the target site if the laser exposure time surpasses the thermal relaxation time of the target tissue. The distribution of spread follows a Gaussian relationship and is expected to be focal.[60] Ultimately, lesion dimensions were determined by the total energy dose, medium used, and tissue characteristics (also see Chapter 3).

Laser Balloon Catheter Ablation

Although a number of catheter designs have been used for laser ablation,[61–64] the prospect of performing AF ablation led to the design of a laser balloon catheter capable of projecting forward a circumferential ring of laser energy (980 nm).[52,65–67] The balloon design has a collapsible profile and was filled with a mixture of radiographic contrast agent and deuterium oxide (D_2O). D_2O was used to minimize self-heating of the balloon by shifting the absorption of wavelengths to greater than 980 nm. The light is transferred from the fiberoptic core with the use of a modified glass fiber tip, through an optically transparent shaft in the balloon, and projected as either 90° or 150° arcs or a 360° ring application onto the distal balloon surface. The emitted light is then circumferentially delivered to the tissue in a uniform and continuous manner without gaps.[52,66,67] Laser energy is delivered via endoscopic visual guidance in regions where balloon contact with tissue created a bloodless environment; an aspect that is critical because lasing directly into blood increased the possibility of char formation.

Real-time endoscopic visualization was achieved using an endoscope positioned at the proximal end of the balloon. The first generation of the endoscopic laser balloon ablation catheter (ELBAC) came in one of the three noncompliant balloon sizes, namely 20, 25, and 30 mm. The second-generation system was designed as a compliant balloon with an adjustable diameter that permits greater circumferential contact and ablation using a single balloon dimension. Furthermore, a 30° adjustable aiming arc is manipulated (rotation and advancement/retraction) to allow the operator to better tailor energy delivery to regions of balloon/tissue contact—very similar to the spot ablation performed during standard point-by-point ablation.[68] A deflectable sheath allowed for left atrial navigation.

In an open-thoracotomy animal model of endocardial access we demonstrated electrical isolation of 19 of 27 PVs with the first-generation system after a single 360° ring application of photonic energy.[66] Complete PVI was achieved in five of the five PVs targeted. Results of pathologic examination revealed no PV stenosis, no pericardial damage, minor lung lesions without pleural perforation, minimal endothelial disruption, and, in the presence of adequate heparinization, no endocardial charring or adherent thrombus. Using a percutaneous technique, Lemery and coworkers also successfully delivered photonic energy to five of the five targeted PVs, with gross inspection revealing endocardial lesions at the ostium in four of the five PVs.[67] The first-generation ELBAC was used clinically in a multicenter experience with 30 paroxysmal AF patients.[69] Using the 20-, 25-, or 30-mm balloon, either the 90° or 150° arc was used to achieve PVI under endoscopic visual guidance. Acutely, 105 of 116 PVs (91%) were successfully isolated. The chronic (12 month) drug-free rate of freedom from AF after a single procedure was 60% (18 of 30 patients). There were no significant PV stenoses, but adverse events included one episode of cardiac tamponade, one stroke without residual defect, and one asymptomatic phrenic nerve palsy.[69] Although this provided the clinical proof-of-principle of performing AF ablation under endoscopic visualization, the ablation procedure proved laborious—the mean procedure time being 334 ± 112 minutes—largely because the 90° and 150° arcs proved relatively cumbersome to be positioned serially so as to achieve a fully encircling lesion set.

Accordingly, the second-generation laser balloon able to deliver the 30° arc/spot lesions was tested preclinically and clinically. An in vivo evaluation of visually guided ablation in acute and chronic porcine models was performed to assess the feasibility and reproducibility of achieving PVI.[70] PV conduction was assessed immediately and more than 30 minutes after ablation in 15 pigs. Chronic lesions in survival animals were remapped at 4 weeks in 10 pigs. In the acute study, 30 of 30 (100%) targeted PVs were electrically isolated, with 29 of 30 (97%) being isolated after placing only the initial circumferential lesion set. In the chronic animals, invasive electrical remapping at 4 weeks revealed that 8 of 10 (80%) PVs remained persistently isolated. The lesions were histologically circumferential in 120 of 120 (100%) PV sections and transmural in 116 of 120 (96.7%) PV sections (average transmurality 99.5%). No esophageal or PN injury was noted.[70] Another comparative preclinical study revealed that laser balloon ablation had a greater chronic isolation rate than standard RF ablation using an electroanatomical mapping system in a porcine model.[71]

Clinical use of the second-generation balloon was first evaluated in a single-center, open-label, nonrandomized trial of safety and efficacy of performing PVI in patients with drug-refractory paroxysmal AF.[70] All PVs were targeted in 27 patients, and successful PVI was achieved in 100% of the PVs after 1.3 attempts/PV–84% of the PVs (85 of 101) were isolated after the initial visually-guided lesion set. The mean fluoroscopy time was 17.3 ± 6.3 min/patient, the mean ablation time was 110.9 ± 29.6 minutes, and the total laser energy delivery time was 65.9 ± 14.9 minutes. To assess the durability of PVI, at 3 months after ablation, all patients were planned for a remapping procedure regardless of intervening symptoms. Of the 23 patients who ultimately agreed to a second procedure, 61 of 68 (90%) PVs continued to remain electrically isolated.[70] This indicated that visually guided point-by-point ablation using the ELBAC resulted in reliable, reproducible, and persistent PVI.

The generalizability was evaluated in a larger study conducted at three sites.[72] In 56 patients, 202 of 206 PVs (98%) were acutely isolated. Furthermore, at 105 ± 44 days post procedure, 52 patients returned for a protocol-mandated PV remapping procedure. At this time, 162 of 189 PVs (86%) remained isolated, translating to 32 of 52 patients (62%) with all PVs remaining isolated. On comparing the operators performing less than 10 versus 10 or more procedures, the durable PVI rate was 73% versus 89% ($P = .011$), respectively. Thus even very early in the learning curve, there was an extremely high rate of durable PVI. After two procedures and 12.0 ± 1.9 months of follow-up, the drug-free rate of freedom from AF was 71.2%. The system was further studied in a large multicenter experience including the first 200 paroxysmal AF patients treated with the laser balloon (33 operators, 15 centers).[73] With this laser balloon, 98.8% (95% confidence interval, 97.8–99.5%) of targeted PVs were isolated using a mean of 1.07 catheters/patient. Fluoroscopy and procedure times were 31 ± 21 and 200 ± 54 minutes, respectively, and these improved with operator experience. There were no instances of stroke, transient ischemic attack, atrioesophageal fistula, or significant PV stenosis. There was a 2% incidence of cardiac tamponade and a 2.5% incidence of PN palsy. At 12 months, the drug-free rate of freedom from atrial arrhythmias after one or two procedures was 60.2% (95% confidence interval, 52.7–67.4%).[73]

In addition to these initial studies with laser balloon-based PVI, a few more recent studies have clarified some of the strengths and limitations of this system. Bordignon and colleagues assessed the effects of low-dose (5.5–8.5 W) versus high-dose (>8.5 W) laser energy on acute and chronic success in 60 paroxysmal AF patients undergoing ablation.[74] After placing a single circular lesion set, acute PVI was achieved in 69% and 89% of the low- and high-dose groups, respectively ($P < .01$). After additional ablation, all PVs were isolated. Procedure time was also shorter in the high-dose group (128 ± 17 versus 154 ± 38 minutes; $P < 0.01$). Furthermore, after a median follow-up of 311 days (range 261–346 days), the chronic success rate was 60% and 83% in the low- and high-dose groups, respectively.

In another study from the same group, 140 paroxysmal AF patients were prospectively randomized (1:1) to PVI using either the laser balloon or cryoballoon systems.[75] The rates of acute PVI (99.6% versus 98.9%, P = not significant), mean procedure times (136 ± 30 versus 144 ± 33 minutes, $P = .13$), and mean fluoroscopy times (21 ± 9 versus. 15 ± 6 minutes, $P < .01$) were similar between the cryoballoon and laser balloon groups, respectively. At 12-month follow-up, 37% and 27% of patients in the cryoballoon and laser groups experienced AF recurrences

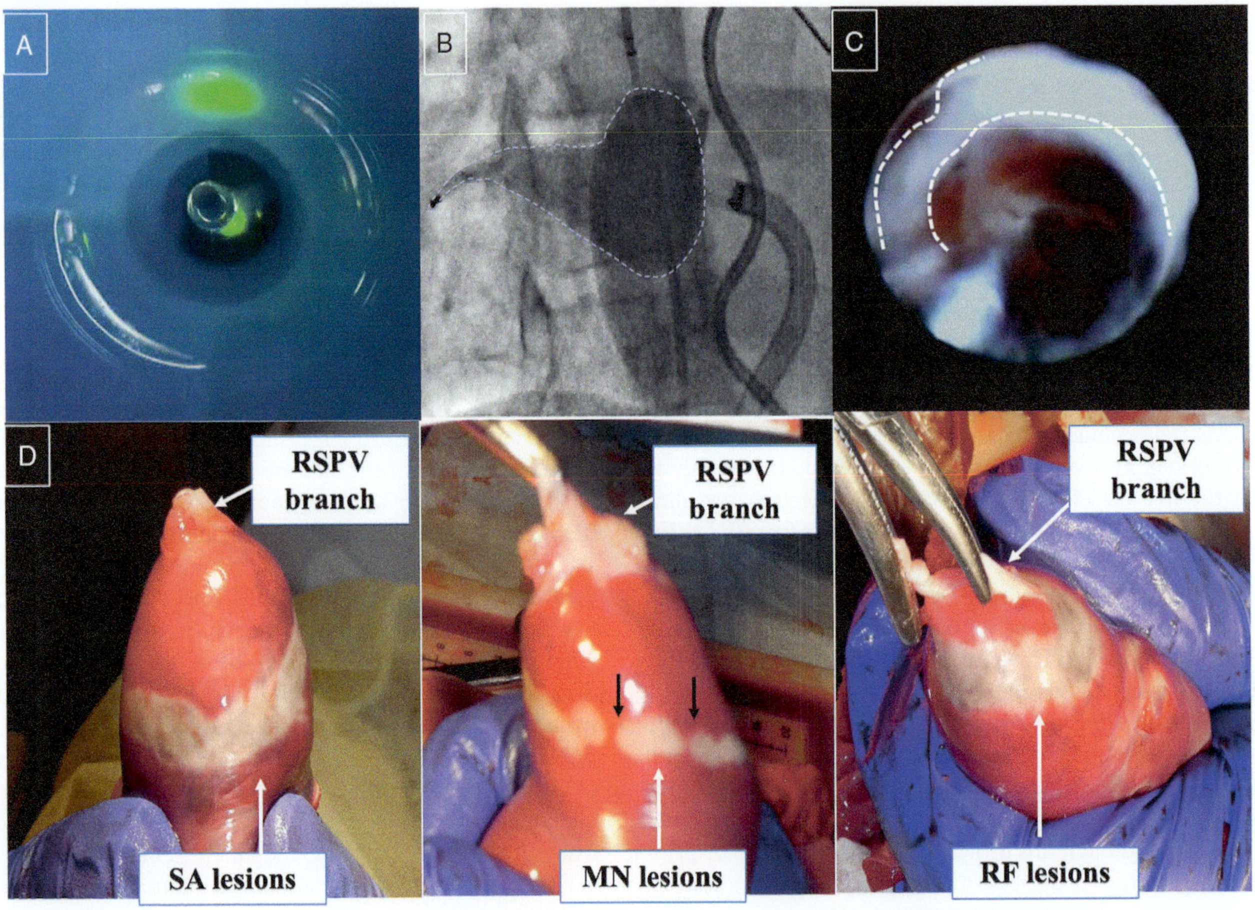

Fig. 17.8 (A) The appearance of endoscopic laser balloon ablation catheter. (B): Fluoroscopic image during left superior pulmonary vein isolation. (C) Demonstration of appearance of isolating lesion set made in semi-automatic mode. The *dotted lines* represent a single continuous lesion created in semiautomatic mode. (D) Gross necropsy views of the RSPV (the vein shown here has been everted with the endocardial surface on the outside). *Left to right,* Continuous lesion set with semiautomated (SA) mode, lesion with manual point-by-point (MN) mode with two endocardial lesion gaps (*white arrows*), and a continuous but more distally placed lesion with radiofrequency ablation (RF). (Adapted from Kuroki K, Reddy VY, Iwasawa J, et al. Pre-clinical evaluation of semi-automated laser ablation for pulmonary vein isolation: a comparative study. *J Cardiovasc Electrophysiol.* 2022. doi:10.1111/jce.15777 15777.)

(P = .18). Phrenic nerve palsies occurred in 5.7% and 4.2% of the cryoballoon and laser balloon patients, respectively.[75] This finding was replicated by the other investigators with a larger number of patients (cryoballoon ablation: n = 1720 and laser: n = 713) in a retrospective study. They reported that the rate of transient phrenic nerve palsy was significantly higher with cryoballoon ablation (3.0%, n = 45) than laser balloon (0.1%, n = 1, P = .004). The rate of persistent phrenic nerve palsy did not significantly differ between the two groups; however a higher rate phrenic palsy recovery was observed after 6 months in laser balloon compared with cryoballoon ablation.[76]

Finally, Wissner et al. compared the standard ELBAC approach of individual PVI (n = 18 patients) with a wide-area isolation approach of performing a single circumferential lesion set encompassing both ipsilateral PVs (n = 20 patients). While PVI was achieved in 97% of PVs using the standard approach, circumferential ipsilateral PVI was feasible in only 2/18 (11%) right PVs and 8/18 (44%) left PVs. Thus while the ELBAC is highly reliable in achieving durable individual PVI, to achieve wide-area isolation, additional improvements in the catheter design are necessary (principally a more deformable balloon able to achieve a greater degree of tissue contact).[77] Unlike the other single-shot device, ELBAC required the operator to rotate the laser arc to sequentially create a series of overlapping arc lesions similar to the approach used in point-by-point radiofrequency ablation. Although this technique allows the operator to tailor energy to different tissue (e.g., more energy anteriorly, and less to the thinner posterior left atrium), the overall procedure time for PVI can be substantial since each of these laser lesions take ~20 seconds (limited to 30°/application) with at least a 30% overlapping.

Accordingly, the third generation of the laser balloon (X3, Fig. 17.8) was introduced to improve ablation efficiency by using a more compliant balloon and a motorized system that rotates the laser arc continuously. The lesion generator is continuously moved around the PV ostium (either clockwise or counterclockwise) at a preset speed (2.25° per second) by an integrated motor. Our preclinical study demonstrated that semi-automated

ELBAC reduced catheter use time by ~50% compared to manual mode. In addition lesion transmurality and circumferentiality were similar between the semi-automated mode and manual point-by-point mode.[78] Gapless and uniform lesion formation by using the semi-automated mode was also demonstrated by another in vivo study.[79]

In a prospective, single-arm pivotal multicenter study, Schmidt et al. enrolled 60 patients and reported the semiautomated mode significantly decreased ablation time (77.3 ± 25.8 versus 173.8 ± 46.6 minutes; $P < .01$), procedural time (103.7 ± 32.3 versus 236.0 ± 52.8 minutes; $P < .01$), and fluoroscopy time (6.9 ± 3.5 versus 35.6 ± 18.2; $P < .01$), compared with the conventional point-by-point mode.[80] The investigators also reported that first-pass acute PVI was achieved in 225 of 228 (98.7%) of these PVs treated with the semiautomated mode, as compared with 206 of 225 PVs (91.6%) with the manual mode. Superior PVs with maximum ostial diameter <24 mm were reported to have high success rates with a single semi-automated mode application.[81] The 6-month and 12-month atrial fibrillation–free rates for X3 were reported as 89.5% and 71.9%, respectively.[80] In comparison with the older generation of ELBAC, X3 had a tendency to achieve durable PVI when assessed during second procedures among the patients with AF recurrence. Tohoku et al. observed that reduced energy application (5–7 W) was the independent factor to predict PV reconnections.[82]

The remaining tasks to advance the use of this technology are further improvements such as the need for a real-time recording system of intracardiac electrograms, a durably structured balloon, and improvement in instruments for visualizing tissue cauterization in a 360° panoramic view. With these and other improvements laser balloon has the potential to develop into an even more optimal device for PVI.[83]

SUMMARY

Pulmonary vein isolation has remained the most effective evidence-based strategy for atrial fibrillation ablation. Laser balloon ablation, in its more recent iteration, achieves rapid antral isolation that is enabled by the motorized movement of the laser arc and a conformable balloon that allows for better antral fit and wider antral lesions. Pulsed field ablation of the pulmonary veins, achieved either via a one-shot device or by focal catheter, represents the newest advance in our decades-long pursuit of durable pulmonary vein isolation. While several legacy energy sources have evolved to become efficient and significantly safer, PFA has started its journey with both these procedural aspects already in its favor. However, much is to be learned from real-world experiences, as PFA technologies are still in their early stages and have yet to be widely available across the world.

In order to improve PV durability, integration with 3D mapping, use of routine intracardiac echocardiography, contact assessment, etc. may play a role beside operator's experience. There remain certain unknowns with PFA, such as the impact of the lack of effective autonomic modulation resulting from sparing of ganglionated plexi. This has potential to limit its efficacy on AF control despite an increase in PVI durability; ongoing studies are needed to provide better insight. Finally, rare adverse events such as coronary spasm with potential for ischemic complications may surface with increasing frequency as newer catheters and sicker patients get exposed to PFA. One must at this time remain both excited and vigilant as we embark on yet another new chapter of pulmonary vein isolation.

REFERENCES

Please refer to the e-book for a complete list of references.

18

Catheter Ablation of Atrial Fibrillation Initiated by Non–Pulmonary Vein Triggers

Li-Wei Lo, Shih-Ann Chen

KEY POINTS

- The incidence of non–pulmonary vein (PV) triggers increases as the atrial fibrillation burden progresses from paroxysmal (10–28%) to nonparoxysmal atrial fibrillation (>50%) and is also prevalent during redo ablation procedures.
- Targeting the non-PV trigger is the Class IIa recommendation in atrial fibrillation ablation beyond pulmonary vein isolation.
- Identifying the non-PV triggers is challenging and can be localized by the P-wave morphology from standard 12-lead ECG, intracardiac electrogram activation sequence, and three-dimensional electroanatomical mapping.
- Accurate localization and mapping are important for non-PV trigger ablation. Possible locations of those triggers include superior vena cava, crista terminalis, right atrial appendage, Eustachian ridge, coronary sinus, tricuspid and mitral annuli, ligament of Marshall, interatrial septum, left atrial posterior wall and appendage, and others.
- A successful ablation usually involves targeting a specific site of origin. Empirical isolation of selected structures (superior vena cava, coronary sinus, and left atrial posterior wall) may be effective but requires more evidence to prove its benefit.

INTRODUCTION

Catheter ablation of atrial fibrillation (AF) has become an established therapy and has a potential to cure this most commonly encountered arrhythmia. It has been reported more than two decades ago that the pulmonary veins (PVs) are a major source of ectopy initiating AF.[1,2] In addition to this main origin, the literature demonstrated the importance of the non-PV (NPV) triggers initiating AF, including from the superior vena cava (SVC), left atrial (LA) free wall (LAFW), crista terminalis (CT), coronary sinus (CS), ligament of Marshall (LOM), left atrial appendage (LAA), and interatrial septum (IAS).[3–8] In our laboratory we found that the NPV triggers are more prevalent in female patients, dilated left atria, very late recurrence after index procedures, after multiple procedures, and with longer AF duration.[9–12] Those with NPV triggers initiating AF also had a worse ablation outcome and a higher recurrence rate.[11] With the development of high-density mapping from three-dimensional (3D) electroanatomical systems, it is now easier and more efficient to identify those NPV triggers. This chapter will highlight the catheter ablation of AF initiated by NPV triggers and summarize the electrophysiologic characteristics, mapping, and ablation strategies in this field.

ELECTROPHYSIOLOGIC CHARACTERISTICS AND INCIDENCE OF NPV TRIGGERS

The incidence of NPV triggers ranged from 10% to 28% in patients with paroxysmal AF and is higher (>50%) in patients with nonparoxysmal AF (Table 18.1).[3,11,13–23] The SVC and LAFW (including the LAA) are the two most common sites of NPV triggers, including 11.3% to 13% of patients with SVC triggers and 10.9% to 11.7% of patients with LAFW triggers.[3,9] In another study, CT was found to be the most common NPV trigger site (3.2%) in 342 patients, whereas the incidences of SVC and LAFW triggers were each 1%.[24] Arruda et al. found an incidence of 12% of SVC triggers in a study of 190 patients.[25] Nevertheless, the existence of NPV triggers should always be kept in mind during AF ablation and presents more often in patients with nonparoxysmal AF and during redo procedures. The different incidences reported in the literature might be secondary to the aggressiveness of the provocation test used. It is possible that the advanced atrial remodeling in patients with nonparoxysmal AF is an important mechanism that increases the incidence of the NPV triggers.[26]

PATHOPHYSIOLOGY OF AF TRIGGERS FROM NPV AREAS

From the viewpoint of histology, an embryonic sinus venosus capable of spontaneous depolarization has been found in specimens from junctional areas encountering different embryonic tissues such as the right atrial (RA)-SVC junction, CT, LOM, and CS ostium.[27,28] SVC cardiomyocytes have distinct action potentials and ionic current profiles that may be responsible for the arrhythmogenic activity of the SVC. The CT, which is an area exhibiting abnormal automaticity, anisotropy, and slow

TABLE 18.1 Summary of the Literature on the Incidences and Characteristics of NPV Triggers in AF Patients Receiving Catheter Ablations

Study Group	Total Patients, N	Patients with NPV, n (%)	Age, y	Males, n (%)	LA Size, mm	Mean Ectopy	NPV Distributions	Procedural Complication Rates, %	Follow-Up Duration, mon	AF Recurrence free rate
Lin et al.[3]	240 (all PAF)	68 (28%)	61 ± 13	43 (63%)	NA	1.1	LAPW (38%), SVC (37%), CT (3.7%), LOM (8.2%), CS ostium (1.4%), IAS (1.4%)	0	22 ± 11	63.2% (Without AAD)
Yamaguchi et al.[13]	75 (all PAF)	17 (23%)	62 ± 8	13 (76%)	37±5	1.1	LA roof (26%), LAPW (5%), LAAW (5%), LOM (5%), LAA (5%), SVC (26%), CT (5%), CS ostium (5%), IAS (11%)	NA	23 ± 10	76%
Rha et al.[14]	37 (PAF/NPAF 29/8) 31 induced AF	8 (25.8%)	NA	NA	NA	1	LAPW (50%), LAAW (21.4%), SVC (26.8%)	NA	NA	NA
Shah et al.[15]	160 (All PAF)	36 (24%)	NA	NA	NA	2.4	Outside PV ostia (46%), LA PW (35%), RA (6%), CS (4%), SVC (4%)	NA	8 ± 6	68% (Without AAD)
Valles et al.[16]	45 (PAF/NPAF 38/7) 39 induced AF	6 (15%)	NA	NA	NA	1	LAPW (17%), SVC (33%), CT (33%), CS (17%).	0	NA	NA
Hung et al.[11]	197 (All NPAF)	21 (20%) PerAF 42 (45%) LS PerAF	55 ± 10 (PerAF), 51 ± 10 (LS PerAF)	167 (85%)	40 ± 6 (PerAF), 44 ± 7 (LS PerAF)	NA	LAAW (24%), LOM (8%), SVC (24%), CT (17%), CS (17%), IAS (13%)	NA	28 ± 23	51% (PerAF), 27% (LS PerAF)
Kurotobi et al.[19]	214 (PAF/ NPAF 170/44)	77 (45%) PAF, 27 (61%) NPAF	62 ± 11 (PAF), 59 ± 11 (NPAF)	153 (71%)	35 ± 5 (PAF), 39 ± 6 (NPAF)	1.36	LAPW (14.3%), Roof (4.6%), SVC (21%), CT (7.4%), MI (6.9%), CS (7.4%), IAS (3.4%),	NA	18.7	72%
Lin et al.[22]	130 (All NPAF)	15 (12%)	NA	NA	NA	1 or more	LAPW (10%), MA/CS (10%) SVC (30%), CT (35%), IAS (18%)	NA	NA	NA
Elayi et al.[23]	48 (All LS PerAF)	18 (37.5%)	61 ± 9	38 (79%)	48 ± 7	1.1	LAA (25%), CS (30%), SVC (10%), CT (15%), IAS (20%)	1 (asymptomatic PV stenosis)	17 ± 5	69% (7 on AAD)

AAD, antiarrhythmic drug; *AF*, atrial fibrillation; *CS*, coronary sinus; *CT*, crista terminalis; *IAS*, interatrial septum; *LA*, left atrial; *LAAW*, LA anterior wall; *LAPW*, LA posterior wall; *LOM*, ligament of Marshall; *LS PerAF*, long-standing persistent AF; *MA*, mitral annulus; *MI*, mitral isthmus; *NPAF*, nonparoxysmal AF; *PAF*, paroxysmal AF; *PerAF*, persistent AF; *PV*, pulmonary vein, *SVC*, superior vena cava.

TABLE 18.2 Suggested Approaches to Provocative Test for NPV Trigger in AF Patients

Steps of Provocation in Different Types of AF
Paroxysmal AF • Isoproterenol 1–4 μg/min • Burst atrial pacing from right atrium and coronary sinus with brief pauses in between each burst. • High-dose adenosine IV bolus (12–18 mg) • If AF induced → Electrical cardioversion to see spontaneous reinitiation of AF • AF is induced for at least twice.
Nonparoxysmal AF • If sinus rhythm during ablation → Induced as paroxysmal AF. • If AF noted and sustained after PV isolation → Identify max CFAE or identify rotor (or depending on the driver identification strategy decided by the operator) and ablate. • AF sustained after ablation → Cardioversion to see if NPV triggers, and then induce as above if required.

AF, Atrial fibrillation; *CFAE,* complex fractionated atrial electrogram; *IV,* intravenous; *PV,* pulmonary vein.

conduction, with an age-related localized remodeling causes a superficial endocardial zone of conduction slowing leading to a reentry.[29] Approximately two-thirds of focal RA tachycardias occurring in the absence of structural heart disease arise along the CT.[30,31] The LOM is a remnant of the left-side SVC and contains nerves, fibrous tissue, and muscle bundles.[8] The Marshall bundle directly connects to the free wall of the left atrium in a complex anatomy. It is catecholamine sensitive and can develop an automatic rhythm under isoproterenol infusion.[32] The musculature within the CS has also been reported to have an arrhythmogenic activity with spontaneous depolarizations induced by catecholamine loading, and complex connections exist between CS and left atrium.[33,34] The trigger may arise from deep within CS musculature and can be recognized by a discrete potential associated with the CS atrial signal both during sinus rhythm and tachycardia.

Moreover, AF is a dynamic state with a natural propensity to persist and progress. Both electrical and structural remodeling happen as the AF sustains for a longer duration. It was demonstrated decades ago in an animal model that AF begets AF, as AF can create self-maintaining mechanisms, with a change in electrical properties of the atrial myocytes.[35] AF itself leads to a marked shortening of the atrial effective refractory period, a reversion of its physiological rate adaptation, and an increase in rate, inducibility, and stability of AF.

In addition, structural remodeling also occurs as the AF sustains for a longer duration. Mary-Rabine and coworkers showed that part of the atrial myocytes displayed a loss of myofilaments, presented with aggregates of small mitochondria in the sarcoplasmic reticulum, and had clusters of accumulated glycogen and lysosomal degeneration.[36] Morillo et al. reported that AF caused an alteration in the ultrastructure of the atria.[37] Such structural remodeling of the atrium causes atrial dilatation. The small increase in the extracellular matrix might also have resulted in an inhomogeneous conduction and electrical uncoupling. It has been demonstrated that focal triggers are more prevalent in the area of diseased atrium with low voltage or border zone of low-voltage areas.[38] Therefore, the prevalence of NPV triggers is higher in those with nonparoxysmal AF or those with recurrence after multiple ablation procedures.

PROVOCATION TEST FOR NPV TRIGGERS

There is no standard provocation test and mapping technique of the NPV triggers. Therefore, the reported incidence of non-PV triggers varies in different laboratories.[3,11,13-23] It is also disputed whether the provocative NPV triggers are related to the clinical ectopies that initiate AF. Table 18.2 shows the provocative test used in our laboratory for both paroxysmal and nonparoxysmal AFs. Antiarrhythmic medications should be discontinued for at least five half-lives before the ablation procedure. During the electrophysiologic study, spontaneous initiation of ectopic beats preceding AF is observed during baseline or after isoproterenol loading.[2-6,10,11] In general, we attempt to find the spontaneous onset of atrial ectopic beats or repetitive episodes of short runs of sustained AF before or after infusion of isoproterenol. Higher-dose isoproterenol (>4 μg/min) should be considered to induce NPV ectopy in the patients who received ablation under deep sedation or general anesthesia. Burst atrial pacing from the right atrium and CS with brief pauses in between each bursts should be performed with pacing cycle length from 350 ms to 250 ms (or shorter). High-dose adenosine (12–18 mg) bolus injection may be considered to provoke the ectopy. If a consistent ectopic focus and atrial activation pattern are demonstrated that induced AF, the site with the earliest and most consistent atrial activation is considered to be the initiating focus of the AF. If AF sustained during the provocation test, an electrical cardioversion should be given to restore sinus rhythm and observe the ectopy that reinitiates AF spontaneously.[39] The method used to provoke AF should be attempted at least twice to ensure the reproducibility.

In patients with nonparoxysmal AF, if patients remain in AF after PV isolation, the subsequent complex fractionated atrial electrogram (CFAE) or rotor ablation is possible to eliminate NPV triggers.[40,41] Some CFAE or rotor may represent the location of NPV triggers and elimination of those sources after PV isolation increased the long-term ablation outcome in nonparoxysmal AF patients. If AF sustained after CFAE or rotor ablation, an electrical cardioversion should be given to restore sinus rhythm and then observe any ectopy that reinitiates AF. Most laboratories still believe that the NPV triggers are important

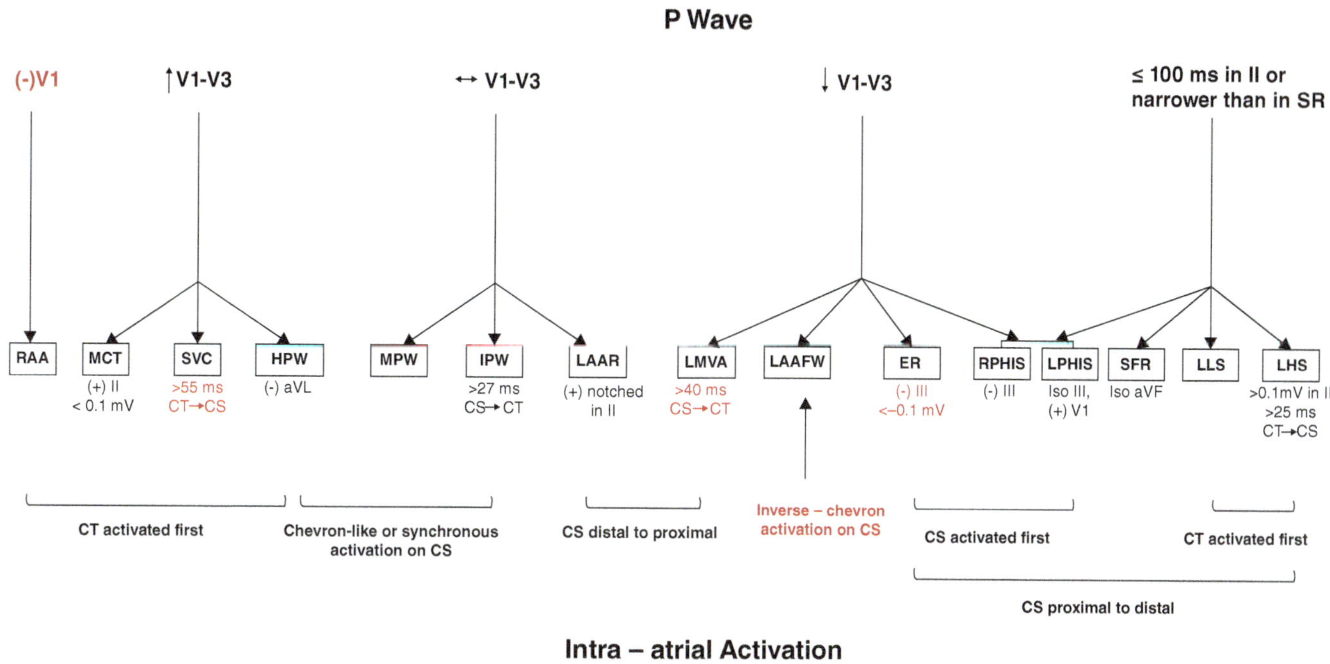

Fig. 18.1 Algorithm for identifying the NPV origin. The first two steps of the algorithm are based on (1) evaluation of P-Wave amplitude changes in the precordial leads and P-wave duration (on the top right) and on (2) intra-atrial activation timing and pattern from the two multipolar catheters (CS and CT, at the *bottom*). The most site-specific characteristics are traced in red and can be used directly to identify the specific site of origin (>95% specificity). *ER,* Eustachian ridge; *HPW,* high posterior wall; *IPW,* inferior posterior wall; *LAAFW,* left atrial appendage free-wall side; *LAAR,* left atrial appendage ridge side; *LHS,* left high septum; *LLS,* left low septum; *LMVA,* lateral mitral valve annulus; *LPHIS,* left para-Hisian site; *MCT,* crista terminalis mid to low; *MPW,* mid-posterior wall; *RAA,* right atrial appendage; *RPHIS,* right para-Hisian site; *SFR,* right septum-fossa region; *SVC,* superior vena cava. (Reproduced with permission from Kubala M, Lucena-Padros I, Xie S, et al. P-wave morphology and multipolar intracardiac atrial activation to facilitate nonpulmonary vein trigger localization. *J Cardiovasc Electrophysiol.* 2019;30:865–876. https://doi.org/10.1111/jce.13899.)

and ablation of those ectopies is required if detected or induced during the procedure (Class IIa recomendation in catheter ablation consensus from the Heart Rhythm Society).[12]

MAPPING AND LOCALIZATION OF THE NPV TRIGGERS

It is sometimes not easy to identify the exact location of the NPV trigger because it may rapidly degenerate into AF. In most patients, triggers can be localized by the information from the standard 12-lead ECG, intracardiac electrogram activation sequence, and 3D electroanatomical mapping data. The strategies used to map the NPV triggers include: (1) Investigating the P-wave morphology from the standard 12-lead ECG when it is available. An ectopic atrial P wave sometimes may be obscured by a coincident QRS–T-wave complex. There is a T-wave substraction algorithm (correlation waveform analysis) that can be used for clarification of the ectopic P-wave morphologyA.[42] (2) Identifying the earliest endocardial activation site and evaluating the activation pattern from the multipolar CS and decapolar catheter placed in right atrium to SVC referenced to the P-wave onset. (3) The 3D electroanatomical activation mapping of the region beyond PVs by high-density mapping catheters (e.g., HD Grid, double spiral catheter, PentaRay/OctaRay catheter, Orion mapping catheter, basket catheter, etc.) guided by P-wave morphology and activation patterns derived from the CS and decapolar catheters.

Therefore, the first step is looking at the p-wave morphology. It has been proposed by Marchlinski and coworkers with an algorithm based on the P-wave amplitude changes in the precordial leads and duration and intracardiac activation timing and pattern from the CS and CT multipolar mapping catheters. Fig. 18.1 shows the algorithm for identifying the NPV origin.[43]

In addition to mapping by multipolar catheters, the NPV triggers can also be evaluated by the endocardial activation sequence of the high RA, His bundle, and CS catheter recordings.[39] In our laboratory, we use this method for localization of the NPV triggers. Fig. 18.2 is the algorithm showing the scheme we used for assessing the origin of the NPV ectopoic activity initiating AF. The accuracy of this algorithm for discriminating ectopy from the SVC or upper portion of the CT from PV ectopy is 100%.[39,44,45] The electrical signals from the right superior PV (RSPV) can be recorded from a contiguous area of the right atrium as a far-field blunt signals, and ectopies from both areas exhibit similar P-wave morphologies. In cases with the ectopy from the upper portion of the CT or from the RA–SVC junction, ectopy from the RSPV should be excluded.[44,45] If far-field blunt signals from the right PV are recorded on the high posteromedial RA wall, the true origin of the ectopy can be differentiated by simultaneous mapping of the SVC and RSPV.[44,45]

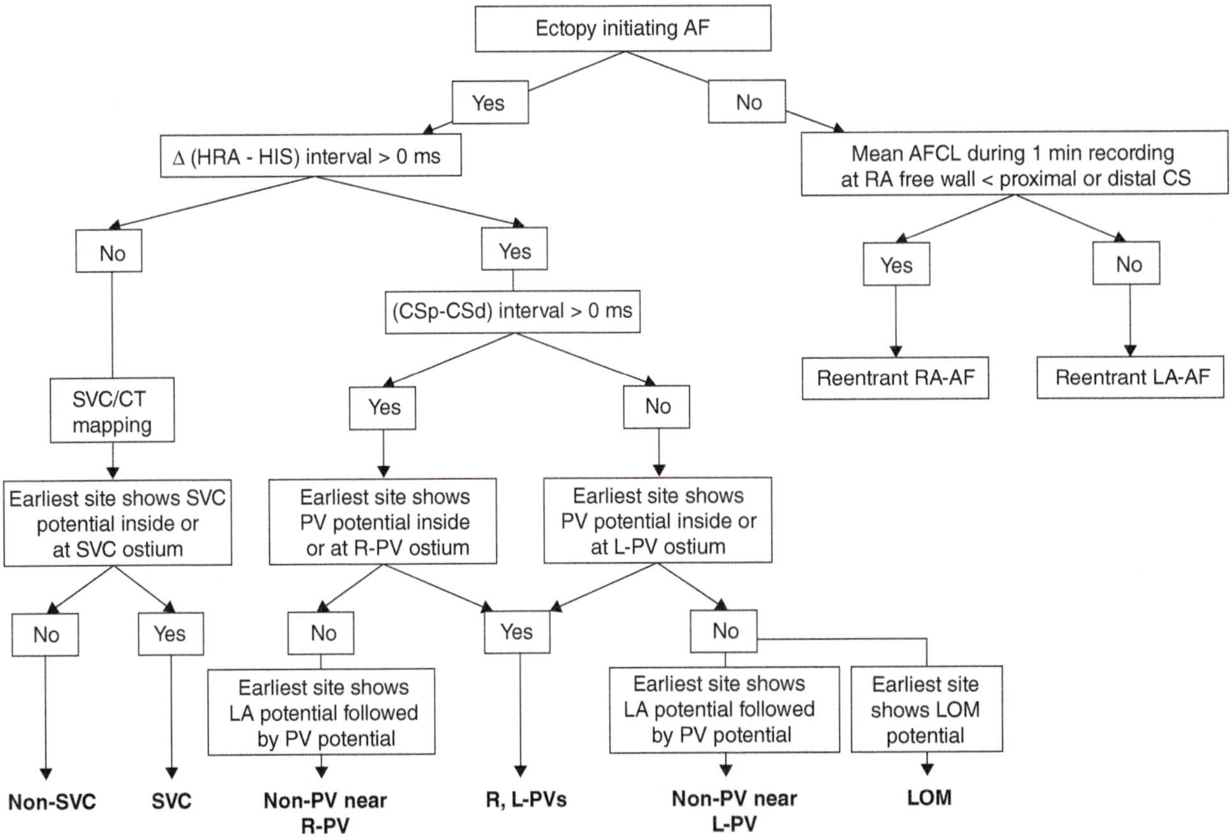

Fig. 18.2 Algorithm showing scheme used in our laboratory for assessing the origin of the non-PV ectoppic activity initiating AF. *AFCL*, Atrial fibrillation cycle length; *CS*, coronary sinus; *CSd*, distal portion of coronary sinus; *CSp*, proximal potion of coronary sinus; *CT*, crista terminalis: *HIS*, His-bundle area; *HRA*, high right atrium; *LA*, left atrium; *LOM*, ligament of Marshall; *L-PV*, left pulmonary vein; *RA*, right atrium; *R-PV*, right pulmonary vein; *SVC*, superior vena cava. (Reproduced with permission from Higa S, Tai CT, Chen SA. Catheter ablation of atrial fibrillation originating from extrapulmonary vein areas. Taipei approach. *Heart Rhythm.* 2006;3:1386–1390.)

In cases with a monophasic positive narrow P wave in lead V_1 or relatively shorter activation time (≤15 ms) preceding the P-wave onset during the ectopy, the ectopy from the IAS is suspected. Simultaneous mappings of the right- and left-sided IAS should be performed to avoid any misdiagnosis.[44,45] If the earliest endocardial activation site is around the posterolateral portion of the mitral annulus or left PV ostium, an LOM potential should be identified by the differential pacing method previously proposed by our laboratory or by a detailed epicardial mapping. Table 18.3 briefly summarizes the diagnostic criteria for the NPV ectopy initiating AF.[45]

NPV TRIGGERS FROM DIFFERENT LOCATIONS

SVC Triggers

SVC is an important and the most common NPV trigger because it originates from embryonic sinus venous tissue and is capable of spontaneous firings. It has been reported that pacemaker activity was identified in some of the SVC cardiomyocytes.[46] In an animal study, the myocardial sleeve of SVC showed evidence of heterogeneous properties and the potential to form a substrate for heterogeneity of electrical coupling.[28] The SVC has been identified as an origin of AF with the observation of repetitive discharges during the onset of AF.[4] Sharp SVC potentials preceding the atrial activity can be found during AF initiation with a higher incidence of intravenous conduction block. Fig. 18.3 shows an example of AF initiating from the SVC. Complex fractionated signals are noted at the electrograms recorded from the SVC. For patients with SVC triggers, an electrical disconnection of the arrhythmogenic SVC and right atrium at the level of the RA–SVC junction is a preferable approach to minimize AF recurrence and SVC stenosis.

It should be noted that the SVC can be divided into three parts—those above, those crossing, and those below the location of the right pulmonary artery, as shown in Fig. 18.4.[47] The SVC ectopy initiating AF is mostly from the second portion of the SVC and was significantly more oval. As it is the narrowest portion of the SVC, isolation should be performed at the third portion (below right pulmonary artery) to prevent stenosis. It is mandatory to perform: (1) SVC angiography, (2) high-density mapping for identifying the sinus node origin, and (3) pacing to check the phrenic nerve location before SVC isolation.

SVC angiography can help us identify the third (proximal) portion of SVC and perform ablation at an appropriate level. Identification of the sinus node location through high-density activation map during sinus rhythm can avoid an unintentional

TABLE 18.3 **Diagnostic Criteria for the NPV Ectopy Initiating AF**

Location	Criteria
AF initiators from RA	Difference in the time interval between the atrial activation at the high RA and His bundle area during sinus rhythm and ectopy of < 0 msec
IVC, SVC	• Positive (SVC) and negative (IVC) P waves in the inferior leads and positive or biphasic P waves in V_1 (SVC) • Earliest ectopic activity in the VC during simultaneous mapping of the VC and right PV • Reversal of the double-potential sequence during ectopy (VC potentials with a rapid deflection-far-field atrial potential sequence; distal-to-proximal venous activation sequence)
CT	• Polarity of the P waves in the inferior leads: upper portion of the CT, positive; middle portion, biphasic; lower portion, negative • Earliest ectopic activity along the CT during simultaneous mapping of the CT, VC, and right PV
CS ostium	• Negative P waves in the inferior leads • Earliest ectopic activity in the CS ostium
AF initiators from LA	Difference in time interval between the atrial activation at the high RA and His bundle area during sinus rhythm and ectopy of > 0 msc
LA free wall or LA appendage	• Atrial potentials with a rapid deflection-PV potential found after the earliest atrial activation
LOM	• Earliest activation site along the vein of Marshall, posterolateral portion of the mitral annulus, or left PV ostium • Reversal of the triple-potential sequence; the LOM potential is earlier than the LA or left PV potentials (LOM-LA-PV potentials sequence)

AF, Atrial fibrillation; *CS*, coronary sinus; *CT*, crista terminalis; *IVC*, inferior vena cava; *LA*, left atrium; *LOM*, ligament of Marshall; *PV*, pulmonary vein; *RA*, right atrium; *SVC*, superior vena cava; *VC*, vena cava. (Reproduced with permission from Higa S, Tai CT, Chen SA. Catheter ablation of paroxysmal atrial fibrillation originating from the non-pulmonary vein areas. In: Huang S, Wood M, eds. *Catheter Ablation of Cardiac Arrhythmias*. Elsevier; 2006:289–304.)

sinus nodal injury.[48] It is safer to isolate SVC during sinus rhythm (compared to during AF) and to target > 1 cm above the SVC orifice. The right phrenic nerve descends vetically along the right brachiocephalic vein and to the right anterolateral surface of the SVC. Then, it travels posterioly when it approaches the SVC-RA junction, with a proximity to the right PVs before reaching the diaphragm. Right phrenic nerve injury is a rare (0.48%) complication of this technique.[49] Although two-thirds of the patients recover completely and nearly one-sixth recover partially, it may occur during ablation of RSPV and SVC isolation. Pacing the right phrenic nerve through a catheter advanced distal to the SVC isolation line and capturing the nerve at twice the capture threshold is recommended during the SVC isolation. Direct visualization of the diaphramatic motion through fluoroscopy, palpitaiton of diaphragmatic excursion or recording of the diaphragmatic CMAP (compuound motor action potential) are potential monitoring strategies during phrenic nerve pacing.

Noteworthy, the ECG pattern may mimic reverse typical atrial flutter in a minority of the patients with AF originated from SVC. It is observed in the patients with a low-voltage zone at the venoatrial junction.[50] The low-voltage zone forms an area where wave break occurs, and this may cause the formation of conduction disturbance and intra-atrial reentry by serving as an anisotropic barrier. This slow conduction zone in the SVC ostium may serve as a buffer for rapidly firing signals in the patients with AF originating from SVC, eventually forming regularly conducting signals with a flutter-like ECG pattern. Fig. 18.5 shows an example of AF originating from the SVC with a surface ECG manifestating as a pseudo-atrial flutter.

CT Triggers

The CT conduction gap is a critical isthmus in RA reentrant arrhythmias like upper and lower loop reentries. It also can be an initiator of AF with the formation of an ectopic activation from the CT. Previous animal studies reported a specific atrial fiber consistently along the border of the CT with slow diastolic depolarizations.[51,52] Therefore, enhanced automaticity can cause a sponatneous depolarization from the CT and subsequently result in an atrial ectopy. A study of noncontact mapping demonstrated the mechanism of CT ectopy in the initiation of paroxysmal AF.[53] Fig. 18.6 shows the AF intiating from CT with the initial ectopic beat causing a reentry in the crista gaps. The wavefront propagated centrifugally from the earliest site of the middle CT. In this subtype of AF, a dominant reentrant circuit in crista gap can be a driver of AF with fibrillatory conductions to the rest of the right atrium.[54] Therefore, the transverse gap conduction in the CT can be an arrhythmogenic source of reentry and also an ectopy that initiates AF. Mostly, a linear ablation on the transverse gap is useful to treat both crista gap–related reentry and to eliminate the ectopy. Block of crista gap after ablation is not able to be identified during sinus rhythm. Thus, pacing from CS can unmask the block of the crista gap after ablation. Intracardiac ultrasound (ICE) is particulary useful to identify the location of CT and help in catheter positioning and ablation during the energy delivery.

Eustachian Ridge, Right Atrial Appendage, and Tricuspid Annulus Triggers

The Eustachian ridge is the inferior extension of the CT that separtes the orifice of the inferior vena cava from the CS. Presence of pacemaker cells, which can be a source of enhanced automaticity have been demonstrated in a previous study.[55] Therefore, it is possible that AF triggers originate from the Eustachian ridge and result in sustained atrial tachyarrhythmias. The RA appendage has remnant autorhythmic tissues and may be a source of atrial arrhythmias. Triggerred activity has been found in RA appendage.[56] However, it is sometimes not easy to

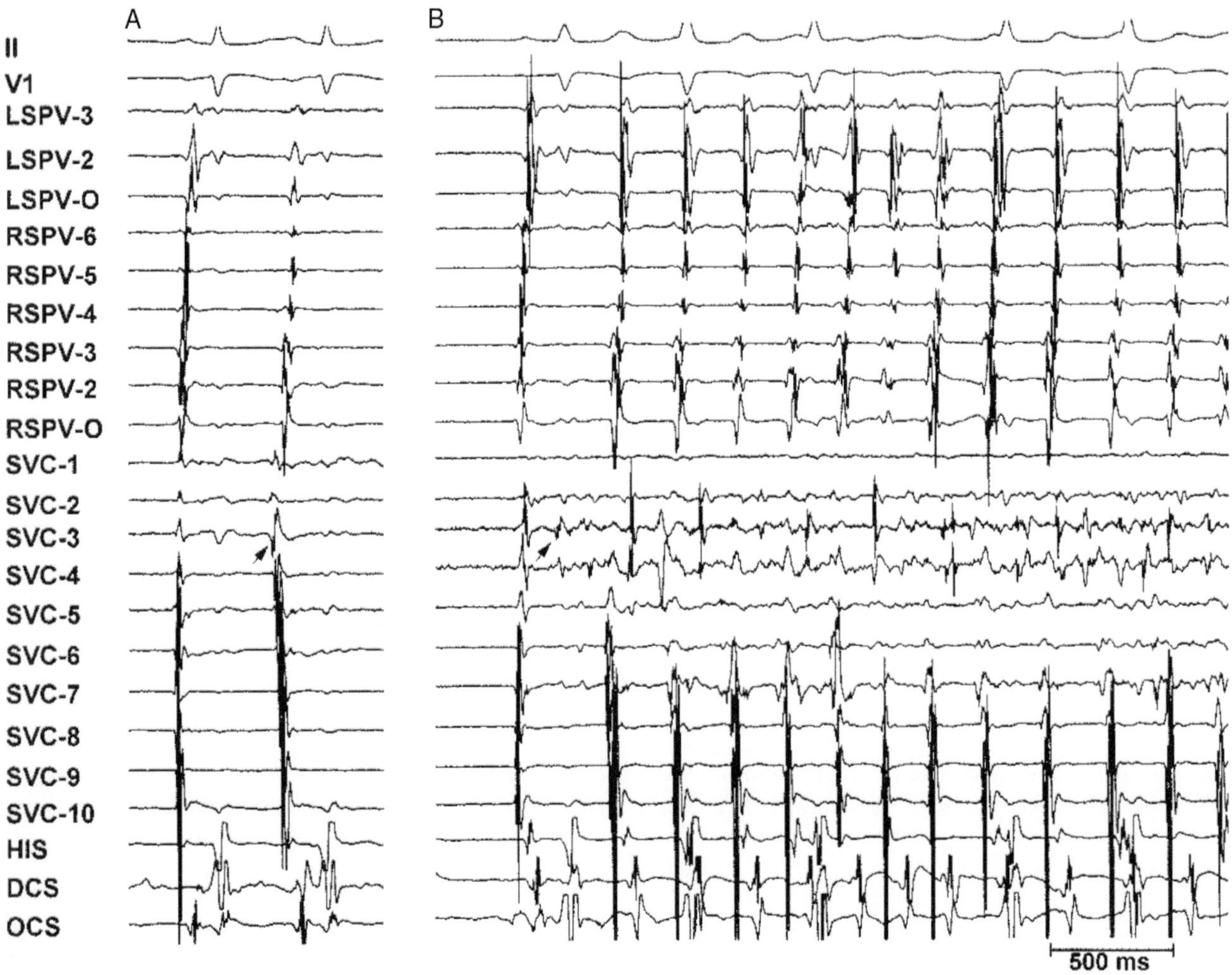

Fig. 18.3 Shows (A) the spontaneous onset of ectopic beats and then (B) the initiation of AF from the third SVC site (SVC-3 *arrow*). There is complex fragmentation in the SVC electrograms, whereas PV, His bundle, and coronary sinus electrogram are more organized. *DCS*, Distal coronary sinus; *His*, His bundle; *LSPV-O*, left superior PV ostium; *OCS*, coronary sinus ostium; *RSPV-O*, right superior PV ostium; *SVC-1*, most distal SVC bipolar recording; *SVC-10*: most proximal SVC bipolar recording. (Reproduced with permission from Tsai CF, Tai CT, Hsieh MH, et al. Initiation of atrial fibrillation by ectopic beats originating from the superior vena cava: electrophysiological characteristics and results of radiofrequency ablation. *Circulation.* 2000;102:67–74.)

reach the appendage focus because of abundant trabeculations. In addition, the blind-ended structure and reduced wall thickness increase the risk of perforation during ablation. Perforation in this region could lead to a severe complication. Preablation contrast injection to deliniate the strucutre or ICE imaging can facilitate manuevering the ablation catheter to a proper location. The RA appendage has been reported as one of the most common RA CFAE sites that lead to a procedural AF termination in patients with persistent AF, which may further support its importance with regard to AF triggers.[57] Triggers from the tricuspid annulus may occasionally be seen as well. In addition to high-density activation maps, positioning a multipolar catheter along the tricuspid annulus can assist the identification of the precise location for an effective ablation.

CS Trigger

The CS is usually considered as beginning proximally at the RA orifice and ending distally at the site of origin of the valve of Vieussens or the great cardiac vein.[58] The myocardial sleeves around the CS are composed of bands of muscle from the LA and RA walls. The length of myocardial sleeve is variable but usually extends almost the legnth of the CS. Evidence suggests that the CS can be a substrate of reentrant AF and the muscle sleeve can be a potential ectopic trigger or may form parts of a reentrant circuit of AF.[59] When mapping the CS, a decapolar catheter can be placed within CS to record the activation. Usually the proximal electrodes are at the CS ostium, the first middle pairs of the elctrodes are positioned before the insertion of the valve of Vieussens, and the distal pairs of the electrodes should be beyond the valve of Vieussens distally. When a focal trigger is recorded with the earliest activation at the proximal ostial electrode, attention should be focused on the RA, LA septum, or CS ostial structure. When a focal trigger with the earliest activation is recorded at the proximal three or four electrode pairs of the CS catheter, one should pay more attention to the trigger originating from an LA structure. If the trigger is located

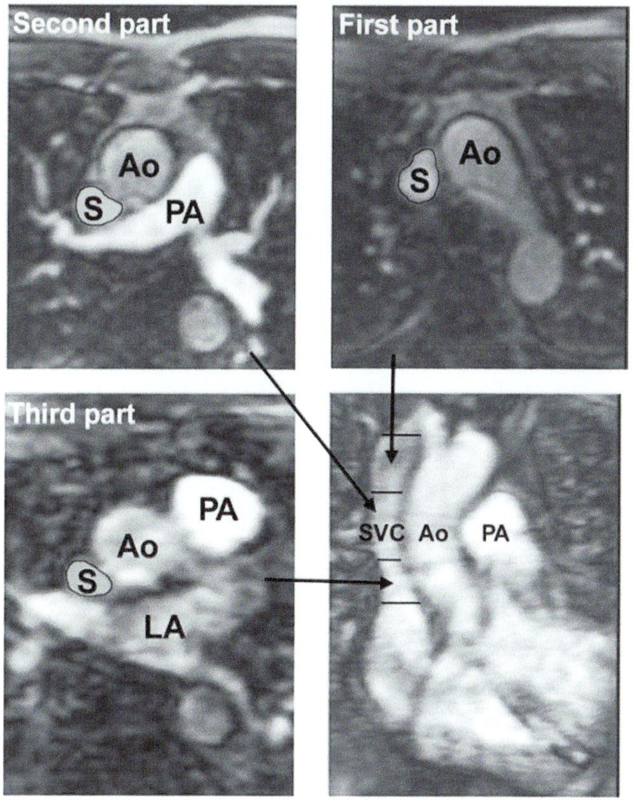

Fig. 18.4 Coronal scout view of the SVC. The SVC is divided into three portions according to the level of the right pulmonary artery. The cross section of the SVC revealed an eccentric and nonround shape. *A,* Aorta; *LA,* left atrium; *PA,* pulmonary artery; *R-PA,* right pulmonary artery; *S,* superior vena cava. (Reproduced with permission from Huang BH, Wu MH, Tsao HM, et al. Morphology of the thoracic veins and left atrium in paroxysmal atrial fibrillation initiated by superior caval vein ectopy. *J Cardiovasc Electrophysiol.* 2005;16:411–417.)

at the level of the valve of Vieussens, a trigger from the LOM should also be ruled out. Since there is no muscle sleeve distal to the valve of Vieussens, a trigger distal to this location suggests an origin from LA structurs.[60] P-wave morphology from the surface ECG may also provide evidence of the ectopic location. Usually the P waves in the inferior leads are negative and we may need to further evaluate the P-wave morphology in the precordial leads to identify whether it is coming from the CS ostium (biphasic/positive P wave in lead V_1, flat to negative P wave in lead V_6) or from the body fo the vessel (positive P wave in lead V1, negative P wave in leads V_{4-5}).

For patients with a CS trigger, an electrical isolation of the arrhythmogenic CS musculature from the atrium by an endocardial and/or epicardial ablation under the guidance of a 3D mapping system is the preferable approach rather than a focal ablation, to minimize AF recurrence.[61] Endocardial ablation should be performed from the LA and the epicardial ablation can be performed within CS with the ablation catheter tip facing the posterosuperior aspect of the CS (toward the LA). Alternative choice is a focal ablation targeting the electrical connections between the LA and the CS, but careful mapping and accurate identification of the connection sites are required and may be time consuming. A low RF energy power is recommended; care must be taken if an inappropriate impedance rise occurs during the CS ablation. In which case the energy application should be stopped immediately to prevent steam pops.

LOM Trigger

The best strategy to detect the LOM trigger is a direct cannulation with a small multipolar catheter into the Marshall vein.[8] Without direct recording, a trigger from LOM might manifest as an early activation in the middle CS. LOM potentials can be manifested when mapping at the left PVs manifesting as double potentials. The first potential is considered to be due to the activation of the LA myocardium far field potential, and the second potential (D2) is due to the activation of PV musculature or LOM tract. LOM potential can be demonstrated by comparing the signals at the CS ostium to D2 interval during sinus rhythm with that during distal CS pacing. If D2 is a PV potential, the CS ostium to D2 interval prolongs during the distal CS pacing, compared to sinus rhythm. An LOM potential is considered when the CS ostium to D2 interval shortens during the distal CS pacing compared to sinus rhythm.[62] The diagram in Fig. 18.7 depicts the concept of the differential pacing. LOM triggers should be considered when the double potentials transform to triple potentials during atrial premature beats at the onset of spontaneous AF. The intracardiac recording in Fig. 18.8A shows an ectopic beat originating from the LOM tract. The LOM potential (arrow) precedes the LA potential (star) and the PV potential (arrowhead). Panel B shows the spontaneous onset of AF from the LOM after isoproterenol infusion. Simultaneous mapping of the LOM and left PV ostia can monitor the successful isolation of both the LOM and left PVs from the LA. Ethanol infusion into Marshall vein through an angioplasty guidewire and balloon catheter has been reported as an adjunctive therapy to the PV isolation.[63] In addition to eliminating the Marshall trigger with ethanol infusion, this technique is also an effective method to create a durable mitral block in the lateral mitral isthmus region.

Recently, numerous studies have been reported that demonstrated that combined catheter ablation and LOM ethanol infusion improves ablation success in patients with nonparoxysmal AF.[64–66] In nonparoxysmal AF patients with LOM triggers and/or refractory mitral flutter, adjunctive LOM ethanol infusion in addition to PV isolation and substrate modification provides a good long-term freedom from AF and atrial arrhythmia. Fig. 18.9 shows an example of AF initiating from the LOM trigger. AF termination happened by ethanol infusion into the LOM (see figure legends for details). A multicenter single-blinded trial from 12 centers in the United States investigating the addition of LOM ethanol infusion to catheter ablation, compared with catheter ablation alone, showed an increased likelihood of remaining free of AF or atrial tachycardia after 6 and 12 months of follow-ups (see the VENUS randomized clinical trial).[65] The Marshall-PLAN trial also demonstrated that systemically targeted anatomical atrial structures (LOM ethanol infusion, PV isolation, and prespecified linear lesions) are feasible, safe, and associated with a high rate of freedom from arrhythmia recurrence at 12 months in patients with persistent AF.[66]

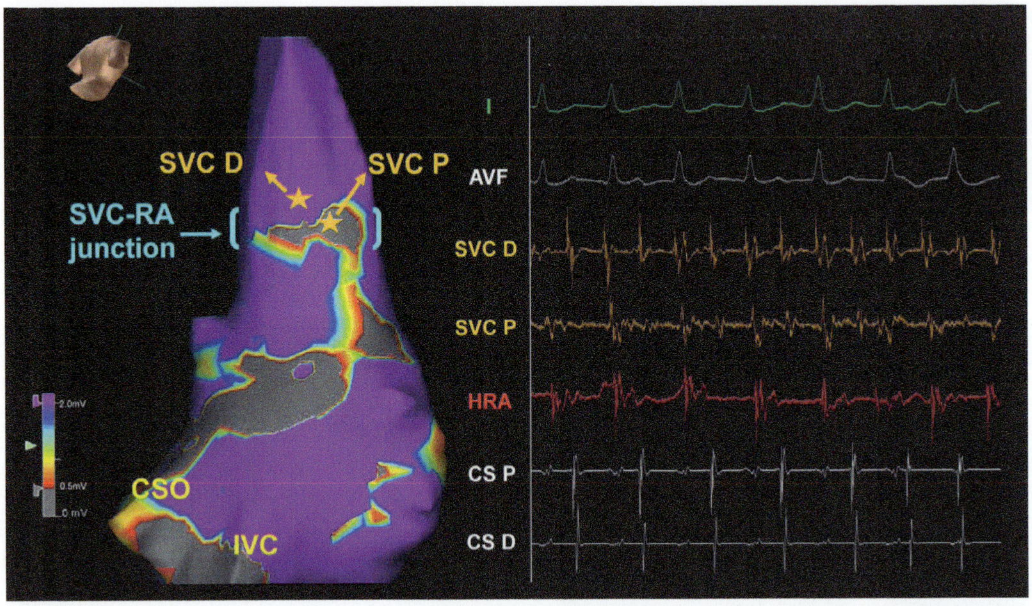

Fig. 18.5 The 3D electroanatomic mapping shows the low-voltage zone in the SVC venoatrial junction with the intracardiac tracing at the SVC-P with the most fractionated electrogram. The low-voltage zone located in the SVC ostium may cause slow conduction and serve as a buffer for rapidly firing signals in the patients with AF originating from the SVC, eventually forming a regularly conducted signal with a flutter-like pattern ECG. *CSD,* Distal bipolar pairs of CS catheter; *CSP,* proximal bipolar pairs of the CS catheter; *HRA,* high right atrium; *SVC D,* distal bipolar pairs of SVC catheter; *SVC P,* proximal bipolar pairs of SVC catheter. (Reproduced with permission from Huang HK, Chang SL, Lin YJ, et al. Atrial fibrillation originating from superior vena cava with atrial flutter-electrocardiogram pattern. *Pacing Clin Electrophysiol.* 2017;40:754–761. https://doi.org/10.1111/pace.13092.)

LA Triggers

The LA posterior wall (PW) is considedred as a similar embryologic origin of the PVs.[67] The substrate can lead to greater spontaneous triggered activity and propulsion of fibrillatory impulses to the atria. If repeated triggers can be identified from the LA PW, focal ablation targeting the earliest activation site can be considered.[3,39] However if attempts to identify the exact location of ectopy still remains refractory to focal ablation, a PW isolation should be considered. The most common strategy for PW isolation is the posterior box lesion set with an application of linear ablation, including roof and inferior lines connecting bilateral PV isolation. The technical difficulty of delivering a durable lines should be considered. A gap over the line may cause an iatrogenic proarrhythmia following ablation. In a recent meta-analysis study, PW isolation as an end point of AF ablation can be achieved in a large proportion of cases with good rates of 12-month freedom from atrial arrhythmia.[68] Although the procedure-related complication rate is low, atrioesophageal fistula is still a potential risk. In another prospective multicenter observational study, PV antral isolation extended to the entire PW demonstrated an acceptable long-term arrhythmia-free survival in nonparoxysmal AF patients.[69] On the other hand, a recent prospective randomized trial conducted in patients with persistent AF convereted to paroxysmal AF by antiarrhythmic medication, the addition of posterior box isolation to PVI did not improve the rhythm control outcome or influence overall safety, while leading to a longer ablation time.[70] Therefore, some suggest that PW isolation may be reserved for select cases with ectopy/drivers identified in the PW or redo ablation procedures.[70–72]

Ectopy coming from LA anterior wall can be observed in a limited number of patients. It has been reported that the pressure from the ascending aorta may compress and stretch the anterior wall of the left atrium and leads to the NPV trigger from aortic encroachment to the left atrium.[73] Fig. 18.10 shows a patient with an aortic encroached area of LA anterior wall with an observation of repeated triggers arising from said area. Termination of AF is noted during focal ablation of this location.

The LAA has been reported as an underrecognized origin of NPV triggers. It may be responsible for up to 27% of patients presenting for repeat ablation procedures.[74] In the BELIEF trial, electrical isolation of LAA improved the long-term outcome in patients with nonparoxysmal AF.[75] However, some conflicting results had been published in other studies suggesting the incidence of true LAA triggers is very low (0.3%).[74] While other studies suggest triggers from the LAA are prevalent only in patients with long-standing persistent AF.[11] The LAA is a large structure and triggers may coming from different region of LAA. The posterior LAA has a close contact with left superior PV and shares the same neighboring myocardium with the coumadin ridge, which harbors the LOM tract. Therefore, one should be very careful with triggers that are coming from the posterior aspect of LAA. A detailed mapping of LAA, coumadin ridge, and left superior PV should be applied. Triggers from the LOM are also characterized by an early breakthough in the mid-CS, which is rare in true LAA triggers.[60] When triggers are coming from the LAA anterior aspect or the LAA body, those are true LAA ectopies. Most of the operators performed focal ablation rather than the LAA electrical isolation to prevent LAA

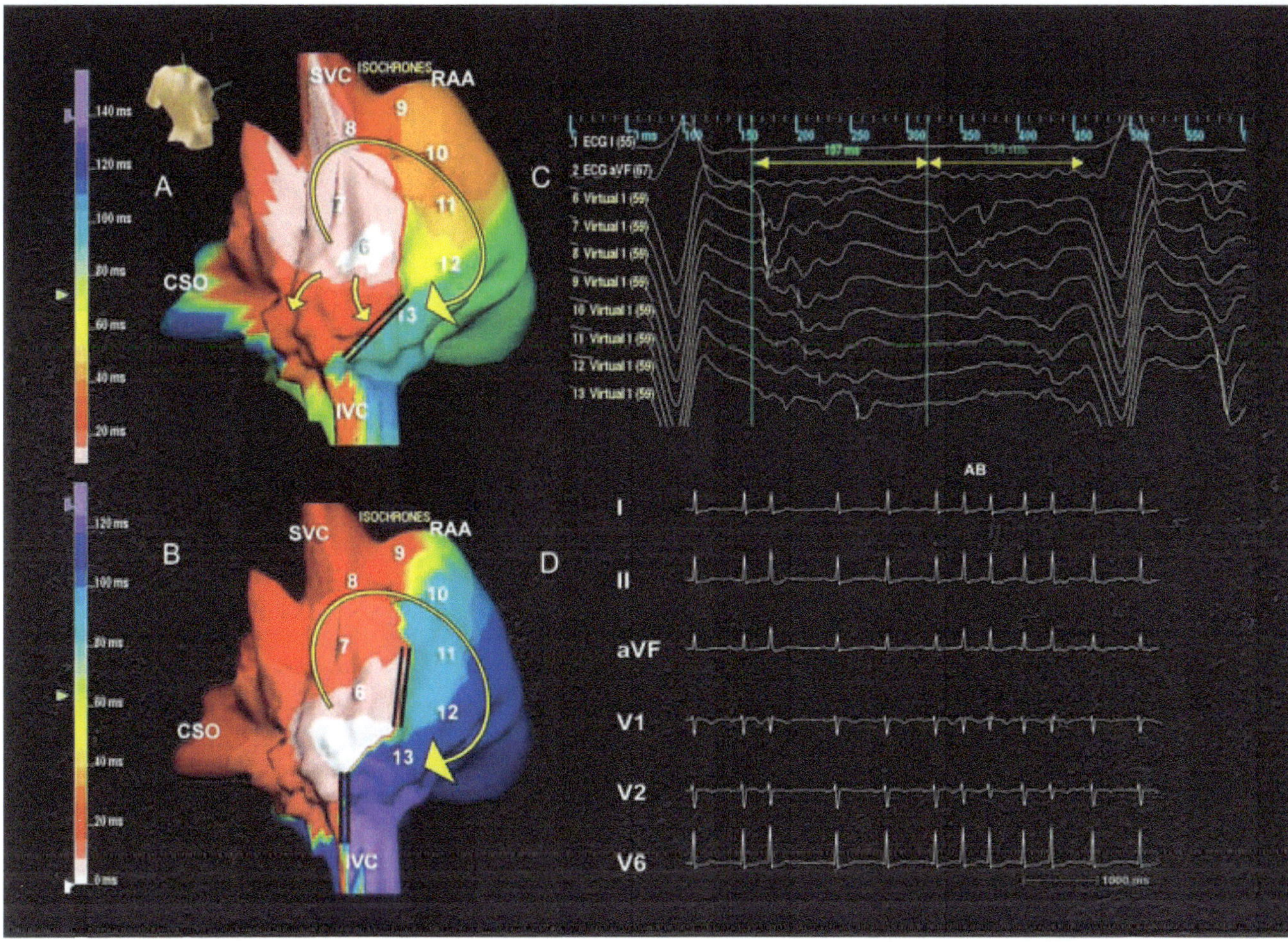

Fig. 18.6 Isochronal maps from the noncontact mapping system show the activation pattern during the initiation of AF. Panels A and B show the isochronal maps for the first two beats initiating a reentry in the modified right posterior oblique view. Panel C is the virtual unipolar electrogram along the activation followed by the ectopy. Panels D shows the surface ECG during the initiation of the AF. The wavefront propagated centrifugally from the earliest site of the middle crista terminalis with unidirectional block occurring in the low crista terminalis and activation spread around the upper crista terminalis to begin a reentry into the second cycle of AF. There is a QS pattern of virtual unipolar electrogram at the ectopic initiating site, followed by a rS morphology from the second cycle and thereafter. *CSO*, Coronary sinus ostium; *IVC*, inferior vena cava; *RAA*, right atrial appendage. (Reproduced with permission from Lin YJ, Tai CT, Liu TY, et al. Electrophysiological mechanisms and catheter ablation of complex atrial arrhythmias from crista terminalis: insight from three-dimensional noncontact mapping. *Pacing Clin Electrophysiol.* 2004;27:1231–1239. https://doi.org/10.1111/j.1540-8159.2004.00614.x.)

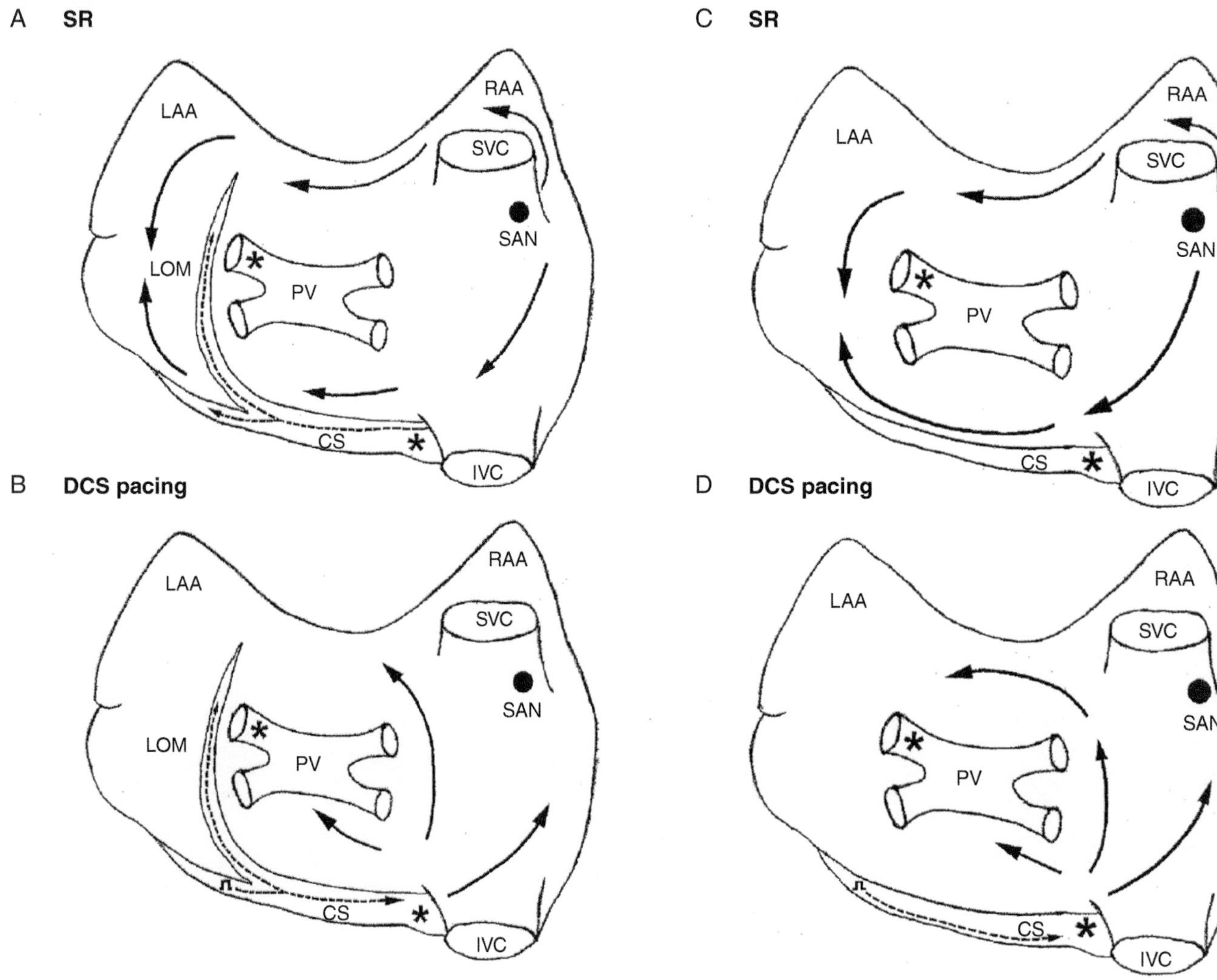

Fig. 18.7 A posterior view of the right and left atria showing the bipolar recording site (*stars*), the stimulating site (Ω), and the location of LOM in patients with (A and B) or without LOM tract (C and D). (A) During sinus rhythm, electrical impulse originates in the region of sinus node. Activation spreads anteriorly around the SVC, preceding right to left across the Bachmann bundle to reach the base of LAA (*solid lines*). The wavefront traverses the posterior left atrium beneath the right PVs (*solid lines*). The LOM tract is activated following activation of the CSO because the LOM is insulated from the left atrial wall (*broken line*). (B) During CS pacing, the activation wavefronts spread simultaneous along the proximal CS and the LOM (*broken lines*), through the CSO, and propagates onto the posterior right and left atria (*solid line*). (C) During sinus rhythm, the electrical impulse originates in the region of sinus node. Activation spreads anteriorly around the SVC, proceeding from right to left across the Bachmann bundle to reach the base of the LAA (*solid lines*). The wavefront traversing the posterior right atrium propagates between the vena cava onto the posterior left atrium beneath the right PVs (*solid lines*). The left superior PV is activated following activation of the base of the LAA. The CSO is activated from the wavefront traversing the posterior right atrium. (D) During distal CS pacing, the activation wavefront spreads along the proximal CS to ostium (*broken line*), and traverses the posterior left atrium to reach the left superior PV (*solid lines*). *IVC*, Inferior vena cava; *LAA*, left atrial appendage; *RAA*, right atrial appendage; *SAN*, sinus node. (Reproduced from Tai CT, Hsieh MH, Tsai CF, et al. Differentiating the ligament of Marshall from the pulmonary vein musculature potentials in patients with paroxysmal atrial fibrillation: electrophysiological characteristics and results of radiofrequency ablation. *Pacing Clin Electophysiol*. 2000;23(Pt. I):1493–1501.)

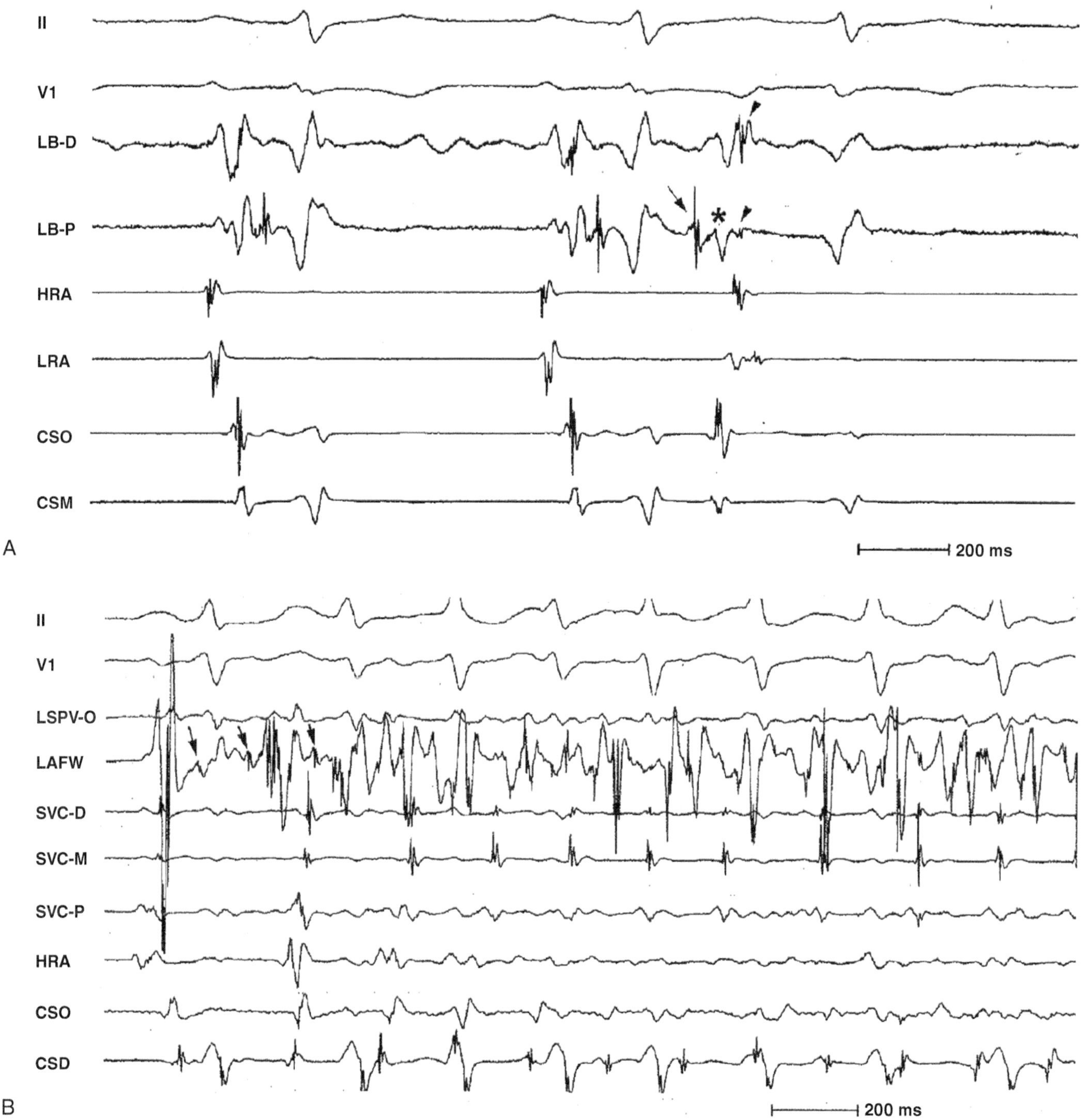

Fig. 18.8 (A) Intracardiac recordings of an ectopic beat originating from the LOM tract. Note that the LOM potential (*arrow*) precedes the LA potential (*star*), and the PV potential (*arrowhead*). (B) Intracardiac tracing shows the spontaneous onset of AF from the LOM after infusion of isoproterenol. Earliest activation of the LOM potential followed by the LA potential is noted in the initiating ectopic beats. *CSD*, Distal CS; *CSM*, middle CS; *LAFW*, LA free wall; *LB-D*, distal portion of lingual branch; *LB-P*, proximal portion of lingual branch; *LAT*, LOM tract; *LRA*, low right atrium; *LSPV-O*, ostium of the left superior PV; *SVC-D*, distal SVC; *SVC-M*, middle SVC; *SVC-P*, proximal SVC. (Reproduced from Tai CT, Hsieh MH, Tsai CF, et al. Differentiating the ligament of Marshall from the pulmonary vein musculature potentials in patients with paroxysmal atrial fibrillation: electrophysiological characteristics and results of radiofrequency ablation. *Pacing Clin Electophysiol.* 2000;23(Pt. I):1493–1501.)

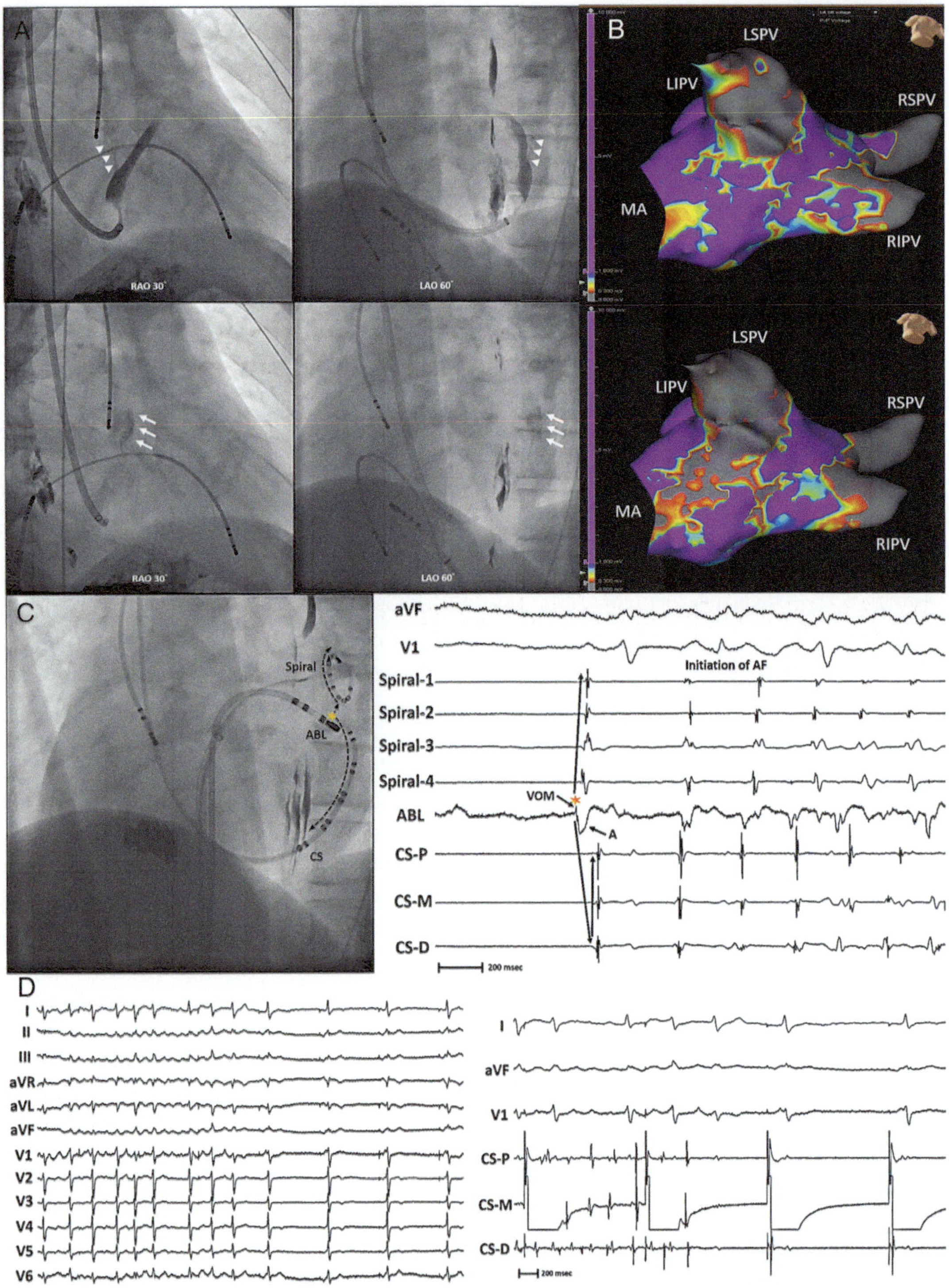

Fig. 18.9 Fluoroscopic images, electroanatomic maps, surface ECG, and intracardiac recordings obtained from a long-standing persistent AF patient with a history of hyperthyroidism, who underwent catheter ablation with a successful termination of AF upon LOM ethanol infusion. (A) Fluoroscopic images in the 30° RAO view (*left*) and 60° LAO view (*right*) of the LOM (*arrowheads*), before (*top*) and after (*bottom*) LOM ethanol infusion. (B) Voltage map recorded before (*top*) and after (*bottom*) LOM ethanol infusion, shown in the inferior posterior view of left atrium. After LOM ethanol infusion, an extensive scar is noted over the inferior and posterior left atrium, extending between the LAA and left PV. (C). Ectopic LOM trigger initiates AF. The spiral catheter is placed in the left superior PV, while the ablation catheter is placed in the left inferior PV to record a double potential. The LOM ectopy, which is recorded from the tip of ablation catheter (*star*), conducts to the left atrium through the left superior PV, and from the distal to the proximal CS because of the LOM is connected to the CS (*dotted line*). (D) AF termination into sinus rhythm at 9 seconds after initiation of a second ethanol infusion into the LOM, with no recurrence by the 46-month follow-up. *ABL*, Ablation catheter; *LAO*, left anterior oblique; *MA*, mitral annulus; *RAO*, right anterior oblique. (Reproduced from Liu CM, Lo LW, Lin YJ, et al. Long-term efficacy and safety of adjunctive ethanol infusion into the vein of Marshall during catheter ablation for nonparoxysmal atrial fibrillation. *J Cardiovasc Electrophysiol.* 2019;30:1215–1228.)

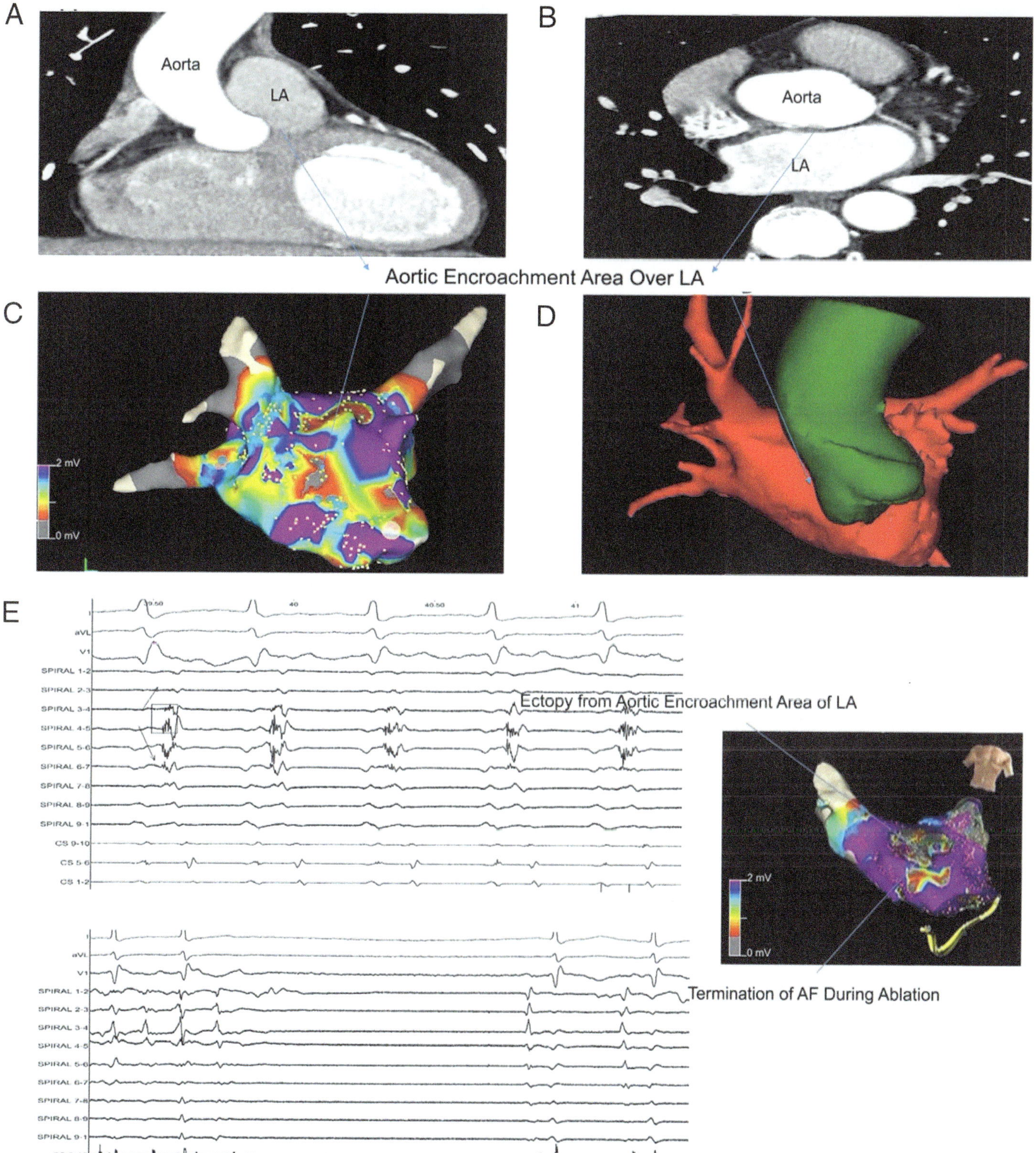

Fig. 18.10 (A) CT scan of aorta and left atrium in sagittal view showing the aortic encroached area. (B) CT scan of aorta and left atrium in coronal view showing aortic encroached area. (C) Low-voltage area depicted in the encroached area from the 3D electroanatomic voltage map of the left atrium. (D) Reconstructed images of aorta and left atrium. (E) Intracardiac tracings of trigger arising from LA anterior wall encroached area and termination of AF to sinus rhythm during ablation. (Reproduced from Allamsetty S, Lo LW, Lin YJ, et al. Impact of aortic encroachment to left atrium on non-pulmonary vein triggers of atrial fibrillation. *Int J Cardiol.* 2017;227:650–655.)

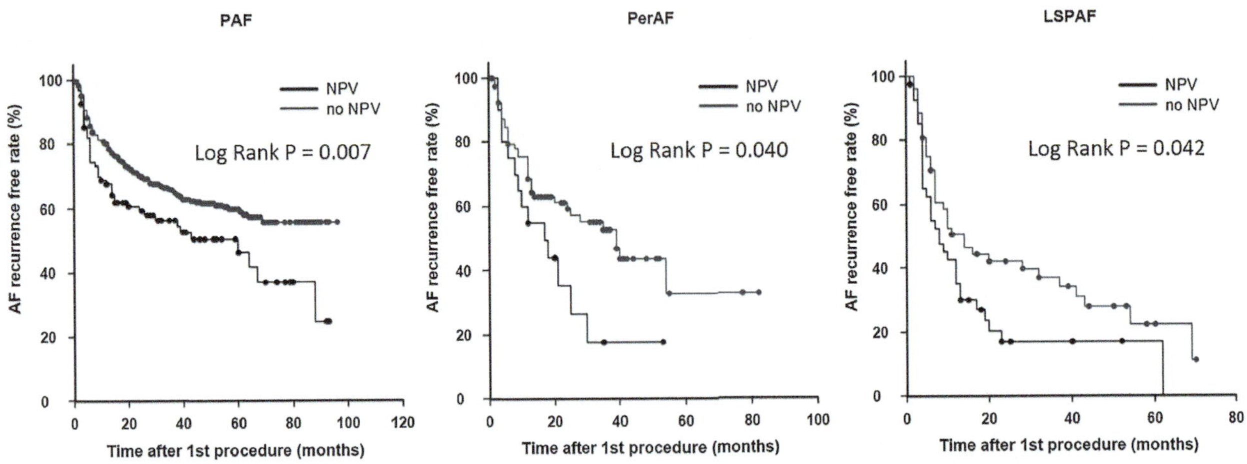

Fig. 18.11 The recurrence rate between patients with and without NPV triggers in three different groups. Kaplan-Meier survival curve demonstrating significant differences in the freedom from the AF recurrence rate between patients with coexisting PV/NPV triggers and PV trigger only after the index procedure in paroxysmal, persistent, and long-standing persistent AF groups. (Reproduced from Hung Y, Lo LW, Lin YJ, et al. Characteristics and long-term catheter ablation outcome in long-standing persistent atrial fibrillation patients with non-pulmonary vein triggers. *Int J Cardiol.* 2017;241:205–211.)

mechanical dysfunction. Routine LAA isolation is performed in some institutes with reports of good result and safety profiles.[74–78] Nevertheless, long-term anticoagulation and/or LA occlusion device implantation should be considered if electrical LAA isolation is performed.

IAS Triggers

For patients with IAS triggers, a focal ablation of the earliest activation site during the ectopy preceding the onset of AF is performed until a complete elimination of the ectopy is achieved.[11,79] It is often located to the muscular portion at the level of the fossa ovalis or limbus. Usually the P-wave duration is narrow during the initiating beat with a negative or biphasic P wave in lead V_1 in atnteroseptal or mid-septal triggers, while a positive lead V_1 P wave is noted in the posteroseptal trigger. In the inferior leads, a positive P wave is noted if the trigger is more anterior, while the P wave is negative when it is originating more posteriorly.[79] Simultaneous mapping of the RA and LA septa is important to achieve a successful localization and ablation of the ectopy.

EFFICACY AND OUTCOME OF CATHETER ABLATION

It is important to understand that there is a lower ablation success and a higher recurrence rate in those with presence of NPV triggers initiating AF during the index procedure.[11] Fig. 18.11 shows the AF recurrence free rate between those with coexisting PV/NPV triggers and PV trigger-only groups in paroxysmal, persistent, and long-standing persistent AF populations, respectively. Moreover, in those with identified NPV triggers, ablation targeting those NPV triggers in addition to PV isolation improved long-term outcomes of both paroxysmal and nonparoxysmal AF ablations.[69,80,81] Therefore, the AF ablation consensus document also recommends NPV ablation as a Class IIa recommendation.[12]

CONCLUSION

NPV triggers represent an important initiating mechanism of atrial tachyarrhythmia and demonstrate an increased incidence as the AF burden progresses from paroxysmal to persistent and long-standing persistent AF. It is also prevalent during redo AF ablation procedures. Accurate localization and mapping of those NPV triggers are important steps and can improve the ablation outcome. Targeting the NPV trigger is also the only Class IIa recommendation of ablation beyond PV isolation in AF. A successful ablation usually involves targeting a specific site of origin. However, for unmappable and infrequent atrial beats originating from uncommon areas, the development of a novel single beat analysis by invasive or noninvasive high-density mapping systems is required. Currently, isolation of selected structures (e.g., SVC, LAA, CS and LA PW, etc.) may be effective, but more evidence is required for empirical ablation beyond PV isolation.

REFERENCES

Please refer to the e-book for a complete list of references.

19

Substrate-Based Ablation of Atrial Fibrillation

Michael Ghannam, Thomas Crawford, Hakan Oral

KEY POINTS

- Atrial substrate modification is required for a successful outcome in a minority of patients with paroxysmal atrial fibrillation (AF) and in most patients with persistent AF.
- Substrate modification is considered when AF persists despite effective elimination of pulmonary vein (PV) arrhythmogenicity by extraostial PV isolation (PVI), antral PVI, or wide-area circumferential ablation.
- Substrate modification strategies include empiric anatomical guided ablation, ablation guided by complex fractionated atrial electrograms or abnormal atrial voltage, or ablation of ganglionic plexi.
- Termination of AF to sinus rhythm or to an atrial tachycardia is considered the most favorable procedural endpoint for substrate modification.
- Complete bidirectional conduction block should be confirmed when linear ablation is performed.

INTRODUCTION

Atrial fibrillation (AF) is a complex and heterogeneous disease.[1] Successful elimination of AF triggers, through pulmonary vein isolation (PVI) and extra-PVI triggers is an effective strategy for many patients, particularly with paroxysmal AF[2,3]; however, the modest success in patients with advanced AF suggests that additional mechanisms contribute to the perpetuation of AF in this population. Classic models describing the interplay between "triggers" and "substrates" for arrhythmia propagation have been long recognized.[4] Over the past few decades, advances in cellular electrophysiology, imaging, computer modeling, and multidomain high-density mapping have yielded key insights into how the atrial substrate contributes to AF propagation. Multiple strategies to identify and target abnormal atrial substrate have been described, both through empiric anatomy-based lesions and through image/electrogram-guided approaches. The purpose of this chapter is to review the rationale for a substrate-based AF ablation approach and examine the clinical considerations of such strategies.

Rationale for a Substrate-Based Ablation Approach

There are two predominant mechanisms of AF that have guided ablation strategies over the decades. The multiple wavelet theory describes AF as a self-perpetuating rhythm independent of focal discharges, allowing constant formation and dispersal of wavelets.[5,6] Critical to the multiwavelet hypothesis is a minimal left atrial (LA) size that can accommodate the wavelength as determined by the product of the conduction velocity and the effective refractory period. The second is a localized source model in which focal areas of reentry or discharges sustain AF. These organized regions result in disorganized fibrillation due to wave-break as the impulses encounter tissue with anisotropy and conduction heterogeneity.[7] These competing mechanisms may not be mutually exclusive, particularly in patients with nonparoxysmal AF.[8]

While a complete model of AF is lacking, atrial structural and electrical remodeling is understood to promote these phenomena. Structural changes in response to AF may be a consequence of a physiologic adaptation to pressure overload and metabolic stress.[9] Atrial biopsy specimens from patients undergoing cardiac surgery show an increase in cell size, loss of sarcoplasmic reticulum and atrial myofibrils, changes in mitochondrial shape, accumulation of glycogen granules, alteration in connexin expression, and increase in extracellular matrix.[10,11] Electroanatomical remodeling facilitates trigger formation, shortening of atrial refractory periods,[12,13] and the promotion of fibrosis.[14] This results in a nonhomogeneous decrease in atrial refractoriness and slowing of intra-atrial conduction.[15] Fibrotic regions can support areas of microreentry[16] including complex, intramural drivers of AF.[17]

Substrate modification may therefore be beneficial to eliminating AF through several mechanisms. Linear lesions and ablation aimed at atrial "debulking" may interrupt the multiple wavelets and reentrant circuits perpetuating AF.[7,18] Additionally, given the lines of evidence linking fibrosis to AF maintenance,[19,20] elimination of the underlying fibrotic substrate through ablation may result in an atrium that is unable to maintain AF (Table 19.1).

ANATOMIC APPROACHES TO SUBSTRATE MODIFICATION

Antral Pulmonary Vein Isolation

In addition to a direct role of the PVs as a source of AF triggers, the atrial tissue around the PVs may harbor complex

TABLE 19.1 Strategies for Substrate Ablation

Ablation Strategy	Targets	Mapping	Substrate Altered	Endpoint
PV isolation	PV antrum	Anatomic with or without 3D mapping	PV arrhythmogenicity CFAEs GPs Microreentry Rotors Debulking	Complete PV and antral electrical isolation
Linear ablation	LA roof Mitral isthmus LA anterior wall Posterior wall isolation	Anatomic with or without 3D mapping	Macroreentry CFAEs Rotors GPs	Conduction block across lines
Electrogram-guided ablation	CFAEs Frequency gradient Focal sources	Electrogram features with or without computerized analysis	Macroreentry Rotors, high-frequency sources GPs	AF termination/slowing Elimination of CFAEs
Autonomics	Parasympathetic ganglionic plexi LOM	High-frequency pacing (plexi) Angiography (LOM)	Autonomics with or without CFAEs	Attenuation of vagal response

3D, Three-dimensional; *AF,* atrial fibrillation; *CFAE,* complex fractionated atrial electrogram; *LA,* left atrium; *LOM,* ligament of Marshall; *PV,* pulmonary vein.

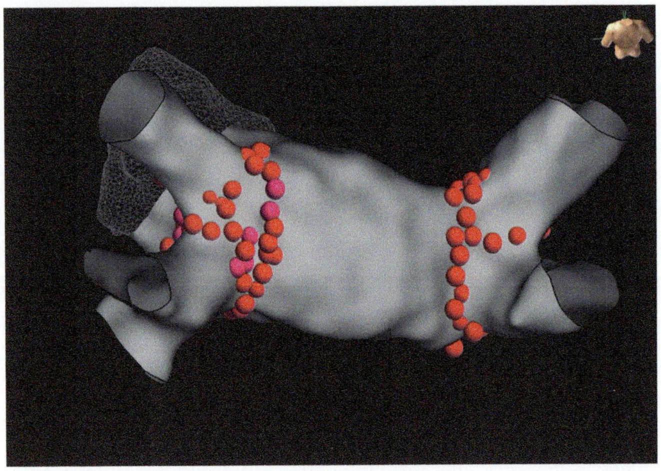

Fig. 19.1 A three-dimensional electroanatomical depiction of the left atrium and the pulmonary veins shown in a right posterior oblique projection with cranial angulation. Two encircling pulmonary vein lesions were created; ablation at the left and right carina was required to achieve electrical isolation. *LAA,* Left atrial appendage; *LIPV,* left inferior pulmonary vein; *RIPV,* right inferior pulmonary vein; *RSPV,* right superior pulmonary vein.

myofibril arrays, ganglionic plexi (GPs), and areas of slow conduction and fractionated electrical activity, which also may contribute to AF. PVI may also result in ablation of anchor points for rotors and can affect the complexity of AF drivers elsewhere in the atrium (Figs. 19.1 and 19.2). Kumagi et al. demonstrated that nearly 50% of atrial sites demonstrating high dominant-frequency and complex fractionated electrograms (CFAEs) remote to the PVIs were reduced after PVI in patients with persistent and paroxysmal AF.[21] Multiple randomized controlled studies have demonstrated the benefits of wide circumferential ablation strategies including antral ablation as compared to more ostial ablation during PVI.[22,23] The PVI–antral junction is also richly innervated with GPs, and neuromodulation of these inputs has been suggested to improve AF ablation outcomes.[24] By extending the encircling lesions outside the PV into the atrial tissue, residual arrhythmogenic foci and GPs may simultaneously be eliminated. This may be supported by observations that many patients who demonstrate PV reconnection nonetheless may attain good ablation outcomes.[25] Detailed discussion on the pathophysiologic basis and clinical aspects of PVI ablation is covered in detail in Chapters 15, 16, 18, and 20.

Linear Ablation

Catheter ablation for AF initially consisted of linear ablation to emulate the Cox surgical maze procedure.[26] Linear catheter ablation was first limited to the right atrium (RA) and had low efficacy. Later, linear ablation was performed in the LA, with various lesion sets being used to anchor venous structures, mitral and tricuspid annuli, or other linear ablation lesions. Linear ablation has been performed both as a stand-alone strategy and as an adjunctive strategy to other ablation techniques targeting the PV antrum and complex electrograms.[27]

Linear ablation has been performed along the roof of the LA between the contralateral superior PVs, along the lateral mitral isthmus between the ostium of the left inferior PV and the lateral mitral annulus, along the LA septum, from the anterior aspect of the right PV antrum to the septal mitral annulus, along the posterior mitral annulus parallel to the coronary sinus, anteriorly between a roofline and anterior mitral annulus, and along the RA aspect of the interatrial septum from the superior vena cava (SVC) to the inferior vena cava (Fig. 19.3).

The original intent of linear ablation for AF was to interrupt macroreentrant circuits.[6,28] Other possible mechanisms by which linear ablation may improve outcomes of AF ablation are interruption of microreentrant circuits, elimination of anchor points for high-frequency sources, and atrial debulking. CFAEs may also be prevalent along the course of linear lesions such as

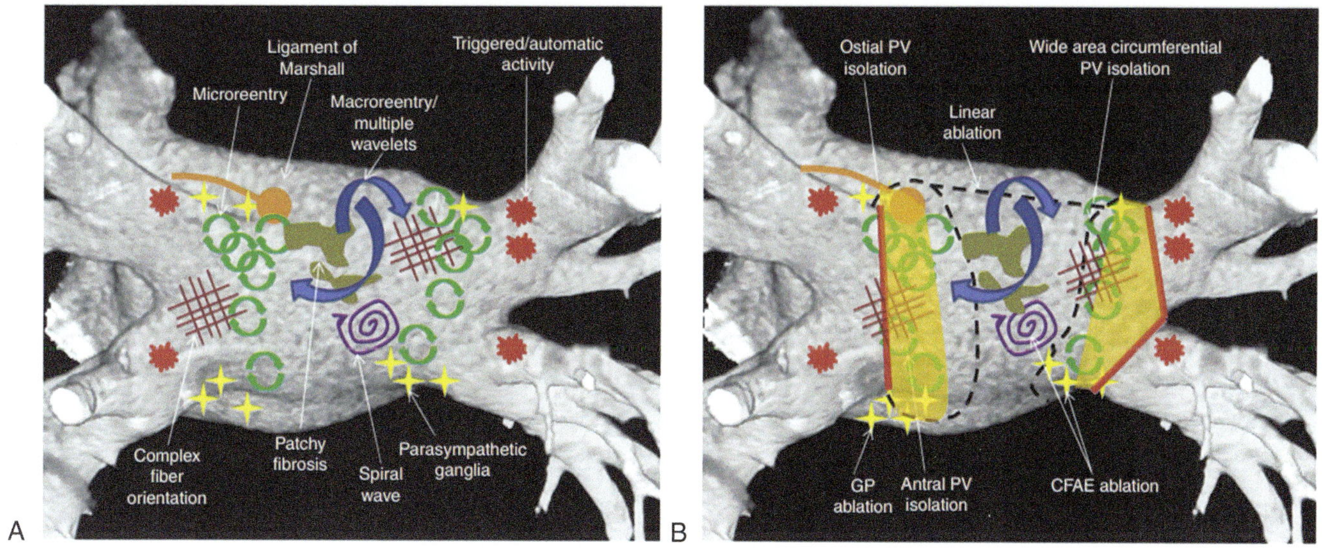

Fig. 19.2 (A) Proposed mechanisms responsible for the initiation and maintenance of atrial fibrillation (posteroanterior atrial view shown). Note the concentrated distribution of critical mechanisms near the pulmonary veins (PVs) and posterior left atrial wall. (B) Potential effects of PV isolation and linear ablation on left atrial substrate for atrial fibrillation. Ostial PV isolation may eliminate PV arrhythmogenicity but little else. Antral (*orange and red highlight*) and wide-area PV isolation may also eliminate arrhythmia mechanisms near the PV. Linear ablation (roofline shown) may interrupt macroreentry circuits with variable collateral effects on fractionated electrograms and autonomics. *CFAE*, Complex fractionated atrial electrogram; *GP*, ganglionic plexi.

the septum or the roof. Finally, autonomic ganglia may be eliminated during linear ablation at certain sites.

Several studies demonstrated that additional linear ablation improves the clinical efficacy of catheter ablation in patients with paroxysmal and persistent AF.[27,29] More contemporary randomized controlled studies, including the STAR AF II trial, did not show that empiric roof and lateral mitral linear ablation conferred benefit over antral PVI in patients with persistent AF.[30] The CLEAR-AF study examined the role of limited linear ablation (PVI + roof line) versus a more extensive linear ablation (PVI + roof line + anterior line) in 214 patients undergoing ablation of persistent AF[31] (Fig. 19.4). While an extensive linear ablation was more likely to result in acute AF termination, this strategy did not improve long-term arrhythmia outcomes.

Linear lesions may be a necessary step in the conversion of AF to sinus rhythm, often through an intermediate step of atrial tachycardia. In a study that used a stepwise ablation strategy including isolation of thoracic veins, ablation of CFAEs, and linear ablation until AF terminated, linear ablation was necessary in more than 80% of the patients with persistent AF for termination.[32] The Alster-Lost-AF trial randomized 124 patients with persistent AF to either PVI or an extensive ablation approach combining CFAE with linear ablation and failed to show benefit of this extensive approach over a strategy of PVI alone.[33]

Ablation Technique

The greatest difficulty with linear or anatomy-based ablation is achieving and confirming complete block across the lesion set. Careful assessment of local electrograms along the length of an ablation set, differential pacing, as well as high-density activation mapping can be useful to assess for conduction block (Table 19.2).

This is particularly difficult for the mitral isthmus line, which may require extensive ablation laterally and within the coronary sinus. With complete isthmus block, widely separated electrograms, usually by more than 100 ms, should be recorded along the length of the ablation line.[34] Pacing the coronary sinus or appendage distal to the ablation line results in proximal-to-distal coronary sinus activation on the septal side of the line. Likewise, coronary sinus pacing proximal to the line results in distal-to-proximal coronary sinus activation lateral to the line. As the pacing site is moved away from the edge of the ablation line (i.e., during differential pacing), the conduction time from the stimulus to the electrograms recorded on the opposite side of the line decreases in the setting of conduction block, but increases in the setting of slow conduction across the line (Fig. 19.5).

Incomplete linear lesions may be proarrhythmic and may lead to refractory atrial flutters that are often highly symptomatic. The use of steerable sheaths may improve the likelihood of achieving linear mitral block with endocardial ablation alone.[35] High-power, short-duration ablation create durable lesions during PVI ablation; however conventional ablation settings (30–40 W for 20–40 seconds) may better allow for effective ablation of thicker tissue with a lower risk of catheter overheating, and may be preferable along the mitral isthmus.[36] Additionally, ablation strategies using automated ablation lesions tagging (Ablation Index CARTO, Biosense Webster, Diamond Bar, CA) may help provide more durable linear lesion sets.[37] Ablation of the vein of Marshall to achieve complete mitral isthmus block is discussed below.

Posterior Wall Isolation

The posterior wall (PW) is a frequent target of ablation for patients with nonparoxysmal AF.[7] The PW shares embryological

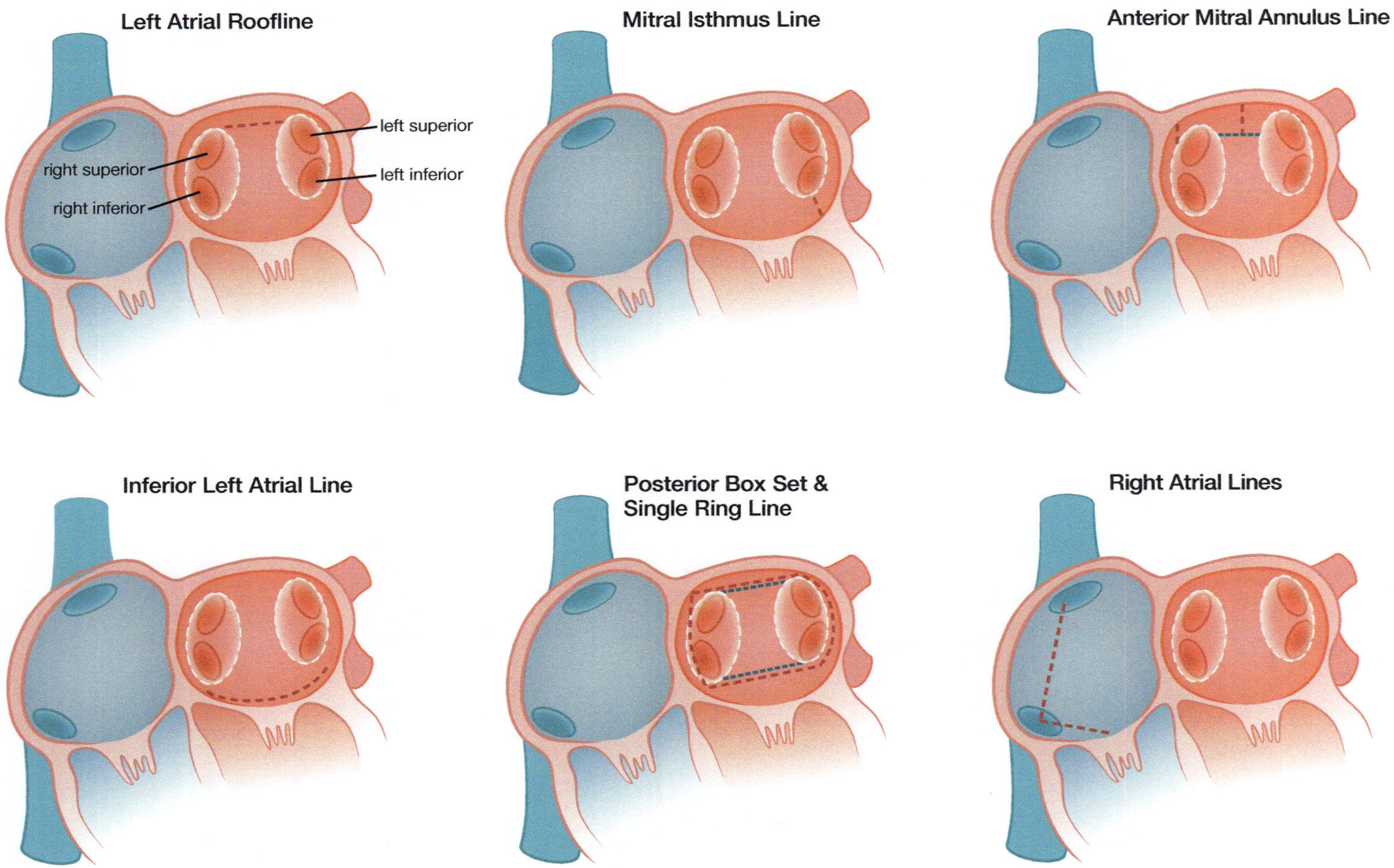

Fig. 19.3 Linear ablation lesions for the left and right atria. The view perspective is anteroposterior. Pulmonary vein (PV) encircling lesions are shown in *blue broken lines,* and linear lesions in *solid red lines.* The posterior box set is shown in blue, and the single-ring lesion set is shown in *red. CVT,* Cavotricuspid isthmus; *LA,* left atrium; *LI,* left inferior; *LS,* left superior; *RI,* right inferior; *RS,* right superior.

origins with the PVs.[38] Additionally, the PW harbors significant conduction heterogeneity due to distinct myocardial fiber orientation as well as unique cellular ion currents not found in other areas of the atrium.[39] The PW is a common source of sustained rotors in both animal and human models.[40] LA wall stress is disproportionately distributed to the PW compared to other areas of the atria, rendering it susceptible to adverse remodeling.[41]

Despite these pathophysiologic findings, clinical data regarding the additive benefit of PW isolation have been mixed. A meta-analysis of 17 studies examining PW isolation in patients with nonparoxysmal AF demonstrated that PW can be achieved in the majority of patients (94.1%; 95% CI, 87.2–99.3%) with a low rate of major complications (0.1%).[42] A contemporary randomized controlled trial by Lee et al. randomized 217 patients with persistent AF to PVI versus PVI with PW isolation, and reported no improvement clinical outcomes including arrhythmia recurrence, repeat ablation, or use of antiarrhythmic medications.[43] A similar lack of efficacy was found in a randomized clinic trial by Pake et al., which included 114 patients with persistent AF partially responsive to antiarrhythmic medications.[44] Last, a randomized clinical trial by Kim et al. failed to show additional benefit of PW isolation in addition to re-isolation of PVI alone in patients undergoing repeat AF ablations who were found to have PV reconnection.[45]

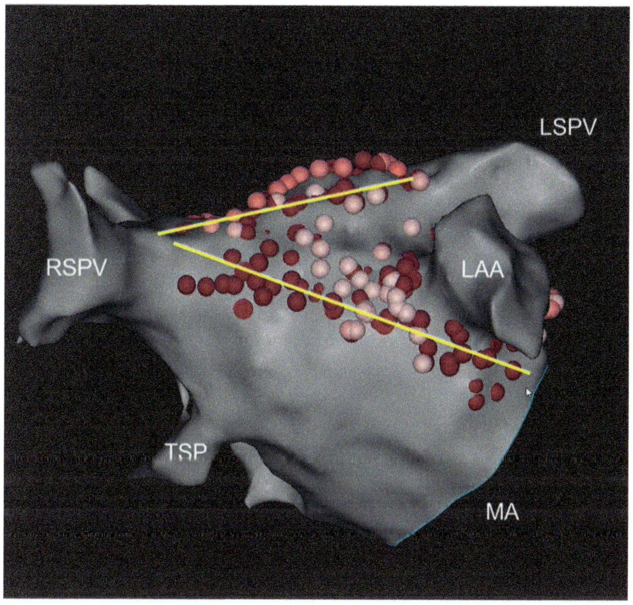

Fig. 19.4 A three-dimensional electroanatomical depiction of the left atrium and the pulmonary veins are shown in right anterior posterior oblique projection with cranial angulation. Two linear lesions sets are shown (*yellow lines*) between the RSPV and LSPV (roof line) and from the MA to the RSPV (anterior line). *LAA*, Left atrial appendage; *LSPV*, left superior pulmonary vein; *M(A)*, mitral annulus; *RSPV*, Right superior pulmonary vein; *TSP*, transseptal puncture.

Challenges to PW isolation include the proximity of the esophagus, which may limit aggressive ablation, as well as difficulty targeting epicardial inputs from the septopulmonary bundle (Fig. 19.7D).[46] Proven isolation of the posterior wall may require multiple procedures to achieve but may improve ablation outcomes.[47] PW isolation rates may also be improved with hybrid epicardial/endocardial techniques,[48] which are covered in detail in Chapter 21.

Ablation Technique

Various techniques to isolate the posterior wall have been described. In the LA box set, the PVs are isolated by antral encircling ablations, and a roofline is created as described previously. A linear lesion is then created between the left and right inferior PV to complete the set.[39] Alternatively, the continuous single-ring linear lesion extends up the ridge between the left PV and the atrial appendage, across the roof, inferiorly along the interatrial septum between the foramen ovale and right PVs, then inferior to the right PV, and lateral across the atrium to meet the start of the line by ascending lateral to the left inferior PVs.[49] Completion of this line isolates the PV and posterior LA wall en bloc.[49] A single-ring technique combined with activation mapping may spare complete ablation along the posterior wall[50] (Fig. 19.6). Frequently, ablation of residual electrograms within a posterior box lesion is required to attain durable

TABLE 19.2 **Assessing Conduction Block Across Linear Ablation Lines**

Finding/Maneuver	Finding Indicative of Complete Block	Comment
Widely split electrograms	>100 ms generally indicates block	Absolute time between electrogram components depends on local conduction velocities Block may be present with shorter times and conduction persistent with longer times
Differential pacing	Pacing site close to edge line produces longer conduction times from stimulus to opposite side of line than pacing at site away from line	Must pace from immediate edge of line
Propagation from pacing adjacent to line	Pacing on either side of line produces two wavefronts, each propagating toward the ablation line from opposite directions	*Roofline:* pace LAA and confirm that posterior wall is activated from caudal to cranial direction *Mitral isthmus line:* pacing CS lateral to line produces proximal to distal CS activation and pacing CS medial to the line produces distal-to-proximal CS activation *Anterior mitral isthmus line:* pacing lateral to line produces atrial septal activation from the posterior and lateral directions *Posterior wall isolation:* entrance and exit block within *box*

CS, Coronary sinus; *LAA*, left atrial appendage.

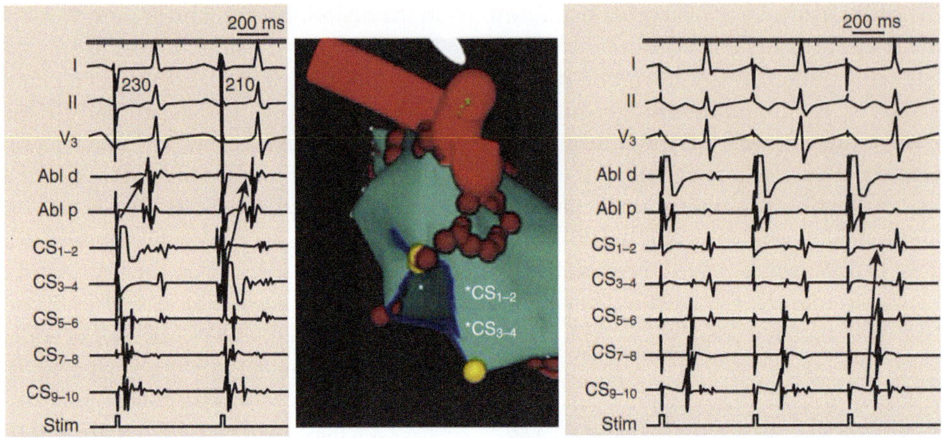

A B

Fig. 19.5 Mitral isthmus block. (A) Differential pacing to assess counterclockwise block across an ablation line in the mitral isthmus. The ablation catheter is positioned medial to the ablation line in the left atrium. Pacing was performed in the coronary sinus, and as the pacing site was switched from the distal electrodes (CS 1–2) to a more proximal pair of electrodes (CS 3–4), the interval between the pacing stimulus and the local electrogram recorded from the ablation catheter shortened from 230 to 210 ms. (B) Clockwise conduction block along the mitral isthmus. Note that atrial activation progresses from the proximal (CS 9–10) to distal (CS 1–2) electrodes during left atrial pacing medial to the ablation line. *Abl d*, Distal bipole of the ablation catheter; *Abl p*, proximal bipole of the ablation catheter; *CS*, coronary sinus; *Stim*, stimulus. (From Morady F, Oral H, Chugh A. Diagnosis and ablation of atypical atrial tachycardia and flutter complicating atrial fibrillation ablation. *Heart Rhythm*. 2009;6:S29–S32.)

isolation (Fig. 19.7A–C). Cryoballoon ablation has also been used to effectively attain PVI and PW isolation (see later). The endpoint for both approaches is the absence or dissociation of electrograms within the lesion box and exit block during pacing from the posterior wall.

Left Atrial Appendage Isolation

LA appendage (LAA) can be a source of triggered activity when challenged with high-dose isoproterenol (up to 30 μg/min for up to 10–15 minutes) in up to 27% of patients presenting for redo ablation procedures.[51] In a conflicting study of 7129 patients undergoing ablation, only 0.3% of cases reported that the LAA was a source of triggered activity.[52] Discrepancies between these series may be due to trigger mapping techniques; however, beyond a source of AF triggers, the LAA can contribute to the substrate supporting AF and frequently harbors focal drivers of AF.[53] Hocini et al. reported that among patients undergoing stepwise ablation for persistent AF, focal reentry involving the LAA occurred in 19% of patients who had focal source of atrial tachycardias.[54] Reentry in the LAA has also been demonstrated in patients without prior ablation.[55] In a study of 113 patients with persistent AF undergoing ablation, the LAA was identified as a driver of AF in 66/113 (58%) of patients.[56]

Support for empiric LAA isolation (LAAI) can be found in the BELIEF trial, which randomized 173 patients to either extensive LA ablation alone or extensive atrial ablation with electrical isolation of the LAA.[57] Clinical efficacy in the LAAI arm was 76% compared with 56% in the standard, albeit extensive LA ablation. Complete LAAI at initial ablation could not be achieved in 13% of patients, and LAA reconnection was noted at repeat ablation in 37% of the patients.

Ablation Technique

To assess progress of LAAI, a multipolar mapping catheter can be placed at the ostium of the LAA. Position of the catheter may be confirmed with a three-dimensional mapping system, intracardiac echo, and/or fluoroscopy (Fig. 19.8). Ablation may be carried out in sinus rhythm or during AF; ablation in sinus rhythm allows for targeting of early potentials in a manner analogous to performing PVI. Preprocedure imaging with contrast-enhanced CT, MRI, or TEE can be used to define the anatomy and exclude preexisting LAA thrombus.[58] Care should be taken not to ablate inside the LAA due to the risk of perforation. The phrenic nerve variably courses along the posterior aspect of the LAA[59] and may lay in close proximity to ablation lesions. High-output pacing (e.g., 20 mA at 10 ms) should be performed to reduce the risk of phrenic nerve injury during ablation. Isolation of the LAA has also been performed with cryoablation or through the creation of linear ablation along the atrial roof, lateral mitral isthmus, and anterior wall[60]; the optimal isolation strategy in terms of clinical efficacy or the implications for LAA thrombus formation are unknown.[61] Given the increased risk for LAA thrombus after isolation, patients should continue on life-long, uninterrupted anticoagulation or be considered for LAA occlusion/exclusion procedures.[62]

Vein of Marshal Alcohol Ablation

The ligament of Marshal (LOM) is the remnant of the left SVC and contains autonomic innervations and myocardial muscle bundles.[63] The LOM arises from the coronary sinus musculature and passes laterally and anterior to the left PVs to join with the ridge between the left superior PV and appendage. The structure then continues for varying lengths medial to the left PVs. The ligament shares muscle fibers with the LA and PV epicardia.

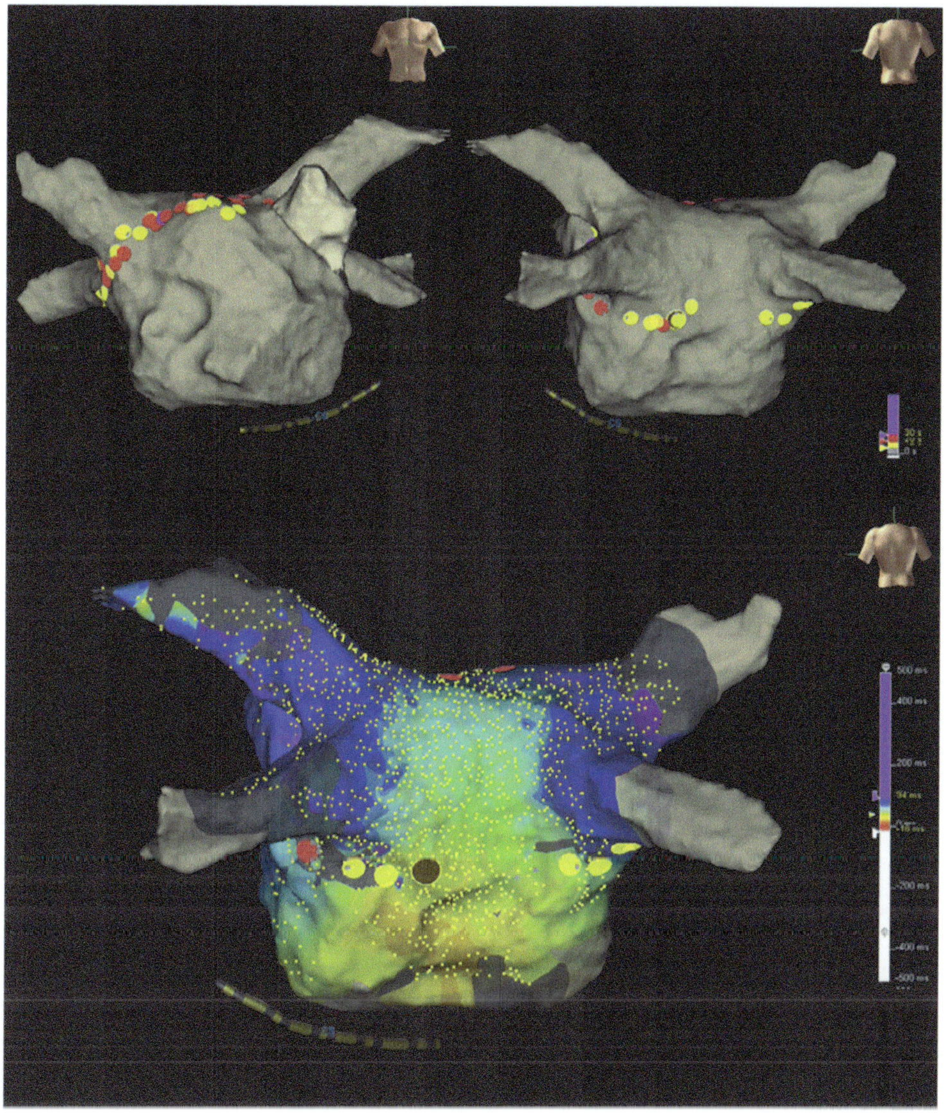

Fig. 19.6 Single ring isolation with esophageal sparing. The three-dimensional electroanatomical depictions of the left atrium are shown; color scale denotes activation mapping during coronary sinus pacing. Ablation was performed beginning anterior to the right pulmonary veins, roof, left pulmonary ridge, and, finally, underneath the pulmonary veins. There is rapid conduction into the posterior wall, with slowing into the pulmonary veins denoting a change in fiber orientation. Ablation at the brown point at the proximal insertion of these muscle bundles into the posterior wall resulted in isolation of the pulmonary veins and posterior wall. (From Mahajan R, Thiyagarajah A, Lau D, et al. Single ring isolation for atrial fibrillation ablation: how to do it and avoid the esophagus. *Heart Rhythm Case Rep.* 2020;6:169–173.)

The ligament contains sympathetic and parasympathetic nerve fibers, and a central vein of Marshall (VOM) that can be visualized with angiography.[64]

Retrograde ethanol injection into the VOM was first described as an adjuvant technique to achieve regional atrial ablation near the left PVs and vagal denervation.[65] Ensuing studies demonstrated it as key target to assist with isolation of the left PVs[66] and to target a spectrum of arrhythmias originating from the lateral mitral isthmus and LA ridge.[67,68] Its role as a target for de novo treatment of persistent AF was demonstrated in the VENUS randomized clinical trial.[69] In this multicenter trial, 350 patients with persistent AF were randomized to catheter ablation alone versus catheter ablation with VOM ethanol infusion. While >95% of patients in both groups underwent a variety of extra-PV ablation (including linear lesions and CFAEs) at the discretion of the operator, the addition of ethanol ablation of the VOM increased the likelihood of freedom from AF after a single procedure (49.2% versus 38%, difference, 11.2% [95% CI, 0.8–21.7%]; $P=.04$) and led to a reduction in the overall AF/AT burden (zero burden in 78.3% versus 67.9%; difference, 10.4% [95% CI, 2.9–17.9%]; $P=.01$). Achieving perimitral block was associated with an increased procedural success rate[70] and should be incorporated into procedural endpoints when performing VOM ablation.

Additional studies have examined the use of ethanol ablation into the VOM as part of empiric anatomy-based lesion set to achieve substrate modification. In the prospective Marshall-PLAN study, 75 consecutive patients with persistent AF

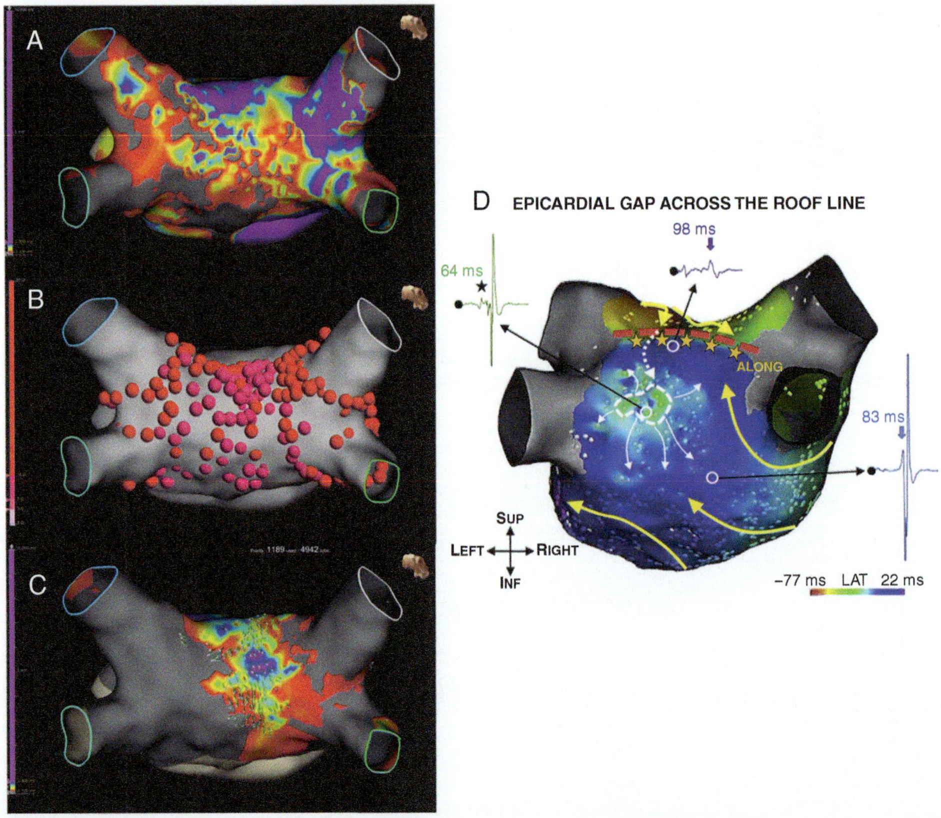

Fig. 19.7 Challenges to posterior wall isolation. (A) The three-dimensional electroanatomical depictions of the left atrium and the pulmonary veins are shown in the posteroanterior angulation; a preablation voltage map is shown with the color scale demonstrating areas of dense scar (gray <0.01 mV) and normal tissue (*purple* >0.5 mV). (B) Extensive ablation was performed around the pulmonary veins, left and right carina, and throughout the posterior wall in a point-by-point fashion. (C) Postablation, a repeat electroanatomical and activation map (*arrows*) was created demonstrating persistent voltage throughout the left atrial roof and posterior wall, with electrical activation proceeding in a cranial-to-caudal fashion through conduction gaps in the roof line. (D) A separate procedure is shown demonstrating epicardial breakthough across a roof line. A roof line ablation (*red dashed line*) was created with widely split electrograms (*purple*) and noncapture with pacing at sites along the line (*yellow stars*), consistent with effective endocardial ablation. High-density activation mapping during left atrial appendage pacing is shown, demonstrating epicardial breakthough near the left inferior pulmonary vein with a fractionated early signal preceding sharper signals locally (*green*) and at remote sites along the posterior wall (*blue*). (D adapted from Pambrun T, Duchateau J, Delglove A, et al. Epicardial course of the septopulmonary bundle: anatomical considerations and clinical implications for roof line completion. *Heart Rhythm*. 2021;18:349–357.)

underwent sequential ablation of predefined anatomical targets including VOM ethanol ablation, epicardial coronary sinus muscle bundle ablation, LA ridge ablation, antral PVI, and linear ablation at the LA roof, lateral mitral isthmus, and the cavotricuspid isthmus.[71] This extensive ablation resulted in single- and multiple-procedure 12-month success rates of 72% and 89%, respectively. Completion of linear block, including across the mitral isthmus, was demonstrated in >90% of patients. While lacking a control group, these outcomes are favorable compared to prior studies of persistent AF ablation.[72,73]

Ablation Technique

The VOM can be identified by coronary sinus angiography in approximately 75% of patients (Fig. 19.9).[74,75] The VOM arises from the posterior aspect of the coronary sinus and is cannulated with a left internal mammary artery guide catheter or a coronary vein subselection catheter (Rapido IC-90; Boston Scientific, Natick, MA). An angioplasty balloon is advanced over a guidewire for selective angiography of the VOM. For ablation, three separate injections of 3 mL of 100% ethanol are given 2 minutes apart. Ethanol injection creates areas of low atrial electrogram voltage on the lateral wall of the LA between the lateral coronary sinus and left PV and anterior to the PV. In addition, the ethanol injection alone produces partial or complete electrical isolation of the left PV in most patients and, depending on the course of the venous tributaries, may impact the roof or posterior atrium as well (Fig. 19.10).

ELECTROGRAM-GUIDED ATRIAL ABLATION

Targeting Atrial Fibrosis

Electroanatomical remodeling facilitates propagation through a variety of mechanisms. Unsurprisingly, the extent of atrial fibrosis has been correlated with worse procedural outcomes after

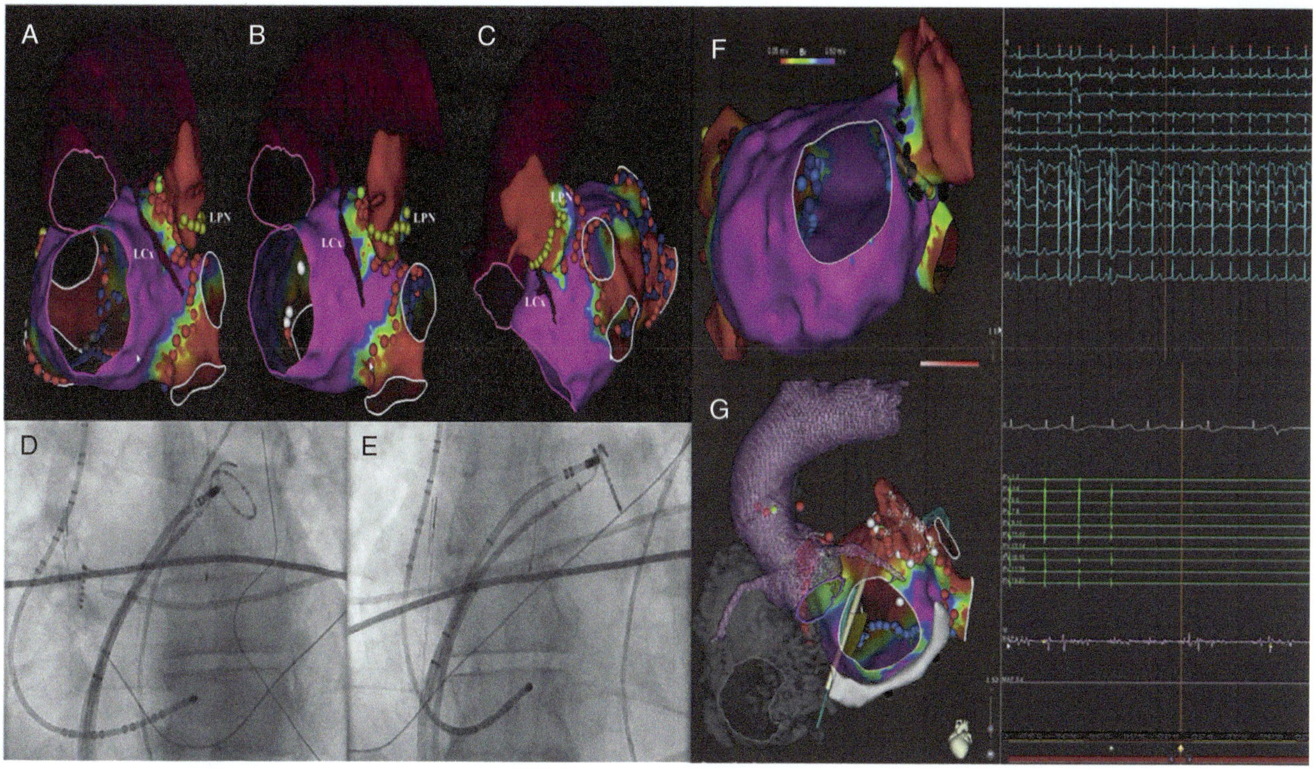

Fig. 19.8 LAA isolation. (A, B) Electroanatomical maps of the LA in anterior and lateral views showing the distance between the LCx coronary artery and the RFA lesions delivered at the anterior edge of the LAA ostium. (C) Electroanatomical maps of the LA in the posterior view showing the distance between the LPN and the RFA lesions delivered at the posterior edge of the LAA ostium. (D, E) The orientation of the circular mapping catheter and the ablation catheter in the shallow LAO view at the level of the LAA ostium and at the level of the earliest LAA activation. (F, G) Electroanatomic maps of patients undergoing LAAEIA with RFA showing AF termination and LAA isolation. (F) Ablation catheter in the inferior aspect of the LAA ostium terminates AF into normal sinus rhythm. (G) Note LAAEI while delivering RFA energy at the anterior wall of the LAA ostium. A Penta Ray catheter is in the LAA, with total electrical silence demonstrating successful LAA isolation. *AF*, Atrial fibrillation; *CT*, computed tomography; *EAM*, electroanatomical mapping; *FAM*, fast anatomical mapping; *ICE*, intracardiac echocardiogram; *LA*, left atrium; *LAA*, left atrial appendage; *LAAEI*, left atrial appendage electrical isolation; *LAO*, left anterior oblique; *LCx*, left circumflex; *LMCA*, left main coronary artery; *LPN*, left phrenic nerve; *PV*, pulmonary veins; *3D*, three-dimensional; *RFA*, radiofrequency ablation. (From Romero J, Natalo A, Di Biaco L. How to perform left atrial appendage electrical isolation using radiofrequency ablation. *Heart Rhythm*. 2018;15:1577–1582.)

AF ablation. In the DECAFF study, late gadolinium-enhanced cardiac magnetic resonance imaging (LGE-MRI) was used to quantify areas of atrial fibrosis in patients undergoing first-time catheter ablation procedures for AF[76] (Fig. 19.11). In this multicenter study, 272 patients underwent quantification of atrial scar. Over a 12-month follow-up period, there was a significant relationship between the percentage of scarred atrial myocardium and the likelihood of arrhythmia recurrence, which persisted despite adjusting for common variables associated with arrhythmia recurrence including the type of AF, heart failure, and LA volume (HR 1.06/%; 95% CI, 1.03–1.09, $P < .001$). Similar findings have been reported in studies using bipolar voltage maps to define atrial scar.[77] In a study of 165 patients undergoing AF ablation, the extent of atrial scar was more predictive of response to PVI-only ablation irrespective of the type of AF (persistent versus paroxysmal) or the number of years since the diagnosis of AF.[78] This suggest that assessing atrial fibrosis (rather than AF subtype alone) may better inform on the appropriate ablation strategy and may help identify patients who may best respond to extra-PVI ablation.

The extent of LGE-MRI defined atrial fibrosis has been correlated well with electroanatomical data confirming low-voltage atrial areas. However, the mechanistic importance of these findings may be called into question, with several studies showing a lack of co-regionality with LGE-MRI–defined scar and the location of AF drivers and rotors.[79,80]

Voltage-Based Ablation

Rolf et al. reported on the use of tailored ablation strategy of substrate modification in patients with paroxysmal and persistent AF.[81] In 178 patients, LA voltage maps were created in sinus rhythm after the completion of PVI. Peak-to-peak voltage cutoffs were used to classify areas as healthy (>0.5 mV), diseased (0.2–0.5 mV), or likely scar tissue (<0.2 mV). Areas with contiguous areas of low-voltage areas (LVAs) were targeted for ablation with the aim of homogenizing the atrial substrate through either targeted ablations or linear lesions as deemed appropriate. Patients with persistent AF had greater rates of LVAs than those with paroxysmal AF (35% versus 10%). Additionally, 26 patients with LVAs who only underwent PVI were included as

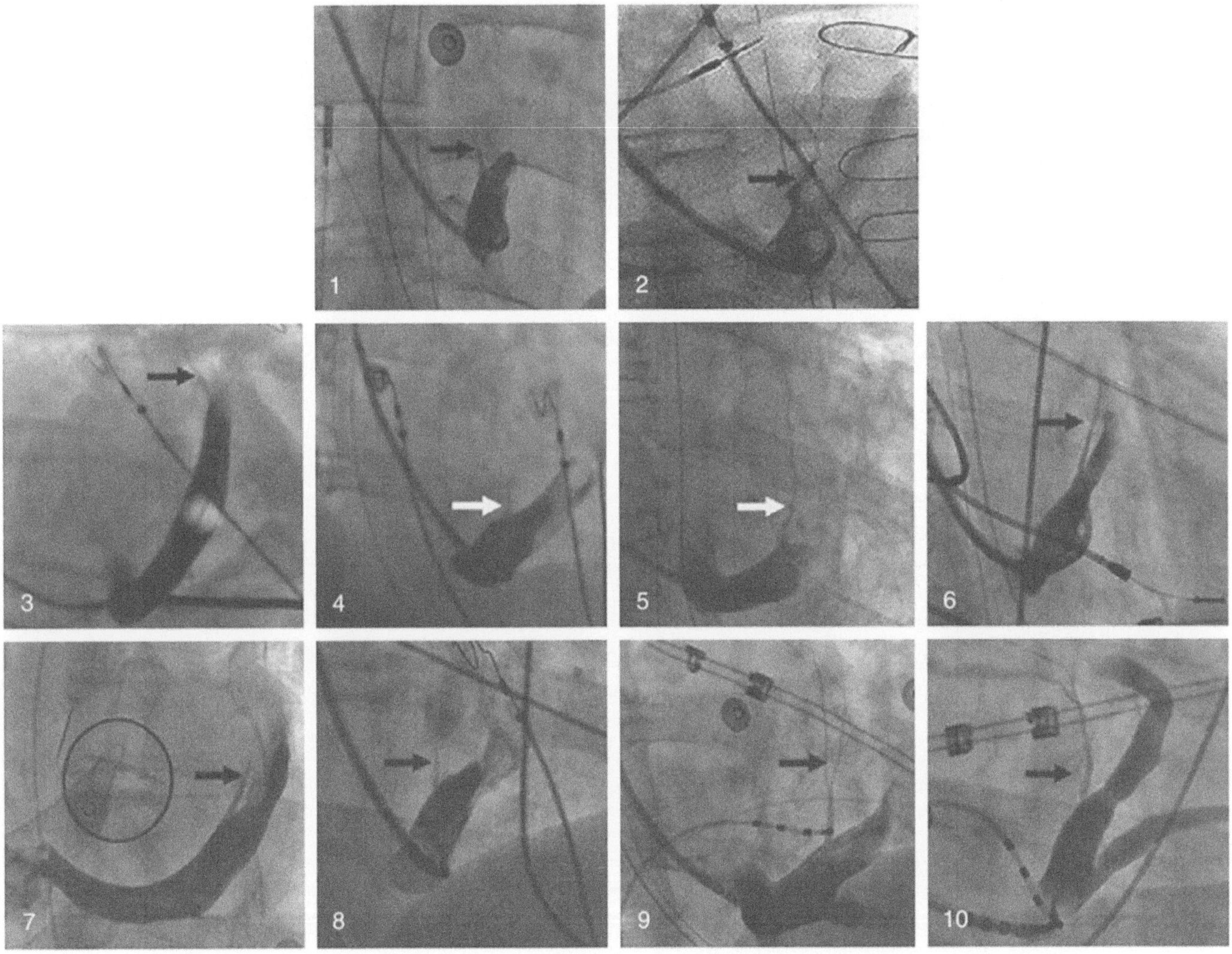

Fig. 19.9 Vein of Marshall subselective venograms in 10 patients (1–6, 8–10). Right anterior oblique fluoroscopic projections (except for patient number 7, left anterior oblique). (From Hwang C, Chen P-S. Ligament of Marshall: why it is important for atrial fibrillation ablation. *Heart Rhythm*. 2009;6:S35–S40.)

a comparison group. Patients with LVAs who did not undergo substrate modification had worse arrhythmia outcomes than those who did undergo additional ablation (12-month freedom from AF/AT 70% versus 27%, log rank $P < .001$); additionally, patients with LVAs who underwent additional ablation had similar outcomes compared to those without LVAs who did not require additional substrate modification. While retrospective, this study suggests that modifying the atrial substrate may lead to similar ablation outcomes compared to patients with less advanced atrial remodeling. An observation study by Yagishita et al. of 201 patients undergoing ablation, using similar definitions of atrial scar and substrate modification approaches, yielded similar results.[82]

In the Box Isolation of Fibrotic Areas (BIFA) study, patients with nonparoxysmal AF underwent a PVI followed by tailored ablation targeting areas fibrotic areas defined by sinus bipolar electrograms <0.5 mV.[83] Rather than using a homogenization approach or the use of linear lesions, fibrotic areas were circumferentially isolated with the endpoint of attaining entrance block confirmed with a circular mapping catheter. Significant areas of fibrotic areas were discovered in 60% of patients, application of this technique resulted in a single-procedure success rate of 72% after 12-month follow-up.

Several randomized controlled studies have examined a voltage-based substrate ablation strategy. Kircher et al.[84] randomized 124 patients to a strategy of conventional versus and LVA-guided ablation. The control group consisted of patients who underwent PVI (paroxysmal AF, n = 37) or PVI and PW isolation and lateral mitral isthmus ablation (persistent AF, n = 25), while the intervention group underwent PVI plus ablation of LVAs through a combination of linear lesions and regional ablation. Patients undergoing tailored LVA ablation had improved ablation outcomes (12-month arrhythmia recurrence off antiarrhythmics, 90% versus 72%, $P = .04$), with similar safety outcomes. In the STABLE-SR trial,[85] 229 patients with nonparoxysmal AF were randomized to a stepwise ablation approach (PVI plus linear ablation and CFAE) versus a strategy of PVI + CTI followed by substrate modification in sinus rhythm. Similar to prior studies, LVAs were seen in only approximately 50% of patients with nonparoxysmal AF who did not require extensive ablation. These two approaches yielded similar ablation outcomes with a nonsignificant trend toward improved outcomes

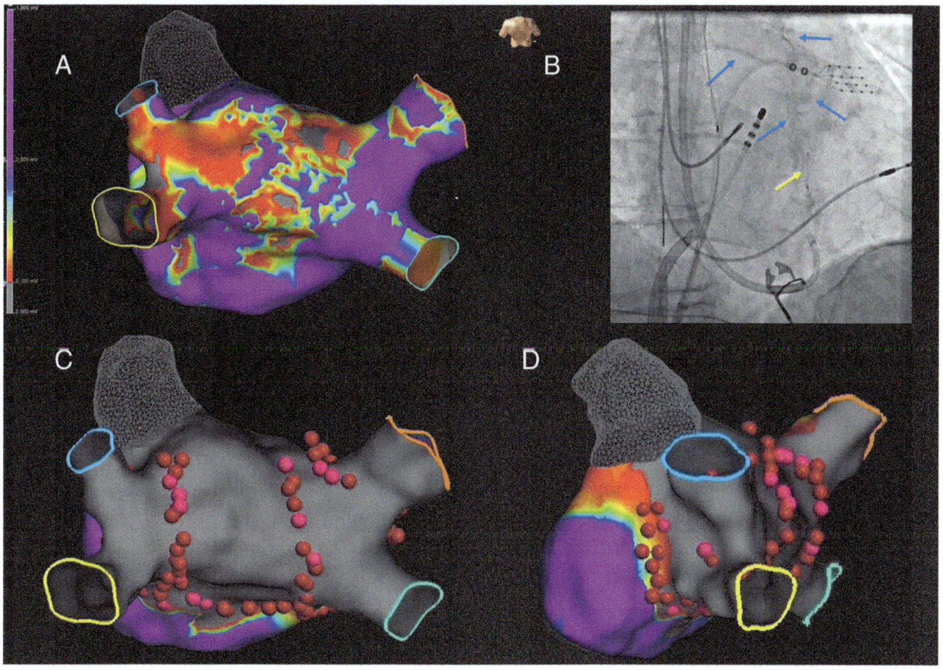

Fig. 19.10 Effects of vein of Marshall (VOM) ethanol ablation. (A) Preablation three-dimensional electroanatomical depiction of the left atrium and the pulmonary veins is shown; color scale denotes dense scar (*red* 0.1 mV, *purple* >0.5 mV). (B) Anterior posterior fluoroscopy is shown; the multipolar mapping catheter is positioned within the LAA. Contrast medium was injected through the lumen of a coronary angioplasty balloon (*yellow arrow*) positioned within the VOM demonstrating tributaries of the vein along the ridge, junction of the LSPV and LA(A) and extending to the atrial roof (*blue arrows*). (C, D) Ethanol ablation through the VOM was performed, along with antral ablation and an inferior linear lesion. A repeat voltage map was attained demonstrating electrical isolation of the pulmonary veins, posterior wall, and mitral isthmus. Due to the effects of alcohol ablation, complete isolation of these structures was attained without the need for extensive endocardial ablation.

in the substrate modification group (HR 0.78; 95% CI, 0.47–1.29, $P = .33$). The STABLE-SR-II[86] trial examined a simplified approach (PVI versus PVI and LVA ablation) with similar results (no additive benefit to LVA ablation) (Fig. 19.12).

The VOLCANO trial randomized 62 patients with paroxysmal AF with LVA discovered after PVI to a strategy of scar homogenization plus trigger mapping/ablation of induced atrial tachycardias versus only trigger mapping and ablation of induced atrial tachycardias.[87] A control group of patients with paroxysmal AF and no areas of LVA were also included. While the presence of LVA was a strong predictor of arrhythmia recurrence, the addition of substrate modification did not improve procedural outcomes.

Mapping and Ablation Technique

One challenge to performing substrate modification vis-a-vis ablation of LVAs is that the electrogram amplitudes are heavily dependent on the measurement technique.[88] Electrode-size, interelectrode distance, the use of multielectrode versus point-by-point mapping, catheter orientation, and mapping system filters, and algorithms have all been shown to influence atrial electrograms.[89–93] Within the same patient, substantial differences in electrogram fractionation and amplitudes have been demonstrated when electroanatomical data are collected in sinus/paced rhythm versus AF.[94,95] The cycle length and direction of wavefront activation when mapping in paced rhythms also lead to substantial changes in the spatial distribution and extent of LVAs, fractionation, and conduction velocities; these changes are exaggerated in patients with persistent AF.[96]

Studies in which LVA modification is performed during sinus rhythm have been reported,[97] but comparative studies to ablation in AF are lacking. Additionally, the ideal cut-off voltage for defining LVAs is unknown. The majority of the aforementioned studies used an voltage cut-off of <0.5 mV; however, abnormal conduction properties have been demonstrated in atrial tissue with greater bipolar voltages (<1.3 mV)[98] and low cutoffs may lack the sensitivity to identify the entirety of the arrhythmogenic substrate. Studies correlating atrial LGE-MRI to electroanatomical mapping have likewise been inconsistent regarding the optimal voltage cutoffs to accurately identify fibrosis.[99–101]

Ablation of Complex Fractionated Atrial Electrograms

An intraoperative epicardial mapping study in humans suggested that areas of CFAEs may indicate sites of slow conduction, conduction block, wavefront collision, or anchor points for reentrant circuits that can perpetuate AF.[102,103] CFAEs may also indicate sites of high-frequency sources (rotors), fibrillatory conduction, and sites of autonomic innervation.[104–106] CFAEs have been targeted for ablation to eliminate both paroxysmal and persistent AF. CFAEs are quite prevalent and can be found at many sites in both atria. The sites that most commonly harbor

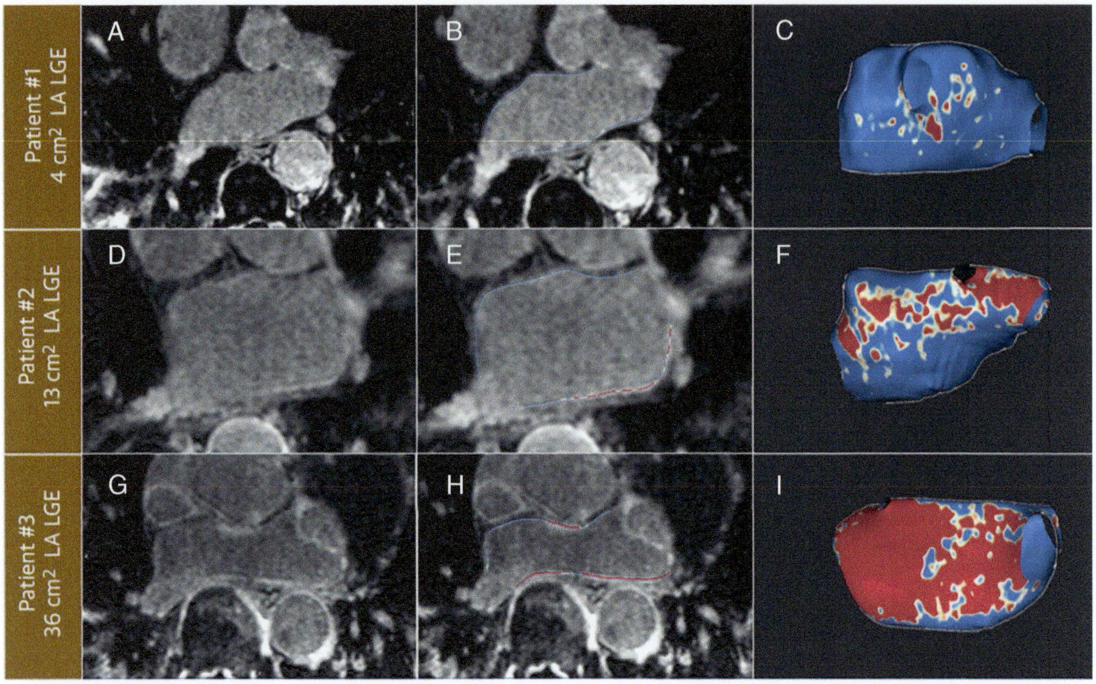

Fig. 19.11 Late gadolinium-enhanced (LGE) magnetic resonance imaging of the atrium. Images from three patients with varying amounts of LGE are shown. (A, D, G) LGE-CMR data, with their respective segmentations based on the degree of enhancement shown in B, E, and H. Three-dimensional reconstructions are shown in C, F, and I. *Blue regions* indicate no uptake, with a color scale from *white*to red showing indicating increased enhancement. (From Bertelsen L, Diederichsne S, Haugan K, et al. *J Am Coll Cardiol Imaging.* 2020;13:1690–1700.)

CFAEs are the interatrial septum, LA roof, LA appendage, near the PVs, and along the crista terminalis in the RA.[107] Clustering of CFAE sites near the PVs appears to be more pronounced in patients with paroxysmal compared with nonparoxysmal forms of AF. CFAEs may be recorded over 38–56% of the LA endocardium.[107–112]

Ablation of CFAEs has been performed in AF. Local energy delivery is continued until there is elimination of the local electrogram, loss of the fractionated high-frequency electrogram components, or increase in the atrial cycle length. In the original description of the technique, an average of 64 ± 36 sites were ablated per patient.[102] The average duration of RF delivery was reported as 36 ± 13 minutes.[112] Antral ablation for PVI targets many of the sites that frequently harbor CFAEs. Antral PVI may greatly reduce the CFAE distribution over the LA endocardium from 56% before to 23% after PVI.[113] For patients undergoing PVI and CFAE ablation, completion of PVI first may reduce the total amount of RF energy delivered. Once CFAEs are eliminated from the LA, the RA may then be mapped. Complex atrial electrograms are also frequently recorded within the coronary sinus. Ablation along the LA endocardium abutting the coronary sinus prolongs LA cycle length in patients with persistent AF. Ablation within the coronary sinus further prolongs atrial cycle length. The techniques for ablation along and within the coronary sinus were described previously. The endpoint for electrogram-guided ablation is termination of AF into sinus rhythm or into an organized atrial tachycardia, elimination of all complex atrial electrograms, or, for patients with paroxysmal AF, noninducibility of AF (Table 19.4). Termination of AF most commonly occurs during ablation at the interatrial septum near the PV ostia and at the atrial roof near the LAA.[114,115]

In the original study by Nademanee et al., ablation of CFAEs without routine isolation of the PVs was reported to result in freedom from AF in 91% of the 121 patients with paroxysmal or chronic AF.[102] AF terminated during ablation in 63% and 95% of the patients without and with infusion of ibutilide, respectively. In a follow-up study of 674 patients, 89% of patients with paroxysmal AF, 85% of patients with persistent AF, and 71% of patients with permanent AF were reported to be in sinus rhythm at 2 years.[105] In a study of 100 patients with chronic AF who underwent CFAE ablation in the LA and the coronary sinus, only 33% and 57% of patients were in sinus rhythm without antiarrhythmic medications after single and repeat procedures, respectively.[112] In a randomized study, ablation of CFAEs after antral PVI was not found to be associated with a superior efficacy to antral PVI alone in patients with persistent AF.[116] However, ablation of CFAEs was limited to a maximum of 2 hours because the goal of the study was to determine whether AF could be terminated within a practical time frame. AF terminated in only a minority of patients in this study, suggesting that ablation of CFAE for up to 2 hours may not have been sufficient to eliminate most of the residual drivers of AF.

CFAE ablation is often incorporated into "stepwise" ablation strategies combining PVI, linear ablation, and CFAE aiming at AF termination. While these approaches have shown encouraging results in retrospective analyses,[72] randomized controlled trials have failed to demonstrate a clear incremental benefit in either paroxysmal or persistent AF ablations.[30,117–120] CFAE

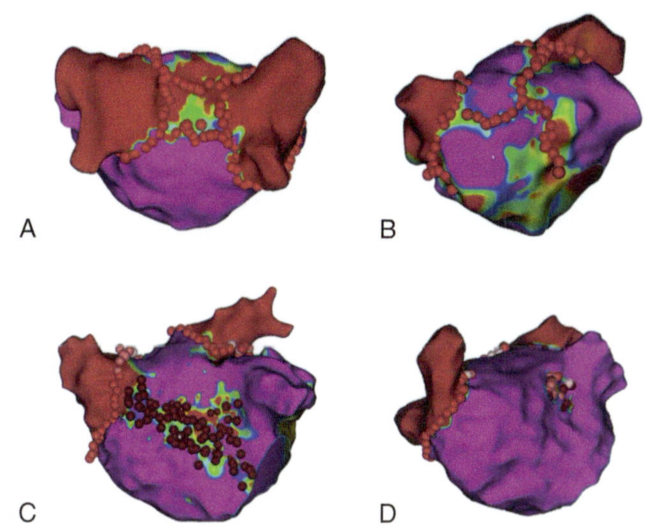

Fig. 19.12 Low-voltage modification of atrial substrate. Substrate modification targeting areas of low atrial voltage can be performed through various methods. Preablation three-dimensional electroanatomic depictions of the left atrium and the pulmonary veins are shown; color scale denotes dense scar (*red* 0.1 mV) to normal tissue (*purple* >0.5 mV). (A) Liner ablation is performed to isolate LVAs within the posterior wall. (B) Left atrial homogenization is performed via complex lesion sets directed over LVA. (C) Anterior substrate is targeting; to avoid creation of additional arrhythmia circuits, lesions were created encompassing LVAs and anchored to antral ablation lesions and the mitral annulus. (D) Focal areas of LVA are targeted at the base of the left atrial appendage. The surrounding tissue demonstrated normal bipolar voltage (*purple*), and therefore extensive linear ablation was not performed. *LVA,* Low-voltage areas. (Adopted from Yang G, Zheng L, Jiang C, et al. *J Am Coll Cardiol EP*. 2022;8:882–891.)

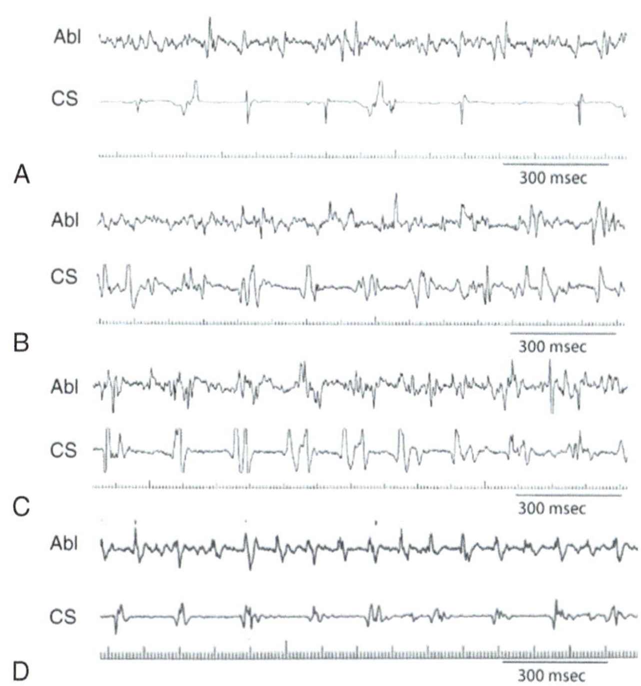

Fig. 19.13 Examples (A–D) of complex fractionated atrial electrograms. *Abl,* Distal bipole of the ablation catheter; *CS,* distal bipole of the coronary sinus catheter. (From Oral H, Chugh A, Good E, et al. Radiofrequency catheter ablation of chronic atrial fibrillation guided by complex electrograms. *Circulation.* 2007;115:2606–2612.)

ablation increases the probability of recurrent atrial arrhythmias in the form of atrial tachycardia or flutter, may prolong the procedure and may result in extensive atrial ablation.[119] Furthermore, termination of AF as an endpoint of ablation has not been predictive of clinical outcome in recent randomized studies,[121] whereas the presence of sinus rhythm before or during ablation was a strong predictor.

Mapping and Ablation Technique

CFAEs are identified during AF by visual assessment or by automated computerized algorithms (Fig. 19.13).[107,108] In the original description by Nademanee et al., CFAEs were defined as (1) atrial electrograms that are fractionated and composed of two or more deflections and/or have perturbation of the baseline with continuous deflections of a prolonged activation complex over a 10-second recording period or (2) atrial electrograms with a very short cycle length (≤120 ms) averaged over a 10-second period.[102] In addition, these electrograms are usually considered to be of low voltage (<0.15 mV). Other electrogram characteristics that have been targeted for ablation are sites with a large (>70 ms) temporal gradient between activation of the proximal and distal ablation bipoles, sites with continuous electrical activity without isoelectric intervals, sites with a cycle length less than the mean LA cycle length, and sites demonstrating centrifugal activation (Figs. 19.14–19.16; Table 19.3).[122]

For automated algorithms, samples of 2.5–10 seconds are acquired.[108,109] For optimal spectral analysis, windows of a 5-second duration or longer are recommended.[110] In addition, automated algorithms incorporate voltage parameters (low voltage <0.1–0.2 mV, high voltage >1.0 mV) and refractory periods of 50–60 ms.[108] Between 70 and 120 points are generally acquired to produce the color-coded map to display electrogram frequency or degree of fractionation.[108,110] There appears to be good agreement between visual and automated CFAE classification; however, more sites are characterized as CFAEs with visual than with automated assessment.

A difficulty in targeting CFAEs is that most may be caused by passive activation and lack specificity to indicate drivers of AF. Several studies have examined methods to increase the yield of CFAE ablation by applying more strict criteria for ablation than previously used. These strategies have included ablating CFAEs with only continuous activity,[97,123] ablation of CFAEs only within LVAs,[124] or ablating CFAEs that display spatiotemporal dispersion[125] (Fig. 19.17). The optimal definition and endpoint of CFAE ablation remain to be seen; under current paradigms, multiple meta-analyses have suggested little incremental benefit of routine CFAE ablation.[126–128] Primary CFAE-guided ablation may lead to excessive and unnecessary ablation in the LA and is usually reserved as an adjunctive step in patients with persistent or long-standing persistent AF who failed anatomy-based approaches.

Ganglionated Plexus Ablation

Fluctuations in autonomic tone have been associated with the initiation of AF in humans and animal models.[129] Vagal stimulation may facilitate spontaneous premature depolarizations in the atria, shorten the atrial and PV ERP, and increase heterogeneity of refractoriness.[130] Activation of the autonomic nervous

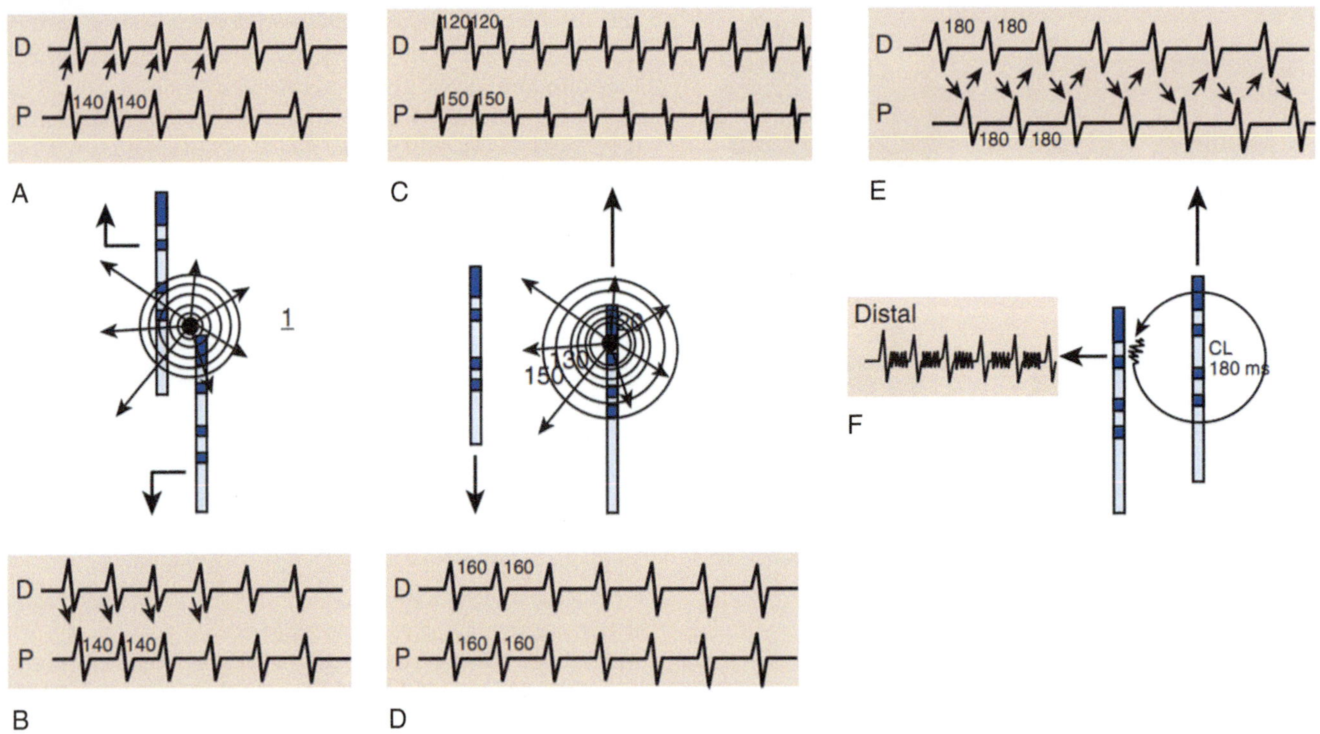

Fig. 19.14 Depiction of electrograms recorded near or at differing hypothetical focal sources. (A) Proximal-to distal activation sequence (*arrows*) consistent with the catheter position relative to a focal source of cycle length (CL) of 140 ms with 1:1 activation of the surrounding tissue. (B) Distal-to-proximal activation sequence. (C) Electrograms recorded with the distal (*D*) catheter bipole positioned over a high-frequency source (shortest cycle length, 120 ms) with a frequency gradient to the surrounding tissue, as indicated by the CL of 150 ms recorded on the proximal (P) bipole. (D) When the catheter is moved away from the source, simultaneous activation at the proximal and distal bipoles is seen, with no discernible difference in CL. (E) Temporal gradient between the proximal and distal bipoles when the catheter is positioned directly over a hypothetical local circuit of CL 180 ms. (F) A fractionated signal is recorded with the distal bipole at a hypothetical zone of slow conduction within the circuit. (From O'Neill MD, Kim KT, Jais P, et al. Ablation strategies in chronic atrial fibrillation. In: Aliot E, Haïssaguerre M, Jackman WM, eds. *Catheter Ablation of Atrial Fibrillation*. Malden, MA: Blackwell Futura; 2008:163–189.)

system may precede and substantiate PV triggers but also affects the underlying atrial substrate[131] through various mechanism including the development of CFAEs,[104] rotor formation,[132] ion channel expression,[133] and the development of atrial fibrosis.[134]

The intrinsic cardiac autonomic system includes autonomic ganglia within epicardial fat pads and the LOM.[135] These GP contain neuronal input from atrial myocardium and the extrinsic autonomic nervous system in addition to cholinergic and adrenergic neurons. In addition, there is an extensive network of interconnecting neurons among the ganglia themselves and between the ganglia and atrial and PV myocardium.[135] GPs that are targeted for endocardial ablation are often located (1) at the anterior aspect of the right superior PV; (2) posteriorly and inferiorly near the right inferior PV; (3) at the left upper PV GP between the LAA and left PVs (Marshall tract plexus); and (4) at the left lower PV GP located in the posterior and inferior aspect of the left inferior PV (Figs 19.18 and 19.19). Because of the proximity of the GP to the PVs, ablation approaches that do not directly target the GPs have been observed to also modify the autonomic substrate. It is postulated that autonomic activation initiates AF by facilitating afterdepolarizations in atrial and PV tissue.[135] In addition, autonomic activation dramatically shortens action potential duration, especially in the PV myocardium. Stimulation of GPs may have remote effects such as PV depolarizations or electrogram fractionation at a distance, suggesting active communication among the ganglia.[135]

Mapping and Ablation Technique

Mapping of GPs is performed by high-frequency stimulation. Mapping can be performed from the cardiac endocardium or epicardium.[136] Typically, stimulation is performed at 20 Hz (1200 beats per minute), at 5–100 V, and with a pulse width of 10 ms.[136,137] This is usually performed under general anesthesia because of poor patient tolerance. Sites showing a vagal response are usually found in the antral regions of the PVs. The locations of the targeted plexi are shown in Table 19.4. Patients in sinus rhythm may develop AF during programmed electrical nerve stimulation. High-frequency stimulation of GPs results in sympathetic and parasympathetic activation; however, the parasympathetic response occurs immediately, whereas the sympathetic response is delayed.[136,137] During AF, a vagal response is defined as atrioventricular (AV) block with a 50% or greater increase in mean RR interval within 5–10 seconds, associated with hypotension or induced AV block of more than 2 seconds' duration

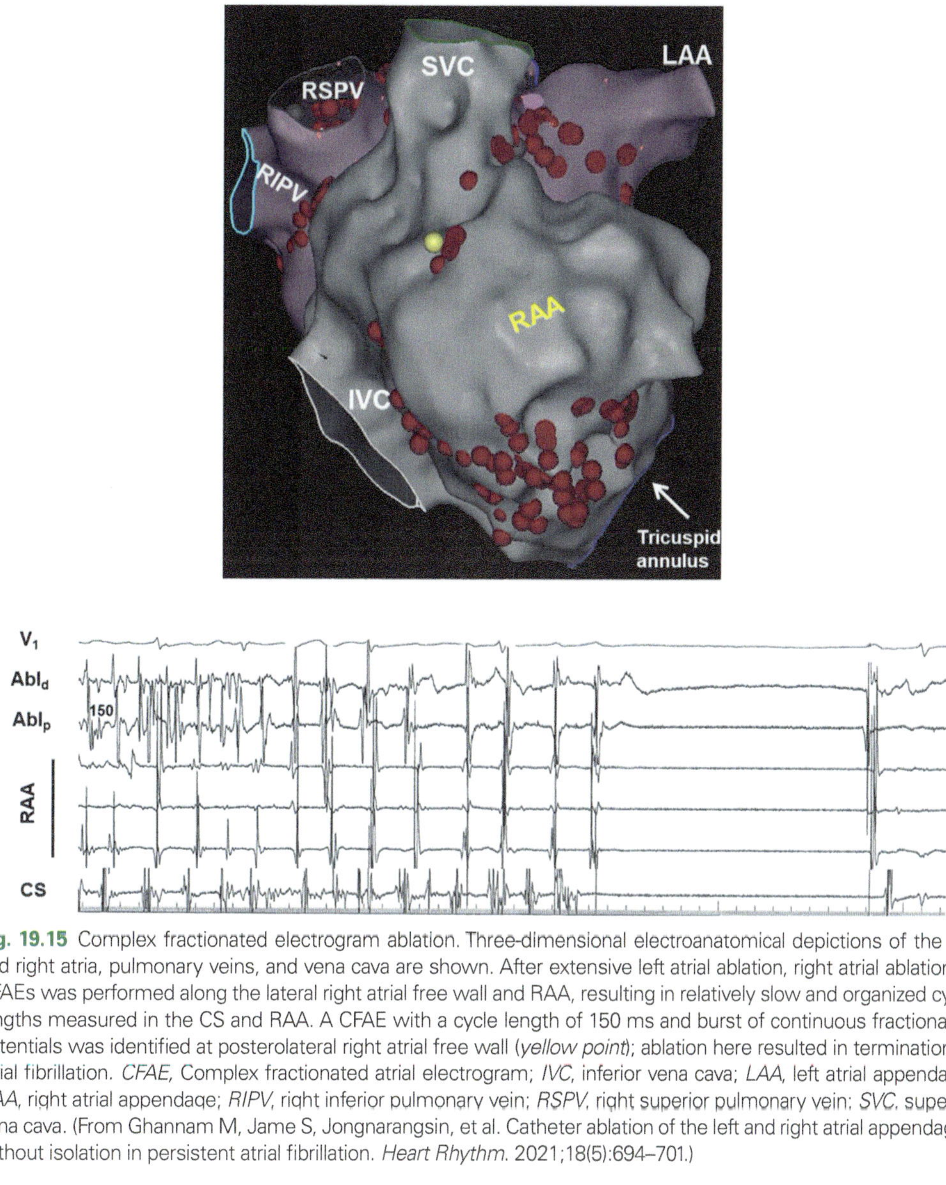

Fig. 19.15 Complex fractionated electrogram ablation. Three-dimensional electroanatomical depictions of the left and right atria, pulmonary veins, and vena cava are shown. After extensive left atrial ablation, right atrial ablation of CFAEs was performed along the lateral right atrial free wall and RAA, resulting in relatively slow and organized cycle lengths measured in the CS and RAA. A CFAE with a cycle length of 150 ms and burst of continuous fractionated potentials was identified at posterolateral right atrial free wall (*yellow point*); ablation here resulted in termination of atrial fibrillation. *CFAE*, Complex fractionated atrial electrogram; *IVC*, inferior vena cava; *LAA*, left atrial appendage; *RAA*, right atrial appendage; *RIPV*, right inferior pulmonary vein; *RSPV*, right superior pulmonary vein; *SVC*, superior vena cava. (From Ghannam M, Jame S, Jongnarangsin, et al. Catheter ablation of the left and right atrial appendages without isolation in persistent atrial fibrillation. *Heart Rhythm*. 2021;18(5):694–701.)

(see Fig. 19.19B).[135,136] Occasionally, GP stimulation results in firing from the adjacent PVs and, rarely, a predominantly sympathetic hypertensive response may occur.[74] Stimulation mapping may fail to induce vagal responses in up to 30% of patients, even when selected for characteristics of vagally induced AF. In patients with positive endocardial and epicardial responses, 5 ± 2.4 sites are usually targeted per patient.[136]

Endocardial ablation is delivered at each site demonstrating a positive response to stimulation. Percutaneous epicardial mapping and ablation for GPs have also been performed.[135,136] Typically, three to eight RF applications are needed per site. The endpoint of ablation is the elimination of all vagal responses within the LA. Occasionally AV block is not seen during ganglia stimulation. AV block is mediated by the vagal output from the crux GP located between the IVC and coronary sinus ostium.[135] Loss of interconnecting neurons from other GP to the crux fat pad may result in failure to elicit vagal responses. A specific order of ablation has been recommended to minimize the loss of vagal response from ablation: first, Marshall tract GP; then, left superior GP, anterior right GP, inferior left GP; and, finally, inferior right GP. The sites for autonomic ablation overlap with those incorporated in PV antral ablation, and PVI results in changes in Holter-derived indices of autonomic tone similar to endocardial and epicardial parasympathetic catheter denervation.[136] Similarly, there may be overlap between the location of CFAEs and GP innervation sites[138]; more studies are needed to understand this relationship and its clinical implications.

RIGHT ATRIAL SUBSTRATE ABLATION

Initial attempts of catheter AF ablation targeted the RA but demonstrated limited benefit from RA linear ablation alone.[139–142] However, it is recognized that RA foci such as the SVC, crista terminalis, and coronary sinus ostium may play a role in initiation of AF.[142,143] Identification of RA arrhythmogenic substrate is challenging as the majority of imaging and electroanatomical studies aimed at identifying arrhythmogenic atrial tissue have primarily focused on the LA.[144,145] Nevertheless, the importance of the

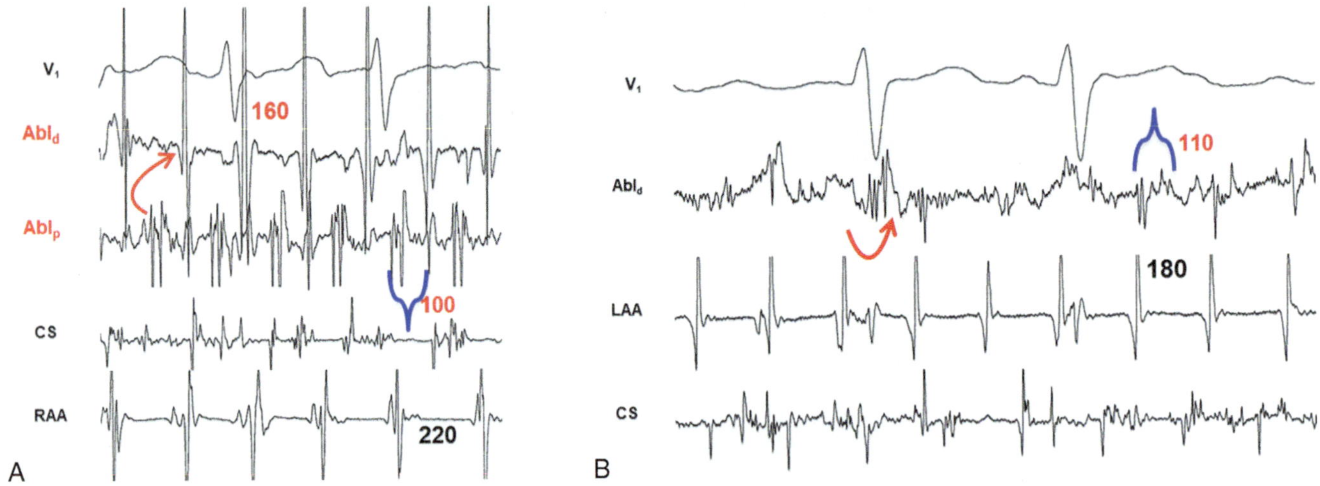

Fig. 19.16 Selective ablation of CFAEs. (A) CFAEs are recorded on the proximal and distal bipoles of an ablation catheter. A temporal gradient accounting for the majority of the AF cycle length was recorded (100 ms compared to a global cycle length of 160 ms); ablation here resulted in termination of AF to atrial tachycardia. (B) Long-duration electrograms are seen on the ablation catheter, accounting for the majority of the AF cycle length (110 ms compared to 180 ms), Ablation here resulted in termination to sinus rhythm. *Abl*, Ablation; *CFAE*, complex fractionated atrial electrograms; *CS*, coronary sinus; *LAA*, left atrial appendage; *RAA*, right atrial appendage. (From Ghannam M, Jame S, Jongnarangsin, et al. Catheter ablation of the left and right atrial appendages without isolation in persistent atrial fibrillation. *Heart Rhythm*. 2021;18(5):694–701.)

TABLE 19.3 Targets for Ablation of Complex Fractionated Atrial Electrograms

Electrogram Feature (Reference)	Definition	Possible Pathophysiology
Complex fractionated atrial electrogram (CFAE)[102]	Atrial electrograms that are fractionated and composed of two or more deflections, and/or have perturbation of the baseline with continuous deflections of a prolonged activation complex over a 10-second recording period, or atrial electrograms with a very short cycle length (≤120 ms) averaged over a 10-second period	Slow conduction Pivot points GPs Rotor Fibrillatory conduction Wave front collision
Continuous electrical activity[107]	Absence of isoelectric intervals for ≥1-second recording period	Focal reentry Anisotropy Summation overlapping electrograms High-frequency depolarization
Temporal activation gradient[114]	>70-ms interval between activation of proximal and distal ablation electrodes	Focal reentry
Frequency gradient[122]	Electrogram cycle length < mean left atrial cycle length	Focal reentry/automaticity or triggered activity
Centrifugal activation [114]	Radial spread of activation from a focus	Focal reentry/automaticity or triggered activity

RA in sustaining AF, particularly in patients with persistent AF, has repeatedly been demonstrated.[146] Recent studies using high-density mapping catheters have shown that potential arrhythmogenic substrate (defined as LVA or corridors of slow conduction) can be detected in the RA in majority of patients undergoing AF procedures.[147] Ablation in the RA is necessary to terminate AF in up to 15–30% of patients.[116] Among patients undergoing FIRM ablation, 20–30% required ablation of RA sources.[40] CFAEs can also be found in the RA; however in a randomized study, routine ablation of CFAEs in the RA was not associated with an improvement in clinical efficacy of LA catheter ablation of AF.[116]

Monitoring RA cycle length in comparison to LA cycle length may be helpful to determine when to proceed with RA ablation during LA ablation of AF. In a study of 113 patients with persistent AF, RA drivers were identified in 36% of patients and who had RA cycle length less than LA cycle length upon completion of LA ablation lesion sets.[56] The RA appendage was the most common site of RA drivers and can be targeted in analogous fashion to the LA appendage (Fig. 19.20). Autonomic innervations are found within the fat pads around the SVC and coronary sinus ostium (crux) and may contribute to arrhythmia mechanisms.

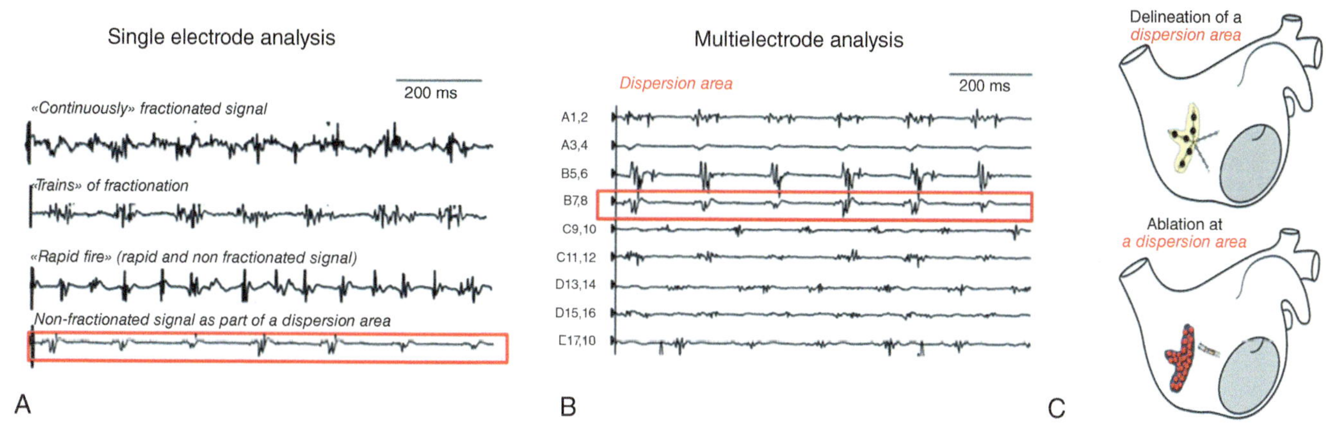

Fig. 19.17 Multipolar electrode analysis of CFAE. (A) Single-electrode analysis of bipolar electrograms from four different regions are shown. Signals highlighted in *red* are nonfractionated with relatively slow cycle length and do not meet conventional criteria as a target of CFAE ablation. (B) Multielectrode analysis of the same signals (*red box*) reveal that these signals are contained within a larger area of CFAEs, demonstrating spatiotemporal dispersion and may be incorporated into ablation strategies (shown in C). *CFAE*, Complex fractionated atrial electrograms. (Adapted from Seitz J, Bars C, Theodore G. *J Am Coll Cardiol.* 2017;69:303–321.)

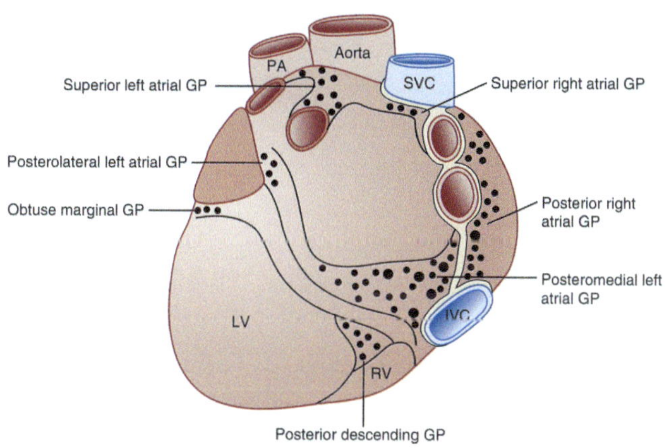

Fig. 19.18 Drawing of a posterior view of the human heart and major vessels illustrating the locations of posterior atrial and ventricular ganglionic plexi (GP). Positions of the superior vena cava (SVC), inferior vena cava (IVC), right ventricle (RV), pulmonary artery (PA), and left ventricle (LV) are shown. (Modified from Armour JA, Murphy DA, Yuan BX, et al. Gross and microscopic anatomy of the human intrinsic cardiac nervous system. *Anat Rec.* 1997;247:289–298.)

ADDITIONAL TECHNIQUES AND FUTURE CONSIDERATIONS

Delayed-Enhanced Magnetic Resonance Imaging–Based Ablation

Assessment of atrial scar through late LGE-CMR can be performed at specialty centers and has been shown to correlate well with histopathologic and endocardial voltage mapping.[148] There are significant technical challenges to producing high-fidelity images of the thin-walled atrium[149] and the optimal image acquisition and processing techniques remain to be described[150] (technical aspects of LGE-CMR and atrial imaging are discussed in detail in Chapter 10). Nonetheless, this technique has been used in high-volume centers with good inter- and intra-observer agreement.[148,151] The aforementioned DECAAF I trial was able to link the amount of LGE-CMR identified scar with postablation outcomes, supporting the validity of an imaging-based approach.[76] Given the known limitations of electroanatomical mapping to identify arrhythmogenic substrates, the use of imaging-guided ablations has been explored in several prospective studies.

The ALICIA trial randomized 155 patients (54% paroxysmal fibrillation) undergoing first-time or repeat ablation at a single-center to a strategy of either PVI alone or PVI plus a CMR-guided substrate modification approach.[152] In the imaging-guided group, a 3D fibrosis map was merged within the navigational system, and areas of CMR-defined fibrosis were targeted through either homogenization, isolation through encirclement of scarred regions, or anchoring of fibrotic lesions to other linear lesions. Extra-PV substrate was identified and ablated in 45/79 (57%) of patients in the CMR-guided ablation group. While a strategy of PVI plus CMR-guided ablation was found to be safe, it did not improve clinical outcomes compared to a PVI-only approach. The DECAAF II trial was multicenter, randomized controlled trial of 843 patients with persistent AF undergoing first-time ablation.[153] Patients were randomized to a strategy of PVI alone–versus PVI and CMR-guided fibrosis ablation through homogenization or encirclement of extrapulmonic atrial fibrosis. Patients undergoing additional CMR-guided ablation experienced a high number of adverse outcomes (2.2% versus 0%, $P = .001$), including ischemic stroke. Like the ALICIA trial, a strategy of PVI plus CMR-guided ablation did not improve clinical outcomes compared to a PVI-only approach.

Despite the multiple lines of evidence linking imaging identified fibrosis to AF substrate, the use of CMR-based ablation in its current form is not supported by trial data. This may relate to the known limitations of the imaging techniques or the multiple approaches and subjective endpoints of fibrosis ablation used in these studies. Last, fibrosis is a heterogeneous entity with varying contributions to arrhythmogenesis based on its texture and spatial distribution[153]; further refinement in CMR imaging may help better identify the critical substrate from bystander regions and could improve the utility of substrate modification approaches.

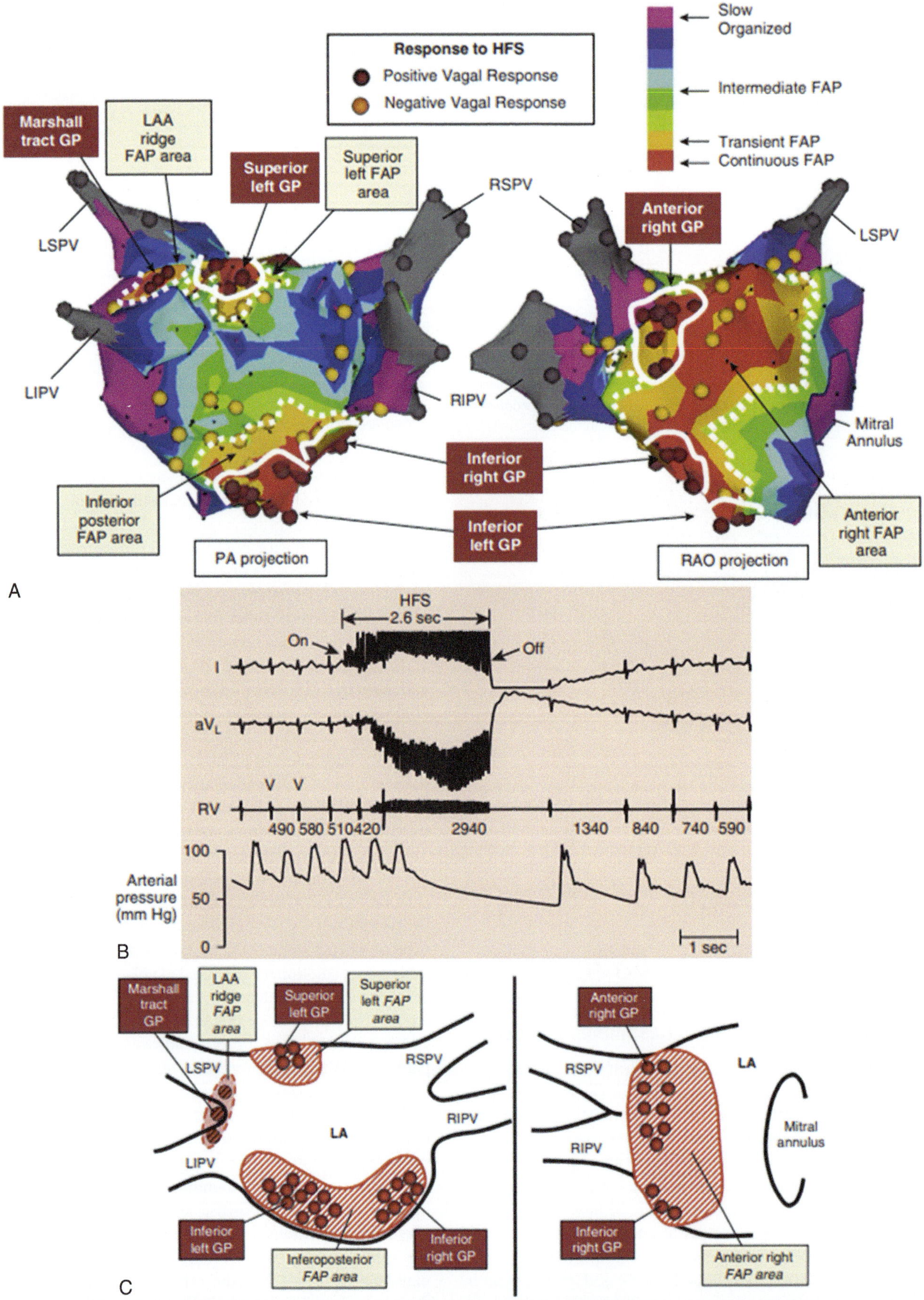

Fig. 19.19 Correlation between locations of fractionated atrial potentials (FAPs) and ganglionic plexi (GP) in patients undergoing catheter ablation of atrial fibrillation. (A) Electroanatomical map of FAP in a patient with

(Continued)

Fig. 19.19, cont'd paroxysmal atrial fibrillation. Electrograms were recorded for 2.5 seconds at each site. Sites exhibiting FAP for the entire 2.5 seconds were classified as continuous FAP and are *red*. Sites with FAP for >0.5 seconds but with organized atrial potentials for the remainder of the 2.5 seconds were classified as transient FAP and are *orange*. Sites exhibiting periods of irregular amplitude, polarity, and cycle length, but not rapid, were classified as intermediate FAP and are *green–light blue*. Sites exhibiting high-amplitude, discrete atrial potentials with average cycle length of 180 ms or more were classified as slow organized atrial potentials and are *purple*. An FAP area was defined as a contiguous area of FAPs (continuous or transient FAP). Four FAP areas were identified: left atrial appendage (LAA) ridge FAP area, superior left FAP area, inferoposterior FAP area, and anterior right FAP area. Sites where endocardial high-frequency stimulation (HFS) produced a vagal response (B) are marked by brown tags, corresponding to the five major GP areas: (1) Marshall tract GP, (2) superior left GP, (3) inferior left GP, (4) inferior right GP, and (5) anterior right GP. HFS failed to produce a vagal response at the sites marked by orange tags. Note that all five GP are located within the four FAP areas (C). (B) Tracings shown from top to bottom are electrocardiogram leads I and aVL, electrogram from the right ventricle (RV), and arterial pressure. During atrial fibrillation, endocardial HFS (cycle length, 50 ms; pulse width, 10 ms) in the posterior left atrium, 2.5 cm inferior to the ostium of the left inferior pulmonary vein (LIPV), results in transient complete atrioventricular block (RR interval, 2940 ms) and hypotension (vagal response), identifying the inferior left GP. C, Schematic representation of the relationship between the FAP areas and GP locations. Red tags indicate sites with a positive HFS response. Red crossed-hatch areas indicate FAP areas. LAA ridge FAP area and Marshall tract GP are located anterior to the left pulmonary veins. All five GP are located within one of the four FAP areas. *LSPV*, Left superior pulmonary vein; *PA*, posteroanterior; *RAO*, right anterior oblique; *RIPV*, right inferior pulmonary vein; *RSPV*, right superior pulmonary vein. (Modified from Nakagawa H, Scherlag BJ, Patterson E, et al. Pathophysiologic basis of automatic ganglionated plexus ablation in patients with atrial fibrillation. *Heart Rhythm*. 2009;6:S26–S34.)

TABLE 19.4 Target Sites for Ablation for Autonomic Ablation

Target Site	Location
RS GP	Anterior to RS PV
RI GP	Inferior and posterior to RI PV
LS GP	Anterior and/or posterior to LS PV
LI GP	Posterior and inferior to LI PV
Ligament of Marshall	Inferior–anterior aspect of left atrial lateral ridge inferior to LI PV

GP, Ganglionic plexi; *I*, inferior; *L*, left; *PV*, pulmonary vein; *R*, right; *S*, superior.

Cryoballoon Ablation for Posterior Wall Isolation and Extrapulmonary Vein Structures

Cryballoon-based ablation to attain PVI has been widely adopted with comparable safety and long-term outcomes as compared to RF ablation,[154] this approach is covered in detail in Chapter 16. The use of cyroballoon ablation in extrapulmonary structures, including ablation for isolation of posterior wall, LAA isolation, SVC isolation, and mitral isthmus and LA roof linear block has been explored primarily through retrospective and single-center series.[155] In the case of posterior wall isolation with cryoballoon, a randomized clinical trial was able to demonstrate improved ablation outcomes with PVI + PW compared to PVI alone in patients with persistent AF.[156] The use of this technique may not be suitable in all patients due to anatomical considerations including the variable course of the phrenic nerve, yet the ability to create large, contiguous lesions may be helpful in patients with advanced atrial substrates requiring extensive ablation.[157]

Ablation of extra-PV structures uses similar safety and monitoring practices as PVI ablation; the balloon is maneuvered to the desired location over the inner-lumen mapping catheter or guidewire to avoid damage from the balloon-tip[158] (Fig. 19.21). Electroanatomical maps can be created to assist with navigation and to monitor lesion efficacy. Close monitoring of esophageal temperature and impairment of phrenic nerve function is recommended during lesion application. There is no consensus on the optimal freeze-application duration or how this should be adjusted over different extrapulmonary structures,[157] though it appears reasonable to use similar protocols utilized for PVI. Nonetheless, in experienced centers, the rates of acute linear block in the LA are high (>90%).[159] Adjuvant radiofrequency may be required, particularly to achieve complete PW isolation.[156] Further prospective trials are needed to fully understand the best practices, safety, and efficacy of substrate-based cryoballoon ablation.

Panoramic Mapping and Ablation of Atrial Fibrillation Drivers

Various activation and phase mapping techniques have been used clinically to identify and ablate AF targets in the form of rotational (rotors) or focal drivers.[160,161] There is a variable relationship between the underlying atrial substrate and the location and number of AF drivers,[99,162,163] though generally a more advanced atrial substrate is supportive of focal drivers of AF.[164] Targeting these drivers alone (without PVI or other anatomic-based approaches) appears to be insufficient in patients with persistent AF[165] and the optimal strategy for mapping and identifying focal drivers remains to be seen. This topic is covered in greater detail in Chapter 18 of the fourth edition.

Endpoints for Substrate-Based Ablation

When antral PVI is used as the primary ablation strategy, elimination of antral potentials and complete PVI is the procedural endpoint. The endpoint of anatomical ablation (linear ablation, PW isolation, LAA isolation) is complete conduction block across the ablation lines. If block cannot be obtained after initial endocardial ablation, high-density mapping can be used to assess for epicardial connections into the PVs, posterior wall, across the mitral isthmus, and roof line, which can be targeted with focal ablation at the insertion site of these connections.[166–169]

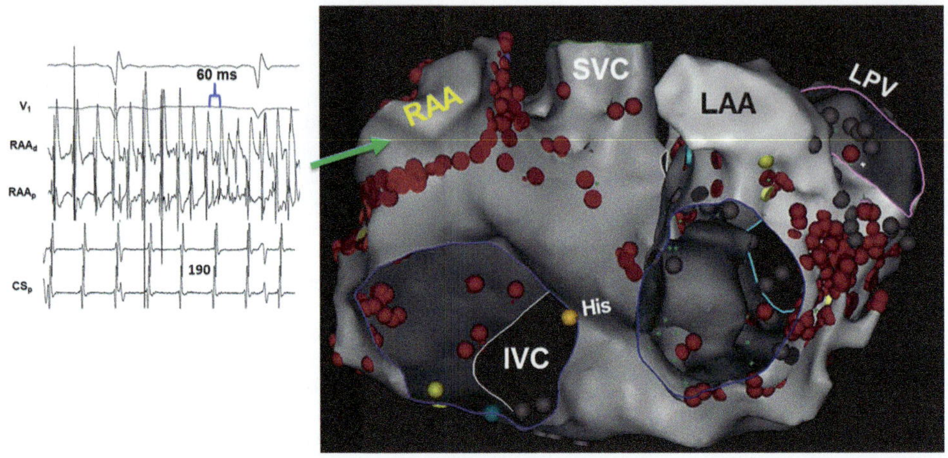

Fig. 19.20 Right atrial appendage ablation: three-dimensional electroanatomical depictions of the left and right atria, pulmonary veins, and vena cava are shown. A stepwise ablation was performed in a patient with long-standing persistent AF. After extensive linear and biatrial CFAE ablation, rapid electrogams (cycle length 60 ms) persisted within the RAA suggesting a driver of AF within this structure. Circumferential ablation around the RAA was performed resulting in termination of AF. *CS*, coronary sinus; *IVC*, inferior vena cava; *LAA*, left atrial appendage; *LPV*, left pulmonary vein; *RAA*, Right atrial appendage; *SVC*, superior vena cava. (From Ghannam M, Jame S, Jongnarangsin, et al. Catheter ablation of the left and right atrial appendages without isolation in persistent atrial fibrillation. *Heart Rhythm*. 2021;18(5):694–701.)

For ablation strategies targeting LVA or CFAEs, the endpoint is typically elimination of all abnormal signals (atrial defragmentation) and/or slowing/termination of AF. While termination and noninducibility of AF is a conceptually appealing goal, the value of aiming for this endpoint is less clearly established. In a long-term follow-up study of patients undergoing a biatrial defragmentation approach, termination of AF during ablation was the sole independent predictor of long-term freedom from arrhythmias.[170] Other studies have shown no improvement in outcomes with AF termination, and a higher complication rate likely related to the extensive ablation required to achieve this endpoint.[171] Likewise, the prognostic value of achieving noninducibility of AF is a matter of debate. The method of reinduction testing (rapid pacing, isoproterenol infusion, adenosine administration, etc.), the definition of noninducibility (>1 minute sustained, >10 minutes sustained, etc.), and the response to AF reinduction (no further ablation, linear ablation, EGM directed ablation, etc.) renders direct comparisons among trials difficult.[172] Noninducibility of AF by high-dose isoproterenol infusion (up to 20–30 μg/min) may be a more clinically useful end point for catheter ablation of AF than noninducibility by rapid atrial pacing. Isoproterenol has a higher specificity (97% versus 72%) and better diagnostic accuracy (83% versus 64%) than rapid atrial pacing for predicting recurrent AF.[173] However isoproterenol is more likely to identify focal triggers of AF rather than mechanisms capable of perpetuating AF.

The ideal endpoints for substrate-based ablation of AF remain unclear. Inadequate elimination of the arrhythmogenic substrate is unlikely to yield success and may create further tachycardia circuits; on the other hand, it is not clear that an extensive ablation is required to attain durable rhythm control, particularly in those who have not clearly demonstrated the need for extra-PVI ablation.

Troubleshooting the Difficult Case

Challenges with PVI are covered in Chapters 15–17, 20, 22. For any ablation strategy, difficulty in catheter navigation may be indicative of the inaccuracy of the electroanatomical map due to a limited number of registered points or patient movement during the case. Preprocedural imaging acquisition with computed tomography or cardiac magnetic resonance imaging may aid in identifying variations in the individual atrial and PV anatomy such as cor triatriatum. Phased-array intracardiac echocardiography has been used to provide accurate two-dimensional imaging and three-dimensional reconstruction of the LA and the PVs. In addition to defining the anatomy, intracardiac echocardiography can confirm catheter tissue contact in real-time.

Inability to create continuous transmural lesions is a common challenge during linear substrate modification. Potential causes are poor catheter stability and insufficient power delivery. Switching to a different catheter or a preformed sheath may be helpful. Steerable sheaths may offer better catheter stability; however, caution should be exercised to avoid myocardial perforation. High-definition mapping catheters can be used to better delineate low-voltage signals in patients with advanced atrial substrates or prior ablation-related scar,[174,175] which can be critical for identifying gaps in linear ablation lesion sets, on incomplete homogenization of abnormal atrial substrate. Esophageal deviation techniques may be used when ablation is required throughout the posterior wall to achieve isolation.[176]

For autonomic ablation, patient discomfort may be an issue during high-frequency stimulation mapping unless the patient is deeply sedated. Prior ablation may interrupt neural interconnections from peripheral sites needed to manifest AV block during stimulation. A specific sequence of ablation has been described previously to minimize this effect. A summary of problems encountered during substrate ablation and possible solutions is given in Table 19.5.

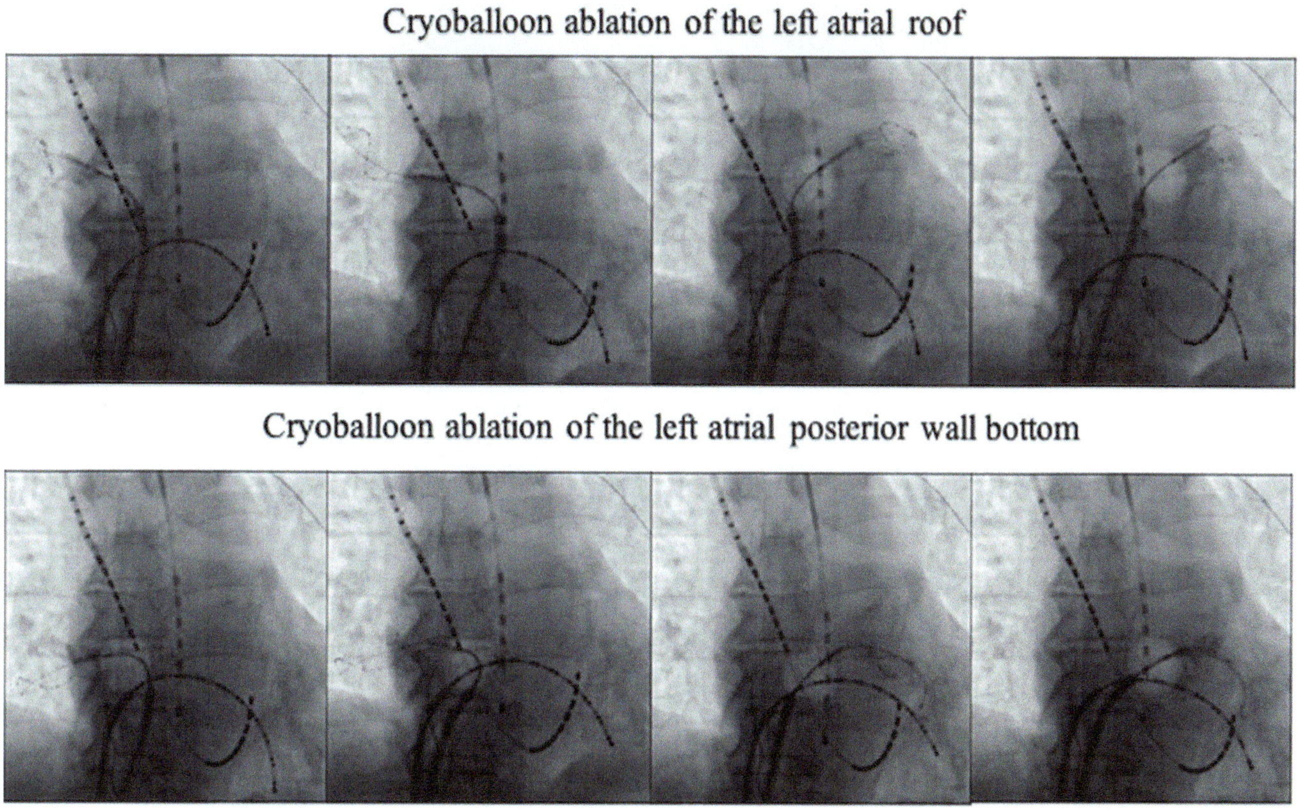

Fig. 19.21 Cryoballoon ablation of the pulmonary veins and posterior wall. Serial fluoroscopic images are shown depicting cryoballoon lesion sites. After application in the superior pulmonary vein, the catheter is dragged along the atrial roof, with overlapping cryoapplication performed along the roof and finally within the contralateral superior vein. This is repeated for the inferior pulmonary veins, and along the atrial posterior wall. (Modified from *J Arrhythm*. 2021;37:1477–1487.)

TABLE 19.5 Troubleshooting the Difficult Case

Problem	Causes	Solutions
Linear Ablation		
Difficult catheter manipulation	Atrial enlargement, difficult anatomy	Change sheath angulation or use steerable sheath
Unable to produce block across lines	Gaps from noncontiguous lesions Nontransmural lesions	Careful mapping of ablation line for gaps, especially near PV ostia and left atrial appendage ridge, create new line parallel to first attempt, epicardial ablation (in CS for mitral isthmus line)
	Tissue edema from preceding ablation	Create new line parallel to first
	Esophagus near ablation lines	Redirect line, monitor esophageal temperature, displace esophagus with TEE probe, displace esophagus with intrapericardial balloon or steerable sheath
Electrogram-Guided Ablation		
CFAE sites difficult to identify	Poor tissue contact	Change sheath
	Variable electrogram characteristics	Average analysis over 5- to 10-second window, use automated algorithm
	Diffuse, extensive CFAE sites	Linear ablation and antral PV isolation
Ablation of GPs		
Unable to elicit vagal reflex with mapping	Prior ablation interrupts neural interconnections	Map for surrogate targets (i.e., fractionated potentials)
	Ganglia remote from endocardial sites	Map epicardial sites
	Patient unresponsive to electrical stimulation	Perform empirical antral PV isolation

CFAE, Complex fractionated atrial electrogram; *CS*, coronary sinus; *PV*, pulmonary vein; *TEE*, transesophageal echocardiography.

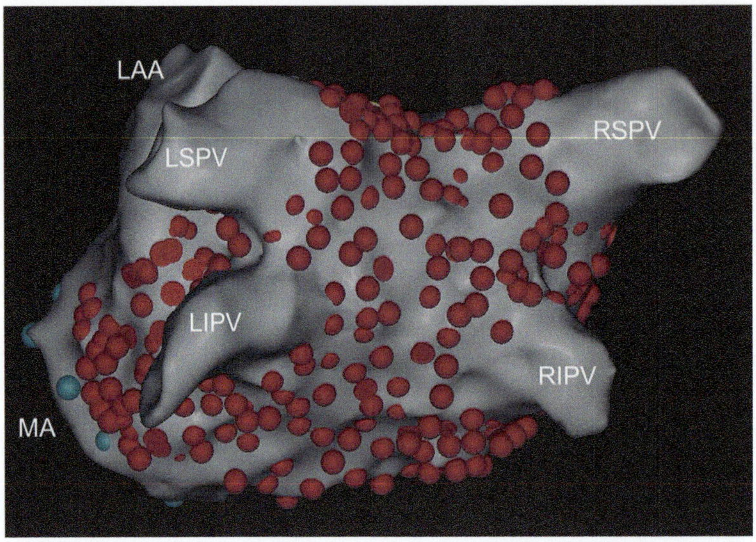

Fig. 19.22 Extensive ablation during atrial substrate modification. Three-dimensional electroanatomical depictions of the left atrium and pulmonary veins is shown. The ablation strategy consisted of an extensive substrate modification approach including empiric anatomic-based lesions (pulmonary vein isolation, posterior wall isolation, and lateral mitral isthmus ablation) and ablation of complex fractionated atrial electrograms. This required ablation throughout the entirety of the posterior wall and inferior wall down to the level of the coronary sinus. Ablation was performed along the lateral mitral isthmus, atrial ridge, and extended to the base of the left atrial appendage to achieve block along the mitral annulus and complete atrial defragmentation.

CONCLUSION

Substrate-based ablation for AF encompasses multiple techniques aimed at eliminating pathologic atrial and autonomic tissues responsible for AF perpetuation. This includes both empiric- and anatomical-based lesion sets as well as tailored ablation guided by local electrograms or imaging data. Clinical trials have failed to identify an optimal approach to substrate ablation, with many studies failing to show benefit compared to PVI alone. Given the inability to reliably distinguish the most critical substrate for AF in each patient, these techniques often demand extensive ablation, prolonging procedure time and entailing additional risks to patients (Fig. 19.22). Incomplete substrate elimination may create new circuits for atrial tachycardia and flutter. Despite these challenges, substrate-based ablation can improve outcomes for many patients, particularly those with nonparoxysmal AF and those with AF that persists despite durable PVI.[177,178] Due to the heterogeneous and multifactorial nature of AF, it is unlikely that one ablation approach will be applicable to all patients, and further efforts to identify tailored substrate ablation strategies may improve the yield of these techniques. Our understanding of the uses and limitations of substrate ablation will continue to evolve alongside our understanding of the complex pathophysiology underpinning AF.

REFERENCES

Please refer to the e-book for a complete list of references.

20

Ablation of Persistent and Long-Standing Persistent Atrial Fibrillation

Jay A. Montgomery, Jamie L. Kowal, Gregory F. Michaud

KEY POINTS

- Ablation of persistent and long-standing persistent trial fibrillation (AF) is a potentially complex procedure that carries a lower success rate than ablation for paroxysmal AF.
- Posterior wall isolation remains the cornerstone of AF ablation in every AF population, with antral isolation having better outcomes than ostial ablation. Further adjunctive ablation comes in many forms.
- Currently, we favor posterior wall isolation, careful attention to low-voltage areas, and strategic use of ethanol injection in the vein of Marshall in the persistent and long-standing persistent AF population.
- Preprocedural predictors of recurrence include longer duration since persistent AF diagnosis, greater than 1 year of continuous AF, elevated APPLE score, and fibrosis on DE-MRI.

INTRODUCTION

Atrial fibrillation (AF) is a growing health epidemic, with more than 33 million people with the disease worldwide.[1] The prevalence is expected to exceed 12 million in the United States alone by 2050.[2] Within this group, the phenotype of AF varies greatly. Most patients with AF present initially with paroxysmal AF, which is currently defined as AF always terminating in 7 days or less, either spontaneously or with intervention (Table 20.1).[3–5] If AF sustains for >7 days, it is defined as persistent AF, and if AF sustains continuously for >1 year, it is defined as long-standing persistent AF.[3,5] Within the persistent AF group, early persistent AF is now defined as sustaining for less than three months.[5] A Canadian registry enrolling before the widespread adoption of catheter ablation for AF showed that after an initial diagnosis of paroxysmal AF, 8.6%, 24.3%, and 36.3% will progress to persistent AF within 1, 5, and 10 years, respectively.[6]

Not surprisingly, clinical classification of AF type by a treating physician can be at odds with more objective implantable device–recorded data, and clinical factors such as heart failure or structural heart disease may play a role in the physicians' assessment of treatment options for patients. In addition, there is significant heterogeneity across each group in terms of AF burden, with patients clinically assigned to either group having no AF or continuous AF during 365 days of monitoring.[7]

While some patients may be predisposed to development of AF due to genetic factors that may lead to shortened atrial refractory periods,[8–10] ectopic foci,[11] or abnormal pulmonary vein (PV) architecture in the absence of identifiable risk factors,[12] others develop AF at an advanced age or after prolonged periods of hypertension, obstructive sleep apnea, obesity, chronic kidney disease, and heart failure.[13–15] In these two scenarios, the existing atrial substrate may be quite different, with the former group displaying uniformly "healthy" atrial tissue (normal atrial voltage by electroanatomic mapping) and the latter extensive atrial scarring early in the natural history of a patient's AF. This heterogeneity of substrate, coupled with the wide variation in arrhythmia burden within each classification of AF (paroxysmal, early persistent, persistent, and long-standing persistent) means that these classifications based on time alone cannot fully predict a given patient's likely benefit from medical or invasive therapies and can only partially guide the optimal treatment strategy.

Catheter ablation for AF is superior to antiarrhythmic drug therapy in maintaining sinus rhythm across many different patient populations.[16–22] In 1998, Haissaguerre et al published the seminal findings that PV triggers often initiate AF, and elimination of these triggers by catheter ablation may eliminate AF in some patients.[23] Nearly twenty years later, PV isolation (PVI) remains the foundation of all widely accepted modern catheter ablation techniques for AF, with an expectation that a single procedure will eliminate paroxysmal AF in approximately 60–70% of patients at 1 year (Table 20.2).[24,25] Interestingly, as technology, technique, and experience have all improved over time, improvements in the availability and usage of ambulatory monitoring has likely led to greater identification of short and subclinical AF episodes, which has contributed to a relative stagnation of AF outcomes through time.[22,26,27]

While AF-free survival for patients with paroxysmal AF undergoing PVI seems to be consistently >50%, outcomes in those with persistent and long-standing persistent AF are generally worse, though results seem to vary by center and in association with other clinical factors.[28–30] For this reason, adjunctive ablation strategies that could be coupled with PVI have been sought for patients with persistent and long-standing persistent AF.

TABLE 20.1 Arrhythmia Diagnostic Criteria and Indications for Ablation

Paroxysmal AF	• AF that terminates within 7 days of onset, spontaneously or with intervention • Class I indication for ablation if symptomatic, refractory to at least 1 antiarrhythmic • Class IIa indication for ablation prior to antiarrhythmic
Persistent AF	• AF sustains for >7 days • Class IIa indication for ablation if symptomatic, refractory to at least 1 antiarrhythmic
Early persistent AF	• AF sustains >7 days but <3 months
Long-standing persistent AF	• AF is continuous AF >12 months in duration • Class IIb indication for ablation if symptomatic, refractory to at least 1 antiarrhythmic
AF recurrence after ablation	• AF or atrial tachycardia (AT) documented to last 30 seconds occurring after a 3-month blanking period
Non–pulmonary vein trigger	• Early atrial depolarizations leading to AF or sustained AT

TABLE 20.2 Key Points for AF Ablation

Ablation Targets	• All ablations for AF should include complete pulmonary vein isolation (PVI) • Patients with persistent AF have worse ablation-free survival than those with paroxysmal AF after PVI • Further ablation may include vein of Marshall ethanol injection, ablation of non–pulmonary vein (PV) triggers, posterior wall ablation/isolation, left atrial appendage electrical isolation or excision, roof or mitral line, cavotricuspid isthmus line, and ablation targeting fibrosis, ganglionic plexi, rotors, or other drivers
Special Equipment	• Electroanatomic mapping (EAM) is strongly recommended • Intracardiac echocardiography, contact-force-sensing catheters, general anesthesia with high-frequency ventilation, and deflectable sheaths can all be useful in achieving durable lesions • Multipolar catheters can be helpful in determining sources of non-PV triggers
Sources of Difficulty	• Achieving durable PVI remains challenging and may be necessary but not sufficient for achieving arrhythmia-free survival in many patients with persistent and long-standing persistent AF • Contact-force and impedance monitoring, adenosine challenge, achieving ablation line unexcitability, and maintaining close lesion spacing may help achieve durable lesions • Posterior wall ablation and isolation can be achieved efficiently and safely in most patients with high power or low flow irrigation lesions of short duration to limit esophageal heating
Predictors of Outcome	• Longer time since persistent AF diagnosis and longer time in continuous AF predict worsened outcome • APPLE score (1 point each for age >65, persistent AF, eGFR <60 ml/min/1.73 m2, LA diameter ≥43 mm, and left ventricular ejection fraction <50%) predicts AF recurrence after ablation with an odds ratio for AF recurrence for scores of 1, 2, or ≥3 equal to 1.73, 2.79, and 4.70 as compared to a score of zero (similar predictive power for repeat ablation) • Delayed-enhancement magnetic resonance imaging (DE-MRI) shows linear correlation between left atrial fibrosis burden and post-ablation recurrence with recurrence rates of 15%, 36%, 46%, and 69% corresponding to <10%, ≥10–<20%, ≥20–<30%, and ≥30% fibrosis of the LA

Over the last 20 years, the most frequently used adjunctive ablative strategies have been the placement of linear ablation lesion sets (typically left atrial roof and mitral lines) and ablation of complex fractionated atrial electrograms (CFAEs).[31–34] When these additional ablation lesion sets were compared to PVI alone in the multicenter STAR AF2 randomized controlled trial (RCT), they showed longer procedure times and a trend toward worse outcomes.[29] Other adjunctive invasive strategies intended to reduce the recurrence of persistent AF include mapping and ablation of non-PV triggers, posterior wall ablation/isolation, cavotricuspid isthmus line placement, left atrial appendage isolation or excision, ablation in areas of fibrosis, ablation of ganglionic plexi, mapping and ablation of rotors, and surgical ablation.[27,35] Rigorous multicenter data is currently limited and/or conflicting for these strategies, as will be discussed below. In addition, all of these techniques require additional time, most require additional expertise, some require extra equipment, and most probably increase procedural risk, with the goal of achieving outcomes similar to what PVI achieves in patients with paroxysmal AF. As such, the 2014 ACC/AHA/HRS guidelines have assigned a Class I indication for catheter ablation of drug-refractory, symptomatic *paroxysmal* AF, a Class IIa indication for drug-refractory, symptomatic *persistent* AF, and a Class IIb indication for drug-refractory, symptomatic *long-standing persistent* AF (Table 20.1).[3,5] The 2019 AHA/ACC/HRS Focused Update expanded indications by assigning a IIb recommendation for selected patients with symptomatic AF and concurrent HF with a reduced left ventricular ejection fraction, citing potential to lower mortality and reduce heart failure hospitalization.[36]

ASSESSMENT OF THE PATIENT WITH PERSISTENT AND LONG-STANDING PERSISTENT AF

Patients with persistent AF may have a wide range of symptomatology, arrhythmia burden, and comorbidities.[7,37,38] Many patients with persistent AF are initially encountered by the electrophysiologist in the outpatient setting, often in the midst of a prolonged episode of AF. A few questions are important to consider when evaluating a patient with persistent or long-standing persistent AF:

- Is the patient symptomatic? Can that be determined if it is unclear?
- Is the patient presenting in sinus rhythm or AF?
- What is the AF burden and how long is the current episode? How long since diagnosis?
- Are other diseases worsened by the presence of AF (i.e. heart failure, sick sinus syndrome, hypertrophic cardiomyopathy)?
- Are there factors precluding certain antiarrhythmic drug therapy (heart failure, coronary artery disease, renal disease, lung disease)?
- Are there factors precluding catheter ablation (high anesthesia risk, intolerance of anticoagulation, left atrial appendage thrombus)?
- Is the patient expected to have open-heart surgery which could potentially be paired with a surgical ablation for AF?

Assessing and Defining Symptomatology

Patients with persistent AF often complain of nonspecific symptoms such as fatigue or exercise intolerance making it difficult to ascertain whether a concomitant problem such as obesity, sleep apnea, or clinical heart failure is the major instigator. In addition, patients are often unaware when AF started and may feel minimal palpitations which may give the false impression that AF is asymptomatic. In that sense, symptomatology attributable to AF may be "in the eye of the beholder." In this circumstance, one should consider direct-current cardioversion (DCCV) with or without an antiarrhythmic medication for the purpose of determining improvement in symptomatology when in sinus rhythm. The patient is encouraged to keep a literal or mental symptom diary for the days and weeks preceding and following cardioversion. Most patients with persistent AF will experience some improvement of symptoms after cardioversion. If a patient with persistent AF experiences no symptomatic improvement with a trial of sinus rhythm, rhythm control is less appealing, given that multiple ablations and/or continuation of antiarrhythmic drugs may be needed to achieve long-term success.[3] Greater than 10% of patients will fail to have even momentary restoration of sinus rhythm, even at 360 J,[39,40] in which case placement of two sets of defibrillator pads (one in anteroposterior configuration and one in anterolateral configuration) connected to two separate external defibrillators can be synchronized and fired simultaneously (by a single operator) with near-universal success.[41,42] We recommend very firm pressure on the two anterior patches (this can best be done from on top of the stretcher or with the bed very low) with dry towels and rubber gloves to ensure no current is leaked through the operator applying pressure. In addition, pretreatment with ibutilide can also be used to aid cardioversion, although caution should be used in patients with heart failure and a low ejection fraction.[43] Of note, amiodarone may raise the defibrillation threshold.[44–46]

Presenting Rhythm

Among patients with a clinical diagnosis of persistent AF, those who present to the electrophysiology (EP) lab in sinus rhythm or who have early conversion to sinus rhythm during the procedure (prior to the completion of the planned ablation) have a significantly greater likelihood of long-term success.[47] This is likely due, at least in part, to the presence of sinus rhythm being a marker of a phenotype, which is likely to have improved outcomes. Arriving to the lab in sinus rhythm, all other things being equal, is statistically more likely in patients with a lower AF burden. Conversion early during the procedure could be a marker of a patient with a more paroxysmal, self-terminating phenotype, which may have terminated even in the absence of ablation. By the same reasoning, a patient with persistent AF who presents to clinic in sinus rhythm may be expected to have better outcomes with ablation than one who does not.

AF Burden and Chronicity

As discussed above, patients with persistent AF are more likely to experience recurrence than those with paroxysmal AF (Table 20.1).[48] Among patients with persistent AF, those classified as persistent AF for >1 year seem to be approximately twice as likely to have recurrence as compared to those <1 year since that diagnosis.[49] Additionally, those with long-standing persistent AF (>1 year of *continuous* AF) have worse outcomes compared to those who have been in AF <12 months.[5]

Disease Processes Exacerbated by AF

When determining how aggressively to treat AF, it is reasonable to consider comorbidities. In patients with heart failure and AF, AF ablation has been associated with an improvement in left ventricular ejection fraction (LVEF) of 8.5% as well as an improvement in 6-minute walk and quality of life as compared with rate control.[50] Additionally, AF ablation compared favorably to atrioventricular (AV) node ablation with bi-ventricular pacing in heart failure patients with significantly greater quality of life, 6-minute walk, and LV ejection fraction in the AF ablation group.[51] Most notably, evidence from the randomized controlled CASTLE-AF trial showed a significant reduction in the primary composite endpoint of death or hospitalization for worsening heart failure (HR 0.62; $P = .007$) among patients with LVEF 35% or less randomized to ablation as opposed to medical therapy (rate or rhythm control) for atrial fibrillation.[52] The study also showed significant reductions in the individual endpoints of all-cause mortality (HR 0.53; $P = .007010$), cardiac mortality (HR 0.49; $P = .007$), and hospitalization for worsened heart failure (HR 0.56; $P = .007004$) in the ablation group. Similar to prior studies, LVEF and 6 minute walk also showed significant improvements in the ablation group. Interestingly, these effects were seen in the setting of a 50% recurrence rate in the ablation group but a reduction in AF burden (rather than complete elimination) to around 25% as opposed to 60% for those receiving medical therapy alone. While the CABANA trial results showed a nonstatistically significant decrease in a composite score of mortality, stroke, bleeding, and cardiac arrest with catheter ablation versus antiarrhythmic therapy in the overall population, subgroup analysis showed that AF ablation reduced mortality by 60% relative to drug therapy in patients with clinical HF at the time of enrollment.[53,54] Conversely, RAFT AF failed to demonstrate superiority of an ablation-based rhythm-control strategy compared to a rate-control strategy in patients with coexistent HF (preserved and reduced EF) for the composite primary endpoint of all-cause mortality and HF events.[55] This is in the context of early trial termination citing lower-than-expected enrollment and event rates with perceived futility based on interim analysis. However the trial did show a trend toward improved outcomes and met several secondary endpoints, not limited to an increased LVEF at 24 months, in the ablation cohort. In a separate evaluation, patients with concurrent persistent or longstanding persistent AF and advanced systolic HF (LVEF ≤ 35%) with at least NYHA class II symptoms and an indication for device therapy (ICD or CRT-D) seemed to demonstrate no significant improvement comparing an ablation strategy to best medical therapy (rhythm or rate control) when evaluating for absolute LVEF improvement.[56] While the ablation cohort did demonstrate an LVEF increase of 8.8% from baseline, the control group experienced a similar improvement despite remaining in sinus rhythm significantly less time as documented by their implanted device. That said, this trial was also prematurely terminated due to futility with follow-up limited to one year. Studies demonstrating LVEF improvement generally realized greater benefits of ablation during the second and third years of follow-up, suggesting that a more robust patient population may need to be studied for a longer duration to draw specific conclusions regarding LVEF improvement.[52] Taken in total, contemporary work demonstrates at least a trend toward improved outcomes with the adoption of an AF ablation-based rhythm-control strategy in patients with baseline heart failure.

In addition, patients with tachy-brady syndrome plagued by symptomatic sinus bradycardia or long postconversion pauses in the setting of needed rate or rhythm control medications for AF may benefit from an early ablative approach in order to avoid or postpone the need for placement of a permanent pacemaker.[5]

Last, observational data suggest that AF ablation is associated with a reduced incidence of stroke or TIA as compared to propensity-matched patients with AF who do not undergo ablation.[57–60] This effect seems to be greater in patients without recurrence of arrhythmia after ablation.[61] However, despite propensity matching, it is possible that the decision to perform ablation and also ablation success may be a marker of a "healthier" patient population who would be less likely to suffer a stroke regardless of ablation. Therefore, a randomized trial will be needed to determine the true effect, if any, that AF ablation has on long-term stroke risk. Notably, recent guidelines state that "a patient's desire to eliminate the need for long-term anticoagulation by itself should not be considered an appropriate selection criterion for AF ablation."[5]

Antiarrhythmic Drug Options

In many patients with persistent AF, antiarrhythmic drug options are limited. Patients with persistent AF and structural heart disease should not be prescribed Class 1c antiarrhythmic medications.[3] In this group, sotalol, dofetilide, dronedarone, and amiodarone are options. For those with heart failure, dronedarone, and to some extent sotalol because of its β-blocker effect and renal elimination, are also contraindicated. In addition patients with poor or fluctuating renal function or serum potassium levels are at elevated risk of torsades de pointes with the Class III antiarrhythmic drugs sotalol and dofetilide. For those who do qualify for a Class III drug, several days of hospitalization for drug loading is recommended. Finally, any patients with advanced lung disease or those with expected lifespan of a decade or more are not ideal candidates for amiodarone, given the risk of long-term, potentially fatal, toxicities.[3] After all of these considerations are taken into account, there is a significant cohort of persistent AF patients with few or no good antiarrhythmic drug options. Despite this, operators should be aware that patients with persistent AF and especially those with long-standing persistent AF may require continuation or initiation of antiarrhythmic drug therapy after ablation to maintain sinus rhythm.

Potential Contraindications to Ablation

Ablation of AF is contraindicated or certainly riskier in certain populations. Given the elevated incidence of periprocedural stroke in the absence of anticoagulation, intraprocedural heparin and oral anticoagulation are recommended for at least 2 months after ablation in all patients, regardless of baseline stroke risk.[3] The 2014 ACC/AHA/HRS guidelines states that "AF catheter ablation should not be performed in patients who cannot be treated with anticoagulant therapy during and following the procedure."[3] In patients with heparin-induced thrombocytopenia or other specific contraindication to heparin, bivalirudin can be used for the acute procedure.

In addition, those with exceptionally high risk of general anesthesia, such as those with advanced lung disease and concomitant morbid obesity, should warrant special consideration and attention prior to referral for ablation. Most patients with chronic IVC filters can safely undergo AF ablation. Fluoroscopy, and occasionally contrast venography, should be used to ensure safe passage of wires and sheaths. Occasionally, chronic thrombus may prevent access through a filter.

Patients with congenital heart disease are at significantly elevated risk of AF, and the risk increases with increasing age.[62–66] Simple congenital heart disease, in which the atrial septum has been repaired, requires extra care to perform transseptal puncture. This has been performed in high-volume centers using intracardiac echocardiography with a high degree of success and few complications.[67,68] AF ablation in complex congenital heart disease, which may include surgical baffles and severely distorted anatomy, should be referred to an operator experienced with these patients[62] (see Chapter 14).

Patients with AF Undergoing Cardiac Surgery

In patients with symptomatic AF who are undergoing cardiac surgery (specifically mitral valve surgery, aortic valve surgery, or coronary artery bypass grafting), concomitant surgical ablation of AF is recommended.[3,5,69] In addition in patients with AF undergoing cardiac surgery, it is reasonable to perform left atrial appendage excision or exclusion, whether or not surgical ablation of AF is performed.[69] While the original Cox-Maze procedure consisted of a cut-and-sew lesion set, the Cox-Maze IV procedure switched to limited atriotomy (often in the setting of mitral valve surgery) with both radiofrequency and

TABLE 20.3 Target Sites

Pulmonary Vein Isolation	• Complete pulmonary vein isolation (PVI) is the cornerstone of any ablation for atrial fibrillation • May be adequate as a stand-alone procedure to achieve control of AF, especially in patients with paroxysmal or early persistent AF • Wide-area circumferential ablation has improved outcomes as compared to ostial PVI
Posterior Wall Ablation/Isolation	• The LA posterior wall is formed from the embryological pulmonary vein (PV) bud • Isolation of the posterior box by placement of roof and inferior lines is difficult and highly susceptible to reconnection • Careful ablation of all signals within the area of the posterior box may be a more realistic approach • Ideal power, irrigation, and time per lesion across the posterior wall requires further study, though short duration lesions are likely desirable
Non–Pulmonary Vein Triggers	• Early atrial depolarizations leading to sustained AF or AT • Typically mapped during high-dose isoproterenol infusion (i.e. 20 mcg/min) • Multipolar catheters can be helpful for rapid localization
Left Atrial Appendage Electrical Isolation	• Mixed results across randomized trials • Stroke risk uncertain with electrical isolation
Right Atrial Ablation	• Ablation of the cavotricuspid isthmus (CTI) is recommended in any patient with history of or induction of sustained CTI-dependent flutter • Further RA ablation as dictated by non-PV trigger mapping
Left Atrial Lines	• Include roof line, lateral mitral line, and anterior mitral line • Consider ablation at these sites if significant scarring is seen in these areas by voltage map or if persistent roof-dependent or peri-mitral flutter is seen • Difficult to achieve acute and chronic linear mitral block
Complex Fractionated Atrial Electrogram Ablation	• Multicomponent atrial electrogram displaying continuous baseline perturbation OR <120 ms cycle length over 10s • Initial positive results; more recent randomized studies without benefit
Ablation of Fibrotic Areas	• Recognized by low-voltage (typically <0.5 mV bipolar) on electroanatomic maps or delayed-enhancement on magnetic resonance imaging (DE-MRI) • Nonrandomized studies suggest benefit of isolation or homogenization of low-voltage areas • 69% recurrence in those with >30% left atrial fibrosis by DE-MRI
Ganglionic Plexus Ablation	• Has been described using high-frequency stimulation to confirm ganglionic plexus (GP) sites or with empiric ablation in typical GP areas • Mixed results across randomized trials
Rotor and Driver Mapping and Ablation	• Rotor: Mapping and ablation of phase singularities and rotational activity during sustained AF • Disparate results across multiple studies • Driver: Mapping sites activating earlier than all neighboring sites in AF. No randomized data
Hybrid Ablation	• May have superior results to endocardial-only ablation, especially for long-standing persistent AF, but carries higher risks

cryoablation performed from both endocardial and epicardial locations, making the procedure shorter and less technically challenging.[69] Because aortic valve and coronary artery bypass surgeries do not necessitate an atriotomy, approaches have been developed which are performed exclusively from an epicardial approach, although these approaches cannot reliably create a contiguous line of ablation down to the mitral valve annulus.[5,69] In patients with persistent and long-standing persistent AF, extensive surgical lesion sets seem to have very good efficacy, though paroxysmal AF patients may not have an added benefit with extensive linear ablation[70–72] (see Chapter 21).

ABLATION STRATEGIES IN PATIENTS WITH PERSISTENT AF

As discussed above, ablation outcomes with PVI become progressively worse moving from paroxysmal to early-persistent, persistent, and long-standing persistent AF.[5] For this reason, PVI-only is a widely accepted first-line catheter ablation strategy for paroxysmal AF, but the "correct" ablation for persistent and long-standing persistent AF is controversial. In this section, we will briefly discuss PVI and several adjunctive ablation techniques, keeping in mind that many of these techniques are discussed more exhaustively in other chapters of this book (Table 20.3). Techniques to circumvent challenging cases are summarized in Table 20.4.

Pulmonary Vein Isolation

PVI remains the cornerstone of all widely accepted strategies for ablation of AF and is recommended as a class I indication during all AF ablation procedures (Fig. 20.1).[3,5] Between 2011 and 2016, several studies showed success rates of 47–82% for ~1 year arrhythmia-free survival (pooled mean 67%) in relatively 'healthy' populations of patients with persistent AF undergoing PVI-only ablation with either radiofrequency or cryoballoon.[73] Notably, many of these studies excluded long-standing persistent AF. In addition, the mean left atrial (LA) size (4.5 cm) may be smaller and LVEF (57%) may be greater than what could

TABLE 20.4 **Troubleshooting the Difficult Case**

Problem	Causes	Solution
Unable to achieve even momentary sinus rhythm	Elevated atrial defibrillation threshold	Use double synchronized defibrillation (two separate generators) and/or concomitant ibutilide infusion
Poor catheter stability	Excessive heart or respiratory motion	Use steerable sheath Use low tidal volume, periodic apnea, or jet ventilation
Posterior box does not maintain isolation and/or roof line will not block	Complex epicardial/endocardial architecture and/or poor catheter contact	Ablate posterior wall in its entirety with short duration lesions
Pulmonary veins are already isolated at the time of redo AF ablation	Nonpulmonary vein triggers are present	Non-PV trigger mapping and ablation Posterior wall isolation

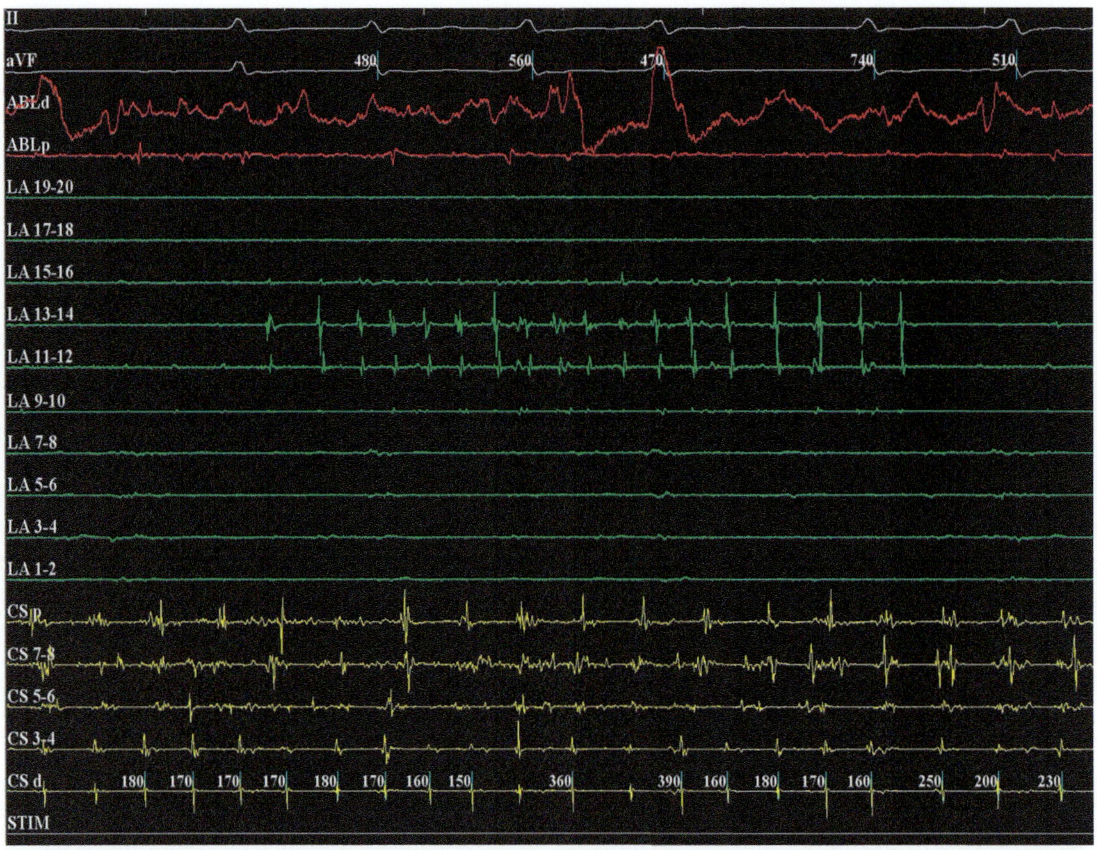

Fig. 20.1 A multispline catheter labeled LA 1–20 (Pentaray, Biosense-Webster, Diamond Bar, CA) is in the left upper pulmonary vein shortly after pulmonary vein isolation has been achieved in a patient with persistent atrial fibrillation. A decapolar catheter is in the coronary sinus (CS), and an ablation catheter (ABL) is at the pulmonary vein antrum. Despite isolation of the vein, a brief, fast run of pulmonary vein tachycardia is seen. This underscores the importance of durable pulmonary vein isolation.

be expected in a real-world long-standing persistent cohort.[73] In fact, among a group of patients with more advanced persistent AF with LA size 5.1 cm and LVEF 50%, a single-procedure success rate of 36% at ~11-month follow-up was reported at a single center.[74] Those with long-standing persistent AF had 20% success.

Some evidence suggests that performing wide-area circumferential ablation around the PVs (rather than ostial ablation) may be more efficacious.[75,76] In a trial by Nilsson et al, this effect appeared to be magnified in persistent AF patients, who had an 85% recurrence rate with ostial ablation, and 48% recurrence with extra-ostial ablation, with allowance for one reablation.[75] Notably, the largest anatomical difference in PVI lines between an ostial approach and wide-area approach is the wider placement of the posterior lines, which isolates a much larger portion of the posterior wall. Our method of ablating posterior to the PVs is described below.

Posterior Wall Isolation/Ablation

During embryologic development, a single embryonic PV arises from the posterior wall and then branches into the four main PVs and their distal branches (Fig. 20.2).[77] As a result, the smooth tissue

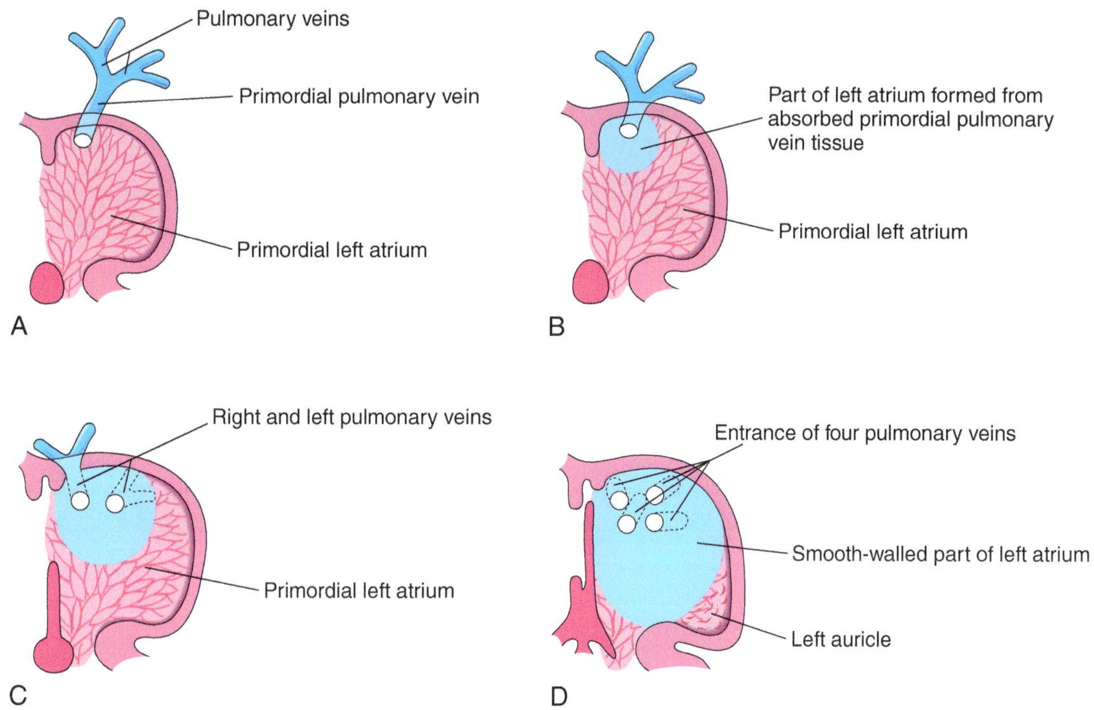

Fig. 20.2 The primordial pulmonary vein interfaces with the primordial left atrium. At 5 weeks' gestation (A), a single, branching primordial pulmonary vein empties into the primordial left atium. The antrum of the vein expands and begins to form part of the left atrial wall while the branchpoint becomes nearer the left atrial cavity. By 6 weeks (C), the right and left veins are arising from two separate ostia, and a larger portion of the left atrial posterior wall is made up of what was initially pulmonary vein tissue. At 8 weeks (D), four separate pulmonary vein ostia are seen. Eventually, most of the left atrium is formed by absorption of the primordial pulmonary vein and its branches. (Figure adapted from Moore KL Persaud TVN, Torchia MG. *The Developing Human.* 10th ed. December 31, 2015; Figure 13-16.)

of the PVs extends into the LA tissue and incorporates the posterior LA wall as well as some of the LA roof and interatrial septum.[78] As such, ablation of the posterior wall has been considered as an additional potential target in AF ablation, and there is compelling but not definitive evidence that ablation and isolation of the left atrial posterior wall may reduce recurrence of persistent AF.

After transitioning from the cut-and-sew Cox-maze III to the primarily radiofrequency and cryoablation Cox-maze IV, the initial lesion set at Washington University in St. Louis included an ablation line connecting the right and left lower pulmonary veins. Later, a roof line connecting the two upper veins was added to complete a posterior box. Among the first 100 patients, recurrence off antiarrhythmic medication was 53% with only an inferior connecting line placement versus 15% in those with a posterior box.[79] A larger follow-up study from the same group revealed an odds ratio of 0.382 for AF/AT recurrence with completion of a posterior box when adjusted for other factors.[80] Several other nonrandomized studies have suggested increased efficacy when PWI is added to pulmonary vein isolation for persistent atrial fibrillation.[81] A recent trial by Aryana et al. randomized 110 patients with persistent and long-standing persistent AF to either PVI only versus PVI plus posterior wall isolation utilizing cryoablation.[82] While adjuvant radiofrequency ablation was required in some portion of the population to create durable PVI and PWI, randomization to PWI resulted in significantly lower rates of recurrent AF (25.5% versus. 45.5%, $P = .007028$) at 12 months without a significant difference in adverse events between groups. More recently, the CAPLA trial showed no benefit to posterior wall box isolation (superior and inferior lines) when added to PVI for persistent AF using RF ablation.[83] In contrast, another recent study suggested that isolation of low-voltage areas within the atrium, including the posterior wall, reduced AF recurrence for patients with persistent AF.[84] While the benefit of posterior wall isolation has conflicting data, the preferred method of ablating the posterior wall also remains unknown. Kumar et al. showed that a standard posterior box by endocardial catheter ablation (roof line connecting the left upper to right upper PV as well as inferior line connecting the left lower to right lower PV) only succeeds in isolating the posterior wall 23% of the time acutely.[85] Of the patients in whom posterior wall isolation was successful but who had re-ablation for AF recurrence, 0 of 5 still had isolation of the posterior wall.[85] Similar findings have been published in which standard posterior box has been used without success in patients undergoing repeat ablation for AF recurrence following de novo ablation with PVI alone.[86,87] Last, investigators in the CAPLA trial found that more than half of patients required ablation within the box, and some failed to achieve isolation.[83] Therefore a standard posterior box via catheter ablation does not seem to be a reliable method using current technologies.

In the LIBERATION study, where posterior wall ablation was diffuse, obligate repeat mapping was performed 3 months after

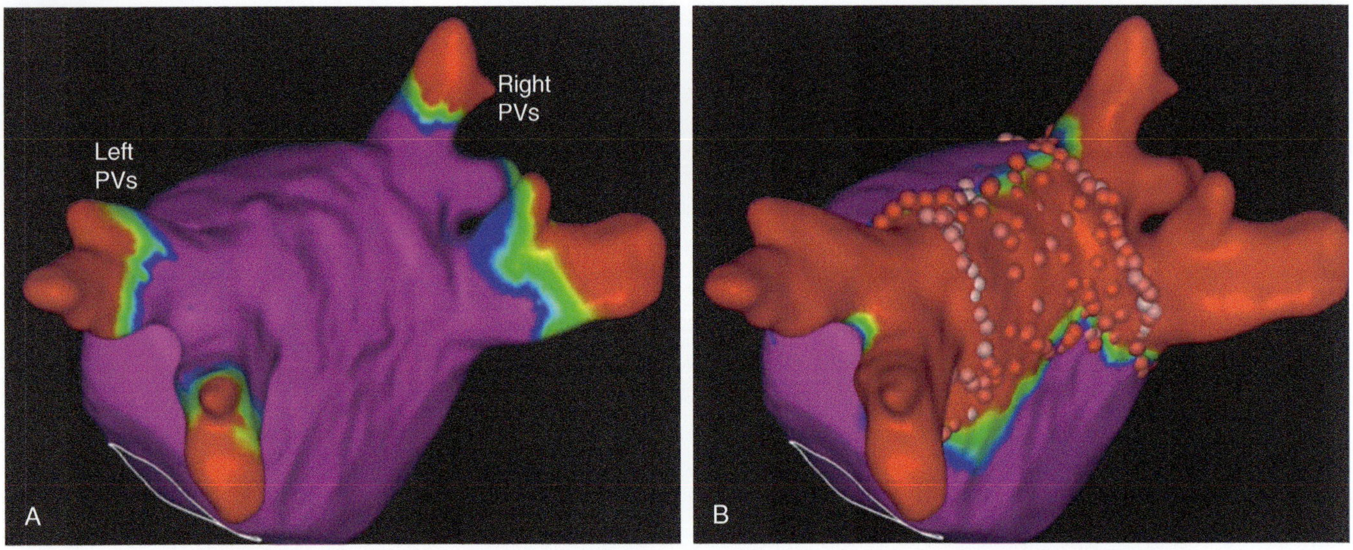

Fig. 20.3 In addition to pulmonary vein isolation, we use a strategy of ablating all local signals across the posterior wall in patients with persistent and long-standing persistent atrial fibrillation. Preablation (A) and postablation (B) voltage maps are shown from a left posterolateral orientation with *purple* corresponding to bipolar voltage >0.5 mV and *red* corresponding to bipolar voltage <0.1 mV. Individual ablation lesions are visible as assigned by Visitag force–time integral (Biosense-Webster, Diamond Bar, CA). After pulmonary vein antral isolation is achieved, all local signals within the area of the posterior box are targeted. Initial roof and inferior lines are not placed, as the goal is to ablate all posterior wall tissue. We prefer using 40–50 W power, 10–20 *g* force, and ~4- to 8-second lesions to limit lesion depth on the posterior wall. Testing for pace-capture after ablation can be helpful to verify adequate lesion delivery. In areas with esophageal heating, lesion duration may be limited to 6 seconds.

the first procedure. This showed that 63% of patients who had PVI and posterior wall ablation had durable isolation of both the PVs and the posterior wall.[88] A more recent retrospective study showed that diffuse posterior wall isolation using a low-flow (2 mL/min), medium-power, short-duration (LF-MPSD) ablation strategy in addition to PVI[89] resulted in very low rates of pulmonary vein reconnection among patients presenting for redo ablation (11.1% in PVI + PWI versus 77.8% in PVI), suggesting that part of any possible benefit may be enhanced durability of PVI. A contingent of electrophysiologists has long advocated posterior wall ablation by moving a multipolar lasso catheter all around the posterior wall and ablating all visible signals until electrical silence is achieved.[88]

We take these data to suggest that posterior wall ablation/isolation is likely not beneficial in patients with persistent and long-standing persistent AF if performed empirically as roof and inferior lines. However targeting posterior wall ablation to patients with posterior wall substrate seems to be beneficial. Additionally, it seems likely that mapping and diffusely ablating all signals on the posterior wall is the most efficacious approach.

The posterior LA is a smooth, thin-walled structure that nearly always directly overlies the esophagus. An ideal ablation strategy would be one that creates transmural lesions across the LA wall but does not heat the adjacent esophageal tissue. Many operators traditionally used low-power settings (~20 W) on the posterior wall with irrigated catheters. However, in recent years relatively high-power settings with shorter lesion duration have become common. For many years, we used a low-flow (2 mL/min) 20–35 W, ~10 seconds per lesion protocol for posterior wall ablation in an effort to attain rapidly effective endocardial ablation without causing deep tissue heating, although more recently have used 50-W standard flow lesions as short as 6 seconds. The important part of both strategies is the short duration, which favors resistive heating at the endocardial surface. The optimal combination of power, duration, and irrigation rate will need to be explored through further study.

Our Method of Pulmonary Vein Isolation With Posterior Wall Ablation

We perform complete isolation/ablation of the posterior wall box using high-power short duration settings in select patients with advanced persistent and long-standing persistent AF, especially if posterior wall substrate is present. After substrate and anatomical mapping is performed using a multispline catheter (Pentaray or Octaray, Biosense-Webster, Diamond Bar, CA), we perform pulmonary vein antral isolation using a deflectable sheath and a contact-force sensing ablation catheter (SmartTouch, Biosense-Webster, Diamond Bar, CA) with typical irrigated settings at 50 W for 8–20 seconds except for posterior to the pulmonary veins, where we ablate for a shorter time. Typically, we ablate at 40–50 W for 4–8 seconds with close monitoring of esophageal temperature and position as well as impedance decrease. Lesions that are distant from the esophagus may occasionally receive a maximum of 10 seconds if contact force and impedance drop are minimal.

We aim for contact force of at least 10 *g* throughout the LA. With this, we aim for impedance decrease of 10 Ω and electrogram diminution, which can usually be achieved with slightly greater contact force of 15–20 *g* if necessary.

After PVI is accomplished, we then target all local signals within the posterior box area (Fig. 20.3) with the same 40–50 W,

4- to 8-second lesions as described above (setting maximal lesion duration at 10 seconds is adequate in most patients). We typically see rapid electrogram diminution at ablation sites. After all local signals seem to be ablated within this region, testing for pace-capture at 10 mA or higher can help ensure adequate lesion delivery has been achieved. This method will require varying amounts of ablation, but overall, the number of lesions required to obtain posterior wall isolation is not excessive (lesions usually less overlapping than along an isolation line) and is often no more time-intensive than placement of a successful roof line, which is effectively created by this strategy anyway. We do not create initial roof and inferior lines, as the goal is to ablate all posterior wall tissue. We never ablate with a transesophageal echocardiography probe in place due to mechanical stenting of the anterior esophageal tissue into the posterior LA, and we adjust the position of an insulated esophageal temperature probe to approximately match the position of the ablation catheter, so that reablation in an area of esophageal heating would only occur after return to baseline esophageal temperature which may be minutes later.

Vein of Marshall Ethanol Infusion

In 1850, John Marshall first described a developmental vestige of the embryonic left superior vena cava that has since become known as the ligament of Marshall. This is an anatomically complex structure which gives rise to the vein of Marshall (VOM), located in the mitral isthmus between the mitral valve annulus and left inferior PV with origination at the mid-proximal coronary sinus (CS). In addition to containing striated cardiac muscle bundles (Marshall bundles) with multiple insertions into the CS musculature and posterior left atrial free wall, the ligament of Marshall was also found to have tracts of sympathetic and parasympathetic innervation that modulate the electrophysiological properties of atrial tissue.[90–92] These findings suggest that the ligament of Marshall may play a role in the genesis and maintenance of adrenergic atrial fibrillation, making it a subject of interest for adjuvant therapy. Given its location on the epicardial surface, however, it is unclear whether conventional endocardial ablation is sufficient for electrical isolation of these structures.[92] To address this challenge, techniques for retrograde balloon cannulation and ethanol infusion in the vein of Marshall have been developed and studied, demonstrating in preliminary evaluation to have local ablative effects, elimination of AF triggers and VOM innervation, and facilitation of more robust mitral isthmus ablation.[93–97]

A recent multicenter randomized clinical trial compared the rhythm-control effectiveness of two ablation strategies in de novo treatment of persistent and longstanding persistent AF: catheter ablation alone or in combination with vein of Marshall ethanol infusion with voltage to quantify the ethanol-induced scar prior to PVI.[96] Of the 343 patients randomized, 185 patients were included in the VOM cohort with successful ethanol injection performed in 83.7% (operators were unable to cannulate the VOM in 30 patients). Freedom from any clinical AT/AF greater than 30 seconds in duration on 1-month continuous monitoring performed at 6 and 12 months was reached in 38% of patients (60/158) randomized to catheter ablation and 49.2% of patients (91/185) randomized to vein of Marshall-catheter ablation ($P = .04$) with an odds ratio of 0.63 (85% CI, 0.41–0.97). While additional research is needed to assess longer-term efficacy, this approach appears promising, not only for as adjunctive therapy for persistent atrial fibrillation but also for mitral isthmus-dependent atrial flutter.

Ablation of Non–Pulmonary Vein Triggers

Isolation of PVs is primarily undertaken with the goal of eliminating the initiating triggers for AF. However non-PV triggers of AF are present in many patients, and they may be more prevalent in patients with reduced ejection fraction.[98–100] When non-PV triggers, induced with isoproterenol infusion, are defined as only those early atrial depolarizations leading to AF or sustained AT (Table 20.3), they have been found in 11% of AF patients with no difference in prevalence across paroxysmal, persistent, and long-standing persistent subtypes.[98] In the same study, 91% of patients had PV triggers, again, with no difference across subtypes. This supports the importance of PVI as the cornerstone of ablation for all types of AF. However there is observational data that ablation of non-PV triggers, including repetitive atrial activity that is not observed to induce AF, reduces recurrence of paroxysmal AF among patients with reduced ejection fraction.[100] Interestingly, another recent randomized trial in paroxysmal AF patients in an Asian population showed that trigger elimination in addition to PVI reduced recurrence rates as compared to stepwise ablation to noninducibility.[101] Contrary to most prior studies, this trial found that 76% of all non-PV triggers were found in the superior vena cava (SVC). Given that a high prevalence of SVC triggers was seen in a prior study in an Asian population, it seems likely that there may be a genetic predilection to SVC triggers in this group.[102] When triggers are found in the SVC or the CS, complete isolation of these structures is recommended. When isolating the SVC, pace mapping for phrenic nerve capture is strongly recommended prior to ablation, to avoid phrenic nerve palsy.

We believe that induction and mapping of non-PV triggers is reasonable in many patients with persistent and long-standing persistent AF, especially at the time of redo ablation if PVs are isolated or if a repetitive PAC is present in sinus rhythm. We place a duo-decapolar catheter along the crista terminalis and into the CS. After PVI and any other planned anatomical ablation (i.e., posterior wall ablation) is complete, we place a multispline catheter into the left atrial appendage and place the ablation catheter into the SVC to record SVC potentials (Fig. 20.4). We infuse isoproterenol at 20 mcg/min for twenty minutes, followed by a 10-minute washout period. We map and ablate any trigger that induces AF and consider ablating repetitive atrial firings that do not induce AF during the challenge (Fig. 20.5). Given the complexities and uncertainties of non-PV trigger mapping, an alternative approach is to perform empiric isolation of the posterior wall, CS, and SVC, which account for a significant proportion of non-PV trigger sites (also see Chapter 18).

Left Atrial Appendage Electrical Isolation

The left atrial appendage (LAA) may serve as both a site of AF triggers as well as AF substrate. Several recent studies have shown an association between left atrial appendage isolation

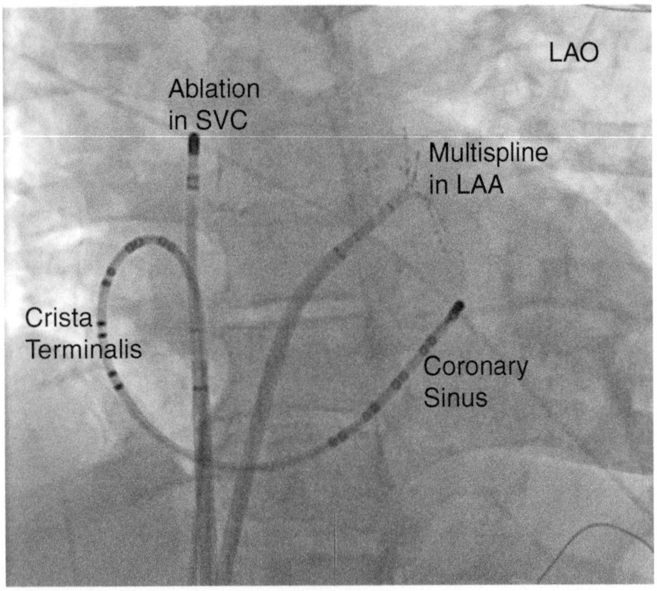

Fig. 20.4 Typical catheter positioning for mapping of non–pulmonary vein triggers. A duodecapolar catheter (Livewire, St. Jude, Symlar, CA) is placed along the crista terminalis and into the coronary sinus. The multispline catheter is placed at the left atrial appendage (LAA) antrum. The ablation catheter is placed into the superior vena cava (SVC) near the upper reaches of visible electrograms. Isoproterenol is infused at 20 µg/min for 20 minutes followed by a 10-minute washout period. Any early atrial depolarization that induces atrial fibrillation or sustained atrial tachycardia is considered a non–pulmonary vein trigger and is targeted for ablation.

and/or excision and improvement in arrhythmia-free survival among patients with persistent and long-standing persistent AF.[103–106] The BELIEF trial randomized patients with long-standing persistent AF to extensive radiofrequency ablation including PV antral isolation, complete posterior wall, CS, and LA roof ablation, ablation of the anterior LA septum, and mapping and ablation of non-PV triggers with or without electrical isolation of the left atrial appendage.[103] This showed 56% arrhythmia-free survival in the group which included LAA isolation versus 28% in the group without LAA isolation (hazard ratio 1.92). However the aMAZE trial randomized 610 patients with symptomatic persistent and long-standing persistent AF in a 2:1 fashion to PVI with versus without LARIAT left atrial appendage occlusion and found no stastically significant improvement in freedom from atrial arrhythmia recurrence.[107] While electrical isolation of the left atrial appendage could logically be expected to impair LAA function (this was seen in 56.5% of patients with LAA isolation in the BELIEF trial), most studies have not described an increased embolic risk,[103–106,108,109] though one published report suggested an increase in stroke, transient ischemic attack, and LAA thrombus in patients with an electrically isolated LAA.[110]

For now, we have not adopted routine LAA isolation for persistent or long-standing persistent AF unless it is part of a hybrid surgical procedure.

Right Atrial Ablation

After the publication of the STAR AF2 trial, there was renewed interest in ablation of the cavotricuspid isthmus in patients with persistent AF in an effort to find an adjunctive ablation strategy that is unlikely to worsen outcomes or safety. Ablation of the cavotricuspid isthmus serves the purpose of likely eliminating typical atrial flutter as well as segmenting the right atrium, which could theoretically reduce sustainability of AF. Data for this are limited, with one study showing no additive benefit of cavotricuspid isthmus ablation when added to PVI plus roof line, mitral line, and complex fractionated electrogram ablation in patients with long-standing persistent AF.[111] It is our current practice to perform ablation of the cavotricuspid isthmus for any patient who has ever had documented or induced sustained atrial flutter during ablation for AF. Further ablation in the right atrium should be guided by the presence of non-PV triggers of AF.

Left Atrial Lines

The original Cox-maze procedure was intentionally designed to leave one-way corridors of conduction through the atria, the idea being that leaving narrow lanes of conduction without the possibility of macroreentry would abolish AF.[112] Application of this idea to standard PVI led to the practice of placing ablation lines across the left atrial roof and also down to the mitral valve annulus (lateral or anterior). In all cases, the lines anchor from one unexcitable structure to another. These lines theoretically serve two purposes: prevention of macroreentry and limiting the expanse of uninterrupted atrial substrate available for fibrillation.

A left atrial roof line is placed from the ablation lines around the left upper PV to the ablation lines surrounding the right upper PV. This line, if complete, prevents roof flutter (macroreentry around the PVs) and electrically distances the superior portion of the posterior wall from the anterior wall.

Two different lines can be placed with the goal of preventing mitral flutter: an anterior mitral line and a lateral mitral line. Anterior mitral lines are often placed from the anterolateral mitral annulus to the right superior pulmonary vein ablation lines but can also link to the left superior vein (coursing anterior to the appendage) or to an intact roof line. Potential drawbacks to the anterior line approach include the relatively long distance of the line and a significant delay of left atrial activation due to the posterior rerouting of conduction.[113] We reserve anterior lines for patients in whom a significant anterior scar is already present. This line can facilitate biatrial flutter, and for this reason, we often anchor the left upper PV (or both upper veins) to remain superior to the RA-LA convergence. A lateral mitral line is placed across the narrowest part of the mitral isthmus linking to the left inferior PV ablation lines. The primary drawback to this approach is the fact that ablation in the CS is very often required to achieve block. If this approach is used, we recommend isolation of the majority of the coronary sinus with ablation directed at local electrograms angled generally toward the left atrium. As mentioned above, ethanol infusion in the vein of Marshall greatly facilitates achievement of acute and durable block with this method.

Early results with both of these approaches suggested improved efficacy among patients with persistent and long-standing persistent AF.[114] However the randomized, multicenter

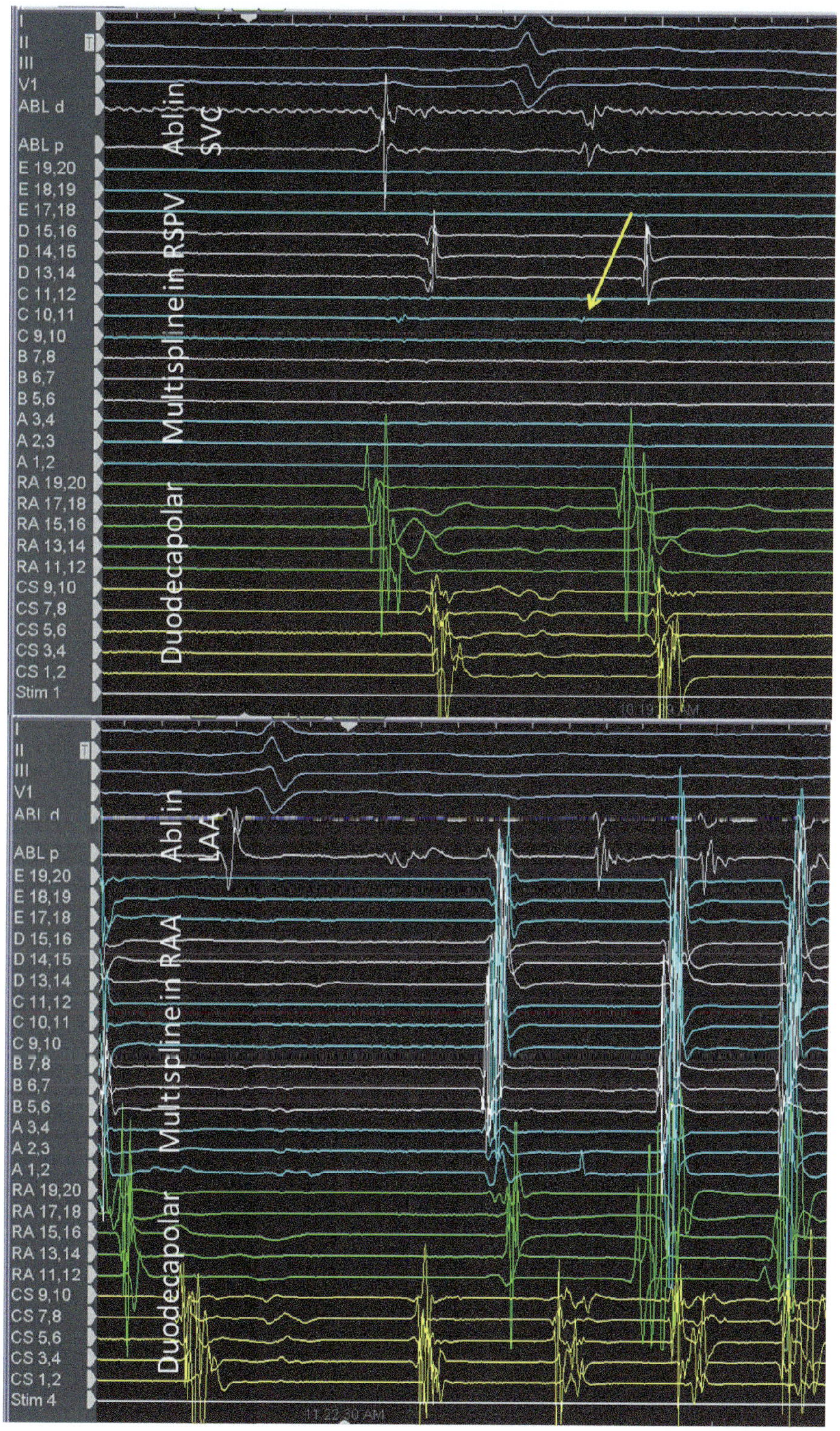

Fig. 20.5 Non–pulmonary vein trigger mapping can be a useful adjunctive ablation strategy in patients with persistent atrial fibrillation. (A), A multispline catheter is in the right superior pulmonary vein (RSPV) antrum, a duodecapolar catheter is looped around the right atrium and into the coronary sinus, and an ablation catheter is placed in the superior vena cava (SVC). The first atrial depolarization is from the sinus node with the earliest activation seen on RA 19,20, followed by the SVC signal on the ablation catheter. The next depolarization (which was later seen to induce AF) is seen earliest on a far-field signal from the RSPV (*yellow arrow*) as well as a local signal on the ablation catheter, next at RA 19,20, followed by a local atrial signal at the RSPV antrum (just outside the ablation line) and the coronary sinus. This suggests an SVC trigger. SVC isolation was performed. Later, a second trigger is seen (B). With the multispline in the right atrial appendage (RAA) and the ablation catheter in the left atrial appendage (LAA), an early depolarization occurs with earliest activation alternating between the LAA and the mid coronary sinus. This induces sustained atrial tachycardia which later degenerated into AF. AF terminated during isolation of coronary sinus musculature. The source of this focal trigger was probably within the ligament of Marshall.

STAR AF2 trial failed to show benefit (and suggested possible worsened outcomes) with placement of roof and mitral lines as compared to an antral PVI-only group.[29] The neutral or reduced efficacy with the addition of roof and mitral lines is probably related to the potential for conduction recovery and proarrhythmia. The left atrial roof and either mitral line location can include thick and anatomically complex tissue, and durable block is often not achieved in many patients. Because of the anatomical location of these lines between two unexcitable structures, conduction slowing, but not block, may stabilize macroreentry in a way that conduction recovery of a PVI line does not.

With our standard posterior wall isolation approach, a roof line is placed by default due to complete ablation of the posterior wall between the pulmonary veins. If roof flutter is observed or a roof line is deemed necessary, this is the approach we recommend for ablation. We recommend a detailed voltage map with a multispline catheter (Pentaray or Octaray, Biosense-Webster, Diamond Bar, CA) and consideration of placement of a mitral line only if significant atrial low voltage is seen across the mitral isthmus, anterior wall, or septum, which seems likely to facilitate peri-mitral flutter, or if mitral flutter is observed or induced during the procedure.

Complex Fractionated Atrial Electrograms

Complex fractionated atrial electrograms (CFAEs) are defined as multicomponent atrial electrograms displaying continuous baseline perturbation OR having a mean cycle length ≤120 ms over a 5-second epoch. While the analysis time interval can be altered by the operator up to 8 seconds, 5- to 6-second intervals are the most widely used as they have been shown to be the most reproducible over time. These sites are thought to be either areas of continuous re-entry or collision zones between fibrillatory waves entering from different directions. Initial studies suggested high efficacy for CFAE ablation in patients with persistent AF.[115,116] However other studies had mixed results, and a meta-analysis of several relatively small studies showed a small benefit (RR 1.15 for PVI-alone versus PVI + CFAE ablation) in 2011.[117] Subsequently, the multicenter STAR AF2 trial showed no benefit for CFAE ablation as compared to PVI or PVI + left atrial lines in patients with persistent AF.[29] At this stage, we do not recommend ablation of CFAEs given evidence of no benefit as well as the increased risk of additive ablation, however certain anecdotal experiences seem compelling to explore ablation of CFAE areas with higher resolution tools (Fig. 20.6) (also see Chapter 19).

Ablation of Fibrotic Areas

Atrial fibrosis reduces electrical coupling, slows electrical conduction, leads to a dispersion of atrial refractory periods, and causes anisotropic conduction, all of which may predispose to AF initiation and maintenance.[118] As such, there is increasing interest in identifying areas of atrial fibrosis as a therapeutic target. There are two primary methods of detecting atrial fibrosis: through delayed enhancement magnetic resonance imaging (DE-MRI) and by using low-voltage areas (LVAs) on electroanatomic maps as a surrogate for fibrosis.

DE-MRI assesses the presence of gadolinium in cardiac tissue 10–20 minutes after injection as a way to discern fibrotic from healthy tissue. The DECAAF study assessed atrial fibrosis burden prior to AF ablation by DE-MRI and showed a strong linear correlation between burden of fibrosis and AF recurrence with 15% recurrence in those with stage I fibrosis and 69% recurrence in those with stage IV fibrosis.[119,120] Leveraging this knowledge, ALICIA trial investigators were the first to integrate DE-MRI images into a 3D fibrosis map merged with an ablation navigation system, finding no added benefit in supplementing PVI with MRI-guided ablation in the 181 patients studied.[121] Notably, investigators excluded patients with a large left atrium, and most participants had paroxysmal AF and a low fibrotic burden. Similar results, however were observed in the recently published DECAAF II trial in which 843 patients with persistent AF were randomized to either PVI alone or a PVI plus MRI-guided ablation.[122] Likewise, there was no significant difference in atrial arrhythmia recurrence between the studied groups. Importantly, the PVI plus fibrosis-guided ablation cohort had a higher rate of safety events, driven primarily by ischemic stroke. Currently available data suggests that DE-MRI guided ablation does not provide benefit as adjuvant therapy to PVI.

A recent randomized trial suggested that a substrate-based strategy using voltage mapping and ablation in addition to PVI led to a reduction in AF recurrence for patients with persistent AF.[123] In this study, patients with persistent AF randomized to undergo PVI alone or PVI plus additional substrate modification (PVI + SM) underwent voltage mapping in sinus rhythm with ablation and/or isolation of low-voltage areas (LVAs, defined as <0.5 mV). This substrate-based approach is not dissimilar to widely accepted methods for ablation of ventricular tachcyardia. Depending on the location and extent of the LVAs, the regions were either connected to an isolated structure (i.e., PVI), isolated with lines en bloc (i.e., the posterior wall), or incorporated into a linear lesion set (i.e., anterior wall of the left atrium). Overall, patients randomized to the tailored approach were less likely to have AF recurrence (35% PVI + SM versus 50% PVI only, HR 0.62, $P = .006$) at 12 months, with 75% of patients having an implantable cardiac monitor. One caveat is that being randomized to the PVI + SM group seemed to improve outcomes even among patients without LVAs (in whom the prescribed therapy was identical in both groups), presumably either due to chance or unintended procedural confounding. Several nonrandomized studies and a smaller randomized study had previously suggested benefit for this approach as well.[118,124,125]

Therefore, while MRI-guided ablation (using current technology) does not appear to be beneficial for persistent AF, endocardial voltage-guided ablation increasingly shows promise for a tailored approach to ablation of persistent AF (Fig. 20.7) (also see Chapter 19).

Ablation of Ganglionic Plexi

The relationship between the autonomic nervous system and AF has been known since Coumel reported AF onset preceded by sinus slowing in 1978.[126] The link between AF and the parasympathetic nervous system was further elucidated through studies showing decreased action potential shortening and reduced

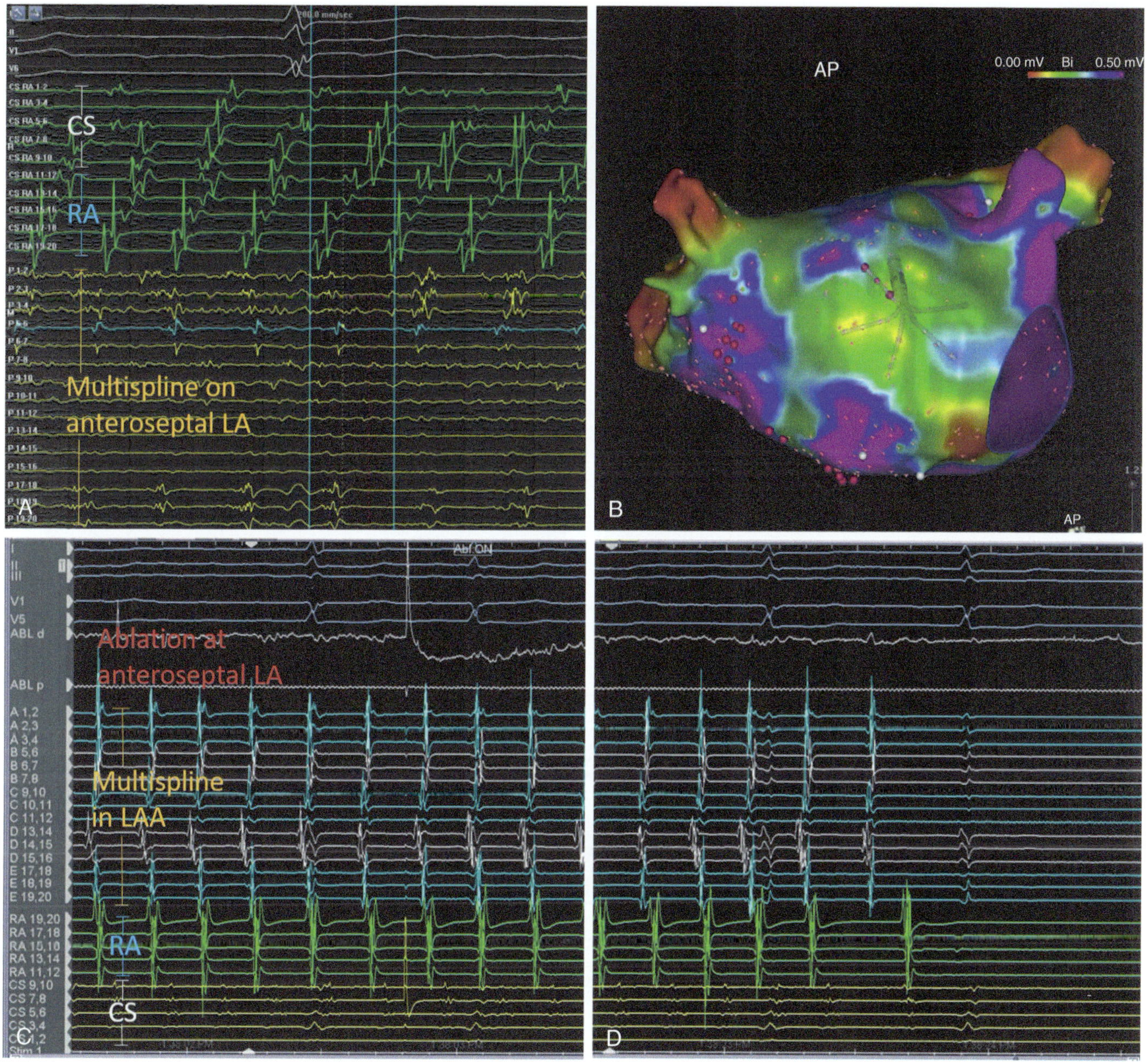

Fig. 20.6 Continuous atrial activity is seen (A) during sustained atrial fibrillation (AF) on several bipoles of a multispline catheter (labeled P1–2, P2–3, etc.) with the catheter placed along the anteroseptal left atrial wall (B). An ablation catheter is then placed at the site of continuous activity, and the multispline catheter is moved to the left atrial appendage (LAA) (C). Ablation at this site is associated with termination of AF after 20 seconds (D). This observation suggests that at least some sites of continuous atrial activity play a role in sustaining AF. Better mapping tools may help differentiate true drivers of AF from incidental collision sites, where ablation could possibly be proarrhythmic.

ability to induce AF by vagal nerve stimulation after ablation of parasympathetic nerve fibers.[127] The interface of these autonomic fibers and the myocardium is focused around the ganglionic plexi (GPs), which consist of a concentrated neural network embedded in the epicardial fat pads along the ligament of Marshall and at the juncture with the great vessels.[128]

The most common GP locations are at the junction of the left superior PV and the LA, at the junction of the left inferior PV and the LA, at the ligament of Marshall, at the junction of the right superior PV and the left atrium, and near the junction of the IVC with the RA.[129–131] These sites can be located in individual patients by applying high-frequency electrical stimulation (typically 16–50 Hz) at typical GP sites with a positive vagal effect defined as an increase in the RR interval and/or sudden decrease in the blood pressure by >20 mm Hg. These sites can then be ablated with effectiveness defined as loss of the vagal effect. Empiric ablation at likely GP sites is feasible and may be associated with improved outcomes, with ablation clustered 1–2 cm outside the LA-PV junction at the left superolateral area (the posterior roof near the left upper PV), the left inferoposterior area (just inferior

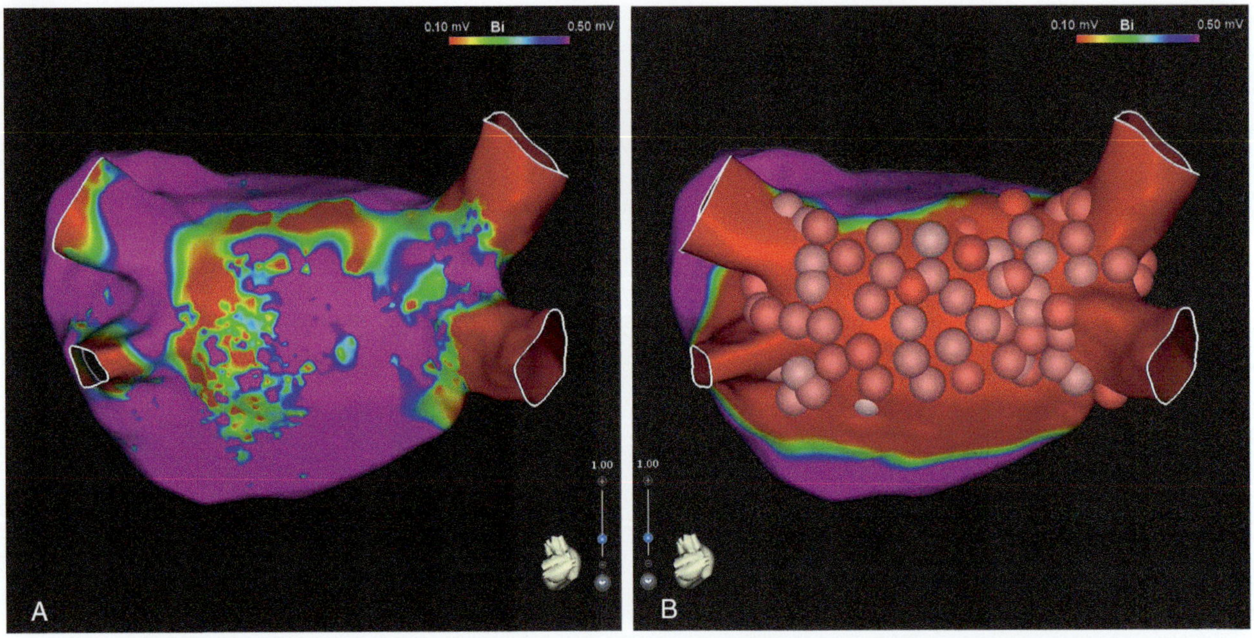

Fig. 20.7 Sustrate-based mapping and ablation can be a useful adjuncts in patients with persistent AF. A left atrial preablation voltage map acquired during sinus rhythm shows significant low voltage across the posterior wall (A). In addition to a pulmonary vein isolation, the posterior wall was isolated en bloc by ablating diffusely with the endpoint of no local electrograms and no pace-capture after ablation (B). Recent data suggest that isolation of low-voltage areas at the time of PVI reduces recurrence of persistent AF.

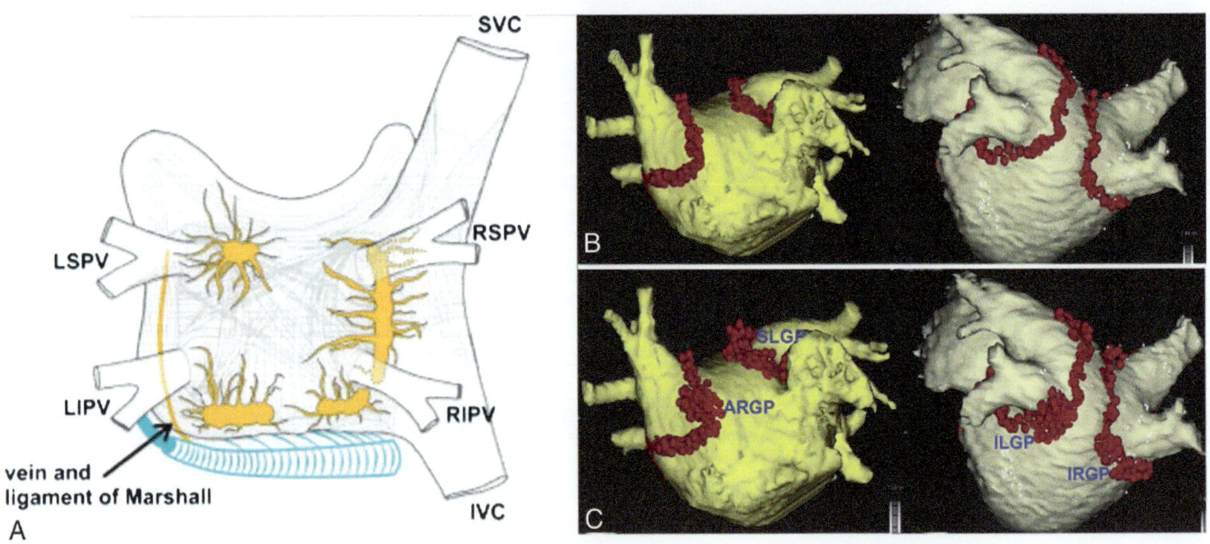

Fig. 20.8 Anatomic sites of ganglionic plexi are shown (A) at the posterior left atrial roof near the left upper pulmonary vein (PV), the left inferoposterior area (just inferior and posterior to the left lower PV), the right superoanterior area (anterior and superior to the right upper PV), and the right inferoposterior area (inferior to the right PV). When empiric ablation of ganglionic plexus sites is performed, pulmonary vein isolation (B) is performed followed by empiric ablation of likely ganglionic plexus locations (C). (Reproduced with permission from (A) Calkins H, Kuck KH, Cappato R, et al. 2012 HRS/EHRA/ECAS Expert Consensus Statement on Catheter and Surgical Ablation of Atrial Fibrillation: recommendations for patient selection, procedural techniques, patient management and follow-up, definitions, endpoints, and research trial design: a report of the Heart Rhythm Society (HRS). *Heart Rhythm.* 2012;9(4):632–696. E21. https://doi.org/10.1016/j.hrthm.2011.12.016, and (B, C) Reproduced with permission from Katritsis DG, Pokushalov E, Romanov A, et al. Autonomic denervation added to pulmonary vein isolation for paroxysmal atrial fibrillation: a randomized clinical trial. *J Am Coll Cardiol.* 2013;62(24):2318–2325. https://doi.org/10.1016/j.jacc.2013.06.053.)

and posterior to the left lower PV), the right superoanterior area (anterior and superior to the right upper PV), and the right inferoposterior area (inferior to the right PV)[132] (Fig. 20.8).

Targeted ablation of GP sites with the goal of reducing AF recurrence has been studied in a few randomized controlled trials. Driessen et al randomized 240 patients (59% with persistent AF) to thoracoscopic ablation (PVI in paroxysmal AF patients, Dallas lesion set in persistent AF patients) with versus without mapping and ablation of GPs as determined by high-frequency stimulation.[133] Despite 100% success in eliminating evoked vagal responses in the GP ablation (GPA) group (only 13% of these responses were eliminated in the control group), no difference in efficacy was seen, and the GP ablation group had more than double the incidence of major complications (19% versus 8%), including major bleeding and pacemaker implantation. In contrast, a study randomizing 264 patients with persistent AF to percutaneous catheter-based PVI plus roof and mitral lines versus PVI plus ablation at GP sites (as determined by high-frequency stimulation) plus CFAE ablation near GP sites showed significantly improved freedom from AT/AF at 3 years in the GP + CFAE ablation group, primarily driven by a lower incidence of atrial flutter in the GP group.[134] Another randomized trial in 242 patients receiving catheter-based therapy for *paroxysmal* AF focused GP ablation only at *likely* GP sites that lie along the PVI lines (high-frequency stimulation was not performed) and showed improved outcomes when GP ablation was added to PVI versus PVI alone or GP ablation alone, though it could be argued that this effect could partly be explained by more extensive PVI ablation.[135] In a more direct comparison of patients undergoing thoracoscopic AF ablation, 102 patients were randomized to receive PVI with and without epicardial GP ablation for paroxysmal and persistent AF.[136] An average 89 ± 26 high-frequency stimulation sites were tested (outside of the PVs and left atrial appendage), identifying a median of 18.5% of GPs as ectopy-triggering. In the GP ablation group, ectopy-triggering GP sites were eliminated with additional targeting of AV dissociating GPs in patients remaining in incessant AF in the procedure. Over a 1-year follow-up, the study showed that GPA did not prevent atrial arrhythmia more than PVI alone, and resulted in a longer procedural time. While there was a larger reduction of antiarrhythmic drug use postablation in the GPA group, medication discontinuation was left to the discretion of the patient rather than being physician or protocol driven.

Taken together, it is not yet clear whether intentional GP ablation will be a useful adjunct for patients undergoing ablation for persistent AF or whether high-frequency stimulation is necessary to locate GP sites.

Rotor and Driver Mapping and Ablation

While AF seems to be *triggered* most commonly by premature beats or atrial runs from the pulmonary veins, AF seems to be *sustained* by a variety of factors, which may include rotor activity, the target of focal impulse and rotor modulation (FIRM).[137] In the FIRM approach, 64-pole basket catheters are placed in the right and left atria with spatiotemporal computational analysis of unipolar and bipolar signals via a proprietary computer program (Topera, Menlo Park, CA). These algorithms identify stable electrical rotors, described as phase singularities with surrounding rotational fibrillatory conduction during sustained AF, which are targeted for ablation.[138] Rotor mapping shares with trigger mapping the idea of targeting the true sources of AF rather than performing a predefined anatomical ablation. However, in a meta-analysis, pooled estimates did not show any therapeutic benefit of PVI + FIRM approach over PVI alone, and the most recent data seem to suggest that this approach is inferior to conventional PVI despite successfully ablating identified rotors.[139–141]

Novel methods have likewise been developed to identify localized intermittent drivers of persistent AF, including *stochastic trajectory analysis of ranked signals* (STAR) mapping. In brief, STAR mapping is a statistical vector mapping approach that uses data from multiple individual wavefront trajectories to identify regions that most often precede activation of neighboring areas, termed early sites of activation (ESA). Data collection is performed by whole-chamber basket catheters or standard multipolar catheters. While analysis has predominantly been retrospective, a prospective single-center validation study has been performed in 30 patients, 27 of whom underwent STAR-guided AF driver ablation after PVI (three patients converted to a rhythm other than AF during PVI).[142–144] During an average follow up of 17.3 ± 10.1 months, 22 of 27 patients (81.5%) remained free from AT/AF off antiarrhythmic therapy after a single procedure. These nonrandomized results provide hope for this method, but a randomized trial evaluating PVI plus STAR mapping versus PVI-only is yet to be presented.

Alternative Approaches

While this text provides separate chapters detailing each of the following approaches, we would be remiss in omitting a brief comment on pulsed-field ablation and hybrid AF ablation (see Chapters 17 and 21). Pulsed-field ablation (PFA) is a novel non–thermal ablative strategy that has garnered significant interest. Published 1-year outcomes of the early feasibility studies suggest that PFA allows the formation of robust stable lesions in patients with paroxysmal atrial fibrillation leading to reduced atrial arrhythmia recurrence at 1-year follow-up.[145] Whether this success will translate to patients with persistent and long-standing persistent atrial fibrillation or refractory atrial flutter is yet to be seen. A small single-arm feasibility study suggests that adjuvant ablation of the left atrial posterior wall and CTI by PFA technology is durable and safe, but ongoing studies will offer more insight.[146]

Surgical ablation for AF (often performed concomitantly with another cardiac surgery) has demonstrated efficacy for patients with persistent and long-standing persistent AF.[70,72] Through these experiences, it has become apparent that a surgical approach can be advantageous for certain aspects of the procedure, such as ligament of Marshall ablation, left atrial appendage ligation, and posterior wall isolation, while an endocardial approach with electroanatomical mapping can be advantageous for other aspects of the procedure, such as ablation of the cavotricuspid isthmus, ablation at the mitral annulus, checking for complete block across linear lesions, and performing "touch-up ablation" across surgically placed lines.[147] Comparing a combined epicardial/endocardial ablation approach consisting of PVI plus posterior wall isolation and cavotricuspid isthmus line to traditional endocardial PVI plus roof and cavotricuspid isthmus lines for patients with drug-refractory persistent or long-standing persistent AF, results of the CONVERGE trial suggest that hybrid ablation offers greater freedom from atrial arrhythmias at 12 months (67.7% patients in hybrid group versus 50% in catheter ablation group, $P = .036$) and overall reduction of AF burden after 18 months of follow-up in the 153 patients studied.[148] While these results are encouraging, hybrid ablation carries greater risks of major and minor bleeding, increased incidence of the need for pacemaker, and increased mortality as compared to historical outcomes from purely endocardial approaches. As such, hybrid ablation should only be performed in experienced centers and probably reserved for patients with symptomatic persistent or long-standing persistent AF.[149]

Ablation to Termination

Intuitively, termination of AF during ablation would seem to be highly correlated with positive outcomes. This is the basis of the "stepwise" approach to AF ablation initially described by the Bordeaux group.[150] While initial outcomes appeared impressive, longer-term follow-up revealed 17% five-year arrhythmia-free survival after one procedure.[151] Interestingly, in the STAR AF2 trial, patients who converted during the procedure had better outcomes than those who did not, but this was driven primarily by patients who converted very early during the procedure (prior to completion of PVI).[47] Furthermore, only 5% of patients who underwent PVI-only ablation had acute termination (as opposed to 40% in the PVI + CFAE and 17% in the PVI + lines groups), but there was no difference in recurrence between these groups. A randomized trial of stepwise ablation to AF termination failed to provide any benefit over PVI alone.[152]

Prior data about the prognostic significance of achieving acute termination has been mixed.[150,151,153] This may suggest that termination of AF early during ablation may be primarily a marker of patients likely to have better outcomes. Alternatively, though most recent data suggest limited overall benefit for CFAE ablation, stepwise ablation, and ablation to termination, better mapping tools may differentiate true drivers of AF from incidental collision sites, where ablation could possibly be proarrhythmic. This idea is supported by the anecdotal experience of termination of persistent AF while ablating at CFAE sites (Fig. 20.6) as well as termination of persistent AF during FIRM ablation, which is reported to be common in some studies[154,155] but not others.[156,157] For now, ablation with the goal of termination of AF is probably unnecessary and may not improve outcomes despite increasing procedure time and possibly complications.

Use of Adenosine

Many randomized and nonrandomized studies have assessed the use of adenosine to assess for dormant PV conduction after ablation due to the ability of adenosine to hyperpolarize injured, depolarized myocardial cells. Conflicting results have caused waxing and waning enthusiasm for this strategy over time. A recent meta-analysis suggests that adenosine-induced PV reconnection after PVI predicts recurrence of AF if the PV reconnection is not targeted for ablation.[158] Furthermore, there was a trend toward improved outcomes in those who had adenosine challenge as compared to those who did not have adenosine challenge. Given this, it is reasonable to perform adenosine challenge to assess for dormant PV conduction after PVI, though it is a Class IIb recommendation in the most recent guidelines.[5]

Predictors of Outcome

While it is not possible to know definitively how an individual patient with persistent AF will respond to ablation, outcomes may be predicted based on clinical factors, detailed assessment of arrhythmia chronicity, and through radiologic evaluation (Table 20.2). Using readily available clinical data, the APPLE score (which assigns points for age >65, persistent AF, eGFR <60 mL/min/1.73 m^2, LA diameter ≥43 mm, and LVEF <50%) has moderate predictive power in determining AF recurrence after ablation.[159] When compared with a score of zero, the odds ratios for AF recurrence for scores of 1, 2, or ≥3 are 1.73, 2.79, and 4.70. This exceeds the predictive power of the CHADS2 and CHA^{2}DS^2-Vasc scores, which were previously shown to predict recurrence. The APPLE score was found to be equally predictive of recurrence in patients presenting for repeat AF ablation.[160]

As mentioned above, patients who have carried the diagnosis of persistent AF >1 year are approximately twice as likely to have recurrence as those <1 year since that diagnosis, and patients in continuous AF for >1 year are likely to have even worse outcomes.[5,49]

DE-MRI has shown a strong, linear correlation between burden of fibrosis and AF recurrence with recurrence rates of 15%, 36%, 46%, and 69% corresponding to <10%, ≥10–<20%, ≥20–<30%, and ≥30% fibrosis of the LA, respectively. A recent review of available data suggests that ablation may be unlikely to succeed in patients with Utah stage IV and those with Utah stage III with diffuse fibrosis.[120]

Defining Success

By convention, recurrence of AF after ablation is defined as 30 seconds of documented AF or atrial tachycardia including atrial flutter. However, a single 45-second AF episode, for example has not been definitively linked to worsened outcomes, per se, and would constitute a radical improvement for a patient with long-standing persistent AF. When counseling patients with persistent AF, complete eradication of AF is not necessarily the expected outcome with a single procedure. However an improvement in quality of life could be attained by converting symptomatic persistent AF to paroxysmal AF with a 1% burden. Accordingly, AF burden on implantable loop recorder, pacemaker, or implantable cardioverter-defibrillator may be an additional relevant outcome in persistent AF trials in the future. Underscoring this point, results of the CIRCA-DOSE study (which used implantable loop recorders in all patients) demonstrate the stark contrast in success when efficacy of ablation is defined in traditional binary terms (time to first recurrence of AF lasting >30 seconds) versus the AF burden (proportion of time an individual is in AF) documented by an implantable loop recorder.[161] In this trial, the incidence of 30 seconds or more of atrial fibrillation after PVI for paroxysmal AF during 12-month follow-up was approximately 53% while the reduction in AF burden was 99.3% compared to the preablation monitoring period. While this level of monitoring may not be cost effective for all patients, having continuous rhythm monitoring for AF burden in future randomized controlled trials comparing persistent AF treatment strategies seems important. Wearable devices may also help bridge this gap.[162,163]

CONCLUSION

Ablation of persistent and long-standing persistent AF is a potentially complex procedure that carries a lower success rate than ablation for paroxysmal AF. Predictors of recurrence include longer duration since persistent AF diagnosis, greater than 1 year of continuous AF, elevated APPLE score, and fibrosis on DE-MRI. Patients with multiple risk factors for recurrence, especially, should be given realistic expectations. PVI remains the cornerstone of AF ablation in every AF population, with antral isolation having better outcomes than ostial ablation. Further adjunctive ablation comes in many forms. Currently, we favor diffuse posterior wall isolation, consideration of ablation lines in patients at high risk for or who demonstrate left atrial flutter, and strategic use of ethanol injection into the vein of Marshall to aid a posterolateral mitral isthmus line.

REFERENCES

Please refer to the e-book for a complete list of references.

21

Epicardial and Endocardial Hybrid Ablation for Atrial Fibrillation

Andy C. Kiser, Jeffrey C. Liu

KEY POINTS

- Isolated catheter ablation of persistent and long-standing persistent atrial fibrillation demonstrates marginal long-term outcomes.
- Technological improvements and minimally invasive techniques enable surgical ablation without sternotomy or cardiopulmonary bypass, but outcomes fall short of the cut-and-sew maze procedure.
- The hybrid approach combines medical, catheter, and surgical therapies either simultaneously or in a staged fashion.
- At a minimum, the therapeutic objectives are electrical isolation of the pulmonary veins and posterior left atrium.
- Collaboration between the surgeon and the electrophysiologist improves patient outcomes.

INTRODUCTION

The Cox-maze III procedure consists of a lesion pattern that divides the atria into appropriate segments to eliminate the reentrant circuits responsible for maintaining atrial fibrillation (AF).[1] The principles of segmentation, specifically pulmonary vein isolation (PVI)[2] and posterior left atrial isolation,[3] remain the cornerstone of all ablative interventions for AF (Fig. 21.1).

Radiofrequency (RF) and cryothermal energy sources have replaced surgical incisions, and transvenous catheters have supplanted sternotomy and cardiopulmonary bypass in treating AF. Endocardial catheter ablation, mainly PVI, and surgical maze-like patterns have become mainstays of interventional treatment of AF. Although catheter and minimally invasive surgical therapies have reduced the invasiveness of ablative AF therapies, independently they fail to meet the superior outcomes of the original "cut-and-sew" procedure.[4–8] Epicardial surgical ablation in conjunction with endocardial catheter ablation, a hybrid ablation procedure, offers the potential advantage of more robust transmural lesion formation, left atrial debulking, and endocardial mapping/ablation of residual arrhythmia circuits. Hybrid AF procedures suggest improved procedural success over isolated epicardial surgical or endocardial catheter ablation procedures for AF, particularly in those with persistent or long-standing persistent AF and those with significant structural heart disease. However, the ideal patient populations that may benefit from hybrid AF ablation and the ideal tools and techniques for a hybrid approach have yet to be determined. This chapter reviews the hybrid ablation procedure including methods of hybrid ablation, available tools, and reported efficacy of the procedure.

CATHETER APPROACH

Since the classic article of Haissaguerre and coworkers[2] demonstrating the role of ectopy originating from PVs as triggers for AF, interventional therapies for AF have predominantly consisted of endocardial catheter-based approaches. Techniques have evolved, moving away from focal elimination of PV tachycardia foci to segmental PVI and ultimately, with the realization that the PV antra were critical to the maintenance of AF, to wide-area circumferential ablation. These approaches work well in paroxysmal AF,[9] especially in the absence of important structural heart disease. However, for patients with structural heart disease and those with persistent and long-standing persistent AF, endocardial lesion patterns have become more complex.[10] Outside of antral PVI, catheter-based lesion sets have become less well defined with significant interoperator variability and endpoints. Catheter-based approaches to these more complex patients have included creation of long linear ablation lesions, with or without an attempt to debulk the left atrium with a posterior wall isolation similar to the Cox-maze procedure. Alternative approaches have included ablation of ganglionic plexi (GP) and attempts to identify critical driver activity in the atria through software signal analysis. More recently, some have moved toward posterior wall isolation rather than focusing on ablation targeted at low-voltage areas (complex fractionated atrial electrograms [CFAEs]) of the left atrium wherever they occur with limited and inconsistent results.[11]

Significant technical advances in catheter ablation technology have paralleled this lesion pattern strategy. High-density automated mapping systems guide lesion placement and map complex tachycardia circuits. Also, with the development of high-flow externally irrigated catheters and contact force sensing technology, consistent catheter contact during lesion

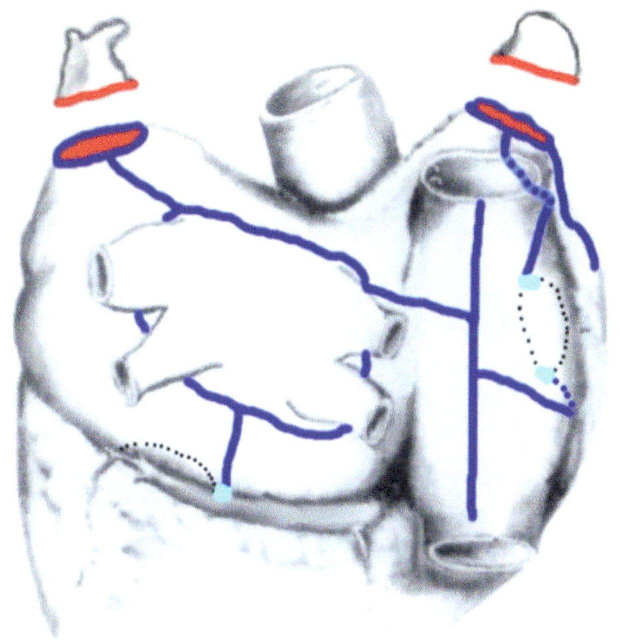

Fig. 21.1 Posterior view of open chest Cox-maze III lesion pattern (*blue:* incision; *aqua:* cryothermal lesions; *red:* appendage excision; *black dots:* tricuspid or mitral valve annulus).

TABLE 21.1 Reported Morbidity Associated With Concomitant Open Surgical Maze II Procedure

First Author	Years of Study	Number of Patients	Reported Morbidity (%)
Isobe[53]	1993–1995	30	10
Jatene[54]	1991–1994	20	20
Takami[55]	1994–1997	50	6
Izumoto[56]	1993–1995	87	24
Gregori[57]	1993–1994	20	5
Kim[58]	1994–2004	127	13
Kosakai[59]	1992–1994	101	14
Szalay[60]	1995–1998	52	15
Sandoval[61]	1993–1995	21	48
Melo[62]	1992–1994	12	66
Kawaguchi[63]	1992–1993	51	14
Cox[64]	1987–1999	346	15
Schaff[65]	1993–1999	221	8
McCarthy[66]	1991–1999	100	6
Arcidi[67]	1993–1999	99	23

placement now makes more durable and consistent lesions with less risk of local tissue charring or steam pops.

Even with the rapid progress made in catheter ablation technology and techniques, success rates remain disappointing to date, especially in the most complex patients who benefit the most from sinus rhythm. Studies with longer than 2-year follow-up report success rates after multiple catheter ablations between 57% and 63% for patients with persistent AF.[12] Success rates should increase as our understanding of the mechanisms of AF develops, along with continuing technological improvements. However, endocardial catheter ablation remains limited by inadequate transmural lesion formation, which is particularly necessary to effectively treat complex patients with nonparoxysmal AF.[13-15] Challenges to endocardial catheter-based transmural lesion formation include fear of iatrogenic collateral injury (in particular with ablation near the esophagus due to fear of atrio-esophageal fistula; phrenic nerve palsy; PV stenosis) as well as an increasing recognition of the importance of epicardial circuits in pathogenesis of AF independent to endocardial activity.[16]

SURGICAL APPROACHES

Approaches to the surgical interventional management of AF emerged from two distinct schools of thought. Surgical approaches to the management of AF in patients undergoing concomitant cardiac surgery, or as a stand-alone procedure, drew from the belief that AF could be managed through atrial debulking and modification of the underlying substrate to minimize the chances of sustained atrial reentry circuits.[1] However, open surgical procedures for AF management, although quite effective, were not broadly adopted due to their associated morbidity (Table 21.1).

Alternative minimally invasive surgical procedures have been developed for patients not requiring concomitant cardiac surgery. Some minimally invasive approaches replicated the maze procedure better than others, with some compromising procedural completeness for less invasive techniques. However, the guiding principles of a surgical therapy for AF remain the same: complete isolation of the four PVs, electrical isolation of the posterior left atrium, management of the left atrial appendage (LAA), and debulking ablation of the right atrium.

The advancement of minimally invasive approaches, with and without the use of cardiopulmonary bypass, has reduced the trauma of the surgical procedure, thereby expanding the number of patients experiencing this therapy. The minimally invasive Cox-maze III/IV[17-19] is perhaps most similar to the original Cox-maze procedure. Performed with cardiopulmonary bypass, the minimally invasive Cox-maze procedure creates a lesion pattern that closely mimics the original maze III pattern (Fig. 21.2) via a right minithoracotomy.

Of 104 nonparoxysmal patients reported, at 3 year,s 92% of the patients were in sinus rhythm and 80% in sinus rhythm without antiarrhythmic drugs (AADs).[17] Complications included only one stroke, and there were no operative deaths. This minimally invasive Cox-maze procedure eliminates the sternotomy and reduces the hospital stay to 4 days. However, the surgery requires cardiopulmonary bypass with or without cardiac arrest.

Alternative minimally invasive techniques do not require the use of cardiopulmonary bypass and use energy sources and devices that consistently create transmural lesions similar to those achieved with an incision. Epicardial off-pump PVI became important with the 1998 report by Haissaguerre and coworkers, which identified the PVs as an important source of triggers to initiate AF.[2] Saltman et al. initially described a bilateral thoracoscopic approach using microwave energy to create

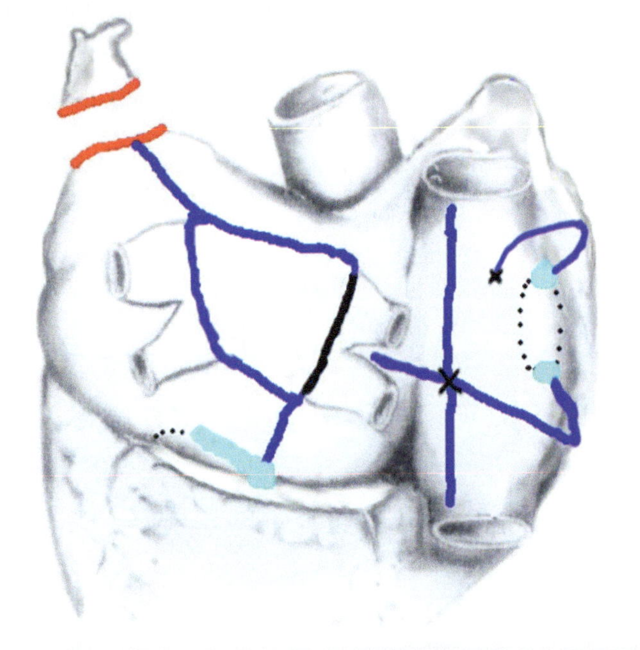

Fig. 21.2 Posterior view of minimally invasive Cox-maze IV lesion pattern as performed via right thoracotomy on cardiopulmonary bypass (*black:* incision; *blue:* radiofrequency lesions; *aqua:* cryothermal lesions; *red:* appendage excision; *black dots:* tricuspid or mitral valve annulus).

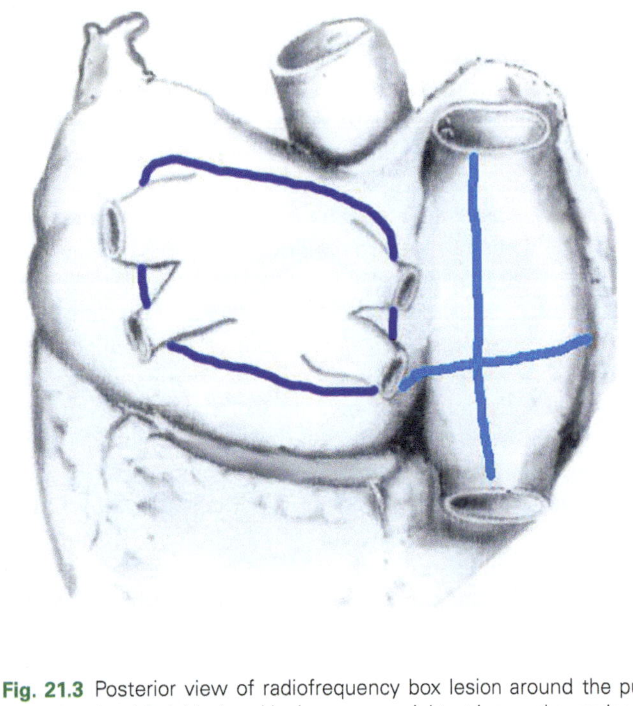

Fig. 21.3 Posterior view of radiofrequency box lesion around the pulmonary veins (*dark blue*) and lesions across right atrium and superior to inferior vena cava (*light blue*).

a box lesion around the PVs.[20] With ablation of the PVs, 62% patients failed to return to AF at 8 months. Pruitt et al. soon followed with a report of 50 patients who were treated using microwave energy via bilateral thoracoscopy to create a box lesion around the PVs, a right atrial lesion to the atrial appendage, and another from the superior to the inferior vena cava (Fig. 21.3).[21] These patients had a rapid return to normal activity and an average hospital stay of 3.7 days. However, late follow-up (mean, 7.6 months) revealed that more than 50% returned to AF with, at endocardial mapping postprocedure, evidence of several PVI failures.[22] However, devices using microwave energy have since been removed from the market.

In the mid-2000s, the bipolar RF clamp was introduced (Fig. 21.4), and in 2005, Wolf et al. described an epicardial off-pump PVI procedure performed via thoracoscopy or minithoracotomy (Fig. 21.5).[23] The initial 27 patients demonstrated promising results, with 91% free from AF at 3-month follow-up. LAA removal contributed to a reduced stroke risk. This

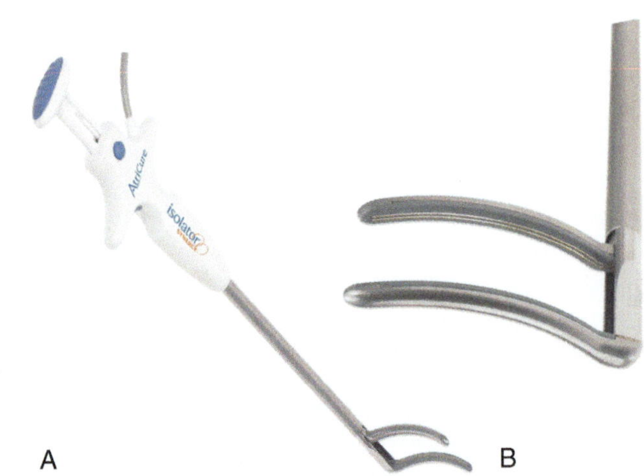

Fig. 21.4 Atricure Isolator bipolar clamp (A) and magnified view (B) of bipolar electrodes.

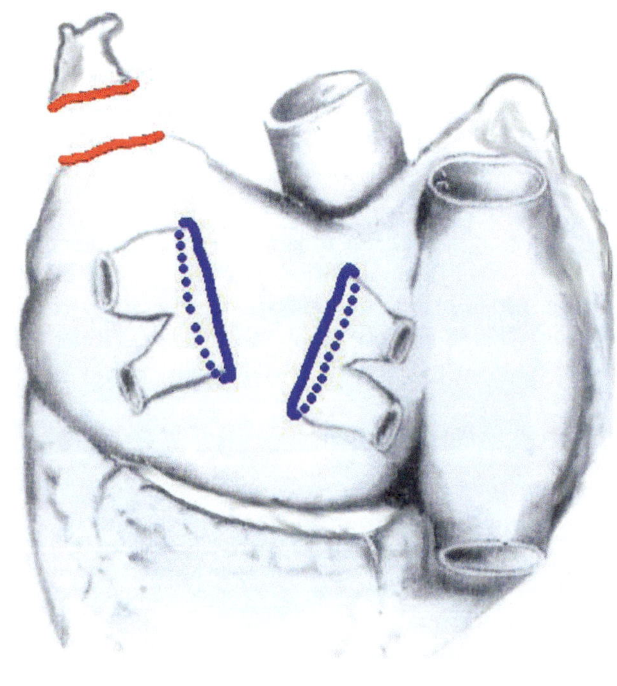

Fig 21.5 Posterior view of Wolf mini-maze lesion pattern (*blue:* radiofrequency lesions [solid in foreground/dotted in background]; *red:* appendage excision).

minimally invasive beating heart procedure opened the door for a less invasive surgical approach but avoided many of the lesions initially described by Cox, specifically lesions connecting to the annulus of the mitral and tricuspid valve.

As the role of GP in the initiation and maintenance of AF become apparent, GP ablation is now also a potential ancillary strategy for surgical AF ablation. Several studies have evaluated the benefit of stand-alone epicardial PVI with GP ablation for the maintenance of sinus rhythm. Edgerton et al. reported outcomes in 52 patients with symptomatic paroxysmal AF.[24] Patients underwent bilateral minithoracotomies with GPs identified by vagal response to high-frequency stimulation. Bipolar radiofrequency clamps were used to isolate the PV antra, and GP ablation was performed. LAA was excised or stapled in 88%. Patients were followed with 24-hour Holter or 2-week monitoring at 6 and 12 months. Average hospital length of stay was 5 days. Three patients required postoperative pacemaker implantation. At 12-month follow-up, 80% of patients were in sinus rhythm. Importantly, Edgerton et al. reported their outcomes based on long-term follow-up with at least 24-hour electrocardiogram (ECG) measurement.

However, the majority of patients in these initial minimally invasive surgical studies had paroxysmal AF. Because endocardial catheter ablation can be highly effective for paroxysmal AF and is a much less invasive procedure, stand-alone epicardial ablation for paroxysmal AF has not gained widespread acceptance. Additionally, some literature suggests that the addition of catheter-based GP ablation may provide a marginal benefit.[25,26] Follow-up studies have demonstrated that surgical PVI alone is insufficient for the treatment of persistent AF.[27]

In those with persistent AF, additional linear ablation to PVI, specifically isolating the posterior left atrium, has shown some benefit.[3] However, the creation of epicardial ablations deep enough to eliminate electrical gaps that may persist near the mitral and tricuspid valve remains difficult, if not impossible, with existing energy sources on the beating heart (Table 21.2). Edgerton et al. developed a beating-heart

TABLE 21.2 Transmurality and Maximum Tissue Ablation Depth for Commercially Available Surgical Ablation Devices

Device	Manufacturer	Energy	Transmurality (%)	Effective Depth (mm)
Coolrail[68]	Atricure	Bipolar RF	91	4
Isolator Clamp[69]	Atricure	Bipolar RF	99	5
EPi-Sense[70]	Atricure	Unipolar RF	15	2
Fusion[71]	Atricure	Bipolar/ unipolar RF	96	6
Cardioblate Clamp[69]	Medtronic	Bipolar CryoFlex *Clamp*	99	5

RF, Radiofrequency.

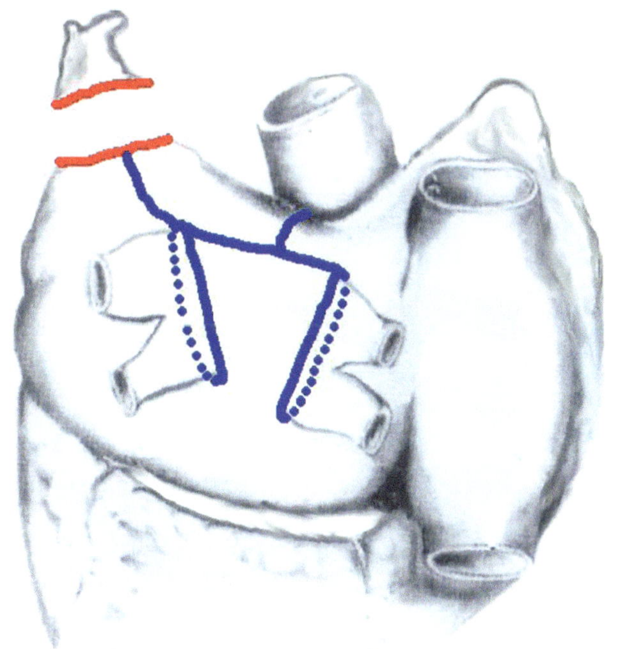

Fig. 21.6 Posterior view of the Dallas ablation lesion set. (*blue:* radiofrequency lesions [solid in foreground/dotted in background]; *red:* appendage excision).

procedure using minimally invasive techniques known as the Dallas lesion set (Fig. 21.6).[7]

This approach connected epicardial ablations to the left fibrous trigone at the aortic valve root. In 30 patients (10 persistent, 20 long-standing persistent), Edgerton et al. described the totally thoracoscopic isolation of bilateral PV antrum using a bipolar RF clamp. Additionally, they interrogated and ablated the GP, excised the LAA, and added a connecting lesion between the PVs at the LA roof, which was also extended to the fibrous aortic valve annulus and to the excised LAA base. Pacing techniques verified conduction block across the roof and anterior trigone lines. Patients were followed for 6 months with ECG and 14- to 21-day auto-triggered monitors. Three (10%) patients required pacemakers. At 6 months, overall success rate was 58% off AADs and 80% with or without AADs, as assessed by long-term (14- to 21-day) event monitoring.

Weimer et al. reported a larger study of 89 patients with paroxysmal (35%), persistent (24%), or long-standing persistent (42%) AF undergoing the Dallas epicardial lesion set.[28] Mean hospital length of stay was 8 days. One patient required conversion to extracorporeal circulation. Freedom from AF and AAD therapy was 71%, 82%, and 90% at 6, 12, and 24 months, respectively, with no difference in those with paroxysmal or persistent AF. However, 5% of patients required subsequent catheter ablation for recurrent AF or atrial flutter.

The minimally invasive, beating heart approach to AF treatment enables real-time interrogation of the surgical ablations because the heart remains electrically active. It is therefore important to interrogate the integrity of the ablation lines to

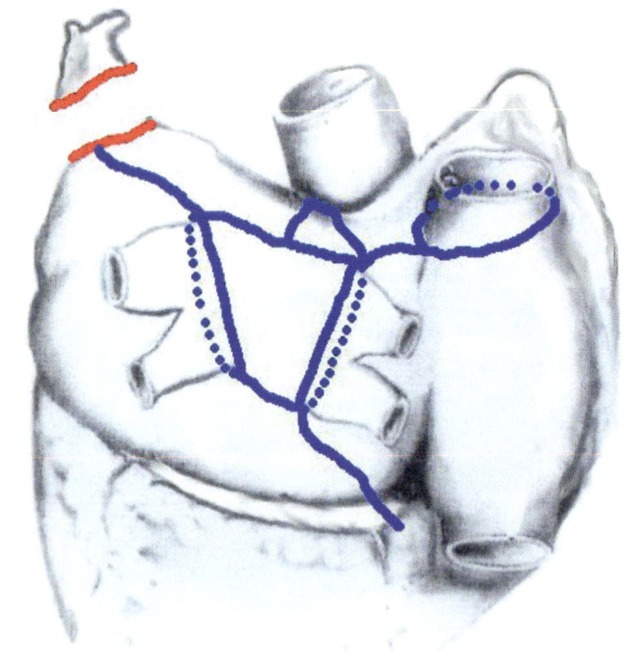

Fig 21.7 Posterior view of five-box ablation lesion pattern (*blue:* radiofrequency lesions [solid in foreground/dotted in background]; *red:* appendage excision).

confirm transmurality and to eliminate gaps. Dialogue continues concerning the validity of lesion interrogation acutely versus delayed lesion interrogation to allow any acute and temporally nonconductive injuries to recover, with evidence that acute vein isolation does not guarantee long-term electrical isolation.[29] The Five-Box Thoracoscopic Maze (Fig. 21.7) procedure described by Sirak critically interrogates the ablation lines to confirm the epicardial electrical isolation of five segments of the left and right atria.[30] Patients fare well with the meticulous thoracoscopic dissection and lesion placement, with an average hospital stay of 3.9 days and 92% freedom from tachyarrhythmias and AADs at 24 months by 7-day event monitoring.[31] Two of the 179 patients required conversion to sternotomy, and 2 patients had catheter ablation of the cavotricuspid isthmus at 13 months and remain in normal rhythm.

Nasso et al. described the use of an alternative surgical technique for PVI through only a right minithoracotomy.[32] In 104 patients, a linear vacuum-assisted unipolar RF ablation catheter was looped around the PVs by way of the transverse and oblique pericardial sinuses using a magnet-tipped introducer. Patients were followed with 24-hour Holter monitoring. Periprocedural complications including one case of intraoperative LA rupture requiring sternotomy for repair, one case of hemorrhagic stroke 4 days postoperative, and one transient ischemic attack in the early postoperative period. At an average 17-month follow-up, 89% were free of AF (96% with paroxysmal AF and 80% with persistent AF). While using only a right thoracic incision provides an advantage for Nasso's approach, the LAA is not addressed.

To evaluate the differences in catheter and surgical ablation for AF, Boersma et al. compared the efficacy and safety of catheter ablation and minimally invasive surgical ablation in 124 patients with drug-refractory AF, left atrial dilatation (> 4 cm), and hypertension in the FAST study.[33] AF was paroxysmal (67%), persistent (33%), or long-standing persistent (8%). The surgical ablation pattern was consistent with the Dallas lesion set as described by Edgerton. Catheter ablation included wide-area linear antrum ablation with PVI guided by a circular mapping catheter. Additional lines were made at the discretion of the electrophysiologist. Patients were followed with ECG and 7-day Holter monitoring at 6 and 12 months. Median length of stay was 5.5 days versus 2 days for surgical or catheter ablation, respectively. In the surgical group, complications included one patient requiring conversion to median sternotomy, one patient requiring pacemaker implantation, six patients with pneumothorax, one with hemothorax, one with stroke, one tamponade, and one rib fracture. In the catheter group, complications included one transient ischemic attack and four groin hematomas. However, at 12 months, freedom from AF longer than 30 seconds in the absence of AADs was 66% in the surgical group versus 37% in the catheter group ($P = .0022$).

HYBRID APPROACH

Independently, surgical or catheter-based therapy has acceptable outcomes for the paroxysmal AF population. But for the long-standing persistent population, neither therapy effectively addresses the existing treatment gap. A hybrid approach combines endocardial and epicardial therapies, taking advantage of the independent strengths of surgical and catheter-based ablation. Catheter-based ablation has the advantage of mapping techniques for ensuring bidirectional electrical isolation of PVs or another linear ablation. In addition, certain areas of the atria (e.g., mitral isthmus, cavotricuspid isthmus) are more accessible from an endocardial approach. Catheter ablation techniques also offer the opportunity for detailed mapping of atypical flutters or atrial tachycardia. However, point-by-point catheter ablation is cumbersome and has questionable durability. Balloon-based "single-shot" catheters (most commonly the cryoballoon) have been developed to overcome point-by-point lesion creation in the veins. Surgical ablation uses an anatomic approach with direct visual guidance but without electrophysiologic guidance. A hybrid ablation procedure may offer significant challenges including multidisciplinary team availability, requirement of a hybrid laboratory, sequence of the procedure, and anticoagulation strategy.

However, the potential benefits of a hybrid approach may outweigh these challenges and address the treatment gap experienced with long-standing persistent AF, specifically in those patients whose outcomes may be more limited with a traditional catheter-based procedure.

Results of Hybrid Ablation Studies

Several studies have considered the potential benefit of a hybrid epicardial and endocardial ablation for the management of AF, many of which Vroomen and Pisson summarized in Table 21.3.[34] Varying ablation tools and lesion sets have been used for hybrid AF ablation. Some surgeons use bipolar RF clamps and a linear

TABLE 21.3 Summary of Nonoverlapping Reports on Hybrid Procedures between 2011 and 2016[34]

First Author	Patients (N)	AF duration (y)	LAD (mm)	(ls)pAF (%)	FU (mon)	FU reached (%)	Monitoring	SR (%) ± AAD
Bisleri[35]	45	7 ± 6	51 ± 10	100	28 ± 2	100	ILR	89/–
Bulava[27]	50	4 ± 3	48 ± 4	100	17 ± 5	100	7-d	94/84
Geld[36]	101	6 ± 6	51 ± 10	83	12	100	24-h	66/37
Gersak[37]	50[b] (45)	5 ± 5	48 ± 1	94	12	70	ILR	88/75
Krul[38]	31	8 (1–25)	47 ± 7	48	12	71	24-h	-/86
La Meir[39]	19	5 (3 8.5)	49 ± 20	74	12	100	7-day	63/37
Mahapatm[40]	15	5 ± 1	52 ± 10	100	16 ± 2	100	24-h	93/87
Muneretto[34]	36	6 (0.5–20)	50 ± 6	100	30 (1–58)	100	ILR	92/78
Pison[15]	78	4 (2–7)	45 (42–48)	63	24 (12–36)	100	7-day	86/74
Richardson[41]	83		49 (42–53)	99	12	95	ILR	71/61
Zembala[42]	27	4 ± 3	46 ± 5	82	12	37	7-day or ILR	0/80
Total	535[b]	–	–	–			–	
Mean		5	49	86	17	89	–	82/70
Gaita[43,a]	33	2 ± 2	51 ± 6	100	128 ± 37	100	Holter	33/27
Total	568[b]	–	–	–	–	–	–	–
Mean		5	49	87	26	89	–	78/66

AF, Atrial fibrillation; *LAD,* left atrial diameter; *(ls)pAF,* long-standing persistent AF; *FU,* follow-up; *SR ± AAD,* sinus rhythm with/without antiarrhythmic drugs; *ILR,* implantable loop recorder; *7-d,* 7-d Holter monitoring; *24-h,* 24-h Holter monitoring. [a]Open concomitant hybrid surgery. [b]Including five patients with only epicardial ablation (not separated in baseline table in the article).

ablation pen via unilateral or bilateral thoracoscopy for the epicardial procedure. Others, more recently, have adopted a transxiphoid approach using a unipolar epicardial vacuum-assisted RF linear ablation catheter (Fig. 21.8) through a pericardioscopic access cannula (EPi-Sense and Subtle Cannula, AtriCure, Mason, OH). In addition to mapping the endocardial electrograms, an electrophysiologist used either cryoballoon or RF ablation technology to complete the endocardial component of the hybrid procedure.

Mahapatra et al. reported their hybrid epicardial and endocardial ablation experience with 15 patients with persistent or long-standing persistent AF. They had failed at least one attempt at endocardial ablation and antiarrhythmic drug therapy.[35] Patients were excluded if they had another indication for cardiac surgery or a prior history of cardiac surgery. Bilateral thoracoscopic off-pump epicardial ablation was performed using the Dallas lesion set. The electrophysiologist confirmed isolation of the PVs and the superior vena cava in the operating room and then, an average of 4 days later, performed an endocardial ablation. During endocardial ablation, SVC isolation was confirmed, a cavotricuspid isthmus line was created, and PV isolation and block across the roof and mitral line were confirmed. Finally, high-dose isoproterenol was used to try to induce dysrhythmias. Any atrial flutter induced was mapped and ablated. If AF was induced, additional complex fractionated atrial electrogram ablation was performed. All patients were treated with amiodarone or dofetilide for 3 months postprocedure. Routine 7-day or 24-hour continuous monitoring was performed. Outcomes were compared to a matched catheter ablation–alone control group. Overall, hospital length of stay in the hybrid group was longer, but otherwise there were no acute complications in either group aside from a tamponade in the catheter-alone group. At 20 months of follow-up, more patients in the hybrid group were free of atrial arrhythmias off antiarrhythmic drugs (87% versus 53%, $P = .04$).

Pison et al. initially reported their experience in 26 patients undergoing hybrid thoracoscopic and transvenous ablation for AF in patients who had either failed prior catheter ablation, had an enlarged left atrial volume (≥29 mL/m^2), or had persistent or long-standing persistent AF.[36] Similar to the studies of Mahapatra, the PVs were isolated at the antra using a bipolar RF clamp. Isolation was confirmed endocardially. In those with persistent AF, a roof line and posterior LA line (box lesion), SVC isolation, and intercaval lines were created. An epicardial and endocardial mitral line was created. A cavotricuspid isthmus line was made in those with a prior history of atrial flutter or flutter during the procedure. Finally, the LAA was excluded in a subset. Patients underwent 7-day continuous monitors at 3, 6, 9, and 12 months postprocedure, and AADs were discontinued at 6 months. Ten of 26 patients had persistent AF, one had long-standing persistent AF, and the remainder had paroxysmal AF. Mean hospital length of stay was 7 days. There were no major complications. At 1-year follow-up, success rate (no atrial arrhythmia >30 seconds without AADs) was 93% in those with paroxysmal AF and 90% in those with persistent AF with two patients requiring redo catheter ablation after the hybrid procedure.

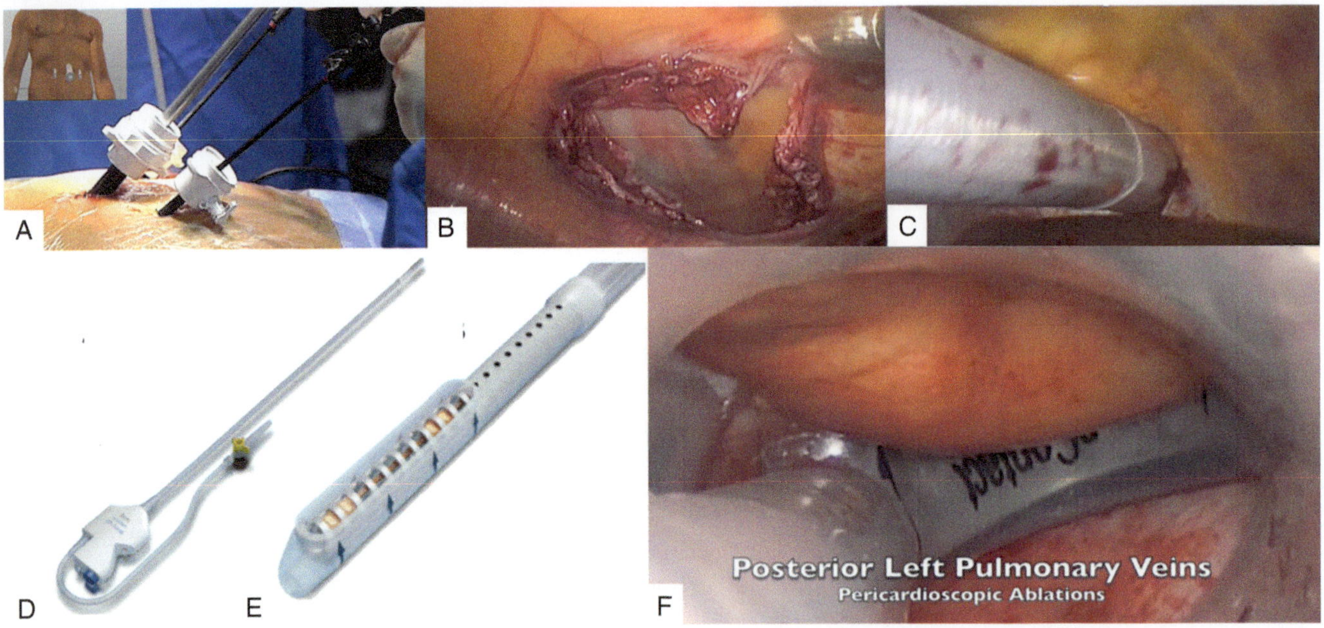

Fig 21.8 Transdiaphragmatic epicardial ablation of the convergent procedure: laparoscopic abdominal access to the diaphragm (A); central diaphragmatic incision exposing the epicardial surface (B); transabdominal cannula insertion into the pericardial space (C); atricure EPi-Sense surgical ablation device (D) and enlarged view of ablation coils (E). Posterior left pulmonary vein ablation using EPi-Sense device (F).

La Meir et al. further examined this patient population with a report comparing a hybrid epicardial and endocardial ablation in 35 patients with epicardial only ablation in 28 patients (45–50% paroxysmal, 18–23% persistent, 31–32% long-standing persistent).[37] Bilateral thoracoscopic epicardial ablation included PVI, roof and inferior LA ablation targeting a posterior "box," and GP ablation. Entrance and exit blocks across the PV and posterior box lines were checked. In the hybrid group of patients, PV isolation and block across the lines were checked endocardially. Induction of AF was performed during endocardial ablation with rapid pacing and/or isoproterenol infusion. In the case of persistent AF, a mitral line was created. Additional SVC isolation was added in those with persistent or long-standing persistent AF and cavotricuspid isthmus ablation was performed in those with a history of typical right atrial flutter or if it became apparent during the procedure. Finally, LAA exclusion was performed in those with an LAA tachycardia or those with CHADS^2 score ≥1. Patients were followed with 7-day continuous monitoring at 3, 6, and 12 months postprocedure. There were no complications including mortality, stroke, or reoperation for bleeding in the two groups. Median length of hospital stay was 3 to 4 days. At 1-year follow-up, success rates free of atrial arrhythmia >30 seconds off AAD therapy were higher in those undergoing hybrid ablation compared to epicardial alone (91% versus 82%, $P = .07$), particularly in those with persistent or long-standing persistent AF.

Pison et al. summarized their groups reports with their overlapping series of 78 patients undergoing hybrid ablation procedure.[38] Epicardial ablation was performed including PVI, posterior box isolation, mitral isthmus ablation, and intercaval lines. These lines were subsequently mapped and completed endocardially as required and a cavotricuspid isthmus ablation was performed endocardially; LAA exclusion was performed in patients with CHADS^2 score of ≥1 or in the presence of LAA tachycardia. Seven-day continuous monitoring was performed at 3 months, 6 months, and 1 year and yearly thereafter. At median follow-up of 24 months, 87% patients were free of AF off AADs (100% for long-standing persistent, 82% for persistent, and 76% for paroxysmal AF). On AAD therapy, freedom from AF was seen in 92% (100% for long-standing persistent group, 85% for persistent group, and 97% for paroxysmal group), although 19 patients (13%) underwent percutaneous endocardial ablation for recurrent AF or LA flutter after the hybrid procedure.

Kurfirst et al. reported their experience of hybrid ablation procedure in 30 patients with persistent and long-standing persistent AF.[39] The epicardial portion of the procedure was performed by a bilateral thoracoscopic approach with PVI, posterior wall box lesion, and ganglionated plexi ablation; the LAA was excluded. Endocardial ablation was performed to complete PVI and posterior box isolation and a mitral isthmus and cavotricuspid isthmus lines were created. Any residual or inducible atrial tachycardia or flutter were mapped and ablated. Patients were followed up at 3, 6, 9, and 12 months by 7-day Holter monitoring. After completion of the hybrid procedure, freedom from AF was 90% without AAD and 93% on drugs.

Bulava et al. further examined the Kurfirst study with a follow-up report on their staged hybrid ablation approach using bilateral thoracoscopic epicardial ablation in 50 patients with long-standing persistent AF and a dilated LA.[40] Epicardial ablation procedure was performed with a bipolar RF ablation clamp and linear ablation pen including PVI, posterior box lesion, a trigone line, ganglionated plexi ablation, and LAA exclusion. Six to 8 weeks after the epicardial procedure, endocardial ablation was performed to confirm and complete the epicardial ablation lines if required. Any induced atrial tachycardia or flutter was mapped and ablated. Follow-up occurred at 3, 6, 9, and 12 months and every 6 months thereafter with 7-day ECG monitoring before each visit. At 1-year follow-up, 94% of the patients were free of atrial arrhythmias with AAD therapy and 84% without AAD therapy.

Muneretto et al. initially described a staged hybrid approach using right-sided thoracoscopy.[41] Bisleri et al. further examined this cohort of 45 patients with long-standing persistent AF surgically treated with an internally cooled vacuum-assisted RF unipolar ablation device (COBRA ADHERE XL, Estech, Sam Ramon, CA) to deliver a continuous lesion encircling the origin of all the PVs ("box" lesion set).[42] An endocardial catheter-based procedure was performed in 30–45 days, and PVI and posterior wall isolation was confirmed or achieved with additional endocardial ablation as needed. Additional ablation addressed CFAEs and cavotricuspid isthmus. All patients were monitored with an implantable loop recorder implanted at the time of the surgery and AF episode duration <5 minutes, and overall burden <0.5% was considered as stable NSR. After a blanking period of first 6 months, over a mean follow-up of 28.4 months, 88.9% patients were free from AF.

In the effort to avoid incisions in the chest and between the ribs, authors evaluated the efficacy of the convergent procedure as initially described by Kiser et al.[43] This hybrid procedure uses pericardioscopic access via a subxiphoid or transdiaphragmatic approach with a unipolar vacuum-assisted linear RF ablation catheter. Gehi et al. reported their experience in a cohort of 101 patients undergoing the convergent procedure hybrid ablation with simultaneous endocardial mapping and ablation.[44] The majority of patients had persistent (47%) or long-standing persistent (37%) AF. The epicardial portion of the procedure used laparoscopic instrumentation and techniques to gain access to the pericardial space through the central tendon of the diaphragm. A cannula inserted into the pericardial space provided an endoscopic view of the epicardial surface, specifically the posterior left atrium, and enabled epicardial ablation using a unipolar, vacuum-assisted RF linear ablation catheter (Fig. 21.8). The epicardial lesion set included antral PV ablation, posterior LA box ablation, and connecting lesions to the coronary sinus (Fig. 21.9). Endocardial ablation, immediately following the epicardial procedure, included completion of antral PVI and mitral isthmus ablation if required. Additional ablation included CFAE-guided ablation, SVC ablation, and cavotricuspid isthmus ablation at the discretion of the electrophysiologist. Any residual atrial flutter or atrial tachycardia was mapped and ablated. Patients were followed at 3, 6, and 12 months with 24-hour Holter monitoring or implantable loop monitor. Complications included two patients with tamponade, two patients with bleeding (one requiring surgical intervention), and two deaths (one atrioesophageal fistula and one sudden and unexplained death at home with unrevealing autopsy). Repeat endocardial ablation was performed in 6% of patients. Including repeat ablation, 12-month arrhythmia free survival was 73% without concomitant antiarrhythmic medications.

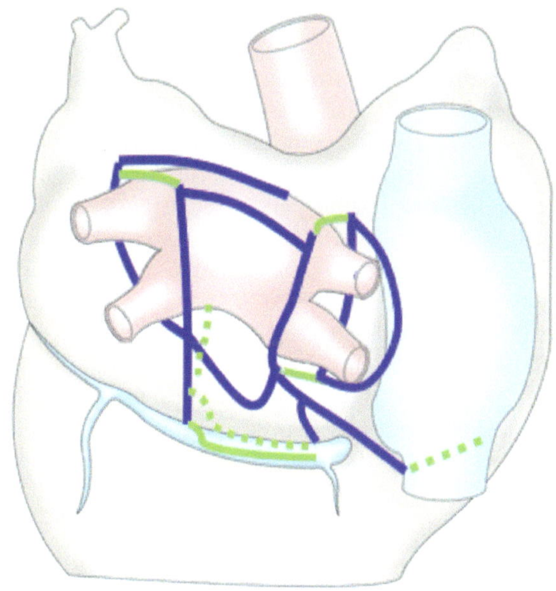

Fig 21.9 Posterior view of the convergent lesion pattern (*blue:* endocardial surgical lesions; *green:* endocardial catheter ablations).

Gersak et al. compiled the experience of four European centers performing combined epicardial and endocardial catheter ablation via the pericardioscopic approach in 73 consecutive patients with persistent or long-standing persistent AF with an average AF duration of >4 years.[45] The lesion set for epicardial ablation included antral PV ablation and posterior LA box ablation. Immediately following epicardial ablation, endocardial mapping/ablation was performed to confirm or achieve isolation of the PVs and the posterior atria. Patients were followed with regular 24-hour Holter monitoring or an implantable loop recorder. Over 1-year follow-up, 4% required repeat endocardial ablation and arrhythmia-free survival was 73%. The authors reported no mortality and one stroke while two patients required conversion to sternotomy. Additionally, one patient demonstrated tamponade; one patient, pericardial effusion; one patient, pleural effusion; and two patients, transfusion.

Civello et al. reported their single-center experience in 104 patients (27% paroxysmal, 30% persistent, 43% long-standing persistent) undergoing hybrid ablation using a transdiaphragmatic approach.[46] Patients were followed with 72-hour Holter at 6 and 12 months postprocedure. At 12 months postprocedure, 73% were in NSR without AAD therapy and 89% with or without AAD therapy. One patient had a cerebrovascular accident, one patient developed PV stenosis, and one patient required drainage of a pericardial effusion, both occurring >7 days postprocedure.

Zembala et al. reported their outcomes using a hybrid ablation technique in 27 patients with persistent AF (5 patients) or long-standing persistent AF (22 patients) and a left atrium with <6-cm diameter.[47] The epicardial portion of the procedure was performed by way of subxyphoid pericardioscopic access through the diaphragm. An irrigated, unipolar, vacuum-assisted RF linear ablation catheter was used through a pericardioscopic access cannula. The epicardial lesion set included a posterior box (roof and low posterior LA lines), antral PV ablation, and connecting lesions to the coronary sinus. Endocardial ablation was performed 15–20 days later. The endocardial lesion set included completion of antral PV isolation, mitral isthmus ablation, and cavotricuspid isthmus ablation. Patients were maintained on AAD therapy for 3 months postablation. Twenty-four-hour Holter monitoring was performed at 6 and 12 months postoperatively. Complications included one patient with tamponade, a second patient requiring sternotomy due to bleeding from an inferior vena cava laceration, and a third patient who died 27 days after discharge of unclear cause. At 6 months postprocedure, 72% of patients were in sinus rhythm, 67% without AAD therapy. At 1 year postprocedure, 80% of patients were in sinus rhythm and off AAD therapy.

In 2020, Wats et al. provided a comprehensive analysis of the convergent procedure.[48] Unlike those reports included in Table 21.3, Table 21.4 included only convergent procedure studies, some of which we have examined here. Most of these studies demonstrated a freedom from any atrial arrhythmia with or without AADs >81% and had follow-up beyond 12 months. When the authors examined freedom from any atrial arrhythmia without AADs, reported outcomes ranged from 58% to 83%. Although most of these reports examined patients undergoing concomitant endocardial and epicardial ablation via a transdiaphragmatic, pericardioscopic approach, surgeons and electrophysiologists began to embrace a subxiphoid approach and a less complex epicardial lesion set that primarily addressed the posterior left atrium (Fig. 21.10). The transition addressed early procedural related complications such as incisional diaphragmatic hernias, esophageal fistulas, bleeding, and death. With expanded experience over time, complications and mortality improved significantly (Table 21.5). Cardiac death, thoracic hernias, and atrioesophageal fistulas have become uncommon occurrences in more modern reports.

The CONVERGE Trial, a multicenter, randomized controlled trial compared the effectiveness of the convergent procedure to catheter ablation alone for patients with persistent or long-standing persistent AF, completed enrollment in 2018.[49] One hundred fifty-three patients from 27 centers in the United States and the United Kingdom participated. At 12-month follow-up with Holter monitor, 67% of the convergent group were free from AF/atrial flutter with no increase or addition of AADs compared to 50% in the catheter ablation group ($P = .0.36$). When the groups were compared without AADs, the convergent group demonstrated an even greater success rate, 53.5% versus 32% ($P = .013$). At 1 year, 94% of convergent patents had ≤5% AF burden. Importantly, posterior left atrial electrical isolation, not performed in the catheter ablation group, which consisted of only PVI + roof line, contributed to the outcome's advantages seen in the convergent group. There were no deaths, atrioesophageal fistulas, or diaphragmatic hernias. Only one patient experienced a stroke and two patients experienced excessive bleeding. Pericardial effusion, commonly expected after intrapericardial surgical procedures, was the most common complication (Fig. 21.11). Both reported and trial complication rates decreased with procedural improvements and as centers gained experience.

The CONVEREGE Trial also emphasized the importance of collaboration between the cardiac surgeon and the electrophysiologist. Makati et al. described best practices and guidelines that reinforce procedural steps and processes that enhancement collaboration and group efficacy.[50] The multidisciplinary convergent team integrates surgeon, cardiologists, nursing, and staff into the pre-, intra-, and postprocedure stages of care with highly effective coordination and communication.

Advantages and Disadvantages of Epicardial Ablation for AF

There are several potential advantages and disadvantages to epicardial ablation techniques for AF. Epicardial ablation offers the opportunity for direct visualization of the atrium and ablation lesions. Even though endocardial ablation technological advances may improve the likelihood of robust antral isolation (e.g., balloon ablation), linear epicardial ablation, particularly in the atrial body, may be more consistent and result in long-standing, transmural, high-quality lesions. Ablation from the direction of epicardium to the endocardium avoids ablation force directed posteriorly toward the esophagus to allow for more aggressive ablation lesions on the posterior LA wall, a potentially critical region for the maintenance of AF, without fear of iatrogenic damage to the esophagus. The LAA can also be managed with direct surgical clipping to mitigate stroke risk and further potentially improve outcomes in freedom for AF as the LAA has independently emerged as an important site of AF triggers.[51] Catheter-based ablation of the LAA resulting in electrical isolation is less desirable due to elevated thromboembolic risk necessitating downstream consideration of LAA occlusive device (Watchman or Amulet) or surgical LAA clipping. However, a stand-alone minimally invasive epicardial approach also has limitations and significant anatomical considerations. Beating heart epicardial ablation does not consistently create lesions that extend to the mitral or tricuspid annulus, leaving an opportunity for iatrogenic circuits causing recurrent AF or flutter. Detailed mapping of ablation lines including antral PVI lines and other left or right atrial lines can be challenging in the operating room but is critical to improving success rates. Surgical epicardial ablation carries sufficiently higher risks than endocardial ablation approaches alone, with the potential for catastrophic complications. However, we have more recently seen a decline in the rate of these complications.

Hybrid (epicardial and endocardial) ablation, either simultaneous or staged, offers significant improvements to a stand-alone epicardial approach. Following epicardial with endocardial ablation offers the opportunity to verify epicardial lesions and approach territories that are inaccessible epicardially. As in endocardial ablation, epicardial ablation often leaves gaps in lines regardless of the surgical device used. Endocardial mapping following epicardial ablation identifies gaps in epicardial ablation lines. Endocardial completion of epicardial ablation lines is typically easier and likely more durable after epicardial ablation than after endocardial ablation alone. Thus, hybrid ablation offers the potential for a more robust ablation pattern and a lower likelihood of iatrogenic flutter. In addition, the electrophysiologist readily maps and ablates arrhythmias encountered during interrogation, such as atrial flutter or atrial tachycardia, and addresses complex fractionated electrograms

TABLE 21.4 **Summary of Convergent Procedure Studies**[48]

Studies	Type	Year	Type of AF (PAF, PsAF, LSPAF)	Timeframe of treatment	No. of Patients	Timing	Mortality	Complications	Follow-up	Freedom from AF ± Antiarrhythmics (%)	Freedom from any Atrial Arrhythmia ± Antiarrhythmics (%)	Freedom from any Atrial Arrhythmia off Antiarrhythmics (%)
Transabdominal without AtriClip												
Kiser et al.	Observational	2011	PAF, PsAF, LSPAF	Jan 2009–May 2010	65	Concomitant	5%	3%	12 mo	–	88%	83%
Zembala et al	Observational	2012	PsAF, LSPAF	Aug 2009–Dec 2011	27	Staged	3.7%	10%	12 mo	80%	–	–
Gehi et al.	Observational	2013	PAF, PsAF, LSPAF	Jan 2009–Dec 2011	101	Concomitant	0%	3%	12 mo	73%	–	–
Civello et al.	Observational	2013	PAF, PsAF, LSPAF	May 2010–Dec 2011	104	Concomitant	0%	5%	12 mo	–	87.5%	72%
Thosani et al.	Observational	2013	PsAF, LSPAF	Jun 2010–Feb 2013	43	Concomitant	0%	0%	6 mo	–	89%	–
Gersak et al.	Observational	2014	PsAF, LSPAF	Jan 2010–Dec 2011	73	Concomitant	0%	7%	12 mo	73%	–	–
Edgerton et al.	Prospective	2016	LSPAF	–	24	Concomitant	14%	7%	24 mo	19%	–	–
Gersak et al.	Observational	2016	PAF, PsAF, LSPAF	Jan 2009–Jul 2013	76	Concomitant and staged	0%	12%	48 mo	–	81%	69%
Zembala et al.	Prospective	2017	PsAF, LSPAF	Jul 2009–Dec 2014	90	Staged	1%	8%	12 mo	–	82%	62%
Kress et al.	Observational	2017	PsAF, LSPAF	Jun 2010–Aug 2014	64	Concomitant	1.6%	7.8%	16 mo	72%	–	
Jan et al.	Randomised	2018	PAF	Jan 2013–Jun 2015	24	Concomitant	0%	12.5%	30.5 mo	–	–	58.3%
Gulkarov et al.	Observational	2019	PsAF, LSPAF	Oct 2013–Mar 2017	31	Concomitant	0%	12.9%	24 mo	71%	52%	–
Gegechkori et al.	Observational	2019	PsAF, LSPAF	Jan 2014–Aug 2016	59	Concomitant	0%	1.6%	12 mo	–	76%	–
Sabzwari et al.	Observational	2019	LSPAF	Feb 2015–Sept 2017	30	–	0%	0%	12 mo	80%	–	63%
Gegechkori et al.	Observational	2019	PsAF, LSPAF	Aug 2016–Oct 2019	64	Concomitant	0%	7.8%	12 mo	–	87.5%	–
Tonks et al.	Observational	2019	PAF, PsAF, LSPAF	Feb 2016–May 2017	36 (25/36 subxiphoid, 13/36 with AtriClip	Concomitant (32/36)	0%	16.7%	12 mo	–	78%	–

LSPAF, long-standing persistent AF; *PAF*, paroxysmal AF; *PsAF*, persistent AF.

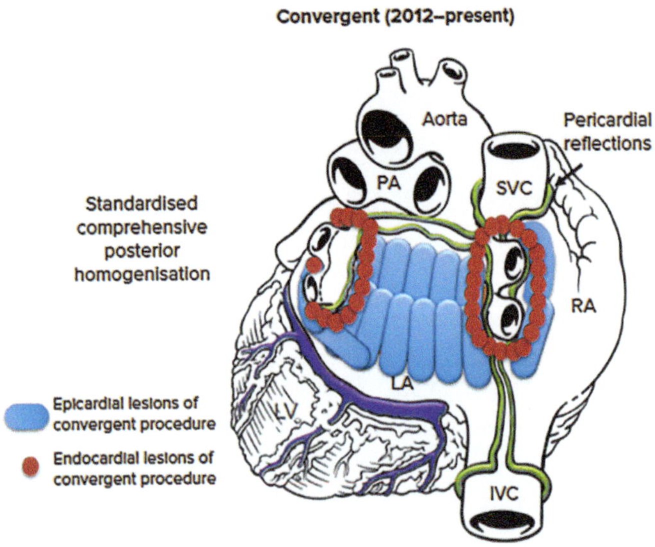

Fig 21.10 Modern convergent procedure ablation pattern.[49] (*Red*, endocardial lesions; *blue*, epicardial lesions). (From DeLurgio DB, Ferguson E, Gill J, et al. Convergence of epicardial and endocardial RF ablation for the treatment of symptomatic persistent AF (CONVERGE trial): rationale and design. *Am Heart J.* 2020;224:182–191. doi:10.1016/j.ahj.2020.02.016.)

TABLE 21.5 Summary of Convergent Procedure Complications[48]

Complications		
Atrioesophageal fistula	6/884	0.7%
Pericardial effusion	10/884	1.1%
Pericardial tamponade	9/884	1.0%
Cardiac death	2/884	0.2%
Unexplained death	2/884	0.2%
Major bleeding	12/884	1.4%
Hematemesis	1/884	0.1%
Stroke	7/884	0.8%
Transient ischemic attack	2/884	0.2%
Pleural effusion	3/884	0.3%
Lung injury	1/884	0.1%
Pulmonary vein stenosis	1/884	0.1%
Transient phrenic nerve palsy	3/884	0.3%
Groin/puncture site complications	2/884	0.2%
Infection	1/884	0.1%

when present. As presented in the studies outlined above, the hybrid approach has demonstrated improved efficacy compared with either an endocardial alone or epicardial alone approach for patients with nonparoxysmal AF. The CONVERGE trial has provided evidence that defines the value of the hybrid approach, especially for patients that are difficult to treat with catheter ablation alone. In fact, the FDA has now approved the EPi-Sense system (AtriCure, Mason, OH), the devices used to create the convergent epicardial lesions, for the treatment of patients with long-standing persistent AF. Patients undergoing hybrid ablation have better outcomes, as discussed previously. Additionally, due to better long-term success rates and fewer repeat ablations, hospital systems find an economic advantage when treating nonparoxysmal AF patients with the convergent procedure over medical management and catheter ablation alone.[52]

Factors Influencing the Success of Hybrid Ablation

Several factors must be considered when building a hybrid ablation program. The approach for epicardial ablation needs to be decided and mastered. Several surgical tools have been developed, each with their advantages and disadvantages. Surgical approaches must be individualized to the patient based on prior surgeries or other anatomical considerations. Ultimately, the comfort level and skill of the cardiac surgeon are the most important factors in choosing an epicardial ablation tool and approach. Hybrid AF ablation changes the working relationship between the electrophysiologist, the cardiac surgeon, and the patient. A multidisciplinary approach benefits all those involved but can bring significant changes to the current working environment. Performing hybrid ablation requires significant changes to the system of patient care. Considerations include the location for the ablation procedure (hybrid surgical

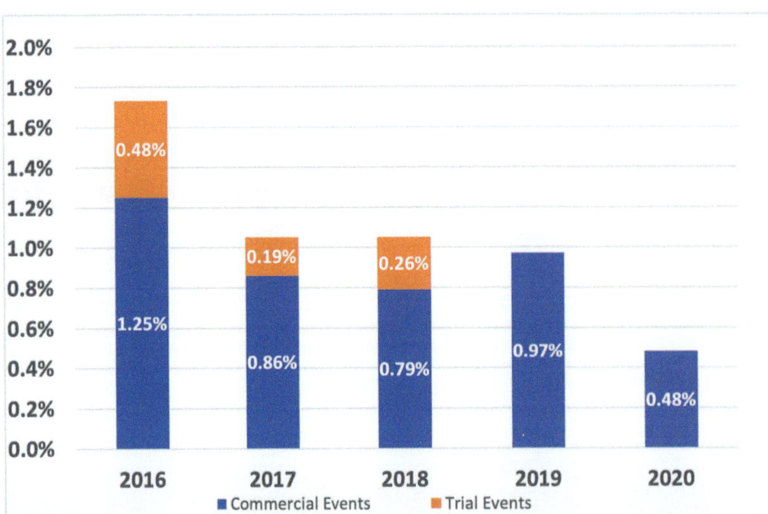

Fig 21.11 Convergent procedure device/procedure-related complication rates.

suite or staged operating room then electrophysiology laboratory), personnel involved during the epicardial and endocardial portions of the procedure (single dedicated team or multiple teams), anesthesia care (dedicated cardiac anesthesia or not), and postoperative care team (cardiac surgery team, electrophysiology team, or a combination). The potential for complications, particularly during the epicardial portion of the procedure, must be considered and a clear plan must be in place to intervene quickly. In addition, communication and planning is critical to preoperative, perioperative, and postoperative care. This includes issues regarding antiarrhythmic drug use, anticoagulant use, and management of any postoperative arrhythmia.

Future Directions in Hybrid Ablation

Although several studies of hybrid AF ablation have demonstrated the potential benefit of this novel technique, there are many unanswered questions that future studies could answer. Varying lesions sets and ablation devices have been used, but the common objective remains antral PVI and left atrium posterior wall isolation. Increasingly, LAA management with surgical clip and/or exclusion is emerging as an important consideration with the hybrid procedure. The value of additional lesions may also be evaluated with future studies. The optimal timing of endocardial ablation remains unanswered. Staged ablation allows for the maturing of the epicardial lesions to better evaluate for gaps in ablation lines. However, simultaneous ablation limits the potential for unstable iatrogenic flutters, which can complicate epicardial only ablation. A study comparing staged with simultaneous epicardial/endocardial ablation could resolve this question. Management of the LAA as a source of both thromboembolization and AF should be considered in future trials that randomize hybrid patients to LAA exclusion. Finally, current studies of hybrid ablation have included patients who are particularly challenging for an endocardial-only ablation, including those with history of prior failed endocardial ablation, severely enlarged atria, or other structural cardiac abnormalities. While the results of the CONVERGE trial have provided evidence supporting the convergent procedure for long-standing persistent patients, more evidence is needed to examine the role of hybrid ablation for paroxysmal and persistent patients.

CONCLUSION

Epicardial AF ablation has come a long way since the initial techniques developed by James Cox. Although the development of epicardial and endocardial ablation techniques had largely occurred in parallel, we are seeing a merging of approaches that offers the potential for significant synergistic benefits. As the potential risks of epicardial ablation have been further mitigate, hybrid procedures may be offered to patients in whom endocardial ablation alone have more limited benefit, including with nonparoxysmal AF, those with significant atrial enlargement, or those with prior failed attempts at endocardial ablation. In these populations, hybrid procedures, the convergent procedure in particular, offers distinct advantages.

REFERENCES

Please refer to the e-book for a complete list of references.

22

Ablation Strategies for Persistent and Long-Standing Persistent Atrial Fibrillation

Jorge E. Romero, Juan Carlos Diaz, Luigi Di Biase

KEY POINTS

- Though pulmonary vein isolation has been demonstrated to be effective in maintaining sinus rhythm in patients with paroxysmal atrial fibrillation (AF), its effectiveness in patients with persistent AF is significantly lower.
- In patients with persistent AF, extrapulmonary vein triggers and atrial substrate play a major role in the initiation and maintenance of the arrhythmia.
- Careful preprocedural planning, as well as the use of adequate radiofrequency and ventilatory settings, can increase procedural efficacy and efficiency.
- Posterior wall isolation, in addition to left atrial appendage electrical isolation and vein of Marshall ablation, may play a significant role in increasing procedural success. The use of other ancillary techniques (superior vena cava isolation, coronary sinus isolation, rotors, and complex fractionated atrial electrogram ablation) is currently not recommended due to the lack of a clearly demonstrated impact on overall atrial arrhythmia recurrence.

INTRODUCTION

Persistent atrial fibrillation (PeAF) is defined as atrial fibrillation (AF) that is continuously sustained for more than 7 days, regardless of whether it terminates spontaneously or requires cardioversion (electrical or pharmacologic). Depending on the duration of the arrhythmia, PeAF can be further categorized as long-standing persistent AF (LSPAF) (i.e., lasting >1 year). Patients with PeAF have a higher risk of stroke and heart failure, decreased quality of life, and higher chance of disease progression and all-cause mortality. Therefore, efforts to reduce progression from paroxysmal AF (PAF) to PeAF and from PeAF to LSPAF or permanent AF are of paramount importance. Catheter ablation (CA) is effective in reducing the risk of arrhythmia recurrence in patients with PeAF and LSPAF,[1] resulting in a reduction in health care costs.[2] Moreover, CA for PeAF is associated with improved cognitive outcomes and a reduction in depressive states, most likely due to an improvement in cerebral perfusion.[3] Consequently, these data demonstrate the importance of achieving adequate rhythm control in patients with PeAF and LSPAF. However, patients with PeAF treated with pulmonary vein isolation (PVI) have a lower procedural success rate than patients with PAF, which has led to significant interest in targeting non-PV triggers and in the development of alternative lesion sets to reduce the risk of atrial arrhythmia recurrence. The different ablation strategies currently used to treat patients with PeAF and LSPAF will be discussed in this chapter.

ANATOMY

The left atrium (LA) is composed of several structures with different degrees of arrhythmic potential for patients with PeAF and LSPAF. These include the pulmonary veins (PVs), the posterior wall (PW), the left atrial appendage (LAA), the coronary sinus (CS), the vein of Marshall (VOM), the LA body, and the vestibule (defined as the smooth portion around the mitral valve).

Pulmonary Veins

The PVs have long been recognized as an important origin of triggers participating in the genesis of PAF[4] and are currently the main target for different CA strategies. In patients with PeAF, PVs are also the main target for ablation, even though their importance in the initiation and maintenance of AF is lower than that observed in PAF. Given the high risk of PV stenosis associated with ostial ablation, wide antral circumferential ablation (WACA) is currently the standard approach for radiofrequency (RF) PVI, as it is associated with a lower risk of arrhythmia recurrence and PV stenosis.[5] From an anatomical standpoint, the PV ostium is defined as the area where the parietal pericardium reflects on the epicardial surface of the LA. From an electrophysiologist's perspective, the PV ostia is the area located beyond the intervenous carina, while the PV antrum is the area that includes the vein and a part of the LA wall, including the intervenous carina (without being in contact with it). Moreover, the pulmonary vein antra are the area where the PVs come into contact with the LA. Thus, WACA should be performed *proximal* to the PV antra (Fig. 22.1).

In most patients, all four PVs have independent ostia, but the left PVs frequently have a common antrum (approximately 25% of patients). Furthermore, in up to one-fourth of patients, an additional vein is present, located most frequently in the right middle position. Normally, all PVs drain into the LA's posterior wall (PW), with

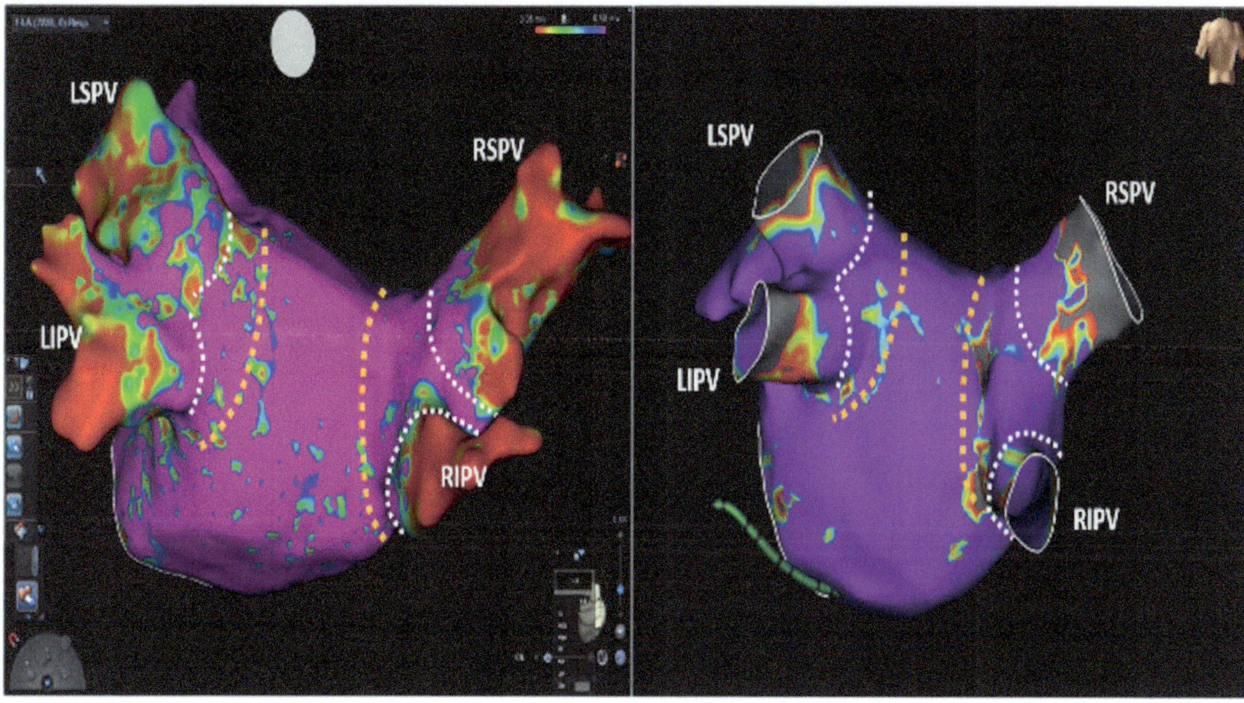

Fig. 22.1 Posterior view of the left atrium using two different 3D mapping systems, Carto (*left*) and EnSite (*right*). The level of the pulmonary vein ostia is demonstrated by a white dashed line. The level of the pulmonary vein antra is marked by a *yellow dashed line*. Note that these yellow lines do not contact the intervenous carina, reducing the risk of pulmonary vein stenosis. *LSPV*, Left superior pulmonary vein; *LIPV*, left inferior pulmonary vein; *RSPV*, right superior pulmonary vein; *RIPV*, right inferior pulmonary vein.

inferior PVs having a more posterior orientation than the superior PVs.[6] Although preprocedural evaluation of PV anatomy using CT scan was initially considered important in reducing adverse events and improving PVI efficacy, there appears to be no difference in outcomes for patients with or without anatomical variations, regardless of whether RF or cryoballoon ablation is performed.[7] Nevertheless, it remains useful to perform image integration, particularly when performing LAA electrical isolation to determine the LAA's ostium position in relation to the left circumflex artery and the phrenic nerve (see later) and to rule out LAA thrombi.

Posterior Wall

The definition of the PW from an anatomical point of view differs significantly from the definition used in electrophysiology (EP). Anatomically, the PW corresponds to the area between a line connecting the inferior PVs to the LA vestibule, while in EP the PW corresponds to the area between the posterior aspect of the right and left PVs, between the superior border of the superior PVs and the inferior border of the inferior PVs. In anatomical terms, this is known as the LA domus since this area is the most superior aspect of the LA in a normal anatomical position. For this chapter, the term *posterior wall* will refer to the EP definition (i.e., the anatomical LA domus, located between the left and right PVs). Similarly, the area between the line connecting the inferior PVs and the LA vestibule (i.e., the anatomical PW) will be referred to as the LA floor.

The PW is of particular interest during CA for AF as it harbors a high number of AF drivers and shares a common embryologic origin with the PVs, leading to similar electrophysiologic properties as those of the PVs. The superior aspect of the PW is thicker than the rest of the LA, with all thickness gradually tapering toward the PV ostia. This increased thickness at the superior aspect is important when performing PW isolation (PWI), as most reconnections occur at this level. Several structures are in close vicinity to the PW: the esophagus (a highly mobile structure separated from the PW only by a fat layer of variable thickness), the descending aorta, and the ganglionated plexi, which have been implicated in arrhythmogenesis. These structures should be considered when performing an ablation in the PW (either during a PWI or a PVI/WACA), as thermal energy transfer to them is possible, leading to irreversible injury.

Importantly, the septopulmonary bundle (SPB) originates in the interatrial groove and runs epicardially through the anterior wall, the PW, and the LA floor. The SPB is of particular importance during PWI, since its epicardial course allows for conduction gaps even when endocardial electrical conduction is abolished.[8]

Left Atrial Appendage

The LAA, a remnant of the embryologic LA, lies between the left PVs and the LA vestibule. The LAA ostium is typically oval-shaped, but its size and shape are highly dependent on LA pressure and the type of AF (being larger and rounder in patients with PeAF than in patients with PAF). When performing ablation, the operator should consider that ostial wall thickness is greater in the anterior (2.5 ± 0.8 mm) and superior (2.4 ± 1.2 mm) parts of the ostium. The ridge separating the LAA from the left PVs should not be considered part of the LAA ostium, and when performing LAA isolation, ablation should not be performed in this area, as it is particularly thick. Instead, ablation should be performed at the same level both in the anterior and in the posterior LAA ostium. Wall thickness can vary significantly, since pectinate muscles traverse the endocardial aspect of the LAA main body increasing thickness to around 1 mm, while the remaining areas may be translucent. This should be considered when manipulating catheters within the LAA, as there is an increased risk of perforation.[9]

Coronary Sinus and Vein of Marshall

Embryologically, the CS forms as the single heart tube divides into the primordial atrium and the sinus venosus, of which the left horn will become the CS (by the 10th week of development) and the right horn will be absorbed by the right atrium (later becoming the smooth intravenous portion).[10] The CS is the largest cardiac vein and comprises the part of the venous system between the CS ostium and valve of Vieussens, which separates the CS from the great cardiac vein (GCV). The CS runs through the left coronary groove and is responsible for most of the venous drainage of the heart (Thebesian veins are responsible for a small proportion of the venous drainage). As such, the CS receives drainage from the GCV, the anterior interventricular vein (which runs through the anterior interventricular septum), the middle cardiac vein (which runs through the posterior interventricular septum), and the lateral veins. A significant number of myocytes are present within the CS, showcasing its role in atrial arrhythmias either as a source of triggers or as an area of focal reentrant mechanisms. In fact, these myocytes are responsible for the electrical connection between the right and left atria (the other two are Bachman bundle and the fossa ovalis). As with all venous systems, there is a high anatomical variability with a few consistent venous branches.

One of the consistent branches is the VOM (present in approximately 92% of CS venograms), an embryological remnant of the left superior vena cava, which originates near the vein of Vieussens and runs through the groove between the LAA and the left PVs.[11] The VOM has also been implicated in atrial arrhythmogenesis. The use of ethanol infusion to produce a line of block in the area drained by the VOM (i.e., the mitral isthmus and anterior portion of the left PVs) has been extensively studied. More recently, a venous connection between the GCV and the LAA, which is different from the VOM, has been described. This vein appears to be an electrical connection between GCV and LAA that may be explained by a myocardial sleeve. Ablation in the CS/GCV can result in inadvertent isolation of the LAA. Likewise, ablation of the GCV/LAA vein may be relevant to achieve LAA electrical isolation (LAAEI) when ablation at the ostial level is challenging.[12]

PATHOPHYSIOLOGY

In patients with PAF, the initiation and maintenance of AF are related to the presence of triggers (most frequently in the PVs), and their elimination plays a major role in the maintenance of sinus rhythm. In contrast, in patients with non-PAF (including PeAF and LSPAF), mechanisms of arrhythmia shift from trigger based to substrate based, in which structural and electrical changes in the LA favor arrhythmia maintenance. Thus, areas of fibrosis/scar, electrogram fractionation, and microreentry increase in prevalence as patients transition from PAF to PeAF and from PeAF to LSPAF. Several strategies have been developed to target these areas, including ablation of complex fractionated atrial electrograms (CFAE), empirical roof and mitral isthmus lines, focal impulse, and rotor modulation (FIRM), scar homogenization, and LA debulking, all of them leading to disappointing results.

Additionally, patients with AF frequently have a higher number of coexisting conditions, which by themselves are associated with a higher risk of disease progression, including hypertension, diabetes, obesity, and obstructive sleep apnea. Thus, patients with non-PAF tend to be older and have larger LA volume indexes and higher number of comorbidities, all of which lead to a higher risk of arrhythmia recurrence even after an initially successful CA. Subsequently, these differences in the pathophysiology between PAF and non-PAF explain the differences in PVI efficacy, as PVs progressively lose their predominant role in arrhythmogenesis.

HOW TO MAP PATIENTS WITH NONPAROXYSMAL AF

Mapping Procedure

After transseptal access has been obtained, mapping should begin with a high-density mapping catheter (Pentarray or Octarray, Biosense Webster; or Advisor HD-Grid, Abbott) through a deflectable sheath (Vizigo, Biosense Webster; or Agilis, Abbott). The goal of high-density mapping is to perform fast anatomical mapping (FAM) of the different LA structures (i.e., the PVs, LAA, mitral annulus, mitral isthmus, posterior and anterior wall, interatrial septum) as well as to obtain local voltage information (to detect areas of low voltage and fibrosis). Noticeably, the voltage map during AF has a better correlation with areas of scar/fibrosis observed in cardiac magnetic resonance imaging than voltage maps obtained during sinus rhythm.[13] The following approach to mapping the LA is recommended:

1. Both anatomical and electrical maps should be created simultaneously. To increase mapping speed and accuracy, ventilation settings should include an inhalation/exhalation ratio of 1:4. This is because mapping is performed automatically at the end of expiration. We also use high-frequency low-tidal-volume (HFLTV) ventilation protocol using a high respiratory rate and low tidal volume to maintain standard minute ventilation levels between 5 and 8 L/min. This is typically achieved with the use of a respiratory rate of around 25–30 breaths/min and a tidal volume of 200 mL (3–3.5 mL/kg).
2. Additionally, if the patient is in sinus rhythm, atrial pacing at a cycle length of 500 or 600 ms will increase the speed of voltage point acquisition.
3. The mapping catheter should be initially inserted in the left PVs. The sheath should remain at the level of the PV antrum and the catheter should be slowly withdrawn, applying alternating

clockwise and counterclockwise rotations to create a 3D anatomy of the vein. The other left PV should then be mapped: if the left superior PV (LSPV) was mapped first, the catheter should be withdrawn to the level of the ostium, and downward flexion accompanied by clockwise rotation will allow insertion into the left inferior PV (LIPV). If the LIPV was mapped first, the catheter should be withdrawn to the ostium and the downward curve withdrawn. Intracardiac echocardiogram (ICE) visualization is particularly helpful in this regard.

4. Once the left PVs have been mapped, the sheath should be slightly withdrawn to the mid-PW. From this point, clockwise rotation of the sheath will allow for engagement with the right superior PV (RSPV) ostium. The sheath should be left at the level of the ostium and the catheter should be advanced with both clock and counterclockwise rotations, to create a three-dimensional anatomy. To engage the right inferior PV, the sheath should be rotated counterclockwise and flexed downward. Again, once engaged the catheter should advance on its own.

After estimating the LA size (by establishing the location of the left and right PVs), the operator should continue mapping the PW (by applying clockwise rotation to the sheath while modifying the downward curve and withdrawing the sheath), the anterior wall (by applying counterclockwise rotation), the LA floor (by applying downward flexion and rotating the sheath with clock and counterclockwise rotations, to cover the entire area), and the interatrial septum (by advancing the catheter to the left PV ostia and withdrawing the sheath to the interatrial septum, after which a strong flexion of the catheter will allow the catheter to bend on itself). Special attention should be given to the left PV ridge separating the veins from the LAA. To map the LAA, the sheath should be advanced to the LAA ostium, and the catheter should advance on its own. If LAA electrical isolation (LAAEI) is planned, the level of the LAA ostium should be carefully mapped by integrating the

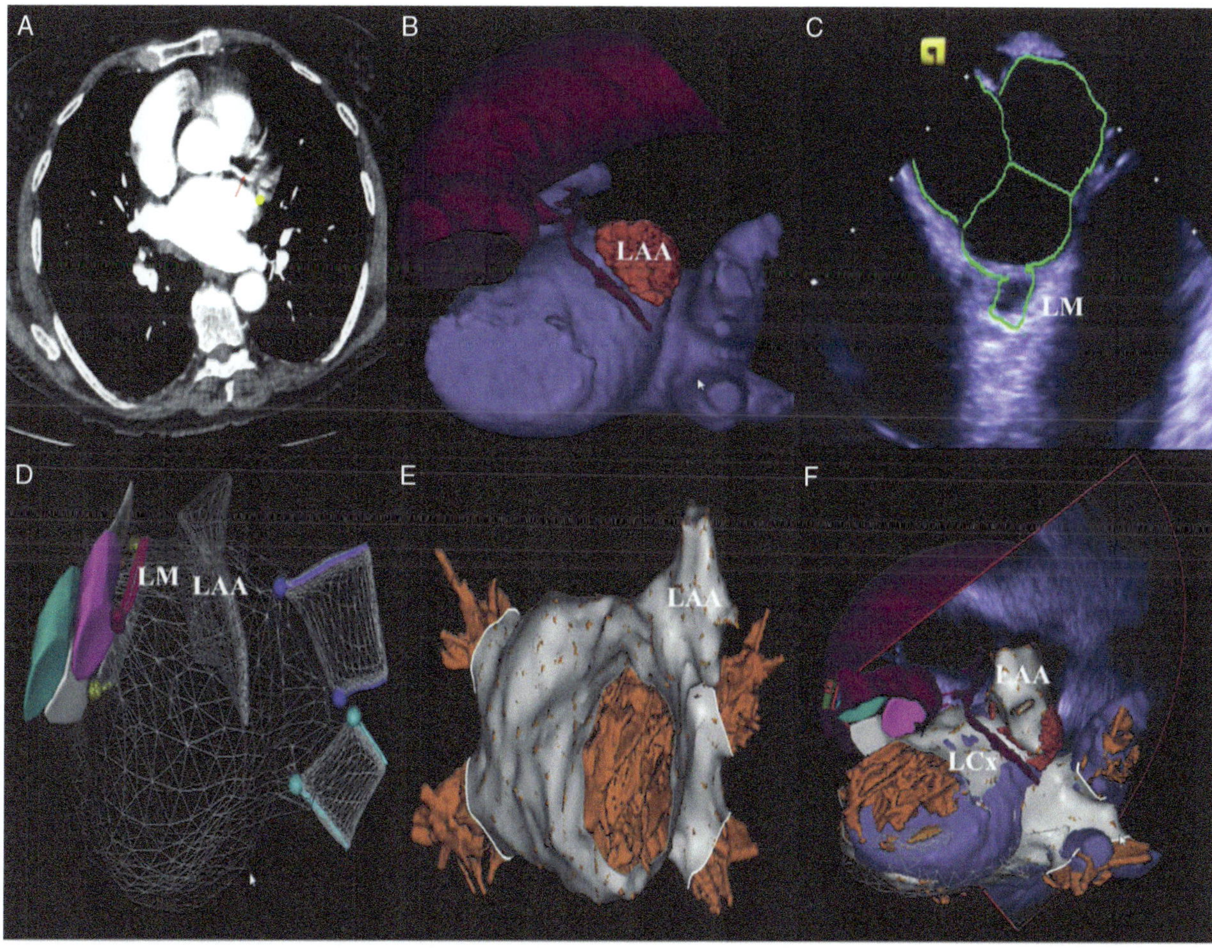

Fig. 22.2 Imaging integration. (A) Preprocedural CT revealing the close anatomical proximity between the anterior aspect of the LAA (*yellow hexagon*) and the LCx coronary artery (*red arrow*). (B) Images exported from the CT scan into the CARTO system for 3D CT reconstruction. Note the relationship between the coronary vessel and the LAA ostium. (C) Short-axis view of aortic coronary cusps and LMCA on ICE. (D) CartoSound anatomic map delineating LA, all four PVs, LAA, sinuses of Valsalva, and LMCA. (E) FAM of the LA and LAA with full volume. (F) Imaging integration of CartoSound reconstruction and FAM with 3D CT reconstruction. *CT*, Computed tomography; *EAM*, electroanatomic mapping; *FAM*, Fast anatomical mapping; *ICE*, intracardiac echocardiogram; *LA*, left atrium; *LAA*, left atrial appendage; *LCx*, left circumflex coronary artery; *LMCA*, left main coronary artery; *LPN*, left phrenic nerve; *PV*, pulmonary veins; *3D*, three-dimensional. (Reproduced with permission from Romero J, Natale A, Di Biase L. How to perform left atrial appendage electrical isolation using radiofrequency ablation. *Heart Rhythm*. 2018;15:1577–1582.)

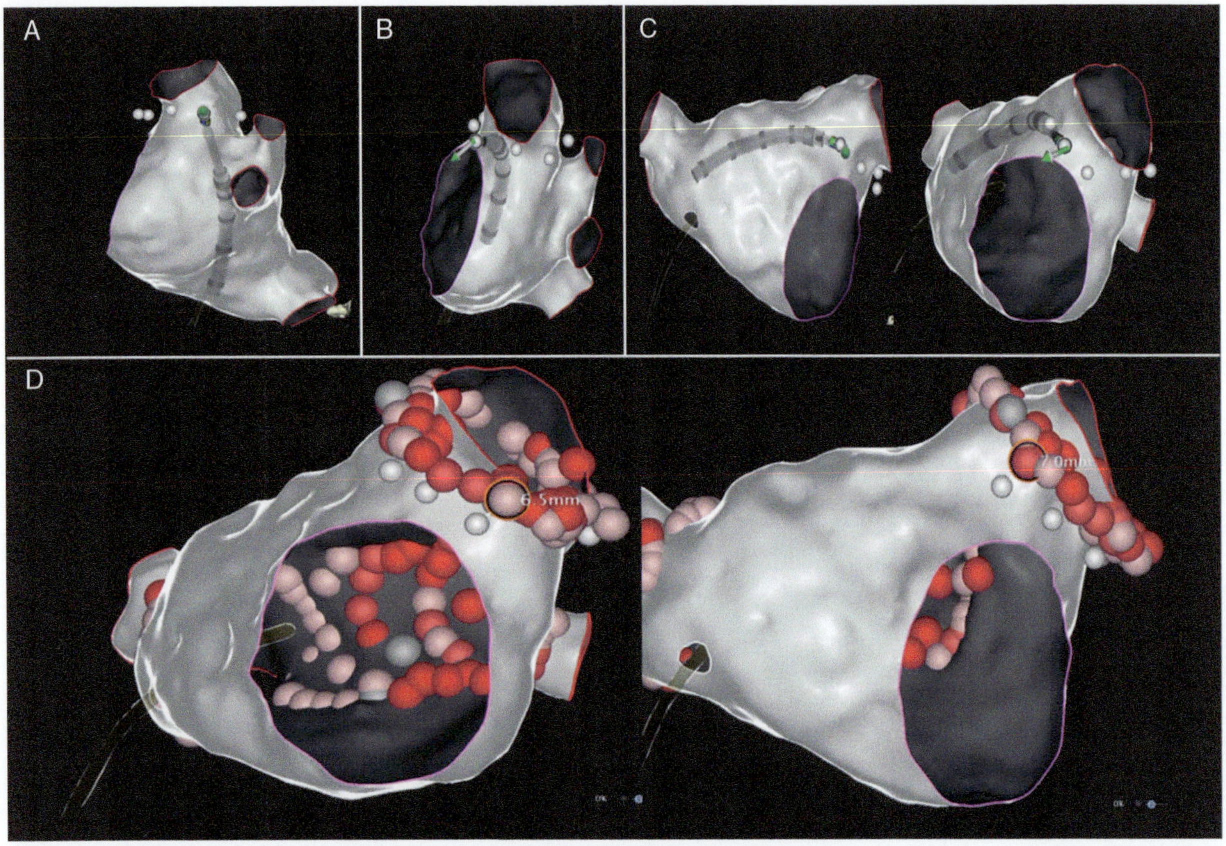

Fig. 22.3 (A) Determining the level of the ostium is fundamental during LAA electrical isolation. The ablation catheter is advanced into the LAA. (B) Pressed against the LAA wall with clock or counterclockwise rotation (depending on whether the posterior or anterior portion of the ostium is mapped, respectively). (C) The catheter is then slowly withdrawn, and the site where the catheter jumps is tagged as the ostial level (*white spheres*). (D) Ablation is done inside the marked LAA ostium (*red spheres*).

information from ICE imaging and electroanatomical mapping (EAM) (Fig. 22.2). By merging these modalities, the anatomy of the LA/LAA is accurately reproduced allowing tracking of the ablation catheter movements.[14]

Typically, the LAA is in proximity to both the left circumflex artery (which runs along the left atrioventricular groove) and the left phrenic nerve (which runs along the posterior wall of the LAA). However, in most cases the left circumflex artery is located at a safe distance from the LAA ostium,[15] and the left phrenic nerve is rarely located at the ostial level (i.e., 4%).[16] Consequently, LAAEI at the ostial level should be safe with a low risk of inadvertent lesions to bystander structures, and ablation within the LAA main body and tip due to minimal wall thickness should be avoided at all costs. To determine the LAA ostial level, the ablation catheter is inserted into this structure and slowly withdrawn while applying clockwise and counterclockwise torque around the ostium. The sites where the catheter "jumps" out of the LAA correspond to the LAA ostium and should be annotated (Fig. 22.3).

ABLATION

Currently, the mainstay strategy for CA of AF is to perform WACA PVI using different energy waveforms including RF, pulsed-field ablation (PFA), and cryoballoon ablation (CBA). However, though PFA and CBA have been used in patients with PeAF, their limitations in targeting areas different from the PVs and PW or performing a focal ablation have made RF the most frequently used energy source to date. To perform RF ablation, the use of contact force (CF) sensing catheters is highly recommended, as it allows for continuous monitoring of adequate tissue contact. In fact, even increasing power will not achieve transmural lesions if a CF of <5 g is used, a constant CF of 10–20 g is encouraged.

Radiofrequency Settings

Currently, there are three types of RF settings used in AF CA:

- Low-power, long-duration (LPLD), in which <35 W of power is used for >20 seconds both the anterior and the posterior walls of the PVs.
- High-power, short-duration (HPSD), in which >40 W of power is used for <20 seconds (generally 10–15 seconds). HPSD relies on rapid resistive heating, creating lesions that are shallower and wider, thus theoretically reducing the risk of damage to adjacent structures and improving lesion overlap. HPSD is associated with a reduction in procedural and ablation time, a higher degree of first-pass isolation, lower

all-atrial arrhythmia recurrence, and a low complication rate.[17]

- Very-high-power, short-duration ablation with the Q-DOT Micro catheter (Biosense Webster), which allows for delivery of up to 90 W for extremely short periods of time (4 seconds). Nonetheless, first-pass isolation without additional touchups is achieved in only 79% of patients.[18]

Improving Catheter Stability: The Importance of Rapid Atrial Pacing and High-Frequency Low-Tidal Volume Ventilation

During ablation, both cardiac (i.e., heartbeat related) and extracardiac (i.e., respiratory related) movements can lead to excessive catheter displacement. As maintaining a constant contact force is crucial to improve acute and long-term clinical outcomes, strategies to reduce catheter movement are of paramount importance during an ablation. Rapid atrial pacing (at a cycle length of 500–600 ms) will increase catheter stability by reducing cardiac movement.

Additionally, catheter stability can be improved by reducing respiratory movement. Jet ventilation (i.e., low tidal volumes with a frequency of 120 cycles per minute) has been used. However, it requires special anesthesia equipment (not readily available) and highly trained operating personnel. Moreover, although the use of jet ventilation does indeed improve catheter stability and arrhythmia-free survival, patients more frequently require vasopressors during the procedure and adjustments to the ventilatory pattern.[19] A simpler approach might be the use of high-frequency low-tidal volume (HFLTV).[20,21] HFLTV involves the use of 200 mL of tidal volume (approximately 2–3 mL/kg) and 30 breaths per minute, as opposed to the standard approach using 6–8 mL/kg and a ventilatory rate of 10–12 breaths per minute. Importantly, HFLTV should only be used during ablation to reduce the risk of hypercarbia. If an end-tidal CO_2 >50 mmHg is present, ablation is stopped, and deep recruitment breaths should be used. When changing ventilatory parameters, respiratory gating should be adjusted accordingly in the 3D mapping system. HFLTV ventilation during catheter ablation of PAF has recently been demonstrated to improve freedom from all-atrial arrhythmia recurrence, AF-related symptoms, and AF-related hospitalizations with shorter procedural times.[22]

Ablation Endpoints

Ablations should be guided by standard lesion quality indexes: if using CARTO 3 ablation index (AI), an AI of 500–550 and 380–400 should be achieved for lesions in the anterior and posterior walls of the LA, respectively.[23] When using the EnSite lesion size index (LSI), an LSI of 5.2 for the anterior and 4 for the posterior portion of the PVs should be achieved.[24] A recent meta-analysis demonstrated significant reductions in procedural times, all-atrial arrhythmia recurrence, acute PV reconnection, and a higher percentage of first-pass isolation when ablation was guided using AI.[25] Additionally, at least 10 Ω of impedance drop for the PW and 15 Ω for the anterior wall should be achieved during ablation, as this is associated with a lower risk of reconnection (Fig. 22.4).[26,27] Finally, the elimination of the negative component of the local unipolar electrogram has also been used as a marker of successful ablation, with RF applications maintained for 2–5 seconds after its disappearance.[28,29]

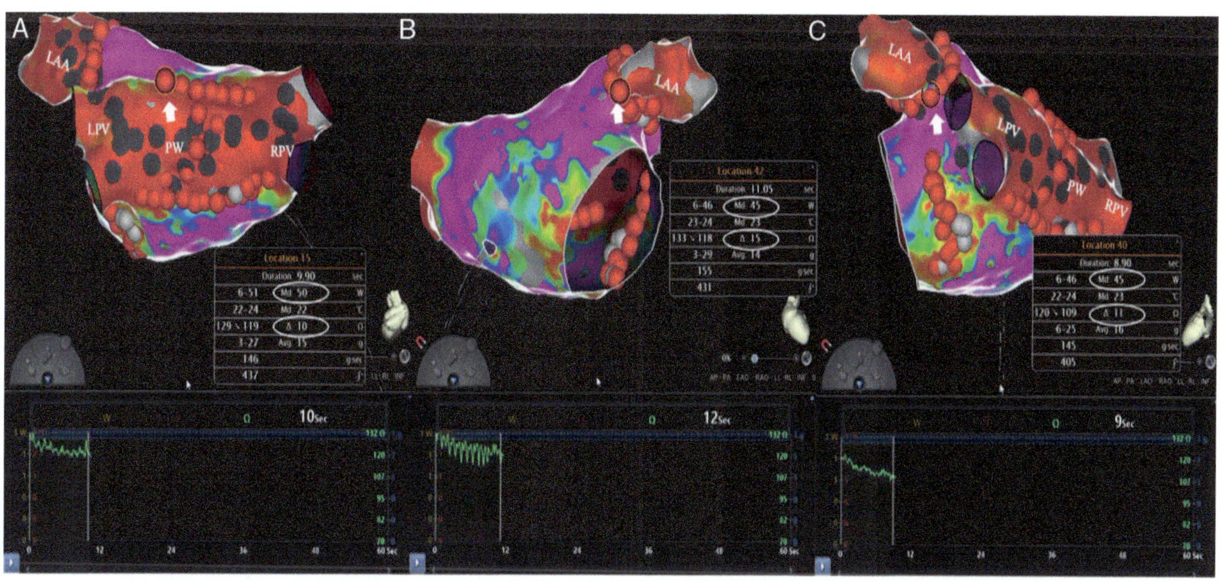

Fig. 22.4 The use of impedance drops can guide ablation, as it reflects transmural lesion formation. (A) For thinner tissues (such as the LA posterior wall) an impedance drop of 10 Ω is associated with transmural lesion formation. (B) For thicker tissues, such as the anterior wall and the anterior LAA ostium, a 15-Ω impedance drop is desirable. (C) As the posterior and inferior portion of the LAA ostium is relatively thin, a 10-Ω impedance drop should be considered.

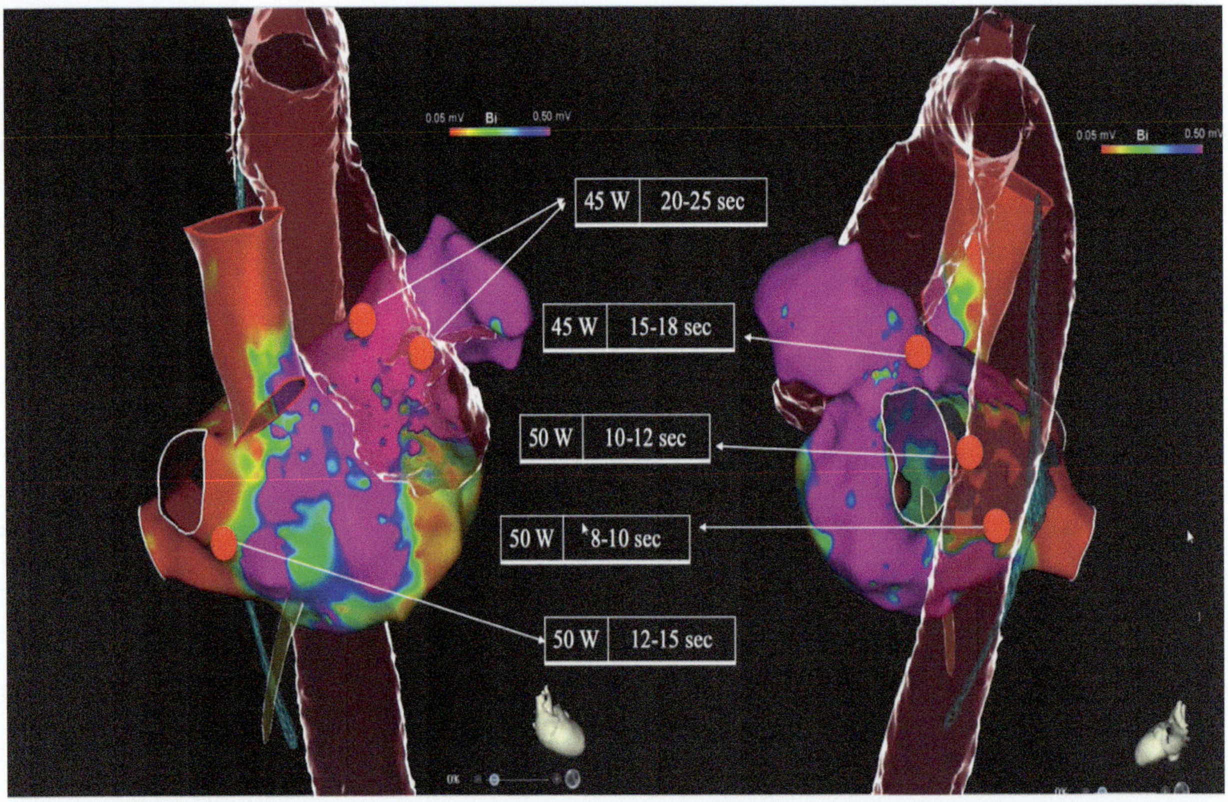

Fig. 22.5 Different high-power settings used. *Left,* During ablation of anterior wall structures, 45 to 50 W can be used. Thicker tissues, such as the anterior portion of the LAA ostium, may require prolonged RF application (up to 25 seconds) to achieve transmurality. *Right,* As tissue thickness is reduced, shorter RF applications should be used. For the PW, 8 to 12 seconds applications can be sufficient to achieve transmurality.

Although HPSD is increasingly being used in EP laboratories worldwide, there are currently no standardized endpoints to guide ablation. Hence, the following multiple endpoints are currently used:

- Lesion index guided (with the same lesion indexes as with LPLD)[30]
- Time guided (with time varying between 5 and 25 seconds per lesion)[17] (Fig. 22.5)
- Unipolar signal guided, in which RF is maintained for 5 seconds after loss of the negative component of the unipolar signal on the RF catheter[29]
- An impedance drop of >10 Ω[31] (Fig. 22.4)

Before definitive randomized clinical trials and standardized ablation endpoints are available, excessive force (>20*g*) and high lesion index values (i.e., lesion indexes which are higher than those recommended for LPLD) should be avoided.

Regardless of the RF settings used, lesions should be contiguous without visual gaps and have a distance of <5.4 mm (from center to center) between each other.[32] If using HPSD, care should be taken to avoid "heat stacking" by not placing closely packed lesions in the PW. In a recent large multicenter study by Costea et al., using data from the prospective REAL-AF registry, the use of 50 W during HPSD AF ablation did not increase freedom from all-atrial arrhythmia or reduce symptoms at 12 months compared to the use of 40 W. However, the 50-W group had a significantly higher rate of first-pass PVI, as well as shorter procedural and total RF times, without increasing procedure-related complications. Given the increased efficacy and improved laboratory efficiency with a similar safety profile compared to 40-W ablation, 50 W could be the preferred choice when performing HPSD PVI.

ANCILLARY TECHNIQUES IN PATIENTS WITH PEAF

Posterior Wall Electrical Isolation

Empirical isolation of the LA PW is frequently performed in patients undergoing ablation for PeAF and LSPAF. From an embryological, anatomical, and electrophysiological standpoint, the PW should be considered an extension of the PVs. A recent meta-analysis by Romero et al. of 10 RCTs comprising 1348 patients demonstrated that after a mean follow-up of 15.7 months, PWI+PVI were not associated with a significant improvement in recurrence of all-atrial arrhythmias when compared to PVI-alone (PVI + PWI: 31.3% [219/698 patients] versus PVI: 35.8% [233/650 patients], RR: 0.84; 95% CI: 0.68–1.05; *P* = .12). Nonetheless, a significant reduction in all-atrial arrhythmias recurrence was observed in patients with nonparoxysmal AF (PVI + PWI: 27.5% [117 of 426 patients] versus PVI: 37.3% [141 of 378 patients]; RR: 0.71; 95% CI: 0.55–0.90; *P* = .006) representing a 29% relative risk reduction and 9.8% absolute risk reduction. Noticeably, only

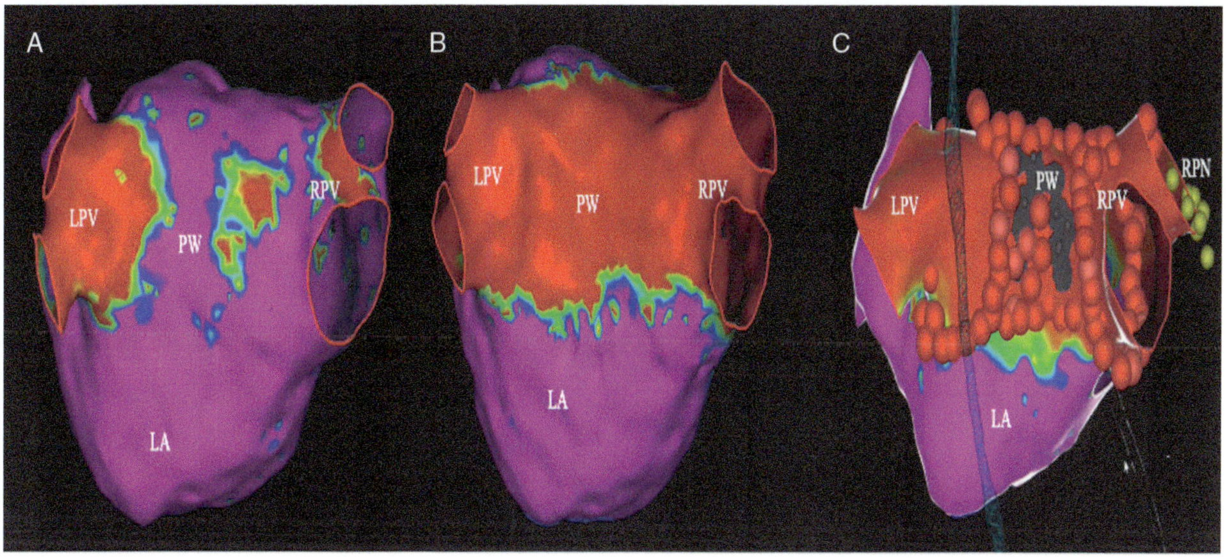

Fig. 22.6 Before (A) and after (B) voltage maps of the PW in a patient undergoing PWI. To achieve this, (C) a superior roof line connecting the superior portion of the left and right PVs, as well as an inferior line, was created. Additionally, EGMs within the PW (probably reflecting the connection sites of the epicardial SPB) are targeted. Both the superior and inferior lines are anchored in the completed WACA of the PVs.

studies using cryoablation have shown significant differences in clinical outcomes.

The main problem when performing PWI is the low rate of durable and complete isolation during follow-up, as different ablation strategies have been used. LA PW isolation can be achieved by linear ablation (*box lesion*). Initially, roof and floor lines are created to connect the superior and inferior PVs, respectively. To minimize the risk of PW reconnection, multiple RF applications are used, especially in thicker areas where RF can be safely used. All potentials identified moving the multielectrode catheter along the PW are sequentially targeted (Fig. 22.6). Using this technique, the reconnection of the whole PW is unlikely and usually limited to areas close to the esophagus where RF energy delivery is limited. The endpoint is to achieve electrical isolation, as documented by the absence of any electrical activity in the PW and demonstrating tissue unexcitability by high-output pacing (20 mA/2 ms).[33,34]

LAA Electrical Isolation

In a series of 987 patients referred for repeat CA, AF triggers originating in the LAA were reported in 27% of patients, either at baseline or after administration of isoproterenol. Moreover, in 8.7% of patients, the LAA was found to be the only source of arrhythmia.[35] LAA firing was assessed only after all the potential sites of reconnection, including the PV antra, the PW, and the septum were checked and targeted if reconnected. Of the patients presenting LAA firing, 43 were not ablated (group 1), 56 received a focal ablation (group 2), and 167 underwent LAAEI guided by a circular mapping catheter and ICE (group 3). After a mean follow-up of 1 year, AF recurred in 74% of group 1 patients, as compared to 68% of group 2 and 15% of group 3 ($P < .001$ for multiple comparisons).[35]

The BELIEF study (Effect of Empirical LAA Isolation on Long-term Procedure Outcome in Patients with Persistent or Long-standing Persistent AF Undergoing Catheter Ablation) was a multicenter randomized clinical trial comparing the outcomes of patients with LSPAF undergoing PVI + trigger ablation (standard approach) against empirical LAAEI + the standard approach. At 12-month follow-up, 25 patients (28%) in the control group and 48 (56%) in the LAAEI group where LAA was isolated were recurrence-free after a single procedure ($P = .001$). During repeat procedures, empirical electrical LAA isolation was performed in all patients. After an average of 1.3 procedures, cumulative success at 24-month follow-up was reported in 49 patients (56%) in the control group and 65 patients (76%) in the LAA isolation group ($P = .003$). Thus, empirical LAAEI improved long-term freedom from atrial arrhythmias without increasing complications.[36]

Several other studies have shown that empirical LAAEI leads to significantly higher freedom from all-atrial arrhythmia recurrence in patients with nonparoxysmal AF, compared to standard ablation alone without an increased risk of acute procedural complications or cerebral thromboembolic events (TEs) as long as oral anticoagulation (OAC) is maintained.[37] At 5-year follow-up, LAAEI was associated with significantly higher freedom from all-atrial arrhythmia recurrence in patients with PeAF and LSPAF (68.9%) when compared to those who underwent standard ablation alone (50.2%; $P < .001$). Acute complication rates were similar between groups (LAAEI 1.3% versus non-LAAEI 0.73%, $P = .36$), with longer procedural times in patients undergoing LAAEI.[38]

Thus LAAEI can be a very safe procedure if the following appropriate technique is used:

- Mapping of the LAA should be performed with the mapping catheter using gentle movements.
- The LAA ostium should be identified as described in previous sections. The LAA ostium lies near to the LMCA and left circumflex (LCx) coronary artery, and although the risk of damaging these vessels when performing LAAEI is minimal, imaging integration with preprocedural CT allows to

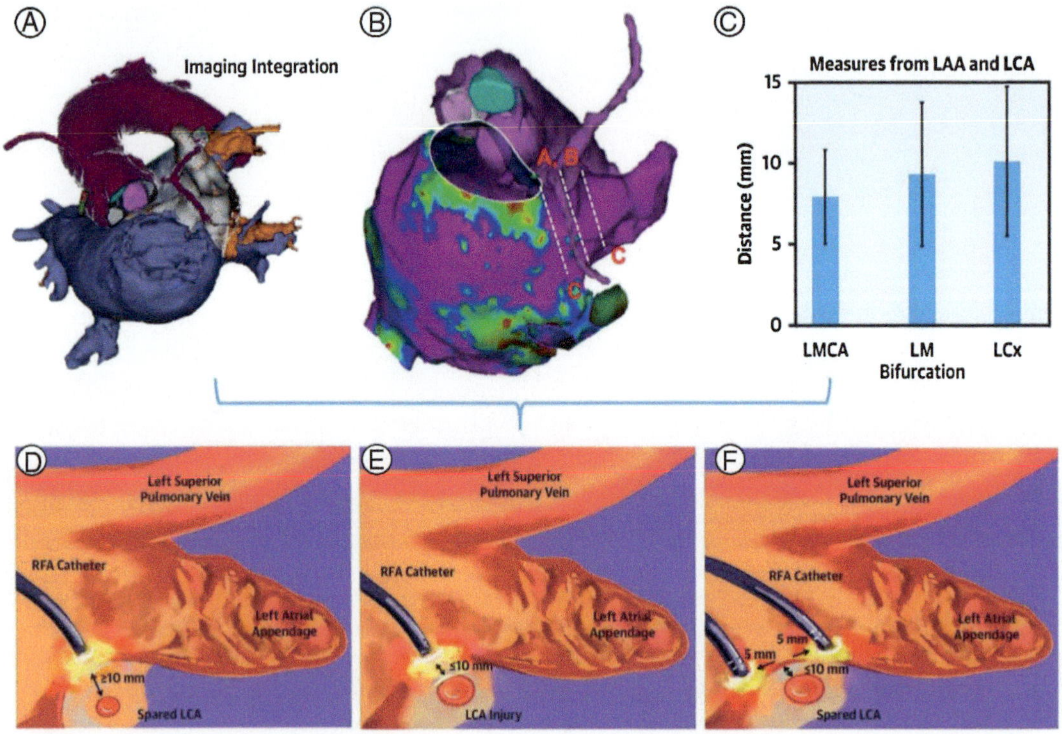

Fig. 22.7 (A) Use of multimodality imaging (CT scan, electroanatomical mapping, and ICE reconstruction) to reduce the risk of coronary artery injury during LAAEI. (B) The distance between the left coronary arteries (i.e., the LMCA, its bifurcation, and the left circumflex artery) and the LAA can be measured. Representations of different locations of the LAA in relation to the left coronary arteries are depicted as *dotted lines* marked A, B, and C. (C) The mean distances from the anterior wall of the LAA ostium to the LMCA, LMCA bifurcation, and LCx were 7.88 ± 2.8 mm, 9.24 ± 4.40 mm, and 10.03 ± 4.56 mm, respectively. (D) When the distance is >10 mm, ablation can be performed without risk of damaging the LCA. (E) A distance of 5 to 10 mm carries a risk of LCA damage during ablation and the ST segment should be continuously monitored. (F) If the coronary artery is located <5 mm away, ablation should not be performed and a different ablation point selected either 5 mm more proximal or moredistal to the LAA ostium. (Reproduced with permission from Romero J, Natale A, Cerna L, et al. Imaging integration to localize and protect the left coronary artery in patients undergoing LAAEI. *JACC Clin Electrophysiol.* 2020;6(2):157–167.).[51]

accurately define the anatomical relationship between the LMCA and LCx and the anterior edge of the LAA ostium. When the distance on cardiac computed tomography between the LAA ostium and left coronary arteries is >10 mm, intraprocedural localization of these vessels may not be necessary (Fig. 22.7).[15] During ablation of the anterior wall of the LAA, monitoring ST-segment for elevation should be performed. Only coronary vasospasm has been reported using cryoballoon ablation for LAAEI.

- LPN mapping with high-output pacing (20 mA/2 ms) should be performed before LAAEI (Fig. 22.8). The LPN is found near the LAA ostium in only 4.5% of patients, and in such cases segmental LAAEI, with posterolateral and anterior mitral isthmus lines, can be performed to avoid LPN injury.[16]
- Cardioversion should be performed before LAAEI to allow for clearer visualization of electrical signals.
- The ablation should be performed at the ostial level, to reduce the risk of inadvertent perforation, left phrenic nerve damage, and coronary artery injury. Importantly, to achieve first-pass LAAEI, the lesions should be delivered slightly beyond the drop-off points inside the LAA where catheter stability and contact force are significantly better. Power should be set to 45 W while maintaining a catheter tip temperature of 42°C for a maximum of 15–18 seconds per ablation site. For the anterior and superior edges of the LAA (which are known to be thicker than the inferior and posterior margins),[39] longer lesions (i.e., 20–25 seconds) are often required, with a target impedance drop of 15 Ω. A medium curve deflectable sheath is used to improve stability and maintain a constant contact force of 15–30g. The ablation catheter should be kept at the level of the LAA ostium and should never be advanced beyond the mapping catheter to avoid inadvertent LAA perforation.[35,40]
- Imaging of the catheter tip with ICE should also be used to monitor catheter stability and real-time lesion formation.
- Several indirect parameters should be used to assess the achievement of transmural lesions, such as >80% electrogram amplitude reduction and catheter tip impedance monitoring, aiming for a 15-Ω drop in the anterior and superior LAA ostial borders and a 10-Ω drop in the posterior and inferior LAA ostium.
- Isolation should be confirmed both by the entrance and exit blocks (Fig. 22.9).

Acute LAA reconnections are frequent (50–70%) and are most commonly found at the anterior and superior margins of the LAA where wall thickness is greater (Fig. 22.10).[39] Therefore, we consider that it is worth assessing for LAA dormant conduction using adenosine or isoproterenol and reassess reconnection after a 30-minute waiting period. High power during LAAEI

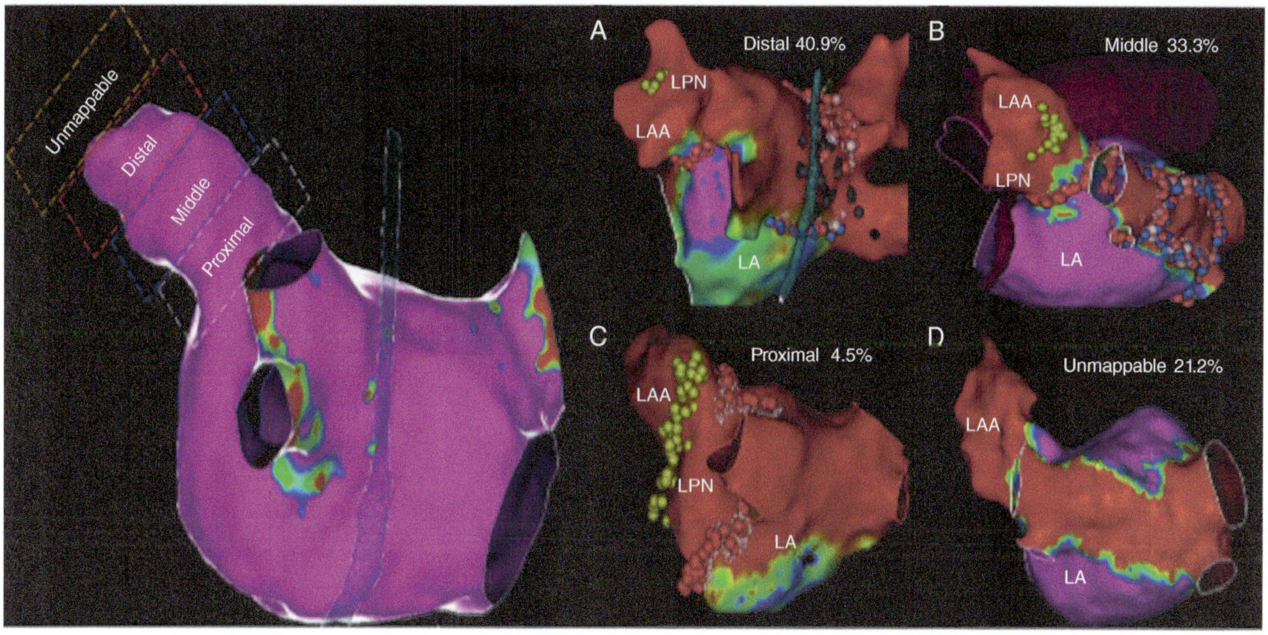

Fig. 22.8 Mapping of the LPN can be used to reduce the risk of inadvertent injury during LAAEI. *Left,* By dividing the LAA into a proximal, middle, and distal third, ablation can be performed. *Right,* In most patients, the LPN is located in the distal (A) or middle (B) third, with only 4.5% of patients having the LPN located in the proximal third (C). In one-fifth of patients, the LPN is unmappable (D).[16]

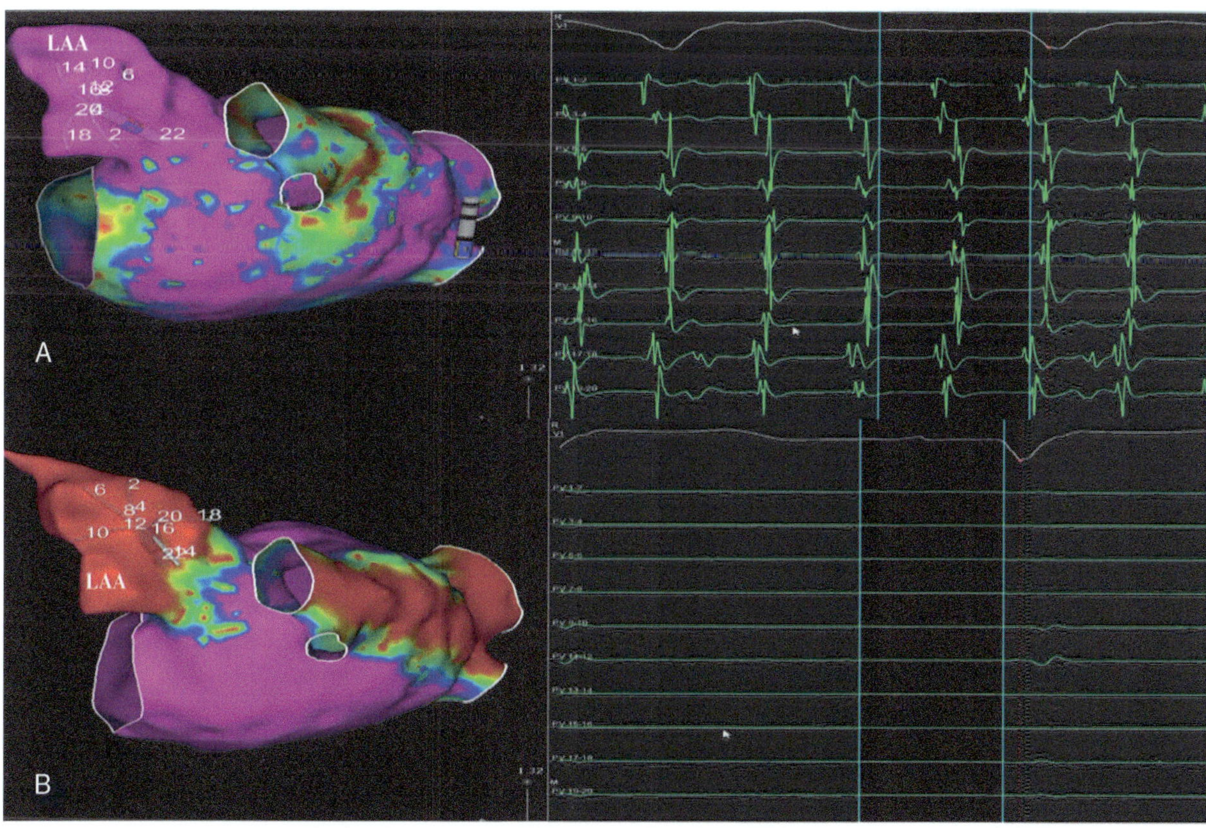

Fig. 22.9 Electrical isolation of the LAA. With the mapping catheter located within the LAA, electrical activity can be continuously recorded during the ablation procedure. (A) Preprocedural voltage maps and EGM within the LAA, demonstrating high-voltage electrograms within the LAA. (B) After LAAEI, ther is no electrical activity recorded by the mapping catheter within the LAA, demonstrating complete LAAEI.

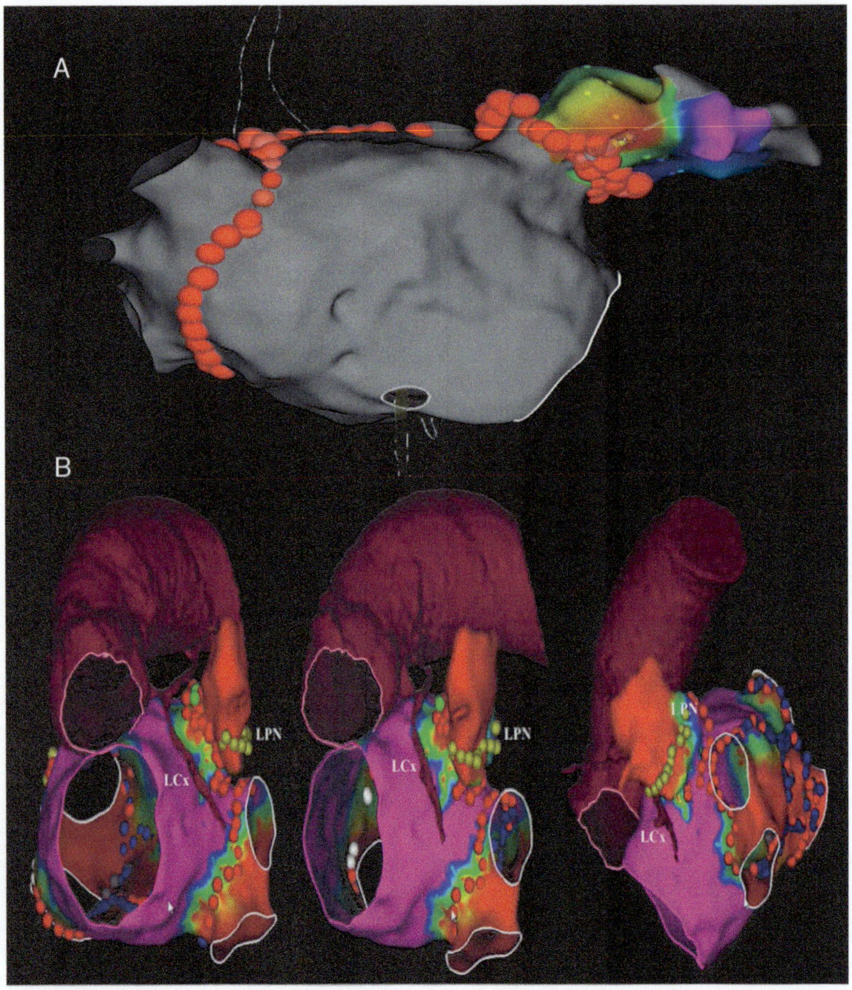

Fig. 22.10 (A) Activation mapping in the LAA to localize conduction gaps. The ablation catheter is being used to map the LAA during sinus rhythm. Most of these acute reconnections are located in the junction of the superior and anterior LAA ostial walls. (B) Final lesions set in a patient with LSPAF. PVI, PWI, and LAAEI were performed after localizing coronary arteries and right and left phrenic nerve.

is useful, as it may overcome the challenges imposed by poor stability and myocardial thickness. The LAA can be acutely and electrically isolated in 93.4 ± 7.2% of cases.[41]

ABLATION OF OTHER STRUCTURES

Vein of Marshall Isolation

The VOM has been identified as an arrhythmic source, as the VOM has muscular sleeves connecting both the CS and the LA. Additionally, the area of the VOM is richly innervated by both adrenergic and parasympathetic nervous systems, facilitating the origin of triggers in this area. However, its location within the ridge between the left PVs and the LAA (an area with significant tissue thickness) as well as its small diameter (which impede direct ablation from within the lumen) make thermal isolation of this structure virtually impossible. The VOM receives blood from the area of the mitral isthmus, which is particularly thick and rich in epicardial muscle fibers. These characteristics make the mitral isthmus and the VOM interesting targets during elimination of reentrant arrhythmias and AF initiated within these structures. Nevertheless, application of RF energy frequently fails to eliminate these epicardial connections.

Recently, techniques aimed at achieving complete elimination of the muscular sleeves within the VOM using ethanol ablation have been found to produce complete abolition of the electrical activity, as well as producing a durable line of block at the mitral isthmus level. In the VENUS trial, VOM ethanol ablation was associated with a lower rate of recurrent atrial arrhythmias at 6 and 12 months.[42] Interestingly, VOM ethanol ablation appears to be associated with a significant improvement in first-pass left PV isolation, as well as a reduction in reconnection of the left PVs.[43] However VOM ethanol ablation is technically demanding and increases fluoroscopy exposure and procedural time.

To perform alcohol VOM ablation, the CS should be cannulated with deflectable sheath. A 6F guiding catheter is then advanced, and a CS venogram in right anterior oblique view should be performed. The VOM is identified as a cranially oriented vein proximal to the valve of Vieussens, posterior to the LAA. Care should be taken to distinguish the VOM from the

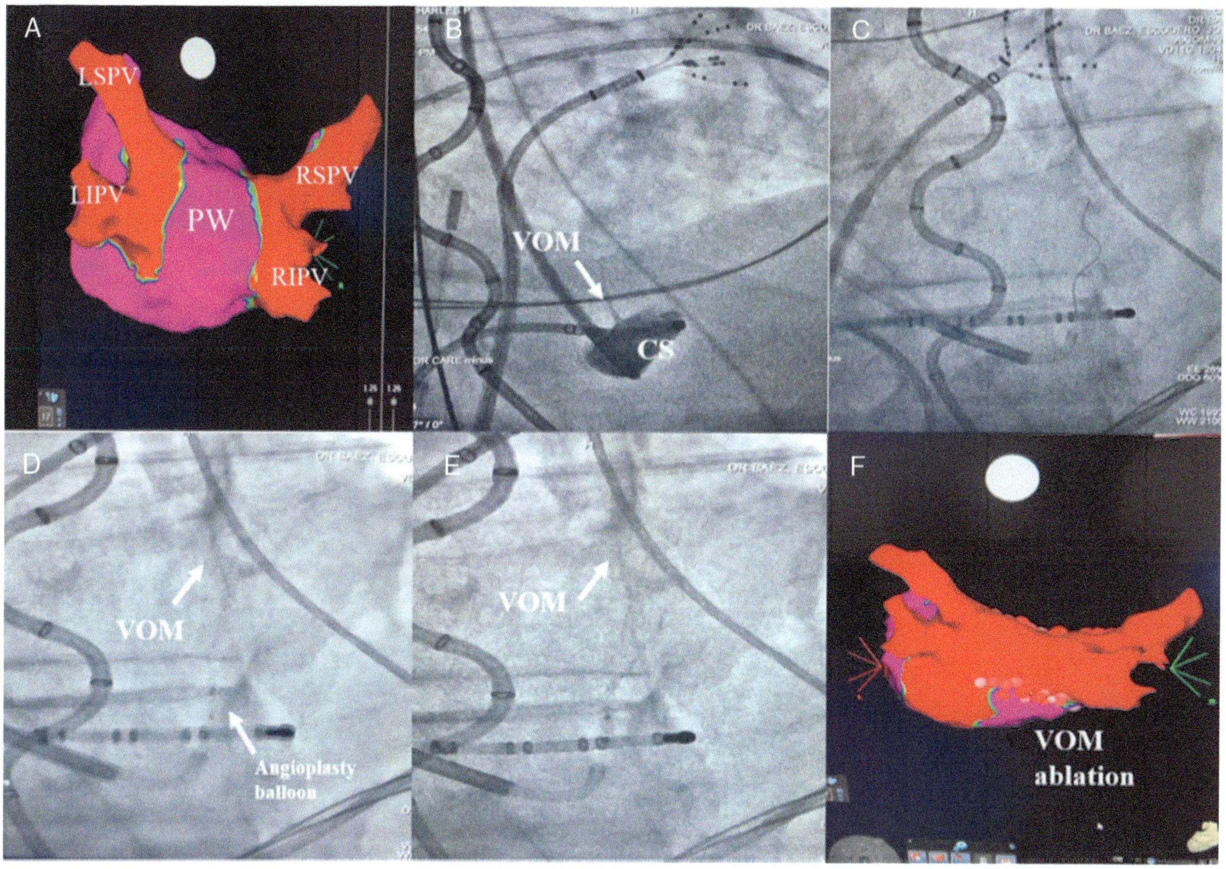

Fig. 22.11 (A) Posterior view of the LA, demonstrating myocardial viability (seen as normal voltage) in the mitral isthmus area. (B) Cannulation and contrast injection at the CS reveals the VOM. (C) Using an angioplasty guidewire, (D) the VOM is selectively cannulated and the vein is occluded with an angioplasty balloon. (E) 1 mL of 95% to 99% ethanol is injected and repeated for a total of two or three applications. (F) Final voltage map, demonstrating complete elimination of myocardial voltage in the mitral isthmus. (Courtesy of Dr. Jose Baez-Escudero.)

TABLE 22.1 Key Points for RF CA of Non-PAF

Mapping	High-density mapping during atrial pacing (at a CL of 600 ms) reduces mapping time while at the same time providing a significant amount of information.
Ablation target	In patients with non-PAF, PVI + PWI should be considered as a standard approach. Use of HFLTV ventilation can result in increased catheter stability, a more stable contact force and reduced procedural times. When using HPSD, avoid excessive force (>20 g) and high lesion indexes particularly in the PW. LAAEI could reduce the risk of arrhythmia recurrence. Procedure related risks are low, and the risk of subsequent TE events can be minimized by proper OAC treatment or LAA occlusion. Select patients can benefit from ablation of the CS or VOM. Low-voltage myocardium-guided ablation may also be needed.
Special equipment	ICE imaging is fundamental for performing fluoroless ablation procedures and provides valuable information during TS puncture as well as identifying anatomic structures during mapping. CARTOSound can be used to tag important anatomical structures, including the CS, PVs, and the esophagus. Deflectable sheaths should be used in all patients to facilitate catheter movement.
Sources of difficulty	Patients with PeAF and LSPAF with recurrence after PVI + PWI have worse clinical outcomes and frequently require mapping and ablation of extrapulmonary triggers.

CA, Catheter ablation; *CS*, coronary sinus; *HFLTV*, high-frequency low-tidal volume; *HPSD*, high-power short-duration; *ICE*, intracardiac echocardiography; *LAA*, left atrial appendage; *LAAEI*, left atrial appendage electrical isolation; *OAC*, oral anticoagulant; *PAF*, paroxysmal atrial fibrillation; *PV*, pulmonary vein; *PVI*, pulmonary vein isolation; *PW*, posterior wall; *PWI*, posterior wall isolation; *RF*, radiofrequency; *TE*, thromboembolic; *TS*, transseptal; *VOM*, vein of Marshall.

LAA vein, which runs *anterior* to the LAA. The VOM should be cannulated using a 0.014" angioplasty guidewire, and a 2-mm coronary balloon inserted into the vein to occlude it. After the guidewire has been removed, 0.5–1 mL of contrast is gently injected into the VOM to avoid dissection due to the high viscosity of the contrast medium and the thin vessel walls; at this point, adequate occlusion of the vein should be assessed (i.e., lack of contrast leakage into collaterals). Once complete occlusion is confirmed, 2–3 mL of 98% ethanol are infused, and repeated. After each injection, progressive staining of the

TABLE 22.2 **Troubleshooting the Difficult Case**

Inadequate or inconsistent contact force	Consider the use of deflectable sheaths. Advance the deflectable sheath until only the two distal electrodes are left outside of the sheath. Consider atrial pacing at a cycle length of 600 ms. Consider the use of HFLTV ventilation.
Avoiding embolic events	Consider uninterrupted/minimally interrupted OAC. Deliver the first UFH dose immediately after femoral access and additional doses after TS access is obtained to maintain an ACT >350 sec.
Unable to achieve PWI	Search for gaps in the ablation line. Consider the possibility of an epicardial connection (i.e., SPB) and ablate the insertion site.
Unable to achieve LAAEI	Consider high power (45 W) for longer duration, particularly in the anterior and superior ostium.

ACT, activated clotting time; *HFLTV,* high-frequency low-tidal volume; *OAC,* oral anticoagulant; *PWI,* posterior wall isolation; *SPB,* septopulmonary bundle; *TS,* transseptal; *UFH,* unfractionated heparin.

atrial tissues on repeat contrast injection is observed. EAM of the LA overlying the area of the VOM will reveal loss of voltage, thus confirming adequate ethanol ablation (Fig. 22.11, Tables 22.1 and 22.2).

Low-Voltage Myocardium-Guided Ablation

The ERASE-AF (Low-Voltage Myocardium-Guided Ablation Trial of Persistent Atrial Fibrillation) randomized clinical trial by Yan Hou et al. concluded that PVI plus individualized ablation of atrial low-voltage myocardium significantly improved outcomes in patients with persistent AF.

Other Triggers (Also See Chapter 18)

Coronary Sinus

The muscular sleeves within the CS can act both as triggers and areas of focalized reentry in patients with non-PAF. Ablation of the distal CS (avoiding the proximal CS, as the His bundle lies near its superior aspect) could reduce the risk of arrhythmic recurrence.[44] Isolation of the CS is usually performed first inside the vessel and then completed from within the left atrium if necessary (Fig. 22.12). We usually begin ablation from the distal CS (lateral LA at about 4 o'clock in the LAO projection), progressing to the septal area anterior to the right inferior PV. The vector of the contact sensing catheter should always be pointing toward the left atrial floor, to reduce the risk of perforation. Continuous monitoring of the PR interval is warranted during ablation along the proximal CS and the low LA septum, since a lesion of leftward extensions of AV nodal tissue may result in PR prolongation and occasionally into AV block. The endpoint is the complete abolition of all CS potentials. Monitoring of the PR interval is crucial in this phase, and RF energy is prompted discontinued in case of PR prolongation. The power setting is 30–35 W lasting up to 10 seconds at this location.

Cavo Tricuspid Isthmus

Empirical cavotricuspid isthmus (CTI) ablation is not associated with a reduction in overall atrial arrhythmia recurrence in patients with AF, with or without a history of typical atrial flutter.[45]

Superior Vena Cava

Although the SVC has been associated with non-PV triggers inducing AF, empiric SVC isolation has not been associated with a reduction in atrial arrhythmia recurrence.[46] Moreover, given the proximity of the SVC to the right phrenic nerve, there is a risk of phrenic nerve paralysis when performing SVC isolation. This has led to a low use of SVC isolation during ablation procedures for PeAF, with only 2.8% of patients receiving this lesion set in a recent study using the NCDR AFib Ablation Registry.[47] Interestingly, patients with paroxysmal AF were more likely to receive SVC isolation than patients with PeAF (5.7% versus 2.8%, $P < .001$). The reported rate of phrenic nerve lesions was very low, with only 0.1% of patients in the PeAF cohort; however, whether this represents the true incidence is yet to be determined, as there is a significant possibility of underreporting. When performing SVC isolation, careful mapping of the trajectory of the right phrenic nerve should be undertaken prior to ablation, using high-output pacing. Ablation should commence from the septal area, as this is farthest away from the phrenic nerve. Although different power settings have been used, the muscular sleeves within the SVC are very thin, and as such little energy is required to produce isolation. Thus, we recommend a power of 35 W using elimination of local potentials as an endpoint. Ablation should initially be avoided in areas where capture of the phrenic nerve is documented.

Rotors and Complex Fractionated Atrial Electrogram

Ablation of CFAE did not result in a reduction in arrhythmia recurrence in the STAR-AF II trial[48] and the EARNEST-PVI trial[49] and thus is currently not recommended. Likewise, ablation of rotors has not demonstrated any role in improving clinical outcomes compared to PVI alone.[50]

FUTURE PERSPECTIVES

Several trials are currently undergoing to evaluate the potential impact of different lesion sets and ablation strategies in patients with PeAF. In the Posterior Wall and/or Left Atrial Appendage Empiric Electrical Isolation for Non-Paroxysmal

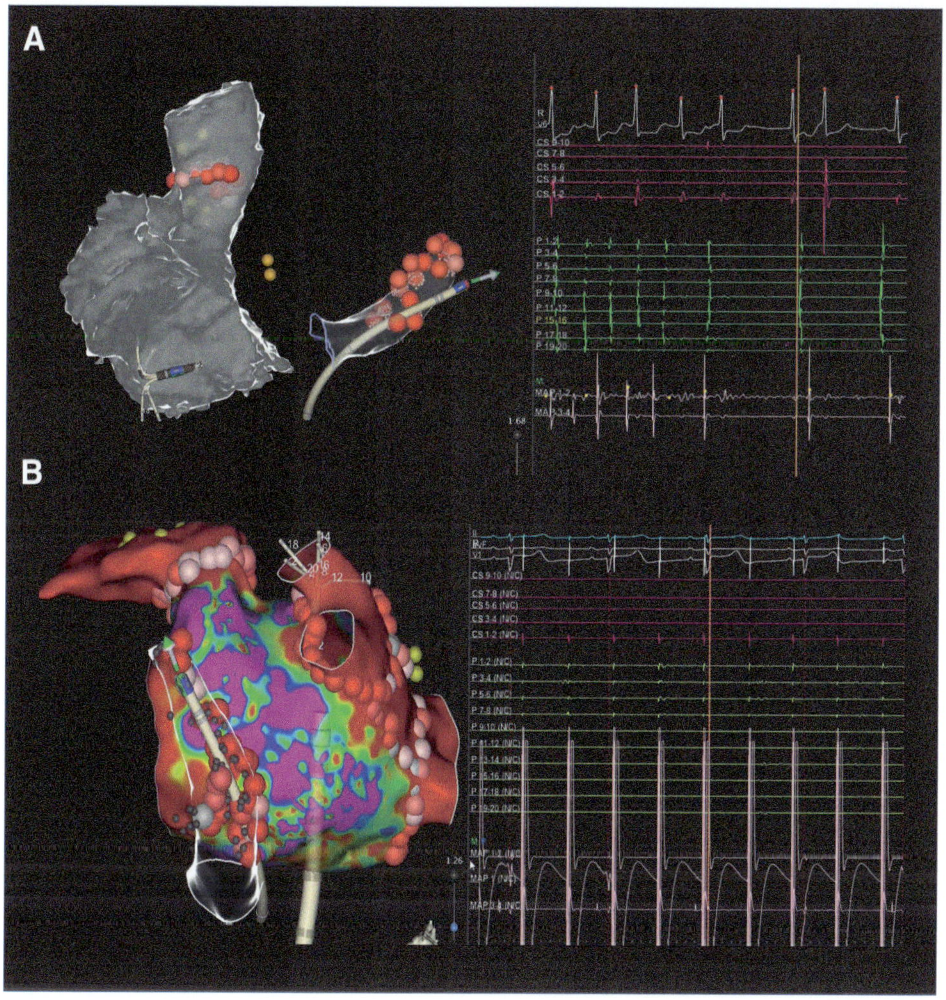

Fig. 22.12 Coronary sinus electrical isolation. (A) After PV and PWI, persistent atrial fibrillation with irregular beats originating from the CS are observed, as hallmarked by early activation of the ablation catheter (*white electrograms*) located within the CS compared to the mapping catheter located within the LA. Ablation from within the CS achieves termination of atrial fibrillation and elimination of the ectopic beats, with significant delay in the CS activation (as observed on the ablation catheter; *white electrograms*) on the next sinus beat (*red arrow*) compared to the mapping catheter located in the LA (*green electrograms*). (B) Additional RF applications from within the CS and from the LA (directly opposite to the CS) are frequently needed to achieve complete CS isolation, as demonstrated by entrance and exit block.

Atrial Fibrillation (The PLEA Trial; NCT04216667), PVI plus PWI, PVI, PWI plus LAAEI plus PVI, PWI, and LAAEI plus CSI will be compared to the standard approach (i.e., PVI alone) in decreasing the incidence of the composite endpoint of all-cause mortality and all-atrial arrhythmia recurrences. The additive value of PWI will also be studied in the STAR AF 3 Trial, which will randomize patients with PeAF into three different groups: PVI, PVI + PWI, and PVI plus CFAE ablation using the CARTO finder software. Both the PIVOTAL and the CRRF-PeAF trial will evaluate the utility of cryoballoon ablation (CBA) in patients with PeAF: in the CRRF-PeAF trial, patients with PeAF will be randomized to PVI using either RF ablation or CBA. In the PIVOTAL trial, the additive value of PWI in patients with PeAF undergoing cryoballoon PVI will be studied. The results of these trials are expected to shed light on the best ablation strategy, as well as the use of alternative energy sources (i.e., cryothermal energy) in the management of patients with PeAF.

CONCLUSION

Patients with non-PAF tend to be sicker, with significant structural and electrophysiologic changes in their atria, which result in lower-than-expected effectiveness of WACA PVI alone as a treatment strategy. Therefore, several adjunctive strategies (including ablation of different structures such as PW, LAA, CS, VOM, and low-voltage areas) could be beneficial for this patient population.

REFERENCES

Please refer to the e-book for a complete list of references.

PART 5

Catheter Ablation of Atrioventricular Nodal Reentry Tachycardia and the Atrioventricular Junction

23

Ablation of Atrioventricular Nodal Reentry Tachycardia and Focal Junctional Tachycardia

Nitish Badhwar, Shana Greif

KEY POINTS

- The mechanism of atrioventricular nodal reentrant tachycardia (AVNRT) is reentry involving fast and slow atrioventricular (AV) nodal pathways.
- The typical slow-fast form of AVNRT is diagnosed by the presence of a long atrium–His bundle (AH) interval (>200 ms) during tachycardia, with the earliest retrograde atrial activation localized at the level of the superior part of the triangle of Koch, just behind the tendon of Todaro (fast pathway or anterior approach to the AV node).
- The atypical fast-slow form of AVNRT has a short AH interval during tachycardia (<200 ms), and early retrograde atrial activation is localized near the coronary sinus ostium (CS os) or in the proximal portion of the CS.
- The atypical slow-slow form of AVNRT has a long AH interval (>200 ms), with early retrograde atrial activation near the CS os or in the proximal portion of the CS similar to the fast-slow form of AVNRT.
- The ablation target for AVNRT is the antegrade or retrograde slow pathway using radiofrequency or cryoablation.
- In the left-sided variant, successful ablation is performed in the inferoseptal mitral annulus (MA), inferolateral MA, or noncoronary aortic sinus of Valsalva.
- Retrograde fast pathway ablation should be considered in typical AVNRT associated with prolonged PR interval (>300 ms) in sinus rhythm and absence of antegrade fast pathway conduction.
- Three-dimensional electroanatomical mapping system is very useful in delineating the His and marking and selecting catheter ablation sites. It improves the safety and efficacy of the procedure.
- The acute success rate is almost 100%, with a 2% (typical) to 5% (atypical) rate of recurrence. The rate of complications (AV block) is ≤0.5%.
- Focal junctional tachycardia and concealed nodoventricular/nodofascicular tachycardia are uncommon causes of paroxysmal supraventricular tachycardia arising from the AV junction region. Diagnostic maneuvers to differentiate them from AVNRT are important as they have a different ablation strategy.

INTRODUCTION

Atrioventricular nodal reentrant tachycardia (AVRNT) is the most common form of paroxysmal supraventricular tachycardia (PSVT). It occurs more frequently in women (65%) than in men, and the initial episode of tachycardia tends to occur at an older age than in patients with atrioventricular (AV) reentrant tachycardia.[1] Patients frequently complain of regular rapid pounding in the neck due to almost simultaneous atrial and ventricular contractions.[2] It can be associated with syncope and rarely cardiac arrest.[3] Sustained AVNRT has been induced during an electrophysiology study performed to investigate the cause of syncope in 2% of the patients. Occasionally, AVNRT can present as incessant tachycardia that can lead to tachycardia-induced cardiomyopathy.[4] AVNRT can trigger atrial fibrillation (tachycardia-induced tachycardia), and inducible AVNRT was noted in 4.3% of the patients presenting for atrial fibrillation ablation. Ablation of AVNRT alone was successful in preventing the recurrence of atrial fibrillation in a small subset of patients.[5]

Most patients with AVNRT present with a narrow-complex tachycardia and no visible P wave or with a P wave at the end of the QRS (pseudo-r′ in V1 or pseudo-S in II, III, aVF) simulating an incomplete right bundle branch block (Fig. 23.1). However, the patient may have a preexisting bundle branch block (Fig. 23.2) or develop a functional bundle branch block due to fast rates that are then maintained by the linking phenomenon. Rate-dependent aberrancy occurs more commonly in the right bundle, though it can also occur in the left bundle. There are electrocardiographic (ECG) features that suggest AVNRT: (a) pseudo s wave in inferior leads and/or pseudo r′ wave in V1; (b) notch in aVL; (c) no retrograde P waves visible during tachycardia; (d) pseudo r′ wave in lead aVR; and (e) notch in lead I.[6] The presence of pseudo-r′ in lead aVR appears to be more accurate than other ECG criteria in one study.[7]

Although most patients have no evidence of structural heart disease, AVNRT can also occur in patients with congenital or acquired heart disease. For example, in patients with an implantable cardiac defibrillator, AVNRT can result in

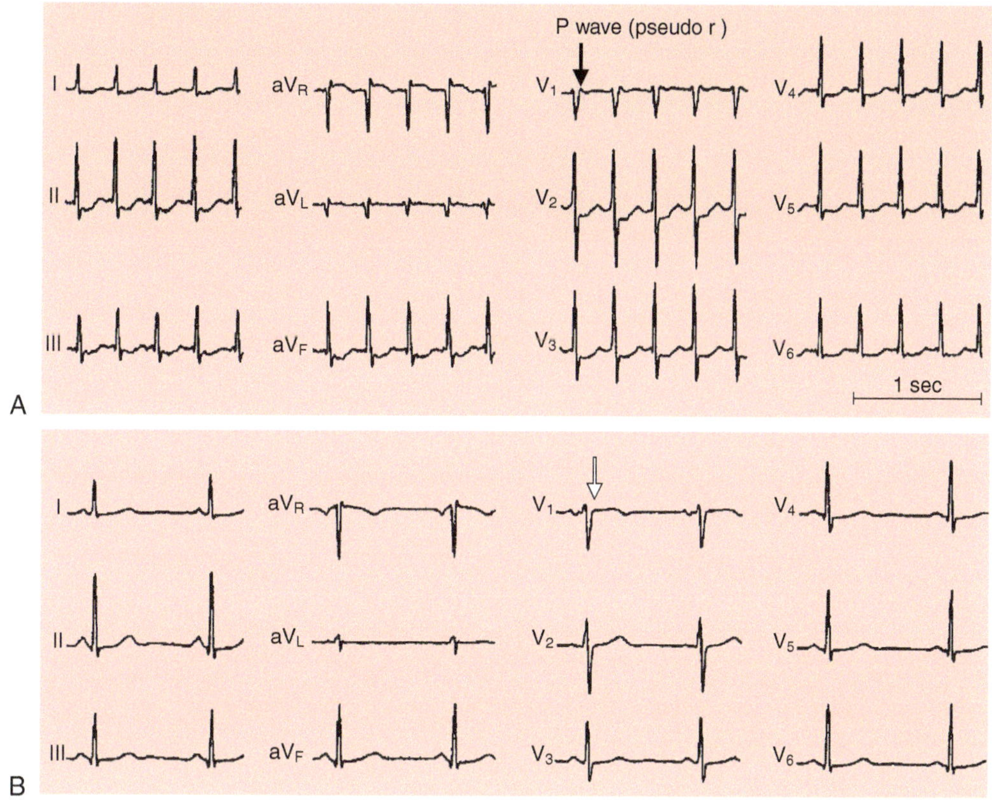

Fig. 23.1 Twelve-lead electrocardiogram of a patient with atrioventricular nodal reentrant tachycardia (AVNRT) during tachycardia and tachycardia termination. (A) AVNRT presenting as narrow complex tachycardia with a pseudo-r′ *(filled arrow)*. (B) On termination of the tachycardia, the r′ is not present *(open arrow)*.

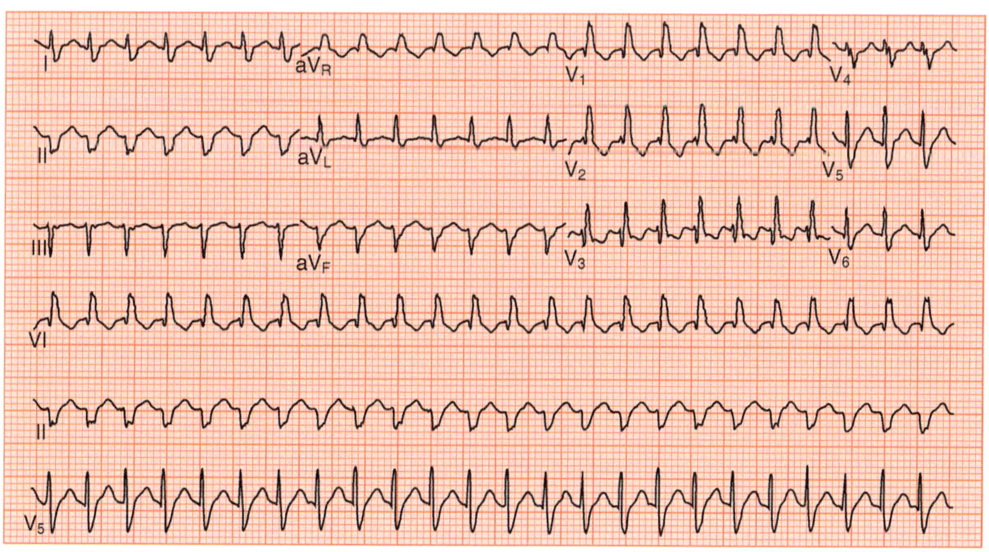

Fig. 23.2 Twelve-lead electrocardiogram of a patient with atrioventricular nodal reentrant tachycardia and preexisting right bundle branch block and left anterior hemiblock.

inappropriate implantable cardioverter-defibrillator therapies (Fig. 23.3).[8] Although a regular tachycardia is the most frequent presentation of AVNRT, some patients develop a regularly irregular tachycardia due to alternating antegrade or retrograde conduction through different slow AV nodal pathways.[9] Even though the rhythm may appear irregular and resemble other arrhythmias, close inspection reveals that the short and long cycle lengths alternate on a consistent basis (Figs. 23.4 and 23.5). Occasionally regularly irregular tachycardia is caused by dual atrioventricular nodal non-reentrant tachycardia (DAVNNT), also termed "double fire."[8] This is characterized by a sinus beat that leads to a consecutive dual anterograde nodal conduction

A

B

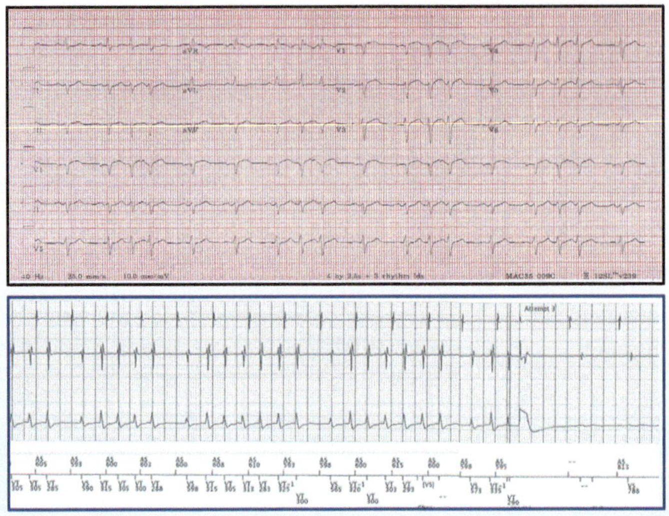

Fig. 23.3 Dual AV nodal nonreentrant tachycardia (DAVNNT) in a patient with ischemic cardiomyopathy resulting in inappropriate implantable cardioverter defibrillator (ICD) shock. (A) 12 lead ECG shows regularly irregular narrow complex tachycardia. Careful analysis of rhythm in lead II shows sinus P waves frequently followed by two ventricular complexes (double fire over fast and slow pathway). (B) ICD interrogation shows atrial electrogram (EGM) on top followed by ventricular EGM and far-field shock ECG on bottom. DAVNNT leads to V>A and fast ventricular rate that falls in the VT zone leading to ICD shock. (From Singh DK, Badhwar N. Implantable cardioverter-defibrillator shock caused by uncommon variety of nonreentrant atrioventricular nodal tachycardia. *Card Electrophysiol Clin.* 2016;8(1):57–60.)

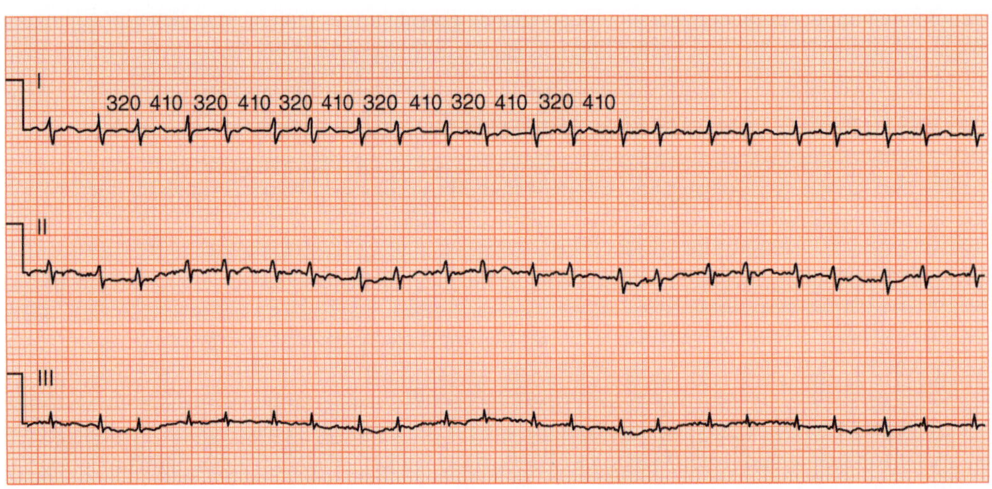

Fig. 23.4 Leads I, II, and III showing a narrow complex tachycardia with alternating cycles lengths of 320 and 410 ms.

via the fast pathway (FP) and slow pathway (SP), which results in two ventricular depolarizations (Fig. 23.3).

Although AVNRT can have a benign course, it can also result in disabling symptoms, especially in elderly patients in whom syncope may be the initial presentation. In addition, patients with AVNRT and coexisting intraventricular conduction disease may develop paroxysmal AV block due to the fast atrial rates (Fig. 23.6).

Catheter ablation eliminates AVNRT in most patients with a low risk of complications. Therefore, it can be offered as a first-line therapy to symptomatic patients and to those who cannot tolerate or do not wish to take antiarrhythmic agents.[1] In addition patients with high-risk occupations may undergo catheter ablation as first-line therapy. This chapter focuses on the electrophysiology, diagnosis, and ablation of AVNRT and FJT.

ANATOMY OF THE ATRIOVENTRICULAR NODE AND ITS INPUTS

The anatomy of the AV node and its relationship with nearby atrial structures and with the His bundle were described by Tawara.[10] The AV node is not a right-sided structure as depicted in most textbooks but is indeed a septal structure located in the AV septum that separated the left ventricle from the right atrium. It is in contact with both the right and the left atria. The

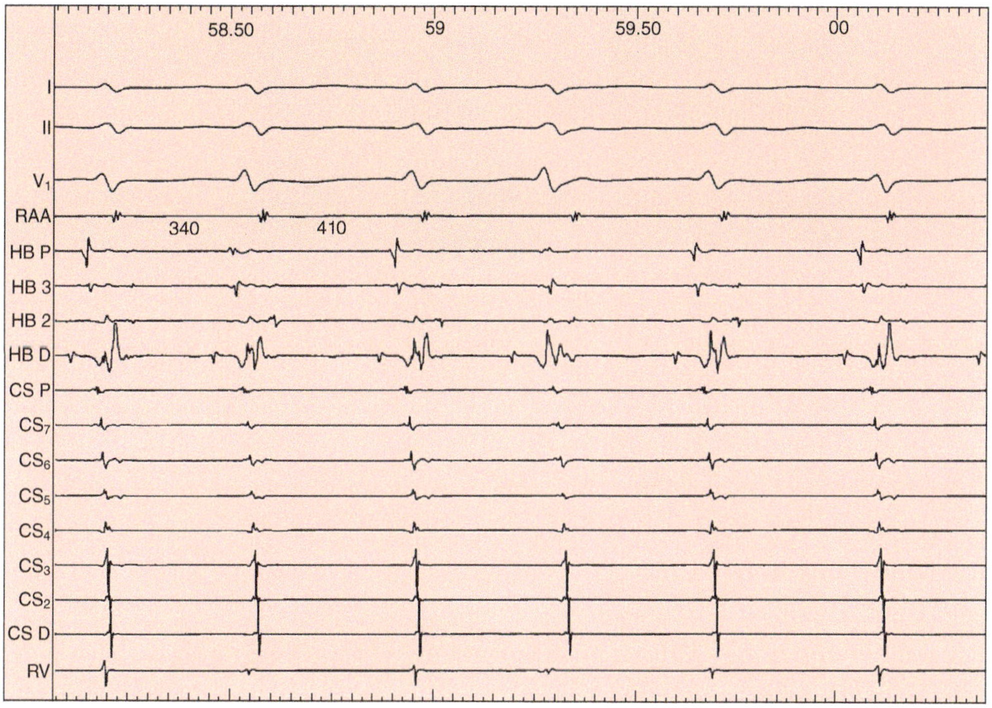

Fig. 23.5 Intracardiac recordings corresponding to the same tachycardia shown in Fig. 21.4. Leads I, II, and V_1 are depicted simultaneously with electrograms from the right atrial appendage (RAA), His bundle (HB), coronary sinus (CS), and right ventricle (RV). During electrophysiology study similar alternating cycle lengths were induced. Please note that the His bundle–atrial interval remains constant but the atrium-His bundle interval oscillates between a faster (190 ms) and a slower (260 ms) conduction over one or more antegrade slow atrioventricular nodal pathways.

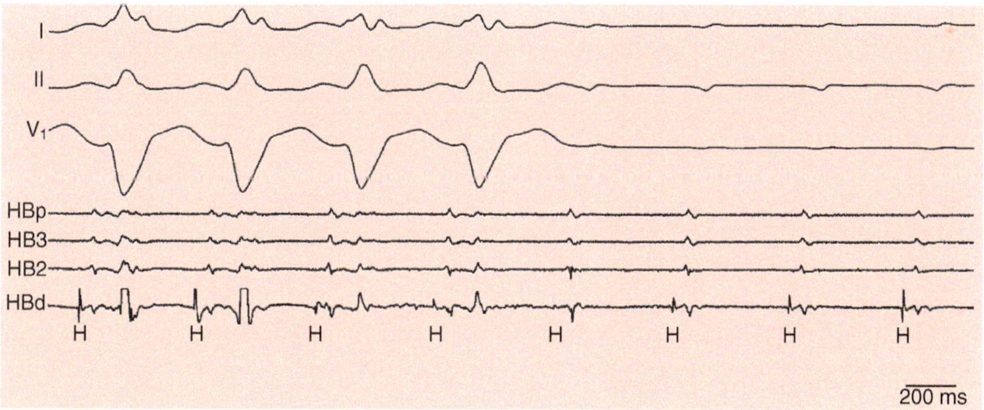

Fig. 23.6 Patient with left bundle branch block and recurrent syncope. Induction of atrioventricular nodal reentrant tachycardia repeatedly resulted in phase 3 or acceleration-dependent paroxysmal atrioventricular block due to block distal to the site where the His bundle (HB) electrogram (H) was recorded.

AV node is not insulated from the surrounding myocardium as it occurs with the His bundle or the right bundle branch.[11,12] Right-sided and left-sided inputs[13] provide activation to the AV node proceeding from both atria. Histologically, the AV node is a discrete structure that can be traced in consecutive sections. It is constituted by specialized myocardium with characteristic immunohistochemistry expressing HCN4, which is the major isoform of the funny channel.[14] The compact AV node is located at the apex of the triangle of Koch. This triangle is bounded by the tendon of Todaro posteriorly, the ostium of the coronary sinus (CS os) inferiorly, and the septal leaflet of the tricuspid valve anteriorly (Fig. 23.7).[15] However, AV nodal tissue extends well beyond the compact AV node. AV nodal conduction is modulated by the sympathetic and parasympathetic nervous system. Therefore, the ability to demonstrate fast and slow AV nodal pathways in the antegrade and retrograde directions varies depending on the autonomic tone. The right coronary artery provides the AV nodal artery in 90% of patients and may run in the subendocardium close to the CS os, which may explain the rare instances of AV nodal block during radiofrequency (RF) ablation in the area of the slow pathway, despite considerable distance from the compact AV node.[16]

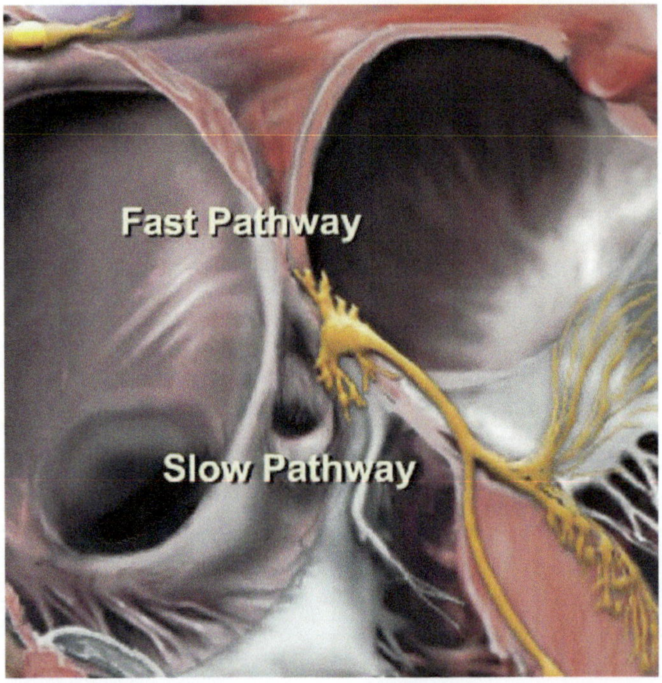

Fig. 23.7 Anatomy of the atrioventricular (AV) junction, including landmarks of the triangle of Koch (bounded by the tendon of Todaro, septal leaflet of the tricuspid valve, and coronary sinus ostium). Usual locations of the fast and slow pathways are labeled. (From Lee KW, Badhwar N, Scheinman MM. Supraventricular tachycardia part I. *Curr Probl Cardiol.* 2008;33:467–546.)

PATHOPHYSIOLOGY

The fundamental studies by Gaskell,[17] His,[18] and Tawara[10] a century ago form the basis for the present understanding of the anatomy and physiology of the AV node. Mines, in 1913,[19] was the first to describe the existence of two regions in the specialized conduction system with different conduction and recovery properties. Moe and associates[20] later demonstrated the existence of two AV nodal pathways underlying AVNRT. The fast AV nodal pathway (β pathway) was found to have a longer refractory period than the slow AV nodal pathway (α pathway). These different electrophysiologic properties facilitate the onset and maintenance of AVNRT. Mendez and Moe[21] found that the two AV nodal pathways located in the upper portion of the AV node in the rabbit communicated with a final lower common pathway. Denes and associates[22] were the first to document the presence of dual AV nodal pathways in patients with and without AVNRT. The initial reported prevalence (10%) of dual AV nodal pathways[23,24] is low compared with present-day findings, probably because electrophysiology studies were initially performed without sedation and therefore under a predominant adrenergic tone. Now under sedation, dual AV nodal pathways are found in most patients, even in those without AVNRT.[24,25] Dual AV nodal pathways can be uncovered using a single atrial extrastimulus of increasing prematurity (AH jump) (Fig. 23.8) or during decremental atrial stimulation (crossover). Nevertheless, the lack of a jump does not rule out the existence of two distinct AV nodal pathways. In this regard, a continuous AV nodal conduction curve is observed in a subgroup of individuals with inducible AVNRT.[26]

Dual AV nodal physiology is a normal behavior of the human AV node. As mentioned previously, the presence of dual AV nodal physiology in itself does not imply the presence of AVNRT. A common misconception is to look for dual AV nodal physiology when AVNRT is suspected and to search for another arrhythmia when a jump is not observed. This simplistic approach can prevent identification of the correct mechanism of the arrhythmia. Consistent with these observations, similar incidences of dual AV nodal physiology in patients with and without AVNRT were found. A jump of 50 ms or longer (with 10-ms decrease in atrial extrastimulus) was present in 83% (417 of 500) of patients *with* AVNRT and in 77% (385 of 500) of patients *without* AVNRT (studied for other reasons); this difference was not statistically significant. The magnitude of the jump, however, was greater in patients with AVNRT (93 ± 7 vs. 61 ± 7 ms, $P < .05$).

If dual AV nodal pathways are present in most individuals with or without AVNRT, what is required to induce AVNRT? One explanation may be the fact that the slow AV nodal pathways are *slower* in patients with AVNRT, as reflected by a greater jump in those with clinical arrhythmia. This may represent an increase of collagen with age, which is supported by experimental studies that facilitate the induction of AVNRT by creating lesions that prevent antegrade activation by the superior approach to the AV node in dogs.[27] A longer conduction time over the antegrade slow pathway allows recovery of excitability of the retrograde limb (fast or slow AV nodal pathway). Anatomic differences may be important because a larger CS os is observed in most patients with AVNRT (Fig. 23.9) and may

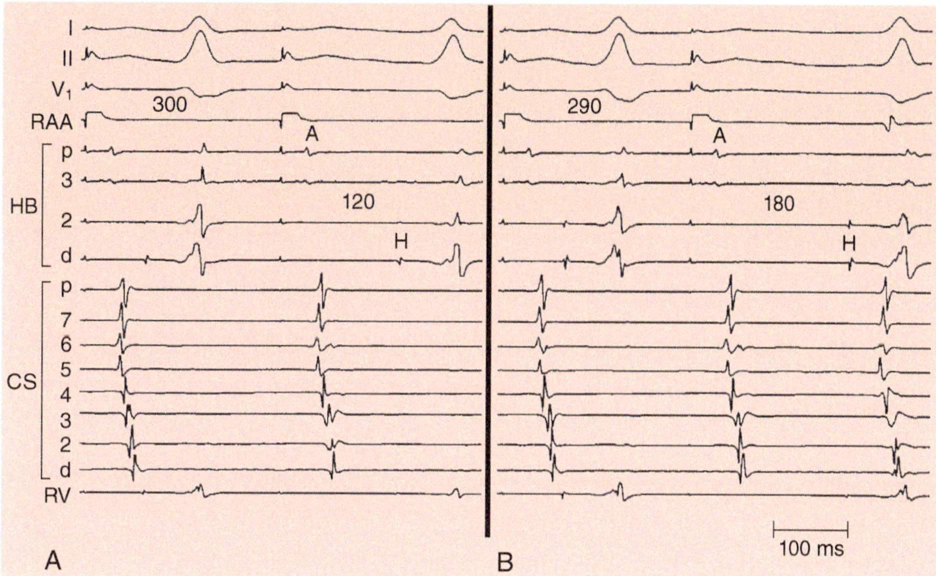

Fig. 23.8 Demonstration of dual atrioventricular (AV) nodal pathways. Single extrastimuli of progressively shorter coupling intervals were delivered from the right atrial appendage (RAA) at a basic drive of 600 ms. A *jump* or sudden increase of the atrium-His bundle interval from 120 ms (A) to 180 ms (B) occurs after shortening of the atrial extrastimulus from 300–290 ms. The atrial extrastimulus in (B) conducts through the slow AV nodal pathway, followed by retrograde conduction through the fast AV nodal pathway to activate the atrium (echo beat). *A,* Atrial electrogram; *CS,* coronary sinus; *d,* distal; *H,* His recording; *HB,* His bundle; *p,* proximal; *RV,* right ventricle.

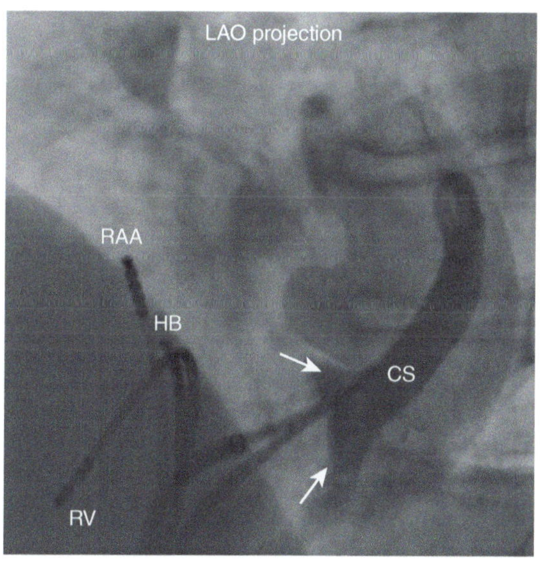

Fig. 23.9 Coronary sinus (CS) angiogram in a patient with slow-fast atrioventricular nodal reentrant tachycardia (AVNRT). Radiograph in the left anterior oblique (LAO) projection of the mapping catheters and angiogram of the CS performed with a pigtail catheter introduced through a preshaped long sheath. *Arrows* show the borders of the CS ostium. A larger CS ostium has been suggested as the anatomic substrate for greater conduction time in the slow pathway of patients with AVNRT. Multipolar catheters are positioned in the CS, right atrial appendage (RAA), His bundle (HB), and right ventricle (RV).

allow for greater conduction time over the slow pathway.[28,29] In fact, the proximal CS is significantly larger in patients with AVNRT than those with AVRT (14.1 ± 5 vs. 9.9 ± 2 mm, *P*< .0001). A cut off of proximal CS greater than 11.2 mm identifies AVNRT with a sensitivity of 92.6% and specificity of 76.9%.[30]

The frequency of premature atrial or ventricular beats and the length of the excitable gap also modulate the frequency and duration of AVNRT. Finally, the coexistence of AVNRT with other arrhythmias, as well as occurrence of familial forms of AVNRT, suggests the possibility of an underlying abnormality.[31–33]

Before the advent of surgical and catheter ablation, the slow and fast AV nodal pathways were believed to be part of the AV node, representing regions with different electrophysiologic properties (i.e., longitudinal dissociation). In fact, several experimental and clinical observations supported an intranodal location of these AV nodal pathways and the reentrant circuit supporting AVNRT.[34–37] In some patients with AVNRT, atrial activation close to the AV node can be dissociated from the reentrant circuit without interruption of the tachycardia (Fig. 23.10).[37,38] This observation suggests that reentry confined to the AV node can sustain AVNRT without atrial involvement. Different degrees of ventriculoatrial (VA) block during AVNRT occur in the upper common pathway, allowing continuation of the tachycardia without retrograde atrial activation.[39] In a similar fashion, the His-Purkinje system and the ventricles are not part of the reentrant circuit. This is demonstrated by episodes of 2:1 AV block with persistence of AVNRT (Fig. 23.11). Block can occur either proximal or distal to His bundle activation. This block is functional and occurs in tachycardias with short cycle lengths, which find the His-Purkinje system refractory. As mentioned before, the presence of concurrent intraventricular conduction abnormalities may even result in paroxysmal AV block during AVNRT (see Fig. 23.6).

Earliest atrial activation during retrograde AV nodal conduction can occur in the upper or lower portion of the triangle of Koch, depending on whether the fast or the slow AV nodal

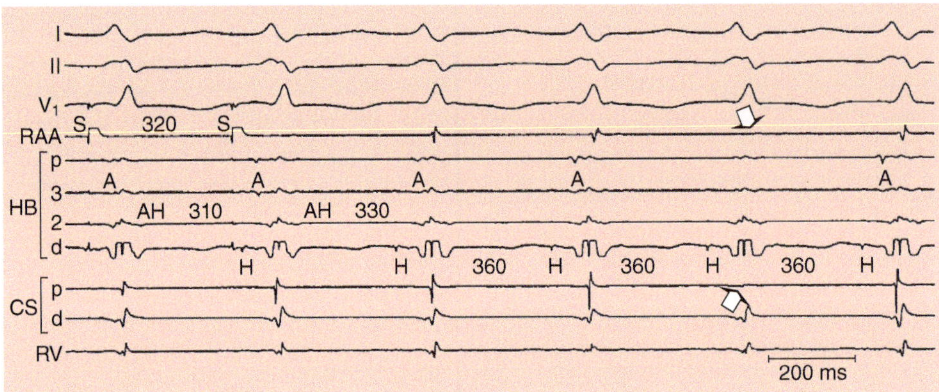

Fig. 23.10 Induction of sustained slow-fast atrioventricular nodal reentrant tachycardia (AVNRT). Rapid atrial pacing at a cycle length of 320 ms results in sustained AVNRT following a critical prolongation of the atrium–His bundle interval (330 ms). The cycle length of the tachycardia was 360 ms. The third tachycardia complex fails to conduct to the atrium *(arrows)* without perturbation of the tachycardia. *A,* Atrial electrogram; *CS,* coronary sinus; *d,* distal; *H,* His recording; *HB,* His bundle; *p,* proximal; *RAA,* right atrial appendage; *RV,* right ventricle. (From Gonzalez MD, Contreras L, Cardona F, et al. V-A block during atrioventricular nodal reentrant tachycardia: reentry confined to the AV node. *Pacing Clin Electrophysiol.* 2003; 26:775–778.)

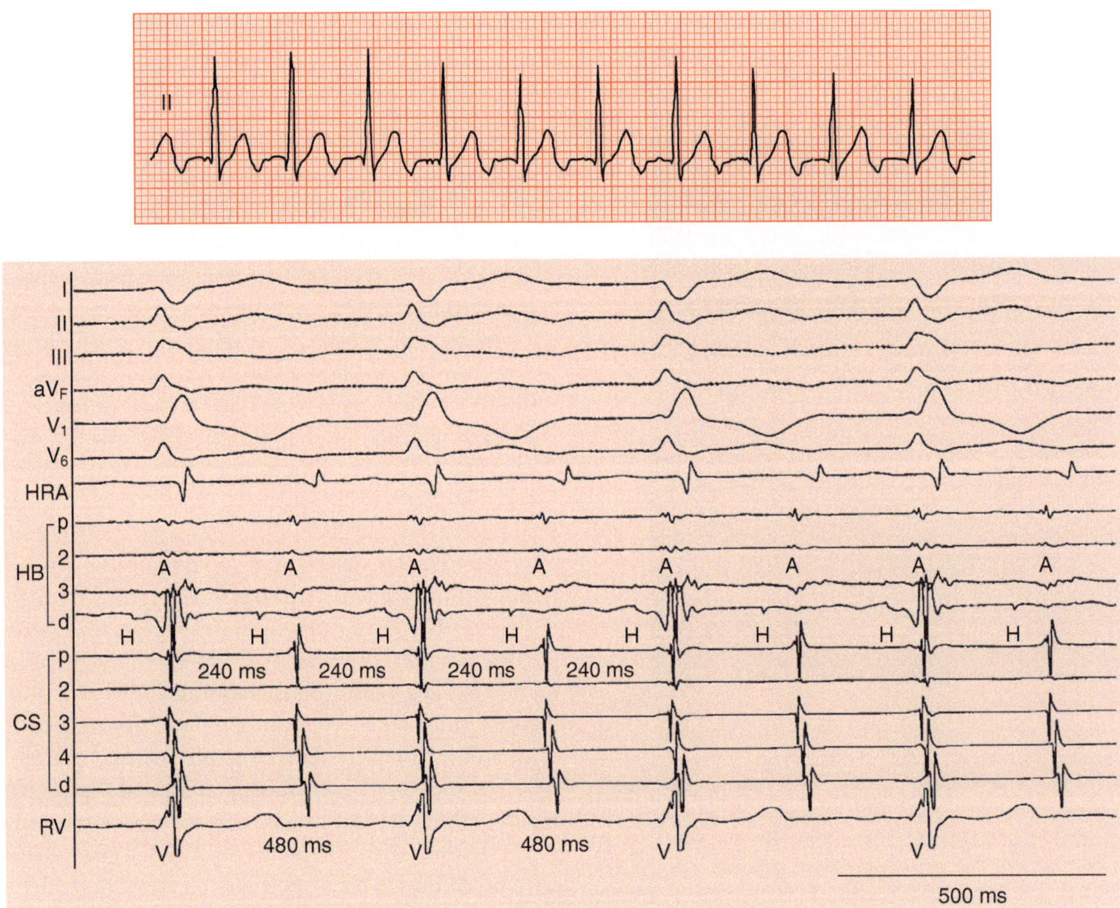

Fig. 23.11 Slow-fast atrioventricular nodal reentrant tachycardia (AVNRT) with 2:1 conduction to the ventricles. At the *top,* a rhythm strip with the characteristic electrocardiographic manifestation of AVNRT with 2:1 atrial-to-ventricular conduction is shown. Negative P waves in inferior leads during tachycardia are the nonconducted atrial depolarizations. These P waves are located equidistant between QRS complexes. The ventricular cycle length in tachycardia doubles the atrial cycle length. Functional block during AVNRT (cycle length, 240 ms) occurs distal to His bundle activation (H) as shown in the *lower panel.* Because ventricular activation occurs almost simultaneously with retrograde atrial activation, the only visible P waves are the nonconducted ones. *A,* Atrial electrogram; *CS,* coronary sinus; *d,* distal; *H,* His recording; *HB,* His bundle; *HRA,* high right atrium; *p,* proximal; *RV,* right ventricle.

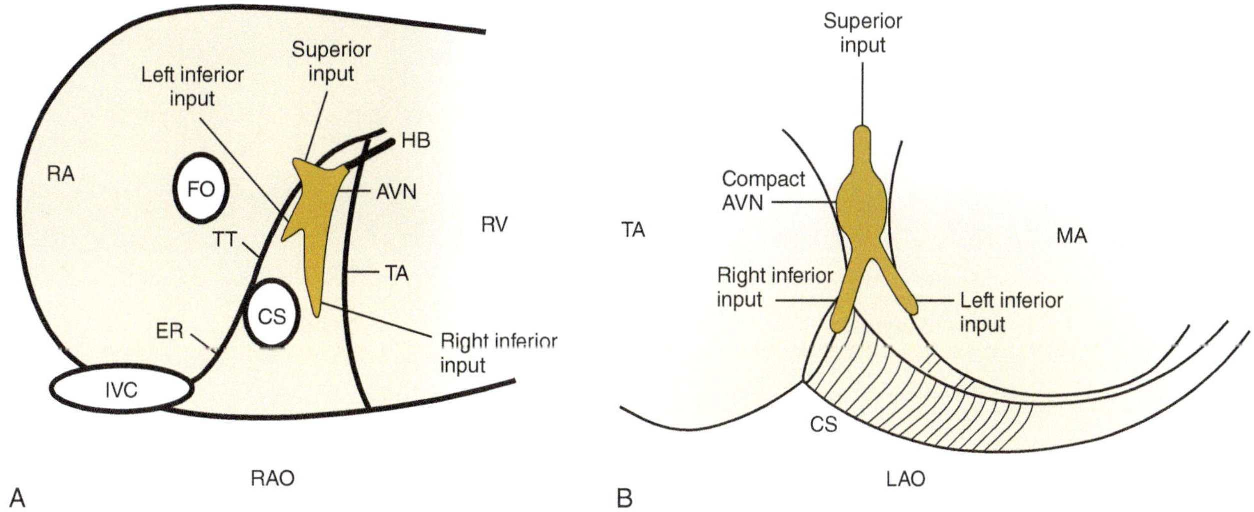

Fig. 23.12 (A) Schematic representation of atrioventricular node (AVN) inside the triangle of Koch as viewed from the right anterior oblique (RAO) projection. The boundaries of the triangle of Koch are defined by the tendon of Todaro (TT), the tricuspid annulus (TA), and the ostium of the coronary sinus (CS). The superior, left inferior, and right inferior inputs are shown. (B) Schematic representation of AVN as viewed from the left anterior oblique (LAO) projection. The AVN is shown above the CS along with the mitral annulus (MA) and the TA. The superior extension (*anterior* in the old anatomic nomenclature) is in contact with both atria. The right inferior input is in contact with the CS. The left inferior input is in contact with the MA. *ER,* Eustachian ridge; *FO,* fossa ovalis; *HB,* His bundle; *IVC,* inferior vena cava; *RA,* right atrium; *RV,* right ventricle. (Modified from Gonzalez MD, Contreras LJ, Cardona F, et al. Demonstration of a left atrial input to the atrioventricular node in humans. *Circulation.* 2002;106:2930–2934.)

pathway is activated.[40] These observations and the results of surgical and catheter ablation of the anterior (superior) or posterior (inferior) approaches to the AV node[41–46] led to the conclusions that the fast and slow AV nodal pathways have an extranodal component and that the perinodal atrium is required to sustain AVNRT.

The original description of the AV node, made by Tawara in 1906,[10] included posterior extensions of the AV node reaching both the mitral and tricuspid annuli. These observations were later confirmed by Becker, Inoue, and Anderson[47,48] (Fig. 23.12). The presence of a left atrial input to the AV node proceeding from the mitral annulus has been demonstrated during electrophysiology study.[13] Therefore in addition to the right-sided superior (anterior) and inferior (posterior) inputs to the AV node, the mitral annulus provides an independent input for activation proceeding from the left atrium[13] (Fig. 23.12). These inputs probably participate in the various forms of AVNRT by providing entrance and exit sites in a reentry that involves the atrium,[49] or they may represent exit points from an intranodal circuit sustaining AVNRT.[37] VA conduction over the slow pathway has been shown to result in earliest atrial activation on the left side of the interatrial septum, which is abolished with ablation of the slow pathway in the right atrium.[50] Consistent with the clinical observation of intranodal reentry,[37,38,51,52] different forms of AVNRT can be contained within the transitional cells of the posterior AV nodal input in a rabbit heart,[53] owing to functional dissociation of cellular activation.[54] Fig. 23.13 depicts possible reentrant circuits that are either contained in the compact AV node or involve the right- and left-sided inputs.

DIAGNOSIS

AVNRT is divided into typical (slow-fast) and atypical (slow-slow, and fast-slow). In a single patient, both these forms may be present at different times during the electrophysiology study. There is no electrophysiologic finding that alone is diagnostic of AVNRT; the diagnosis is made on the weight of typical features and the exclusion of atrial tachycardia, focal junctional tachycardia (FJT), concealed NVT/NFT, and septal accessory pathway mediated tachycardia.

An initial careful baseline electrophysiologic (EP) study is required before any ablation procedure. The presence of a concealed accessory AV pathway should be ruled out before induction of the tachycardia by performing para-Hisian and differential ventricular pacing.[55,56]

Atrial pacing will demonstrate dual AV nodal physiology (Box 23.1) in approximately 85% of patients with AVNRT.[22,23,25,26,40] Conversely, the absence of verifiable dual AV nodal physiology does not rule out AVNRT.

Prolongation of the AH interval to more than 200 ms during decremental atrial pacing is usually indicative of conduction over the slow pathway.[22,57,58] This frequently manifests as a paced PR interval greater than the PP interval such that the paced atrial depolarization conducts, not to the next QRS, but to the second QRS following the pacing stimulus (Fig. 23.14) and is referred to as crossover. During atrial extrastimulus testing, dual AV nodal physiology is typically manifested by a jump of 50 ms or longer in the A2H2 interval following a shortening in the A1A2 interval by 10 ms (see Fig. 23.8). When two atrial extrastimuli are delivered, a jump from fast to slow-pathway

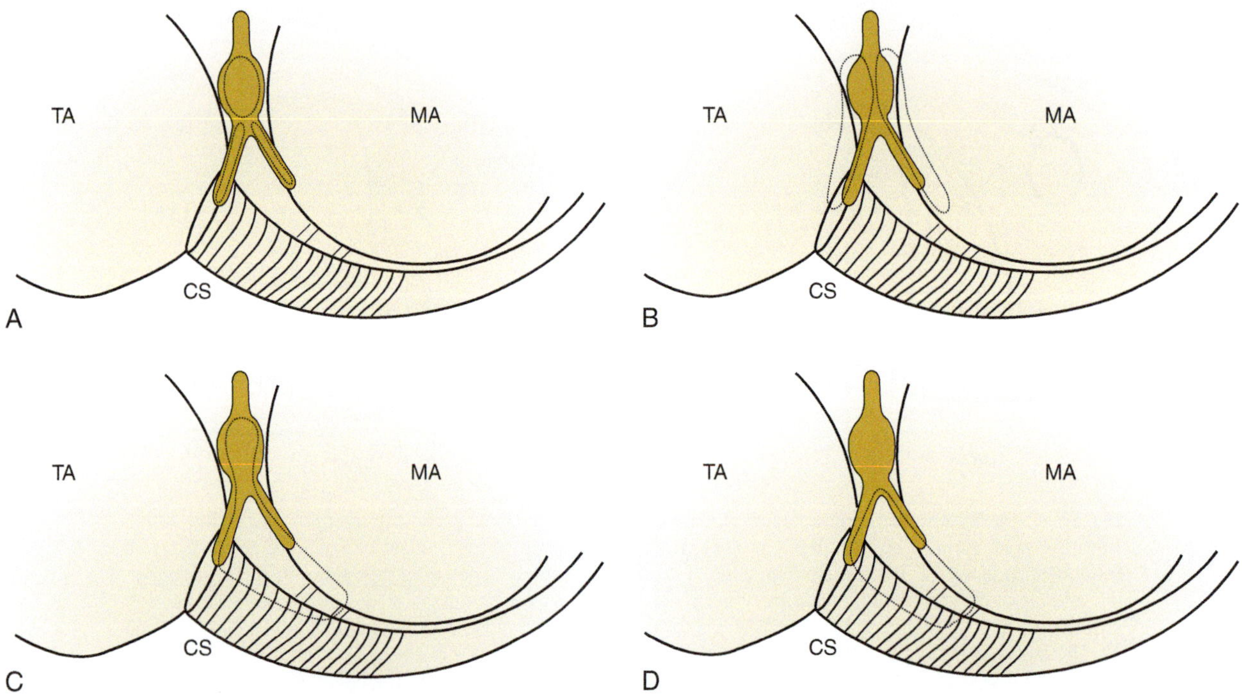

Fig. 23.13 Hypothetical reentrant circuits underlying different forms of atrioventricular nodal reentrant tachycardia (AVNRT). (A) Reentry *(broken lines)* confined to different segments of the AV node without participation of the atria. (B) Reentry involving atrial tissue and different segments of the compact AV node and its inputs. (C) Reentry involving the musculature of the coronary sinus connecting both inferior inputs and the compact AV node. This circuit has been proposed to describe slow-fast AV nodal reentry. (D) Reentry similar to that in C without involvement of the compact AV node. This circuit has been proposed to describe slow-slow and fast-slow AV nodal reentry. Within a given reentrant circuit, opposite wavefronts will give rise to different forms of AVNRT. *CS,* Coronary sinus; *MA,* mitral annulus; *TA,* tricuspid annulus.

BOX 23.1 Diagnostic Criteria of Atrioventricular Nodal Reentrant Tachycardia

Slow-Fast

Dual AV nodal physiology in most (85%) but not all cases

Long AH interval (>200 ms) during tachycardia

Initiation tachycardia dependent on critical AH interval during antegrade slow-pathway conduction

Earliest retrograde atrial activation in tachycardia posterior to the tendon of Todaro, posterior and to the left of the His bundle near apex of triangle of Koch

Ventricular postpacing interval > 115 ms longer than TCL

Late ventricular extrastimuli that advance His bundle activation also advance retrograde atrial activation and reset the tachycardia. Absence of a lower common pathway in most patients

Exclude atrial tachycardia and reciprocating tachycardia by appropriate maneuvers

Slow-Slow

Same as for slow-fast variant except for early retrograde atrial activation near the CS ostium*

Initiation dependent on critical HA interval during retrograde slow-pathway conduction

At identical cycle length, the HA interval during ventricular pacing is usually longer than that observed during tachycardia (lower common pathway)

VA interval during ventricular pacing at TCL minus VA interval during tachycardia > 85 ms

Fast-Slow

Short AH interval during tachycardia (<200 ms)

Inverted P waves in inferior leads during long-RP tachycardia

Initiation dependent on critical HA interval during retrograde slow-pathway conduction

Early retrograde atrial activation near the CS ostium or in the proximal portion of the CS

At identical cycle length, the HA interval during ventricular pacing is usually longer than that observed during tachycardia (lower common pathway)

AH interval during atrial pacing at TCL > 40 ms longer than AH interval in tachycardia

Exclude atrial tachycardia and reciprocating tachycardia by appropriate maneuvers

Left Sided

Same as for slow-fast variant except for the following:

- Inability to eliminate 1:1 slow-pathway conduction from right atrium or CS
- Late atrial extrastimulus from mitral annulus that resets tachycardia
- Short HA interval (<15 ms) may be present
- Double response to atrial extrastimulus may be present

AH, Atrium-His bundle; *AV,* atrioventricular; *CS,* coronary sinus; *HA,* His bundle-atrial; *TCL,* tachycardia cycle length.

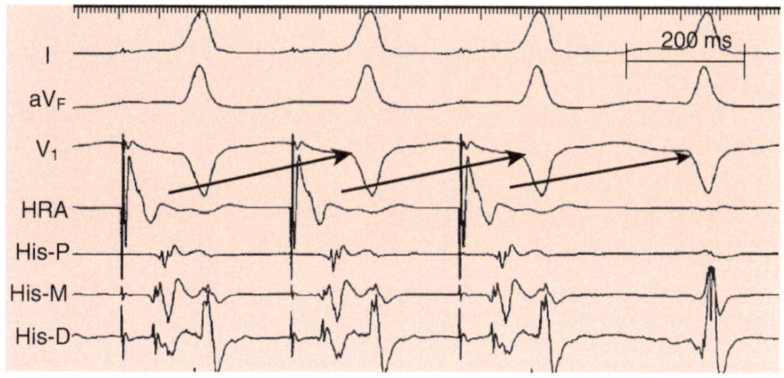

Fig. 23.14 Antegrade slow-pathway conduction during atrial pacing at 280 ms. The PR interval is 340 ms and therefore exceeds the PP interval (crossover). The stimulus conducts, not to the following QRS, but to the second QRS as indicated by the *arrows*. *D,* Distal; *HRA,* high right atrium; *M,* mid; *P,* proximal.

BOX 23.2 Features of Dual Atrioventricular Nodal Physiology and Slow-Pathway Conduction

Dual AV Nodal Physiology

>50 ms increase in A2H2 interval with ≤10 ms decrease in A1A2 interval

>50 ms increase in AH interval with 10 ms decrease in atrial pacing rate

AV interval longer than AA interval during atrial overdrive pacing (crossover)

Abrupt change in slope of AV nodal conduction curve without *jump* (children especially)

Double response (two ventricular responses to a single atrial activation due to simultaneous fast- and slow-pathway conduction)

Slow-Pathway Conduction

AH interval > 200 ms

Earliest retrograde atrial activation near coronary sinus ostium (exclude accessory pathway)

A1A2, Coupling interval of a single atrial extrastimulus after a basic atrial pacing drive; *A2H2,* AH interval following the atrial extrastimulus; *AH,* atrium-His bundle interval; *AV,* atrioventricular.

conduction is defined as an increase in the A3H3 interval of 50 ms or more in response to a decrement of 10 ms in the A2A3 interval (A1A2 being constant).[58] The induction of AV nodal echo beats is an indication of dual AV nodal physiology. The diagnosis of retrograde dual AV nodal physiology is made based on jumps but is mainly dependent on changes of earliest atrial activation site (Box 23.2) from near the His bundle area (retrograde fast pathway) to proximal CS region (retrograde slow pathway).[40] Retrograde His bundle-atrial (HA) interval jumps, and retrograde slow, antegrade fast AV nodal echo beats, may be seen.

Induction of AVNRT is dependent on achieving a critical AH interval[26] for typical slow-fast AVNRT; this requires exclusive antegrade slow-pathway conduction, which can be achieved by atrial extrastimulus testing or atrial burst pacing near the Wenckebach cycle length. If antegrade slow-pathway conduction cannot be achieved because short antegrade fast-pathway refractoriness, S3 stimulation, burst atrial pacing, or ventricular stimulation with or without isoproterenol may be required. If retrograde fast-pathway conduction is absent during ventricular pacing (VA block or earliest retrograde atrial activation at proximal CS) or by lack of echoes or AVNRT following antegrade slow-pathway conduction, isoproterenol infusion should be given.[55] It is important to remember that retrograde block over the fast AV nodal pathway may be due to mechanical trauma of the fast pathway by the catheter recording His bundle activity, which can be minimized by advancing the catheter to the ventricle.

Slow-Fast Variant

The typical form, or slow-fast variant, is the most common form of AVNRT. Atypical AVNRT (fast-slow and slow-slow) was noted in 6.4% of the cases of AVNRT in a multicenter series.[59]

The antegrade limb of the tachycardia is the slow AV nodal pathway, with an AH interval longer than 200 ms (Table 23.1).[60] A short VA (measured from the surface QRS to the earliest

TABLE 23.1 Classification of Atrioventricular Nodal Reentrant Tachycardia Types

Variable	HA	VA (His)	AH/HA	Earliest Retrograde Atrial Activation
Typical AVNRT	≤70 ms	≤60 ms	> 1	Superior septum
Atypical AVNRT	>70 ms	> 60 ms	Variable	Inferior septum

Atypical AVNRT has been traditionally classified as fast-slow (His-atrial >70 ms, ventriculoatrial >60 ms, atrial-His/His-atrial <1, and atrial-His <200 ms) or slow-slow (His-atrial >70 ms, ventriculoatrial >60 ms, atrial-His/His-atrial >1, and atrial-His >200 ms). Intermediate unclassified types may also exist. AH = atrial-His interval; AVNRT = atrioventricular nodal re-entrant tachycardia; HA = His-atrial interval; VA = ventriculo-atrial interval measured from the onset of ventricular activation on surface ECG to the earliest deflection of the atrial activation on the His bundle electrogram. (Reproduced with permission from Katritsis DG, Josephson ME. Classification of electrophysiological types of atrioventricular nodal re-entrant tachycardia: a reappraisal. *Europace.* 2013;15:1231–1240.)

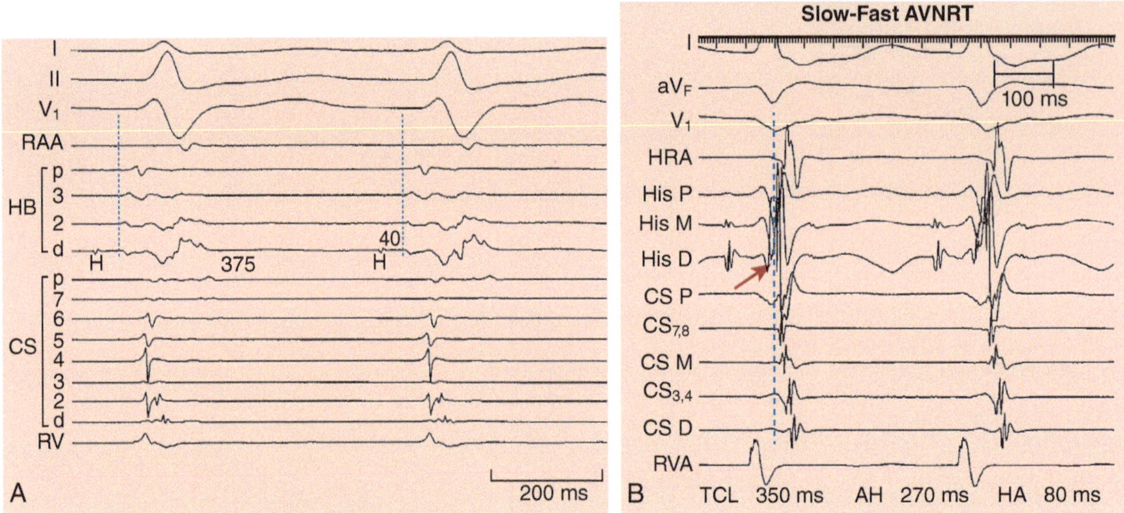

Fig. 23.15 Two examples of slow-fast atrioventricular (AV) nodal reentry. (A) Atrial activation precedes ventricular activation during slow-fast atrioventricular nodal reentrant tachycardia. Using close bipolar electrodes, earliest atrial activation (*dotted lines*) recorded close to the proximal portion of the His bundle precedes ventricular activation. In the absence of these recordings, atrial activation would appear to be simultaneous to ventricular activation. (B) Intracardiac electrograms recorded during slow-fast AV nodal reentry. The earliest atrial activity (*arrow*) is recorded on the His catheter and is approximated by the vertical line. Atrial activation in the coronary sinus (CS) is concentric. The tachycardia cycle length (TCL) is 350 ms, atrium–His bundle (AH) interval is 270 ms, and His bundle-atrial (HA) interval is 80 ms. *D/d,* Distal; *H,* His recording; *HB,* His bundle; *HRA,* high right atrium; *M,* mid; *P/p,* proximal; *RAA,* right atrial appendage; *RV,* right ventricle; *RVA,* right ventricular apex.

intracardiac atrial electrogram) time of less than 60 ms excludes reciprocating tachycardias using a concealed AV accessory pathway.[26] However, atrial tachycardias (AT) with 1:1 AV conduction over the slow AV nodal pathway can have a short VA time, simulating AVNRT. The VA relationship in AT shows significant change after atrial overdrive pacing (AOD) during SVT as compared to AVNRT.[61] Ventricular overdrive pacing during SVT leads to VAV response in typical AVNRT as compared to VAAV response in atrial tachycardia.[62]

Induction of slow-fast AVNRT is usually accomplished by atrial extrastimuli or rapid atrial stimulation. Adrenergic stimulation (isoproterenol, 1–4 μg/min) may be needed. Inducibility of AVNRT sometimes occurs only after the infusion of isoproterenol has been discontinued. Occasionally, atropine, 1–2 mg, with or without catecholamine infusion is necessary for AVNRT induction. Regardless of the maneuver used, induction of slow-fast AVNRT from the atrium requires antegrade block over the fast AV nodal pathway, with antegrade conduction over the slow AV nodal pathway allowing retrograde conduction over the fast AV nodal pathway. Less commonly, ventricular stimulation can also induce slow-fast AVNRT. Local atrial activation near the exit site of the fast AV nodal pathway (superior aspect of the triangle of Koch) can be recorded using closely spaced electrodes (Figs. 23.15 and 23.16). The site of earliest retrograde atrial activation is critical to differentiate slow-fast from slow-slow AVNRT because the HA intervals can overlap in these two forms of tachycardia. A contemporary conceptualization of the reentry circuit for slow-fast AVNRT is shown in Fig. 23.13C. In this model, retrograde atrial activation through the fast pathway activates both the left and right sides of the atrial septum. The wavefront of right atrial activation fails to penetrate into the triangle of Koch because of block along the Eustachian ridge.[25] The left atrial wavefront, however, activates the CS myocardium and propagates to the CS os and inferior triangle of Koch between the os and the tricuspid valve. The wavefront then ascends the

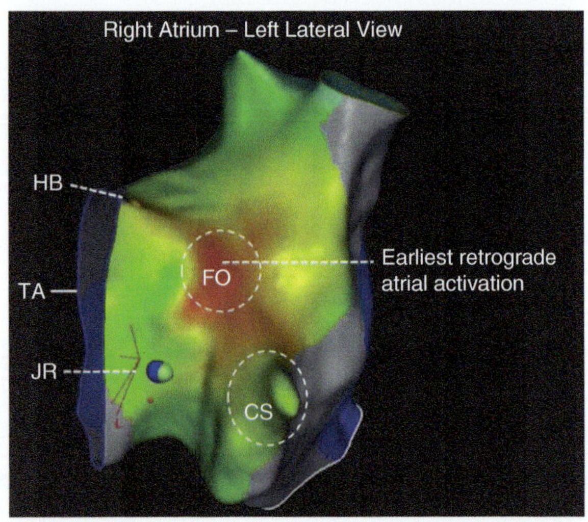

Fig. 23.16 High-density mapping using a multipolar close electrodes catheter (PentaRay) of the triangle of Koch, proximal coronary sinus, and fossa ovalis during slow-fast AVNRT. The right atrium is viewed from the left lateral projection. Earliest retrograde atrial activation is recorded in the region of the fossa ovalis (FO), posterior to the site where the His bundle electrogram was recorded and the tendon of Todaro (not shown). *HB,* His bundle; *TA,* tricuspid annulus; *CS,* coronary sinus; *JR,* site where junctional rhythm was induced in sinus rhythm during RF energy delivery.

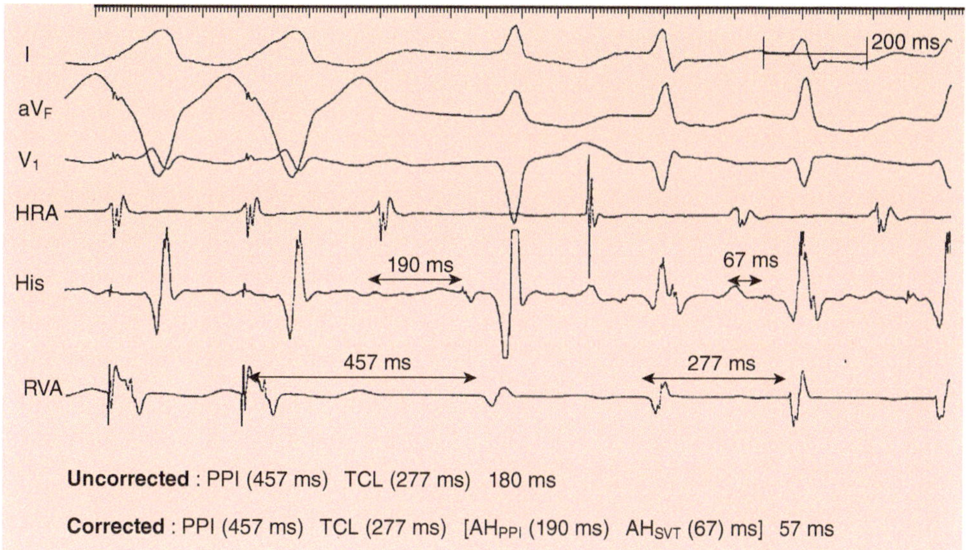

Fig. 23.17 Correction of ventricular post pacing interval (PPI) for atrium–His bundle (AH) interval prolongation in the return cycle. Overdrive ventricular pacing that captures the atrium is terminated with continuation of a narrow complex tachycardia. The ventricular postpacing interval is long compared with the tachycardia cycle length (TCL) (difference > 115 ms) consistent with atrioventricular (AV) nodal reentry. The AH interval in the return cycle is prolonged (190 ms) compared with that in tachycardia (67 ms) because of concealed or decremental conduction in the AV node. After correction for this AH prolongation, the difference between the postpacing interval and the tachycardia cycle length is < 115 ms (57 ms), consistent with AV reciprocating tachycardia. The patient underwent successful ablation of a concealed posteroseptal pathway. *CS,* Coronary sinus; *D,* distal; *HA,* His bundle-atrial bundle; *HRA,* high right atrium; *M,* mid; *P,* proximal; *RVA,* right ventricular apex; *SVT,* supraventricular tachycardia.

atrial septum in the triangle of Koch to activate the fast pathway and complete the circuit.[25] In this conceptualization, the right inferior extension comprises the anterograde slow pathway, and the fibers crossing the superior tendon of Todaro comprise the retrograde fast pathway.[25] Ablation within the CS or left atrium is necessary when the left inferior extension or left atrial myocardium provides the critical portion to the reentry circuit rather than the right inferior extension.

Slow-Slow Variant

In this form of reentry, a slow AV nodal pathway is used as the antegrade limb, and another slow AV nodal pathway as the retrograde limb. Reentry using both the right and left inferior AV nodal inputs has been proposed.[25] The electrocardiogram during tachycardia may show characteristic negative P waves in inferior and precordial leads, typical of earliest retrograde atrial activation in the proximal CS (Fig. 23.18).[63] This tachycardia can be induced by atrial or ventricular stimulation and frequently requires administration of isoproterenol. As previously mentioned, although the HA interval is usually longer than that recorded during slow-fast AVNRT, an overlap in the HA intervals between these two forms of AVNRT is frequently observed (see Table 23.1).[25]

The earliest site of retrograde atrial activation was found in the right atrium near the anterior edge of the CS os or just inside the CS (mean distance from the os, 1.5 ± 0.5 cm) (Fig. 23.18). The earliest site of retrograde atrial activation near the CS os is what characterizes slow-slow AVNRT, and not the HA interval. Short HA intervals may also occur and are typically attributed to long conduction times in the lower common pathway, almost offsetting the longer HA times. Neither the antegrade nor retrograde fast pathway is necessary for this reentrant circuit and therefore may be absent.

Characteristic of the slow-slow form of AVNRT is the presence of a lower common pathway. In other words, there is a portion of the AV node that is distal to, and not part of, the reentrant circuit that sustains the tachycardia. The presence of a lower common pathway is demonstrated by comparing the HA interval during tachycardia with the earliest atrial activation site, with the HA interval observed during ventricular pacing at the same cycle length as the tachycardia.[60] In patients with slow-slow AVNRT, the HA interval during ventricular pacing (measured from the end of the His bundle deflection) is longer than that recorded during tachycardia (Fig. 23.19).

As in the slow-fast form, preexcitation of the atrium during slow-slow AVNRT only follows ventricular extrastimuli that advance retrograde His bundle activation (Fig. 23.20). However, because of the presence of a lower common pathway, retrograde His bundle activation needs to be advanced more than 15 ms before retrograde atrial activation is also advanced. By contrast, during AV reentrant tachycardia, late ventricular extrastimuli can advance retrograde atrial activation even when retrograde His bundle activation is not altered, as long as ventricular activation near the earliest atrial activation site is advanced.

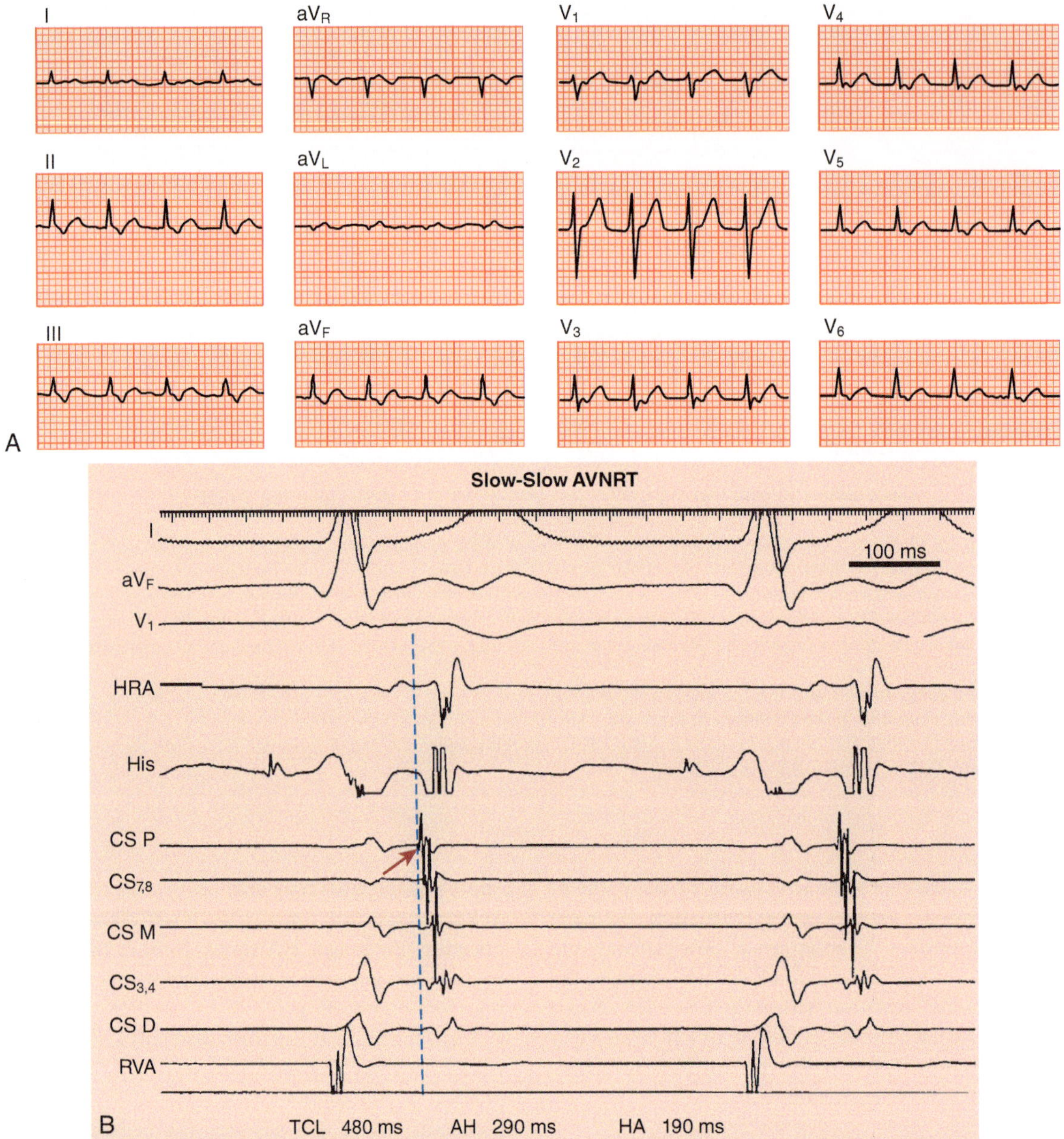

Fig. 23.18 Slow-slow atrioventricular (AV) nodal reentry. Surface electrocardiogram showing slow-slow AV nodal reentry with the P wave in the ST segment. (A) the P wave is inverted in the inferior leads. (B) Surface electrocardiographic leads I, aVF, and V1 along with intracavitary electrograms. *AH,* Atrium-His bundle; *AVNRT,* atrioventricular nodal reentrant tachycardia; *CS,* coronary sinus; *D,* distal; *HA,* His bundle-atrial bundle; *HRA,* high right atrium; *M,* mid; *P,* proximal; *RVA,* right ventricular apex. Earliest retrograde atrial activation is recorded in the proximal coronary sinus (*arrow*).

Fast-Slow Variant

The fast-slow form of AVNRT is the least common form of AVNRT. Similar to slow-slow AVNRT, the complete reentry circuit is not fully understood. In fast-slow AVNRT, it is assumed that the fast AV nodal pathway is used as the antegrade limb and one or more slow AV nodal pathways as the retrograde limb, with the assumption that this arrhythmia is the reversal of the typical slow-fast circuit. However, this simplified concept has been challenged by the concept that fast-slow reentry may represent reentry within the right and left inferior AV nodal inputs but in a direction opposite to that of slow-slow AVNRT.[25] The electrocardiogram during tachycardia may show a PR interval that is shorter than the RP interval (long-RP tachycardia) (Fig. 23.21A). The AH interval is less than 200 ms,[60] with P waves inverted in inferior leads (see Table 23.1). The HA interval is longer than the AH interval because of retrograde conduction over the slow AV nodal pathway.

Similar to the slow-slow form, fast-slow AVNRT can be induced by atrial or ventricular stimulation, frequently during administration of isoproterenol. In some patients, AVNRT

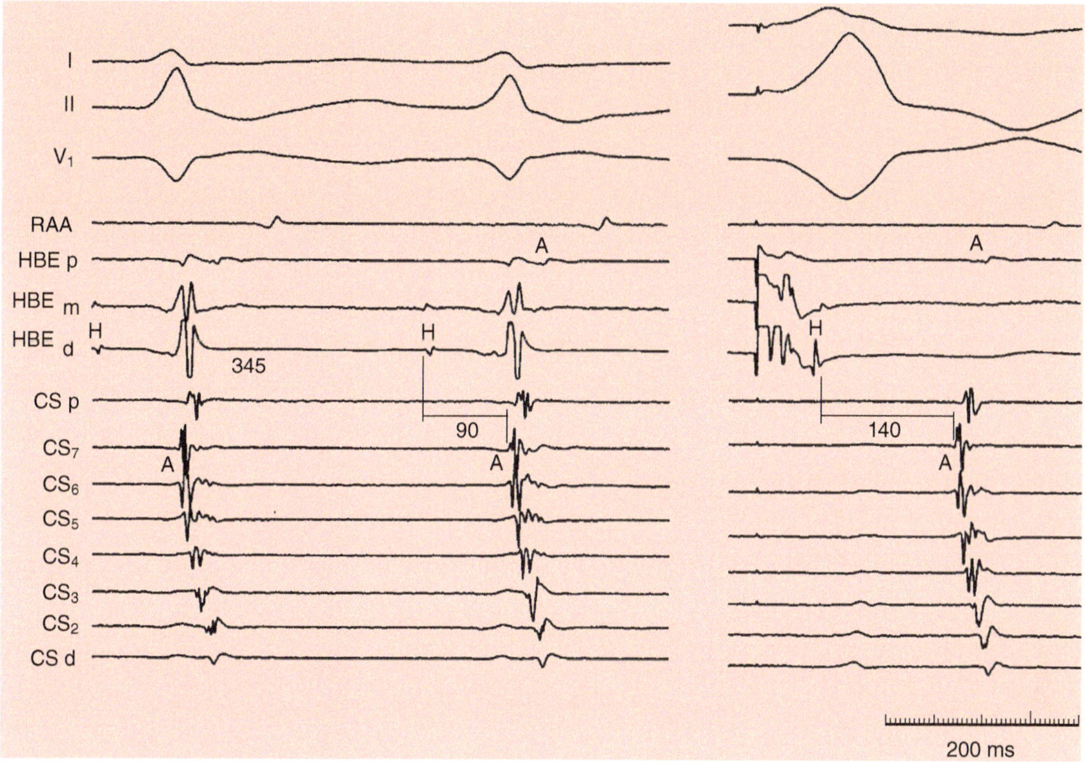

Fig. 23.19 Demonstration of a lower common pathway in atrioventricular (AV) nodal reentrant tachycardia using a retrograde slow AV nodal pathway. *Left,* The His bundle-atrial (HA) interval during tachycardia measured to the earliest atrial activation site in the proximal coronary sinus (CS_7) is 90 ms. *Right,* During ventricular stimulation at the tachycardia cycle length (345 ms), the HA interval is 140 ms, consistent with a common lower pathway distal to the reentrant circuit supporting the tachycardia. *d,* Distal; *HBE,* His bundle electrogram; *m,* mid; *p,* proximal; *RAA,* right atrial appendage. (From Curtis AB, Gonzalez MD. Supraventricular tachycardia. In: Naccarelli GV, Curtis AB, Goldschlager NF, eds. *Electrophysiology Self-Assessment Program.* Bethesda, MD: American College of Cardiology; 2000.)

is induced only by ventricular stimulation. Earliest retrograde atrial activation is close to the CS os (Fig. 23.21B).[25]

Left-Sided Variant

The left-sided variant has been reported to occur in up to 1.5–2% of patients undergoing ablation for AVNRT.[25,64] There are no pathognomonic surface or intracardiac electrocardiographic findings for the left-sided AVNRT variant. Similarly, there are no clinical characteristics differentiating between these patients and those with more common forms of AVNRT.[64] This includes typical slow-fast AVNRT using a left inferoseptal input[64,65] or left inferolateral input.[66] Rarely it can involve a fast-slow type of AVNRT using a superior slow pathway requiring ablation superior to His or noncoronary aortic sinus of Valsalva.[67] The diagnosis is confirmed not only by electrophysiologic findings consistent with AVNRT but also with successful slow-pathway ablation from the left atrium after failure of right atrial ablation. Late atrial extrastimulus from the mitral annulus that resets the tachycardia can identify the successful site of ablation.[66] The presence of a short HA interval (≤15 ms) and the occurrence of antegrade double response to atrial pacing are sometimes noted in patients with this AVNRT variant.[25] The AH intervals and TCLs are longer in the left-sided variant than in right-sided slow-fast AVNRT.[64]

DIFFERENTIAL DIAGNOSIS

The diagnosis of AVNRT requires exclusion of alternative mechanisms. These include orthodromic AVRT, atrial tachycardia, concealed NFT/NVT and JT (Tables 23.2 and 23.3).

VA times determined during pacing in sinus rhythm from the base and apex of the right ventricle can help identify the presence of an accessory pathway. With this maneuver, pacing from the base of the right ventricle will produce a shorter VA time than apical ventricular pacing in the presence of an accessory pathway. By contrast, the VA times are shorter when pacing from the right ventricular apex when retrograde conduction occurs through the AV node.[55] In sinus rhythm, para-Hisian pacing can also differentiate between retrograde conduction over the AV node versus retrograde conduction over a septal accessory pathway.[56] It should be remembered that para-Hisian pacing may fail to demonstrate retrograde conduction over accessory AV pathways located at other sites.

Orthodromic reciprocating tachycardia can be excluded when the VA time is less than 60 ms, which is common in

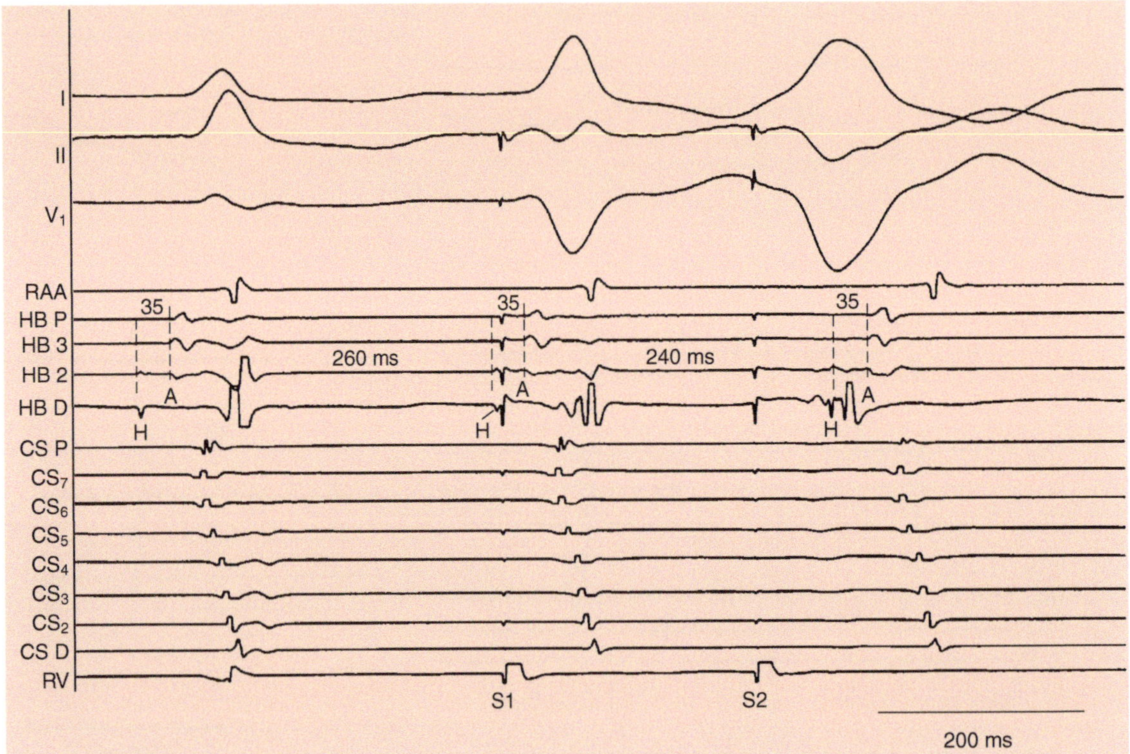

Fig. 23.20 Entrainment of slow-fast atrioventricular nodal reentrant tachycardia (AVNRT) using double ventricular extrastimuli. S_1 *peels back* the refractory period of the right ventricle, which in turn allows S_2 to capture the right ventricle and advances retrograde His bundle activation. This maneuver is frequently required in AVNRT with short cycle lengths in which the ventricular effective refractory period is reached before His bundle activation can be advanced. Note that S_2 advances both retrograde His bundle and atrial activations with constant His bundle-atrial intervals (35 ms), consistent with absence of lower common pathway. The sequence of atrial activation following S_2 is identical to that observed during tachycardia. *CS,* Coronary sinus; *D,* Distal; *HB,* His bundle; *P,* proximal; *RAA,* right atrial appendage; *RV,* right ventricle.

typical or slow-fast AVNRT.[26] The response after ventricular overdrive pacing (VOD) is an additional maneuver to differentiate different forms of SVT. During ventricular pacing with 1:1 V-A conduction and atrial entrainment, both AVNRT and orthodromic AVRT lead to a VAV response as opposed to VAAV response during AT.[62] The VA interval during ventricular pacing is more than 85 ms longer than the corresponding VA interval during tachycardia in atypical AVNRT.[68,69] In addition the difference between the ventricular post pacing interval (PPI) and TCL is more than 115 ms.[69] Correction of the PPI may be needed to account for rate-related prolongation of the return AH interval–Δ = [PPI-(AH return-AH supraventricular tachycardia)-TCL] (Fig. 23.17).[70] Corrected PPI-TCL < 110 ruled out AVNRT in this study.[70] Capture of the A during initial beats of VOD that show fusion argue for orthodromic AVRT vs AVNRT during which A is only captured by nonfused ventricular beats.[71] The observation of antegrade His activation during VOD confirms diagnosis of orthodromic AVRT and rules out AVNRT.[72] His overdrive pacing during SVT has also been shown to reliably differentiate AVNRT (capture of A after two beats) from accessory pathway mediated tachycardia (capture of A during first two beats).[73] Change in VA with bundle branch block (BBB) can be used to differentiate septal pathway mediated AVRT from AVNRT. No change in VA time is noted in AVNRT with BBB. RBBB leads to increase in VA time (up to 25 ms) in AVRT using anteroseptal pathway and LBBB increases the VA time (up to 25 ms) in AVRT using posteroseptal pathway.[74] Variability of VA interval by more than 10 ms and stabilization of VA after 3 beats during initiation of short or long RP tachycardia is consistent with a diagnosis of atypical AVNRT (as compared to orthodromic AVRT).[63]

Preexcitation of the atrium during AVNRT only follows ventricular extrastimuli that advance retrograde His bundle activation (Fig. 23.20). However, because of the presence of a lower common pathway, retrograde His bundle activation needs to be advanced more than 15 ms before retrograde atrial activation is also advanced. By contrast, during AV reentrant tachycardia, late ventricular extrastimuli (basal location preferred over apical location) can advance retrograde atrial activation even when retrograde His bundle activation is not altered (V on His), as long as ventricular activation near the earliest atrial activation site is advanced. Delay of retrograde atrial activation and termination of SVT by V on His during SVT rules in diagnosis of orthodromic AVRT and rules out AVNRT. Bystander accessory pathway is diagnosed when the atrial activation advanced by V on His is different from that during tachycardia.

Atrial tachycardias that originate in perinodal structures are not uncommon. Thus atrial activation sequence may be

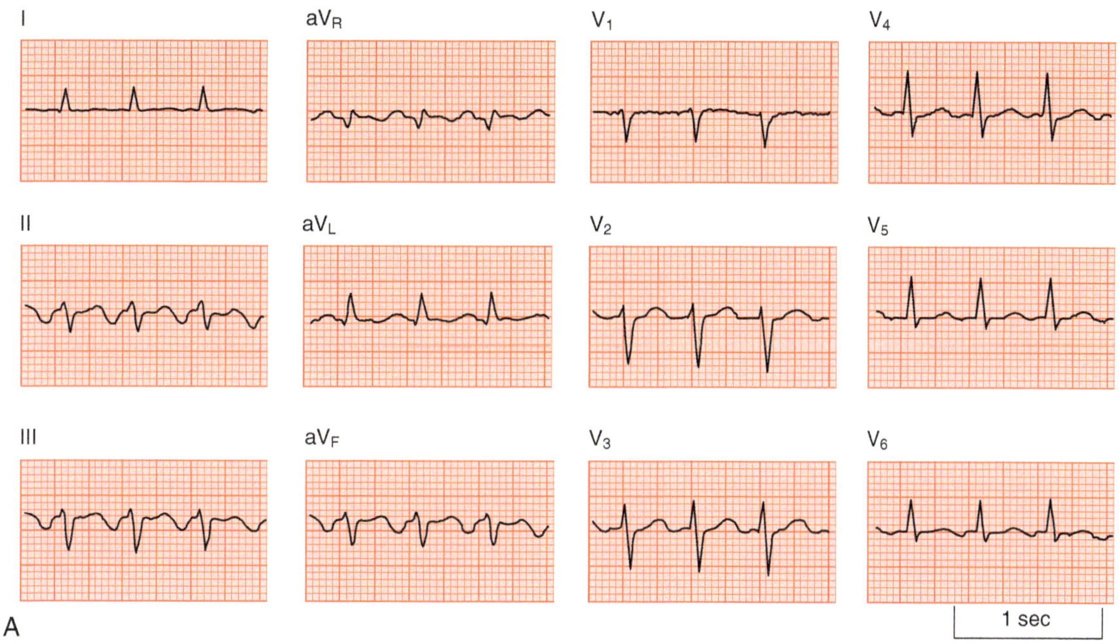

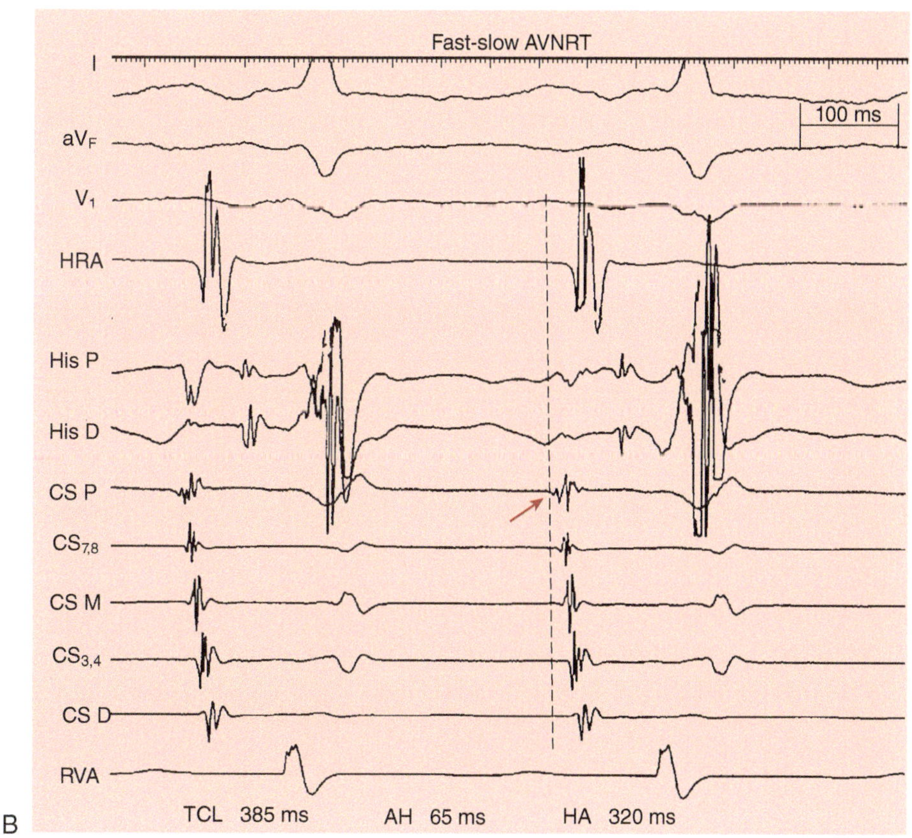

Fig. 23.21 (A) Electrocardiogram during fast-slow atrioventricular (AV) nodal reentrant tachycardia. Negative P waves in inferior and precordial leads are recorded before the QRS complexes with a PR shorter than the RP interval, giving rise to a long-RP tachycardia pattern. (B) Intracardiac electrograms recorded during fast-slow AV nodal reentry. Note that the earliest atrial activation *(vertical dotted line and arrow)* occurs at the proximal coronary sinus (CS P). The tachycardia cycle length (TCL) is 385 ms, the atrium-His bundle (AH) interval is 65 ms, and the His bundle-atrial (HA) interval is 320 ms. *D,* Distal; *HRA,* high right atrium; *M,* mid; *RVA,* right ventricular apex; *TCL,* tachycardia cycle length.

TABLE 23.2 Differential Diagnosis: Atrioventricular Nodal Reentry, Orthodromic Reciprocating Tachycardia, and Atrial Tachycardia[a]

Maneuver	PS ORT	AVNRT	AT
Para-Hisian pacing in sinus rhythm[56]	No change in VA with loss of His capture	Increased VA with loss of His capture	Increased VA with loss of His capture
VA pacing ventricular base versus pacing ventricular apex in sinus rhythm[55]	VA shorter pacing base	VA shorter pacing apex	VA shorter pacing apex
His overdrive pacing during tachycardia[73]	Capture A within 2 beats	Capture A after 2 beats	Capture A after 2 beats
Late ventricular extrastimulus delivered during tachycardia	Advance atrial activation if ventricular electrogram close to location of accessory pathway is also advanced	Advance atrial activation only if retrograde His bundle activation is advanced	Unable to advance atrial activation unless His is advanced
Δ Ventricular PPI and TCL and sequence of activation post pacing[69,62]	<115 ms unless decremental conduction, VAV response (pseudo VAAV in decremental pathway)	>115 ms, VAV response (pseudo VAAV response in atypical AVNRT)	VAAV response
Δ VA during ventricular pacing at TCL and VA during tachycardia[69]	<85 ms	>85 ms (atypical AVNRT)	Variable; VA conduction may be absent
Δ VA with BBB[74]	Up to 25 ms with RBBB in anteroseptal pathway, Upto 25 ms with LBBB in posteroseptal pathway	None	None
Antegrade His activation during VOD performed in tachycardia[72]	Yes	No	No
Retrograde VA conduction	Non decremental except in slowly conducting APs (e.g., PJRT)	Decremental	Decremental
Atrial and ventricular pacing at TCL	1:1 conduction present	Wenckebach conduction may occur	1:1 antegrade conduction present; VA block may be present
VA dissociation during tachycardia	Not possible	Possible	Possible
VA interval in tachycardia[26]	>60 ms (50 ms in pediatric patients)	<60 ms Typical AVNRT, >60 ms in atypical AVNRT	May be longer or shorter than 60 ms
VA linking[61]	Yes	Yes	No
Variation in VA interval > 10 ms at onset of tachycardia[63]	No	Yes (atypical AVNRT)	Yes

AP, Accessory pathway; *AT,* atrial tachycardia; *AVNRT,* atrioventricular nodal reentrant tachycardia; *BBB,* bundle branch block; *HA,* His bundle-atrial; *ORT,* orthodromic reciprocating tachycardia; *PJRT,* permanent form of junctional reciprocating tachycardia; *PPI,* post pacing interval; *PS,* posteroseptal; *TCL,* tachycardia cycle length; *VA,* paced ventricular electrogram to atrial electrogram; *VA,* ventriculoatrial interval; *VAAV,* ventriculo-atrial-atrio-ventricular; Δ, difference between.

[a]This table assumes that there is a single arrhythmia mechanism and no bystander or multiple accessory atrioventricular pathways.

TABLE 23.3 SVT With VA Dissociation

	Focal Junctional Tachycardia	AV Nodal Reentry	Nodofascicular/ Nodoventricular Tachycardia
Initiation with critical AV nodal delay	–	+	+
Effect of late APD in SVT: termination or reset	–	+	+
Early APD in SVT advances His	+	–	–
Response to AOD during SVT	AHHA	AHA	AHA
His-refractory VPD during SVT: termination or reset	–	–	+
CL change with ipsi BBB vs narrow QRS	–	–	+
Anterograde His with RV VPD	–	–	+

AV, Atrioventricular; *APD,* atrial premature depolarization; *SVT,* supraventricular tachycardia; *AOD,* atrial overdrive pacing; *VPD,* ventricular premature depolarization; *CL,* cycle length; *ipsi BBB,* ipsilateral bundle branch block.

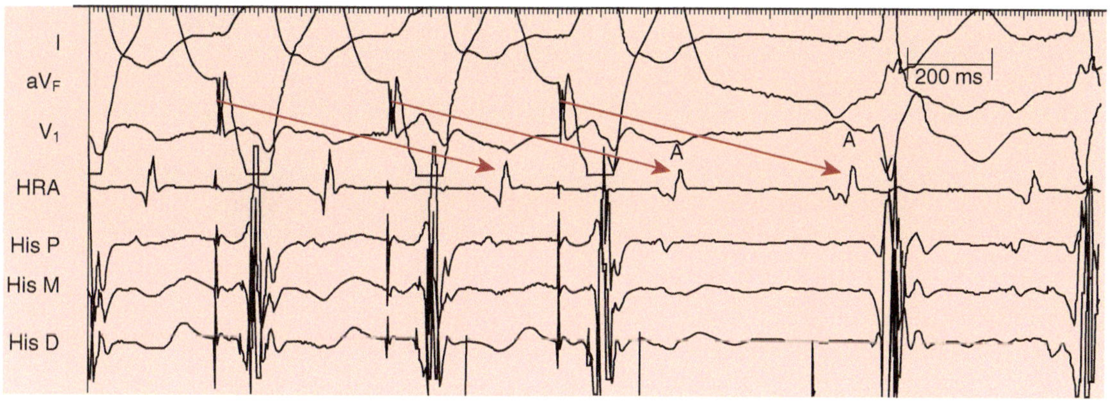

Fig. 23.22 Pseudo VAAV (ventriculo-atrial-atrio-ventricular) response to the termination of ventricular overdrive pacing during atrioventricular nodal reentry. Because of very long retrograde conduction times, the atrial electrogram during ventricular pacing is associated, not with the preceding ventricular complex, but with two complexes before *(arrows)*. This pattern may be confused with the response of atrial tachycardia to ventricular overdrive pacing. *HRA,* High right atrium; *M,* mid; *P,* proximal; *V,* ventricular electrogram.

identical to that of slow-fast AVNRT and right ventricular pacing. An atrial tachycardia can be diagnosed when there is variability in the VA interval during tachycardia (lack of VA linking). In patients with AT, atrial overdrive pacing during tachycardia from two different sites (high right atrium and coronary sinus) shows significant difference in VA interval of the first return beat of tachycardia after cessation of pacing.[61] Ventricular pacing at a rate faster than the rate of the tachycardia typically accelerates the atrial rate to that of the pacing rate with concealed entrainment. The presence of a VAAV sequence of activation following rapid ventricular pacing suggests an atrial tachycardia as the mechanism.[62] However, atypical AVNRT and permanent form of junctional reciprocating tachycardia (PJRT) with a decrementally conducting retrograde accessory pathway can lead to pseudo VAAV response to rapid ventricular pacing (Fig. 23.22). This happens when the retrograde VA interval exceeds the paced RR interval and atrial activation precedes ventricular activation during tachycardia.

For long-RP tachycardias, comparing the AH intervals between tachycardia and atrial pacing at the TCL can differentiate among AVNRTs (difference, >40 ms), atrial tachycardia (difference, <20 ms), and reciprocating tachycardias (difference, >20 but <40 ms).[75]

Differentiation of junctional tachycardia from slow-fast AVNRT may be difficult.[76,77] Both tachycardias have a short and constant HA conduction interval with earliest retrograde atrial activation near the apex of the triangle of Koch (fast-pathway region, behind the tendon of Todaro). An automatic JT can be differentiated from AVNRT by the response to premature atrial contractions (PACs) introduced during or before AV junctional refractoriness (Fig. 23.23).[76] A PAC introduced during AV junctional refractoriness cannot penetrate to the automatic focus and therefore cannot alter the tachycardia. By contrast, a junctional refractory PAC may advance, delay the following beat of tachycardia by conduction in the slow pathway in AVNRT or terminate tachycardia (Fig. 23.25).[77] PACs introduced before AV junctional refractoriness may advance the immediately following beat and continue an automatic tachycardia but must terminate AVNRT because of collision of the antegrade PAC wavefront and retrograde tachycardia wavefront in the fast pathway.

ATRIOVENTRICULAR NODAL REENTRY AND ATYPICAL PRESENTATIONS

Irregular AVNRT that can be misdiagnosed as atrial fibrillation on surface electrocardiograms is an uncommon presentation of this arrhythmia. Alternating conduction over two slow AV nodal pathways with different conduction times can give rise to alternating short-long cycles during tachycardia.[71,78] In addition double-response tachycardia can occur with each sinus beat conducting over both the fast and slow pathways to produce an apparently irregular cycle length, which may be confused with atrial fibrillation.[8] Similarly, intermittent functional block distal or proximal to the His bundle can give origin to periods of AVNRT with 1:1 AV relationship alternating with 2:1 AVNRT (see Fig. 23.11). The electrocardiogram during tachycardia could be mistaken for an atrial tachycardia.[79] The distinctive characteristic of 2:1 AVNRT is the location of the nonconducted P wave centered between the preceding and following QRS (see Fig. 23.11). Older individuals with underlying AV nodal disease can present with a symptomatic AV nodal reentrant arrhythmia but with a rate below 100 beats per minute. Despite a lower rate than that required to make a diagnosis of tachycardia, the mechanism of this arrhythmia is identical to that observed in younger patients with AVNRT. These older patients tend to be quite symptomatic despite the relatively slow rate, probably owing to almost simultaneous atrial and ventricular contraction. Slow AVNRT has been described in older patients with a prolonged PR interval (262 ± 54 ms) at baseline.[80] All patients underwent slow-pathway ablation. The AV Wenckebach cycle length prolonged from 522 ± 90 ms at baseline to 666 ± 48 ms after ablation. Only one patient required a permanent pacemaker due to

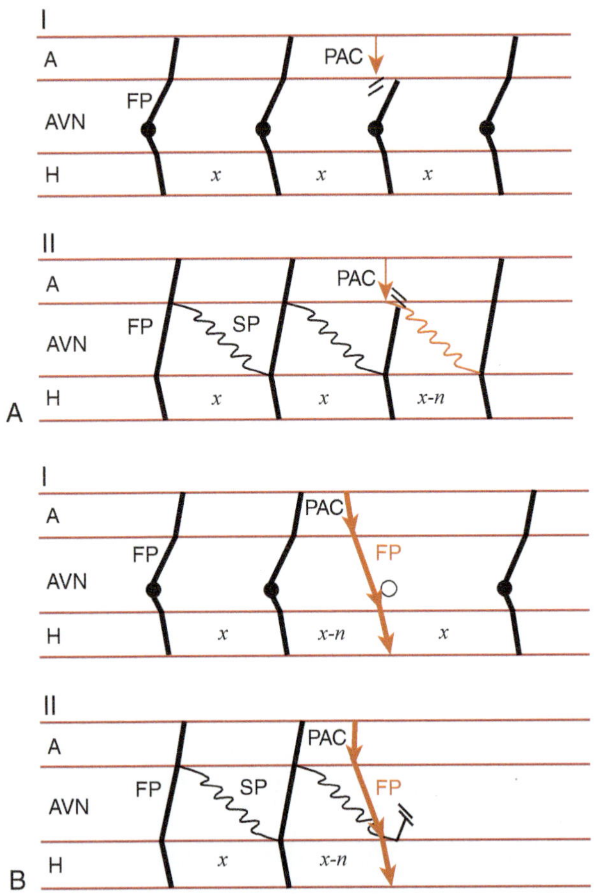

Fig. 23.23 Atrial extrastimulus testing to differentiate atrioventricular nodal (AVN) reentry from an automatic junctional tachycardia. (A) Response to premature atrial complex (PAC) delivered when the AV junction is refractory (local atrial activation from PAC occurs at or after His activation). *(I)*, Response in junctional tachycardia. A PAC delivered at a time the junctional focus has already depolarized the AVN and is unable to influence the immediate or the next junction beat. *Solid circles* represent junction focus; *black lines* show conduction through AVN, His (H), and atrium (A). *(II)*, Response in AVN reentry tachycardia (AVNRT). A similarly timed PAC cannot influence the immediate next beat but can influence the following (*x-n*) beat of AVNRT by conduction through the slow pathway. *Black lines* show conduction through AVN, H, and A, and *red lines* show PAC and its response. Although this figure shows advancement of the next beat (*x-n*), delay of the next beat or termination of tachycardia is also specific to AVNRT. The *orange arrow* indicates PAC. (B) Response to PACs delivered before AV junctional refractoriness. *(I)*, Response in junctional tachycardia. The *open circle* represents the anticipated junctional tachycardia beat timing if no PAC was delivered. An early PAC advances the immediate junctional tachycardia beat and His timing by AV nodal fast-pathway activation, and junctional tachycardia continues. *(II)* Response in AVNRT. An early PAC may advance the immediate His by activation of the AV nodal fast pathway. However, that makes the fast-pathway refractory and unavailable for retrograde conduction, terminating the AVNRT circuit. The *orange arrow* indicates PAC and its response. *A*, Atrium; *FP*, fast atrioventricular node pathway; *H*, His; *SP*, slow atrioventricular node pathway; *x* and *x-n*, HH intervals. (From Padanilam BJ, Manfredi JA, Steinberg LA, et al. Differentiating junctional tachycardia and atrioventricular node re-entry tachycardia based on response to atrial extrastimulus pacing. *J Am Coll Cardiol.* 2008;52:1711–1717.)

an AV Wenckebach cycle length of 710 ms after ablation. The arrhythmia rate is slower, likely because of an underlying AV nodal disease, and thus their risk of AV block after ablation is probably higher than for others with AVNRT.

AV NODAL REENTRY AND OTHER ARRHYTHMIAS

Atrial fibrillation is often associated with AVNRT. In a study of 629 patients undergoing atrial fibrillation ablation, 27 (4.3%) had inducible AVNRT.[5] These patients were younger than those without AVNRT, and ablation limited to AVNRT was associated with reduction of clinical recurrences of atrial fibrillation. Among 409 patients with atrial fibrillation, AVNRT was inducible in seven (1.7%), and the ablation was limited to the AVNRT in five (1.2%), with lower recurrence of atrial fibrillation. Among patients with paroxysmal atrial fibrillation, those with no identifiable pulmonary vein triggers appear more likely to have AVNRT (11%) than those with pulmonary vein triggers (2%).[81] It has also been reported that ablation of the slow pathway decreases vulnerability to pacing-induced atrial fibrillation in patients presenting with AVNRT. In 21–25% of patients with idiopathic ventricular tachycardia, AVNRT is also inducible, which is not the case in patients with ventricular tachycardia associated with structural heart disease.[31,32] A comprehensive electrophysiology study is necessary during the evaluation of patients with atrial and ventricular arrhythmias to assess for inducibility of AVNRT, and as in the case of atrial fibrillation, its potential role as the trigger of the clinical arrhythmia.

JUNCTIONAL TACHYCARDIA

Junctional tachycardia (JT) will be referred to as focal junctional tachycardia in this chapter (also known as junctional ectopic tachycardia, JET, or automatic JT) to differentiate it from reentrant forms of tachycardia involving the AV node (AVNRT, and rare forms identified in the past as junctional reentrant tachycardia). JT is encountered rather infrequently in adult patients except during administration of beta-agonist agents or other stimulants. It is a common finding after cardiac surgery, during adrenergic stimulation, ischemia, or as a manifestation of digoxin toxicity.[82] It is encountered more frequently in children than in adults. It can also be seen after slow pathway ablation for AVNRT. Clinically, JT has a similar presentation to focal atrial tachycardias, either intermittent bursts or incessant. It is frequently symptomatic like AVNRT due to the simultaneous AV systole leading to cannon A waves in the jugular veins, as well as systolic pulmonary vein flow reversal.

JT is very sensitive to catecholamines suggesting abnormal automaticity as one of the underlying mechanisms. Initiation with rapid atrial or ventricular pacing suggests triggered activity as another possible mechanism. This is further supported by the fact that JT may occasionally terminate with adenosine administration or carotid sinus massage. Programmed electrical stimulation has not been shown to be helpful with the induction or termination of JT, which strongly argues against reentry.

The typical ECG during JT shows evidence of AV dissociation (Fig. 23.24). It is an important differential diagnosis of supraventricular tachycardia (SVT) with ventriculoatrial (VA)

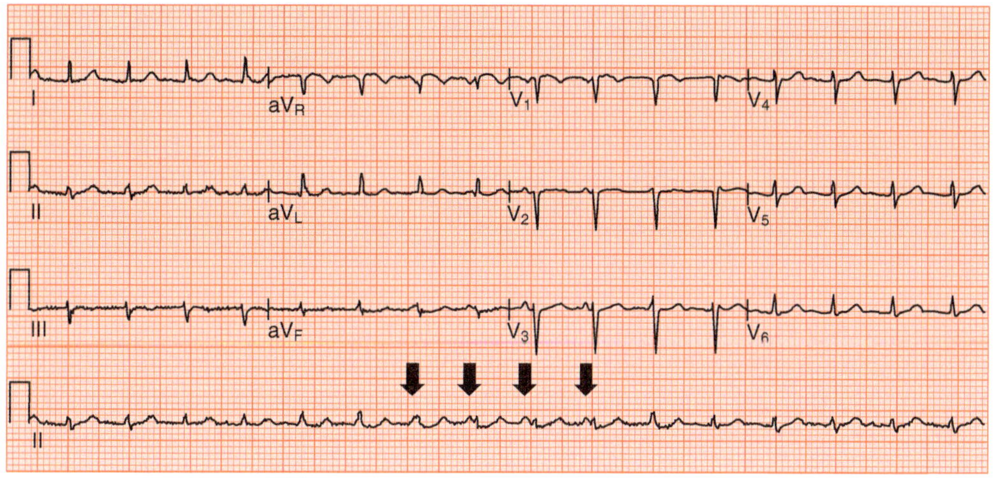

Fig. 23.24 Electrocardiogram during junctional tachycardia. Sinus P waves are recorded *(solid arrows)* that are dissociated from junctional tachycardia.

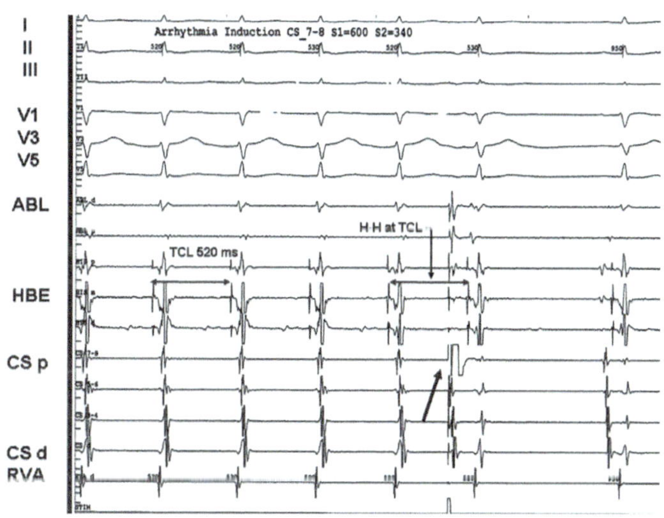

Fig. 23.25 Late PAC delivered during A on V supraventricular tachycardia from the CS proximal electrode terminates tachycardia without affecting the next V (suggesting the AV junction is committed). This is diagnostic for AV nodal reentrant tachycardia and argues against junctional tachycardia. (From Viswanathan MN, Scheinman MM, Badhwar N. Narrow complex tachycardia: what is the mechanism? *Cardiac Electrophysiol Clin.* 2010;2(2):203–207.)

block or dissociation. The other differential diagnoses include atrioventricular nodal reentrant tachycardia (AVNRT) with upper common pathway block and concealed nodofascicular (NF)/nodoventricular (NV) tachycardia (that uses an accessory pathway inserting from the AV node to fascicle or the ventricle).[39]

The diagnosis of typical AVNRT is mainly supported by the initiation with atrial premature stimulation and the need for a critical A-H interval for initiation. PACs given from the CS ostium can help differentiate AVNRT from JT. Insertion of late PACs at a time when the septal A is committed (i.e., has already been depolarized by the tachycardia) will advance or delay the timing of the next His, or terminate tachycardia in patients with AVNRT,[77] but not those with JT (Fig. 23.25). Insertion of an early PAC during tachycardia can capture the His and V via the fast pathway; this will not affect JT that will continue (Fig. 23.23) but will terminate AVNRT since it uses retrograde fast pathway that has now been antegradely engaged by the early PAC.[76] It is possible that PACs during tachycardia could advance the immediate His electrogram over the fast pathway without terminating the tachycardia and switch the sequence of activation from slow-fast to slow-slow AVNRT (antegrade double AV nodal response), or terminate and reinitiate the tachycardia mimicking a response considered as diagnostic of JT.

Atrial overdrive pacing (AOD) during tachycardia can also be used to differentiate JT from AVNRT.[83] After cessation of AOD, an AHHA response is seen in patients with JT (Fig. 23.26) as compared to AHA response in AVNRT. An important caveat to this maneuver is that AOD can terminate tachycardia and re-initiate AVNRT with the "double fire" phenomenon (conduction over fast and slow AV nodal pathways resulting from a single atrial depolarization). If the SVT is reliably induced with atrial extrastimuli, the relationship of an initiating extrastimulus to first tachycardia beat can also differentiate AVNRT from JT. In AVNRT (reentrant mechanism) there is an inverse relationship between the initiating extrastimulus to the first tachycardia beat. The opposite finding is seen in patients with JT (triggered mechanism).[84]

The diagnosis of concealed orthodromic NVT/NFT is supported by the following findings: (1) initiation with atrial or ventricular premature stimulation; (2) evidence of preexcitation during rapid atrial pacing; (3) bundle branch block resulting in a change in tachycardia cycle length; (4) advancement of the timing of the next His or tachycardia termination with a ventricular premature depolarization (VPD) delivered when the His bundle is refractory; and (5) dissociation of atrium from SVT.[85] Table 23.3 lists electrophysiologic findings and response to diagnostic maneuvers in EP lab in patients with JT, AVNRT, and concealed NVT/NFT.

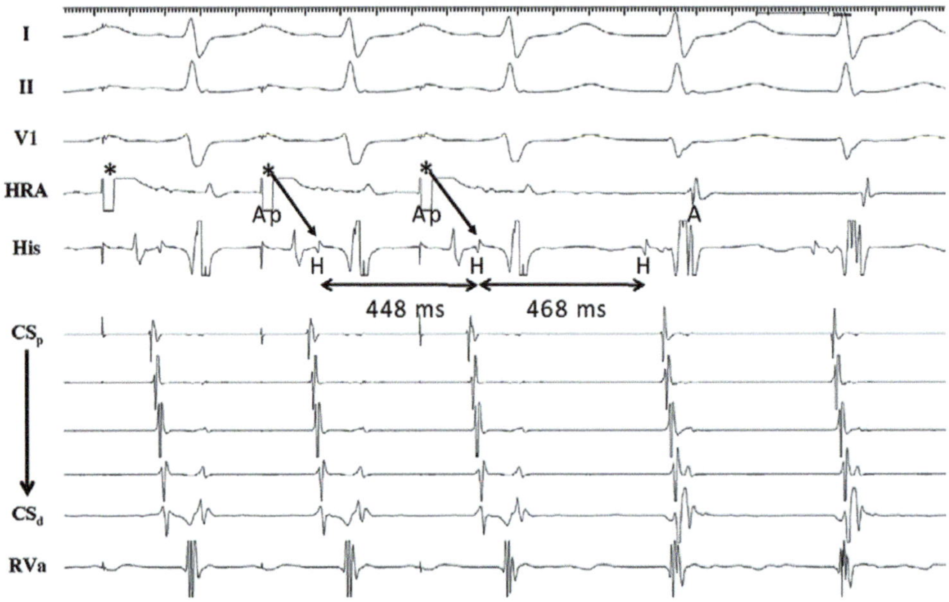

Fig. 23.26 Atrial overdrive pacing during junctional tachycardia. The junctional tachycardia cycle length is 468 ms. Atrial overdrive pacing is performed at 448 ms. The H-H intervals are shown, demonstrating the last advanced His signal. After cessation of pacing, an AHHA response is observed. *Solid arrows* represent conduction down the fast pathway of the AV node. *Ap,* atrial pace; *CS,* coronary sinus; *HRA,* high right atrium; *RVa,* right ventricular apex. (From Fan R, Tardos JG, Almasry I, Barbera S, Rashba EJ, Iwai S. Novel use of atrial overdrive pacing to rapidly differentiate junctional tachycardia from atrioventricular nodal reentrant tachycardia. Heart Rhythm. 2011;8:840–844.)

ABLATION

Slow Pathway Ablation

After atrial fibrillation, AVNRT is the most commonly treated arrhythmia with catheter ablation, followed by atrial flutter and AVRT.[1] A recent randomized trial, and observational studies, as well, have provided evidence that catheter ablation is the treatment of choice for symptomatic patients, by substantially reducing hospitalization, improving quality of life, and reducing costs.[1]

The initial treatment strategy for typical AVNRT involved modification of AV nodal conduction with ablation of the fast pathway at the anterosuperior aspect of the triangle of Koch. This approach carried a higher risk of AV block resulting in long-term pacing requirements due to damage of the compact AV node and His bundle located in that region. In the early 1990s, the treatment strategy for AVNRT shifted toward ablation of the slow pathway at the posteroinferior aspect of the triangle of Koch, which was shown to be a more effective approach with a lower risk of AV block for all variants of AVNRT.[46] The slow pathway can be targeted for ablation by an anatomical approach, electrogram-guided approach and 3D mapping-based approach. The targets for slow-pathway ablation are given in Box 23.3.

BOX 23.3 Targets for Slow-Pathway Ablation

Anatomic Guidance

Tissue between CS ostium and tricuspid annulus at the level of CS ostium (rightward inferior input)

Proximal CS musculature (connection with leftward inferior input through the LA-CS connections)

Increased risk of AV block: area triangle of Koch, superior to the CS ostium

A/V ratio = 1:10–1:3

Electrogram Guidance

Slow-pathway activation potentials

Earliest retrograde atrial activation near CS (slow-slow and fast-slow AVNRT only)

3D Mapping Guidance

Low voltage bridge

Turn around point in sinus rhythm when mapping with HD catheter in posteroseptal region

A/V, Atrial-to-ventricular; *AV,* atrioventricular; *AVNRT,* atrioventricular nodal reentrant tachycardia; *CS,* coronary sinus; *LA,* left atrium.

Anatomical Approach

The initial target for slow pathway ablation is the isthmus between the tricuspid annulus and CS os, corresponding to the rightward inferior AV nodal extension.[43,44,46,86] The most common site for effective ablation of the slow pathway is immediately anterior to or at the edge of the CS os (Fig. 23.27).[25,87–89] Ablation at this site is successful in eliminating AVNRT in approximately 95% of cases. If the initial ablation lesion is not successful, then the ablation catheter can be repositioned slightly more superiorly towards the apex of the triangle of Koch. In some cases, successful ablation requires ablation inferior to the CS os, superior to the CS os, or within the proximal CS. It should be remembered, however that ablation at more superior sites along

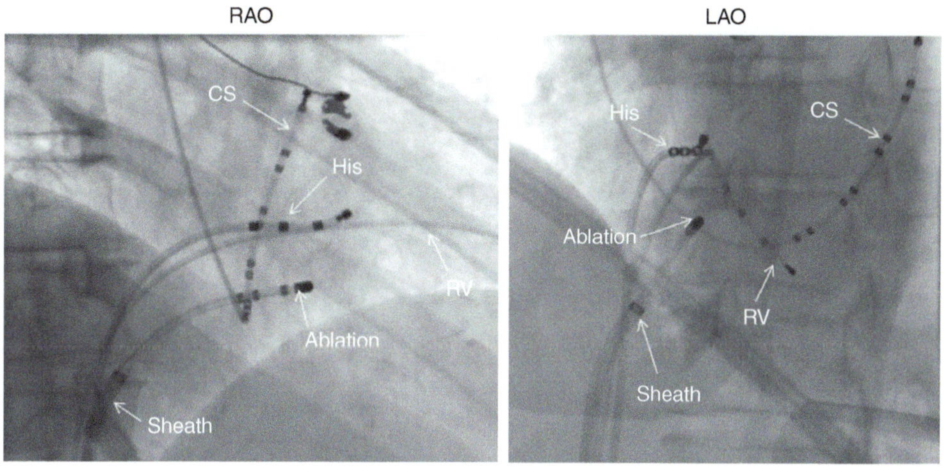

Fig. 23.27 Catheter position for radiofrequency slow-pathway ablation. The tip of the ablation catheter is between the coronary sinus ostium (CS os) and the tricuspid valve in the right anterior oblique (RAO) view. In the left anterior oblique (LAO) view, the tip of the ablation catheter is just posterior (septal) to the His catheter at the level of the CS os. Note the angled sheath supporting the ablation catheter. *RV,* Right ventricle.

the tricuspid annulus is associated with an increased risk of AV block.

Positioning of the catheters is best performed during sinus rhythm because the atrial and ventricular electrogram components are more easily discerned. The right anterior oblique view is especially useful for positioning catheters because it displays Koch's triangle en face. The angle of the left anterior oblique view should be adjusted so that the His catheter is perpendicular to the fluoroscopic plane. The ablation catheter should have a distal electrode 4 mm in length. The length of the deflecting segment of the ablation catheter that has proved most effective has ranged from 2 to 3 inches (D–F curves). The use of a long sheath with slight distal septal angulation often enhances catheter reach and stability. When using a sheath, it is important to keep the curves of the sheath and catheter coaxial. The ablation catheter is advanced into the right ventricle, moved inferiorly and medially so that it lies anterior to the CS os (Fig. 23.27). The ablation catheter is then withdrawn toward the tricuspid annulus until the distal pair of electrodes records a small atrial deflection and a large ventricular deflection (Figs. 23.28, A, B). Clockwise torque will move the sheath and catheter toward the septum. The atrial electrogram at successful sites may show multiple components. The A/V ratio recorded from the distal electrode pair in sinus rhythm may range from approximately 1:10–1:3.

Electrogram-Guided Approach

Ablation of the slow pathway can also be guided by identification of discrete electrical potentials that are thought to represent activation of the slow pathway. These slow pathway potentials have been described as sharp and rapid or slow and broad signals, occurring after the local atrial activation near the CS os. Slow pathway potentials are usually observed in the middle between the atrial and ventricular electrograms when mapping at the midanteroseptum region. Mapping more inferiorly shows the slow pathway potential approaching the atrial signal, and where it merges with the atrial signal signifies the optimal site of slow pathway ablation. Similar potentials may be observed in patients with or without AVNRT, as well as at sites distant from the location of the slow pathway. In order to distinguish slow pathway potentials, mapping should be limited to the posterior septum. Additionally, atrial pacing maneuvers can be performed to demonstrate a lower amplitude and more delayed recording of the slow pathway potential with more rapid rates of stimulation, consistent with decremental AV nodal conduction properties. Haïssaguerre et al.[44] and Jackman et al.[46] each described an electrogram-guided approach to ablation of the slow pathway. Both approaches, although they use different activation potentials, reduce the number of RF current applications by identifying critical components of the reentrant circuit. Jackman et al described a sharp late potential following a low-amplitude atrial signal near the CS os during sinus rhythm and suggested that this potential represents the atrial connection of the slow AV nodal pathway.[46] Consistent with this concept, during retrograde slow AV nodal conduction, the sequence is inverted, and the sharp potential precedes the atrial electrogram. This potential is usually recorded anterior to or just inside the CS os (Fig. 23.28B). The slow potential described by Haïssaguerre et al. is usually recorded at slightly more superior sites, although the locations where these two potentials can be recorded frequently overlap.[90,91] These potentials may represent activation of transitional cells as they approach the AV node or activation of the rightward inferior extension of the AV node.[10,48,91]

3DElectroanatomical Mapping Approach

A more recent approach that has emerged uses 3D electroanatomical voltage mapping to identify the slow pathway. Voltage

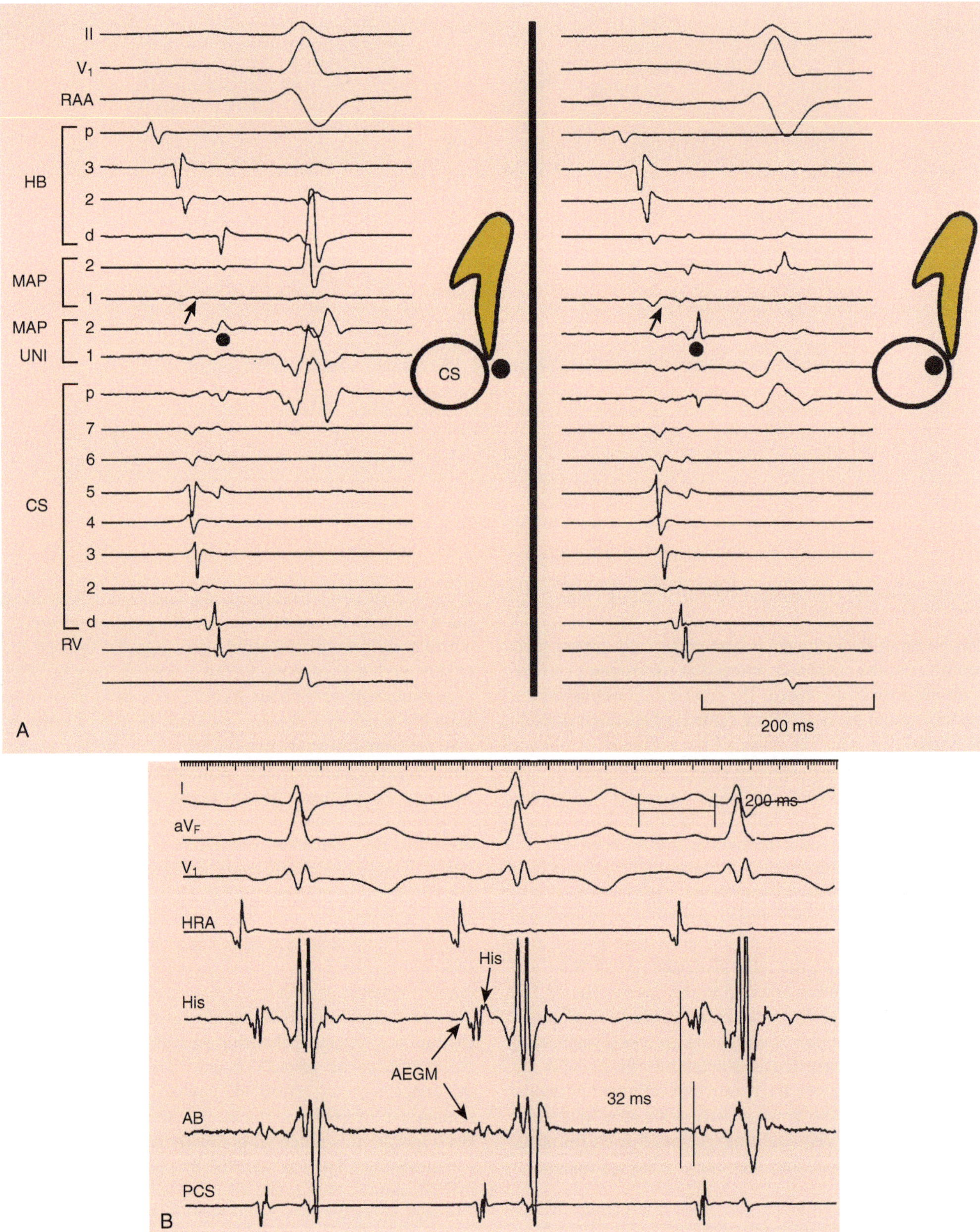

Fig. 23.28 (A) Electrograms recorded near the coronary sinus ostium and the rightward posterior (inferior) extension of the atrioventricular (AV) node. Bipolar and unipolar (UNI) recordings obtained from the mapping catheter (MAP) just before ablation of the slow AV nodal pathway. Late activation potentials *(closed circles)* believed to represent slow-pathway activation and the following local atrial activation *(arrows)* are recorded in front of the anterior edge of the coronary sinus ostium (CS, *left*) and just inside the coronary sinus *(right)*. (B) Intracardiac electrogram at site of successful slow-pathway ablation by the anatomic approach. The atrial electrogram (AEGM) on the ablation catheter (AB) is fractionated and has a 1:8 amplitude ratio compared with the ventricular electrogram. The difference in time of onset from the atrial component of the His electrogram to the onset of the atrial component of the ablation electrogram *(vertical lines)* is 32 ms. *d*, Distal; *HB*, His bundle; *HRA*, high right atrium; *p*, proximal; *PCS*, proximal coronary sinus; *RAA*, right atrial appendage; *RV*, right ventricle.

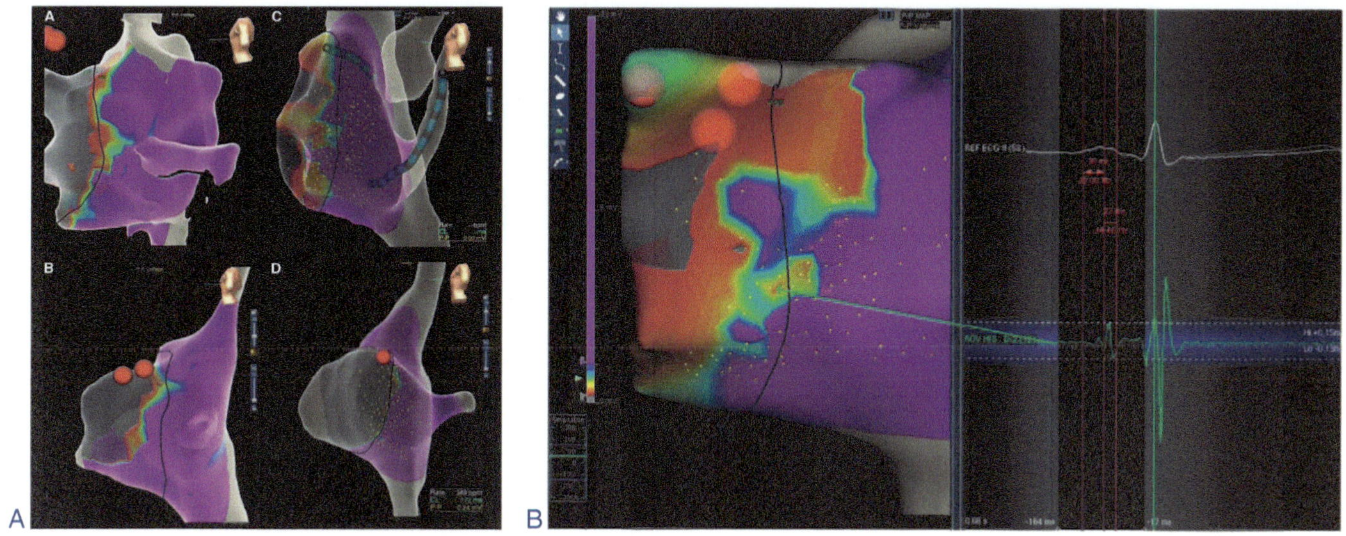

Fig. 23.29 A. Three-dimensional reconstruction of the right atrium and coronary sinus using the Navix mapping system (Abbott) to identify low voltage bridges between the tricuspid annulus on the left and the septum on the right. This image shows: A) Type I low-voltage bridges at voltage gradient mapping of Koch's triangle. B) Type II low-voltage bridges at voltage gradient mapping. C) A "double bridge" case, with a low-voltage bridge extension in a mid-septal location and another appendage in the lower part of Koch's triangle, at the coronary sinus ostium level. D) Voltage gradient map of Koch's triangle in a control patient that does not show voltage bridge. B. Typical "hump-and-spike" electrogram (length and amplitude) recorded inside a type I bridge that is the ideal target for cryoablation. (From Drago F, Battipaglia I, Russo MS, et al. Voltage gradient mapping and electrophysiologically guided cryoablation in children with AVNRT. *Europace.* 2018;20(4):665–672.)

mapping in the area of interest within and around the Triangle of Koch during sinus rhythm or atrial pacing can reveal areas of high voltage that are connected together by areas of low voltage. These low-voltage bridges are associated with function of the slow pathway and may be directly targeted for ablation. In order to optimize visualization of the low-voltage bridge, the voltage map gradient should be adjusted with the high-voltage range set to 1.5–2.0 mV and the low-voltage range incrementally adjusted until the low voltage bridge becomes apparent.[92,93]

This strategy provides direct visualization of the slow pathway and a more targeted approach to ablation, rather than empirically relying on anatomical landmarks or electrogram characteristics. Low-voltage mapping can be particularly useful when the slow pathway is not found in the commonly expected location. It has been increasingly used in the pediatric population, in whom the triangle of Koch is typically a smaller structure, and the risk of AV block is more detrimental (Figs. 23.29A, B).[94] Utilization of 3D electroanatomical mapping also allows for decreased procedure and fluoroscopy times. High-definition catheters are also being used with the 3D mapping system to map the triangle of Koch in sinus rhythm and during tachycardia. This can potentially identify the slow pathway turn around point that can be a more precise target for successful elimination of AVNRT with minimal risk of AV block.[95]

Atypical AVNRT: Slow-Slow and Fast-Slow Variants

Ablation for slow-slow and fast-slow AVNRT targets the slow AV nodal pathway that is used for retrograde conduction, which is often separate from the slow AV nodal pathway associated with antegrade conduction. Localization of the retrograde slow AV nodal pathway is guided by the site of the earliest retrograde atrial activation during AVNRT or ventricular pacing. This site is typically located between the tricuspid annulus and CS os in fast-slow AVNRT and along the anterior aspect of the proximal CS in slow-slow AVNRT (Fig. 23.30).[96] For slow-slow AVNRT, elimination of both antegrade and retrograde slow-pathway conduction is recommended to prevent recurrences of fast-slow and slow-fast AVNRT.[25] Mapping and ablation can be performed during tachycardia or during ventricular pacing to help identify the retrograde slow AV nodal pathway in patients with slow-slow or fast-slow AVNRT. Retrograde fast-pathway conduction is often weak in the setting of slow-slow AVNRT, therefore the retrograde slow pathway can often be targeted at the site of earliest retrograde atrial activation during ventricular pacing. This site is frequently found on the anterior aspect of the proximal CS.

Mapping is initially performed in the lower portion of the triangle of Koch, between the CS os and the tricuspid annulus, followed by mapping in the proximal portion of the CS. The site of earliest retrograde atrial activation is targeted for ablation. If ablation is performed in the proximal CS, low power (20 W) is initially used. The energy output is progressively increased while the impedance is monitored. Successful ablation results in elimination of retrograde conduction over the slow AV nodal pathway (Fig. 23.30).

Patients with slow-slow or fast-slow AVNRT frequently lack retrograde conduction over the fast AV nodal pathway.

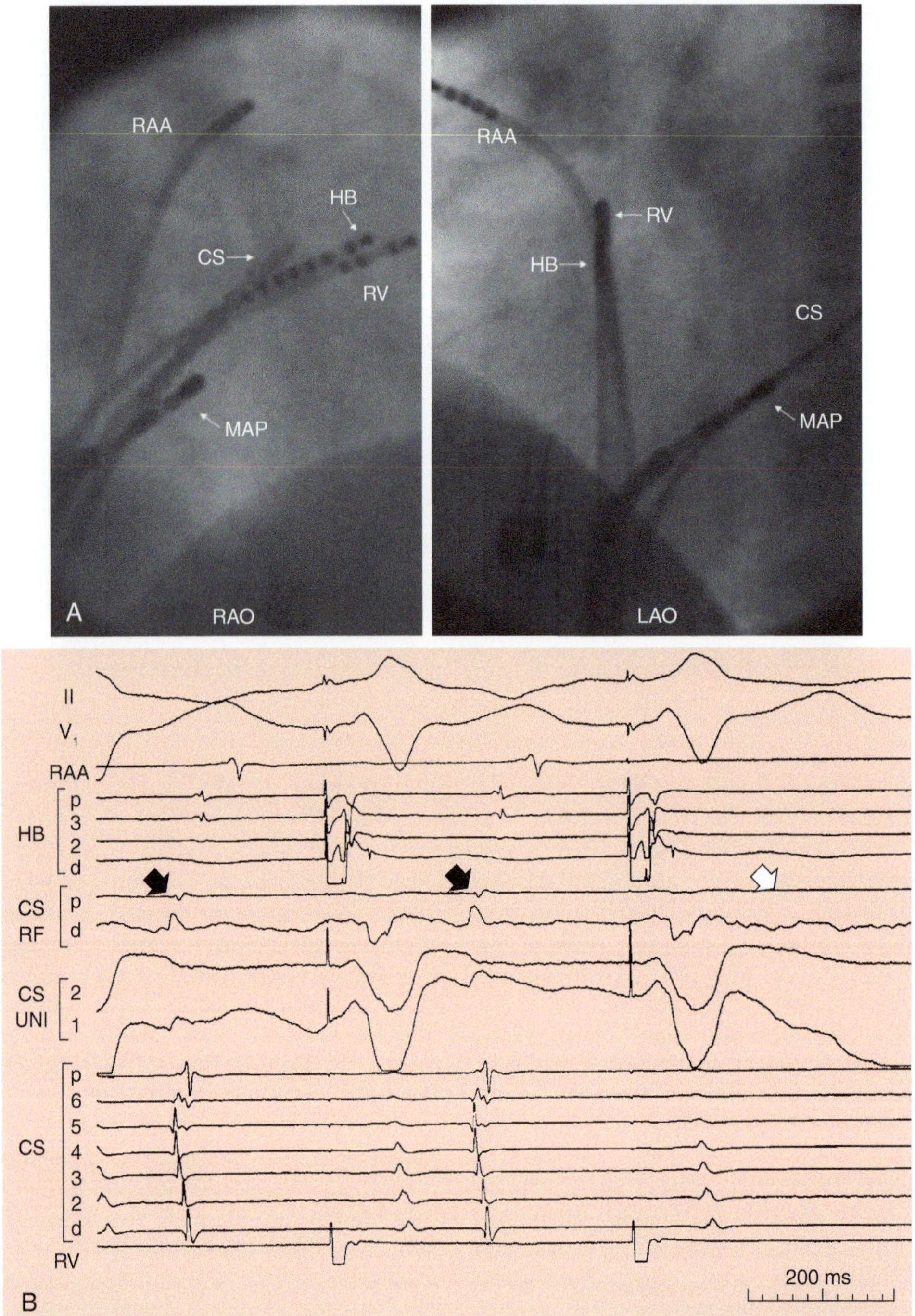

Fig. 23.30 (A) Site of earliest retrograde atrial activation during ventricular pacing in a patient with slow-slow atrioventricular nodal reentrant tachycardia. Radiographs in the right anterior oblique (RAO) and left anterior oblique (LAO) projections show the position of the mapping catheter (MAP) inside the proximal portion of the coronary sinus, about 1.5 cm from the ostium. Multipolar catheters are positioned in the coronary sinus (CS), right atrial appendage (RAA), His bundle (HB), and right ventricle (RV). (B) Retrograde block of slow atrioventricular (AV) nodal pathway conduction during radiofrequency current ablation. During delivery of radiofrequency current through a catheter in the proximal coronary sinus, the first two ventricular paced complexes are followed by retrograde conduction through the slow AV nodal pathway *(solid arrows)*. Retrograde block over the slow AV nodal pathway is observed following the third ventricular paced complex *(open arrow)*. *d,* Distal; *p,* proximal; *UNI,* unipolar.

Therefore during RF current application, junctional beats may have no retrograde conduction to the atrium, preventing assessment of AV nodal function during delivery of energy. In these patients, short applications of RF energy are delivered and AV nodal conduction between applications is evaluated. Alternatively, overdrive atrial pacing may allow continuous monitoring of antegrade AV conduction during ablation. In a multicenter study of RF ablation of conventional slow pathway

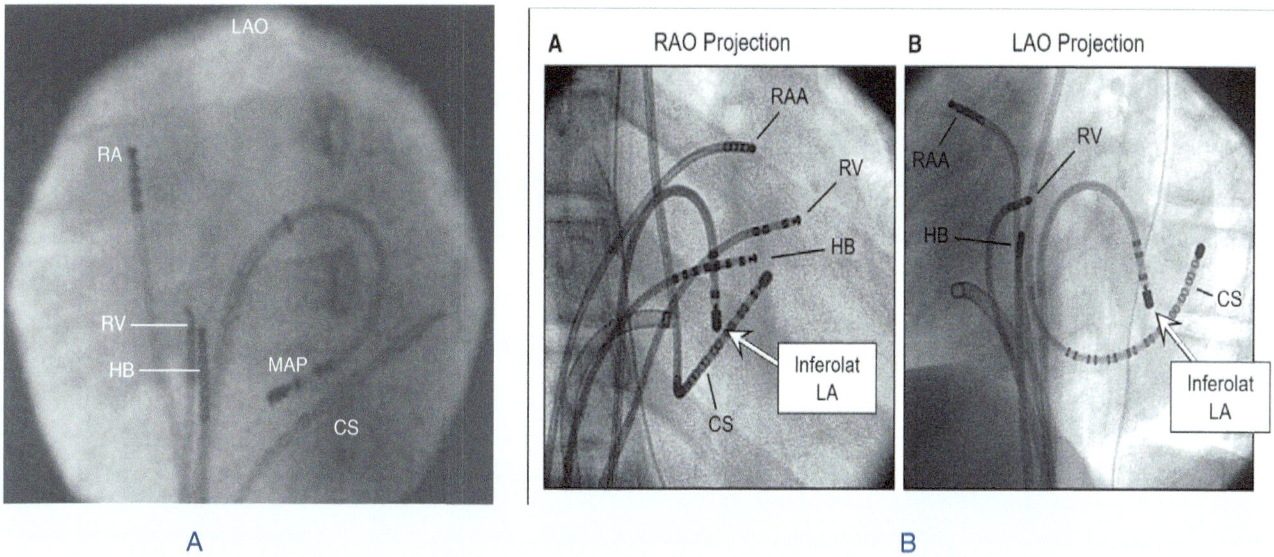

Fig. 23.31 Successful ablation sites in the left atrium in two patients with typical AVNRT using the left sided slow pathway as the antegrade limb. (A) Radiograph in left anterior oblique (LAO) projection showing successful mapping catheter (MAP) position at the inferomedial mitral annulus. The mapping catheter was introduced into the left atrium through a preformed sheath following transseptal puncture. (B) Catheter position in RAO and LAO projections showing the mapping catheter position (*arrow*) at the inferolateral mitral annulus. Resetting with the latest atrial extrastimulus was performed at these sites. Other catheters are positioned at the right atrial appendage (RA, RAA), His bundle region (HB), anterobasal right ventricle (RV), and coronary sinus (CS). (Modified from Lockwood D, Nakagawa H, Jackman WM. Electrophysiological characteristics of atrioventricular nodal reentrant tachycardia: implications for reentrant circuits. In: Zipes DP, Jalife J, eds, *Cardiac Electrophysiology: From Cell to Bedside*. 5th ed. Philadelphia, PA: Saunders Elsevier; 2009:615–646.)

region in 113 patients with atypical AVNRT (3 were left sided) that was compared to conventional slow pathway region ablation in age and sex matched typical AVNRT patients, the recurrence rate at 3 months was 5.6% in atypical and 1.8% in typical group. No additional ablation was done, and no AV block was noted.[97]

Left-Sided AVNRT

In approximately 2% of cases, extensive ablation at the inferior triangle of Koch fails to eliminate slow pathway conduction. In these cases, the left inferior extension of the AV node should be considered as the source of the anterograde slow pathway. The leftward inferior extension of the AV node can usually be effectively ablated at the roof of the CS, 1–3 cm from the CS os, or from the left inferior septal or inferoseptal mitral annular region (Fig. 23.31A).[65] An even rarer form of the left-sided variant of AVNRT has been described with the leftward inferior extension of the AV node located at the inferolateral mitral annulus (Fig. 23.31B).[66] In those cases, the anterograde slow pathway of the circuit can be localized by assessing the resetting response to left atrial extrastimuli during tachycardia. This is performed by delivering a single late atrial extrastimulus at different sites near the inferolateral mitral annulus while demonstrating unchanged morphology of the retrograde atrial signal and reproducible advancement of the next His bundle signal by at least 5 ms with subsequent resetting of the tachycardia cycle length, indicating engagement of the anterograde slow pathway without engagement of the retrograde fast pathway. The site at which this response was observed with the latest atrial extrastimulus is considered to be the atrial insertion of the anterograde slow pathway and targeted for ablation (Fig. 23.32).[64–67] Junctional rhythm is usually noted during ablation at these sites. These sites can be reached from the transseptal or retrograde aortic approaches. Another left sided variant of slow-slow or fast-slow AVNRT uses a superior slow pathway that manifests as earliest A at the His position during atypical AVNRT. This can be successfully ablated in the right atrium (superior to the His) or noncoronary aortic sinus of Valsalva (Fig. 23.33).[67]

RADIOFREQUENCY ABLATION

RF current is delivered from the distal 4-mm-tip electrode of the mapping-ablation catheter toward a pair of dispersive electrode pads placed over the posterior thorax. Larger-tip or irrigated electrodes are not necessary because of the superficial location of AV nodal tissue. Impedance is carefully monitored, and RF energy is halted for any sudden drop or rise in impedance or any evidence of AV or VA block. Catheter position is continuously monitored by fluoroscopy or real-time 3D catheter localization. It is advisable to use low power initially (20–30 W) to test for unwanted effects such as prolongation of the AH interval. After 15 seconds, the power can be gradually increased up to 50 W, with a target temperature

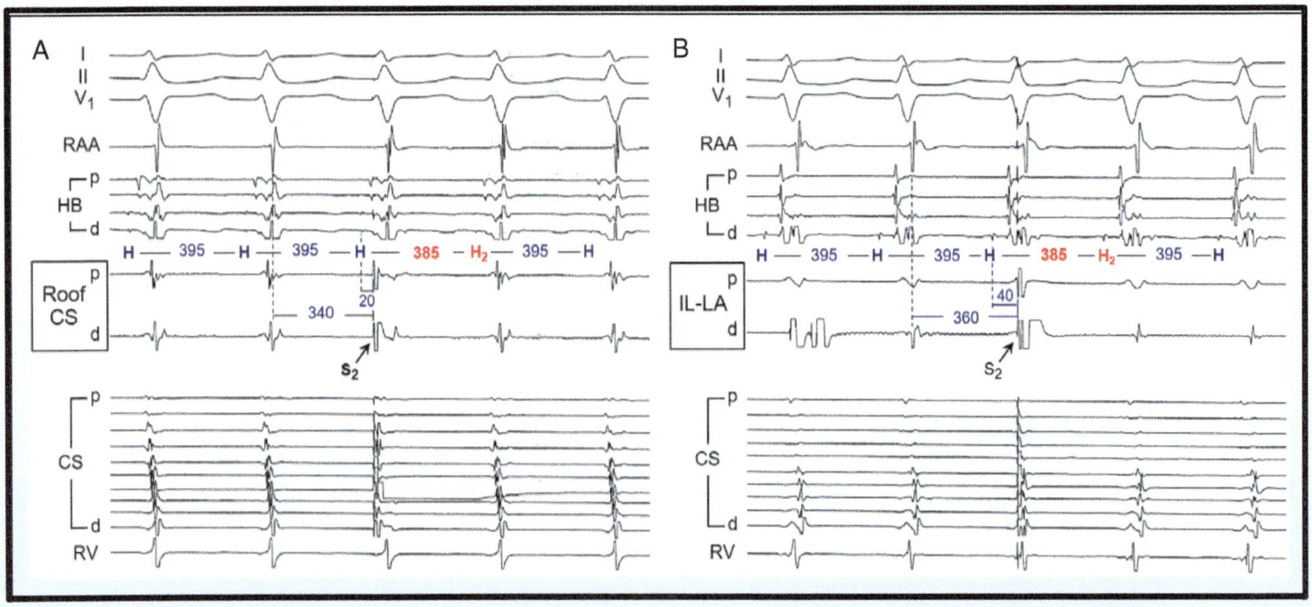

Fig. 23.32 Resetting technique for localizing the atrial end of the inferolateral left atrial slow pathway forming the anterograde limb of the slow/ fast reentrant circuit. (A) During slow/fast atrioventricular nodal reentrant tachycardia with constant cycle length 395 ms, an atrial extrastimulus was delivered to the mapping catheter (roof coronary sinus [CS]) at the roof of the coronary sinus, 4 cm from the ostium, 340 ms after the right atrial appendage (RAA) potential, and 20 ms after the His bundle (HB) potential. The extrastimulus did not prevent retrograde activation of the fast pathway as the timing and morphology of atrial activation in the His bundle electrogram were not changed (A-A = 395 ms in the HBp electrogram). The atrial extrastimulus advanced the next His bundle potential (H_2) by 10 ms (H-H_2 = 385 ms in the HBd electrogram). The advanced His Bundle potential (H_2) was followed by a similar 10 ms advance in atrial activation and a subsequent H_2-H interval equal to the tachycardia cycle length (395 ms in the HBd electrogram), indicating resetting of the tachycardia cycle length (ie, resetting the tachycardia). (B) When a later atrial extrastimulus (360 ms after the RAA potential and 40 ms after the HB potential) was delivered from the mapping catheter in the inferolateral left atrium (LA) close to the mitral annulus (arrow, S_2), after retrograde atrial activation had occurred (A-A = 395 ms in the HBp electrogram), the next His bundle potential (H_2) was advanced by 10 ms (H-H_2 = 385 ms in the HBd electrogram), thus resetting the tachycardia (10-ms advance in atrial activation and a subsequent H_2-H interval equal to the tachycardia cycle length of 395 ms). The resetting of the tachycardia with such a late atrial extrastimulus suggests this site is located close to the atrial end of the slow pathway forming the anterograde limb of the reentrant circuit. II, V1 indicates electrocardiographic leads II and V1; d, distal; and p, proximal. (From Stavrakis S, Jackman WM, Lockwood D, et al. Slow/fast atrioventricular nodal reentrant tachycardia using the inferolateral left atrial slow pathway: role of the resetting response to select the ablation target. *Circ Arrhythm Electrophysiol.* 2018;11(9):e006631.)

of 55–60°C for 30–60 seconds. Rarely the duration of RF application may be extended up to 90–120 seconds. Energy is limited to 20–30 W in the proximal CS. A few lesions are usually sufficient to eliminate AVNRT induction. An accelerated junctional rhythm at a slower rate (cycle length > 350 or 400 ms) is typically observed within a few seconds of effective RF ablation of the slow AV nodal pathway (Fig. 23.34A).[98-101] Although not specific for slow pathway ablation, the development of an accelerated junctional rhythm is strongly indicative of a successful ablation site. If this rhythm is not observed within 10–20 seconds of an ablation lesion, ablation should be stopped, and the ablation catheter repositioned as the absence of an accelerated junctional rhythm during ablation suggests an unsuccessful ablation site. The occurrence of successive rapid junctional beats (cycle length <350 ms) may be a sign of damage to the His bundle and should prompt cessation of RF delivery. Other signs of damage to the compact AV node or His bundle necessitating immediate termination of RF delivery include development of AV block, prolongation of the PR interval, or retrograde VA block during junctional rhythm (Fig. 23.34B). In rare cases, successful ablation of slow AV nodal pathway conduction can be achieved in the absence of junctional beats during RF energy application.[102] A junctional rhythm is not always observed during ablation of the fast-slow or slow-slow variants of AVNRT. In addition rapid junctional rhythm at cycle lengths shorter than the 1:1 conduction rate of the fast pathway can manifest functional retrograde block. If these characteristics remain, the catheter is repositioned, and RF current is applied at a different position. In a study involving 387 patients with AVNRT and 385 successful ablations out of 692 RF applications, the sensitivity and specificity of

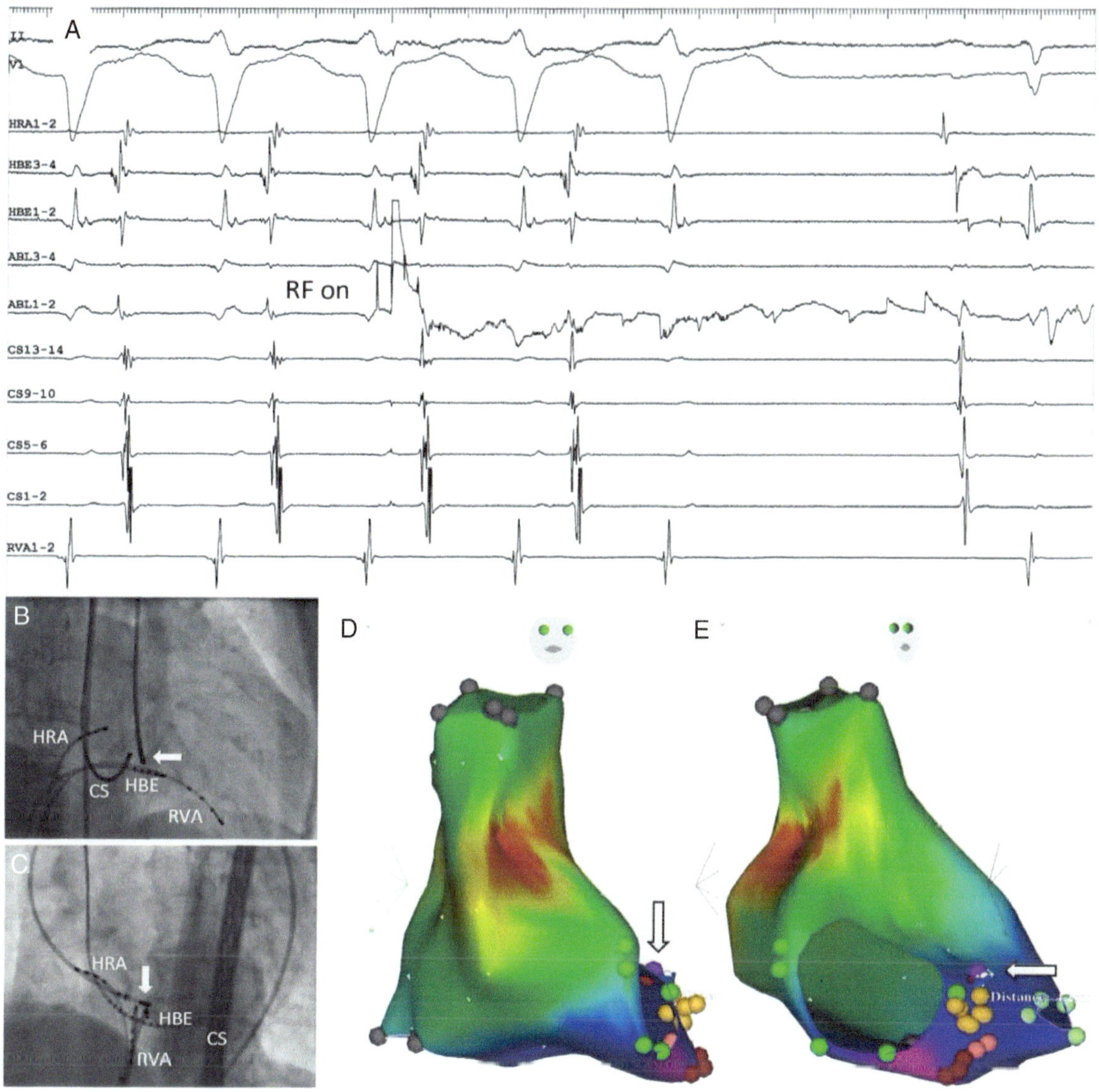

Fig. 23.33 Intracardiac recordings during tachycardia immediately before and after successful radiofrequency (RF) delivery (A) and fluoroscopic views showing the position of catheters (B and C) and CARTO activation maps of the right atrium and noncoronary aortic cusp (noncoronary sinus of Valsalva [NCSV]) during sinus rhythm (D and E) in the right and left anterior oblique views, respectively, at the successful ablation (ABL) in NCSV. (A) The atrial electrogram at ABL1-2 precedes the onset of the atrial electrogram at the His bundle electrogram (HBE) by 4 ms. The tachycardia ended 1.3 seconds after the onset of radiofrequency delivery followed by no junctional rhythm. (B and C) The *white arrows* point to the tip of the ablation catheter at the site of successful ablation. CS indicates coronary sinus catheter; HRA, high right atrium; and RVA, right ventricular apical catheter. (D and E) The distance between the site of successful ablation (purple tag and open arrows) and the nearest HB (yellow tags) measured 4.7 mm. (From Kaneko Y, Naito S, Okishige K, et al. Atypical fast-slow atrioventricular nodal reentrant tachycardia incorporating a "superior" slow pathway: a distinct supraventricular tachyarrhythmia. *Circulation.* 2016;133:114–123.)

junctional rhythm as a sign of success were 99.5% and 79.1%, respectively, with a positive predictive value of 55.5%.[89] In another study, junctional ectopy was seen more frequently (100% vs. 65%) and for a longer duration (7.1 ± 7.1 vs. 5.0 ± 7.0 seconds) during successful versus unsuccessful RF applications.[99] After each RF current application, programmed atrial stimulation, rapid atrial pacing, or both are performed to determine the presence or absence of slow-pathway conduction or inducible AVNRT. A recent multicenter study in patients with typical and atypical AVNRT showed noninducibility of the arrhythmia, usually after ablation-induced junctional rhythm, and despite isoproterenol challenge, is the most credible endpoint for success. Induction of a junctional rhythm during ablation was a sensitive but not a specific marker of success and residual dual AV nodal conduction was not predictive of recurrence.[103]

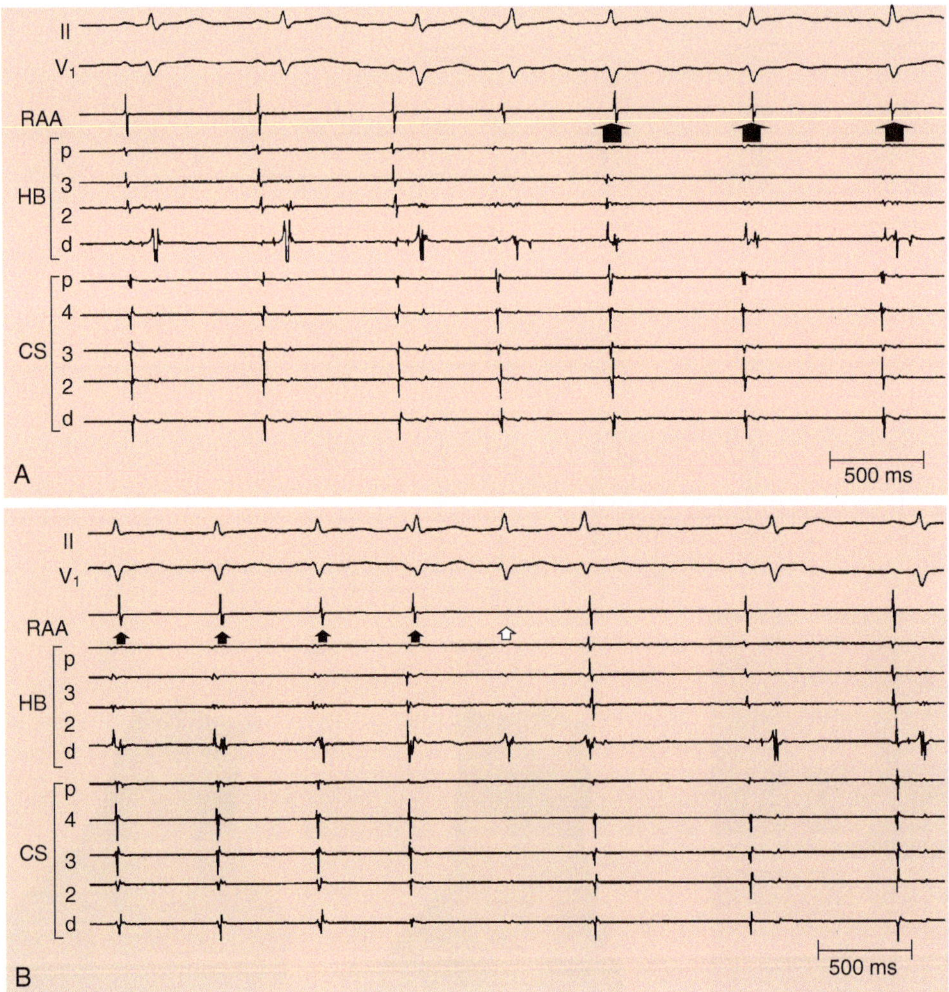

Fig. 23.34 (A) Induction of a junctional rhythm during radiofrequency application between the tricuspid annulus and the ostium of the coronary sinus (CS). One-to-one retrograde conduction over the fast atrioventricular (AV) nodal pathway *(arrows)* implies preserved normal AV nodal function during energy delivery. (B) Retrograde block over the fast AV nodal pathway during radiofrequency application. One-to-one retrograde conduction over the fast AV nodal pathway during catheter ablation *(filled arrows)* is followed by sudden retrograde block manifested by absence of atrial activation *(open arrow)*. Rapid discontinuation of energy application resulted in preservation of AV nodal conduction. *d,* Distal; *HB,* His bundle; *p,* proximal; *RAA,* right atrial appendage.

CRYOABLATION

The target for cryoablation of the slow pathway is similar to that for RF energy, except that with cryoablation the successful sites are often more superior toward the compact AV node than with RF ablation (Fig. 23.35). It is not unusual that the cryoablation catheter must be positioned midway between the CS and the site of the His bundle recording, a position considered to be of high risk in RF ablation. The 6-mm-tip or the 8-mm-tip catheter has proved more effective than the original 4-mm-tip catheter (see Table 23.4). Catheter stability during cryoablation is afforded by ice adherence to the tissue, heralded by the loss of electrograms at the distal electrode. At this point, atrial pacing is begun to assess slow-pathway conduction either by repeated extrastimulus testing or by atrial pacing at a cycle length just above the AV Wenckebach cycle length. If slow-pathway conduction is eliminated within 20–30 seconds, the ablation is continued for a full 4 minutes at −60°C or below.

Cryomapping can be performed initially by reducing the electrode temperature to −30°C and monitoring for slow-pathway block.[104,105] This allows for more rapidly reversible effects, but the superficial tissue cooling with cryomapping may provide false-negative findings; that is, cooling at lower temperatures may be successful at sites of cryomapping failure. Either cryomapping or cryoablation may be initiated during AVNRT with very little chance of catheter movement due to ice adherence to the tissue. Fluoroscopy is not needed to check the position of the catheter once tissue adhesion has occurred, significantly shortening fluoroscopy time.[106–108]

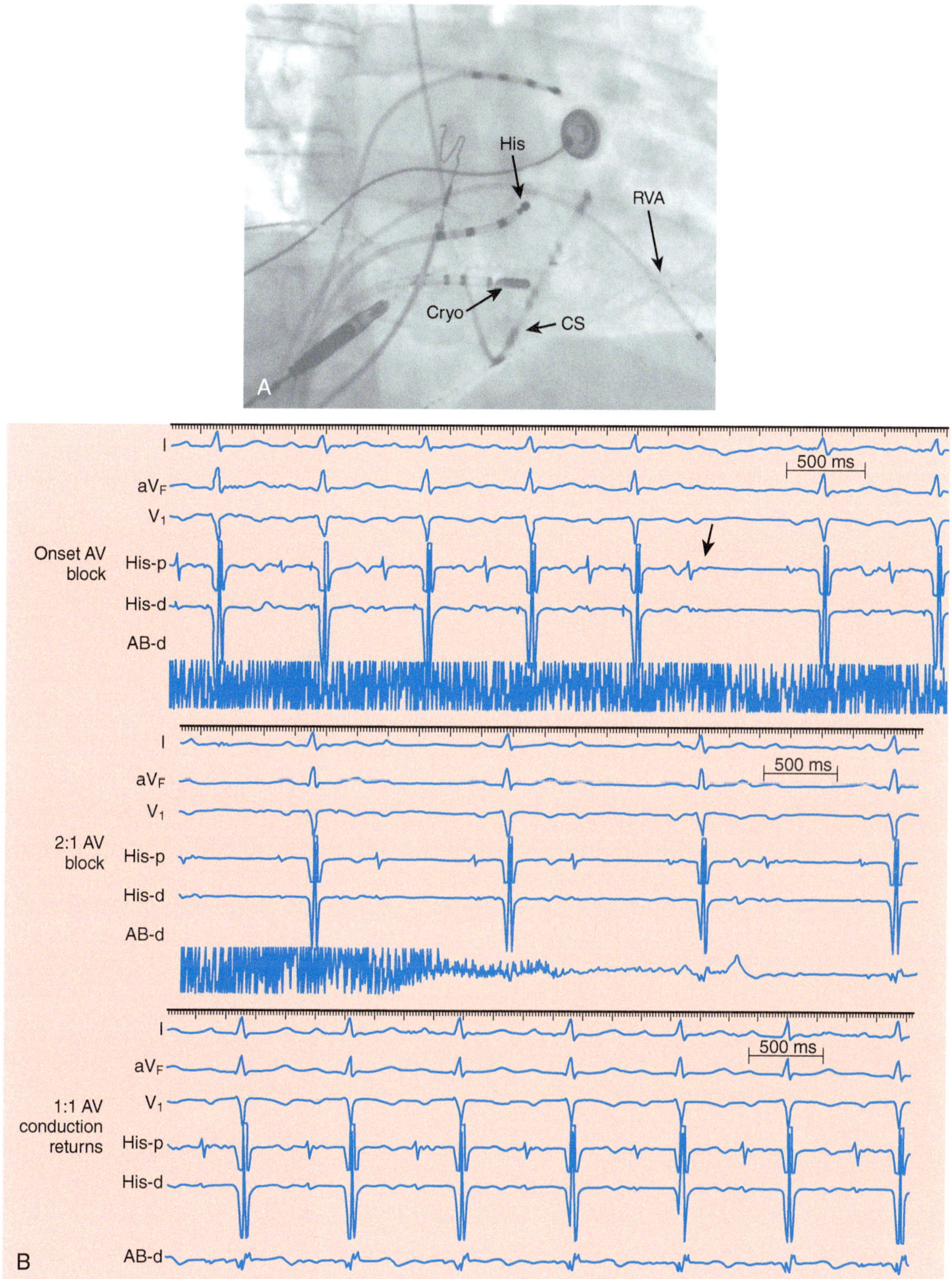

Fig. 23.35 (A) Right anterior oblique view of cryoablation catheter (Cryo) position for slow-pathway ablation. The ablation tip is about halfway between the estimated location of the coronary sinus ostium (CS os) and the His recording. Energy delivery at more inferior sites failed to terminate slow-fast atrioventricular (AV) nodal reentry in this patient. Although this site would be considered at high risk of producing AV block with radiofrequency energy, the need for cryoablation at this superior location is not unusual. In this patient, ablation here resulted in slow-pathway elimination without altering antegrade AV conduction. (B) Transient AV block during slow-pathway cryoablation. *Top,* Tachycardia was terminated by the cryoenergy; however during the ongoing ablation, there is slight atrium-His bundle interval prolongation followed by AV block *(arrow). Middle,* Cryoablation is immediately discontinued, as evidenced by the return of the electrograms on the distal ablation electrodes (AB-d) as the ice investing the electrode melts. There is 2:1 AV block on termination of the ablation. *Bottom,* One minute after termination of cryoablation, 1:1 AV conduction resumes. The patient had no adverse effects from the ablation procedure, and AV nodal reentry was no longer inducible. *d,* Distal; *p,* proximal; *RVA,* right ventricular apex.

TABLE 23.4 Clinical Studies on Cryoablation for Atrioventricular Nodal Reentrant Tachycardia

Author/year	No. of Patients	F/U (months)	APS Cryo	Rec Cryo	Tip (mm)	APS RF	Rec RF	*P*
Zrenner et al. 2004	200	8.1	97%	8%	4	98%	1%	.03
Friedman et al. 2004	103	6	91%	6%	4	—	—	
Kimman et al. 2004	63	13 ± 7	93%	10%	4	91%	9%	NS
Collins et al. 2006	117	12	98%	8%	4	100%	2%	NS
Jensen-Urstad et al. 2006	75	12.7	99%	5%	6	—	—	—
Papez et al. 2006	53	8.1 ± 7.0	96%	12%	4	96%	6%	NS
Gaita et al. 2006	87	27 ± 13	96%	10%	4	—	—	N/A
Gupta et al. 2006	71	2.2 + 0.4	85%	20%	4	97%	6%	0.01
De Sisti et al. 2007	69	18 ± 9	87%	28%	6	—	—	—
Avari et al. 2008	80	10.7	97%	3%	6	95%	2%	NS
Bastani et al. 2009	312	22.4 ± 12.7	99%	5.8%	6	—	—	—
Chan et al. 2009	80	13.6	98%	9%	6	95%	1%	NS
Deisenhofer et al. 2010	509	6	97%	9%	6	98%	4%	0.029
Schwagten et al. 2011	274	51.6 ± 30	97%	11%	4	96%	5%	NS
Rodriguez-Entem et al. 2013	119	8.3 ± 1.4	98%	15%	6	100%	3.4%	0.027
Chaumont C et al. 2020	409	36.8 ± 26	98%	9.2%	6	99%	2.7%	
Olshausen et al. 2021	91	60	95%	11%	6			Largest atypical AVNRT cryoablation study with long-term recurrence similar to typical AVNRT (8.8%)

APS, Acute procedural success; *F/U*, follow-up; *N/A*, not applicable; *NS*, not significant; *RF*, radiofrequency.

During cryoablation, the conduction properties of the fast and slow AV nodal pathways are continuously checked using atrial stimulation. Continuous monitoring of the AH interval is important because the lesion becomes larger than indicated by cryomapping or early in the stages of therapeutic ablation.[105] A useful maneuver is to pace the atrium at cycle lengths 10–20 ms longer than the Wenckebach cycle length during cryoablation to identify incipient damage to the AV node. Ablation should be immediately discontinued if high-grade block occurs, there is dramatic prolongation of the Wenckebach cycle length (by about 100 ms), or Wenckebach block occurs at cycle lengths longer than 500 ms. Termination of AVNRT during tissue cooling, abolition of 1:1 AV conduction over the slow AV nodal pathway, and inability to reinduce AVNRT are markers of success. It is important to note that no junctional rhythm is elicited during cryoablation. It is useful to reassess the status of slow-pathway function and AVNRT inducibility 30–45 minutes after the final cryoablation lesion, because acute recovery is more common than with RF ablation.

The choice between cryoablation and RF ablation needs to be determined on an individual basis. Patients with previous ablation near the fast AV nodal pathway region and those with a short distance between the compact AV node and the roof of the CS os may benefit from cryoablation because of their higher risk of AV block. Another subgroup of high-risk patients includes those with a prolonged AH interval in the basal state.

END POINTS OF ABLATION

Prior to ablation it is necessary to establish end points to assess for ablation success. In the setting of easily inducible tachycardia at baseline, ablation is considered successful if the tachycardia cannot be reinduced, with and without administration of isoproterenol, and there is no further evidence of dual AV nodal physiology (Box 23.4). However, complete elimination of all slow pathway conduction is not always required to be considered a successful ablation, and single echo beats may still be observed. Residual dual AV nodal physiology with single echo beats within a 30 ms decrement in atrial extrastimulus pacing without inducible tachycardia can still be an endpoint for successful ablation.[109–112] Further ablation is recommended if two or more echo beats occur or if single echo beats are observed over a wider window of extrastimulus coupling intervals. Ablation endpoints are less clear when sustained tachycardia cannot be reliably induced at baseline. In these cases, alternative signs of effective slow pathway ablation would have to be relied upon. As previously mentioned, loss of dual AV nodal physiology or

BOX 23.4 End Points for Radiofrequency Delivery

Tachycardia rendered noninducible with and without isoproterenol challenge
Elimination or modification of slow-pathway function

- Elimination of atrium-His bundle (AH) interval jumps
- Elimination of 1:1 antegrade conduction over the slow atrioventricular (AV) nodal pathway
- Retrograde ventriculoatrial block through the slow AV nodal pathway (fast-slow and slow-slow)
- Increase in AV Wenckebach CL
- Decrease in fast pathway ERP cycle length

Slow junctional rhythm during ablation
AH interval jump with single echoes only (previously inducible) over a short window of S2 (30 ms)
Fast-pathway injury (AV block)
PR interval prolongation (persistent)
Transient antegrade AV block after radiofrequency (caution warranted for further ablation)

single echo beats within a 30 ms decrement in atrial extrastimulus pacing can serve as a successful endpoint. During ablation, the occurrence of a slow junctional ectopic rhythm can be indicative of an effective radiofrequency ablation lesion. However, it should be noted that junctional beats are not typically observed during cryoablation of the slow pathway. Successful slow pathway ablation would result in an increase in the AV Wenckebach cycle length, due to the absence of slow pathway conduction to maintain 1:1 conduction beyond the block cycle length of the fast pathway. Additionally, the effective refractory period of the fast pathway can become shorter after successful slow pathway ablation. This phenomenon is thought to be related to the electrotonic interactions between the fast and slow pathways, and therefore improved fast pathway conduction after the removal of the electrotonic effect that the slow pathway might exert on the fast pathway.

It has been suggested that if AVNRT is easily induced at baseline without the use of isoproterenol, there is no need administer this drug after ablation to confirm noninducibility.[113] However, sedation and anesthesia change the balance of the autonomic nervous system over time and the conditions found at the beginning of the procedure may be different than the one after the ablation. Therefore it is often recommended to give isoproterenol after ablation and perform atrial and ventricular stimulation during and following drug administration. Reassessment of tachycardia non-inducibility or alternative endpoints of successful ablation is typically repeated after a 30-minute waiting period following the last ablation lesion.

Complications

Complications related to AVNRT ablation are relatively uncommon (Table 23.6). The most significant complication of AVNRT ablation is AV block. Procedure-related AV block ultimately requiring implantation of a permanent pacemaker has been reported in 0–0.9% of cases. Predictors of acute AV block include ablation superior to the CS os, greater number of delivered RF lesions, worsening of anterograde AV conduction during ablation, occurrence of junctional rhythm with retrograde VA block during ablation, and occurrence of a fast junctional ectopic rhythm during ablation. Risk of late AV block is higher in patients with transient AV block during the procedure and in those with baseline PR prolongation who undergo ablation with complete elimination of slow pathway conduction.[114] Late development of AV block has also been observed with patients receiving pacemaker months to years after ablation, although this is rarer than periprocedural AV block. Patients who underwent late pacemaker implantation were noted to be older and to have had a longer duration of the ablation procedure.[115] It should be noted, however that it may be difficult to distinguish procedure-related AV block from unrelated AV block when it develops much later after ablation. Other reported rare complications of AVNRT ablation include pericardial effusion, pulmonary embolism, and vascular injury such as groin hematoma.

PREVENTING ATRIOVENTRICULAR BLOCK DURING CATHETER ABLATION

AV block from slow-pathway ablation may occur because of direct injury to the compact AV node or fast pathway, especially with anatomical variants in which the compact AV node or fast pathway is inferiorly displaced. In addition unrecognized damage to the AV nodal artery or preexisting fast-pathway dysfunction (intrinsic or from previous ablation) may also contribute to the development of AV block.

Several strategies have been suggested to minimize the risk of procedure-related AV block (Table 23.5). The most important method is close attention to anterograde and retrograde AV conduction during ablation and immediate discontinuation in the event of any junctional beats with VA block or evidence of worsening anterograde AV conduction including PR prolongation. Atrial pacing faster than the junctional rhythm rate during ablation allows for continuous assessment of antegrade conduction in cases of doubt. Rapid junctional rhythm (cycle length less than 350 ms) has been described as an indicator of impending AV block and also warrants withdrawal of ablation.[100] The risk of AV block increases with more superior ablation sites, limiting ablation to sites no higher than the level of the CS os may also help avoid AV block. However, AV block can occur at more inferior sites or even within the CS, such as with anatomical variants with inferiorly displaced compact AV node or fast pathway, or with damage to the AV nodal artery, as previously mentioned.[116] Gradual energy titration starting with low-energy levels has been recommended to avoid potentially harmful energy diffusion and reduce the risk of irreversible AV block.[117]

3-dimensional mapping can be utilized to maintain a sufficient distance between the ablation sites and the position of the His. Mapping would first be performed and any sites where His signals are recorded would be marked. With the His sites marked on the map, their distance from potential targets for ablation can be monitored.

Pace mapping of the triangle of Koch has been described to localize and avoid ablation near the antegrade fast pathway,

TABLE 23.5 **Preventing Atrioventricular Block**

Method	Description	Comment
Ablation sites below triangle of Koch	Inferior to level of CS roof	Standard practice
Monitor retrograde junctional conduction	Discontinue RF for loss of 1:1 retrograde conduction	Standard practice
Monitor for rapid junctional rhythm[100]	Discontinue RF for junctional rhythm < 350 ms	Not prospectively tested
Δ AA timing His and ablation recordings[147]	Difference in timing between AEGM His and AEGM ablation site > 20 ms	Not prospectively tested
Pace mapping triangle of Koch[118]	Identify site on septum producing shortest stimulus to His time and avoid ablation there	Not prospectively tested
Overdrive atrial pacing	Pace atrium faster than junctional rate to monitor antegrade conduction	Not prospectively tested
Gradual power titration[117]	Start at 5 W and increase power by 5 W every 5 seconds until junctional rhythm, then increase power by 10 W for total RF for 120 seconds	Not prospectively tested
3D mapping	Mark distance from ablator to His and avoid ablation within 10 mm	Not prospectively tested
Ablation end point	Non inducible and single echo over (over narrow window) is acceptable	Not prospectively tested
Cryoablation	6 mm tip	Extremely low incidence of AV block

AA, Atrial-atrial interval; *AEGM*, atrial electrogram; *AV*, atrioventricular; *CS*, coronary sinus; *RF*, radiofrequency; *Δ*, difference.

thereby reducing the risk of AV block.[118] This strategy is particularly useful in the setting of absent anterograde fast pathway conduction, or when the anterograde fast pathway is located abnormally close to the slow pathway. Atrial pacing is performed from at least three sites in the triangle of Koch including the anteroseptal, midseptal, and posteroseptal regions. The stimulus to His interval is recorded by pacing the atrium at each site, and the site of the shortest stimulus to His interval is assumed to be the insertion site of the anterograde fast pathway. Ventricular pacing is similarly performed from the adjacent anteroseptal, midseptal, and posteroseptal regions in the right ventricle to localize the site of the retrograde fast pathway. When the anterograde fast pathway is localized to the anteroseptal region, then conventional slow pathway ablation can be performed. When the anterograde fast pathway is localized to the midseptal region, ablation is limited to the posteroseptal region with the longest atrial to His interval. When the antegrade fast pathway is localized to the posteroseptal region or is absent, then retrograde fast pathway ablation in the anteroseptal region can be performed.

OUTCOMES OF SLOW PATHWAY ABLATION

Radiofrequency Ablation Outcomes

The acute success rate for radiofrequency slow-pathway ablation for AVNRT has been reported as 97–100% in large series (Table 23.6). Randomized trials have shown equivalent outcomes using the anatomical and electrogram-guided approaches, although the electrogram-guided approach may have a lower incidence of residual slow-pathway function.[119] Recurrence of AVNRT after initially successful ablation have been reported in approximately 2–5% of patients and is higher in atypical AVNRT. AVNRT recurrences following radiofrequency ablation typically occur within the first days up to a year after ablation. Predictors of long-term success of AVNRT ablation include occurrence of more junctional beats during ablation or complete elimination of slow pathway conduction and dual AV nodal physiology, however these findings are not consistent.[109–112,120–122]

Cryoablation Outcomes

Available clinical data on cryoablation of the slow pathway have reported acute success rates of 85–99% with recurrence rates of 3–28% (Table 23.4).[123–127] Most AVNRT recurrences following cryoablation have been noted to occur relatively late between 1-6 years after ablation. A recent study of 409 patients showed similar acute success of cryoablation (98.8%) and radiofrequency ablation (99.3%). Recurrence in long-term follow-up was higher with cryoablation (9.2%) as compared to radiofrequency ablation (2.7%).[128]

Retrograde Fast-Pathway Ablation

Early catheter ablation techniques for the treatment of AVNRT that were directed at the fast pathway region resulted in a significant incidence of PR prolongation and AV block (20% in one study). Traditional slow pathway ablation was found to be both highly successful and safer regarding the risk of AV block and is the accepted and guideline-recommended method of AVNRT treatment.[1]

Approximately 3% of patients undergoing ablation for AVNRT have PR prolongation at baseline.[129–134] Patients with delayed conduction or prolonged refractoriness of the fast AV nodal pathway have an increased risk of AV block after ablation of the slow AV nodal pathway. However, several reports have documented a lack of detrimental effect of catheter ablation in such patients, despite preexisting abnormal AV conduction.[129–134] The lack of effect of slow AV nodal pathway ablation despite an abnormal fast AV nodal pathway may be explained

TABLE 23.6 **Contemporary Results for Radiofrequency Slow-Pathway Ablation**

Study	No. of Patients	Approach	Acute Success (%)	Recurrence Rate (%)	AV Block (%)	Complication Rate (%)	Comments
Gonzalez et al. 2017	500	Combined anatomic and EGM guided	100	1.5	0.2	0.2, AV block; 0.4, pulmonary embolism	
Topilski et al. 2006[31]	901	Anatomic	97	2.8	3.4 transient AV block; 0.8 permanent AV block (pacemaker)	4, AV block (2 with pericardial effusion)	Two catheter (single diagnostic and ablation) approach used in 65% of patients
Kihel et al. 2006[143]	76	Combined anatomic and EGM guided	99.6	0.7	0	1.8, pericardial effusion and pulmonary embolus	Same results <75 and >75 years old
Rostock et al. 2005[144]	578	Anatomic	100	2.5	0.7 all PPM	Only AV block reported	Same results <75 and >75 years old
McElderry and Kay 2006[89]	2333	Anatomic	99	1.7	0.2	0.5, AV block (3 with pericardial tamponade)	3 AV block in last 2283 patients
Estner et al. 2005[121]	506	Combined anatomic and EGM guided	98.8	5.2	0.9 AV block requiring pacemaker	Only AV block	Younger age only risk of recurrence
Efromidis et al. 2009[119]	228	Randomized to anatomic or EGM guided	100, both approaches	1.7, both approaches	0.9 AV block, both approaches	Only AV block	Prospective randomized trial
Feldman et al. 2010.[112]	1419	Combined anatomic and EGM guided	98.1	1.5	0.07	Only AV block	Age < 20, female and large echo window (85 ms) predicted recurrence
Katritsis et al. 2018[97]	113	Anatomic and EGM guided	100	5.6% (3 month follow up)	0	0	Retrospective multicenter study

AV, Atrioventricular; *EGM*, electrogram; *PPM*, permanent pacemaker.

by several factors. One possibility is that in these patients, the left atrial (mitral annulus) input preserves AV nodal conduction despite damage to the right-sided inputs.[13] Another possibility is that, before ablation, conduction through the posterior inputs (slow AV nodal pathway) prolongs the refractory period of the anterior input (fast AV nodal pathway) because of concealed retrograde conduction of the fast pathway.[133] Nevertheless slow-pathway (SP) ablation was associated with a 3% incidence of acute AV block and a 12% incidence of late AV block in patients with dual AV nodal physiology at baseline.[129] Selective retrograde fast-pathway (FP) ablation was performed in AVNRT patients with prolonged PR interval at baseline and absence of dual AV nodal physiology. This approach was associated with persistent intraprocedural AV block in one of 10 patients (10%); however there was no late AV block reported.[129]

Ablation of the retrograde fast pathway can be considered in select patients with AVNRT in whom antegrade fast-pathway conduction is absent or severely impaired. These patients can be identified by a markedly prolonged PR interval greater than 300 ms at baseline, baseline AH interval 140 ms or greater, AH jump that occurs at long pacing cycle length 600 ms or longer, and/or initiation of typical AVNRT at long coupling intervals greater than 400 ms.[135,136] It is interesting to note that anterograde and retrograde FP conduction can be dissociated in these patients and this discordance (weak antegrade and robust retrograde FP conduction) contributes to the ease of initiating AVNRT. Pursuing standard SP ablation in these patients presents a high risk of advanced AV block requiring pacemaker insertion. Retrograde FP ablation should be considered in these patients to preserve antegrade conduction through the AV node.

The fast pathway can be targeted by positioning the ablation catheter to record the maximal amplitude of the His potential, and then withdrawing the catheter toward the atrium with a clockwise torque to obtain a large atrial electrogram and smaller ventricular electrogram while the His potential decreases to the minimal amplitude or disappears (<0.1 mV). This is posterior and superior to location of standard His catheter. There was no acute or long-term AV block using this approach for retrograde fast pathway conduction in 53 patients with typical AVNRT. AH prolonged from 79 ± 19 ms–145 ± 37 ms. Acute success rate was 96%, retrograde FP block was noted in 72% of the cases and recurrence rate was 6% at 12 ± 7 months.[137] Attempts at targeting retrograde fast pathway may be refined by mapping the site of earliest retrograde atrial activation in this area during AVNRT or ventricular pacing. Initial ablation was started 3–5 mm posterior and superior to the target site and 3D mapping was used to mark the His position and ablation lesions (Fig. 23.36).[136] Radiofrequency energy is delivered at the target site starting at low-energy levels (5–10 W). Energy delivery is withdrawn when there is impedance rise, PR prolongation greater than 30–50%, high-grade AV block, or rapid junctional rhythm with VA block. Additional lesion was applied anterior superior and posterior inferior to successful site. Endpoints of retrograde fast pathway ablation are noninducibility of AVNRT and VA block.[136] Table 23.7 shows the long-term safety and efficacy of retrograde FP ablation in rendering typical AVNRT noninducible in patients with prolonged PR interval and absence of antegrade FP conduction.

ABLATION OF JUNCTIONAL TACHYCARDIA

Patients with junctional tachycardia are often quite symptomatic and if left untreated may develop heart failure particularly if their tachycardia is incessant. Beta-blockers, propafenone, sotalol and amiodarone have been used for medical treatment with variable success. Catheter ablation is an effective alternative when medical therapy fails or is not preferred. The initial report of ablation for JT by Gillette et al[138] is of two cases 3 and 6 months old using direct current shocks in the area of His recording, both resulted in AV nodal block, followed by pacemaker implants with one resuming AV conduction 3 days later. Hamdan et al[139,140] reported their experience with RF ablation for FJT. They targeted the site of earliest retrograde atrial activation when VA conduction was present during JT. It is often useful to introduce a premature ventricular beat during tachycardia that will pull the ventricular electrogram away allowing the earliest A to be clearly seen that can be targeted for ablation. In the absence of VA conduction and hence an atrial target site, sequential RF applications should be made in the posterior septum (slow pathway region) followed by RF applications in the midseptum and anteroseptum respectively if tachycardia persists. Ablation was successful in 14/17 patients; one patient had transient AV block and one patient had persistent AV block requiring pacemaker. Atrial overdrive pacing to assess AV conduction can be performed during ablation to minimize risk of AV block.[141] Another technique is mapping the perinodal region and applying radiofrequency catheter ablation at the site where catheter manipulation resulted in tachycardia termination. This requires very minute catheter movements to be certain that the catheter is still at the same site at which mechanical termination occurred and use of 3D mapping is very useful.[139] Unipolar recording on the ablation catheter can be used to identify the successful site. Unipolar recording that shows shorter HV interval during FJT as compared to sinus rhythm and has a rS recording denotes unsuccessful site in the proximal His bundle that can lead to AV block. Unipolar recording on the ablation catheter that has a similar HV interval during FJT and sinus rhythm with a qS signal during FJT signifies a successful site at the distal His Bundle.[142] The use of 3D mapping system is strongly recommended in these patients to "tag" the His location and measure the distance from this to the ablation site.

Cryoablation may be required if the focus is very close to the His location (i.e., <5 mm). Cryoablation allows to assess safety and efficacy of ablation in mapping mode (−30°C) that is reversible prior to full ablation (-70°C) that is permanent. Law et al reported their experience in six patients (aged 7–36 years) with FJT who underwent cryomapping and ablation during FJT using a 3D mapping system.[143] Cryomapping resulting in transient AV block in one patient in whom no ablation was performed. Five patients had elimination of the tachycardia with cryoablation (4 were just posterior to His location and one near CS os). Collins et al[144] reported their experience with RF (17) and cryoablation (27) in patients with FJT (aged 2.5 weeks to 38 years). Success rate was equivalent, 82% for RF ablation and 85% for cryoablation with recurrence rates of 13% and 14%, respectively. Three patients developed complete heart block, all of them with RF ablation. Cryoablation has become the preferred ablation technique in pediatric patients.

AV junction ablation and pacing is a last resort therapeutic alternative in patients with incessant symptomatic JT who fail pharmacologic therapy and selective catheter ablation of JT focus. This should be accompanied with biventricular pacing or physiological pacing to avoid harmful long-term effects of right ventricular pacing.[145,146]

TROUBLESHOOTING THE DIFFICULT CASE

As previously stated, before proceeding to ablation, the operator should be confident of the diagnosis of AVNRT. This requires eliminating as a possibility orthodromic reentrant tachycardia, atrial tachycardia with 1:1 AV conduction, FJT and concealed NFT/NVT. Most cases of AVNRT can be successfully eliminated by delivering RF energy between the tricuspid valve annulus and the CS os. Securing good catheter contact is extremely important to modify conduction over the slow AV nodal pathway. When ablation at these sites is unsuccessful, alternative sites of ablation should be considered. Ablation within the proximal CS can be particularly beneficial when application of RF current in the usual position between the tricuspid annulus and the CS os does not result in an accelerated junctional rhythm. Only after failing

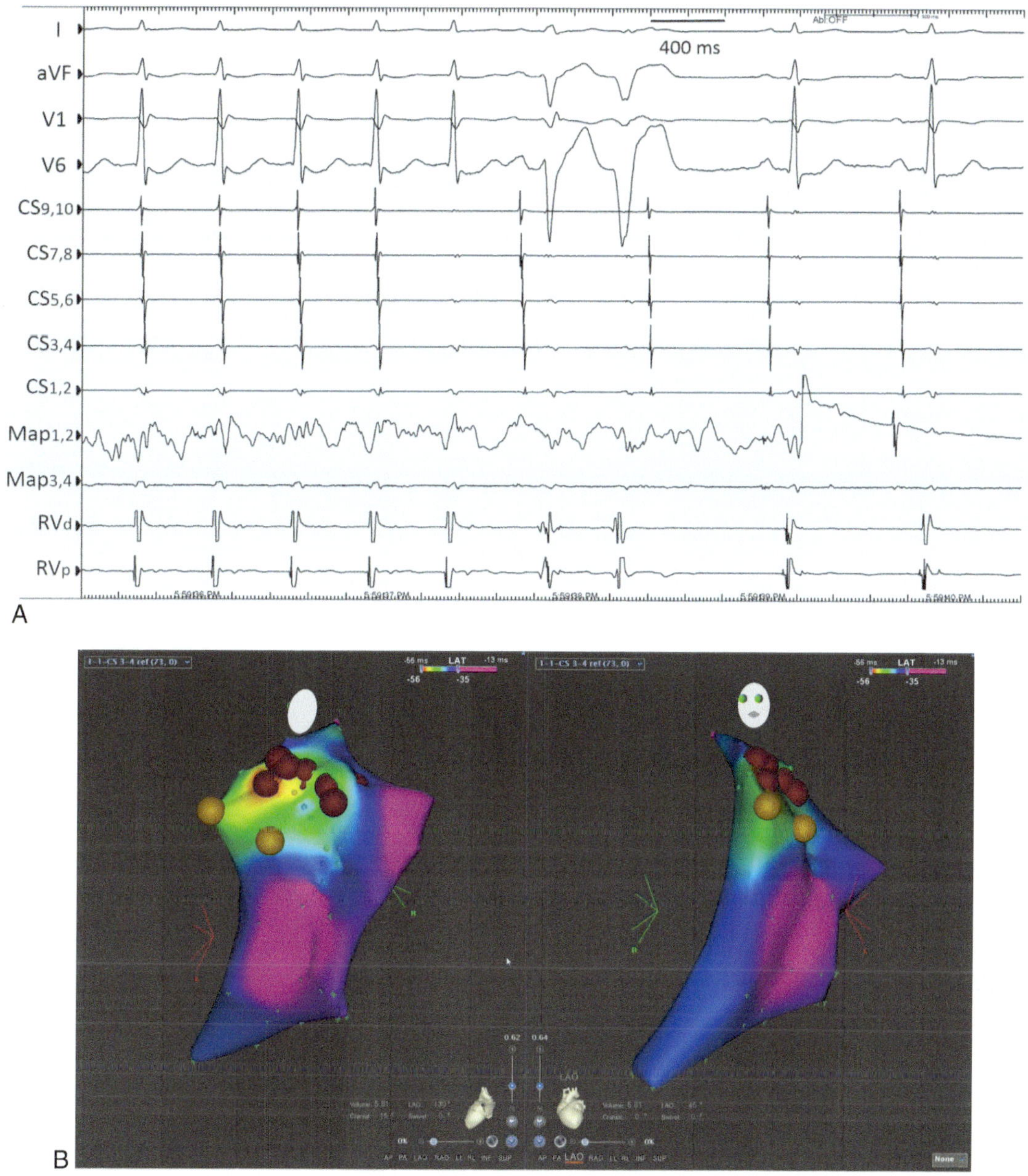

Fig. 23.36 Retrograde fast-pathway ablation in a patient with prolonged PR interval. (A) Termination of AVNRT in the retrograde FP during ablation. This image shows the intracardiac electrograms during application of RF energy directed at the FP exit site. Note that termination of tachycardia occurs with a V but no A electrogram. AVNRT, atrioventricular nodal reentry tachycardia. (B) Activation map of the atrial septum and sites of radiofrequency application. The *left panel* shows an LPO view of the atrial septum. The color scale represents atrial activation times during AVNRT. The region around the anterior septum is quickly activated over a 21-ms range. The *yellow dots* represent sites where His bundle recordings were noted. The *red dots* represent sites of RF lesion application targeting the retrograde fast pathway. *AVNRT,* Atrioventricular nodal reentry tachycardia. (From Tuohy S, Trulock KM, Wiggins NB, et al. Should fast pathway ablation be reconsidered in typical atrioventricular nodal re-entrant tachycardia? *J Cardiovasc Electrophysiol.* 2019;30:1569–1577.)

to eliminate slow-pathway conduction at these sites, ablation in the inferior portion of the mitral annulus can be considered and more rarely higher in the triangle of Koch. Ablation above the superior edge of the CS os is associated with an increased risk of AV block (Table 23.8). Induction of AV nodal reentry is infrequently a problem. AV nodal reentry is usually greatly influenced by autonomic tone. Reduced sedation, hyperventilation, isoproterenol, and atropine may facilitate induction. Catheter stability is sometimes problematic but is usually remedied by the use of a long sheath with slight septal angulation. The use of a catheter with adequate *reach* adds to catheter stability. At times, a large Eustachian ridge may prevent the ablation catheter from achieving a septal position. In this case, turning the angled sheath anteriorly and

TABLE 23.7 Retrograde Fast Pathway Ablation for AVNRT in Patients With Prolonged PR Interval

Study	No. of Patients	Ablation Approach	Baseline PR Interval (ms)	AVB	Success	Comments
Varotto et al. 1996[148]	1	Retrograde FP activation mapping and fluoroscopic anatomy in sinus rhythm	240	0	100%	No long-term AV block RF ablation
Reithmann et al. 1998[149]	5	Retrograde FP activation mapping and fluoroscopic anatomy in tachycardia and sinus rhythm	210–330	0	100	No long-term AV block RF ablation 80% VA block
Verdino et al. 1999[135]	3	Retrograde FP activation mapping and fluoroscopic anatomy in sinus rhythm	310–458	0	100%	No long-term AV block RF ablation
Reithmann et al. 2006[129]	10	Retrograde FP activation mapping and fluoroscopic anatomy in sinus rhythm	289 ± 66	1	100	No long-term AV block RF ablation
Linton et al. 2012[150]	1	EGM based and fluoroscopic anatomy in sinus rhythm	418	0	100	No long-term AV block Cryo ablation
Sato et al. 2011[151]	1	Retrograde FP activation mapping and 3D anatomy in sinus rhythm	312	0	100	No long-term AV block RF ablation
Touhy et al. 2019[136]	5	Retrograde FP activation mapping and 3D anatomy during tachycardia	230–415	0	100	No long-term AV block RF ablation VA block in 80%

3D, Three-dimensional; *EGM,* electrogram; *FP,* fast pathway; *RF,* radiofrequency.

TABLE 23.8 Troubleshooting the Difficult Case

Problem	Causes	Solution
Difficult to induce AVNRT	Retrograde fast AV nodal pathway block due to catheter manipulation	Avoid catheter contact with the fast AV nodal region
	Increased vagal tone due to sedation	Administer isoproterenol and/or atropine
	Similar fast- and slow-pathway refractoriness	Atrial burst pacing, programmed atrial and ventricular stimulation, isoproterenol, atropine
Poor catheter stability	Prominent Eustachian ridge	Use long sheath with septal angulation, apply clockwise torque
Prolonged AH interval before ablation	Absence or prolonged conduction over fast pathway	Ablate retrograde fast pathway (slow-fast variant), cryoablation of slow pathway (reversible), advise patient of risk of AV block
No junctional rhythm during ablation	Poor catheter contact	Unusual slow-pathway location
		Use long/adjustable/angled sheath or long-reach catheter, assess for slow-pathway function (possible ablation without junctional rhythm)
		Ablate below CS, in proximal CS, above CS (risk of AV block) or left atrium
Change to different form of AVNRT	Multiple slow pathways	May require ablation of retrograde slow-pathway function, ablate both rightward and leftward inferior extensions
VA block during junctional rhythm	Ablation near compact AV node, AV nodal artery, or anomalous fast-pathway location	Ablate inferiorly, start very low energy or use cryoablation, map ablation stimulus to His time or His AEGM to ablation AEGM times
	Slow-slow variant (absent retrograde fast pathway function)	Confirm variant, ablation during atrial pacing
Nonspecific end points	Poorly inducible tachycardia	Assess for modification of slow-pathway function, AV nodal conduction curves after junctional rhythm
	Absence of dual AV nodal physiology	Monitor for junctional rhythm and inducibility, assess for alteration AV and VA conduction properties

AEGM, Atrium electrogram; *AH,* atrium-His bundle; *AV,* atrioventricular; *AVNRT,* atrioventricular nodal reentry tachycardia; *CS,* coronary sinus; *VA,* ventriculoatrial.

then directing the catheter posteriorly allows the catheter to negotiate around the obstacle. Intracardiac ultrasound can be helpful in positioning the sheath and catheters in patients with difficult anatomy. If no junctional rhythm is apparent with RF ablation between the tricuspid annulus and the CS os, mapping of the proximal CS may identify slow-pathway potentials and provide successful ablation. As noted earlier, patients with absent or poor antegrade fast-pathway function are at risk of heart block after slow-pathway ablation. The status of the antegrade fast pathway should be documented before ablation. If fast-pathway function is poor and the decision is to proceed with ablation, AV conduction must be closely monitored during ablation. Cryoablation is probably safer than RF ablation in these patients. A summary of common problems encountered during ablation of AVNRT, and possible solutions is given in Table 23.8.

ACKNOWLEDGMENTS

We would like to acknowledge the contributions by Mario D. Gonzalez, Javier E. Banchs, Talal Moukabary, and Jaime Rivera, who are the previous authors of this chapter.

REFERENCES

Please refer to the e-book for a complete list of references.

24

Ablation of Challenging/Difficult Atrioventricular Nodal Reentry Tachycardia

Rachel M. Kaplan, Bradley P. Knight

KEY POINTS

- Anatomical challenges to slow-pathway ablation can include vascular access and congenital anomalies, most commonly a persistent left superior vena cava.
- Alterations in slow-pathway anatomy, including left-sided extensions, may require different ablation approaches.
- Diagnostic challenges can include differentiating atypical forms of atrioventricular nodal reentry tachycardia (AVNRT) from septal accessory pathways and differentiating junctional tachycardia from typical AVNRT.

INTRODUCTION

As with most procedures, ablation of the slow atrioventricular (AV) nodal pathway for atrioventricular nodal reentry tachycardia (AVNRT) can be straightforward or challenging. Every aspect of the procedure, from vascular access to diagnosis to monitoring during ablation, can pose a specific challenge to accomplishing a safe and effective ablation. This chapter reviews potential challenges at various points of the procedure and provides advice and examples on how to manage each one (Table 24.1).

ANATOMICAL CHALLENGES

Vascular Access

Vascular access is the cornerstone of endocardial catheter-based procedures. Typically, the femoral veins are used, though access via the internal jugular vein used to be commonplace for insertion of a coronary sinus (CS) catheter. This approach can be used in the rare patient without venous access from the lower body. Such patients include those with an occluded inferior vena cava due to extensive prior clotting/clotted filter or unusual congenital defects with an absence of a true inferior vena cava. In such patients, all catheters must be inserted from the upper body and access the heart via the superior vena cava. Consideration should be given to using the fewest number of catheters possible. Access can be obtained both from the internal jugular veins and the subclavian veins, ideally by an experienced operator to reduce the risk of pneumothorax. An example of an ablation catheter at the slow-pathway position from the right internal jugular vein is shown in Fig. 24.1.

Large Coronary Sinus and Persistent Left-Sided Superior Vena Cava

A persistent left-sided superior vena cava (PLSVC) is a congenital anomaly that is encountered commonly in the electrophysiology lab. In fact, PLSVC is the most common thoracic venous anomaly.[1] PLSVC is often considered by electrophysiologists with regard to device implantation but poses an additional challenge in AVNRT ablation as well. The PLSVC drains into the CS , resulting in a CS that is larger than normal because of the increased blood return. Additionally, PLSVC is often undiagnosed unless detected incidentally on other chest imaging or when the large CS is noted on echocardiography. Electroanatomical mapping can be helpful to delineate the size of the CS and provide a visual estimation of its size relative to the right atrium. The approach to ablating the slow pathway in a patient with a large CS ostium, however, is not much different than the standard electroanatomical approach targeting a site just outside the mid to lower third of the CS ostium. An example of a large CS due to PLSVC during ablation of AVNRT is shown in Fig. 24.2. The larger size and blood flow from such a CS can affect catheter stability when the ablation catheter is at the slow pathway. In such cases, long, steerable guide sheaths may be helpful to maintain stability and avoid sliding into the large CS.

Congenital Heart Disease and Pediatric Patients

Pediatric patients can pose additional challenges in AVNRT ablation. Multiple access points in the same femoral vein may be difficult in very small patients (<20–25 kg). Instead, using more veins with a single access in each may enable multiple catheters in the heart despite individually small veins. For example, a single access in each of the right femoral vein, left femoral vein, and right internal jugular vein can be an alternative to having all three catheters in the right femoral vein (as is common in larger children and adults).

Specific forms of congenital heart disease can affect the location of the AV node and the slow pathway. In ostium primum atrial septal defects and complete atrioventricular canal defects,

TABLE 24.1 Key Challenges and Possible Solutions

Difficult Challenge	Possible Solutions
No IVC access	Consider internal jugular venous access.
Large coronary sinus/persistent left SVC	Use 3D mapping to delineate CS ostium and visualize catheter stability.
Altered slow-pathway location due to complex congenital heart disease	Consider imaging (preoperative and/or intraoperative) and high-density mapping to delineate location of AV node/His and slow pathway.
Unclear diagnosis	Perform additional maneuvers to determine AVNRT vs septal accessory pathways or junctional tachycardia.
Atypical form of AVNRT	Ablate slow pathway.
Prolonged PR interval at baseline	Monitor conduction carefully. Accept single echo beat as endpoint. Inform patient prior to the procedure of increased risk for pacemaker.
No VA conduction at baseline	Use isoproterenol to improve conduction. Consider atrial pacing during ablation though may not be able to see junctional beats as a result.
Ineffective ablation lesions due to stability	Consider use of a different sheath or even steerable sheath if stability is the problem.
Ineffective ablation lesions despite appropriate stability, heating, and position	Consider left-sided slow-pathway extensions. Target similar electrogram signals on the left side of the septum.

3D, three-dimensional; *AV*, atrioventricular; *AVNRT*, atrioventricular nodal reentry tachycardia; *CS*, coronary sinus; *IVC*, inferior vena cava; *SVC*, superior vena cava; *VA*, ventriculoatrial.

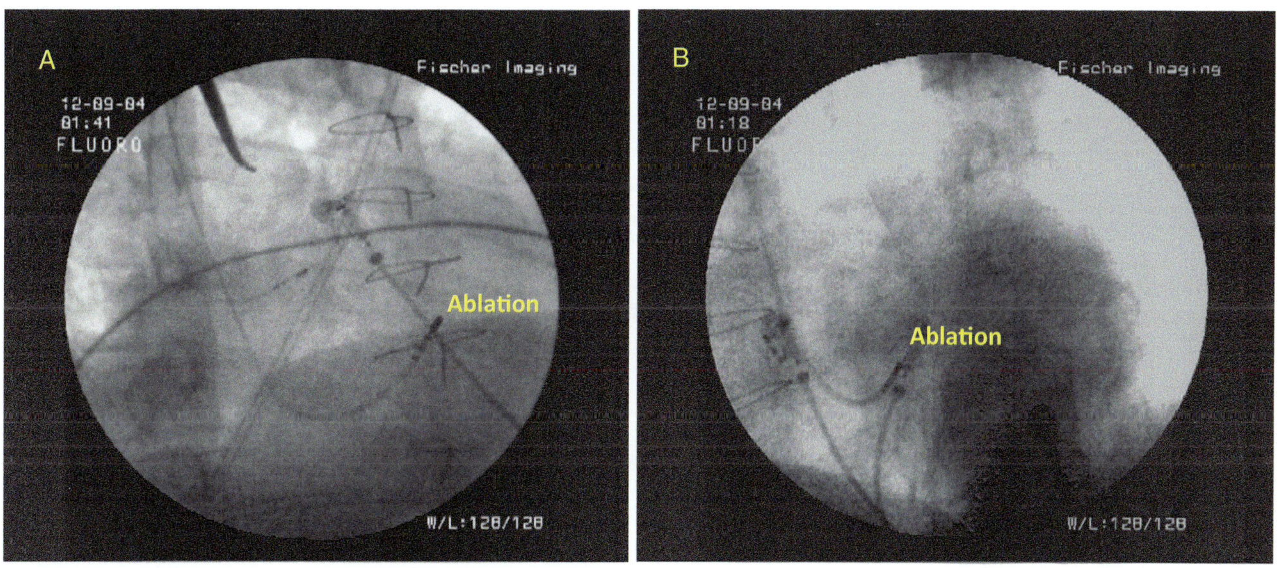

Fig. 24.1 Fluoroscopic images of an ablation catheter positioned at the slow pathway from right internal jugular venous access in right anterior oblique (A) and left anterior oblique (B) views.

the AV node is displaced inferiorly with its upper border at the ostium of the coronary sinus. The location of the slow pathway can be variable and mapping the His and fast pathway carefully is important to delineate the specific patient's anatomy and therefore where ablation may be performed safely. In D-transposition of the great arteries, while the AV conduction system is not malpositioned by the defect itself, the Mustard surgical repair procedure alters the relative position of those structures. Often, the triangle of Koch and slow-pathway region end up within the pulmonary venous atrium, and thus ablation in that location may require either retrograde systemic arterial access or trans-baffle puncture.[2] Single-ventricle physiology can be due to multiple different congenital lesions and can cause difficulty with accessing the appropriate structures. Careful electroanatomical mapping and consideration of intracardiac echocardiography may be helpful in specific patient cases. The use of focal cryoablation rather than radiofrequency energy is more common in pediatrics in an effort to avoid heart block in such young patients.

Nonfluoroscopic Approaches

Ablation with minimal or no fluoroscopy has become increasingly popular in recent years. While the focus for this trend is often on the benefits toward the operator (e.g., not having to wear lead), in some patient populations such as pregnant women, fluoroless approaches have made ablation for rhythms like AVNRT feasible and safe without exposing the woman or fetus to radiation. With the increased use of three-dimensional

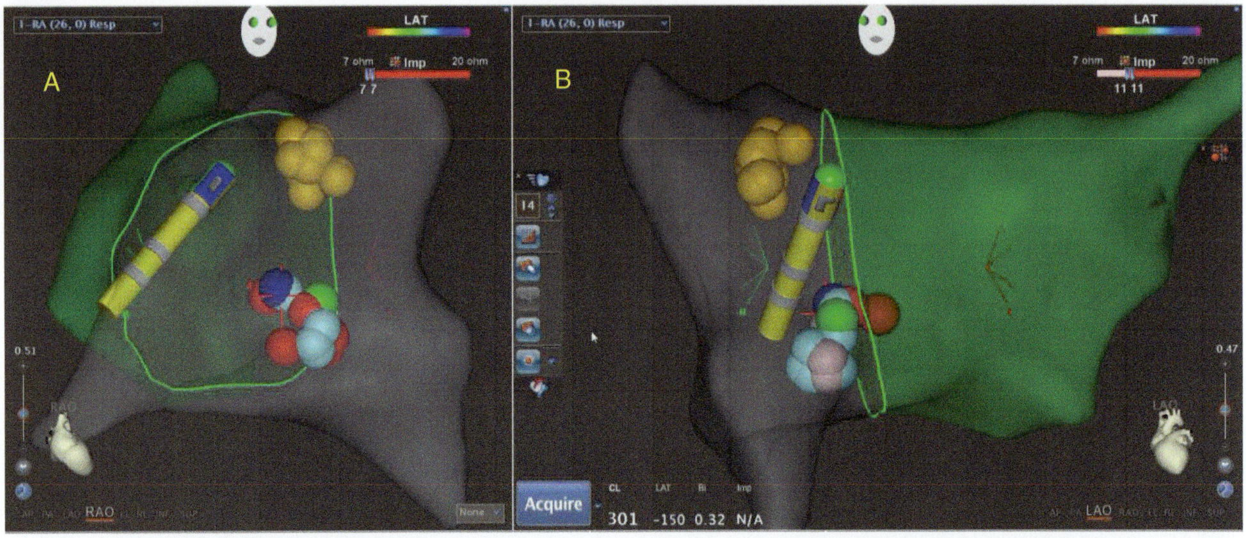

Fig. 24.2 Electroanatomical maps from CARTO of slow-pathway ablation in a patient with persistent left superior vena cava in the right anterior oblique view (A) and left anterior oblique view (B). The enlarged coronary sinus is shaded *green*. *Yellow spheres* denote His recordings. Ablation lesions are shown in the multicolored spheres at the slow-pathway site, inferior to the His cloud.

(3D) electroanatomical mapping in most patients, the operator's comfort level with primarily (or exclusively) using mapping can increase. One major difference is in the initial creation of the map. In mapping systems that are magnet based, only certain catheters can be used to create geometry on the map (e.g., an ablation catheter or specially designed mapping catheter that has the requisite magnet). In more open-platform, impedance-based systems, the map can be created with standard diagnostic electrophysiology catheters. In either case, the appropriate catheter can be used to start making geometry of the inferior vena cava so that additional catheters may be advanced along that same path to reach the heart without requiring fluoroscopy (Fig. 24.3).

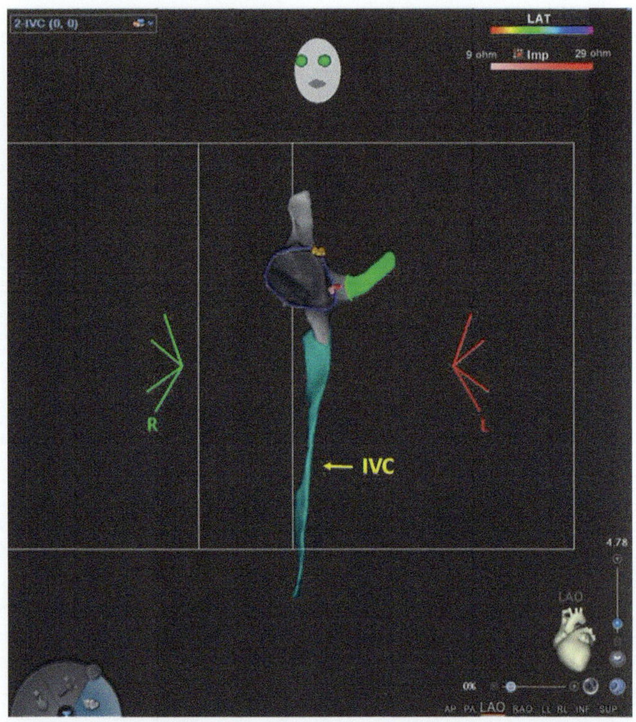

Fig. 24.3 Electroanatomical map of the path through the inferior vena cava up to the heart using the CARTO mapping system.

DIAGNOSTIC CHALLENGES

Atypical Forms of AVNRT

The most common type of AVNRT, termed "typical" AVNRT, involves conduction down the slow pathway and retrograde conduction up the fast pathway. This results in a tachycardia with a short septal VA time <70 ms, which narrows the diagnosis. However, other combinations of nodal pathway conduction can result in more complicated forms of AVNRT to diagnosis (see Chapter 23). While "atypical" AVNRT can refer to any of those, including both antegrade and retrograde conduction along slow or intermediate pathways, the most common atypical AVNRT involves antegrade conduction down the fast pathway and retrograde conduction up the slow pathway. The resulting tachycardia has a longer septal VA time (>70 ms) and can pose more of a challenge to accurately diagnose. Ventricular overdrive pacing can demonstrate the diagnosis if able to be clearly performed. Fig. 24.4 shows ventricular overdrive pacing of a supraventricular tachycardia (SVT) with septal VA time >70 ms. The tachycardia is entrained, with a V-A-H-V response. Careful measurements must be made to accurately identify the last entrained atrial electrogram (EGM) to avoid the mistake of reporting a V-A-A-H-V response and diagnosing an AT. The measured PPI-TCL is 204 ms and stimulation to atrial EGM minus ventricular-to-atrial EGM of 200 ms. Both of these findings are consistent with AVNRT. In some cases, though, this maneuver is not feasible under the conditions present during the procedure and the diagnosis can be harder to confirm. Once atypical AVNRT is confirmed, ablation is targeted at the slow

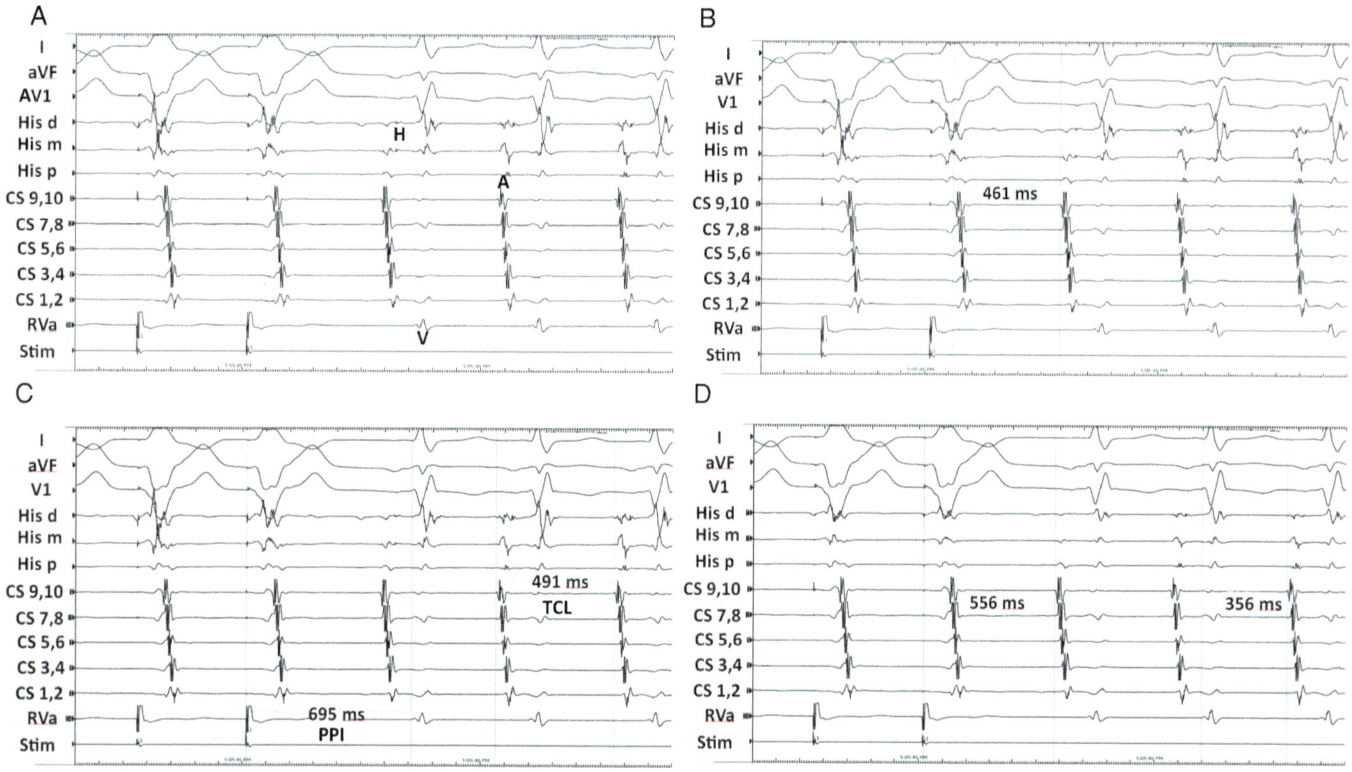

Fig. 24.4 Ventricular overdrive pacing of atypical atrioventricular nodal reentry tachycardia (A) with atrial electrogram (EGM) (*A*), His (*H*), and ventricular EGM (*V*) denoted. (B) Measurements demonstrating the last entrained atrial electrogram and confirming the presence of a V-A-H-V response. (C) Measurements of post-pacing interval (PPI) and tachycardiac cycle length (TCL). (D) SA (stimulus to atrial EGM) time of 556 ms, and VA (ventricular EGM to atrial EGM) time of 356 ms.

pathway in the same manner as with typical AVNRT. In some cases, patients who previously underwent slow-pathway modification for typical AVNRT can present years later with recurrent SVT, which can be due to atypical AVNRT. As before, the slow pathway is again targeted in those patients.[3]

Differential Diagnosis of Atypical AVNRT

Differentiating SVTs with long septal VA times is a substantial part of understanding the mechanisms of these arrhythmias. A clear diagnosis should ideally be identified prior to starting ablation; however, qualities of the tachycardia may impede a straightforward diagnosis. The tachycardia may terminate with each attempt, have too much variation in the cycle length, or not be sufficiently sustained. Other observations may be helpful in clarifying the diagnosis. For example, para-Hisian pacing during sinus rhythm can help elucidate the presence of retrograde conduction up a septal accessory pathway. In cases where attempts at ventricular entrainment consistently terminate the tachycardia, the onset of pacing can still provide useful information. Entrainment with fusion on the surface electrocardiogram demonstrates the presence of an accessory pathway. In tachycardias that are sustained, His-refractory premature ventricular beats can be delivered, which may be able to prove the diagnosis of orthodromic reciprocating tachycardia. This maneuver in particular can be helpful in distinguishing a decremental septal pathway such as that seen in permanent junctional reciprocating tachycardia from atypical AVNRT. In some cases where atrial tachycardia is suspected, mapping of the earliest atrial activation leads to the AV node. Such a finding should raise suspicion for AVNRT as the diagnosis and further attempts should be made to clarify the etiology of the arrhythmia before starting ablation. In any case where ablation is not having the expected effect, consideration should be given to confirming that the working diagnosis is correct.

Differentiating Junctional Tachycardia and Typical AVNRT

Junctional tachycardia can involve retrograde VA conduction, resulting in an intracardiac EGM pattern that mimics typical AVNRT. Junctional tachycardia in isolation is uncommon in adults, but it occurs more often in the presence of isoproterenol as might be used following slow-pathway ablation. In that scenario, it is important to accurately differentiate junctional tachycardia from recurrent AVNRT as the latter indicates that further ablation on the slow pathway is still necessary. Two maneuvers using atrial pacing can be used to clarify the diagnosis. Atrial overdrive pacing can be used in a similar way that ventricular overdrive pacing is used for initial diagnosis. If the tachycardia continues after atrial overdrive pacing, then observation of the EGM sequence can result in either an atrial-His-atrial (A-H-A) response or atrial-His-His-atrial (A-H-H-A) response. In junctional tachycardia, atrial overdrive pacing suppresses the tachycardia and when it resumes, it does so with a His signal; this results in an A-H-H-A response. In typical AVNRT, atrial overdrive pacing entrains the tachycardia and the last paced beat conducts antegrade down the slow pathway and then retrograde up the fast, leading to an A-H-A response.[4] A second maneuver is the delivery of His-refractory premature atrial complexes (HRPACs). In this case, if the HRPAC affects the tachycardia in any way (advancing His, delaying His, or termination), this excludes junctional tachycardia.[5]

BASELINE ELECTROPHYSIOLOGIC CHALLENGES

Prolonged Baseline PR Interval

Patients with a long PR interval at baseline may be at higher risk for complete heart block during or after slow-pathway ablation. In these patients, either the fast pathway is significantly diseased or it is entirely absent. A number of studies, each of which is relatively small, have demonstrated conflicting findings, with some showing up to a 9% need for permanent pacemaker in follow-up to others without significant increase in long-term complications of conduction system.[6–9] One factor associated with needing permanent pacing was the complete elimination of the slow pathway rather than allowing single AV nodal echo beats after ablation. The latter is an accepted endpoint for slow-pathway ablation in all patients and certainly of particular importance in this population.[10] Atrioventricular conduction must be carefully monitored in all patients during slow-pathway ablation but may be particularly challenging when the PR is prolonged, especially if there are bursts of ectopy that may be difficult to follow in real-time or premature atrial beats that do not conduct physiologically.

Absence of Retrograde Conduction at Baseline

Some patients do not have retrograde conduction under baseline conditions, particularly when receiving sedation during a procedure. As previously noted, careful monitoring of atrioventricular conduction is essential during slow-pathway ablation. However, in patients without baseline retrograde conduction, junctional beats would not have an associated atrial activation. In those cases, one could not determine if there was development of heart block from ablation. There are several options to address this issue. One is that the use of β-agonism such as occurs with isoproterenol infusion may improve conduction and the patient may gain retrograde conduction. Low-dose isoproterenol can often be effective at improving conduction in this manner without leading to an excessive tachycardia response that may make catheter stability during ablation a concern.

A second option is to pace the atrium during ablation. Atrial pacing enables a clear view of atrioventricular conduction during ablation but may suppress the junctional ectopy that one desires to see during slow-pathway ablation. A third option is to use cryoablation rather than radiofrequency ablation. Cryoablation provides a more reversible lesion if heart block develops and consequently is associated with a lower risk of heart block during AVNRT ablation. It is, however, associated with a higher rate of recurrence. A meta-analysis of cryoablation compared to radiofrequency ablation for AVNRT found a significantly higher freedom from recurrence within 1 year in patients who had radiofrequency ablation (96.5% versus 90.9% for cryoablation, odds ratio = 0.40, 95% confidence interval 0.28–0.58, $P < .001$).[11] As mentioned above, cryoablation is commonly used in pediatric electrophysiology labs but is less frequently used in adults. It can be a helpful tool for ablation close to the His or after trying all other options to optimize retrograde conduction for slow- pathway ablation.

WHEN YOUR ABLATION DOES NOT SEEM TO BE WORKING

In some cases, despite ablation in the anatomically appropriate locations for the slow pathway, no junctional beats are seen. Sometimes the problem is stability at the site of the slow pathway or contact with the region. In those cases, switching to a different curve of ablation catheter or exchanging the guide sheath for a steerable one may be the key to achieving good stability and making an effective lesion. Other times, stability and contact are not the issue, but rather the ablation is not having the expected result on the slow pathway. Often, the operator will continue to evaluate and ablate at sites more superiorly and may begin encroaching on the location of the His. At ablation sites close to the His, cryoablation can be used instead of radiofrequency to reduce the risk of permanent damage to the His/AV node if heart block does occur. Some patients, however, have altered slow-pathway extensions that may require ablation from different approaches rather than simply getting closer to the His. The left-sided slow-pathway extension has been described and is estimated to occur in 1–1.5% of patients.[9,12] In these cases, ablation from the left side may be required to sufficiently modify the slow pathway so that it cannot support reentrant tachycardia.

Ablation of Left-Sided Slow-Pathway Extension

A transseptal or retrograde aortic approach may be used to reach the left side of the septum. In the case shown in Fig. 24.5, the patient had a known patent foramen ovale that the ablation catheter easily crossed. When positioned on the left side, a similar signal is targeted with an atrial-to-ventricular ratio of 1:4–1:8 (Fig. 24.6). Ablation is performed directly opposite the right-sided lesions, as shown on the electroanatomical map in Fig. 24.7. Ablation at this site resulted in junctional beats and noninducibility thereafter. While junctional beats are an expected finding of ablation on the slow pathway, their presence alone is not sufficient to conclude that the ablation was effective. Pacing maneuvers must be repeated, including on isoproterenol infusion, to confirm that the slow pathway has been modified and can no longer support tachycardia. In the case shown in Fig. 24.8, numerous junctional beats were seen with ablation on the left side (A, electrograms; B and C, catheter position). However, AVNRT remained easily inducible (D). In fact, in that case, further ablation had to be performed on the right side before AVNRT was no longer able to be induced.

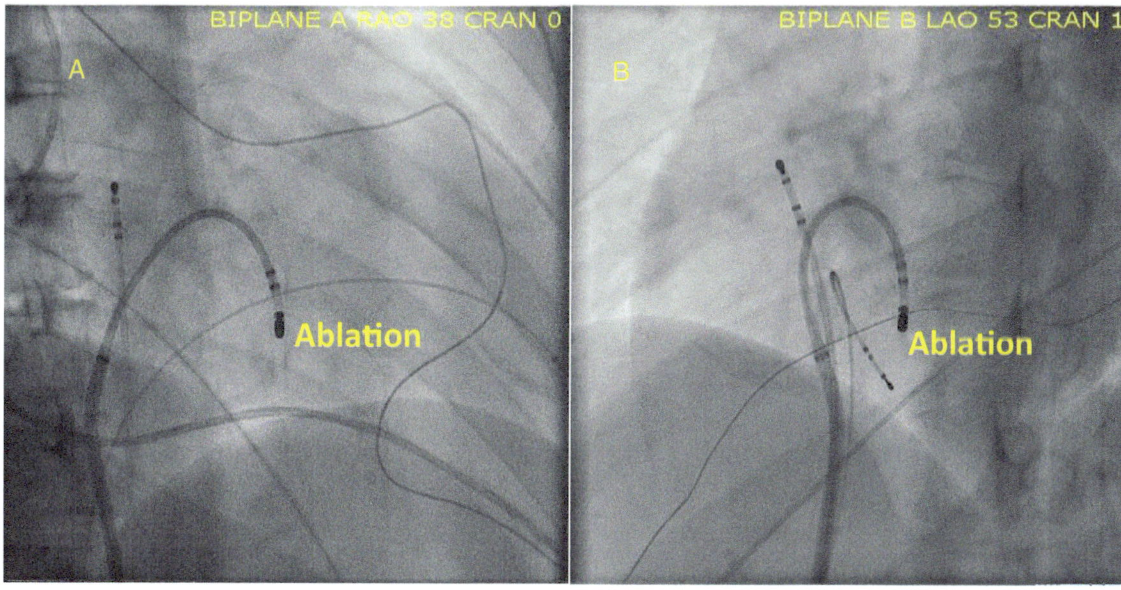

Fig. 24.5 Fluoroscopic images of ablation catheter through a patent foramen ovale and positioned on the left-sided slow pathway in the right anterior oblique (A) and left anterior oblique (B) views.

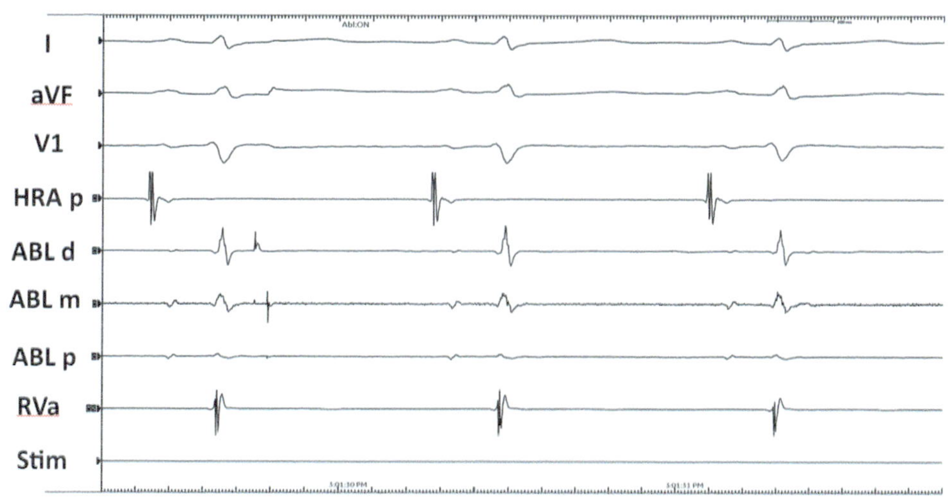

Fig. 24.6 Electrograms of successful ablation site of the left-sided slow-pathway extension. The signals on distal ablation demonstrate a 1:8 ratio of atrial and ventricular electrogram.

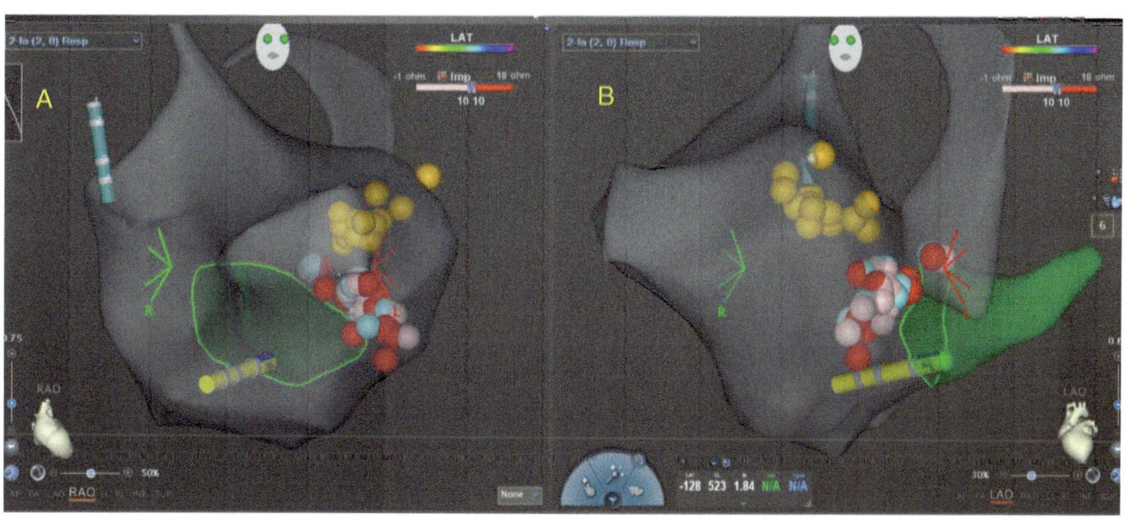

Fig. 24.7 Electroanatomic map made with CARTO showing right anterior oblique (A) and left anterior oblique (B) views of the ablation lesions on the right and left sides of the septum. His cloud is represented by the *yellow spheres*.

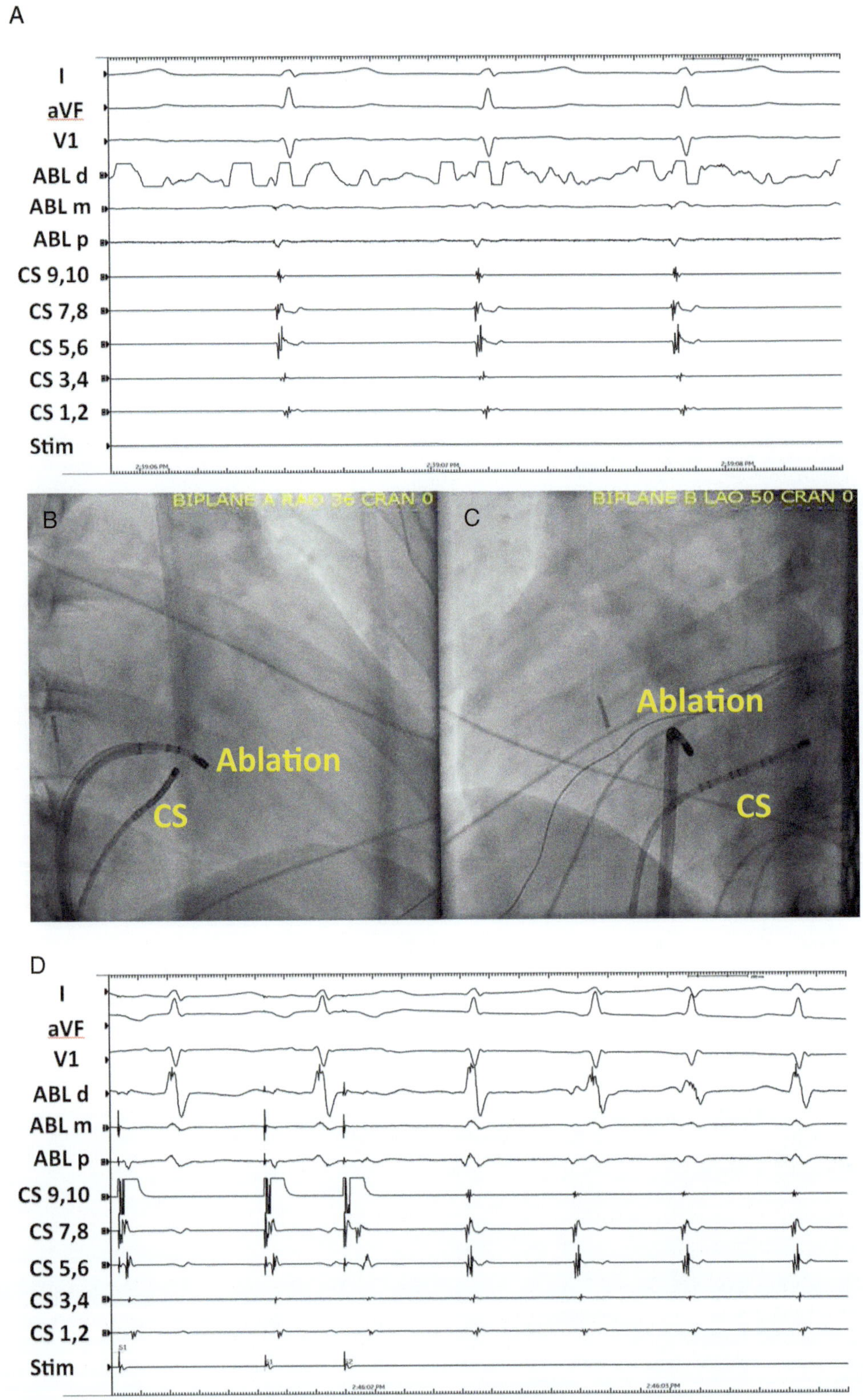

Fig. 24.8 (A) Ablation of left-sided slow pathway with junctional beats during ablation; fluoroscopic position of the ablation catheter in the right anterior oblique view (B) and left anterior oblique view (C). (D) Despite numerous junctional beats, atrioventricular nodal reentry tachycardia was still inducible after left-sided ablation.

Recurrent AVNRT After "Successful" Prior Ablation

Recurrent tachycardia after an apparently successful ablation is frustrating to both the patient and the electrophysiologist. The first step should be confirmation of a recurrent arrhythmia. Then at the second electrophysiology study, careful attention should be paid to all maneuvers performed. Possible etiologies for recurrent arrhythmia despite prior ablation can include incorrect initial diagnosis and not performing sufficient ablation on the slow pathway. In cases where the His and the slow pathway are not far apart, the first operator may have done only as much ablation as was felt safe to avoid heart block. Cryoablation rather than radiofrequency energy may be considered and referral to a more experienced operator or a left-sided approach as described above may be useful in those scenarios.

CONCLUSION

Many different factors can provide challenges to a successful slow-pathway ablation for AVNRT (Table 24.1). Anatomical considerations, from vascular access to the location of the slow pathway in various congenital anomalies, may require advanced preparation, imaging, and laboratory setup to optimize chances of success. Establishing a clear diagnosis, particularly in cases of atypical AVNRT, is important. Monitoring VA (or AV) conduction during slow-pathway ablation can be challenging, but the methods described in this chapter can assist in those cases to ensure safe ablation is being performed. Last, consideration of left-sided slow pathway ablation may help modify the slow-pathway without encroaching on the compact AV node and His bundle region in some patients.

REFERENCES

Please refer to the e-book for a complete list of references.

25

Ablation/Modification of Atrioventricular Junction for Heart Rate Control of Permanent Atrial Fibrillation

Ting-Tse Lin, Jien-Jiun Chen, Lian- Yu Lin, Shoei K. Stephen Huang

KEY POINTS

- Mapping uses a combined anatomy- and electrogram-guided approach.
- The target of right-sided approach is just proximal to or below the His bundle electrode position on the fluoroscopic view or at the proximal His location. The target of the left-sided approach is just below the aortic valve at the septal site where a His potential can be recorded. If the His potential is not recorded at the upper septal site, it may be recorded in the noncoronary sinus cusp.
- Sources of difficulties include inability to record the His potential and failure of the right-sided approach.
- Successful atrioventricular (AV) junction ablation allows 100% biventricular pacing with cardiac resynchronization therapy in patients with atrial fibrillation and reduced ventricular function.
- His bundle pacing or left bundle branch area pacing is a novel promising technique to deliver resynchronized therapy in atrial fibrillation patients undergoing AV junction ablation.
- AV node modification is not recommended because of lack of benefits and yet at higher risks of developing complete AV block as well as failure of rhythm control.

INTRODUCTION

Atrial fibrillation (AF) has become a worldwide health issue not only because it is the most common cardiac arrhythmia seen in clinical practice but also because it is highly correlated with a significant morbidity and mortality, including the risk for stroke, dementia, heart failure (HF), and overall mortality.[1–4] While both rate and rhythm control strategies are widely used, early rhythm control therapy was associated with a lower risk of adverse cardiovascular outcomes than the usual care.[5] However, it is difficult to maintain sinus rhythm for all AF patients. The traditional way of attaining ventricular rate control is the use of atrioventricular (AV) nodal blocking agents including β-blockers, nondihydropyridine calcium channel blocker, digitalis, and sometimes amiodarone. The lenient rate control was acceptable as an initial approach, defined as a resting rate <110/min regardless of HF status (with the exception of tachycardia-induced cardiomyopathy) and <80/min for patients with symptoms or deteriorated systolic function.[6,7] In patients with severe symptoms in whom drug therapy fails or drug discontinues as a result of adverse effects, ablation of the AV node and permanent pacing are effective in controlling the ventricular rate.[8] This chapter describes the techniques of radiofrequency (RF) catheter ablation for ventricular rate control in patients with long-lasting or permanent AF. For rhythm control strategy, please see Chapters 15 to 22.

COMPLETE ATRIOVENTRICULAR JUNCTION ABLATION

General Consideration

Rate reduction, allowing adequate time for ventricular filling and avoiding rate-related ischemia, may result in improved hemodynamics in patients with AF. Therefore, complete AV junction ablation provides an effective way to control the ventricular rate during AF. AV junction ablation in conjunction with permanent pacemaker implantation provides highly effective control of heart rate and improves symptoms in selected patients, such as tachycardia-bradycardia syndrome, drug-refractory atrial tachyarrhythmias, and even permanent AF patients with cardiac resynchronization therapy (CRT), who have not received adequate biventricular pacing to improve the heart function as a result of an irregular rapid ventricular rate. This technique has been termed *ablate and pace*. Since 1982, AV junction ablation has remained an important treatment option for refractory atrial arrhythmias. Early works on AV junction ablation were achieved by direct-current (DC) shock.[9,10] At present, RF energy has completely replaced DC shock as the energy source for catheter ablation of the AV junction. RF ablation of the AV node with His-bundle pacing (HBP) can cause a rise in pacing thresholds and loss of capture because of current shunting to His lead and compact lesion.[11,12] Cryoablation seems to offer theoretical advantages over RF ablation, and cryoablation of the AV junction has also been reported.[13] Forty-four patients with HBP underwent AV junction ablation using cryoablation (first 22 patients) and RF ablation (following 22 patients). Acute success was 100% with both strategies. Median procedural duration was significantly longer for cryoablation (50 minutes) compared with RF ablation (36 minutes). The rise of capture threshold (>1V) was comparable in both groups with all of the ablation lesions being within 6 mm of the His lead tip. During follow-up, four patients receiving cryoablation required a redo procedure and none with RF ablation. Cryoablation does not offer any advantage over RF ablation for AV junction ablation in patients with HBP and tended to require more redo procedures.[14]

AV junction ablation could be performed after or before the permanent pacemaker implantation. A frequently used approach is to perform AV junction ablation via the femoral vein immediately following permanent pacemaker implantation, but some operators prefer ablation followed by pacemaker insertion since the ablation procedure might damage or dislodge the permanent pacing leads. The latter procedure needs two venous punctures and catheters: one to perform the ablation and one to pace the right ventricle temporarily. However, one study enrolling 70 patients showed that device implantation before RF ablation of the AV junction is feasible and safe.[15] An alternative strategy is to implant the permanent pacemaker for 6 to 8 weeks before the ablation procedure. This approach is safest in terms of acute lead dislodgement and allows proper anticoagulation if a left-sided approach or DC cardioversion is required during the ablation procedure. Recently, AV junction ablation through the superior vena cava has been proposed. Ablation procedure during permanent pacemaker implantation through the pocket by using the same subclavian or axillary vein access could be achieved successfully and safely with a significant reduction in procedure and laboratory occupancy time.[16–18]

Before AV junction ablation is performed, appropriate ventricular backup pacing by a temporary electrode catheter at the right ventricular (RV) apex or a permanent pacemaker must be ensured. For patients with a permanent pacemaker implanted before ablation, care should be taken to ensure effective pacing during ablation because interaction between RF energy and the pacemaker may occur. The RF skin patch should be placed as far away as possible from the pacemaker generator location. The pacemaker should preferably be set to VOO mode at 40 to 50 beats/min to avoid oversensing and inappropriate inhibition of pacing during RF energy delivery. If VVI mode is set and if inappropriate inhibition does occur, placing a donut-shaped magnet over the pulse generator could reprogram pacing mode to VOO immediately. Ventricular asystole or extreme bradycardia may occur during RF energy application because of destruction of the AV junction and inhibition of the permanent pacemaker by RF energy. Turning off the RF power supply restores pacemaker activity. After ablation, permanent pacemakers should be interrogated to assess for alterations in pacemaker programming or changes in pacing or sensing thresholds. The pacemaker is often set at a higher rate (80–90 beats/min) in the first 1 to 2 months post AV junction ablation to reduce the risk of sudden cardiac death (discussed later).[6]

Mapping and Ablation

For the ablation procedure, an approach from the right side is usually tried first.[19] The anatomy of the AV node and conduction system is reviewed in Chapters 6 and 23. The most common approach is right-sided with access via the femoral vein.

AV junction ablation is performed under the guidance of fluoroscopy and intracardiac electrograms. The ablation catheter is positioned, under fluoroscopy, at the compact node region, which is located at the atrial midseptal region, just proximal and inferior to the His bundle catheter position. In a left anterior oblique view, clockwise twist of the catheter will ensure its contact with the septal aspect of the tricuspid annulus (Fig. 25.1). When positioned over 1 o'clock on the tricuspid valve annulus in the left anterior oblique view, a His bundle electrogram will be clearly observed in between the atrial and ventricular signals. The AV node locates over the apex of the triangle of Koch and does not have a characteristic electrogram. Typically, it is not the size of the His potential, but its relationship to the size of atrial and ventricular electrograms (Fig. 25.2). Ablation of the AV conduction system as proximally as possible would increase the chance of the escape rhythm to emerge. Ablation at the site of maximal His recording often produces right bundle branch block only. Therefore, the catheter should be withdrawn toward the atrium to record an A/V ratio of 1:1 or 1:2 and a small His electrogram, usually <0.15 mV in amplitude. An atrial position with an A/V ratio of 1:2 to 1:5 favors the His bundle ablation, and a very small or absent atrial signal suggests that the catheter is probably too far into the ventricle and a right bundle branch potential rather than the His bundle is recorded.[20] In addition, the catheter tip may need to be deflected slightly inferiorly to follow the course of the AV conduction system. One report mapped the AV node by using electrograms on both proximal and distal bipoles of the ablation catheter. The report found that the presence of His and atrial electrograms on the distal bipole, and the absence of ventricular electrogram on the proximal bipole, could improve the accuracy of AV junction ablation and avoid right bundle branch injury.[21] Some advocate use of unipolar electrograms recorded from the tip electrode of the ablation catheter to recognize the most proximal His recording. Here, the His potential shows an entirely negative (QS) morphology, reflecting the entire His activation proceeding away from the electrode.[20] During AF, mapping may be complicated by variable atrial electrogram amplitudes and obfuscation of the His electrogram by the continuous atrial activity (Fig. 25.3, Video 25.1). If feasible, cardioversion to sinus rhythm may allow better demonstration of the His potential. With standard 4-mm-tip ablation electrodes, RF is delivered for a total duration of 60 seconds at 50 to 60 W with target temperatures of 55°C to 65°C. One study showed that a temperature range of 60°C ± 7°C was required to achieve permanent AV nodal block, whereas at lower temperature, an accelerated junctional rhythm is seen. The development of an accelerated junctional rhythm within 5 seconds and the appearance of AV nodal block within 30 seconds of RF onset were both highly characteristic of successful target sites (Fig. 25.4; see Video 25.1).[22] It is highly advisable to carefully map and ensure catheter stability to avoid delivering ineffective lesions. Multiple ineffective deliveries may produce tissue edema and damage, which obscure the

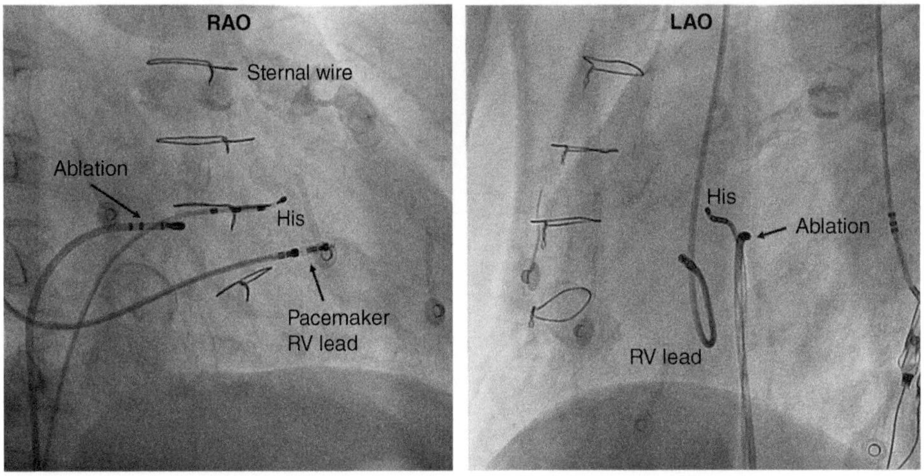

Fig. 25.1 Standard right-sided approach for ablation of the atrioventricular junction. Right anterior oblique (RAO) and left anterior oblique (LAO) fluoroscopic views showing the ablation catheter aligned with the proximal His catheter (His) along the septum. *RV,* Right ventricle.

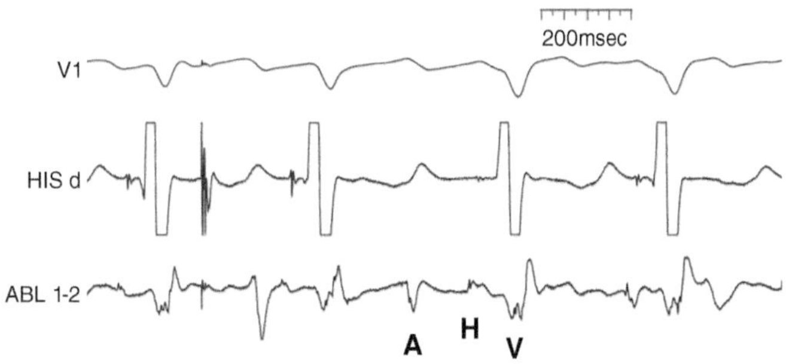

Fig. 25.2 Surface electrocardiographic leads and electrograms from the distal His catheter (HIS d) and distal ablation catheter (ABL 1-2) showing an atrial (A)–to–ventricular (V) electrogram ratio of 1:1.5 and a small His potential (H).

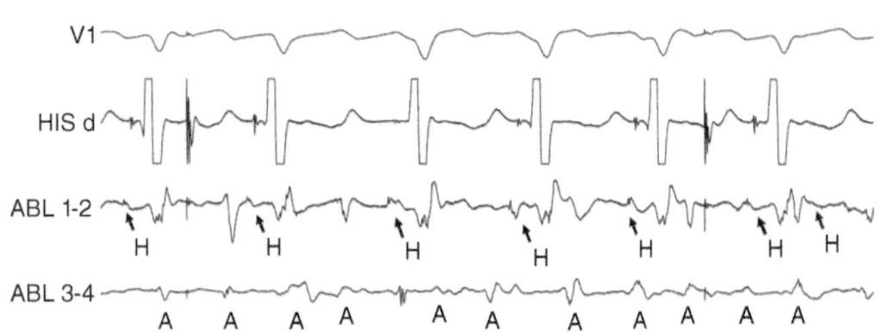

Fig. 25.3 Mapping of the His bundle in atrial fibrillation. The irregular atrial electrograms (*A*) may obscure the His recording (*H*). In addition, variation in the amplitude of *A* complicates the estimation of the atrial-to-ventricular electrogram ratio. The proximal ablation catheter (ABL 3-4) showed only A electrogram. *ABL 1-2,* Distal ablation catheter; *HIS d,* distal His catheter.

His recording and distance the ablation catheter from the target tissue. Typically, effective AV junction ablation is usually marked by accelerated junctional rhythm followed by slowing of the ventricular response and emergence of a paced ventricular rhythm. It is essential to wait for at least 30 minutes to ensure that the AV block is permanent.

Cryoablation of AV junction is an alternative energy modality. Cryoablation can be delivered using the 9F 8-mm FreezorMax 5 ablation catheter (CryoCath Technologies Inc., Montreal, Canada). Without prior mapping, −80°C freezes is applied to achieve the effective AV junction ablation, especially when reaches within 20 seconds. If this is not the case, the freeze can be interrupted for repositioning to obtain better tissue contact. The freeze is also aborted if it does not result in AVB or significant slowing of AF response within 1 minute. Otherwise, applications are continued for 240 seconds.[14]

A left-sided retrograde approach via the femoral artery is used if the approach from the right side of the heart is undesirable or unsuccessful,[19,23] which occurs in about 5% of patients. The left-sided portion of the His bundle emerges on the septum just below the aortic valve (Fig. 25.5). A right-sided His bundle catheter may act as a fluoroscopic reference. The target is a signal with atrial and ventricular potentials and the largest His bundle electrogram. After the aortic valve is crossed with a tight curve on the ablation catheter, the curve can be maintained on the catheter while it is rotated toward the septum and withdrawn toward the aortic valve. Alternatively, the ablation catheter can be straightened and directed toward the inferior apical septum, then withdrawn toward the right-sided His bundle catheter until the His potential is recorded beneath the noncoronary aortic cusp. A His electrogram is recorded at the site of ablation. The His potential must be differentiated from the left bundle branch recording. In older patients with aortic disease or peripheral arterial disease, the AV node can be approached through a transseptal puncture from the right atrium. The ablation catheter is directed to the left ventricle and placed under the aortic valve. The left-sided His activation should occur essentially at the same time as the right-sided His. The left bundle branch is typically recorded 1 to 1.5 cm inferior to the optimal His bundle recording site. The left bundle branch recording is identified by a potential-to-ventricular electrogram interval of 20 ms or less and an A/V ratio of 1:10 or less. Electrogram recordings and catheter positions for the left conduction system are discussed in Chapter 32. In rare circumstances in which standard right-sided and left-sided approaches are both unsuccessful, energy delivery in the noncoronary or right aortic

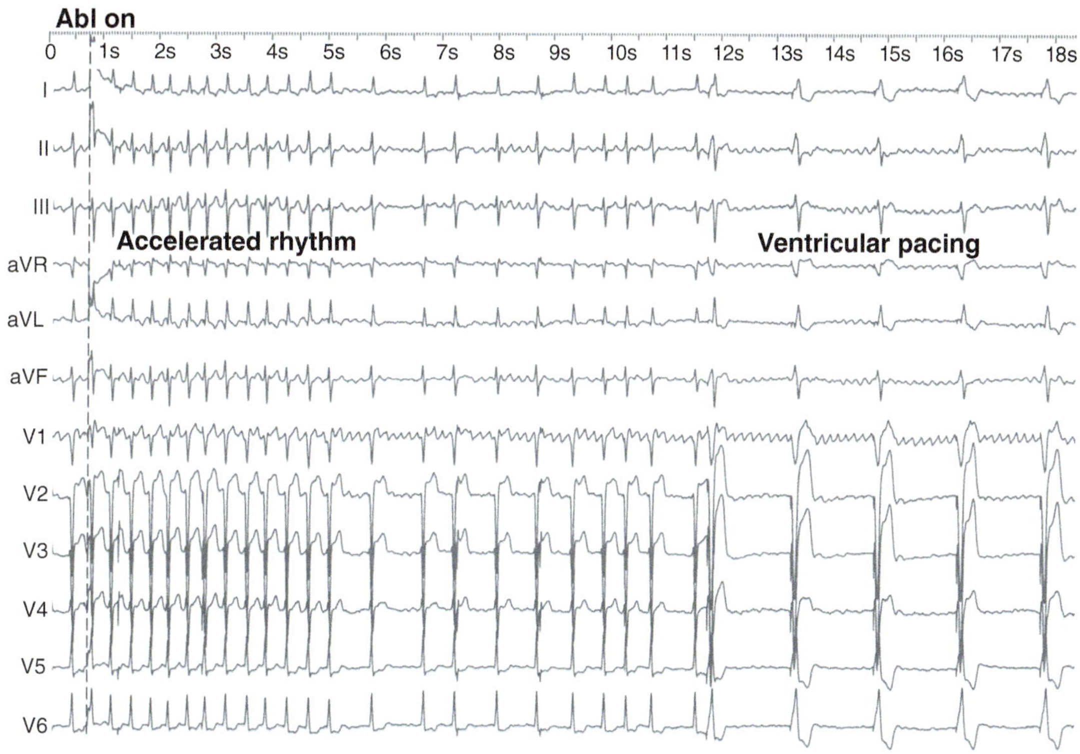

Fig. 25.4 Successful ablation usually starts with accelerated junctional rhythm, followed by complete heart block within 15 seconds after radiofrequency delivery. Note the ventricular pacing after heart block. *Abl on,* Delivery of ablation energy.

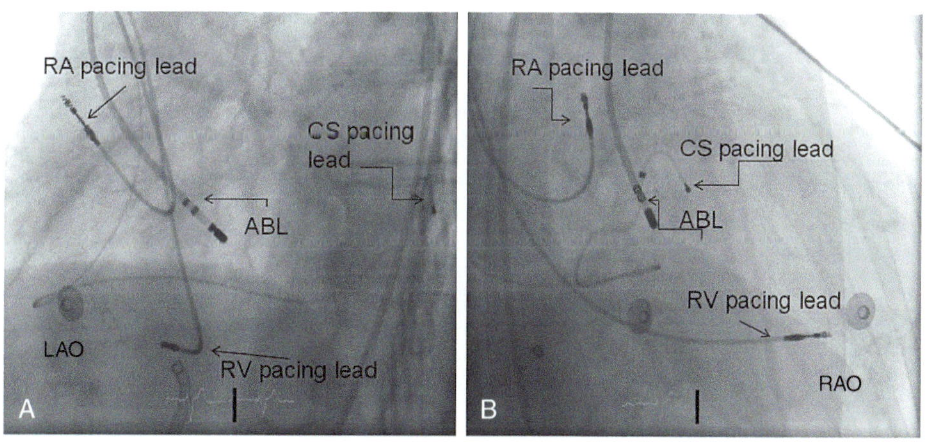

Fig. 25.5 Atrioventricular junction ablation with a left-sided approach in a patient with a CRT device. Left anterior oblique (LAO) (A) and right anterior oblique (RAO) (B) fluoroscopic images of catheter position during ablation. The ablation catheter (ABL) was just below the aortic valve. This patient already has a biventricular device, and no other catheter, except the ablation catheter, is required. The ablation catheter can record the atrium–His-ventricular electrogram. *CRT,* Cardiac resynchronization therapy; *CS,* coronary sinus; *RA,* right atrium; *RV,* right ventricle.

cusp where the His bundle potential is recorded may lead to complete AV block.[24]

In patients with preexisting complete bundle branch block, ablation of the contralateral bundle branch results in complete heart block. Mapping and ablation of the bundle branches are described in Chapter 32. Complete heart block may also result from ablation of both fast- and slow-pathway inputs to the AV node (Fig. 25.6). The targets for ablation are listed in Box 25.1.

ATRIOVENTRICULAR JUNCTION ABLATION IN PATIENTS UNDERGOING CARDIAC RESYNCHRONIZATION THERAPY DEVICE IMPLANTATION

In recent years, implantation of a CRT device is an expanding and effective therapy in symptomatic HF patients with prolonged QRS duration (preferably ≥150 ms with left bundle branch block [LBBB] and low left ventricular ejection fraction

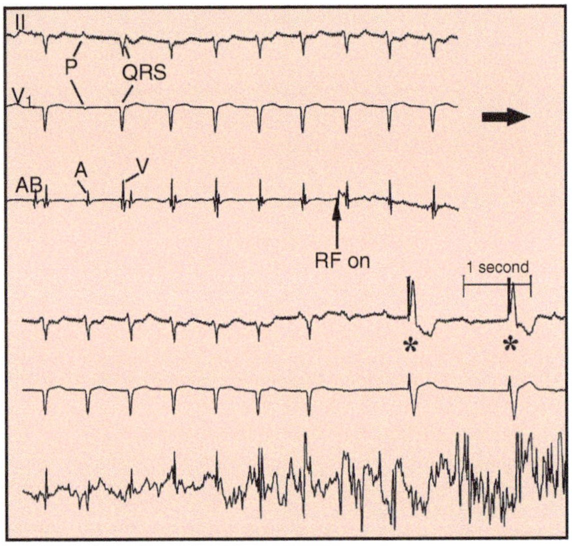

Fig. 25.6 Induction of complete heart block by ablation of the fast- and slow-pathway atrioventricular (AV) nodal inputs. Electrocardiographic leads II and V1 and the ablation (AB) electrograms are shown in this continuous tracing. A clear His recording could not be obtained in this patient. This recording was made after attempts at ablation of the proximal His bundle by anatomical guidance resulted only in fast-pathway ablation and a very long PR interval of 600 ms. At the start of the tracing, there is a blocked P wave in sinus rhythm, revealing the very long PR interval. With radiofrequency (RF) energy delivery to the slow-pathway region (RF on), there is a development of complete AV block and a ventricular paced rhythm (*asterisks*). *A*, Atrial electrogram; *P*, P wave; *QRS*, QRS interval; *V*, ventricular electrogram.

BOX 25.1 Targets for Ablation

Distal Atrioventricular Node–Proximal His Junction (Right-Sided Approach)

Recording from the ablation distal bipole electrode:
Small His electrogram (≤0.15 mV)
A/V ratio 1:1 or ≥1:2
QS morphology with unipolar His recording

Left-Sided His Bundle (Left-Sided Approach)

H-V interval >30–40 ms
A/V ratio about 1:5 to 1:10
Site <1–1.5 cm below aortic valve, on the septum

Compact Atrioventricular Node

Site proximal and slightly inferior to His catheter in the triangle of Koch
Midseptal, posteroseptal for AV node modification and more anterior approach for permanent AV block
A/V ratio 1:1–1:2

Bundle Branches

Right Bundle Branch

Absent or minimal atrial electrogram
BB-V interval <30–35 ms

Left Bundle Branch

A/V ratio ≤1:10
BB-V interval ≤20 ms
Site about 1–1.5 cm below aortic valve, on the septum

AV, Atrioventricular; *A/V ratio*, atrial-to-ventricular electrogram amplitude ratio; *BB*, bundle branch; *BB-V ratio*, bundle branch–to-ventricular; *H-V*, His-to-ventricular.

[LVEF ≤35%]).[25,26] Long-lasting or permanent AF is a common arrhythmia in HF patients, and there were significant benefits of CRT in AF patients with HF.[27,28] A trial involving 36,935 HF patients treated with CRT showed the greatest magnitude of reduction in mortality in patients with biventricular pacing exceeding 98% of all ventricular beats.[29] For patients with <98% biventricular pacing, the most frequent cause of nonresponders was inappropriately programmed long AV delay, followed by atrial tachyarrhythmias and premature ventricular complexes. One meta-analysis, including 7495 patients with 22.5% AF patients, found a higher all-cause mortality in AF patients than in patients with sinus rhythm, and the risk of nonresponse to CRT was also higher in AF patients.[30] In addition, failure of CRT was associated with new-onset AF during follow-up. One systematic review showed that CRT and AV junction ablation was associated with a substantial reduction in all-cause mortality and improvements in New York Heart Association (NYHA) functional class compared with CRT without AV junction ablation in patients with HF.[31] Another meta-analysis showed that in patients with permanent AF undergoing CRT implantation, AV junction ablation tended to reduce mortality and improved clinical response only when it was applied to patient with <90% of biventricular pacing.[32] Furthermore, compared with rate-slowing drugs, AV junction ablation alone was not associated with additional improvements in heart function, in NYHA functional class, exercise capacity, and quality of life.[32] In patients with an existing CRT, AV junction ablation could be added in those patients with incomplete (<90–95%) biventricular capture due to AF. Holter monitoring may help assess the percentage of biventricular pacing and the cause of incomplete capture. Therefore, both American College of Cardiology (ACC)/American Heart Association (AHA)/Heart Rhythm Society (HRS) and European Society of Cardiology (ESC) guidelines suggest that AV junction ablation will allow near 100% ventricular pacing with CRT in patients with AF and LVEF ≤35% (Class 2A recommendation, level of evidence B).[33,34]

On the other hand, AV junction ablation plays an important role in patents with uncontrolled heart rate irrespective of QRS duration. In a randomized, prospective Ablate and Pace in Atrial Fibrillation (APAF) trial, CRT plus AV junction ablation for patients with symptomatic permanent AF is superior to RV apical pacing in reducing the clinical manifestations of HF whether they met the requisites of guideline for CRT implantation or not.[35] In the APAF-CRT trial, 133 patients with severe symptomatic permanent AF, narrow QRS and at least one HF hospitalization within 1 year, CRT plus AV junction ablation was superior to pharmacological therapy in reducing mortality (mortality 11% in CRT + ablation versus 29% in drug) during a mean follow-up of 4 years.[36] Currently ESC guidelines recommend to implant CRT plus AV junction ablation in patients with reduced EF (Class I recommendation, level of evidence B). For patients with mid-range ejection fraction (EF), there is evidence that after AV junction ablation for rate control, CRT is superior to RV pacing in improving symptoms but not mortality and hospitalization (Class 2A recommendation, level of evidence B). For those with preserved EF, RV pacing should be considered first (Class 2A recommendation, level of evidence B) rather than CRT (Class 2B recommendation, level of evidence C).[34]

Permanent HBP or left bundle branch area pacing (LBBAP) is a promising novel technique for delivering cardiac resynchronization in AF patients undergoing AV junction ablation.[37,38] A small observational study showed that AV junction ablation, followed by permanent His bundle pacing with a single RV lead, might significantly improve echocardiographic measurements and NYHA classification in AF patients with narrow QRS, who have HF with preserved or reduced LVEF.[12] One recent single-center retrospective study comparing outcomes in patients with HBP and LBBAP undergoing AV junction ablation showed that AV junction ablation in the presence of an LBBAP lead is associated with a higher success rate, fewer procedural and fluoroscopy times, and fewer acute and chronic lead-related complications. In addition, an acute rise in threshold was noted in eight cases (14.5%), and four (8%) developed exit block after AV junction ablation in HBP patients. For HF patients with reduced EF, both conduction system pacing methods improved LVEF from the mean of 37% to 46% during follow-up.[38] In general, the potential benefit of HBP and LBBAP depends on the ability to achieve a narrow QRS complex that is similar to the native QRS complex, rather than on the LVEF. Further study is needed to confirm the beneficial effects of both approaches.

ATRIOVENTRICULAR JUNCTION ABLATION PLUS PACING VERSUS PRIMARY CATHETER ABLATION IN DRUG-REFRACTORY ATRIAL FIBRILLATION

In recent years, primary catheter ablation of certain types of AF has evolved rapidly in many hospitals throughout the world.[6,7,39] The details of catheter ablation for AF are reviewed in Chapters 15 to 22. For symptomatic, drug-refractory AF patients, the decision to attempt primary catheter ablation or AV junction ablation plus pacemaker may be uncertain due to various factors for consideration (see later). One multicenter trial (PABA-CHF) enrolled 81 AF patients to compare the efficacy of primary AF ablation to that of AV node ablation and pacemaker implantation.[40] The result showed that patients in the primary ablation group had greater improvement in EF, exercise capacity, and quality of life. Another observation study with 1000 AF patients also showed better survival rates with pulmonary vein isolation compared with AV junction ablation over a 7-year follow-up.[41] A recent systemic review incorporating seven randomized controlled trials in 425 patients showed that even in patients with persistent AF and HF, the primary catheter ablation group was associated with a greater improvement in EF, exercise capacity, and symptoms of HF.[42] However, the efficacy of catheter ablation for paroxysmal AF is around 70–80% in 2 years but much lower for persistent AF with a longer duration. The efficacy depends on the length of follow-up, the experience of operator, the underlying substrates, the age of the patient, the size of the atrium, and other factors. In additin, multiple ablation procedures are required to achieve a higher success rate, with each procedure carrying a risk of complications.[43] Therefore, for the strategy of AF control, one should consider various factors, including the duration and severity of AF, atrial size, and the patient's comorbidities.

OUTCOMES AND COMPLICATIONS OF AV JUNCTION ABLATION

The overall acute success rate for AV junction ablation is essentially 100% in recent reports.[44–46] A recurrence of AV conduction occurs in about 5% of patients. To compare cryoablation with RF for AV junction ablation, the rate of AV re-conduction requiring a redo procedure is significantly higher in patients received cryoablation.[14] Regarding outcomes of hospitalization for HF, the change of LVEF, and mortality, there are no significant difference after long-term follow-up between these two different energy modalities. A systematic review by Chatterjee and colleagues showed that AV junction ablation significantly improves symptoms and quality of life in patients with drug-refractory AF compared with pharmacotherapy alone.[47] With regular R-R intervals after AV junction ablation, the cardiac output and overall cardiac performance, as well as exercise capacity, can be improved.[48,49] A meta-analysis of clinical outcomes after AV junction ablation and pacing in 1181 patients in 21 studies demonstrated improvements in quality of life, EF, and exercise time.[8]

Complications directly related to the ablation procedure itself are rare, especially with right-sided procedures. Of these, there have been some concerns that AV junction ablation and pacemaker insertion may predispose patients to an increased risk of sudden cardiac death. The risk is highest in the days and few weeks after the procedure in patients paced at <70 beats/min, reduced left ventricular function, symptomatic HF, and a history of ventricular arrhythmias.[50] The proposed mechanism of sudden death is bradycardia-dependent prolongation of the QT interval.[51,52] QT interval prolongation decreases over time and is overcome by setting the ventricular pacing rate to a minimum of 80 or 90 beats/min for the first 1–2 months following ablation, then reducing it to a conventional 60–70 beats/min.[51] In addition, alterations in pacemaker function are common during RF delivery, which include inhibition of pacing, asynchronous pacing and induction of pacemaker-mediated tachycardia.[34,43] Interference may be enhanced in unipolar pacing systems. Problems persisting after termination of RF delivery are uncommon but include persistent reset mode requiring reprogramming, elevation of pacing or sensing thresholds, and direct damage to pacemaker leads.[34] For these reasons, permanent pacemakers should be thoroughly evaluated both before and after ablation.

In patients with permanent AF and HF, pharmacological rate control is often adopted to manage HF symptoms. Although AV junction ablation plus CRT carries risk of procedures, the "ablate and pace" strategy has been shown to reduce symptoms of HF and hospitalization for HF compared with drug therapy.[35] Furthermore, in patients with symptomatic, permanent AF and a narrow QRS who were hospitalized with HF within 1 year, AV junction ablation plus CRT significantly reduced the all-cause mortality rate when compared with drug therapy during 4-year follow-up.[36] The benefit during the initial years was mostly

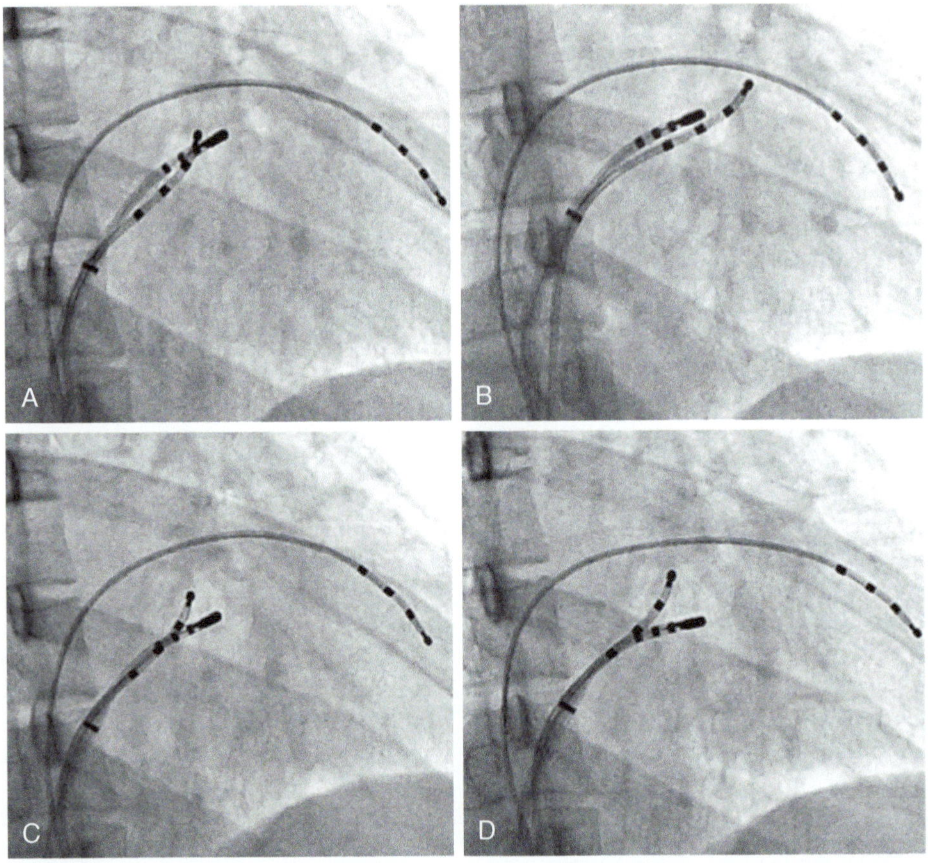

Fig. 25.7 Right anterior oblique views of ablation catheter positions to create a linear lesion perpendicular to the estimated course of the His bundle when the His bundle cannot be recorded. (A–D) The ablation catheter is moved superiorly to inferiorly, with the His catheter as reference. Complete heart block was achieved at the site in D.

attributable to fewer hospitalizations and a benefit in all-cause mortality was observed during the late years. Importantly, a reduction in all-cause death was observed in patients with preserved EF, with no significant interaction between mortality and EF. This trial supports ablation plus CRT as a first-line therapy in patients with permanent AF and narrow QRS who were hospitalized for HF, regardless of their baseline EF.[36]

TROUBLESHOOTING THE DIFFICULT CASES

AV junction ablation is usually a simple and straightforward procedure. The most common problem encountered is the inability to record a clear His potential. This may result from an intramyocardial course of the His bundle or from obfuscation of the His by scar or fibrosis (e.g., from prior surgery). In this instance, localization of the His bundle may be facilitated by use of a separate multipolar mapping catheter. A systematic search of the septum inferiorly and superiorly at variable extents into the ventricle often reveals its location. Pacing from the distal ablation electrodes at high output may identify areas of QRS narrowing, identifying His capture. If this is as a result of an inability to differentiate it from atrial signals during AF, it may help perform internal or external DC cardioversion so that mapping can be performed in sinus rhythm. By cardioversion, even if brief, the His may become apparent. However, proper anticoagulation or transesophageal echocardiography to exclude left atrial thrombus should be considered. Moreover, the inability to record His is a frequent problem after delivery of multiple ineffective lesions to the target area. The resulting edema and tissue damaging may physically distance the ablation catheter from the target tissue. This problem is best avoided by careful mapping and selective RF delivery only to favorable sites with stable catheter positions. Another effective His bundle ablation site may be identified by using unipolar electrogram recordings, particularly if a QS morphology is present.[53]

If the His still cannot be identified by any means, anatomically based lesions may be attempted from the right side of the heart before left-sided ablation is attempted. In this instance, the use of irrigated-tip RF or large-tip catheters (either RF or cryothermal energy) may compensate for the absence of precise mapping. A line of lesions on the septum perpendicular to the course of the His bundle may be effective (Fig. 25.7).

Despite clear His recordings, RF lesions may fail to induce heart block. This typically results from unstable catheter positions or poor tissue contact. The use of long preformed sheaths with septal angulation can be helpful, especially in the setting of enlarged cardiac chambers. The use of irrigated-tip or large-tip catheters coupled with high-output generators is sometimes necessary. Alternatively, the use of cryocatheter to generate cryolesion may overcome the problem of catheter instability

TABLE 25.1 **Troubleshooting the Difficult Case**

Problem	Cause	Solution
Inability to record His potential	• Intramyocardial course or His obscured by scar or fibrosis	• Mapping with multipolar catheter • Pace map from ablation catheter for His capture (QRS narrowing) • Create anatomically based linear lesion perpendicular to His • Left-sided approach (ablate from upper septum of left ventricle or noncoronary cusp) • Target compact AV node or AV nodal inputs
	• Acute tissue edema from ineffective RF lesions • His obscured by atrial activity in AF	• Careful initial mapping and catheter instability to limit ineffective lesions • If feasible, cardiovert AF
Ineffective RF delivery	• Poor tissue contact	• Use preformed sheath; change catheter reach, curve, or stiffness • Overdrive ventricular pacing to reduce cardiac motion • Left-sided approach
	• Intramyocardial course, insufficient lesion size	• Use irrigated RF or large-tip catheter with high-output generator • Left-sided approach–Ablate right and left bundle branches separately
Loss of pacing during ablation	• Pacemaker inhibition from EMI • Pacemaker reset mode • Displacement of temporary pacemaker wire	• Program VOO or asynchronous pacing • Check battery status before ablation • Careful catheter manipulation; use screw in temporary pacemaker wire, temporary pacing from ablation catheter advanced into right ventricle

AF, Atrial fibrillation; *AV*, atrioventricular; *EMI*, electromagnetic interference; *RF*, radiofrequency energy.

and poor tissue contact at the AV junction (see Chapter 2). If heart block cannot be achieved from the right ventricle, the left ventricular approach should be tried. If this also fails to target the compact AV node, ablation to target individual bundle branch or AV nodal inputs could be attempted. Common problems related to AV junctional ablation and their solutions are listed in Table 25.1.

ATRIOVENTRICULAR JUNCTION MODIFICATION

AV junction modification without causing complete AV block can also be achieved by catheter ablation but is now rarely used in clinical practice. It has been reported that selective ablation of the slow pathway of the AV node results in an increase in AV refractoriness and therefore decreases the ventricular rate.[54,55] In practice, the technique is similar to that used for treating AV nodal reentrant tachycardia. Ablation is begun in the slow-pathway region of the low posteroseptal right atrium during AF. It is delivered at sites with A/V ratios of 1:4 to 1:10. While the ventricular response is monitored, lesions are delivered in incremental steps superiorly toward the midseptal area. The endpoint is reduction of the ventricular response to <100 beats/min, ideally to between 60 and 80 beats/min. At this point, an isoproterenol or atropine challenge may be administered and ablation continued until the heart rate is <120 beats/minduring the pharmacologic stress.[56] AV junction modification leads to satisfactory ventricular rate control in 25–85% of patients.[54–57] The ventricular rhythm remains irregular and the sudden fall in ventricular rate may be arrhythmogenic. This technique has been largely abandoned because of the high incidence of AV block and polymorphic ventricular arrhythmias, both of which may occur days after the procedure.[58] These problems are overcome by the presence of a permanent pacemaker, the avoidance of which is the primary benefit of AV junctional modification. One clinical trial showed that complete AV node ablation and pacemaker insertion brings a more substantial improvement in exercise capacity, quality of life, and left ventricular ejection fraction than AV junction modification alone.[59] In addition, there have been consistent benefits of complete AV junction ablation and CRT or conduction system pacing in the literature, with no reported superiority of the AV node modification approach.[60]

A new approach for atrioventricular conduction modulation by ablation at a distance from AV node was testified, which showed 88% of successful AVN modulation and no case of persistent high-degree AVN block during the 1-year follow-up.[61] The procedure was performed during sinus rhythm. Electroanatomical activation mapping of the right atrium was performed during ventricular stimulation to identify the right atrial breakthrough, which was presumably the main atrial insertion of the AV node. The primary ablation line was postulated as a semicircumferential line with a diameter of at least 1.5 cm from breakthrough point. The line was divided into three segments (i.e., upper, middle, and lower part). The irrigated-tip ablation catheter with contact force-sensing technology was used with the delivery of a power of 25 W. Conduction intervals and atrioventricular block cycle length were frequently measured after each ablation segment. Modulation was considered successful if two endpoints were fulfilled: (1) an increase in atrioventricular block cycle length >50 ms and (2) atrioventricular block cycle length exceeding 450 ms. If the primary ablation line was not successful, additional applications were delivered inside the ablation line. The success of modulation after initial ablation was achieved in 58% of patients and 42% needed second ablation. The new approach AV node modulation showed a high success rate and no risk of AV block could be. If results are unsatisfactory, subsequent AV junction ablation and pacemaker implantation are still considered for the "pace and ablate" strategy.

REFERENCES

Please refer to the e-book for a complete list of references.

PART 6

Catheter Ablation of Accessory Atrioventricular Connections

26

Ablation of Free Wall Accessory Pathways

Varun Malik, Mark J. Davies, Jeremy P. Moore

KEY POINTS

- The atrioventricular (AV) annulus is mapped for atrial or ventricular accessory pathway (AP) insertion sites or the AP itself.
- Ablation targets include the earliest site of atrial or ventricular activation by the AP, sites of AP potentials, and sites of electrogram polarity reversal (left free wall APs).
- Special equipment includes preformed sheaths (especially for the transseptal approach), multielectrode halo or electroanatomical (including high-density) mapping catheters, and steerable sheaths (especially for the right free wall). Catheter navigation systems are useful, and electroanatomical mapping may play an important role in fluoroscopic radiation reduction.
- Open window mapping, using an automated algorithm to define local activation (high-density mapping catheters), can rapidly define the location of the accessory pathway, potentially reducing procedural times and fluoroscopic doses.
- Sources of difficulty are misdiagnosis of atrioventricular nodal reentry with eccentric atrial activation or atrial tachycardia as orthodromic reciprocating tachycardia, catheter stability (especially with right free wall APs), AP insertion sites away from the annulus, multiple insertion sites, and epicardial APs.

Free wall locations are the most common sites for accessory pathways (APs) in clinical practice. Left free wall APs are the most common, accounting for 50–60% of all APs. Right free wall APs account for 10–20%.[1] Each pathway location presents distinct challenges to the electrophysiologist. Left free wall APs are highly amenable to ablation and have the highest success rates with the lowest incidences of recurrence. However, the left heart is less accessible, necessitating either an arterial (retrograde) or, more commonly, a transseptal approach. In contrast, right free wall APs are readily approached from conventional venous access but have the lowest success rates and highest incidences of recurrence.

ANATOMY

There are several important anatomical differences of the tricuspid and mitral annuli that need to be taken into consideration during AP mapping and ablation.[2–4] The hinge of the mitral atrioventricular (AV) annulus is well formed with a distinct cord of fibrous tissue around the annulus (Fig. 26.1A). This formation of fibrous tissue is interposed between the atrial and ventricular myocardia. On the ventricular side of the mitral annulus, basal cords of ventricular myocardium may descend in a curtain-like fashion from the mitral hinge to insert into the trabeculations on the ventricular wall. These cords restrict catheter manipulation beneath the valve during attempts at left free wall AP ablation using a retrograde aortic approach (Fig 26.2). In the limited human histologic descriptions of left free wall APs, the atrial connection can usually be discretely identified and located near the annulus.[2,3] These pathways then traverse the annulus on its epicardial aspect and may cross at variable depths within the epicardial fat pad (Fig. 26.1B). The ventricular insertion usually branches into multiple connections with the ventricle that may be displaced away from the annulus and towards the apex.[2,3] The histologically determined length of an AP is typically 5–10 mm, with a maximal diameter of 0.1–7 mm.[5] The left-sided epicardial AV groove is shallow but contains the left circumflex artery near the annulus and the coronary sinus (CS) more remote from the annulus. Although the CS is useful for quickly mapping the mitral valve area, it runs an average of 10–14 mm on the atrial side of the true annulus.[6] This separation from the annulus is more pronounced in the proximal 20 mm of the CS. Therefore, during catheter mapping, the CS location and electrograms are best regarded as gross estimates of the true AP location on the annulus. The anterior limit of the left free wall is anatomically well demarcated by the aortomitral valve continuity, which rarely contains AP connections. The exact location of this continuity is difficult to recognize by fluoroscopy alone. The posterior limit of the left free wall is anatomically continuous with the posteroseptal area and is arbitrarily defined on fluoroscopy.

In contrast to the mitral annulus, the tricuspid valve annulus (TVA) is less well formed and frequently discontinuous.[2,3] The right atrial and right ventricular myocardia tend to overlap or fold over one another as they insert on the tricuspid annulus (see Fig. 26.1B). Right free wall APs may cross discontinuities in the less-distinct fibrous annulus or skirt the epicardial aspect

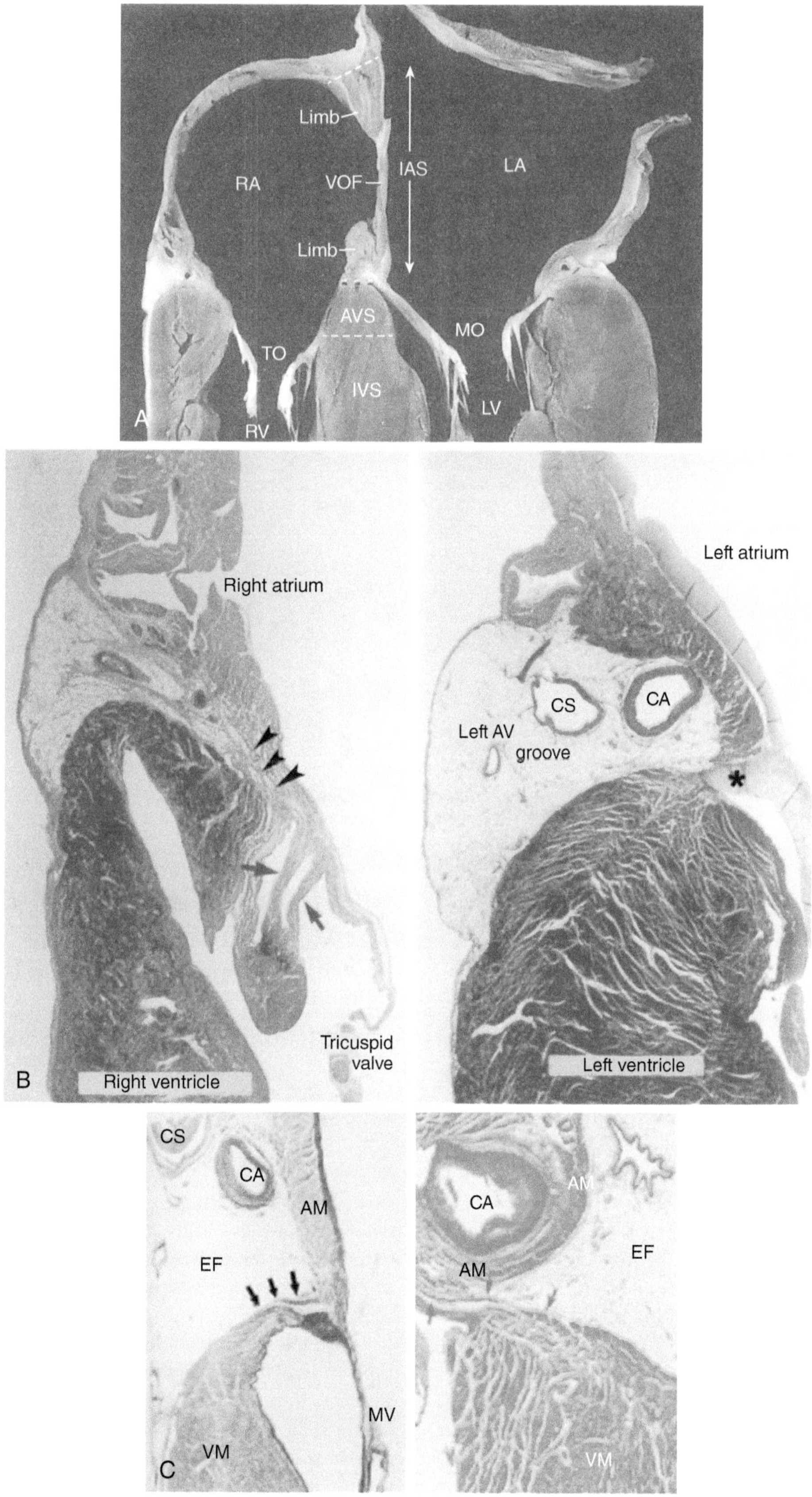

Fig. 26.1 (A) Gross histologic section demonstrating a cross section of the atrioventricular (AV) valves along the free walls. Note the more apical position of the tricuspid valve orifice (TO) compared with the mitral valve orifice (MO). (B) Histologic sections of the tricuspid *(left)* and mitral valve *(right)* annuli through the free walls. Along the tricuspid annulus, the atrial and ventricular myocardium folds over one another, separated by a poorly defined fibrous component *(arrowheads)*. The *arrows* show two cords supporting the base of the valve

(Continued)

leaflet. *Right*: The distinct fibrous component to the mitral annulus creates a well-formed hinge *(asterisk)* for the mitral valve and separates the atrial and ventricular myocardia. Note the relation of the circumflex coronary artery (CA) and coronary sinus (CS) to the mitral annulus. (C) Histologic sections of the mitral annulus in patients with a left posterior accessory pathway *(left)* and a left lateral accessory pathway *(right)*. In each case, the accessory pathways *(arrows)* cross in the epicardial fat pad (EF) on the epicardial aspect of the annulus fibrosus. Note the distant location of the CS to the accessory pathway *(left)*. *Right:* atrial myocardium (AM) encircles the circumflex CA. *AVS,* Atrioventricular septum; *IAS,* interatrial septum; *IVS,* interventricular septum; *LA,* left atrium; *limb,* limbus; *LV,* left ventricle; *MO,* mitral valve orifice; *RA,* right atrium; *RV,* right ventricle; *TO,* tricuspid valve orifice; *VM,* ventricular myocardium; *VOF,* foramen ovale. (A from Classification and terminology of cardiovascular abnormalities. In: Emmanouilides GC, Riemenschneider TA, Allen HD, eds. *Moss and Adams' Heart Disease in Infants, Children, and Adolescents: Including the Fetus and Young Adult.* Baltimore: Williams & Williams; 1995:115. B from Ho SY, Anderson RH. Anatomy of accessory pathways. In: Farre J, Moro C, eds. *Ten Years of Radiofrequency Catheter Ablation.* Armonk, NY: Futura; 1998:149–163. C from Becker A, Anderson R, Durrer D, et al. The anatomic substrates of Wolff-Parkinson-White syndrome: a clinicopathologic correlation in seven patients. *Circulation.* 1978;57:870–879.)

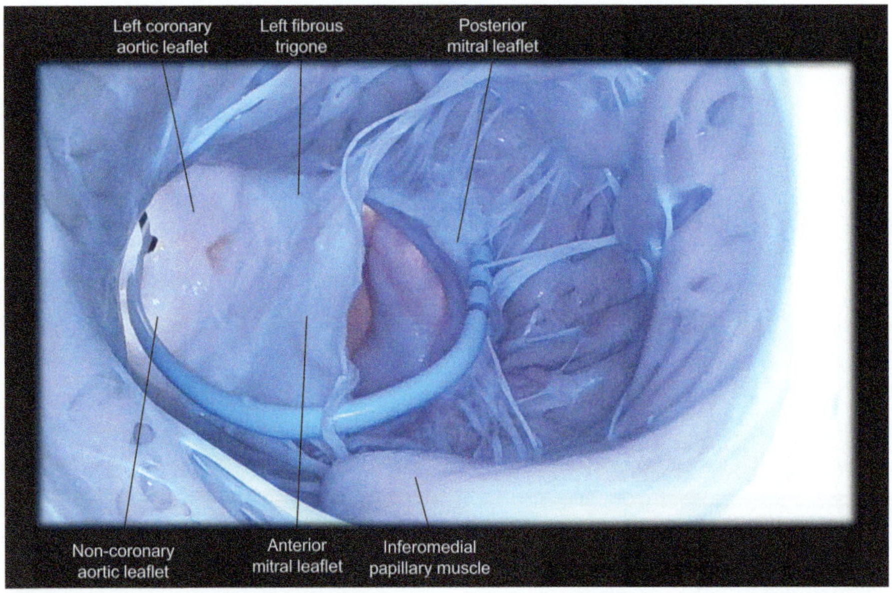

Fig 26.2 Apical (endoscopic) view of the mitral valve and its apparatus of a cadaveric human heart. The trabeculae as well as the mitral subvalvular apparatus can easily be seen. The anterior (*left of the image*) and posterior mitral valve leaflet (*right of the image*) have been labeled, as well as the inferomedial papillary muscle. A catheter (*light blue*) has been placed into the heart using the retro aortic approach and curled onto the mitral valve (MV) annulus. Indeed, as depicted (and inadvertently), the catheter appears to have traversed between the chordae supporting the anterior mitral valve leaflet as well as the subvalvular structures of the posterior mitral valve leaflet at its tip. This demonstrates the difficulty of catheter manipulation as well as the potential risk to the subvalvular mitral valve apparatus from this approach.

of the annulus, as do left free wall APs.[2,3] The less-developed tricuspid annulus and acute angulation of the tricuspid leaflets toward the ventricle make catheter positions along the right free wall unstable. Fluoroscopic definition of the right free wall is difficult because there are no clear landmarks for guidance.

Because of the association of Ebstein anomaly with right-sided APs, the anatomy of this condition merits special consideration.[7] In this disorder, the apically displaced tricuspid valve leaflets are tethered to the ventricular wall at variable distances from the annulus. This contributes to catheter instability during mapping of the tricuspid annulus. Although not anatomically displaced, the true tricuspid annulus may be poorly developed, with extensive discontinuities of the fibrous architecture.[3] Electrograms recorded from the annulus in Ebstein anomaly may be of low amplitude and fragmented owing to the disorganized tissue.[8] This fragmentation adds to the difficulty in mapping the tricuspid annulus in this condition. There are often several APs in Ebstein anomaly, which may traverse the epicardial aspect of the annulus or pass subendocardially through gaps in the fibrous annulus.[2,3]

A complete description of free wall accessory AV connections must also include those resulting from connections of the ventricle to the coronary sinus (CS) musculature, the ligament of Marshall, and the atrial appendage. Mahaim-type atriofascicular connections are described in Chapter 29. The venous wall of the CS is surrounded by a continuous sleeve of atrial myocardium that extends 25–51 mm from the CS ostium.[9] This muscle is continuous with the right atrial myocardium proximally but is usually separated from the left atrium by adipose tissue. This separation may be bridged by strands of striated muscle producing electrical continuity between the CS musculature and the left atrium. These connections, which can be broad and very extensive, are reported in up to 80% of hearts in autopsy series.[9] Electrical continuity of the CS musculature with the ventricle is less common, but it may provide the substrate for reciprocating tachycardias.[10] Ventricular connections may result from CS musculature extensions over the middle cardiac vein, posterior cardiac vein, or AV groove branch of the distal left circumflex artery. Ventricular connections with the CS are described in 3–6% of hearts at autopsy.[10] Sun and associates[10] reported that 36% of patients (most with previously failed ablation) who had left posterior or left posteroseptal AV connections actually used the CS musculature as the intermediary between the atrium and ventricle in reciprocating tachycardias.

The ligament of Marshall is a vestigial fold of pericardium that carries the vein of Marshall from its origin as a branch of the CS to its termination near the left superior pulmonary vein. It marks the location of the embryonic left superior vena cava. This structure may also contain bundles of muscle fibers that are continuous with the CS musculature. These fibers may end blindly or insert directly into the left atrial musculature at the inferior interatrial pathway.[11] With proximal connections between the CS musculature and the ventricle, the ligament of Marshall can support AV reciprocating tachycardia.[11]

Another unusual form of AV connection is a direct epicardial muscular continuity between the atrial appendage and the ventricle.[12–14] There are several reports of connections between the right atrial appendage and ventricle, whereas left atrial appendage connections have been less commonly described.[14] The developmental basis for these connections is unknown. Because of epicardial ventricular insertions more than 1 cm apical to the annulus and atrial origins within the atrial appendage, endocardial mapping of the annulus for these APs can be perplexing.[12,13] For left-sided connections, mapping of the anterior coronary venous branches may demonstrate the earliest ventricular activation.[14] At surgical division of one such right-sided connection, a broad band of myocardium under the epicardial fat pad was noted from the base of the atrial appendage to the base of the right ventricle.[12] Case reports describe successful catheter ablation of these connections from the right atrial appendage.[13]

PATHOPHYSIOLOGY

Diagnosis

As with APs at other locations, free wall APs may participate in reciprocating tachycardias or undergo bystander activation during tachycardias mechanistically unrelated to the presence of the AP. Free wall APs have been associated with specific electrophysiologic characteristics.[15] Compared with septal and left free wall locations, right free wall APs are less likely to demonstrate retrograde conduction, to participate in reciprocating tachycardias, and to be associated with inducible atrial fibrillation.[15] Pathways in the right free wall may be more likely to demonstrate decremental anterograde conduction than those in other locations. Compared with right free wall pathways, left free wall APs are more likely to demonstrate decremental retrograde conduction and have longer retrograde refractory periods.[15] Right-sided pathways may worsen cardiac function by activating the RV early and causing a functional left bundle branch block (LBBB).[16]

Surface electrocardiogram (ECG) localization of manifest free wall APs is imperfect and becomes less accurate if minimal preexcitation is present (QRS <120 ms).[17] ECG algorithms for AP localization are most accurate for the diagnosis of left free wall APs compared with all other locations, achieving at least 90% sensitivity and almost 100% specificity.[17–21] In using any localization algorithm, one must be aware of the portion of the QRS complex on which the algorithm is based. Some algorithms use only the first 20–60 ms of the delta wave, whereas others are based on the morphology or polarity of the entire QRS complex.[19–22] Provided that significant preexcitation is present, all left free wall APs should demonstrate a positive delta wave in V_1, with the R wave > the S wave (R > S) in lead V_1 or V_2 at the latest (Fig. 26.3). A negative delta wave in lead I, aVL, or V_6 is pathognomonic of a left lateral pathway. As the pathway location moves from posterior to lateral to anterior, the delta

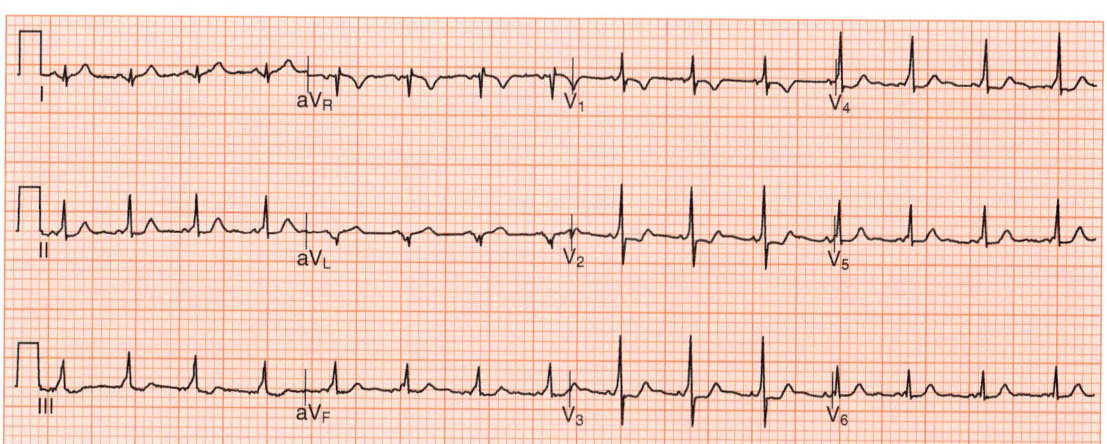

Fig. 26.3 Twelve-lead electrocardiogram in sinus rhythm from a patient with a manifest left lateral accessory pathway. The positive delta wave in V_1 with R > S wave indicates a left free wall location. The negative delta waves in leads I and aV_L are pathognomonic of a left free wall position. The positive delta waves in leads II, III, and aVF suggest a position anterolateral on the annulus.

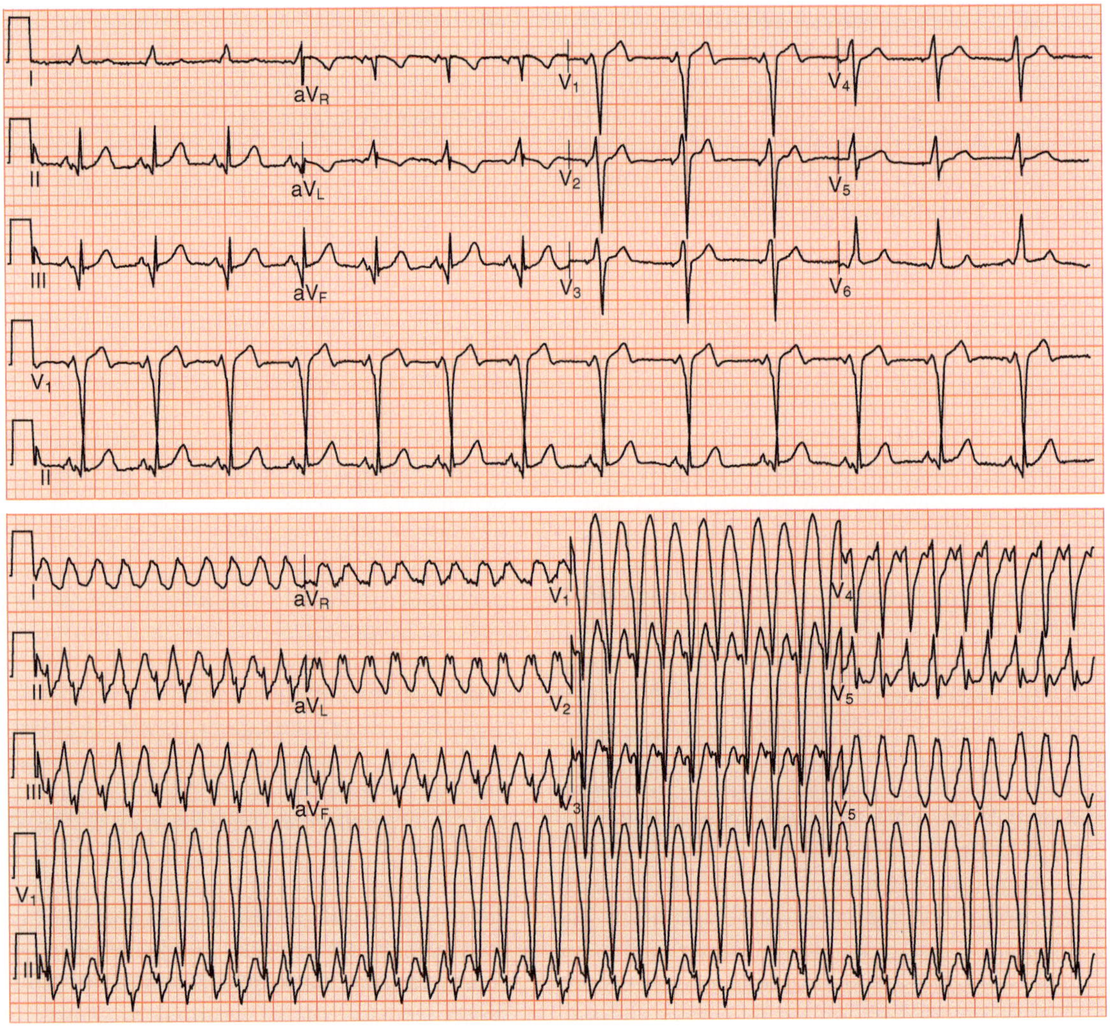

Fig. 26.4 (A) Twelve-lead electrocardiogram (ECG) in sinus rhythm from a patient with a manifest right free wall accessory pathway. The delta wave is positive in lead V_1; however, the transition to R > S wave in the precordial leads does not occur until V_5, indicating a right free wall location. The delta waves are negative in leads II, III, and aVF, indicating a position inferiorly on the right ventricular free wall. (B) ECG from the same patient during antidromic reciprocating tachycardia using the right free wall pathway. The QRS complex is fully preexcited.

waves in the inferior leads, especially aVF and III, change from negative to isoelectric to positive in polarity. The ratio of the dominant amplitude in limb leads II and III can predict if a left free wall pathway is anterior lateral or posterior lateral. If the ratio II/III is >1, the pathway is likely anterior, and if it is <1, it is likely posterior.[23]

As opposed to left free wall APs, the ECG diagnosis of right free wall APs is the least accurate and least consistent among algorithms,[17–19,21] with a sensitivity of 80–90% and a specificity of 90–100%. Confusion may arise in the interpretation of a positive delta wave in V_1 as indicating a left-sided AP (Fig. 26.4). This finding is diagnostic of a left free wall AP only if R is > S; a positive delta wave with R < S in V_1 is consistent with a right free wall AP or a minimally preexcited left free wall AP. A negative delta wave in V_1 is consistent with a septal AP. Therefore, most algorithms identify right free wall APs by a positive initial delta wave in V_1 but a late transition to R > S in the precordial leads at V_3 or later, coupled with leftward orientation to the initial delta wave, such as delta wave positivity in lead I or aVL.[19–21] As the pathway location moves from the right superior free wall to the right middle and right inferior free wall, the delta wave in inferior leads aVF and II changes from positive to isoelectric to negative.[19–21] A useful algorithm for AP localization that is based on the initial 20 ms of the delta wave is shown in Fig. 26.5.

A study comparing several algorithms was not able to duplicate the accuracy of the original articles. Wren et al.[24] looked at the accuracy of seven well-known algorithms[19–22,25–27] to predict AP location in children. In 100 children aged 3.8–17 years (mean age 11.7 years), the accuracy of prediction was 30–49% for exact location and 61–68% including adjacent locations. The algorithms were least accurate in predicting midseptal or right anteroseptal AP locations. The accuracy of algorithms may vary with ECG lead position, degree of preexcitation, patient body habitus, heart rotation, and prior QRS abnormalities.

The location of the AP can also be inferred from the surface ECG by the polarity of the retrograde P waves during

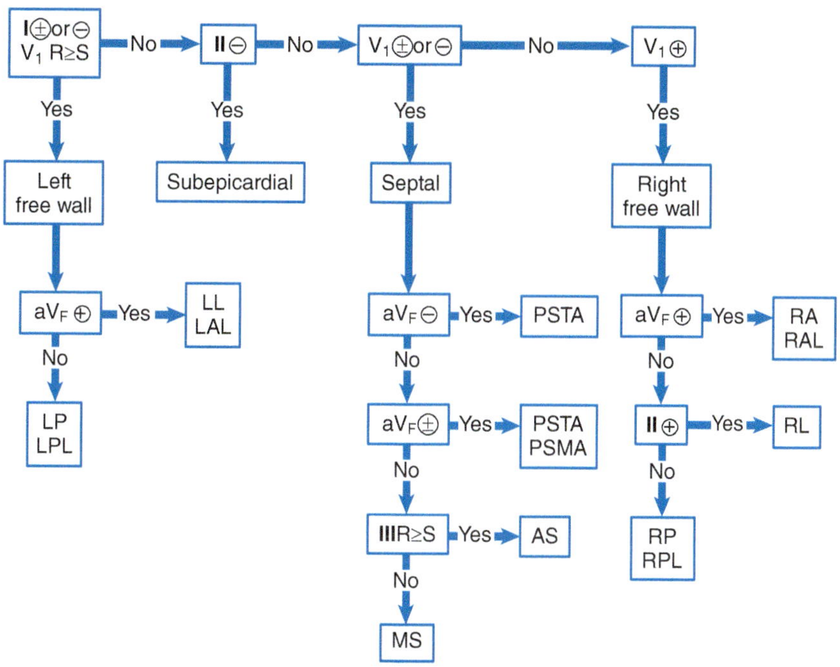

Fig. 26.5 Algorithm for accessory pathway localization by surface electrocardiogram (ECG). This algorithm is based on the polarity of the first 20 ms of the delta wave. Left free wall pathways are readily identified by an isoelectric or negative delta wave in lead I or an R > S wave in V_1. Note that with right free wall pathways, the initial component of the delta wave is positive in V_1 but with R < S wave. Right free wall pathways are identified by a late transition to R > S usually in V_3 or later. *AS,* Anteroseptal; *LAL,* left anterolateral; *LL,* left lateral; *LP,* left posterior; *LPL,* left posterolateral; *MS,* midseptal; *PSMA,* posteroseptal mitral annulus; *PSTA,* posteroseptal tricuspid annulus; *RA,* right anterior; *RAL,* right anterolateral; *RL,* right lateral; *RP,* right posterior; *RPL,* right posterolateral. (From Arruda MS, McClelland J, Wang X, et al. Development and validation of an ECG algorithm for identifying accessory pathway ablation site in Wolff-Parkinson-White syndrome. *J Cardiovasc Electrophysiol.* 1998;9:2–12.)

orthodromic reciprocating tachycardia (ORT).[28,29] A negative P wave in lead I is highly suggestive of a left free wall location, with a 95% positive predictive value.[29] A negative P wave in lead V_1 is highly suggestive of a right-sided AP. The presence of a positive retrograde P wave in lead I suggests a right free wall AP with a positive predictive value of 99%.[29] For either right or left free wall APs, the presence of negative P waves in all three inferior leads indicates an inferior location, whereas positive P waves in these leads indicate a superior location. Isoelectric or biphasic P waves in any of the inferior leads suggest a middle free wall location.[28]

At electrophysiologic testing, the hallmark of any ORT is the demonstration of obligatory 1:1 atrial and ventricular activation to maintain tachycardia (Box 26.1).[30] The diagnosis of ORT using a free wall AP also requires an eccentric atrial activation sequence earliest along the right or left atrial free wall. Coupled with such an eccentric atrial activation sequence, ORT is highly suggested by demonstration of the shortest QRS-to-atrium time of ≥60 ms, constant ventricle-to-atrium times despite changes in the tachycardia cycle length, and the ability to advance atrial activation by a premature ventricular stimulus delivered during His bundle refractoriness.[30] The last finding indicates the presence of an AP but does not prove participation in the tachycardia. A preexcitation index >70 ms is consistent with a left lateral AP.[31] The preexcitation index is the difference between the tachycardia cycle length and the longest coupling interval of a right ventricular apical premature

BOX 26.1 Diagnostic Criteria

Orthodromic Tachycardia

Obligatory 1:1 AV relationship with earliest atrial activation on AV free wall
- Shortest V-to-A time ≥60 ms
- Constant V-to-A conduction times despite TCL variations
- Advance atrial activation during His refractoriness (proves pathway presence but not participation in tachycardia)
- Preexcitation index >70 ms (left lateral AP)
- Ipsilateral bundle branch block prolongs His- (or V-) to-A time (and usually TCL) by ≥35 ms[a]
- Reproducible tachycardia termination by premature ventricular stimuli during His refractoriness without conduction to atrium[b]

Antidromic Tachycardia

Obligatory 1:1 AV relationship with earliest ventricular activation on free wall
- QRS morphology in tachycardia consistent with maximal preexcitation
- Tachycardia QRS morphology reproduced by atrial pacing near pathway insertion
- Each limb of tachycardia circuit supports conduction at TCL
- Advance ventricular activation by atrial extrastimuli near insertion with advancement of subsequent His and atrial activation
- Changes in V-to-His interval precede changes in TCL
- Exclusion of ventricular tachycardia and bystander participation, especially AV nodal reentry (His-to-A time in tachycardia ≤70 ms consistent with AV nodal reentry)

[a]Proves free wall AP-mediated tachycardia.
[b]Proves AP-mediated tachycardia.
A, Atrium; *AP,* accessory pathway; *AV,* atrioventricular; *His,* bundle of His; *TCL,* tachycardia cycle length; *V,* ventricle.

stimulus that advances the atrium.[31] *Diagnostic* of participation of a free wall pathway is prolongation of the QRS-to-atrium (or His-to-atrium) time during reciprocating tachycardia (and usually of the tachycardia cycle length as well) by 35–40 ms or longer with ipsilateral bundle branch block.[30,32] Left anterior fascicular block also prolongs the QRS-to-atrium time in patients with left free wall APs.[32] Coupled with an eccentric atrial activation sequence, the ability to reproducibly terminate the tachycardia with a premature ventricular stimulus delivered during His bundle refractoriness but that does not result in atrial activation also proves an ORT. Parahissian pacing techniques consistently indicate the presence of retrograde conduction over right free wall APs.[33] The response of left free wall APs to parahisian pacing is more complex. In about 25% of cases of left free wall APs, parahissian pacing is consistent with retrograde conduction over only the AV node. His capture may lead to a paradoxical shortening of the ventricle-to-atrium times, with left lateral APs because of the more rapid activation of the left free wall through the His-Purkinje system than occurs with septal ventricular capture alone.

The diagnostic features of antidromic reciprocating tachycardia are given in Box 26.1. Preexcited reciprocating tachycardias may use the AV node or a second AP as the retrograde limb. There are no surface ECG features that are diagnostic of antidromic tachycardia, but the diagnosis is excluded by demonstration of an atrial-to-ventricular relationship other than 1:1. Antidromic reciprocating tachycardias account for around 5% of AVRT and give rise to broad complex QRSd ≥120 ms.

Differential Diagnosis

ORTs using free wall APs must be differentiated from atrial tachycardias arising from near the atrioventricular (AV) valve annuli or CS musculature.[34] Differentiation between atrial tachycardia and ORT is best accomplished by dissociating the ventricles from the tachycardia using entrainment maneuvers. The demonstration of a V-A-A-V response after termination of ventricular pacing that entrains the atrium excludes an ORT and confirms an atrial tachycardia.[35] The ability to initiate the tachycardia with ventricular pacing, initiation with a critical AV or ventriculoatrial (VA) interval, and advancement of the same atrial activation sequence with premature ventricular stimuli during His refractoriness are all consistent with an ORT rather than AV nodal reentry.[30]

About 6% of cases of AV nodal reentry tachycardia (AVNRT) are associated with an eccentric atrial activation sequence that is earliest in the posterior or distal CS, with even the shortest VA times being longer than 60 ms (Fig. 26.6).[36] This pattern is easily confused with ORT using a left-sided concealed AP, both at electrophysiologic testing and on the surface ECG, because the retrograde P wave during AVNRT is negative in leads I and aVL and positive in V_1. The eccentric atrial activation sequence is usually demonstrated with ventricular pacing as well. The keys to the diagnosis of AVNRT with eccentric atrial activation are (1) demonstration of dual AV nodal physiology, (2) ability to also induce *typical* AV nodal reentry with concentric atrial activation or variable patterns of retrograde atrial activation in most

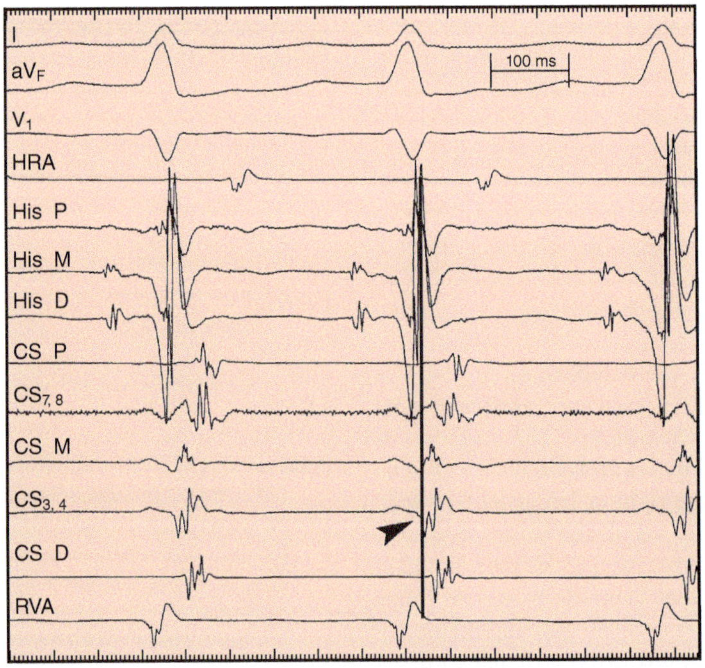

Fig. 26.6 Eccentric retrograde atrial activation during atrioventricular (AV) nodal reentrant tachycardia. The middle cardiac cycle is annotated, with ventricle-to-atrium (V-A) activation times indicated by the *vertical line*. The earliest atrial activation occurs in the next most distal bipole (*arrowhead*, CS 3,4) in the coronary sinus (CS) and there is also reversal of polarity between CS 3,4 and CS M bipoles. Indeed, this tachycardia was rendered noninducible by slow-pathway ablation. In this example, the V-A times are short for reciprocating tachycardia (and thus consistent with AV node reentry), but V-A times can also be long with an eccentric activation sequence in AV node reentry. *D*, Distal; *HRA*, high right atrium; *M*, mid; *P*, proximal; *RVA*, right ventricular apex.

TABLE 26.1 **Multivariate Predictors of Successful Left Free Wall Ablation Sites by the Transaortic Approach**

Study	AP Potential	EGM Stability	Delta-V Interval (ms)	A Amplitude	Local AV Interval (ms)	Local VA Interval (ms)	Best Positive Predictive Value (%)
Hindricks et al. 1995[42]	+	—	Value not specified	— (variable; performed during pre-excited AF)	—	—	70
Bashir et al. 1993[43]	+	—	10	—	—	—	20–25
Chen et al. 1992[41]	+	<10% change in EGM amplitude	0	A >1 mV	—	—	62
Cappato et al. 1994[44]	+	—	≤0	A/V ratio ≥0.1	≤40	—	87
Xie et al. 1996[45]	+	—	0	—	30	≤30	67
Villacastín et al. 1996[39]	+	—	—	—	—	Pseudo disappearance	59

A, Atrial electrogram; *AP,* accessory pathway; *AV,* atrium-to-ventricle; *Delta,* delta wave onset; *EGM,* electrogram; *V,* ventricular electrogram; *VA,* ventricle-to-atrium; —, not reported.

patients, (3) absence of retrograde VA conduction without isoproterenol, (4) inability to advance the atrium with premature ventricular stimuli during His refractoriness (may require left ventricular pacing), (5) demonstration of only decremental retrograde VA conduction, and (6) ability to dissociate the atrium and ventricle from the tachycardia.[36] Standard slow pathway modification or ablation in the region of the posteroseptal right atrium eliminates this tachycardia.

The differential diagnosis of an antidromic tachycardia includes ventricular tachycardia or a supraventricular tachycardia with passive activation of a bystander AP. Ventricular tachycardia should be diagnosed by the dissociation of the atrium from the tachycardia or a variable His-to-atrium timing relationship without alteration of the tachycardia cycle length. Antidromic tachycardia is diagnosed by demonstrating an obligatory 1:1 atrium-to-ventricle relationship during tachycardia, reproduction of tachycardia QRS morphology by atrial pacing at the presumed AP insertion site, and advancement of the ventricular *and* subsequent atrial activation by a premature atrial stimulus near the AP site (Table 26.1).[30]

The presence of a bystander AP is best recognized by dissociation of AP conduction from the tachycardia. The demonstration of a His-to-atrium interval of ≤70 ms indicates AV nodal reentry with bystander AP rather than an antidromic reciprocating tachycardia.[30]

BOX 26.2 **Target Sites**

Left Free Wall

Presumed AP potential
- Delta-VEGM ≤0 ms (anterograde conduction)
- VEGM–AEGM ≤40 ms (retrograde conduction)
- AEGM–VEGM ≤40 ms (anterograde conduction)
- AEGM amplitude >0.4 mV
- QRS–AEGM interval ≤70 ms (retrograde conduction)
- Isoelectric VEGM–AEGM interval ≤5 ms (retrograde conduction)
- Site of AEGM polarity reversal (in tachycardia)

Right Free Wall

Presumed AP potential
- Delta-VEGM ≤ −10 ms
- AEGM amplitude >1 mV
- AEGM–VEGM ≤40 ms (anterograde conduction)
- QRS–AEGM interval ≤70 ms (retrograde conduction)
- Isoelectric VEGM–AEGM interval ≤5 ms (retrograde conduction)

AEGM, Atrial electrogram; *AP,* accessory pathway; *Delta,* delta wave onset; *QRS,* QRS onset; *VEGM,* ventricular electrogram.

MAPPING

The most widely used approaches to mapping of free wall APs rely on identification of the earliest ventricular activation during anterograde AP conduction and earliest retrograde atrial activation during ORT or retrograde eccentric conduction (Box 26.2). However, mapping based on electrogram morphology rather than timing can be performed in some situations. Both unipolar and bipolar recordings are helpful. Unipolar recordings from the electrode tip provide information on local activation through electrogram timing and morphology. Bipolar recordings from the distal electrode pair reflect timing and more clearly demonstrate the electrogram components and AP potentials. Three-dimensional computer mapping has become the standard imaging tool for mapping APs and for marking the best sites to return to if catheter stability is poor, mechanical pressure (transiently) disrupts pathway conduction (bump termination) or pathway conduction returns shortly after ablation has been transiently successful.

Left Free Wall Accessory Pathways

Mapping of left free wall APs is facilitated by multielectrode recordings from a CS catheter; however, the anatomical distance

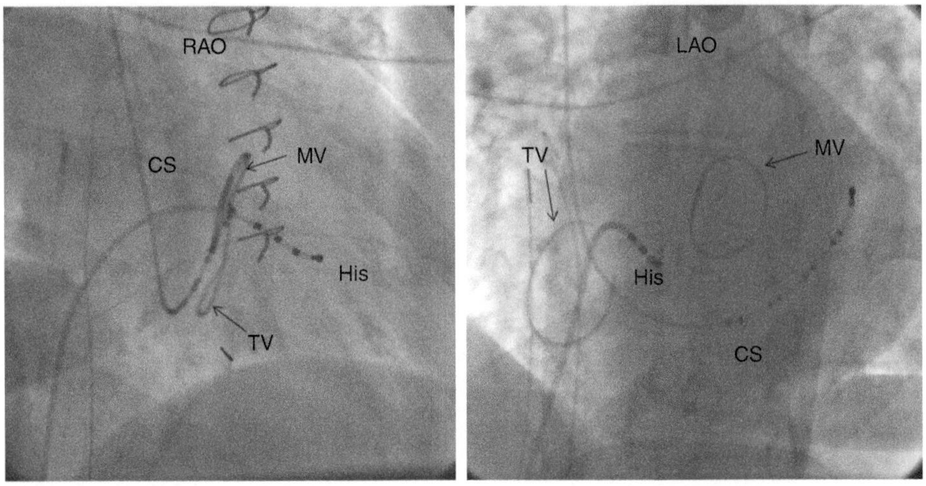

Fig. 26.7 Fluoroscopic position of tricuspid (TV) and mitral (MV) valve annuli as defined by valvuloplasty rings. Note the separation of the mitral valve annulus from the coronary sinus catheter (CS) in the left anterior oblique (LAO) view. *RAO,* Right anterior oblique.

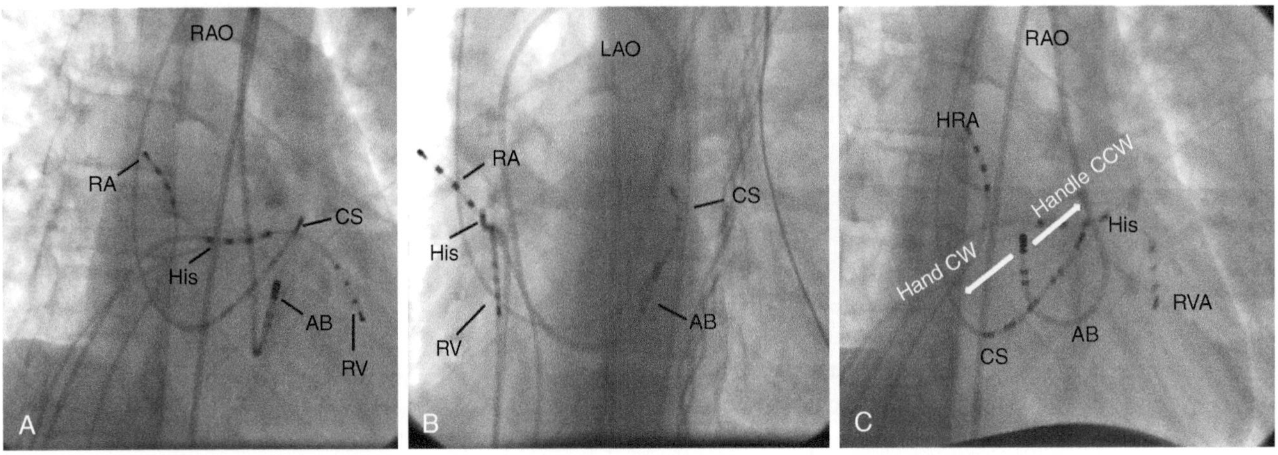

Fig. 26.8 Catheter positions in right anterior oblique (RAO) (A) and left anterior oblique (LAO) (B) views for ablation of left free wall accessory pathway by the retrograde transaortic approach. (C) Catheter-tip motion in response to torque on the handle once in mapping position. *AB,* Ablation catheter; *CCW,* counterclockwise; *CS,* coronary sinus catheter; *CW,* clockwise; *His,* His bundle catheter; *RA,* right atrial catheter; *RV,* right ventricular catheter.

from the true mitral annulus limits the accuracy of CS mapping alone to identify target sites for ablation (Fig. 26.7). Left free wall APs can be ablated without the use of CS catheters (single catheter technique), but the CS catheter is standard, along with right atrial, His, and right ventricular catheters.[37,38] Mapping and ablation may be performed via the transaortic (retrograde) approach or transseptal (anterograde) approach. The transaortic approach is directed at sites beneath the mitral annulus and therefore targets the AP ventricular insertion. For the transaortic approach, the catheter is always prolapsed across the aortic valve to prevent perforation of the leaflets or entry into the coronary arteries. The catheter readily crosses the aortic valve, with the D curvature of the deflected catheter tip opening to the right of the fluoroscopy screen (anteriorly) in the right anterior oblique view. After entering the left ventricular cavity, the curvature is maintained on the catheter tip, and the catheter is rotated in a counterclockwise direction to turn the catheter tip posteriorly toward the annulus (Fig. 26.8 and Video 26.1 on Expert Consult). The catheter can then be opened slightly to engage a subannular position, or it can be withdrawn to cross over the annulus into the left atrium. The catheter tip is either moved incrementally in steps beneath the annulus or made to slide along the mitral annulus for mapping before being dropped down beneath the annulus for energy delivery (see Fig. 26.8). It is often difficult to achieve stable catheter positions for the far lateral and anterior mitral annulus with the transaortic approach and the subvalvular apparatus can make catheter manipulation challenging.

The transseptal approach has become the preferred method at mapping the atrial side of the annulus or the mitral annulus itself. As opposed to the transaortic approach, in which the ablation electrode is perpendicular to and beneath the annulus, the transseptal approach is directed at positions on or above the annulus, with the electrodes parallel to the annulus (Fig. 26.9).[1,39] After passing through the atrial septum, the catheter is directed laterally with a large sweeping

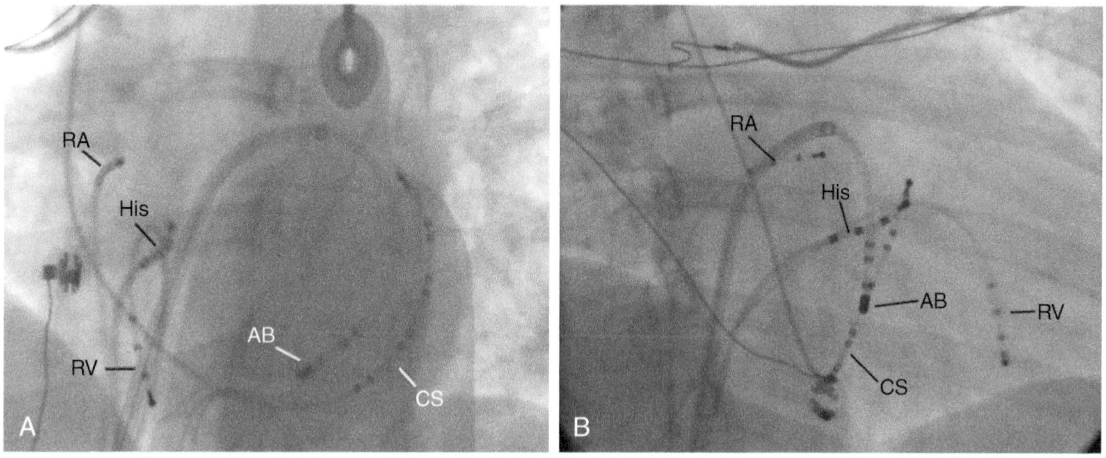

Fig. 26.9 Catheter positions for transseptal approach to ablation of left free wall accessory pathway. (A) Left anterior oblique view showing the preformed transseptal sheath (Daig SL2 Swartz Sheath) crossing the foramen ovale and used to position the ablation catheter (AB) along the proximal mitral annulus. From this position, the ablation catheter can be easily advanced to move proximally on the annulus and withdrawn to move distally. (B) Right anterior oblique view of catheter positions. The ablation catheter has been moved slightly more distally. Note that the tip of the ablation catheter is slightly on the ventricular side of the coronary sinus catheter (CS). *His*, His bundle catheter; *RA*, right atrial catheter; *RV*, right ventricular apical catheter.

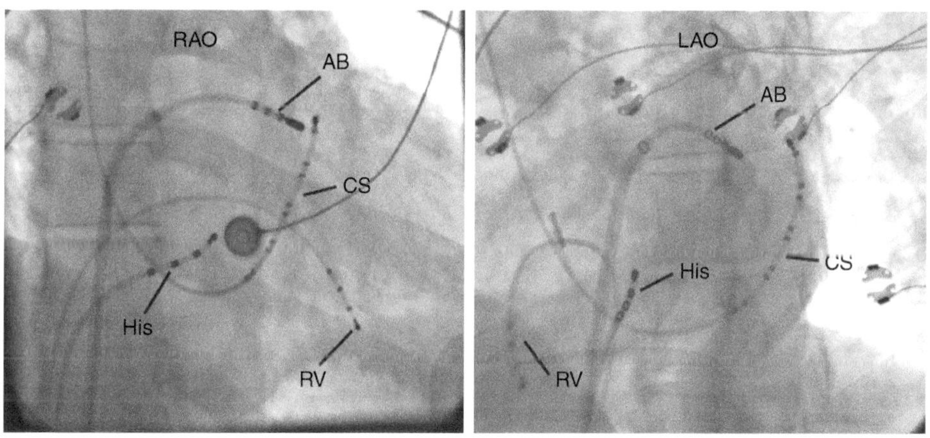

Fig. 26.10 Transseptal approach to ablation of a left anterior accessory pathway. Turning the sheath and catheter in a counterclockwise direction allows advancing the tip into the left ventricle. By advancing the sheath, the superior aspect of the annulus is reached. The ablation catheter is then straightened and withdrawn to map the annulus. *AB*, Ablation catheter; *CS*, coronary sinus catheter; *His*, His bundle catheter; *LAO*, left anterior oblique; *RAO*, right anterior oblique; *RV*, right ventricular apical catheter.

curve to direct the tip back toward the atrial septum. With the aid of preformed sheaths, the catheter tip is made to slide along the annulus by advancing and withdrawing the catheter (see Fig. 23.9 and Video 26.2 on Expert Consult). Anterior mitral valve positions are readily reached with the transseptal approach (Fig. 26.10). Although ability to maneuver the catheter is greater, catheter stability may be more problematic than with the transaortic approach.

The decision regarding use of the transaortic or transseptal approach is based on physician familiarity and certain patient characteristics. Because the two approaches are complementary, it is best for the physician to be familiar with both techniques. The transseptal approach is favored in the presence of peripheral vascular disease, aortic valve disease or prosthesis, or small ventricular chambers. In children weighing <30 kg, the transaortic approach may be associated with frequent valve trauma.[40] The transseptal approach provides better access to far lateral and anterolateral AP locations. The transseptal approach may be contraindicated in the presence of distorted cardiac anatomy such as congenital heart disease, pneumonectomy, kyphoscoliosis, or severe dilation of the aorta or right atrium. Intracardiac or transesophageal echocardiography (TEE) would be necessary for these cases.

The characteristics of electrograms at successful ablation sites have been studied extensively for left free wall APs.[39,41–45] Most of these data are derived from early experience with

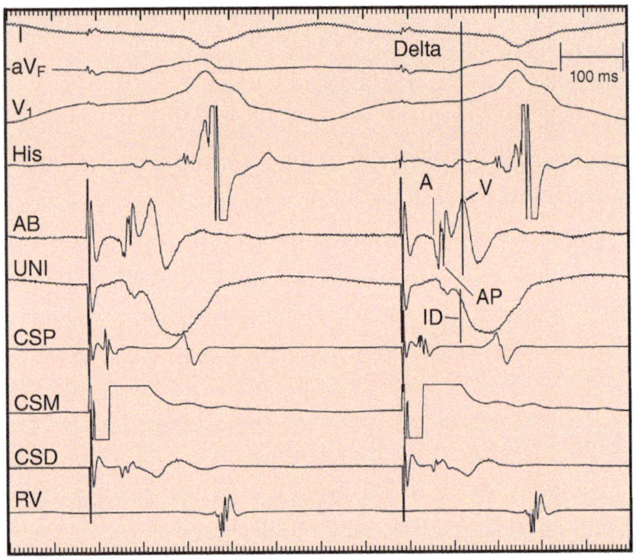

Fig. 26.11 Mapping anterograde left free wall accessory pathway (AP) activation during pacing from the middle coronary sinus (CSM). The onset of the delta wave (*Delta*) is marked by the *vertical line* on the surface electrocardiographic leads *(top three tracings)*. On the bipolar distal ablation electrodes (AB), the onset of the local atrial electrogram (A) and the onset of local ventricular electrogram (V) are marked. The local atrium-to-ventricle (A-V) interval is 25 ms, and the peak of the local bipolar ventricular electrogram coincides with delta wave onset (Delta-V = 0). The intrinsicoid deflection (ID) of the unipolar electrogram (UNI) precedes delta wave onset by approximately 5 ms. The unipolar ventricular ablation electrogram is entirely negative (QS morphology) and fuses with the atrial electrogram. A discrete high-frequency electrogram between the atrial and ventricular components represents a possible AP potential. *CSD,* Distal coronary sinus; *CSP,* proximal coronary sinus; *RV,* right ventricle.

ablation by the transaortic approach and have not been reproduced for the transseptal approach. Five electrogram characteristics have been described as useful in predicting successful ablation sites when mapping anterograde AP activation by the transaortic approach: (1) delta-to-ventricle (V) interval, (2) atrial electrogram amplitude, (3) electrogram stability, (4) local AV electrogram interval, and (5) presence of a presumed AP potential. The delta-to-V interval should be measured from the onset of the delta wave to the peak or intrinsicoid deflection of bipolar mapping electrograms.[42,43,46] For unipolar electrograms, the maximal negative *dV/dt* reflects local ventricular activation.[46] The absence of a QS morphology in the unipolar electrogram indicates a site with a <10% chance of ablation success. Pacing from near the AP insertion should also accentuate the degree of preexcitation. For left free wall APs, a delta-to-V time of ≤0 ms is usually recorded at successful ablation sites, with average intervals of only 2–10 ms (Fig. 26.11).[41,43,47]

The atrial electrogram amplitude at successful sites should be >0.4–1 mV, or the atrial-to-ventricular (A/V) ratio should be >0.1 by the transaortic approach. The small atrial electrogram amplitude indicates the subannular position of the catheter. The absence of any atrial electrogram suggests a position too far from the annulus. For transseptal mapping, an A/V ratio equal to 1 is sought along the mitral annulus.[38] Greater and lesser ratios indicate atrial and ventricular displacement of the catheter, respectively. Electrogram stability is defined as <10% change in the atrial and ventricular electrogram amplitudes or A/V ratio >5–10 cardiac cycles.[41,43,45]

The transaortic approach usually provides good catheter stability because the catheter is "wedged" beneath the mitral valve. Conventionally, for the transseptal approach, stability can be assessed by consistent electrogram amplitudes, catheter motion concordant with the CS catheter (on fluoroscopy), and when on the atrial side of the annulus, consistent PR segment elevation on the unipolar electrogram.[13] The last finding also indicates sufficient catheter contact with the atrial myocardium. In the modern era, catheters that recognize tissue contact with the catheter (contact force) are extremely helpful. Local AV intervals of ≤40 ms should be sought, with average intervals of 25–50 ms reported for successful ablation sites (see Fig. 26.11).[44,45] The AV intervals for left free wall APs are longer than for other AP locations, and the times at successful sites overlap with those at unsuccessful sites. The local AV times alone therefore have limited specificity in identifying successful ablation sites for left-sided APs.

Finally, the recording of a presumed AP potential has been used to define appropriate ablation sites. The ability to record AP potentials may be influenced by the catheter approach used to map the annulus. Presumed AP potentials are defined as discrete, high-frequency potentials that occur between the atrial and ventricular electrograms and at least 10 ms before the onset of the delta wave (see Fig. 26.11).[39,41,42,44,48] The amplitude of AP potentials ranges from 0.5 to 1 mV.[41] The validation of a signal as a true AP potential is a tedious process and is not always practical in the clinical setting. It is probably for this reason that AP potentials are reported at 35–94% of successful ablation sites and at up to 72% of unsuccessful sites.[41,42,44,48,49] The recording of larger AP potentials in the CS than along the mitral annulus suggests the presence of an epicardial AP.[50]

For mapping of retrograde AP conduction during ORT or ventricular pacing, electrogram characteristics reported to identify successful sites include catheter stability, presence of a presumed AP potential, continuous electrical activity, and the local VA interval.[39,41,45] These data are derived largely from studies using the transaortic approach. Catheter stability is defined the same as for mapping of anterograde conduction. The presence of a presumed AP potential is reported at only 37–67% of successful ablation sites during retrograde AP conduction mapping.[39,41,45] It is possible that AP potentials are obscured by the large ventricular electrogram with the transaortic approach. The QRS onset-to-local atrial electrogram (QRS-A) interval is usually about 70 ms in the absence of a left ventricular conduction delay (Fig. 26.12).[39,41] The local VA interval at successful ablation sites is typically 25–50 ms.[39,41,45] At very short VA intervals, the atrial electrogram may be inscribed on the terminal portion of the ventricular electrogram. Continuous electrical activity (<5-ms isoelectric interval between V and A electrograms) and the pseudo-disappearance of the atrial electrogram into the ventricular electrogram are manifestations of extremely short VA times.[39,43] One group has reported successful ablation

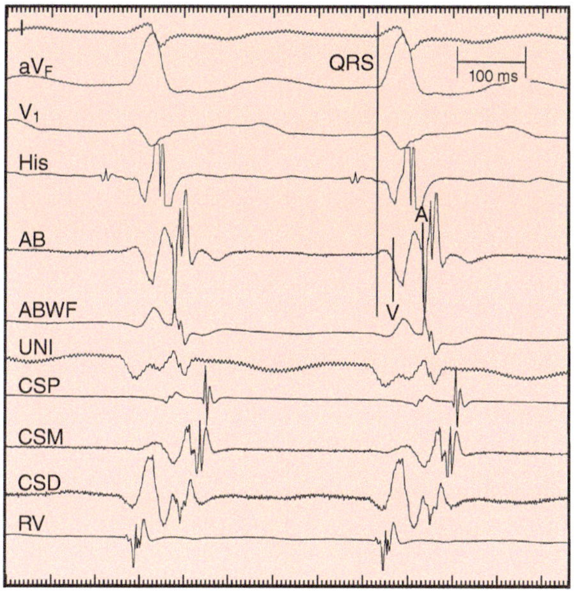

Fig. 26.12 Electrograms from successful ablation site during mapping of retrograde accessory pathway (AP) conduction in orthodromic reciprocating tachycardia. The distal coronary sinus is earliest on this catheter. The QRS onset (QRS) to local atrial electrogram (A) interval on the ablation catheter is 68 ms and is shown by the *vertical line*. The local ventricular (V)-to-atrial interval on the ablation electrodes is 40 ms. *AB,* Ablation catheter; *CSD,* distal coronary sinus; *CSM,* middle coronary sinus; *CSP,* proximal coronary sinus; *His,* His bundle catheter; *RV,* right ventricle; *UNI,* unipolar electrogram.

by pace mapping beneath the mitral annulus with the ablation catheter and measuring the stimulus-to-atrial times recorded on the CS catheter.[51] The site producing the shortest stimulus-to-atrial interval should be at the ventricular insertion of the AP. The average stimulus-to-atrial interval at successful sites was 46 ± 15 ms.[51]

The predictive accuracy of any single electrogram characteristic for identifying a successful ablation site rarely exceeds 30%. The electrogram must satisfy three or four criteria to achieve 60–80% predictive values.[43,48] Multivariate predictors of successful ablation sites are given in Table 26.1.

One problem with mapping retrograde atrial activation times is the difficulty in discriminating between atrial and ventricular components of the electrograms. This problem may be addressed in several ways. One method is to compare the electrogram recorded on the ablation catheter while simultaneously pacing the atrium and the ventricle with the electrogram recorded during ventricular pacing alone (Fig. 26.13).[52]

Another approach to unmasking distinct components of anterograde and retrograde electrograms exploits the oblique course of AP conduction across the AV annulus.[53] For left free wall APs, the ventricular insertion is usually more proximal in the CS than the atrial insertion.[53,54] When the ventricular insertion of the AP is activated by a wavefront conducting in the same direction as the oblique AP propagation, the VA intervals recorded on mapping electrodes are short and may overlap (Figs. 26.14 and 26.15). By reversing the direction of wavefront activation, the local VA intervals may be prolonged if conduction over the AP backtracks past ventricular sites previously activated. The same separation of components of anterogradely conducted electrograms is possible by reversing the direction of activation of the atrial AP insertion. For left lateral APs, pacing of the basal posteroseptal right ventricle provides counterclockwise activation of the ventricular insertion (from the left anterior oblique perspective), whereas pacing of the high right ventricular outflow tract near the pulmonic valve provides clockwise activation of the ventricular insertion. Because the ventricular AP insertion tends to be more proximal along the CS than the atrial insertion, the VA intervals are typically prolonged by clockwise activation with right ventricular outflow tract pacing. A change in local VA times of >15 ms is considered to represent a significant change in the activation wavefront. For reversing atrial activation wavefronts of left free wall APs, CS pacing proximal and distal to the site of earliest retrograde atrial activity is used. For anterograde mapping, pacing distal to the atrial insertion should provide a counterclockwise activation wavefront and the longest AV intervals. The target sites are AP potentials or just to the side of the earliest site of atrial or ventricular activation predicted to be the mid-AP site by changes in the local electrogram times. Note that this technique does not target the sites of the shortest AV or VA times, which may spuriously indicate AP location because of pathway slant.

A useful technique for ablation of left free wall pathways from the transseptal approach is to identify the point of atrial electrogram polarity reversal when mapping the annulus.[55] This vectorial technique obviates the need to measure VA intervals. Through transseptal access, the ablation electrode bipole is oriented parallel to the axis of the annulus. Wide-bandpass electrogram filtering is set to 0.5–500 Hz to accentuate the directional characteristics of the electrogram polarity. The bipole is then moved proximally and distally, parallel to the annulus, during ORT, and the polarity of the atrial electrogram is noted. With the tip electrode negative and the proximal electrode positive, the atrial electrogram will be predominantly negative at catheter positions on the annulus proximal to the atrial insertion (Fig. 26.16). At positions distal to the atrial insertion, the direction of the atrial activation wavefront is reversed relative to the bipole, and the atrial electrogram is predominantly positive. The point at which the atrial electrogram becomes isoelectric marks the atrial insertion and the site for ablation. The positive predictive value of electrogram reversal for identifying the successful ablation site is 75%.[55] To be effective, this technique requires that the mapping bipole remain parallel with the axis of atrial activation on the annulus.

Right Free Wall Accessory Pathways

Mapping and ablation of right free wall APs is more difficult than for left-sided APs because of the absence of a venous structure paralleling the tricuspid annulus and because of catheter instability. To facilitate rapid localization of right free wall APs, it is often useful to employ a circular multi-electrode halo catheter positioned near the tricuspid annulus

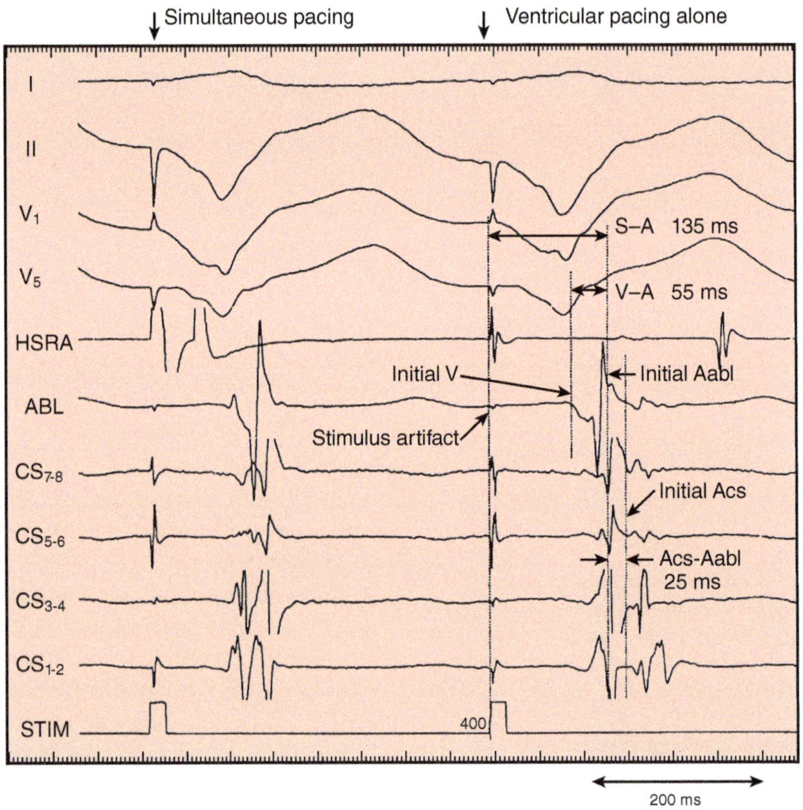

Fig. 26.13 Use of simultaneous atrial and ventricular pacing to discriminate components of mapping electrograms in a patient with left-sided accessory pathway. The penultimate beat of the drive train comprises simultaneous atrial and ventricular pacing (labeled). The atrial electrogram is advanced relative to the ventricular electrogram and precedes it. No electrical activity follows the ventricular activation in this beat. The last beat of the drive comprises only ventricular pacing. Retrograde conduction over the accessory pathway is evident by atrial activation now following the ventricular electrograms. By comparing the electrograms from the two cardiac cycles, the atrial and ventricular components of the electrograms are more apparent. *Aabl,* Onset local retrograde atrial electrogram on the ablation catheter; *ABL,* ablation; *Acs,* onset local atrial electrogram recorded on the coronary sinus; *CS1-2,* distal coronary sinus; *CS7-8,* proximal coronary sinus; *HSRA,* high septal right atrium; *S-A,* interval between stimulus artifact (Stim) and local atrial electrogram; *V-A,* interval between local ventricular and atrial electrograms. (From Nakao K, Seto S, Iliev II, et al. Simultaneous atrial and ventricular pacing to facilitate mapping of concealed left-sided accessory pathways. *Pacing Clin Electrophysiol.* 2002;25:922–928.)

(Fig. 26.17). Use of this catheter, or rarely, of 2 F mapping catheters positioned in the right coronary artery represents the closest equivalent to a CS mapping for the right side of the heart.[8] Catheter mapping from the subclavian or right internal jugular approach is sometimes more productive than from the femoral approach. As for transseptal access to the left side of the heart, the use of preformed or steerable sheaths to direct the ablation catheter to specific locations on the tricuspid annulus is helpful. The sheaths allow for placement of the mapping catheter parallel to the annulus for mapping, as with the transseptal approach to left APs (see Fig. 26.17 and Video 26.3 on Expert Consult).

Because of the relative infrequency of right free wall APs, multivariate analyses of electrogram characteristics specific to this site that predict successful ablation are not available. Presumably, the stability and AP criteria defined for left APs are applicable. For ablation along the tricuspid annulus, a 1:1 A/V ratio is usually sought.[47,56] Most series have also used retrograde local VA times of 40 ms or less as a criterion for radiofrequency (RF) delivery. The timing of local ventricular activation before delta wave onset is usually earlier than for left APs (Fig. 26.18). Haïssaguerre and colleagues[47,56] found that the local ventricle preceded delta wave onset by 18 ± 10 ms for right APs and 2 ± 6 ms for left APs at successful sites. The average local AV time was 28 ± 7 ms for right-sided APs. In children, the local AV times were 11–26 ms, with delta-to-V electrogram intervals of 28–52 ms at sites of successful right free wall AP ablation in five patients.[57] If it is difficult to discriminate the components of the local electrograms, reversal of the activating wavefronts may be useful, as described earlier.[53] For right free wall APs, opposing ventricular wavefronts are produced by pacing the right ventricle near the annulus, anterior and posterior to the site of earliest retrograde AP conduction. Opposing atrial activation

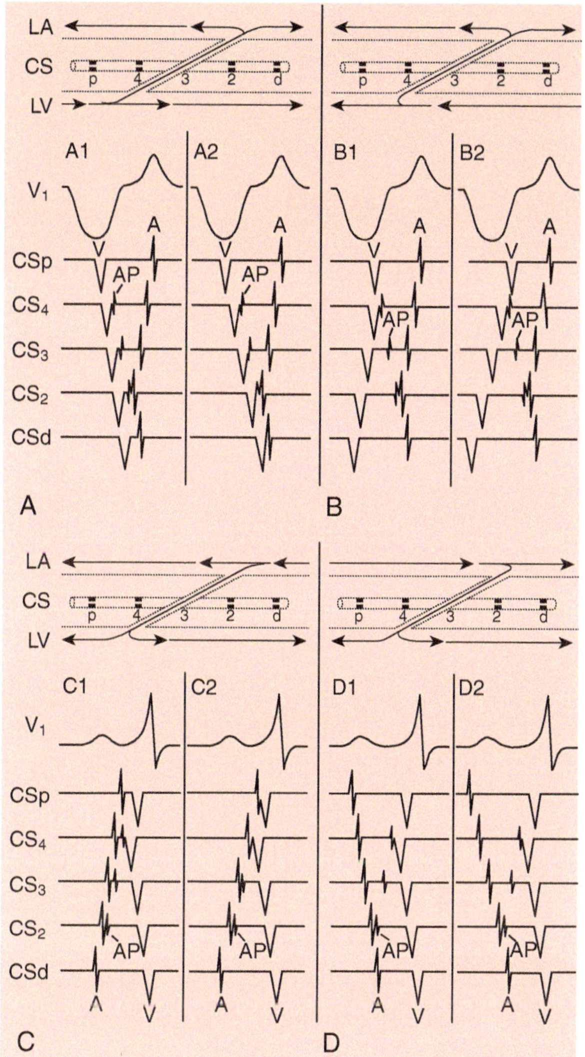

Fig. 26.14 Activation of oblique accessory pathways. Schematic of anterograde and retrograde activation of an oblique left free wall accessory pathway (AP) from opposing directions. (A, B) Activation of the ventricular insertion from the proximal-to-distal and distal-to-proximal directions, respectively. (C, D) Activation of the atrial insertion from the distal-to-proximal and proximal-to-distal directions, respectively. Note the separation of the components of the electrograms when the AP is activated from the direction opposite to the direction of conduction over the pathway. *A,* Atrial potential; *CS,* coronary sinus; *d,* distal; *LA,* left atrium; *LV,* left ventricle; *p,* proximal; *V,* ventricular potential. (From Kenichiro O, Gonzalez M, Beckman K, et al. Reversing the direction of paced ventricular and atrial wavefronts reveals an oblique course in accessory AV pathways and improves localization for catheter ablation. *Circulation.* 2001;104:550–556.)

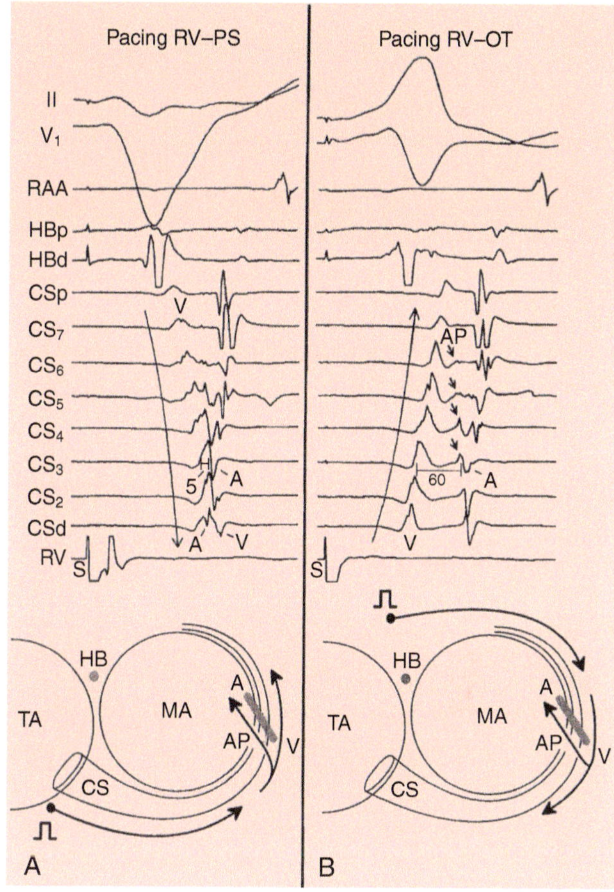

Fig. 26.15 Reversing the direction of activation of the ventricular insertion in a patient with a left lateral accessory pathway (AP). The schematics show the presumed pathway orientation and wavefront propagation. When activated from proximal to distal by right ventricular posteroseptal (RV-PS) pacing (A), the coronary sinus (CS) electrograms overlap considerably. When activated from distal to proximal by right ventricular outflow tract (RV-OT) pacing (B), there is greater separation of the electrogram components and definition of an AP potential. *d,* Distal; *HB,* His bundle; *MA,* mitral annulus; *p,* proximal; *RAA,* right atrial appendage; *S,* stimulus artifact; *TA,* tricuspid annulus. (From Kenichiro O, Gonzalez M, Beckman K, et al. Reversing the direction of paced ventricular and atrial wavefronts reveals an oblique course in accessory AV pathways and improves localization for catheter ablation. *Circulation.* 2001;104:550–556.)

is produced by pacing on either side of the presumed atrial insertion.

Of the about 10% of right free wall APs where TVA mapping and ablation is unsuccessful, the atrial insertion site may be off the annulus. Chen et al.[58] studied 11 patients who had failed right free wall AP ablations using both temperature-controlled and irrigated catheters, guided by electrophysiologic and fluoroscopic mapping along the tricuspid annulus. Electroanatomical mapping was performed in the right atrium during ORT, or with ventricular pacing. The earliest atrial activation representing the insertion site of the AP was found to be separated from the TVA by an average of 14.3 ± 3.9 mm, and the local activation time was 27.8 ± 17.0 ms earlier than the earliest TVA point. RF ablation (RFA) with an irrigated catheter at the earliest site successfully ablated all of these previously failed pathways (Fig. 26.19).[58]

Electroanatomical Mapping

For both right and left free walls, AP electroanatomical mapping systems of electrical activation is optional because of the discrete area of interest. However, in efforts to minimize radiation exposure and prevent deterministic/stochastic effects,

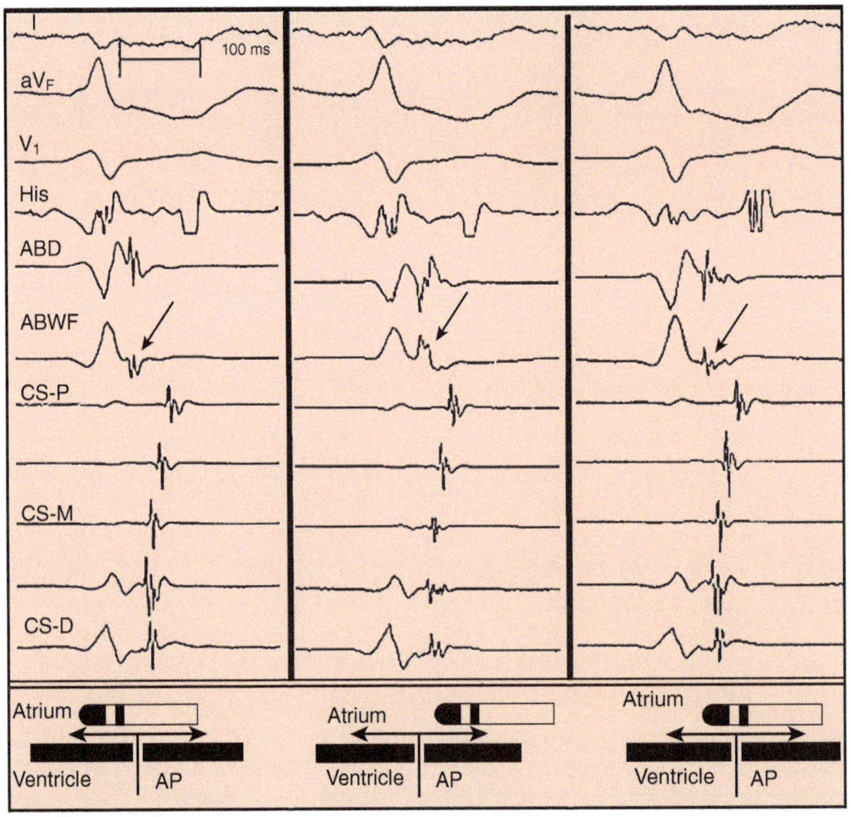

Fig. 26.16 Atrial electrogram polarity reversal during mapping of orthodromic reciprocating tachycardia using a left free wall accessory pathway. *Left,* During reciprocating tachycardia, the distal bipolar ablation electrograms are displayed with standard (ABD) filtering at 30–500 Hz and wide filtering (ABWF) at 0.5–500 Hz. Here, the electrode is parallel to the annulus and proximal to the site of atrial accessory pathway (AP) insertion. The atrial component of the ABWF electrogram *(arrow)* is negative. *Middle,* The distal electrode pair has been moved distal to the site of the AP insertion, represented by the positive atrial component to the ABWF electrogram. *Right,* When the electrode pair is directly over the atrial insertion of the AP, the atrial component to the ABWF electrogram is isoelectric as the wavefront spreads away from the electrode pair in two opposing directions. The schematics at the *bottom* of the tracings illustrate the relation of the electrodes to the atrial insertion site. *CS,* Coronary sinus; *D,* distal; *M,* mid; *P,* proximal.

electroanatomical mapping systems have gained popularity, especially in pediatric patients as a result of dramatic reduction in fluoroscopic exposure to near-zero levels.[57,59,60] One study used the novel imaging tool CARTO UNIVU (Biosense-Webster, Diamond Bar, CA), an advanced imaging module for CARTO 3 (Biosense-Webster) system that allows integration of fluoroscopic images with three-dimensional electroanatomical maps in pediatric patients who underwent left-sided AP ablation.[60] The authors reported a significant reduction in fluoroscopic time (0.1 versus 8.4 min, $P < .05$), fluoroscopy dose (0.5 versus 132 mGy, $P < .05$), number of catheters used (two versus three, $P < .05$), and number of vascular accesses (two versus three, $P < .05$) compared with controls, who underwent left-sided AP ablation using the CARTO 3 system. Importantly, there were no complications, and the long-term success rate was 97% at a median follow-up of 9.6 months.[60] The catheter navigation and registration capabilities of computerized systems are also very helpful because they allow the operator to precisely return to sites of interest (Fig. 26.20). Electroanatomical mapping is also useful if a right free wall pathway is off the annulus.[58]

Last, while electroanatomical mapping of accessory pathways has conventionally used point-by-point registration (and subsequent manual annotation of signals into either atrial, ventricular, or accessory pathway), the era of high-density mapping has permitted the emergence of a newer method to facilitate rapid and automatic annotation of electrical activation signals in order to define the accessory pathway. Open window mapping, as the name suggests, uses a window centered on the local signal with extension of the region of interest (or window) on either side to allow signals (wherever they arise, from the atrial or ventricular aspect of the annulus) indiscriminately. The maximal dV/dt is then automatically annotated (to differentiate near-field from far-field electrograms, which are also present within the region of interest). In doing so, the

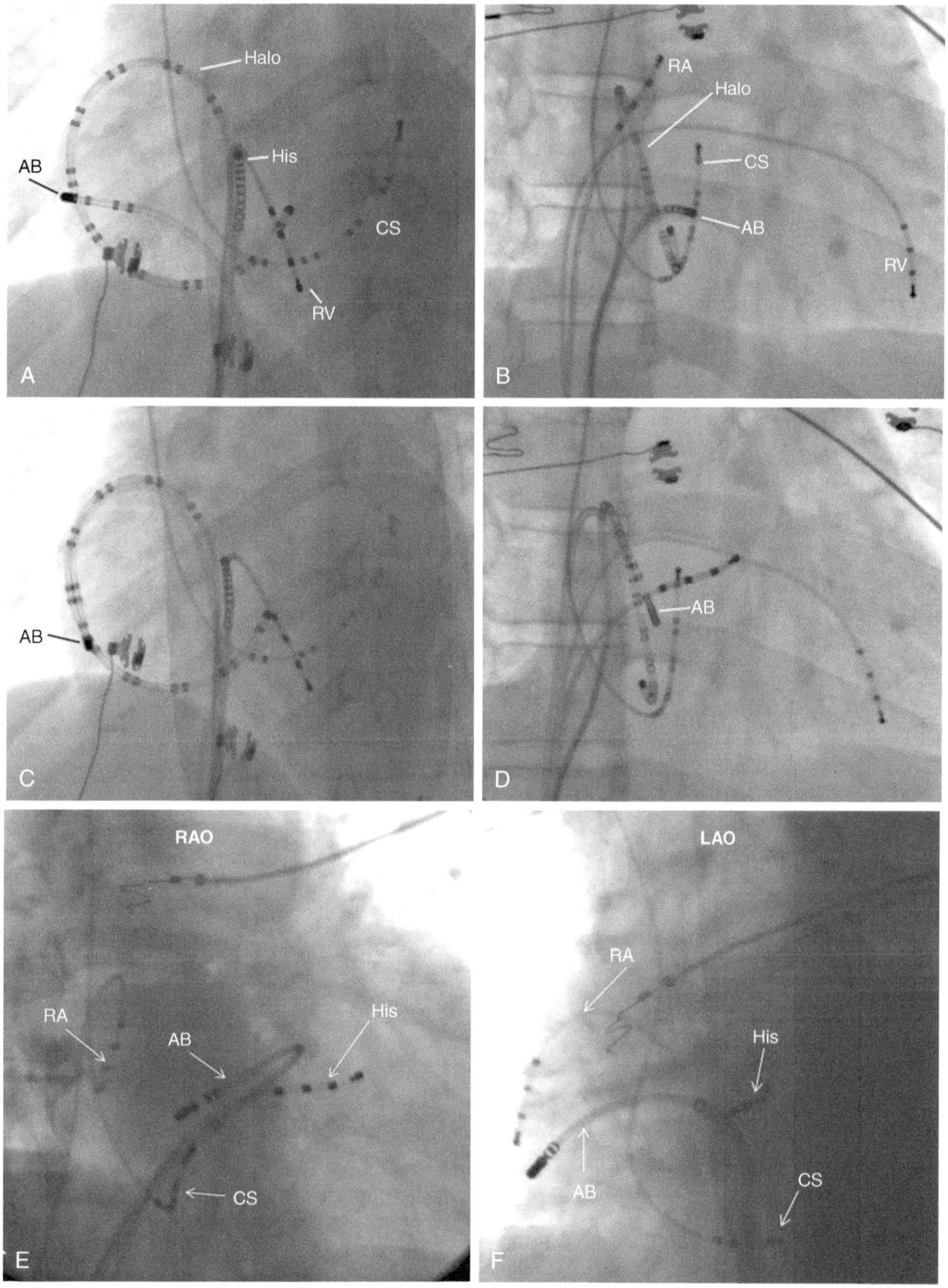

Fig. 26.17 Catheter positions for ablation of a right free wall accessory pathway. (A) Left anterior oblique (LAO) 40-degree view showing the 20-electrode halo catheter parallel to the tricuspid annulus and the ablation (AB) catheter near electrodes 11 and 12 along the free wall. The His, right ventricular apical (RV), and coronary sinus (CS) catheters are shown. (B) Right anterior oblique (RAO) 30-degree view of the same catheter positions as in A, except that the His bundle catheter is replaced by a right atrial (RA) catheter. Note that the ablation catheter tip is to the ventricular side of the halo catheter. (C) LAO 40-degree view with the ablation catheter now placed parallel to the tricuspid annulus. (D, RAO 30-degree view of catheter positions in C. (E, F) Ablation of right free wall accessory pathway with ablation catheter (AB) positioned under the tricuspid annulus. A Daig SR3 sheath is used to direct the catheter into the ventricle and under the annulus. In this patient, catheter positions on the atrial aspect of the annulus were unstable or unsuccessful. The accessory pathway was ablated at this site. An irrigated catheter was needed because of excessive temperatures with low-energy deliveries with a standard catheter.

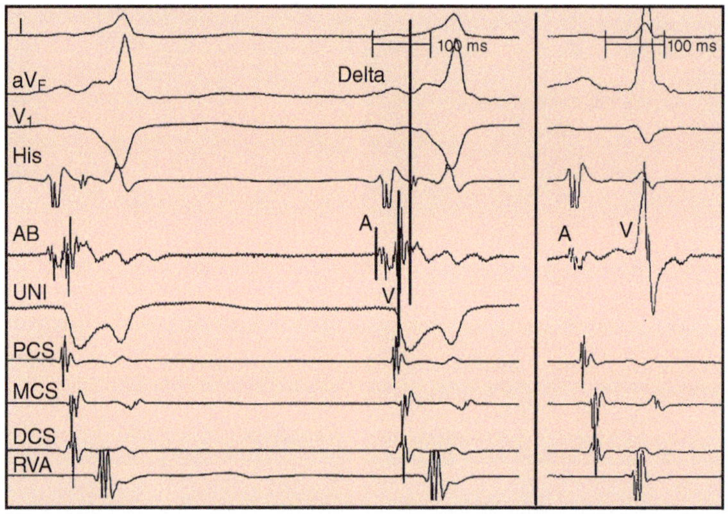

Fig. 26.18 Electrograms from the site of successful ablation of a right free wall accessory pathway. *Left,* On the distal ablation bipole (AB), there is continuous electrical activity with the local ventricular electrogram (V) preceding the delta wave (*Delta*) onset by 25 ms. The local atrial (A)-to-ventricular (V) electrogram interval is 38 ms. The unipolar distal ablation electrogram (UNI) has a QS morphology. *Right,* After ablation, the ablation electrogram shows prolongation of the atrioventricular times, but the morphology of the local atrial electrogram is unchanged. *DCS,* Distal coronary sinus; *MCS,* middle coronary sinus; *PCS,* proximal coronary sinus; *RVA,* right ventricular apex.

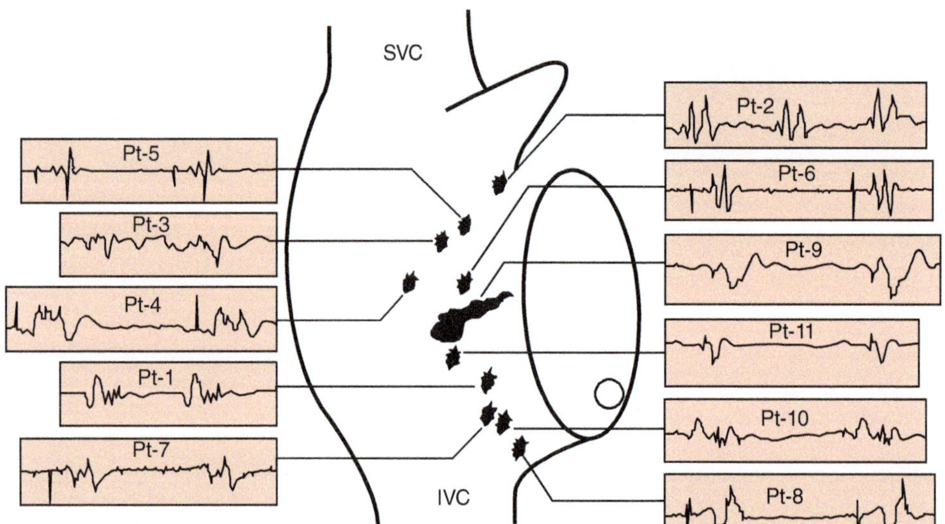

Fig. 26.19 Ablation sites in the body of the atrium away from the tricuspid valve annulus. Schematic representation of the distribution of target sites and their electrograms (paper speed = 100 mm/s) of all patients with an accessory pathway (AP) on the right-sided free wall. Nine patients presented an isolated deflection between ventricular electrogram and the atrial electrogram in their target electrograms, most probably suggesting an AP potential, and the remaining two showed ventriculoatrial fusion (patients 5 and 6). The average atrioventricular ratio in all the target sites is approximately 1.5. Patient 9 exhibited an AP with a wide branching in the right atrium. *IVC,* Inferior vena cava; *SVC,* superior vena cava. (From Chen M, Yang B, Ju W, et al. Right-sided free wall accessory pathway refractory to conventional catheter ablation: lessons from 3-dimensional electroanatomic mapping. *J Cardiovasc Electrophysiol.* 2010;21:1317–1324.)

"leak" along the annulus can be detected easily and therefore targeted (Fig. 26.21). It may be helpful to perform this with the pathway either fully preexcited (to avoid fusion) or during ORT. This technique confers advantages over conventional point-by-point methods by removing the reliance on subjective annotation of signals.

Ablation

Before ablation, it is essential to obtain the most stable catheter position possible. Catheter dislodgment before completion of the ablation lesion may transiently suppress AP function increasing chance of recurrence. Catheter stability is enhanced using preformed or steerable sheaths and catheters

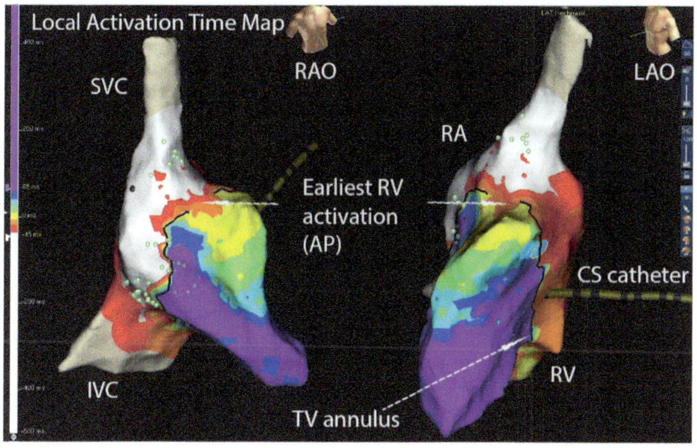

Fig. 26.20 Use of an electroanatomical catheter navigation system for ablation of a right free wall accessory pathway. Right anterior oblique (RAO; *left*) and left anterior oblique (LAO; right) representations (akin to fluoroscopic views). Signals and catheters are registered, and ablation lesions can be annotated. This map depicts the anatomy of the right atrium (RA) and ventricle (RV), as well as the superior vena cava (SVC) and inferior vena cava (IVC) and the TV annulus (*black free-form line* depicting an early-meets-late line of block). His signal (*light blue dots*) is annotated, as is the coronary sinus (CS) catheter shadow (*in yellow*). Earliest RV activation (across AP) marked by local activation (LAT) mapping (ms). The colors indicate antegrade activation of the accessory pathway (AP; *white arrows*) across the TV annulus on the right free wall (*from white-purple*). These maps allow easy anatomical registration of the regions of interest (His, AP, and TV) as well as the location of the catheters within the heart in real time and can therefore facilitate the operator to return to these areas quickly as required, reducing the need for fluoroscopy. Mapping was performed using a 16-electrode mapping catheter (Advisor HD Grid Sensor Enabled, Abbott Laboratories, Il) using the EnSite Precision system (Abbott laboratories, Il). (Courtesy Mr R Kutieleh and Professor P Sanders, Centre for Heart Rhythm Disorders, University of Adelaide.)

with sufficient curvature or reach to access the target site. With ventricular pacing to entrain reciprocating tachycardias, the ablation catheter is less subject to dislodgment on termination of the arrhythmia due to continued overdrive pacing at a similar rate to the tachycardia. Adequate sedation should be established before RF delivery to minimize patient movement in response to pain. Marking of the catheter site with electroanatomical mapping systems or by fluoroscopy may allow return to successful sites despite catheter dislodgment (see Fig. 26.22).

Standard 4-mm tip nonirrigated RF catheters are usually adequate for free wall APs. The target temperatures for right and left free wall APs is typically 60°C–65°C.[61] Favorable ablation sites should not be abandoned until temperatures >50°C–55°C are achieved. For impedance monitoring, a 5- to 10-Ω decrease in impedance usually signifies adequate tissue heating. The energy needed to reach the target temperature varies with catheter location. Low blood flow positions beneath the mitral or tricuspid annulus may require little energy because of the absence of convective cooling. Loss of AP function should occur within 1–6 seconds after RF energy delivery.[62] Longer times to success may be associated with higher recurrence rates.

Endocardial cryoablation is effective for free wall AP ablation and offers the advantage of complete catheter stability because of adherence to the tissue during ablation.[63] Another advantage of cryoablation is cryomapping, where the tip temperature is

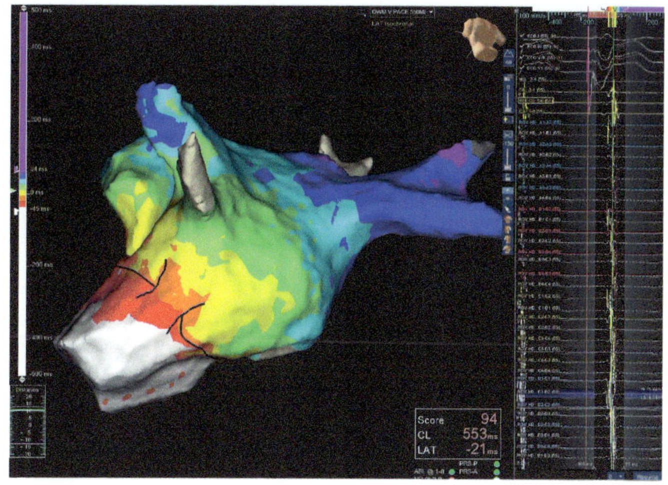

Fig. 26.21 Open window mapping of a concealed left free wall accessory pathway during ventricular pacing (cycle length 550 ms). Activation of the left atrium (*from white to purple*) is seen via a left free wall channel (AP) across the mitral annulus. Marked on the electroanatomical map as *a pair of black intersecting lines* across the mitral annulus (*black ring*). Targeted radiofrequency ablation at this site was successful. Mapping was performed using a 16-electrode mapping catheter (Advisor HD Grid Sensor Enabled, Abbott Laboratories, Il) using the EnSite Precision system (Abbott laboratories, Il). (Courtesy Mr R Kutieleh and Professor P Sanders, Centre for Heart Rhythm Disorders, University of Adelaide.)

progressively lowered to −30°C for a maximum of 60 seconds, allowing assessment of the lesion's results while the effects are still reversible. Large-tip (6 or 8 mm) cryoablation catheters should be used to minimize the likelihood of AP recurrence. If the cryoapplication results in sudden loss of AP conduction in 10–30 seconds, the lesion may be continued for 240–360 seconds with a target temperature of −70°C to −80°C.[64,65] Additional lesions may be applied to achieve a freeze-thaw-freeze effect. One study assessed the time to effect (TTE), that is, the time interval between the onset of cryomapping at −30°C and the disappearance of AP conduction.[66] The authors demonstrated that during a mean follow-up of 20 months, the AP recurrence rate was significantly lower at 6% if the TTE was within 10 seconds of reaching −30°C, compared with 38.5% when the TTE was longer than 10 seconds.

Irrigated-tip ablation catheters have now become standard practice although their initial use was restricted to resistant APs that failed conventional RF ablation.[67] Irrigated catheters, by cooling the tip, allow delivery of higher power and therefore create larger lesions.[67] In a study of irrigated catheter use for AP that failed conventional RF ablation, using a temperature cutoff of 50°C (which is higher than the usual cutoff of 42–48°C) with 50 W maximal power (outside the CS) and 20–30 W within the CS safely eliminated 94% of APs after failed conventional RF delivery.[67]

In one study involving 41 pediatric patients who underwent RFA of APs using an open-irrigation catheter, the procedural success rate was 95% after the first procedure, with no complications and no AP recurrence at 12 months.[68] Power was titrated up to 30 W for right-sided APs, 40 W for left-sided APs, and 20 W within the coronary sinus.[68] A 5- to 10-Ω impedance drop

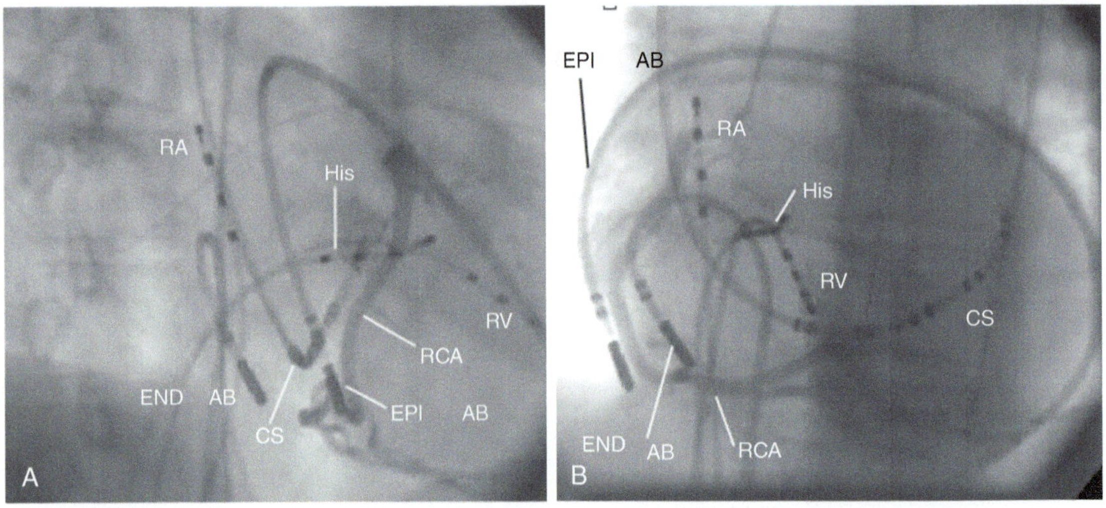

Fig. 26.22 Percutaneous epicardial catheter approach to ablation of an epicardial right inferior free wall pathway. (A) In this right anterior oblique view, the epicardial ablation catheter (EPI AB) enters the pericardial space from subxiphoid access and encircles the heart from posterior to anterior to reach the site of successful ablation. Attempts at ablation from the endocardial ablation catheter (END AB) failed. The right coronary artery (RCA) is visualized by angiography and is very near the epicardial ablation catheter. (B) Same catheter positions shown in left anterior oblique view. *CS,* Coronary sinus; *His,* His bundle catheter; *RA,* right atrial catheter; *RV,* right ventricular catheter.

is typically recommended. Ablation catheters with contact force sensing may further improve safety and success rates by providing real-time catheter tip–tissue contact information.

After successful ablation, thorough electrophysiologic testing should be undertaken to document the complete elimination of AP function and to exclude other mechanisms of tachycardias. Adenosine has shown to unmask dormant AP conduction after apparent successful catheter ablation in about 8–12% of the cases.[69,70] The likely mechanism is AP membrane potential hyperpolarization. Adenosine-induced dormant AP conduction is associated with a higher risk of clinical recurrence and, hence, necessitates additional ablation for complete elimination of AP conduction.[70]

Epicardial left free wall APs may require ablation from within the CS (Table 26.2).[50,56,67,71–74] Epicardial APs account for 4% of all left free wall APs and 10% of failed ablations.[50] Before CS ablation, CS angiography may be used to delineate the anatomy, exclude diverticulum, and assess possible damage to the CS from the ablation. Also, coronary angiography may be performed to determine the proximity of the ablation site to the left circumflex artery. Much of the published experience used non–temperature-controlled (power-controlled) ablation in a small series of patients (see Table 26.2). Mural thrombus in the CS was reported in one series.[56] For temperature-controlled RF within the CS, a cutoff up to 60°C with power limits of 20–30 W (non-irrigated catheters) have historically been used.[67] For resistant epicardial APs, irrigated RFA within the CS is more effective and thus the conventional approach. For irrigated catheters, maximal power of 20–30 W (50°C temperature cutoff) delivered for 60 seconds is suggested.[67] No complications were reported in

TABLE 26.2 Catheter Ablation of Left Free Wall Accessory Pathways From Within the Coronary Sinus

Study	Energy Type	No. of Patients	Maximal Power	Target Temperature	Duration (sec)	Success (No./Total) [%]	Complications
Wang et al. 1992[71]	RF	5	Not reported	Power control	—	5/5 [100%]	Not reported
Haïssaguerre et al. 1992[56]	RF	7	30 W	Power control	60	6/7 [85%]	CS mural thrombus (2 patients)
Giorgberidze et al. 1995[72]	RF	5	Not reported	Power control	—	3/5 [60%]	None
Langberg et al. 1993[50]	RF	2	28 ± 9 W	Power control	—	2/2 [100%]	Not reported
Cappato et al. 1994[73]	RF	6	Not reported	Power control	—	6/6 [100%]	None
Yamane et al. 2000[67]	Irrigated RF	7	30 W maximum	50°C	60	7/7 [100%]	Stenosis of cardiac veins (2 patients)
Gaita et al. 2002[74]	Cryoablation	1	NA	−75°C	240	1/1 [100%]	None

CS, Coronary sinus; *NA,* not applicable; *RF,* radiofrequency; —, not reported.

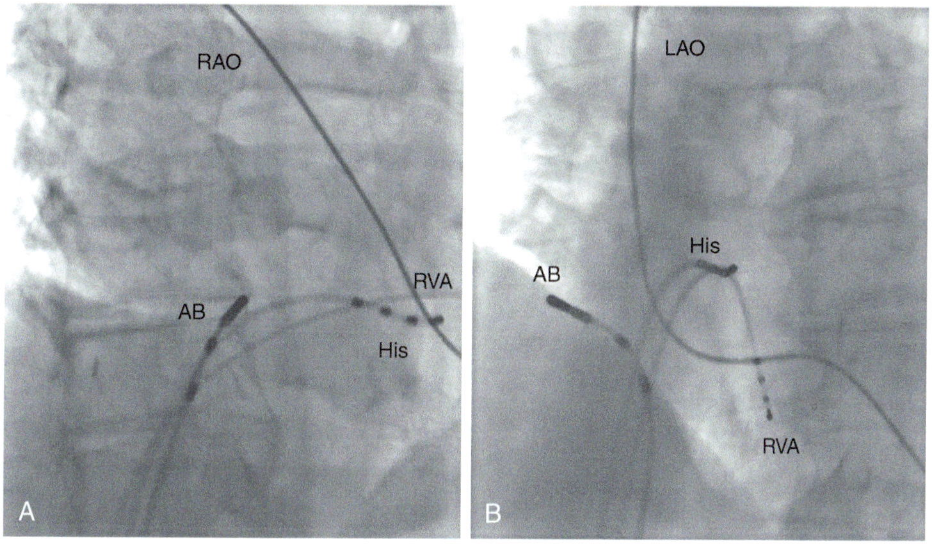

Fig. 26.23 (A, B) Stereotaxis magnetic ablation catheter (AB) navigation for ablation of a right free wall pathway. The catheter is very stable along the middle free wall tricuspid annulus despite the absence of a preformed sheath. *His,* His bundle catheter; *LAO,* left anterior oblique; *RAO,* right anterior oblique; *RVA,* right ventricular apex.

TABLE 26.3 Results of Transseptal Ablation for Left Free Wall Accessory Pathways

Study	No. of Patients	Success (%)	Complications (%)	Recurrence (%)	Cross Over (%)[a]	Fluoroscopy Time (minutes)	Procedure Time (hours)	Comments
De Ponti et al. 1998[76]	388	96	1.2	1.2	2	—	—	Complication rate includes ablation of atrial tachycardias
Swartz et al. 1993[38]	76	97	2	2	0	63 ± 47	4.9 ± 2.2	Complication rate includes other pathway locations
Fisher and Swartz 1992[55]	26	100	0	0	0	25 ± 10.5	2.8 ± 0.9	Vectorial 3D mapping
Yip et al. 1997[77]	49	92	4	4	4	22.5 ± 15.2	1.7 ± 0.05	Preformed transseptal sheaths
Manolis et al. 1995[78]	31	100	0	3	0	76 ± 48	5.4 ± 1.9	*W sign* used for mapping

3D, Three-dimensional.
[a]Cross over to transaortic approach.

this small series of patients with use of this strategy. Cryoablation in the CS has also been described.[74] Right and left epicardial APs may also be ablated by direct epicardial mapping achieved by percutaneous pericardial access (Fig. 26.22).[75]

The use of robotic and magnetic navigation systems for free wall AP ablation theoretically improves catheter stability (Fig. 26.23) and maneuverability, but superiority over manual ablation has not been demonstrated.

CLINICAL RESULTS

Left Free Wall Accessory Pathways

The rates of success for left free wall AP ablation are the highest of any AP location and are typically in excess of 90% (Table 26.3).[38,55,76–88] In the largest reported single-center series, 96% of 388 patients with left free wall APs were successfully ablated via a transseptal approach.[76] The recurrence rates for left free wall APs are the lowest of any location, at 2–5%.[38,55,76–78] Recurrences are more likely with concealed APs, delivery of transiently effective pulses due to catheter instability, or the need for more than five lesions to achieve acute success.[62,79–81] Historic success rates for ablation by either transaortic or transseptal approaches were similar in direct comparison (Table 26.4).[82–88] These studies usually reported similar total procedure times, fluoroscopy times, and rates of crossover to the other approach. Overall, complication rates also appeared to be similar, but some studies have found a trend toward a higher rate of complications with the transaortic approach.[84,86]

TABLE 26.4 Comparison of Transaortic and Transseptal Ablation Procedures

Study	Approach	No. of Patients	Success (%)	Recurrence (%)	Complications (%)	Cross Over (%)[a]	Procedure Time [Range]	Fluoroscopy Time (minutes) [Range]	Comments
Deshpande et al. 1994[82]	TA	42	95	—	4.7	4.7	244 ± 82 minutes	51 ± 22	—
	TS	58	75	—	3.4	24	268 ± 88 minutes	53 ± 22	—
Lesh et al. 1993[83]	TA	89	85	—	6.7	12	220 ± 13 minutes	44 ± 4	—
	TS	33	85	—	6.1	12	205 ± 13 minutes	45 ± 5	—
Natale et al. 1992[84]	TA	49	88	4	4	6	—	42 ± 29	—
	TS	31	100	0	0	0	—	34 ± 18	—
Saul et al. 1993[85]	TA	50	40	—	—	14	3.3 [2–9.5] hours[a]	52 (18–259]	Pediatric patients
	TS	13	100	—	—	0	4.3 [2–6] hours[a]	58 [14–197]	—
Manolis et al. 1994[86]	TA	50	87	11	8	10	7.1 ± 2.4 hours[a]	121 ± 81[a]	—
	TS	23	96	4	0	17	5.5 ± 2.1 hours[a]	81 ± 57	—
Vora et al. 1997[87]	TA	13	100	16	8	0	—	38 ± 30[a]	Nonrandomized pediatric patients
	TS	36	100	0	3	0	—	61 ± 45	—
Montenero et al. 1996[88]	TA	10	100	—	—	—	—	45 ± 10	Pediatric patients
	TS	18	100	—	—	—	—	23 ± 1	—
Luria et al. 2001[110]	TA	23	87	4	0	13	156 ± 58 minutes[b]	37 ± 25[b]	Single catheter for both approaches
	TS	21	90	5	0	5	119 ± 39 minutes	22 ± 21	—

TA, Transaortic approach; *TS*, transseptal approach; —, not reported.
[a]Cross over to other approach.
[b]$P < .05$ transaortic versus transseptal.

TABLE 26.5 Success Rates for Right Free Wall Accessory Pathways[a]

Study	No. of Patients	Acute Success (%)	Recurrence (%)	Comments
Calkins et al. 1999[89]	92	90	14	Power-controlled ablation
Swartz and coworkers 1993[38]	12	67	16.7	Power-controlled ablation
Jackman et al. 1991[90]	14	100	9	Power-controlled ablation
Lesh et al. 1992[79]	21[b]	80	11.8	Power-controlled ablation
Haïssaguerre et al. 1994[47]	32	93.7	11	—
Drago et al. 2002[57]	21	95	0	Pediatric series with electroanatomical mapping

[a]Non–Ebstein anomaly series.
[b]Number of accessory pathways.

In comparative trials, there are no features that predict the success of one approach or the other.[83] Because the techniques are complementary, it is to the operator's advantage to be familiar with both, allowing crossover should one approach fail. Because arterial access is required for the retrograde transaortic approach, vascular complications may be more common with this technique.[84,86] The success rates for ablation of concealed left APs by the transaortic approach are lower in some reports, possibly because of the smaller atrial electrograms recorded with this approach.

Right Free Wall Accessory Pathways

The success rates for right free wall AP ablation are the lowest of any AP location, averaging about 90%, ranging from 66% to 100% (Table 26.5).[38,47,79,89,90] In the largest series of 92 patients with right free wall APs, the success rate was 90%.[89] The lower success rate is attributed to either catheter instability, or if the pathway is off the TV annulus in the main body of the atrium.[58] The recurrence rates are higher for right free wall APs than for other locations, ranging from 9% to 16.7% (see Table 26.5).[38,47,79,89,90] Indeed, the right free wall location is a predictor of recurrence in some studies.[89] The success rates are lower still for patients with Ebstein anomaly. In the largest reported series of 100 such patients, 52 had right free wall APs.[91] The initial success rate for these pathways was 79%, with a 32% recurrence rate. In another report of 21 patients with Ebstein anomaly, only 76% of patients had elimination of all right-sided APs.[8] In these patients, acute success was predicted by a body surface area ≤1.7 m^2, presence of only a mild degree of tricuspid regurgitation, and only a mild severity of Ebstein anomaly.[91] Of these, only body surface area was predictive of long-term success.

Complications

The complication rate for the transaortic approach to left-sided APs ranges from 0% to 8% and is typically <4%.[38,55,76–78,82–88] Half of all complications are vascular related because of arterial access and include hematomas, dissections, pseudoaneurysms and arteriovenous fistulas.[92,93] Routine use of vascular ultrasound to obtain access has been shown to reduce these complications.[94] Almost unique to the transaortic approach is damage to the aortic or mitral valvular apparatus. Aortic valve trauma occurs in up to 30% of pediatric patients undergoing a retrograde ablation technique.[40] Aortic leaflet perforation and catheter entrapment in the mitral valve apparatus have been reported.[95,96] The latter may require transesophageal echocardiography to direct the extraction, and surgical removal has been necessary. By removing the CS catheter, the mitral annulus may be relaxed, facilitating catheter removal. Dissection or thrombosis of the left main coronary artery has resulted from catheter trauma or energy delivery in the artery.[97] There is a reported 2% risk for thromboembolic events because of thrombus formation on the catheter (despite anticoagulation) or dislodgment of aortic debris.[98] A 1.5% risk for tamponade, stroke, pericardial effusion, or cardiac perforation is reported for ablations at all locations. The risk for complications is higher for patients older than 65 years.[99]

The reported incidences of complications with the transseptal approach are 0–6% in adults and 0–25% in pediatric series.[38,55,76–78,87,100,101] The transseptal approach greatly reduces the incidence of vascular complications but introduces potential complications arising from atrial septal puncture. In a large series of transseptal procedures performed in the catheterization laboratory, the incidence of major complications related specifically to transseptal access was 1.3% and included tamponade (1.2%), embolization (0.08%), and death (0.08%).[102] It should be noted that in this series, a Brokenborough needle was

TABLE 26.6 Troubleshooting the Difficult Case

Problem	Causes	Solution
Misdiagnosis	Atrioventricular nodal reentry with eccentric atrial activation	Demonstrate only decremental retrograde conduction, dissociate atrium and/or ventricle from tachycardia
	Atrial tachycardia near atrioventricular annulus or from CS musculature	Dissociate ventricle from tachycardia
No early or favorable target sites	Poor catheter mobility	Use preformed sheaths or halo catheter, change catheter reach or stiffness
	CS distant from mitral annulus	Map mitral annulus directly
	Unable to discriminate component electrograms	Map AP conduction in opposite direction, change approach of mapping catheter (e.g., transaortic to transseptal), reverse direction of AP activation wavefront, map electrogram polarity reversal, simultaneous pacing
	Long AP conduction times	Map electrogram polarity reversal or shortest times with electroanatomical mapping system
	Epicardial AP location	Map CS and venous branches, map right coronary artery, epicardial mapping by pericardial access, map atrial appendages or ventricle apical to atrioventricular annulus
	Ligament of Marshall connection	Map left atrium anterior to left superior pulmonary vein
	Ebstein anomaly	Simultaneous atrial and ventricular pacing or atrial or ventricular premature stimuli to separate fractionated electrograms, map right coronary artery, use computerized mapping system
Unsuccessful energy delivery	Poor catheter stability and/or contact	Use preformed sheaths, change catheter curvature, reach, or stiffness; change catheter approach to ablation site (e.g., femoral to subclavian/jugular vein for right-sided AP); rapid pacing during ablation; use cryoablation; switch to irrigated catheter and consider contact force sensing mechanisms.
	Low temperatures with radiofrequency ablation	Improve catheter contact; use high-output generator and large-tip catheter (if using nonirrigated catheters)
	Low-current delivery with radiofrequency ablation	Lower system impedance (additional skin patches); use irrigated or cooled radiofrequency catheter; use cryoablation
	Epicardial AP	Ablation in CS or tributary with cryoablation or cooled radiofrequency; percutaneous epicardial ablation
	Wrong location	Continued mapping, map polarity reversal, map AP conduction in alternate direction, map for epicardial AP, consider unusual AP location

AP, Accessory pathway; *CS*, coronary sinus.

used with fluoroscopic and pressure guidance only. There have been refinements to transseptal procedures, such as the use of imaging (transoesophageal or intracardiac echocardiography) to better visualize the puncture site, radiofrequency/electrified wires, radiofrequency needle-tipped wires, and needle-tip wires. These newer techniques improve both safety and efficiency.

There are limited reports of ablation within the CS. To date, only mural thrombus or venous branch stenosis has been reported.[56] However, there remain the risks for perforation, catheter adhesion, and coronary artery injury. Indeed, it is important to recognize the close anatomical relationship of the MV annulus and CS to the circumflex artery to avoid thermal injury. In a study of 24 children with coronary sinus APs, 2 of 24 developed coronary artery injury from RF in the proximal CS (both were for posteroseptal AP).[103]

Complications from right free wall AP ablation are rare and are less common than for other AP locations.[38,47,79,90,104] Cardiac perforation may rarely occur, as may pulmonary embolism. Stenosis of a marginal right coronary artery branch has been reported in a child with Ebstein anomaly.[105] Mapping of the right coronary artery can lead to arterial injury or thrombosis.

TROUBLESHOOTING THE DIFFICULT CASE

The most common causes of failed AP ablations are (1) inability to access the target site (25% of cases), (2) catheter instability (23%), (3) mapping errors because of oblique AP orientation (11%), (4) epicardial AP (8%), and (5) recurrent atrial fibrillation (3%).[106] These problems and possible solutions are listed in Table 26.6. Misdiagnosis of the arrhythmia mechanism is more common for left than for right free wall APs. For left free wall APs, the diagnosis of ORT may be mimicked by AV nodal reentry with eccentric atrial activation or by atrial tachycardias arising from the CS musculature or the ligament of Marshall.[11,34,36] These arrhythmias can be recognized by the presence of decremental retrograde conduction only and by the ability to dissociate the ventricle from the tachycardia. It should be noted that during retrograde AV nodal conduction in patients without APs, the far lateral to anterolateral CS is frequently activated in a distal-to-proximal sequence.[107] This occurs due to rapid conduction over the Bachmann bundle into that region of the left atrium and may be confused with retrograde conduction over an AP. Para-Hisian pacing maneuvers validate the presence of retrograde right free wall AP conduction with consistency, but left free wall APs may be missed.[33]

Difficulties with mapping may occur if no favorable ablation sites are found. If both anterograde and retrograde AP conduction are present, it may be useful to map conduction in the opposite direction to that which is problematic (i.e., map retrograde conduction if anterograde mapping fails).[106] Most APs have an oblique course, and the atrial and ventricular insertions can be several centimeters apart. If no early anterograde or retrograde sites are found for left free wall APs in the CS, direct mapping of the mitral annulus should be performed because the CS is usually anatomically removed from the course of the AP. It is possible to place multielectrode halo catheters along the mitral annulus through transseptal access for difficult cases. Altering the direction of AP anterograde or retrograde activation may make the electrogram components more apparent and reveal AP potentials.[53] This approach can be used for right free wall APs as well.

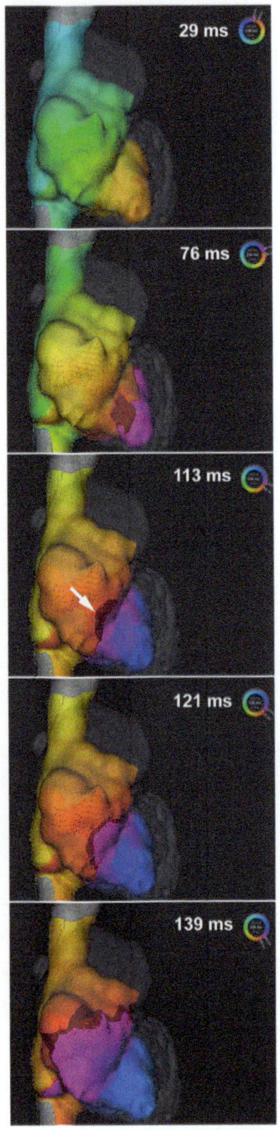

Fig 26.24 Open window mapping of a concealed right atrial free wall accessory pathway in Ebstein anomaly. Local activation time demonstrated earliest transition from the right ventricle to the atrium (*white arrow*). This area was targeted with successful radiofrequency ablation and no further inducible orthodromic AVRT. Map was produced using the 64-electrode Intellamap Orion catheter on the Rhythmia HD system (Boston Scientific, MA).

Changing the approach of the mapping catheter to access sites of interest may be needed. For left APs, changing from transaortic to transseptal mapping, or vice versa, may be helpful. For right-sided APs, changing from the femoral to a subclavian or internal jugular approach can be attempted. If the AP demonstrates slow anterograde or retrograde conduction, the usual timing criteria used to identify successful ablation sites may not be applicable. In such cases, the earliest activation sites should be sought. Mapping of electrogram polarity reversal is particularly helpful in this situation because this technique is independent of electrogram timing.[55] The use of 2 F multielectrode catheters to map the CS branches or the right coronary artery can be tried.[108] For complex cases, the use of electroanatomical mapping systems can be valuable. These systems can give insights into the complete AP activation course as with open window mapping techniques. Fig. 26.24 demonstrates ventriculo-atrial activation over a concealed right

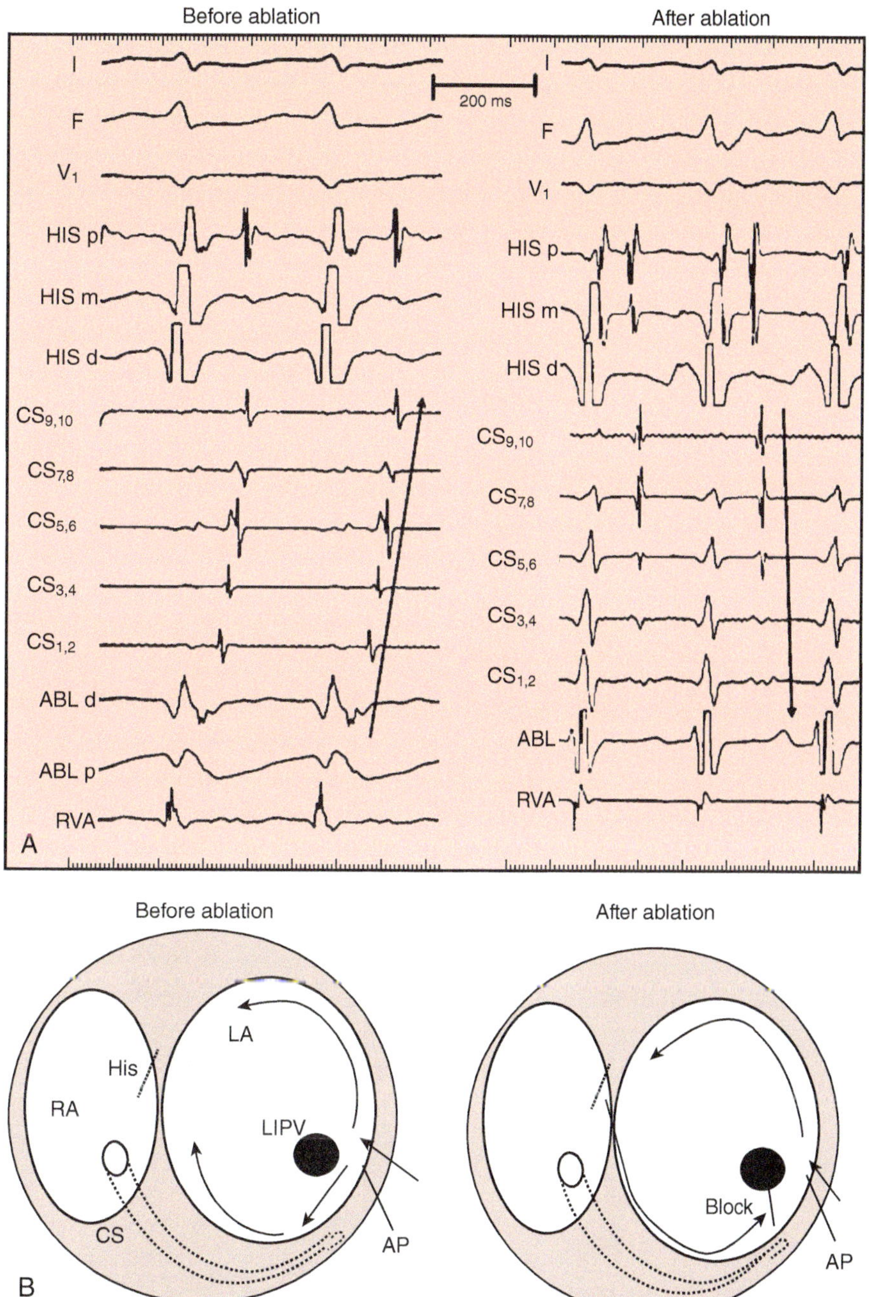

Fig. 26.25 Intraatrial conduction block after radiofrequency energy delivery for left lateral accessory pathway (AP). (A) Electrograms and surface electrocardiogram tracings in orthodromic reciprocating tachycardia with earliest atrial activation in the distal coronary sinus (CS 1,2). After ablation, the tachycardia cycle length is unchanged at 310 ms, but ventricle-to-atrium (VA) times are prolonged, and the atrial activation is earliest in the proximal His electrogram (HIS p). The CS is now activated from proximal (CS 9,10) to distal. (B) Schematic illustration of the reentry circuits before and after ablation. Before ablation, there is left atrial activation which radiates proximally and distally from the AP insertion *(arrows)*. After ablation, intraatrial block results in left atrial activation only distally from the AP insertion. The wavefront crosses over the roof of the left atrium to the atrial septum and then conducts proximal to distal in the CS. The ablation catheter recorded a VA time of 40 ms distal to the site of block, and the tachycardia was terminated with ablation to this site. *I, F, V_1,* Surface ECG leads; *ABL d,* ablation distal; *ABL p,* ablation proximal; *His,* His bundle; *LA,* left atrium; *LIPV,* left inferior pulmonary vein; *RA,* right atrium; *RVA,* right ventricle.

free wall AP in Ebsteins anomaly (Video 26.4 on Expert Consult). The occurrence of frequent atrial fibrillation may preclude mapping, especially for retrograde-only APs. In such cases, small incremental doses of ibutilide (0.1 mg to maximum of 1–2 mg) may prevent atrial arrhythmias without altering AP conduction.

Poor catheter mobility and stability are the most common reasons for failed AP ablations.[106] Catheter stability can be enhanced by using preformed sheaths, steerable sheaths, or different catheter curvatures and shaft stiffness, or by changing the approach to the ablation site (e.g., transaortic to transseptal, or from femoral to jugular access). Slower pacing or the use of cryothermal energy may also stabilize the catheter during ablation. The use of robotic catheter navigation systems may potentially enhance catheter stability (see Fig. 26.22).

RFA may also fail because of the inability to deliver sufficient current or to achieve satisfactory temperatures at the target site. If low current delivery is a problem, cooled ablation electrodes can be used.[67] If satisfactory temperatures cannot be reached despite full energy delivery, poor catheter contact is likely. The use of contact force to deliver ablation lesions greatly assists with this issue.

The inability to ablate an AP from endocardial approaches may suggest an epicardial location.[50] Further attempts at endocardial ablation slightly away from the annulus may occasionally be successful for pathways inserting off the annulus.[58] Left free wall epicardial APs may be recognized by earliest activation times or large AP potentials recorded in the CS or in a venous tributary. Coronary muscular connections to the ventricle are typically mapped to the proximal middle cardiac vein or a posterior venous branch.[10] Ablation within the CS or venous branch may be necessary. For these applications, cryoablation provides the greatest safety, followed by irrigated-tip RFA and, finally, noncooled RFA. Epicardial mapping and ablation through percutaneous pericardial access provides another approach to epicardial AV connections.[76,109]

Intraatrial conduction block without alteration of AP conduction after ablation delivery may occur in 6.9% of attempts at left free wall AP ablation.[110] In this situation, the resulting abrupt change or reversal of the retrograde atrial activation sequence may be misinterpreted as the appearance of a new arrhythmia (Fig. 26.25). Careful mapping along the CS distal to the ablation site will reveal persistent sites of early atrial activation.

Rarely, a concealed retrograde accessory pathway may have a single ventricular insertion site with two discrete atrial insertion sites. In such cases, during AVRT the retrograde atrial activation sequence may change from eccentric to midline (or vice versa) after successful ablation of one atrial insertion site or may exhibit beat-to-beat variability in retrograde atrial activation sequence without alteration in the tachycardia cycle length. Identification and ablation of the ventricular insertion site, or the separate discrete atrial insertion sites, result in successful composite treatment.[111]

ACKNOWLEDGMENTS

We would like to acknowledge the contributions by Richard K. Shepard and Santosh K. Padala, who are the authors of the previous edition.

REFERENCES

Please refer to the e-book for a complete list of references.

27

Ablation of Posteroseptal Accessory Pathways

James P. Daubert

KEY POINTS

- Posteroseptal accessory pathways (APs) are not true septal pathways but are located in the complex inferior pyramidal space involving the right atrium, right ventricle, left ventricle, left atrium, and coronary sinus and its branches.
- Mapping often needs to be performed in multiple regions, including the septal tricuspid annulus, septal mitral annulus, proximal coronary sinus, and normal and abnormal branches of the coronary sinus including the middle cardiac vein, posterior cardiac vein, and possibly coronary sinus diverticula.
- Targets for catheter ablation are similar to other APs including anterograde or retrograde AP potentials, earliest local ventricular activation during preexcited rhythm, and early atrial activation during orthodromic atrioventricular (AV) reentrant tachycardia—or possibly during ventricular pacing—but may also include coronary sinus muscular extension potentials analogous to AP potentials for these epicardial accessory connections.
- Equipment potentially needed for these mapping and ablation procedures include precurved or deflectable sheaths for positioning along the tricuspid annulus, equipment for transseptal puncture (intracardiac echocardiography, transseptal needles and sheaths, and guidewires), preformed or deflectable sheaths for transseptal access, balloon occlusion angiographic catheters for coronary sinus venography, 4-mm-tip or irrigated radiofrequency catheters, or possibly cryoablation catheters for ablation adjacent to coronary arteries.
- Potential challenges include the very complex anatomical relationships; adjacent AV conduction system; the need for mapping along the tricuspid valve, mitral valve, and coronary sinus in many procedures before selecting an ablation target; oblique AP angulation as in other regions; abnormal anatomy such as coronary sinus diverticula; and proximity to coronary artery branches such as the right coronary artery or AV nodal artery.

ANATOMY

Accessory pathways (APs) are located around the tricuspid or mitral atrioventricular (AV) valves with the exception of the aortomitral continuity in the left anterior septal aspect of the heart. Posteroseptal APs are the second most common variety of AV connection encountered clinically after left free wall APs. In general, they exhibit somewhat negative delta waves in the frontal plane electrocardiogram (ECG) leads and an early transition on the precordium (often in V_2). Neighbors of the posterior septal AP include left posterior free wall APs along the mitral annulus (MA), true midseptal APs along the tricuspid annulus (TA), and right posterior APs along the TA. Posteroseptal APs exhibit very complex anatomy consisting of several subtypes. Although the term *posteroseptal* is firmly entrenched in the electrophysiologic vocabulary, cardiac anatomists have long protested that these pathways are not truly septal in location.[2–4] Furthermore, from a true anatomical perspective, this region could be considered inferior rather than posterior.[5] As opposed to most left free wall APs, which anatomically lie epicardial to a well-defined annulus fibrosis, tricuspid and posteroseptal APs lack the same robust annulus fibrosis as shown in Fig. 27.1. Like other APs, they are now understood to course obliquely across the AV annulus rather than transversely, and this is appreciated in Fig. 27.1 with the atrial ventricular aspects of the AP residing in different sections (A and C, respectively). Fig. 27.2A illustrates relevant right atrial (RA) endocardial anatomical relationships of posterior septal APs. The triangle of Koch is defined by the tendon of Todaro (TT), the septal leaflet of the tricuspid valve, and the coronary sinus (CS) orifice (see Fig. 27.2A). The His bundle resides in the apex near the central fibrous body (asterisk) and the compact AV node outlined in yellow according to its typical location. Posterior septal pathways lie inferior (termed somewhat inaccurately as posterior) to the roof of the CS or within the CS ostium or proximal extent (about 2 cm)[6] or along the

Disclosures are Abbott, Acutus Medical, Affera, Biosense, Biotronik, Boston Scientific, Farapulse, Medtronic, Microport, Phillips, Syneos, and Vytronus for consulting, advisory boards, events committees, DSMB, steering committees, lecture honoraria, and research grants. None relate to royalties, stock or stock options, or speakers bureaus.

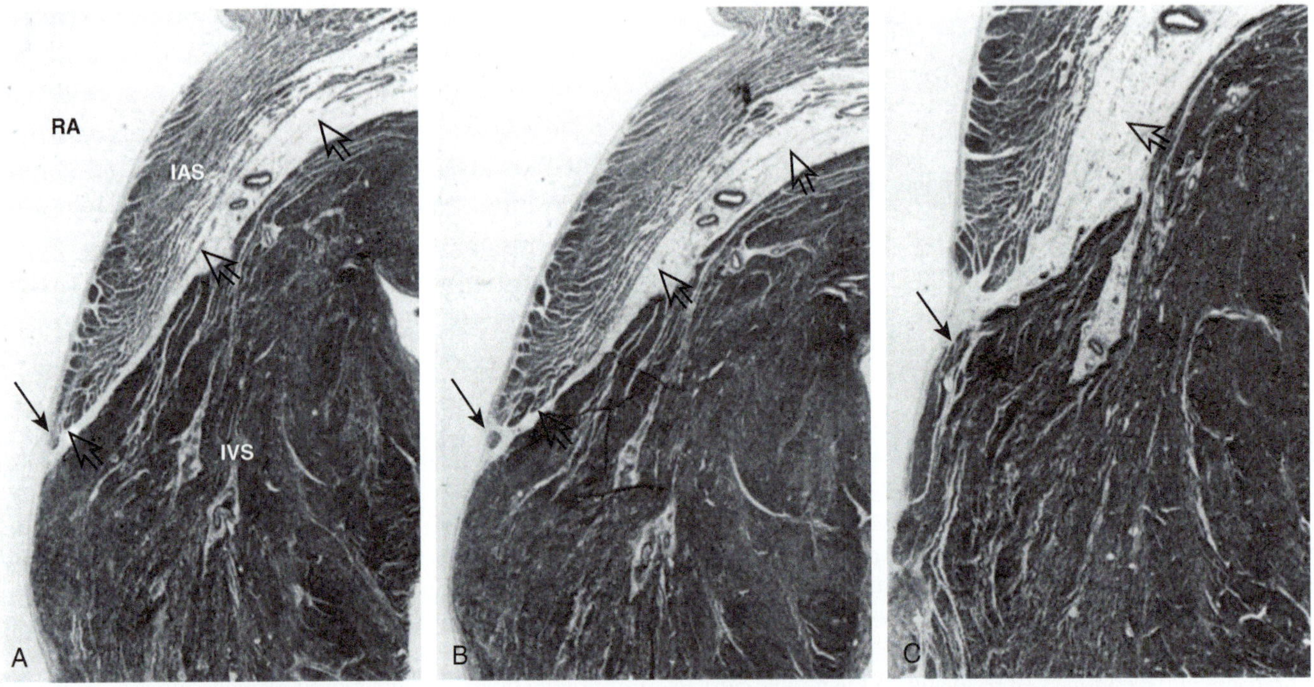

Fig. 27.1 Histologic section showing a right posteroseptal accessory pathway. Sections from a patient with Ebstein anomaly and preexcitation consistent with a right posterior septal AP taken just posterior to the coronary sinus. Labels identify the interatrial septal myocardium (IAS), epicardial fat (*open arrow*), interventricular septum (IVS), and AP (*solid arrow*). The pathway was about 3 mm in diameter at the atrial insertion (A), coursed throughout the epicardial fat without a notable annulus fibrosis (B) and inserted into the endocardial side of the ventricular tissue (C) slightly more anteriorly. The oblique nature of the pathway is evident by the three separate sections showing it. (Modified from Becker AE, Anderson RH, Durrer D, Wellens HJ. The anatomical substrates of Wolff-Parkinson-White syndrome. A clinicopathologic correlation in seven patients. *Circulation*. 1978;57:870–879.)

posterior (inferior) septal aspect of the MA. It can easily be appreciated that these pathways are challenging in view of their proximity to the normal conduction system. Moreover, differentiating atrioventricular reentrant tachycardia (AVRT) caused by a posteroseptal AP from AV node reentry, wherein the earliest A can be mapped to a very similar area, may pose additional challenges. Patients, especially those with congenital anomalies, exhibit considerable variation in Koch triangle and location of the AV node. Fig. 27.2B illustrates this variation with a large CS orifice and small triangle of Koch. Fig. 27.2C–E further shows sections through the septal region demonstrating the AV node giving rise to the bundle of His and the relationships of the AV nodal artery. Because the TA lies slightly more apical than the MA and the interatrial septum slightly leftward to the interventricular septum, one must recall that the RA is anatomically juxtaposed with the left ventricle (LV) in this region. The inferior pyramidal space is not true septal territory and has anatomical relationships with the CS and AV nodal artery.

Epicardial accessory AV connections are an important subgroup of posteroseptal APs. The various endocardial as well as epicardial pathways are illustrated in Fig. 27.3. Pathway type 1 (see Fig. 27.3) is an endocardial connection between the RA and right ventricle (RV). Pathway type 2 is RA to LV; this portion of the LV is termed the *posterior superior process*. Pathway 3 refers to an endocardial left atrial (LA) to LV AV connection. Pathway type 4, an epicardial one, depicts a muscular connection between the LV and CS musculature in the middle cardiac vein; similar pathways can occur in slightly more distal coronary venous branches such as the posterior cardiac vein. Last, pathway type 5, another epicardial one, portrays a CS diverticulum, an anatomical anomaly, electrically connecting the LV and the CS musculature of the diverticulum.

PATHOPHYSIOLOGY

APs in the posterior septal region can exhibit all of the same pathophysiologic processes as other APs, plus some other unique ones as well. When manifest (i.e., exhibiting anterograde conduction), the surface QRS is a fusion of AP-generated ventricular muscle activation and activation over the His-Purkinje system. A rare but critical exception arises when anterograde AV nodal–His block occurs.[7] Needless to say, this rare circumstance should be elucidated before ablating the AP! Pathways in the posterior septal region are not as apt to be concealed (retrograde only), accounting for only 10–13% of posteroseptal APs compared with 30% of left free wall ones.[8–10]

Analogous to other AP locations, patients possessing posteroseptal APs may be asymptomatic, that is, thus far free from

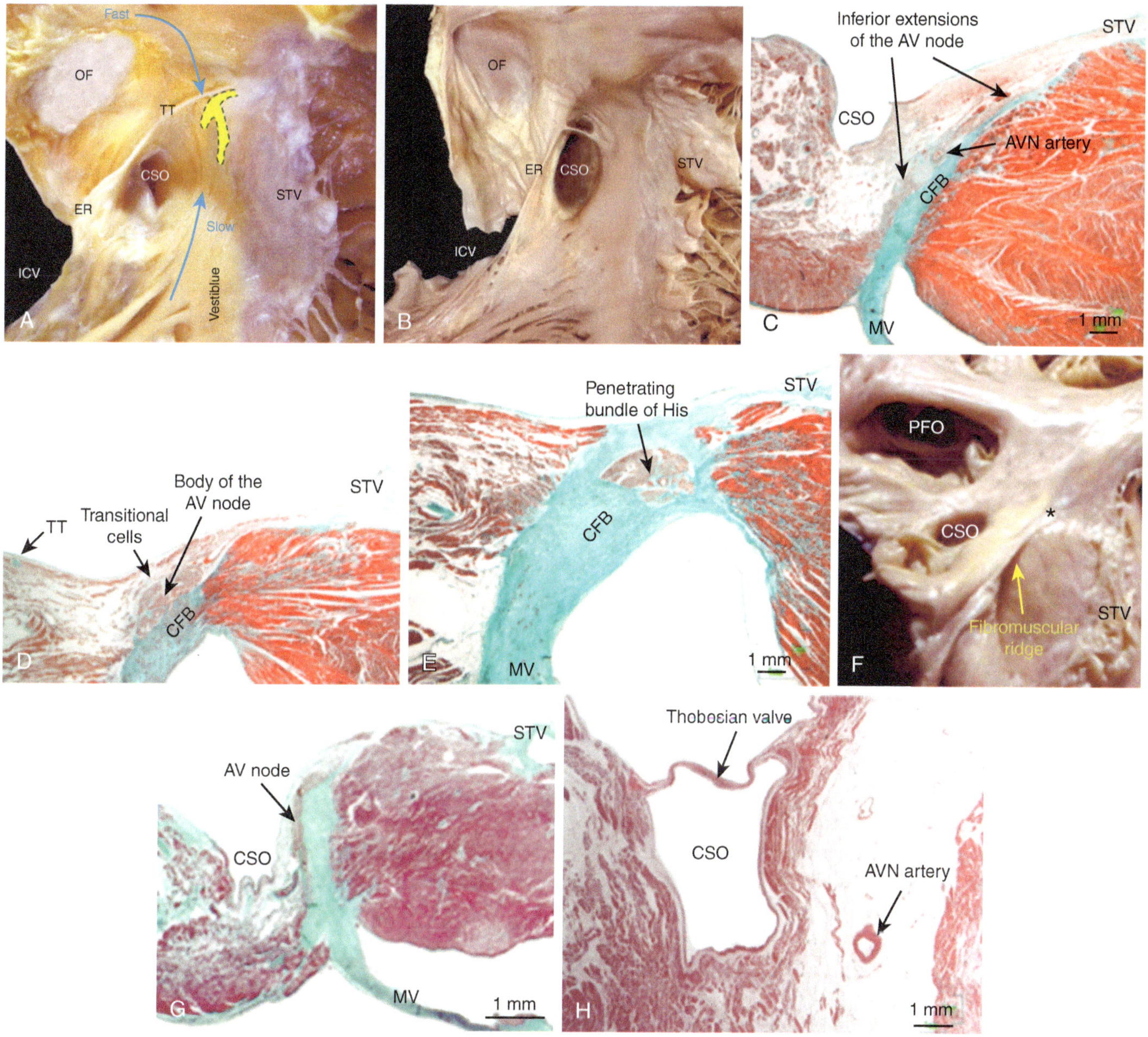

Fig. 27.2 The triangle of Koch. (A) This dissection is viewed right anterior oblique and shows portions of the right atrium with the borders of the triangle of Koch. The putative location of the AV node is shown in yellow along with the fast and slow pathways. See text for details. (B) Another example with a larger coronary sinus ostium and smaller triangle. (C, D, E) Histologic sections with similar orientation to panel A through the coronary sinus ostium and inferior extensions of the AV node, body of the AV node, and penetrating bundle of His. (F, G) Dissection from a heart with Ebstein anomaly. Note the smaller triangle of Koch and abnormal septal leaflet with the AV node at the level of the coronary sinus ostium in this example. (H) Sagittal section through the mouth of the coronary sinus showing the proximity of the AV node artery to the endocardium and the triangle of Koch. ∗, Central fibrous body; *AVN* artery, atrioventricular nodal artery; *CFB*, central fibrous body; *CSO*, coronary sinus ostium; *ER*, Eustachian ridge; *ICV*, inferior cava vein; *MV*, mitral valve; *OF*, oval fossa; *PFO*, patent foramen ovale; *STV*, septal leaflet of the tricuspid valve; *TT*, tendon of Todaro. (From Sánchez-Quintana D, Doblado-Calatrava M, Cabrera JA, Macías Y, Saremi F. Anatomical basis for the cardiac interventional electrophysiologist. *Biomed Res Int*. 2015;2015:547364.)

known or suspected arrhythmias. In the asymptomatic patient, the physician needs to consider the rare chance of cardiac arrest occurring in the future and implement risk stratification.[11–14] A survey of pediatric electrophysiologists found that most lean toward ablation for patients with asymptomatic APs unless they are in a high-risk location for AV block.[15]

As for other APs, the most common arrhythmia produced by posteroseptal APs is orthodromic AVRT. A common mode of induction consists of a spontaneous or stimulated premature atrial beat that blocks (in a bidirectionally conducting AP) anterogradely, conducts slowly down the AV node, and then reenters the AP retrogradely (Fig. 27.4).

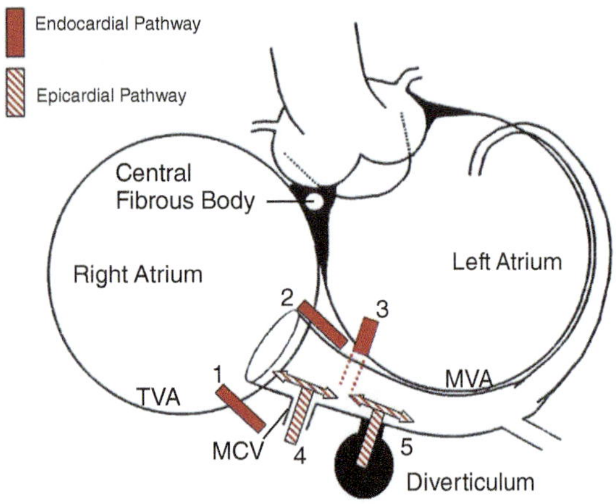

Fig. 27.3 Schematic showing complex anatomy and different anatomical subtypes of accessory atrioventricular connections in the posteroseptal region. A short-axis schematic of the heart is shown. Five anatomical types of posteroseptal accessory pathways are shown. See text for details. *MCV,* Middle cardiac vein; *MVA,* mitral valve annulus; *TVA,* tricuspid valve annulus. (Reproduced with permission from Brado J, Hochadel M, Senges J, et al. Outcomes of ablation in Wolff-Parkinson-White-syndrome: data from the German Ablation Registry. *Int J Cardiol.* 2021;323:106–112.)

Posteroseptal APs were notably absent in the Duke, Maastricht, and French publications collating true antidromic AVRT cases, that is, pathways using the AV node as the retrograde circuit.[16–19] (Posterior septal pathways may exhibit other preexcited tachycardias such as those using a second, retrogradely conducting AP. Conversely, in a large multicenter pediatric series including 1147 patients, antidromic AVRT was rarer than in adults (2.6% versus 8–10%). In this pediatric series, posteroseptal APs evidently did participate in antidromic AVRT circuits. Atrial fibrillation with preexcitation over posterior septal AP may be symptomatic or lead to sudden cardiac arrest.

Most pathways (about 75%) exhibiting the phenotype of permanent junctional reciprocating tachycardia (PJRT) are located in the posterior septal region.[20–23] *Permanent* denotes that these arrhythmias tend to be incessant because of the relatively slow rate. Owing to the long retrograde conduction time, they fall under the "long-RP" classification. Fig. 27.5 shows electrocardiographic and electrogram data from a left posteroseptal, epicardial, decremental retrograde-only AP with incessant (long-RP), slow AVRT. Notably, this patient did exhibit a mild, tachycardia-induced cardiomyopathy that resolved with successful catheter ablation. Tachycardia-induced cardiomyopathy has been observed in nearly a quarter of PJRT patients in one large series.[21] Notably, tachycardia is not the only mechanism for ventricular dysfunction. Posteroseptal APs, and right free wall ones, occasionally develop ventricular dysfunction secondary to a dyssynchronous contraction pattern engendered by the left bundle branch block (LBBB)-like conduction pattern.[24] By eliminating preexcitation, catheter ablation can resolve this cardiomyopathy.

Demographically, it is well appreciated that AV nodal reentrant tachycardia (AVNRT) is more common in female patients and APs slightly more common in male patients; one study[25] showed that the main increase in prevalence of APs was for pathways located in the left posterior septal region.

Two other electrocardiographic phenomena, relating to depolarization and repolarization, respectively, are noteworthy. Preexcitation over a posteroseptal AP presents a "pseudo-infarct" pattern in the inferior leads because of the negative delta waves inferiorly. When preexcitation is eliminated, cardiac repolarization remains abnormal, typically exhibiting T-wave inversion inferiorly—a process called *cardiac memory*. Resolving over a period of several months, cardiac memory is relatively conspicuous for posterior septal pathways.[26,27]

Ebstein anomaly is another important association with posterior septal APs. Indeed, Wolff-Parkinson-White (WPW) syndrome may be demonstrated as a concomitant diagnosis in up to 10% of Ebstein anomaly patients.[28–31] In Ebstein anomaly, the posteroseptal location is second most frequent behind the right free wall group. In a multicenter series, 19 of 34 Ebstein patients displayed multiple pathways, especially the combination of a right free wall and a posterior septal one.[29]

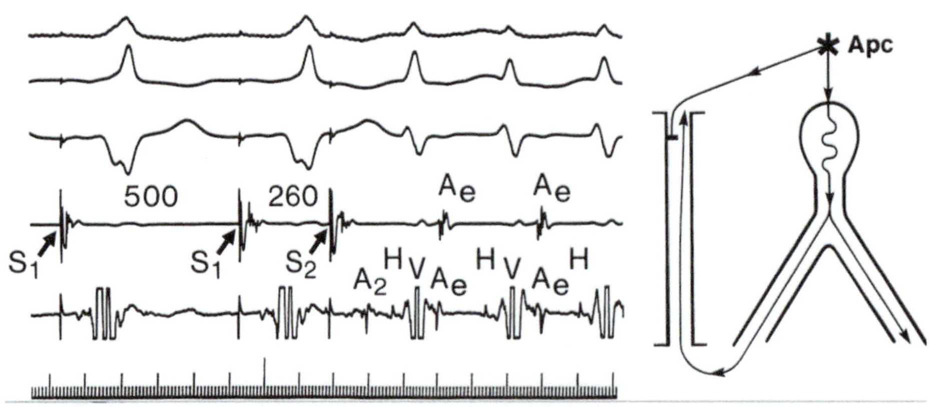

Fig. 27.4 Schematic of accessory pathway and AV node and induction of orthodromic atrioventricular reentrant tachycardia with an atrial premature contraction (Apc). See text for details. (Modified from Bhatia A, Sra J, Akhtar M. Preexcitation syndromes. *Curr Probl Cardiol.* 2016;41:99–137.)

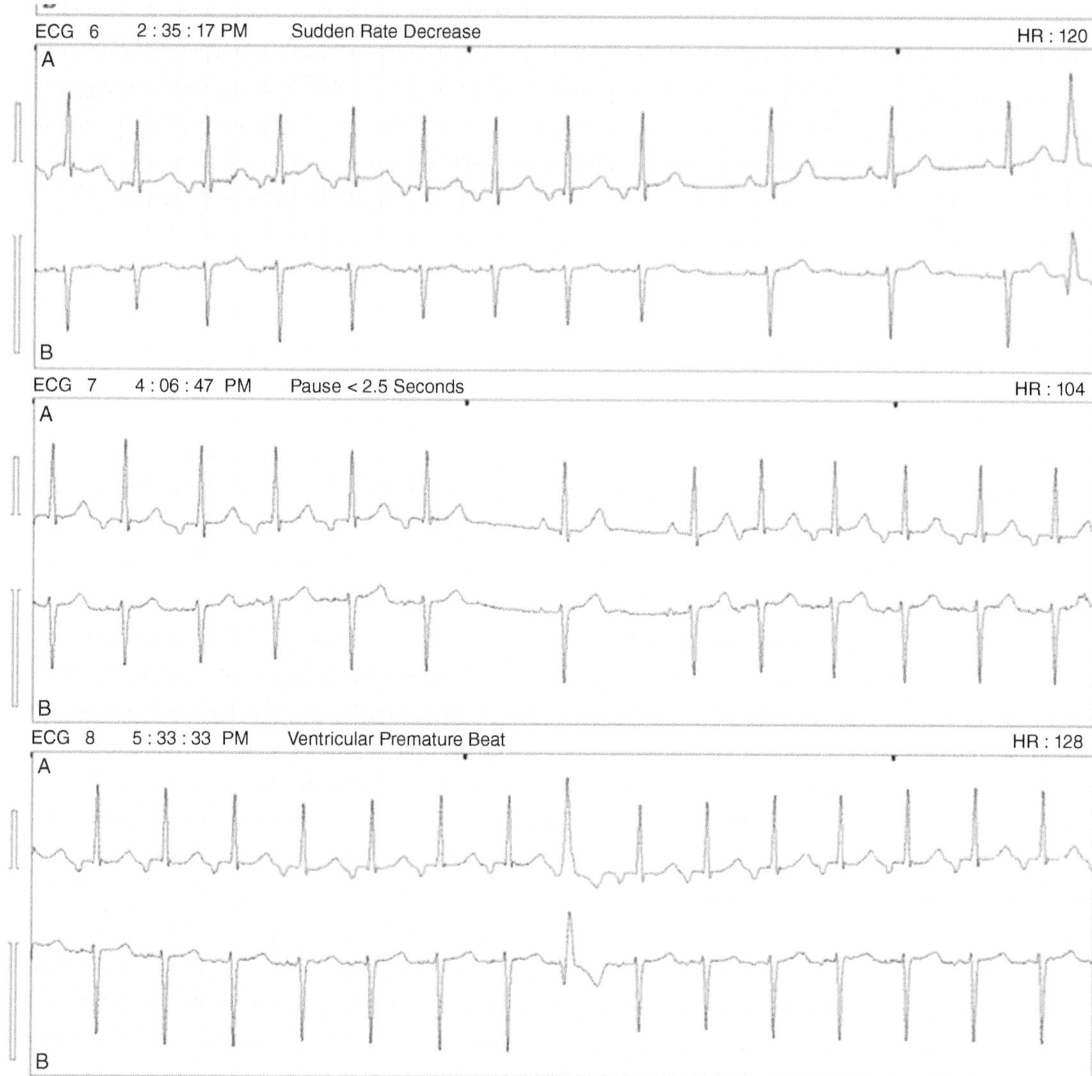

A

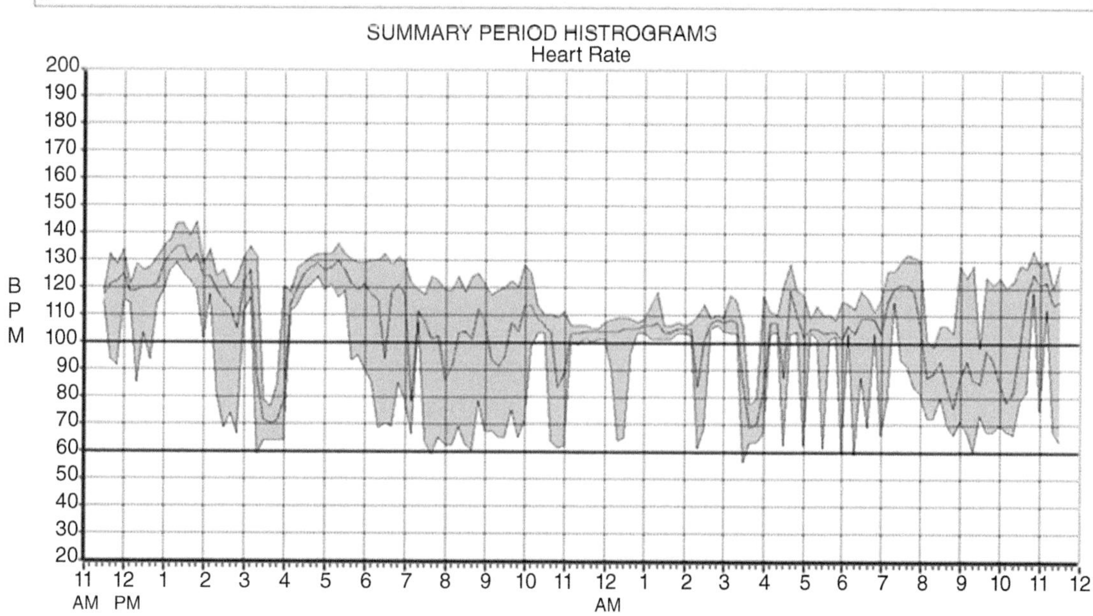

B

Fig. 27.5 Permanent junctional reciprocating tachycardia case. (A) The incessant nature of the tachycardia with cessation for two sinus beats and resumption; note termination in retrograde AP limb; also note advancement with PVC that is almost definitely fused. (B) Holter-derived heart rate trend depicting a high burden of relatively slow SVT. A tachycardia-cardiomyopathy had developed.

(Continued)

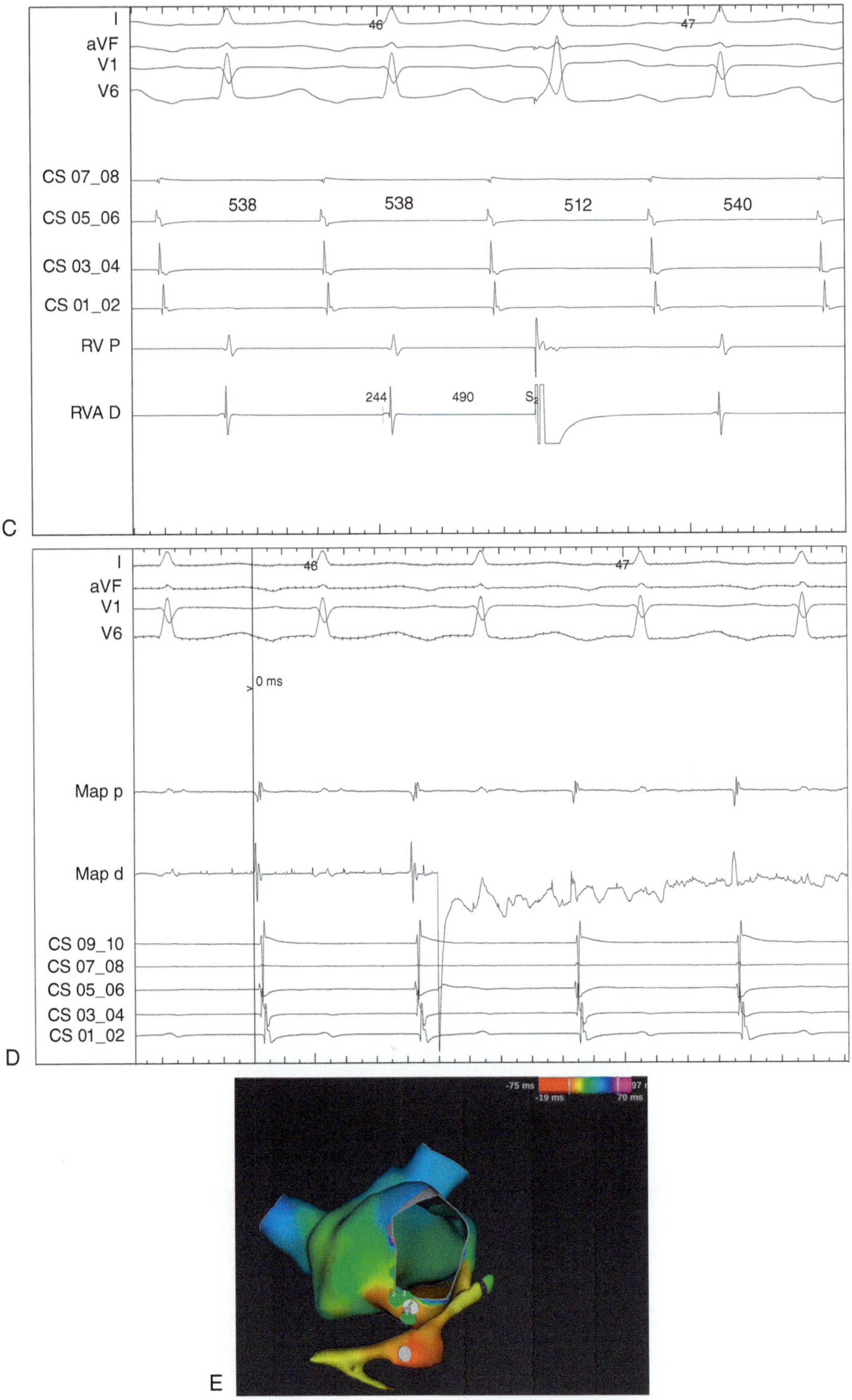

Fig. 27.5, cont'd (C) His-refractory PVC advancing the next A confirming AVRT (versus AVNRT or AT). (D, E) Electrograms and electroanatomical map, respectively, of the earliest A mapped to a broad-necked diverticulum of the CS 2 cm from the ostium; this is pathway type 5 in Fig. 24-6; SVT terminated here; this site was earlier than the mitral annulus by ~ 20 ms where ablation failed, and ever earlier than the tricuspid annulus. Video shows the propagation map from the CS diverticulum spreading both proximally and distally in the CS and connecting with the inferior left atrium near the earliest site mapped on the mitral annulus.

ARRHYTHMIA DIAGNOSIS AND DIFFERENTIAL DIAGNOSIS

Let us first consider the differential diagnosis for tachycardias associated with a posteroseptal AP, and then the preexcitation pattern as it relates to posteroseptal versus other APs. As noted, the most commonly observed arrhythmia is orthodromic ARVT. The usual differential diagnosis applies when confronted with a narrow QRS, regular tachycardia, namely AVNRT, (orthodromic) AVRT, and atrial tachycardia; automatic junctional tachycardia should not be neglected. Dissociation of the atrium and ventricle excludes AVRT. Armed with intracardiac recordings, bolstering the surface P-wave timing, and examining the earliest atrial activation, the diagnosis is sometimes nearly obvious. For example, supraventricular tachycardia (SVT) with CS distal to proximal activation makes AVRT using a left lateral AP highly likely. In addition, the cycle length or ventriculoatrial (VA) interval changes associated with ipsilateral bundle branch block when present provide a clear diagnosis of a free wall AP's involvement in a tachycardia[32] (see Key Points and Tables 27.1 and 27.2). Importantly, posteroseptal APs may exhibit an intermediate degree of VA interval prolongation with LBBB (Fig. 27.6). Among posteroseptal APs, Haïssaguerre et al. correlated LBBB-related VA prolongation with a positive delta wave in V_1, indicative of an LV insertion.[33]

Conversely, because of the concentric pattern (i.e., midline atrial activation) with orthodromic AVRT using a posteroseptal AP, retrograde AV nodal activation is not easily excluded. Although atrial recordings at the CS ostium should be earliest in AVRT via a posteroseptal AP, it can be similar with retrograde slow pathway activation, and for right posteroseptal APs, the His atrial and CS proximal atrial may be nearly tied. Further challenging the clinician, recall that retrograde AV nodal activation may appear eccentric because of left-sided AV nodal exits (from either the fast or a slow pathway).[34–36]

Next steps in diagnosing a narrow QRS, 1:1 SVT reside with the stimulator. Maneuvers during tachycardia comprise programmed single ventricular extrastimulus and ventricular entrainment. Pacing during sinus rhythm includes differential pacing (base versus apex) or para-Hisian pacing. The key principles to understanding the different response centers around the situation in AVRT where a ventricular stimulus is potentially able to engage the retrograde AP at a time when the His bundle has just conducted anterogradely. This cannot occur in AVNRT or atrial tachycardia (except for the theoretical use of a bystander retrograde AP). Advancing the timing of the retrograde atrial with a His-refractory premature ventricular complex (PVC) or with surface QRS fusion during entrainment (fusion referring to orthodromic activation via His plus ventricular pacing) are two manifestations of the same phenomenon. Should a His refractory PVC advance the A during SVT, the presence of an AP is proved. Recently, a rule to apply to earlier, non-His refractory PVCs has been described[37] (Fig. 27.7). Another principle relates to ventricular pacing being able to engage an AV AP earlier when pacing from near its insertion (more basally in general, but also theoretically in the LV for a left-sided one) as opposed to the mode of retrograde engagement of the AV node via the right bundle branch, which terminates in the RV apical septal region (see Table 27.1). Comparing VA or His-to-atrial intervals during SVT and during pacing relies on the concept that in AVNRT anterograde activation of the ventricle occurs concurrently with retrograde conduction to the atrium, whereas in AVRT there is sequential activation (ventricular-AP-atrial-AV

TABLE 27.1 Diagnostic Criteria Part I: Differentiating Posteroseptal Orthodromic Atrioventricular Reciprocating Tachycardia From Atrioventricular Nodal Reentrant Tachycardia or Atrial Tachycardia

Maneuver	Orthodromic AVRT	AVNRT	AT
Development of BBB[87]	Lengthening the TCL by 35 ms indicates ipsilateral free wall AP[a]	No significant change in TCL	No significant change in TCL
Development of LBBB	Lengthening the tachycardia VA by 5–30 ms consistent with posteroseptal AP	No consistent change in VA interval	No significant change in VA interval
Development of RBBB	Minimal change in VA consistent with posteroseptal AP	No significant change in VA interval	No significant change in VA interval
VA dissociation	Disproves AVRT	2:1 block below His not uncommon; 2:1 block above His in LCP rare; VA dissociation very rare	2:1 and other non-1:1 AV conduction is common
Ventricular entrainment[88]	V-A-V response	V-A-V response	V-A-A-V response[b]; or dissociation of the As from the Vs.

AV, Atrioventricular; *AVNRT*, atrioventricular nodal reentrant tachycardia; *AVRT*, atrioventricular reentrant tachycardia; *AP*, accessory pathway; *AT*, atrial tachycardia; *BBB*, bundle branch block; *LBBB*, left bundle branch block; *LCP*, lower common pathway of the atrioventricular node; *RBBB*, right bundle branch block; *TCL*, tachycardia cycle length; VA, ventricular-to-atrial interval.

[a]Prolongation of the HV interval could theoretically lengthen the tachycardia CL.

[b]Knight et al. use the terms A-V and A-A-V to describe the events the last ventricular stimulus, but common parlance uses V-A-V and V-A-A-V (Knight BP, Zivin A, Souza J, et al. A technique for the rapid diagnosis of atrial tachycardia in the electrophysiology laboratory. *J Am Coll Cardiol*. 1999;33:775–781).

TABLE 27.2 Diagnostic Criteria Part II: Differentiating Posteroseptal Orthodromic Atrioventricular Reciprocating Tachycardia From Atrioventricular Nodal Reentrant Tachycardia

Maneuver	Posteroseptal Orthodromic AVRT	AVNRT
Para-Hisian pacing[89]	No change in Stim-A with loss of His capture; or change in atrial activation sequence	Increased Stim-A with loss of His capture; identical atrial activation sequence
PVC during His refractoriness[90]	Advances atrial activation[a]; delays atrial activation; or terminates tachycardia without conduction to atrium[b]	Unable to advance or delay atrial activation[c]
Delta HA interval[91]	$HA_{pace} - HA_{svt} < -10$ ms (i.e., more negative)	$HA_{pace} - HA_{svt} > -10$ ms (less negative or positive number)
Preexcitation index[92]	10–70 ms; overlaps with right free wall, anteroseptal and left free wall; left free wall not <50 ms	Usually > 100 ms
Difference between ventricular PPI and TCL[93]	<115 ms	>115 ms
Corrected difference between ventricular PPI and TCL[94]	<110 ms	>110 ms
Difference between VA during ventricular pacing at TCL and VA during tachycardia	<85 ms	>85 ms
VA pacing at ventricular base versus pacing at ventricular apex[95]	VA shorter with pacing of base	VA shorter with pacing of apex
Ventricular entrainment without fusion[96]	Acceleration of A to PCL within 1 beat of fully paced morphology	Acceleration of A to PCL in ≥2 beats of fully paced morphology
Ventricular entrainment with fusion[97]	Atrial timing altered; or a fixed SA interval is established within the transition zone (fusion, i.e., before fully paced morphology)	Atrial timing not altered; No fixed SA interval established when fusion present

AVNRT, Atrioventricular nodal reentrant tachycardia; *AVRT*, atrioventricular reentrant tachycardia; *PCL*, pacing cycle length; *PPI*, postpacing interval; *Stim-A*, ventricular stimulus-to-atrial electrogram interval; *SA*, stimulus to atrial; *SVT*,supraventricular tachycardia; *TCL*, tachycardia cycle length; *VA*, ventricular-to-atrial interval.

[a]Demonstration of PVC advancing the tachycardia (i.e., left column, under AVRT) is consistent with AVRT and proves the existence of an accessory pathway (AP), but theoretically the rhythm could be AVNRT or atrial tachycardia (AT) with a bystander AP.

[b]Perturbing the atrium with a PVC during His refractoriness and advancing the next His (i.e., advancing the tachycardia) does prove existence of an AP and participation in the tachycardia as does delaying the atrial activation (i.e., that it is AVRT).

[c]Failure of a premature ventricular complex (PVC) to affect the tachycardia (i.e., right column, under AVNRT) is consistent with atrioventricular nodal reentrant tachycardia (AVNRT) but does not exclude atrioventricular reentrant tachycardia (AVRT).

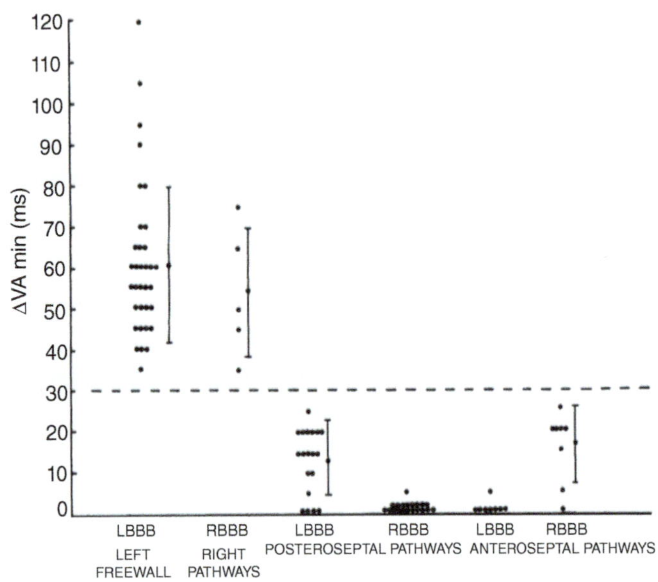

Fig. 27.6 Change in VA interval (QRS onset to local A) during atrioventricular reentrant tachycardia with occurrence of bundle branch aberrancy. See text for details. (From Kerr CR, Gallagher JJ, German LD. Changes in ventriculoatrial intervals with bundle branch block aberration during reciprocating tachycardia in patients with accessory atrioventricular pathways. *Circulation.* 1982;66:196–201.)

node-His) with pacing, it is sequential from ventricular to atrial over either the AVN or the AP (see Table 27.1). Finally, para-Hisian pacing evaluates whether atrial activation timing is dependent on or independent of His bundle activation (see Table 27.1). The actual change in stimulus to A (at the proximal CS) with loss of His bundle capture compared with His bundle capture was recently quantified for nodal conduction versus AP conduction while previously it was nebulously "different." A delta Stim-A of less than 37 ms indicated presence of an AP while a change of more than 51 ms ruled out a non-decremental septal AP.[38]

Posteroseptal APs can participate in wide QRS tachycardias of several types. In addition to a narrow QRS morphology, orthodromic AVRT can exhibit bundle branch block aberrancy as discussed earlier and in the Key Points. Antidromic AVRT using the AP anterogradely and the His bundle–AV node retrogradely was not observed for posteroseptal Aps in three of four large series but was seen in one pediatric series.[16–19,39] However, pathway-to-pathway tachycardias, that is, using a second AP as the retrograde limb, were noted. Either of these tachycardias will be wide, have a slurred QRS onset, and have regular cycle length; some SVT versus ventricular tachycardia (VT) ECG criteria will classify these as VT since they resemble VT by having a myocardial activation

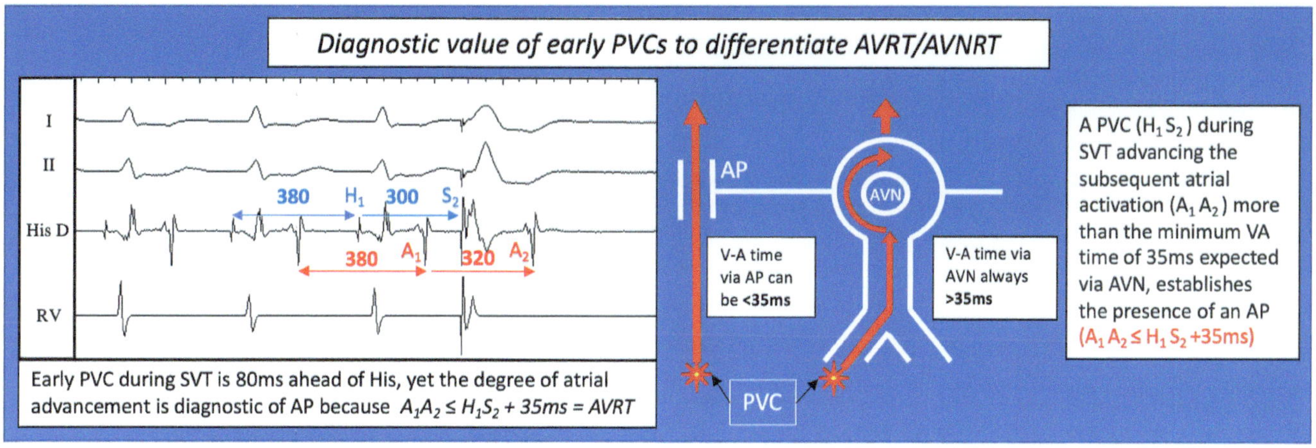

Fig. 27.7 Early premature ventricular complex role in differentiating atrioventricular reentrant tachycardia from atrioventricular nodal reentrant tachycardia. See figure and text. (From Shah AN, Field J, Clark BA, et al. Diagnostic utility of early premature ventricular complexes in differentiating atrioventricular reentrant and atrioventricular nodal reentrant tachycardias. *Heart Rhythm.* 2022.)

pattern rather than a bundle branch to Purkinje rapid activation mode. Other algorithms may prove more accurate for detecting preexcitation versus VT.[40] Other preexcited tachycardias include atrial flutter, atrial tachycardia, or atrial fibrillation as well as, more rarely, AV node reentry with a bystander AP.

Turning to preexcitation, differentiating posteroseptal APs from neighboring ones can be difficult as can be expected from the anatomy. Challenges include the proximity to the AV conduction system and possible need to consider multiple locations. Predicting the location of an AP before electrophysiologic study has great value in preprocedural planning. Understanding the likelihood that a pathway is left-sided or near the conduction system modifies informed consent and optimizes selection of catheters and sheaths. Fortunately, a number of algorithms have been designed that use the 12-lead ECG and examine the axis of the delta wave or the polarity of the QRS morphology through certain leads (see Chapter 26).

The first attempt at classification and ECG localization was published in 1945 by Rosenbaum et al., who divided preexcitation patterns into either LV or RV pathways.[41] In type A, or LV pathways, the delta wave was upright in all precordial leads. In type B, or RV pathways, the delta wave was negative, with prominent S waves in the right precordium.

In 1987, Milstein et al. reported an algorithm that used previously described ECG features of AP locations and refined these features with an analysis of 97 patients with a single known AP.[42] Their algorithm used the polarity of delta waves, the presence of isoelectric periods in certain leads, or an LBBB-like pattern (Rosenbaum B) to localize single pathways to one of four locations: right lateral, left lateral, anterior septal, and posterior septal. Milstein et al. tested their algorithm on the ECGs of 141 patients with WPW who had invasive AP location verification and reported an accuracy of 90–91%. Two other algorithms, both published in 1995, attempted more specific anatomical localization dividing AP locations into eight or nine zones and reporting >90% accuracy.[43,44]

Fig. 27.8 shows one of the most commonly used algorithms for determining the ventricular insertion of an AP developed by

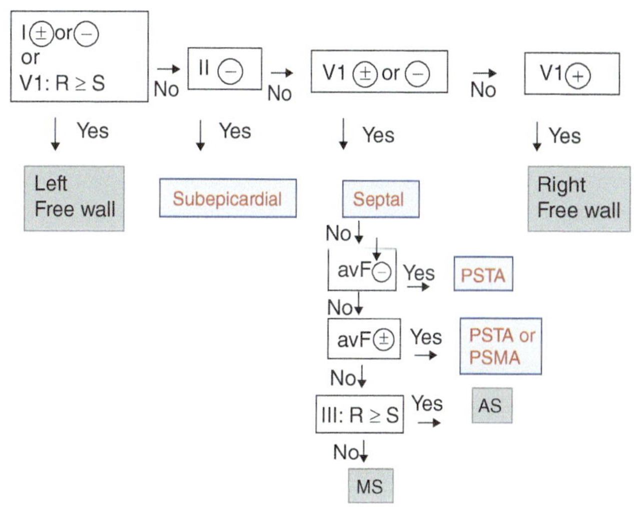

Fig. 27.8 ECG algorithm for localizing AP by preexcitation. Details regarding right and left free wall AP delineation are omitted. See text for details. (Modified from Arruda MS, McClelland JH, Wang X, et al. Development and validation of an ECG algorithm for identifying accessory pathway ablation site in Wolff-Parkinson-White syndrome. *J Cardiovasc Electrophysiol.* 1998;9:2–12.)

the Oklahoma team.[45] It focuses on the initial 20–40 ms of the delta wave. First, left free wall pathways are identified by a negative or isoelectric delta wave in lead I and/or a dominant R wave in V_1 (R > S). Next, relevant to the posteroseptal space, a negative delta in II classifies the AP as subepicardial (middle cardiac vein, CS-associated diverticulum, or possibly left posterior cardiac venous branch); subsequent data disclose that a negative delta wave in II is specific for subepicardial pathways, but the finding has only moderate sensitivity of 68%, that is, absence of it does not rule out the middle cardiac vein (MCV) region.[46] If the findings for neither left free wall nor subepicardial pathways are present, the septum or right free wall is implicated. The next branch point considers V_1, and if positive, the right free wall is the site, but if negative or isoelectric, the pathway should be septal. Note that the right free wall APs have a positive delta wave but an overall negative QRS in V_1 and a transition at V_3 or later. Breaking down the septal pathways (V^1 isoelectric or negative), the algorithm considers aVF: negative pointing to posteroseptal TA, isoelectric compatible with posteroseptal TA or MA, and positive characteristic of midseptal or anteroseptal site. Subepicardial APs, the most inferior or posterior, have negative delta waves in II, III, and aVF; next most inferiorly, the posteroseptal TA negative (or isoelectric) in aVF and III but not II. On the other hand, the most anteriorly located (anteroseptal) APs have positive delta waves in II, III, and aVF; the midseptal and posteroseptal MA are intermediate.

Since multiple algorithms have been published, each emphasizing slightly different ECG features, and at times contradicting each other, it is important to know which is most reliable. In 2015, Maden et al. reviewed 207 patients who had undergone successful ablation for WPW and compared the algorithms by D'Avila, Chiang, and Arruda.[47] Predictive accuracy was 72.4% with D'Avila, 71.5% with Chiang, and 71.5% with Arruda—all significantly less than the reported accuracy from the initial publications but useful nonetheless. Although all three algorithms had similar accuracy, Maden et al. noted that the Arruda algorithm best predicted both sidedness for an AP and the likelihood of septal location. Furthermore, if wrong, the Arruda algorithm was most likely to predict a location adjacent to the actual pathway. For this reason, this remains the preferred algorithm by most. A double transition, increasing R wave in V_2, but loss of R wave in V_3, may identify a right posteroseptal AP when present[48] (Fig. 27.9). Somewhat at odds with this observation, another study found this precordial signature more often in CS-related APs, perhaps owing to slightly different groups and exclusively q waves in V_1 in the first study.[49]

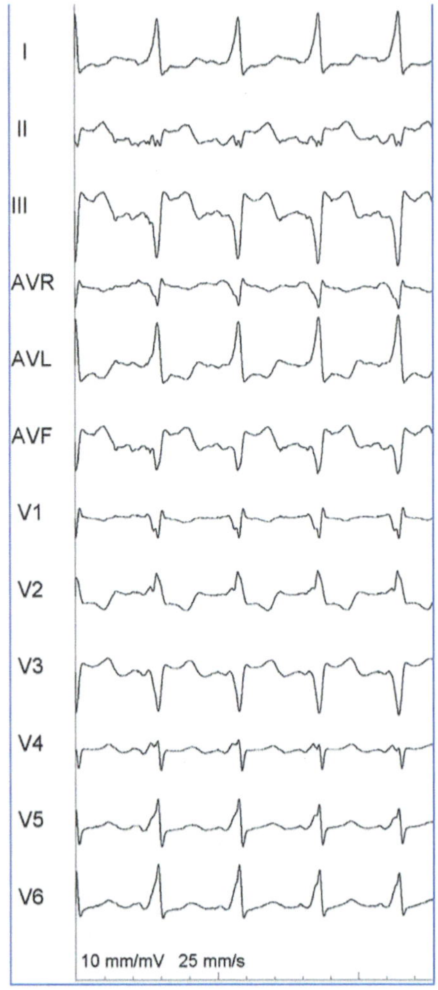

Fig. 27.9 Reverse pattern break or "double transition." In this scenario, R in V_1 > R in V_2 > R in V_3. It may indicate a right posteroseptal AP especially if q in V_1 but other reports indicate an epicardial CS related AP might be present. (See text for more details. (From Bera D, Mukherjee SS, Narasimhan C, et al. Precordial reverse pattern break: a predictor of posteroseptal accessory pathways ablatable from the proximal coronary sinus. *Heart Rhythm.* 2022;19:1386–1388.)

Other algorithms have focused on the polarity of a retrograde P wave for patients who have 12-lead ECGs of narrow-complex regular tachycardia. In 1997 Tai et al. examined 406 patients and reported that for narrow-complex short RP tachycardia, a pseudo-R′ prime in lead V_1 in conjunction with pseudo-S waves in the inferior leads was pathognomonic for AVNRT.[50] In addition, a positive P wave in V_1 predicted a left-sided pathway. Delineating the retrograde P wave from the T wave can be challenging, though. Thus, Rostock et al. used a computer model to remove the T wave during narrow-complex tachycardia and reported that a positive P wave in V_1 also predicted a left-sided pathway, with further refinement in pathway location provided by observing the P wave polarity in leads I, aVR, and aVL.[51] For the retrograde P waves generated by either right or left posteroseptal APs, lead I is isoelectric, and aVR and aVL are positive; the authors found that left septal pathways, like other left-sided APs, had positive P waves in V_1, whereas right septal APs had negative P waves in V_1.

MAPPING

Following a diagnosis of preexcitation (anterograde AP conduction) or AVRT (and a plan for ablation), the pathway needs to be located. Regarding anterograde AP conduction, the aforementioned section helps one noninvasively identify a likely posteroseptal AP, but algorithm-derived location needs invasive confirmation and substantial fine-tuning before ablation. Similarly, with AVRT and a retrograde-only AP, noting an early atrial on the proximal CS recording is only a start. In general, given the anatomical complexity, one should have a low threshold for exploring all the possible locations before ablating unless very convincing and ideal targets are identified. The TA is usually the starting point unless an extremely strong suspicion of a left septal AP is present. If an AP has bidirectional conduction, it should be mapped in both directions, as it may in reality be two separate APs. Intertwined with this concept is the important fact that most APs cross the annulus obliquely, so the anterograde and retrograde insertion sites on the annulus will differ to a surprising degree; the site of AP potentials correlates more closely with the site of successful ablation.[52–54] When mapping either the TA or MA, it is advisable to map its entirety to detect a second AP; at

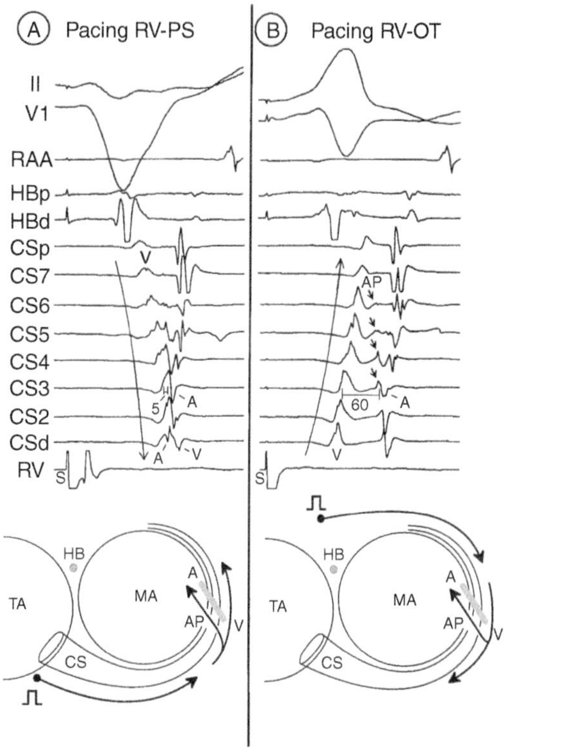

Fig. 27.10 Differential ventricular pacing. This shows the effect on the timing of local V, AP, and A intervals when the ventricular pacing site is altered reversing the direction of the wavefront from counterclockwise (A) along the mitral annulus to clockwise (B). The local VA time increased dramatically, making it easier to appreciate the AP potential. The pathway conducted obliquely with the ventricular end located more posteriorly. *CS*, Coronary sinus; *HB*, His bundle; *MA*, mitral annulus; *RAA*, right atrial appendage; *TA*, tricuspid annulus. (From Otomo K, Gonzalez MD, Beckman KJ, et al. Reversing the direction of paced ventricular and atrial wavefronts reveals an oblique course in accessory AV pathways and improves localization for catheter ablation. *Circulation*. 2001;104:550–556.)

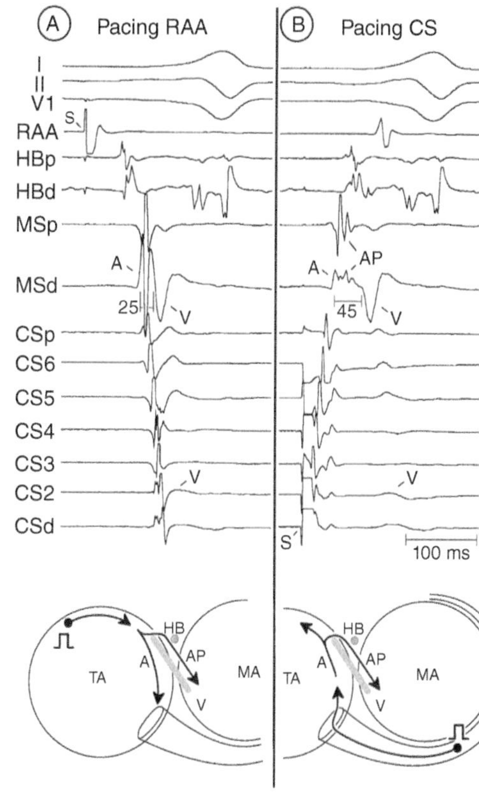

Fig. 27.11 Differential atrial pacing. With reversal of the direction of atrial activation from clockwise (pacing from the RAA) to counterclockwise (pacing from CS), the local AV at the site of earliest ventricular activation increased from 25 to 45 ms, illuminating an oblique AP pathway with the atrial end situated more anteriorly than the ventricular insertion. *CS*, Coronary sinus; *HB*, His bundle; *MA*, mitral annulus; *RAA*, right atrial appendage; *TA*, tricuspid annulus. (From Otomo K, Gonzalez MD, Beckman KJ, et al. Reversing the direction of paced ventricular and atrial wavefronts reveals an oblique course in accessory AV pathways and improves localization for catheter ablation. *Circulation*. 2001;104:550–556.)

"late" points the mapping can proceed quickly and with less detail. Conversely, multiple sites, with smaller incremental steps, need to be sampled when more promising findings emerge. For mapping the atrial insertion, or more accurately retrograde AP conduction, AVRT is ideal because one cannot confuse retrograde AV nodal conduction with AP conduction (since the AV node–His activates anterogradely). On the other hand, with RV pacing, the atrium may be activating via retrograde AV nodal conduction or via retrograde AP conduction or both. Simply ablating at the earliest site risks AV nodal block. Similarly, the operator needs to ensure that preexcitation is present when mapping the anterograde ventricular insertion. Differential pacing, that is reversing the activation wave front by pacing from different directions from the AP insertion along the annulus, should be strongly considered to temporally separate the atrium and ventricle and make the AP potential more apparent than it would be in AVRT or pacing at other sites (Figs. 27.10 and 27.11). If AVRT is not inducible (neither at baseline nor with isoproterenol), differential ventricular pacing or ventricular pacing during adenosine (seeking to block the AV node, and not the AP) should be considered.

A practical and pervasive problem is differentiating atrial, ventricular, and AP potentials. In proximity to the AP, these can be fused; multiple component atrial or ventricular electrograms, however, spawn confusion. Evaluating the signals in sinus rhythm, versus ventricular (or atrial) pacing or AVRT, can aid the discriminative efforts. Deliberately recording further toward the atrial and/or toward the ventricular aspect of the annulus often elucidates the identity of the different signal components. Perhaps most critical, but often omitted, AP potential validation is illustrated in Fig. 27.12. The principle rests on changing the timing of the atrium or the ventricle usually with respect to the AP potential or observing what happens with AP block.

Putting these concepts together, if anterograde AP conduction is present, this can quickly be mapped in sinus rhythm or during atrial pacing if necessary for elicitation of preexcitation noting the timing of local ventricular activation relative to the delta wave onset and the possible presence of an AP potential.

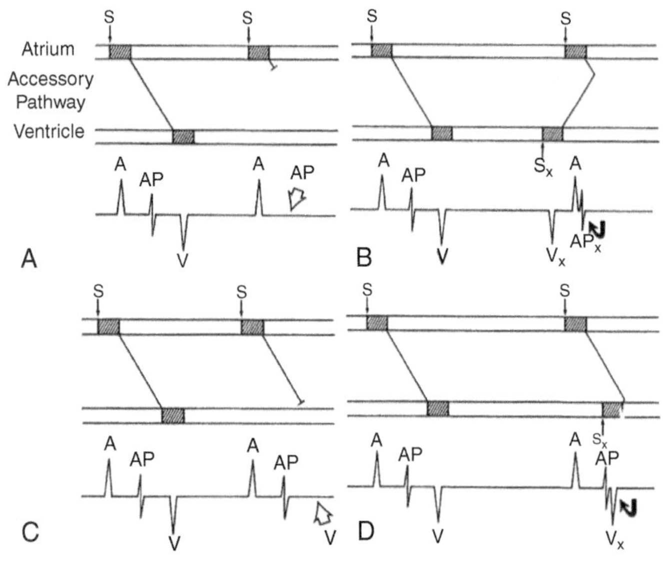

Fig. 27.12 Validation of AP potentials. This schematic illustrates potential methods for confirming the identity of AP potentials. (A) A stimulus at coupling interval shorter than the AP refractory period (2nd S) leads to block between the A and AP; note the absence of an AP and V. (B) A ventricular premature stimulus is introduced early enough that it advances the AP potential but late enough that it does not change the local A. (C) Similar to panel A, introduction of a premature stimulus or a stimulus at CL shorter than the AP refractory period (2nd S) leads to block, but in this case, block is between the AP and V with loss of the V but no change in the AP potential. (D) A late ventricular premature stimulus is introduced late enough that it does not change the local A or the AP potential but advances the V potential. (From Jackman WM, Friday KJ, Yeung-Lai-Wah JA, et al. New catheter technique for recording left free-wall accessory atrioventricular pathway activation. Identification of pathway fiber orientation. *Circulation.* 1988;78:598–611.)

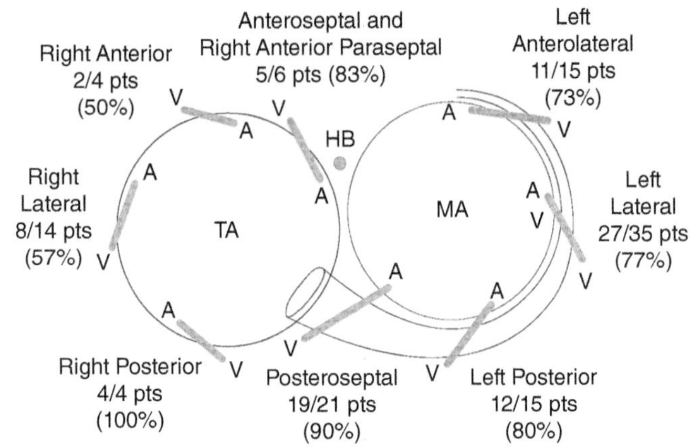

Fig. 27.13 Observed direction for oblique accessory pathways in different anatomical locations; 114 APs were mapped to eight anatomical regions. The relative orientation of atrial and ventricular insertions is depicted. *A*, Atrial end; *HB*, His bundle; *MA*, mitral annulus; *TA*, tricuspid annulus; *V*, ventricular end. See text for details. (From Otomo K, Gonzalez MD, Beckman KJ, et al. Reversing the direction of paced ventricular and atrial wavefronts reveals an oblique course in accessory AV pathways and improves localization for catheter ablation. *Circulation.* 2001;104:550–556.)

Next, depending on the approximate AP location and expected pathway orientation (Fig. 27.11), atrial pacing on either side of the apparent AP location can be performed to temporally separate the local atrial and ventricular signals and allow identification of the AP potentials (see Fig. 27.11). Validation of the AP potentials should be strongly considered (see Fig. 27.12). Then, before ablation, the location (if present) of the atrial insertion should be assessed with AVRT and with differential ventricular pacing (see Fig. 27.10).

In the typical setting of an oblique AP orientation (see Fig. 27.13), common mapping approaches may prove inaccurate, such as stimulus to delta, which may locate the atrial insertion but not where the AP traverses the annulus. Similarly, recording the shortest VA interval could be found at a site of modestly early atrial activation with relatively late ventricular activation.[33]

Bipolar electrograms are most commonly used, but the additive value or preeminence of unipolar recordings for AP localization has often been noted. Simmers et al. analyzed 1230 unipolar ablation catheter signals in 35 patients with anterograde AP conduction.[55] When an AP potential was believed present, unipolar signal characteristics featuring a short local AV interval of 30 ms or less along with catheter stability was usually successful (76%), whereas absence of these two qualities predicted dismal success rate of 1%. For bipolar signals, only an AP potential predicted success, and its presence carried a 48% likelihood. When the same signals were analyzed without regard for AP potentials, unipolar signals with minimal local initial positivity of 0.1 mV or less, along with short local AV interval of 30 ms or less as well as catheter stability, yielded a 63% success; absence of these features characterized a rarely successful site (7%). Barlow et al. stressed a unipolar QS pattern for mapping during either anterograde or retrograde conduction. Specifically, a QS was identified at 90% of successful sites, but also at 75% of transiently successful sites and even 55% of unsuccessful sites; conversely, when the QS pattern was absent, success was rare (8%).[56] It should be acknowledged that identification of retrograde atrial signals in unipolar recordings is often challenging. The timing of local activation for a bipolar signal is complex and varies with the electrogram morphology and electrode size and spacing but should generally be taken as the peak (especially for a simple one-deflection waveform) and not the onset. Cross-referencing the unipolar rapid deflection facilitates choice of the bipolar activation time (Fig. 27.14). In addition to using AP potential recordings and unipolar electrogram morphology, mapping for the earliest local ventricle with respect to the delta wave onset is advisable. The average local ventricle-delta was 19 ± 6 ms for right posteroseptal versus 12 ± 5 ms for left posteroseptal pathways in one series, less than right free wall APs but more negative than left free wall ones.

Another approach recently put forward uses a so-called open mapping window, not trying to discern atrial from AP from ventricular electrograms but rather letting the mapping system catalogue them all and demonstrate the earliest breakout site (Fig. 27.15). This approach acknowledges that without very careful validation operators can err on identifying the source of the electrogram. Using varying thresholds for early meets late can identify the actual conduction across the annulus by

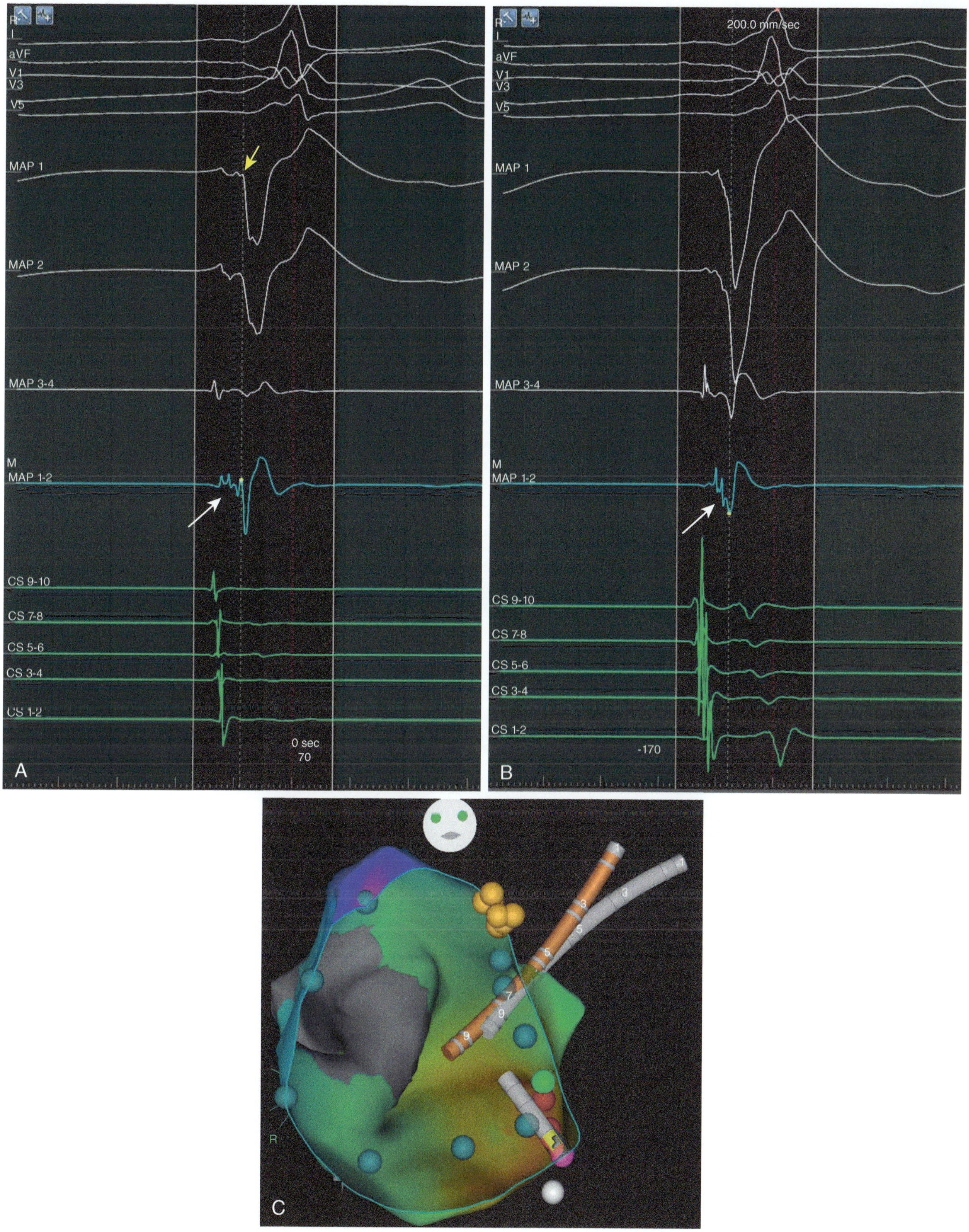

Fig. 27.14 Bipolar and unipolar electrograms illustrated in epicardial posteroseptal AP. Bipolar and unipolar electrograms illustrated an epicardial posteroseptal accessory pathway. (A, B) Preexcited sinus rhythm tracings from surface leads (I, aVF, V_1, V_3, and V_5), coronary sinus (CS), and ablation catheter in middle cardiac vein (MCV) are shown. The *dotted vertical line* is at delta wave onset. Map 1 and map 2 are unipolar; map 1-2 and map 3-4 are bipolar. Note the late activation of the ventricular activation in the body of the CS in panel B. Note the accessory pathway (AP)-like potential (*white arrow*) or CS muscular extension seen in panel A and slightly later in panel B. The map catheter is at *green dot* (C) proximal to mid-MCV and at *pink dot* (B) (one or two components) deeper in MCV. After the small A, then probable AP potential, note the steeply negative intrinsic deflection without preceding positive potential (no r wave) in unipolar map 1 in panel B. A tiny r wave precedes the negative deflection in panel A (*yellow arrow*). The AP potential is 15–20 ms before delta wave onset, and the rapid QS in unipolar is 10–15 ms before the delta wave onset.

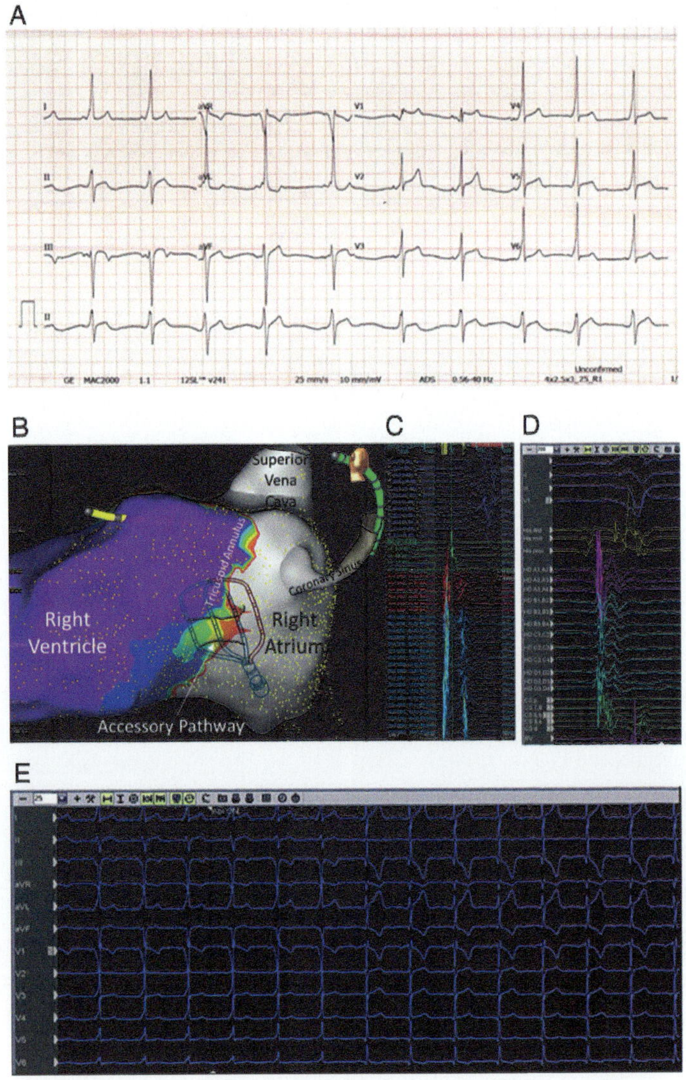

Fig. 27.15 Open window mapping. (A) Preexcited 12-lead suggesting posteroseptal AP. (B) High-density map made with multielectrode catheter of the right atrium, tricuspid annulus (TA), and right ventricle. (C) Electrograms recorded via electroanatomical mapping system. (D) Electrograms near TA seen on recording system. (E) During ablation, preexcitation is eliminated. (Reproduced with permission from Frisch DR. High-density mapping of a posteroseptal accessory pathway using open-window mapping. *J Innov Card Rhythm Manag.* 2021;12:11–13.)

the AP. This methodology can be used with any of the three main electroanatomical mapping systems.[57–60] When compared to conventional mapping (n = 61), the dual chamber or open mapping (n = 50) resulted in fewer RF lesions and lower fluoroscopy dose.[59]

Some clues can suggest whether the successful site will reside along the posteroseptal TA, within the CS or its branches, or across on the (left) posteroseptal MA (Table 27.3). If the ostial CS atrium precedes the His atrium during AVRT by more than 25 ms, this favors a left posteroseptal AP. Sorting out the sharp (local CS musculature) from the lower-frequency, far-field LA signal in the CS recordings can also identify subtypes of posteroseptal APs. With epicardial insertions, the sharp (high slew rate), local CS signals or CS muscular extensions that are in essence AP potentials (see Fig. 27.14) will precede the low-frequency, far-field LA signal in the CS recordings. The same sequence typically occurs with right endocardial APs (because of RA-to-CS connections) (see Table 27.3).[61] A recently described pacing maneuver may help determine the need for a left- versus right-sided ablation approach for posteroseptal APs.[62] The theoretical basis relates to the similarity between LBBB and RV apical pacing and the effect on VA interval during ORT for left-sided APs. The VA during pacing minus the VA during ORT was >40 ms for APs inserting in the LA and < 40 for those inserting in the RA.

TARGET SITES

Table 27.4 summarizes the characteristics of desirable ablation sites. Succinctly, the ablation site should be selected to be highly likely to be successful, the best available site based on the information available, and unlikely to cause harm (principally to the

TABLE 27.3 Predictors of Ablation Site for Posteroseptal Accessory Pathways

Right Endocardial Favored	CS Branch Likely	Left Endocardial Favored
Difference between VA at His and earliest VA in CS <25 ms	Difference between VA at His and earliest VA in CS <25 ms	Difference between VA at His and earliest VA in CS >25 ms
Long-RP tachycardia	Earliest retrograde atrial activation in ORT at proximal to middle CS	Earliest retrograde atrial activation in ORT at middle CS
Negative delta wave in V1[33]	Negative delta wave in II	R > S wave in V1
Earliest VA <15 mm from CS os	Earlier A in CS or branch than TA or MA	Earliest VA >15 mm from CS os
Sharp/blunt CS EGM at earliest retrograde site[61]	Sharp/blunt CS EGM at earliest retrograde site[61]	Blunt/sharp CS EGM at earliest retrograde site
Change in VA with LBBB <15 ms[67]	Change in VA with LBBB variable	Change in VA with LBBB >15–30 ms

CS os, Coronary sinus ostium; *EGM*, electrogram; *LBBB*, left bundle branch block; *MA*, mitral annulus; *ORT*, orthodromic reciprocating tachycardia; *TA*, tricuspid annulus; *VA*, ventricular-to-atrial interval.

TABLE 27.4 Target Sites for Ablation

Feature	Caveats and Nuances
Stable Catheter Electrograms and Position by Fluoroscopy and Electroanatomical Map	
Contact force > 5–10*g*	If contact force catheter used
Not within 5 mm of coronary artery	Consider coronary angiography in MCV or CS diverticulum.
Not above roof of CS or with upward deflection in CS	To minimize AV node injury - For midseptal pathways (i.e., not posteroseptal) needing ablation between His and CS os select ventricular aspect; consider cryoablation.
Anterograde Conduction, "Ventricular Insertion"	
Accessory pathway potential	- Consider use of differential atrial pacing to separate A, APP, and V. - Optimally validated by programmed stimulation
Local V to delta	- Minus 20 ms (local V earlier than delta) for right posteroseptal - Minus 5–15 ms for left posteroseptal - Timing of local V confirmed by unipolar rapid deflection - Consistent selection of delta wave onset critical - Presumes correct identification of A, AP, and V - Earliest V may identify ventricular insertion, but with pathway oblique orientation ablation may be unsuccessful.[33,61]
Unipolar distal QS	Sharp rapid negative deflection without preceding positive deflection is ideal.[62]
Retrograde Conduction, "Atrial Insertion"	
Accessory pathway potential	- Consider use of differential ventricular pacing to separate V, APP, and A. - Optimally validated by programmed stimulation
Earliest local A	- Presumes correct identification of V, AP, and A - Earliest A may identify atrial insertion but with pathway oblique orientation ablation may be unsuccessful.[33,61]
Fused V and A	Nonspecific, depends on direction of activation wave front[61]

A, Atrial; *APP*, accessory pathway potential; *AV*, atrioventricular; *CS os*, coronary sinus ostium; *MCV*, middle cardiac vein; *V*, ventricular.

AV and/or a coronary artery). Ablating at the first acceptable site is an inferior strategy because ablation will render the interpretation of electrograms even more challenging. The axiom "measure twice, cut once" is apt for AP ablation (see Table 27.4).

ABLATION

AP ablation is a Class I indication in patients with symptomatic SVT and a Class IIa indication in asymptomatic patients with preexcitation provided that the AP has high-risk characteristics or that the patient has a high-risk occupation or activity.[63]

The mapping and identification of an optimal site of ablation are detailed in the "Mapping" and "Target Sites" sections. Following this, it is important to have also considered other elements to successfully eliminate the AP, including catheter type, sheath, energy source, ablation settings, ventilation and anesthesia, cardiac rhythm, and monitoring for success and complications. Anatomical data, although limited in number, suggest that APs are relatively thin structures measuring a few millimeters.[5,6] Accordingly, a 4-mm electrode ablation catheter, capable of creating a 5- to 6-mm deep lesion,[64,65] is usually sufficient for ablating such a structure, unless the AP is subepicardial. Tissue heating is resistive or ohmic immediately adjacent to the catheter and then conductive for deeper tissue. Temperature-guided ablation modes allowed development of a typically successful electrode (and thus hopefully tissue) temperature to permanently ablate the structure (above about 50°C)[66] while minimizing higher temperatures associated with increased coagulum formation.[10,67] Whereas larger electrode tips create larger lesions (provided higher power is delivered to maintain current density), this is usually not required; furthermore, the larger electrode hampers accurate mapping. Irrigated radiofrequency (RF) electrode catheters offer advantages in several scenarios, including deeply located APs, in anatomical settings exhibiting low blood flow thus limiting convective cooling (e.g., under valve leaflets), or within the CS or especially its branches, and to minimize coagulum and thus avoid cerebral embolism when ablating in the left heart. Saline irrigation increases convective surface cooling, keeps electrode temperature low, increases the volume of the resistive heating zone, creates the highest temperatures several millimeters deep to the electrode, and thus generates deeper lesions. Caution should be used near the conduction system or coronary arteries, however. In seeking to avoid needing to change catheters, an irrigated catheter is a reasonable choice for a posteroseptal AP,[68,69] given the potential need for a mitral annular, CS, or MCV approach. However, irrigated RF might be disadvantageous if the AP in actuality were midseptal because of the possible heightened risk of AV nodal injury. A small randomized study found no difference with respect to success, duration of RF or fluoroscopy, or complications for solid- versus irrigated-tip catheters.[70] Contact force (and irrigated) catheters have become standard for atrial fibrillation, but it is not clear that these are necessary for AP ablation, although obviously excellent contact is critical. When physicians mapped the TA and MA blinded to contact force, the right posteroseptal region featured the second worse contact force with 69% of sites having <5g of contact force despite long sheaths.[71] When ablating in the MCV or other venous branches, coronary angiography is recommended, and irrigated RF or cryoablation (see later) is preferable. For irrigated RF in the CS, a starting power of 20 W and uptitration based on impedance and effect is reasonable; the impedance cutoff may need to be increased to 150 or 200 Ω. In addition, manually increasing irrigation flow above that dictated by the energy may prove efficacious. For standard or irrigated RF ablation, at the TA, MA, or proximal CS, a starting power of 30 W is appropriate.

OUTCOMES

In a meta-analysis, the overall first procedure success rate for AP ablation (overall) was 90.9%, with a 7% recurrence rate and 8% repeat ablation frequency; some of the series were from the early 1990s, and the success rate improved over time to some degree.[72] In a large multicenter series, posteroseptal APs were associated with the second-lowest success rate (90% versus 88% for right free wall and 95% for left free wall), highest recurrence rate (8% versus 7% for right free wall and 3% for left free wall), and a high complication rate significant for 3% AV block.[73] A recent single-center, pediatric series of anterior and midseptal AP pathway ablations found an impressive 0% risk of complete AV block or pacemaker implantation, though two (~1%) of patients had transient second-degree AV block with one having persistent first-degree AV block. However many patients had recurrence requiring repeat ablation, and cryoenergy was used for more than half of the group.[74] In Jackman's single-center series, posteroseptal APs had the lowest success rate (93% versus 100% for other locations) and highest recurrence rate (14%, similar to 13% for right free wall and much higher than left free wall at 5%). In a more contemporary, state-of-the-art series from Oklahoma, overall acute success was impressive at 99%; recurrences remained relatively high for posteroseptal APs (10.1%) and anteroseptal APs (14.7%) yet had declined for right free wall APs (2.8%) and remained low for left free wall APs (2.2%).[75]

COMPLICATIONS

Complications of posteroseptal AP ablation include those possible for any catheter procedure or catheter ablation.[76] Complications especially relevant to these anatomical locations include AV block, coronary artery injury, cardiac perforation or tamponade, coronary venous injury, occlusion or perforation, and inadvertent cavotricuspid isthmus block (confusing activation sequence interpretation).[77] AV block occurred in 1 of 43 (2.3%) posteroseptal AP patients in Jackman's early series (in a patient with congenital heart disease)[9] and in 3 of 98 (3.1%) posteroseptal AP cases in Calkins' multicenter series.[73] It is important to note that when accelerated junctional beats occur during slow pathway ablation, the presence of retrograde atrial activation is reassuring, yet when a retrograde AP is present, the reassurance would be potentially false. A recent administrative database study noted a trend toward declining volume of AP ablation overall and that most hospitals performing AP ablation performed very few; incredibly, six or more AP ablations per year positioned a hospital in the highest tertile. Moreover, hospital volume by tertile was inversely related to complication frequency. Considering low versus high tertile complication rates, tamponade incidence varied from 0% to 0.72%, from 0.3% to 0.6% for AV block requiring a pacemaker, and from 0.9% to 2.8% for any complication. AP location was not available in this database. In the Swedish National Ablation Registry, AP ablations remained relatively steady between 2006 and 2015, while AF ablations increased markedly.[78] A German ablation registry recorded data from 2007 to 2010 and included 12,566 patients undergoing AP ablation. The risk of complications for septal APs was 9.1% compared to 3.9% and 2.0%, respectively, for right and left free wall ones. Analogously, AV node injury requiring a pacemaker was reported in 2.9% of septal APs vs 1.2% in right-sided and 0% in left-sided ones.[76]

In a consecutive, single-center series of 508 patients over 14 years, the average complication rate for AP ablation was 3.5% and declined over time; recurrence rates were intermediate for posteroseptal (lower than right free wall but higher than left free

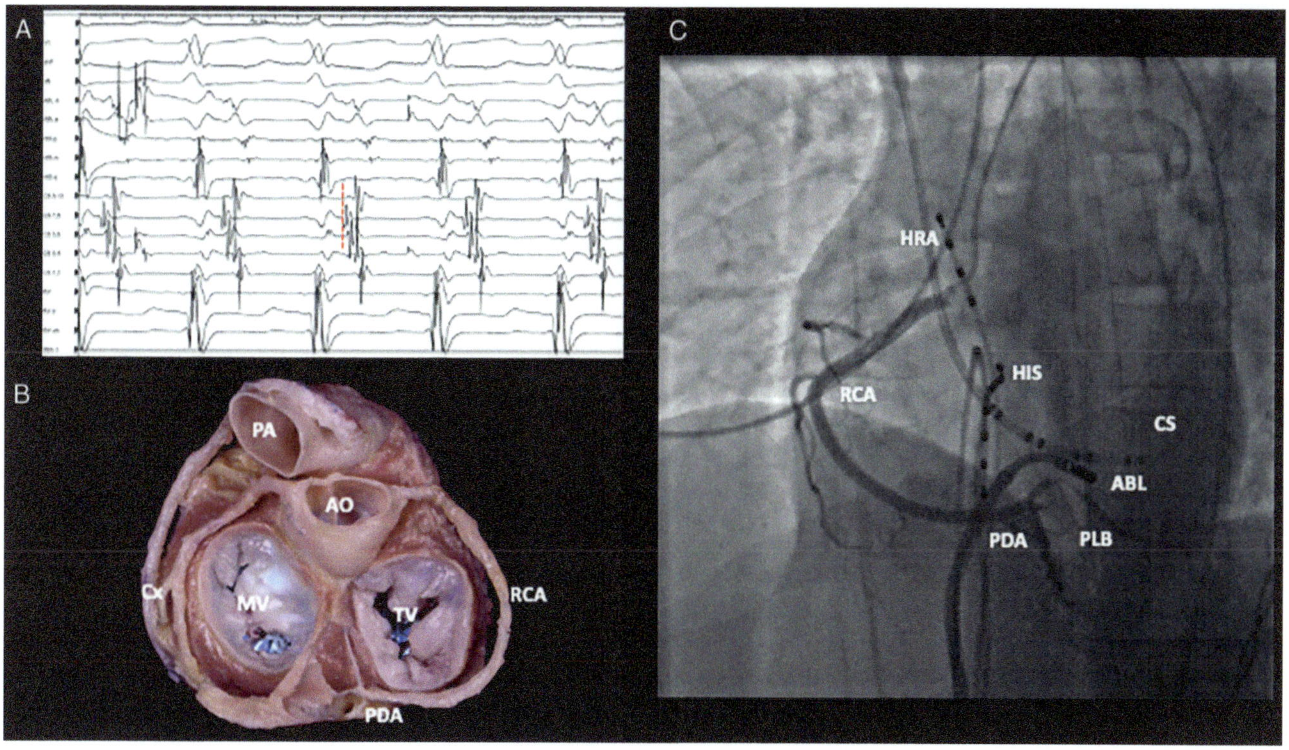

Fig 27.16 Importance of coronary angiographic imaging prior to ablation of posteroseptal accessory pathways. (A) Posteroseptal pathway with earliest atrial activation (*red dotted line*) at CS 7,8 (CS catheter not fully engaged into CS). (B) Complex anatomy of this region from a posterior view. (C) LAO angiographic view of the ablation catheter near the site of successful ablation in close proximity to the PLB of the RCA. *ABL*, Ablation catheter; *AO*, aorta; *CS*, coronary sinus catheter; *CX*, circumflex artery; *HIS*, bundle of his catheter; *HRA*, high right atrial catheter; *MV*, mitral valve; *PA*, pulmonary artery; *PDA*, posterior descending artery; *PLB*, posterior lateral branch; *RCA*, right coronary artery; *TV*, tricuspid valve.

wall).[79] Regarding transseptal versus retrograde approaches, an early series found a similar success rate (85%) and complication rate (~6%) for both.[80] Coronary artery dissection and aortic valve injury, although rare, only occur with retrograde catheterization. The greater experience with transseptal catheterization owing to atrial fibrillation ablation has likely increased the success rate and reduced the complication rate for this approach at most centers.

Thermally induced coronary artery injury may occur during AP ablation along the TA or MA but is most worrisome in the posteroseptal space, especially in the CS branches[81,82] (Fig 27.16). Indeed, in a compilation of 61 cases of coronary artery injury from ablation (1992–2017), posteroseptal APs were the most common location at 35.6% with the cavotricuspid isthmus second at 19.3%.[83] The most informative and largest experience comes from Oklahoma where coronary angiography was performed in 169 consecutive epicardial posteroseptal AP ablations.[82] Notably, a coronary branch was usually within 2 mm of the ablation site (59%), reasonably close (3–5 mm) in 16%, and safely away (>5 mm) in 25%. Ablation when the coronary was <2 mm caused harm in half the cases. Cryoablation, less likely to injure the coronary,[84] was used in 26 patients having a coronary branch within 5 mm of the ablation target with a lower but reasonable success of 65%, and a higher recurrence rate (23% versus 10%). Another smaller series found the posterolateral branch (of the RCA or circumflex) to be on average 2 mm from the CS or its branch at the closest location.[79]

TROUBLESHOOTING THE DIFFICULT CASE

A well-founded, thorough approach to diagnosis, electrocardiographic pathway location and mapping will less often result in puzzlement and/or an initially unsuccessful ablation. Nevertheless, correct interpretation of electrograms remains challenging, and certain reminders may help when the electrophysiologist encounters an impasse (Table 27.5). Taking a step back and verifying the criteria used to establish the diagnosis (SVT type) and evidence for AP location are warranted. One should consider whether multiple pathways are present (different site of atrial pacing or induction of atrial fibrillation and evaluating pattern[s] of preexcitation), whether one AP has been eliminated leaving another, or if residual preexcitation is caused by a fasciculoventricular one (not needing ablation). Tachycardia may need to be reinitiated and reevaluated. Another map or multiple maps (during pacing from more than one atrial or ventricular site or perhaps preferably during

TABLE 27.5 Troubleshooting the Difficult Case

Problem	Causes	Solution
Is the diagnosis accurate?	SVT type Accessory pathway location Preexcitation variant? Anatomical variant	Revisit diagnosis of AVRT versus AVNRT versus AT. Revisit ECG algorithm. Consider multiple APs (differential atrial pacing; induce atrial fibrillation). Consider fasciculoventricular AP as cause of preexcitation. Consider Ebstein, or is CS anomaly present?
Unable to find suitable ablation site	Consider possible epicardial pathway Misinterpretation of signals	Map in coronary sinus and branches; perform CS venography. Change pacing site in A or V[61]; change pacing from A to V or vice versa; examine signals in SR.
Poor catheter stability	Excessive respiratory motion; intermittent airway obstruction Excessive cardiac motion Suboptimal catheter characteristics	Nasal or oral airway during moderate sedation; conversion to general anesthesia to control respiration or allow use of apnea Pace during mapping and ablation. Use other curve if asymmetric curve catheter; use more or less sheath if using preformed sheath; use preformed sheath if only using short sheath; use deflectable sheath; change catheter regarding reach, stiffness, contact force, and/or curvature; and change approach (transseptal to retrograde aortic or vice versa).
Failure despite good electrogram characteristics	Poor catheter contact Oblique pathway Low temperature (nonirrigated) Low power delivery Not close enough Reevaluate electrograms	Improve contact with sheath, different catheter, or approach; use contact force catheter. Map during pacing from alternate sites. Improve contact, reduce impedance, and use higher-output generator. Use irrigated RF (especially in CS or branch). Map in opposite chamber or in CS/branch. Use unipolar signals to cross-validate.
Recurrent atrial fibrillation	Spontaneous or degeneration from AVRT	Map during A or V pacing instead of AVRT; give lowest necessary dose of intravenous ibutilide or procainamide to minimize chance of eliminating preexcitation.

A, Atrial; *AP*, accessory pathway; *AT*, atrial tachycardia; *AVNRT*, atrioventricular nodal reentrant tachycardia; *AVRT*, atrioventricular reentrant tachycardia; *CS*, coronary sinus; *ECG*, electrocardiogram; *RF*, radiofrequency; *SVT*, supraventricular tachycardia; *V*, ventricular.

AVRT) should be made. As emphasized, for posteroseptal APs, one needs to consider the TA, CS, CS branches, a possible CS diverticulum, and the MA for mapping and ablation. In a vast systematic experience between 1989 and 2005, Jackman's group evaluated 904 patients who had undergone prior unsuccessful ablation. Incorrect mapping (60%) was the predominant cause for failure; second most common was technical or anatomical challenge such as proximity to a coronary or low power caused by a venous branch; unusual AP location was least common.[75]

REFERENCES

Please refer to the e-book for a complete list of references.

28

Catheter Ablation of Superoparaseptal ("Anteroseptal") and Midseptal Accessory Pathways

John M. Miller, Tanyanan Tanawuttiwat, Takeki Suzuki, Siddharth P. Shah

KEY POINTS

- Diagnosis of superoparaseptal ("anteroseptal") and midseptal accessory pathways (APs) is made on the basis of an electrocardiographic pattern (if overt preexcitation is present) and evidence of midseptal/superoparaseptal AP insertions during intracardiac mapping studies.
- Orthodromic reciprocating tachycardia (ORT) using a midseptal AP must be differentiated from atrioventricular (AV) nodal reentry and septal or para-Hisian atrial tachycardias.
- Mapping of superoparaseptal APs is used to locate the site with the earliest anterograde ventricular activation near or anterior/lateral to the His bundle recording, the earliest anterograde ventricular activation-to-delta wave interval (15–40 ms pre-delta), and earliest retrograde atrial activation in the region of the His bundle recording during ORT. Recording a discrete AP potential is very helpful but not always achievable and must be distinguished from the His potential.
- Mapping of midseptal APs is used to locate the site of the earliest anterograde ventricular activation between the coronary sinus (CS) ostium and the His recording location, the earliest anterograde ventricular activation-to-delta wave interval (15–25 ms pre-delta), and the earliest retrograde atrial activation between the CS ostium and the His recording location during ORT. Left midseptal connections are rare.
- The ablation target can be the site of earliest anterograde ventricular activation or retrograde atrial activation on the AV annulus. Recording the AP potential can verify the correct target. Pathways typically traverse the AV groove at a slant, with atrial insertions generally located "clockwise" to ventricular insertion sites in the left anterior oblique view.
- Use of long preformed or deflectable vascular sheaths may be helpful; electroanatomical mapping systems are often useful to "tag" sites of interest, and cryoablation may be useful or even preferred. Effecting deeper tissue damage, such as with cooled/irrigated radiofrequency ablation, is rarely needed.
- Sources of difficulty include lack of catheter stability, proximity to elements of the normal conduction system with risk of heart block, catheter-induced mechanical block of pathway conduction, and accelerated junctional rhythm (narrow QRS) during ablation that can be mistaken for elimination of preexcitation.

Atrioventricular (AV) accessory pathways (APs) are thin fibers, usually composed of typical myocardial cells, that allow electrical communication between atrium and ventricle extrinsic to the normal AV node–His bundle axis. The clinical expression of these pathways ranges from simply causing an abnormal electrocardiogram; to forming an integral component of a macroreentrant circuit incorporating atrial and ventricular myocardium, AV node and His bundle, and the AP (AV reciprocating supraventricular tachycardia [SVT]); to functioning as an alternative pathway for transmission of rapid atrial tachyarrhythmias such as flutter and fibrillation to the ventricles. Symptoms may range from none to occasional mild palpitations to severe palpitations accompanied by dyspnea, chest discomfort, lightheadedness, and even syncope or cardiac arrest from rapidly conducted atrial fibrillation.

Since its introduction in the late 1980s, catheter ablation of APs has become a relatively routine matter in most electrophysiology laboratories. However, ablation of pathways in the so-called anteroseptal and midseptal locations can be a challenge for even experienced operators because of the proximity of these pathways to the normal cardiac conduction system (AV node and His bundle). Inadvertent injury to these structures resulting in the need for permanent pacing, especially in a young patient, is a significant adverse outcome. Fortunately, techniques have been developed to decrease the likelihood of this complication. This chapter discusses the relevant anatomy of these pathways and the use of techniques to achieve optimal outcomes.

ANATOMY AND NOMENCLATURE

Older nomenclature of septal pathways has undergone modification. A reexamination of the anatomy of the AV junctions has suggested that the terminology used in the original descriptions

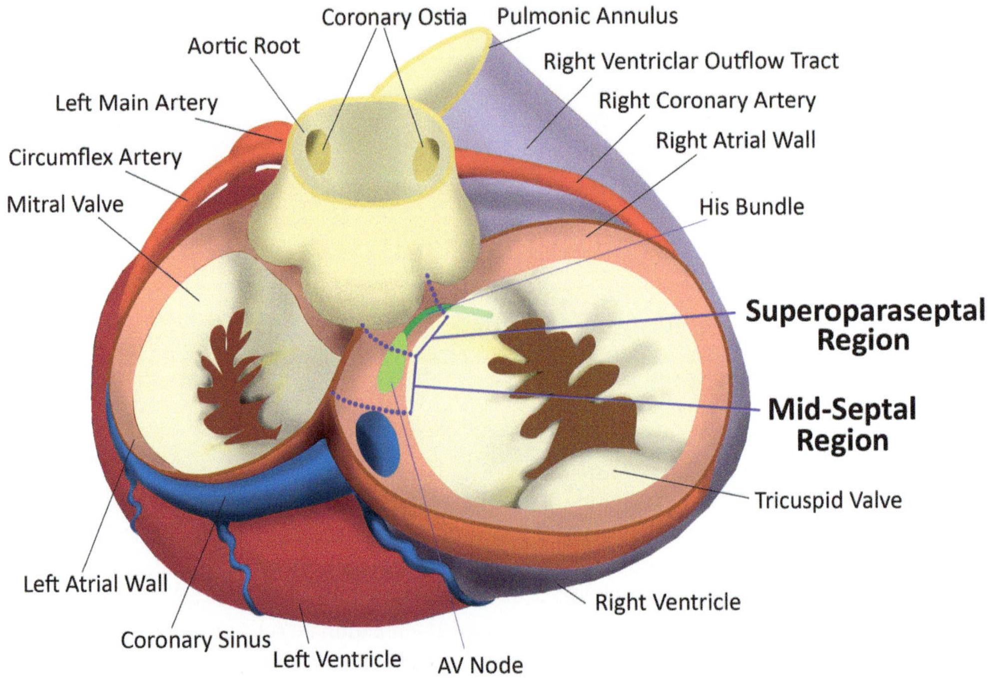

Fig. 28.1 View of atrioventricular (AV) groove from above with most of the atrial muscle removed; the right atrial rim has been rendered semi-transparent to reveal structures beneath. Note the small dimensions of the actual atrial septum (*dashed line*). True septal ("midseptal") pathways have an atrial insertion on the right or left side in this region, in which the AV node resides. Pathways in the region of the His bundle, previously called anteroseptal, in fact have free wall and not septal atrial insertions (hence "superoparaseptal" pathways).

of AP locations was anatomically inaccurate and, in some cases, frankly misleading. A reclassification of cardiac electrophysiologic anatomy has been developed to try to correct these antiquated but ingrained terms.[1] In addition, a more complete understanding of the anatomy of the atrial and ventricular septa has resulted in a "shrinking" of the atrial septum: most trainees conceive of the atrial septum as a relatively large disk comprising the intersection of two spheres (atria) compressed together. In fact, the true muscular atrial septum is much smaller, consisting of a relatively thin rim of atrial tissue surrounding the fossa ovalis.[2–4] This has implications for how precisely one must position a needle and catheter to safely puncture the septum for left atrial access and for evaluation and ablation of the pathways under consideration in this chapter.

In the old vernacular, "anteroseptal" pathways were regarded as being located in the apex of Koch triangle, connecting the atrial and ventricular septa in the region of the His bundle. In the anatomically accurate nomenclature, these pathways are more properly regarded as *superoparaseptal,* because there is no atrial septum in the region anterior to the His recording location (atrial walls are separated here by the aortic root; Fig. 28.1). These connections are, thus, right free wall, paraseptal pathways. Posteriorly, pathways in the region of the ostium of the coronary sinus (CS), which previously were called "posteroseptal," are in fact *posterior paraseptal,* because the CS itself is, by definition, entirely posterior to the atrial septum. Pathways located between these two boundaries of the septum have been called "midseptal" or "intermediate septal," but, because they are the only truly septal interconnections, they may simply be called *septal.* Further complicating the situation is the fact that the AV valves are not isoplanar; the tricuspid valve is slightly inferiorly displaced relative to the mitral valve such that a portion of the medial right atrium is juxtaposed to subaortic left ventricular muscle, rather than right ventricle.

In the discussion that follows, we will consider that superoparaseptal ("anteroseptal") APs are located in the apex of Koch triangle at a site from which a small His potential can usually be recorded. True septal or midseptal APs are located in the floor of Koch triangle, between the His recording location and the anterior portion of the CS ostium.

DIAGNOSIS AND DIFFERENTIAL DIAGNOSIS

Superoparaseptal Accessory Pathways

Superoparaseptal APs comprise 6–7% of all APs in most large series. About 80% of these APs exhibit anterograde conduction, and 20% are retrograde-only conducting ("concealed"); only about 5% conduct exclusively in the anterograde direction. Because these pathways connect the right atrial and right ventricular paraseptal free walls in a region that is cephalad, or superior, as well as anterior to most of the rest of the ventricular mass, an anterogradely conducting pathway manifests positive delta waves in the inferior leads (II, III, and aVF) and the lateral precordial leads (V_3 through V_6); negative delta waves are present in lead V_1 (Fig. 28.2) and often in V_2.[5] Leads I and aVL have positive delta waves (negative in aVR). During ORT, the

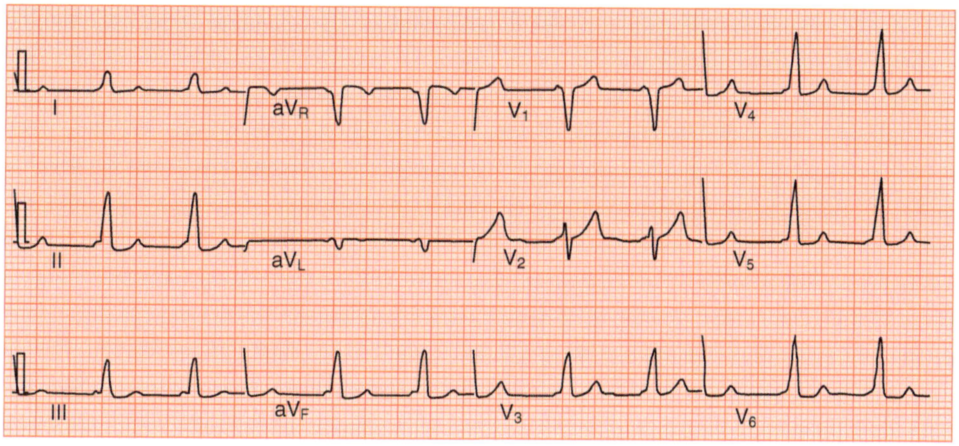

Fig. 28.2 Electrocardiogram of superoparaseptal accessory pathway with anterograde conduction, showing a very short PR segment and positive delta waves in 1, 2, 3, aVF, and lateral precordial leads.

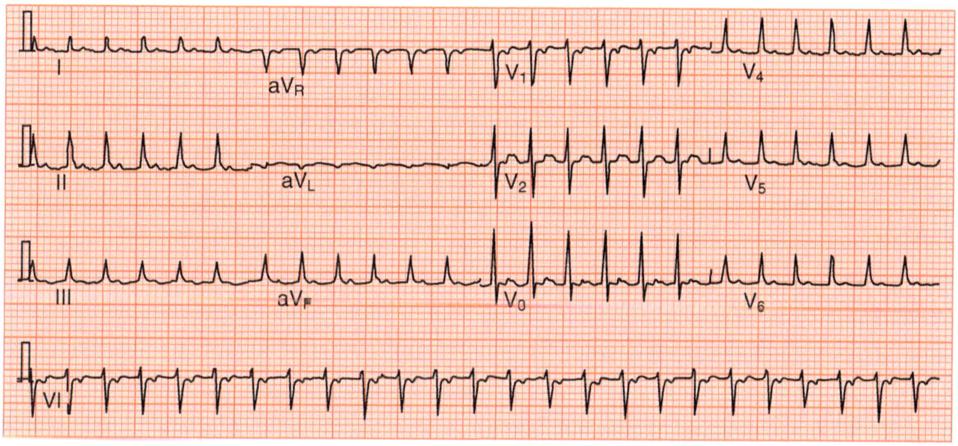

Fig. 28.3 Electrocardiogram of supraventricular tachycardia incorporating a retrogradely conducting superoparaseptal accessory pathway. Note the positive P waves in the inferior leads with negative P wave polarity in leads aVR and V_1.

P wave is typically situated in the early portion of the ST segment; although retrograde, it is usually positive in the inferior leads, because much of the atrial mass is located caudad from the atrial insertion (Fig. 28.3).

Midseptal Accessory Pathways

Midseptal pathways account for 5% or less of all APs in most series. Approximately 85% of midseptal APs show anterograde conduction (15% are retrograde only), with only about 4% conducting anterograde only. These APs connect atrium and ventricle in a complex region that can give rise to slightly different delta wave polarities in different individuals. A typical preexcitation pattern has predominantly positive delta waves in leads I, II, aVL, and V_2 through V_6, with leads III and aVF usually having predominantly negative delta waves, and aVR and V_1 having isoelectric delta waves. Variations in this pattern, especially in the inferior leads and in V_2, have been reported. During ORT, because of the more posterior location of the pathway's atrial insertion (near the compact AV node), the P wave is usually inverted in the inferior leads. Multiple APs are present in up to 25% of patients with midseptal APs.

Electrophysiologic Testing

The electrophysiologic diagnosis of supraventricular tachycardia (SVT) incorporating a superoparaseptal or midseptal pathway is usually relatively straightforward (Table 28.1); however, the atrial activation sequence during SVT may resemble that of normal AV nodal output (unlike the situation with left or right free wall APs, in which the atrial activation sequence during SVT is eccentric). This similarity of atrial activation can provide a diagnostic challenge in some cases. Standard diagnostic techniques, including introduction of ventricular premature extrastimuli during His refractoriness in an episode SVT, should be used to define the tachycardia mechanism. In some cases, such as when the ventricular-to-atrial interval is very short or SVT is nonsustained or noninducible, other techniques must be used to establish the presence of an AP. These include para-Hisian pacing, differential site ventricular pacing (basal versus apical), comparison of His-to-atrial (HA) intervals, use of single ventricular extrastimuli, and ventricular overdrive pacing during (entrainment of) SVT, including inspection of phenomena observed during initiation of SVT and of pacing during SVT.

TABLE 28.1 **Diagnostic Criteria**

Surface ECG: Sinus Rhythm (in Presence of Preexcitation)	
Superoparaseptal APs	• Delta waves predominantly positive in leads I, II, III, aVL, aVF, and V_3 through V_6; negative in aVR and V1, and often in V_2
Midseptal APs	• Delta waves predominantly positive in I, II, aVL, and V_2 through V_6; negative in III and aVF; negative or isoelectric in aVR and V_1
Surface ECG: Orthodromic SVT	
	• P waves in ST segment; positive in I and positive (superoparaseptal) or negative (midseptal) in II, III, aVF
Intracardiac Recordings and Electrophysiologic Testing	
General principles	• Retrograde atrial activation independent of His activation • Premature ventricular extrastimulus during His refractoriness can advance or delay anticipated atrial activation, or terminate tachycardia without causing atrial activation • ΔHA interval ($HA_{ventricular\ pacing}$ - HA_{SVT}) < 0 distinguishes orthodromic SVT from AV nodal reentry • Advancement of timing of atrial activation with overdrive ventricular pacing while QRS is fused • After entrained ventricular pacing during SVT, PPI-TCL <115 ms and SA-VA <85 ms • Para-Hisian or differential site ventricular pacing useful to prove existence of pathway, confirm its elimination following ablation (if normal retrograde AV node/His conduction intact)
Superoparaseptal APs	• Earliest anterograde ventricular activation at or anterior to/rightward of His recording location • Earliest retrograde atrial activation in His bundle recording or slightly lateral on tricuspid annulus • Small (<0.1 mV) His deflection in ablation recording • Sensitivity to mechanical block by catheter manipulation
Midseptal APs	• Earliest anterograde ventricular and retrograde atrial activation between His and coronary sinus ostium • May exhibit "decremental" conduction properties (anterograde or retrograde)

AP, Accessory pathway; *AV*, atrioventricular; *ECG*, electrocardiogram; *ΔHA*, difference in His-to-atrial interval; *SVT*, supraventricular tachycardia; *PPI*, postpacing interval; *TCL*, tachycardia cycle length; *SA*, stimulus-to-atrial interval; *VA*, ventriculoatrial interval.

Pacing from a location near the His bundle (para-Hisian pacing) can distinguish conduction over an AP from that over the AV node, as follows: at low pacing outputs, ventricular capture occurs, whereas at higher outputs, the His bundle/proximal right bundle branch are also captured with the adjacent ventricular myocardium, resulting in a narrower QRS. If a septal AP is present, the stimulus-to-atrial interval will be identical regardless of whether the His is captured, because these APs typically conduct more rapidly than the AV node does. If there is no AP, the stimulus-to-atrial interval is longer with ventricular-only capture than when the His is captured, because with ventricular pacing the impulse must travel some distance using relatively slow myocyte-myocyte conduction before it encounters elements of the His-Purkinje network to begin activating it retrogradely. With His capture, the impulse need only traverse the AV node to activate the atrium (Fig. 28.4).[6] This technique can be used to assess whether the AP has been successfully ablated (Fig 28.5).

Using a principle similar to that of para-Hisian pacing, comparison of the stimulus-to-atrial intervals observed with right ventricular apical versus basal stimulation can demonstrate the presence of an AP. The apex, though physically more distant from the atrium than the ventricular base, is nonetheless *electrically* closer because of the proximity of the distal right bundle branch to the pacing site. Entry into the rapidly conducting His-Purkinje system allows a shorter stimulus-to-atrial interval during pacing from the apex than from the base. From the base, the impulse must again travel relatively slowly for some distance through ventricular myocardium before it engages the His-Purkinje system. However, in the presence of an extranodal AP, pacing from the base results in a shorter stimulus-to-atrial interval compared to apical stimulation since the AP makes the base electrically closer to the atrium as well as physically (Fig. 28.6). Fixed-rate pacing or extrastimuli during SVT can be used.[7] This technique can also be used to confirm successful AP ablation.

Comparison of the HA intervals observed during SVT and during ventricular pacing at the SVT cycle length can distinguish AV nodal reentry from septal pathway–dependent ORT. The HA interval during ORT should be longer than the HA interval during ventricular pacing. The His bundle and atrium are activated in series during ORT but in parallel (AV node and AP simultaneously) during pacing. However, the HA during AV nodal reentry should be the same as or slightly shorter than that during pacing, because the His bundle and atrium are activated in parallel during SVT but in series during pacing (the opposite of the situation in ORT).[8]

Similarly, overdrive right ventricular apical pacing at a cycle length slightly faster than that of SVT (entrainment of SVT) can distinguish atypical AV nodal reentry from ORT using a septal AP. If AV nodal reentry is the SVT diagnosis, the stimulus-to-atrial interval during ventricular pacing will exceed the QRS-to-atrial interval by more than 85 ms, and the postpacing interval will exceed the SVT cycle length by more than 115 ms. In ORT using a septal AP, these intervals are less than the cutoff values noted. This distinction occurs because the pacing site is remote from the SVT circuit in AV nodal reentry but near or within it in ORT.[9] Although this criterion was meant

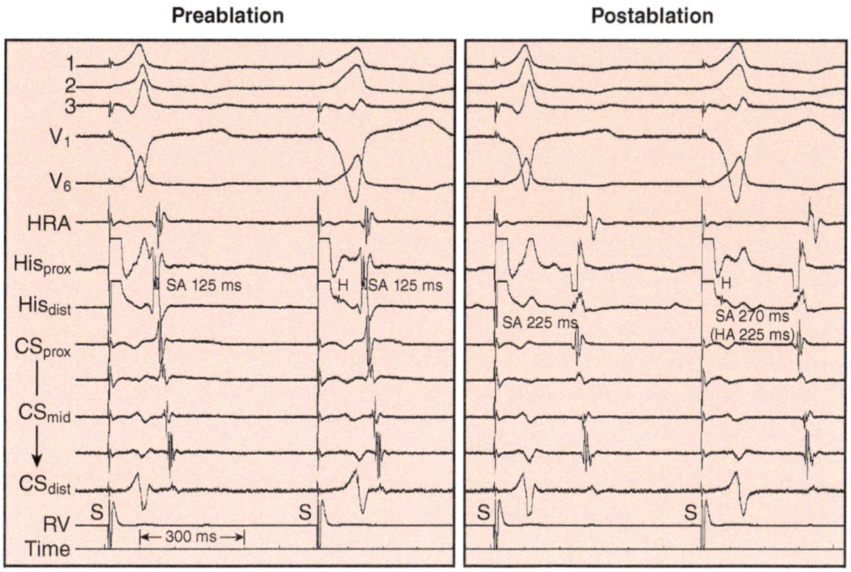

Fig. 28.4 Para-Hisian pacing. In this and subsequent figures, surface leads 1, 2, 3, V_1, and V_6 are shown with intracardiac recordings from high right atrium (HRA), His bundle proximal (prox) and distal (dist) electrode pairs, coronary sinus (CS), and right ventricle (RV) near the His recording location. *S*, Stimulus artifact; *H*, His deflection. Para-Hisian pacing is shown before (*left*) and after ablation (*right*). On each panel, the first complex shows His and ventricular capture, the second ventricular capture only. Before ablation, the stimulus-atrial (S-A) interval is the same regardless of whether His capture occurs because the accessory pathway is the preferred path of conduction. In the complex on the right, the apparent "H-A" interval is shorter than the S-A interval during His capture, indicating that atrial activation is occurring independent of AV nodal conduction. After successful ablation, retrograde conduction requires His activation; the S-A interval is longer than before ablation and increases further in the absence of His capture (complex on the right) since with pure ventricular pacing it takes longer to get to the His bundle. Once the His is activated as shown, the H-A time is the same as the S-A time during His capture.

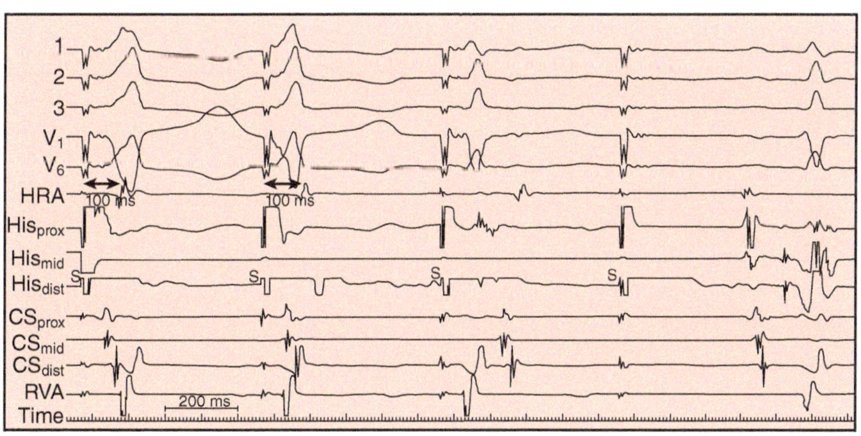

Fig. 28.5 Para-Hisian pacing revealing presence of pathway after apparently successful radiofrequency application. Four stimuli from the His region result in (*left* to *right*) ventricular capture, His and ventricular capture, pure His capture, and no capture. The two complexes on the left have identical stimulus-atrial (S-A) intervals indicating lack of dependence on His conduction for atrial activation (i.e., accessory pathway present). A sinus complex at the right confirms the pure His capture complex, which has a longer S-A than either of the first two complexes, confirming the persistence of the pathway.

for and tested in long RP tachycardias, we have not seen it give misleading results in more typical septal pathways. The first few cycles of pacing should also be evaluated: if the timing of atrial activation is advanced with pacing at a time when ventricular fusion is present on the ECG, this shows that an extranodal pathway is present (since fusion signifies anterograde His bundle activation).[10]

Midseptal APs occasionally present additional nuances. In some cases, these pathways have demonstrated so-called decremental conduction properties (cycle length–dependent prolongation of conduction intervals). Especially in the absence of overt preexcitation, this feature could cause confusion by suggesting conduction only through the AV node, rather than the presence of an AP.[11]

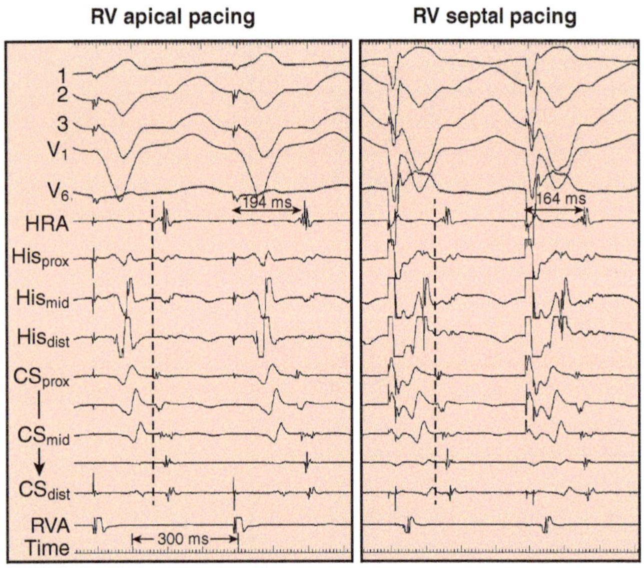

Fig. 28.6 Differential site pacing. *Dashed lines* denote onset of atrial activation. *Left*, RV apical pacing yields a stimulus-HRA time of 194 ms, whereas RV basal pacing yields a stimulus-HRA interval of 164 ms, indicating the presence of an extranodal pathway. *CS*, Coronary sinus; *H*, His deflection; *RVA*, right ventricular apex; *S*, stimulus artifact.

MAPPING AND ABLATION TECHNIQUES

Superoparaseptal Accessory Pathways

Ablation of APs in the region of the His bundle may be successfully and safely accomplished using the same techniques used for APs in other locations (Table 28.2). In the presence of preexcitation, the ventricular insertion site can be targeted by searching for the earliest site of ventricular activation during sinus rhythm; atrial pacing usually is not necessary to attain maximum preexcitation, because the ventricular insertion of the AP is relatively close to the sinus node. Electrogram characteristics at successful ablation sites include (1) a ventricular activation time that precedes the surface ECG delta wave onset by 15–40 ms; (2) a sharp "QS" deflection on the unipolar electrogram of the ablation electrode; (3) a sharp AP potential that are sometimes quite large (Fig. 28.7); and (4) an almost continuous recording incorporating atrial-AP-ventricular components (Fig. 28.7). Differentiation of atrial from ventricular components of a complex recording can usually be accomplished by introducing atrial extrastimuli or burst pacing that block in the AP. Pre-delta wave activation times are longer (i.e., earlier) in right-sided than in left-sided APs in general, and especially so with superoparaseptal APs.[12] The site with the longest (earliest) pre-delta time should be sought; for example, even if the pre-delta time in the first site sampled is 15 ms, ablation should not be performed there until multiple other nearby sites have been sampled, none of which has a longer interval. Fluoroscopically, this can be very close to the His bundle recording site (Fig. 28.8). It is important to distinguish the AP potential from the His recording; repeated bursts of pacing or premature stimuli will usually accomplish this (Fig. 28.9). It is also critical to correctly define the onset of the surface ECG delta wave (earliest of all 12 leads).

TABLE 28.2 Target Sites for Ablation

Superoparaseptal APs	*Ventricular insertion site (in presence of preexcitation):* • Ventricular activation time that precedes surface ECG delta wave onset by 15-40 ms • Sharp "QS" deflection on the unipolar electrogram of the ablation electrode • Presence of a sharp AP potential between atrial and ventricular electrograms, preceding delta wave onset • Nearly continuous recording with atrial-AP-ventricular components • Small (<0.1 mV) His deflection present (may be obscured by ventricular electrogram) *Atrial insertion site (in presence of retrograde conduction):* • Presence of a sharp AP potential between ventricular and atrial electrograms • Earliest atrial electrogram • Small (<0.1 mV) His deflection present
Midseptal APs	*Ventricular insertion site (in presence of preexcitation):* • Ventricular activation time that precedes the surface ECG delta wave onset by 15–40 ms • Sharp "QS" deflection on the unipolar electrogram of the ablation electrode • Presence of a sharp AP potential between atrial and ventricular electrograms, preceding delta wave onset • Nearly continuous recording with atrial-AP-ventricular components *Atrial insertion site (in presence of retrograde conduction):* • Presence of a sharp AP potential between ventricular and atrial electrograms • Earliest atrial electrogram

AP, Accessory pathway; *ECG*, electrocardiogram.

During ORT, the site with a demonstrated AP potential is the ideal target site; failing that, the site with the earliest atrial electrogram activation is a reasonable target. Due to pathway slant, it is possible that the atrial electrogram at a site with an AP potential may be later than another site with the earliest atrial electrogram (in which case, the former site is usually preferred [Fig. 28.10]). In addition, it is important to distinguish between the site with the *shortest local ventricular-to-atrial interval* and the site with the *earliest atrial activation time*; they are often the same site, but if they are not, the site with the earliest atrial activation time is preferred. The ventricular and atrial electrograms may be almost fused during SVT or ventricular pacing; introduction of premature ventricular extrastimuli during either pacing or SVT may separate the electrogram components, allowing the operator to correctly assess the timing of atrial activation as well as relative electrogram amplitudes. Also, during SVT, the amplitude of the His bundle electrogram in the ablation recording can be assessed. The AP can be safely ablated if the His deflection is less than 0.2 mV in amplitude, though there is probably less chance of injury if it is smaller still.

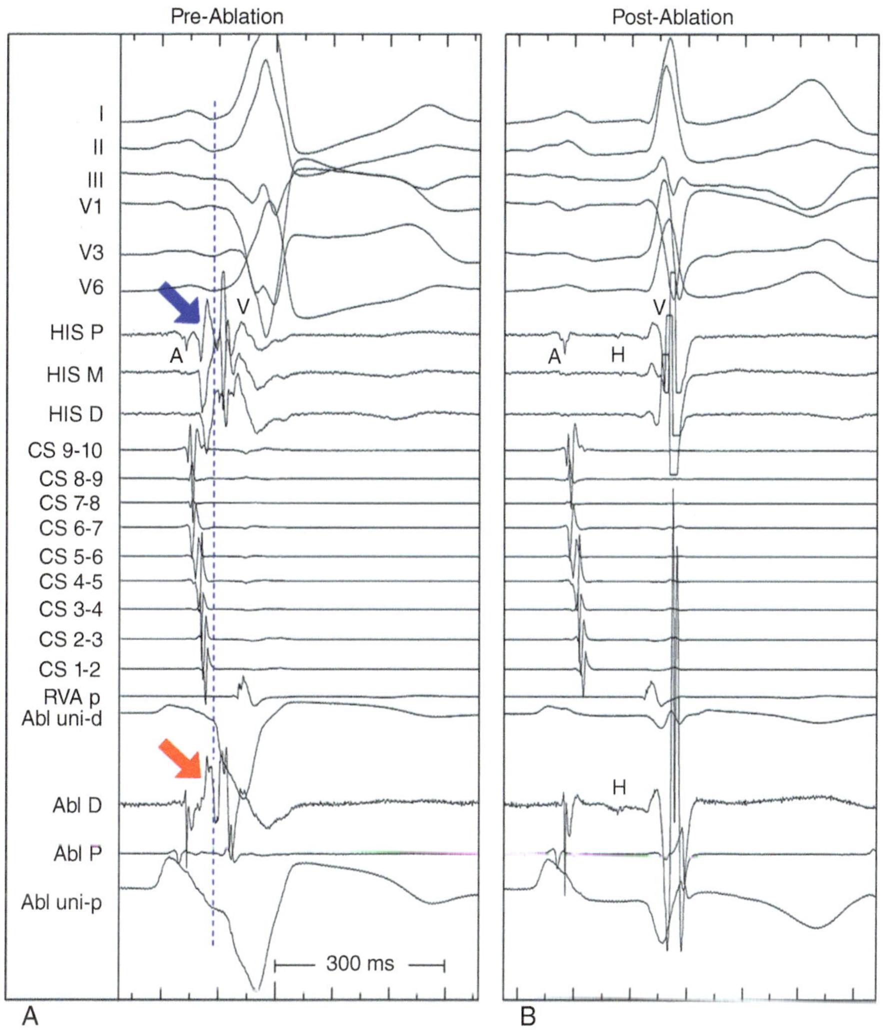

Fig. 28.7 Site of superoparaseptal accessory pathway ablation. The *dashed line* indicates the onset of the delta wave. Note the large deflection of an accessory pathway potential in the His recordings (*blue arrow*) as well as the ablation distal recording (Abl D, *red arrow*), which is absent after ablation. Also note the sharp negative deflection in the distal unipolar electrogram with a small atrial electrogram. The His potential (H) is evident only in the postablation recording. *A*, Atrial electrogram; *Abl*, ablation catheter; *CS*, coronary sinus; *H*, His deflection; *RVA*, right ventricular apex; *S*, stimulus artifact; *uni*, unipolar electrogram; *V*, ventricular electrogram.

Ordinarily, one should ablate on the ventricular aspect of the annulus if this site affords stable catheter-tissue contact; this is because the His bundle (on the ventricular side) has an insulative fibrous sheath protecting it somewhat, while the (unprotected) AV node is on the atrial side. Atrial sites (ratio of atrial to ventricular electrogram amplitudes >0.4) may yield successful ablation but with a slightly higher risk of injury to the normal conduction system. A long vascular sheath may help stabilize the position of the catheter tip regardless of whether an atrial or a ventricular site is chosen. Some operators prefer to ablate with a catheter introduced from the internal jugular vein approach, either positioning the catheter tip on the atrial aspect or advancing it slightly across and beneath the tricuspid annulus to ablate from the ventricular aspect.[13]

It is worth spending extra time to "fine-tune" the ablation site, ensuring both the best possible timing and the morphology of the ablation electrogram as well as catheter tip stability. Delivering as few ablation applications as possible (and, consequently, doing as little damage as possible) is an important goal when ablating in the vicinity of the AV node and His bundle. Mapping systems that can "tag" or track the location of mapping or ablation sites may be useful in guiding the operator either toward more favorable sites or away from sites that are less attractive. Locations of His potential recordings can also be tagged on the mapping system as areas to avoid ablating if possible. If the best ablation site is very close to the His bundle recording site, the His recording catheter can occasionally be advanced slightly into the ventricle, leaving the insulated portion of the catheter as a potential physical barrier overlying the His bundle itself. Due to pathway slant, the atrial insertion in right-sided and septal APs is usually located in a "clockwise" direction from the ventricular insertion site (left anterior oblique view). This can be used to good advantage by targeting the atrial insertion that may be several millimeters further

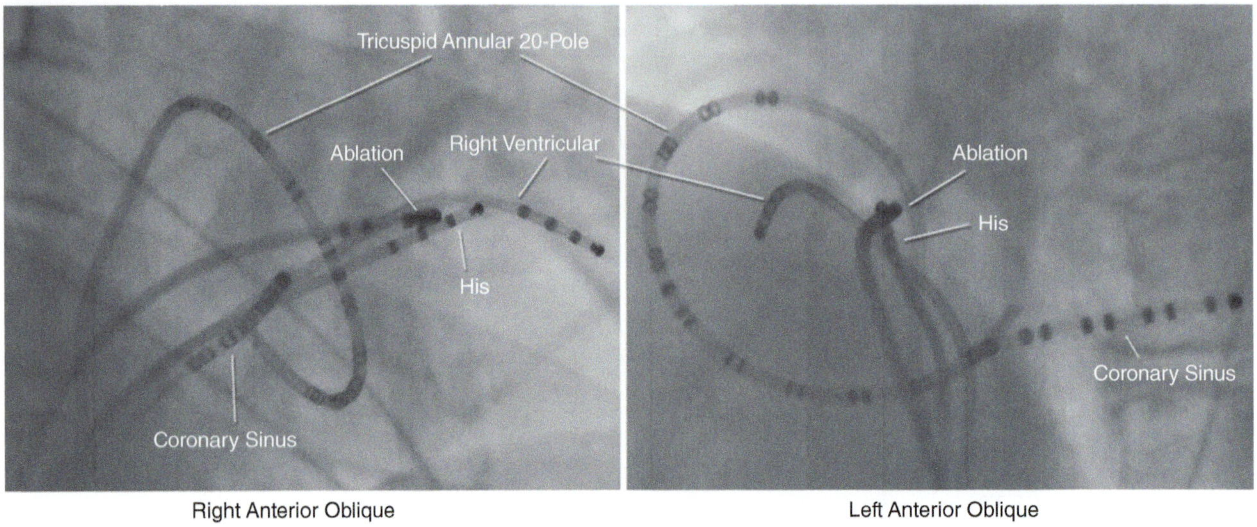

Fig. 28.8 Fluoroscopic images of superoparaseptal accessory pathway ablation site. Catheters and views as labeled; note the near-superimposition of the ablation catheter and His recording electrodes. Ablation at this site was successful without injury to the His bundle.

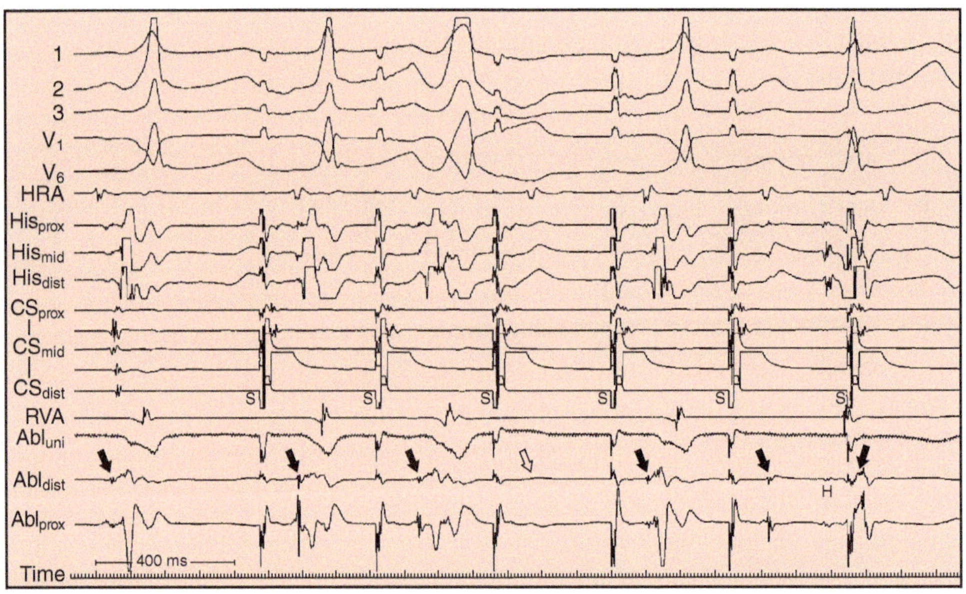

Fig. 28.9 Proof of accessory pathway potential recording. *Dark arrows* indicate AP potential; *white arrow*, its absence. A sinus rhythm complex is followed by a burst of pacing from the coronary sinus, resulting in conduction over the AP after the first two stimuli but not the third stimulus, that captures atrium but blocks in the AP (hence no AP potential; this proves the potential was not atrial in origin). The fourth stimulus is like the first, but the fifth stimulus blocks distal to the AP (thus, it is not ventricular in origin). A small His potential (H) is seen in the ablation recording, indicating the proximity to the normal conduction system (as well as that the AP potential is not the His spike).

away from the conduction system than the ventricular insertion (Fig. 28.11).

Once a site has been chosen for ablation, radiofrequency (RF) energy delivery should begin at relatively low power (30 W) and low temperature (50°C–60°C) settings but with firm catheter contact. Poor contact may result in only minimal damage but with edema formation that then distorts electrograms and may lead to an increased physical barrier to subsequent effective energy delivery. If preexcitation is present, ablation may be attempted during sinus rhythm or during atrial pacing. Unsuccessful energy applications should be stopped after no more than 15 seconds; continued energy delivery at such sites is unlikely to be beneficial but may have already caused damage to the AV node or His bundle that may be difficult to discern as long as preexcitation persists. It is useful to try to ensure that normal AV node–His conduction is still intact after one or two failed energy deliveries. Use of higher energies, or of large-tip catheters capable of causing more extensive damage, is generally not needed in ablation of these APs; the cause of ablation failure in this setting is almost always incorrect localization or poor/inconsistent catheter–tissue contact, and not inability to make a large enough area of damage with a

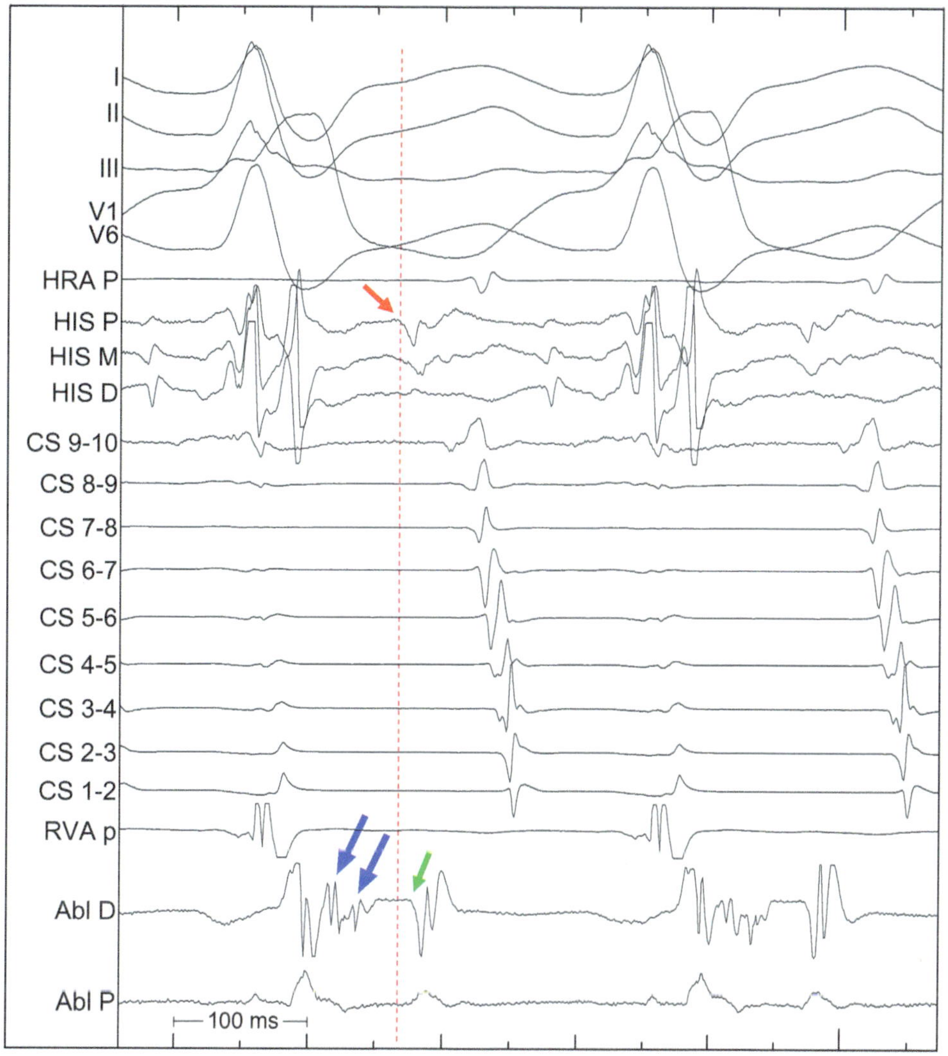

Fig. 28.10 Accessory pathway (AP) potential vs earliest site of atrial activation. Two complexes of SVT are shown; the *dashed line* shows onset of earliest atrial activation in standard catheters, at proximal His recording (*red arrow*). However, signals consistent with AP potential are seen in the AblD channel (*blue arrows*) while the atrial electrogram at this site (*green arrow*) is later than at the His proximal site. Ablation at this site eliminated SVT; note that there is no His potential seen in this channel, signifying it was not only a more effective ablation site than the site of earliest atrial activation but also a safer one.

standard-sized RF lesion. In addition, large-tip catheters (i.e., 8 mm) degrade the accuracy of mapping since sampling is done over a larger area.

For nonseptal concealed APs, ablation is usually performed during ventricular pacing so that loss of AP conduction can be readily monitored. However, use of this method for ablation of pathways in the vicinity of the AV node and His bundle could result in inadvertent damage to these structures that would not be evident until after cessation of pacing (when it may be too late). Alternative methods for ablation of concealed APs in this region include ablation during sinus rhythm, during SVT, and during atrial-entrained SVT. Ablation during sinus rhythm has the advantage of allowing monitoring for either PR prolongation or accelerated junctional rhythm, indicating damage to the normal conduction system and prompting cessation of energy delivery. However, AP ablation success cannot be assessed until ventricular pacing is performed after cessation of RF delivery. Ablation during SVT allows monitoring of both normal conduction and ablation success (SVT terminates retrogradely once the AP is eliminated). However, the sudden change in heart rate associated with successful ablation and cessation of SVT can lead to ablation catheter displacement and incomplete ablation. With ablation during atrial-entrained SVT, atrial pacing is performed during sustained SVT at a rate slightly faster than the SVT cycle length while ablation energy is delivered. When AP conduction is eliminated, SVT terminates (as indicated by a change in atrial activation sequence) but the heart rate does not change; therefore, the likelihood of catheter movement is decreased, and complete ablation is facilitated (Fig. 28.12). Because this method allows monitoring of efficacy (AP ablation) and safety (normal AV conduction) and addresses the problem of catheter movement, it is preferred.

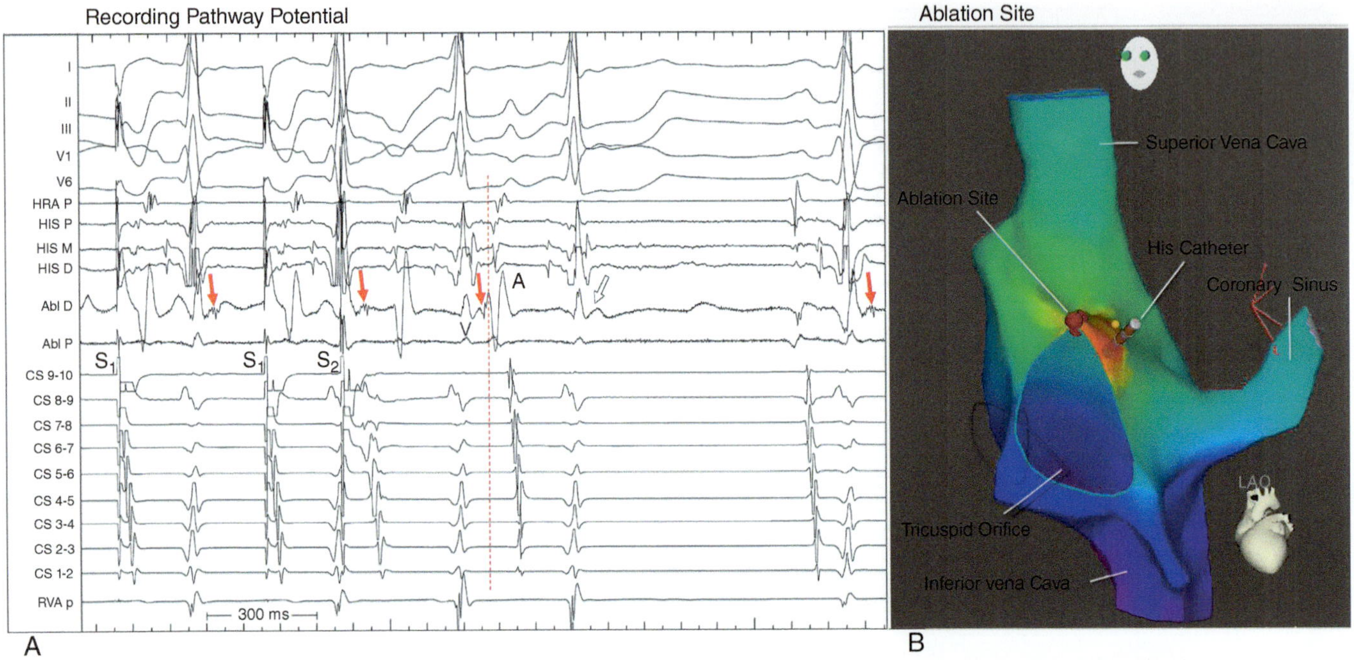

Fig. 28.11 Concealed superoparaseptal pathway. (A) With atrial pacing (S1) and extrastimuli (S2), a small deflection (*red arrow*) follows the ventricular electrogram in the ablation recording (Abl D) and occurs between the ventricular and earliest atrial electrograms (indicated by *dashed line*) on a single orthodromic echo complex. This potential is likely an accessory pathway recording, since it occurs during the echo complex but not when an atrial recording is absent (*white arrow*, fourth QRS complex). Further, it cannot be an atrial recording, since it is separate from other atrial recordings, during drive complexes and cannot be ventricular, since it is absent on the fourth complex. (B) Electroanatomical activation map of right atrium during SVT. The earliest site of activation, corresponding to recordings in panel A, is about 5 mm lateral to the His bundle location (*orange dots, catheter icon*). Ablation here eliminated pathway conduction almost instantly without endangering normal AV conduction. At a prior ablation procedure, anterograde conduction had been eliminated with ablation more medially, distal to the His recording site. This discrepancy between anterograde and retrograde pathway insertions indicates a slanted pathway course.

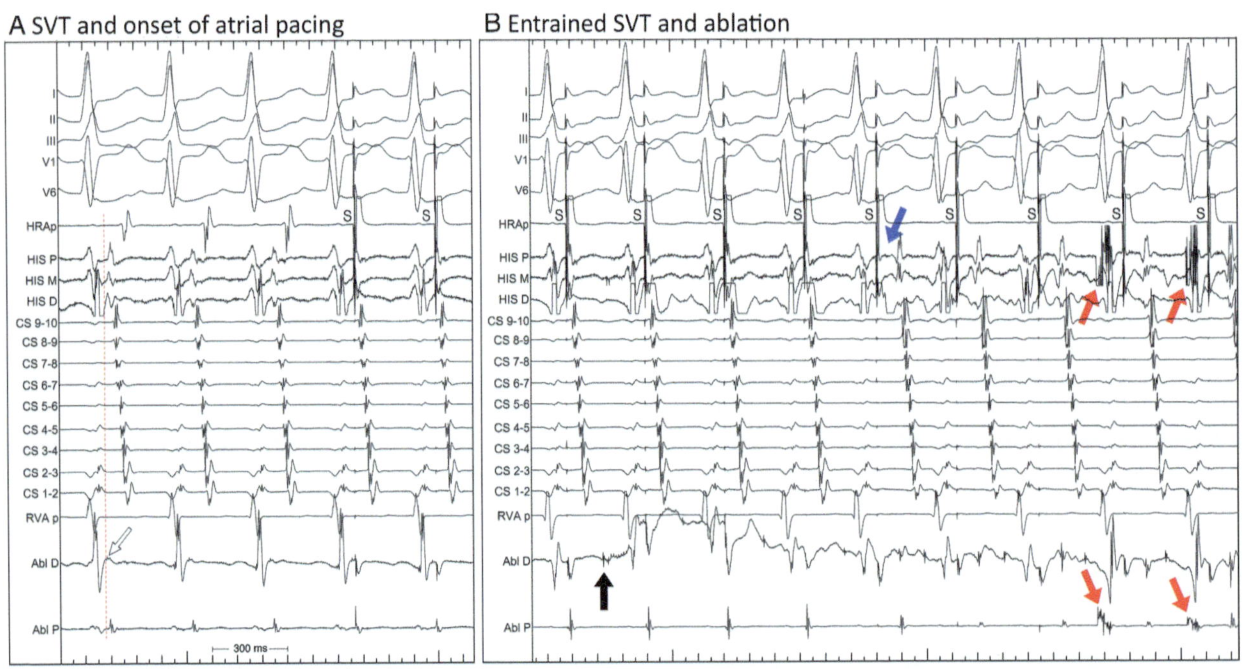

Fig. 28.12 Entrained atrial pacing during ablation. (A) Three complexes of SVT are shown, after which atrial pacing from high right atrium (HRA) begins (S). (B) A few seconds later, pacing continues, about 10 ms shorter than the SVT cycle length. Radiofrequency energy is started (*black arrow*), and a few cycles later, an abrupt change in the atrial activation sequence (*blue arrow*) to fully paced signifies interruption of the accessory pathway, while a constant heart rate facilitates maintenance of catheter position at the target. *Red arrows* show electrical artifact from catheter–catheter contact (proximal ablation electrodes and proximal His electrodes).

TABLE 28.3 **Troubleshooting Difficult Cases**

Problem	Causes	Possible Solutions
Pathway block during mapping	• Catheter trauma of superficially located pathway	• Careful catheter manipulation • If catheter remains in same location that caused block, ablate • Move catheter away from site • Administer isoproterenol/epinephrine • Wait up to 1 hour for recovery • Pace-match delta wave
Accelerated junctional rhythm during RF application	• Heating of AV node	• Stop RF application immediately • Reposition catheter prior to another RF application • Atrial overdrive pace during RF application to ensure intact normal conduction; stop RF delivery if PR prolongs
Right bundle branch block during RF application	• Catheter positioned too distally	• Reposition catheter
Unable to successfully ablate at site of earliest atrial activation in SVT	• Poor catheter contact • Incorrect location on right side • Left-sided atrial or ventricular pathway insertion	• Vascular sheath; alter approach (switch to SVC or femoral vein) • Continue mapping (especially 5-10 mm laterally on tricuspid annulus) • Map LA/LV septum; LVOT; noncoronary sinus of Valsalva
Large His potential in best ablation recording	• True para-Hisian pathway	• Use cryomapping to test sites before ablation • Advance His catheter so that insulated shaft "shields" His bundle from ablation energy • Map noncoronary sinus of Valsalva; LA/LV septum; LVOT

AV, Atrioventricular; *LA*, left atrium; *LV*, left ventricle; *LVOT*, left ventricular outflow tract; *RA*, right atrium; *RF*, radiofrequency; *SVC*, superior vena cava; *SVT*, supraventricular tachycardia.

Cryomapping and ablation have been introduced as techniques to avoid unwanted damage to the AV node and His bundle.[14] With cryomapping, the catheter tip is first cooled to 0°C at potential ablation sites; if AP conduction is lost without damage to the normal conduction elements, the catheter tip temperature can be decreased to −80°C for cryoablation. Cold-induced attenuation of normal pathway conduction may be hard to appreciate because preexcitation is near-maximal in sinus rhythm or with right atrial pacing; instead, if CS pacing results in a greater degree of normal conduction (less preexcitation), application of cold to the AV node or His bundle will result in an increase in preexcitation. Such areas should be noted as sites at which ablation definitely should not be performed.

TROUBLESHOOTING THE DIFFICULT CASE

Successful ablation of superoparaseptal APs poses particular challenges (Table 28.3). These APs are by definition close enough to the His bundle that a small His potential is usually recorded in the ablation signal (or sometimes first becomes evident after successful ablation). Inadvertent damage to the His bundle is the primary hazard in ablating these APs. Additional potential difficulties include AP sensitivity to catheter trauma and accelerated junctional rhythm during RF energy delivery.[15]

These pathways are often very superficial (toward the endocardial surface), and catheter trauma results in transient block of pathway conduction in one or both directions in up to 38% of cases (Fig. 28.13).[16] If this occurs, and the catheter has moved ("grazed" the pathway as it was passing by), one can wait and hope that pathway conduction resumes. This may take up to 30 minutes or longer, if pathway conduction resumes at all during the study. Isoproterenol/epinephrine has been used by some to try to facilitate resumption of conduction; although this has been reported to be successful, the additional waiting time may have been responsible for return of AP conduction, rather than the medication, and there are no randomized controlled studies of isoproterenol/epinephrine in this setting. If the catheter tip is still at the site at which trauma interrupted AP conduction, one can proceed with ablation despite lack of return of conduction after a reasonable waiting period (10–15 minutes). Use of mapping systems that allow tagging of sites on a three-dimensional rendering of the heart may be helpful in this regard, but only if sites with acceptable electrogram characteristics were designated as such before catheter-mediated loss of AP conduction. If catheter-induced AP block occurs and one is uncertain as to whether the catheter is still at the site that caused mechanical block, it may be appropriate to move the catheter well away from the site (i.e., its continued presence may be causing ongoing mechanical block). In this situation, tagging of the site with a mapping system can be very helpful: if conduction returns after the catheter is moved away, the tagged site facilitates repositioning of the catheter tip back to the same site. An additional technique that is occasionally helpful is pace-mapping on the annulus to replicate the delta wave contour[17]; we have found that for the best match, atrioventricular pacing or sinus rhythm with tracked ventricular pacing with an AV interval set to match that during

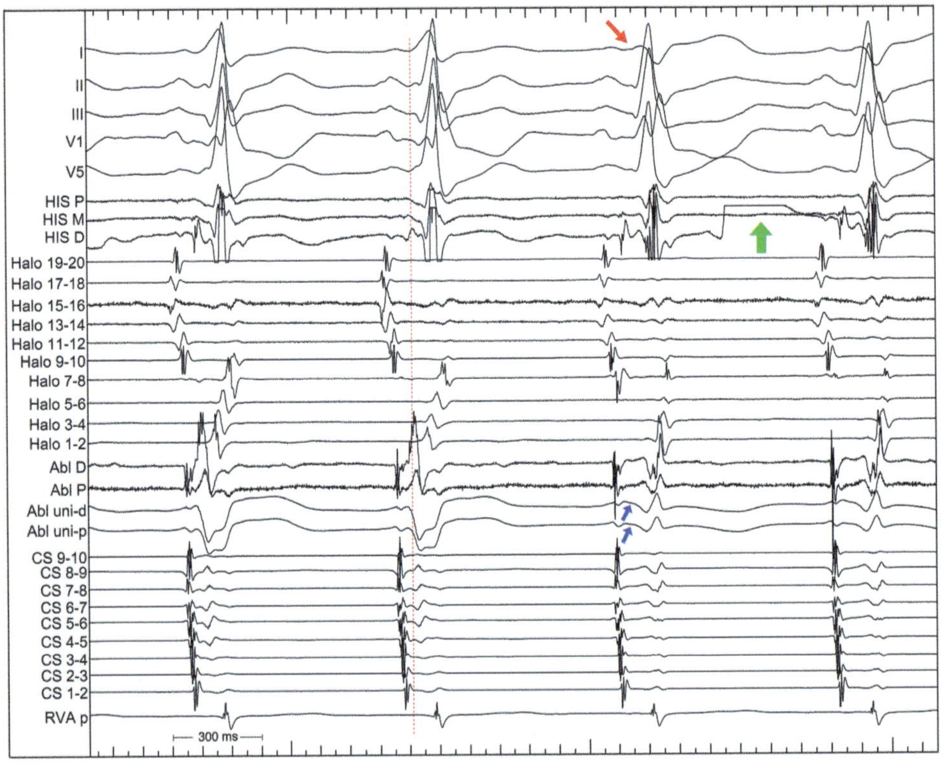

Fig. 28.13 Mechanical block in mid-septal accessory pathway due to catheter manipulation. The first two complexes show preexcitation; the last two do not, due to catheter trauma. *Red arrow* shows absence of delta wave in lead 1; *blue arrows* show corresponding changes in the ablation recording. Minor movement of the His recording catheter (*green arrow*) may have caused the trauma. *A*, Atrial electrogram; *Abl*, ablation catheter; *CS*, coronary sinus; *H*, His deflection; *RVA*, right ventricular apex; *S*, stimulus artifact; *uni*, unipolar electrogram; *V*, ventricular electrogram.

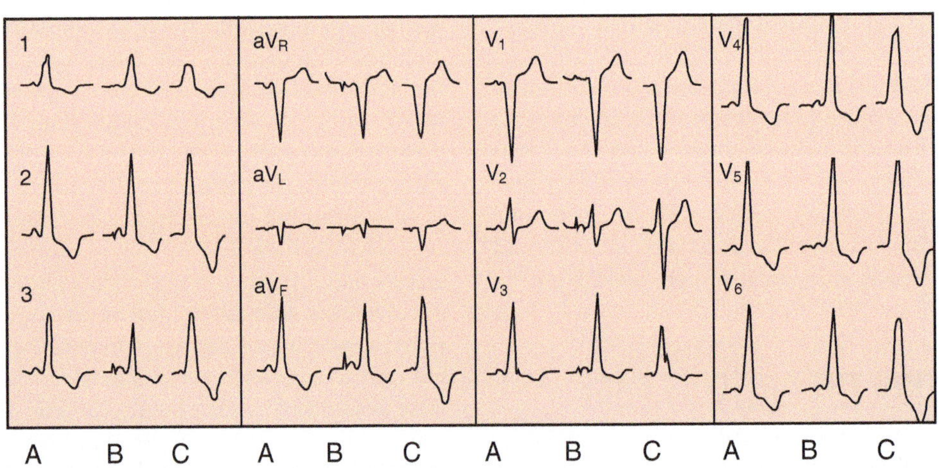

Fig. 28.14 Pace-matching of the delta wave after pathway trauma. During mapping, both anterograde and retrograde pathway conduction ceased and did not reappear after 20 minutes. Pacing the tricuspid annulus to match the delta wave was then used to guide ablation. All 12 ECG leads are shown: (A) prior to pathway trauma; (B) (bolder tracings for emphasis), atrioventricular pacing with an AV interval to match that of preexcited complexes; and (C) ventricular pacing only at the same site as in B. Note the closer match when AV pacing is used.

preexcited sinus rhythm should be used (Fig. 28.14). We have successfully used this technique in several cases of traumatic loss of preexcitation, when pathway conduction has not resumed after 15–20 min.

Accelerated junctional rhythm during RF energy delivery (Fig. 28.15) occurs in up to 5% of patients[18] and results from heating of the His bundle. Accelerated junctional rhythm typically results in a narrow QRS complex on ECG, a finding that

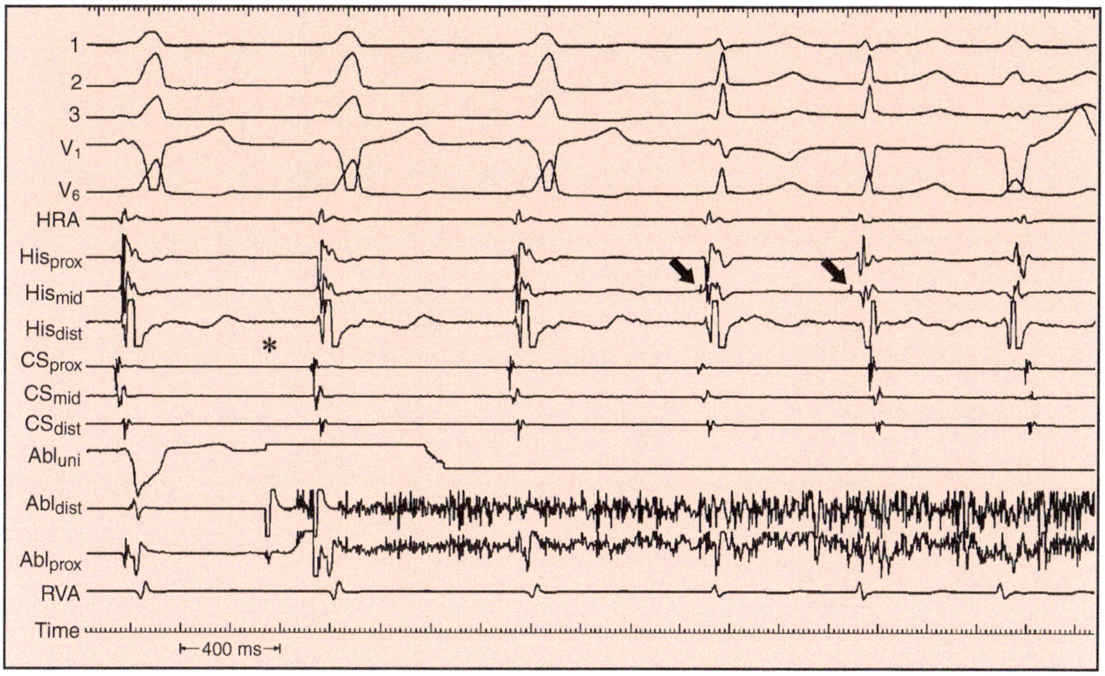

Fig. 28.15 Accelerated junctional rhythm during ablation attempt (superoparaseptal accessory pathway [AP]). Radiofrequency (RF) delivery is begun at the *asterisk*; the next two preexcited beats are followed by two narrow QRS complexes but not due to AP ablation. Instead, these are accelerated junctional complexes caused by heating of the His bundle (*arrows*). RF application was stopped just after the end of the recording. The AP was eventually ablated with preservation of normal atrioventricular conduction.

may erroneously suggest that the AP has been successfully ablated and that energy delivery should continue. In fact, this is exactly the wrong thing to do, because the His bundle may be incurring damage. The operator has only seconds to discontinue RF energy delivery before the His bundle is irreversibly damaged. If energy delivery continues, progressive acceleration of the junctional discharge rate may occur, as during intentional His bundle ablation. This can provide an important warning to the operator if the danger has not already been appreciated. Fortunately, as noted above, the His bundle itself is contained within a fibrous sheath that is somewhat protective against ablation. Of note, cryoablation does not result in accelerated junctional rhythm; absence of this rhythm during cryoablation should not be interpreted as lack of risk of damaging the normal conduction system.

Para-Hisian pathways represent a subgroup of the superoparaseptal pathways that are more closely related to the His bundle itself (His deflection >0.1 mV).[19] Despite this proximity to the His, these APs can still be ablated successfully without incurring His bundle injury, perhaps because of the insulative effect of the fibrous sheath surrounding the His bundle. Some authors have observed inappropriate sinus tachycardia shortly after ablation of APs in this location, presumably due to alteration of parasympathetic tone caused by the ablation.[20] This is self-limited and requires no treatment.

Rare cases have been reported in which superoparaseptal APs could be ablated only at sites other than the expected apex of Koch triangle. These sites have included the left ventricular outflow tract[21] and the noncoronary sinus of Valsalva (Fig. 28.16).[13,22] If several attempts at ablation in the expected right ventricular region have failed to interrupt AP conduction, or repeatedly resulted in accelerated junctional rhythm, one should evaluate other, less common ventricular insertion sites such as these.

On some occasions, RF application results in AV block, but in the AV node; this appears to be a vagal effect rather than direct damage to the AV node, that is >1 cm away from the ablation site.

Using the techniques described, superoparaseptal pathways can be successfully ablated in more than 95% of patients, with about 1% risk of heart block or other significant complications. Right bundle branch block occurs in up to 10% of cases.[18] Cryoablation has been less successful on long-term follow-up than RF ablation (up to 20% recurrence after hospital discharge)[14]; whether this is due to an inherent inferiority of cryoablation or simply less familiarity with the technique is not clear. Assessment of successful ablation includes standard techniques (i.e., lack of preexcitation at rest or with decremental atrial pacing, lack of any retrograde conduction, or conduction only over the AV node with cycle length–dependent prolongation of conduction time or demonstration of His dependence of retrograde conduction [Fig. 28.17]). Para-Hisian pacing and differential-site right ventricular pacing can also be used (see earlier discussion).

Midseptal Accessory Pathways

The principles of ablation of midseptal APs are similar to those for superoparaseptal APs (Fig. 28.18). Care should be taken to

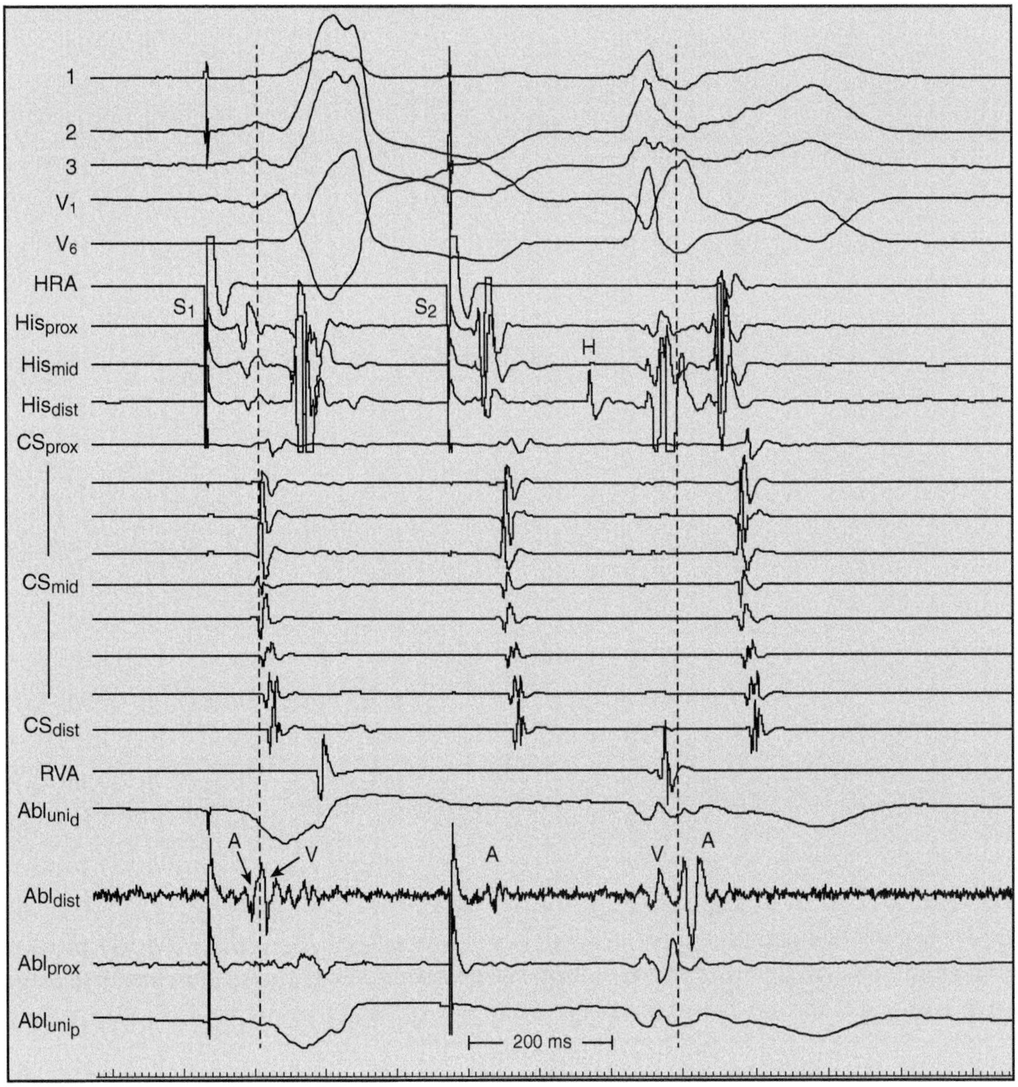

Fig. 28.16 Mapping in the noncoronary aortic sinus of Valsalva. Two complexes are shown, with atrial pacing (S1) resulting in a preexcited QRS (with atrial [A] and ventricular [V] components shown) and a premature complex (S2) blocking in the pathway, conducting with right bundle branch block pattern, followed by a pathway echo (also labeled). The ablation recording does not have a His potential (H), shown in the His recording.

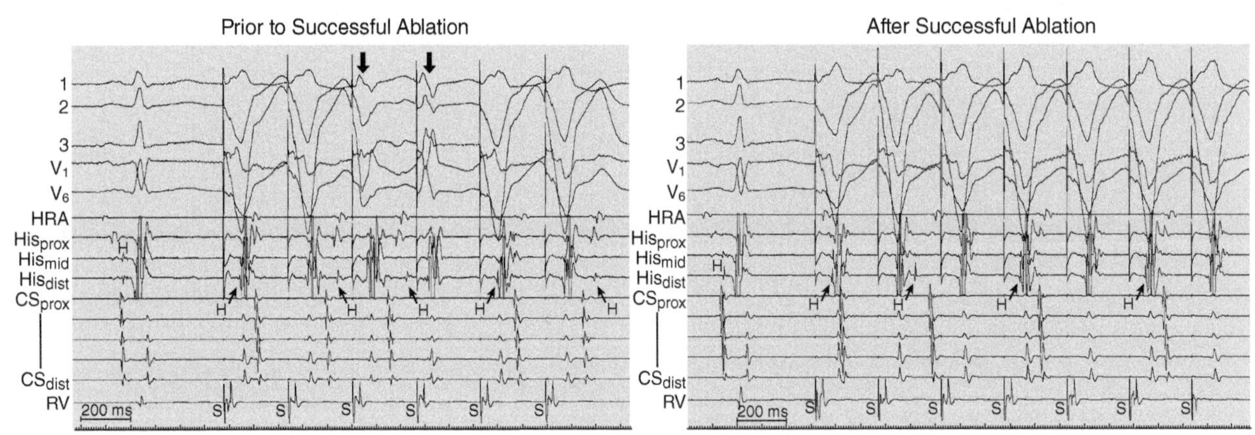

Fig. 28.17 Use of burst ventricular pacing to demonstrate His dependence or independence of atrial activation. *Left*, Prior to successful ablation, burst ventricular pacing (S) yields retrograde His potentials (H, *thin arrows*). The atrial recording follows the first His potential but precedes the second, third, and fifth His potentials, indicating an accessory pathway to activate the atria. *Large arrows* denote fused or conducted QRS complexes (echoes). *Right*, After successful ablation, each atrial complex is preceded by a His; not all ventricular complexes result in His activation, but no atrial activation occurs without a preceding His potential.

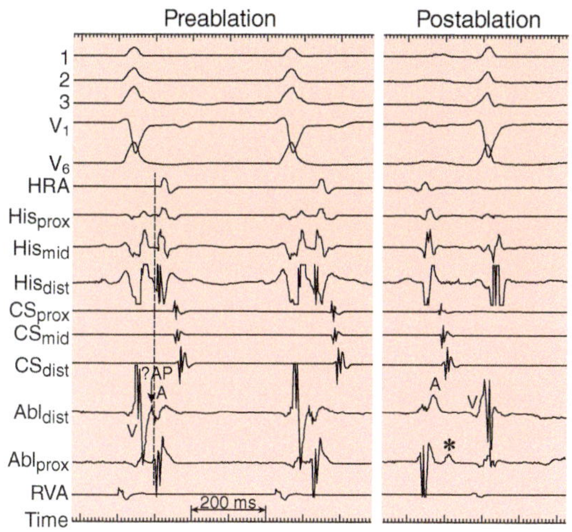

Fig. 28.18 Site of midseptal accessory pathway (AP) ablation. *Left,* Supraventricular tachycardia incorporating a retrogradely-conducting midseptal pathway having earliest atrial activation in the distal ablation (Abldist) recording followed by the His region. The Abldist also shows a possible AP potential between ventricular and atrial components (*small arrow*). After ablation, the ablation recordings do not show a His potential but a deflection similar to some so-called slow AV nodal pathway recordings is seen (*asterisk*).

ablate on the ventricular side of the annulus, to avoid AV nodal damage (Fig. 28.19). Midseptal APs are successfully ablated in about 98% of cases, with an approximately 1% risk of complete AV block, although transient AV block may occur in up to 5% of patients. Junctional rhythm during RF delivery is seen in up to 50% of cases.[18] When this is encountered, pacing the atrium at a rate faster than the junctional rhythm is helpful to ensure consistency of normal AV conduction; if energy delivery is stopped immediately upon observing PR prolongation or nonconducted P waves, normal conduction is almost always preserved.

Occasionally, ablation of midseptal APs is not successful after several RF applications on the tricuspid annulus. In most cases, this is due to poor site selection or poor electrode–endocardial contact at an appropriate site. Ablation at any site that results in some damage but not enough to be effective (especially when repeated) can result in edema that acts as a physical and electrical barrier to additional energy delivery to the target tissue. In this case, the electrogram is degraded (lower amplitude, lower frequency; Fig. 28.20). In some cases, ablation can be successful only if it is performed from the left side of the septum. Clues to the presence of a left midseptal AP are absence of sites with pre–delta wave intervals in excess of 10 ms if preexcitation is present, absence of an AP potential at all sites on the tricuspid annulus, and relatively long local ventricular-to-atrial intervals (>60 ms) on the tricuspid annulus. Left-sided ablation may be performed using the retrograde aortic or the trans-septal approach. The surface ECG preexcitation pattern is not specific enough to suggest the necessity of a left-sided approach.[18]

APs in both superoparaseptal and midseptal regions can be safely and successfully ablated using only two electrode catheters (an ablation catheter and a right ventricular for assessing retrograde conduction). Most operators prefer to use additional catheters for fluoroscopic (coronary sinus) and electrical (His bundle) reference.

Recurrence of AP conduction after apparently successful ablation occurs in up to 15% of right-sided APs, including superoparaseptal and midseptal APs.[23] Poor catheter stability is the most common cause (suboptimal ablation due to poor contact), although in the case of APs near the AV node and His bundle, operator timidity (unwillingness to deliver adequate energy to the area for fear of causing heart block) may be responsible for incomplete ablation. Common problems encountered in the ablation of septal pathways and their solutions are listed in Table 28.3.

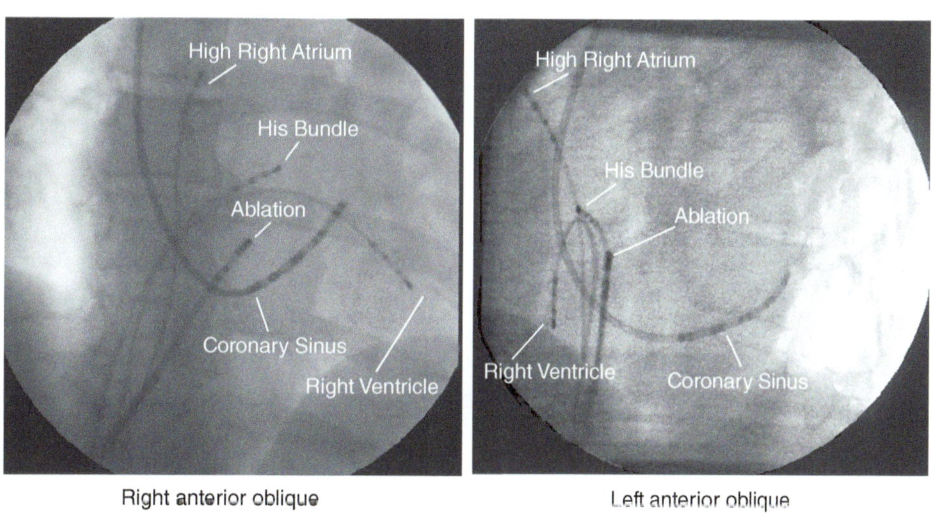

Fig. 28.19 Fluoroscopic images of midseptal accessory pathway ablation site. Catheters and views are as labeled. The ablation catheter is situated between the coronary sinus ostium and His recording electrodes, in the region of the compact atrioventricular (AV) node. Ablation at this site was successful without damaging the AV node.

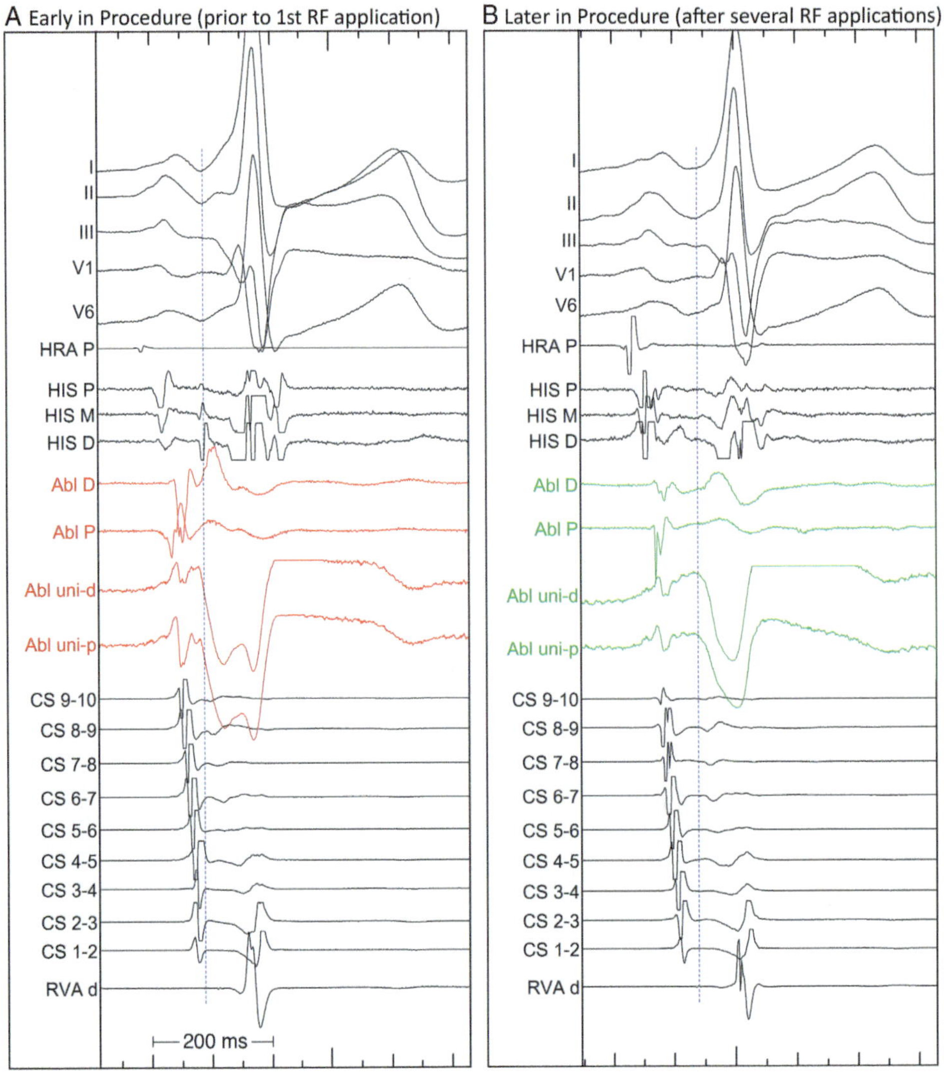

Fig. 28.20 Degradation of signals with multiple radiofrequency (RF) applications targeting a mid-septal pathway. *Blue dashed lines* indicate onset of the surface ECG delta wave. (A) Early in the procedure, good signal quality is present on ablation catheter recordings (in *red*, that earlier than delta wave, QS on Abl uni-d). RF application at this site did not eliminate preexcitation (seconds after onset of RF delivery, catheter movement occurred). Subsequent RF applications at the same site transiently eliminated the delta wave but catheter movement after a few seconds precluded full efficacy. (B) Later in the procedure, electrograms from the ablation site (in *green*) are still relatively early compared to the delta wave but appear to be more far-field (lower amplitude and frequency). Note less preexcitation than in A due to some pathway damage.

SUMMARY

Ablation of APs in the region of the normal conduction system presents special challenges to the electrophysiologist. Although differentiation of AP-related SVTs from atrial tachycardias and AV nodal reentry can sometimes be difficult, the major challenge remains avoidance of damage to the AV node and His bundle that would require permanent pacing. Fortunately, this complication can usually be avoided by careful attention to catheter positioning and monitoring of normal AV conduction.

REFERENCES

Please refer to the e-book for a complete list of references.

29

Ablation of Atriofascicular Accessory Pathways and Variants

Mohamed Bassiouny, Mohamed H. Kanj, Patrick Tchou

KEY POINTS

- Atriofascicular accessory pathways are decrementally conducting accessory pathways that are most commonly located along the right free wall, connecting the atrium to the right bundle branch.
- They participate in antidromic tachycardia with a left bundle branch block morphology, antegrade conduction over the accessory pathway, and retrograde conduction over the atrioventricular node or another accessory pathway.
- The most effective method for ablating the atriofascicular pathway involves mapping and ablating the discrete *M* potential along the tricuspid annulus.
- Sources of difficulty include catheter instability and prolonged transient loss of accessory pathway conduction because of mechanical trauma during mapping. Locating the atrial insertion may be time consuming, and ablating the ventricular insertion is more challenging because of extensive arborization.
- Long and steerable sheaths may help stabilize the catheter along the tricuspid annulus, and three-dimensional mapping systems may guide ablation.

ATRIOFASCICULAR ACCESSORY PATHWAYS

In 1938, Dr. Ivan Mahaim first described nodoventricular fibers that connected the atrioventricular (AV) nodal region to the ventricular myocardium.[1] The description was histologic, and no physiologic properties were reported. More recently, in the early 1980s, slowly conducting AV accessory pathways (AP) with AV node-like decremental properties participating in antidromic tachycardia were postulated to be nodoventricular fibers.[2–4] However, others also identified right lateral APs having similar properties that were independent of the AV node.[5] Nevertheless, the eponym *Mahaim fibers* became widely adopted to describe all atypical APs with decremental conduction properties instead of the initially defined anatomical fibers. In the early 1980s, the most prevalent thought was that nodoventricular pathways, possibly those described by Mahaim, were the predominant cause of these types of antidromic reentry arrhythmia.[2,3] They had the potential to be involved in reentrant pathways or in "bystander" activation of the ventricles during supraventricular tachycardia such as AV nodal reentry.[4] In the late 1980s, independent publications from two different groups questioned this concept,[6,7] with further case reports demonstrating that these types of antidromic tachycardia were using AV as opposed to nodoventricular pathways in their reentrant circuits. With additional publications from other groups, it became apparent that the majority (>90%) of reentry tachycardias involving slowly conducting atypical pathways were in fact attributed to atriofascicular, or the less frequent AV pathways with decremental conduction and a separate atrial origin from the AV node.[5–9] Thus, the term *Mahaim pathway* fell out of favor, and instead the more precise description of atypical decrementally conducting pathways that also includes the correct anatomy is now preferred.[10] Interestingly, a lateral AV connection with an AV node-like structure, which most likely represented an atriofascicular pathway, was described by Dr. Stanley Kent in 1914; however, he misinterpreted the structure as parts of the then-postulated normal conduction system.[8]

ANATOMY

The atriofascicular pathway consists of a long, insulated fiber with decremental conduction properties that connect atrial tissue to the distal His-Purkinje network. This differentiates it from other slowly conducting AV pathways that insert directly into the myocardium rather than into the normal His-Purkinje system (HPS). It acts as a parallel conductive system that is structurally and physiologically similar to the AV node and the His-bundle. It almost always originates from the right atrial free wall along the tricuspid valve annulus, where slow potentials similar to those at the AV node can be occasionally recorded (Fig. 29.1). A single left-sided atriofascicular accessory pathway has been reported.[9] However, the majority of decremental pathways that originate outside the right atrium are AV pathways. They arise from the left atrium and can insert into the left ventricle along the mitral annulus,[11,12] the mitral annulus–aorta junction,[13] or into the myocardium abutting the left coronary cusp.[14]

When mapping an atriofascicular pathway, a His-like structure can be frequently identified along the tricuspid annulus and is characteristic of such pathways. Decremental conduction typically occurs through a structure between the atrial tissue

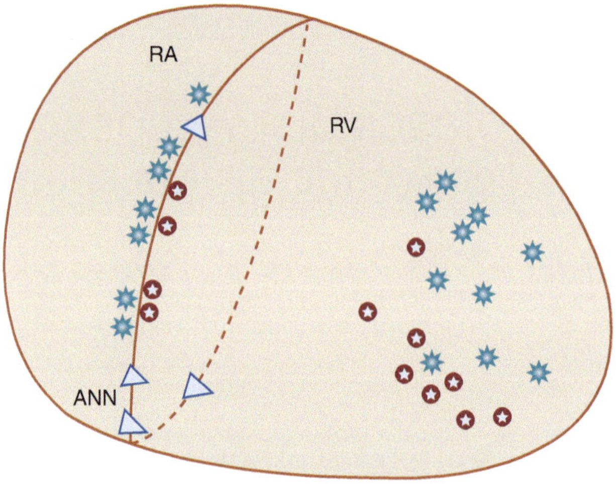

Fig. 29.1 Schematic illustration of the anatomy of anterograde decrementally conducting pathways in the right anterior oblique view. The origins and insertions of atriofascicular (*blue stars*), long atrioventricular (*stars in red circle*), and short atrioventricular pathways (*blue triangle*) are depicted. The tricuspid annulus is represented by the brown line. *ANN,* Tricuspid annulus; *RA,* right atrium; *RV,* right ventricle. (From Haïssaguerre M, Warin JF, Le Metayer P, et al. Characteristics of the ventricular insertion sites of accessory pathways with antegrade decremental conduction properties. *Circulation.* 1995;91:1077–1085.).

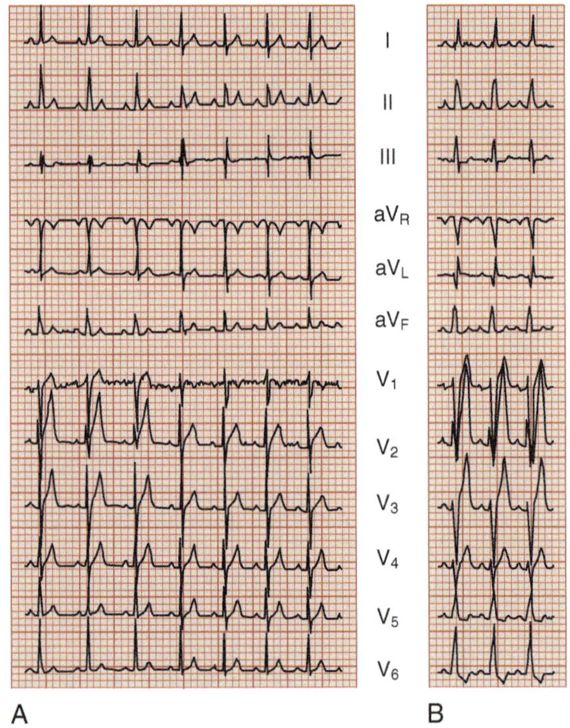

Fig. 29.2 (A) Twelve-lead electrocardiogram showing subtle preexcitation in the form of rsR = pattern in lead III in the first three beats, and absent septal q in leads I and V_5-V_6 in all QRS complexes. (B) Manifest preexcitation after intravenous verapamil that predominantly affected the atrioventricular node, leading to ventricular activation predominantly over the decrementally conducting accessory pathway. (From Sternick EB, Timmermans C, Sosa E, et al. The electrocardiogram during sinus rhythm and tachycardia in patients with anterograde conduction over Mahaim fibers. The importance of an "rS" pattern in lead III. *J Am Coll Cardiol.* 2004;44:1626–1635.)

and the His-like structure. The distal insertion of the pathway is usually located several centimeters from the tricuspid valve, at the distal right bundle (RB) branch or its branching Purkinje fiber, toward the apical third of the right ventricular free wall (see Fig. 29.1). Extensive arborization via the Purkinje network is common and suggested by the presence of a QS pattern on unipolar electrograms or sharp potentials fusing with the earliest bipolar ventricular potentials over a wide area of ventricular tissue. However, simultaneous activation via local His-Purkinje network may be an alternative explanation.[15]

PATHOPHYSIOLOGY

Atriofascicular pathways are associated with unique tachyarrhythmias given their characteristic anatomy and electrophysiologic properties. The AP provides the substrate for AV reentry tachycardia by acting as the antegrade limb, whereas the AV node–HPS or another AP acts as the retrograde limb. Typically they are not capable of retrograde conduction, and to date there is only one report of an atriofascicular pathway participating in both antidromic and orthodromic reentry tachycardia.[16] Retrograde conduction block of atriofascicular pathways occurs near the atrial insertion.[15] This facilitates initiation of AV reentry tachycardias with premature ventricular beats as they block retrogradely in the atriofascicular AP and conduct up the AV node–HPS allowing for reentry to occur. As with other types of APs, atriofascicular accessory pathways may preexcite the ventricle during an atrial tachycardia or participate in a figure-of-8 manner with a coexisting orthodromic reentry or AV nodal reentry.

Atriofascicular pathways are mostly right sided, with a few exceptions, inserting in the right bundle branch (RBB) or its distal Purkinje fibers, giving rise to a QRS with a left bundle branch block (LBBB) morphology during antidromic AV reentrant tachycardia. However, identifying atriofascicular pathways during sinus rhythm may be challenging as their slow antegrade decremental conduction leads to minimal and sometimes no preexcitation in sinus rhythm. Similar to the native AV node–HPS, they are sensitive to autonomic changes, adenosine,[17–19] and occasionally verapamil,[7] leading to variations in the amount of preexcitation depending on the degree of their contribution to ventricular activation. In addition, similar to the AV node, there have been reports of atriofascicular pathways with dual conduction properties leading to tachycardia because of a 1:2 response or beat-to-beat variation in the antidromic AV reentry tachycardia cycle length.[20,21]

DIAGNOSIS

12-Lead Electrocardiogram

The diagnosis of atriofascicular pathways can be challenging in sinus rhythm, as preexcitation can be absent at baseline because of faster conduction along the AV node compared with the AP.[17,22,23] However, subtle preexcitation can be detected in approximately 60% of patients in the form of an absence or a decrease of the septal q in leads I and V_5-V_6 and the presence of an rS pattern in lead III (Fig. 29.2).[16,24] Day-to-day variation in the degree of preexcitation is common and does not necessarily reflect an AP with a long refractory period.[24] Sinus

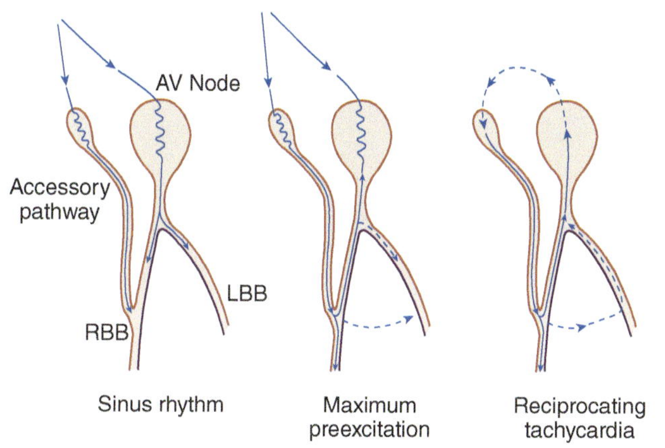

Fig. 29.3 Schematic illustration of the pathophysiology of atriofascicular pathways. In sinus rhythm, conduction is faster down the atrioventricular (AV) node–His Purkinje system, which contributes to the majority of ventricular activation. During maximal preexcitation, more decremental conduction occurs in the AV node compared with the accessory pathway, and ventricular activation occurs via the accessory pathway. Reciprocating tachycardia is initiated when sufficient conduction delay in the accessory pathway allows enough time for recovery of the retrograde AV node conduction to complete the circuit. *LBB,* Left bundle branch; *RBB,* right bundle branch. (From Leitch JW, Klein GJ, Yee R. New concepts on nodoventricular accessory pathways. *J Cardiovasc Electrophysiol.* 1990;1:220–230.)

tachycardia or rapid atrial pacing, especially pacing the atrium near the pathway versus pacing from the coronary sinus, can manifest the preexcited QRS morphology, as conduction decrements more significantly down the AV node and preferential AP conduction occurs to the ventricles. The conduction scenarios showing varying degrees of preexcitation are schematically illustrated in Fig. 29.3.

Classically, the maximally preexcited QRS, either achieved with rapid atrial pacing or during antidromic tachycardia, is similar to a typical LBBB: R wave in V_1 is minimal or absent (rS, or QS), precordial R wave transition is beyond lead V_4, and an R in limb lead I. The QRS is usually less than 150 ms in duration as the atriofascicular pathway allows for more rapid activation of the ventricles through a close connection to the HPS. For the same reason, the initial QRS forces are typically rapid, especially in the anterior chest leads, with absence of a delta wave that is classically seen with pathways that insert into the myocardium near the annuli. The QRS typically shows left-axis deviation. However, the frontal axis can vary widely between −75 and +60 degrees. This variation is dictated by the location of ventricular insertion as well as the retrograde conduction properties of the RBB (see later discussion).[15,25,26]

Electrocardiogram (ECG) criteria can suggest a decrementally conducting AV pathway and help differentiate it from ventricular tachycardia (VT), which allows for a more thorough intracardiac electrophysiologic evaluation.[22] However, it cannot distinguish between atriofascicular mediated tachycardia and supraventricular tachycardia (SVT) with LBBB aberration, as both can have a typical LBBB pattern.[22,27] In addition, in one study the maximally preexcited QRS width or axis during antidromic tachycardia could not predict the location of the atriofascicular AP.[28]

Intracardiac Electrograms

During Sinus Rhythm

A three-component electrogram: an atrial component A, a His-Purkinje–like potential, sometimes referred to as an M potential, and a ventricular component V can frequently be identified near the proximal (atrial) insertion along the tricuspid annulus. The M potential is a His-like potential, which represents depolarization of the bundle forming the distal portion of the atriofascicular pathway that inserts into the distal RBB or its Purkinje branches. In sinus rhythm, ventricular activation is predominantly over the AV node and His bundle, minimizing any ventricular preexcitation. Atrial pacing close to the origin of the AP can manifest the preexcitation as fusion occurs between ventricular activation over the AP and the His bundle (Fig. 29.4).

The distal (ventricular) insertion of atriofascicular pathways occurs at the distal RB or its branches located in the anterior right ventricular free wall. During more rapid atrial pacing, ventricular activation may occur preferentially over the atriofascicular pathway because of greater conduction slowing in the AV node. Similar to the AV node, decremental conduction in the atriofascicular pathway occurs in the proximal segment of the AP between the atrial insertion and the M potential.

Induction of Antidromic Atrioventricular Reentrant Tachycardia

This tachycardia can be induced via atrial stimulation, ventricular stimulation, or both. Induction with atrial stimulation can be achieved with burst atrial pacing or with the administration of atrial extrastimuli. It requires anterograde block in the AV node and conduction over the AP with subsequent retrograde conduction over the AV node. This occurs when the refractory period of the AP is shorter than the refractory period of the AV node anterogradely. It also requires retrograde AV node conduction to recover sufficiently for the reentry to occur. Thus isoproterenol may be needed for induction. Initiation of tachycardia may be more readily achieved when atrial stimulation is closer to the AV node than the AP, such as from the coronary sinus, which allows more time for the AV node to recover and facilitate retrograde conduction.

In many cases, the AV node has more decremental properties than the atriofascicular pathway as revealed with rapid atrial pacing, atrial premature stimuli, or after the administration of intravenous adenosine. The A-His interval prolongs more than the A-M interval. The HV interval gradually shortens and the QRS widens and assumes an LBBB pattern as it becomes more preexcited because of increasing activation of the ventricle via the AP. Maximal preexcitation occurs when there is retrograde activation of the His bundle with reversal of distal RB, proximal RB, and His activation sequences. Antidromic AV reentry tachycardia is typically initiated after such reversal of RB and His activation (Fig. 29.5).

Because initiation of tachycardia with atrial stimulation requires the AV node to block during atrial pacing while the AP still conducts, it is not always a reliable means of initiating the tachycardia, and in some cases it is not feasible to initiate the

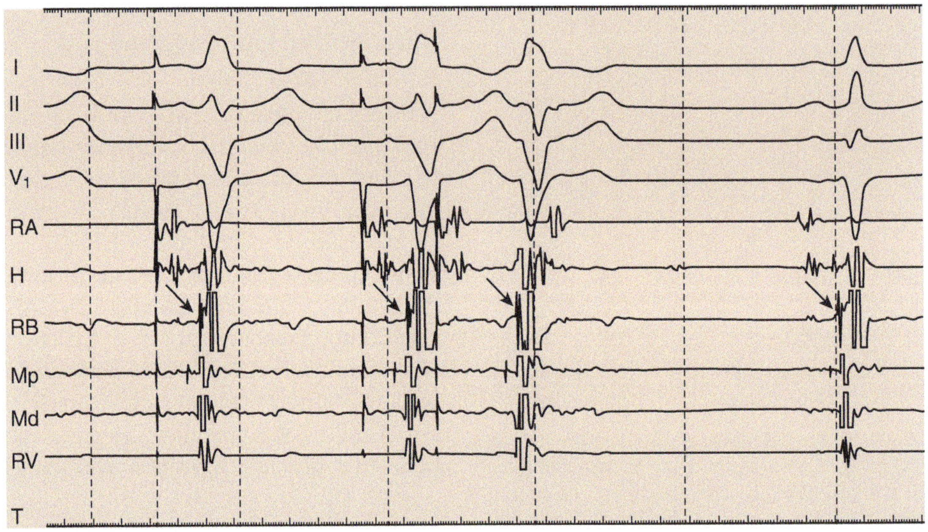

Fig. 29.4 Changes in degree of preexcitation over an atriofascicular pathway with atrial pacing. During atrial pacing at a slow drive train fusion is noticed between ventricular activation over the accessory pathway and the atrioventricular node–His Purkinje system. Maximal preexcitation is seen with delivery of an atrial premature beat that leads to more prolongation in the A-RB (right bundle) than the A-M (Mahaim potential) intervals with reversal of the RB-H activation sequence. Notice that preexcitation is minimized in sinus rhythm after a long pause, as conduction down the AV node recovers and becomes more rapid. The M potential is seen during atrial pacing with fusion or during maximal preexcitation as well as during SR with very subtle preexcitation. *d,* Distal; *p,* proximal; *RA,* right atrium; *RV,* right ventricle.

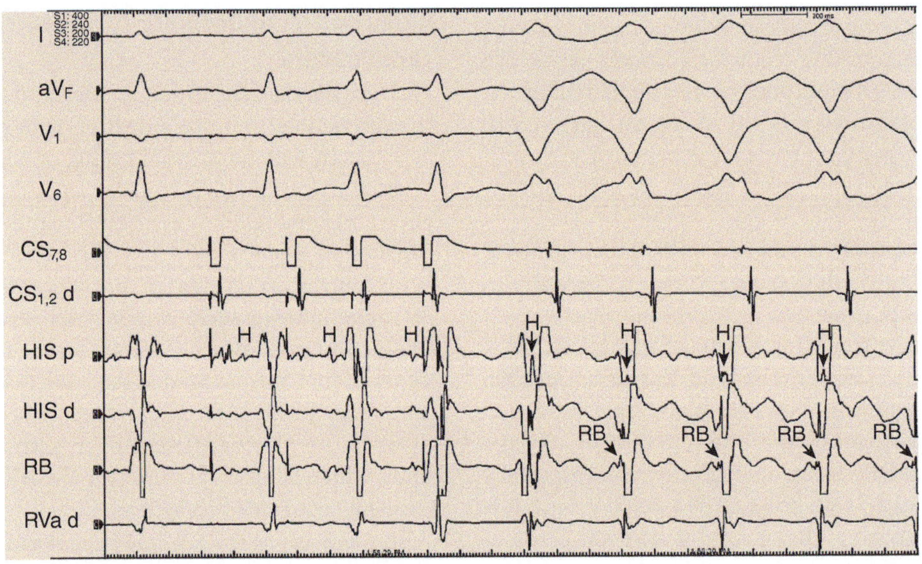

Fig. 29.5 Initiation of antidromic atrioventricular (AV) reentry tachycardia with atrial premature stimuli. AV reentry tachycardia using an atriofascicular pathway for anterograde conduction and the right bundle branch (RB), His bundle, and AV node for retrograde limb is initiated after three shortly coupled atrial premature stimuli. The AH interval progressively prolongs, the HV interval shortens, and the QRS widens. Tachycardia begins after maximal preexcitation is reached with the third premature stimulus that blocks anterogradely in the AV node and conducts down the accessory pathway. Notice that the earliest ventricular activation is at the region of the distal RB, which precedes His bundle activation. *CS,* Coronary sinus; *d,* distal; *p,* proximal.

tachycardia. However, because these APs typically have conduction block in the retrograde direction, ventricular stimulation can almost always initiate the reentry circuit. Thus, initiation of tachycardia is frequently easier to accomplish with ventricular pacing. With ventricular pacing, one only needs to achieve sufficient retrograde activation delay via the normal HPS-AV node axis that would allow reentry into the ventricle to occur via the AP. This delay can be achieved either via slowing in the AV node when sufficiently short retrograde H-H intervals can be achieved or by delay in retrograde HPS activation because of retrograde RBB block when a sufficiently short premature ventricular beat impinges on the HPS refractoriness (Figs. 29.6 and 29.7). In some cases, tachycardia can only be induced via ventricular stimulation. Davidson et al.[29] reported on two patients

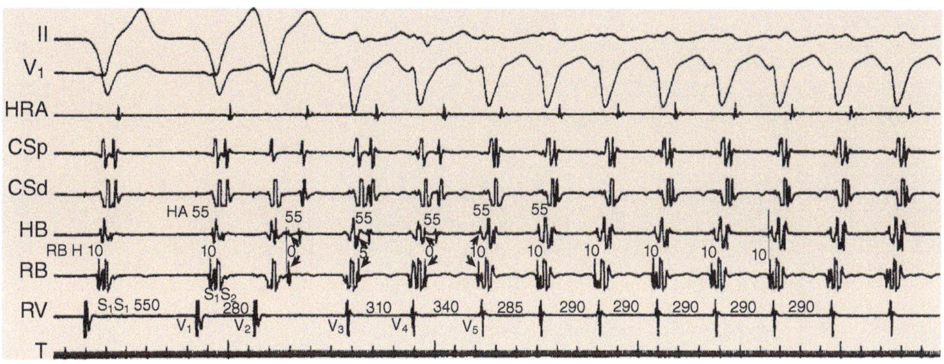

Fig. 29.6 Initiation of antidromic atrioventricular (AV) reentry tachycardia using an atriofascicular bypass tract with ventricular premature stimulation causing retrograde right bundle branch block (RBBB). A premature ventricular stimulus causes retrograde conduction block or delay in the right bundle branch. The impulse then travels transeptally to reach the His retrogradely over the left bundle branch leading to a prolonged V-H interval. Tachycardia is initiated as the impulse goes up the AV node to the atrium, then down the accessory pathway and retrogradely over the His-Purkinje fibers. The tachycardia cycle length and VH shorten on the fourth beat as the retrograde RBBB resolves. Now the right bundle deflection precedes the H instead of occurring simultaneously. These changes in cycle length implied direct involvement of the bundle branches in the tachycardia circuit, whereas the constant HA confirms that atrial activation during ventricular pacing and tachycardia occurred via the atrioventricular node. *CS*, Coronary sinus; *d*, distal; *HB*, His bundle; *HRA*, high right atrium; *p*, proximal; *RV*, right ventricle. (From Tchou P, Lehmann MH, Jazayeri M, Akhtar M. Atriofascicular connection or a nodoventricular Mahaim fiber? Electrophysiologic elucidation of the pathway and associated reentrant circuit. *Circulation.* 1988;77:837-848.)

with no evidence of preexcitation during sinus rhythm at baseline or even with atrial pacing maneuvers. However, an antidromic AV reentry tachycardia using an atriofascicular pathway was readily induced with ventricular stimulation and ablated along the lateral tricuspid annulus in both patients. This was believed to be because of fast conduction over the AV node and slower conduction over the AP. In addition, the refractory periods of the pathways were longer than the respective refractory periods of the AV nodes, thus preventing initiation of tachycardia with atrial premature stimulation.

Electrophysiologic Evaluation During Tachycardia

Both the atrium and ventricle are essential parts of the macroreentrant circuit. The earliest retrograde atrial activation is typically found along the mid atrial septum at the region of the fast AV node pathway unless another AP is used as the retrograde limb. The AV interval is often more than 150 ms during antidromic tachycardia caused by the decremental conduction properties of the AP.[30] The earliest ventricular activation is characteristically located along the right ventricular anterior-lateral free wall near the distal third toward the apex. Direct insertion of the atriofascicular pathway into the distal RBB or its fascicles leads to rapid simultaneous activation of both His and ventricle and a very short V-H interval (16 ± 5 ms).[15] The V-H interval is shorter during antidromic tachycardia than the HV interval in sinus rhythm. This is because of the fact that His and the ventricle are simultaneously (instead of sequentially) activated via the RB. The V-H (and V-A) interval may prolong in the setting of transient retrograde right bundle branch block (RBBB), which may occur as a result of mechanical trauma during catheter manipulation or with ventricular premature beats. In this situation, the tachycardia cycle length increases as conduction has to pass across the interventricular septum via the myocardium, up the left bundle, to reach the His bundle then the AV node and atrium (see Figs. 29.6 and 29.7). The His bundle–atrial (HA) interval remains constant as the final segment of the retrograde limb from the His-bundle to the atrium remains unchanged. Antidromic AV reentry tachycardia with retrograde RBBB is usually initiated with ventricular premature beats from the RV that block retrogradely in the RBB but conducts transeptally up the LBB to the His bundle and up the AV node (Figs. 29.6 and 29.7). Because of anterograde penetration of the RBB, subsequent reentrant beats then continue to maintain the retrograde RBBB by a concealed conduction phenomenon, whereby serial anterograde and retrograde conduction in the RBBB are blocked by a mechanism of interference.[31] Resolution of the retrograde RBBB is typically associated with an acceleration of the tachycardia cycle length accompanied by a shorter ventriculoatrial (VA) interval (see Figs. 29.6, 29.7). This resolution of retrograde RBBB has been demonstrated to occur through the migration of the site of retrograde block toward the His bundle.[32] Minor changes in QRS morphology, axis, and duration may occur as a result of the retrograde RBBB (see Fig. 29.7B, note change in QRS durations). In the absence of RBBB, rapid retrograde conduction over the RB to the His bundle may allow for anterograde left ventricular activation over the left anterior fascicle and fusion with transseptal activation leading to a narrower QRS sometimes with a more inferior axis.[25] Ventricular activation during tachycardia with or without retrograde RBBB is schematically illustrated in Fig. 29.8.

A late atrial premature stimulus delivered in the lateral right atrium during preexcited tachycardia that advances or delays the following ventricular activation without affecting the septal atrial activation around the AV node confirms the presence of an atriofascicular AP.[6,23,33,34] Active involvement in the tachycardia can be confirmed by maintenance of the ventricular, HPS,

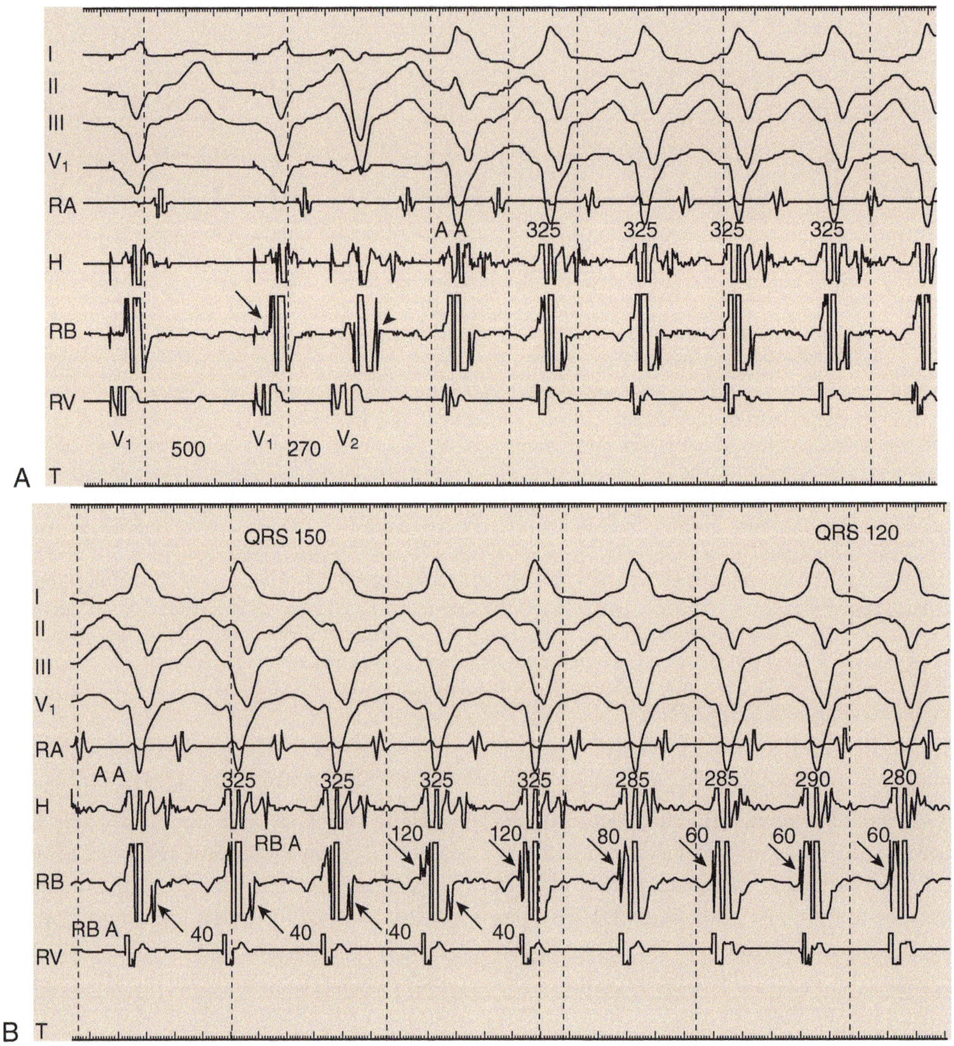

Fig. 29.7 Ventricular premature simulation initiates antidromic atrioventricular (AV) reentry tachycardia over an atriofascicular accessory pathway with retrograde right bundle branch block (RBBB). (A) Retrograde RBBB occurs with a premature ventricular stimulus, which provides sufficient delay as impulse crosses across the interventricular septum, then up the left bundle branch to the His and AV node. By the time the atrium is retrogradely activated the accessory pathway anterograde conduction has recovered and the antidromic reentry tachycardia is initiated. (B) Gradual migration of the site of retrograde RBBB is seen in this figure. In the first three beats, the local activation of the proximal part of the right bundle (RB) (*upward arrow*) occurs late with an RB-A interval of only 40 ms as it is activated anterogradely after the impulse reaches the His region. As the site of retrograde block gradually migrates proximally, the distal end of the RB (*downward arrow*) is activated earlier and can be seen gradually marching ahead of the local ventricular electrogram. As the block resolves, the RB allows for more rapid retrograde activation and the distal RB-A interval as well as the tachycardia cycle length shorten. *RA,* Right atrium; *RV,* right ventricle.

and atrial activation sequence and timing after resetting the tachycardia. Cycle length oscillation following the extrastimulus is common and characteristic of decrementally conducting APs (Fig. 29.9). His refractory premature atrial beats typically advance the next ventricular activation and reset the tachycardia; however, in 15% of cases they delay the next ventricular activation.[35] By contrast, failure to influence the tachycardia with a late atrial premature beat does not constitute sufficient evidence to rule out the presence of an atriofascicular AP as the pacing location may be far away from the origin of the AP and would not allow the premature beat to preexcite the reentrant circuit. Alternatively, the premature atrial beat may decrement in the pathway in such a manner as to obscure any changes in the cycle length of ventricular activation. Electrophysiologic features of atriofascicular accessory pathways are summarized in Box 29.1.

1:2 Atrial to Ventricular Conduction Over an Atriofascicular Pathway

In addition to participating in antidromic AV reentry tachycardia, atriofascicular pathways may rarely present with tachycardia secondary to 1:2 atrial to ventricular conduction over the accessory pathway similar to that reported with dual AV nodal physiology[20] (Fig. 29.10). Different explanations were postulated

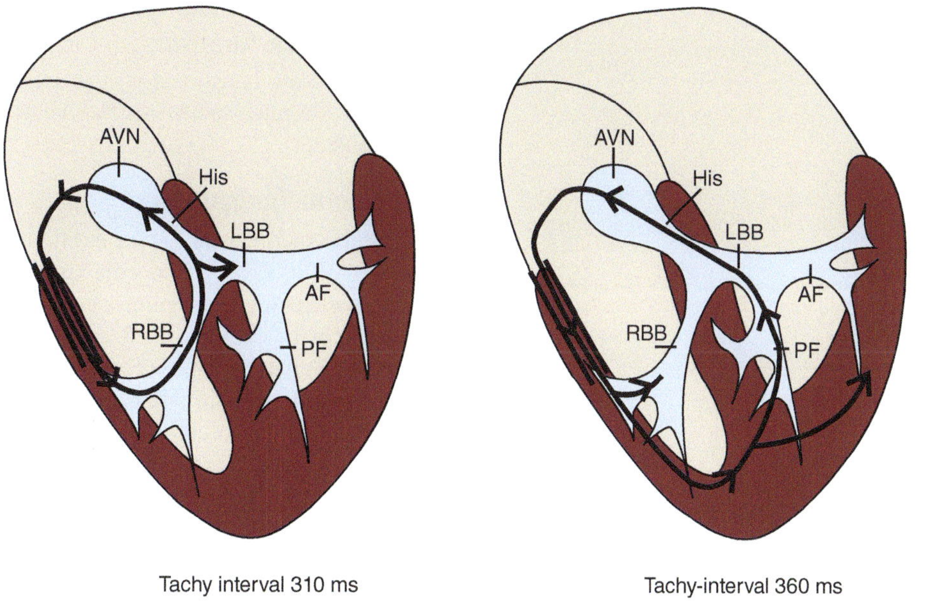

Fig. 29.8 Prolongation of antidromic atrioventricular reentry tachycardia cycle length as a result of increase in the VA interval in the setting of transient retrograde right bundle branch block (RBBB). *Left,* Reentrant circuit with retrograde conduction via the right bundle (RB). Note that the circuit is shorter than that seen when there is retrograde RBBB as shown (*right*). In addition, with retrograde conduction via the RB, the impulse can spread to the left bundle branch when it reaches the His bundle level. From there, it can spread down the LB fascicles to activate the lateral myocardium earlier than intramyocardial conduction from the right ventricle. This earlier activation is as a result of the faster conduction of His-Purkinje system tissue when compared with myocardial tissue. Thus with the shorter reentrant circuit, QRS durations of the beats can be somewhat narrower and sometimes show a more inferior axis. *AF,* Anterior fascicle; *AVN,* atrioventricular node; *PF,* posterior fascicle. (Modified from Sternick EB, Timmermans C, Rodriguez LM, et al. Effects of RBBB on the antidromic circus movement tachycardia in patients with atriofascicular pathways. *J Cardiovasc Electrophysiol.* 2006;17:256-260.)

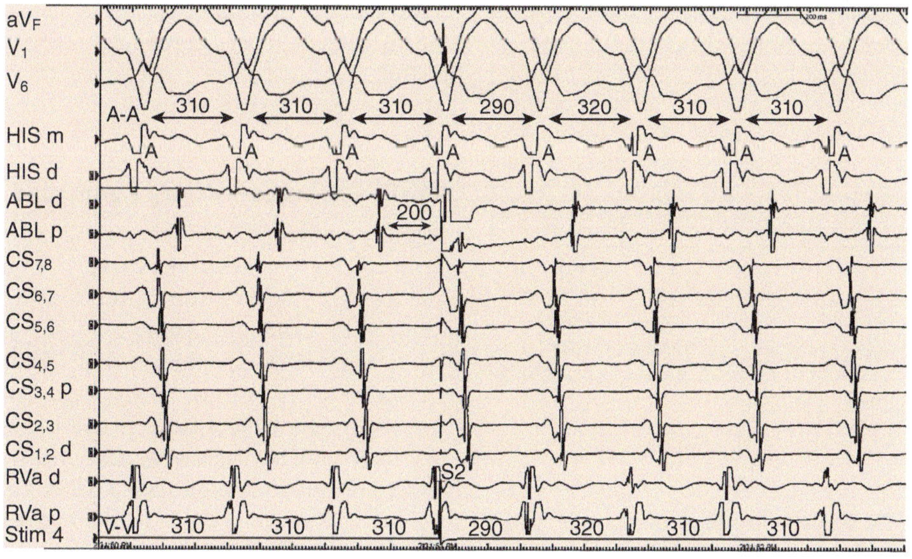

Fig. 29.9 Confirmation of active participation of an atriofascicular bypass tract in atrioventricular (AV) reentry tachycardia. An atrial extrastimulus delivered from the high right atrium (HRA) during preexcited tachycardia that does not affect the atrial activation at the AV nodal region (His catheter), advances the following ventricular, His, and atrial activation with identical QRS morphology, activation sequence, and timing. *ABL,* Ablation catheter; *CS,* coronary sinus; *d,* distal; *m,* mid; *p,* proximal.

BOX 29.1 Electrophysiologic Features of Atriofascicular Accessory Pathways

General Properties

- Obligatory unidirectional conduction in the anterograde direction
- Decremental conduction in the proximal segment of the accessory pathway between A and M potentials.
- Nondecremental conduction in the distal segment of accessory pathway with constant M to RB and V intervals.
- Atrial pacing may prolong the AH interval more than the AM interval with gradual shortening of the HV interval.
- Earliest ventricular activation during preexcitation is at the apical RV anterior wall, which precedes local ventricular activation along the tricuspid annulus.
- Commonly sensitive to isoproterenol, adenosine, and occasionally to verapamil.

Features of Antidromic Atrioventricular Reentry Tachycardia Using an Atriofascicular Accessory Pathway

- The atrium and ventricle are essential parts of antidromic macroreentrant circuit with obligatory 1:1 AV relationship
- Long AV intervals >150 ms during preexcited tachycardia
- Earliest ventricular activation near the RV apex
- RB activation precedes His (except with retrograde RBBB, in which case His precedes proximal RB)
- Rapid simultaneous activation of both His and ventricle with short VH interval (5–25 ms) except in patients with retrograde RBBB (>80 ms)
- Increased VH and VA intervals with transient retrograde RBBB, possibly with minor changes in QRS morphology, duration, and axis.
- A late PAC during AV node refractoriness that advances the V and the subsequent H and A with the exact activation sequence and timing confirms the active participation of an atriofascicular pathway in AV reentry tachycardia.
- Stimulus to QRS can be prolonged during entrainment of a reentry tachycardia involving a decrementally conducting accessory pathway despite pacing from within the reentry circuit, leading to PPI that is longer than the TCL.
- VH is shorter during SVT than during RV pacing at a similar cycle length, because of simultaneous activation of V and His during tachycardia and sequential activation during pacing.
- HA is equal during SVT and RV pacing at a similar cycle length

A, Atrium; *AH*, atrial-to-His bundle interval; *AM*, atrial-to-Mahaim potential interval; *AV*, atrioventricular; *LBBB*, left bundle branch block; *PAC*, premature atrial extrastimulus; *PPI*, postpacing interval; *RB(B)*, right bundle branch (block); *RV*, right ventricular; *SVT*, supraventricular tachycardia; *TCL*, tachycardia cycle length; *V*, ventricle; *VA*, ventricular-to-atrial interval; *VH*, ventricular-to-His bundle interval.

including longitudinal dissociation in the atriofascicular pathway similar to dual AV nodal pathways, distal division into two fibers with different conduction times, or less likely two closely located accessory pathways with markedly differing conduction times.

DIFFERENTIAL DIAGNOSIS

Antidromic AV reentrant tachycardia involving an atriofascicular pathway must be differentiated from other wide QRS complex tachycardias with LBBB type of QRS morphology.

Supraventricular Tachycardia With Left Bundle Branch Block Aberrancy

The tachycardia is associated with normal or prolonged HV interval with anterograde His-bundle activation that precedes RB activation.

Ventricular Tachycardia

Ventricular tachycardia can be easily differentiated from antidromic AV reentry tachycardia involving an atriofascicular pathway when VA dissociation occurs, which may occur spontaneously or be demonstrated by delivering a ventricular premature stimulus that blocks retrogradely to the atrium without terminating the VT. In addition, fusion beats with atrial pacing and atrial extrastimuli are possible without terminating VT, whereas during antidromic AV reentry tachycardia, the same premature atrial beat will advance (or delay) the next tachycardia beat with the same QRS morphology or terminate it. Although fusion is theoretically possible with an extremely slow tachycardia having markedly prolonged conduction in the atriofascicular pathway, such has not been seen by the authors nor reported in the literature.

Bundle branch reentrant VT (BBRVT) typically has an LBBB morphology with an HV interval that is comparable to that seen during sinus rhythm or somewhat prolonged. The H and RB activations show an anterograde sequence. Because this tachycardia tends to have a rapid rate, there is usually VA dissociation. However, when BBRVT has 1:1 VA conduction, late atrial premature beats will not be able to advance the next ventricular beat. Early atrial extrastimuli can potentially advance a slow tachycardia, with similar QRS morphology and His, RB, and ventricular activation sequence. When the cycle length of the LBBB QRS tachycardia prolongs in association with retrograde RBBB, one can exclude focal or reentrant VT as this phenomenon is characteristic of antidromic reentry related to a right-sided AP.

Wolff-Parkinson-White Syndrome

Rapidly conducting AV pathways do not exhibit notable decremental anterograde conduction, and therefore patients commonly demonstrate preexcitation during sinus rhythm especially with right-sided pathways. They are frequently capable of retrograde conduction and predominantly present with orthodromic AV reentry tachycardia. Antidromic tachycardia occurs in only 10% of patients and is characterized by a short AV interval, ventricular activation that is earliest along the tricuspid or mitral annulus, and a wider QRS complex. The QRS tends to have a more slurred onset in the anterior chest leads as a result of slower conduction through the periannular myocardium as opposed to the rapid deflection seen in a typical LBBB QRS pattern.

Decremental Atrioventricular Pathways

The majority of decremental AV pathways insert several centimeters from the tricuspid annulus via a long, insulated bundle of fibers into the right ventricle free wall. However, shorter decremental accessory pathways that insert into the myocardium immediately contiguous to the tricuspid annulus have

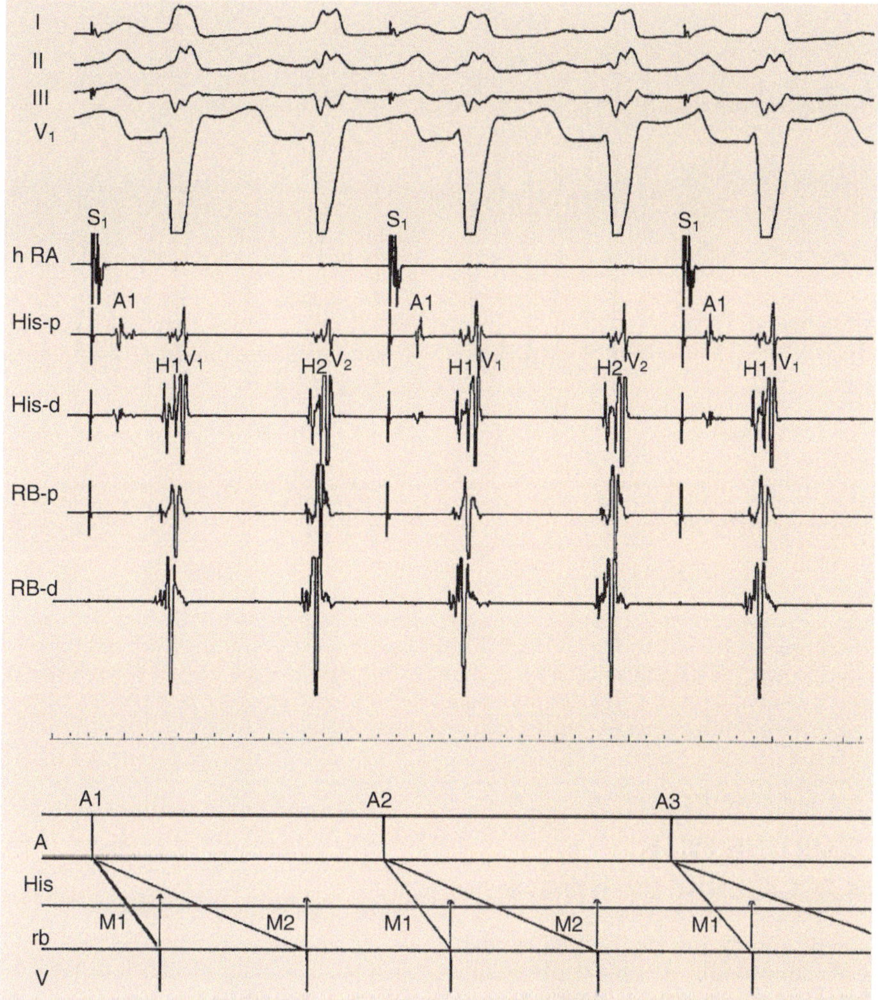

Fig. 29.10 Atrioventricular conduction (1:2) over an atriofascicular pathway. Each atrial stimulus gives rise to two ventricular complexes with a short VH interval and retrograde activation over the right bundle branch from distal to proximal suggestive of dual anterograde conduction over an atriofascicular accessory pathway. *d*, Distal; *p*, proximal; *RA*, right atrium. (From Sternick EB, Sosa EA, Scanavacca MI, Wellens HJ. Dual conduction in a Mahaim fiber. *J Cardiovasc Electrophysiol.* 2004;15:1212–1215.)

been reported. Less commonly. we have even encountered left lateral decremental pathways that insert along the mitral annulus, and recently a left-sided decremental pathway inserting at the outflow region by the left coronary cusp.[14] The pathophysiology is also very similar to atriofascicular pathways, but the maximally preexcited QRS of right-sided AV pathways typically shows an LBBB morphology with a wider QRS duration (165 ± 26 vs. 133 ± 10 ms) and broad r waves (>40 ms) in V_2-V_4 (Fig. 29.11). The further the ventricular insertion is from the RB, the longer is the VH interval, as activation has to go through the more slowly conducting myocardial tissue. Short AV pathways are characterized by a longer VH interval during antidromic AV reentry tachycardia (46 ± 22 ms), compared with long AV (37 ± 9 ms) and atriofascicular pathways (16 ± 5 ms).[15]

Nodoventricular/Nodofascicular Pathways

Retrogradely conducting ventricular-nodal pathways have been demonstrated to participate in narrow QRS tachycardia in some case reports.[9,36–38] However, participation of an anterogradely conducting nodoventricular pathways in a reentrant tachycardia is controversial. Several criteria would have to be satisfied to demonstrate that such a wide QRS tachycardia indeed involves the AV node, the nodoventricular or nodofascicular pathway, and retrograde conduction via the His bundle. (See Atriofascicular Pathway Variants.)

Fasciculoventricular Accessory Pathways

These types of APs are bystanders and have not been demonstrated to participate in reentry tachycardia. They present with a minimally preexcited QRS and a normal PR interval. Rapid atrial pacing and atrial extrastimuli are associated with prolongation of the AH interval with a relatively fixed, short HV interval, and minimal changes in the degree of preexcitation (see following text). Pure His bundle pacing or ectopic/escape junctional beats can easily differentiate atriofascicular from fasciculoventricular pathways, as it normalizes the QRS of the former but not the latter.

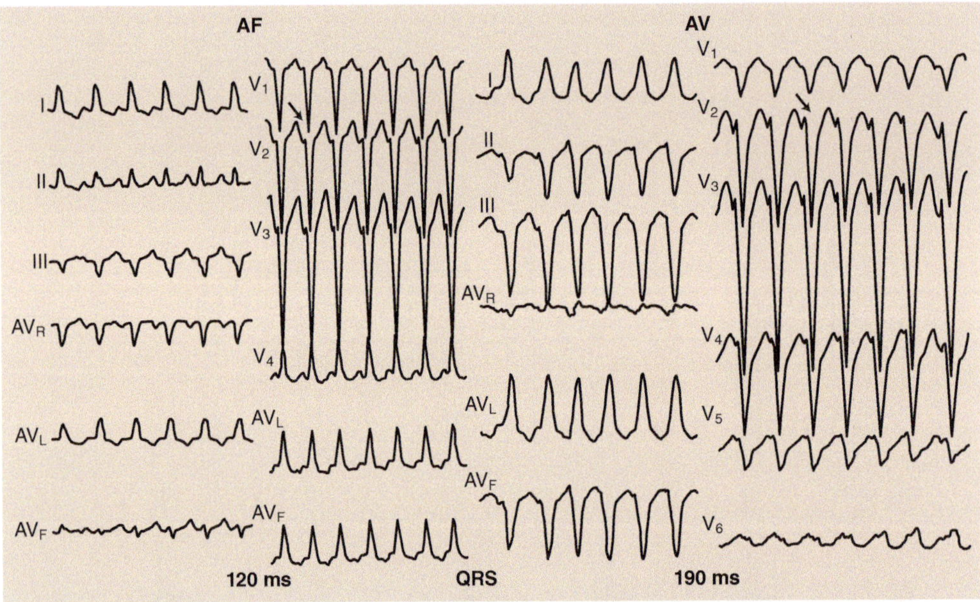

Fig. 29.11 Twelve-lead electrocardiogram of a patient with atriofascicular (AF) accessory pathway (*left panel*) and another with atrioventricular (AV) accessory pathway (*right panel*) during maximal preexcitation. AV pathways have longer QRS duration and broader R waves in the anterior leads (*arrow*). (From Haïssaguerre M, Warin JF, Le Metayer P, et al. Characteristics of the ventricular insertion sites of accessory pathways with anterograde decremental conduction properties. *Circulation.* 1995;91:1077–1085.)

ATRIOVENTRICULAR NODAL REENTRY TACHYCARDIA COEXISTING WITH ATRIOFASCICULAR ACCESSORY PATHWAYS

Because fast and slow pathways are considered normal anatomic structures of the AV node, dual AV nodal physiology commonly coincide with atriofascicular or slowly conducting long AV APs. Differentiating antidromic AV reentrant tachycardia (AVRT) from AV nodal reentry as the driver of the tachycardia circuit may be complex, and theoretically they both can coexist as a figure-of-eight type reentry with the common limb being the retrograde fast nodal pathway. When the tachycardia shows only partial preexitation of the ventricle through the AP, that is, there is ventricular fusion, the driver of the tachycardia is AV nodal reentry. However, when the tachycardia is fully preexcited, the determination of which circuit is driving the tachycardia can be difficult. Depending on the electrophysiologic properties of the AP and the slow/fast AV nodal pathways there are three possible scenarios:

1. Both antidromic AV reentry as well as preexcited AV nodal reentry can occur, and the circuits are capable of conducting at the cycle length of the tachycardia (Fig. 29.12). However, one can have a slightly shorter cycle length and be considered the driver of the tachycardia. In this scenario, ablation of the faster driving circuit at a location outside the common pathway would result in shifting of the tachycardia to the other circuit with only a minor change in the tachycardia cycle length.
2. Both circuits can maintain tachycardia but at different cycle lengths. This scenario can appear where AV nodal reentry tachycardia may be the driver, but after ablating the slow pathway, antidromic AV reentry tachycardia can be sustained, but it occurs at a longer cycle length. If the cycle lengths have a great enough difference, fusion of ventricular activation can be seen. Conversely, the AV reentry tachycardia can be the driver, but after ablating the AP, a narrow QRS AV nodal reentry would occur at a longer cycle length.
3. Only AV nodal reentry is capable of maintaining conduction at the presenting tachycardia cycle length. In this scenario, intermittent narrow QRS complexes are expected to be seen during tachycardia, as conduction across the AP undergoes a Wenckebach pattern. After the AP blocks, the AV nodal reentry tachycardia may continue as a narrow QRS tachycardia because of retrograde penetration of the AP blocking further anterograde conduction. AV nodal reentry will certainly continue with a narrow QRS at the same cycle length, without evidence of preexcitation, following ablation of the AP. In this scenario, the AP may still be able to support antidromic AVRT at a slower tachycardia cycle length (TCL) than the presenting tachycardia.

Therefore, the question of whether an AP is a bystander is more complex than a yes/no type answer. For ablation purposes, unless the AP is clearly incapable of participating in a tachycardia of concern (scenario 3), the best approach is to ablate the accessory pathway first, then address whether AV nodal reentry tachycardia remains an inducible tachycardia. In scenario 3, one should ablate the slow pathway first, and then test to see if the AP can maintain any tachycardia.

MAPPING

Mapping of atriofascicular APs can be challenging as identification of the atrial insertion with ventricular pacing is limited by lack of retrograde conduction, whereas mapping of the

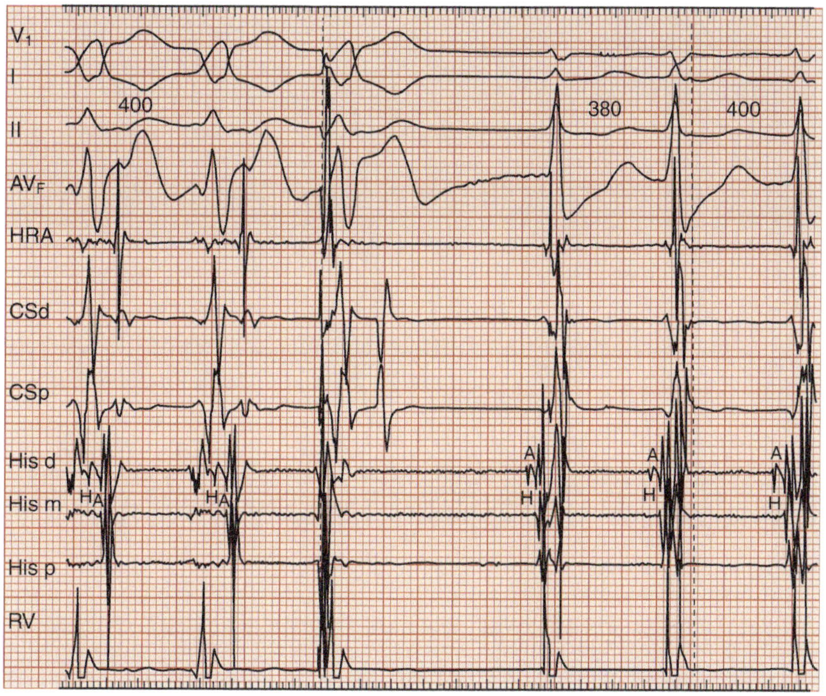

Fig. 29.12 Transformation of a preexcited tachycardia into a narrow complex atrioventricular (AV) nodal reentry tachycardia with a premature atrial stimulus. A premature atrial stimulus delivered from the HRA during a preexcited tachycardia blocks in the accessory pathway anterogradely and uncovers an AV nodal reentry. Notice the longer HA interval (40 ms versus 25 ms) during preexcited tachycardia compared with AV nodal reentry. This confirms that both antidromic atrioventricular reentry tachycardia and AV nodal reentry can occur in this patient and can sustain at similar cycle lengths. *CS*, Coronary sinus; *d*, distal; *m*, mid; *p*, proximal; *RV*, right ventricle. (From Grogin HR, Randall JL, Kwasman M, Epstein LM, Schamp DJ, Lesh MD, Scheinmann MM. Radiofrequency catheter ablation of atriofascicular and nodoventricular Mahaim tracts. *Circulation.* 1994;90:272–281.)

ventricular insertion can be difficult because of arborization. Various strategies have been developed to successfully map and ablate atriofascicular pathways.

MAPPING OF ACCESSORY PATHWAY ALONG THE TRICUSPID ANNULUS

Identification of the M Potential

The most effective method for identification of atriofascicular pathways involves locating the M potential along the tricuspid annulus.[15,23,33,39–42] Mapping should be done during preexcited ventricular activation with right lateral atrial pacing to favor conduction via the AP or during antidromic tachycardia involving the pathway. At times, the preexcitation and the M potential may be visible even during sinus rhythm. Right atrial pacing may be preferred as it reduces the risk of catheter shift with termination of the tachycardia. The use of preformed or steerable sheaths is highly recommended to improve catheter stability and tissue contact. A three-dimensional mapping system can be very helpful for locating the AP especially in case of catheter shift with tachycardia termination or AP conduction block because of mechanical trauma (see the following text).

Mapping typically begins along the anterolateral free wall of the right atrium because it is the most common origin of atriofascicular pathways and its variants. The M potential may vary in amplitude and frequency, thus careful and thorough but gentle (to avoid mechanical trauma) mapping of the tricuspid annulus is often needed to locate it (Fig. 29.13). The site of successful ablation can be identified by simultaneous recording of an atrial (A) electrogram, a sharp accessory pathway or M potential, as well as a ventricular (V) electrogram on the distal electrode of the mapping catheter. Unlike standard AV pathways, local ventricular activation along the tricuspid annulus is delayed, occurring after the onset of the QRS and after the activation of the RV apex (see Fig. 29.13). In some circumstances, the M potential may not be visible along the tricuspid annulus. In these cases, one can search for the M potential in the region between the early right ventricular activation site and the tricuspid annulus. Identification of the M potential is paramount in achieving a successful ablation.

CATHETER-INDUCED MECHANICAL CONDUCTION BLOCK

Atriofascicular pathways are typically superficial and are subject to intermittent conduction block with mechanical trauma near the atrial insertion (Fig. 29.14). By serially applying pressure at different sites along the tricuspid annulus via the tip of the catheter, the AP can be located at the site of loss of preexcitation or at the site of termination of antidromic tachycardia.[23,43,44] However, we believe that this technique should be used sparingly

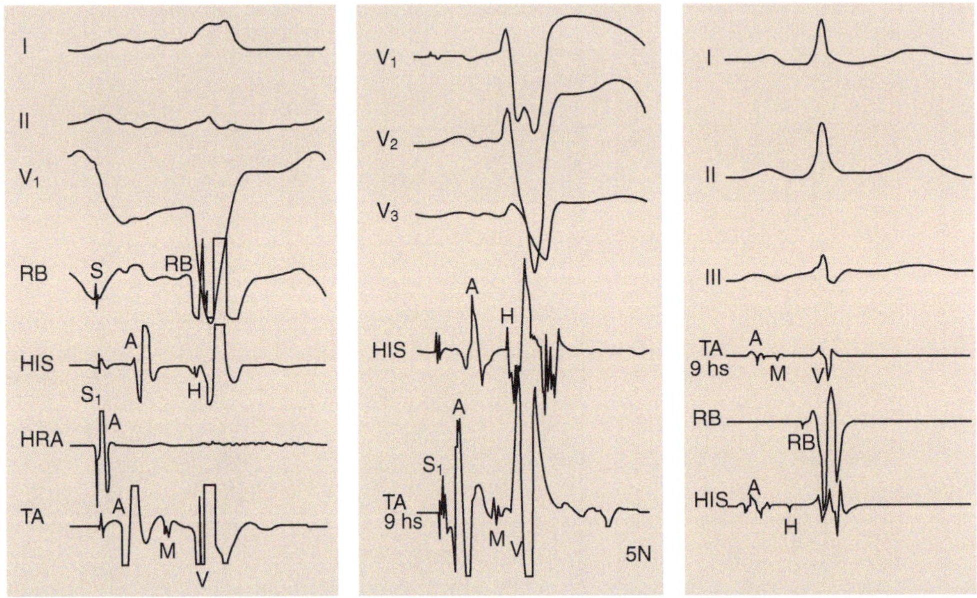

Fig. 29.13 Variation in the amplitude and duration of the accessory pathway (*M,* Mahaim potential) at the site of successful ablation in three different patients. Note earlier QRS onset and ventricular activation at the right bundle electrograms compared with the ventricular activation at the tricuspid annulus electrogram showing the M potential. *HRA,* High right atrium. (From Sternick EB. Mahaim fiber tachycardia: recognition and management. *Indian Pacing Electrophysiol J.* 2003;3:47–59.)

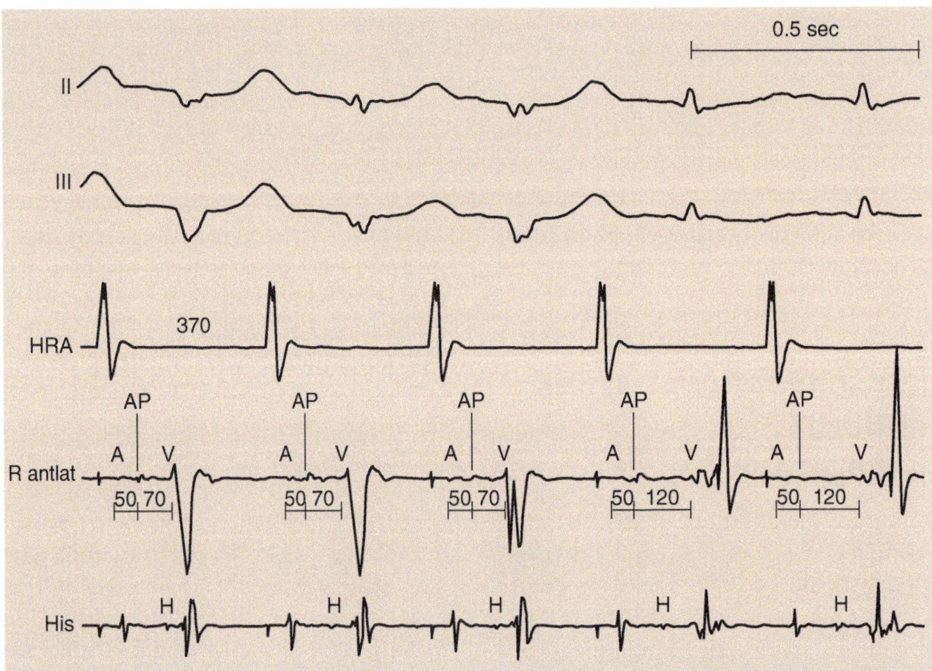

Fig. 29.14 Mapping of an atriofascicular pathway by catheter-induced mechanical trauma during right atrial pacing. Conduction block or delay in the accessory pathway distal to the accessory pathway (AP) potential because of intentional mechanical pressure via the mapping catheter, at a subannular location along the anterolateral tricuspid valve, leads to prolongation of the AP-V interval, normalization of the HV interval, and loss of preexcitation as ventricular activation proceeds via the AV node-His Purkinje system (last two beats). Surface electrocardiogram leads are II and III. Intracardiac recordings are from high right atrium (HRA), mapping catheter in right anterolateral tricuspid annulus (R antlat), and bundle of His. (From Cappato R, Schluter M, Weib C, et al. Catheter-induced mechanical conduction block of right-sided accessory fibers with Mahaim-type preexcitation to guide radiofrequency ablation. *Circulation.* 1994;90:282–290.)

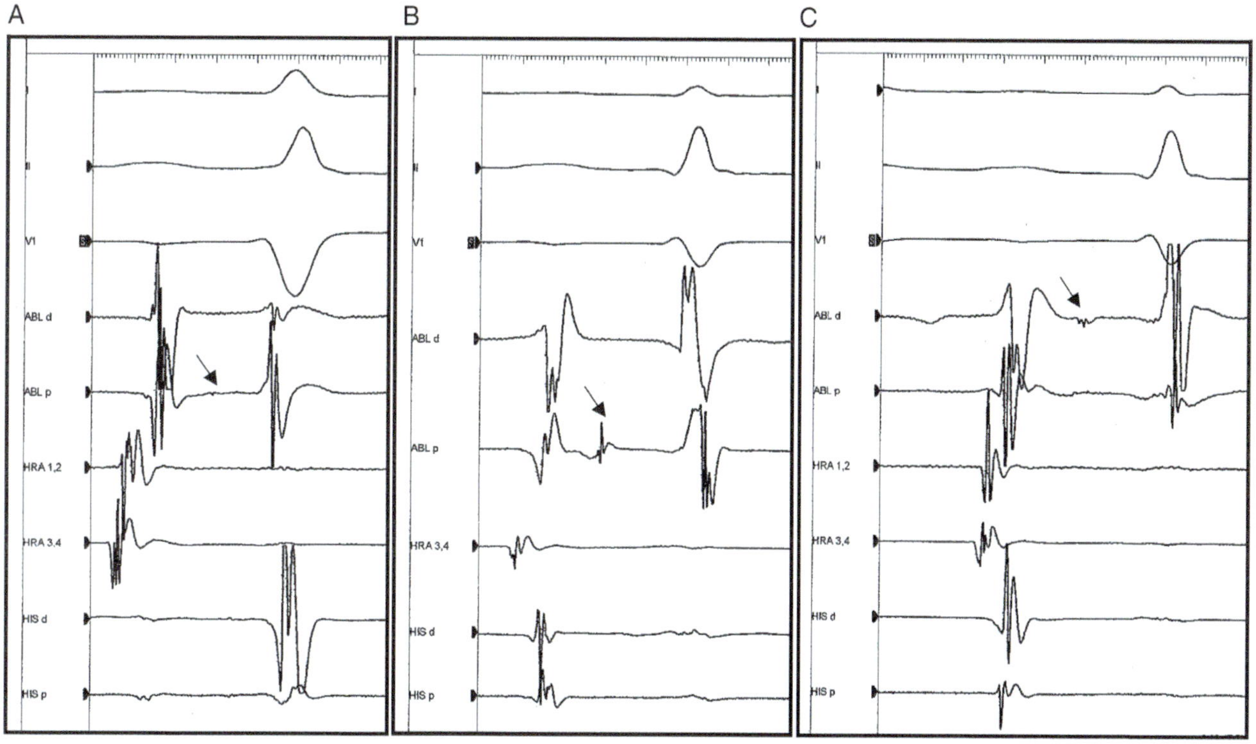

Fig. 29.15 (A) Baseline: a small AP potential (*arrow*) is recorded at the lateral part of the tricuspid annulus at mid distance between A and V on the proximal electrode of the ablation catheter. (B) After mechanically induced catheter trauma to the AP, a large AP potential (*arrow*) is recorded on the proximal electrode of the ablation catheter. (C) After repositioning of the catheter, a small AP potential is recorded on the distal electrode of the ablation catheter (*arrow*). Note the normal QRS configuration in panels B and C compared with the left bundle branch block pattern in panel A. (From Belhassen B, Viskin S. Successful ablation of right atriofascicular pathway guided by pathway potential recording despite catheter-induced mechanical pathway trauma. *Pace*. 2011; 34:e118–e121.)

because of the inaccuracy of this method, for minor delays in recognition of conduction block may lead to misidentification of the AP location as the catheter moves to a different location. In addition, conduction block from mechanical trauma can last for hours making confirmation of the successful ablation very challenging and time consuming. Nevertheless, inadvertent mechanical trauma to the pathway on the ventricular side may still preserve the presence of the M potential more proximally along the tricuspid annulus, even when preexcitation can no longer be elicited (Fig. 29.15). Thus, ablation guided by the M potential can still be performed successfully.[45] We strongly recommend the use of electroanatomical mapping in conjunction with this method to help track the catheter location as conduction block in the AP will terminate the tachycardia and may lead to inadvertent catheter movement.

IDENTIFICATION OF THE ATRIAL INSERTION

Shortest Stimulus to the Fully Preexcited Ventricular Electrogram

The atrial insertion site could also be identified as the site of shortest stimulus to the fully preexcited ventricular interval during constant atrial pacing.[17,40,46] The closer the atrial stimulation site is to the pathway, the shorter is the stimulus to QRS interval. An RV activation site can similarly be used as a surrogate for the preexcited QRS. Difficulty in stabilizing the catheter along the tricuspid annulus at a constant distance during rapid pacing, inconsistency in capturing the atrium in certain locations, and in identifying multiple regions with similar stimulus-to-QRS intervals that may be related to changes in the conduction velocity over the pathway with changes in the autonomic tone complicate this technique. Often a three-dimensional activation mapping system is used to aid in visual representation of the stimulus to ventricular activation interval. Pacing should be done at low amplitude to avoid capturing a wide area of atrial myocardium, and intracardiac echocardiography (ICE) or contact force-sensing catheters are often helpful to check for tissue contact and annular location.

Atrial Extrastimulus During Antidromic Tachycardia

The response to atrial extrastimuli during antidromic tachycardia could aid in locating the atrial insertion site.[17] Mapping the tricuspid annulus and locating the area on the annulus where the latest premature atrial extrastimulus occurred, which without affecting the activation of the atrial tissue surrounding the AV node can reset the tachycardia, advancing the next QRS and His, identify the area closest to the atrial insertion of the pathway. The technique is technically challenging and time consuming and has the same limitations as mapping with the shortest stimulus to preexcited QRS technique. A three-dimensional mapping system and often ICE are highly recommended.

IDENTIFICATION OF THE VENTRICULAR INSERTION

Targeting the distal ventricular insertion is difficult because it often extends over a large area.[15] Mapping involves identifying sites with a QS pattern on unipolar electrograms or sharp potentials fusing with the earliest bipolar ventricular potentials.[46] Pace mapping has been rarely used to identify areas with a paced QRS complex that exactly matches the maximally preexcited or antidromic tachycardia QRS morphology and duration.[47–49] In preexcited tachycardia associated with decrementally conducted APs that do not insert into the HPS, such mapping can more readily identify a successful ablation site. Typically, these insertions are closer to the AV annulus and there is minimal arborization of the ventricular insertion site. This technique can also be helpful when attempting to ablate a decremental AP during atrial fibrillation.[48]

ABLATION

Radiofrequency (RF) ablation of atriofascicular pathways and its variants is highly effective, with a success rate of 90–100%.[17,19,25,35,42,43] The catheter ablation procedure usually requires venous access only as the pathway is most commonly right sided. The standard approach is through the femoral vein, although an internal jugular venous access may occasionally be helpful in some difficult cases. Long and steerable sheaths can help in stabilizing the catheter near the tricuspid annulus. Rarely left-sided decremental APs may be encountered and require arterial or transseptal access or epicardial ablation via the distal coronary sinus–anterior interventricular vein (see the following text). Steerable RF ablation catheters, with or without an irrigated tip, are used for mapping and ablation, guided by fluoroscopy in the left anterior oblique view.

The outcome of ablation is dependent on the mapping technique used. Identifying and ablating the M potential is the gold standard and is associated with a 100% success rate when achieved.[15,23,33,40,41] The ablation catheter is maneuvered along the tricuspid annulus to locate the M potential during right atrial pacing or antidromic AV tachycardia. RF energy can be delivered from the atrial or ventricular aspect of the tricuspid annulus depending on catheter stability. Ablation is preferably performed during atrial pacing or sinus rhythm to avoid catheter shift that may occur with termination of an antidromic tachycardia. Ablation can also be performed during preexcited atrial fibrillation; however, mapping of the AP potential is usually not possible at the level of the tricuspid annulus as a result of the interference from the irregular atrial electrograms, and is usually performed more distally at a subannular location closer to the ventricular insertion (Fig. 29.16).[42,48] Alternatively, catheter-induced mechanical trauma can be used to identify the location of the AP along the tricuspid annulus guided by loss of the preexcitation.[43] If possible, we recommend performing cardioversion and mapping and ablating in sinus rhythm or during atrial pacing targeting the M potential at the tricuspid annulus.

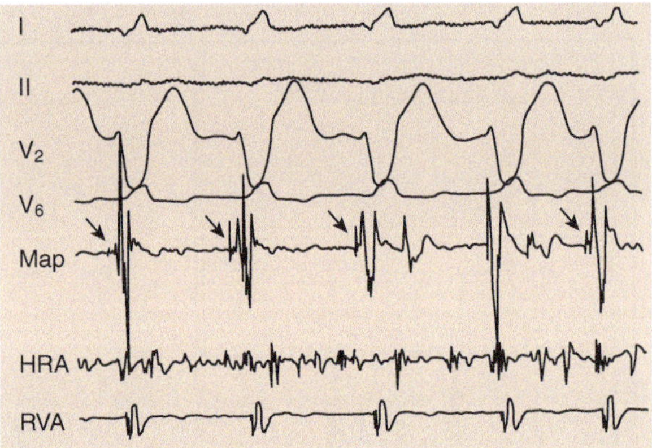

Fig. 29.16 Mapping and ablation of the distal part of the accessory pathway during preexcited atrial fibrillation. At the successful ablation site, a regular sharp potential is seen preceding the QRS by 20 ms. It is separated from the local ventricular electrogram by a fixed interval on the mapping catheter at a location close to the ventricular insertion at the apical right ventricular free wall. *HRA*, High right atrium; *Map*, mapping catheter; *RVA*, right ventricular apex. (From Kottkamp H, Hindricks G, Shenasa H, et al. Variants of preexcitation-specialized atriofascicular pathways, nodofascicular pathways, and fasciculoventricular pathways: electrophysiologic findings and target sites for radiofrequency catheter ablation. *J Cardiovasc Electrophysiol.* 1996;7:916–930.)

Loss of preexcitation is expected within a few seconds of application of RF energy at the optimal ablation site. To avoid tissue edema that may limit the ability to ablate the AP, energy delivery should be interrupted and further mapping performed if preexcitation persists. RF energy application in the region of the M potential will often result in an automatic rhythm with a morphology similar to that of the antidromic tachycardia or maximally preexcited QRS.[23,40,50] This phenomenon is comparable to the accelerated junctional rhythm seen while ablating the slow AV nodal pathway (Fig. 29.17), and similarly is absent if cryothermal applications are used for ablation. Persistence of preexcitation during this automatic rhythm should not be misinterpreted as inaccurate location. In fact, it is a sign of a good location for energy delivery and is associated with a successful outcome.[50] We recommend energy delivery until no more automatic rhythm is seen during ablation. Recurrence is more common with the use of catheter-induced mechanical trauma for mapping. In a study involving 11 patients, catheter-induced mechanical trauma was used to identify the location of the AP in eight patients: six during atrial pacing and two during atrial fibrillation. Despite multiple RF energy applications, preexcitation recurred within 12 hours in all six patients who were ablated with this mapping technique, necessitating a repeat ablation.[43] In another study, four of five patients with atriofascicular pathways had immediate recovery of conduction within less than 1 minute of mechanical trauma, allowing for immediate ablation with a long-term success rate of 75%. One patient had prolonged conduction block as a result of mechanical trauma leading to termination of the procedure without delivering any ablation lesion.[44]

The atrial insertion site is often targeted when the M potentials cannot be located. However, this technique is often complicated and time consuming. A higher number of RF applications are commonly needed to achieve conduction block with this

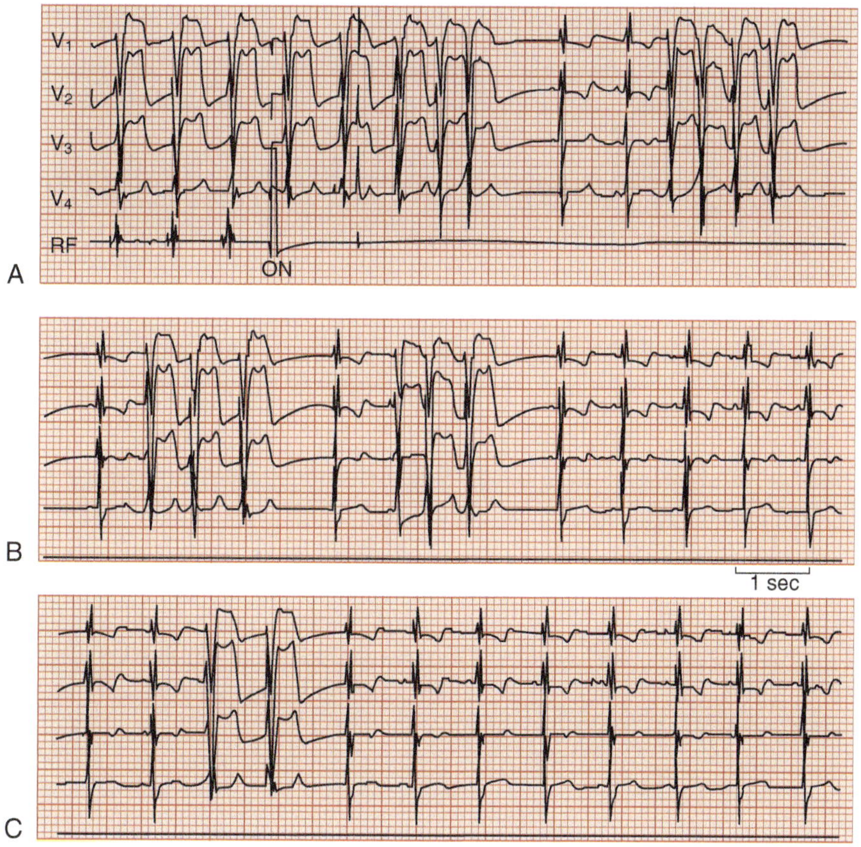

Fig. 29.17 Automatic tachycardia during radiofrequency ablation of a decrementally conducting accessory pathway. Runs of automatic tachycardia with a QRS morphology that is similar to that of the preexcited rhythm are triggered by radiofrequency (RF) ablation of the *M* potential. (A) The frequency and rate of automatic tachycardia are high initially. (B) It progressively decreases as the RF application is continuously delivered. (C) The automatic tachycardia stops as the accessory pathways is successfully ablated. (From Sternick EB, Gerken LM, Vrandecic MO, et al. Appraisal of Mahaim automatic tachycardia. *J Cardiovasc Electrophysiol.* 2002; 13:244-249.)

technique, compared with targeting the *M* potential, suggesting lower accuracy.[17,42,45]

Ablation of the ventricular end of the AP is possible despite the large area on insertion, but it is complex and less successful.[15,47,51] Injury of the right bundle is not uncommon with this approach and theoretically may be proarrhythmic by prolonging the reentry circuit, as the impulse has to cross the septum and use the left bundle for retrograde conduction.

TROUBLESHOOTING THE DIFFICULT CASE

Catheter Stability and Tissue Contact

Mapping and ablation of the atriofascicular pathways along the tricuspid annulus by targeting the *M* potential can be challenging. Stabilizing the ablation catheter at that location may be difficult, especially when mapping is performed during antidromic tachycardia as a result of the vigorous movement of the annulus and risk of catheter movement with termination of the tachycardia. The acute angle needed to reach this location when a femoral approach is used can also affect catheter stability. The use of a long precurved sheath or a steerable sheath can be helpful. In addition, the use of ICE and contact force monitoring catheters can help ensure adequate tissue contact.

When faced with a challenging case, we recommend the use of three-dimensional electroanatomical mapping to mark the location of the AP during antidromic tachycardia, which can be verified and ablated in sinus rhythm or during atrial pacing to improve stability. Simultaneous pacing of the right atrium and the right ventricle can be used to lessen the rocking motion of the lateral tricuspid annulus during ablation. Alternative approaches such as using the internal jugular vein for access, which will allow the catheter to reach the tricuspid annulus with less curvature, should be considered. Another option is cryoablation, as tissue contact is maintained once the temperature drops and the catheter freezes to the tissues.

Difficulty Identifying the M Potential

In cases where the M potential cannot be found along the tricuspid annulus, the atrial or ventricular insertion sites may be targeted. As mentioned before, the atrial insertion site could be identified during constant atrial pacing as the site of shortest stimulus to fully preexcited ventricular activation, to the right ventricular electrogram, or during antidromic tachycardia via the response to atrial extrastimulus. These methods are often complex, time consuming, and less accurate. Use of a three-dimensional activation mapping system may improve precision.

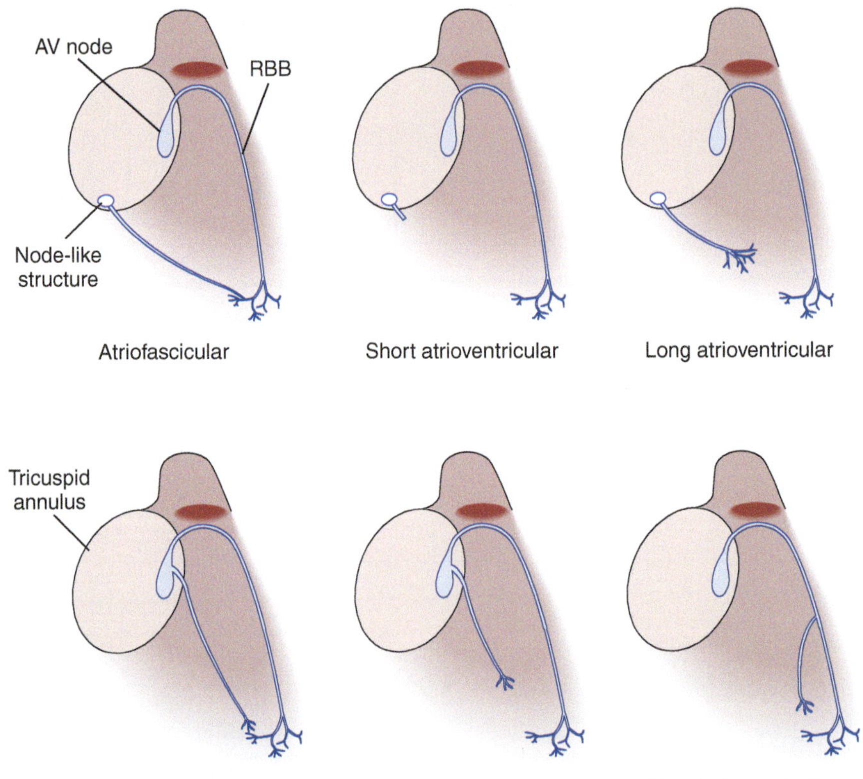

Fig. 29.18 Schematic illustration of the anatomy of atriofascicular pathways and their variants. *AV,* Atrioventricular; *RBB,* right bundle branch. (From Sternick EB, Wellens HJJ. Historical notes and classification of variants of ventricular preexcitation. In: *Variants of Ventricular Preexcitation.* Malden, MA: Blackwell Futura; 2006:1–6.)

Another alternative method would be to target the ventricular insertion; however, these pathways typically manifest a wide early activation area, and extensive ablation may be needed to achieve conduction block. Incomplete ablation at the insertion site theoretically may be proarrhythmic by facilitating antidromic tachycardia occurrence because of slower conduction into the His bundle induced by the ablation. Use of serial application of mechanical trauma along the tricuspid annulus is not advisable. The technique is imprecise and is associated with a higher failure rate.[43,44] Prolonged but transient conduction block that last for several hours commonly occurs, with recurrence of preexcitation after the termination of the procedure.

Loss of Accessory Pathway Conduction Because of Mechanical Trauma

Atriofascicular pathways and its variants are prone to mechanical trauma. Despite careful catheter maneuvering, prolonged conduction block may occur with relatively mild trauma. As mentioned before, three-dimensional electroanatomical mapping may help locate the AP by identifying the last catheter location before conduction block and loss of preexcitation. Ablation may be performed at this site after recovery of AP conduction, which may require several hours of waiting. Ablation may be delivered at this site if recovery of conduction does not occur in a reasonable amount of time, but this approach has a much lower success rate. Confirmation of immediate procedural success is problematic if ablation is performed before recovery of conduction.

ATRIOFASCICULAR PATHWAY VARIANTS

This entity includes various APs that share common electrophysiologic properties with an atriofascicular pathway. They typically exhibit decremental antegrade conduction, and except for nodoventricular/nodofascicular pathways, they almost never conduct retrogradely. They are best categorized based on their origination and insertion site rather than their conduction properties (Fig. 29.18). They include accessory AV pathways, accessory nodoventricular/nodofascicular pathways, and fasciculoventricular pathways. They most commonly insert on the right side, leading to preexcitation with an LBBB morphology. Left-sided decremental pathways are rare exceptions and present with tachycardias with an RBBB morphology. Despite being rare, it is important to distinguish the various types of APs with decremental conduction, as their diagnosis requires special electrophysiologic testing and not all require ablation therapy.

ATRIOVENTRICULAR PATHWAYS WITH DECREMENTAL CONDUCTION

Decrementally conducting AV pathways are divided into two categories: short and long.

Short Decremental Atrioventricular Pathways

Short AV pathways are most commonly found more laterally at the right free wall. Both the atrial and ventricular insertions are close to the tricuspid valve annulus. The distal insertion is

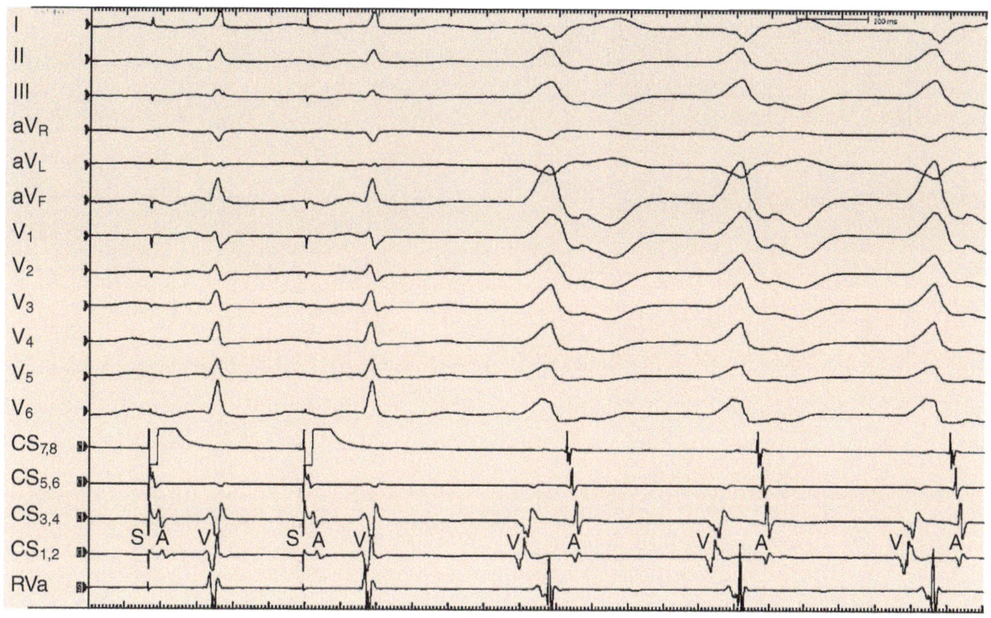

Fig. 29.19 Initiation of antidromic atrioventricular (AV) reentry tachycardia with burst pacing from the coronary sinus at a cycle length of 440 ms. The last paced beat leads to a double activation pattern, with a narrow QRS complex (second QRS) secondary to conduction down the His-Purkinje system (HPS) and a wide QRS complex (3rd QRS) with right bundle branch block morphology secondary to conduction down a slow decremental left anterior lateral accessory pathway. Antidromic AV reentry initiates as the long conduction time down the accessory pathway allows the HPS to recover and conduct retrogradely to complete the reentry circuit.

typically more localized than those of the long AV and atriofascicular pathways and can be located at the base of the RV away from the right bundle and HPS.

Prolongation of conduction across the AP by more than 30 ms with rapid pacing is consistent with decremental properties.[52] As with atriofascicular pathways, short AV pathways typically only conduct anterogradely. They sometimes respond to lidocaine and are less sensitive to adenosine.[53] The preexcited QRS has a less typical LBBB pattern and a wider QRS than those seen with atriofascicular and long AV pathways. During antidromic AV reentry tachycardia or maximal preexcitation with rapid atrial pacing over a short AV pathway, the His potential commonly falls within the QRS and the VH interval is long in duration (46 ± 22 ms) because of the distance from the ventricular insertion to the RB. It can prolong further with retrograde RBBB.

Short decremental AV pathways can be mapped and ablated near the tricuspid annulus by identifying the earliest ventricular activation during atrial pacing.[15]

Iatrogenically acquired decremental AV pathways that develop after RF ablation of nondecremental WPW pathway have been reported.[54] Decremental conduction was defined as 30 ms or more cycle length–dependent prolongation of the P-delta interval. Those cases were adenosine sensitive and were more commonly located along the coronary sinus. Repeat ablation successfully eliminated those pathways.

Long Decremental Atrioventricular Pathways

The anatomy and pathophysiology of long AV pathways are very similar to those of atriofascicular APs. They consist of long insulated fibers that insert away from the tricuspid annulus at the middle of the right ventricular free wall. The only difference is that the distal insertion is more separated from the right bundle branch by regular myocardium. A His-like structure can be usually identified near the annulus, and extensive arborization of the ventricular insertion over a wide area is also common.[15]

Similar to atriofascicular pathways the 12-lead ECG usually shows no or minimal preexcitation at rest that widens with more rapid heart rates. The maximally preexcited QRS classically has an LBBB morphology as the vast majority of these pathways are right sided. The main difference between long AV and atriofascicular pathways is the longer ventricular-His (VH) interval (37 ± 9 ms versus 16 ± 5 ms) during antidromic AV reentry tachycardia or maximal preexcitation with rapid atrial pacing.[15]

Long decremental AV pathways are mapped and ablated near the tricuspid annulus by targeting the M potential similar to those found with atriofascicular pathways.

LEFT-SIDED DECREMENTAL ACCESSORY PATHWAYS

Although decrementally conducting pathways are predominantly right sided, left-sided bypass tracts can be occasionally encountered. They are mostly atrioventricular APs and can insert along the mitral annulus, the mitral–aortic junction,[13] and even the left coronary cusp[14] or the greater cardiac vein.[55] Only a single left atriofascicular pathway has been previously described.[9]

Left-sided pathways have similar electrophysiologic properties as right-sided pathways and have been associated with antidromic AV reentry tachycardia with an RBBB pattern, when the pathway has a lateral ventricular insertion (Figs. 29.19, 29.20,

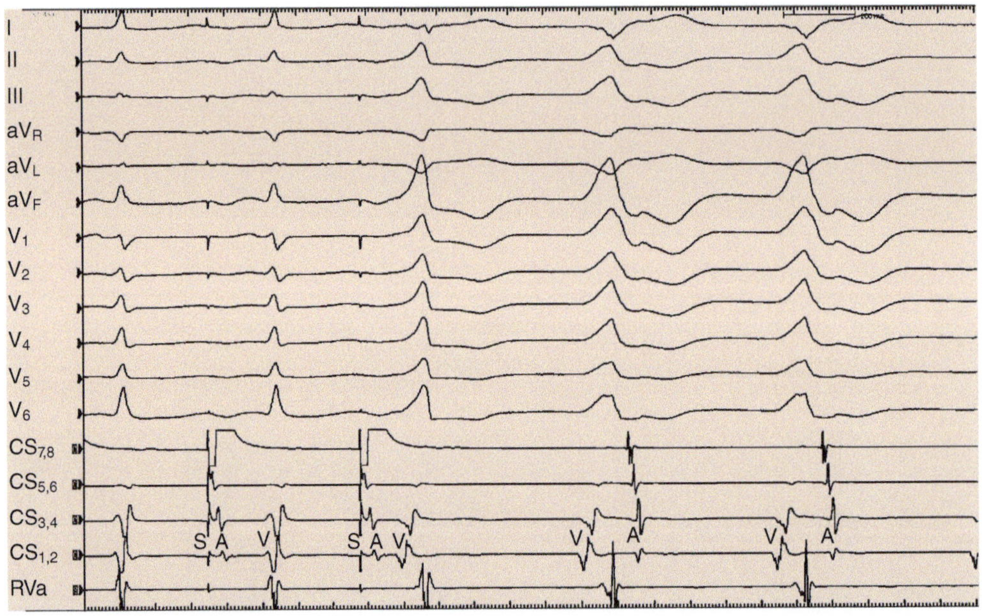

Fig. 29.20 Initiation of antidromic atrioventricular (AV) reentry tachycardia with 1–2 AV response with coronary sinus burst pacing. Both atrial paced beats conduct with a 1–2 AV response. The third QRS complex is a result of fusion between the slow decremental conduction down the left anterior lateral accessory pathway from the first atrial paced beat and conduction down the HPS from the second paced beat. Antidromic AV reentry is initiated with slow decremental conduction from the second atrial paced beat.

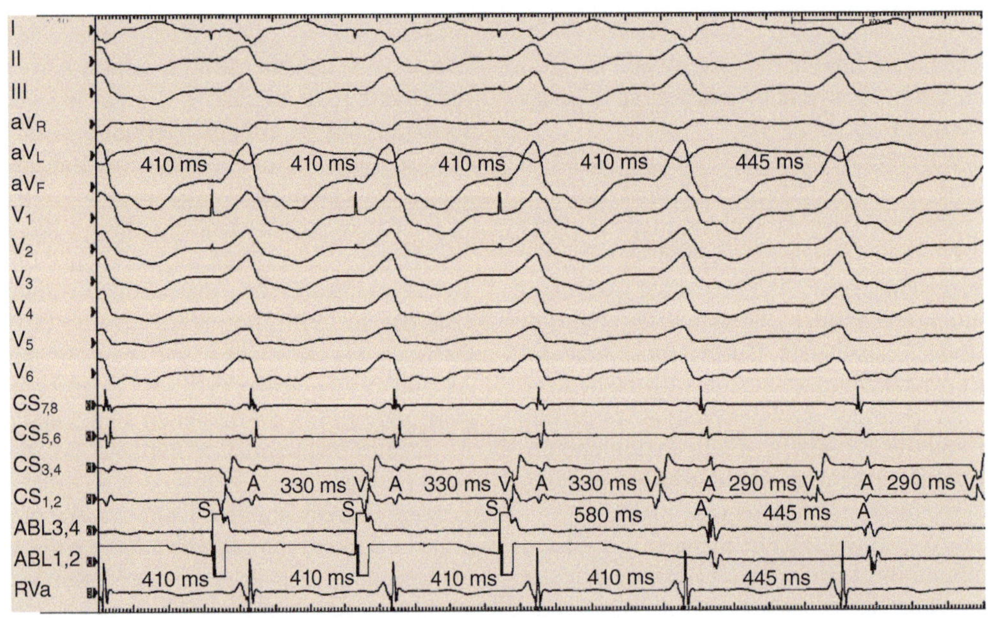

Fig. 29.21 Concealed entrainment of the antidromic atrioventricular (AV) reentry tachycardia with burst pacing from the left atrium near the anterior lateral mitral valve annulus. Tachycardia accelerates from 445 ms to the pacing cycle length of 410 ms with burst pacing. The Stim-V exceeds the tachycardia cycle length. The QRS morphology with burst pacing is exactly similar to the tachycardia morphology denoting concealed entrainment. *ABL*, Ablation catheter; *CS*, coronary sinus.

29.21, and 29.22), or an LBBB pattern, when myocardial insertion is more septal or near the aortic cusp (Fig. 29.23). Initiation of the tachycardia with atrial premature beats depends on a critical difference in the refractory periods of the AP and the AV node causing anterograde block to occur in the AV node but not in the AP with atrial pacing. Delay in the AP conduction allows enough time for recovery of retrograde conduction through the AV node. Very rarely, tachycardia can be initiated following a 2:1 AV conduction with a single atrial stimulus triggering two ventricular responses (see Fig. 29.20). As with right-sided pathways, tachycardia can frequently be more readily initiated by pacing from the ventricle near the AP insertion. Near concealed entrainment with a postpacing interval (PPI) > TCL can be observed with pacing from the atrium near the AP insertion (see Fig. 29.21).

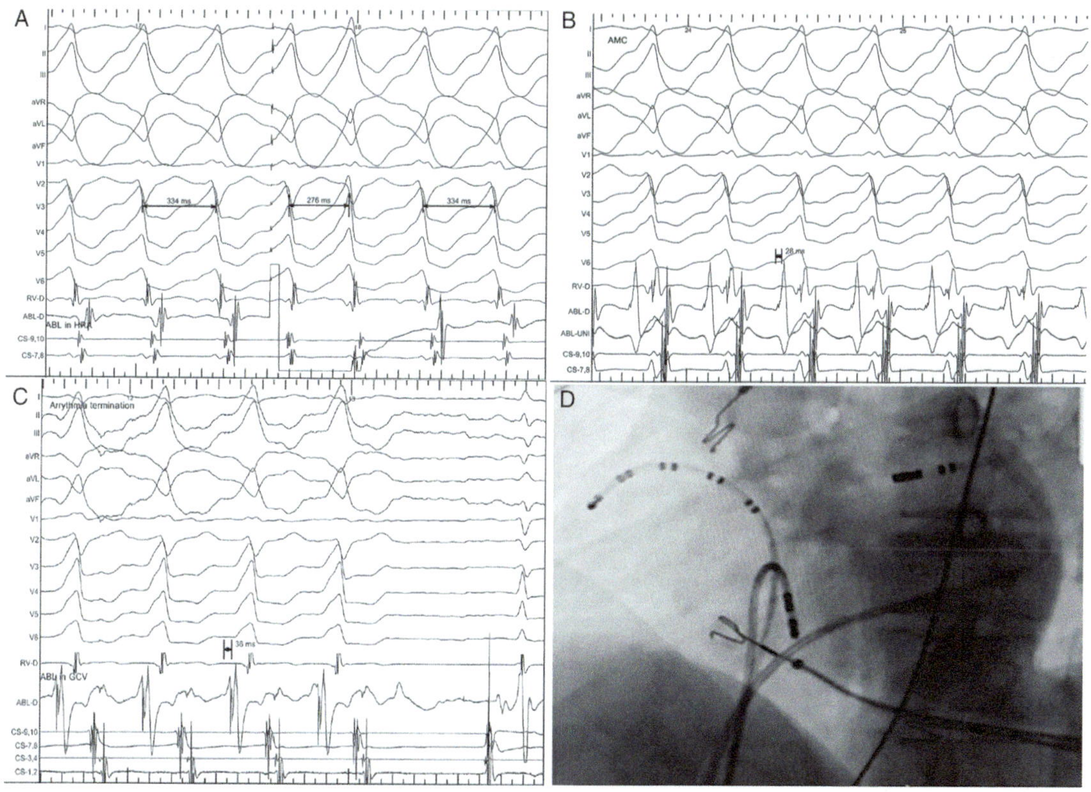

Fig. 29.22 (A) Wide-complex tachycardia with a slow-rise delta wave, R wave in V1 with "pattern break" appearance in V2. A single His-synchronous atrial extrastimulation (from ablation catheter) during arrhythmia results in advancement of ventricle, confirming antidromic AVRT and excluding VT. (B) Through retrograde aortic approach, the earliest endocardial ventricular activation time (−24 ms) recorded at the aortomitral continuity. (C) Intracardiac recording at the site of successful ablation. The ablation catheter recorded a sharp electrogram that preceded the QRS onset by about 36 ms along the greater cardiac vein–anterior interventricular vein junction. (D) The LAO fluoroscopic view of catheter positions. The irrigated ablation catheter was placed in greater cardiac vein / anterior interventricular vein junction. The decapolar catheter was placed in the right atrium. (From Emkanjoo Z, Madadi S, Kamali F. Catheter ablation of an antidromic atrioventricular reentrant tachycardia using a slow, decrementally conducting accessory pathway in the great cardiac vein. *Pacing Clin Electrophysiol.* 2021;44:389-394.)

Ablation of the left-sided pathway can be achieved by mapping the earliest ventricular activation during maximal preexcitation with atrial pacing or during antidromic AV reentry tachycardia. The insertion is commonly localized near the annulus and far from the His-Purkinje system. Occasionally endocardial ablation can be challenging, and epicardial ablation along the greater cardiac vein may be required (see Fig. 29.23). In that case, the QRS morphology on 12-lead ECG showed an R wave in V_1 with a slow rise of initial portion of the QRS and "pattern break" appearance in V_2. Earliest endocardial activation was noted along the aortomitral continuity; however, ablation there was unsuccessful. The accessory pathway was successfully ablated along the greater cardiac vein–anterior interventricular vein junction.

NODOVENTRICULAR AND NODOFASCICULAR ACCESSORY PATHWAYS

Mahaim et al. were the first to histologically describe myocardial fibers connecting the AV node region to the septal ventricular crest and conjectured about their functional significance.[1] Physiologically functioning nodoventricular or nodofascicular pathways appear to be the least common type of atypical decremental pathways. They are postulated to connect the AV node to the ventricular tissue near the tricuspid annulus along the midseptum (nodoventricular) or the HPS along the right bundle or the left posterior fascicle (nodofascicular).

Nodoventricular/nodofascicular pathways were proposed to conduct antegradely and derive decremental conduction properties from their origin in the AV node.[56] However, the majority of antidromic reentry tachycardias that were first believed to be caused by such pathways were actually most likely atriofascicular pathways. Currently, the ability of nodoventricular/nodofascicular pathways to participate in antidromic reentry tachycardia remains controversial despite some case reports suggesting the presence of such a pathway participating in a reentrant tachycardia.[57] Several criteria would have to be satisfied to demonstrate that such a wide QRS tachycardia indeed involves the AV node, the nodoventricular or nodofascicular pathway, and retrograde conduction via the His bundle. The wide QRS tachycardia circuit must be independent of atrial activation. Thus, a firm demonstration of VA dissociation would be one requirement. For nodoventricular pathways, entrainment from the ventricle at a site near the early activation of the preexcited tachycardia showing fusion and a PPI close to the tachycardia cycle length would

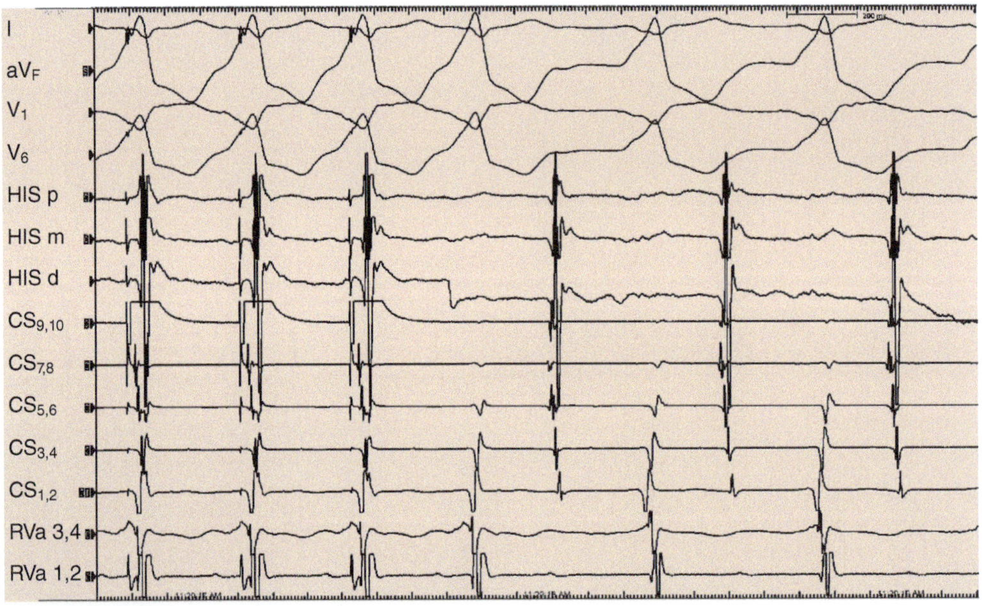

Fig. 29.23 Initiation of antidromic atrioventricular (AV) reentry tachycardia using a left-sided decrementally conducting atrioventricular accessory pathway inserting into the left coronary cusp with burst pacing from the CS at a cycle length of 340 ms. The last paced beat conducts anterogradely down the accessory pathway with left bundle branch block morphology and initiates an antidromic AV reentry with retrograde conduction over the slow AV node pathway.

demonstrate participation of ventricular tissues in the reentrant circuit. The VH interval during tachycardia should be similar to or longer than VH during RV apical pacing. In contrast, the VH interval during a nodofascicular reentrant tachycardia should be short and less than the VH during RV apical pacing. Atrial pacing, via either a single beat or burst pacing, which results in termination of the tachycardia without advancing the QRS or preexciting the retrograde His, would prove AV nodal involvement of the reentrant circuit. Lastly, overdrive atrial pacing during tachycardia that conducts with a similar QRS morphology as the preexcited tachycardia would exclude VT and confirm participation of an anterogradely conducting nodoventricular/nodofascicular pathway in the tachycardia.

By contrast, participation of ventricular nodal pathways in narrow QRS tachycardia with VA dissociation is well documented.[9,36-38] The atrium is not a prerequisite for the maintenance of a reentry tachycardia using this type of pathways, as the upper turning point is at or just below the AV node (Fig. 29.24).

In this situation, the differential diagnosis includes AV nodal reentry or junctional tachycardia with retrograde block to the atrium. A His-refractory PVC that terminates the tachycardia or advances/delays the next His and QRS and resets the tachycardia can exclude AV nodal reentry and junctional tachycardia and confirm the mechanism of the SVT.[36-38] AV nodal reentry and junctional tachycardia with VA block can also be excluded if the PPI during ventricular overdrive pacing is close to TCL or if entrainment from the RV near the accessory pathway insertion shows fixed fusion (see Fig. 29.24). Finally, catheter-induced ipsilateral BBB may also assist in the diagnosis, as it may be associated with prolongation of the HA interval and the cycle length of the tachycardia involving a concealed nodofascicular or nodoventricular pathway because of involvement of the HPS in the reentrant circuit, but such is not the case in AV nodal reentry or junctional tachycardia. However, this may not occur if the AP originates at a site along the septum where right bundle and left bundle activation wave fronts typically collide during sinus rhythm.

MAPPING AND ABLATION

Successful ablation of manifest nodoventricular/nodofascicular pathways has been reported by targeting the slow AV node (AVN) pathway region.[57] Alternatively, one can ablate the earliest ventricular activation during atrial pacing with maximal preexcitation or during antidromic tachycardia involving a nodoventricular pathway.

Ablation of concealed nodoventricular pathways is more challenging than other atypical APs because of the proximity to the AV node, which increases the risk of complete heart block with ablation. RF energy has been used in the majority of reported cases, but cryoablation is another option. Several techniques have been developed to map and ablate the distal part of the accessory pathway, especially in patients presenting with narrow complex tachycardia. Mapping the midseptum and ablating the distinct AP potential have been previously reported,[9] but it may be hard to differentiate it from the RB potential. A more elegant way to identify the distal insertion is to target the site at which maximum advancement of the His potential can be achieved with a single extrastimulus with a fixed coupling interval during orthodromic tachycardia.[37,38] Alternatively, performing a PPI map by entraining the tachycardia at various locations along the midseptum can identify the ventricular insertion as the site where near concealed entrainment occurs with the shortest stimulus-His and the shortest PPI.[36]

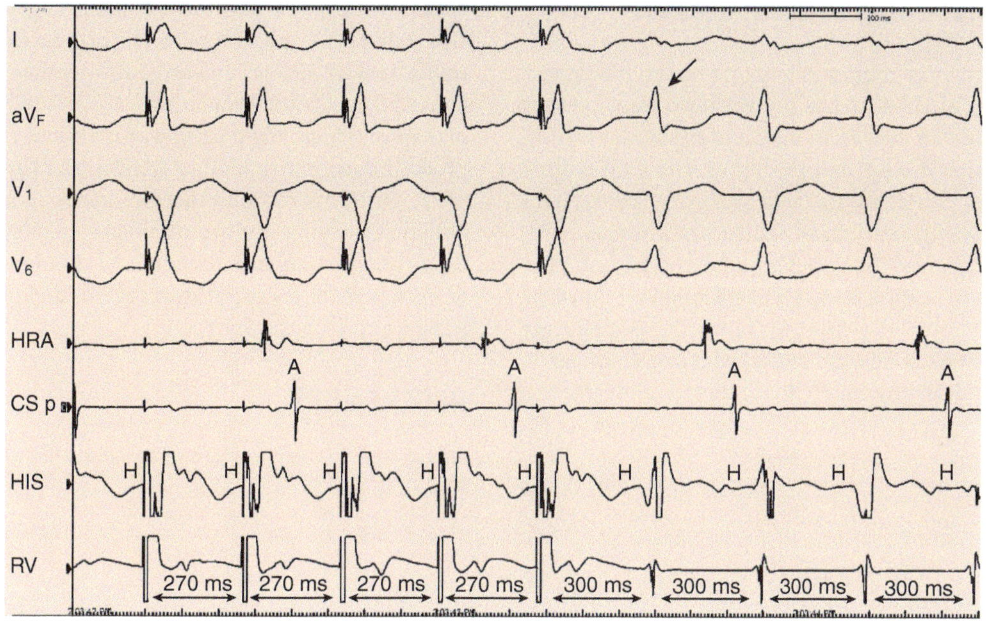

Fig. 29.24 Entrainment of a narrow-complex tachycardia with ventriculoatrial dissociation confirms the participation of a ventriculonodal accessory pathway in tachycardia. Manifest entrainment with a QRS morphology that is close to that of the tachycardia (constant fusion) is seen with pacing from the right ventricle within the reentrant circuit. The postpacing interval at the pacing site is equal to the tachycardia cycle length with a similar QRS morphology and HV timing. The first unpaced QRS (*arrow*) is at the cycle length of pacing showing that a large part of the ventricle is in the orthodromic arm of the entrainment activation. These observations confirm the participation of a ventriculonodal pathway in the tachycardia and excluding atrioventricular nodal reentry or junctional tachycardia. *CS*, Coronary sinus; *HRA*, high right atrium; *p*, proximal; *RV*, right ventricle.

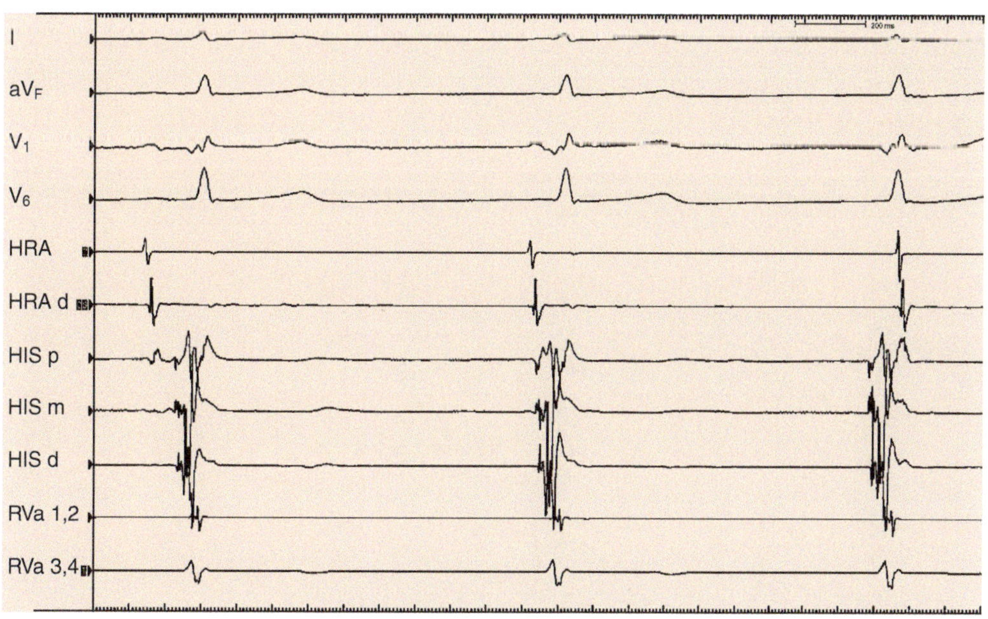

Fig. 29.25 Surface electrocardiogram and intracardiac electrograms in a patient with a fasciculoventricular bypass tract. The first beat is a sinus beat conducting with normal PR and A-H intervals and short HV interval. The second and third beats are junctional extrasystoles conducting with the same short HV interval and fixed degree of preexcitation. *d*, Distal; *HRA*, high right atrium; *m*, mid; *p*, proximal; *RV*, right ventricle.

FASCICULOVENTRICULAR ACCESSORY PATHWAYS

This is a rare form of AP that has not yet been implicated in reentry tachycardia, but acts as an innocent bystander leading to minimal preexcitation, left axis deviation with a QRS duration of 90–120 ms.[2,58] Although these pathways are referred to as *accessory pathways,* they may well be just a variant early branching of the HPS into the upper septal myocardium. Electrophysiologic features include normal PR and AH intervals and short HV intervals (<35 ms). Atrial pacing is classically associated with AH prolongation and a fixed degree of preexcitation and short HV interval.[59] Preexcitation may increase if conduction delay occurs in the HPS below the origin of the pathway and decrease with increased HV intervals if delay occurs within the pathway. A fixed degree of preexcitation and a short HV interval with His bundle pacing or junctional rhythms (Fig. 29.25) can easily differentiate fasciculoventricular APs from atriofascicular and AV APs, as well as other forms of APs in which His pacing or junctional rhythm will lead to predominant ventricular activation over the His-Purkinje network, with loss of preexcitation and increase in HV interval. Differentiation is important as fasciculoventricular pathways do not require ablation or medical therapy. The fast conducting property of these pathways is not conducive to generating a reentrant tachycardia.

REFERENCES

Please refer to the e-book for a complete list of references.

30

Ablation of Challenging/Difficult Accessory Pathways

Satoshi Higuchi, Christopher C. Cheung, Adam Oesterle, Henry H. Hsia, Joshua D. Moss, Melvin M. Scheinman

KEY POINTS

- The first step in approaching the difficult accessory pathway ablation is to exclude cognitive failure and establish the correct diagnosis via appropriate pacing techniques.
- Special techniques and technologies may be required to identify accessory pathway potentials, the presence of multiple pathways, and the course of oblique pathways.
- Nonconventional strategies are sometimes needed to achieve optimal anatomical positioning and stability, including the use of deflectable sheaths, alternative energy sources, and access to the coronary venous system or epicardial surface.

INTRODUCTION

The objective of this chapter is to outline problems that may be encountered during the mapping and ablation (ABL) of accessory pathways (APs) and to describe our approach to several difficult and illustrative cases.[1,2] In each example, the patient underwent multiple prior unsuccessful procedures, and a thorough understanding of fundamental electrophysiology in combination with innovative approaches was critical to ultimately achieving success. Specific factors highlighted include the presence of multiple pathways, a pathway with decremental conduction properties, and the need for epicardial access.

COMMON CHALLENGES IN ACCESSORY PATHWAY MAPPING/ABLATION

Accessory pathways (APs) are remnants of incomplete separation of the atrial and ventricular myocardium by the annulus fibrosus in the process of cardiogenesis. These myocardial bridges allow for electrical conduction, which can facilitate early ventricular activation in the case of anterograde conduction and the arrhythmogenic substrate for AV reentrant tachycardia (AVRT). Catheter ABL of AV pathways has become the first-line therapy for arrhythmia associated with APs, such as AVRT and preexcited atrial fibrillation.[3,4] A number of case series have reported initial success rates to be highest for left-sided pathways (95%) and lower for right-sided pathways (88%) and septal connections (89%).[5-13] However, primary success can be occasionally elusive, resulting in the need for lengthy or sometimes repeat procedures. In approaching a patient with prior unsuccessful catheter ABL, several contributing factors should be considered during procedural planning:

1. Misdiagnosis of the tachycardia: no AP present, or bystander AP
2. Localization error: AP present and participatory in tachycardia but localized incorrectly
3. Unusual AP location: AP present and participatory, and localized correctly, but in an unusual or atypical location for conventional catheter access
4. Difficult to ablate or high risk of AV node injury: AP present and participatory in tachycardia, and localized correctly to a generally common anatomical site, but challenging or high risk to apply effective ABL energy
   - For example, stable electrode-tissue contact (catheter instability, poor tissue contact, or difficult access to the target site) can be difficult to maintain for right-free wall APs (see Chapter 26).
   - Ablation of anterior-septal or mid-septal APs adjacent to the AV node and/or His bundle carry a high risk of iatrogenic injury (see Chapters 27 and 28).

1. MISDIAGNOSIS OF THE TACHYCARDIA

Orthodromic AVRT using a posterior-septal AP can be misdiagnosed as slow/slow AVNRT, and vice versa. Most such diagnostic errors can be prevented by delivering ventricular extrastimuli synchronized to His refractoriness during SVT. Delivering the ventricular extrastimuli from the basal posterior-septal RV in closer proximity to the ventricular insertion of the AP can best separate the diagnoses of AVNRT from atrioventricular reciprocating tachycardia.[14,15]

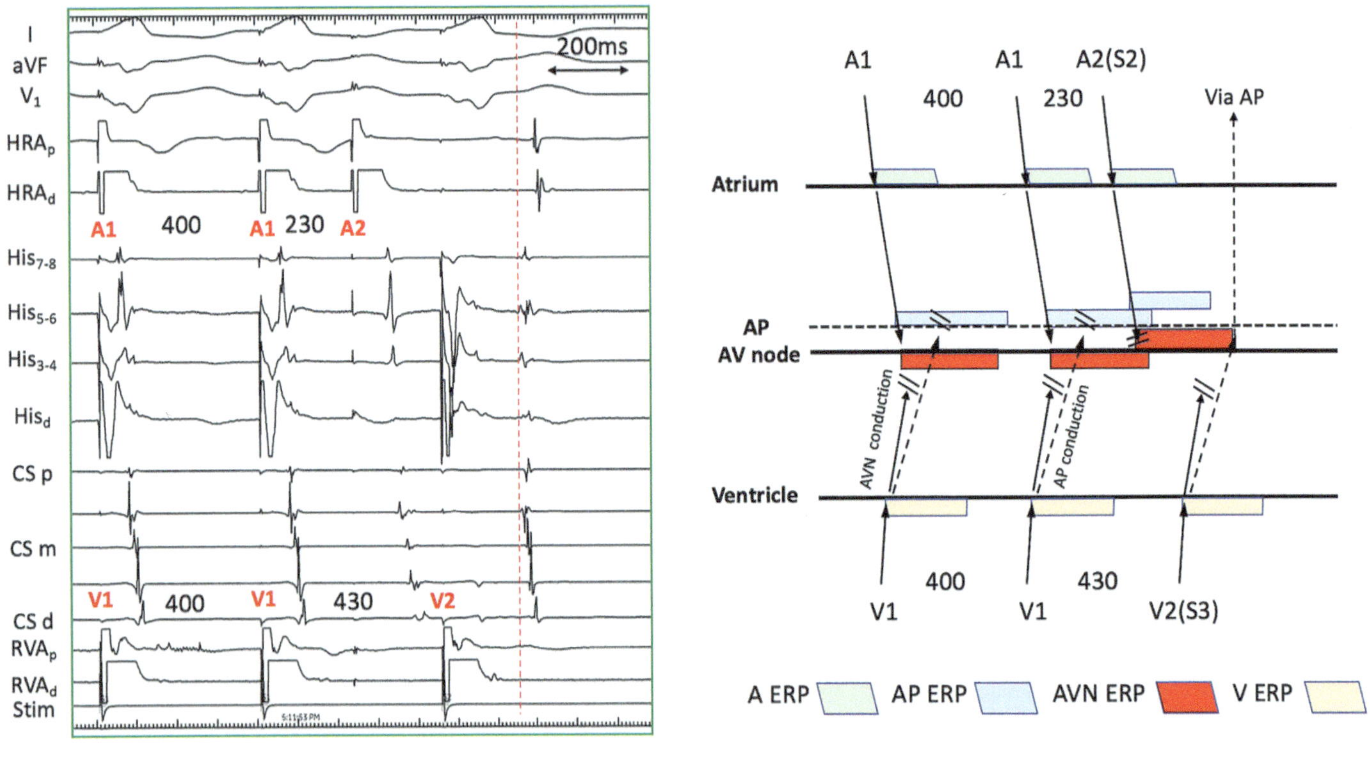

A B

Fig. 30.1 Sequential dual-chamber extrastimulation. (A) The eight-beat drive train of simultaneous AV pacing (A1V1, 400 ms) is followed by a stimulated atrial complex (A2, 230 ms) when the AV node is refractory, followed by a stimulated ventricular complex (V2, 430 ms). (B) Diagram of (A), retrograde activation of the AP (indicated by the dashed arrow) is observed because the refractory period of the AV node is extended beyond that of the AP by delivery of A2 at the AV nodal ERP. This extension of the AV node–refractory period results in a blocked retrograde stimulus at the level of the AV node after V2 delivery, thereby allowing for retrograde conduction exclusively over a posterior left atrial accessory pathway. *A2,* Programmed atrial stimulus; *A ERP,* atrial effective refractory period; *AP,* accessory pathway; *AV,* atrioventricular; *AVN,* atrioventricular node; *CS,* coronary sinus; *ERP,* effective refractory period; *HRA,* high right atrium; *RVA,* right ventricular apex; *Stim,* stimulation; *V2,* programmed ventricular stimulus; *V ERP,* ventricular effective refractory period; *X d, m, p,* the distal, mid, proximal electrode pairs of the relevant catheter.

Para-Hisian pacing can also help distinguish a septal AP from the slow AV nodal pathway.[16]

Long RP tachycardia using a decremental AP can also be misdiagnosed as fast/slow AVNRT (see Case 2). In particular, identification of a slowly conducting concealed AP, with a retrograde effective refractory period (ERP) longer than the retrograde ERP of the AV node, can be challenging, since ventricular stimulation may result in either nodal conduction alone or a fused atrial complex from retrograde conduction over both the AV node and the AP. Sequential dual-chamber extrastimulation, in which a ventricular extrastimulus (V2) is delivered after delivery of an atrial extrastimulus (A2) during AVNERP, may result in retrograde conduction block in the AV node while still allowing retrograde conduction over the AP (Fig. 30.1).[17]

Multiple tachycardia mechanisms, such as AVNRT or atrial tachycardia with a bystander AP, can also be a source of misdiagnosis. In Case 2, the importance of careful assessment with ventricular pacing studies during tachycardia (including delivery of His-refractory premature ventricular complexes and ventricular overdrive pacing) is emphasized.

2. LOCALIZATION ERROR

The most common cause of ABL failure is likely to be inaccurate pathway localization, with energy application at incorrect and ineffective sites. Factors related to both the operator and the AP itself can contribute:

1. Operator-related factors
   - Misinterpretation of electrophysiologic data, by failure or inability to recognize earliest atrial or ventricular activation sequence or AP potentials
   - Incomplete mapping, a point of particular relevance to posterior-septal APs, when careful mapping of the coronary sinus (CS) and left side of the septum is essential
2. AP-related factors
   - Distorted low-amplitude electrograms due to prior ABL attempts
   - Oblique APs
   - Multiple APs

For AP localization (mapping), identification of the site of earliest atrial and/or ventricular activation during retrograde and/or anterograde conduction, respectively, is critical. Often, however, the local bipolar electrograms can consist of multiple

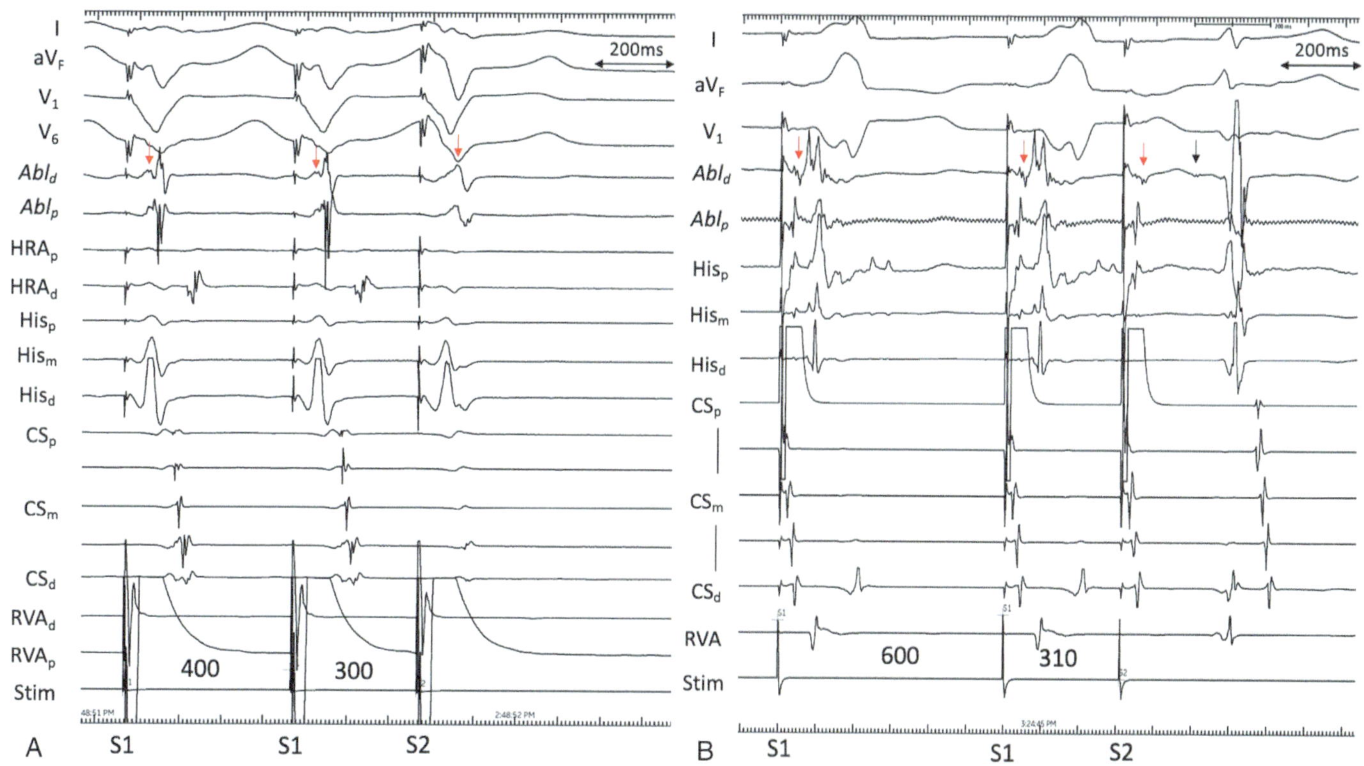

Fig. 30.2 Separation of local atrial and ventricular complexes. (A) Mapping of the atrial insertion in a patient with anterior-septal AP. The ablation catheter is located at the noncoronary cusp. A six-beat drive train of ventricular pacing (400 ms) followed by ventricular extrastimuli (300 ms) results in retrograde conduction block in the AP. Note that on the distal pair of the ABL catheter, there were continuous complexes during the drive train obfuscating distinct A and V signals. In contrast, after a ventricular extrastimuli, only the ventricular complex is observed, suggesting that the ventricular signal precedes the atrial components. (B) Mapping of the ventricular insertion in another patient with anterior-septal accessory pathway. The ablation catheter is located in the para-Hisian region of the tricuspid annulus. A six-beat drive train of atrial pacing (600 ms) followed by an atrial extrastimuli (310 ms) results in conduction block in the AP but anterograde conduction over the AV node. The *red arrows* indicate the atrial complexes. Note that His bundle electrogram is found following the atrial extrastimuli (*black arrow*). *A2,* Programmed atrial stimulus; *Abl,* ablation catheter; *A ERP,* atrial effective refractory period; *AP,* accessory pathway; *AV,* atrioventricular; *AVN,* atrioventricular node; *CS,* coronary sinus; *ERP,* effective refractory period; *HRA,* high right atrium; *RVA,* right ventricular apex; *Stim,* stimulation; *V2,* programmed ventricular stimulus; *V ERP,* ventricular effective refractory period; *X d, m, p,* the distal, mid, proximal electrode pairs of the relevant catheter.

continuous potentials comprising atrial, ventricular, and AP components. Appropriate interpretation of local potentials may also be hindered by the presence of overlapping electrograms, often seen with multiple APs and right free wall pathways, or distorted, low-amplitude fractionated atrial electrograms near the site of a prior unsuccessful radiofrequency (RF) ABL attempt. Delivery of a ventricular and/or atrial extrastimulus to promote retrograde/anterograde AP refractoriness can facilitate the separation and identification of atrial and ventricular components (Fig. 30.2). Burst pacing at a rate that achieves 2:1 AP conduction can also be deployed. A bipolar EGM alone may be misleading, particularly with the more widely spaced bipoles and/or larger electrodes on some mapping and ABL catheters—a sharp potential may represent activation several millimeters away from the electrode of interest. The use of a unipolar electrogram in conjunction with the bipolar electrogram can therefore be effective, with the presence of a QS pattern on the unipolar EGM at the site of earliest activation or a sharp AP potential on the unipolar EGM.

The possibility of both (1) an oblique AP course, with atrial and ventricular insertions located at different sites along the AV groove or (2) multiple APs must also be considered.

OBLIQUE ACCESSORY PATHWAYS

Jackman and colleagues previously demonstrated in a series that APs had an oblique course in 99 of 114 (87%) patients.[18–20] Given the oblique or slanted nature of the pathway, the ventricular insertion sites did not correspond to the site of earliest retrograde atrial activation across the valvular annuli during ventricular pacing or orthodromic tachycardia, and/or the atrial insertion sites did not correspond to the site of earliest anterograde ventricular activation during preexcitation. For most APs along the mitral annulus (posterior-septal and left free wall APs), the direction from ventricular insertion to atrial insertion follows a counterclockwise orientation (when viewed in the left anterior oblique projection, Fig. 30.3).[16,20,21] In contrast, for many of the APs along the tricuspid annulus, their

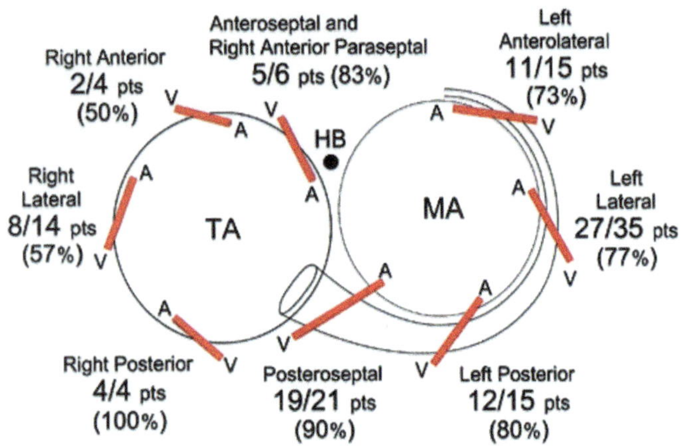

Fig. 30.3 Orientation of oblique course in eight anatomical regions. Most APs along the mitral annulus (posteroseptal and left free wall pathways) take the direction from ventricular insertion to atrial insertion in a counterclockwise orientation. In contrast, many of the APs along the tricuspid annulus (anteroseptal and right free wall pathways) take the direction from ventricular insertion to atrial insertion in a clockwise orientation. Hence, the ventricular insertion of anteroseptal and right anterior paraseptal APs is often located toward the right free wall, allowing distance from compact AV node. *A*, Atrial end of AP; *AP*, accessory pathway; *HB*, His bundle; *MA*, mitral annulus; *TA*, tricuspid annulus; *V*, ventricular end of AP. (Adapted from Otomo K, Gonzalez MD, Beckman KJ, Nakagawa H, Becker AE, Shah N, et al. Reversing the direction of paced ventricular and atrial wavefronts reveals an oblique course in accessory AV pathways and improves localization for catheter ablation. *Circulation.* 2001;104(5):550-556.)

direction from ventricular insertion to atrial insertion follows a clockwise orientation. Importantly, the ventricular insertion for anterior-septal and right anterior paraseptal APs can be located toward the right free wall, allowing effective ABL away from the septum and reducing the risk of AV block. In cases with oblique pathways, localizing the proper ABL target should be based on:

1. Identification of the atrial or ventricular insertion site on their corresponding side of the annulus using differential site pacing maneuvers, or
2. Ablation at the midportion of the pathway itself, as identified by an AP potential.

A key technique to identify an oblique AP course is to perform differential atrial pacing (pacing at two separate sites close to the annulus but on opposite sides of the site of earliest anterograde ventricular activation) and differential ventricular pacing for retrograde atrial activation. In a single AP with an oblique course, differential ventricular pacing can elicit two different local V-A intervals at the site of the earliest retrograde atrial activation. Ventricular pacing from the direction of the ventricular insertion (a "concurrent" ventricular wavefront) results in a shorter local V-A interval at the site of earliest atrial activation, and ventricular potentials and AP potentials may overlap given wavefront propagation over both tissues in the same direction (Fig. 30.4A, C, E). In contrast, pacing from the opposite side of the ventricular insertion results in ventricular wavefront propagation away from the AP shortly after activation of its ventricular end, with a reversal of the wavefront propagation direction over the AP itself (a "countercurrent "wavefront). That results in an increase in the local V-A interval and helps expose the AP potential, separating it from local ventricular activation (Fig. 30.4B, D, F).

In the presence of an oblique course, the shortest local V-A interval may not occur at the site of the most optimal target. With a concurrent ventricular wavefront, ventricular activation initially precedes the atrial activation close to the atrial insertion of the AP (CS_2 EGM in Fig. 30.4A, C). However, the local V-A interval can shorten progressively beyond the atrial insertion of the AP due to parallel wavefront propagations along the annulus (CS_d EGM in Fig. 30.4A, C, E). The shorter (or even negative) local V-A interval beyond the atrial insertion of the AP may explain the location of the fractionated atrial EGMs in many patients with prior failed ABL procedures.

Localizing the correct atrial and ventricular insertions of oblique APs can be challenging, particularly for those with prior ABL given fractionated signals after energy delivery. Therefore, targeting an exposed AP potential may allow for the highest rate of ABL success. Identifying an AP potential requires pacing maneuvers to prove the potential is not part of the either atrial or ventricular complex.[22-25] A key technique is again delivery of ventricular extrastimuli as shown in Fig. 30.5 to demonstrate:

1. A premature ventricular depolarization advances the local ventricular electrogram but did not affect the potential of interest (thereby demonstrating it is not part of the ventricular electrogram) (Fig. 30.5A).
2. An earlier premature ventricular depolarization captures the potential of interest without affecting the atrial complexes, proving that it is not part of the atrial potential (Fig. 30.5B).

A new technique for accurate AP localization is "open window mapping" using a high-resolution three-dimensional electroanatomical mapping system.[26-28] While traditional high-density mapping can be limited by the need for manual scrutiny and reannotation of signals of the chamber of interest, open window mapping automatically annotates the presumed local signal without reference to whether it represents atrial, ventricular, or AP depolarization. The technique relies on three components: (1) a high-density multielectrode mapping catheter, (2) inclusion of atrial and ventricular signals in the same window of interest, and (3) automatic annotation to the local signal with maximal dV/dt. Conduction is then visualized over the entire course of atrioventricular or ventriculoatrial conduction, and the center of the pathway can be targeted for ABL (Fig. 30.6). This technique can be particularly valuable for signals with complex deflections or in the context of slanted or oblique pathways, where short local VA or AV intervals can occur at annular sites distant from the AP based on the direction of the wavefront.

Multiple Accessory Pathways

Multiple APs are typically located unilaterally; their reported incidence is 3–15%.[29-38] Several reports suggest a higher incidence in patients with right free wall and posterior-septal AV connections,[29,32,35,36] possibly related to the presence of multiple discontinuities in the tricuspid annulus fibrosus.[39,40] Multiple APs provide the substrate for complex reentrant circuits, potentially resulting in multiple atrial wavefronts and the

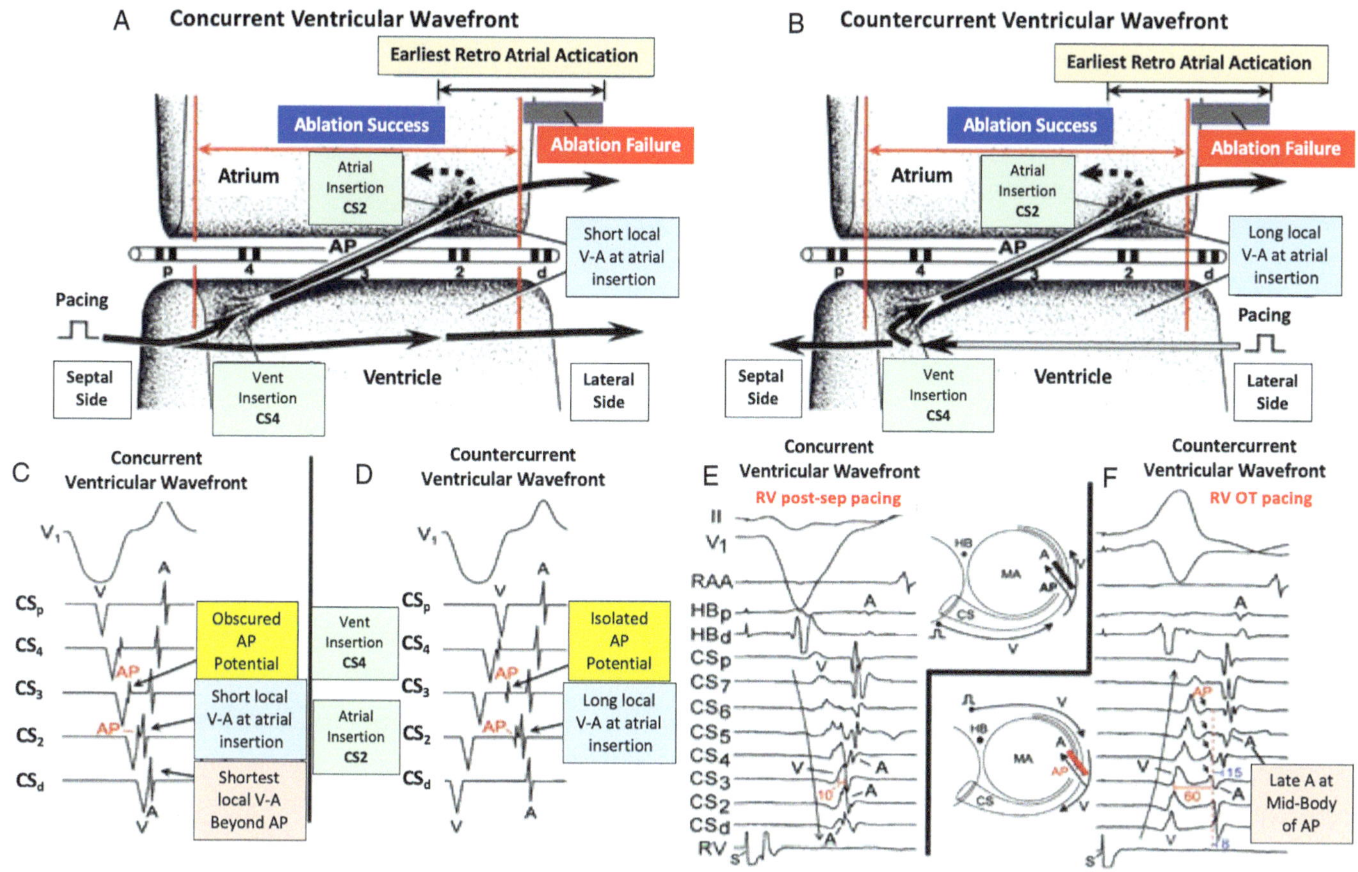

Fig. 30.4 Effects of the oblique course in a left free wall AP for two different pacing sites. (A) Ventricular pacing that produces ventricular activation and AP activation propagating simultaneously in the same direction (concurrent direction). (B) Ventricular pacing from the opposite side, reversing the direction of the ventricular wavefront (countercurrent direction). Note that during retrograde AP conduction, atrial activation propagates rapidly in the same direction as the AP due to the parallel atrial fiber orientation. This rapid atrial propagation may cause bipolar intracardiac electrograms to identify "earliest" retrograde atrial activation over a wide range, extending beyond the atrial insertion of the AP ("Earliest" Retro Atrial Activation). Radiofrequency applications in the distal half of this region (*blue hatched area*) are likely to fail to eliminate AP conduction. (C) Concordant ventricular wavefront results in an artificially short local V-A interval at the site of earliest atrial activation and the ventricular potential, overlapping and masking the AP activation potential. (D) Countercurrent ventricular wavefront increases the local V-A interval along the length of the AP, exposing the AP potential and the atrial activation sequence. (E) Concordant ventricular wavefront produced by RV posterior septal pacing. (F) Countercurrent ventricular wavefront produced by RV outflow pacing. Note the V-A interval along the AP is increased, unmasking the AP potential and the ventricular activation sequence. *A*, Atrial end of AP; *A2*, programmed atrial stimulus; *Abl*, ablation catheter; *A ERP*, atrial effective refractory period; *AP*, accessory pathway; *AV*, atrioventricular; *AVN*, atrioventricular node; *CS*, coronary sinus; *ERP*, effective refractory period; *HB*, His bundle; *HRA*, high right atrium; *MA*, mitral annulus; *RVA*, right ventricular apex; *Stim*, stimulation; *TA*, tricuspid annulus; *V*, ventricular end of AP; *V2*, programmed ventricular stimulus; *V ERP*, ventricular effective refractory period; *X d, m, p*, the distal, mid, proximal electrode pairs of the relevant catheter. (Modified from Nakagawa H, Jackman WM. Catheter ablation of paroxysmal supraventricular tachycardia. *Circulation*. 2007;116(21):2465-2478.)

development of atrial fibrillation during AVRT. Multiple APs should be suspected with the following observations during the electrophysiologic study:

1. Different patterns of preexcitation during atrial pacing or atrial fibrillation, characterized by different delta wave morphologic and ventricular activation patterns
2. Different patterns of atrial activation during ventricular pacing or orthodromic reciprocating tachycardia
3. Preexcited tachycardia using a second AP (not the AV node) as the retrograde limb of the circuit
4. Mismatch between the atrial and ventricular ends of the AP, as assessed by comparing antidromic and orthodromic reciprocating tachycardia, exceeding that expected for an oblique pathway (mismatch distance, >1 cm)
5. Change from orthodromic to antidromic reciprocating tachycardia, or vice versa[30,36]

Some APs cannot be identified during the baseline study and become evident only after successful interruption of the more dominant pathway (see Case 1). A multipolar catheter along the mitral or tricuspid annulus provides detailed information on

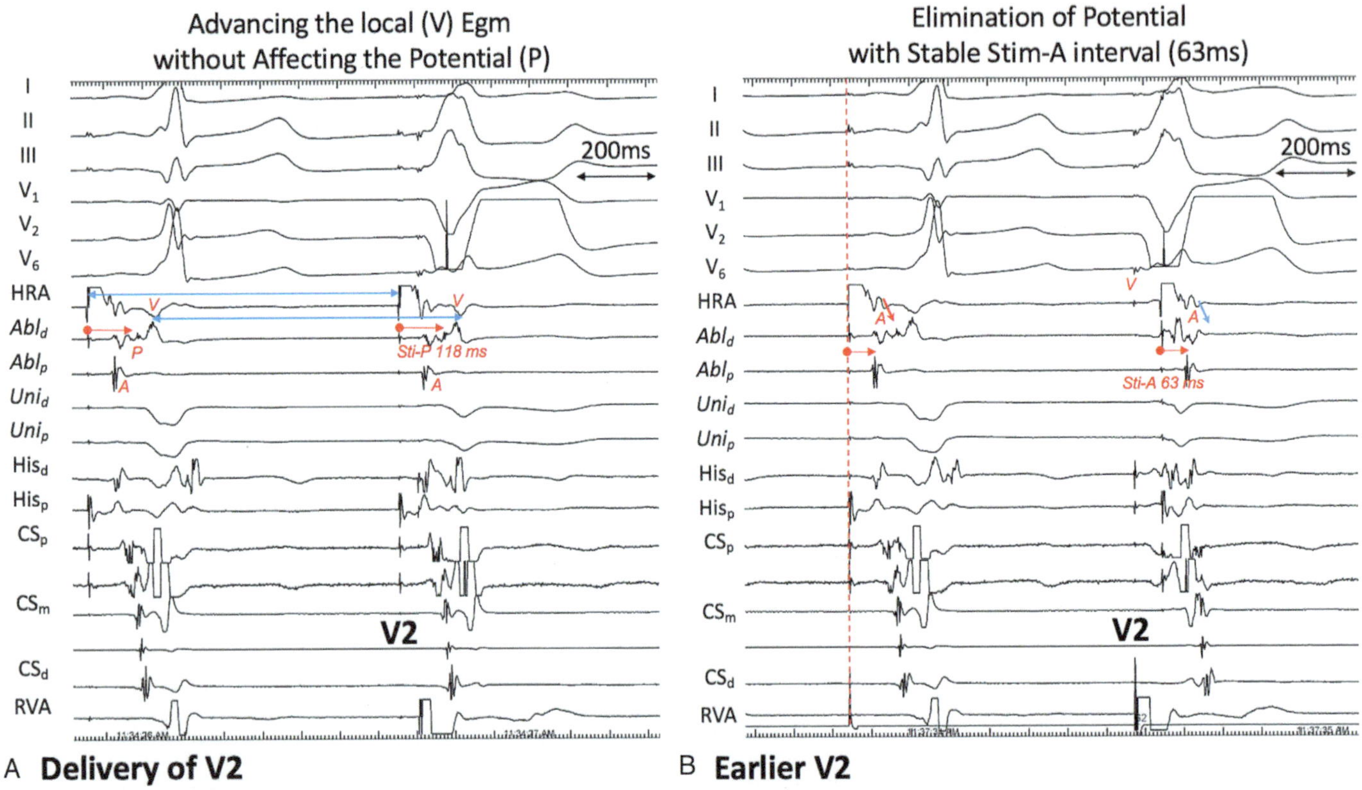

Fig. 30.5 Validating an AP potential. Intracardiac electrogram showing the response to a delivery of ventricular extrastimuli during atrial pacing. An isolated sharp potential (P) is recorded by the distal electrodes of the ABL catheter. (A) Delivery of a ventricular extrastimulus (V2) shortly after stimulated atrial complex. Advancement of the ventricular complex without change in potential shows that potential is not part of the ventricular complex. (B) Delivery of earlier V2 shows fused atrial complex without the potential (*blue arrow*); hence, the potential (*red arrow*) is not part of the atrial complex. *A2,* Programmed atrial stimulus; *Abl,* ablation catheter; *A ERP,* atrial effective refractory period; *AP,* accessory pathway; *AV,* atrioventricular; *AVN,* atrioventricular node; *CS,* coronary sinus; *ERP,* effective refractory period; *HRA,* high right atrium; *RVA,* right ventricular apex; *Stim,* stimulation; *V2,* programmed ventricular stimulus; *V ERP,* ventricular effective refractory period; *X d, m, p,* the distal, mid, proximal electrode pairs of the relevant catheter.

VA timing in addition to atrial and ventricular activation patterns at multiple sites, facilitating recognition of subtle activation changes. If such changes such as prolongation of local VA time or changes in surface delta-wave morphology are unrecognized, RF applications may be erroneously considered ineffective. Energy application at a site of optimal electrogram timing and morphology but with apparent failure should therefore raise suspicion of the presence of multiple APs, and commitment to a full-duration application should be undertaken at such a site with careful scrutiny of local VA timing or delta-wave morphologic changes. Meticulous remapping along the AV junction should then be undertaken to identify a distinct second AP.

3. UNUSUAL AP LOCATION

Pericardial Access for Epicardial Mapping and Ablation

Mapping of the posterior-septal APs using the CS or its tributaries as part of the AP connection can be challenging since the posterior-septal pyramidal space is the junction of five chambers (right atrium, right ventricle, CS, left atrium, and left ventricle). Most reported epicardial APs occur adjacent to a CS diverticulum, the middle cardiac vein (MCV), or the great cardiac vein.[41] Percutaneous pericardial access for epicardial mapping and ABL may be considered when endocardial mapping/ABL at these sites is unsuccessful (see Case 3).

Fibrous Trigone (Aorto-Mitral Continuity Ablation)

The aorto-mitral continuity and fibrous trigone have been considered to be an area with only fibrous valvular tissue, without myocardium. However, a number of APs have been mapped and successfully ablated in this region, suggesting that muscular fibers may potentially cross what is otherwise thought to be a predominantly fibrous structure.[42,43] APs that cross the fibrous trigone are rare but form a particular challenge for mapping and ABL. It is important to consider such an AP when mapping along the traditional portions of right and left AV rings does not reveal a distinct site of earliest activation, or when diagnostic maneuvers are suggestive of a left or right anterior-septal AP but multiple early sites are found.[42] Careful mapping in the outflow tracts or the sinuses of Valsalva (rather than the traditional AV ring) may reveal the ventricular insertion, which on the left side can localize at

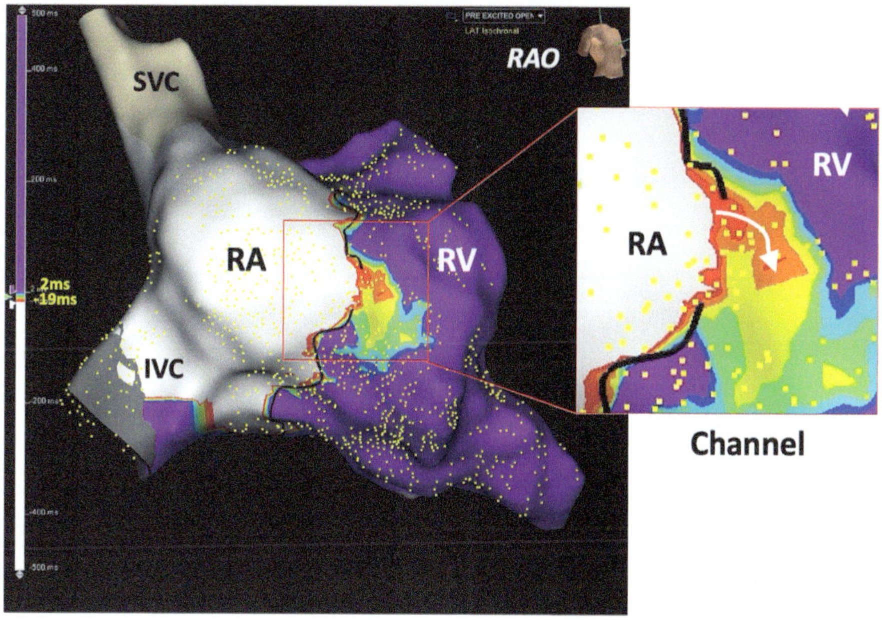

Fig. 30.6 Open window mapping technique. High-density open window mapping of retrograde conduction over a right free wall AP. Ventricular activation during sinus rhythm, demonstrating ventricular insertion at the lateral right ventricle. Electrograms recorded at a high-density mapping catheter are automatically annotated as maximum dV/dt. The *white arrow* indicates the direction of activation across the AP. Ablation at this site immediately eliminated the accessory pathway conduction. *AP,* Accessory pathway; *IVC,* inferior vena cava; *RA,* right atrium; *RAO,* right anterior oblique; *RV,* right ventricle; *SVC,* superior vena cava.

the aorto-mitral continuity.[43] Ablation of these pathways can be challenging due to the proximity of the atrial insertion to the AV node as well as the anatomically unusual site of the ventricular insertion. They can sometimes be targeted in the right or left coronary cusp as well.

Atrial Appendage-to-Ventricular APs

The atrial appendage-to-ventricular pathway is a recognized variant, most frequently on the right side. This type of AP has an epicardial course connecting the atrial appendage and the ventricular base, and ABL at endocardial sites may be ineffective. Features suggestive of this AP variant are as follows:

1. A preexcitation (anterograde conduction) pattern indicative of a right anterior or anterolateral AP
2. Earliest ventricular activation recorded more than 1 cm apical to the tricuspid annulus
3. Retrograde atrial signals in the right atrial appendage earlier than those along the tricuspid annulus
4. A relatively long VA conduction time during tachycardia, consistent with a long epicardial AP course
5. Failed or transient loss of pathway conduction with RF delivery at the tricuspid annulus

Epicardial elimination of an atrial appendage-to-ventricular pathway has been reported using a percutaneous subxiphoid approach.[44] In the previous series of 10 APs mapped via the epicardium, three were right atrial appendage-to-ventricular APs.[45] All three were successfully ablated using an epicardial approach. Another prior report demonstrated a left atrial appendage-to-LV and two bi-atrial appendage connections in three children, all refractory to endocardial ABL and all with very short ERPs.[46] High-energy delivery may be required to achieve a permanent AP elimination with an endocardial approach, and an epicardial approach can be used for those appendage-to-ventricular pathways that remain refractory to endocardial ABL.

CHALLENGING CASE PRESENTATION

Case 1: Diagnosis and Ablation of a Case With Complex Dual Accessory Pathways

A 41-year-old woman with a long-standing history of palpitations was referred for evaluation after two prior failed ABL procedures for supraventricular tachyarrhythmia (SVT). The first ABL targeted the slow pathway region for a presumed diagnosis of atypical AVNRT. A second procedure involved extensive ABL over the inferior septum and the posterior right and left atria (and CS). No evidence of anterograde preexcitation was found either at baseline or in response to atrial overdrive pacing.

During right ventricular (RV) pacing, the VA interval, defined by the time from the QRS onset to the CS proximal electrograms, suddenly prolonged from 194 ms to 260 ms with a change in the atrial activation pattern (the earliest atrial activation shifted from the proximal CS to the lateral high right atrium [HRA]) (Fig. 30.7). Two regular narrow QRS tachycardias: SVT-1A ("short RP tachycardia") with the earliest atrial electrogram recorded by the proximal CS electrodes and SVT-1B ("long RP tachycardia") with the earliest atrial electrogram recorded by the HRA were induced and alternations between SVT-1A and SVT-1B occurred throughout the study. Fig. 30.8 shows the conversion from a "long RP" SVT-1B (cycle

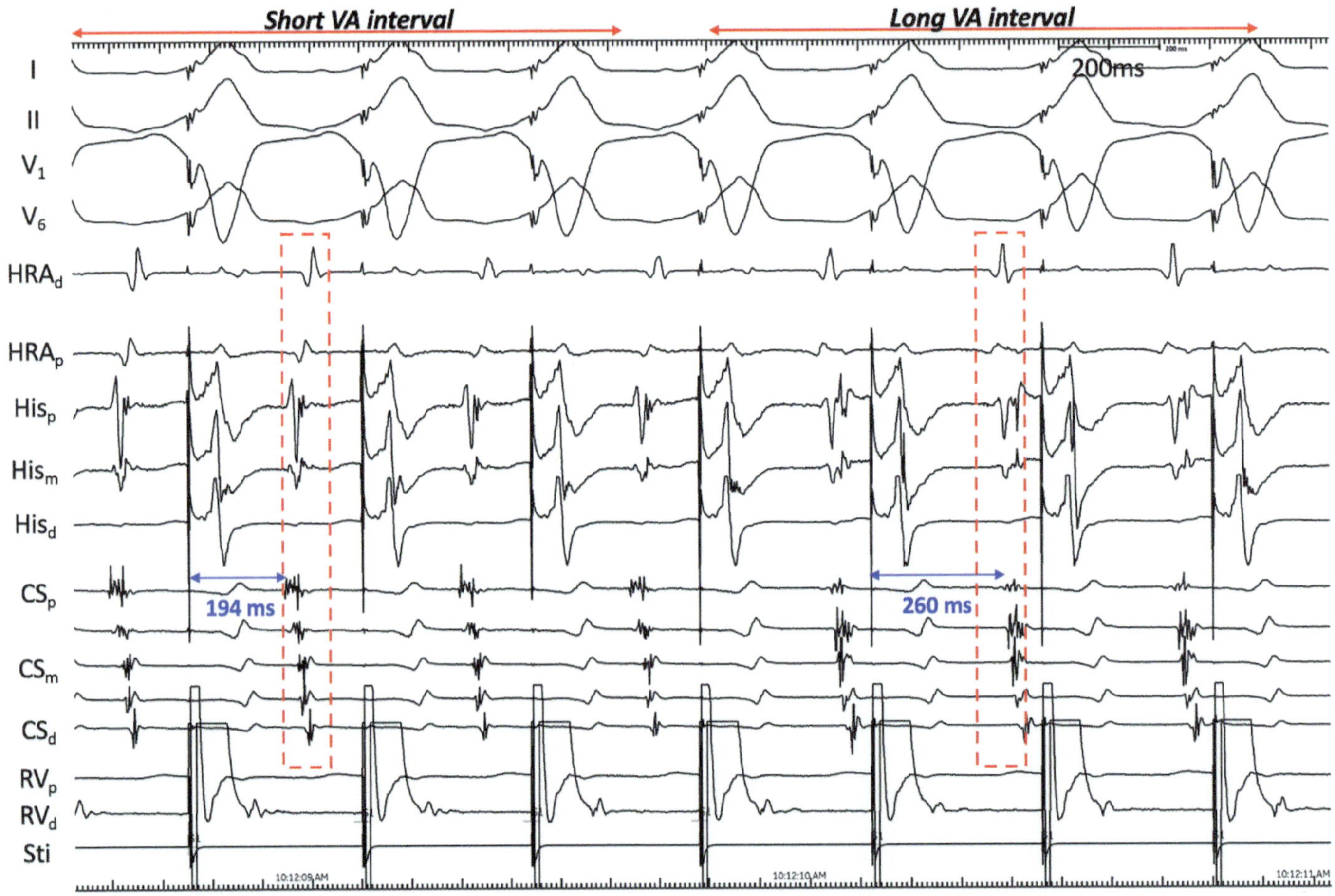

Fig. 30.7 Right ventricular (RV) overdrive pacing during sinus rhythm. The ventriculo-atrial (VA) interval defined by the time from the QRS onset to the CS proximal electrograms suddenly prolonged from 194 ms to 260 ms with a change in the atrial activation pattern (the earliest atrial activation shifted from the proximal CS to the lateral HRA). *A*, Atrial end of AP; *A2*, programmed atrial stimulus; *Abl*, ablation catheter; *A ERP*, atrial effective refractory period; *AP*, accessory pathway; *AV*, atrioventricular; *AVN*, atrioventricular node; *CS*, coronary sinus; *ERP*, effective refractory period; *HB*, His bundle; *HRA*, high right atrium; *MA*, mitral annulus; *RVA*, right ventricular apex; *Stim*, stimulation; *TA*, tricuspid annulus; *V*, ventricular end of AP; *V2*, programmed ventricular stimulus; *V ERP*, ventricular effective refractory period; *X d, m, p*, the distal, mid, proximal electrode pairs of the relevant catheter. (Adapted from Higuchi S, Po SS, Howell SJ, Scheinman MM, Hsia HH. Atrial activation detour: a tale of alternating tachycardias. *JACC Clin Electrophysiol.* 2022;8(9):1173–1184.)

length [TCL] 395 ms) to a "short RP" SVT-1A (TCL 340 ms) in response to a spontaneous premature atrial complex (PAC). SVT-1B with the earliest atrial activation at HRA and later at the proximal CS (QRS to proximal CS 210 ms), suggested the presence of a right lateral AP. Following a PAC that preexcited the septum (His), the earliest atrial activation during SVT-1A was on the septum (QRS to proximal CS 155 ms) along with a shorter TCL. The transition from SVT-1B to SVT-1A in response to a PAC argued against the involvement of decremental APs.

A steerable duo-decapolar catheter (Livewire, Abbott) was then positioned along the tricuspid annulus (TA). A His-refractory premature ventricular complex (PVC) advanced the next atrial signals by 40 ms and converted SVT-1A (TCL 343 ms) to SVT-1B (TCL 408 ms) (Fig. 30.9). The VA interval prolonged from 163 ms to 228 ms (measured to the proximal CS), along with a 65-ms increase in the TCL. However, the earliest atrial activation located at the low right atrium (bipolar TA1–2) remained constant at 142 ms during both SVTs. The prolongation of the TCL by 65 ms equals the interval prolongation between the QRS onset and CS proximal electrograms, suggesting that the atrium was part of the circuit and excluded the participation of concealed nodo-ventricular or nodo-fascicular APs. With His-refractory PVCs, both SVTs reproducibly terminated without conducting to the atrium, confirming the participation of an AP in the tachycardia circuits.

Having defined the mechanism of the SVTs, an ABL catheter (NaviStar ThermoCool SmartTouch, Biosense Webster, Inc.) was introduced into the right atrium via a deflectable sheath (Agilis NxT, Abbott) and the TA was mapped to localize the atrial insertion of the AP. Detailed mapping inside the

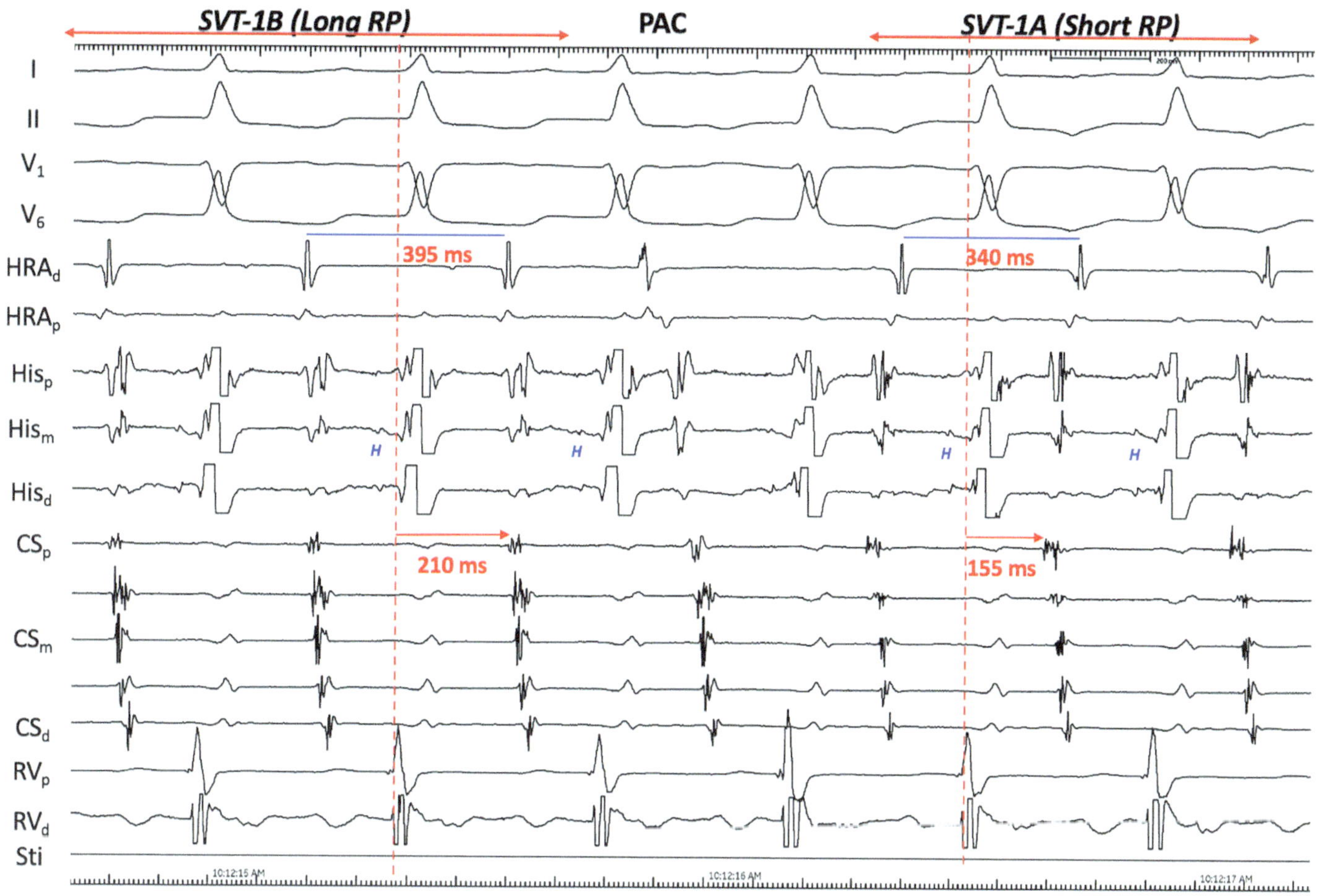

Fig. 30.8 Conversion from SVT-1B into SVT-1A. Intracardiac electrogram recordings showing conversion from SVT-1B (long RP tachycardia, TCL 395 ms) to SVT-1A (short RP tachycardia, TCL 340 ms) by a spontaneous PAC. The atrial activation was earliest at the lateral HRA with septal atrial conduction block and a clockwise atrial activation around the tricuspid annulus and late activation at the septum (QRS onset to the proximal CS 219 ms). Following a PAC that preexcited the septal (His) atrium and resolution of the block, the right atrium is activated early at the septum (QRS onset to the proximal CS 150 ms) along with a shorter SVT cycle length. *A*, Atrial end of AP; *A2*, programmed atrial stimulus; *Abl*, ablation catheter; *A ERP*, atrial effective refractory period; *AP*, accessory pathway; *AV*, atrioventricular; *AVN*, atrioventricular node; *CS*, coronary sinus; *ERP*, effective refractory period; *HB*, His bundle; *HRA*, high right atrium; *IVC*, inferior vena cava; *MA*, mitral annulus; *PVC*, premature ventricular complex; *RVA*, right ventricular apex; *Stim*, stimulation; *SVC*, superior vena cava; *SVT*, supraventricular tachyarrhythmia; *TA*, tricuspid annulus; *TCL*, tachycardia cycle length; *V*, ventricular end of AP; *V2*, programmed ventricular stimulus; *V ERP*, ventricular effective refractory period; *X d, m, p*, the distal, mid, proximal electrode pairs of the relevant catheter. (Adapted from Higuchi S, Po SS, Howell SJ, Scheinman MM, Hsia HH. Atrial activation detour: a tale of alternating tachycardias. *JACC Clin Electrophysiol.* 2022;8(9):1173–1184.)

middle cardiac vein (MCV) and CS did not show any early atrial signals during either form of SVT. Both SVT-1A and SVT-1B exhibited the same earliest atrial recordings located at the posterior-septal TA (outside the CS) (Fig. 30.10). The local electrogram recordings at the earliest atrial activation site consisted of multicomponent, split potentials, with spontaneous alternations between SVT-1A and -1B. The first and earliest signals (red arrows: 97 ms) remained fixed and represented either an AP potential and/or part of the earliest local atrial signal. The second component (black arrows) varied with the changes in the right atrial activation pattern between the two SVTs. These findings were best explained by SVT-1A and -1B having the same retrograde conducting pathway, but with intra-atrial conduction block (white block) that resulted in a detour in the atrial activation sequence.

During sinus rhythm, a sharp potential was recorded at the earliest retrograde atrial activation site on the posterior-septal TA (Fig. 30.11). A single ventricular extrastimulus delivered while the atrium was refractory resulted in no change in the potentials (blue arrows in Fig. 30.11A), proving that this potential was not part of the ventricular signal. An earlier ventricular extrastimulus resulted in an earlier activation of this potential relative to the local atrial signals (by 11 ms), along with a possible reversal in the signal polarity (Fig. 30.11B). Following an even earlier spontaneous PVC, the potential (blue arrows) appeared before the local atrial EGM (red arrows) without any changes in

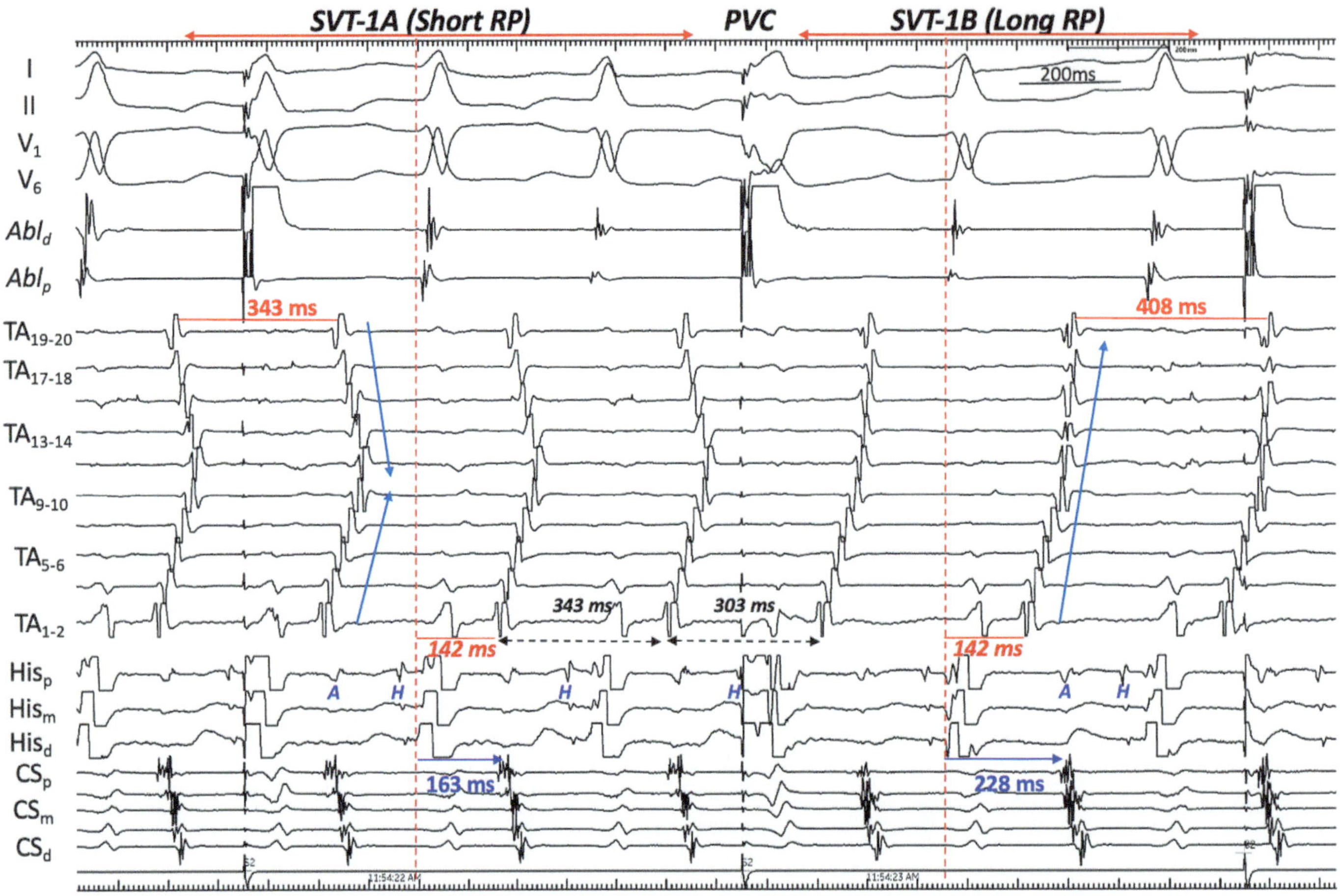

Fig. 30.9 Conversion from SVT-1A into SVT 1B. (A) Twelve-lead ECG showing SVT-1A (short RP tachycardia) and SVT-1B (long RP tachycardia). The *red solid lines* represent retrograde P waves. (B) Intracardiac electrogram recordings showing conversion from SVT-1A (TCL 343 ms, "short RP") to SVT-1B (TCL 408 ms, "long RP") by a His-refractory PVC. Following the ventricular extrastimulation, the VA interval defined by the time from the QRS onset to the proximal CS recordings prolonged from 163 ms to 228 ms, along with a 65-ms increase in the TCL. Note that the His-refractory PVC advances the next atrial signals by 40 ms at the bipolar TA 1-2 electrodes. *A*, Atrial end of AP; *A2*, programmed atrial stimulus; *Abl*, ablation catheter; *A ERP*, atrial effective refractory period; *AP*, accessory pathway; *AV*, atrioventricular; *AVN*, atrioventricular node; *CS*, coronary sinus; *ERP*, effective refractory period; *HB*, His bundle; *HRA*, high right atrium; *MA*, mitral annulus; *PVC*, premature ventricular complex; *RVA*, right ventricular apex; *Stim*, stimulation; *SVT*, supraventricular tachyarrhythmia; *TA*, tricuspid annulus; *TCL*, tachycardia cycle length; *V*, ventricular end of AP; *V2*, programmed ventricular stimulus; *V ERP*, ventricular effective refractory period; *X d, m, p*, the distal, mid, proximal electrode pairs of the relevant catheter. (Adapted from Higuchi S, Po SS, Howell SJ, Scheinman MM, Hsia HH. Atrial activation detour: a tale of alternating tachycardias. *JACC Clin Electrophysiol.* 2022;8(9):1173–1184.)

any of the other atrial signals (Fig. 30.11C). These findings suggested that this (blue) potential was also distinct from the atrial signals and therefore confirmed the presence of an AP potential.

Delivering a RF energy (30 W) at the site of earliest atrial activation on the posterior-septal TA with the AP potential recordings resulted in SVT elimination. After a 60-second RF delivery on the first RF application, the second component of the potentials (blue arrows) recorded by the ABL catheter during sinus rhythm disappeared, suggesting the elimination of the AP potential. Following this RF application, SVT-1A and -1B were no longer inducible. Moreover, cavotricuspid isthmus block was observed. However, a new SVT-2 (TCL 328 ms) was initiated with the earliest atrial activation inside the proximal CS followed by a counterclockwise activation sequence along the TA (Fig. 30.12). SVT-2 was reproducibly reset by ventricular extrastimuli with QRS fusion without any change in the atrial activation sequence, indicating involvement of an AP in the reentrant circuit. The earliest sharp signals (QRS onset–potential interval 90 ms) with multicomponent fractionated electrograms were recorded inside the CS, suggesting a different atrial insertion from that during SVT-1A and -1B (outside the CS). RF energy delivered at the second site resulted in immediate arrhythmia termination within 1.1 seconds and the elimination of the early potential. Further ventricular stimulation demonstrated VA block, and no other arrhythmias were inducible. She has remained arrhythmia free without any symptoms for

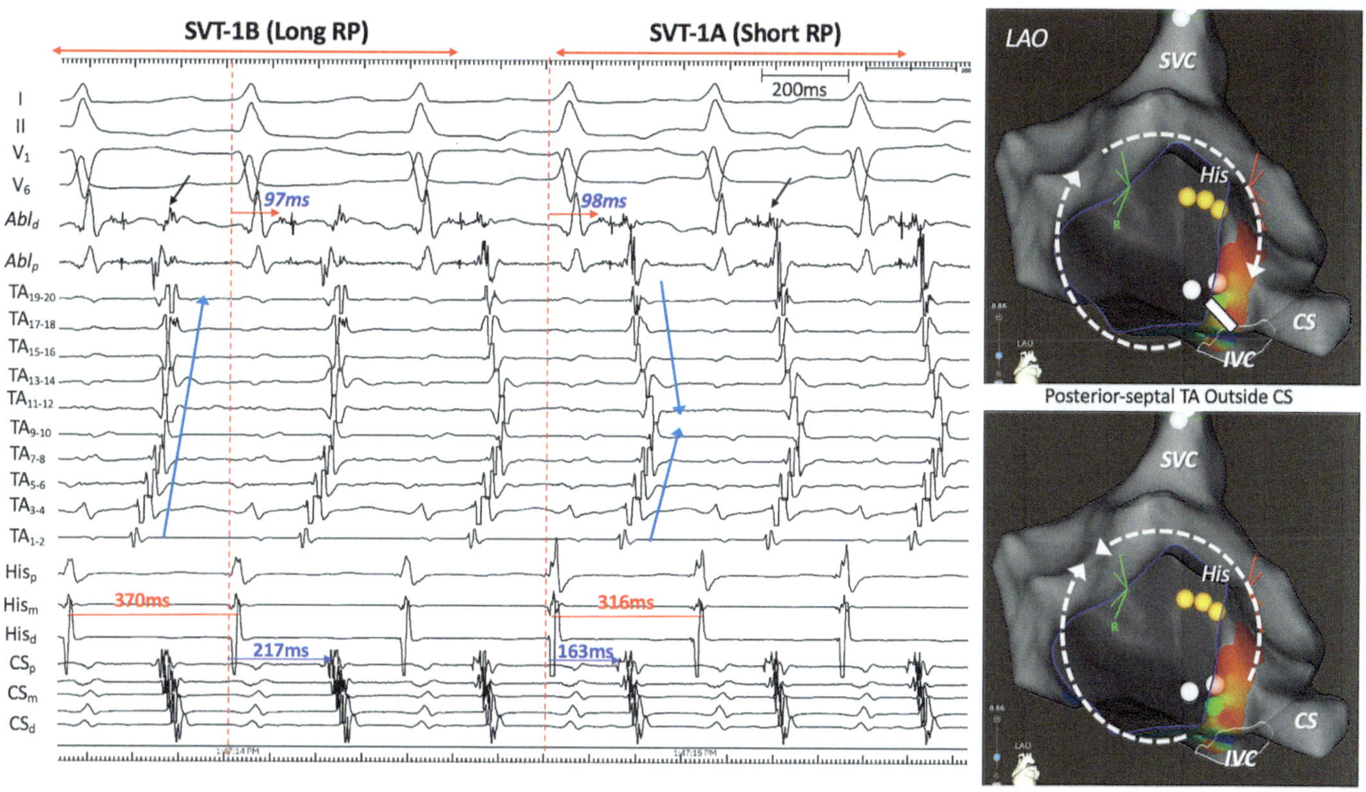

Fig. 30.10 Electrogram alternations during SVT-1A and SVT-1B. (A) Intracardiac recordings showing the earliest local electrograms recorded by the ABL catheter during SVT-1A and SVT-1B. Note that the earliest potentials (*red arrows*) are constant (QRS onset-potential interval 97 ms), while the second component (*black arrows*) alternates between the SVTs. (B) Left anterior oblique (LAO) view with the *red dots* on the posterior-septal TA (outside CS) representing the sites that exhibited the earliest local potentials. The *yellow dots* represent the His bundle. *A*, Atrial end of AP; *A2*, programmed atrial stimulus; *Abl*, ablation catheter; *A ERP*, atrial effective refractory period; *AP*, accessory pathway; *AV*, atrioventricular; *AVN*, atrioventricular node; *CS*, coronary sinus; *ERP*, effective refractory period; *HB*, His bundle; *HRA*, high right atrium; *IVC*, inferior vena cava; *MA*, mitral annulus; *PVC*, premature ventricular complex; *RVA*, right ventricular apex; *Stim*, stimulation; *SVC*, superior vena cava; *SVT*, supraventricular tachyarrhythmia; *TA*, tricuspid annulus; *TCL*, tachycardia cycle length; *V*, ventricular end of AP; *V2*, programmed ventricular stimulus; *V ERP*, ventricular effective refractory period; *X d, m, p*, the distal, mid, proximal electrode pairs of the relevant catheter. (Adapted from Higuchi S, Po SS, Howell SJ, Scheinman MM, Hsia HH. Atrial activation detour: a tale of alternating tachycardias. *JACC Clin Electrophysiol*. 2022;8(9):1173–1184.)

6 months, and her impaired left ventricular function improved after the ABL.

Case 1: Discussion

Catheter ABL of AVRTs using a posterior-septal AP can be challenging.[47] We described a complex case of posterior-septal AP with two distinct retrogradely conducing APs as well as a functional septal right atrial conduction block, likely associated with prior extensive RF ABL in that region.

In the present case, three different retrograde atrial activation sequences along the TA (a chevron pattern in SVT-1A, a clockwise pattern in SVT-1B, and a counterclockwise pattern in SVT-2) were observed. We interpreted those findings to suggest that one AP located on the posterior-septal TA was responsible for both SVT-1A and -1B and a second AP in the proximal CS was responsible for SVT-2. Mapping was complicated by the alternating SVTs with variable shifts in the atrial activation patterns and tachycardia rates. Our conclusion related to the presence of two distinct pathways rested on (1) the same earliest atrial activation for both SVT-1A and -1B, (2) identification of an AP potential for SVT-1A and -1B with the elimination of both by a single ABL, and (3) the immediate elimination of SVT-2 at a distinctly different location within the CS. The AP involvement with two different atrial insertions (SVT-1A, 1B: outside the CS and SVT-2: inside the CS) might be explained by two different APs with the second AP (inside CS) being discovered only after the successful elimination of the first AP (outside CS) or a single broad AP with separate fibers/branches, covering both the outside and inside of the CS.

Another interesting observation was the finding that changes in both the SVT-1A and -1B cycle lengths as well as the VA intervals were related to the changes in the atrial activation sequences. While SVT-1A and -1B used the same retrograde AP, intermittent functional conduction block or slowing in the posterior-septal TA region resulted in different atrial activation sequences

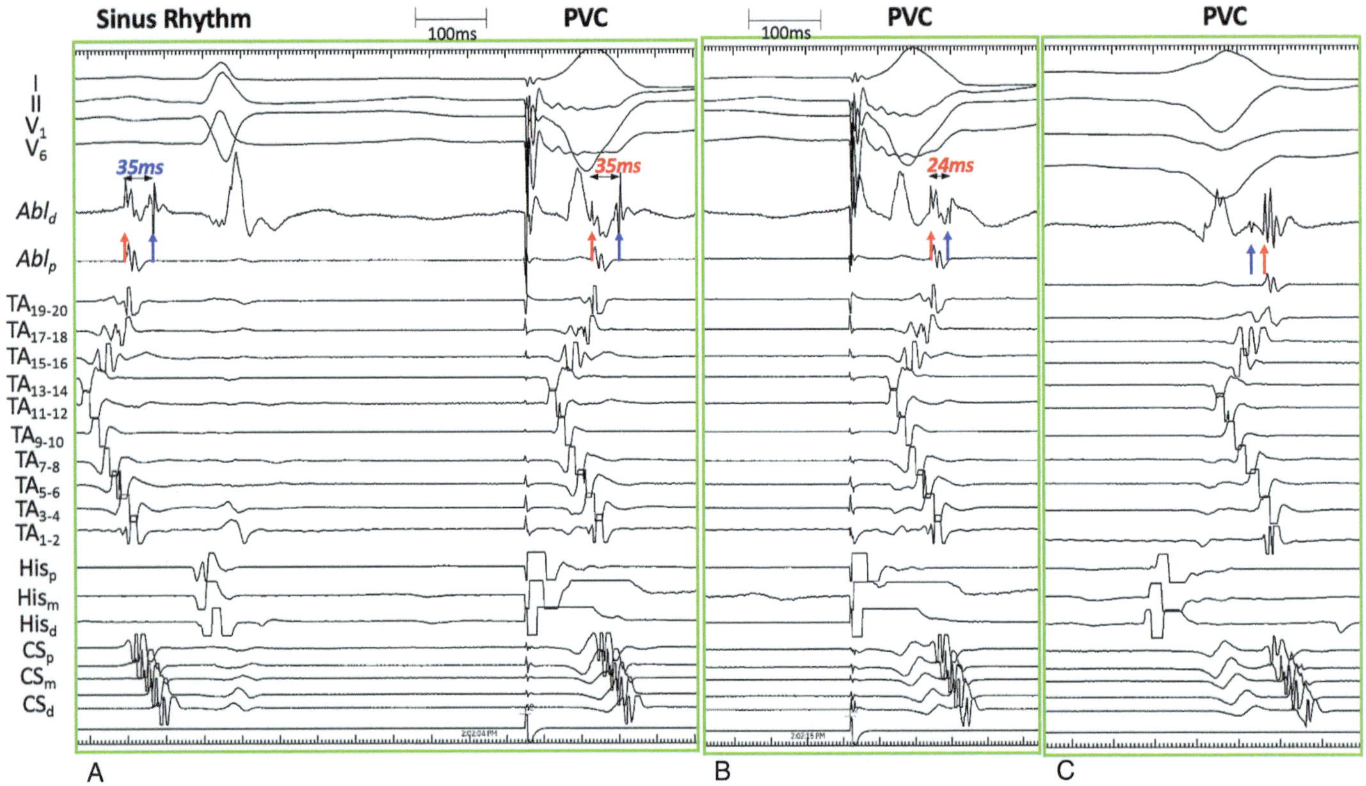

Fig. 30.11 Evidence of an accessory pathway potential. Intracardiac electrogram showing the response to a delivery of ventricular extrastimuli during sinus rhythm at the site in Fig. 30.2. (A) During sinus rhythm, an atrial (*red arrows*) and another potential (*blue arrows*) are recorded by the distal electrodes of the ABL catheter. A ventricular stimulus delivered when the local atrium is refractory results in no change in the second potentials (*blue arrows*), proving that this potential is not part of the ventricular signal. (B) An earlier ventricular extrastimulus is associated with earlier activation of the second potential (*blue arrows*) relative to the local atrial signals (11 ms). (C) Following a spontaneous PVC, the second potential (*blue arrows*) appears before the first potential (*red arrows*) without changes in any other atrial signals. (B, C) Suggests that this (*blue*) potential was also distinct from the atrial signals and therefore confirms the presence of an AP potential. *A*, Atrial end of AP; *A2*, programmed atrial stimulus; *Abl*, ablation catheter; *A ERP*, atrial effective refractory period; *AP*, accessory pathway; *AV*, atrioventricular; *AVN*, atrioventricular node; *CS*, coronary sinus; *ERP*, effective refractory period; *HB*, His bundle; *HRA*, high right atrium; *MA*, mitral annulus; *PVC*, premature ventricular complex; *RVA*, right ventricular apex; *Stim*, stimulation; *TA*, tricuspid annulus; *V*, ventricular end of AP; *V2*, programmed ventricular stimulus; *V ERP*, ventricular effective refractory period; *X d, m, p*, the distal, mid, proximal electrode pairs of the relevant catheter. (Adapted from Higuchi S, Po SS, Howell SJ, Scheinman MM, Hsia HH. Atrial activation detour: a tale of alternating tachycardias. *JACC Clin Electrophysiol.* 2022;8(9):1173–1184.)

from the same AP (Fig. 30.13). Notably, the local atrio-Hisian (AH) intervals recorded by the His proximal bipolar electrodes (125 ms) and the interval between the QRS onset to the earliest atrial electrogram in low lateral right atrium (142 ms) were constant during both SVT-1A or -1B. Those findings suggested that conduction over the AV node–His bundle axis as well as the path from the ventricle to the atrial insertion site were constant during SVT-1A and -1B (blue solid arrows in the Fig. 30.13). The intra-atrial conduction detour, therefore, was the only determinant that gave rise to the changes in both tachycardia rates and VA intervals between SVT 1A and 1B (red solid arrows in the Fig. 30.13). A His-refractory PVC with retrograde AP conduction resulted in an early local atrial activation that induced functional counterclockwise conduction block, allowing for a longer path and atrial detour toward the AV node (Fig. 30.9). Alternatively, a spontaneous PAC preexcited the atrial septum during SVT 1B with resolution of the counterclockwise conduction block (Fig. 30.8). The right atrial detour was "bypassed" and the septum was then activated early resulting in a faster SVT 1A with a different atrial activation pattern.

It has been well described that changes in the VA interval may occur with the development of bundle branch block ipsilateral to the AP site (Coumel law),[48,49] but less appreciated are the effects of the changes in the atrial activation pattern/conduction time on the VA interval and cycle lengths of the SVT. Although prior reports have demonstrated atrial activation detours and TCL changes associated with ABL-mediated conduction block, our findings differed from the prior reports which described the changes in the atrial activation patterns associated with a "fixed" conduction block in the setting of a single AP.[50–52] The challenging situation associated with "intermittent" functional conduction block in the present case required detailed and comprehensive electrophysiological maneuvers to obtain a proper diagnosis and successful ABL outcome.

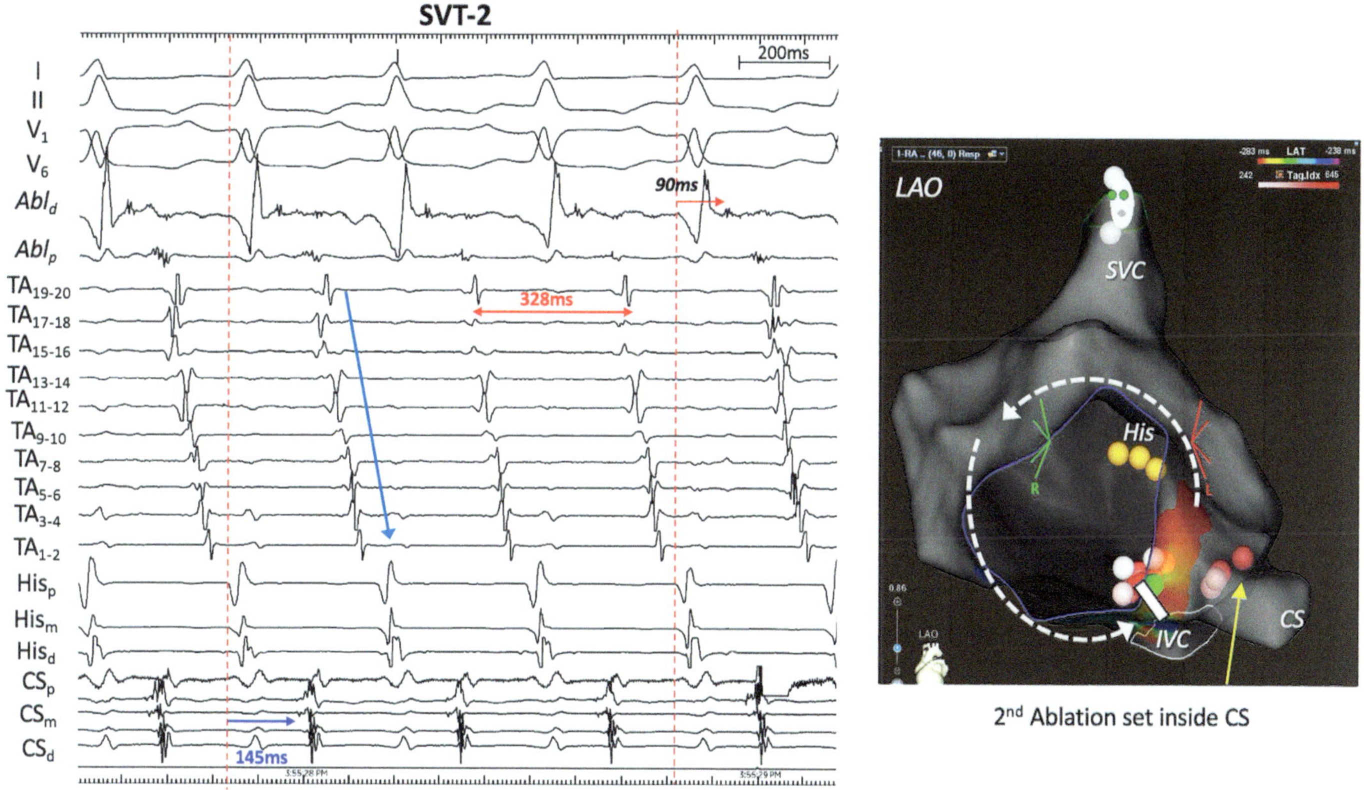

Fig. 30.12 The earliest atrial signals during SVT-2. (A) Twelve-lead ECG showing SVT-2. The *red solid lines* represent retrograde P waves. (B) An intracardiac electrogram showing SVT-2 (TCL 328 ms, short RP), which was induced after the first radiofrequency ablation on the posterior-septal TA. Following the atrial signals in the proximal CS, the subsequent atrial conduction travels along the TA in a counterclockwise direction. Note that the earliest atrial local signals recorded by the ABL catheter exhibit multiple fractionated electrograms. (C) LAO view with the *red dots* representing the site of the earliest atrial electrograms. The *yellow dots* represent the His bundle. *A*, Atrial end of AP; *A2*, programmed atrial stimulus; *Abl*, ablation catheter; *A ERP*, atrial effective refractory period, *AP*, accessory pathway; *AV*, atrioventricular; *AVN*, atrioventricular node; *CS*, coronary sinus; *ERP*, effective refractory period; *HB*, His bundle; *HRA*, high right atrium; *IVC* = inferior vena cava; *LAO*, left anterior oblique; *MA*, mitral annulus; *PVC*, premature ventricular complex; *RVA*, right ventricular apex; *Stim*, stimulation; *SVC*, superior vena cava; *SVT*, supraventricular tachyarrhythmia; *TA*, tricuspid annulus; *TCL*, tachycardia cycle length, *V*, ventricular end of AP; *V2*, programmed ventricular stimulus; *V ERP*, ventricular effective refractory period; *X d, m, p*, the distal, mid, proximal electrode pairs of the relevant catheter. (Adapted from Higuchi S, Po SS, Howell SJ, Scheinman MM, Hsia HH. Atrial activation detour: a tale of alternating tachycardias. *JACC Clin Electrophysiol*. 2022;8(9):1173–1184.)

Finally, SVT-2 was associated with a counterclockwise peritricuspid atrial activation sequence. We hypothesized that prior ABLs at the posterior-septal TA might have produced a clockwise cavotricuspid isthmus block resulting only in the counterclockwise atrial activation pattern (see Fig. 30.13). This case highlighted a complex anatomy with variable conduction delays/block in the posterior-septal right atrial region, especially in patients with a prior ABL.

Troubleshooting for Case 1: Complex Dual Accessory Pathways

Problems	Causes	Solutions
Multiple atrial activation sequences and rates during SVTs	• Dual accessory pathways • Intermittent functional Intraatrial conduction block due to prior ABLs	***Diagnosis*** • Use of a duo-decapolar catheter along the tricuspid annulus to record detailed atrial activation[1,22] • Analyze the earliest atrial activation during different atrial activation *Same: Single AP with intraatrial conduction delay* *Different: Dual APs* • Deliver His-refractory PVCs to confirm participation of APs in the circuit ***Ablation*** • Validate and target AP potentials[19–21]

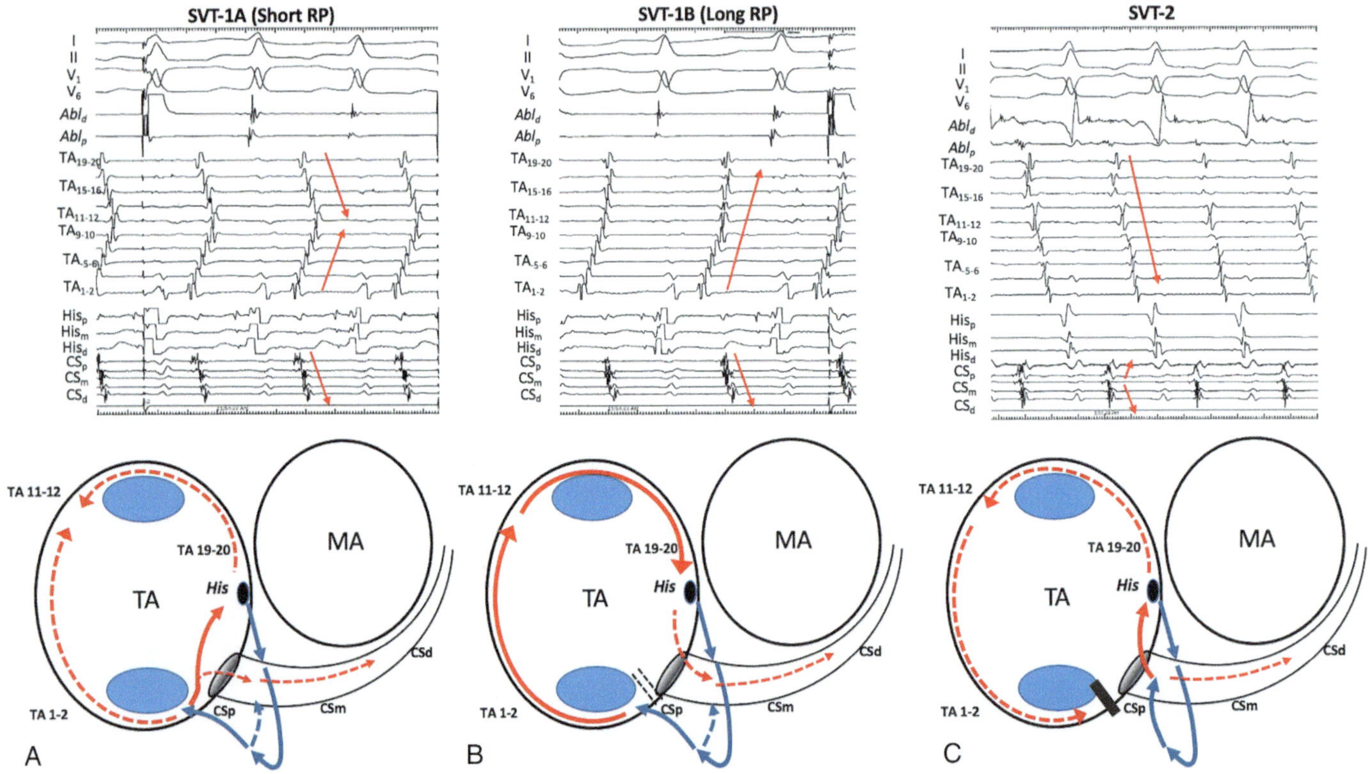

Fig. 30.13 Schema of the potential mechanism. (A) SVT-1A (short RP). During SVT-1A, the reentrant circuit uses an atrial insertion of the AP on the posterior-septal TA (outside CS) followed by atrial conduction localized at the posterior-septal region with simultaneous atrial activation of the medial and lateral TA. (B) SVT-1B (long RP). During SVT-1B, the reentrant circuit uses the same atrial insertion as that during SVT-1A, but the subsequent wavefront travels along the TA in a clockwise direction. Note that the counterclockwise conduction block or slowing at the posterior-septal TA results in depolarization of the proximal CS via the clockwise conduction along the TA. This intra-atrial conduction delay allows for a prolongation of both the SVT cycle as well as VA interval (QRS onset to the CS proximal electrograms). (C) SVT-2. During SVT 2, the reentrant circuit uses a different atrial insertion from that during SVT-1A and -1B (inside the CS). Following a breakthrough at this atrial insertion, a clockwise cavotricuspid isthmus block results in counterclockwise TA activation. The *solid lines* represent active conduction, while the *dotted lines* represent passive conduction (bystander) in the reentrant circuits. The *red lines* represent conduction in the atrium. *A*, Atrial end of AP; *A2*, programmed atrial stimulus; *Abl*, ablation catheter; *A ERP*, atrial effective refractory period; *AP*, accessory pathway; *AV*, atrioventricular; *AVN*, atrioventricular node; *CS*, coronary sinus; *ERP*, effective refractory period; *HB*, His bundle; *HRA*, high right atrium; *MA*, mitral annulus; *RVA*, right ventricular apex; *Stim*, stimulation; *TA*, tricuspid annulus; *V*, ventricular end of AP; *V2*, programmed ventricular stimulus; *V ERP*, ventricular effective refractory period; *X d, m, p*, the distal, mid, proximal electrode pairs of the relevant catheter. (Adapted from Higuchi S, Po SS, Howell SJ, Scheinman MM, Hsia HH. Atrial activation detour: a tale of alternating tachycardias. *JACC Clin Electrophysiol*. 2022;8(9):1173–1184.)

Case 2: Diagnosis and Ablation of a Case With a Decremental Accessory Pathway

A 25-year-old man presented with frequent episodes of a narrow-complex tachycardia characterized by a long RP interval and P wave that was negative in both the inferior and lateral leads (Fig. 30.14). He underwent electrophysiologic studies showing evidence of a posterior-septal AP and underwent three ABLs directed over the proximal CS as well as the posterior left and right atria. Of note, the tachycardia was no longer inducible after each procedure. However, the same tachycardia recurred, and he was referred for repeat ABL.

During the repeat study, retrograde decremental VA conduction during RV pacing was observed with the earliest atrial signal (A) at the bipolar electrode at the CS proximal (CS os). SVT was easily inducible with both atrial and ventricular burst pacing and programmed stimulation. The TCL was 480–490 ms with a septal VA time of 204 ms. The difference in the AH interval during SVT compared with pacing at the same cycle length was 25 ms. A His-refractory PVC delivered from the posterior-septal basal RV advanced the next A while comparable PVCs delivered from elsewhere in the RV failed to reset the tachycardia (Fig. 30.15). The post pacing interval-TCL was greater than 150 ms. The earliest A was located 2 cm into the CS during orthodromic reciprocating tachycardia (ORT), consistent with a slowly conducting decremental AP in proximal CS. RF ABL at the earlier atrial

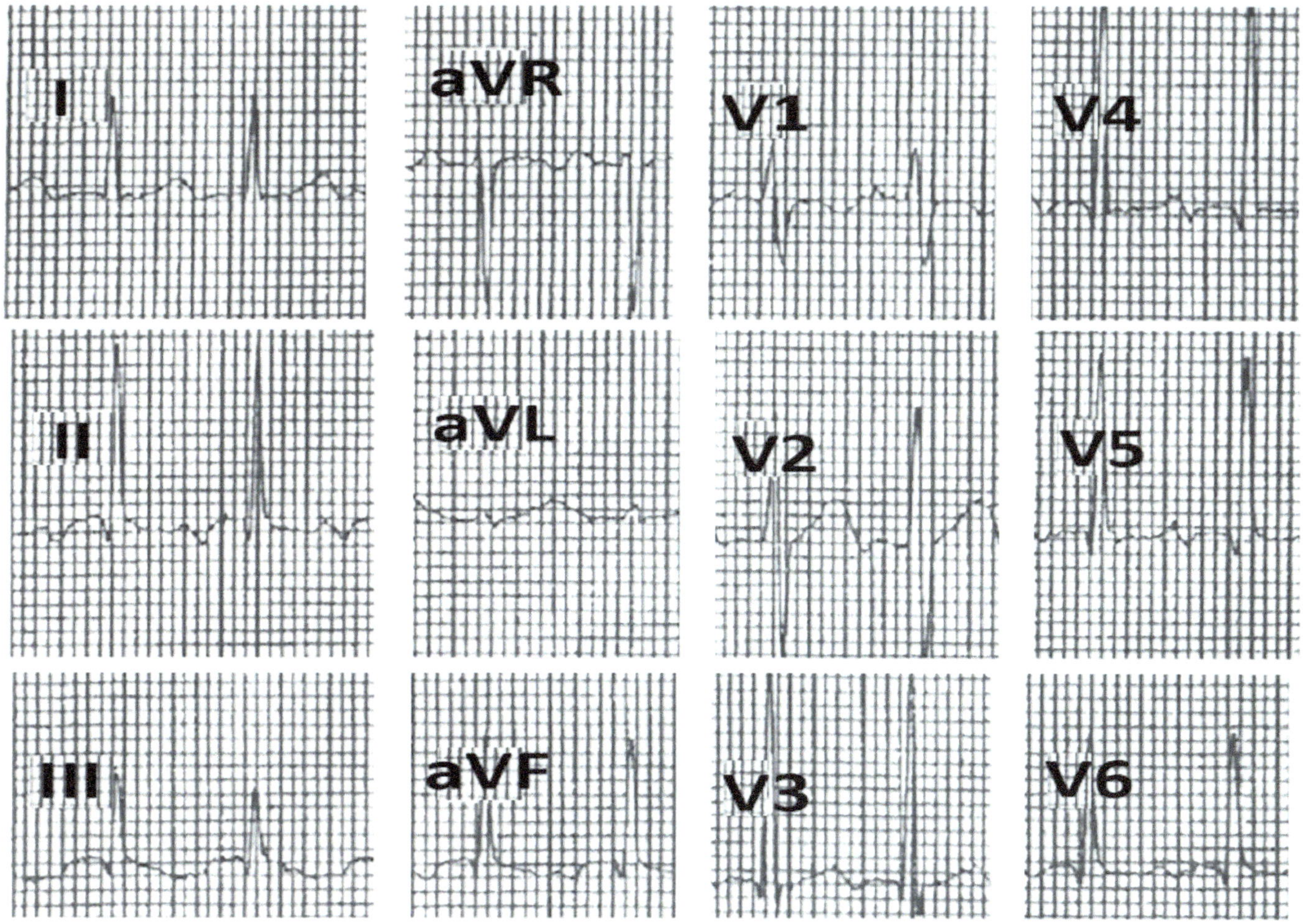

Fig. 30.14 Surface 12-lead electrocardiograms during the supraventricular tachycardia. (Modified from Oesterle A, Lee AC, Voskoboinik A, Moss JD, Vedantham V, Walters TE, et al. Electrophysiologic approach to diagnosis and ablation of patients with permanent junctional reciprocating tachycardia associated with complex anatomy and/or physiology. *J Cardiovasc Electrophysiol.* 2020;31(12):3232–3242.)

recordings in the CS 2 cm distal from the CS ostium resulted in termination of the ORT after 12 seconds, but the tachycardia was reinducible. Repeated mapping during ORT (more proximal in the CS) demonstrated a small earliest isolated potential preceding the atrial electrogram 1 cm into the CS (black arrows in Fig. 30.16). The RF application at this site led to immediate tachycardia termination and SVT was no longer inducible. Moreover, a conduction block from the potential to the atrium appeared following SVT termination suggesting that the potential was not part of the atrial Egm (Fig. 30.16). The isolated potential was also observed after the QRS during sinus rhythm. This was best explained by the disarticulation of the CS musculature from the atrium. The isolated "late" potential was depolarized via the slow retrograde AP conduction from the left ventricle during sinus rhythm with the disconnection between AP atrial insertions and CS musculature. Further RF application at the root of the CS ostium resulted in progressive prolongation of the interval from the QRS to the potential until the potential disappeared (Figs 30.16 and 30.17), suggesting that the potential was independent of the ventricular signal and confirming that the potential was an AP potential. We hypothesized that the pathway took a serpiginous course within the wall of the CS with probable multiple connections to the left atrium. We surmised that the prior ABL procedures failed because they were not directed at the root of the CS at which point the pathway originated over the CS. The patient remains without any symptoms after a follow-up of 17 years.

Case 2: Discussion

Proper differentiation of atypical (fast-slow) AVNRT from the permanent form of junctional reciprocating tachycardia (PJRT) may prove difficult. Michaud et al. described the utility of the postpacing interval (PPI)-TCL measurements as well as the difference in the RV stimulus–atrial electrogram (SA) interval during tachycardia resetting versus the VA interval during SVTs (SA-VA interval).[53] However, exceptions to these rules may occur as witnessed in our series,[2] which may require the use of specialized pacing techniques such as sequential dual-chamber extrastimulation (Fig. 30.1)[17] to prove the presence of pathway

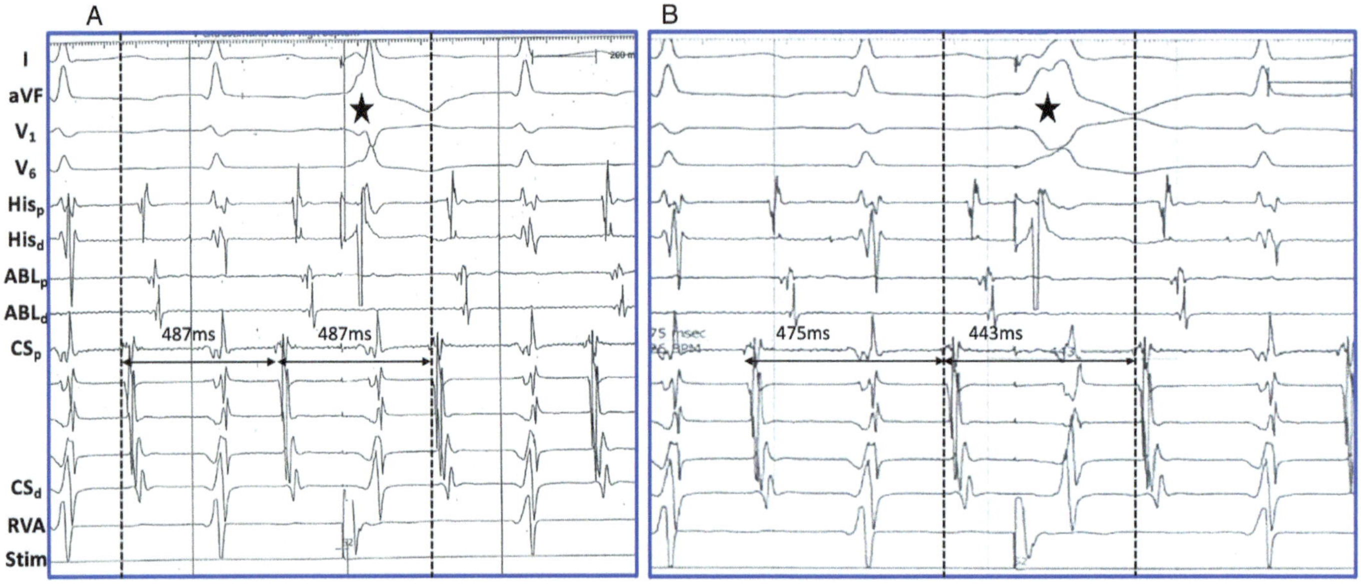

Fig. 30.15 His-refractory premature ventricular contractions. (A) His-refractory premature ventricular contraction (PVC) (*black star*) from the body of the right ventricular (RV) has no effect on the subsequent atrial depolarization. (B) His-refractory PVC (*black star*) from the posterior basal RV septum advances the subsequent atrial depolarization. *A*, Atrial end of AP; *A2*, programmed atrial stimulus; *Abl*, ablation catheter; *A ERP*, atrial effective refractory period; *AP*, accessory pathway; *AV*, atrioventricular; *AVN*, atrioventricular node; *CS*, coronary sinus; *ERP*, effective refractory period; *HB*, His bundle; *HRA*, high right atrium; *MA*, mitral annulus; *RVA*, right ventricular apex; *Stim*, stimulation; *TA*, tricuspid annulus; *V*, ventricular end of AP; *V2*, programmed ventricular stimulus; *V ERP*, ventricular effective refractory period; *X d, m, p*, the distal, mid, proximal electrode pairs of the relevant catheter. (Modified from Oesterle A, Lee AC, Voskoboinik A, Moss JD, Vedantham V, Walters TE, et al. Electrophysiologic approach to diagnosis and ablation of patients with permanent junctional reciprocating tachycardia associated with complex anatomy and/or physiology. *J Cardiovasc Electrophysiol*. 2020;31(12):3232–3242.)

conduction. From a diagnostic standpoint, two features should be noted in this case. First, His-refractory PVCs delivered from the RV near the putative atrial insertion site reset the tachycardia while PVCs from the apex did not, which is an important maneuver to prove the presence of a pathway. In addition, the difference in the AH interval between the SVT vs. atrial pacing during sinus rhythm at the same rate was 25 ms. In patients with AVNRT, this difference would be expected to be greater than 40 ms.[54,55] During PJRT, the AH interval is a true interval reflecting the sequential anterograde activation of the atrium and then the His bundle over the AV node and should be similar to the AH interval when pacing at the TCL. On the contrary, during intranodal tachycardias such as atypical AVNRT or ORT using a nodo-fascicular pathway, the AH interval is a pseudo-interval reflecting the simultaneous activation of the atrium and His bundle and therefore would be paradoxically shorter than the AH interval when pacing at the TCL or during sinus rhythm. Furthermore, a concealed left nodo-ventricular pathway should also be considered as part of the differential diagnoses. The latter pathways show features of a retrograde pathway and may have a potential inscribed between the V and A during the tachycardia.[56] However, the left nodo-ventricular pathways have a single discrete potential, which differs from what was described in our report.[56,57]

In summary, our patient presented with classic features of PJRT[58] with an atrial insertion site in the posterior septum. Histologic examinations from a patient with PJRT showed evidence of an AP that wound around the CS and was well explained by our findings.[59] Pathways in this region may present special problems. First, these pathways may show early near-simultaneous activation over the CS as well as the contiguous regions of the posterior septal right or left atrium. Sun et al. have emphasized the importance of searching for a common origin of these pathways from connections involving the walls of the middle or posterior cardiac veins which act as conduits from the ventricle to the muscular coats of the CS and connections to the adjacent right and left atria.[60] As they pointed out, it is very difficult to completely disarticulate the extensive connections between the CS myocardial coat and the atria, and emphasized the importance of catheter recordings to locate the intermediary CS connections between the atria and ventricles in order to achieve successful ABL. In our case there was no effort made to disarticulate the muscular connections between the CS and atria but instead targeted the discrete potentials within the CS. This case nicely illustrates both the diagnostic and therapeutic challenges associated with pathways in the posterior-septal region.

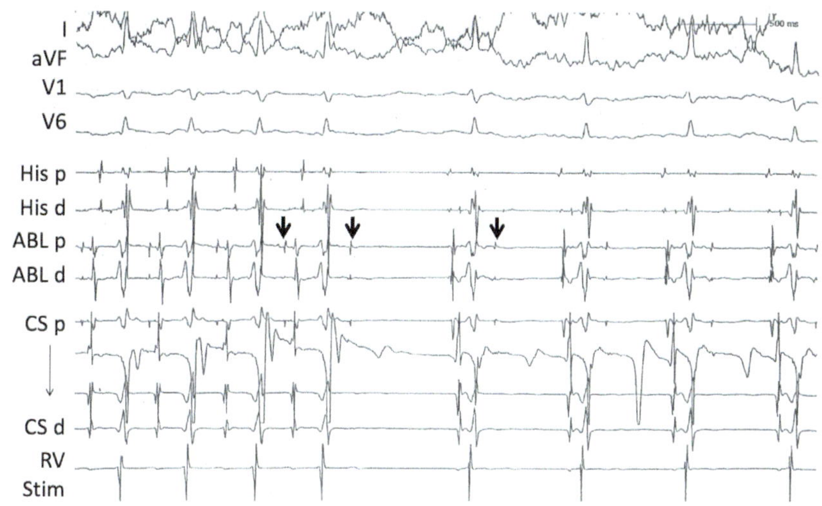

Fig. 30.16 Intracardiac electrogram showing the earliest isolated potential during the tachycardia. During ablation at the earliest site in the CS, tachycardia terminates with block from the potential (*arrow*) to the atrium and the potential is also observed after the QRS during sinus rhythm. *A*, Atrial end of AP; *A2*, programmed atrial stimulus; *Abl*, ablation catheter; *A ERP*, atrial effective refractory period; *AP*, accessory pathway; *AV*, atrioventricular; *AVN*, atrioventricular node; *CS*, coronary sinus; *ERP*, effective refractory period; *HB*, His bundle; *HRA*, high right atrium; *MA*, mitral annulus; *RVA*, right ventricular apex; *Stim*, stimulation; *TA*, tricuspid annulus; *V*, ventricular end of AP; *V2*, programmed ventricular stimulus; *V ERP*, ventricular effective refractory period; *X d, m, p*, the distal, mid, proximal electrode pairs of the relevant catheter. (Modified from Oesterle A, Lee AC, Voskoboinik A, Moss JD, Vedantham V, Walters TE, et al. Electrophysiologic approach to diagnosis and ablation of patients with permanent junctional reciprocating tachycardia associated with complex anatomy and/or physiology. *J Cardiovasc Electrophysiol.* 2020;31(12):3232–3242.)

Troubleshooting for Case 2: A Decremental Accessory Pathway

Problems	Causes	Solutions
Long RP tachycardia: PJRT with long PPI-TCL interval (>115 ms)	AP with decremental retrograde VA conduction	***Diagnosis*** • Ventricular pacing from the RV base (near the putative atrial insertion site)[38,39] • Analyze the AH interval during sinus rhythm/atrial pacing vs SVT o $AH_{(A\ pacing)} - AH_{(SVT)} > 40$ ms o AH interval during an SVT < during sinus rhythm likely AVNRT[55,56] • Sequential dual-chamber extrastimulation[17] ***Ablation*** • Target the AP potential (inside the CS)[19–21]

Case 3: Diagnosis and Ablation of a Case With an Epicardial Accessory Pathway

A 48-year-old woman with a history of Wolff-Parkinson-White (WPW) syndrome presented with recurrent palpitations. She had undergone multiple attempts at catheter ABL, with transient suppression and recurrence of preexcitation shortly after each prior ABL attempt. The prior ABL sites included mid-septal and posterior-septal sites in both the right and left atria.

The patient presented for a repeat catheter ABL. Her baseline electrocardiogram demonstrated preexcitation, with a QRS transition between V_1 and V_2, a positive delta wave in lead II, and positive-negative deflections in leads III and aVF (Fig. 30.18). In the electrophysiology lab, quadripolar catheters were placed at the His and RV apex and a decapolar catheter was positioned in the CS. Preprocedural imaging had demonstrated stenosis of the CS ostium that was suspected to be the result of prior ABL.

The baseline AH interval was 69 ms and His-ventricle (HV) interval was 0 ms (Fig. 30.19A). Atrial pacing from the distal CS at a cycle length of 280 ms resulted in the maximal preexcitation and intermittent anterograde AP block, with more positive delta waves inferiorly (Fig. 30.19B). Ventricular pacing at a cycle length of 500 ms demonstrated 1:1 VA conduction with a VA time of 130 ms and earliest atrial activation recorded on the CS 7, 8 bipole, positioned just inside the CS ostium (Figs. 30.20 and 30.21). Electrophysiologic maneuvers failed to induce any sustained supraventricular tachycardia. Transseptal access was obtained, and a 3.5-mm deflectable, irrigated ABL catheter (TactiCath, Abbott) was advanced into the left atrium and left ventricle for additional mapping. Low-amplitude electrograms were noted along the posteromedial mitral annulus, likely due to prior ABLs. A broad area of early left atrial activation was identified during RV pacing, simultaneous with that on the CS 7, 8 bipole. RF applications were delivered at sites with early

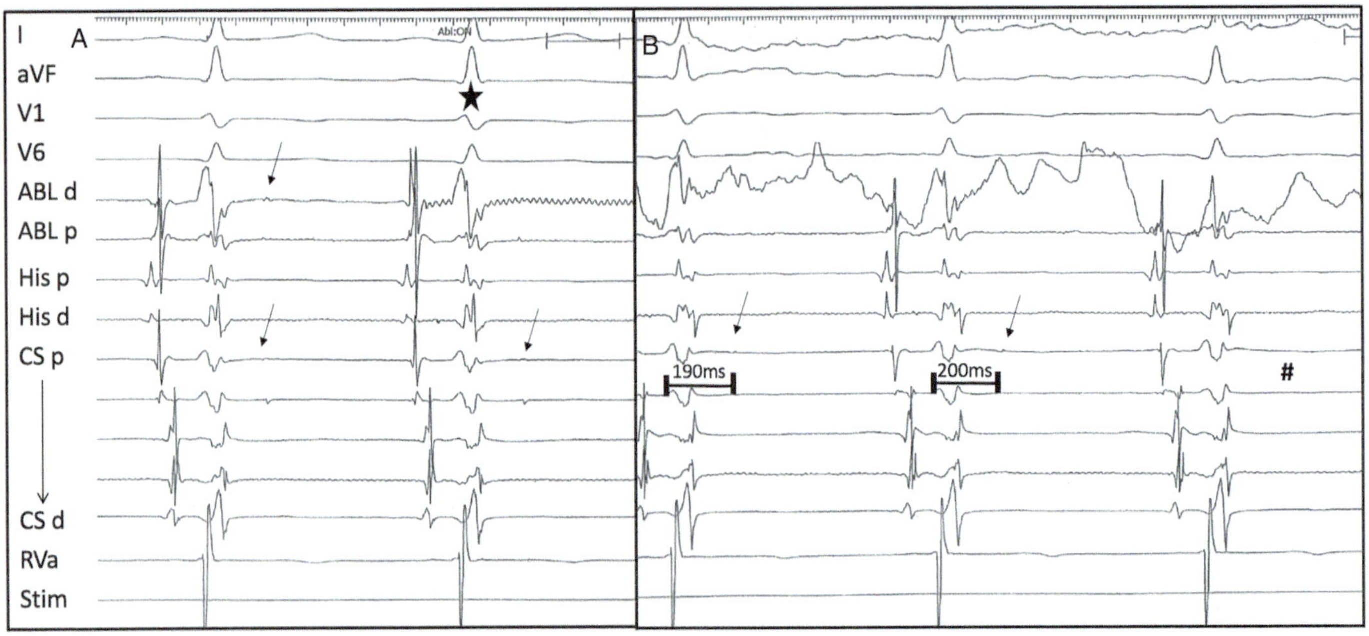

Fig. 30.17 CS potential. (A) Intracardiac electrogram showing an isolated late potential (*black arrows*) with ablation (*black star*) during sinus rhythm at the earliest potential location in the proximal CS. (B) With the ablation, the ventricular to potential time prolonged before the potential disappeared (#), demonstrating that the potential is independent of the ventricular signal and confirming it is an AP potential. *A*, Atrial end of AP; *A2*, programmed atrial stimulus; *Abl*, ablation catheter; *A ERP*, atrial effective refractory period; *AP*, accessory pathway; *AV*, atrioventricular; *AVN*, atrioventricular node; *CS*, coronary sinus; *ERP*, effective refractory period; *HB*, His bundle; *HRA*, high right atrium; *MA*, mitral annulus; *RVA*, right ventricular apex; *Stim*, stimulation; *TA*, tricuspid annulus; *V*, ventricular end of AP; *V2*, programmed ventricular stimulus; *V ERP*, ventricular effective refractory period; *X d, m, p*, the distal, mid, proximal electrode pairs of the relevant catheter. (Adapted from Oesterle A, Lee AC, Voskoboinik A, Moss JD, Vedantham V, Walters TE, et al. Electrophysiologic approach to diagnosis and ablation of patients with permanent junctional reciprocating tachycardia associated with complex anatomy and/or physiology. *J Cardiovasc Electrophysiol.* 2020;31(12):3232–3242.)

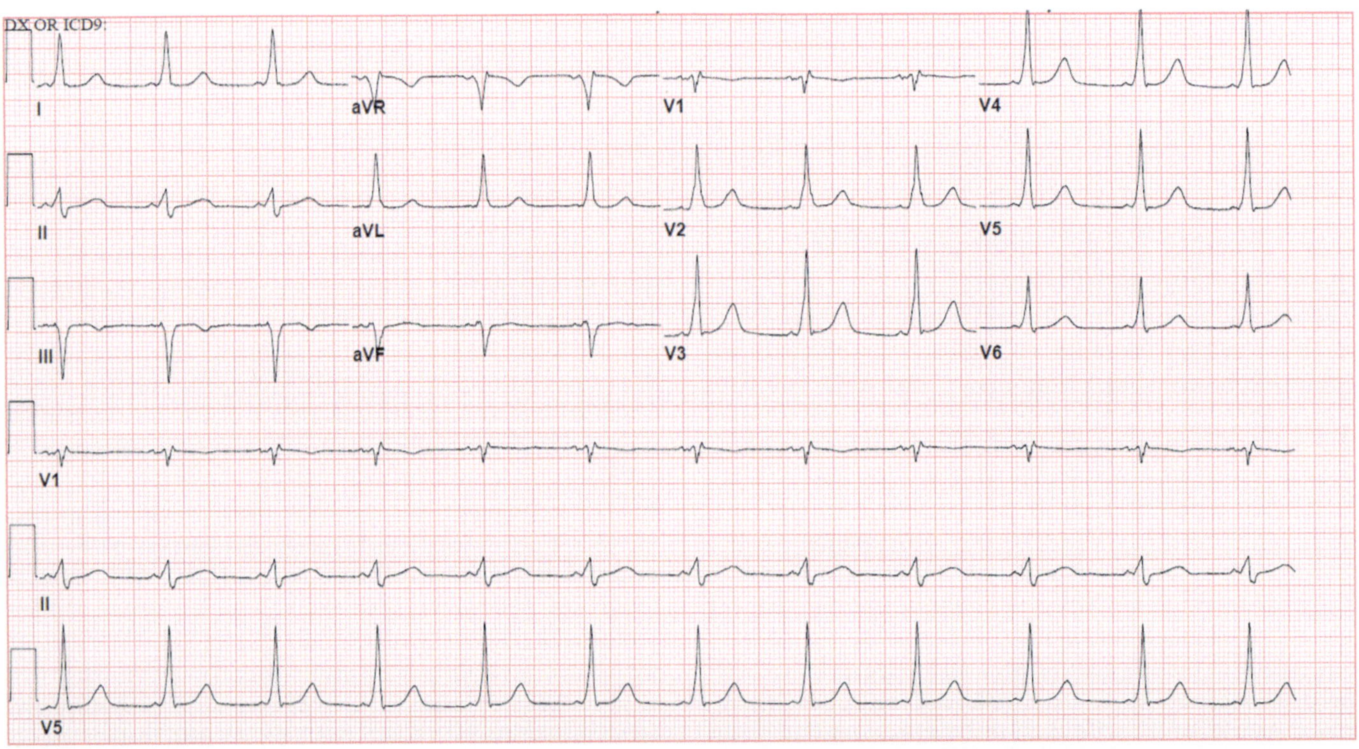

Fig. 30.18 Baseline 12-lead electrocardiogram demonstrating preexcitation.

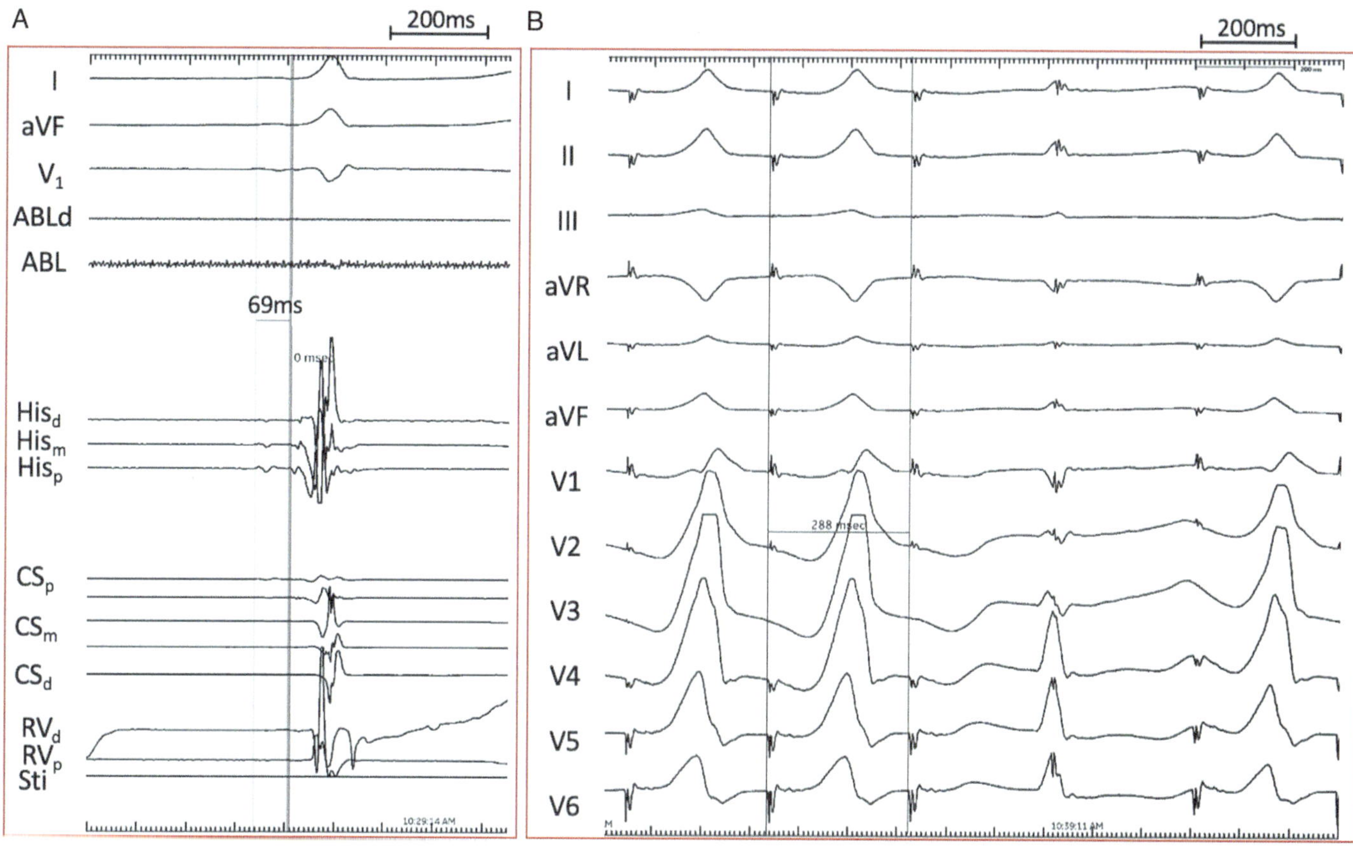

Fig. 30.19 Baseline intracardiac electrograms (A) and maximal preexcitation (B) during pacing from the distal coronary sinus with intermittent block in the accessory pathway. Note the proximal to distal HB activation sequence. *A*, Atrial end of AP; *A2*, programmed atrial stimulus; *Abl*, ablation catheter; *A ERP*, atrial effective refractory period; *AP*, accessory pathway; *AV*, atrioventricular; *AVN*, atrioventricular node; *CS*, coronary sinus; *ERP*, effective refractory period; *HB*, His bundle; *HRA*, high right atrium; *MA*, mitral annulus; *RVA*, right ventricular apex; *Stim*, stimulation; *TA*, tricuspid annulus; *V*, ventricular end of AP; *V2*, programmed ventricular stimulus; *V ERP*, ventricular effective refractory period; *X d, m, p*, the distal, mid, proximal electrode pairs of the relevant catheter.

atrial activation without any effect. Similar atrial timing during RV pacing was noted along the right postero-septum, and several lesions were delivered resulting in a slow junctional rhythm but had no effect on the AP conduction (Fig. 30.21).

Using a micropuncture needle, a subxiphoid pericardial puncture was performed, and a steerable sheath and the ABL catheter were positioned for epicardial mapping. The ABL catheter was maneuvered to the basal crux, opposite the CS 7, 8 bipole (Fig. 30.22). There was a complex three-component electrogram at this site during sinus rhythm (Fig. 30.22A), and ventricular pacing immediately adjacent to this site resembled maximal preexcitation (Fig. 30.22B), with inferiorly directed QRS complexes. Coronary angiography demonstrated no large coronary artery branches in close proximity to the site of interest. ABL applications were delivered (35 W), with the loss of pr-excitation within 2 seconds (Fig. 30.23). There was no recurrent preexcitation during an adenosine-mediated AV block or following a prolonged waiting period, and the patient has had no recurrence of similar symptoms after 10 months.

Case 3: Discussion

We present a challenging case of an AP in a patient with multiple prior failed ABL attempts. The baseline ECG was suggestive of a posterior- or mid-septal AP, and the maximum preexcitation during atrial pacing was suggestive of an even more anterior site. Endocardial mapping showed a broad area of the early retrograde atrial activation posterior-septally on both the right and left sides. After several unsuccessful endocardial applications, epicardial mapping demonstrated a markedly early and complex three-component signal at the basal crux, and the AP conduction was successfully eliminated there.

Accessory pathways are epicardial structures but are typically accessible from the endocardium when positioned immediately adjacent to the tricuspid or mitral valve annulus or within the CS.[61] However, prior ABL attempts in this case may have resulted in endocardial scar, limiting both the ability to visualize the electrograms and deliver energy from the endocardium. Epicardial access is a safe and alternative approach for AP ABL, particularly when endocardial approaches have failed.[61,62] In a case series of 21 patients referred for epicardial AP ABL, epicardial ABL was successful in 6 patients and helped guide a successful subsequent endocardial ABL in another two patients.[61] Other case reports have demonstrated a successful epicardial ABL of posterior-septal APs, with tissue histology confirming the epicardial location of the pathway.[62]

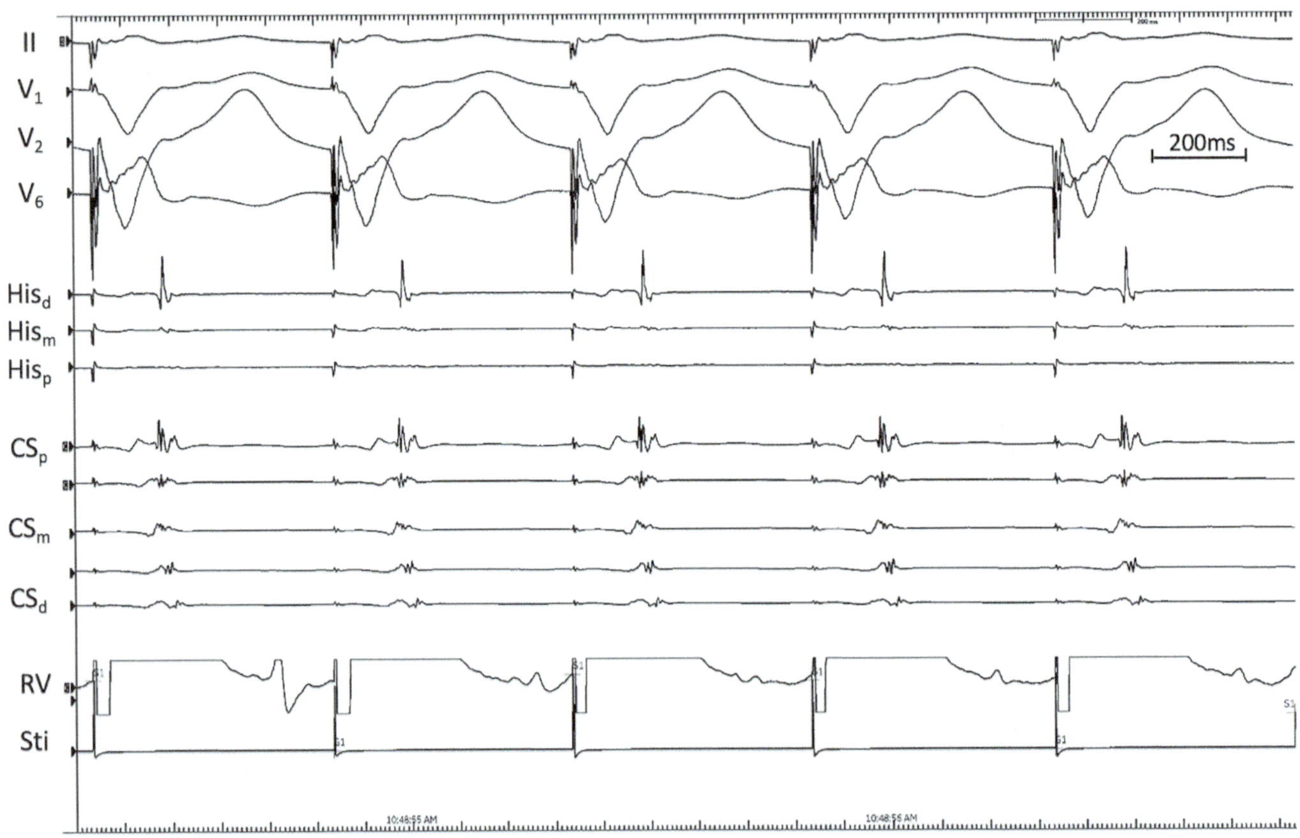

Fig. 30.20 Ventricular pacing demonstrated the earliest atrial activation at CS 7, 8. *A*, Atrial end of AP; *A2*, programmed atrial stimulus; *Abl*, ablation catheter; *A ERP*, atrial effective refractory period; *AP*, accessory pathway; *AV*, atrioventricular; *AVN*, atrioventricular node; *CS*, coronary sinus; *ERP*, effective refractory period; *HB*, His bundle; *HRA*, high right atrium; *MA*, mitral annulus; *RVA*, right ventricular apex; *Stim*, stimulation; *TA*, tricuspid annulus; *V*, ventricular end of AP; *V2*, programmed ventricular stimulus; *V ERP*, ventricular effective refractory period; *X d, m, p*, the distal, mid, proximal electrode pairs of the relevant catheter.

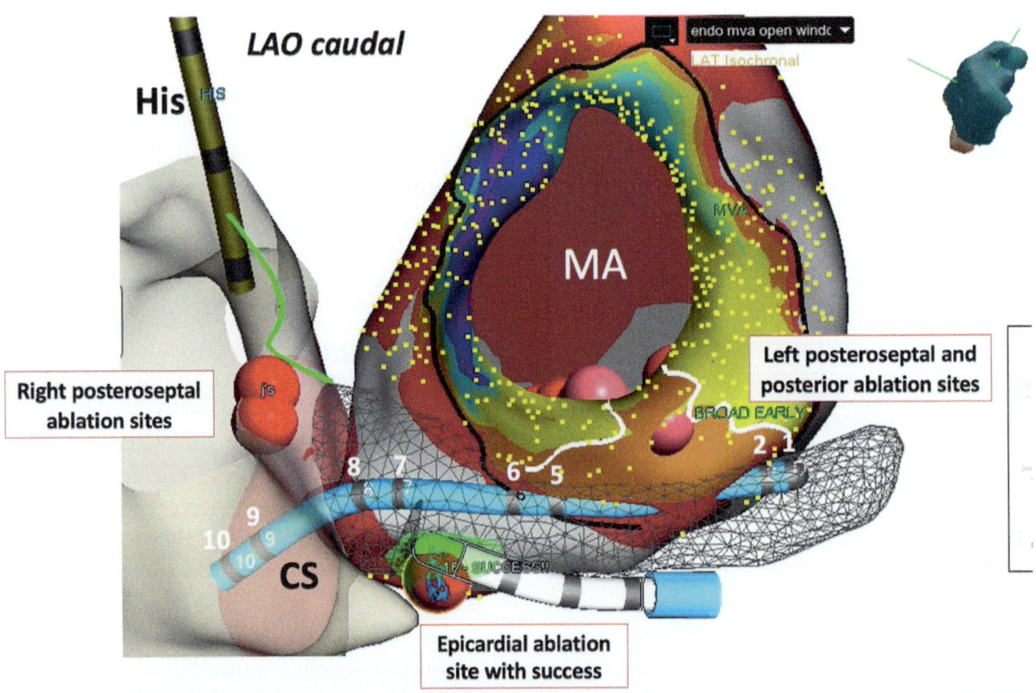

Fig. 30.21 Electroanatomical map demonstrating the right posteroseptal, left posteroseptal and posterior, and epicardial ablation sites (epicardial sites adjacent to the earliest activation along the CS catheter). *CS*, Coronary sinus; *LAO*, left anterior oblique; *MA*, mitral annulus.

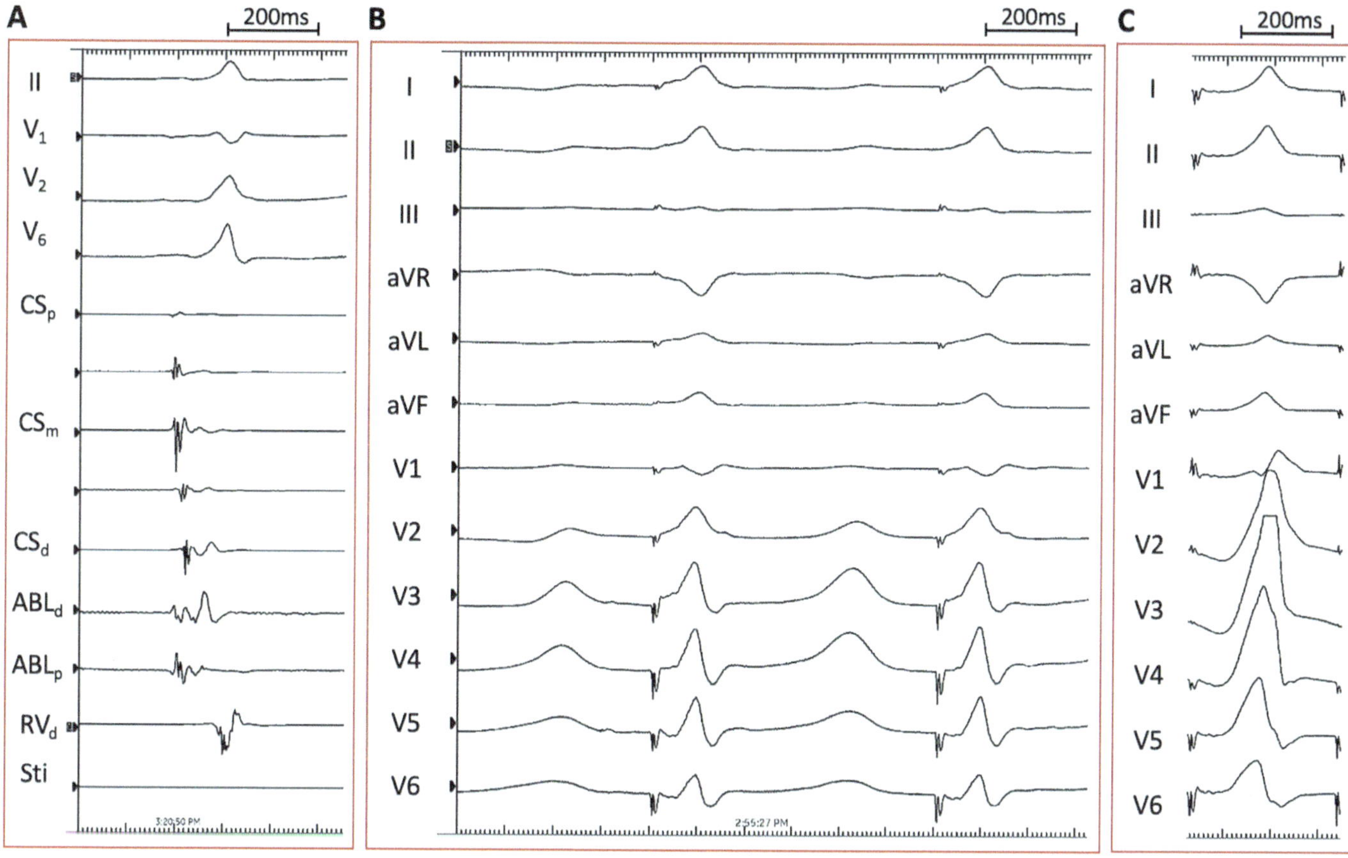

Fig. 30.22 Complex electrograms at the epicardial ablation site (A), with ventricular pacing from the epicardium, immediately ventricular to the early activation site (B), demonstrating a QRS morphology resembling the maximal preexcitation (C). *A*, Atrial end of AP; *A2*, programmed atrial stimulus; *Abl*, ablation catheter; *A ERP*, atrial effective refractory period; *AP*, accessory pathway; *AV*, atrioventricular; *AVN*, atrioventricular node; *CS*, coronary sinus; *ERP*, effective refractory period; *HB*, His bundle; *HRA*, high right atrium; *MA*, mitral annulus; *RVA*, right ventricular apex; *Stim*, stimulation; *TA*, tricuspid annulus; *V*, ventricular end of AP; *V ERP*, ventricular effective refractory period; *X d, m, p*, the distal, mid, proximal electrode pairs of the relevant catheter.

As the CS is itself an epicardial structure, ABL of posterior-septal APs within the CS and associated diverticula can be a strategy to achieve AP block.[63,64] In a cohort of 110 patients with posterior-septal APs, Pascale et al. reported 13 patients (12%) in whom ABL from within the CS was necessary.[65] CS access was not pursued in our case due to preexisting stenosis at the CS ostium noted on preprocedural imaging, likely the result of a prior ABLs. In cases where access to the CS is not practical, an epicardial approach has been successful.[66] As in this case, the lack of a discrete site of early atrial activation should prompt additional mapping in adjacent structures, including the epicardial space.

Analysis of the surface ECG delta-wave polarity typically assists with the septal AP localization and procedural planning. A negative delta wave in at least two inferior leads is suggestive of a posterior-septal AP, with APs localized to the CS and/or associated diverticula typically manifesting deep negative delta wave in all three inferior leads.[66] Anterior-septal AP activation typically results in a positive delta wave in the inferior leads, with progressive loss of the positive deflection (beginning with lead III, then aVF) for pathways in mid-septal space. In this case, prior ABLs and cardiac rotation may have resulted in the misleading ECG, with inferiorly directed positive delta waves, particularly during periods of maximum preexcitation. This was more consistent with a mid- or even anterior-septal location. A slanted pathway with more disparate atrial and ventricular insertion sites should also be considered, particularly when targeting an AP near the AV node or His bundle; in this case, however both early anterograde and retrograde activation were mapped posteriorly.

Troubleshooting for Case 3: An Epicardial Accessory Pathway

Problems	Causes	Solutions

Diffusely early endocardial activation	Epicardial AP	• Detailed mapping in the posterior septum region
		• Additional mapping in adjacent structures:
		  ○ Left atrium via a transseptal puncture
		  ○ Inside the coronary sinus[66]
		  ○ Middle (posterior) cardiac vein[64]
		  ○ CS diverticulum[65]
		  ○ Epicardial basal crux[62,66]

Stenosis at the CS ostium	Prior CS ABL	

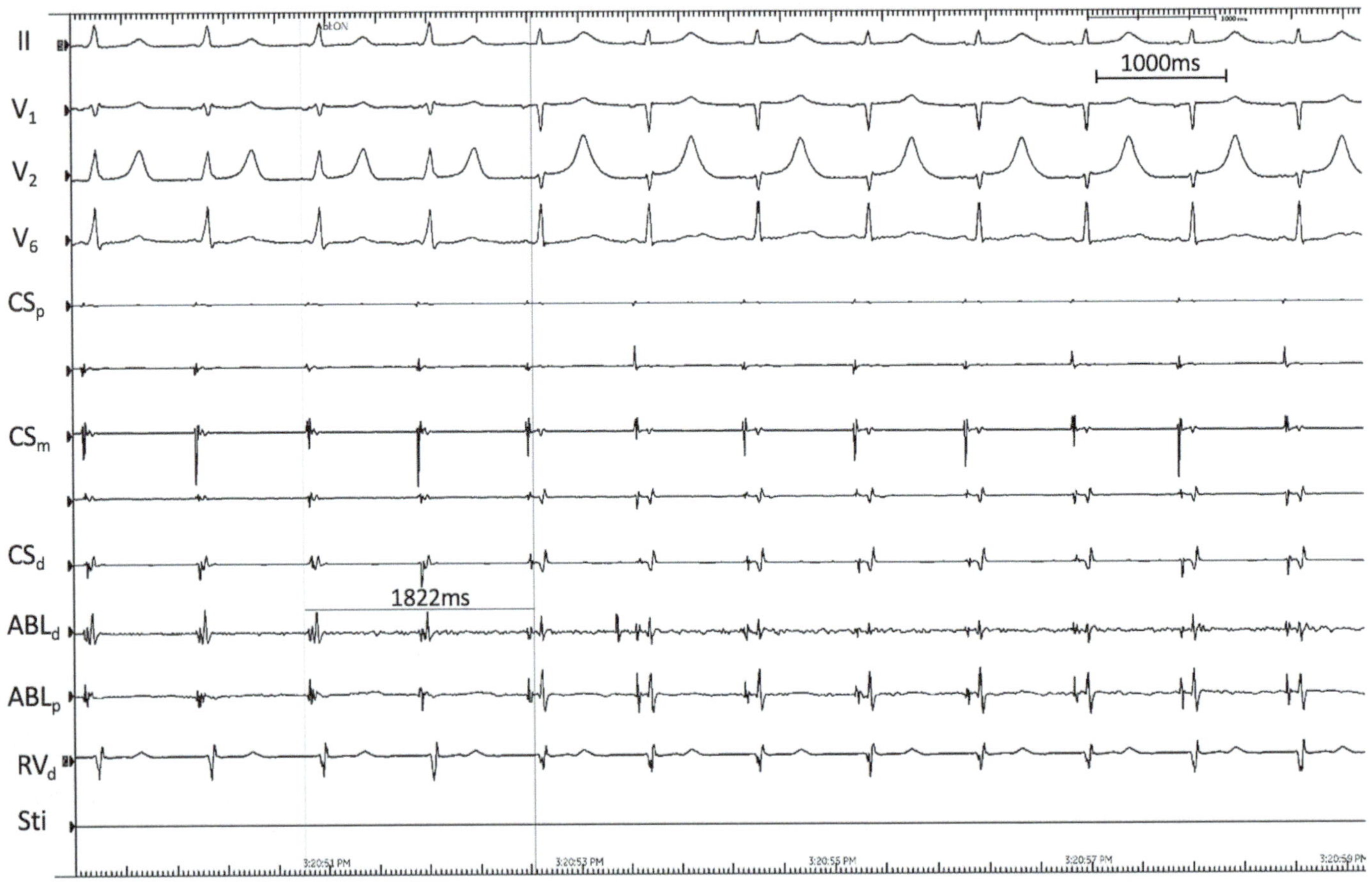

Fig. 30.23 Radiofrequency ablation with cessation of the accessory pathway conduction within 2 seconds of starting the energy delivery. *A*, Atrial end of AP; *A2*, programmed atrial stimulus; *Abl*, ablation catheter; *A ERP*, atrial effective refractory period; *AP*, accessory pathway; *AV*, atrioventricular; *AVN*, atrioventricular node; *CS*, coronary sinus; *ERP*, effective refractory period; *HB*, His bundle; *HRA*, high right atrium; *MA*, mitral annulus; *RVA*, right ventricular apex; *Stim*, stimulation; *TA*, tricuspid annulus; *V*, ventricular end of AP; *V ERP*, ventricular effective refractory period; *X d, m, p*, the distal, mid, proximal electrode pairs of the relevant catheter.

CONCLUSION

The approach to the patient with a challenging AP ABL involves, first, an appreciation of the anatomic landscape (i.e., oblique Aps), APs that traverse the annulus in unusual locations (i.e., connections from myocardial bridges from appendages to ventricular myocardium), and the specifics of localizing atrio-fascicular APs. Second, an appreciation of the presence of multiple APs may serve to confound traditional approaches. Third, an appreciation is needed of the role of special pacing maneuvers for decremental Aps, including the role of simultaneous atrial and ventricular pacing, as well as an appreciation of the value of pacing the ventricle at the site of earliest atrial activation. Finally, the role of advanced electroanatomical mapping technology serves to both minimize trauma to APs and facilitate and enhance the accuracy of mapping.

REFERENCES

Please refer to the e-book for a complete list of references.

PART 7

Catheter Ablation of Ventricular Tachycardias

31

Ablation of Ventricular Outflow Tract Tachycardias

Jackson J. Liang, Sanjay Dixit

KEY POINTS

- Ventricular outflow tract tachycardias originate from the right or left ventricular (LV) outflow tracts, aortic cusps, pulmonary artery, and the corresponding epicardium (LV summit region).
- The mechanism underlying outflow tract arrhythmias is usually triggered activity, and the site of origin is focal. Activation mapping during arrhythmia is optimal to identify the site of earliest activation as the target for ablation.
- Mapping of outflow tract tachycardias is often enhanced by the use of electroanatomical mapping systems. Computed tomography, intracardiac echocardiography, and coronary angiography are important adjuncts for mapping and ablation of coronary cusp, intramural, and epicardial sites of origin.
- A comprehensive understanding of the anatomy of the outflow tract region, including the neighboring anatomical structures, is necessary to maximize safety and efficacy of ablation of outflow tract ventricular arrhythmias.
- Challenges to ablating outflow tract tachycardias include mapping and ablation of noninducible tachycardias and ablation of tachycardias originating from regions that are difficult to target due to anatomical constraints (including the LV summit region, para-Hisian, and/or intramural location).
- There is an increasing recognition that idiopathic ventricular arrhythmias can also originate from the basal inferior septum, and catheter ablation can be effective in eliminating these arrhythmias.

Ventricular tachycardias (VTs) most frequently occur in patients with structural heart disease. However, approximately 10% of VTs occur in patients with normal electrocardiogram (ECG), echocardiogram, and coronary angiography results and hence are considered to be *idiopathic VTs (IVTs)*.[1]

IVTs have been classified based on the ventricle of origin, ECG morphology (QRS configuration and axis), clinical pattern of the tachycardia (repetitive, nonsustained, or sustained), evidence of catecholamine dependency, and response to pharmacologic agents.[1,2] In general, the clinical history, combined with the response of the arrhythmia to programmed stimulation, adenosine, verapamil, and propranolol, may help differentiate among different types of IVTs.

This chapter will summarize the mechanism and common clinical presentations of idiopathic outflow tract tachycardias (OTVTs) and provide an in-depth description regarding the anatomical and electrocardiographic localization of these arrhythmias and current state of ablation strategies.

MECHANISM

The most common origins of IVTs are the right and left ventricular outflow tracts (RVOT, LVOT). In earlier experiences, the majority of OTVTs originated from the RVOT (70%) and, less frequently (20%), from the aortic cusps. However, in the more recent reports, OTVTs appear to be equally distributed between the RVOT and aortic cusps. In a minority of patients (10%), the site of origin can be the basal LV, pulmonary artery, or the LV epicardium.[3,4]

Idiopathic OTVTs usually exhibit one of three clinical phenotypes: repetitive monomorphic premature ventricular contractions (PVCs; most common), nonsustained monomorphic VT, or exercise-induced sustained VT (least common). Considerable overlap may occur among the three phenotypes. For example, patients with only repetitive monomorphic PVCs may develop salvos of nonsustained or sustained VT during exercise or isoproterenol infusion. The observation that ablating one phenotype at a discrete site eliminates the other two phenotypes of arrhythmia suggests that the three phenotypes are representative of the same focal cellular process.[5]

The signature characteristic of idiopathic OTVTs is termination following administration of adenosine or verapamil.[6,7] Lerman and colleagues elegantly demonstrated that the mechanism underlying most idiopathic OTVTs is triggered activity mediated by catecholamine-induced delayed afterdepolarizations.[8–10] Catecholamine stimulation of the β-adrenergic receptor results in an increase in intracellular cyclic adenosine monophosphate (cAMP) and $I_{ca,L}$ activities, resulting in spontaneous oscillatory release of Ca^{2+} from the sarcoplasmic reticulum that activates a transient inward current (I_{ti}), giving rise to delayed afterdepolarizations. Because activation of adenylyl cyclase and $I_{ca,L}$ is critical for the development of cAMP-mediated triggered activity, this arrhythmia is sensitive to a variety of electropharmacologic perturbations such as β-blockers, calcium channel blockers, vagal maneuvers, and adenosine.[11] The effect of adenosine on VT (with rare exceptions) is mechanism specific, terminating only ventricular arrhythmias that are due to cAMP-mediated triggered activity.

Clinical Presentation

According to a population-based study from the Mayo Clinic that analyzed patients from Olmstead County who were diagnosed with IVTs between 2005 and 2013, it would appear that the incidence of IVTs in the general population has increased over time.[12] These arrhythmias are most commonly observed in the third to sixth decades.[5,12,13] Sustained IVT occurs with equal distribution between men and women, while symptomatic PVCs are more frequently present in women.[12] Interestingly, RVOT arrhythmias show a predilection for females, whereas those originating in the aortic cusps tend to be more common in men. In two large series (including one from the authors' institution), 70% of patients with RVOT VT were women, whereas approximately 70% of patients with aortic cusp VTs were men.[3,4]

The most common clinical phenotype of idiopathic OTVTs is repetitive monomorphic PVCs. Palpitations are the most common symptom (48–80%) and are usually experienced as isolated forceful heart beats resulting from the increased stroke volume associated with the beat following the PVC (post exrtrasystolic potentiation). Fatigue and low energy are also common symptoms seen in patients with at least moderate burden of PVCs. This may be due to ineffective ventricular contraction during PVCs resulting in a reduced cardiac output. Lightheadedness may be observed in 25–50% of patients, while true syncope is rare (10%). The latter usually occurs in patients with ventriculoatrial conduction and may be a result of baroreceptor reflex activity.

Exercise testing induces VT in approximately 70% of patients who present with sustained IVT but in only 10% of patients whose clinical presentation is repetitive monomorphic PVCs. In the former group, sustained VT is typically observed either during exercise or in the recovery phase.[14] This observation can be mimicked with pharmacologic agents as well. Thus, in these patients, the clinical arrhythmia can be induced during isoproterenol infusion as well as during isoproterenol washout period. This highlights the evanescent nature of triggered activity–mediated arrhythmias.

Other scenarios that provoke these arrhythmias include physical or emotional stress, anxiety, and stimulants such as caffeine. In females, IVTs occur more often during the premenstrual and perimenopausal periods and with gestation, suggesting a role for hormonal influence.[15]

Idiopathic OTVTs have a benign course in most patients, suggesting that the underlying pathophysiologic process is not progressive and that the tachycardia does not represent an early manifestation of an occult cardiomyopathy. This finding has been confirmed during long-term follow-up studies in patients with RVOT tachycardias.[16] However, there are two exceptions to this general rule. First, patients with a high burden of ventricular arrhythmia can develop a reversible form of LV cardiomyopathy.[17] Walters et al. showed in a swine model of PVC-mediated cardiomyopathy that desynchrony due to bigeminal pacing (from both the RV apex or LV epicardium) over 14 weeks resulted in marked reduction of LV ejection fraction and evidence for increased ventricular fibrosis on histologic examination.[18] Consistent with this observation, Bogun et al. found that a PVC burden >24% was associated with development of PVC-induced cardiomyopathy.[19] However, arrhythmia burden alone may be a poor predictor of future development of cardiac dysfunction, since patients with a lower burden of arrhythmia (16% ± 4%) have also been shown to develop cardiomyopathy, while some patients with an higher PVC burden (33% ± 13%) can maintain normal LV function over extended follow-up periods. Thus, there may be other factors involved in the development of cardiac dysfunction in patients with OTVT. Longer QRS duration of ectopic beats and greater LV dyssynchrony may be associated with greater decline in LV ejection fraction.[18] Nevertheless, in patients with OTVT who develop true tachycardia-mediated cardiomyopathy, suppression of the clinical arrhythmia, either pharmacologically or by ablation, is associated with improvement of LV function.[19,20] Thus, it is good clinical practice to monitor cardiac function with annual echocardiograms in asymptomatic patients with PVC burden exceeding 5%. Interestingly, while LV function may normalize after elimination of PVCs, myocardial fibrosis and LV dyssynchrony may persist.[21] Interestingly, work from a canine PVC cardiomyopathy model by Tan et al. suggested that neural remodeling (extracardiac sympathetic hyperinnervation and sympathetic neural hyperactivity) may persist even after PVC elimination and recovery of LV function.[22] As such, is it possible that not all PVC-induced structural and neural changes are fully reversible, and thus early prophylactic ablation therapy may be beneficial.[21] Another clinical scenario that is not uncommon is the development of OTVTs in patients with underlying structural heart disease. This is particularly challenging in patients with arrhythmogenic right ventricular cardiomyopathy (ARVC), where the appearance of OTVTs may be a manifestation of the underlying disease, and the prognosis of the arrhythmia in these patients is less benign than for the typical OTVT population. Suspicion for ARVC may arise if the arrhythmias manifest multiple ECG morphologies including different axis and precordial transition patterns. Algorithms have also been developed to improve differentiation between idiopathic OTVTs versus those occurring in the setting of ARVC.[23,24] Signal-averaged ECG, cardiac magnetic resonance imaging (MRI), and electroanatomical voltage mapping may be helpful to diagnose ARVC in patients presenting with RVOT VT. In one study, voltage and local electrogram abnormalities on electroanatomical maps were helpful in differentiating idiopathic RVOT tachycardia from RVOT tachycardia due to subclinical ARVC. In these patients, the voltage / electrogram abnormalities correlated with fibrofatty myocardial replacement seen on endomyocardial biopsy specimens obtained from these locations.[25]

ANATOMICAL SUBSTRATE

Most patients with idiopathic OTVT have demonstrated lack of gross structural heart disease as evidenced by ECG, echocardiography, radionuclide imaging, and cardiac angiography. However, in patients with RVOT VTs that were initially thought to be idiopathic in nature, studies using MRI have shown structural defects including the presence of focal wall thinning, abnormal systolic wall motion, and focal fatty infiltration, findings not appreciated using conventional imaging.[26,27] The most common site of abnormality in most cases was the RV free wall. However, the abnormal substrate in these studies did not consistently correspond with the site of arrhythmia origin, and subsequent studies have shown a considerably lower prevalence of such abnormalities (approximately 10%).[28] Investigators have also conducted RV biopsies in patients with RVOT tachycardias, which have shown a wide spectrum of findings ranging from normal tissue to myocardial atrophy and fibrofatty replacement consistent with ARVC.[25] Importantly, during electroanatomical mapping, identification of areas manifesting fractionated electrograms and voltage abnormalities consistent with scar can serve as target locations for obtaining endomyocardial biopsy to increase the diagnostic yield in patients with suspected ARVC, myocarditis, and/or cardiac sarcoidosis who present with OTVTs.[25]

Idiopathic OTVT may also occur in patients with other unrelated cardiac diseases, including patients with history of coronary disease. In such patients, the presence of an old infarction that is anatomically distinct from the OT region signifies the coexistence of two unrelated processes. Ellis et al. reported the presence of unrelated structural heart disease in 43% of patients (42/97) who underwent ablation of an idiopathic OTVT. In that series, patients with idiopathic OTVT and unrelated structural heart disease were more likely to have the source of the arrhythmia ablated from the coronary cusps or basal LV region compared with patients without structural heart disease in whom the arrhythmia most commonly arose from the RVOT.[29] Additionally, the OT region has been increasingly recognized to be involved in arrhythmogenesis in patients with Brugada syndrome. Pappone et al. have shown that in high-risk Brugada syndrome patients undergoing ablation, ajmaline infusion frequently precipitates type 1 Brugada ECG pattern by enhancing conduction abnormalities in the underlying electrophysiologic substrate (area of low bipolar voltage manifesting abnormal electrograms) and worsens RV function along the RVOT anterior free wall. Their experience also showed that endocardial and epicardial ablation can eliminate the Brugada ECG pattern and render patients noninducible for VF.[30]

ANATOMY OF THE OUTFLOW TRACTS

A comprehensive understanding of the anatomical relationship between the structures in the outflow tract region is crucial to successful localization and ablation of these arrhythmias[31] (also see Chapter 6). In the thoracic cavity, the cardiac orientation is such that the RVOT, and particularly its free wall, is the most anterior structure (Fig. 31.1). The superior aspect of the RVOT crosses the anterior aspect of the LVOT such that its anteriormost extension together with the pulmonic valve lies almost left of the aortic valve (Fig. 31.2). The pulmonic valve annulus lies superior to the aortic annulus, and the aortic valve is tilted right in the horizontal plane such that the left coronary cusp (LCC) typically lies superior (cranial) to the right coronary cusp (RCC) and noncoronary cusp (NCC). The RCC is in close proximity to the RVOT region; it is because of this anatomical relationship that successful ablation of OTVT originating from the superior and "septal" RVOT can sometimes be accomplished from the RCC, and vice versa, making interpretation of previous studies describing sites of origin based on successful elimination site more challenging to interpret.[32] In fact, the structure immediately anterior to the aortic valve is the posterior muscular infundibular portion of the RVOT. Importantly, the penetrating bundle of His resides in the membranous interventricular septum directly underneath the NCC.

The classic understanding of outflow tract and great artery junction is that there is an abrupt termination of ventricular myocardium at the level of the semilunar valves. However, it has now been established that myocardial sleeves extend into the aorta and pulmonary artery for variable distances (Fig. 31.3).[33–35] The outflow tract–great artery junction is complex in terms of both its development and histology with multiple tissue types interfacing in this region (arterial smooth muscle, cardiac muscle, collagen, and valve tissue). In the pulmonic valve region, the myocardial sleeves can extend symmetrically across the valve cusps from few millimeters to more than 2 cm into the pulmonary artery.[33] The myocardial extensions above the aortic valve are significantly different from those observed in the pulmonic valve. At the base of the RCC, the LV myocardium is closely opposed to the aortic wall with myocardial sleeves running in parallel to the base of the cusp. By contrast, the LCC is separated from the LV myocardium by a thick band of fibrous tissue interspersed with strands of ventricular myocardium.[36]

Fundamental to the understanding of IVTs arising near the aortic and mitral valve is the concept of the "LV ostium" (Fig. 31.4).[36,37] The LV ostium is best described as an elliptical opening at the base of LV and is covered by a tough fibrous structure, which is perforated by the aorta anteriorly and the mitral valve posteriorly. The aorta is joined to the LV ostium at an angle of approximately 30° above the horizontal plane with the NCC being most inferior, the LCC most superior, and the RCC most anterior and in direct contact with the LV ostium. The aortic valve itself has a central location at the base of the heart and LV ostium with relationships to all other valves and cardiac chambers. The RCC is positioned immediately posterior to the infundibular aspect of the RVOT. Caudally, the RCC is continuous with the anterior LVOT, and at the level of valve insertion, there is either a true physical continuity or very close proximity to myocardial tissue from either the LVOT or the posterior RVOT.[32] The NCC lies posterior and to the right of the RCC, and as such it has no anatomical relationship with any ventricular myocardium.[38] Instead, the NCC lies adjacent to the interatrial septum and has relations to both the right and left atria. This may explain why ventricular arrhythmias rarely originate from the NCC. The commissure between the RCC and

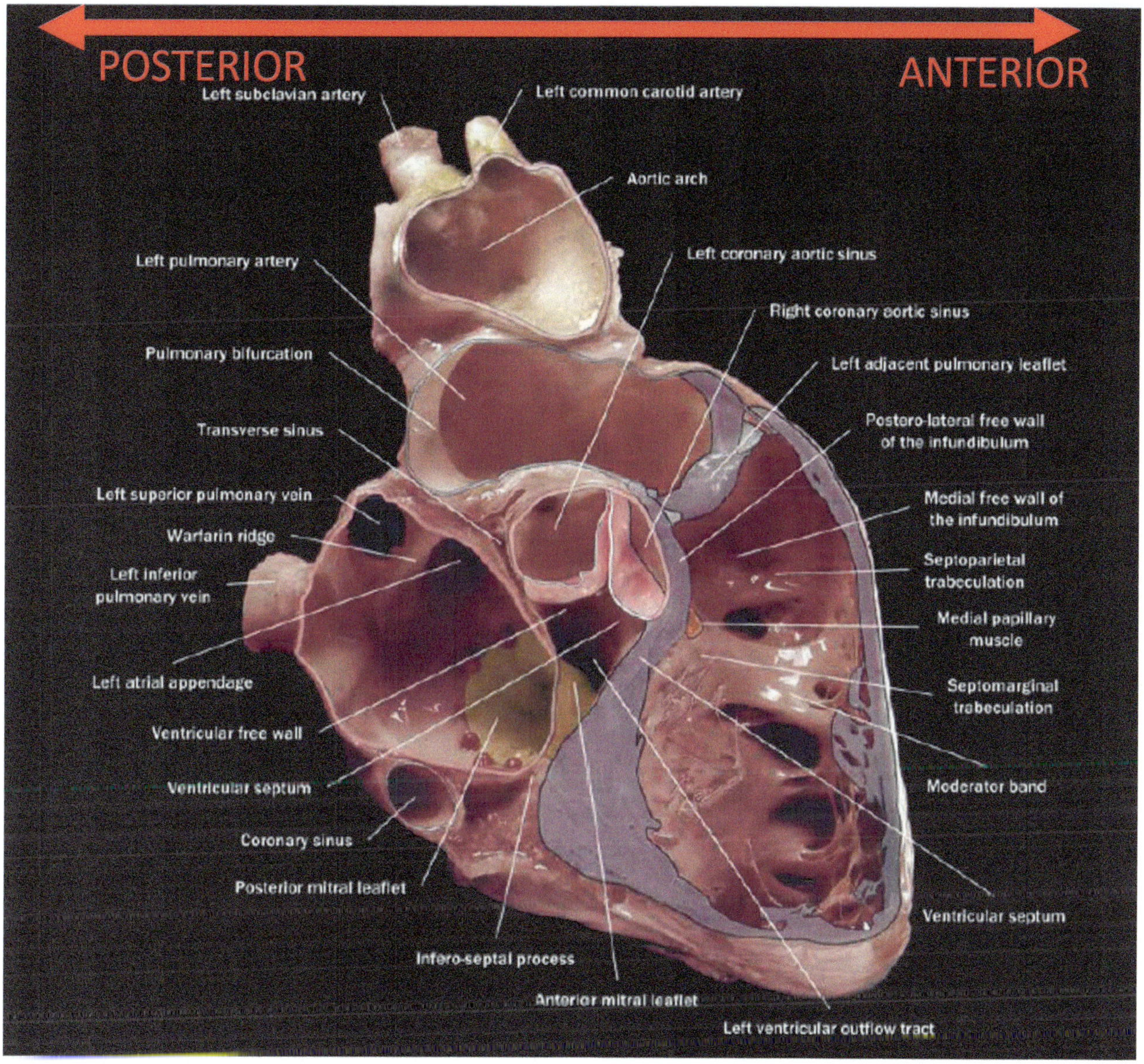

Fig. 31.1 Sagittal section of the right ventricle viewed from the right direction. The right ventricular outflow tract (RVOT) is the anterior-most structure in the heart. (Reproduced with permission from Mori S, Shivkumar K. *Atlas of Cardiac Anatomy*. Vol. 1. Cardiotext Publishing; 2022.)

NCC forms part of the membranous interventricular septum and is the location of the penetrating bundle of His. The LCC lies superior, posterior, and to the left of the RCC. The commissure between the LCC/RCC is immediately posterior and caudal to the distal RVOT. Myocardial tissue is present in the LCC but not to the same extent as in the RCC. In addition the LCC is usually separated from the LVOT by connective tissue (also see Chapter 6, Fig. 6.31). The LV summit is an interesting entity, and this region is being increasingly recognized as source of epicardial IVTs.[39] The LV summit is the triangular epicardial aspect of the most superior portion of the LV extending cephalad to the aortic portion of the LV ostium and is bounded by the origin of the left anterior descending artery (LAD) and left circumflex coronary artery (LCx).[37] The base of this triangle is defined by the first septal perforator of the LAD and this triangular region is bisected by the anterior interventricular vein (AIV) (see Chapter 6, Fig 6.32). As will be discussed later, the close proximity of the epicardial coronary vessels make it particularly challenging to target IVT originating from the LV summit region.

Within the OTVT region, the sources of these arrhythmias show a predilection for certain locations (Fig. 31.5). In one study, approximately 80% of RVOT tachycardias were localized to the superior anteroseptal aspect just below the pulmonic valve.[40] Similarly, LVOT tachycardias have been found to originate from a narrow location that includes the LCC and RCC, the bordering aspects of LV ostium (septal para-Hisian, aortomitral continuity [AMC], and the superior mitral annulus) and the adjoining LV summit region. Thus, in the entire outflow tract region, almost 90% of idiopathic tachycardias seem to originate from a fairly narrow

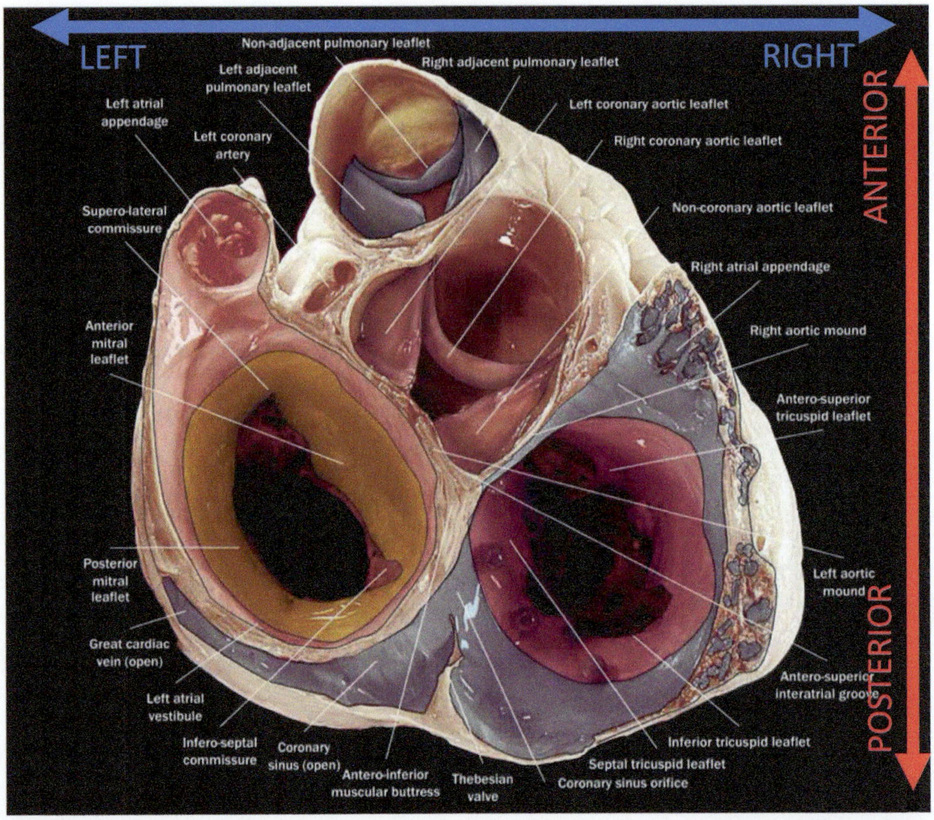

Fig. 31.2 Coronal section of the heart viewed from a superior direction. The RVOT courses anteriorly and leftward as it ascends, such that distally the anterior aspect of the pulmonic valve is leftward of the aortic valve. (Reproduced with permission from Mori S, Shivkumar K. *Atlas of Cardiac Anatomy*. Vol. 1. Cardiotext Publishing; 2022.)

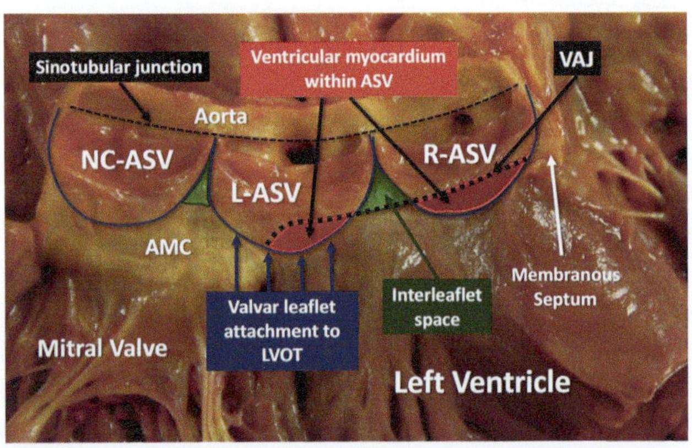

Fig. 31.3 Aortic root anatomy. Gross dissection of the aortic valve with a sagittal cut made between the right (R) and noncoronary (NC) aortic valvar leaflets. The noncoronary aortic sinus has been pulled to the left (L) with the photograph taken from a left posterior oblique view with respect to the heart position within chest. The aortic root is bounded superiorly by the sinotubular junction (*black dashed line*) and inferiorly by the nadirs of the attachments of the semilunar aortic valvar leaflets (*blue line*). The ventriculoarterial junction (VAJ) is demarcated with a *thick black dotted line*. Regions where ventricular myocardium may be identified within the aortic sinus of Valsalva (ASV) are shown in red. The interleaflet spaces are shown in green. *AMC*, Aortomitral continuity; *LVOT*, left ventricular outflow tract. (From Cheung JW, Anderson RH, Markowitz SM, Lerman BB. Catheter ablation of arrhythmias originating from the left ventricular outflow tract. *JACC Clin Electrophsyiol.* 2019:5(1):1–12.)

anatomical zone. This observation raises an interesting question about why this location is predisposed to triggered activity. It is conceivable that this may be related to its embryologic origin (from the neural crest cells). However, it remains unclear whether this tissue is naturally present in all individuals and manifests arrhythmias in a selected few or whether it is only seen in those patients who subsequently develop OTVTs. Alternatively, predisposition to OTVTs may be the result of an acquired inflammatory process, such as subclinical myocarditis, which can itself cause ventricular ectopy, or result in fibrosis that can disrupt the perivalvular tissue, thus isolating myocardial cell groups, which in turn may develop abnormal resting or threshold membrane potentials promoting abnormalities of impulse formation (triggered activity and/or abnormal automaticity).

DIAGNOSIS

Electrocardiographic Patterns and Anatomical Localization

Because OTVTs have a focal source and occur in patients with structurally normal hearts, their site of origin can usually be predicted by standard 12-lead ECG. However, given the narrow

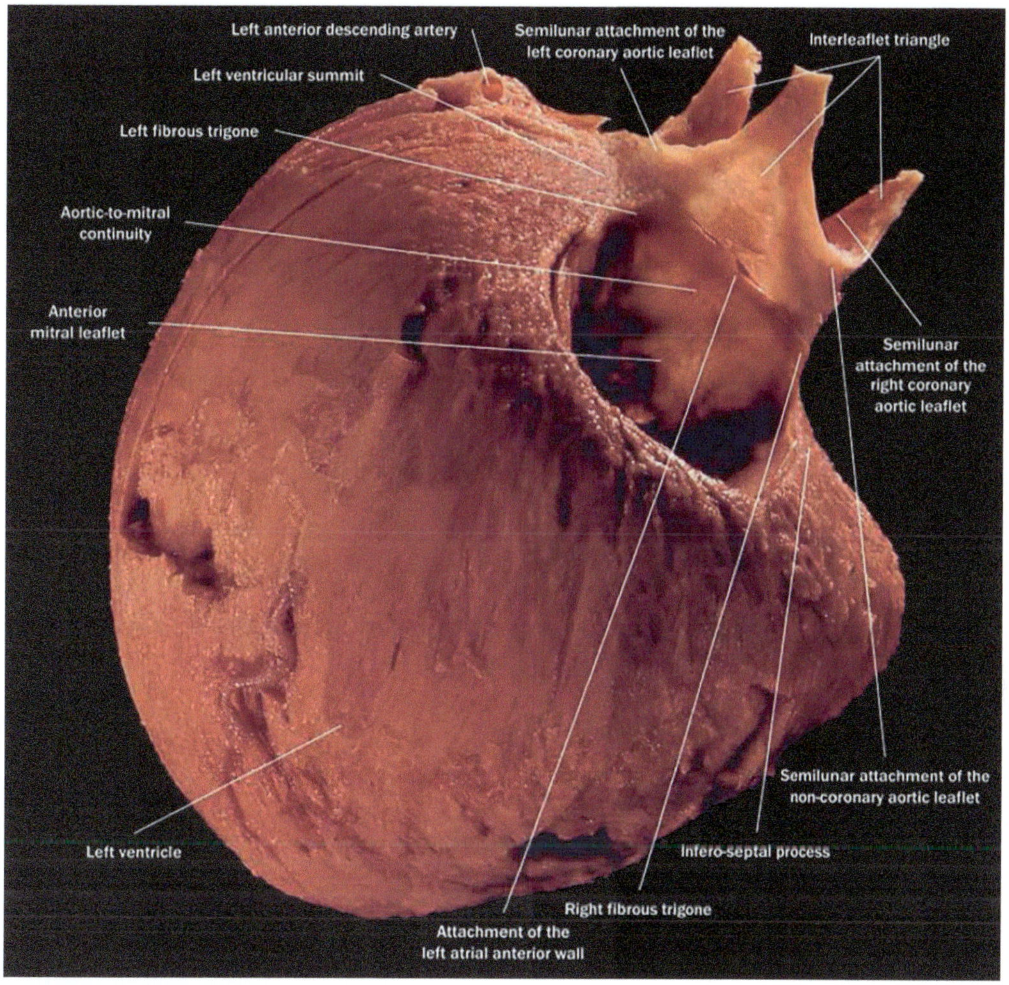

Fig. 31.4 Left ventricular ostium and aortic root. (Reproduced with Permission from Mori S, Shivkumar K. *Atlas of Cardiac Anatomy. Anatomical Basis of Cardiac Interventions, Vol. 1.* Hopkins, Minnesota: Cardiotext Publishing, LLC; 2022.)

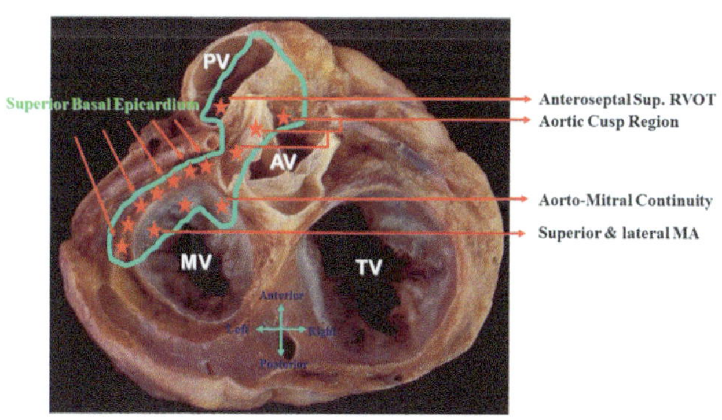

Fig. 31.5 Coronal section of the heart viewed from superior direction. The area outlined in *green* highlights the region of the heart in the RVOT and LVOT where idiopathic ventricular arrhythmias usually originate. (Courtesy of Dr. Samuel Asirvatham, MD.)

anatomical zone from which OTVTs originate, coupled with anatomical variations (especially with regard to the heart position within the chest cavity), ECG overlap between adjacent sites exists and accurate localization requires invasive mapping. Nevertheless, understanding ECG patterns of OTVTs is a useful tool for arrhythmia localization and procedure planning.

The classic ECG profile of RVOT tachycardia is a left bundle branch block (LBBB) pattern with inferior axis evidenced by tall R waves in leads II, III, and aVF and QS complexes in aVR and aVL.[41] Fig. 31.6 shows common sites of origin of OTVTs in relation to the precordial leads V_1–V3 and limb lead I. Because lead V_1 is a unipolar right-sided lead, tachycardias originating from the anterior (free wall) RVOT propagate posteriorly and away from V_1, creating a predominantly negative or LBBB pattern. Tachycardias originating further posteriorly and leftward (septal aspect) in the RVOT region while still having an LBBB pattern usually manifest a small R wave preceding the large S wave in lead V_1. Because of the continuity between the posterior RVOT and the anterior LVOT, a similar small R wave (preceding the S wave) in lead V_1 can be seen with tachycardias originating in the RCC region. Further posterior or leftward from the RCC sits the LCC, and tachycardias originating from this location usually manifest either equal-sized R and S waves or a larger R than S wave in lead V_1. The AMC region is the next leftward location to the LCC, but it sits more anterior and tachycardias originating from this region show more prominent R waves, which are preceded by a small q wave. In the authors' experience, this qR pattern in lead V_1 together with inferiorly

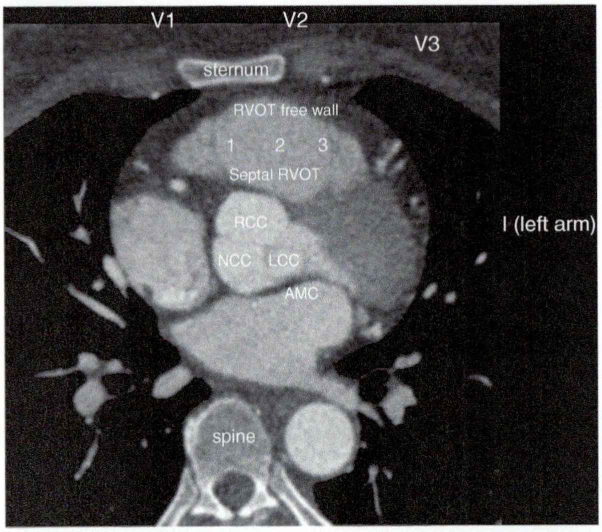

Fig. 31.6 Relationship between outflow tract anatomy and electrocardiogram morphology. The RVOT free wall is the most anterior structure, immediately beneath the precordial leads V_1–V_3. As such, arrhythmias originating from the RVOT free wall are predominantly negative across the precordium. Moving posteriorly toward the spine (from septal RVOT to RCC, LCC, aortomitral continuity, and superior mitral annulus, the activation wavefront moves increasingly more toward the precordial leads resulting in more positivity in V1 and earlier precordial transition. The RVOT site 1 is the most leftward, thus generating a positive complex in lead I, while RVOT site 3 is the most rightward and generates a negative complex in lead I. *LCC,* Left coronary cusp; *RCC,* right coronary cusp; *RVOT,* right ventricular outflow tract. (From Liang JJ, Han Y, Frankel DS. Ablation of outflow tract ventricular tachycardia. *Curr Treat Options Cardio Med* 2015:17:363.)

directed axis is pathognomonic of tachycardia origin from an AMC location. Beyond the AMC is the top of mitral annulus, and tachycardias originating from this region usually manifest large monophasic R waves in lead V_1.

Other leads can also be helpful in localizing OTVTs. The ratio of QRS complexes in leads aVR and aVL was found to be useful in predicting the relatively superior or inferior location of the tachycardia source within the outflow tract region. In general, leads aVR and aVL being located at the respective shoulders usually manifest prominent negative (QS) complexes for OTVTs. However, for tachycardias originating at a lower level in the RVOT (near the His-bundle region), complexes in lead aVL become progressively less negative or even isoelectric to positive, whereas complexes in lead aVR remain negative. Conversely, when the source of the tachycardia is leftward and in the superior most aspect of the outflow tract (such as above the pulmonic valve), complexes in lead aVL may be more negative than complexes in lead aVR. Similarly, the ratio of R waves in leads II and III can also help differentiate more superior from inferior location of tachycardia sources within the outflow tract region. Interestingly, for OTVTs, QRS complexes in leads II and III are usually mirror images of those in leads aVR and aVL respectively.

Although the 12-lead ECG is extremely helpful in localizing the site of origin of OTVTs, it is important to verify accurate ECG lead position because even minor changes in the location of certain leads can substantially alter the morphology of QRS complexes recorded by those leads. This is particularly true for precordial leads V_1 and V_2 as well as limb lead I. It is not uncommon for precordial leads V_1 and V_2 to be misplaced an intercostal space higher or lower than their standard location (fourth intercostal space). Similarly, the electrodes for limb lead I can sometimes be displaced from the shoulder to the nearby upper chest area. These lead displacements are particularly common during exercise test protocols (done to evoke outflow tract ventricular arrhythmias) or during electrophysiology study (to accommodate the precordial defibrillation pads). Such minor changes in lead placement have been shown to alter the morphology of QRS complexes significantly, which in turn can affect the accuracy of the ECG to localize the site of origin of the clinical arrhythmia.[42] Thus, superior displacement of precordial leads V_1 and V_2 can result in reduced R-wave amplitude and R/S ratio, whereas inferior displacement of these leads can increase R-wave amplitude and the R/S ratio. It is thus conceivable that in a case where VT is originating from cusp region, if leads V_1 and V_2 are misplaced superiorly resulting in reduced R-wave amplitude and lower R/S ratio of QRS complexes, then the tachycardia origin may be erroneously predicted to the RVOT region. Similarly, for tachycardias originating in RVOT, if leads V_1 and V_2 are misplaced inferiorly, then because of increased R-wave amplitude and R/S ratio, the source may be erroneously predicted to the cusp region. It was also found that anterior displacement of the upper limb leads from shoulders to the adjacent upper chest/torso can significantly reduce the R-wave amplitude and/or even reverse the QRS polarity in limb lead I. This alteration in QRS morphology can influence one's ability to distinguish anterior/leftward accurately from posterior/rightward location of the tachycardia source in the superior RVOT region.

Clinical Arrhythmias From RVOT

To characterize electrocardiographic patterns of RVOT tachycardias, a numbering system has been created that divides the RVOT into nine distinct anatomical sites (Fig. 31.7*A*).[43,44] Sites 1–3 are

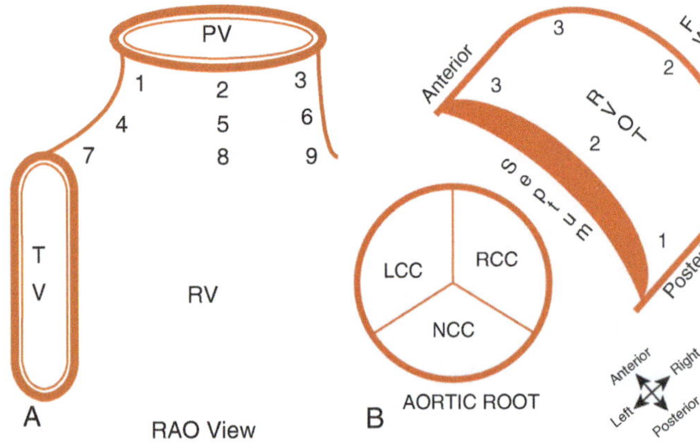

Fig. 31.7 Schematic representation of the right ventricular outflow tract (RVOT). (A) Locations of the nine standard mapping sites along the septal RVOT are shown in right anterior oblique projection (RAO). Sites 1–3 represent the first row of sites underneath the pulmonic valve in an anterior to posterior orientation. (B) The RVOT in a coronal projection depicting sites 1–3 along the septal and the free-wall aspects of the superior RVOT. Site 1 is posterior and rightward relative to site 3, which is anterior and leftward; site 2 is between these. The QRS complex morphology in multiple leads can help localize tachycardia origin from these sites. See text for details. *FW,* Free wall; *LCC,* left coronary cusp; *NCC,* noncoronary cusp; *PV,* pulmonic valve; *RCC,* right coronary cusp; *RV,* right ventricle; *TV,* tricuspid valve.

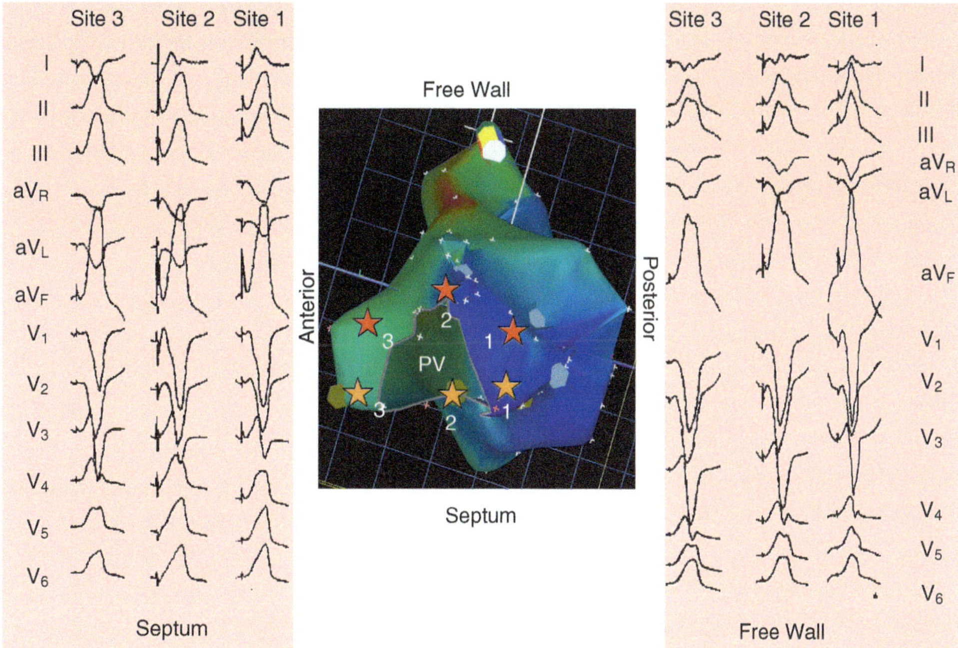

Fig. 31.8 Twelve-lead electrocardiogram pace maps from sites 1–3 along the septum and free-wall aspects of the right ventricular outflow tract (RVOT). Sites were tagged on an electroanatomical shell (CARTO; Biosense Webster, Diamond Bar, CA) displayed in the center of the figure in a coronal projection. The pace maps from septal RVOT sites 1–3 are shown to the left of the shell and those from the free-wall sites 1–3 are shown to the right of the map. Pace maps from all sites displayed left bundle branch block morphology with an inferior frontal plane axis. The R waves in the inferior leads (II, III, and aV^F) were taller and narrower for pace maps from septal sites as compared with the corresponding free wall sites. In addition the precordial QRS transition was later for free wall sites compared with septal locations. Transition from anterior to posterior sites over both the septal and free wall aspects of the RVOT resulted in increasing R-wave amplitude in lead I.

the most superior anatomical sites below the pulmonic valve in a posterior to anterior orientation. Sites 4–6 and 7–9, are respectively, the two rows below from an outflow to inflow orientation. This numerical site classification from 1 to 9 is applied separately to the septal and free-wall aspects of the RVOT.

The vast majority of RVOT arrhythmias arise from its most superior aspect, just below the pulmonic valve. Therefore, the ECG characteristics of these anatomical sites were studied in detail in 14 patients with structurally normal hearts.[44] Under guidance with an electroanatomical mapping system, a 4-mm mapping catheter was carefully positioned serially at sites 1–3 in both the RVOT septum and free wall (Fig. 31.7, B) and pace mapping from each site was performed. Fig. 31.8 shows pace maps from all six superior RVOT sites. Pace maps from septal sites manifested monophasic R waves in the inferior leads, which were taller and narrower in comparison with those over the corresponding free wall sites. The duration of the R wave in lead II was specifically analyzed, and at septal sites this was found to be significantly shorter when compared with R wave at corresponding free wall locations. In addition, the contour of the R wave in the inferior leads was helpful in differentiating between pace maps of septal and free wall locations in the superior RVOT. Typically, R waves from free wall sites demonstrated characteristic *notching*, which was uncommon in corresponding septal locations (Fig. 31.8). The precordial QRS transition also was helpful in distinguishing septal from free wall locations in the superior RVOT. In this series, the combination of late precordial transition (at or beyond lead V_4) and notching of the R wave in the inferior leads was found to be a sensitive and specific ECG criterion for identifying tachycardias originating from the free wall aspect of superior RVOT.

The QRS morphology in limb lead I can be helpful in distinguishing anterior or leftward locations from posterior or rightward locations in the superior RVOT region. Lead I manifests a positive polarity (R wave) for pace maps and tachycardias originating from posterior or rightward locations (site 1), whereas for pace maps and tachycardias originating from anterior or leftward aspect of the superior RVOT (site 3), complexes in lead I manifest negative polarity (QS pattern). This applies to both the septal and free wall aspects (Fig. 31.9). Site 2, midway between the anterior and posterior RVOT, typically displays either a biphasic or a multiphasic QRS pattern in limb lead I (see Fig. 31.9). Table 31.1 summarizes the ECG criteria to localize arrhythmias in the superior RVOT origin.

In older reports, the site of origin of RVOT tachycardia was infrequently (approximately 4–6%) found to be above the plane of the pulmonic valve.[31,32,44,45] However, subsequent studies have suggested that the incidence of supravalvular foci from the pulmonary artery may actually be higher than previously thought.[46–48] The myocardial sleeves extending beyond the pulmonic valve into the pulmonary artery are the likely source of such supravalvular foci. In that context it is interesting to note that while Hasdemir et al. previously reported a 17% incidence of suprapulmonic muscular sleeves

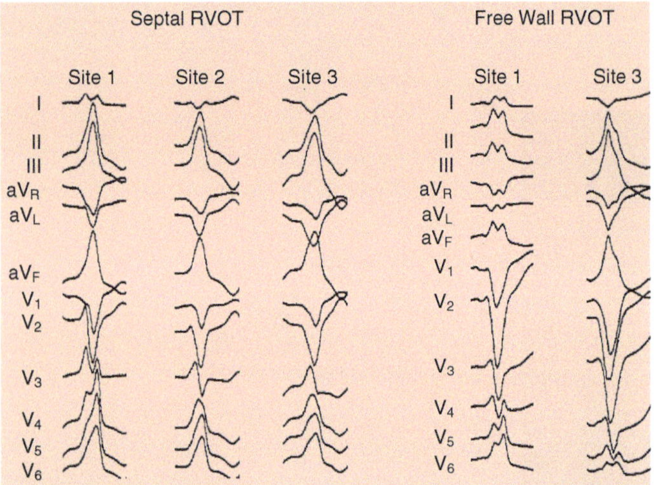

Fig. 31.9 Electrocardiogram (ECG) morphologies of tachycardias that were successfully ablated in the superior right ventricular outflow tract (RVOT). The left-hand side of the figure displays the 12-lead ECG morphology of characteristic septal RVOT tachycardias from sites 1 through 3, whereas the right-hand side of the figure displays the ECG morphology of characteristic free-wall RVOT tachycardias from sites 1 and 3. Tachycardias originating from free wall show notching in the inferior leads and late precordial transition (≥V_4). In comparison, tachycardias originating from septal RVOT have earlier precordial transition and lack notching of the R wave in the inferior leads. For both septal and free-wall tachycardias, lead I helps distinguish anterior (leftward) from posterior (rightward) location. See text for details.

in autopsied hearts, Gami et al. subsequently reported a much higher (73%) incidence. Using electroanatomical voltage mapping and intracardiac echocardiography (ICE), Liu et al. have also demonstrated that sleeves of myocardial tissue extended above the pulmonic valve in approximately 90% of patients.[33,34] These supravalvular tachycardias have been shown to manifest LBBB morphology with intermediate, right, or vertical frontal plane axis and a precordial transition by V_2 or later. Compared with RVOT tachycardias arising below the pulmonic valve, tachycardias from the pulmonary artery may have greater R-wave amplitude in the inferior leads. Another clue supporting suprapulmonic valve origin is a taller R wave in lead III compared with lead II, which is likely due to more leftward orientation of suprapulmonic valve compared with infrapulmonic valve location in the RVOT (Fig. 31.2). However, because of considerable overlap, there are no unique characteristic ECG features that can consistently and reliably differentiate the source of OTVT as being from above or below the pulmonic valve. Lead I can be helpful in differentiating between RCC versus a suprapulmonic valve site of origin. Due to the fact that the distal RVOT and pulmonic valve are situated relatively leftward of the aortic root and RCC, tachycardias originating in the latter location manifest a relatively large R wave in lead I.[49] Ablation of suprapulmonic sites of origin was usually performed within 5–21 mm above the pulmonic valve. At the successful ablation sites, a low-amplitude, sharp (or multicomponent), presystolic electrical potential (preceding the QRS onset by 28.2 ± 2.9 ms) with simultaneous activation in bipolar and unipolar recordings was usually noted during the clinical arrhythmia.[48,50] In sinus rhythm, the

TABLE 31.1 Diagnostic Criteria

RVOT source	LBBB pattern; R-wave transition after V_3; tall R in leads 2, 3, aV_F
• Septal	• Absence of notching in leads 2, 3, aV_F; precordial transition < V_4
• Free wall	• Presence of notching in leads 2, 3, aV_F; precordial transition ≥ V_4
• Anterior sites	• Negative lead 1
• Posterior sites	• Positive lead 1
Coronary cusps	Strongly inferior axis; precordial transition earlier than in NSR
• Left coronary cusp	• *m* or *w* pattern in V_1
• Right coronary cusp	• QS or rS pattern in V_1
• Left–right junction	• QS pattern, with notching on downstroke, in V_1
Aortomitral continuity	RBBB, inferior axis, qR pattern in V_1
LV summit	Inferior axis, delayed upstroke in lead 2, QS in lead 1, R/S ratio in V_2 < 1

LBBB, Left bundle branch block pattern; *LV*, left ventricle; *NSR*, normal sinus rhythm; *RBBB*, right bundle branch block pattern; *RVOT*, right ventricular outflow tract.

successful ablation site usually manifested a small far-field atrial signal. In one study, a standard 4-mm-tip radiofrequency (RF) catheter was used for pulmonary artery OTVT ablation; in this series the investigators delivered power for up to 60–90 seconds using a temperature cut-off at 55°C.[50] In another study, a 3.5-mm-tip open irrigated catheter was used with maximum power delivery of 40 W, temperature not to exceed 43°C, a flow rate of 20 mL/min, and lesion duration of 60 seconds.[48] While some operators have not infrequently performed ablation from above the pulmonic valve to eliminate OTVTs, our clinical experience has suggested otherwise and we have been able to successfully target almost all RV OTVTs (including in patients underoing repeat ablation after failed prior attempts) below the pulmonic valve or the adjoining location in the RCC.

Clinical Arrhythmias From Basal LV

In the authors' experience, idiopathic arrhythmias originating from the basal LV constitute approximately 10–20% of OTVTs. The basal LV includes the septum, inferior, anterior, and lateral walls bordering the mitral valve. The aortic valve is typically positioned at 30° angle superior to the mitral valve in close proximity to this region and is a part of the LV ostium (as discussed earlier). When targeting tachycardias originating from the basal LV, it is helpful to create a detailed electroanatomical map of this region at the outset. For this we primarily use ICE (specifically with CARTOSOUND, Biosense Webster, Diamond Bar, CA) to generate the initial shell of the RVOT, LVOT, aortic cusps, and basal LV, which guides further mapping and ablation. In centers where ICE is not routinely used for OTVT ablation procedures, orthogonal fluoroscopy can also be helpful in creating the electroanatomical map and guide ablation (Fig. 31.10).

To develop ECG criteria for basal LV tachycardias, distinct basal LV anatomical sites in a series of patients with structurally normal hearts were systematically pace mapped. These sites included the

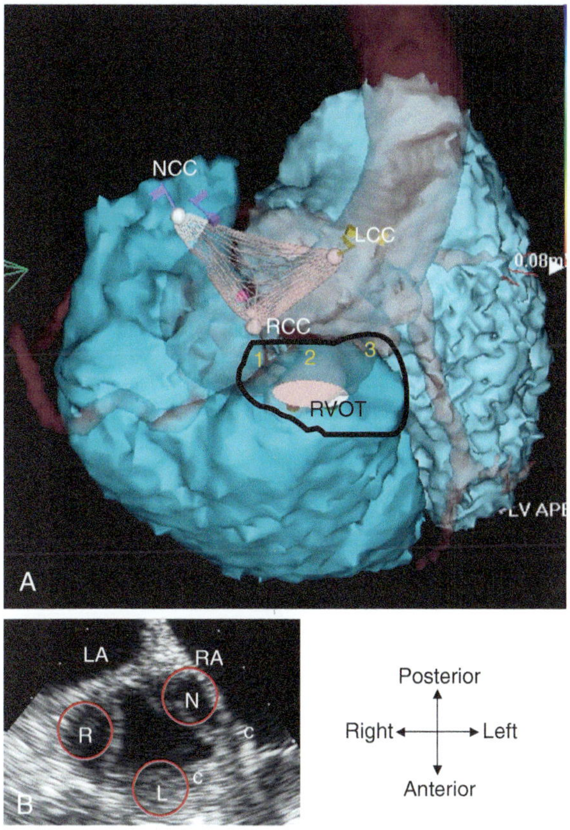

Fig. 31.10 Computed tomography angiogram of the outflow tract region in a coronal view depicting the relationship between the superior right ventricular outflow tract (RVOT) and aortic cusps. The posterior septal and anterior septal RVOTs (sites 1 and 3) are in close proximity to the RCC and LCC, respectively (A). Accurate anatomical localization of the aortic cusp is also facilitated by ICE (B). *LA,* Left atrium; *L/LCC,* left coronary cusp, *N/NCC,* noncoronary cusp; *RA,* right atrium; *R/RCC,* right coronary cusp.

septal para-Hisian region, AMC, superior, superolateral, and lateral mitral annulus (Fig. 31.11).[3] Pace maps from the septal para-Hisian region showed a relatively narrow QRS duration (mean 134 ± 28 ms), and this region had a characteristic pattern in V_1 of initial negative forces (QS or rS) albeit with an early precordial transition (reversal of Q/R ratio ≤ V_2). Compared with this location, the slightly more leftward AMC region manifested a small q wave followed by a larger R-wave (qR) pattern in lead V_1; this pattern, in the authors' experience, is pathognomonic for tachycardias originating from this location. In addition, from both septal para-Hisian and AMC locations, pace maps manifested predominantly positive complexes (R or Rs) in limb lead I.

In comparison, pace maps from lateral basal LV sites (superolateral and lateral mitral annulus) demonstrated a wider mean QRS duration (mean 182 ± 1 ms), and a right bundle branch block (RBBB) morphology in lead V_1 (monophasic R waves) and either no precordial transition or late appearing s wave (≥V_5; for inferolateral basal LV sites). The lateral basal LV sites typically manifested predominantly rS or QS complexes in limb lead I (Fig. 31.11).

In summary, with the exception of left para-Hisian sites, which consistently demonstrated LBBB morphology and early precordial transition patterns, pace maps from all other locations in the basal LV manifested RBBB morphology. In addition a qR morphology in lead V_1 together with an inferior axis was pathognomonic for pace maps from AMC locations (Fig. 31.11).

In a consecutive series of 122 patients who underwent ablation of idiopathic OTVT at our center, the arrhythmia was localized to the basal LV in 12 patients as follows: septal para-Hisian region in two, AMC in four, superior mitral annulus in three, and superolateral mitral annulus in three. Representative ECG morphologies of these tachycardias are depicted in Fig. 31.12. The criteria for localizing idiopathic basal LV tachycardias are summarized in Table 31.1.

Clinical Arrhythmias From the Aortic Cusps

Idiopathic ventricular arrhythmias that can be successfully ablated from within the coronary cusps have been increasingly recognized.[51–53] As mentioned earlier, the aortic valve is the central structure of the outflow tract region and has direct relations to all other cardiac chambers. This association is the key to understanding why successful ablation of OTVTs manifesting diverse morphologies suggesting origin in the septal RVOT, basal LV, GCV (great cardiac vein), etc. may still be accomplished from the cusp region and vice versa. This relationship is advantageous in balancing feasibility, efficacy, and safety while mapping and ablating various OTVT morphologies from the cusp region.

Similar to the aforementioned approach in the RVOT and basal LV region, we have also assessed the ECG characteristics of pace maps and clinical tachycardias arising from the aortic cusp region in a cohort of 20 patients with structurally normal hearts.[54] Using a retrograde approach, the mapping catheter was positioned in each aortic cusp and pacing was performed. The 12-lead ECG of pace maps from each location were then analyzed to identify unique features. Accurate catheter localization in the cusp region was guided by orthogonal fluoroscopy, ICE, and electroanatomical mapping. It was found that precordial lead V_1 was the most useful ECG lead to distinguish between the aortic cusps. Pace maps from the RCC consistently produced a negative vector in lead V_1 with a QS or rS pattern, whereas pace maps from the LCC produced an overall positive vector in V_1 that manifested either "rs" morphology or had multiphasic components resembling an M- or a W-shaped QRS complex (Fig. 31.13). In addition, the mean QRS duration was shorter in LCC pacing (142 ms; range, 108–180 ms) compared with RCC pacing (164 ms; range, 141–241 ms). The vector, amplitude, and ratio of the inferior leads did not distinguish RCC from LCC morphology. As noted earlier, the NCC lies adjacent to the interatrial septum and has relations to both atria, and therefore mapping in the NCC typically revealed a prominent atrial electrogram with or without a very small ventricular electrogram, and pacing from this cusp resulted in exclusively atrial capture. The ECG features of coronary cusp VTs are listed in Table 31.2. Lead I can be helpful in differentiating sites of origin within the cusps: lead I tends to be positive for arrhythmias from the RCC and negative for those from the LCC. Importantly, the accuracy of pace mapping from the cusp region can be limited in some patients by presence of preferential conduction via strands of myocardium leading to different exit sites and QRS morphologies.

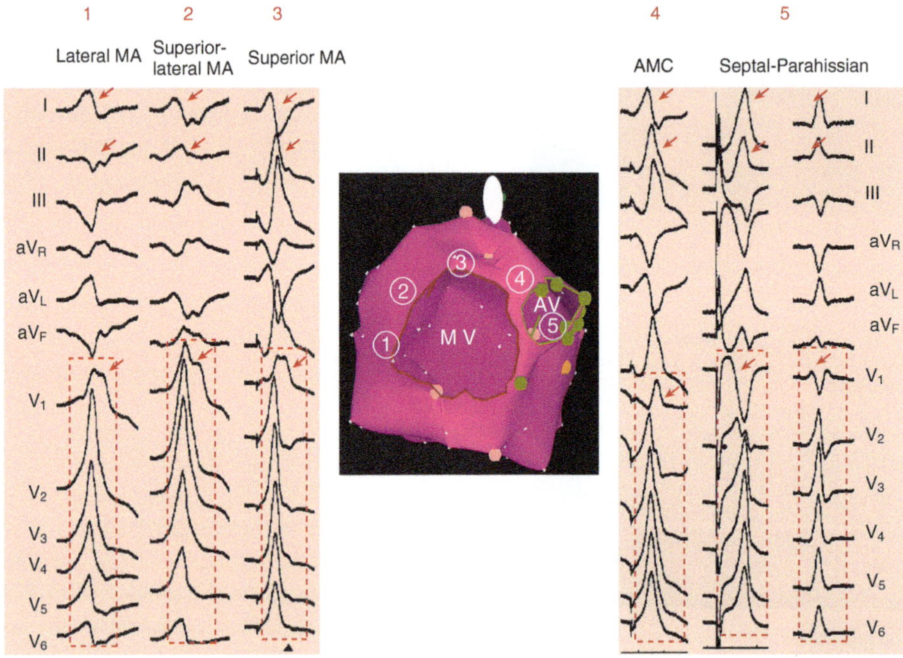

Fig. 31.11 Pace maps from various basal left ventricle sites. In a lateral-to-medial distribution, paced sites included the lateral, superolateral, and superior mitral annulus (MA), the aortomitral continuity (AMC), and the septal para-Hisian region (sites numbered 1–5). Electroanatomical map of basal LV in superior posteroanterior projection is shown in the center. QRS morphology in leads I, II, V_1 (*arrows*) and precordial transition pattern (*rectangles*) can help distinguish the anatomical sites. *AV*, Aortic valve; *MV*, mitral valve. See text for details.

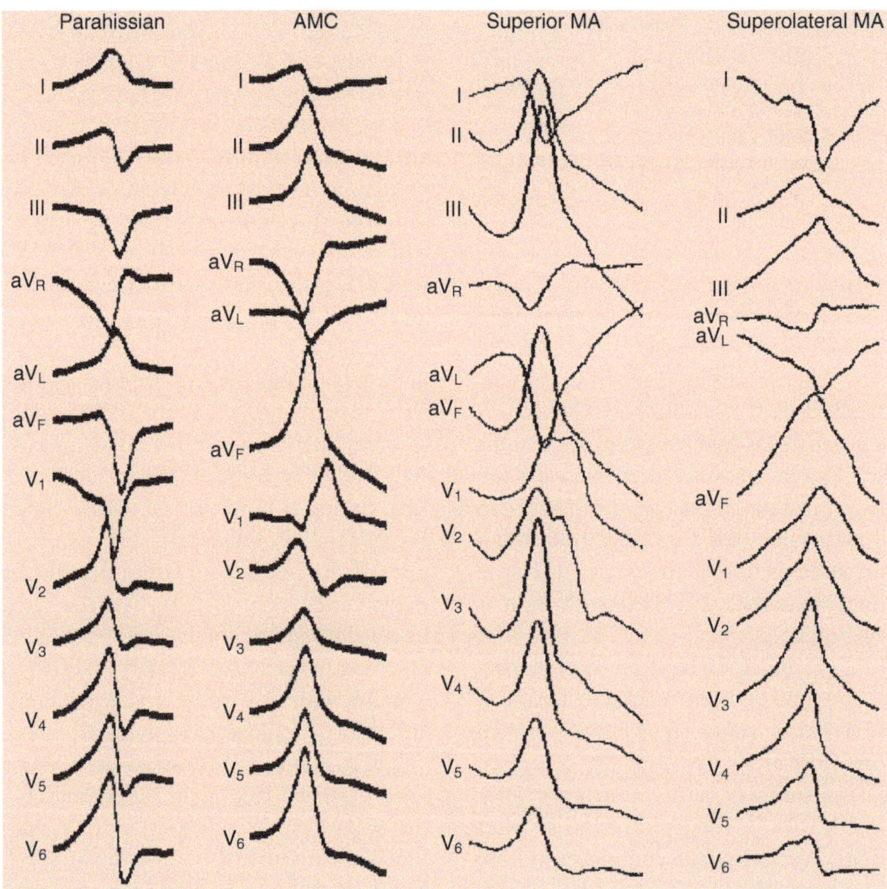

Fig. 31.12 Typical electrocardiogram morphologies of idiopathic basal left ventricle tachycardias from the septal para-Hisian region, aortomitral continuity (AMC), superior mitral annular (MA), and superolateral MA locations. QRS morphology in leads V_1 and I combined with the ratio of QRS in leads II/III and the precordial transition pattern can reliably distinguish medial from lateral mitral annular site of origin. See text for details.

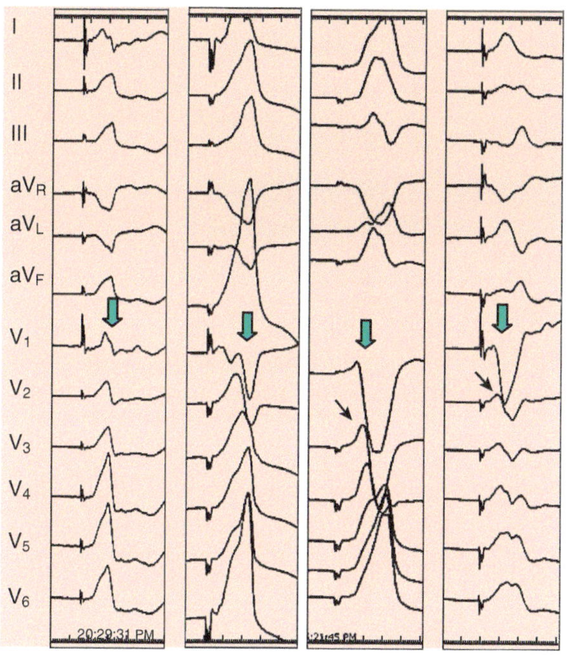

Fig. 31.13 Pacing morphologies from the left coronary cusp (*left*) and right coronary cusp (*right*). For left coronary cusp pacing, the first example (*left*) shows an M-shaped pattern in V_1, whereas the second one is more W-shaped (*arrows*). In both cases, V_1 has a multiphasic QRS pattern with a precordial transition by lead V_2. The two examples of right coronary cusp pacing show a left bundle branch block in V_1 and a later precordial transition ($\geq V_3$).

Interestingly, a common site of origin for cusp tachycardias is the common commissure between the RCC–LCC, and arrhythmias arising from this location manifest additional unique features. In a series of 19 patients with idiopathic outflow tract, VTs successfully ablated from the RCC–LCC commissure (as confirmed by real-time visualization with ICE and merging of preacquired computed tomography angiography with the electroanatomical shell), we found that VAs arising from this location manifested a QS pattern in lead V_1 with notching on the downward deflection.[55] Furthermore, at the site of successful ablation from this location, the intracardiac electrogram showed a distinct low-amplitude presystolic activation during

TABLE 31.2 Target Sites for Ablation

RVOT source	Sites with late diastolic/presystolic potentials 15–50 ms before QRS onset; sharp QS in unipolar recording; perfect pace map match
Coronary cusps	Sites with late diastolic/presystolic potentials 15–80 ms before QRS onset (with isoelectric segment between potential and QRS); QS in unipolar recording; pace maps may have multiple-paced morphologies; delayed signal in NSR that reverses during PVC
Other sites (GCV/AIV, AMC, LV summit)	Sites with late diastolic/presystolic, often fragmented potentials 15–50 ms before QRS onset; QS in unipolar recording; perfect pace map match

AIV, Anterior interventricular vein; *AMC,* aortomitral continuity; *GCV,* great cardiac vein/anterior interventricular vein; *LV,* left ventricle; *NSR,* normal sinus rhythm; *RVOT,* right ventricular outflow tract.

VA, which reversed during sinus rhythm (Fig. 31.14). Although in our experience the 12-lead ECG is helpful in localizing cusp tachycardias, it can nevertheless be influenced by the overall orientation of the aortic root vis-à-vis the LV. This is especially so with age-related changes such as unfolding of the aortic arch that can alter the orientation of the aortic root, as reported by Maeda et al., who used cardiac MRI to identify these changes and correlated the influence of that on pace maps obtained from different sites in the LVOT.[56] In this study, older age was associated with increased angle of the aortic root and decreased aortoventricular septal angle as seen on cardiac MRI. Furthermore, the LCC tended to be more cranial relative to the RCC in older patients compared to younger patients. This in turn significantly influenced the QRS morphology of pace maps (and possibly arrhythmias) originating from the cusp region. Specifically, the R-wave amplitudes tend to be greater when pace mapping from the LCC (versus the RCC) in older patients, whereas in younger patients this difference was not significant.[56] Liao et al. have shown that in OTVT cases with LBBB-type pattern in V_1, the presence of an abrupt V_3 transition (R-wave amplitude in lead V_3 >3 times greater than that in lead V_2) is highly predictive of site of origin from the septal margin of the LV summit, and that ablation from the interleaflet triangle just below the RCC–LCC junction was often successful in eliminating these arrhythmias.[57]

Clinical Arrhythmias From the Epicardial LV Summit

In a small subset of patients with idiopathic OTVT, the site of origin may be midmyocardial or epicardial. The most common location for these tachycardias is the LV summit region.[39] The LV summit is defined as the triangular portion of the epicardial LVOT with the apex at the bifurcation between the LAD and the CAAs and the base formed by an arc connecting the first septal perforator branch of the LAD with the CCA. The LVS is bisected by the great cardiac and anterior interventricular vein in two regions, one closer to the apex of the triangle and one at the base of the triangle. These anatomical definitions are based on orthogonal fluoroscopy, ICE and intraprocedural coronary angiography.[58] Although tachycardias originating from this location share many ECG features with other OTVTs, they may manifest a QS pattern in lead I (seen in 30%), delayed time to reach the peak or nadir of QRS complexes, and early precordial R-wave transition (at or before V_3 in 70% of patients).[59] In a study that analyzed ECG features of clinical VT arising from the epicardial and endocardial aspects of the anterobasal LV, two or more of the aforementioned ECG features accurately distinguished epicardial from endocardial site of origin of clinical VT originating from this LV location.[60] Additionally, Hayashi et al. recently reported the presence of a precordial "pattern break" in lead V_2 (abrupt loss of R-wave amplitude in V_2 compared to V_1 and V_3), which was found in cases where the site of origin of the arrhythmia was adjacent to the AIV sulcus (Fig. 31.15).[61] In patients presenting with LV summit arrhythmias, percutaneous epicardial ablation is frequently unsuccessful due to the proximity of the coronary vessels and the presence of epicardial fat. In our experience, epicardial ablation is more successful for arrhythmias arising from the basal and lateral aspect of the LV summit region than the apical and septal aspect. We have found

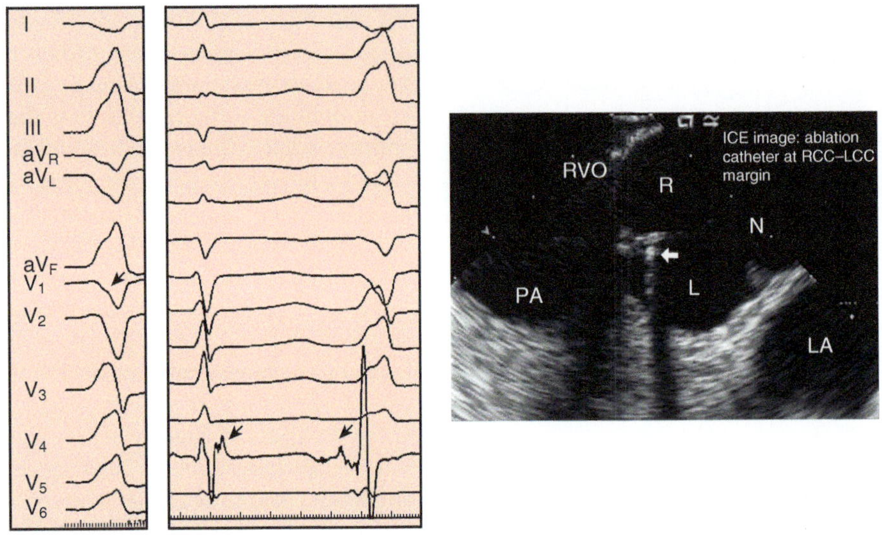

Fig. 31.14 Morphology of ventricular arrhythmia originating at the commissure between the right and left coronary cusps. V_1 has a unique pattern with QS morphology and a notch on its downslope (*arrow*). Typically, at the site of early activation, a late potential is seen during sinus rhythm (*arrow*) that reverses to become early presystolic signal during tachycardia (*arrow*). On the right-hand side, an ICE image showing the mapping catheter at the commissure between the right and left coronary cusps. *L,* Left coronary cusp; *LA,* left atrium; *N,* noncoronary cusp; *PA,* pulmonary artery; *R,* right coronary cusp; *RVO,* right ventricular outflow tract.

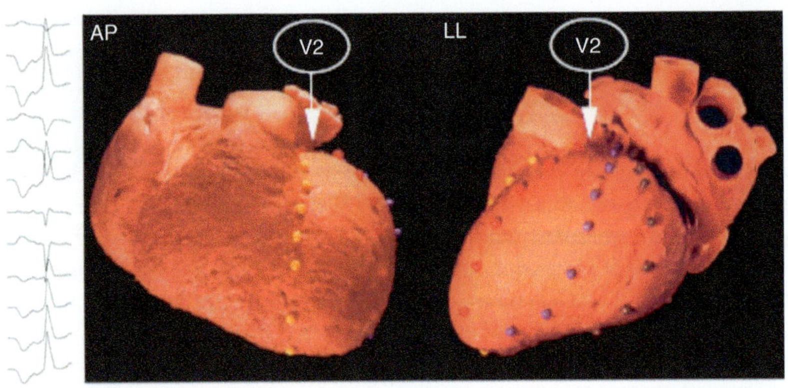

Fig. 31.15 V_2 pattern break. QRS morphology showing V_2 pattern break (*left panel*). The unipolar lead V_2 is located anatomically opposite to the anterior interventricular sulcus. *AP,* Anterior-posterior view; *LL,* left lateral view. Images from UCLA Cardiac Arrhythmia Center-Wallace A. McAlpine Collection. (Courtesy: K. Shivkumar, MD, PhD, as adapted from: Hayashi T, Santangeli P, Pathak RK, et al. Outcomes of catheter ablation of idiopathic outflow tract ventricular arrhythmias with an R wave pattern break in lead V_2: a distinct clinical entity. *J Cardiovasc Electrophysiol.* 2017;28:504-514.)

the following ECG characteristics to be predictive of a lateral and/or basal arrhythmia site of origin in the LV summit region: (1) Q-wave ratio >1.85 in aVL/aVR; (2) R/S ratio >2 in lead V_1; and (3) absence of q-waves in lead V_1.[59] Tachycardias manifesting two or more of these ECG features were more likely to be successfully ablated from the epicardium.

Intramural LVOT Arrhythmias

There has been increasing recognition of LVOT tachycardias originating from intramural foci. In a single center study, Yamada et al. reported that over 20% of all patients undergoing ablation for LVOT arrhythmias had a presumed intramural source originating from the basal LV between the AMC and epicardial LV summit.[62,63] In these studies, the ECG characteristics of intramural LVOT arrhythmias tended to be closer to the ECG morphology of arrhythmias arising from the endocardium of the AMC region rather than epicardial LV summit. Specifically, intramural LVOT arrhythmias had a maximum deflection index (MDI) in the precordial leads which fell between the MDI values for epicardial and endocardial LVOT arrhythmias. Additionally, compared to epicardial LV summit foci, intramural foci had a smaller R-wave amplitude ratio in lead II compared to lead III, smaller Q-wave amplitude ratio in aVL versus aVR, earlier local ventricular activation time in relation to the QRS onset at the His-bundle region, and later ventricular activation time in relation to the successful ablation site.[63] Importantly, the AMC itself is not a muscular sturcutre; thus, PVCs exiting from this region may actually originate from a deeper tissue component that ultimately is in contuation with the midmyocardial aspect of the LV summit.

Differentiating RVOT From Aortic Cusps Site of Origin

One of the challenges in the mapping and ablation of OTVTs is the ability to distinguish those arising from cusp region from those originating in the RVOT. Although the RVOT is superior and anterior to the aortic cusp region, the RCC, RCC–LCC junction, and the bordering LCC are in close proximity to its anterior septal aspect. Not surprisingly, there is significant overlap in the ECG characteristics of tachycardias arising from these locations. Nonetheless, the 12-lead ECG when carefully analyzed can still provide important clues that can be helpful in distinguishing RVOT from cusp tachycardias.

Amplitude and Duration

Ouyang and associates were one of the first to study the distinguishing ECG features between the RVOT and the aortic cusps tachycardias.[53] They found that the R-wave duration in V_1 and V_2 was greater in aortic cusp VTs compared with RVOT VTs. They also reported that an R-wave duration ≥50% of total QRS width or R/S amplitude ratio ≥30% in leads V_1 or V_2 strongly favored tachycardia origin from aortic cusps.

Precordial Transition

The precordial R-wave transition is another important ECG parameter that can be helpful in distinguishing RVOT from aortic cusp origin. Our group as developed an algorithm based on precordial transition pattern seen during clinical arrhythmia versus sinus rhythm to differentiate tachycardias arising from RVOT versus the cusp region.[64] The R- and S-wave amplitude and duration, as well as the QRS duration in leads V_2 and V_3, were measured during both sinus rhythm and the arrhythmia (PVC/nonsustained VT). A transition ratio was then calculated by computing the percentage R wave during arrhythmia $(R/R + S)_{VT}$ divided by the percentage R wave in sinus rhythm $(R/R + S)_{SR}$ (Fig. 31.16A). We found a V_2 transition ratio ≥ 0.6 to predict a cusp origin with 95% sensitivity and 100% specificity. The advantage of this algorithm is that it takes into account subjective variation in the patient's body habitus, cardiac rotation, respiratory variation, and ECG lead positioning by measuring precordial transition during the PVC/VT relative to the SR precordial transition. However, we acknowledge that calculating a V_2 transition ratio can be cumbersome. Therefore, a more practical clinical tool for accurately localizing these arrhythmias is to assess whether precordial transition during the PVC/VT occurs before or later than that in sinus rhythm. When the precordial transition of the clinical arrhythmia occurs later than the precordial transition in sinus rhythm, then that excludes a cusp source of the tachycardia with 100% accuracy (Fig. 31.16, *B*). This approach presumes that there is no underlying bundle branch block during native conduction.

Treatment of Outflow Tract Ventricular Arrhythmias

The decision to treat medically and/or ablate OTVTs depends on the frequency and severity of symptoms and patient preference. The initial drug of choice is usually a β-blocker. Calcium channel blockers, such as verapamil and diltiazem, may also be considered and can act synergistically with β-blockers. These arrhythmias show variable response to antiarrhythmic drug therapy and all classes of membrane specific antiarrhythmic drugs may decrease the arrhythmia burden although the degree of reduction is unpredictable. Acute termination of OTVTs can be achieved by several means. The initial step is to increase vagal tone by Valsalva maneuvers or by application of carotid sinus pressure. If these strategies are ineffective, an intravenous dose of adenosine (6–24 mg) or verapamil (10 mg) or lidocaine (dose calculated by body weight) can be effective to terminate VT.[9]

Catheter ablation of idiopathic OTVTs in symptomatic patients is usually considered when β-blockers, calcium channel blockers, or antiarrhythmic drugs are not effective, not tolerated, or not desired.[65] In addition, in patients with PVC-mediated cardiomyopathy, ablation therapy may be considered the first line of treatment because this offers the most effective method for arrhythmia suppression while avoiding antiarrhythmic drug therapy in this vulnerable patient population with limited drug options. A challenging treatment dilemma is asymptomatic patients with normal ventricular function who have a high burden of ventricular arrhythmia and so may be at risk of developing PVC-induced cardiomyopathy. The typical approach is to monitor these patients closely with serial ambulatory ECG monitors and echocardiograms as discussed earlier, and intervene aggressively should they develop cardiac dysfunction.

In patients with apparently idiopathic OTVT and structurally normal heart on echocardiogram, it is important to rule out presence of scar and cardiomyopathy. One series by Ghannam et al. identified MRI scar in 25% of patients with apparently idiopathic PVCs referred for ablation and found that the presence of scar predicted long-term risk of VT, independent of LVEF.[66] In patients with apparently idiopathic OTVAs in whom scar on MRI is present, suggesting underlying NICM, programmed ventricular stimulation can be considered to risk stratify long-term risk of sudden death. In patients with scar who are inducible for sustained VT after elimination of OTVT, risks and benefits of ICD implantation should be discussed on an individualized basis.

Mapping of Ventricular Outflow Tract Tachycardias. The choice of mapping strategy begins with careful review of the 12-lead surface ECG. For OTVTs with LBBB morphology and late precordial transition (>V_4 and/or later than the precordial transition during sinus rhythm), the RVOT should be mapped first, whereas for arrhythmias manifesting RBBB morphology, mapping can begin in the aortic cusps and/or LVOT. If the ECG morphology is suggestive of an epicardial LV summit origin, the GCV/AIV should be mapped as well, and this can be accomplished by either positioning a separate recording catheter in this location and/or advancing the ablation catheter. Although the GCV–AIV region can be challenging to access, in the authors' experience, a long sheath in the proximal or mid-CS can facilitate catheter advancement to this location. Smaller-caliber multipolar catheters can also be helpful to map in this location (EP Star; Baylis Medical, Mississauga, ON, Canada; Map-iT; Access Point Technologies EP, Rogers, MN).

In the past, a 4-mm nonirrigated tip mapping/ablation catheter was typically used for targeting RVOT tachycardias and the majority of basal LV tachycardias and a 3.5-mm open-irrigated

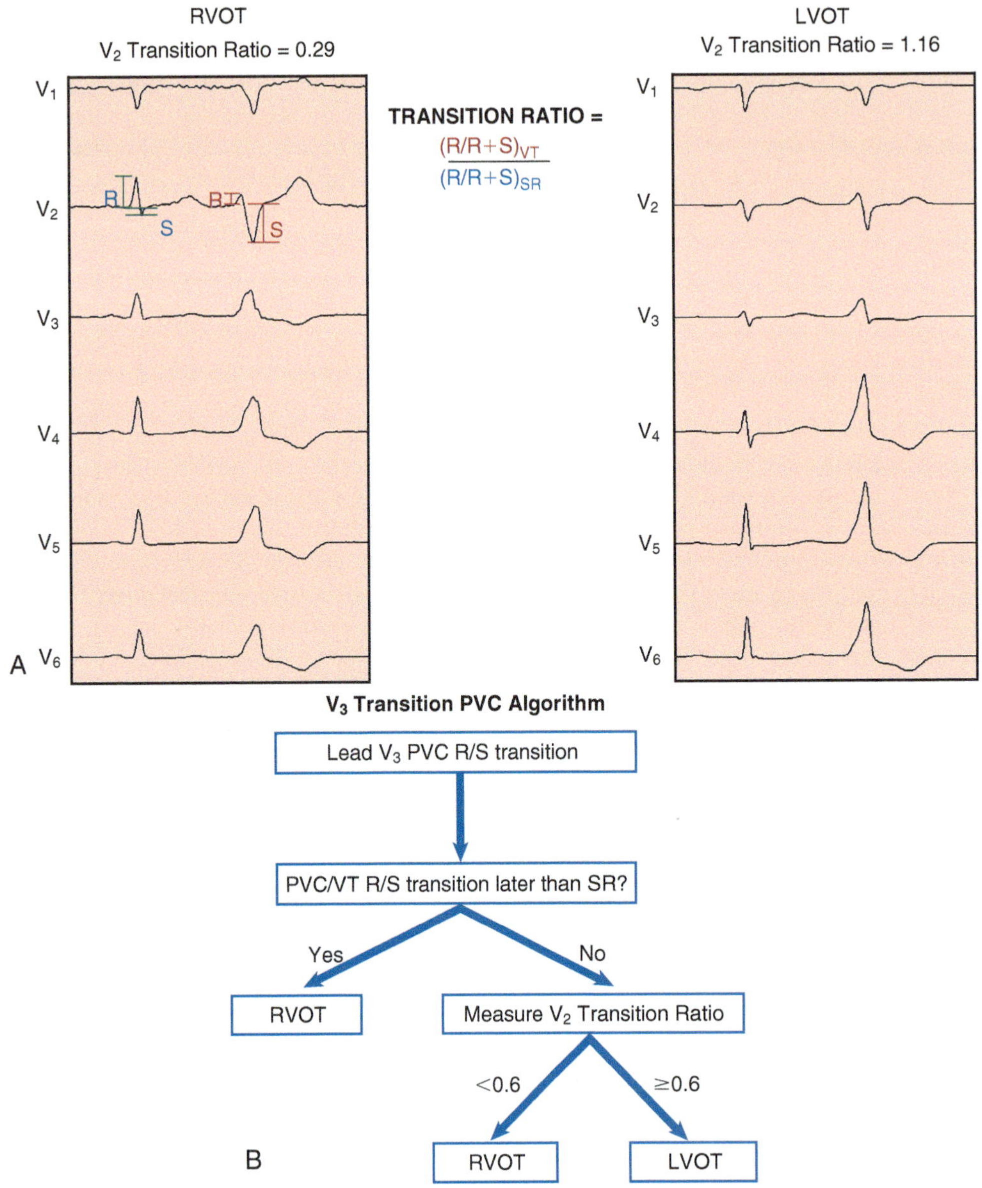

Fig. 31.16 (A) Calculating V_2 transition ratio. *Left,* An example of a patient with a right ventricular outflow tract tachycardia (RVOT). *Right,* An example of a patient with left ventricular outflow tract tachycardia (LVOT). In each panel a normal sinus beat is followed by a premature ventricular complex (PVC). Measurements of the R- and S-wave amplitudes (mV) are performed for both the normal sinus beat (*blue*) and the PVC (*red*). The V_2 transition ratio is calculated using the following formula: $[B/(B + C)_{VT}]/[E/(E + F)_{SR}]$ (A). Consistent with V_2 transition ratio calculation, precordial transition of the left panel PVC occurred later compared with sinus rhythm, thus predicting a right-sided site of origin while precordial transition of the right panel PVC occurred earlier compared with sinus, suggesting a left-sided origin. Diagnostic algorithm for outflow tract ventricular tachycardia (VT) with transition in lead V_3 (B). If the PVC transition (R > S) occurs later than sinus rhythm, the PVC origin is the RVOT (100% specificity). If the PVC transition occurs at or earlier than the sinus transition, the V_2 transition ratio is measured. If the transition ratio is <0.6, then RVOT origin is likely. If the transition ratio is ≥0.6, then LVOT origin is likely (sensitivity 95%, specificity 100%). See text for details.

tip catheter was preferred for the cusp region and for ablating in the GCV–AIV location. In the latter location, due to the low blood flow and limited confines, it is not uncommon to encounter very high impedances at baseline (before power delivery). This can be overcome by resetting the power delivery parameters. Despite these modifications however in our experience it is difficult to deliver more than 20 W of power for a sustained period from this location. These days, regardless of the case setting, the open irrigated catheter platform is used in most, if not all, cases and energy delivery is customized based on the tachycardia site of origin.

The procedure is usually begun by creating a detailed electroanatomical shell of the chamber of interest. In the ideal scenario, mapping is performed while the patient is having frequent arrhythmia since this allows creation of the chamber geometry together with electrical activation of each point relative to a

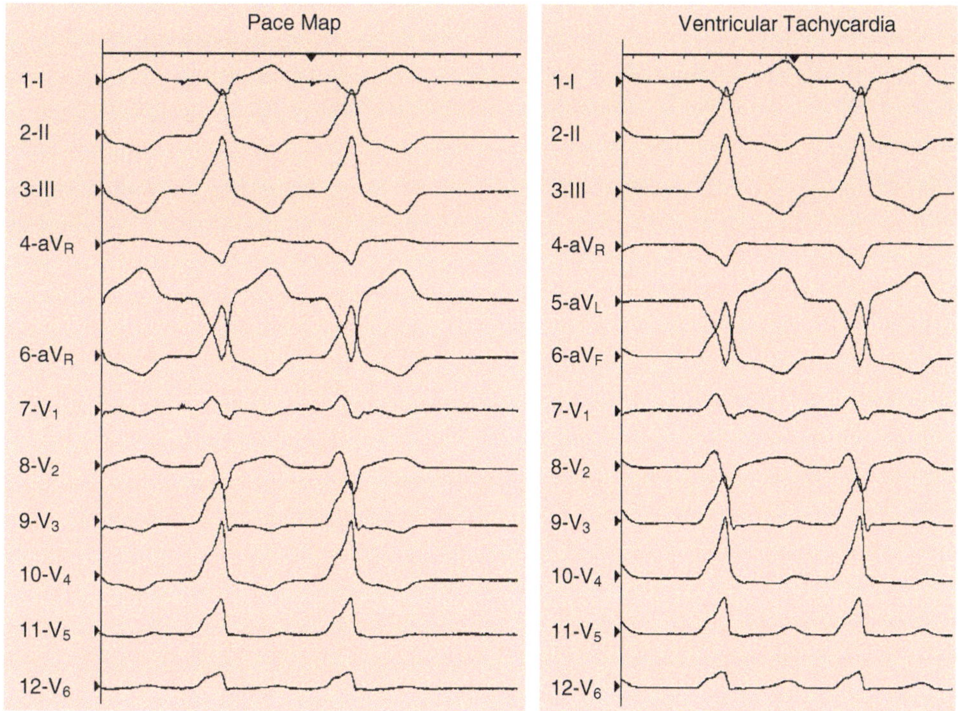

Fig. 31.17 Pace mapping left coronary cusp arrhythmia. *Right,* Clinical ventricular tachycardia from the left coronary cusp is depicted. *Left,* Pace map at the diastolic threshold from the successful site of ablation within the cusp resulted in identical QRS morphology. (Courtesy Dr. Enrique Rodriguez.)

reference. It is important to identify important anatomical landmarks during creation of the electroanatomical map. When mapping the RVOT, the His signal, tricuspid annulus, outflow tract, and pulmonic annulus are defined. When mapping the LVOT and particularly the AMC and aortic cusps, the use of ICE can be especially helpful to define the anatomy. In addition, the electroanatomical map can be integrated with the shell of the chamber of interest created using CARTOSOUND technology (Biosense Webster, Diamond Bar, CA), which allows for rapid and accurate creation of the outflow tract region including the valves. It is important to point out that catheter location at the same position can differ significantly during sinus rhythm versus tachycardia beats. Therefore, if the electroanatomical map is constructed during tachycardia, at critical locations (earliest site and location demonstrating the best pace map) additional points during sinus beats should also be acquired. These can be retained on the original map as *floating* or *location*-only points, which prevents shell distortion. The advantage of this approach is that if the tachycardia terminates and becomes noninducible during mapping or after the first ablation, then the points marked during sinus rhythm at this location can serve as targets for additional lesions. While a point-by-point contact mapping with the ablation catheter has been typically used for idiopathic OTVT ablation, multielectrode catheter platforms such as the Pentaray, DecaNav (both by Biosense Webster), HD Grid (Abbott, Chicago, IL), or Orion (Boston Scientific, San Jose, CA) can also be used for this purpose. Their advantage is the ability to rapidly acquire a much higher-density map in the area of interest. Their disadvantage includes lesser maneuvarability and the propensity to cause ventricular ectopy during mapping. Moreover, since a separate ablation catheter is also required, the use of multielectrode catheters can add significantly to the overall procedure cost. For these reasons, we tend to favor using the ablation catheter alone for targeting OTVTs. Contact force sensing technology is another modality that has been found to improve the success of catheter ablation in different arrhythmia scenarios, and nowadays we use it frequently for ablating OTVTs.[67–69]

In patients with spontaneous arrhythmia, the site of origin is determined by activation mapping. At the site of earliest activation, the local bipolar electrogram recorded from the distal electrode usually precedes the QRS onset of the clinical arrhythmia by >15 ms and the unipolar electrogram records a QS signal. Typically pace mapping from such a location should produce an exact match (all 12 ECG leads) of the clinical tachycardia. Fig. 31.17 shows an example of a pace map from the successful ablation site in the LCC, which replicates exactly the clinical arrhythmia. In the absence of spontaneous arrhythmia, a variety of maneuvers can be helpful, including ventricular or atrial burst pacing, incremental isoproterenol infusion, aminophylline, calcium, phenylephrine or epinephrine infusion. Isoproterenol infusion is typically used and titrated to achieve a 20–30% increase in the sinus rate. In a small subset of patients, increased burden of arrhythmia becomes manifest during isoproterenol washout.[8] In some cases, despite these maneuvers, only rare PVCs can be induced. In these cases, pace mapping can be helpful.[70] The key to success when pace mapping is to pay special attention in making sure that the ECG match is as perfect as possible including subtle features such as notches within the QRS complexes across multiple leads. To help quantify this

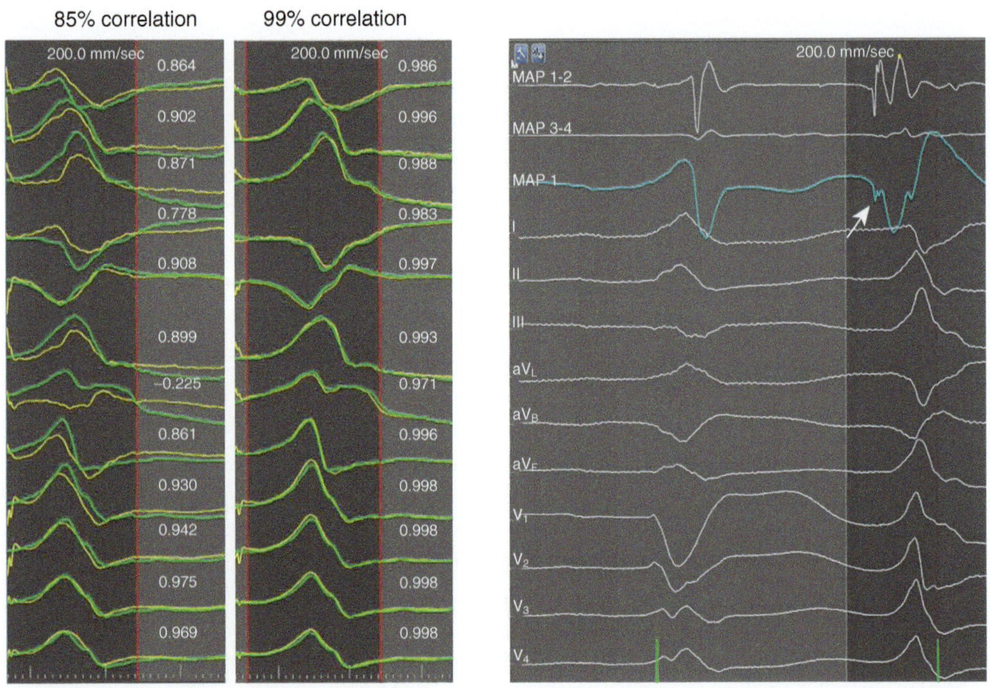

Fig. 31.18 Automated quantification of pace maps to the clinical arrhythmia. In this patient with infrequent PVCs, pace mapping was performed using an automated algorithm (PaSO; Biosense Webster, Diamond Bar, CA). *Left,* Increasing degree of correlation with the best pace map having a 99% match to the clinical PVC (the clinical PVC in *green* and the pace maps overlay in *yellow*). *Right,* Activation at the site of 99% pace map during a spontaneous clinical PVC. This showed an early bipolar activation (−46 ms) and the unipolar signal showed *QS* morphology (*arrow*). Ablation at this site was successful.

comparison, automated algorithms have been developed which may be helpful. Fig. 31.18 shows an example of the use of automated quantification of pace mapping using the PASO module (CARTO, Biosense Webster) in a patient with rare PVCs.

Holter and event monitoring can be helpful to quantify arrhythmia burden throughout the day, which can guide scheduling of the ablation procedure accordingly based on when highest ventricular arrhythmia burden is expected so as to increase likelihood of procedural success. The procedure is typically performed under conscious sedation, titrated in such a manner to keep the patient comfortable while not suppressing the arrhythmia mechanism (delayed after depolarization mediated triggered activity). Identification of clinical triggers can also be helpful, especially for patients with infrequent arrhythmia in whom it is not likely to be spontaneous or readily inducible at the time of ablation.

ABLATION

We typically perform ablation in the outflow tract region using irrigated-tipped ablation catheters with power levels titrated from 20–40 W in order to achieve 10–15 Ω impedance drop over a 60- to 90-second duration. The preferred catheter irrigant is normal saline. Because the arrhythmia source is focal and usually superficial, ablation at successful sites usually results in early termination of the arrhythmia (≤15 seconds; sometimes preceded by increase in arrhythmia frequency likely due to stimulatory effect of RF energy in proximity to the arrhythmia focus).[3,40] If ablation does not result in early termination of the arrhythmia (<30 seconds), RF delivery is stopped and additional mapping is continued to find the next ideal location where the aforementioned protocol is repeated. Previously, ablation in the cusp region was typically performed with lower power settings (10–35 W) and shorter lesion durations (30–60 seconds) due to fear of damage to coronary arteries and aortic root perforation. However, there has been increasing recognition that longer and higher-power lesions can be safely delivered from this location. We have recently demonstrated that prolonged duration ablation (up to 5 minutes) using incremental power delivery ranging from 20–45 can be safely delivered from both within and below the aortic cusp region to successfully target intramural and LV summit OTVTs that are refractory to conventional ablation. However, when using this approach it is imperative to monitor tissue–catheter contact and live lesion creation with ICE in order to minimize the risk of excessive energy delivery leading to "steam pop"[71] (Fig. 31.19).

Mapping and ablation in the aortic cusps are greatly complemented by the use of ICE with or without CARTOSOUND as discussed earlier. This tool provides real-time confirmation of catheter position and visualization of the coronary ostia. Coronary angiography was previously frequently used to delineate the ostium of the left main coronary artery when targeting arrhythmias in the LCC or the commissure between the RCC and LCC. However, as shown by Hoffmayer et al., the combination of ICE with electroanatomical mapping is a suitable alternative to

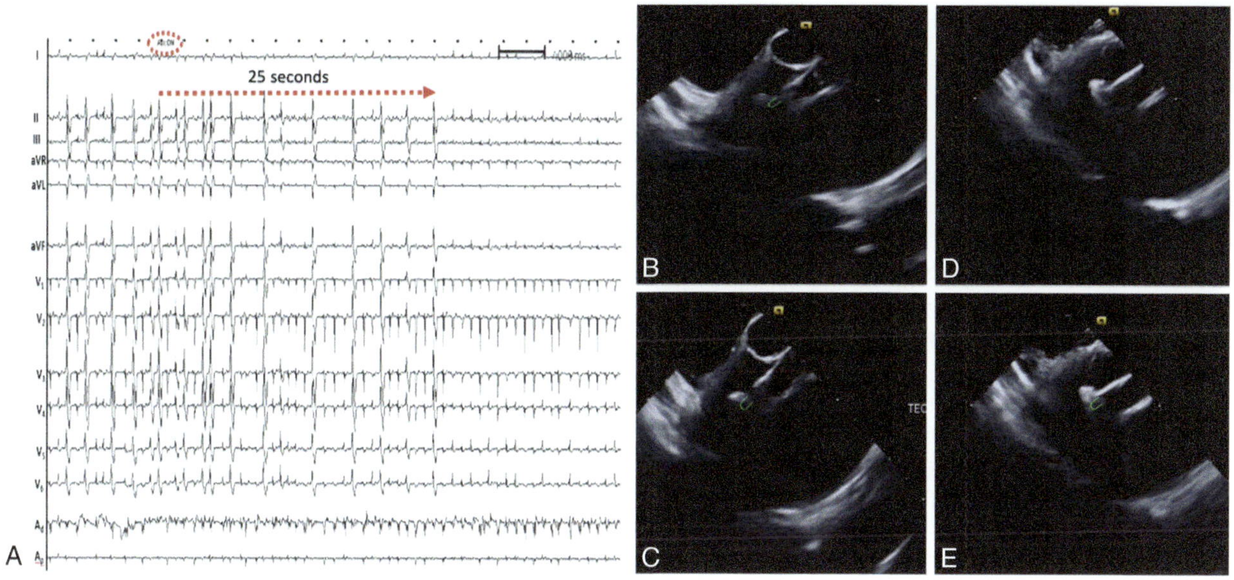

Fig. 31.19 Intracardiac echocardiography visualization of lesion formation during ablation. (A) The electrocardiogram shows start of energy application (dotted red oval) and delayed suppression of premature ventricular complexes (after 25 s of radiofrequency delivery) from subvalvular left ventricular outflow tract (B). Catheter tip is visualized in this location by intracardiac echocardiography, and lesion formation is demonstrated after 30 s (B), after 1 min (C), after 2 min (D), and after 3 min (E). (From Garg L, Daubert T, Lin A, et al. Utility of prolonged duration endocardial ablation for ventricular arrhythmias originating from the left ventricular summit. *JACC Clin Electrophysiol* 2022:8(4):465-476.)

coronary angiography to guide safe ablation in the aortic root.[72] At the present time we are using ICE (with CARTOSOUND technology) to identify left main ostium and have largely done away with performing coronary angiography before ablating arrhythmias from the aortic cusp region.

It is important nevertheless to understand the anatomy of the coronary arteries in relation to the OT region as several cases of iatrogenic coronary artery injury have been reported during catheter ablation in this region. The LAD artery frequently comes in close proximity to the leftward posterior aspect of the distal RVOT and may be injured during aggressive ablation in this region especially when ablating above the pulmonic valve. One helpful clue of the possibility of proximity to the LAD while mapping in the posterior aspect of the superior RVOT near the pulmonic valve is the recording of far-field atrial signals. These signals, when present, likely originate from the tip of the neighboring left atrial appendage (LAA). CTA and autopsy studies have described the anatomical relationship between the LAA and the LV summit region, and there have been case reports of successful LV summit PVC ablation from the LAA.[73-76] Importantly, the junction between the LAA and posterior RVOT is in close proximity the LAD bifurcation and direct visualization of the coronary arterial system with either coronary angiography or ICE should be done prior to delivery of RF energy from these locations.[77] The LAD can also potentially be compromised when ablating in the lower anterior RVOT region, which typically abuts the early part of mid LAD (after the first septal perforator).[78] Ablation in this location can sometimes be useful for successfully ablating LV summit arrhythmia focus, which demonstrates earliest activation in the anterior interventricular vein.[79]

Caution needs to be exercised when the arrhythmia focus is localized to basal septum in the LVOT or entrance of the RVOT, because these locations are in close proximity to the penetrating bundle of His. If a prominent His deflection is recorded at the site of earliest activation and/or best pacemap, our practice is to defer ablation due to the high risk of causing AV block.[40] In these cases, cryoablation may also be considered.

Ablation of epicardial and intramural IVTs in the outflow tract region requires special consideration. Epicardial IVTs usually arise from the LV summit, and because this location is in proximity to the AMC, LCC, and the superior mitral annulus, early electrical activity can be recorded from these sites as well although the signal at these locations appears *far-field* (recordings lack sharp deflections). In addition the pace maps from these locations are a poor match of the clinical tachycardia.[80] The ideal ablation site for these arrhythmias is usually found either by mapping the coronary venous system and its branches, or by percutaneous epicardial approach.[81,82] For mapping the distal coronary venous system (GCV and AIV), it is helpful to use a long sheath to facilitate catheter manipulation to the appropriate location. In the authors' experience some of these idiopathic epicardial VTs can be successfully ablated from the GCV. However, because this location is in close proximity to large epicardial vessels, coronary angiography should be performed before energy delivery. Idiopathic epicardial VT sources near the AIV can be more challenging to ablate for two reasons: (1) this vessel is difficult to map because of its caliber and acute takeoff from the GCV and (2) it is adjacent to the LAD artery. In some cases, the AIV region can be approached from the endocardium on anterior septal aspect of the RVOT under the pulmonic valve. A catheter in this location when visualized fluoroscopically in the left anterior oblique projection appears to be significantly leftward.[79] However, it is important to recognize that the mid LAD is very close to this location, so coronary angiography should be preformed before delivering energy. Another option especially for tachycardia source around the GCV is to deliver energy from the cusp region or the basal LV endocardium (AMC and superior mitral annulus). The ability to achieve a reasonable pace map (~90% match) of the clinical arrhythmia at lower energy outputs (~5 mA) from these alternative locations suggests relative proximity of the arrhythmia focus. However, successful ablation from these locations usually requires higher energy delivery (up to 40–50 W) for longer duration (2–5 minutes).[83] In the authors' experience, if the idiopathic epicardial arrhythmia focus cannot be targeted from the GCV–AIV region or the alternative options (RVOT, cusp region, and/or basal LV), then approaching it via *direct percutaneous pericardial access is usually not successful because of the close proximity of this location to the left coronary arteries and the presence of epicardial fat both of which limit effective energy delivery.*[79] In cases where elimination of VA is difficult due to the presence of a deep intramural focus, longer-duration ablation lesions may be necessary. In our experience, up to 3–5 minutes of continuous ablation may be required to achieve elimination of tachycardia in some of these cases. When doing so, it is important to pay close attention to impedance changes during energy delivery as well as constantly monitor lesion creation with ICE visualization. Other alternatives include sequential unipolar, simultaneous unipolar, or bipolar ablation.[84] Ablation with a needle-tipped catheter can also be effective for cases with deep intramural arrhythmia foci.[85] Alcohol infusion in septal branches of the coronary venous system has also been shown to be effective for targeting some of these arrhythmias.[86] For patients with epicardial LV summit foci which are in close proximity to coronary vessels, surgical cryoablation or endoscopic robotic epicardial ablation or myocardial ethanol injection under direct visualization have been performed.[87–91] Furthermore, there are ongoing investigations examining alternative treatment modalities including external beam ablation, magnetically directed metallic nanoparticles, and pulsed-field electroporation for targeting challenging arrhythmias.[92–95]

CLINICAL OUTCOMES AND COMPLICATIONS

Catheter ablation of idiopathic OTVT has become a popular approach in the management of these arrhythmias. With increased appreciation for the complex anatomy of the outflow tract facilitated by the use of advanced mapping techniques including ICE, ablation can be done safely and successfully in the vast majority of these patients. A large multicenter study has previously reported acute success rate of 84% and long-term arrhythmia suppression rates (mean follow-up duration: 1.9 years) of 85% and 71% on and off antiarrhythmic medications, respectively.[96] More recently, Hayashi, et al. examined trends in OTVT ablation over a 16-year-period at the authors' center and found our overall procedural and clinical success rates to be 86% and 87%, respectively. This study showed that over the 16-year period, there was an increase in the procedural volume of OTVT ablations and especially those originating from the LVOT (including the LV summit and cusp region). The study also found that over time there was improvement in single procedure efficacy which likely reflects more effective lesion creation aided by increasing use of ICE and contact force-sensing technology. Interestingly, over this 16-year period, procedure-related complication rate remained consistently low (2%).[97]

Catheter ablation of idiopathic OTVT can be safely performed without complication in most patients. In the authors' experience, the most frequent complications during OTVT ablation pertains to vascular access. Another less common but potentially serious complication is the development of pericardial effusion which in our experience can occur in ~1.5% of cases and typically requires pericardiocentesis. Damage to conduction system in the form of bundle branch block or atrioventricular block can also occur infrequently during mapping and ablation of these arrhythmias. Other serious events that are even rarer include development of aortic regurgitation (during retrograde catheter access across the valve and/or ablation in the cusp region), pulmonic regurgitation (during ablation in the superior RVOT or proximal pulmonary artery), or damage to the left coronary artery and its branches (as previously discussed in this chapter).[78,98,99] Furthermore, there has been a recent recognition that silent cerebral embolic events may occur, in patients undergoing left-sided ablation particularly when a retrograde aortic approach is chosen.[100] While the clinical significance of silent brain emboli as seen on MRI remains unclear, in order to minimize possibility of this occurring, operators should always carefully visualize the ascending aorta and aortic valve with echocardiography before advancing an ablation catheter and preferentially select a transseptal approach in patients with significant atherosclerotic aortic disease or aortic valve calcification. Furthermore, a therapeutic ACT (≥300 seconds) should be maintained while mapping and ablating in the LV and aortic cusp region. The results of the STROKE-VT study suggested that the use of direct oral anticoagulants after ablation may result in lower clinical cerebrovascular events and asymptomatic cerebrovascular events seen on MRI compared to aspirin.[101] Even prior to the publication of this study, our routine practice has been to prescribe direct oral anticoagulant therapy for 2–4 weeks in patients undergoing left-sided ablation including the OTVT population.

TROUBLESHOOTING THE DIFFICULT CASE

The most common challenges encountered and potential solutions for mapping and ablation of idiopathic outflow tract VTs are listed in Table 31.3.

Challenges related to infrequency of arrhythmia and/or lack of inducibility during the ablation procedure have been previously discussed in this chapter. Another scenario that is not uncommon is when a broad area of early activation is observed at the presumed site of origin. However, this implies that the true tachycardia source may be in an adjacent location. So, for example, an arrhythmia source in the right coronary cusp region can manifest a broad area of early activation in the superior septal RVOT. Similarly, LV summit source can manifest a

TABLE 31.3 Troubleshooting Difficult Cases

Problem	Causes	Possible Solutions
No inducible tachycardia/PVCs	Sedation Random variability	Withdraw sedation; administer isoproterenol/epinephrine; aminophylline Reschedule on another occasion
Inability to find presystolic sites in RVOT	Incomplete mapping of RVOT Source located outside RVOT	More detailed RVOT mapping, including PA Explore other areas (aortic cusps, GCV/AIV)
No sites with presystolic activity	Incomplete mapping of GCV/AIV LV summit site Intramural site	Use of sheath to facilitate access to GCV/AIV Epicardial mapping; surgical cryoablation Surgical cryoablation
Concern for causing coronary artery injury	Optimal ablation site near coronary artery or ostium	Forego ablation; surgical cryoablation

AIV, Anterior interventricular vein; *GCV,* great cardiac vein/anterior interventricular vein; *LV,* left ventricle; *PA,* pulmonary artery; *PVCs,* premature ventricular complexes; *RVOT,* right ventricular outflow tract.

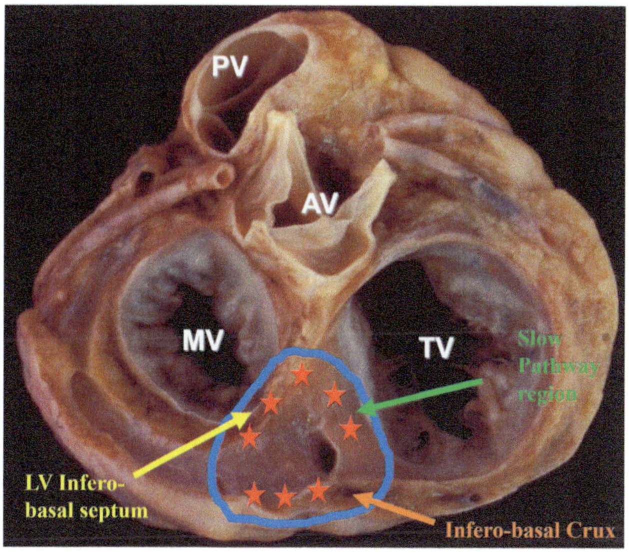

Fig. 31.20 LV inferobasal septal ventricular arrhythmias. Coronal section at the level of the tricuspid and mitral valves showing the regions of the LV inferobasal septum (*yellow arrow*), slow pathway region (*green arrow*) and inferobasal crux (*orange arrow*).

broad area of early activation in the endocardial aspect of the LVOT region. Thus, *diligent mapping of neighboring structures and meticulous analysis of electrograms, including unipolar signal recordings as well as pace maps, are the key to successful ablation.*

When the site of earliest activation is in the coronary cusps or the epicardium, visualization of the coronary arteries using ICE or coronary angiography are recommended to better define the proximity to major epicardial vessels. Although the ostium of the left main coronary artery can be readily visualized with ICE, it does not adequately define the vessel's course distally beyond the ostium. It is therefore recommended to perform left coronary angiography before ablating outflow tract arrhythmias from the GCV–AIV location or via percutaneous epicardial access. In cases where lesions are delivered relatively close to a coronary vessel (5–10 mm), coronary angiography should be repeated after lesion delivery to assess vessel patency postablation. If the ventricular arrhythmia source appears in close proximity to the His-bundle region, then care has to be exercised during RF energy delivery (lesser power over shorter duration while monitoring for conduction changes such as PR prolongation). Cryothermy can also be considered for these locations, although the cryo catheter can be more challenging to manipulate and is not visualized accurately on all electroanatomical mapping platforms.

As discussed earlier, idiopathic epicardial OTVTs can be challenging to ablate. These often arise from the LV summit. In the authors' experience, the majority of these VTs can be successfully ablated usually from basal LV endocardium (AMC region) or sometimes above the aortic cusp region and occasionally the septal RVOT. Meticulous mapping for obtaining earliest activation/best pace map should be performed from all aspects including the septal RVOT, cusp region, AMC, superior mitral annulus, and the GCV–AIV before energy delivery. Of note, in cases where a septal intramural arrhythmia focus is suspected and a septal perforator branch of the AIV is seen, multielectrode microcatheters (EP Star; Baylis Medical, Mississauga, ON, Canada; Map-iT; Access Point Technologies EP, Rogers, MN) or mapping wires (VisionWire, Biotronik, Berlin, Germany) can be used to subselect these coronary venous branches. Although the target branches themselves may be too small to advance an ablation catheter, these microcatetheters and wires can be visualized fluoroscopically as well as on the electroanatomical map, and this location can then be targeted aggressively from the adjacent endocardial locations.

Another challenge when ablating OTVTs pertains to preferential conduction from the source that can result in more than one exit site. While this phenomenon can occur anywhere in the outflow tract, it is particularly common when ablating in the septal RVOT and the coronary cusps. Often, ablation at a site with reasonably early (approximately 15–20 ms) local activation and perfect pace map modifies the arrhythmia QRS morphology without suppressing the frequency.[102] In these cases, the site of origin is likely to be intramural with preferential conduction through adjacent structures, and successful ablation requires either targeting individual exit sites sequentially or more penetrating transmural lesions (often with long-duration lesions) from one location.

BASAL INFEROSEPTUM: SITE OF ORIGIN FOR IDIOPATHIC VAs

While the majority of idiopathic VAs originate from the OT region, there has been increasing recognition of the *basal inferoseptum* (BIS) as another site of origin of these arrhythmias (Fig. 31.20).[103–105] Li et al. reported their approach of successfully ablating idiopathic VAs originating from the BIS of the LV below the left-sided conduction system in seven patients with the observation of transient junctional rhythm during ablation that was seen in three of these cases.[103] Arrhythmias originating from this region typically manifest a RBBB morphology with positive precordial concordance or LBBB morphology with early precordial transition (by precordial leads V_2 or V_3), with leftward and superior axis. Another location that has been observed to be a less common source of idiopathic VAs is the *inferior basal crux* region, and arrhythmias arising from this location can share ECG features with those originating from the LV BIS. We have recently reported ECG findings that can be helpful in distinguishing between the two locations. In our experience the following features were highly predictive of the arrhythmia source being from the LV BIS: (1) presence of small r waves in inferior leads, (2) R/S ratio <1 in V_1, (3) MDI <0.55, (4) QRS notching in lead II, and (5) narrower QRS duration (Fig. 31.21). The first three of these five features were the most likely to be different for VA arising from the LV BIS versus the inferobasal crux region. However, prior to delivering energy in the LV BIS region, we recommend mapping from pertinent adjacent locations and particularly the parahisian region in the RV. The latter can also be a source of idiopathic VAs, and in our experience, the slow pathway (SP) region can sometimes be the target location for these arrhythmias (Fig. 31.22). Characteristic ECG features of idiopathic VAs successfully targeted from the SP region include discordance in QRS axis in between inferior limb leads II (usually predominantly positive forces) and III (usually predominantly negative forces) and LBBB morphology with variable precordial transition patterns (between leads V_2–V_4) (Fig. 31.21).[106] When targeting this location with RF energy, junctional ectopy is commonly seen during energy delivery (observed in 75%), and sometimes additional cryothermy may be necessary. Regardless of the approach, ablation outcomes for VAs targeted from the SP region are excellent with 92% patients in our series experiencing acute clinical success and only one patient needing a pacemaker for temporary heart block.

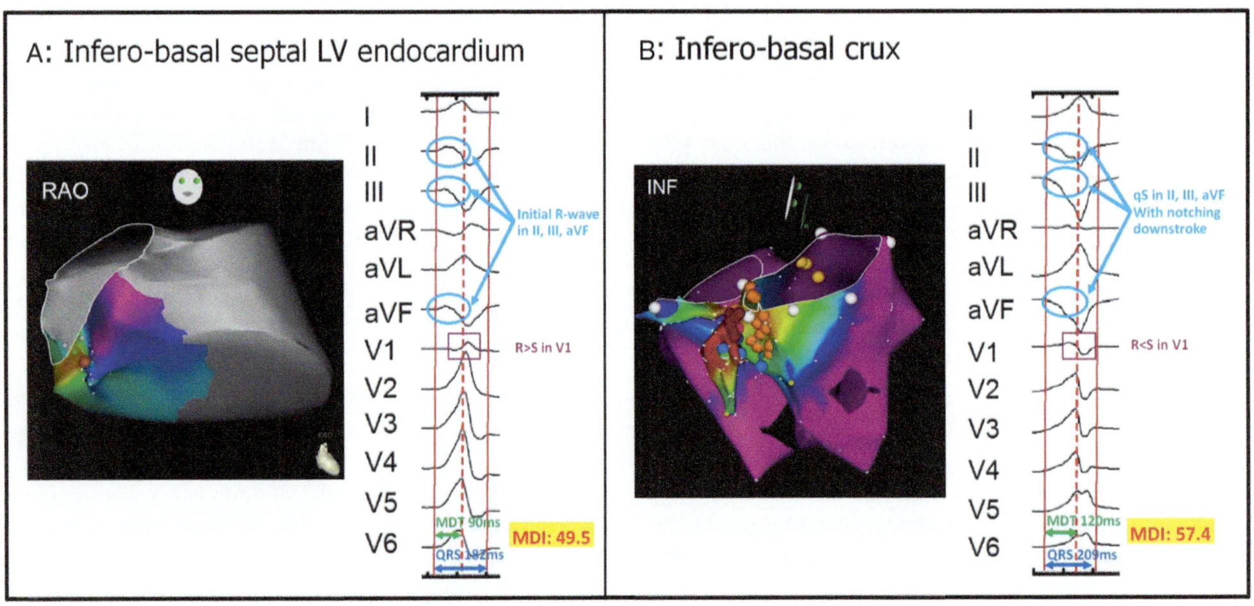

Fig. 31.21 Electrocardiographic features of idiopathic VAs from the basal inferoseptal LV endocardium versus the inferobasal crux. Electrocardiographic (ECG) features that differentiate successful ablation from the basal inferoseptal left ventricular (LV) endocardium (A) versus from the epicardial inferobasal crux (B). Note that basal inferoseptal left ventricular endocardium ventricular arrhythmias are more likely to have initial R-wave (or isoelectric period) in the inferior leads, R>S in lead V_1, narrower QRS duration, and lower maximum deflection index (MDI) value (often with MDI <0.55). *INF,* Inferior; *RAO,* right anterior oblique. (From Liang JJ, Shirai Y, Briceno DF, et al. Electrocardiographic and electrophysiologic characteristics of idiopathic ventricular arrhythmias originating from the basal inferoseptal left ventricle. *JACC Clin Electrophysiol* 2019:5(7):833-842.)

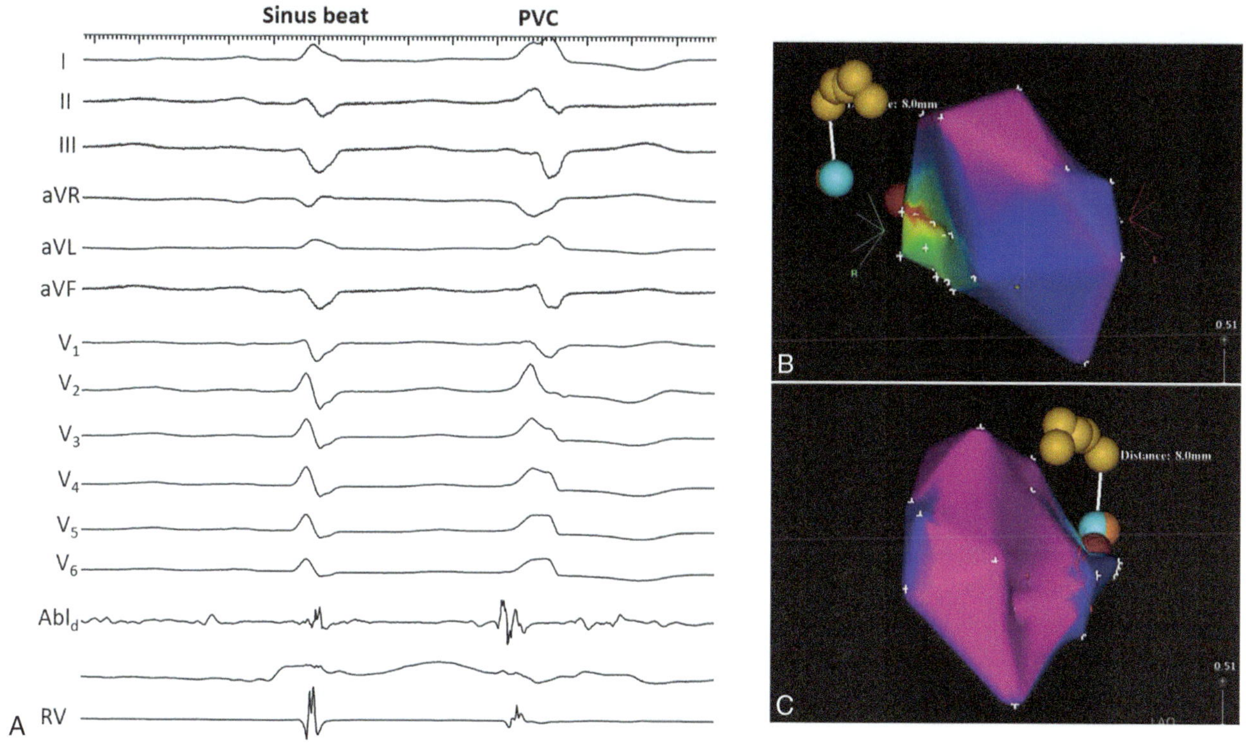

Fig. 31.22 Example of premature ventricular complex (PVC) that was successfully ablated from the slow pathway region. (A) During sinus rhythm the local electrogram has an atrial and a ventricular component and during PVC the local activation at this location precedes QRS by 35 ms. (B, C) Electroanatomical maps in right and left anterior oblique orientations, respectively. In these panels, *yellow dots* represent His-bundle recording locations and *blue dot* represents successful ablation site, which is the slow pathway regionand is about 8 mm from the the closest His-bundle recording. It is not uncommon to observe junction rhythm during radiofrequency energy application in this location.

CONCLUSION

Idiopathic OTVTs constitute an important and frequently encountered clinical arrhythmias. The underlying mechanism is usually triggered activity, and hence the site of origin is typically focal. Although these arrhythmias are usually not life threatening, they can often be quite symptomatic. In a minority of patients these can lead to tachycardia-mediated LV dysfunction. Although pharmacologic therapy can be helpful in the management of these arrhythmias, catheter ablation is often the preferred strategy because it is curative and safe in the majority. The key to successful ablation of OTVTs is accurate localization of the arrhythmia source. This can be achieved by careful analysis of the 12-lead ECG, which provides important preprocedural clues on the site of origin. Additional localization is achieved by careful activation and pace mapping of the outflow tract region, which is facilitated by the use of electroanatomical mapping, advanced imaging, and ICE.

REFERENCES

Please refer to the e-book for a complete list of references.

32

Ablation of Idiopathic Left and Right Ventricular and Fascicular Tachycardias

Akihiko Nogami, Yuki Komatsu, Hiroshi Tada

KEY POINTS

- The mechanism of idiopathic mitral and tricuspid annular ventricular tachycardias (VTs) is mostly nonreentry (triggered activity or automaticity).
- Mitral annular VT has a right bundle branch block (RBBB) pattern and monophasic R or Rs in leads V_2–V_6. Catheter ablation of mitral annular VT is highly successful.
- Tricuspid annular VT exhibits a left bundle branch block pattern, R (r) in lead I, and the presence of an R (r) in lead aVL. Catheter ablation eliminates approximately 90% of VTs arising from the free wall portion of the tricuspid annulus but only 57% of those from the septal portions.
- Activation mapping seems to be most useful for ablation of papillary muscle VTs. They typically do not exhibit any recordings of diastolic potentials during sinus rhythm or VT. Catheter ablation can be challenging at times because catheter stability is difficult due to papillary muscle contractions. Successful catheter ablation usually requires intracardiac echocardiography to visualize the direct contact with the papillary muscle.
- VTs originating from the crux of the heart are rare and may arise by a focal mechanism from the epicardium; they may be induced with ventricular stimulation, and often require isoproterenol (catecholamine sensitive). Ablation may be performed within the proximal coronary sinus or proximal middle cardiac vein, or by an epicardial approach.
- The mechanism of verapamil-sensitive idiopathic left fascicular VT is reentry.
- Verapamil-sensitive left fascicular VT can be classified into six subtypes: (1) left posterior septal fascicular VT that exhibits RBBB configuration and left-axis deviation; (2) left posterior papillary muscle fascicular VT that exhibits RBBB and superior right-axis deviation; (3) left anterior septal fascicular VT that exhibits RBBB, right-axis deviation, and Rs pattern in V_5–V_6; (4) left anterior papillary muscle fascicular VT that exhibits RBBB, right-axis deviation, and deep S waves in V_5–V_6; (5) upper septal fascicular VT that exhibits a narrow QRS configuration and normal or right-axis deviation; and (6) reverse type VT of left posterior fascicular VT that exhibits Qr or rSr morphology in V1 and inferior axis.
- Ablation targets for left fascicular VT are the diastolic potential in the VT circuit or the presystolic fused Purkinje potential at the VT exit. The success rate of ablation is greater than 90% for left posterior fascicular VT.
- The mechanism of nonreentrant fascicular VT is abnormal automaticity from the Purkinje system. It is difficult to distinguish this VT from verapamil-sensitive left fascicular VT by 12-lead electrocardiogram. The ablation target is the earliest Purkinje activation during VT. The recurrence rate after ablation for nonreentrant fascicular VT is much higher than that of verapamil-sensitive reentrant left fascicular VT.

Sustained monomorphic ventricular tachycardia (VT) is most often related to myocardial structural heart disease, including healed myocardial infarction and cardiomyopathies. However, no apparent structural abnormality is identified in approximately 10% of all sustained monomorphic VTs in the United States[1] and 20% of those in Japan.[2] These VTs are referred to as "idiopathic." Idiopathic VTs usually occur in specific locations and have specific QRS morphologies,[3–8] whereas VTs associated with structural heart disease have a QRS morphology that tends to indicate the location of the scar. Idiopathic VT comprises multiple discrete subtypes that are best differentiated by their mechanism, QRS morphology, and site of origin. The most common idiopathic VT originates from a focus in the outflow tract of the right ventricle (RV) (see Chapter 31), and its mechanism is most likely triggered activity. In idiopathic left VT, the following six types exist: left ventricular (LV) outflow tract VT, VT from the mitral annulus, papillary muscle VT, VT arising from ventricular crux, verapamil-sensitive left fascicular VT, and nonreentrant fascicular VT (Box 32.1). This chapter focuses on the assessment and nonpharmacologic treatment of nonoutflow idiopathic left and right VTs and left fascicular VTs.

MITRAL ANNULAR VENTRICULAR TACHYCARDIA

Mitral annular VTs are found in 5% of symptomatic, idiopathic VTs/premature ventricular complexes (PVCs)[9–11] and occur with equal frequency in both sexes or with a male predominance (male, 53–69%). Mitral annular VTs were noted in 5% of all cases of idiopathic VT in some studies[9,10]; however, they have been shown in up to 49% of idiopathic repetitive monomorphic VTs arising from the left ventricle (LV).[11]

BOX 32.1 Classification of Left and Right Ventricular and Fascicular Tachycardias

Outflow Tract VTs *(triggered activity, reentry, or automaticity)*
- Left ventricular outflow tract, aortic sinus of Valsalva, or epicardial summit VT
- Right ventricular outflow tract or pulmonary artery cusp VT

Mitral Annular VT *(triggered activity, reentry, or automaticity)*
- Anterolateral, anteromedial (aortomitral continuity), lateral, posterior, or posteroseptal mitral annular origin

Tricuspid Annular VT *(triggered activity, reentry, or automaticity)*
- Posterior–posterolateral, anterior–anterolateral, posteroseptum, anteroseptal (para-Hisian), or midseptal tricuspid annular origin

Papillary Muscle VT *(triggered activity, reentry, or automaticity)*
- Left posterior papillary muscle, left anterior papillary muscle, or right papillary muscle origin

VT Arising From Ventricular Crux *(triggered activity, reentry, or automaticity)*
- Middle cardiac vein approach or epicardial approach

Left Ventricular Reentrant Fascicular VTs *(reentry)*
- Left posterior septal fascicular VT
- Left posterior papillary muscle fascicular VT
- Left anterior septal fascicular VT
- Left anterior papillary muscle fascicular VT
- Left upper septal fascicular VT
- Reverse type VT of left posterior fascicular VT

Nonreentrant Fascicular VT *(triggered activity or automaticity)*
- Left Purkinje origin
- Right Purkinje origin

VT, Ventricular tachycardia.

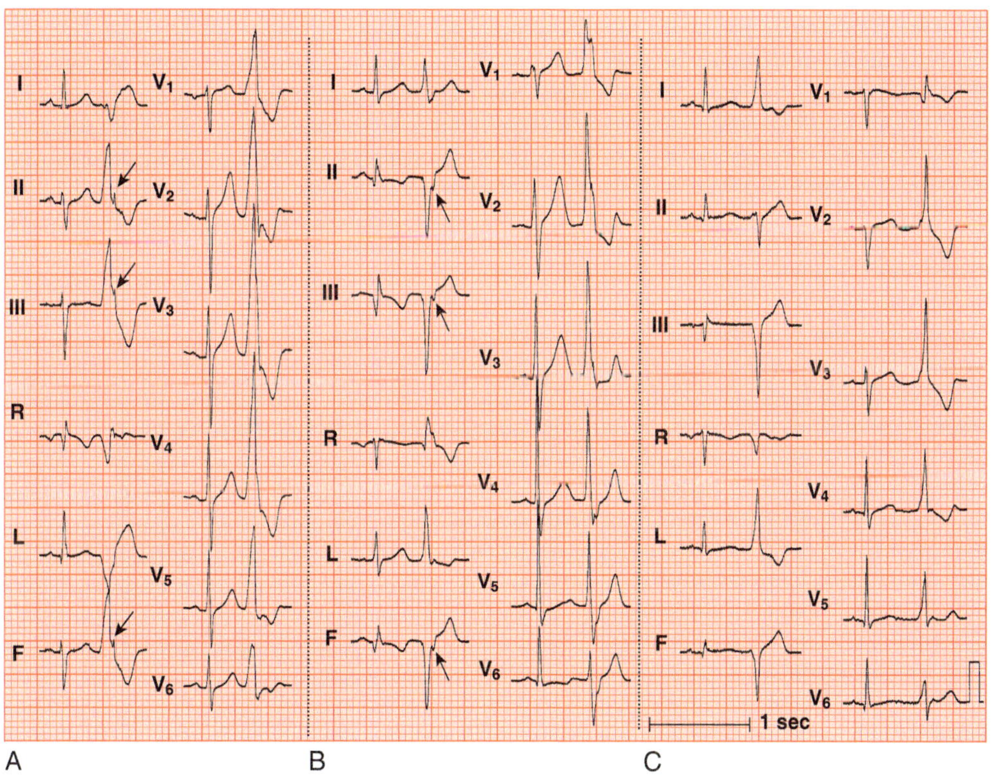

Fig. 32.1 Representative 12-lead electrocardiograms of premature ventricular complexes originating from the anterolateral (A), posterior (B), and posteroseptal (C) portions of the mitral annulus. The *arrows* indicate notching of the late phase of the QRS complex in the inferior leads. (From Tada H, Ito S, Naito S, et al. Idiopathic ventricular arrhythmia arising from the mitral annulus: a distinct subgroup of idiopathic ventricular arrhythmias. *J Am Coll Cardiol.* 2005;45:877–886.)

Pathophysiology

Classification

Mitral annular VT can be classified by the anatomical location. The majority originate from the anterolateral portion of the mitral annulus and, less commonly, the lateral, posterior, or posteroseptal annulus (Fig. 32.1).[9–11] The anterior and anteromedial portion of the mitral annulus, which is the region of the aortomitral continuity (AMC), may also be the origin of the VT.[12] However, the AMC is a fibrous structure and unlikely to be the true site of arrhythmia origin, with the actual site of origin being surrounding or deeper (LV summit) muscle fibers.

Mechanism

The mechanism of this arrhythmia appears to be nonreentry, and it may be a triggered activity based on the response to adenosine, verapamil, and pacing maneuvers. It has been proposed that a remnant of the atrioventricular (AV) conduction system close to the AMC, such as a dead-end tract,[13] might be important in the genesis of the nonreentrant mechanism for the tachycardia. The close proximity of the anterolateral mitral valve to the right ventricular (RV) outflow tract, LV outflow tract, and LV epicardial myocardium near the left coronary cusp suggests that idiopathic VT from these sites could likely originate from a single focus, with different exit points or activation of alternate pathways between the VT focus and an exit point, making assessment of the true site of origin challenging.[9]

Diagnostic Criteria

Surface Electrocardiogram

The electrocardiogram (ECG) in mitral annular VT has a right bundle branch block (RBBB) pattern and a monophasic R or Rs in leads V_2–V_6 (see Fig. 32.1).[9] Further, an ECG analysis can precisely distinguish among the different subtypes by the polarity of the QRS complex in the inferior and lateral leads. In anterolateral VTs, the polarity of the QRS complex in leads I and aVL is negative and positive in the inferior leads. Posterior VTs and posteroseptal VTs have a negative polarity in the inferior leads and positive polarity in leads I and aVL. VT arising from the free wall portion of the annulus, such as an anterolateral VT or posterior VT, has a longer QRS duration (sometimes also described as a delta-wave–like morphology) and notching in the late phase of the R wave/Q wave in the inferior leads. This feature is not observed in posteroseptal, anterior, or anteromedial VTs. Notching of the late phase of the QRS complex in the inferior leads and widening of the QRS complex observed in these VTs may result from phased excitation from the LV free wall to the RV.[9] Posterior VTs have a dominant R in V_1, whereas posteroseptal VTs have a negative QRS component in V_1 (qR, qr, rs, rS, or QS). The Q-wave amplitude ratio of lead III to lead II is greater in posteroseptal VTs than in posterior VTs. Anterior and anteromedial VTs arising from the AMC region exhibit an absence of S waves in lead V_6 and RBBB or left bundle branch block (LBBB) with an early transition as noted in aortic cusp VTs (Fig. 32.2). A proposed algorithm to predict the precise focus of a VT/PVCs originating from the mitral annulus is shown in Fig. 32.3.

Mapping and Ablation

Catheter ablation using radiofrequency (RF) energy to cure patients with mitral annular VT is associated with a high success rate because of the focal origin of this form of VT. The 12-lead ECG is a useful initial guide to localize the site of the origin of the tachycardia. Intracardiac mapping to select the optimal site for ablation includes activation mapping (Fig. 32.4). At successful ablation sites, both atrial and ventricular potentials are recorded, and their ratio is usually <1.[9]

Some patients have a potential noted before the local ventricular electrogram. When ablating VTs from the basal LV inferoseptum, approach to the ostium of the coronary venous system may be considered (Fig. 32.5).[14]

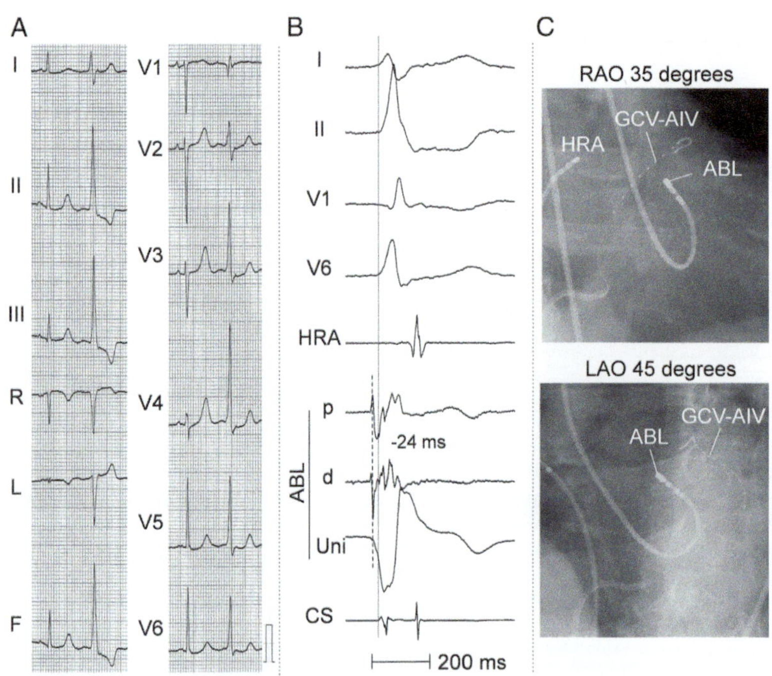

Fig. 32.2 A representative case of a successful ablation of a ventricular tachycardia originating from the aortomitral continuity. (A) A 12-lead electrocardiogram. No notching of the QRS complex was found. (B) Intracardiac recordings. During the premature ventricular complex, a distinct local activation recorded by the ablation catheter (ABL) preceded the onset of the QRS complex by 24 ms. (C) Radiographs obtained in the right anterior oblique (RAO) 35 degrees and left anterior oblique (LAO) 45 degrees projections showing the ablation sites. The distal electrode of the ablation catheter was positioned at the aortomitral continuity just beneath the aortic valve. *AIV,* Anterior interventricular vein; *CS,* coronary sinus; *d,* distal; *GCV,* great cardiac vein; *HRA,* high right atrium; *p,* proximal; *Uni,* unipolar electrogram.

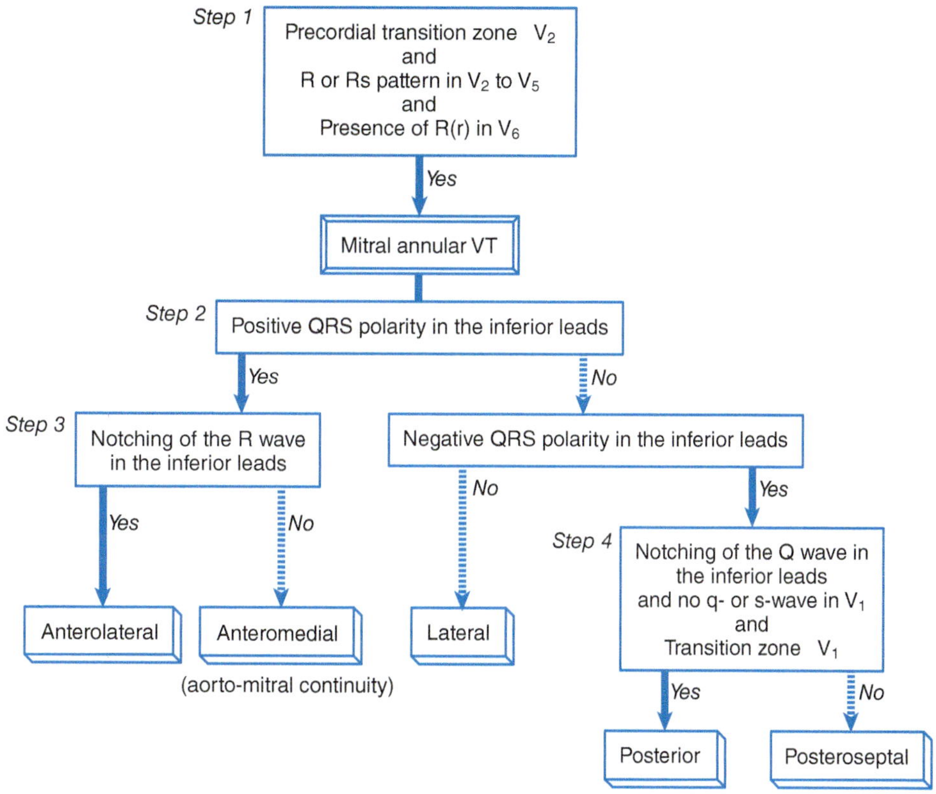

Fig. 32.3 Proposed algorithm to predict the precise focus of a ventricular tachycardia/premature ventricular contractions originating from the mitral annulus based on the QRS wave configuration in 12-lead electrocardiogram recordings. *VT,* Ventricular tachycardia. (From Tada H, Ito S, Naito S, et al. Idiopathic ventricular arrhythmia arising from the mitral annulus: a distinct subgroup of idiopathic ventricular arrhythmias. *J Am Coll Cardiol.* 2005;45:877–886.)

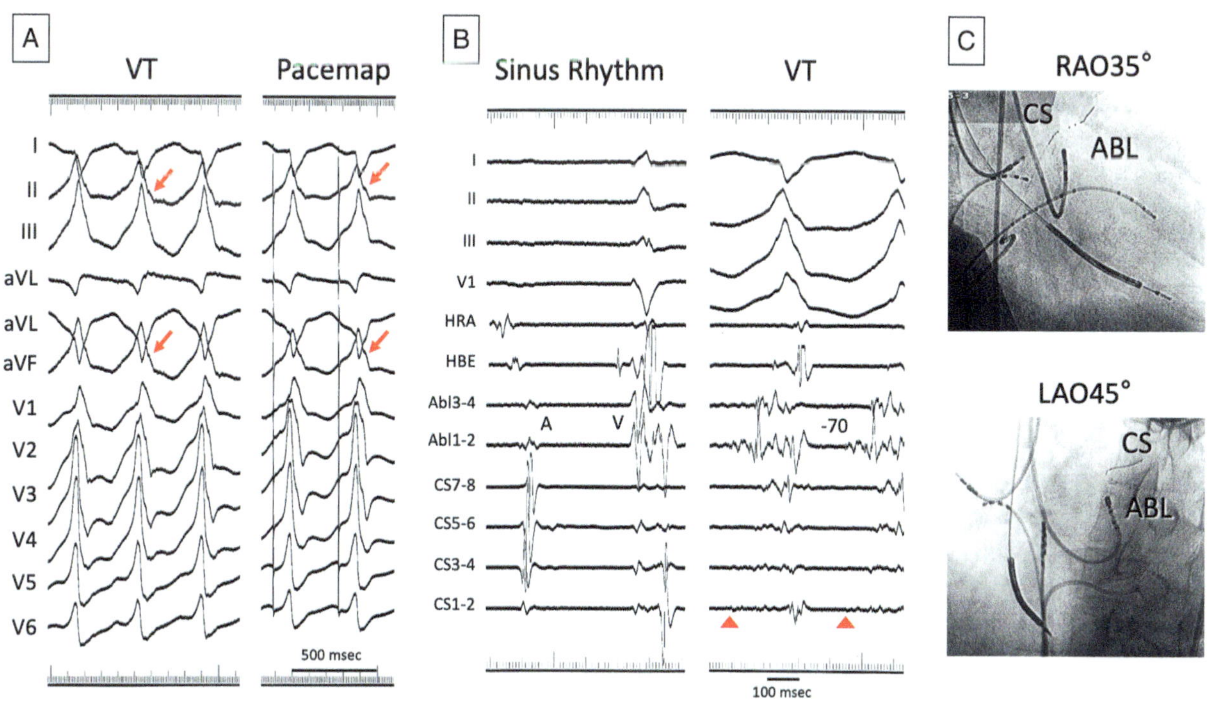

Fig. 32.4 A representative case of successful ablation of a ventricular tachycardia originating from the anterolateral portion of the mitral annulus. (A) QRS morphology showed right bundle branch block configuration, inferior axis with a notching in the late phase of the R wave in inferior leads (*arrows*), and negative polarity in lead I. An excellent pace map was obtained at the successful ablation site. (B) Intracardiac recordings during sinus rhythm and VT at the success site. A low-amplitude potential (*arrowhead*) was recorded at the distal electrode in the coronary sinus (CS). A presystolic potential preceding the QRS onset by 70 ms was recorded by the ablation catheter (ABL) that was placed at the opposite site of the CS distal electrode. (C) Fluoroscopic images in the right anterior oblique (RAO) and left anterior oblique (LAO) showing the catheter positions.

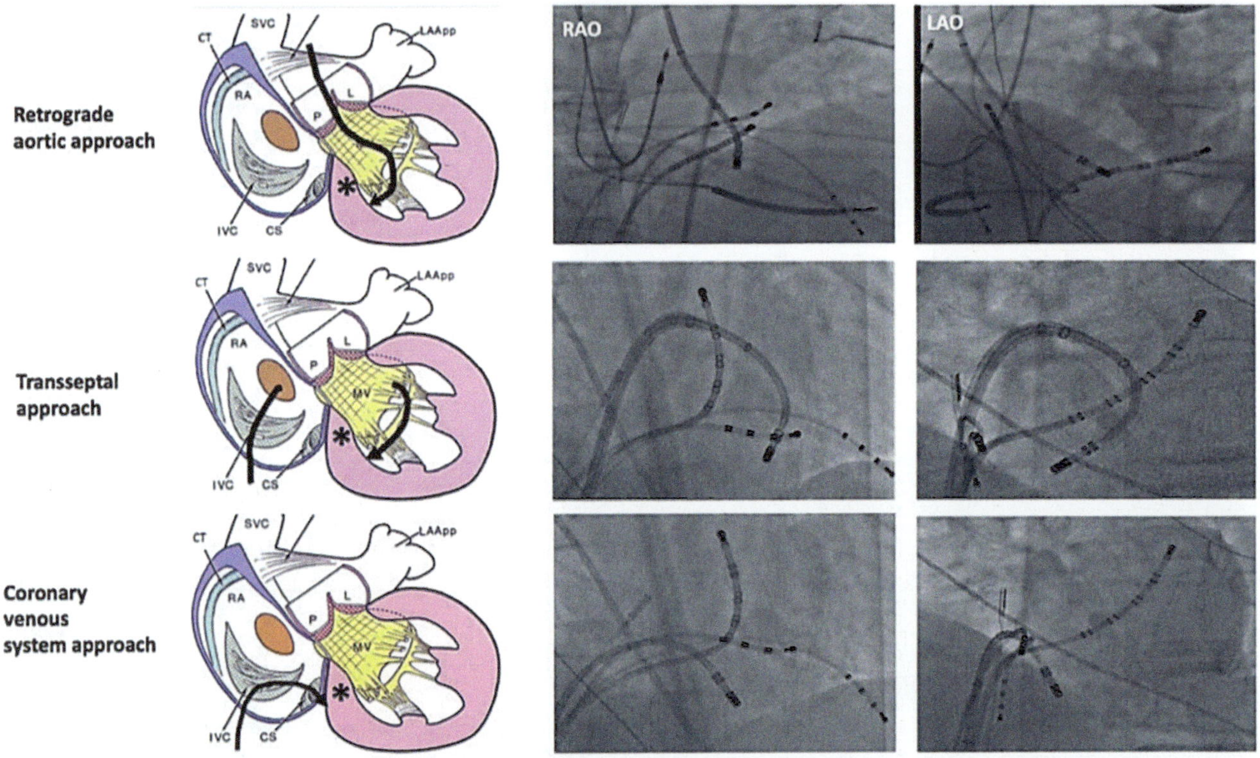

Fig. 32.5 Approaches to the basal crux VTs. *Top*, Retrograde aortic approach. *Middle*, Transseptal approach. *Bottom*, Coronary venous approach. Ablation catheter was placed in the middle cardiac vein. Note the proximity of the ablation catheter in the lower two panels. (From UCLA Cardiac Arrhythmia Center—Wallace A. McAlpine Collection.)

Santangeli and colleagues[15] reported right atrial approach for ablation of ventricular arrhythmias (VAs) arising from the left posterior-superior process of the LV (PSP-LV). The PSP-LV is the most inferior and posterior aspect of the basal LV that extends posteriorly to the plane of the tricuspid valve and is anatomically adjacent to the inferior and medial aspect of the right atrium (RA) (Fig. 32.6). Ventricular tachyarrhythmias originating from the PSP-LV can be mapped and ablated from the RA opposite to the earliest endocardial site in the LV (Fig. 32.7).[15]

Success and Recurrence Rates

Catheter ablation is highly successful with ablation delivered at the site of the earliest ventricular activation or sites with a 12/12 pace-map match. However, there was a recurrence rate of 8% in one series.[11] Most cases may be successfully ablated by an endocardial approach, but ablation in the coronary venous system, specifically the great cardiac vein, has been described.[12] Comparing the morphology of the coronary sinus (CS) ECG with that at the site of ablation on the mitral annulus may be helpful for determining the optimal ablation site.

Ablation of the PSP-LV from the adjacent RA tissue has a theoretical risk of injury to the AV node or septal artery with resulting AV block. However, these complications were not observed in the previous report.[15] Of five patients who underwent RA approach for ablation of VAs arising from the PSP-LV, cryoablation was performed in two and RF energy in the remaining three patients.

TRICUSPID ANNULAR VENTRICULAR TACHYCARDIA

Tricuspid annular VTs are found in 8% of all the cases of idiopathic VTs/PVCs (including right- and left-sided VT/PVC)[16] and approximately 5% of all patients with a right-sided VT origin.[17] Previous study reported that tricuspid annular VT arising from the free wall portion is more common in males than in females (male/female ratio, 1.83), whereas the incidence of that arising from the septum is distributed almost equally between males and females.[18]

Pathophysiology

Classification

Tricuspid annular VT can be classified by the anatomical location. Septal sites were more common than free wall sites in a previous study (74%)[16] but less common in the series presented by another group (43%).[17] Of the septal locations, the majority were anteroseptal or para-Hisian (72%).[16]

Mechanism

The mechanism of this arrhythmia appears to be nonreentrant based on the findings that it typically occurs spontaneously and cannot easily be induced by pacing maneuvers.

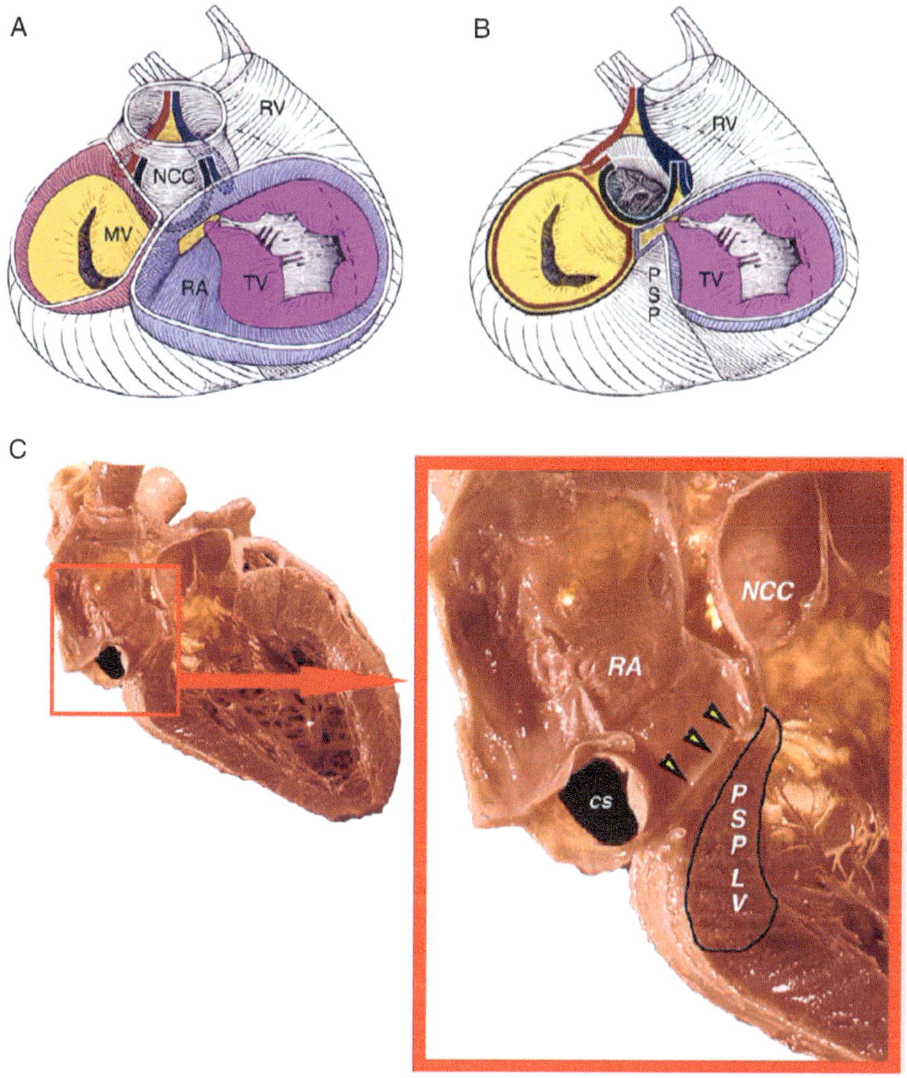

Fig. 32.6 Anatomical description of the posterior–superior process (PSP) of the left ventricle (LV). (A) A diagram of the heart showing the ventricular inflow after partial resection of the atria. The inferior wall of the right atria (RA) lies above and lateral to the PSP-LV medial to the insertion of the septal leaflet of the TV and insertion of the MV to the LV ostium. The coronary sinus (CS) orifice is medial to the inferomedial recess of the RA and not shown in this picture. (B) After further removal of the RA, the PSP-LV is exposed. At the apex of the triangle is located the membranous septum and the right fibrous trigone below the insertion of the noncoronary sinus. (C) An attitudinal cut of the heart through the LVOT axis and magnified in D. (D) The PSP-LV below the noncoronary cusp. The most superior aspect is opposite to the insertion of the RA, and more lateral one can see the ostium of the CS. This anatomical relationship allows mapping of the PSP-LV from the RA. *LVOT,* left ventricular outflow tract; *MV,* mitral valve; *NCC,* noncoronary cusp; and *TV,* tricuspid valve. (From Santangeli P, Hutchinson MD, Supple GE, et al. Right atrial approach for ablation of ventricular arrhythmias arising from the left posterior-superior process of the left ventricle. *Circ Arrhythm Electrophysiol.* 2016;9:e004048.)

Diagnostic Criteria

Surface Electrocardiogram

All VT/PVCs arising from the tricuspid annulus demonstrate an LBBB QRS morphology and positive QRS polarity in leads I, V_5, and V_6 (Fig. 32.8). No negative component of the QRS complex is found in lead I. The R wave in lead I is usually greater because the tricuspid annulus is more rightward and inferior to the RV outflow tract. A positive component (any r or R) is recorded in lead aV_L in 95% of patients, and the overall polarity in aV_L is positive in 89%.[16]

Among all tricuspid annular VTs, the QRS duration and Q-wave amplitude in each of leads V_1–V_3 were greater in VT/PVCs arising from the free wall of the tricuspid annulus compared with the septum. The septal VTs have an early transition in the precordial leads (V_3), narrower QRS complexes, and Qs in lead V_1 with the absence of notching in the inferior leads, whereas the free wall VTs are associated with a late precordial transition (>V_3), wider QRS complexes, absence of Q waves in lead V_1, and notching in the inferior leads (the timing of the second peak of the notched QRS complex in the inferior leads

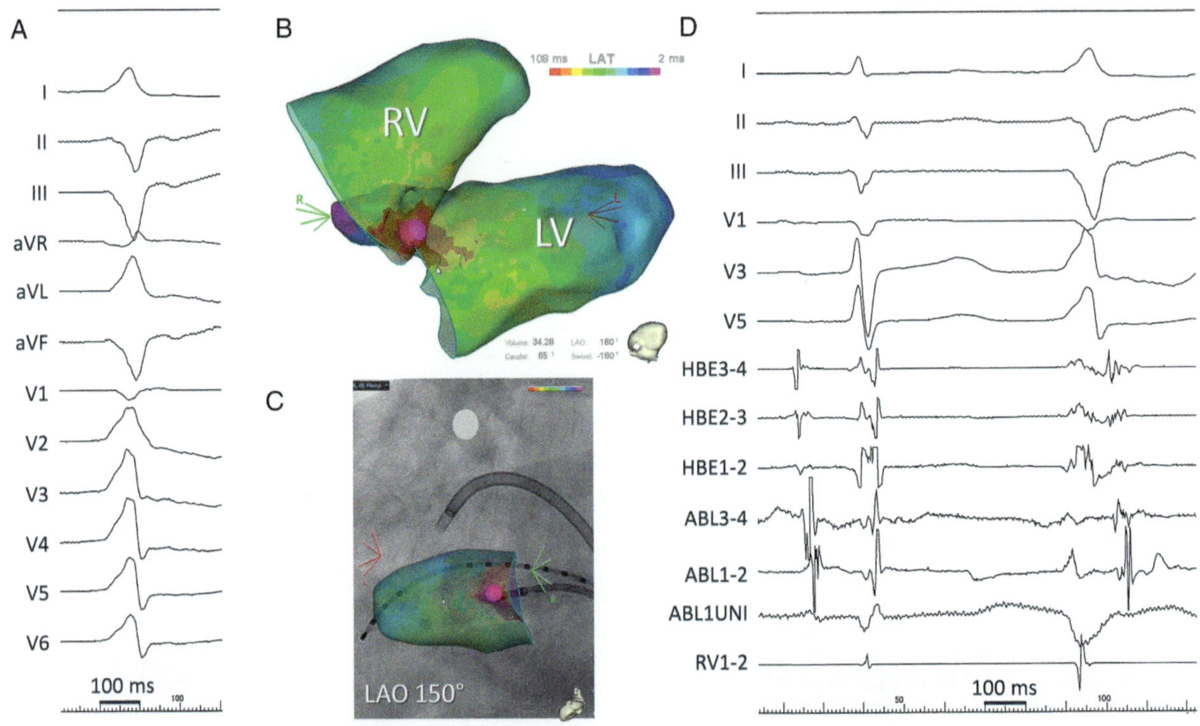

Fig. 32.7 Right atrial approach for ablation of ventricular arrhythmias arising from the left posterior-superior process of the LV. (A) 12-lead ECG during premature ventricular contraction (PVC). (B) Electroanatomical map demonstrating earliest endocardial activation in the posterior–superior process of the left ventricle (LV). Tag indicates the ablation site in the right atrium (RA). (C) Ablation catheter position at RA opposite to the earliest endocardial site in the LV. (D) Intracardiac electrogram during sinus rhythm and PVC. Electrogram during PVC demonstrating a smaller far-field ventricular and a larger atrial signals at the successful ablation site. *ABL*, ablation catheter; *HBE*, His bundle electrogram; *LAO*, left anterior oblique view; *LV*, left ventricle; *RA*, right atrium; *RV*, right ventricle.

corresponds precisely with the LV free wall activation).[16] A proposed algorithm to predict the precise focus of a VT/PVCs originating from the tricuspid annulus is shown in Fig. 32.9.

Mapping and Ablation

The 12-lead ECG is a useful initial guide to localize the site of origin of the tachycardia. Intracardiac mapping to select the optimal site for ablation (Fig. 32.10) includes activation mapping and pace mapping. At successful ablation sites, both atrial and ventricular potentials are recorded, and their ratio is usually <1.[16] VTs originating from near the His bundle have a similar ECG and electrophysiologic characteristics as those from the right coronary cusp or noncoronary cusp adjacent to the membranous septum (Fig. 32.11)[19,20] Therefore, when RV mapping shows the earliest ventricular activation near the His bundle, mapping in the right coronary cusp and noncoronary cusp should be added to identify the origin and the safest location. Confirmation of the distance between the ablation site and His-bundle recording site is important to avoid impairing AV conduction during RF energy applications.

There are two approaches to the tricuspid annulus: direct approach, in which a catheter is placed directly into the tricuspid annulus from the right atrial side; and inverted approach, in which a catheter is inserted into the RV and placed between the valve leaflet and the myocardium into the annulus. The direct approach is usually successful but may cause damage to the valve.

Success and Recurrence Rates

In one series,[16] RF catheter ablation was more often successful for the free wall (90%) than the septal (57%) group. The low success rate in the septal tricuspid annular group was thought to be caused by concern for impairing AV conduction with RF ablation. This is in contrast to the 100% acute success rate in another series.[17]

Complications

In the case of catheter ablation of tricuspid annular VTs originating from anterior or middle septum, careful attention has to be paid because of its proximity to the AV node and His-bundle region.

PAPILLARY MUSCLE VENTRICULAR TACHYCARDIA

Idiopathic VAs that originate from papillary muscles account for 4–12% of idiopathic VAs.[21] Syncope and cardiac arrest are rare, but several cases of PVCs from papillary muscles triggering ventricular fibrillation (VF) have been reported.[22,23] Frequent papillary PVCs can also induce cardiomyopathy.[24]

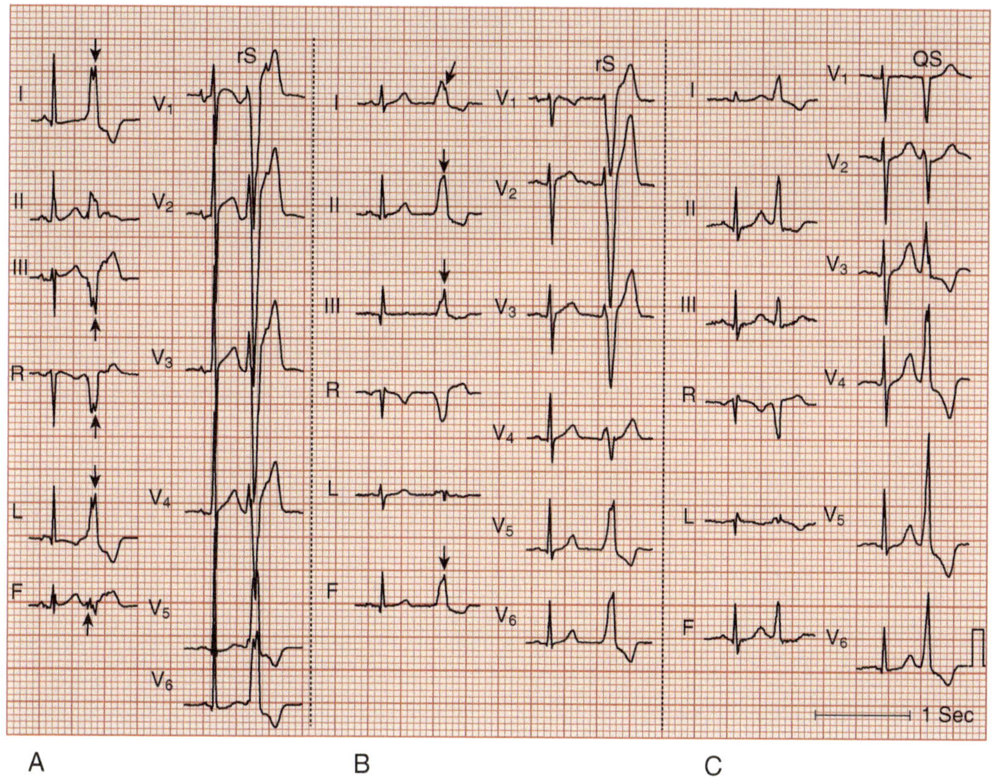

Fig. 32.8 Representative 12-lead electrocardiograms of premature ventricular contractions originating from the (A) posterolateral, (B) anterior, and (C) anteroseptal portions of the tricuspid annulus. The *arrows* indicate the second peak of the notched QRS complex in the limb leads. (From Tada H, Tadokoro K, Ito S, et al. Idiopathic ventricular arrhythmias originating from the tricuspid annulus: prevalence, electrocardiographic characteristics, and results of radiofrequency catheter ablation. *Heart Rhythm.* 2007;4:7–16.)

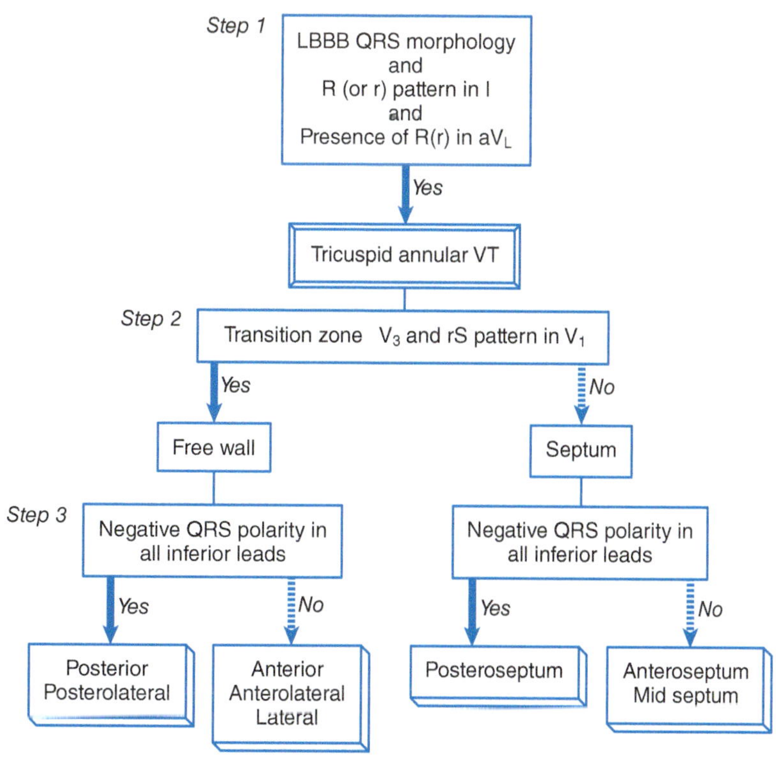

Fig. 32.9 Proposed algorithm to predict the precise focus of ventricular tachycardia/premature ventricular complexes originating from the tricuspid annulus based on the QRS configuration in 12-lead electrocardiogram recordings. *LBBB,* Left branch bundle block; *VT,* ventricular tachycardia.

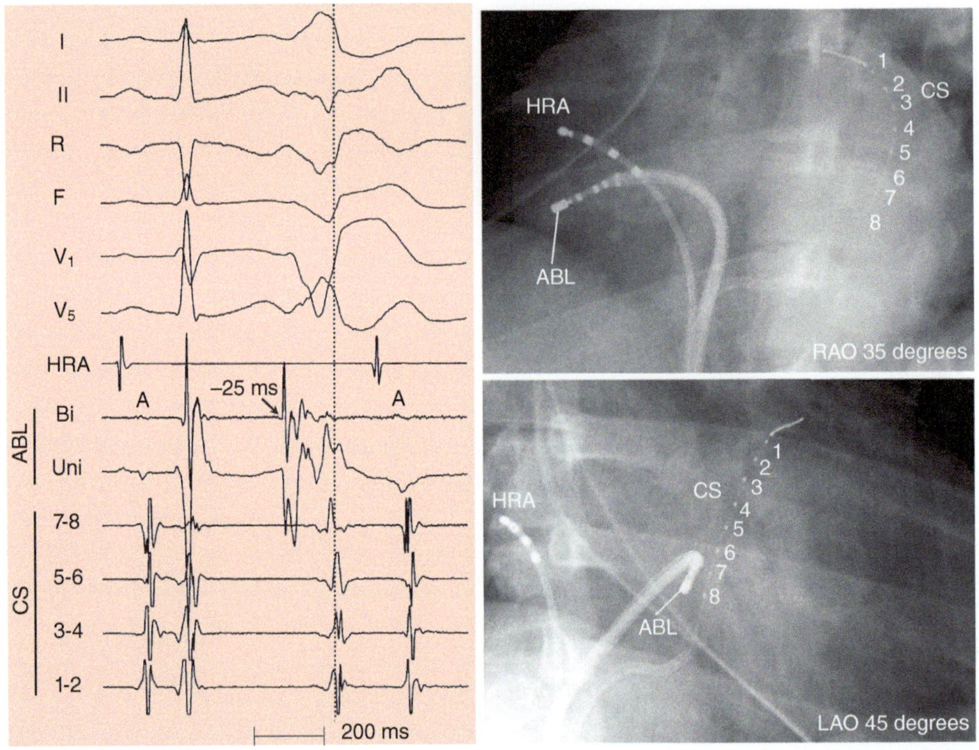

A B

Fig. 32.10 Site of the successful ablation of a premature ventricular complex (PVC) originating from the inferolateral portion of the tricuspid annulus. (A) Intracardiac recordings. During the PVC, a ventricular potential recorded by the ablation catheter (ABL) preceded the onset of the QRS complex by 25 ms *(arrow)*. The timing of the second peak of the notched QRS complex corresponded precisely with that of the activation of the left ventricular free wall *(dotted line)*, which was recorded with the catheter within the coronary sinus (CS). (B) Radiographs obtained in the right anterior oblique (RAO 35 degrees) and left anterior oblique (LAO 45 degrees) projections showing the ablation sites. The distal electrode of the ablation catheter was positioned at the inferolateral portion of the tricuspid annulus. *A*, Atrial activation; *Bi*, bipolar electrogram; *Dist*, distal; *HRA*, high right atrium; *Prox*, proximal; *Uni*, unipolar electrogram. (From Tada H, Tadokoro K, Ito S, et al. Idiopathic ventricular arrhythmias originating from the tricuspid annulus: prevalence, electrocardiographic characteristics, and results of radiofrequency catheter ablation. *Heart Rhythm*. 2007;4:7–16.)

Pathophysiology

Classification

The chordal apparatus of both mitral leaflets inserts into two groups of papillary muscles. The anterior papillary muscle and posterior papillary muscle arise from the middle to apical aspect of the anterior or inferior wall of the LV, respectively (Fig. 32.12). Papillary muscle VAs originate more commonly from the posterior papillary muscle than from the anterior papillary muscle and are less likely to be sustained.[25]

Mechanism

Papillary muscle VTs appear to be based on a focal (nonreentrant) mechanism.[26] Papillary muscle VT is often exercise induced and often catecholamine sensitive, requiring isoproterenol or epinephrine for induction.[24,26]

Diagnostic Criteria

Surface Electrocardiogram

VTs from the papillary muscles have an RBBB pattern with a precordial transition between leads V_2 and V_5 (Fig. 32.12). VAs originating from the posterior papillary muscles exhibit a superior axis, and those from the anterior papillary muscles show an inferior axis. The V_1 morphology of posterior papillary muscle VTs typically has a qR morphology or R compared with an rsR′ for fascicular VTs and will notably have an absence of Q waves in leads I and aVL.[27] Knowledge of ECG characteristics help identification of papillary muscle VAs, as there are similar morphologies from other LV sites including the LV anterior and posterior fascicles, LV septum, and mitral annulus. The papillary muscle VAs manifest distinct QRS morphology in lead V_1 (Rr, R with slurred downstroke, and RR) with a short intrinsicoid deflection (Fig. 32.13).[28] In addition, the QRS width is significantly wider in papillary muscle arrhythmias compared with left fascicular VTs.[27] Papillary muscle VT may exhibit multiple QRS morphologies, with subtle changes seen spontaneously or during ablation. These subtle morphologic changes are thought to be from preferential conduction to different exit sites or multiple regions of origins within the complex structure of the papillary muscles (Fig. 32.12).[25]

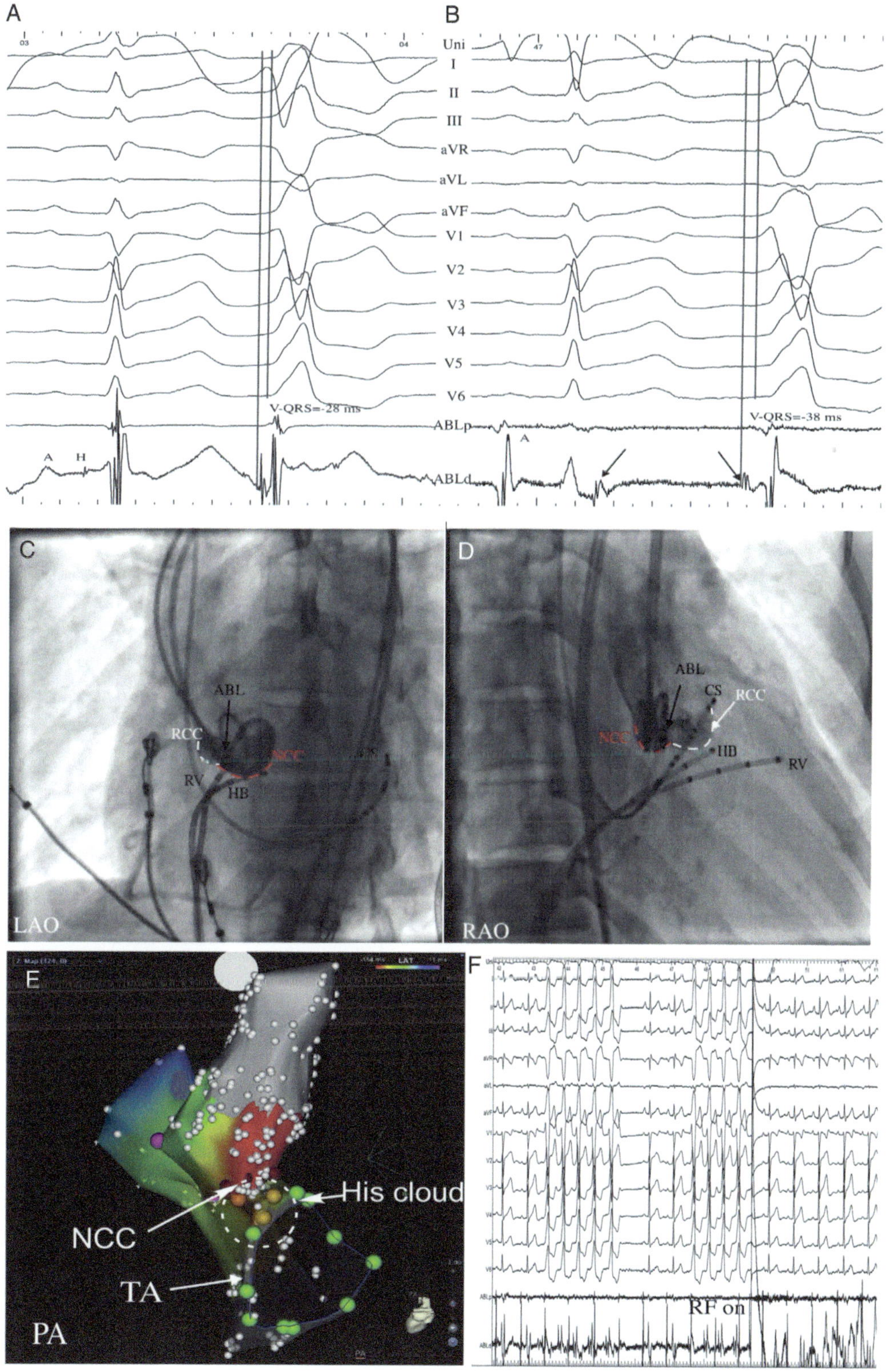

Fig. 32.11 A case of nonsustained VT that was successfully ablated at the NCC contiguous to the RCC. (A) A potential preceding the QRS onset of VT by 28 ms was recorded at the His bundle (HB) region. (B) Two components were recorded at the NCC site opposite to the HB region, with the discrete potential (arrow) following the far-field electrogram. Presystolic potential was observed during VT. (C, D) Fluoroscopic images of the mapping catheter at the successful ablation site in the right anterior oblique (RAO) and left anterior oblique (LAO). (E) Activation map of VT in the PA view. (F) RF ablation suppressed nonsustained. *ABL*, ablation catheter; *NCC*, noncoronary cusp; *RCC*, right coronary cusp; *RV*, right ventricle; *TA*, tricuspid annulus. (From Wei HQ, Guo XG, Liu X, et al. Safety and efficacy of catheter ablation of ventricular arrhythmias with para-Hisian origin via a systematic direct approach from the aortic sinus cusp. *Heart Rhythm*. 2018;15:1626–1633.)

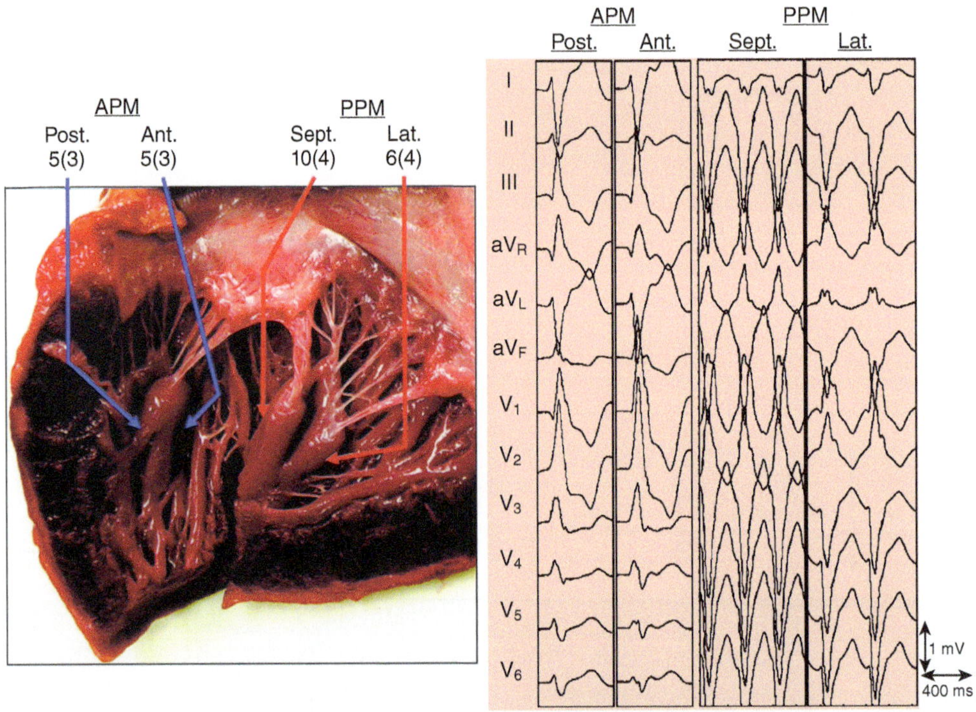

Fig. 32.12 An autopsy specimen of the human heart exhibiting the distribution of the successful ablation sites *(left)* and representative 12-lead electrocardiograms exhibiting the differences in the QRS morphology of the ventricular arrhythmias successfully ablated between both sides of the APMs in the same patient *(right)*. *APM,* Anterior papillary muscle; *PPM,* posterior papillary muscle. (From Yamada T, Doppalapudi H, McElderry HT, et al. Electrocardiographic and electrophysiological characteristics in idiopathic ventricular arrhythmias originating from the papillary muscles in the left ventricle: relevance for catheter ablation. *Circ Arrhythm Electrophysiol.* 2010;3:324–331.)

Mapping and Ablation

Activation mapping seems to be most useful in the ablation of papillary muscle VTs. Intracardiac echocardiography (ICE) is able to not only assess the exact location of the focus but also visualize the adequacy of catheter contact during ablation. ICE may allow targeting various segments such as base, body, and tip of the papillary muscles (Fig. 32.14).[29] The papillary muscle VAs may originate more frequently from the distal portion of the papillary muscles.[30]

RF catheter ablation can be challenging at times because catheter stability is difficult to achieve as a result of papillary muscle contractions. In addition, the myocardium at the base of the papillary muscles is relatively thick. The creation of a deep lesion may be necessary for long-term success because of the distance between the VT origin and endocardial surface.[31]

Detailed three-dimensional reconstruction of the ventricles, papillary muscles, image integration by ICE, magnetic resonance imaging, and/or multidetector computed tomography assists with site of origin localization.[32] The use of contact sensing ablation catheters is also useful to control the power of RF ablation. However, efforts to increase contact force on the papillary muscles may often lead to dislodgement of catheter. Although both transseptal and retrograde approaches to the left ventricle can be used, conversion from transseptal to retrograde approach should be considered when ablation via transseptal access is not successful. This may be due to different alignment of the ablation catheter to the papillary muscles resulting in an improved stability. A relatively wide area (approximately half) of the papillary muscle circumference and multiple ablation lesions may need to be targeted because of the potential for a deep intramural focus with multiple exits.[25] Cryoablation has been used when conventional RF ablation has failed and may be an effective alternative approach because of the improved catheter-tip stability.[32]

Success and Recurrence Rates

During follow-up after ablation, freedom from the recurrence of papillary muscle VAs is 65–82%.[29,30] The recurrence of VAs is not impacted by the site of origin (tip, body or base) on the papillary muscles or the contact force during ablation[29] but is most likely caused by poor catheter stability.[27]

Complications

Gradual titration of the power, careful manipulation of the catheter, and detailed observation using real-time ICE imaging are important to avoid any complications. Postablation follow-up should include echocardiography to rule out mitral regurgitation.[32] Although its incidence appears to be low despite extensive ablation on the papillary muscles, caution should still be kept in mind.

VENTRICULAR TACHYCARDIA ARISING FROM THE CRUX OF THE HEART

VAs may originate from the crux of the heart.[33–36] Crux VTs were found in 18 patients (1.8%) of 1021 cases with idiopathic VTs/

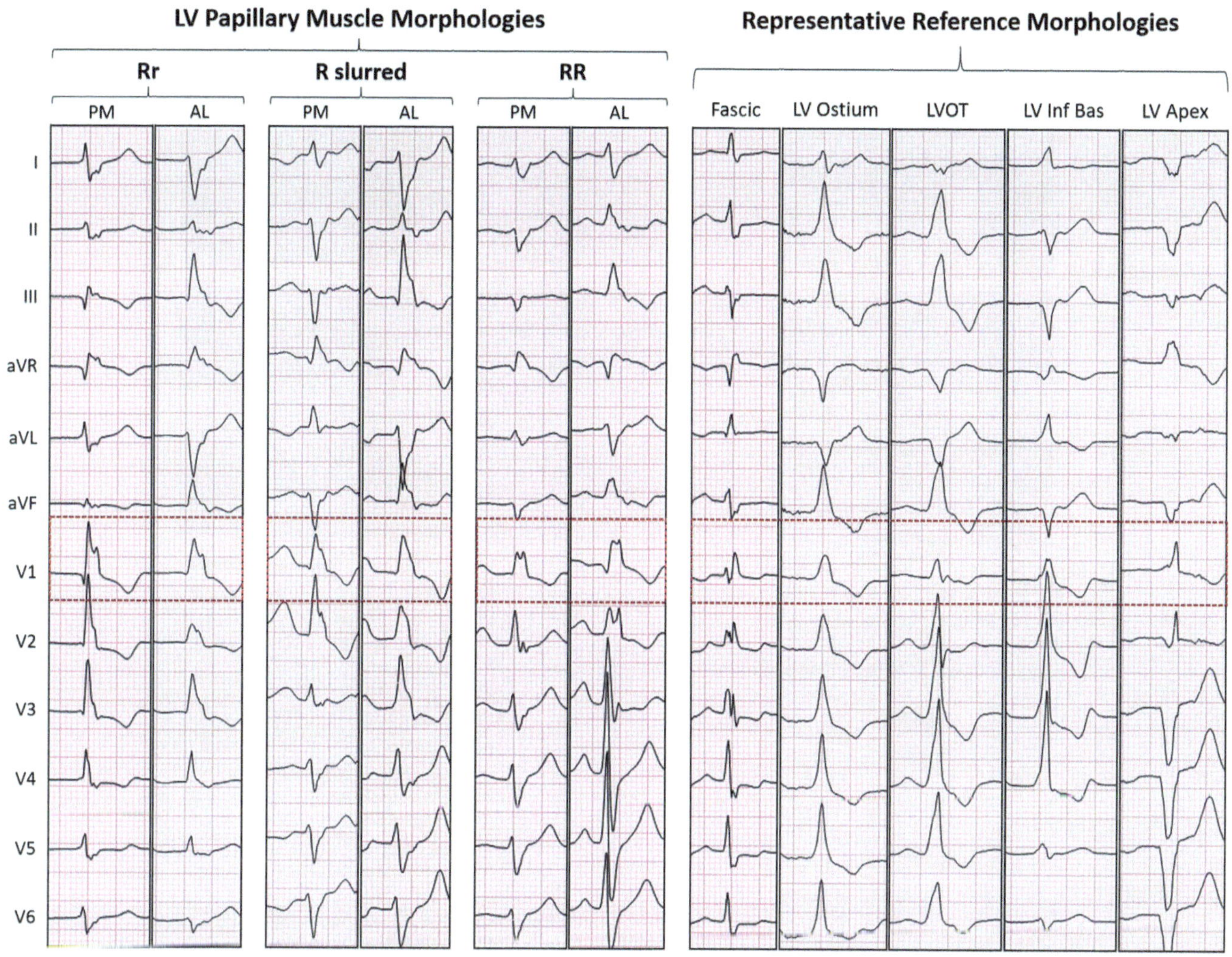

Fig. 32.13 QRS morphologies of PVCs originating from the posteromedial and anterolateral papillary muscles (*left*) and those from various other common LV sites (*right*). PVCs from the papillary muscles exhibit the Rr, R with a slurred downstroke, and RR patterns in lead V1 (red rectangle), which is distinctly different from those from the other LV sites. *PM*, Posteromedial; *AL*, anterolateral; *Fascic*, fascicular; *LV*, left ventricular; *LV Inf Bas*, left ventricular inferior base; *LVOT*, left ventricular outflow tract; *PVC*, premature ventricular complex. (From Briceño DF, Santangeli P, Frankel DS, et al. QRS morphology in lead V1 for the rapid localization of idiopathic ventricular arrhythmias originating from the left ventricular papillary muscles: a novel electrocardiographic criterion. *Heart Rhythm.* 2020;17:1711–1718.)

PVCs undergoing RF catheter ablation.[33] Of these, 15 patients (83%) had sustained VT and three required an implantable cardioverter defibrillator implantation because of syncope.

Pathophysiology

Anatomy

The cardiac crux is a pyramidal space of the posteroseptal region, which is formed by the AV annulus and interventricular groove, and it represents the confluence of all four cardiac chambers and the CS in their nearest proximity and has a pyramidal space. The basal crux area lies in close proximity to the ostium of the MCV, whereas the apical crux area lies near the posterior interventricular artery, more inferior and epicardial compared with the basal crux area.

Classification

Crux VT can be classified into two main groups by the anatomical location using fluoroscopic images and 3-dimensional activation maps: those with apical crux VT and those with basal crux VT.[33] Basal crux VTs were defined as those VTs with a successful ablation region in the proximal CS or proximal middle cardiac vein (MCV) within 2 cm of the MCV ostium. Apical crux VTs were defined as those VTs that the earliest activation or successful ablation region was in the middle MCV, >2 cm from the MCV ostium or epicardial space near these MCV areas.

Mechanism

This type of VT appears to have a focal mechanism from the epicardium and is initiated with programmed stimulation or burst pacing from the RV, and often requires isoproterenol (catecholamine sensitive).[33,36]

Diagnostic Criteria

Surface Electrocardiogram

The ECG demonstrates a superior axis and QS pattern in leads II and III and a maximum deflection index, determined by the analysis of the QRS complex,[37] of ≥0.55 (Fig. 32.15). Most patients

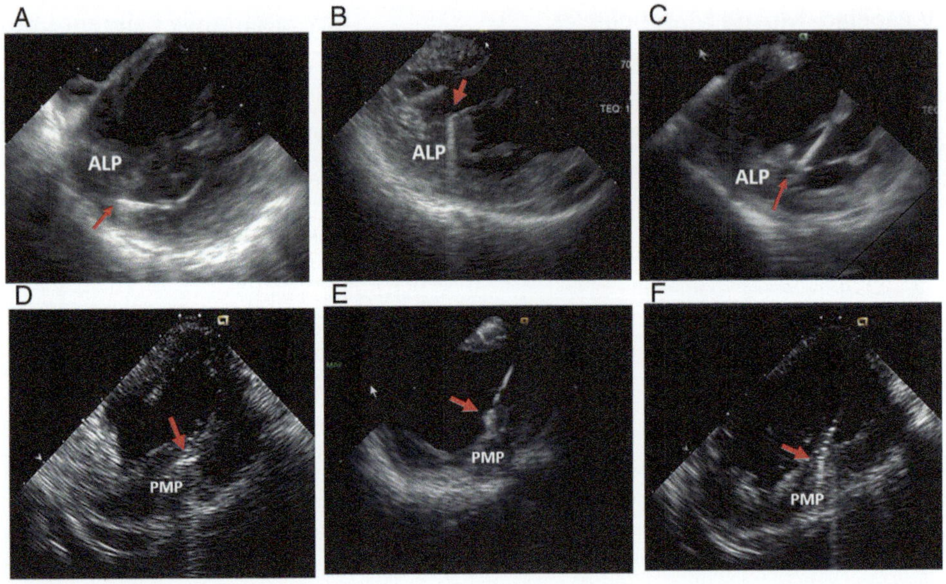

Fig. 32.14 Ablation catheter is visualized by ICE during ablation of VAs originating from the anterolateral and posteromedial papillary muscles. Arrows indicate the position of ablation catheter at base (A), body (B), and tip (C) of ALP; and at base (D), body (E), and tip (F) of PMP. *ALP*, anterolateral papillary muscle; *PMP*, posteromedial papillary muscle. (From Lin AN, Shirai Y, Liang JJ, et al. Strategies for catheter ablation of left ventricular papillary muscle arrhythmias: an institutional experience. *JACC Clin Electrophysiol.* 2020;6:1381–1392.)

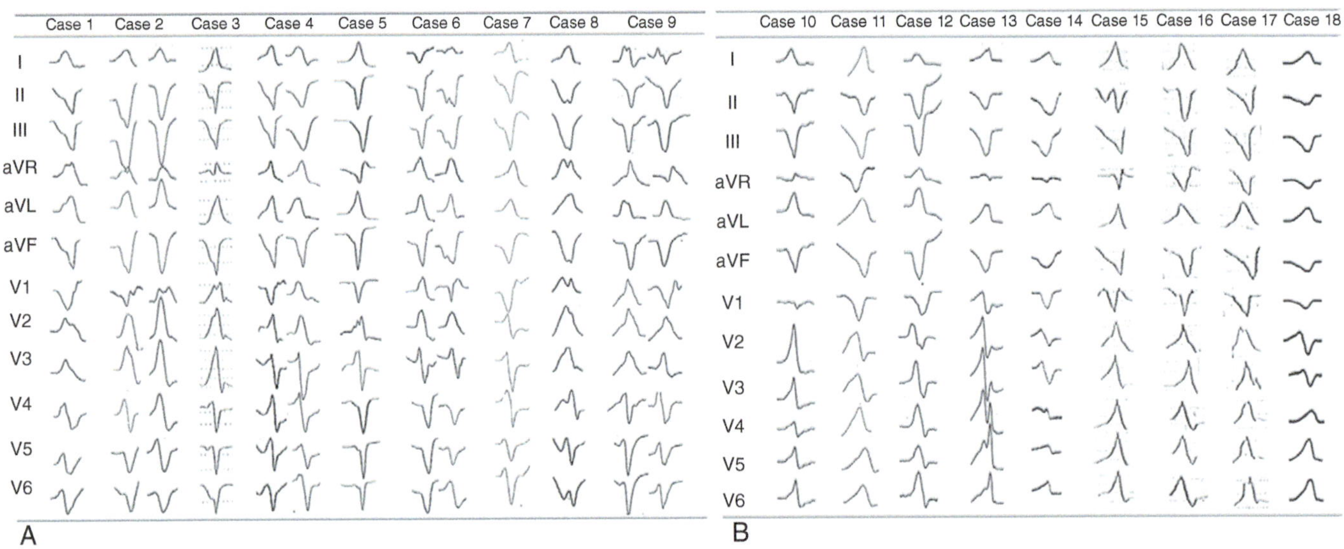

Fig. 32.15 Twelve-lead electrocardiograms of ventricular tachycardias (VTs) originating from the crux of the heart in 18 patients. (A) VTs arising from the apical crux. (B) VTs arising from the basal crux. (From Kawamura M, Gerstenfeld EP, Vedantham V, et al. Idiopathic ventricular arrhythmia originating from the cardiac crux or inferior septum: epicardial idiopathic ventricular arrhythmia. *Circ Arrhythm Electrophysiol.* 2014;7:1152-1158.)

(89%) had an R > S wave in V_2 and pseudo-delta wave duration of >34 ms.[33] In apical crux VTs, V_6 exhibited either a QS or rS pattern, and aVR presented with an R > S wave in most cases. Those with an RBBB pattern had a prominent R wave in V_1 with a transition to an rS or qS pattern in V_6. Those with an LBBB pattern had an early transition in V_2 with a late transition to an rS or qS in V_6. Furthermore, the QRS morphology often changed spontaneously from an RBBB to LBBB in 44% of the patients with apical crux VTs. On the other hand, basal crux VTs were either negative or isoelectric in V_1, positive in V_6, and had an early transition in V_2.

It is important for ablation procedural planning to differentiate the basal crux VTs from the basal inferoseptal LV endocardium. The basal inferoseptal LV endocardial VTs more likely to exhibit an initial small R wave in the inferior leads, narrow QRS width, and lower maximum deflection index compared to the basal crux VT (Fig. 32.16).[38]

Mapping and Ablation

Activation mapping and pace mapping in the CS or MCV are used for the determination of ablation sites. For apical crux VTs, the success rate of RF catheter ablation within the MCV is low, and VT recurrence is high.[33] However the success rate of epicardial ablation over the cardiac crux is high. In basal crux VTs, the success rate of RF catheter ablation within the CS or MCV

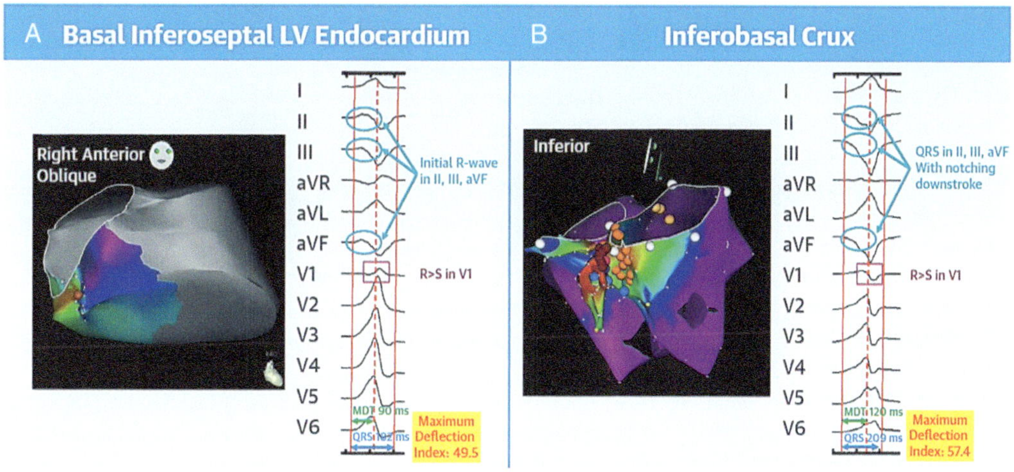

Fig. 32.16 Electrocardiographic features that differentiate successful ablation from the basal inferoseptal LV endocardium (A) versus from the inferobasal crux (B). Note that basal inferoseptal LV endocardium arrhythmias have initial R-wave (or isoelectric period) in the inferior leads, R>S in lead V1, narrower QRS duration, and lower maximum deflection index (MDI) value (often with MDI <0.55). (From Liang JJ, Shirai Y, Briceño DF, et al. Electrocardiographic and electrophysiologic characteristics of idiopathic ventricular arrhythmias originating from the basal inferoseptal left ventricle. *JACC Clin Electrophysiol.* 2019;5:833–842.)

is high, and VT recurrence is relatively low.[33,35] The epicardial approach for the basal crux is challenging because of the existence of pericardial fat and coronary vessels at the basal crux, which often precludes the effective ablation from the epicardium.

Complications

Perforation of the CS or impairment of a coronary artery (posterior descending artery) may occur with catheter ablation from the CS or MCV or if a percutaneous epicardial approach is performed.

REENTRANT LEFT FASCICULAR VENTRICULAR TACHYCARDIA

Pathophysiology

Classification

Verapamil-sensitive fascicular VT is the most common form of idiopathic left VT. It was first recognized as an electrocardiographic entity in 1979 by Zipes and colleagues,[39] who identified the following characteristic diagnostic triad: (1) induction with atrial pacing; (2) RBBB and left-axis configuration; and (3) manifestation in patients without structural heart disease. In 1981 Belhassen and colleagues[40] were the first to demonstrate the verapamil sensitivity of the tachycardia, a fourth identifying feature. Ohe and colleagues[41] reported another type of this tachycardia, with RBBB and a right-axis configuration, in 1988. Lastly, our group reported the upper septal fascicular VT variant.[42–44] According to the QRS morphology, we classified verapamil-sensitive left fascicular VT into five subtypes (Fig. 32.17),[45] namely: (1) left posterior septal fascicular VT that exhibits RBBB configuration and left-axis deviation (Fig. 32.18A); (2) left posterior papillary muscle fascicular VT that exhibits RBBB and superior right-axis deviation (northwest axis) (Fig. 32.18B); (3) left anterior septal fascicular VT that exhibits RBBB, right-axis deviation, and Rs pattern in V_5–V_6 (Fig. 32.18C); (4) left anterior papillary muscle fascicular VT that exhibits RBBB, right-axis deviation, and deep S waves in V_5–V_6 (Fig. 32.18D); and (5) upper septal fascicular VT that exhibits a narrow QRS configuration and normal or right-axis deviation (Fig. 32.19).[42–44] Left posterior septal fascicular VT is most common and left upper septal fascicular VT is very rare. Left upper septal fascicular VT sometimes occurred after previous catheter ablation of other fascicular VTs.[43,44] Papillary muscle fascicular VTs involve the Purkinje network lying around the papillary muscles.[45] The papillary muscle fascicular VTs and "papillary muscle VT" (VT from myocardium of the papillary), are basically different entities, while there must be some overlap making identification challenging.

Recently, we reported on patients with a new type of verapamil-sensitive LV fascicular VT with distinctive surface ECG and electrophysiologic characteristics that appear to share a reentrant circuit in the reverse direction of the left posterior septal fascicular VT.[46] The 12-lead ECG of this VT exhibited Qr or rSr morphology in V1 with an early precordial transition and inferior-axis (Fig. 32.20). This VT showed verapamil sensitivity and the majority of the patients also had a common-type left posterior septal fascicular VT as well.

Substrate and Anatomy

The anatomical basis of this VT has provoked considerable interest. Some data suggest that the VT may originate from a false tendon or fibromuscular band in the LV.[47–50] Suwa et al.[48] described a false tendon in the LV of a patient with idiopathic left VT in whom the VT was eliminated by surgical resection of the tendon. Using echocardiography, Thakur and colleagues[49] found false tendons extending from the posteroinferior LV to the basal septum in 15 of 15 patients with idiopathic left VT but in only 5% of control patients. In contrast, Lin and colleagues[51] reported that the fibromuscular band was a common echocardiographic finding In the papillary muscle fascicular VTs, Purkinje network in the fibromuscular

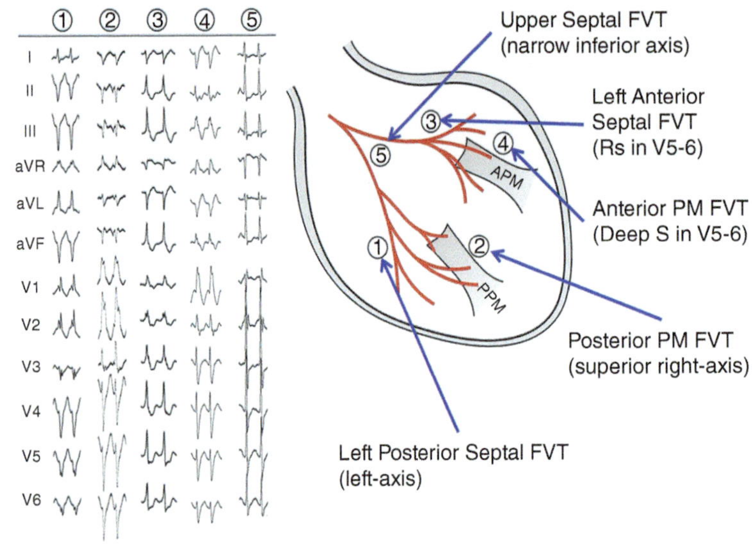

Fig. 32.17 Classification of verapamil-sensitive left fascicular ventricular tachycardia (FVT). According to the QRS morphology and site of successful ablation, verapamil-sensitive left FVT can be classified into five subtypes. Left posterior septal FVT is the most common type and exhibits right bundle branch block (RBBB) and left-axis deviation. Left anterior septal FVT exhibits RBBB and right-axis deviation. Upper septal FVT, which is the most uncommon variant of FVT, exhibits a narrow QRS configuration and normal or right-axis deviation (northwest axis). Whereas left posterior septal FVT exhibits left-axis deviation, left posterior papillary muscle FVT exhibits superior right-axis deviation (northwest axis). Whereas left anterior septal FVT exhibits Rs pattern in V5-6, left anterior papillary muscle FVT exhibits deep S waves in V5-6. *APM*, anterior papillary muscle *PPM*, posterior papillary muscle. (From Komatsu Y, Nogami A, Kurosaki K, et al. Fascicular ventricular tachycardia originating from papillary muscles: Purkinje network involvement in the reentrant circuit. *Circ Arrhythm Electrophysiol.* 2017;10. pii:e004549.)

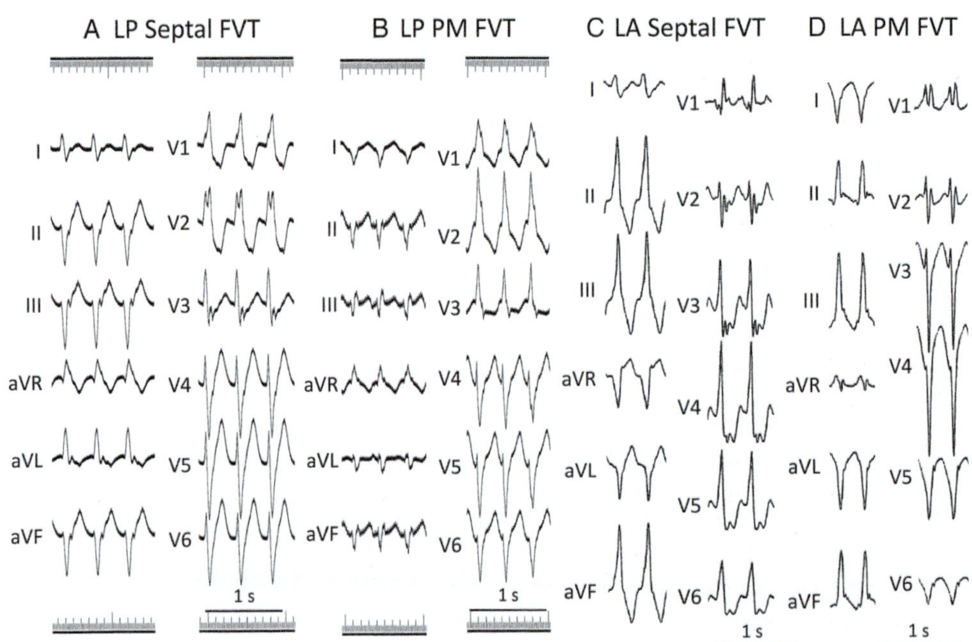

Fig. 32.18 Twelve-lead electrocardiograms of verapamil-sensitive left fascicular VTs. (A) Left posterior septal fascicular VT. (B) Left posterior papillary muscle fascicular VT. (C) Left anterior septal fascicular VT. (D) Left anterior papillary muscle fascicular VT. *FVT,* Fascicular ventricular tachycardia; *LA,* left anterior; *LP,* left posterior; *PM,* papillary muscle.

bands near papillary muscles can be the substrate of the VT. An autopsy specimen of the human heart shows the anatomical connection between the anterior and posterior papillary muscles (Fig. 32.21), and the possible electrical connection between them may explain the changes in QRS axis during ablation of papillary muscle fascicular VTs.[45] Haïssaguerre et al. proposed three kinds of Purkinje reentry VTs;[52] bundle branch reentry, fascicular ventricular tachycardia, and distal Purkinje-muscle reentry. The distal Purkinje-muscle reentry is the papillary muscle fascicular VTs, which contain more distal

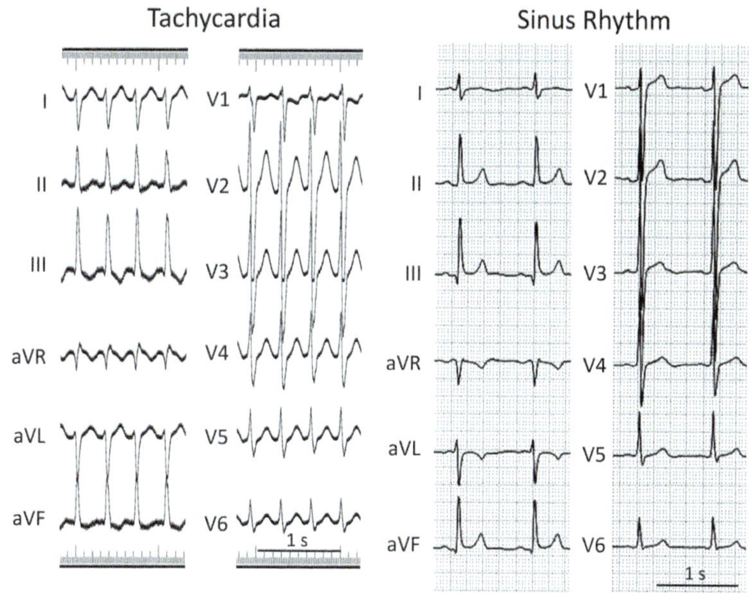

Fig. 32.19 Twelve-lead electrocardiograms of upper septal fascicular VT. Tachycardia on the left and sinus rhythm on the right. (From Talib AK, Nogami A, Nishiuchi S, et al. Verapamil-sensitive upper septal idiopathic left ventricular tachycardia: prevalence, mechanism, and electrophysiological characteristics. *J Am Coll Cardiol EP.* 2015;1:369–380.)

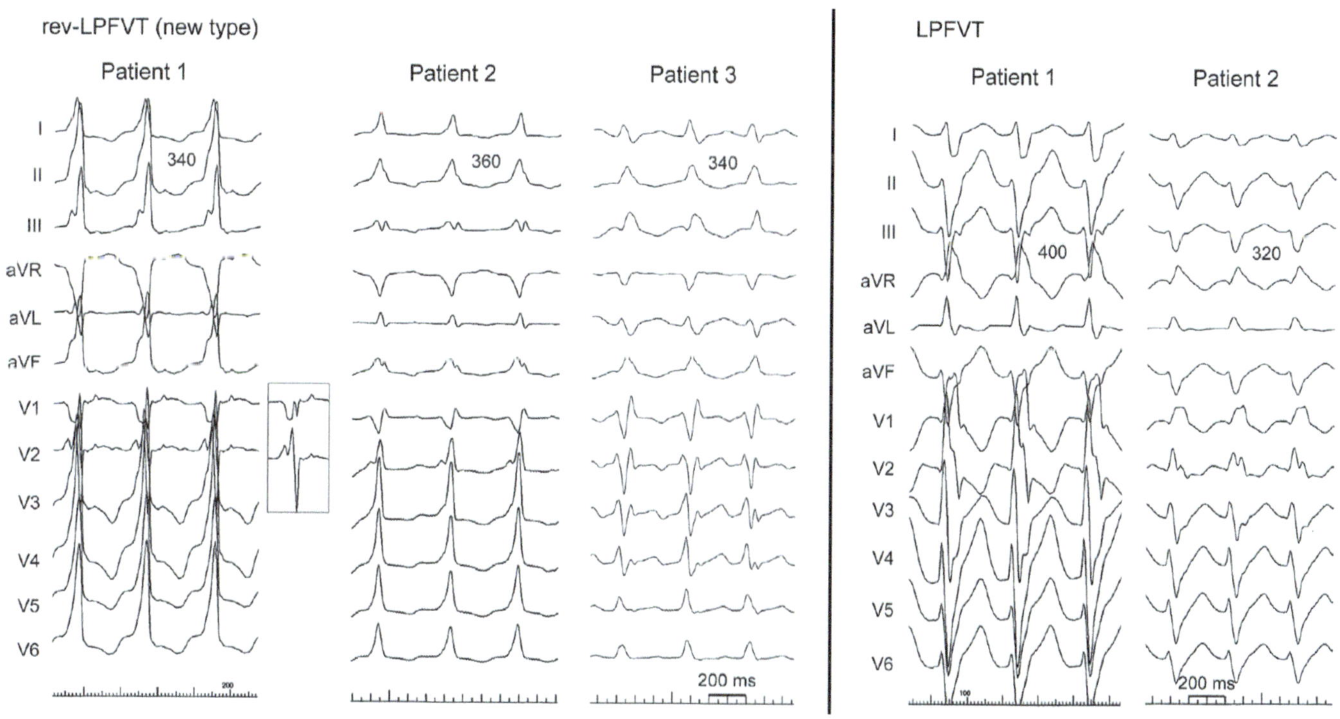

Fig. 32.20 Twelve-lead electrocardiograms of reverse-type left posterior fascicular VT. Two of three patients with reverse-type left posterior fascicular VT (*left*) also had common left posterior septal fascicular VT (*right*). *LPFVT,* Left posterior fascicular ventricular tachycardia; *rev,* reverse type. (From Phanthawimol W, Nogami A, Haruna T, et al. Reverse-type left posterior fascicular ventricular tachycardia: a new electrocardiographic entity. *JACC Clin Electrophysiol.* 2021;7:843–854.)

Purkinje network in the fibromuscular bands near papillary muscles (Fig. 32.22).

Mechanism

The mechanism of verapamil-sensitive left VT is reentry because it can be induced, entrained, and terminated by programmed ventricle or atrial stimulation. To confirm the mechanism and its reentry circuit, our group performed LV septal mapping using a multipolar linear electrode catheter (Fig. 32.23).[53] In 15 of 20 patients (75%), two distinct potentials, P1 and P2, were recorded during the VT at the midseptum (Fig. 32.24). Although the mid-diastolic potential (P1) was recorded earlier

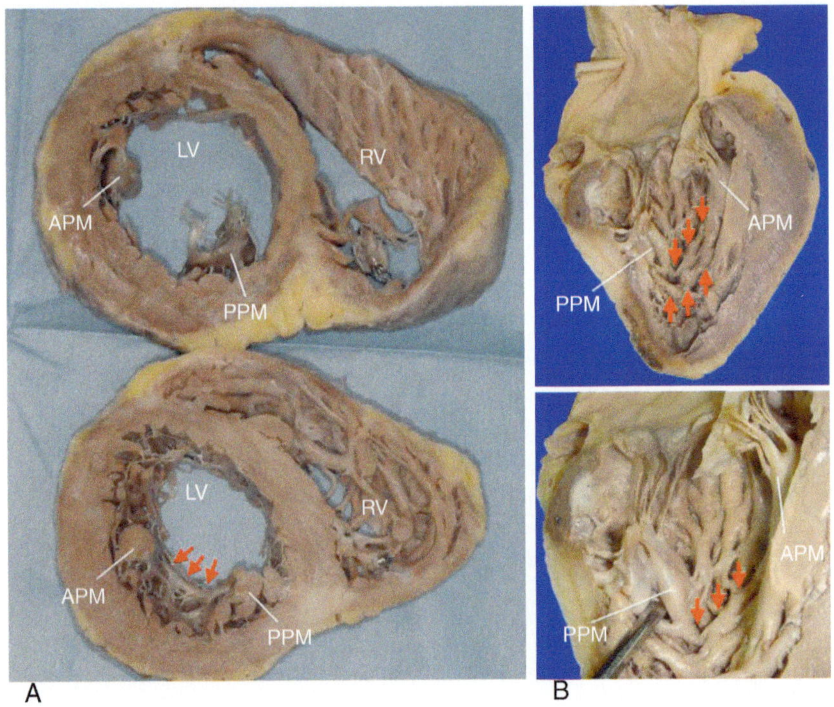

Fig. 32.21 An autopsy specimen of the human heart illustrating the myocardial structure between the anterior papillary muscle (APM) and posterior papillary muscle (PPM). As shown in this anatomical dissection, there is a possibility of anatomical and electric connection between the APM and PPM (*arrows*). *LV*, Left ventricle; *RV*, right ventricle. (From Komatsu Y, Nogami A, Kurosaki K, et al. Fascicular ventricular tachycardia originating from papillary muscles: Purkinje network involvement in the reentrant circuit. *Circ Arrhythm Electrophysiol.* 2017;10. pii:e004549.)

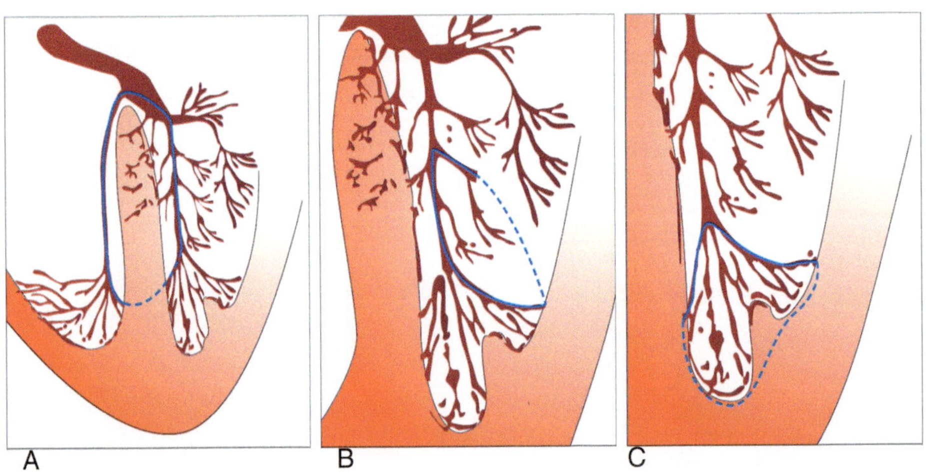

Fig. 32.22 Schematic representation of Purkinje reentry. Pathways are shown at decreasing geometric scales: (A) bundle branch reentry, (B) fascicular ventricular tachycardia, and (C) distal Purkinje–muscle reentry. An increasing length is ascribed to the muscular component (slower conductor; *dotted line*) when the Purkinje rapidly conducting component (*bold line*) decreases in size. (From Haissaguerre M, Vigmond E, Stuyvers B, et al. Ventricular arrhythmias and the His-Purkinje system. *Nat Rev Cardiol.* 2016;13:155–166.)

from the proximal rather than the distal electrodes, the fused presystolic Purkinje potential (P2) was recorded earlier from the distal electrodes. During sinus rhythm, recording at the same site demonstrated P2, which was recorded after the His bundle potential and before the onset of the QRS complex, suggesting P2 as potentials of left posterior fascicle (LPF). The sequence of the P2 during sinus rhythm was the reverse of that seen during VT. Entrainment pacing from the atrium or ventricle captured P1 orthodromically and reset the VT (Fig. 32.25). Although P1 has proved to be a critical potential in the VT circuit, whether the LPF (P2) is involved in the retrograde limb of the VT circuit was controversial.[50,54–56] Morishima and colleagues[55] reported a case with negative participation of the proximal LPF (P2) to the LPF VT circuit. Selective capture of LPF (P2) by a sinus

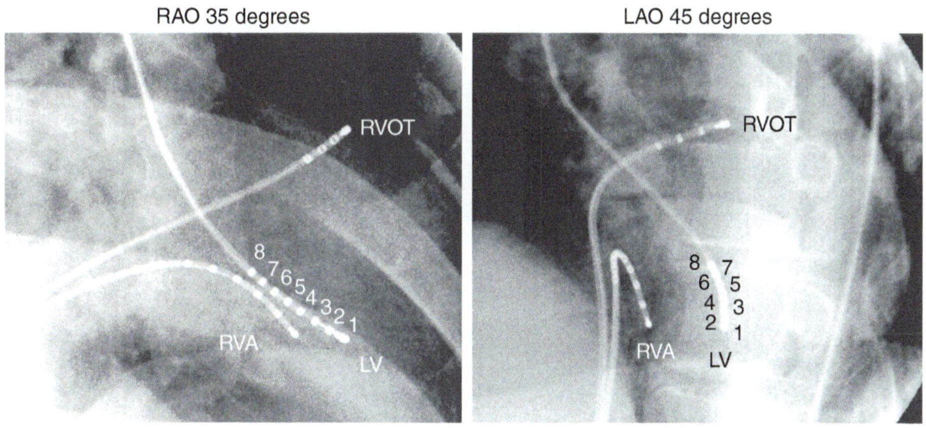

Fig. 32.23 Representation of an octapolar linear electrode catheter positioned at the left ventricular septum as viewed fluoroscopically in the right anterior oblique (RAO) and left anterior oblique (LAO) projections. The distance between electrodes 1 and 8 of the octapolar electrode catheter was approximately 25 mm. *LV,* Left ventricle; *RVA,* right ventricular apex; *RVOT,* right ventricular outflow tract. (From Nogami A, Naito S, Tada H, et al. Demonstration of diastolic and presystolic Purkinje potential as critical potentials on a macroreentry circuit of verapamil-sensitive idiopathic left ventricular tachycardia. *J Am Coll Cardiol.* 2000;36:811–823.)

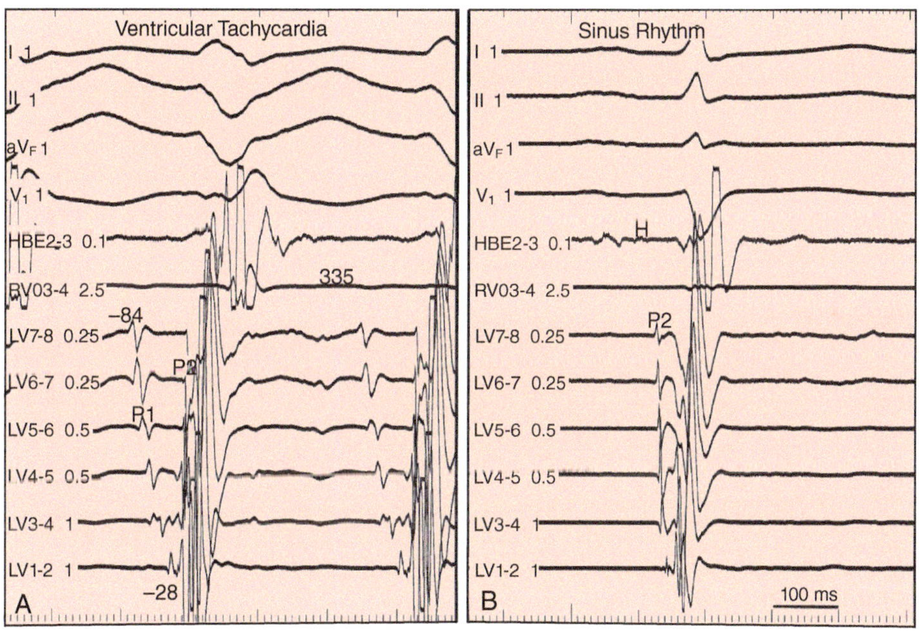

Fig. 32.24 Intracardiac recordings from an octapolar electrode catheter. (A) During left posterior fascicular ventricular tachycardia, a diastolic potential (P1) and a presystolic Purkinje potential (P2) were recorded. Whereas P1 was recorded earlier from the proximal rather than the distal electrodes, P2 was recorded earlier from the distal rather than the proximal electrodes. (B) During sinus rhythm, recording at the same site demonstrated the P2, which is now recorded before the onset of the QRS complex and is earliest on the proximal electrodes. *1–2,* distal bipole; *7–8,* proximal bipole; *H,* His; *HBE,* His bundle electrogram; *LV,* left ventricle; *RVO,* right ventricular outflow. (From Nogami A, Naito S, Tada H, et al. Demonstration of diastolic and presystolic Purkinje potential as critical potentials on a macroreentry circuit of verapamil-sensitive idiopathic left ventricular tachycardia. *J Am Coll Cardiol.* 2000;36:811–823.)

complex did not affect the cycle length of VT, suggesting P2 as a bystander (Fig. 32.26A). And the postpacing interval after the entrainment from LV septal myocardium was equal to the cycle length of VT, suggesting LV septal myocardium as the retrograde limb (Fig. 32.26B). Maeda and colleagues[56] also reported a case of LPF (P2) in a bystander circuit of LPF VT. Although RF energy application at the site with P1 and P2 changed the activation sequence of P2 and the surface QRS morphology, VT did not terminate and the cycle length and activation sequence of P1 remained unchanged (Fig. 32.27).

Circuit Diagram of Left Fascicular VTs

The hypothesized circuit of LPF VT is depicted in Fig. 32.28A. In this circuit, P1 fiber is connecting to the distal portion of LPF with a turnaround. There is decremental properties and verapamil sensitivity between P1 fiber and myocardium. P2 represents the

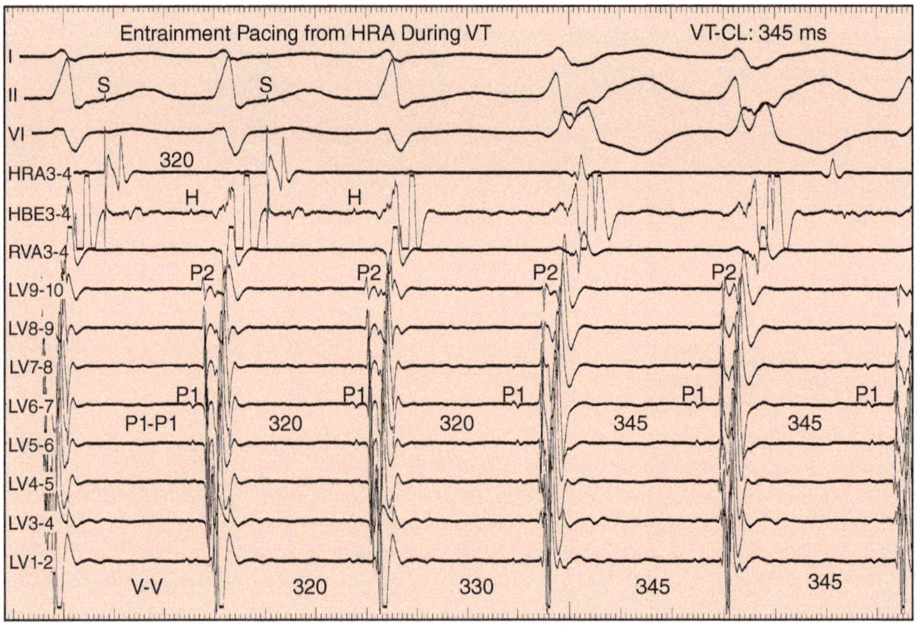

Fig. 32.25 Intracardiac recordings during entrainment pacing from the high right atrium (HRA) during left posterior fascicular ventricular tachycardia (VT). Right atrial pacing (CL: 320 ms) during VT (CL: 345 ms) resulted in a narrowing of the QRS width without VT interruption. Whereas the diastolic potential (P1) was orthodromically captured, the presystolic Purkinje potential (P2) was antidromically captured. The activation sequence of P2 was identical to that observed during sinus rhythm. *CL*, Cycle length; *H*, His; *HRA*, high right atrium; *HBE*, His-bundle electrogram; *LV*, left ventricle; *S*, pacing stimulus.

activation of the LPF, and it is a bystander during VT. P1 represents the anterograde limb of the circuit in VT and LV septal muscle is the retrograde limb. During sinus rhythm, the activation goes from P2 to P1 at the point of the fusion; therefore, P1 is buried in the local ventricular activation. Liu and colleagues[57] first proposed this schematic diagram of LPF VT (Fig. 32.29). Although the basic concept of the circuit is similar to ours, their diagram also explains why P1 is not always recorded during VT. In our series,[53] P1 could be recorded in 75% of the patients during the VT. They also reported that P1 was detected in 64% of the patients. They described that a slow conduction zone is connecting the ventricular myocardium and proximal P1; in the cases with a recorded P1 during VT, the P1 fiber is parallel and adjacent to the LPF and the connection between P1 and the LPF (P2) is located at a more distal portion of the LPF. On the other hand, in the cases without a recorded P1, the P1 fiber may be short in length or nonparallel in orientation to the LPF, or both.[57]

The circuit of the LAF VT was shown in Fig. 32.28B. In this circuit, P1 fiber is connecting to the distal portion of LAF with a turnaround. There is decremental properties and verapamil sensitivity between P1 fiber and myocardium. P2 represents the activation of the LAF. During VT, the anterograde limb is the P1, and the retrograde limb is the LV muscle.

The circuits of posterior and anterior papillary muscle fascicular VTs are presumed to be smaller than the septal types and located distally.

We hypothesized the potential VT circuits that mediate the left upper septal fascicular VT, as shown in Fig. 32.28C. We propose the existence of a left middle fascicle (or left septal branch) in this circuit where P1 represents retrograde conduction within the left middle fascicle while P2 represents activation of the LPF. LPF is the dominant anterograde limb of the reentrant circuit for this VT. While His and RBB are the bystanders, they are activated almost at the same time as the LAF and LPF which explains why VT exhibits an almost similar QRS configuration to that during sinus rhythm. Therefore, P1 is the common retrograde limb of the VT circuit and represents an important ablation target. This left middle fascicle might exclusively conduct retrogradely, because most patients do not exhibit septal q waves before ablation, and there is typically no change in QRS morphology after successful RF ablation.[43]

The hypothesized VT circuit in reverse-type LPF VT is depicted in Fig. 32.30B. VT circuit of common LPF VT is shown in Fig. 32.30A for comparison. During a reverse-type LPF VT, the LV superior-middle septum is activated first displaying a centrifugal activation pattern. Importantly, the ventricular septal propagation is the antegrade limb of the reentrant circuit while P1 potential is the retrograde limb of the reentrant circuit, which is buried in the local ventricular electrogram. Superior turnaround of the circuit in the common LPF VT is still unsolved (Fig. 32.30A). If the circuits of LPF VT and reverse-type LPF VT are completely reversed, the intramural site at the earliest activation during reverse-type LPF VT may be the superior turnaround of the LPF VT circuit. Nevertheless, further electrophysiologic investigation is needed to confirm this.

Diagnostic Criteria

Surface Electrocardiogram

The 12-lead ECG of left posterior septal fascicular VT exhibits left-axis deviation (Fig. 32.18A),[53] and the left posterior

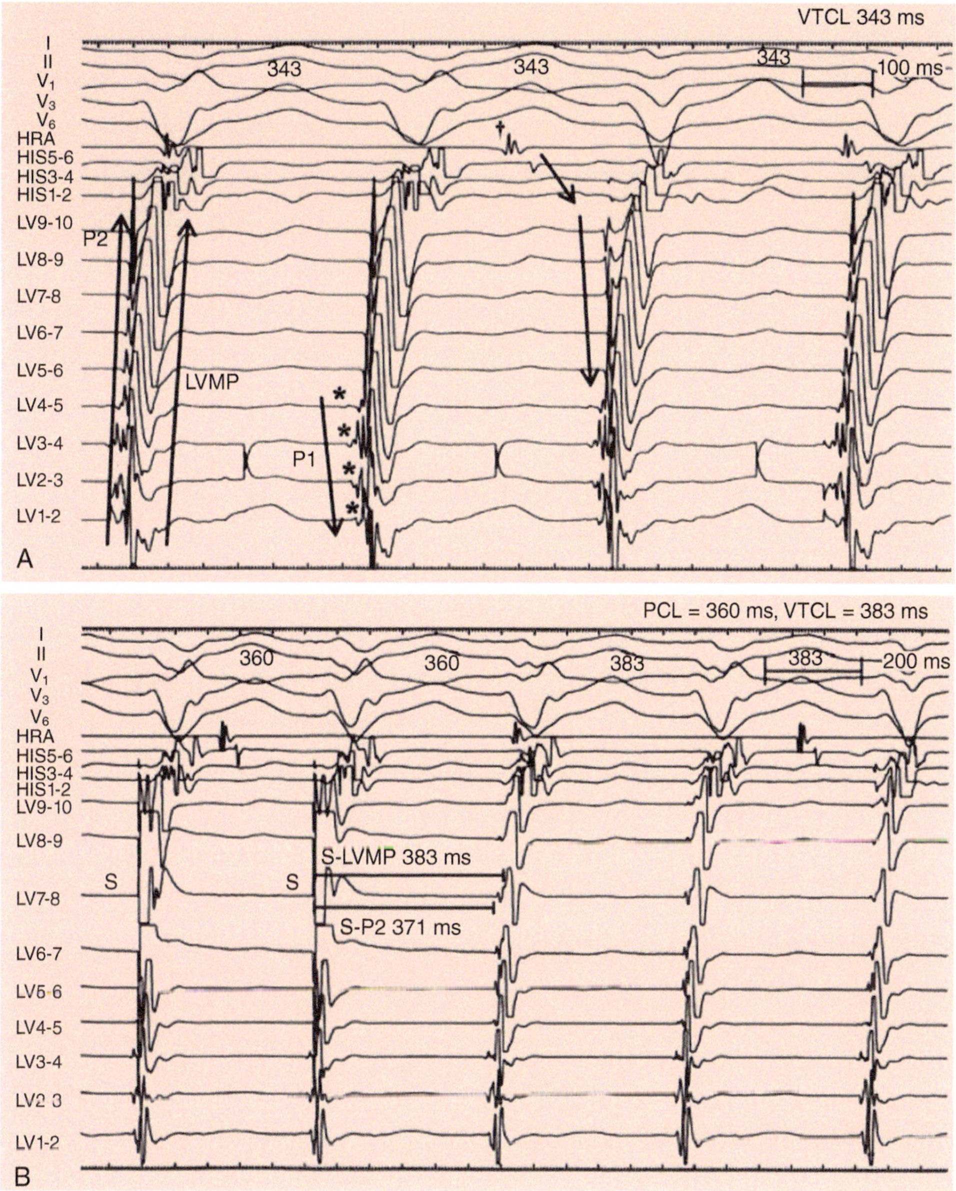

Fig. 32.26 Negative participation of the proximal left posterior fascicle to the ventricular tachycardia (VT) circuit. (A) Three sequences of potentials were recorded at the left posterior septum during verapamil-sensitive idiopathic left VT: diastolic Purkinje potentials (P1) propagating from base to apex (*asterisks*) and presystolic left posterior fascicular potentials (P2) and systolic left ventricular myocardial potentials (LVMP) propagating in the reverse direction. Note that selective capture of the left posterior fascicle by a sinus beat (dagger) did not affect the cycle length of VT. (B) During entrainment pacing from LV 7–8, both P2 and LVMP were simultaneously captured. Although the postpacing interval of LVMP was equal to VTCL, the postpacing interval of P2 was shorter than VTCL. *CL,* Cycle length; *HRA,* high right atrium; *LPF,* left posterior fascicle; *LVP,* left ventricular myocardium potential; *PCL,* pacing cycle length; *S,* pacing stimulus. (From Morishima I, Nogami A, Tsuboi H, Sone T. Negative participation of the left posterior fascicle in the reentry circuit of verapamil-sensitive idiopathic left ventricular tachycardia. *J Cardiovasc Electrophysiol.* 2012;23:556–559.)

papillary muscle fascicular VT exhibits superior right-axis deviation (northwest axis) (Fig. 32.18B).[45] The uncommon type of this VT is a left anterior fascicular (LAF) VT whose QRS morphology exhibits an RBBB configuration and inferior axis.[41,58] Left anterior septal fascicular VT exhibits Rs pattern in V_5–V_6 (Fig. 32.18C), and left anterior papillary muscle fascicular VT exhibits deep S waves in V_5–V_6 (Fig. 32.18D).[45,58] In our series of six cases with LAF VT,[58] the mean cycle length of the VT was 390 ± 62 ms, and the mean electrical axis during the VT was 120 ± 16 degrees.

Another type of VT is an upper septal fascicular VT, whose QRS morphology exhibits a relatively narrow QRS configuration and normal or right-axis deviation (Fig. 32.19).[42–44] This type of VT sometimes occurs after previous catheter ablation of other fascicular VTs. Of 12 patients with upper septal VT,

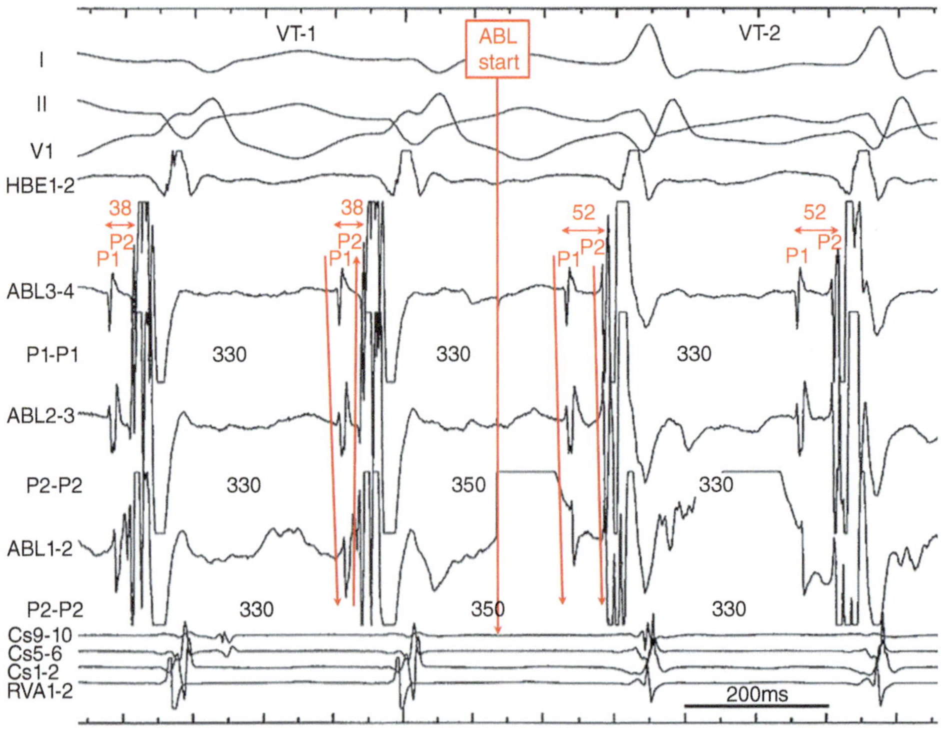

Fig. 32.27 Left posterior fascicle (P2) as a bystander circuit of left posterior fascicular VT. During VT-1, a diastolic potential (P1) and presystolic potential (P2) were recorded at the midseptal area near the left posterior fascicle (LPF). Immediately after RF energy application at this site, the VT–1 transitioned to VT-2. When VT-1 transitioned to VT-2, the QRS complexes reflected a more basal exit site with the same tachycardia cycle length. During VT-2, the activation sequence of P2 changed, while the activation sequence of P1 remained unchanged (*arrows*). The P1-P1 interval also remained unchanged during VT-1 and VT-2. *Cs*, Coronary sinus; *HBE*, His-bundle electrogram; *RVA*, right ventricular apex. (From Maeda S, Yokoyama Y, Nogami A, et al. First case of left posterior fascicle in a bystander circuit of idiopathic left ventricular tachycardia. *Can J Cardiol.* 2014;30:e11–e13.)

six patients (50%) had one or two previous ablations for other fascicular VT. However another six patients did not have a previous ablation, and this tachycardia was their de novo arrhythmia.[43] In most of the patients with upper septal fascicular VT, QRS configuration during sinus rhythm exhibits an S wave in lead I and Q waves in leads III and aVF, suggesting conduction delay at the LPF area (Fig. 32.19).[43]

The 12-lead ECG of reverse type of left posterior septal fascicular VT is very unique, which exhibited Qr or rSr morphology in V1 with an early precordial transition and inferior-axis (Fig. 32.20).[46]

Intracardiac Electrograms and Differential Diagnosis

With left posterior septal fascicular VT, the earliest ventricular activation is recorded from the apical septum, and diastolic potentials are recorded from the midseptum (Fig. 32.24). His activation follows QRS onset by 5–30 ms.[53] During sinus rhythm, recording from the same site demonstrates the Purkinje potentials after the His-bundle potential and before the onset of the QRS complex.

With left anterior fascicular septal VT, the earliest ventricular activation is recorded from the anterolateral LV (Fig. 32.31A), and diastolic Purkinje potentials are recorded from the midseptum (Fig. 32.31B). It may be difficult to distinguish between interfascicular VT[59] (bundle branch reentry tachycardia type B) and verapamil-sensitive left anterior fascicular VT (intrafascicular VT).[58] Interfascicular VT circuit mostly uses the LAF as the anterograde limb and the LPF as the retrograde limb. Recordings of His-bundle potential and LPF during VT is important. Interfascicular VT usually has a His-bundle potential recorded in the diastolic phase during the VT, and the His activation precedes activation of the left bundle to produce an RBBB QRS morphology. In idiopathic reentrant fascicular VTs, the H-V interval is shorter (or negative) and follows left fascicular activation.

The differential diagnosis includes supraventricular tachycardias with bifascicular block or aberrancy. If there is retrograde ventriculoatrial conduction during the tachycardia, it mimics AV nodal reentry tachycardia or AV reciprocating tachycardia. The response of these tachycardias to verapamil and the ability to initiate and entrain them by atrial pacing may also lead to diagnostic confusion. To avoid a misdiagnosis, measurement of a shorter H-V interval during the tachycardia than in sinus rhythm is important. And an earlier potential than the His-bundle potential is recorded during the left fascicular VT from the LV septum where the left bundle potential is recorded during sinus rhythm.

VT can be slowed or terminated by the intravenous administration of verapamil; however it is unresponsive to adenosine or Valsalva maneuvers. Importantly, verapamil is not the only effective drug. Lidocaine, β-blockers, and Class

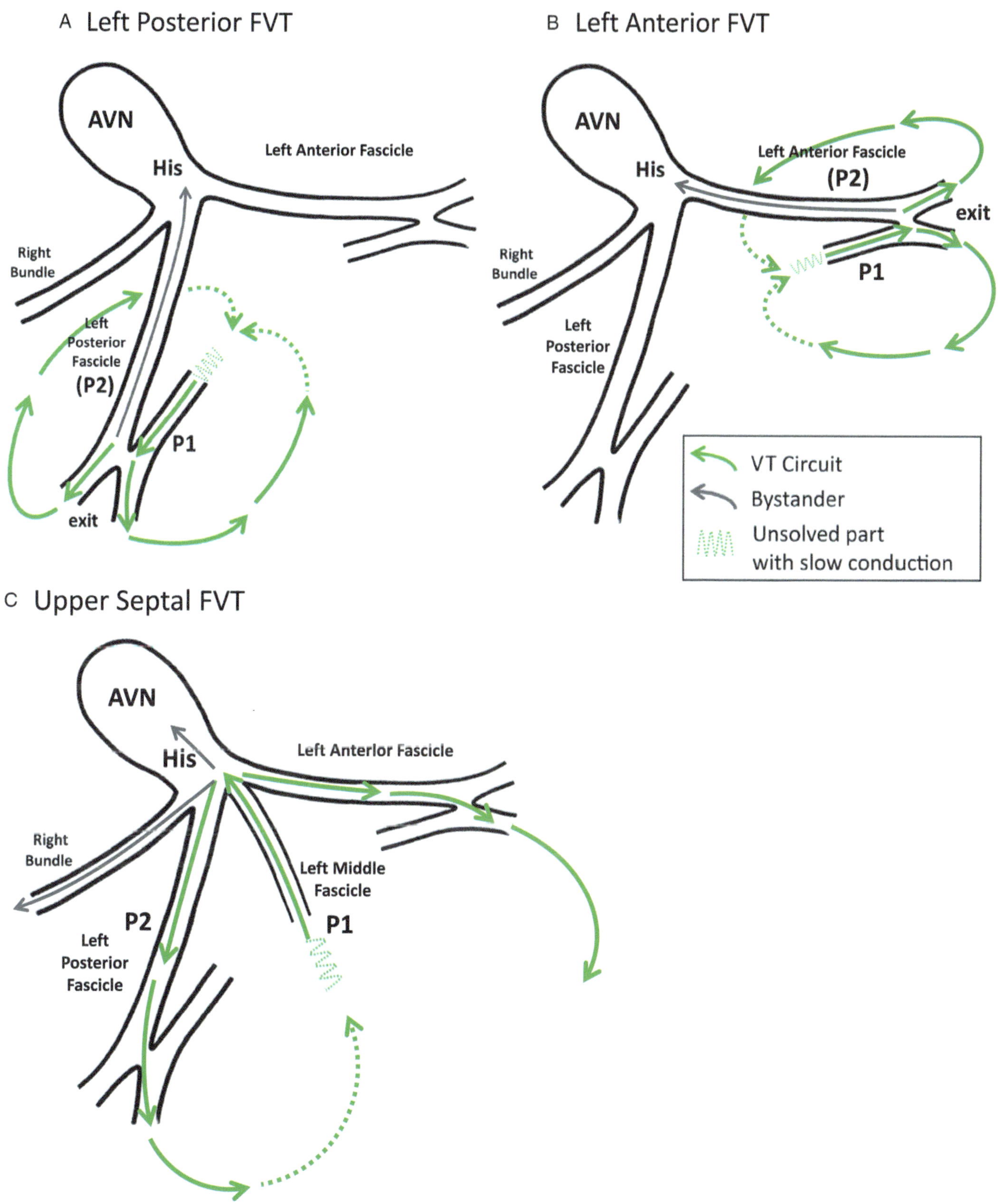

Fig. 32.28 Schematic diagram of the reentrant fascicular VTs. (A) Left posterior fascicular VT. The antegrade limb was P1, and the retrograde limb was the septal myocardium. P2 (left posterior fascicle) is a bystander. The reentrant circuit of VT can involve the Purkinje network around the papillary muscles. (B) Left anterior fascicular VT. (C) Upper septal fascicular VT. In this circuit, the left middle fascicle (left septal branch) is the retrograde limb and the antegrade limb is the left posterior fascicle. *AVN*, Atrioventricular node; *LAF*, left anterior fascicle; *LPF*, left posterior fascicle; *RB*, right bundle.

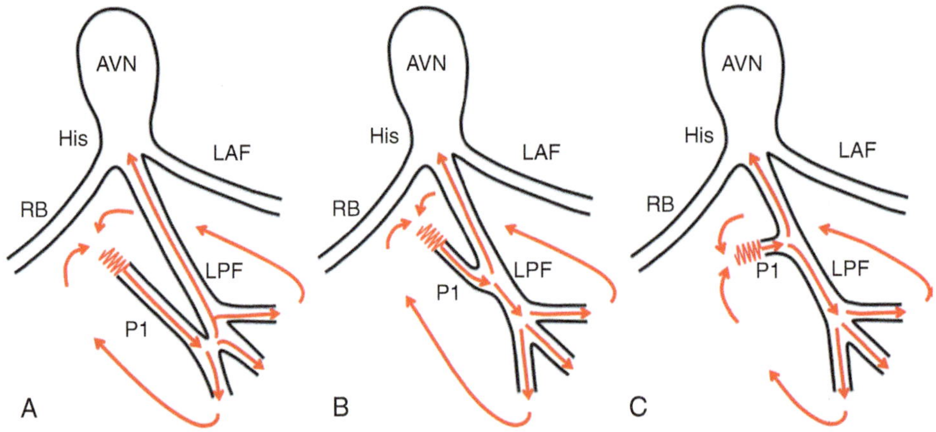

Fig. 32.29 Schematic diagram of the left posterior fascicular ventricular tachycardia (LPF-VT) reentry circuit. The reentry circuit of LPF-VT includes ventricular myocardium, a part of the LPF, a P1 fiber, and a slow conduction zone connecting the ventricular myocardium and proximal P1. (A) In the cases with a recorded P1 during LPF-VT, the P1 fiber is parallel and adjacent to the LPF, and the connection between P1 and the LPF (P2) is located at a more distal portion of the LPF. (B) The P1 fiber is parallel and adjacent to the LPF, but short, and the connection between P1 and the LPF (P2) is located at the middle or proximal portion of the LPF. C, In the cases without a recorded P1, the P1 fiber may be short in length or nonparallel in orientation to the LPF, or both. *AVN*, Atrioventricular node; *LAF*, left anterior fascicle; *LPF*, left posterior fascicle; *RB*, right bundle. (From Liu Q, Shehata M, Jiang R, et al. Macroreentrant loop in ventricular tachycardia from the left posterior fascicle: new implications for mapping and ablation. *Circ Arrhythm Electrophysiol.* 2016;9:e004272.)

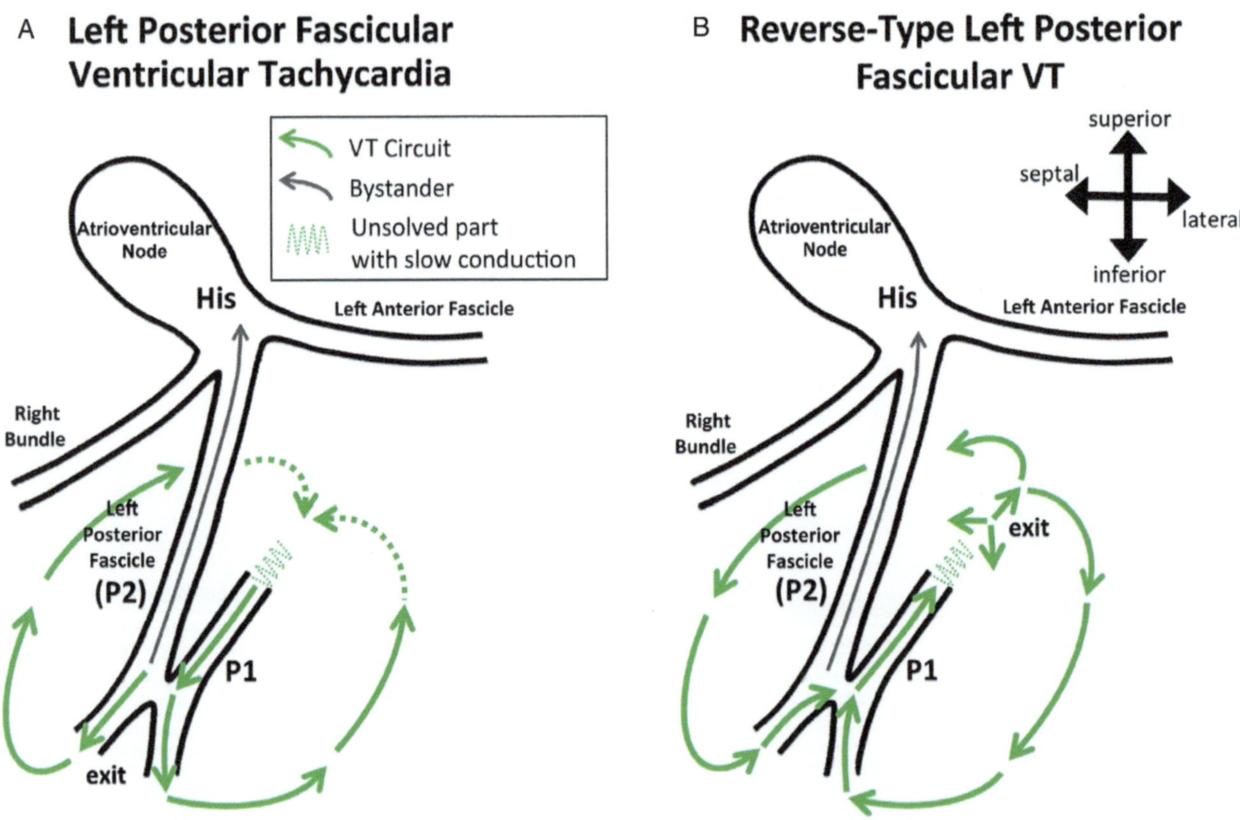

Fig. 32.30 Hypothesized circuit of reverse-type left posterior fascicular VT. (A) Left posterior fascicular VT. (B) Reverse-type left posterior fascicular VT. *His,* His bundle. (From Phanthawimol W, Nogami A, Haruna T, et al. Reverse-type left posterior fascicular ventricular tachycardia: a new electrocardiographic entity. *JACC Clin Electrophysiol.* 2021;7:843–854.)

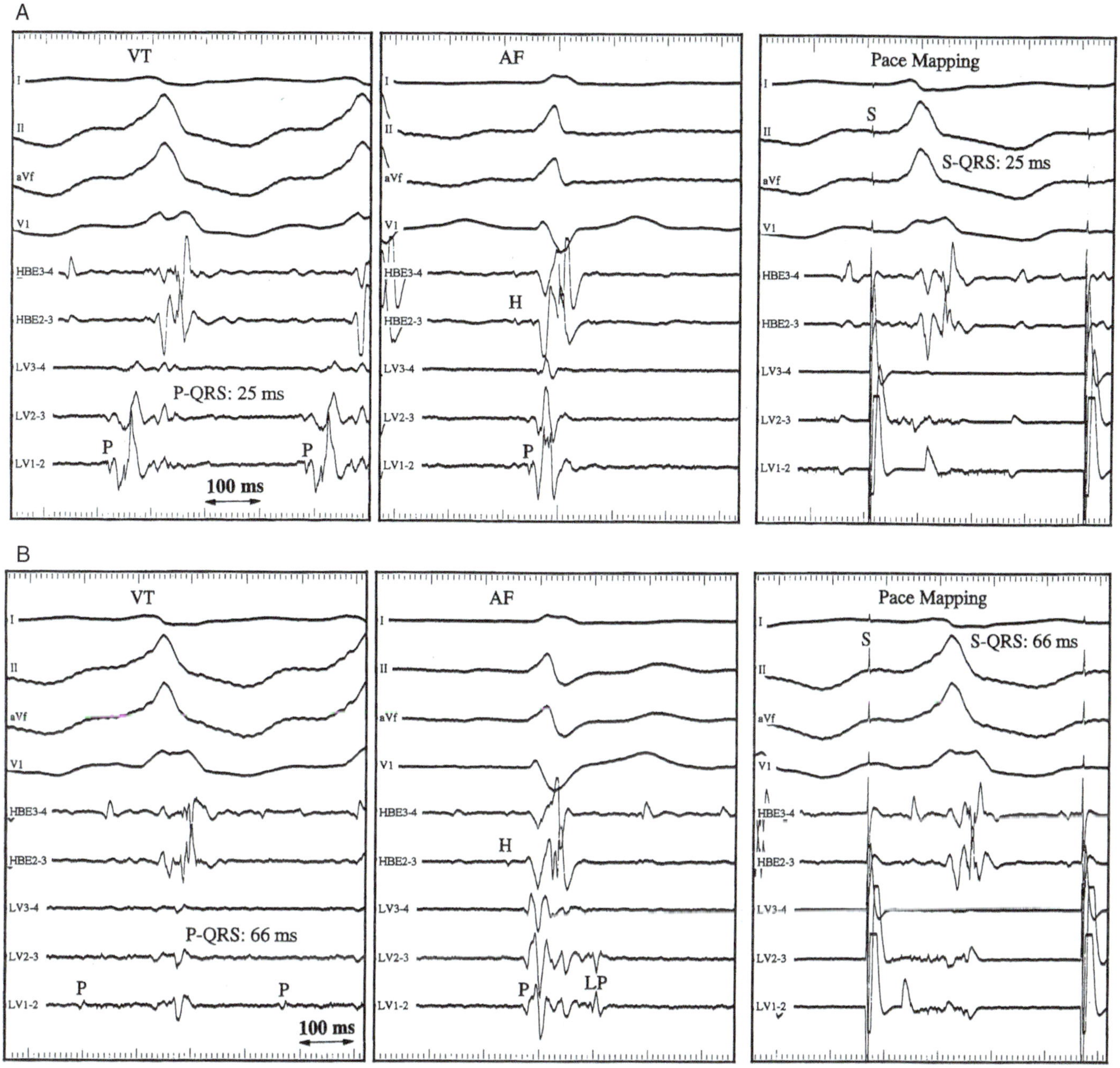

Fig. 32.31 Intracardiac electrograms during left anterior fascicular VT. (A) The earliest ventricular activation is recorded from the anterolateral LV. Pace mapping at that site produced a similar QRS complex with an interval between the pacing stimulus and QRS (S-QRS) of 25 ms, equal to the P-QRS interval during the VT. The radiofrequency current delivered at that site terminated the VT; however the VT was still induced. (B) During the VT, diastolic Purkinje potentials are recorded from the midseptum. Purkinje potential (P) preceded the QRS (P-QRS) by 66 ms. During basal rhythm (atrial fibrillation [AF]), a Purkinje potential was recorded before the His-bundle potential (H), and a late potential (LP) was also recorded after the QRS complex. Pace mapping at that site produced a similar QRS complex with an interval between the pacing stimulus and QRS (S-QRS) of 66 ms, equal to the P-QRS interval during the VT. The radiofrequency current delivered at that site terminated the VT and suppressed the reinduction of the VT. *HBE*, His-bundle electrogram; *LV*, left ventricle. (From Nogami A, Naito S, Tada H, et al. Verapamil-sensitive left anterior fascicular ventricular tachycardia: results of radiofrequency ablation in six patients. *J Cardiovasc Electrophysiol.* 1998;9:1269–1278.)

IA/C drugs might be also effective. Rare cases of adenosine responsiveness occur, but only if the VT shows catecholamine dependency.

The diagnostic criteria for idiopathic left fascicular VTs are given in Table 32.1.

Mapping and Ablation

RF catheter ablation may be considered a potential first-line therapy for patients with idiopathic VT because these VTs can safely be eliminated by ablation in a high percentage of patients.

TABLE 32.1 Diagnostic Criteria for Idiopathic Left Fascicular Ventricular Tachycardias

	Verapamil-Sensitive Left Fascicular Tachycardia	Nonreentrant Fascicular VT (Verapamil Insensitive)
Characteristic surface ECG appearance	• RBBB and left-axis configuration (left posterior septal fascicular VT: most common) • RBBB and superior right-axis configuration (left posterior papillary muscle fascicular VT) • RBBB and inferior axis configuration; Rs in V5–6 (left anterior septal fascicular VT) • RBBB and inferior axis configuration; rS/QS in V5–6 (left anterior papillary muscle fascicular VT) • Narrow QRS and inferior axis configuration (upper septal type which sometimes appears after the previous RFCA for another fascicular VTs) • Qr or rSr morphology in V1 and inferior axis (reverse type of left posterior fascicular VT)	• RBBB and either a left- or right-axis deviation • Faster VT is prone to exhibit wider QRS
Electrophysiologic findings	• Tachycardia dependence on left ventricular fascicular macro-reentry • Diastolic potentials (P1) and presystolic Purkinje potentials (P2) preceding ventricular activation • In reverse type of left posterior fascicular VT, P1 and P2 buried within the QRS • Changes in tachycardia rate preceded by similar changes in Purkinje and diastolic potentials • His activation follows QRS onset (short positive H-V in some types) • Induction and entrainment with ventricular and/or atrial pacing	• Mechanism of tachycardia consistent with abnormal automaticity from Purkinje system • Induction by exercise or catecholamines • Unable to induce or entrain by ventricular stimulation • Transient suppression by adenosine and with overdrive pacing or faster supraventricular rhythm
Drug response	• Responsive to lidocaine, β-blockers, and Class IA/C drugs • Verapamil-sensitive termination or slowing of tachycardia caused by conduction slowing or block in abnormal Purkinje system • Papillary muscle fascicular VT is also verapamil sensitive, but less sensitive	• Responsive to lidocaine, β-blockers, and Class IA/C drugs • No response to verapamil

ECG, Electrocardiogram; *H-V*, His-to-ventricular; *RFCA*, radiofrequency catheter ablation; *RBBB*, right bundle branch block; *VT*, ventricular tachycardia.

Left Posterior Septal Fascicular VT

Conventional LV septal mapping using a multipolar electrode catheter is useful in patients with LPF VT.[53] Two distinct potentials, P1 and P2, can be recorded during the VT from the midseptum (Fig. 32.24). Because the diastolic potential (P1) has been proved a critical potential in the VT circuit, this potential can be targeted to cure the tachycardia. Nakagawa and colleagues[60] first reported the importance of Purkinje potentials in the ablation of this VT, and Tsuchiya and colleagues[61] reported the significance of a late diastolic potential. However, the successful ablation sites identified by these two research groups were different. Whereas Nakagawa's ablation sites were at the apical–inferior septum of the LV, Tsuchiya's ablation sites were at the basal septal regions close to the main trunk of the left bundle branch. These findings suggest that any P1 during VT can be targeted for catheter ablation. The apical third of the septum is usually targeted to avoid the creation of LBBB or AV block (Fig. 32.32).

Using the retrograde aortic approach, the ablation catheter in LV is rotated toward the septum, then the curvature is opened, allowing the tip of the catheter to fall toward the inferior septum toward the apex. When transseptal approach is used, U-curved tip of the ablation catheter is manipulated to be in good contact with the septum. In a previous study,[53] P1 was recorded during VT in 15 of 20 patients (75%). RF ablation was successfully performed at this site in all 15 patients. During energy application, the P1-QRS interval was gradually prolonged, and the VT was terminated by block between P1 and QRS (Fig. 32.33). After termination of the tachycardia, the P1 was noted to occur after the QRS complex during sinus rhythm, whereas the P2 was still observed before the QRS complex (Fig. 32.34). After successful ablation, P1 occurred after the QRS complex, with an identical activation sequence to that observed during the VT. When the distal segment of P1 is ablated, the P1 activation proceeds orthodromically around the circuit and subsequently blocks from a proximal to distal direction during sinus rhythm. The P1 that appears after ablation exhibits decremental properties during atrial pacing or ventricular pacing, or both, and the intravenous administration of verapamil significantly prolongs the His-to-P1 interval during sinus rhythm (Fig. 32.34). Pace mapping at the successful ablation site is usually not good because the selective pacing of P1 is difficult and there is an antidromic activation of the proximal P1 potential. Pace mapping after successful ablation is sometimes better than before ablation because the antidromic activation of P1 is blocked.[62]

In the remaining 5 of 20 patients (25%), the diastolic potential (P1) could not be detected, and a single fused P2 was recorded only at the VT exit site.[53] Successful ablation was performed at this site in all five patients. According to the diagram by Liu and colleagues,[57] the P1 fiber in such cases might be short in length or nonparallel in orientation to the LPF, or both (Fig. 32.29C). The targets for catheter ablation are given in Box 32.2.

Left Posterior Papillary Muscle Fascicular VT

Diastolic Purkinje potential (P1) is recorded at the posterior papillary muscles or between the posterior papillary muscle and the

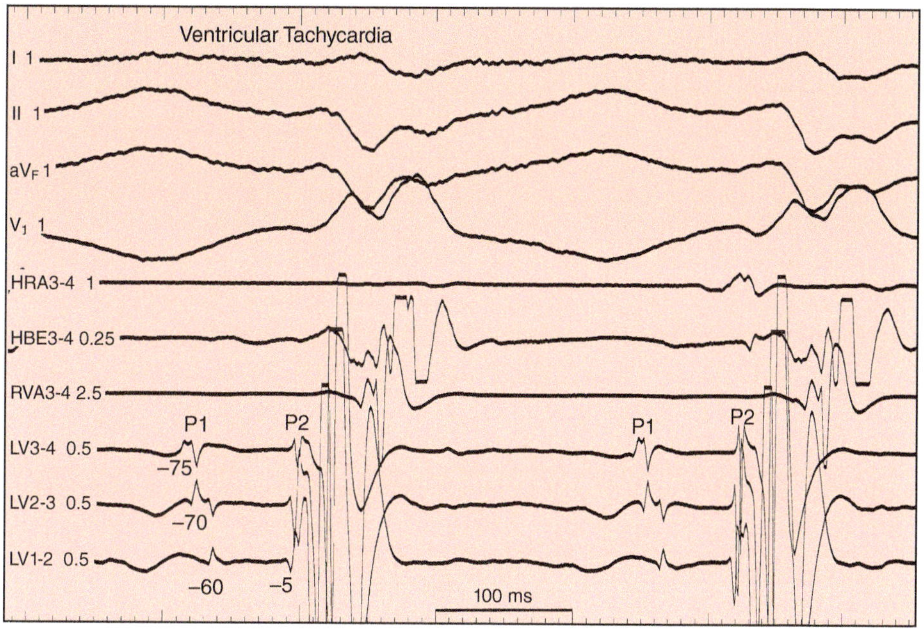

Fig. 32.32 Recordings from the site of successful ablation during left posterior fascicular ventricular tachycardia (VT). A diastolic potential (P1) and presystolic Purkinje potential (P2) were recorded in the midseptal area. The proximal two electrodes of the ablation catheter (LV) recorded the diastolic potential (P1) 15 ms earlier than the distal pair of electrodes. *HBE,* His-bundle electrogram; *HRA,* high right atrium; *LV,* left ventricle; *RVA,* right ventricular apex. (From Nogami A, Naito S, Tada H, et al. Demonstration of diastolic and presystolic Purkinje potential as critical potentials on a macroreentry circuit of verapamil-sensitive idiopathic left ventricular tachycardia. *J Am Coll Cardiol.* 2000;36:811–823.)

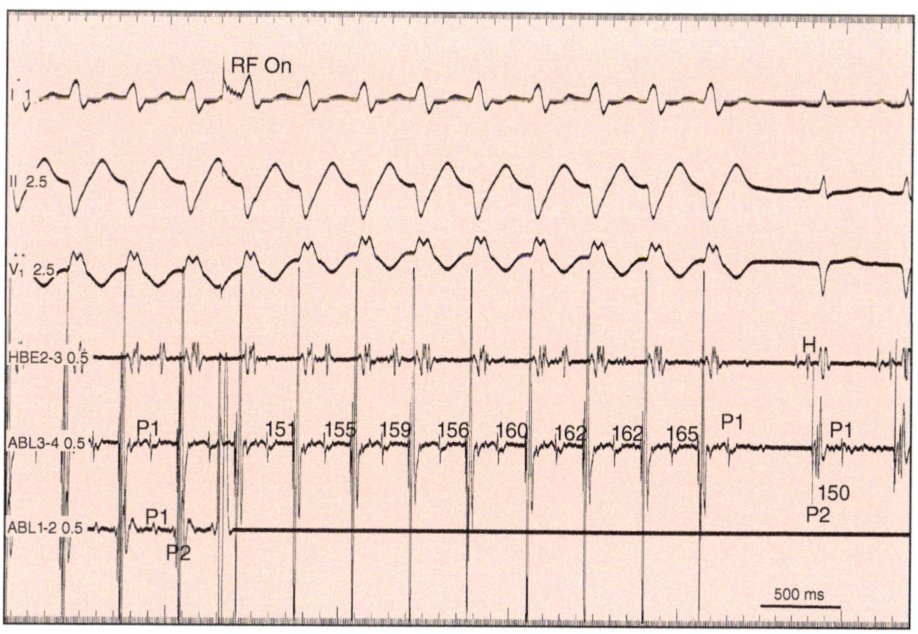

Fig. 32.33 An application of radiofrequency current delivered (RF on) during left posterior septal fascicular ventricular tachycardia (VT). During the energy application, the P1-QRS interval gradually prolonged, and the VT was terminated by block between P1 and QRS. After the ablation, the P1 occurred after the QRS complex during sinus rhythm. *ABL,* Ablation catheter; *H,* His recording; *HBE,* His-bundle electrogram. (From Nogami A, Naito S, Tada H, et al. Demonstration of diastolic and presystolic Purkinje potential as critical potentials on a macroreentry circuit of verapamil-sensitive idiopathic left ventricular tachycardia. *J Am Coll Cardiol.* 2000;36:811–823.)

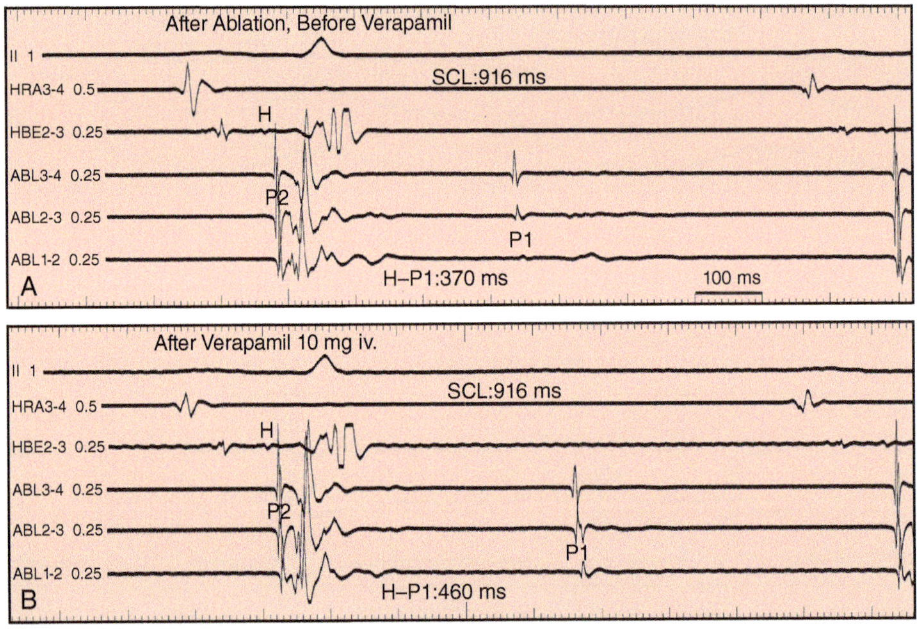

Fig. 32.34 Verapamil sensitivity of P1, which occurred after the QRS complex. A, The His-P1 (H-P1) interval during sinus rhythm was 370 ms. B, The H-P1 interval prolonged after the intravenous administration of 10 mg of verapamil. *ABL,* Ablation catheter; *HBE,* His-bundle electrogram; *HRA,* high right atrium; *SCL,* sinus cycle length. (From Tada H, Nogami A, Naito S, et al. Retrograde Purkinje potential activation during sinus rhythm following catheter ablation of idiopathic left ventricular tachycardia. *J Cardiovasc Electrophysiol.* 1998;9:1218–1224.)

BOX 32.2 Targets for Ablation

Verapamil-Sensitive Left Fascicular VT

- For septal fascicular VT, diastolic Purkinje potential (P1) in the anterograde limb of the VT circuit (middle septum). The earliest diastolic potential (P1) is not needed. The distal third of P1 potentials is usually targeted to avoid the creation of LBBB or atrioventricular block (P1 – QRS = 28–130 ms). If diastolic potential (P1) could not be recorded, presystolic fused Purkinje potential (P2) at the VT exit (apical septum).
- During papillary muscle fascicular VT, diastolic Purkinje potential (P1) is recorded at the posterior or anterior papillary muscle or between papillary muscle and the septum. Ablation of this potential is highly effective for suppressing this VT. However ablation at the left posterior or anterior papillary muscle regions often changes the QRS morphology and cycle length of the VT.
- A perfect QRS match during pace mapping is not needed.
- Anatomical approach can be performed if the diagnosis of verapamil-sensitive fascicular VT is correct and VT was not inducible. Anatomical approach includes linear ablation to transect the involved middle to distal left fascicular network.
- For reverse-type posterior septal fascicular VT, ablation to diastolic P1 potential during common posterior septal fascicular VT also suppress the reinduction of reverse posterior septal fascicular VT.

Nonreentrant Fascicular VT (Verapamil Insensitive)

- The earliest Purkinje potential during VT.
- Site of perfect QRS match during pace map; however the best pace map site does not always represent the successful ablation site.

LBBB, Left bundle branch block; *VT,* ventricular tachycardia.

septum during VT. Ablation of the diastolic potential is highly effective for suppressing this VT. Fig. 32.35 shows the example of RF catheter ablation of left posterior papillary muscle fascicular VT.[45] VT exhibited RBBB configuration and superior right-axis deviation, and the posterior papillary muscle region were ablated in the initial procedure. Recurred VT exhibited similar cycle length and QRS morphologies in the chest leads; however, electrical axis changed to horizontal. At the successful ablation site in the repeat procedure, both diastolic and presystolic Purkinje potentials (P1 and P2) were sequentially recorded during VT. The successful ablation site was located on the posterior papillary muscles, which was confirmed by real-time ICE image.

Left Anterior Septal Fascicular VT

Fig. 32.31A shows the intracardiac recording from the VT exit (anterolateral wall). The Purkinje potential preceded the QRS (P-QRS interval) by 25 ms during the VT, and pace mapping at that site produced a similar QRS complex with an interval between the pacing stimulus and QRS (S-QRS) of 25 ms, equal to the P-QRS interval during VT. RF current delivered at this site terminated the VT; however, the VT was still induced. Catheter ablation at the earliest ventricular activation was unsuccessful. Then, the ablation catheter was positioned in the midseptal area, where the diastolic Purkinje potential was recorded during VT (Fig. 32.31B). Pace mapping at that site produced a similar QRS complex, with an S-QRS interval of 66 ms, equal to the P-QRS interval during the VT. RF current delivered at this site terminated the VT and suppressed reinduction of VT. In our series,[58] the Purkinje potential preceded the QRS during VT by 56–66 ms, and catheter ablation at these sites was successful.

Left Anterior Papillary Muscle Fascicular VT

LV endocardial mapping during LAF VT identified the earliest ventricular activation in the anterolateral wall of the LV (Fig. 32.36). RF current delivered to this site suppressed the VT. In our series,[58] the fused Purkinje potential was recorded at that site and preceded the QRS complex by 20–35 ms, with pace mapping exhibiting an optimal match between the paced rhythm and clinical VT.

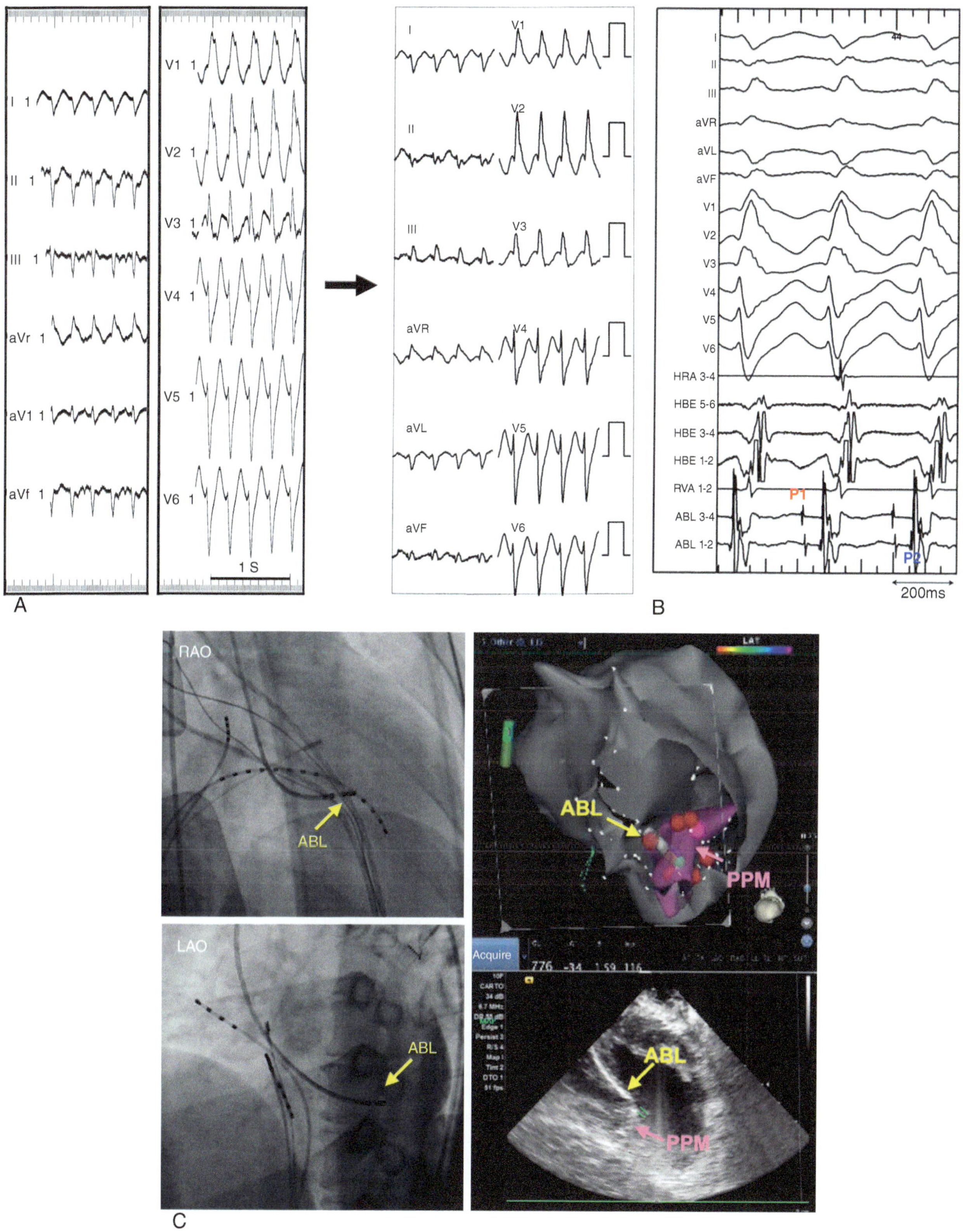

Fig. 32.35 Catheter ablation of posterior papillary muscle fascicular ventricular tachycardia (VT). (A) VT exhibited right bundle branch block (RBBB) configuration and superior right-axis deviation (northwest axis), and the left posterior fascicular region and posterior papillary muscle region were ablated in the initial procedure. The patient had recurrent VT exhibiting RBBB configuration and horizontal axis. (B) At the successful ablation site in the repeat procedure, both diastolic and presystolic Purkinje potentials (P1 and P2) were sequentially recorded during VT. C, The successful ablation site was located on the posterior papillary muscles (PPM), which was confirmed by real-time intracardiac ultrasound image. *ABL*, Ablation catheter; *LAO*, left oblique projections; and *RAO*, right oblique projections. (From Komatsu Y, Nogami A, Kurosaki K, et al. Fascicular ventricular tachycardia originating from papillary muscles: Purkinje network involvement in the reentrant circuit. *Circ Arrhythm Electrophysiol.* 2017;10. pii:e004549.)

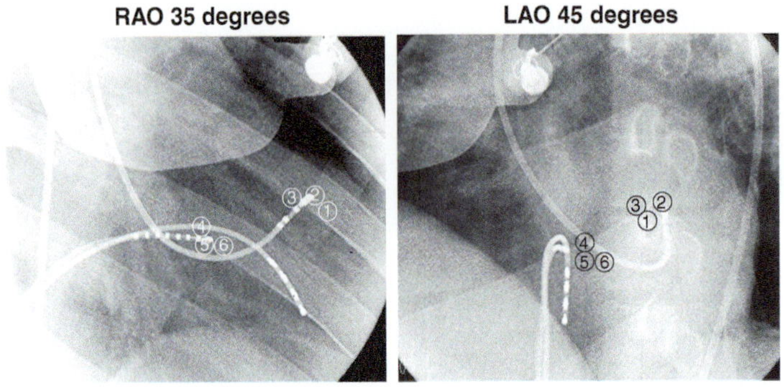

Fig. 32.36 Successful ablation sites for left anterior fascicular ventricular tachycardias (VTs). Patients 1–3 are the left anterior papillary muscle fascicular VT, and patients 4–6 are left anterior septal fascicular VT. Left anterior papillary muscle fascicular VT was successfully ablated at the earliest ventricular activation site in the anterolateral wall of the LV (patients 1–3). In the left anterior septal fascicular VT (patients 4–6), ablation at the VT exit site was unsuccessful and the ablation was successful at the mid-anterior septum of the left ventricle. *LAO,* Left oblique projections; *RAO,* right oblique projections. (From Nogami A, Naito S, Tada H, et al. Verapamil-sensitive left anterior fascicular ventricular tachycardia: results of radiofrequency ablation in six patients. *J Cardiovasc Electrophysiol.* 1998;9:1269–1278.)

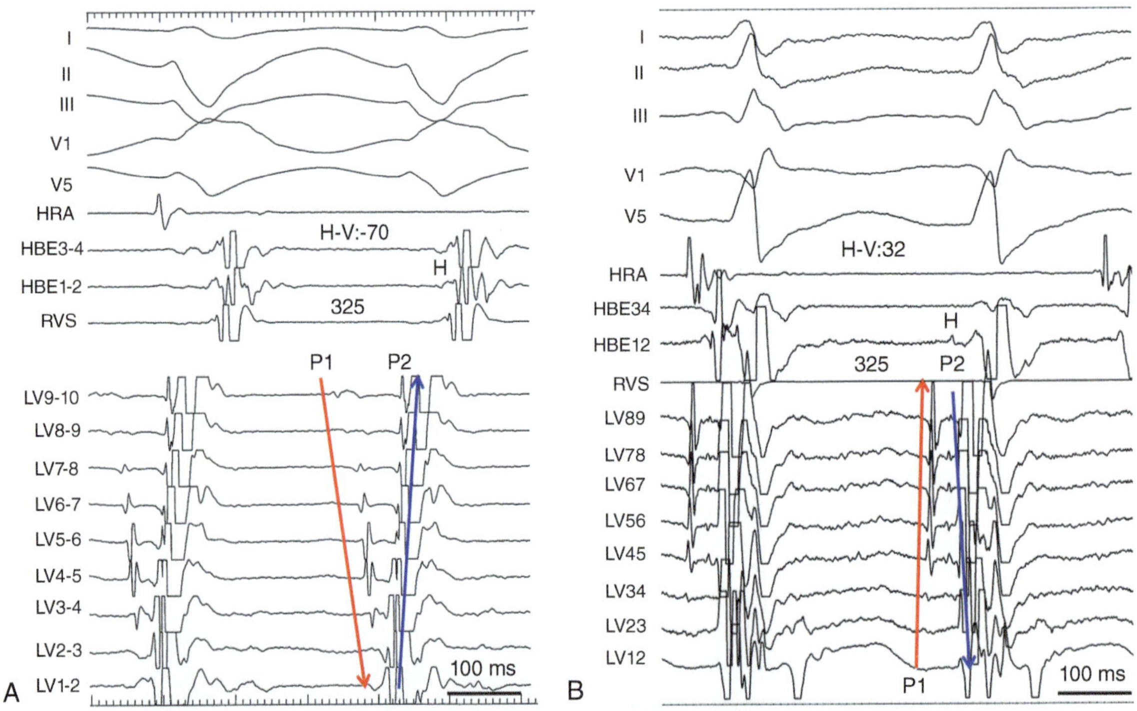

Fig. 32.37 Upper septal fascicular ventricular tachycardia (VT) after the ablation of posterior septal fascicular VT. (A, B, Intracardiac recording during common left posterior fascicular (LPF) VT (A) and upper septal fascicular VT (B), demonstrating the activation sequence of the diastolic potential (P1) (*red arrows*) and presystolic Purkinje potential (P2) (*blue arrows*) during each rhythm. C, Ablation catheter was positioned at upper-middle septum of the left ventricle. D, The diastolic P1 preceded the onset of the QRS by 52 ms. Entrainment from this site resulted in concealed fusion and postpacing interval–ventricular tachycardia cycle length difference of 5 ms and an interval between the pacing stimulus and QRS onset of 52 ms, equal to the P-QRS interval during VT. *ABL,* Ablation catheter; *H,* His-bundle potential; *HBE,* His-bundle electrogram; *HRA,* high right atrium; *LV,* left ventricle; *P1,* diastolic potential; *P2,* presystolic Purkinje potential; *RVS,* right ventricular septum; *S,* stimulation artifact; *VTCL,* VT cycle length. (From Talib AK, Nogami A, Nishiuchi S, et al. Verapamil-sensitive upper septal idiopathic left ventricular tachycardia: prevalence, mechanism, and electrophysiological characteristics. *J Am Coll Cardiol EP.* 2015;1:369–380.)

Left Upper Septal Fascicular VT

Fig. 32.37A, B shows intracardiac recordings during common LPF VT and upper septal fascicular VT which appeared few years later after two ablations for LPF VT.[43,44] During common LPF VT, a diastolic potential (P1) and presystolic potential (P2) were seen. Whereas P1 was recorded earlier from the proximal than from the distal electrodes, P2 was recorded earlier from the distal than from the proximal electrodes. His-bundle potential was recorded after the onset of the QRS complex (negative H-V interval). During upper septal fascicular VT, P1 was

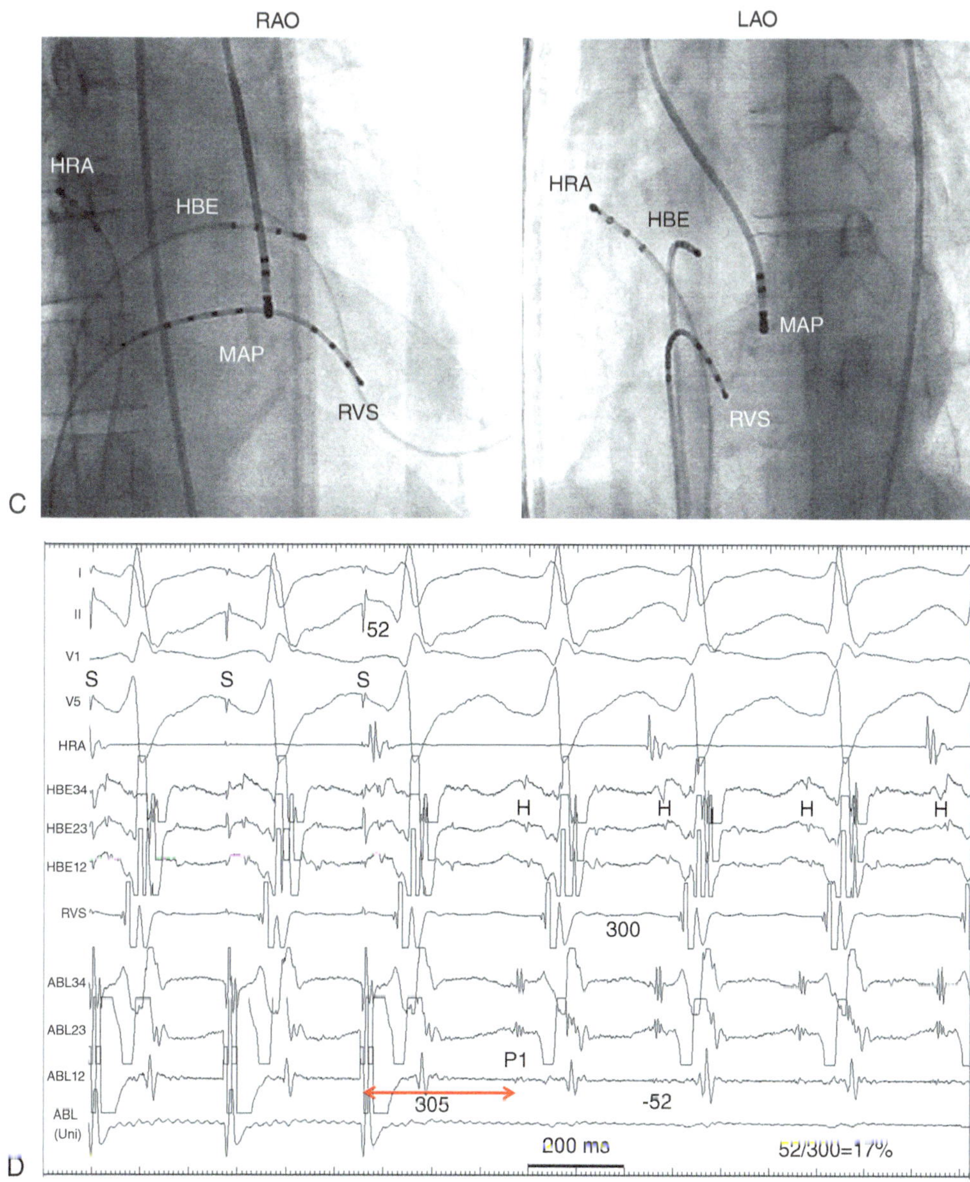

Fig. 32.37, cont'd

recorded earlier from the distal than from the proximal electrodes, whereas P2 was recorded earlier from the proximal than from the distal electrodes, similar to that during sinus rhythm. His-bundle potential preceded the onset of the QRS complex by 32 ms, which was shorter than that during sinus rhythm. An ablation catheter was positioned at the upper-middle ventricular septum (Fig. 32.37C) where the diastolic P1 preceded the onset of the QRS interval by 52 ms. Entrainment from this site resulted in concealed fusion and postpacing interval—ventricular tachycardia cycle length difference of 5 ms and an interval between the pacing stimulus and QRS onset of 52 ms, equal to the P1-QRS interval during VT (Fig. 32.37D). VT was slowed and terminated by RF energy application at this site within a few seconds and VT became noninducible.

Reverse Type of Left Posterior Fascicular VT

Fig. 32.38 shows intracardiac recordings during sinus rhythm, reverse-type LPF VT, and during common LPF VT in the same patient.[46] Entrainment pacing from the atrium during reverse-type LPF VT captures the conduction system and exhibits constant and progressive fusion (Fig. 32.39). The last captured QRS complex was the one after the next QRS complex and exhibited no fusion. During reverse-type LPF VT, the earliest ventricular activation was recorded at the LV superior-middle septum (Fig. 32.38B, arrowhead). While there was no presystolic Purkinje potential before QRS, fragmented P1 and spiky P2 potentials were seen within the QRS. Captured P1 by atrial stimulation reset the VT, but advanced P2 by sinus activation did not.[46] Catheter ablation aiming P1 potential during common LPF VT (Fig. 32.38C) suppressed not only LPF VT but also reverse-type LPF VT.

RF Energy Delivery and the End Point of Ablation

For verapamil-sensitive idiopathic left fascicular VT, RF energy is delivered using maximum power of 50 W. If the VT is terminated or slowed within 15 seconds, additional current is applied

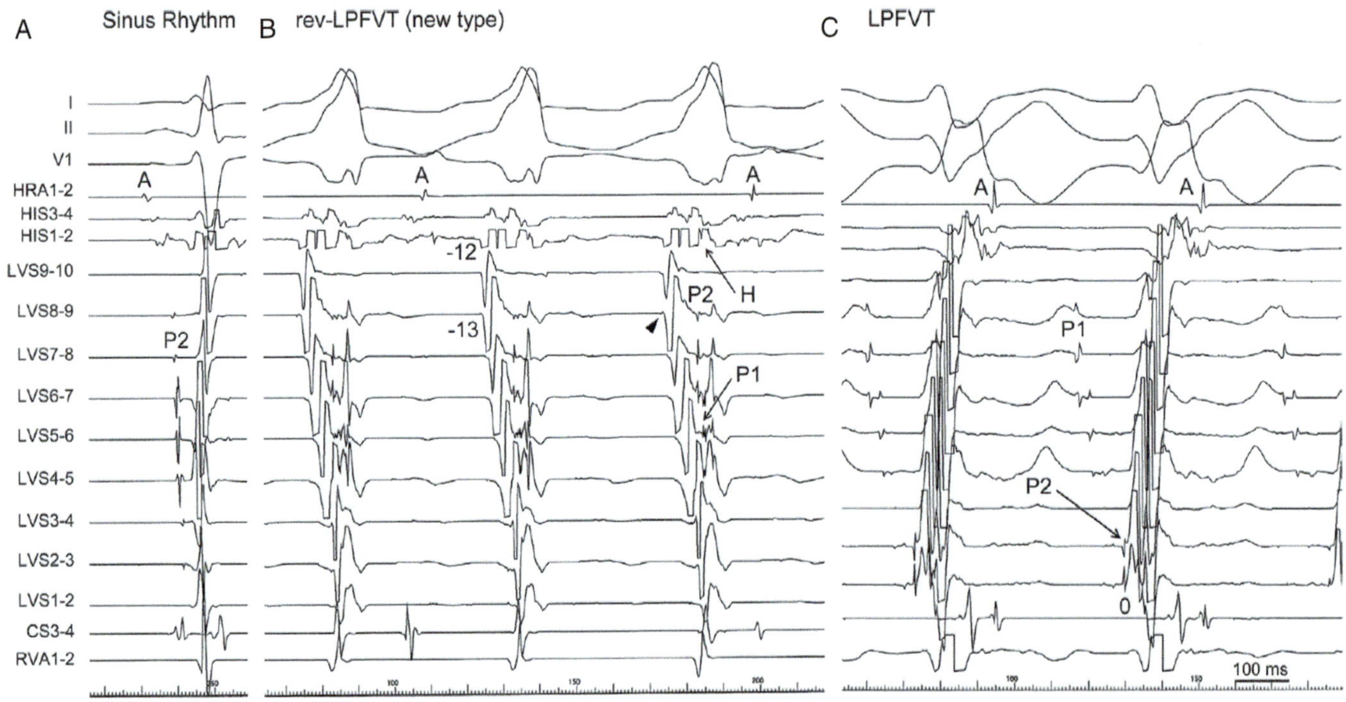

Fig. 32.38 Intracardiac recording in a patient with reverse type left posterior fascicular VT. (A) During sinus rhythm. (B) During reverse-type left posterior fascicular VT. (C) During left posterior fascicular VT. *A*, Atrial potential; *H*, His bundle potential; *HIS*, his bundle electrogram; *LPFVT*, left posterior fascicular ventricular tachycardia; *LVS*, left ventricular septum. (From Phanthawimol W, Nogami A, Haruna T, et al. Reverse-type left posterior fascicular ventricular tachycardia: a new electrocardiographic entity. *JACC Clin Electrophysiol.* 2021;7:843–854.)

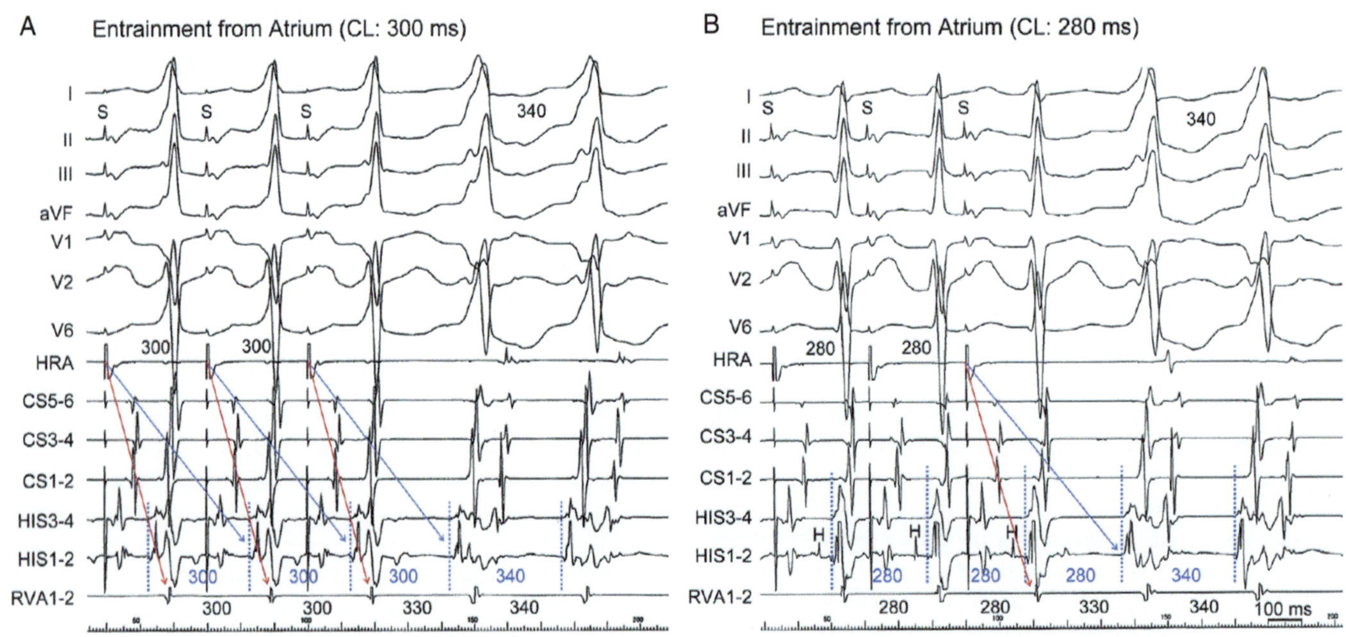

Fig. 32.39 Atrial entrainment during reverse type left posterior fascicular VT. (A) Atrial entrainment pacing (300 ms) showing constant fusion of the QRS complex. Although atrial pacing directly captured the right ventricular apex (*red arrows*), it also captured the anterior ventricular septum (HIS1-2) of the subsequent QRS complex (*blue arrows*). *Red arrows* indicate antidromic capture, and *blue arrows* indicate orthodromic capture. The final captured QRS complex exhibited no fusion. (B) During atrial entrainment pacing (280 ms), His potential appeared before the QRS complex, and the QRS complex became narrower (progressive fusion). *CS*, Coronary sinus; *HIS*, His-bundle electrogram; *HRA*, high right atrium; *RVA*, right ventricular apex; *S*, pacing stimulus. (From Phanthawimol W, Nogami A, Haruna T, et al. Reverse-type left posterior fascicular ventricular tachycardia: a new electrocardiographic entity. *JACC Clin Electrophysiol.* 2021;7:843–854.)

for another 60–90 seconds. If the initial RF current is ineffective, ablation is directed to a more proximal site with the earlier diastolic potential (P1). If the mid-diastolic potential (P1) cannot be detected, RF current is applied at the VT exit site showing a single fused presystolic Purkinje potential (P2). With upper septal fascicular VT, RF energy is delivered for 30–60 seconds during sinus rhythm to avoid AV block. Catheter ablation is performed in this region using a low-power output (i.e., 20 W), which can gradually be increased while carefully monitoring for development of a junctional rhythm or AV block.

After the ablation, programmed stimulation should be repeated. Other than the noninducibility of VT, there are several electrophysiologic findings that can serve as end points of RF applications for LPF VT. After ablation of the distal attachment between P1 and ventricular muscle, P1 appears after the QRS complex (Fig. 32.33 and Fig. 32.34). However, this phenomenon is not sufficient for an end point because this only indicates conduction block in the direction from the left septal ventricular muscle to P1 only. This unidirectional block can be seen during the baseline state[63] or after an insufficient RF application.[62] Creation of residual unidirectional conduction from P1 to the septal ventricular muscle might induce incessant form of nonsustained VT after ablation.[62] Additional RF applications at the same area can successfully create bidirectional block and suppress the VT. To confirm the creation of bidirectional block between P1 and the ventricular muscle, atrial pacing with various cycle lengths is used after the ablation. If there is residual conduction from P1 to the ventricular muscle, a PVC (i.e., ventricular echo beat) with a similar QRS morphology as that observed during the VT can be observed repeatedly.

Success and Recurrence Rates

In the authors' experience, the success and recurrence rates are 97% and 4%, respectively, for LPF VT; 90% and 11%, respectively, for LAF VT; and 100% and 2.5%, respectively, for left upper septal fascicular VT. Recurrence of papillary muscle fascicular VTs after ablation is higher than septal fascicular VTs.[45]

Complications

Aside from the complications that may result from any LV electrophysiologic procedure (e.g., thromboembolism, damage to the femoral artery, valve damage, ventricular perforation), the only complication that has been associated with catheter ablation of idiopathic left VT has been LBBB and AV block. Tsuchiya and colleagues[61] reported that two patients (12.5%) had transient LBBB after ablation in their series of 16 patients. They targeted the left basal septum, and the LBBB disappeared within 10 minutes without VT recurrence. In the authors' experience, only one (0.5%) of 198 patients had a transient AV block. This patient had an LPF VT, and the diastolic potential (P1) at the midseptum was targeted for the ablation. Before the ablation, the patient had catheter-induced RBBB. AV block disappeared immediately after discontinuation of the RF energy delivery.

Troubleshooting the Difficult Case

Common problems encountered with left fascicular VT ablation, and their solutions are given in Table 32.2. Inability to induce VT reliably is a formidable obstacle to successful ablation. Isoproterenol facilitates induction of sustained VT in 60–70% of those patients without inducible sustained VT at baseline. In some patients, the administration of small doses of class Ia/c drugs enhances the slow conduction at the specialized Purkinje tissue and facilitates induction of stable sustained VT. If the VT is not inducible, the possibility of nonreentrant fascicular VT has to be always kept in mind.[64] Catheter mapping sometimes mechanically suppresses the

TABLE 32.2 Troubleshooting the Difficult Case (Verapamil-Sensitive Reentrant Fascicular Ventricular Tachycardia)

Problem	Causes	Solution
Unable to induce VT	• Adrenergic dependency • Insufficient slow conduction • *Bump* phenomenon during mapping • Nonreentrant fascicular VT (misdiagnosis)	• Use isoproterenol • Give small dose of class Ia/Ic drug • Find ventricular echo beat with a similar QRS morphology as that observed during the VT • Use pace mapping and the anatomical (linear) approach • Map PVCs with a similar QRS morphology as that observed during the VT
Unable to find a good electrogram	• Poor catheter contact	• Improve the contact with a different catheter or approach (trans-aortic/-septal, U-curve technique), use catheter with contact force sensor
Unable to find a diastolic potential during VT	• VT circuit with short and/or perpendicular P1 branch	• Ablate the earliest P2 with good pace map
Poor catheter stability	• Excessive heart motion during the VT • Papillary muscle fascicular VT • Frequent ventricular premature beats during the RF energy application	• Ablate during sinus rhythm or overdrive pacing, change catheter reach and stiffness, use cryoablation • Use intracardiac echo • Use cryoablation • Use verapamil IV (after which the noninducibility of VT becomes invalid as an end point) • Use cryoablation or overdrive pacing

IV, Intravenous; *PVC*, premature ventricular complex; *RF*, radiofrequency energy; *VT*, ventricular tachycardia.

conduction in the VT circuit ("bump" phenomenon). In such cases, a ventricular echo beat during sinus rhythm or atrial pacing is useful. If PVCs with a similar QRS morphology to that observed during the VT are repeatedly seen, activation mapping can be performed. If no ventricular echo beats are inducible, the empirical anatomical approach can be an effective strategy for ablation of LPF VT.[65] First, the VT exit site is sought by pace mapping during sinus rhythm, and RF energy is delivered to that site. Second, a linear lesion is placed at the midseptum, perpendicular to the long axis of the LV, approximately 10–15 mm proximal to the VT exit. During anatomical linear ablation, P1 suddenly appears after the QRS complex if the ablation site is on the descending limb of the VT circuit. This anatomical approach is also useful in patients in whom diastolic Purkinje potentials cannot be recorded during VT. Fig. 32.40 and Video 32.1 (see Video 32.1 on Expert Consult) show activation mapping during VT. Although the earliest myocardial activation site was observed at the inferoapical septum, diastolic potentials could not be recorded. RF energy application to this exit site was ineffective. A linear RF lesion approximately 10 mm proximal to the VT exit was also ineffective; finally, more proximal linear RF application successfully suppressed the VT.

There are several possibilities when an acceptable electrogram (P1) cannot be found at the LV septum: (1) poor catheter contact with the septum; (2) the limitation of ablation catheter for the electrogram recording;[66] and (3) VT circuit with short and/or perpendicular P1 branch(see Fig. 32.29C).[57] If catheter contact is poor, electrode catheter and/or manipulation approach (retrograde aortic or transseptal; straight or U-curved) should be used. If good Purkinje potential cannot be recorded even with good contact, the electrode size of the ablation/mapping catheter should be considered. A small electrode can identify a small potential missed by a large electrode because of the cancellation effect.[67] This fact has been elucidated in case reports of fascicular VT, in which the tip of ablation catheter (3.5-mm size) did not detect the P1 potential, which was clearly recognized by a mapping catheter with 1-mm size electrode.[68,69] Recently, we reported the importance of not only small electrode size but also wide spacing for the recording of Purkinje potential (Fig. 32.41).[66]

If ablation catheter stability is poor during the VT because of excessive heart motion, RF energy can be delivered during sinus rhythm. However, even during sinus rhythm, frequent PVCs (with a similar QRS morphology to the VT) and VT are sometimes induced during the RF energy application. In such cases, overdrive pacing or intravenous administration of verapamil is effective for suppressing the PVCs and VT during RF energy application. However, after such an infusion, noninducibility of the VT becomes invalid as an end point for the ablation. Cryoablation of left fascicular VT has been reported in a selected population.[70] Cryoablation is effective given the superficial nature of the reentrant circuit and may offer the advantages of no induction of PVCs and extreme catheter stability

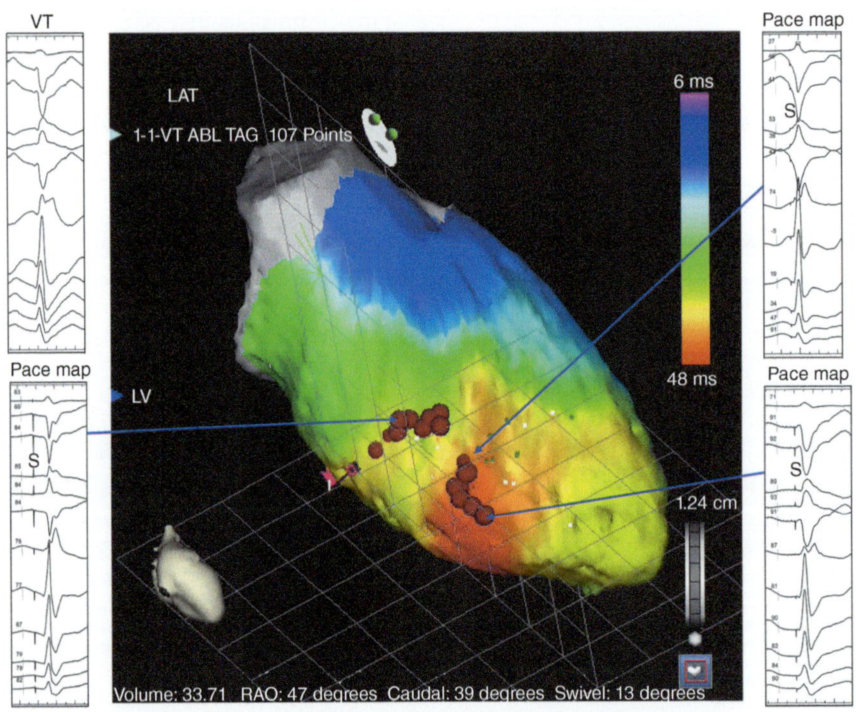

Fig. 32.40 Anatomical approach when diastolic Purkinje potential cannot be recorded during ventricular tachycardia (VT). Whereas the earliest myocardial activation site was observed at the inferoapical septum, diastolic potential could not be recorded (see Video 32.1 on Expert Consult). First, radiofrequency (RF) energy was delivered to the exit site, but that was ineffective. Second, a linear RF lesion approximately 10 mm proximal to the VT exit was created, but that was also ineffective. Finally, more proximal linear lesion successfully suppressed VT induction. *LAT,* Lateral projection; *LV,* left ventricle; *RAO,* right anterior oblique projection.

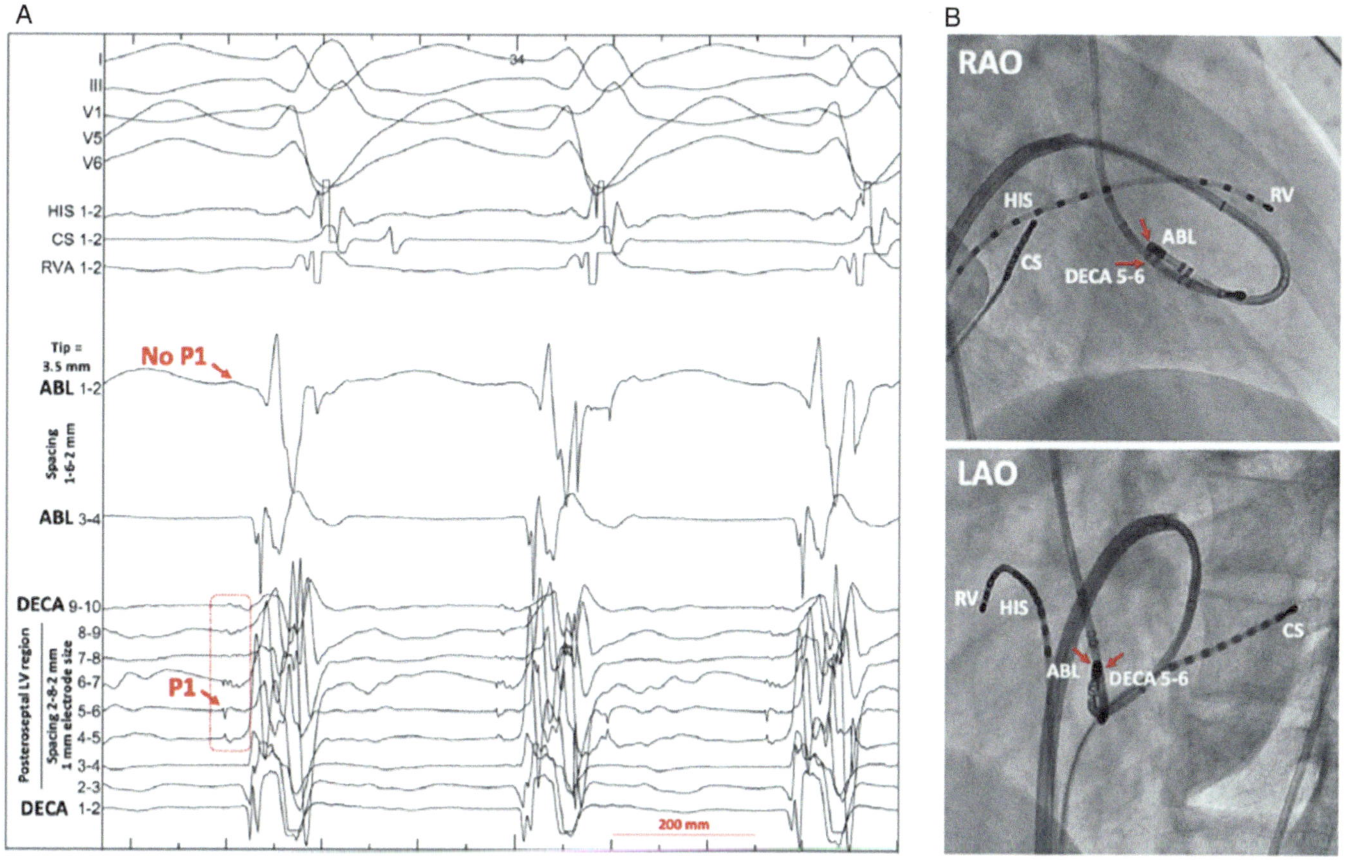

Fig. 32.41 Purkinje potential recorded by variable electrode size and interelectrode spacing. (A) Diastolic Purkinje potential (P1) was detected by multipolar electrode catheter with 1-mm electrodes but was missed by the tip of ablation catheter (ABL) in the same position. (B) Fluoroscopic right anterior oblique (RAO) and left anterior oblique (LAO) views; the position of the ablation catheter was manipulated to be in direct contact with the septum and parallel to multipolar electrode catheter, thus reducing the chance of P1 being not recognized by the ablation catheter because of poor or angled contact with the septum. *CS*, Coronary sinus; *HIS*, His bundle; *RV*, right ventricle; *RVA*, right ventricular apex. (From Naeemah QJ, Nogami A, Komatsu Y, et al. Effect of interelectrode spacing on measurements of Purkinje potential during fascicular ventricular tachycardia. *JACC Clin Electrophysiol*. 2022;8:530–532.)

during ablation. ICE is useful for ablation of papillary muscle fascicular VT.[45]

NONREENTRANT FASCICULAR VENTRICULAR TACHYCARTDIA

Clinical and Electrophysiologic Characteristics

Another type of fascicular VT is the nonreentrant tachycardia from the Purkinje system[64] (Box 32.1). This VT is classified as propranolol-sensitive automatic VT.[1] Although this VT is usually observed in patients with ischemic heart disease,[71] it is also observed in patients with structurally normal hearts.[72,73] Nonreentrant fascicular VT from the LV can present with an RBBB configuration and either a left- or right-axis deviation on the 12-lead ECG, depending on the origin (Fig. 32.42). It is difficult to distinguish this VT from reentrant fascicular VT by 12-lead ECG. This VT can be induced by exercise and catecholamines (e.g., isoproterenol and phenylephrine); however, it cannot be induced or terminated by programmed ventricular stimulation. Although this VT is responsive to lidocaine and β-blockers, it is usually not responsive to verapamil. This can be used as a differentiation from verapamil-sensitive fascicular VT. This VT is transiently suppressed by adenosine and with overdrive pacing. Slow nonreentrant fascicular VT can also be suppressed by faster sinus rhythm (Fig. 32.42C). The clinical and electrophysiologic characteristics of this VT have not been well defined.[64,74] Gonzalez and colleagues[72] reported the electrophysiologic spectrum of Purkinje-related VT in eight patients and showed the mechanism to be consistent with abnormal automaticity or triggered activity in five patients. The 12-lead ECG during VT in these patients showed RBBB with left-axis deviation. A distinct His deflection was recorded with an H-V interval during VT that was shorter than that during sinus rhythm. The authors speculated that this VT arises from a fascicular focus at some distance from the myocardial site of origin of the VT based on the varying ECG morphologies and a poor response to catheter ablation. Our group reported 11 patients (2.8%) with idiopathic nonreentrant fascicular VT among 530 idiopathic VT patients without structural heart disease.[64] All patients had monomorphic VT (cycle

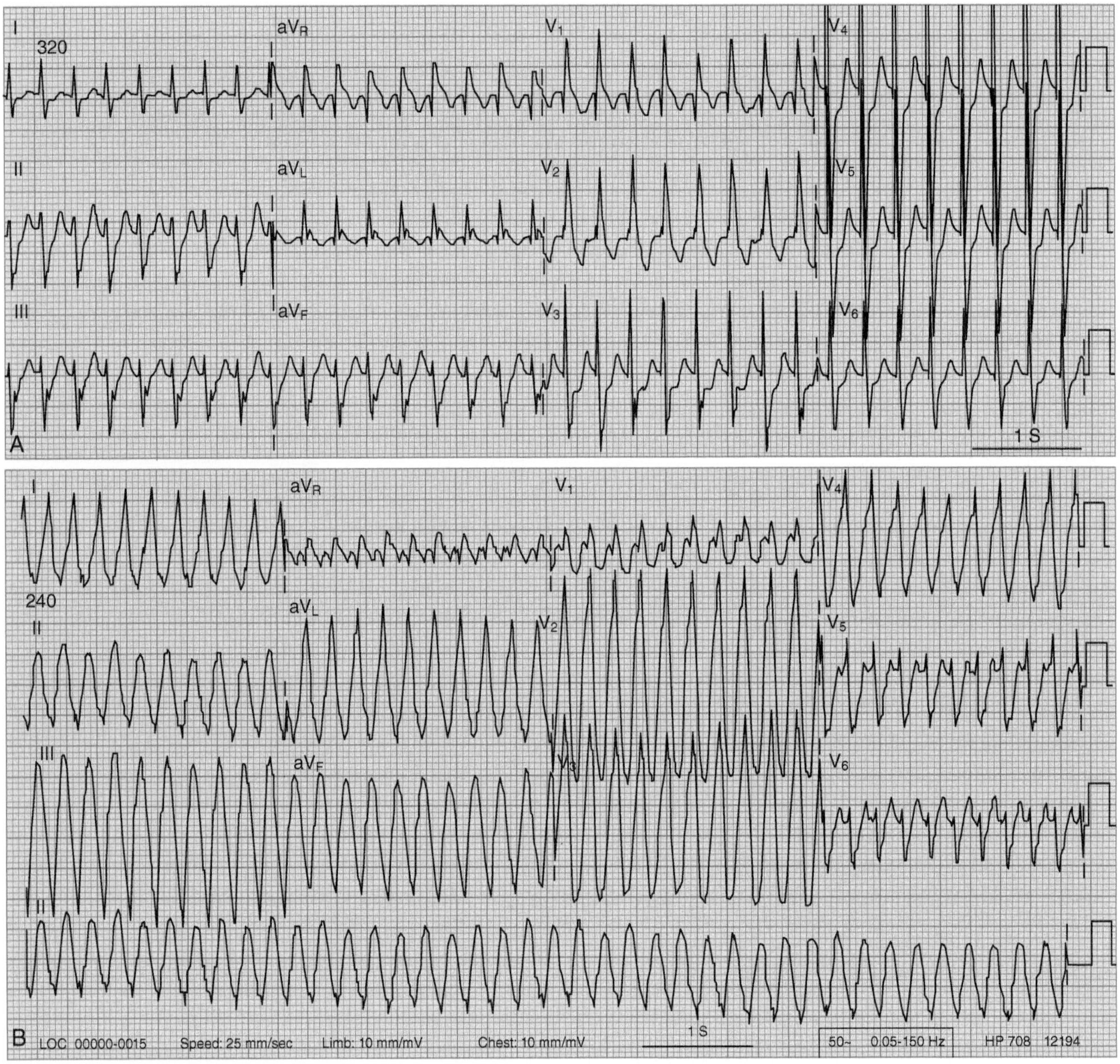

Fig. 32.42 Some 12-lead electrocardiograms (ECGs) of nonreentrant fascicular ventricular tachycardias (VTs) from the left posterior fascicle. (A) This VT presents with right bundle branch block (RBBB) and left-axis deviation. It is difficult to distinguish the nonreentrant fascicular VT from verapamil-sensitive left posterior fascicular VT by 12-lead ECG. (B) This VT also presents with an RBBB and a left-axis deviation; however the cycle length of VT is shorter and the QRS interval is wider than in A. (C) The QRS interval during this slow VT with an RBBB configuration and left-axis deviation is very narrow and was transiently suppressed by faster sinus rhythm.

length: 337 ± 88 ms) with a relatively narrow QRS (123 ± 12 ms), and they did not respond to verapamil. VT exhibited RBBB and superior-axis configuration in 11 patients (73%), inferior axis in three (20%), and LBBB and superior-axis configuration in one (7%). Clinical VT spontaneously occurred in three patients (20%), and it was induced in five (33%) using isoproterenol infusion or burst pacing. In four patients (27%), isolated PVCs, with an identical morphology to the clinical VT, were induced. In the remaining three patients (20%), all the aforementioned protocols failed to induce VT/PVC, thus pace map–guided ablation was performed. In patients with sustained monomorphic VT, overdrive pacing was performed from the RV; however, VT could not be entrained (Fig. 32.43). This finding proves that this VT is a nonreentrant tachycardia.

Monomorphic PVCs have been shown to initiate VF in patients with no structural heart disease[74,75] and ischemic heart disease.[76,77] However, the difference in the clinical and electrophysiologic characteristic between VF triggered by PVC from Purkinje system and monomorphic nonreentrant fascicular VT has not been determined.

Mapping and Ablation

The ablation target of nonreentrant fascicular VT is the earliest Purkinje activation during VT, whereas that of

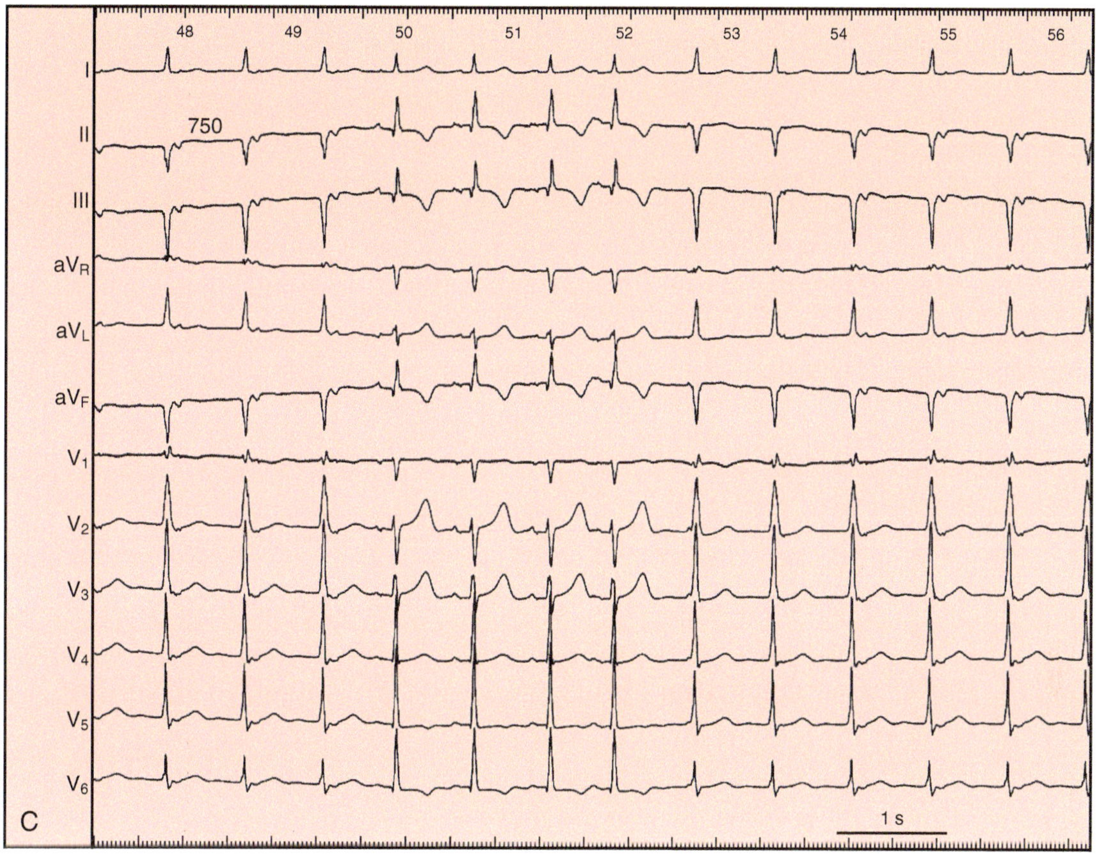

Fig. 32.42, cont'd

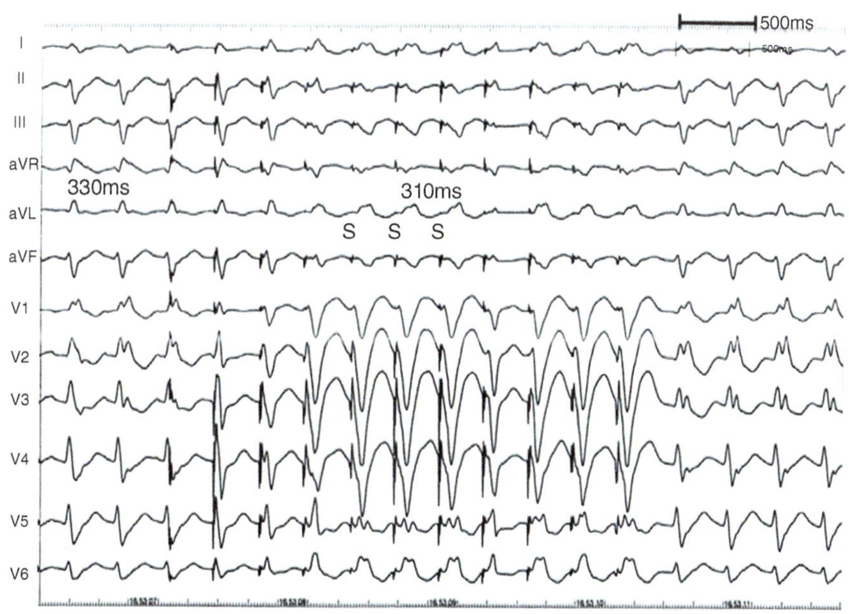

Fig. 32.43 Some 12-lead electrocardiograms showing absence of constant fusion by right ventricular overdrive pacing during nonreentrant fascicular ventricular tachycardia (VT). Pacing cycle length was 310 ms, whereas VT cycle length was 330 ms. This finding proves this ventricular tachycardia with right bundle branch block and superior-axis configuration is a nonreentrant tachycardia. (From Talib AK, Nogami A, Morishima I, et al. Non-reentrant fascicular tachycardia: clinical and electrophysiological characteristics of a distinct type of idiopathic ventricular tachycardia. *Circ Arrhythm Electrophysiol.* 2016;9. pii:e004177.)

verapamil-sensitive reentrant fascicular VT is not necessarily the earliest Purkinje activation. Fig. 32.44A and Video 32.2 (on Expert Consult) show the mapping and ablation of the nonreentrant VT from the distal Purkinje system of the left posterior fascicle. Presystolic Purkinje potentials were recorded from various sites in the LV, but the earliest Purkinje potential was recorded at the basal inferior wall. The Purkinje potential preceded the QRS during VT by 70 ms, and the recording at the same site demonstrated a fused Purkinje potential during sinus rhythm (Fig. 32.44B, C). Pace mapping at this site produced an identical QRS complex, with an S-QRS interval of 70 ms, equal to the P-QRS interval during the VT (Fig. 32.44D). RF current delivered to this site suppressed the VT. In our series of nonreentrant fascicular VTs,[64] a high-frequency presystolic Purkinje potential was recorded during VT and/or PVC, preceding the QRS by 25 ± 16 ms. Nonreentrant fascicular VT usually originated from the left posterior fascicle and less commonly from the left anterior fascicle and RV Purkinje network.

Pace map will be helpful, but the best pace map site does not always represent the successful ablation site. Fig. 32.45 shows that despite obtaining a perfect pace map match at the third of the LV septum, VT could not be terminated. However, RF application at a more proximal part (i.e., the middle third of the LV septum) successfully terminated VT within 4 seconds after RF energy application delivered though pace mapping did not match clinical VT.[64]

Success and Recurrence Rates

The authors' experience includes 15 patients with idiopathic nonreentrant fascicular VT.[64] In all patients, VT and PVC were suppressed by catheter ablation; however, the true acute success rate is unclear because this VT is difficult to induce. VT recurrence was observed in four patients (27%), and among them, three underwent pace map–guided ablation during the first session. A second ablation with activation mapping guidance eliminated the VT during the 88 ± 8-month follow-up. Catheter ablation guided by activation mapping appears effective, whereas pace map–guided approach is less efficacious.

Complications

The complication that has been associated with catheter ablation of nonreentrant fascicular VT has been LBBB and AV block. In verapamil-sensitive fascicular VTs, the creation of LBBB or AV block as the complication is quite rare because the ablation target is the diastolic Purkinje potential (P1) during VT, and the abolition of the normal Purkinje or fascicular potential (P2) during sinus rhythm is not needed.

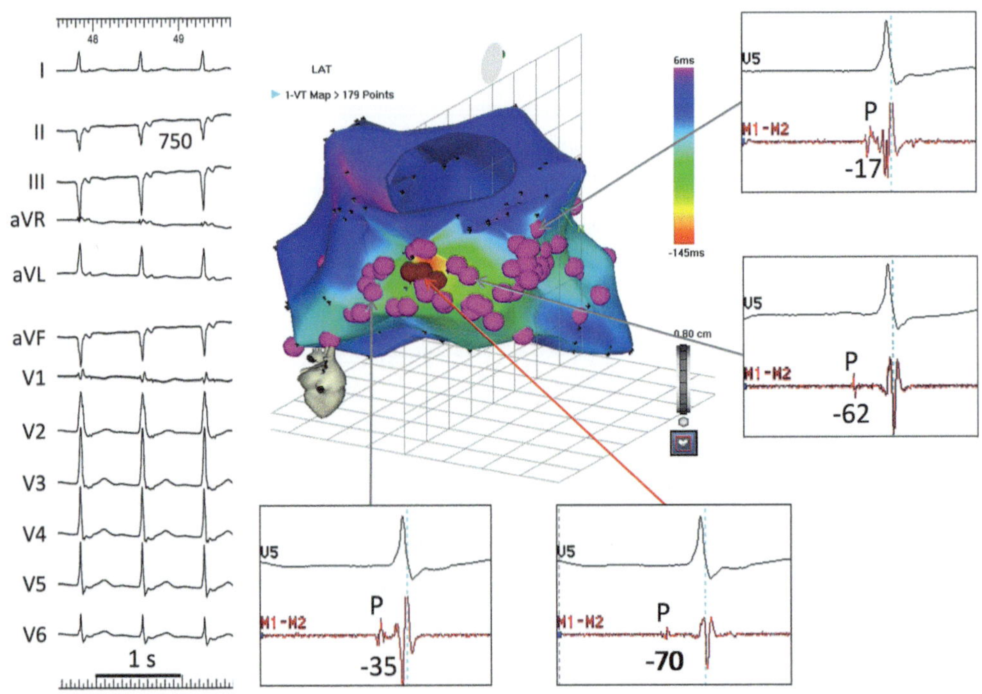

A

Fig. 32.44 Ablation of the nonreentrant fascicular ventricular tachycardia (VT) with right bundle branch block morphology and left-axis deviation. (A) Electroanatomical mapping during VT (see Video 32.2 on Expert Consult). All tags indicate the sites with the presystolic Purkinje potential during VT. The earliest Purkinje potential was recorded at the basal inferior wall *(red tags)*, and radiofrequency current delivered to this site suppressed the VT *(red arrow)*. (B) The Purkinje potential preceded the QRS during VT by 70 ms. (C) The recording at the same site demonstrated a fused Purkinje potential during sinus rhythm. (D) Pace mapping at this site produced an identical QRS complex, with an S-QRS interval of 70 ms. *ABL*, Ablation catheter; *CS*, coronary sinus; *HBE*, His-bundle electrogram; *HRA*, high right atrium; *LAT*, local activation time; *RAO*, right anterior oblique projection; *RVA*, right ventricular apex.

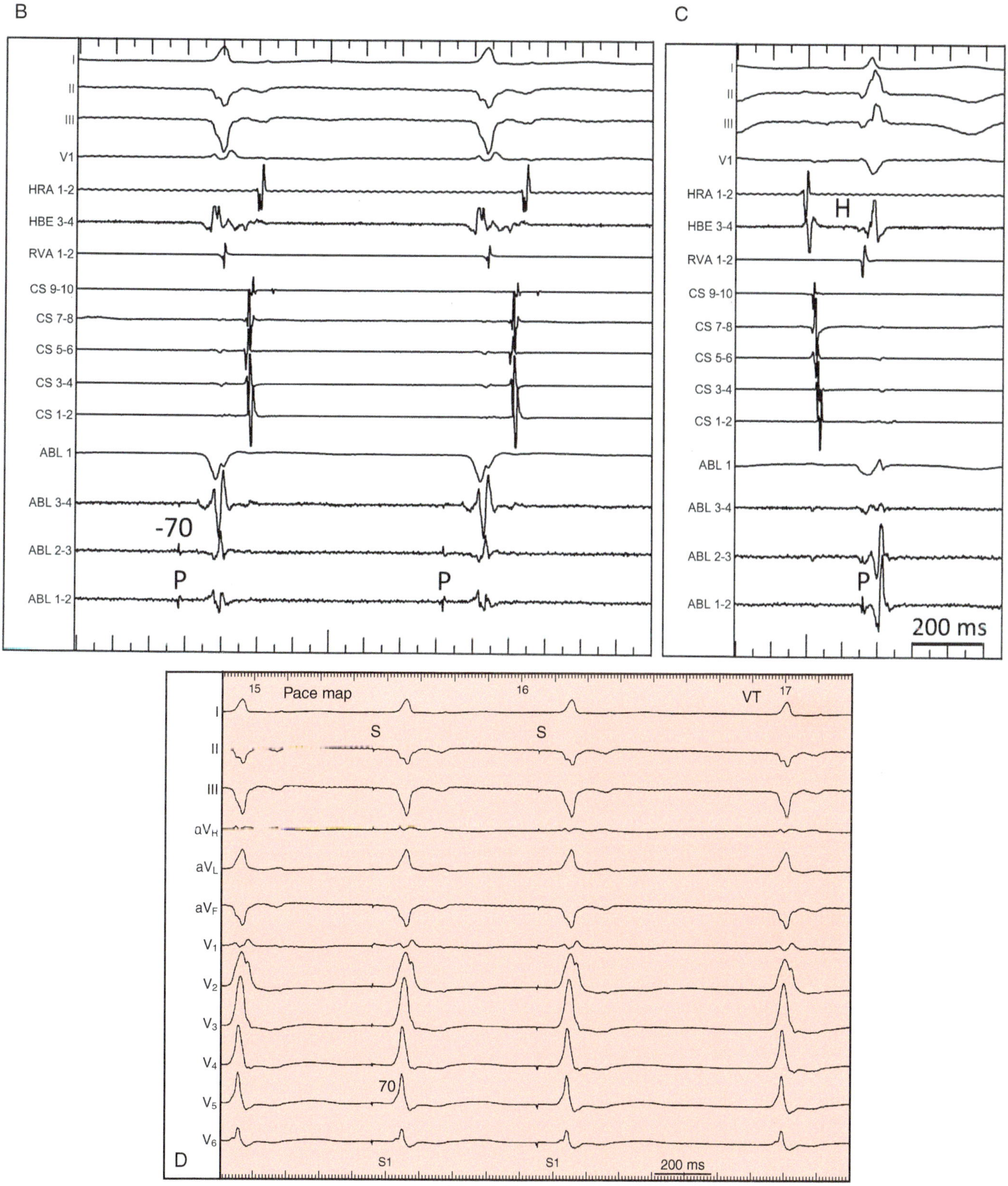

Fig. 32.44, cont'd

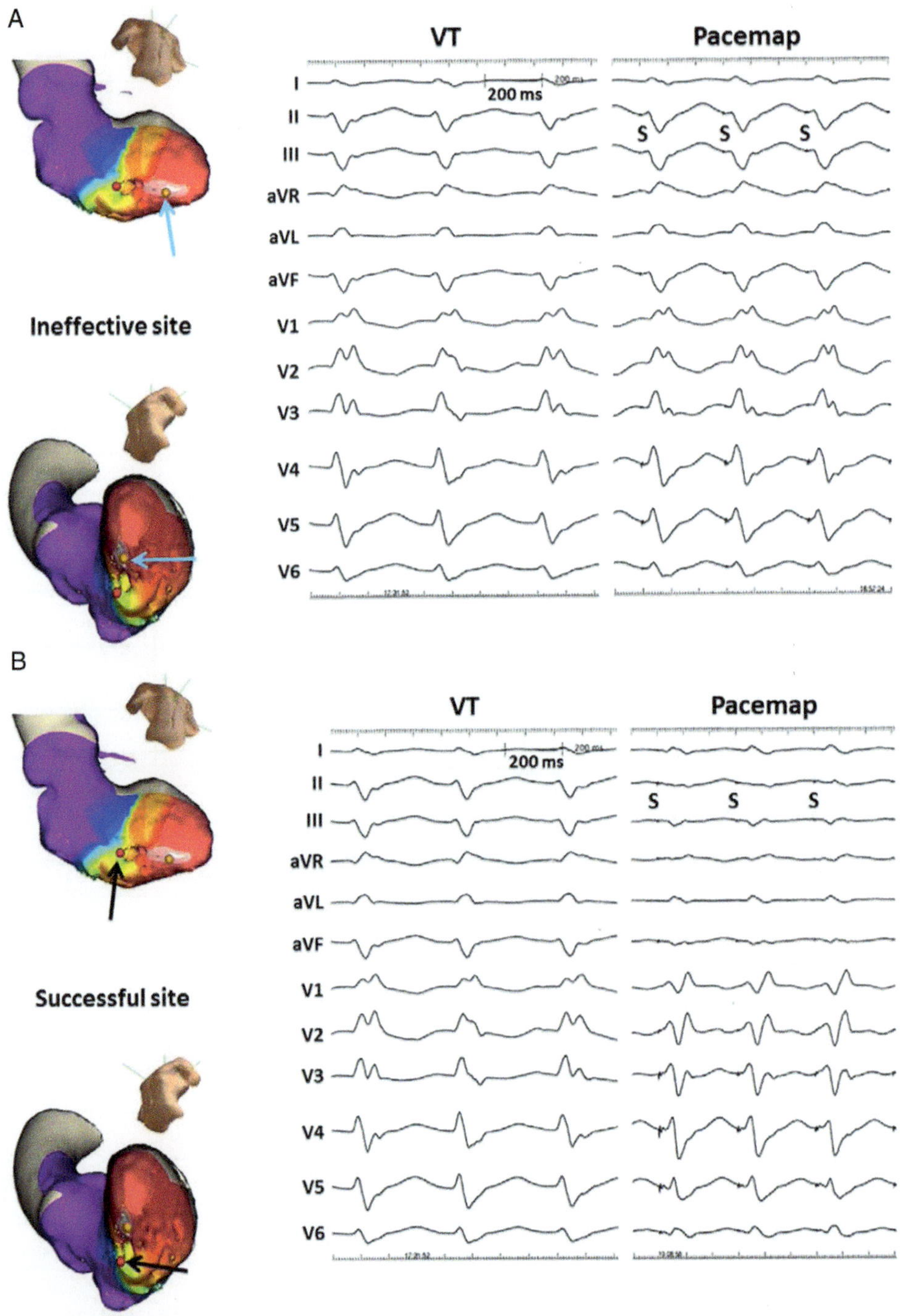

Fig. 32.45 Discrepancy between a good pace map site and the successful ablation site. (A) Ablation of the apical third of the inferior left ventricular septum, where an excellent pace map was obtained, could not suppress the VT. (B) Ablating the mid-third of the left ventricular septum eliminated the VT in 4 s, despite a poor pace map at that site. *VT*, Ventricular tachycardia; *S*, stimulus. (From Talib AK, Nogami A, Morishima I, et al. Non-reentrant fascicular tachycardia: clinical and electrophysiological characteristics of a distinct type of idiopathic ventricular tachycardia. *Circ Arrhythm Electrophysiol.* 2016;9. pii:e004177.)

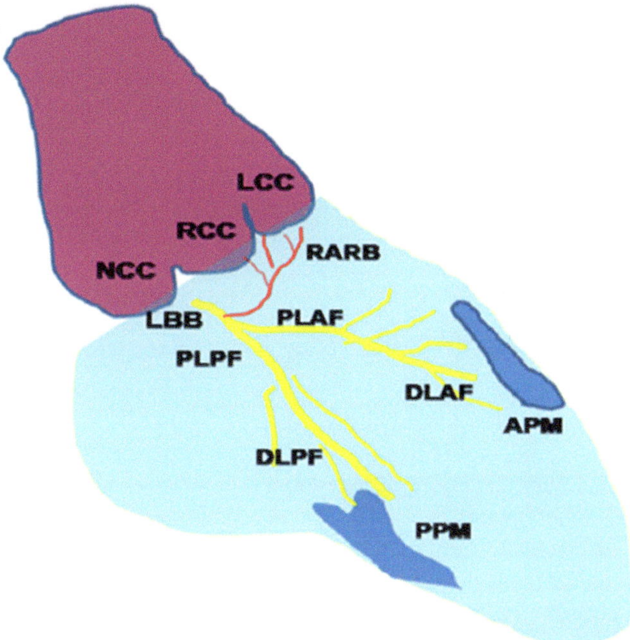

Fig. 32.46 Schematic demonstration of the PLAF, RARB, and RCC. *APM*, Anterior papillary muscle; *DLAF*, distal left anterior fascicle; *DLPF*, distal left posterior fascicle; *LBB*, left bundle branch; *LCC*, left coronary cusp; *NCC*, noncoronary cusp; *PLPF*, proximal left posterior fascicle; *PPM*, posterior papillary muscle; *RCC, RARB*, retro-aortic root branch; right coronary cusp. (From Zhang J, Li K, Ding Y, et al. Terminal end of retro-aortic root branch: An unrecognized origin for "proximal left anterior fascicle" premature ventricular complexes with narrow QRS duration. *Heart Rhythm*. 2022: S1547-5271(22)01967-1.)

By contrast, abolition of a portion of the Purkinje network is usually necessary to suppress the nonreentrant fascicular VT. If the VT arises from a more proximal portion of the fascicle, there is a potential risk for creating LBBB or AV block by ablation. Rodriguez and colleagues[73] reported nonreentrant fascicular VT with an RBBB configuration and right-axis deviation in whom LAF block occurred after the ablation. Lopera and colleagues[71] reported two nonreentrant fascicular VT cases with ischemic heart disease in whom complete AV block occurred after successful ablation of VT. To avoid creation of LAF block for nonreentrant fascicular VA from LAF, Chen and colleagues[78] recommended alternative approach from right coronary cusp for VA from proximal LAF. Purkinje potential was recorded at right coronary cusp both during VA and sinus rhythm, and VA was successfully eliminated by RF application at right coronary cusp. Recently, Zhang and colleagues[79] speculated that exact origin of these VAs was the terminal end of a discrete branch of the left fascicular system (Fig. 32.46) and named the "retro-aortic root branch." This branch seems to be dead-end tract,[13] which starts on the crest of the ventricular septum after the bifurcation of the bundle branches and reaches the aortic root where it fades out.

CONCLUSION

Previous studies have revealed that idiopathic left and right monomorphic VTs and fascicular VTs involving the His-Purkinje system are composed of multiple discrete subtypes that are best differentiated by their mechanism, drug effect, VT morphology, and successful ablation site. Recognition of the heterogeneity of VTs and their unique characteristics should facilitate appropriate diagnosis and therapy.

REFERENCES

Please refer to the e-book for a complete list of references.

33

Ablation of Ventricular Tachycardia in Coronary Artery Disease

Haris M. Haqqani, David J. Callans

KEY POINTS

Mechanism

- The basic mechanism of postinfarct monomorphic ventricular tachycardia (VT) is reentrant myocardial excitation through surviving myocyte bundles within the infarct scar.

Diagnosis and Mapping

- The diagnosis is made by excluding supraventricular and preexcited causes of broad complex tachycardia. Activation, entrainment, and substrate-mapping techniques may all be required to localize critical VT circuit components.

Ablation Targets

- The basic critical target for ablation of postinfarct VT is the narrow diastolic isthmus constrained by unexcitable scar regions as well as by functional barriers. Presystolic and mid-diastolic electrograms are recorded from isthmus sites during tachycardia, and their involvement in VT can be proven by entrainment mapping. For unmappable VT, baseline rhythm correlates of isthmus sites need to be defined by electrogram analysis and pacing. This process is called substrate mapping and localizes the infarct scar and border zone, sites of slow conduction with good pace maps, and sites of late-activating isolated potentials associated with wavefront deceleration.

Special Equipment

- Electroanatomical mapping systems are required for defining substrate, tagging critical target sites, and recording ablation lesion delivery. Preoperative scar imaging and integration into the mapping system may be helpful. Multipolar catheters with narrow-spaced bipoles allow for high-density mapping and have improved visualization of both VT circuits and the underlying substrate. Second-generation open irrigated ablation catheters and contact force sensing have improved the biophysics of lesion delivery and have the potential to allow safer creation of larger lesions with lower thromboembolic risk.

Sources of Difficulty

- Hemodynamic instability and inability to map VT in patients with advanced structural heart disease make these procedures challenging. Multiple inducible VT morphologies are the rule. Effective lesion delivery within dense scar may be difficult with currently available energy sources.

INTRODUCTION

The development of sustained monomorphic ventricular tachycardia (VT) is one of the most significant known complications after a prior myocardial infarction (MI). Regardless of the hemodynamic tolerability of any index episode of VT in this setting, patients with a healed MI scar and significant left ventricular (LV) systolic dysfunction have substantially reduced survival and derive a significant prognostic benefit from implantable cardioverter-defibrillator (ICD) placement, even before developing clinical VT.[1] It is clear, however, that ICDs are deployed primarily for sudden death risk mitigation and should not be considered a treatment for VT. High-voltage ICD shocks for recurrent VT can lead to significant morbidity and mortality, and repeated delivery of antitachycardia pacing (ATP) may also be associated with adverse outcomes.[2] Present-day medical therapy is incompletely effective in preventing ICD therapy and comes with the risk of significant adverse effects and additional extracardiac toxicity in the case of amiodarone.[3,4] Unfortunately, few meaningful breakthroughs in antiarrhythmic drug development have occurred in recent times.

In this light, catheter ablation assumes an important role in the overall management of VT in ischemic cardiomyopathy (ICM) patients. Although a prognostic benefit has been suggested in some trials and although the prevention of ICD shocks may itself lead to improved survival, the primary goal of the procedure is to improve quality of life through the prevention of VT recurrences and ICD therapies without antiarrhythmic drug side effects.[4–8]

ANATOMY

Multiple intracardiac mapping studies have confirmed that the electrophysiologic mechanism of the vast majority of monomorphic VT in the setting of prior MI is reentry.[9–11] As clearly demonstrated in the early seminal surgical studies, and confirmed subsequently by entrainment mapping and ultra-high-density activation mapping, critical portions of

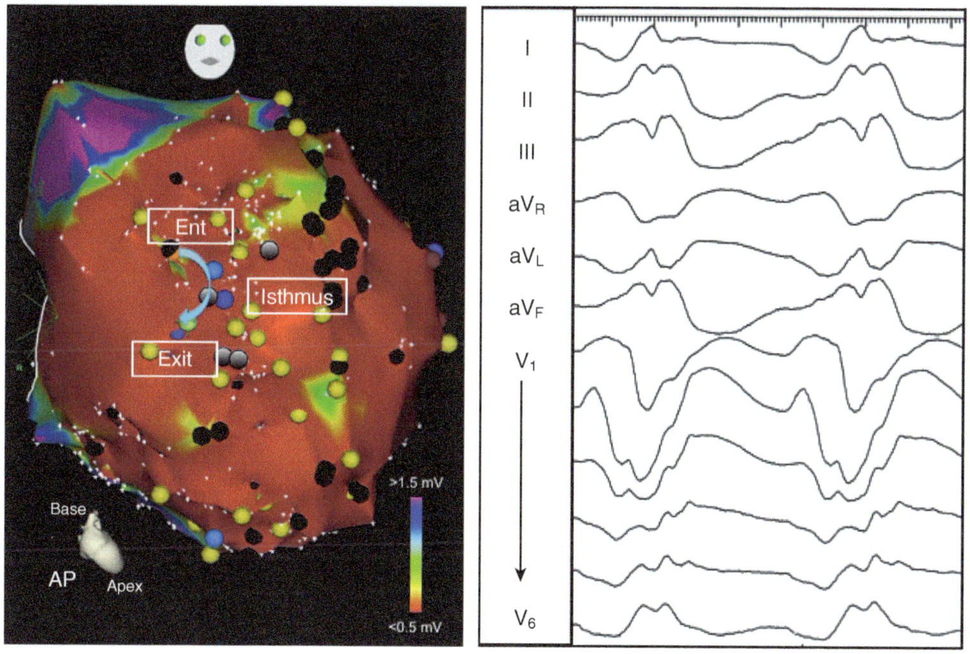

Fig. 33.1 Relationship of infarct scar to ventricular tachycardia (VT) circuit. The electroanatomical endocardial left ventricular substrate map of a 68-year-old man with severe ischemic cardiomyopathy after three infarctions is shown. A large confluent anteroseptal infarct is demonstrated with the red zones corresponding to bipolar voltage <0.5 mV. The circuit components of the monomorphic VT pictured were defined with entrainment and mapped to within the dense infarct core.

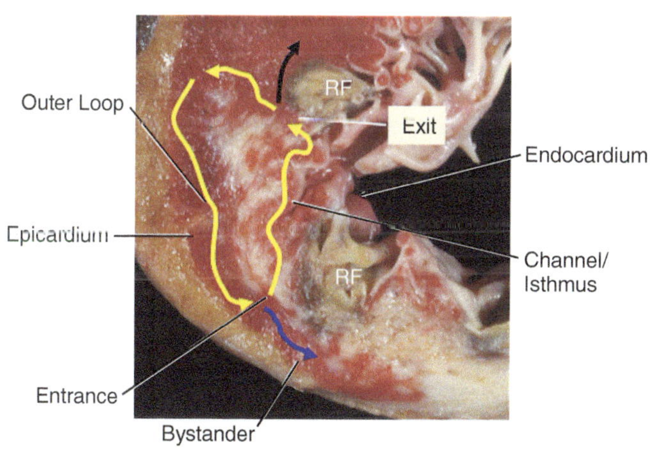

Fig. 33.2 Gross pathologic specimen demonstrating typical postinfarct macroscopic scar heterogeneity with islets of surviving myocardium visible within the dense infarct core. The scar is seen to extend contiguously from the subendocardium with relative epicardial sparing. Putative ventricular tachycardia circuit components have been labeled in addition to two radiofrequency ablation lesions. (Courtesy of Dr W. Stevenson.)

the reentry circuitry of postinfarct VT reside within a healed myocardial infarct scar, usually a large and confluent one[11–13] (Fig. 33.1). Such scars are often associated with advanced LV remodeling, areas of dyskinesis and aneurysm formation, and significant LV systolic dysfunction. Infarct scar formation and remodeling is not a uniform amorphous process; instead, structural and ultrastructural heterogeneity within scar regions is universal (Fig. 33.2). Collateral formation, endoluminal perfusion, acute reperfusion therapy, and ongoing collagen turnover all contribute to the formation of surviving (predominantly subendocardial) myocyte bundles of varying diameter interlaced in networks through the dense infarct core. These bundles are separated by insulating sheets of collagen that alter wavefront propagation through scar in a manner conducive to the establishment of reentrant tachyarrhythmias. Lipomatous metaplasia also occurs frequently and with variable distribution in post-MI scars, and this may also modulate arrhythmogenicity.[14] The extent of electrically active ventricular scar and degree of LV systolic dysfunction in ischemic cardiomyopathy patients are important determinants of arrhythmic risk.[15,16] Sustained monomorphic VT is more likely seen in those with larger infarct scars. The advent of primary prevention medical therapy and earlier, more effective acute reperfusion therapy with primary percutaneous intervention have altered infarct scar characteristics. Patchy fibrosis is now seen more frequently, and aneurysm formation has become uncommon. This has altered the frequency and characteristics of VT seen in the chronic phase after MI with more rapid VT seen in such patients.[17] It remains unclear whether the reduced late VT incidence expected with smaller healed infarcts will be balanced by an increased prevalence of VT as long-term post-MI survival improves.

It should be borne in mind that not all patients with reentrant VT and coronary artery disease have an MIt ventricular scar, and some may instead have a coexisting nonischemic dilated cardiomyopathy. Such patients tend to have basal VT morphologies as well as the frequent epicardial and intramural septal VT exits typical of that substrate, in direct contrast to postinfarct ICM patients whose pathology and VT circuitry characteristically lie in the subendocardial layer.[18]

PATHOPHYSIOLOGY

Disorders of conduction or disorders of repolarization (or both) may form the basis of the electrophysiologic substrate in any arrhythmogenic disease, but in the postinfarct context, abnormalities of conduction have been far better characterized. Myocardial necrosis at the time of the initial infarction and replacement of lost myocytes with collagen-based fibrous tissue leads to an overall reduction in the number and density of gap junctions between surviving cells within an infarct scar. Thus, even though they are capable of generating recordable action potentials, these myocytes are poorly coupled electrically. Not only does this lead to a slowing of wavefront conduction velocity in the scar but also, due to impedance mismatch, a greatly increased likelihood of conduction failure producing unidirectional block. Additionally, electrical propagation is significantly more affected in the transverse direction orthogonal to myofiber axis due to an amplification of normal nonuniform anisotropy by layers of collagen between myocyte bundles. This slow, discontinuous wavefront conduction within an infarct scar sets up the ideal milieu for the establishment of reentrant excitation, with the constrained diastolic isthmus usually located within the core of the scar.[19] The exit of the VT wavefront from this isthmus occurs at the scar border zone where inscription of the surface QRS commences, although the latter can often be remote from isthmus.[11] The wavefront then propagates through the ventricle surrounding the scar, often in a figure-of-eight dual-loop configuration, prior to reentering the protected isthmus within the scar again. The diastolic corridor may in some cases be constrained between dense infarct scar and an anatomical barrier such as a valve annulus or a surgical conduit.[20,21] Evidence that supports reentry as the dominant mechanism of postinfarct VT is summarized in Box 33.1 with some examples in Fig. 33.3.

The contribution of functional barriers to the complete VT reentrant circuit have been underestimated but older resetting studies and recent ultra-high-resolution activation mapping studies confirm their importance, particularly at the entrance to and exit from the diastolic corridor.[22–24] Approximately 40% of VTs have isthmuses that are shared with a second VT.[25,26]

Recently, Callans et al. extended prior animal work and found that human postinfarct VT is also characterized by significant repolarization heterogeneity, with circuit sites having consistently shorter unipolar activation–recovery intervals (postulated to be due to potassium channel beta subunit *KCNE4* upregulation) than noncircuit scar sites.[27] These sites may form the target of novel therapeutic approaches to VT, including gene therapy. Additionally, Srinivasan et al. showed that if VT-specific sites are examined using an extrastimulus protocol, significant prolongation and spatial dispersion of repolarization are seen.[28]

The anatomical substrate in the postinfarct patient can be inferred from the presence of Q waves on the surface ECG, demonstrated by scar imaging techniques such as late gadolinium enhancement (LGE) on magnetic resonance imaging (MRI) or even visualized directly during surgical subendocardial resection. However, the electrophysiologic substrate can really only be defined by the use of invasive catheter-based electrode recordings at an electrophysiology study (EPS).

At EPS, the induction of sustained monomorphic VT with the use of programmed stimulation implies that the electrophysiologic substrate for VT exists although this does not necessarily predict the presence of spontaneous clinical VT since specific triggers such as ventricular ectopy, heart failure, or changes in autonomic tone are required for this to occur.[29,30] Additionally, at EPS, catheter-based electrode recordings from the infarct region show characteristic abnormalities reflective of the loss of functioning cardiomyocytes and the slow and discontinuous wavefront conduction present in ventricular scar. As recorded by standard 3.5-mm-tip mapping catheters (which usually have a 1-mm ring electrode 1 mm farther back along the shaft), normal ventricular myocardial bipolar electrograms (EGMs) are sharp, biphasic or triphasic signals of >1.5 mV peak-to-peak amplitude, ≤70-ms duration, and/or >0.046 amplitude:duration ratio[31,32] (Fig. 33.4). A loss of cardiomyocyte mass in the scar results in attenuation of the bipolar EGM amplitude with dense scar showing bipolar voltage <0.5 mV and regions of bipolar voltage between 0.5 and 1.5 mV typically being seen in the scar border.[33,34] Slow conduction in the infarct scar causes prolongation of the local bipolar EGM with multiple low-amplitude deflections (Fig. 33.5). Such EGMs are called fractionated and are defined by a bipolar voltage <0.5 mV, a duration of >133 ms, and/or an amplitude:duration ratio of <0.005[35] (Fig. 33.4). The multiple deflections of fractionated EGMs have been shown to each correspond to delayed activation of surviving islands of myocytes separated by dense collagen sheets within the field of view of the recording electrode.[36] When activation of a discrete surviving myocyte bundle is sufficiently delayed, a low-amplitude isolated late potential (ILP) may be recorded following an isoelectric interval after the larger initial, usually far-field, ventricular EGM (Figs. 33.4 and 33.5). Such a bundle may form an anatomically constrained conducting channel in the scar that has the potential to serve as the protected diastolic isthmus of a VT circuit[37] (Fig. 33.5).

BOX 33.1 Evidence Supporting Reentry as the Major Mechanism of Post-infarct VT

- Induction and termination with programmed ventricular stimulation
- Site-specificity of induction
- Direct relationship between coupling interval of the initiating extrastimulus and the onset of the first beat of VT
- Continuous electrical activity related to VT onset and perpetuation recorded by an electrode near the slow zone
- Recording of mid-diastolic potentials that cannot be dissociated from VT
- Extrastimulus-mediated resetting of VT with fusion
- Entrainment of VT with overdrive pacing
- Electroanatomical activation map of the ventricle containing >90% of the VT cycle length
- Termination of VT with global noncapture from a nonpropagated extrastimulus

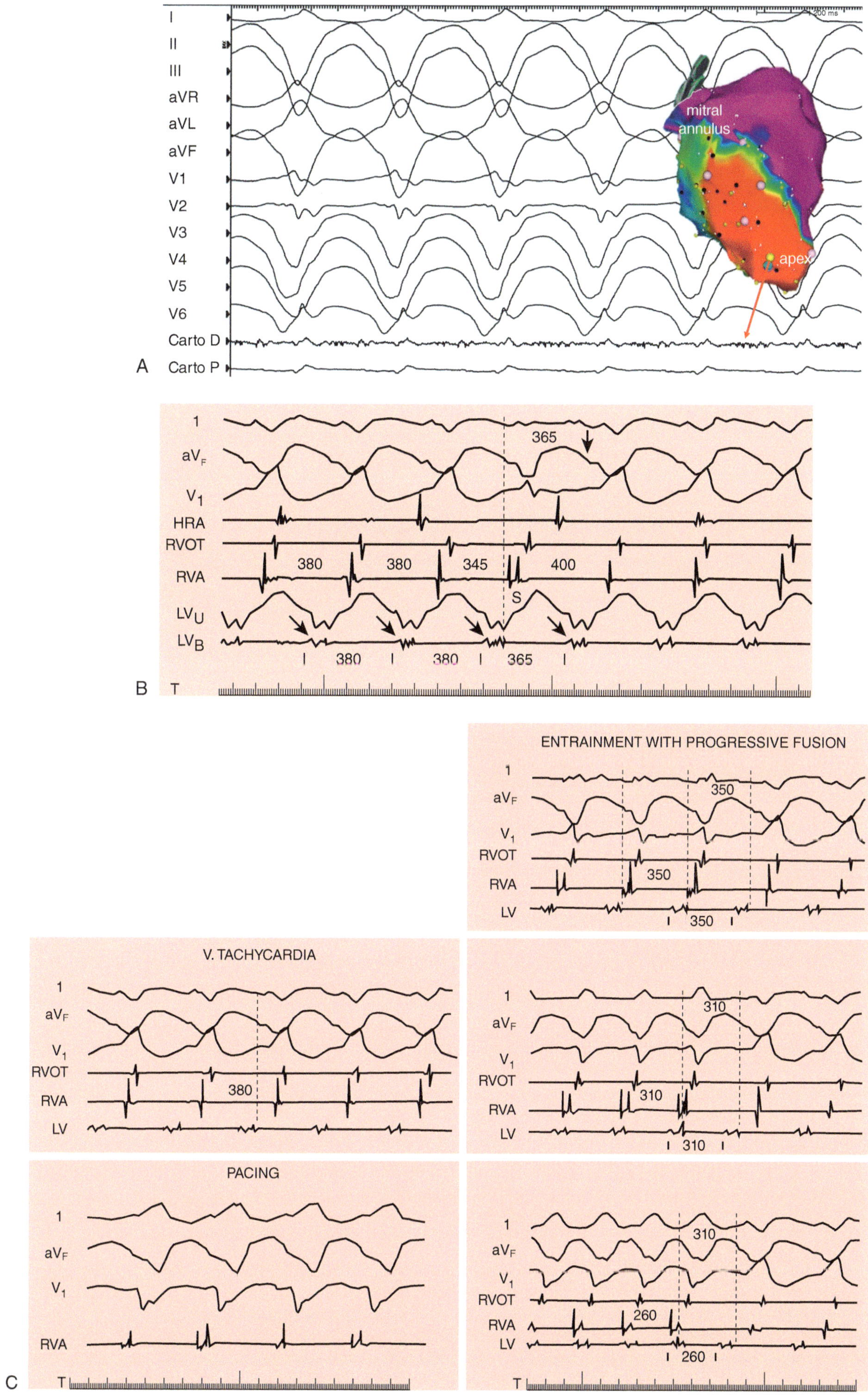
A
I
II
III
aVR
aVL
aVF
V1
V2
V3
V4
V5
V6
Carto D
Carto P
200 ms
mitral annulus
apex
B
1
aVF
V1
HRA
RVOT
RVA
LVU
LVB
T
365
380
380
345
400
S
380
380
365
C
V. TACHYCARDIA
380
PACING
ENTRAINMENT WITH PROGRESSIVE FUSION
350
350
350
310
310
310
310
260
260
RVOT
RVA
LV

Fig. 33.3 Observations supporting a reentrant mechanism for ventricular tachycardia (VT) in the setting of healed infarction. (A) Continuous electrical activity: Electrogram recordings from the infarct left ventricular (LV) septum postinfarct (d) and (p) during sinus rhythm and VT. Continuous activity is demonstrated in the LV recording during VT. This is consistent with a reentrant mechanism, with activation of some portion of the circuit throughout the entire cycle length, all within the field of view of a single recording site. (From Josephson ME. *Circulation.* 1978;57:659, American Heart Association.) (B) Resetting with fusion: Surface ECG and intracardiac recordings during VT. A single extrastimulus is delivered from the right ventricular (RV) apex after the inscription of the LV electrogram at the site of origin and the onset of the surface QRS. Nonetheless, surface fusion is observed, and the tachycardia is reset—i.e., the return cycle beat occurs earlier in time (345 + 400 ms < 380 + 380 ms) than it would have without the extrastimulus. This is inconsistent with a focal mechanism and suggests reentry within a circuit with a distinct entrance and exit site. (From Almendral JM. *J Am Coll Cardiol.* 1986;8:294.) (C) Entrainment with progressive fusion: Surface ECG and intracardiac recordings during VT, RV apical pacing and entrainment at three different cycle lengths. Entrainment at faster cycle lengths changes the nature of the surface ECG fusion to more greatly resemble the paced QRS morphology. (From Almendral JM. *Circulation.* 1986;77:569, American Heart Association.)

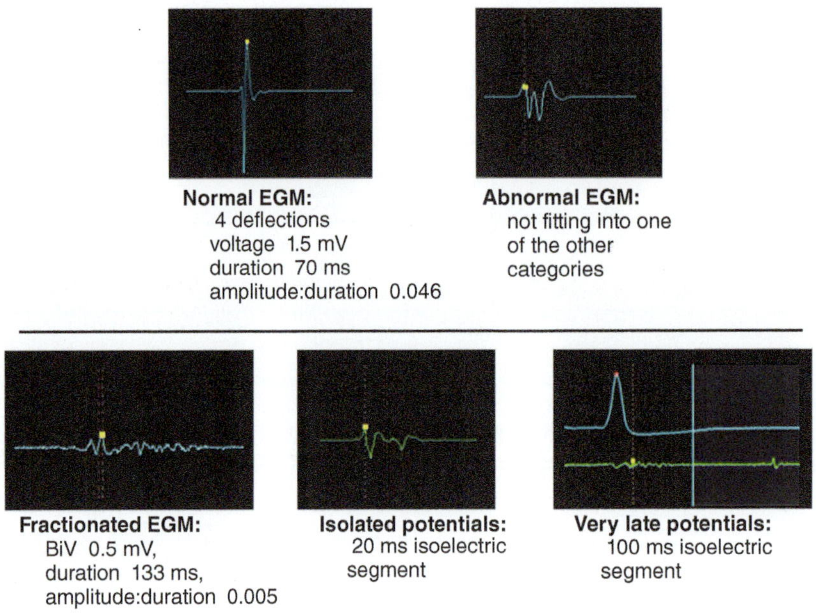

Fig. 33.4 Examples of normal and scar-related ventricular electrograms. See text for details.

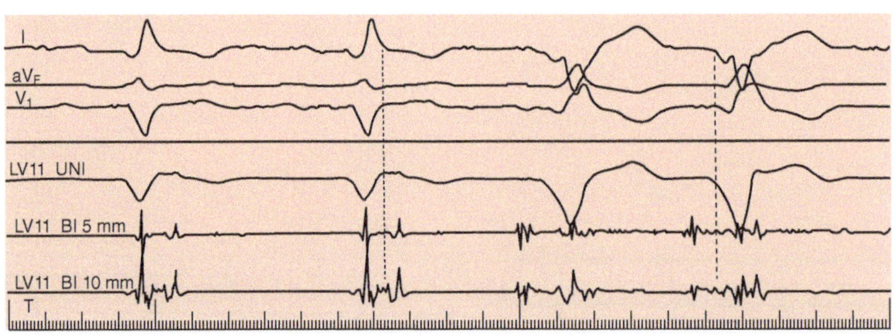

Fig. 33.5 Electrogram recording from a ventricular tachycardia (VT) circuit site. Three surface ECG leads are shown with three intracardiac recordings from a catheter positioned within the infarct zone. During sinus rhythm, a fractionated, multicomponent signal is recorded; the final component of this electrogram is recorded after the end of the surface QRS. During VT (final two beats of the tracing), diastolic potentials are observed, preceding the QRS by 90 ms. (From Josephson ME. *Clinical Cardiac Electrophysiology: Techniques and Interpretations.* 2002.).

In the setting of coronary disease, polymorphic VT may suggest the presence of acute ischemia.[38] There may be multiple operative mechanisms, including abnormal automaticity, Purkinje fiber mediated reentry, or triggered activity from diastolic calcium overload in compromised but still viable cells.[39] Polymorphic VT does not require the presence of a healed anatomical infarct substrate as it can occur in patients with no prior ventricular scar presenting with acute coronary syndromes for

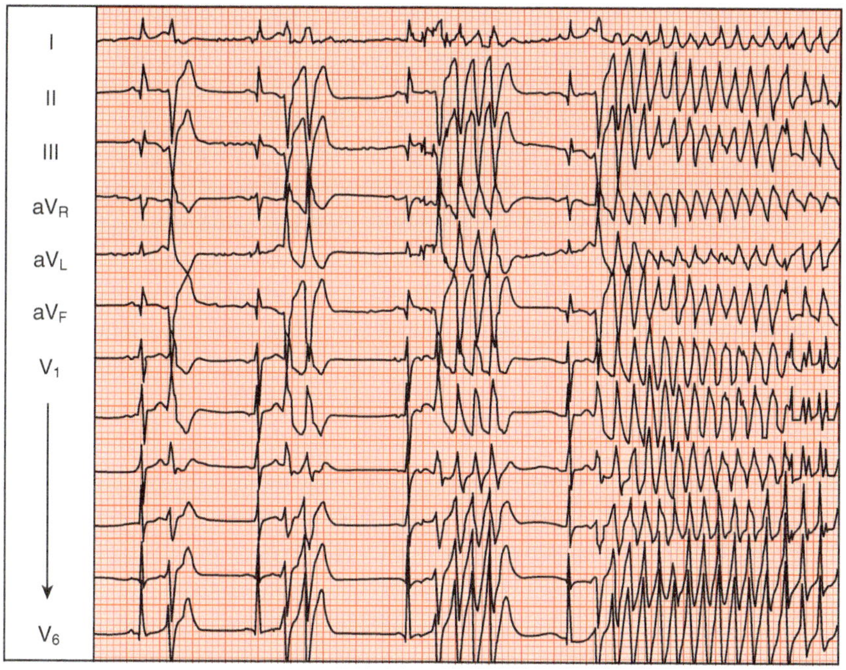

Fig. 33.6 Polymorphic ventricular tachycardia (PVT) in a 41-year-old man who underwent cprpnary artery bypass graft surgery after presenting late with inferior myocardial infarction on the background of severe triple-vessel disease and ejection fraction 33%. Recovery was uncomplicated until day 8 when he began to have multiple recurrent bursts of PVT degenerating to ventricular fibrillation (VF), requiring cardioversion and resuscitation. Each burst of PVT/VF was triggered by an identical premature ventricular contraction with right bundle branch block morphology and left superior axis suggestive of posterior papillary muscle origin.

the first time. It may occur in the very early phase of infarct repair and remodeling where Purkinje fiber triggers at the border of the necrotic zone may be important in its initiation[40] (Fig. 33.6).

ARRHYTHMIA DIAGNOSIS AND DIFFERENTIAL DIAGNOSIS

The vast majority of patients with sustained postinfarct VT can be diagnosed by a 12-lead ECG recorded at the bedside during tachycardia. It is almost axiomatic that a broad-complex tachycardia in the setting of a patient with a prior MI is VT, but multiple published algorithms have been suggested to help exclude the other less likely differential diagnoses, namely supraventricular tachycardia with aberrant conduction (including atrial flutter with 1:1 conduction), preexcited tachycardia, paced tachycardias, and artifact[41–43] (Fig. 33.7).

The diagnostic criteria for postinfarct scar-related VT are listed in Box 33.2. The diagnosis of myocardial scar-related VT hinges on the demonstration of atrial, AV nodal, and His-Purkinje dissociability from the tachycardia (which excludes all forms of supraventricular, preexcited, and fascicular tachycardias, including bundle branch reentry VT). Such proof can be obtained at the bedside with the surface 12-lead ECG or in the laboratory during EPS with pacing maneuvers. In the presence of a dual-chamber ICD system, the presence of ventriculoatrial dissociation on ICD interrogation is essentially conclusive. The diagnosis of VT can also be strongly suggested in patients with single-chamber ICDs as stored EGM morphology in tachycardia should be different than the sinus rhythm morphology. However, right bundle branch block (RBBB) aberrance during SVT can alter the wavefront vector by which the sensing bipole in the right ventricle (RV) is activated and hence also change the ICD EGM morphology.[44] Such ICD intracardiac EGMs may be useful in matching induced VTs to clinical arrhythmias as well as potentially even in pace mapping[45] (Fig. 33.8). The latter maneuver may be the only mapping option in the uncommon scenario in which no VT is inducible at EPS in a patient in whom there are no 12-lead ECG recordings of clinical VT.

PERIPROCEDURAL CONSIDERATIONS

Until recently, catheter ablation for postinfarct VT has generally been used as a near-last resort treatment option, typically reserved for the patient with multiple ICD shocks refractory to repeated device reprogramming who has exhausted all antiarrhythmic drug options, including amiodarone. With improvements in mapping and ablation, the procedure has increasingly been offered at an earlier stage in the natural history, and recent data suggests that this may increase the efficacy of postinfarct VT ablation.[7,8,46] Several large randomized trials have shown that early catheter ablation around the time of secondary prevention ICD insertion, or after the first shock, reduces the incidence of subsequent arrhythmia events.[5–8] The Ventricular Tachycardia Ablation versus Escalation of Antiarrhythmic Drugs (VANISH)

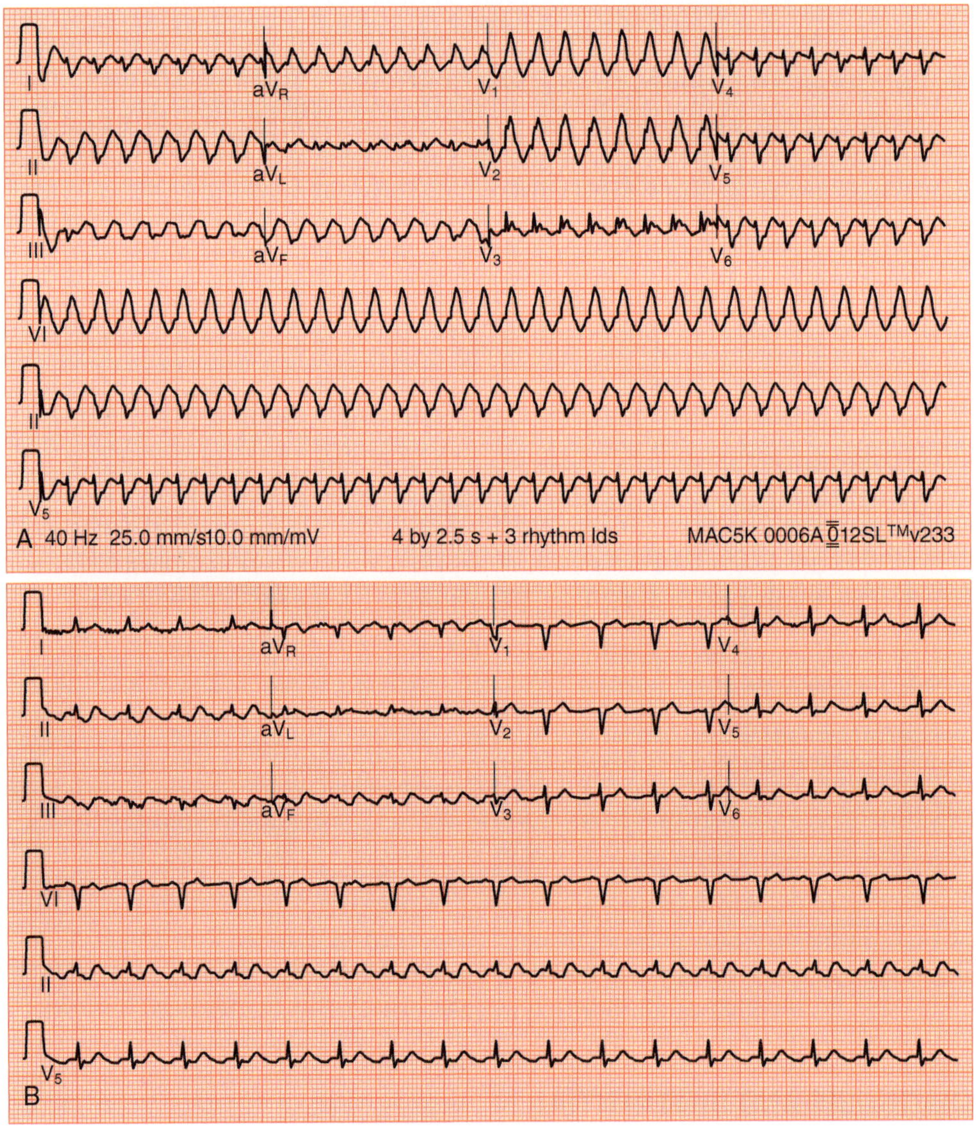

Fig. 33.7 Atrial flutter with 1:1 conduction misdiagnosed as ventricular tachycardia (VT). The first ECG was recorded when an older woman without structural heart disease presented to the emergency department with chest pain. She had a history of atrial fibrillation, and was treated with propafenone. A wide-complex tachycardia with a QRS morphology and axis consistent with VT is shown. The second ECG, however, shows atrial flutter with a narrow QRS; the atrial flutter cycle length is identical to the cycle length of the wide complex tachycardia. She was treated with catheter ablation of atrial flutter and continuation of propafenone.

BOX 33.2 Diagnostic Criteria for Postinfarct VT

- Broad-complex tachycardia with demonstrable atrial and AV nodal dissociation
- Surface QRS morphology inconsistent with SVT or preexcited tachycardia (e.g., negative precordial concordance, QS complex in V_6)
- Surface QRS width in VT narrower than conducted basal rhythm QRS complex
- Sinus rhythm HV interval longer than during tachycardia (except bundle branch reentry)
- Dissociation of His-Purkinje activation from VT (except bundle branch or interfascicular reentry)
- V-V interval precedes and predicts H-H interval during cycle length wobble
- Atrial overdrive pacing changes or narrows QRS complex and/or results in an A-V-V-A response if tachycardia continues after cessation of pacing

study of ICM patients with recurrent VT despite antiarrhythmic drug use showed a significant benefit of catheter ablation over escalation of drug therapy in reducing the composite primary outcome measure of death, VT storm, and appropriate ICD shock.[4] However, catheter ablation in the context of these often very sick ICM patients can be challenging and hazardous, with major complication rates of up to 5–8% described.[7,47–49] Thus, careful preoperative patient assessment and meticulous periprocedural risk management are vital to optimize safety and efficacy.

Preprocedural planning begins with a careful review of all clinical arrhythmia data from 12-lead ECGs, telemetry strips, and stored ICD EGMs. The number and likely exits of all clinical VTs are determined. The patient's clinical condition is assessed with respect to their ability to tolerate a prolonged

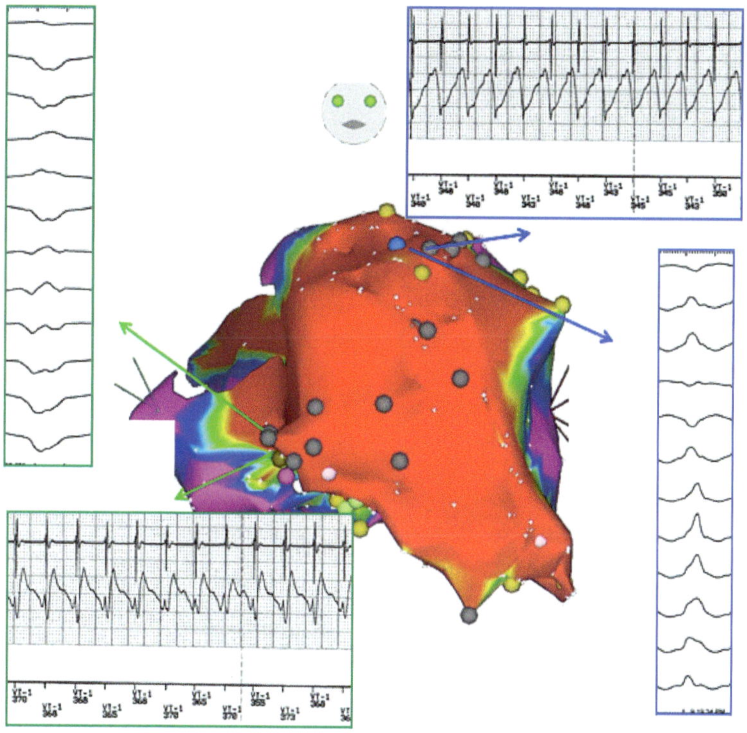

Fig. 33.8 Electrograms recorded during implantable converter-defibrillator (ICD) therapy correlate with different ventricular tachycardia (VT) morphologies. The electroanatomical voltage map from a patient with a large anteroseptal infarction is shown in the anteroposterior projection and displays points of very low bipolar voltage (<0.5 mV) in red, corresponding to the dense scar zone, while *purple* corresponds to normal myocardium (bipolar voltage >1.5 mV). Depicted are two clinical VT morphologies with their recorded ICD electrograms. In the *top green panel* is the surface 12-lead ECG of an atypical left bundle branch block morphology VT, which exits the scar at its mid-inferoseptal aspect. Its accompanying ICD electrograms are displayed in the *lower green panel* with the local tip bipolar electrogram shown in the top channel while the bottom channel shows the far-field RV coil to ICD pulse generator electrogram. These electrograms are seen to have a completely different morphology to the ICD recordings from the right bundle branch block morphology VT (which exits at the opposite aspect of the scar) displayed in the *blue boxes*.

procedure, often with multiple VT inductions and significant intravascular fluid loading. Heart failure decompensation and myocardial ischemia in particular must both be reversed as much as possible before commencing ablation. The PAINESD score provides a useful risk assessment tool and can help in selecting those patients who may require consideration of periprocedural mechanical circulatory support (MCS).[50,51] The presence of peripheral arterial disease is an important comorbidity from the viewpoint of both retrograde transaortic vascular access and potential hemodynamic support options such as an intra-aortic balloon pump (IABP). It should be noted that recent data suggests the possibility of a potentially lower cerebral embolic risk with transseptal LV access compared to retrograde transaortic access.[52] The status of all coronary bypass grafts and stents should be ascertained and myocardial revascularization completed as appropriate. Prior cardiac surgery will generally preclude unrestricted percutaneous pericardial access for catheter ablation (due to the presence of dense adhesions or bypass grafts), but this is a lesser problem in postinfarct VT patients given the accessibility of the majority of VT circuits and the arrhythmogenic substrate with endocardial ablation. Prior valvular surgery is an important consideration, with mechanical prosthetic valves in the aortic and mitral positions precluding retrograde and transseptal access to the LV, respectively. The rare situation of dual mechanical prosthetic valves may require transapical or interventricular septal access to the "no-entry ventricle."[53,54] Additionally, the recent description of trans-right atrial access to the LV by the creation of an iatrogenic Gerbode defect provides an elegant and less disruptive option in these difficult cases.[55]

Oral anticoagulation needs to be carefully considered and, if possible, usually withheld before scar-related VT ablation. This is because even a planned exclusively transseptal approach may require additional retrograde or epicardial access and/or IABP placement.

A preoperative echocardiogram is performed to quantify LV size and systolic function as well as to assess for the presence of intracardiac thrombus. It should be noted that the latter is not an absolute contraindication to an endocardial ablation attempt, particularly with laminated chronic thrombi, though these may hinder catheter access to arrhythmogenic subendocardial regions.[56,57]

Conscious sedation may be preferred for this procedure over general anesthesia wherever possible due to improved hemodynamics, in both VT and sinus rhythm, as well as easier VT induction. There are data to support a lower risk of hemodynamic decompensation during the procedure with conscious sedation compared to general anesthesia.[50] However, patient tolerance is an important consideration in these often protracted and difficult procedures, and administration of conscious sedation by specialist anesthetic staff allows for close patient monitoring, precise adjustment of sedation depth, and early general anesthetic induction if required. A urinary catheter is of use to monitor fluid balance adequately in the face of large fluid loads from open-irrigated catheters as well as to warn of reduced peripheral and splanchnic perfusion and impending cardiogenic shock.

A detailed assessment of the anatomical substrate is important to properly plan the procedure and anticipate potential challenges. This begins with the 12-lead ECG, which may provide useful information on infarct location both in sinus rhythm and in VT. Regional wall motion abnormalities on echocardiography, with or without the use of acoustic contrast or speckle tracking strain imaging, may define the infarct scar satisfactorily. However, the current gold standard for scar imaging is LGE on MRI. The superb soft tissue contrast and resolution provided by this imaging modality can provide a detailed assessment of scar architecture and can be used for image integration with the electroanatomical mapping system. This may help identify likely VT isthmus locations and improve the efficiency and potentially the efficacy of the procedure.[58] Patients with ICDs can be scanned at experienced centers with the appropriate safety precautions.[59] Susceptibility artifact from the pulse generator and leads remains an issue, although newer MRI technologies such as wideband LGE may reduce this also.[60] Patients who cannot undergo MRI may have scar imaging performed with positron emission tomography (PET) and/or multidetector computed tomography (CT) to obtain a high-resolution metabolic scar map that can also be used for image integration.[61,62]

Intraprocedural imaging is an important consideration in VT ablation, where it is needed for defining substrate, tagging ablation targets, tracking lesion location, and monitoring for complications. While fluoroscopy and electroanatomical mapping are deployed universally due to widespread availability and ease of use, ICE has been used increasingly for VT ablation procedures. It allows for real-time scar imaging, visualization of catheter contact, and lesion formation, in addition to assisting with transseptal or percutaneous pericardial access if this is required.[63] Another benefit of ICE is its unique ability to provide real-time monitoring for complications such as stream pop, thrombus formation, and cardiac perforation. This is particularly useful in VT ablation as hypotension frequently occurs during these procedures and ICE can rapidly exclude tamponade as a cause of this. Additionally, ICE is the main online imaging modality that allows visualization and ablation of endocavitary structures such as the papillary muscles, which can be involved in infarct scars.[64] Future options for intraprocedural imaging in VT ablation may include interventional MRI technologies that will allow for more definitive online substrate mapping and accurate assessment of lesion formation with thermography.

MAPPING STRATEGIES

Fundamentally, the aim of mapping VT (or any arrhythmia) is to define the electrophysiologic mechanism and to localize the critical arrhythmogenic components that may be targeted by catheter ablation. For focal VTs, the critical arrhythmogenic site is the point source of origin, and this can be localized with precision using activation mapping and pace mapping alone. In activation mapping, the goal is to localize the site with the earliest presystolic activation time before the QRS is inscribed. Pace mapping relies on the principle that pacing at the site of origin of a tachycardia should theoretically recapitulate the QRS morphology perfectly. Both of these techniques are ideally suited to mapping the site of origin of focal VTs, the majority of which occur in the absence of structural heart disease.

In the postinfarct context, however, the vast majority of VT is due to macroreentry through the infarct scar and, as with any reentrant circuit, terms such as "site of origin" and "earliest" are meaningless. The goal of mapping reentrant VT is to define the narrowest part of the reentrant circuit (the diastolic isthmus) where it is most susceptible to interruption with ablation lesions. In reentry, activation mapping can be used to define the boundaries and direction of rotation of the circuit, with progressively earlier signals mapped further proximally in the protected diastolic corridor. The use of the three-dimensional electroanatomical systems aids in visualization of such activation maps. However, there are several challenges that can affect the routine deployment of activation mapping of scar-related VT, and for this reason, postinfarct VT is often mapped by its response to overdrive pacing (entrainment mapping).

Once vascular access has been obtained and diagnostic catheters have been placed in the heart, VT is induced with programmed stimulation or by catheter manipulation during electroanatomical map creation. Recent data suggest, however that the mechanical effects of catheter manipulation during substrate mapping may indeed reduce VT inducibility.[65] Induced VTs are analyzed for cycle length and/or morphology match to clinical VTs and are assessed as to whether they are mappable by conventional activation and entrainment mapping. In addition to hemodynamic tolerability, the other criteria required to make VT mappable are listed in Box 33.3. Mappable VTs comprise the minority of VTs induced in ICM patients, although most patients have at least one mappable VT morphology.[66] With mappable VTs, ascertainment of circuit components and ablation of critical targets occur during tachycardia. This allows for assessment of the response to radiofrequency energy delivery, with immediate or early VT termination during lesion delivery being an encouraging sign of elimination of that VT.

Unmappable VTs are those that do not allow for entrainment mapping to be performed, often but not exclusively due to hemodynamic compromise. Strategies that may help make nontolerated VTs mappable include the use of inotropes or mechanical circulatory support with IABP or percutaneous LVAD.[67] Substrate mapping approaches can be used for

BOX 33.3 Requirements for VT to Be Mappable

- VT is reproducibly inducible.
- VT is sustained.
- VT is monomorphic.
- VT cycle length is regular.
- VT is hemodynamically tolerated.
- VT does not transition to other morphologies.
- VT does not terminate or change morphology/rate with overdrive pacing.

genuinely unmappable VTs and are considered further later. In general, a combination of mapping strategies is used for most scar-related VT ablation procedures.

Activation Mapping

Using a meticulous point-by-point approach, de Chillou et al. performed three-dimensional contact activation mapping of 33 tolerated VTs in 21 patients.[68] Either single- or dual-loop macroreentrant circuits were demonstrated as the mechanism for all VTs, with protected diastolic isthmuses bounded by parallel conduction barriers such as myocardial scar or valve annuli. Various fractionated and mid-diastolic EGMs were recorded from such regions with a 3.5-mm-tip ablation catheter. Isthmus dimensions measured 18–41 mm in length and 6–36 mm in width and linear ablation across these isthmuses treated VT effectively, with a low 10% recurrence rate at 16 ± 8-month follow-up. While this important study contributed to the mechanistic understanding of postinfarct VT, until recently, routine point-by-point activation mapping of the entire VT circuit was impractical, time-consuming, unnecessary, and, in isolation, usually unhelpful to precisely define the narrowest portion of the protected diastolic pathway. Annotation of long-duration, multicomponent fractionated and double potentials during activation mapping was particularly difficult and mid-diastolic potentials may not have represented critical isthmuses but rather passively activated bystander cul-de-sacs or outer loops.

However, multipolar mapping has changed the landscape of activation mapping in VT. The advent of an ultra-high-resolution electroanatomical mapping system revolutionized the ability to perform activation mapping with rapid acquisition and automatic annotation of tens of thousands of EGMs from very narrowly spaced bipoles located on a 64-electrode mini-basket catheter.[69] Human cases and detailed studies with this mapping system in large animal models of postinfarct VT have led to a reappraisal of much of the physiology of VT circuits.[24] In particular, the central diastolic conduction isthmus, previously considered to represent the zone of slow conduction in this form of reentry, has been shown to have normal conduction velocity in most cases. The necessary conduction delay to allow for reentry seems to occur due to wavefront curvature around the functional barriers at the entrance to and exit from these isthmuses[24] (Fig. 33.9).

The most definitive activation mapping study of human VT was recently performed by Tung et al. in 89 scar-related VT patients undergoing 97 procedures.[11] Using multipolar catheters with improved automated EGM analysis, 151 VT circuits were mapped in detail with the majority (83%) exhibiting transmural

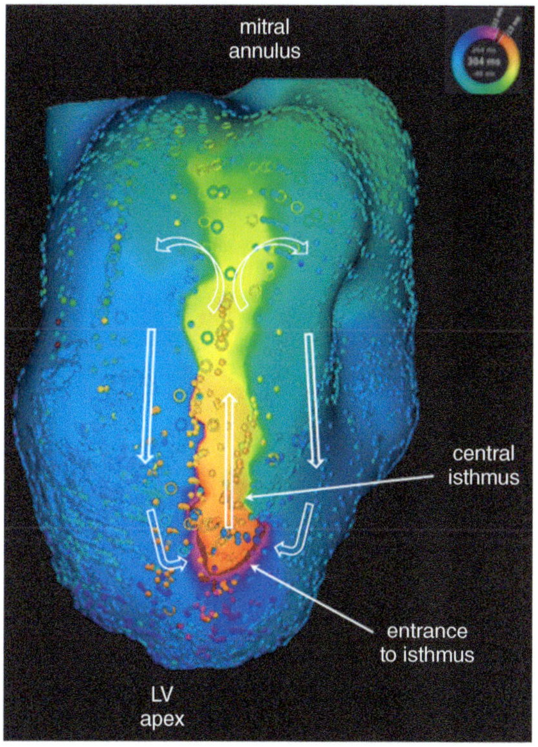

Fig. 33.9 An ultra-high-density activation map of ventricular tachycardia (VT) in a porcine anterior myocardial infarction model showing figure-of-eight reentry. At least some of the barriers constraining the central isthmus are functional. Conduction slowing due to wavefront curvature can be appreciated by isochronal crowding at the entrance to the central isthmus. Conduction velocity within the isthmus is normal.

activation on simultaneous endocardial-epicardial activation maps. With higher-resolution mapping, the mean VT isthmus dimensions were unsurprisingly assessed as smaller than prior studies at 17 × 10 mm.

Entrainment Mapping

In addition to confirming reentry as the arrhythmia mechanism, entrainment mapping allows for rapid and precise delineation of all the components of a reentrant VT circuit. This is true whether the conduction barriers that constrain the reentrant wavefront are determined anatomically or functionally or both. The principles of entrainment were first described by Waldo et al. using the example of typical cavotricuspid isthmus–dependent atrial flutter following which they made similar observations in reentrant VT.[70] These concepts were then extended by multiple other investigators to develop the criteria for entrainment mapping of VT circuit components.[71–73]

Fundamentally, entrainment mapping seeks to answer two basic questions. First, is a particular site located within the reentrant VT circuit? Second, is it within a narrow, constrained diastolic isthmus where the circuit may be vulnerable to interruption with ablation? These questions are answered at each site by analysis of the response to ventricular overdrive pacing (Fig. 33.10).

After mappable VT is induced, the surface 12-lead QRS morphology is examined to obtain a first approximation of the likely region of reentrant wavefront exit from the scar. Detailed analysis

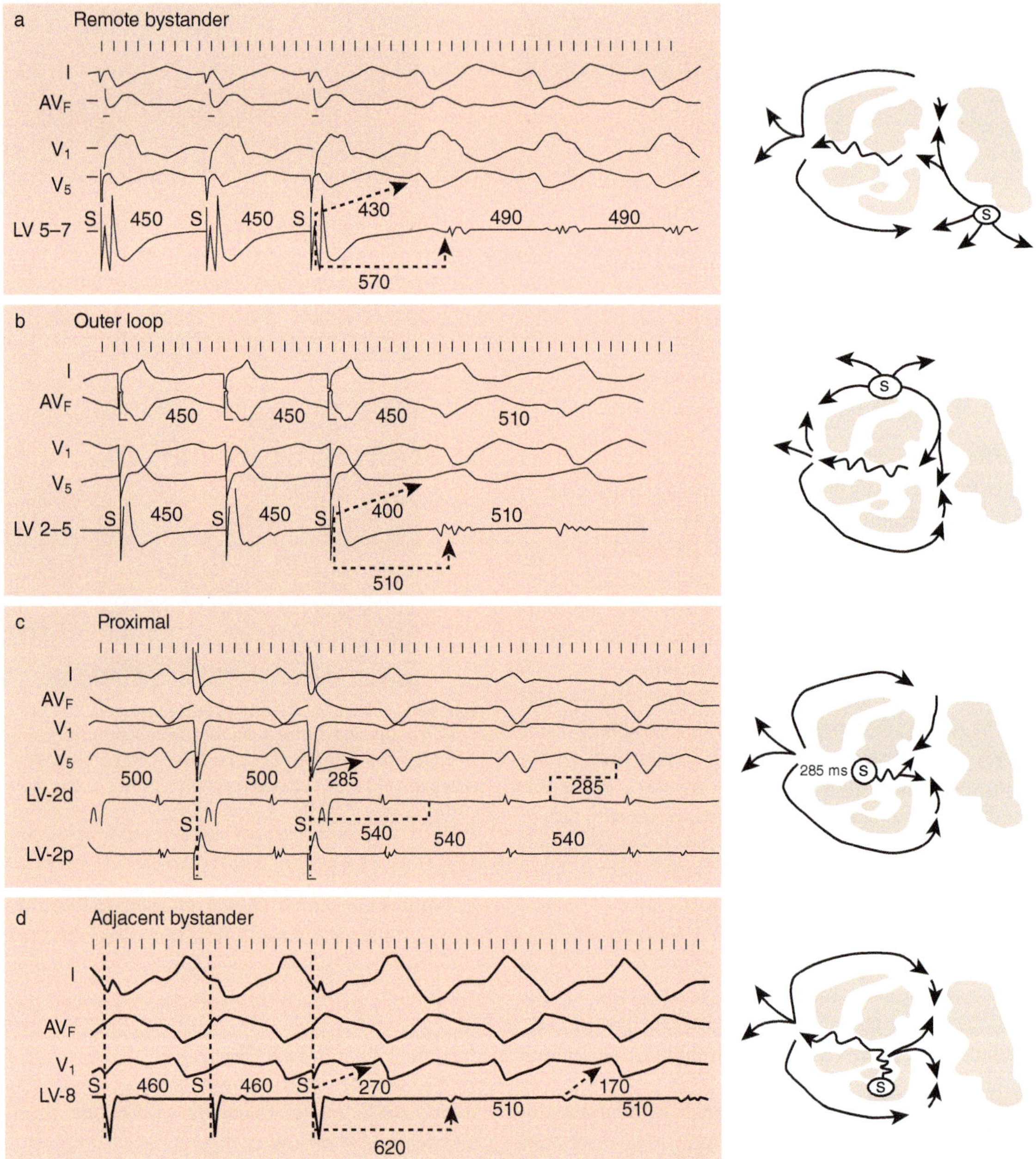

A

Fig. 33.10 (A) Computer model of ventricular tachycardia (VT) within unexcitable infarct scar (*gray stippled areas, right panels*), demonstrating the response to entrainment with pacing at different sites within the circuit. The circuit is depicted as a "figure-of-eight" activation using a central common pathway with slow conduction. Pacing from remote bystander areas (A) will show some degree of fusion, and the return cycle is longer than the VT cycle length (by twice the conduction time from the site to the VT circuit). Pacing from outer loop sites (B) will show manifest entrainment, as the pacing site has access to recruit areas away from the circuit, as it is not bounded by the infarct. Pacing from sites within the central pathway (C) demonstrates concealed entrainment with a stimulus to ECG equal to the electrogram to QRS during VT; the return cycle measured at this electrogram is equal to the VT cycle length. Pacing from adjacent bystander sites (D) result in concealed entrainment, but the return cycle is longer than the VT cycle length (by twice the conduction time from the site to the VT circuit). (From Stevenson WG. Catheter ablation of ventricular tachycardia. In: Zipes DP, Jalife J, eds. *Cardiac Electrophysiology: From Cell to Bedside*. 3rd ed. Philadelphia: WB Saunders Company; 2004:1091.) (B) Algorithm for ablation of scar related ventricular tachycardia. *LV*, Left ventricle; *PES*, programmed electrical stimulation; *PPI*, postpacing interval; *RBB*, right bundle branch; *RV*, right ventricle; *TCL*, tachycardia cycle length. (C) Algorithm to determine catheter position relative to a reentry circuit. *S*, Stimulus; *EG*, electrogram; *CF*, concealed fusion.

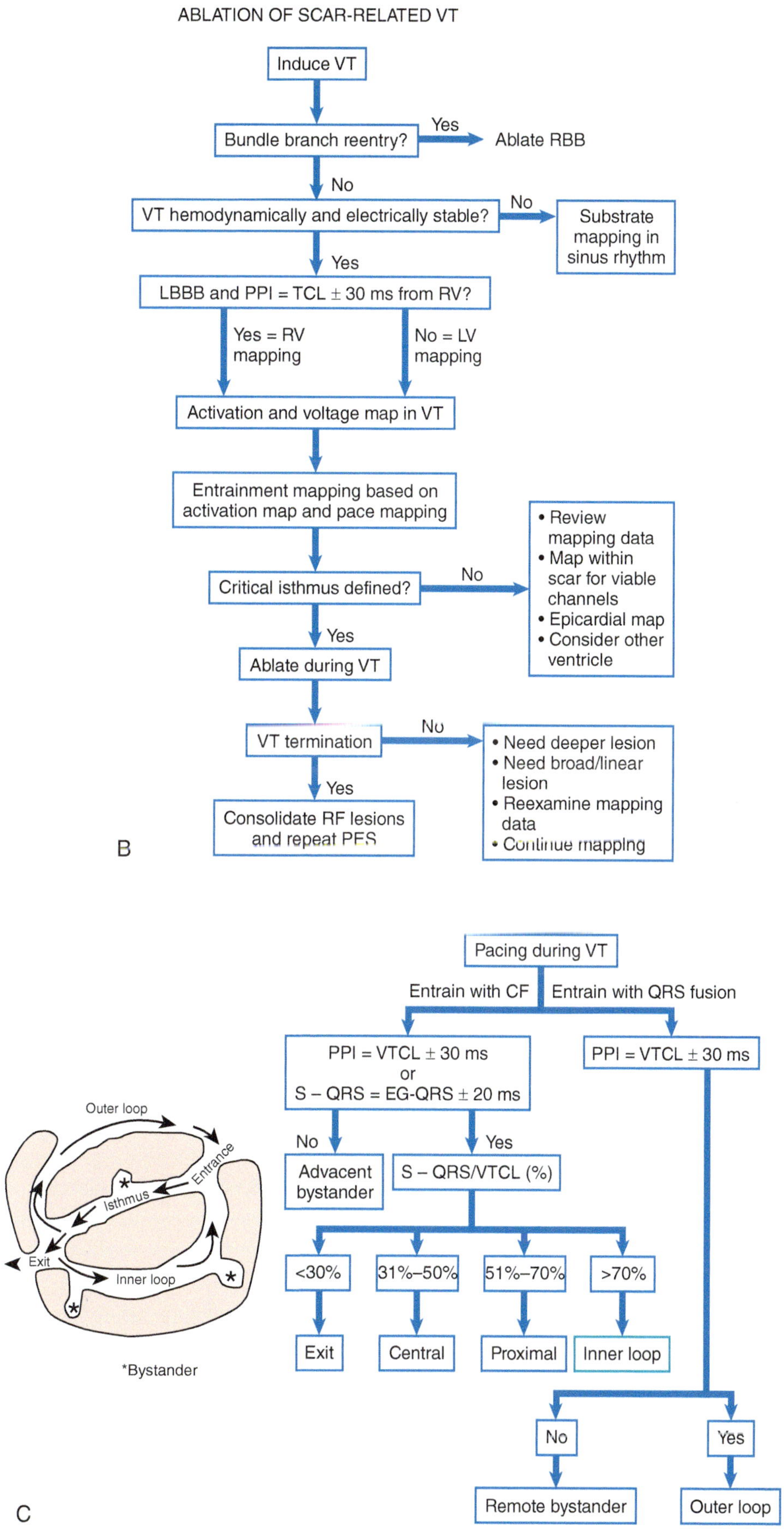

Fig. 33.10, cont'd.

TABLE 33.1 Regions of VT Exit Suggested by 12-Lead QRS Morphology

ECG Characteristic	Region of VT Exit
Bundle branch morphology:	
Left	LV septum or right ventricle
Right	Free wall of LV
Frontal plane axis:	
Superior	Inferior or inferoseptal/lateral LV
Inferior	Anterior or anteroseptal/lateral LV
Right	Lateral LV or apex
Precordial transition (R > S):	
Early	Basal LV
Late	Apical LV
Concordant positive	Mitral annular
Concordant negative	Apex
QRS upstroke:	
Slurred with pseudo-delta	Epicardial
Precordial transition pattern break	Epicardial

ECG, Electrocardiogram; *LV*, left ventricle (ventricular); *VT*, ventricular tachycardia.

of the QRS morphology in various postinfarct VTs was first performed in the seminal intraoperative mapping study by Miller et al.[74] More recently, a frontal-plane QRS axis–based algorithm from Andreu et al. was accurate in localizing VT exit in a 17-segment LV model in 82% of VTs in 108 scar-VT patients, 77 of whom had post-MI VT.[75] Various combinations of surface ECG parameters that allow for VT localization are summarized in Table 33.1. The roving mapping catheter is placed farther back in the scar from the suggested exit zone where a systematic search is conducted for mid-diastolic potentials (MDPs). These may be recorded from the critical central isthmus or from adjacent bystander sites (where ablation would be ineffective). Entrainment mapping seeks to determine how such potentials relate to the VT circuit. The relative activation time of such potentials is much earlier than the presystolic potentials targeted in focal VT ablation. It should be noted that such very early activity may occur within the QRS complex of the preceding beat, particularly in very broad complex VTs where the QRS width is half or more of the VT cycle length. It is common for a larger far-field ventricular EGM to be recorded along with a MDP.

Overdrive pacing is then performed at a cycle length ~20 ms faster than the VT at the minimum output that reliably captures the potential, although high outputs (~10 mA at 2 ms) are frequently necessary in dense scar. Pacing is then ceased and the VT is confirmed to continue at its previous cycle length and with unaltered morphology (Fig. 33.11). If VT terminates with pacing, the pacing train is examined closely to see if VT terminated

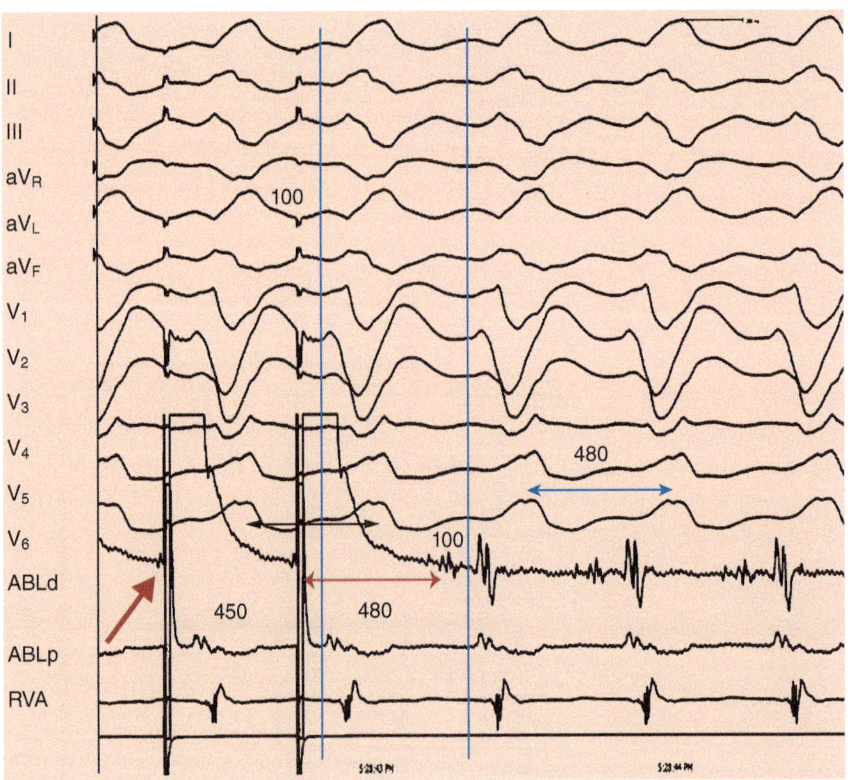

Fig. 33.11 Characteristics of the "perfect map" for ablation of ventricular tachycardia (VT). The optimal single ablation site for VT has the following characteristics: (1) entrainment from the site will produce an exact match of the spontaneous VT QRS in all 12 leads, (2) the return cycle (the duration from the pacing stimulus to the first nonpaced beat, measured at the pacing site) will equal the VT cycle length both 480 ms in this example, and (3) the stimulus to QRS will equal the electrogram to QRS both equal to 100 ms. With multicomponent fractionated signals it can be difficult to know with certainty which component has been locally captured by pacing, and hence where to measure the return cycle length. In this case the *arrowhead* shows the component of the fractionated electrogram which is not captured orthodromically, and hence the horizontal red calipers measure the return cycle to the second component.

with a nonpropagated stimulus that did not result in global ventricular capture. Such sites are highly predictive of successful ablation.[76] Pacing needs to continue long enough for the establishment of entrainment which is confirmed by acceleration of the entire chamber (including all the VT circuit components) to the paced cycle length with constant fusion at that cycle length and progressive fusion at faster cycle lengths. When pacing from outside the protected isthmus, manifest fusion occurs as a result of the antidromic paced wavefront colliding (fusing) with the prior tachycardia (or orthodromic paced) wavefront, with a new paced orthodromic wavefront continuing the tachycardia through the normal VT exit site. If pacing and collision occur within the constrained diastolic corridor inside the scar, it will not be manifest on the surface ECG. Such fusion is said to be concealed. The terms *concealed entrainment* and *entrainment with concealed fusion* (ECF) are used interchangeably to denote this phenomenon. Accordingly, after cessation of overdrive pacing and confirmation that pacing did transiently accelerate the tachycardia before its resumption with unchanged rate and morphology, the surface ECG is examined in minute detail for a notch-perfect QRS match between overdrive pacing and VT (Fig. 33.11). A good pace map match between the two is not sufficient and indicates manifest fusion, implying that the pacing site was not located in a protected corridor.

After confirmation of ECF, the EGM on the distal bipole of the mapping catheter is examined to determine the postpacing interval (PPI) from the last pacing stimulus to the MDP that was captured by pacing. If the pacing site is recording an MDP that is located within the reentry circuit, it should take one VT cycle length for the last paced wavefront to propagate orthodromically through the circuit and return to the pacing site. Thus, for sites located in the VT circuit, the PPI should match the tachycardia cycle length (TCL). While conventionally a PPL–TCL difference of up to 30 ms is taken as being compatible with being within the circuit due to decremental conduction at faster pacing rates, sites with smaller PPI–TCL differences are closer to the circuit (Fig. 33.11).

If both ECF and a small PPI–TCL difference are observed, then this is strong evidence that not only is the pacing site located within the reentrant VT circuit but also it is inside the constrained diastolic isthmus where ablation may interrupt it. During entrainment, all orthodromically captured circuit components should have an identical relationship as during VT. Thus, the stimulus–QRS time (S-QRS) is measured and compared to the mid-diastolic electrogram–QRS time (EGM-QRS). This difference should be close to zero for diastolic isthmus sites but will be longer for adjacent bystander sites connected to the central isthmus (Figs. 33.10C and 33.11). The S-QRS time is then compared to the TCL to determine how proximal the pacing site is in the diastolic isthmus. Sites with S-QRS <30% of the TCL are near the exit end of the isthmus, whereas sites with S-QRS of 51–70% of the TCL are close to the entrance. Central sites in the isthmus have in-between values for the S-QRS time (Fig. 33.10C).

The ability of entrainment mapping to identify sites where VT can be terminated with radiofrequency (RF) ablation was tested comprehensively in the seminal study of Stevenson et al.[73] They found that ECF alone was insufficient to predict VT termination as sites that are attached to the diastolic pathway, including inner loops and blind ending cul-de-sacs, and may also display ECF. By looking at the PPI and S-QRS, they showed that 25% of sites exhibiting ECF were actually bystander sites that were not involved in the reentrant circuit. The presence of MDP combined with ECF and optimal PPI and S-QRS intervals predicted a 35% incidence of VT termination compared with 4% when they were absent. This was confirmed by Bogun et al., who found the positive predictive value of ECF alone for ablation termination to be 54% but this increased with the addition of PPI and S-QRS criteria, particularly in combination with the presence of MDP that could not be dissociated from VT.[77] This group later showed that of these criteria, ECF with S-QRS matching EGM-QRS performed best in predicting successful ablation.[78]

Ablation at a perfect entrainment mapping site may not result in VT termination for a number of reasons. First, the entrainment map may not be perfect with subtle manifest QRS fusion being missed or inaccurate measurement of PPI-TCL or S-QRS intervals. With tight definitions for optimal PPI-TCL (<10 ms) and S-QRS (within 10 ms of EGM-QRS) in addition to ECF, El-Shalakany et al. showed consistent termination of VT with a single lesion at sites where all three criteria were met.[72] Second, RF energy delivery may not result in effective lesion formation due to various factors such as poor contact or poor electrothermal coupling in dense scar. Third, the width of the critical diastolic isthmus may be broader than the volume of an ablation lesion. And finally, an intramural or epicardial isthmus may lie deeper than the maximum depth of an RF ablation lesion.

Entrainment mapping is the most powerful technique for mapping VT circuits, but despite its precision and utility, there are several limitations. The requirement for VT to be mappable is the first of these (Box 33.3), and other techniques must be used for unmappable tachycardias. Overdrive pacing can terminate, accelerate, or transform the VT into another tachycardia, particularly if suboptimal sensing by the stimulator results in inappropriately early introduction of the first pacing stimulus. The local EGMs (usually MDPs) at the sites where entrainment mapping is performed must be able to be captured by pacing and must be of sufficient amplitude to discern among background noise so as to allow for PPI and S-QRS measurement. The local and far-field components of EGMs must be distinguishable lest errors be made in PPI and S-QRS determination.[79] Generally speaking, EGM components that are visible on the distal mapping catheter bipole during pacing are not immediately local EGMs (Fig. 33.11). Even when they are of reasonable amplitude, MDPs can be lost in the pacing channel artifact after cessation of pacing, making PPI determination difficult. When artefact in the recording channel from saturation of the amplifiers precludes PPI measurement on the distal tip bipolar electrode pair, assessment of the PPI can be achieved by comparing two cycles after cessation to twice the TCL, or by using the N + 1 difference method as described by Soejima et al. in which the S-QRS is measured to the second beat following

BOX 33.4 Entrainment and Activation Mapping of Ablation Targets

Candidate sites are located in dense infarct core (bipolar voltage <0.5 mV) or in the scar-border zone (bipolar voltage 0.5–1.5 mV), with mid-diastolic potentials inscribed <70% of cycle length before QRS onset.

Overdrive pacing from target sites results in:

- Acceleration of VT to paced cycle length
- Continuation of VT after cessation of pacing
- Concealed surface QRS fusion (100% pace map)
- PPI = VT cycle length (±30 ms)
- S-QRS = EGM-QRS (±20 ms)
  - Sites producing VT termination with nonpropagated stimulus and non-global capture
  - Sites with continuous electrical activity recorded on mapping catheter
  - Sites where mid-diastolic potentials are recorded that cannot be dissociated from VT

BOX 33.5 Common Substrate Mapping Targets

Candidate sites are located in dense infarct core (bipolar voltage <0.5 mV) or in the scar-border zone (bipolar voltage 0.5–1.5 mV).

- Sites of prolonged (>40 ms) S-QRS during pace mapping
- Sites of perfect pace map match, especially if long S-QRS seen also
- Sites of perfect pace map which initiate tachycardia after cessation of pacing
- Sites of pacing with multiple, abrupt transition exits are produced during pacing
- Higher-voltage channels located between islands of very dense or unexcitable scar
- Core of putative VT machinery within dense scar, susceptible to en bloc isolation
- Isolated late potentials during sinus rhythm, ventricular pacing or extra-stimulus delivery
- Entrance to scar channel (defined by increasingly delayed connected isolated late potentials)
- Decrement of isolated late potentials to one or more extrastimuli (DEEP mapping)
- Deceleration zones on isochronal late activation mapping (usually not in latest isochrones)
- Omnipolar mapping to delineate zones of wavefront conduction slowing

S-QRS, Stimulus-QRS.

pacing cessation.[80] Alternatively, measuring the PPI using the signal on the proximal shaft bipolar electrode pair appears to be a reasonably close approximation.[81] Finally, pacing at high outputs to allow for capture within dense scar may result in a large virtual electrode that also captures far field tissue, potentially obscuring entrainment mapping data or resulting in artefactually shorter postpacing return cycles. This problem may theoretically be exacerbated by the use of bipolar pacing with anodal stimulation at higher outputs, although this seems not to be of any practical significance in the modern era of small, closely spaced bipole electrodes.

The characteristics of candidate sites that may be targeted in the ablation of mappable reentrant scar-related VT appear in Box 33.4.

The largest recent study of entrainment mapping by Shirai et al. suggested that in 62% of mappable postinfarct VTs, endocardial LV entrainment alone was able to identify the isthmus.[82]

Substrate Mapping Approaches for Unmappable VT

While delineating the circuit of a stable VT by entrainment mapping and terminating it early during the delivery of RF energy represents the ideal procedural outcome in scar-related VT ablation, in practice this occurs uncommonly. Even patients whose clinical VT is hemodynamically tolerated frequently have multiple other unmappable morphologies. On average, around one-third of patients have exclusively mappable VTs only and around one-fifth of patients have exclusively unmappable VTs induced.[66,83] Successful ablation in such circumstances relies on finding the footprints of the VT circuit (or circuits) in sinus rhythm. This process is known as substrate mapping (Box 33.5). Substrate mapping is examined in detail in Chapter 36.

The development of an effective procedural strategy to cope with unmappable postinfarct VT borrowed conceptually from the most definitive form of substrate ablation, namely surgical subendocardial resection (SER). Survivors of surgery had a >90% rate of freedom from recurrent VT.[84] This established the obligate relationship between the VT circuit and the infarct scar and its surrounding border zone.[85] At operation, even if VT was noninducible or unmappable, the surgeon could visualize the nature and extent of the infarct zone and plan a resection incorporating the dense infarct core and surrounding border zone.[86] The challenges confronted in attempting to emulate this procedure with a percutaneous catheter-based approach were considerable.

Defining ventricular scar with the use of endocardial catheter recordings in postinfarct patients was first performed by Josephson and colleagues at the University of Pennsylvania more than three decades ago. Cassidy et al. recognized the effect of myocardial fibrosis on bipolar EGM amplitude and duration.[35] This formed the basis for the more detailed definition of dense scar and scar border-zone in the seminal substrate ablation study of Marchlinski et al.[33] With the use of narrowly spaced bipolar electrodes (4-mm-tip electrode, 2-mm ring electrode, and 1-mm interelectrode spacing) and an electroanatomical mapping system, they were able to map the geometry of the infarct scar in sufficient resolution to allow for substrate-based ablation of unmappable VTs. Their voltage definitions (>1.5 mV bipolar peak-to-peak amplitude for normal ventricular myocardium and ≤0.5 mV for dense infarct scar) were arrived at through statistical analysis of endocardial recordings from both postinfarct and control patients and were later validated in radiologic and animal studies (Fig. 33.12). In a porcine model of anterior MI, Callans et al. were able to show that the pathologically defined infarct scar exhibited bipolar voltage ≤1.0 mV.[34] In both human and animal postinfarct studies, the zones of low bipolar voltage tend to be sharply demarcated from normal ventricular myocardium.

While there are no systematic human pathologic data, isolated autopsy findings strongly suggest that the zone of bipolar voltage <1.5 mV does correlate with infarct scar.[87,88] This is corroborated by fibrosis imaging using LGE on cardiac MRI,

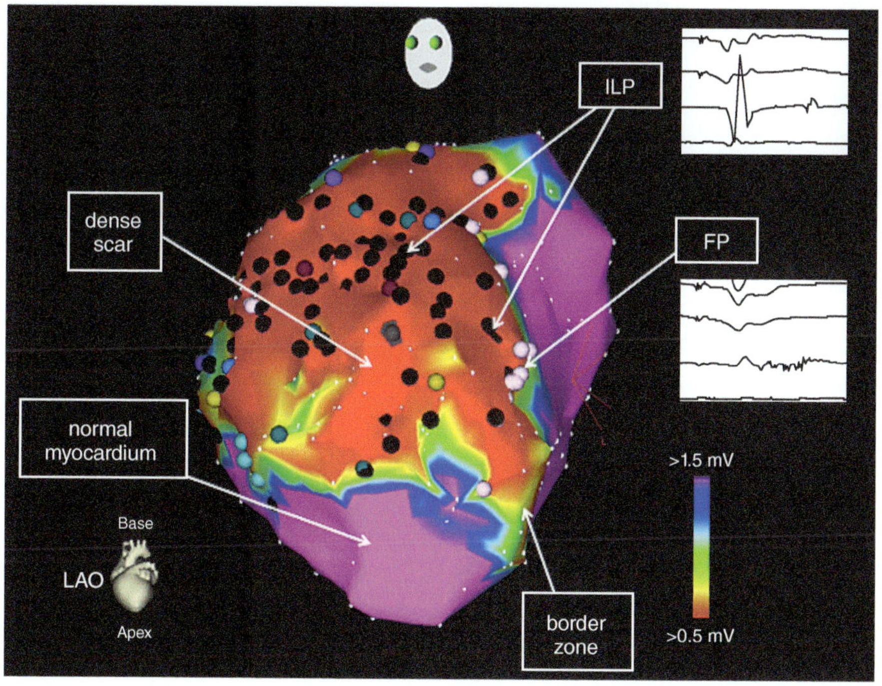

Fig. 33.12 Electroanatomical substrate mapping in a 63-year-old man with large prior anteroseptal infarction with aneurysm formation and an ejection fraction of 20%. The LV endocardium is mapped in sinus rhythm to define the infarct scar and displayed in left anterior oblique (LAO) projection. In this color scheme, is confluent areas of *red* correspond to the dense infarct (bipolar voltage < 0.5 mV), *purple* corresponds to normal tissue (bipolar voltage > 1.5 mV), and the border zone in the "rainbow" of colors in between. Isolated potentials (ILP) are annotated with *black dots* and fractionated potentials (FP) with light pink dots.

where the zone of bipolar voltage >1.54 mV has been shown to best correlate with infarct scar as defined by this technique[89] (Fig. 33.13). The ability to integrate MRI-defined substrate into the electroanatomical mapping system has the potential to increase the efficiency of the substrate mapping process, even potentially in patients with ICDs in situ.[90,91] Perez-David et al. were able to improve the utility of LGE imaging by signal intensity mapping to look at the heterogeneity within infarct scars.[92] They showed that these heterogeneous regions corresponded to electrophysiologically defined conduction channels within the scar and that such regions were found much more frequently in spontaneous VT patients (88%) than in matched control ICM patients with no clinical arrhythmias (33%, $P < .001$).

While signal voltage defines the extent and heterogeneity of ventricular scarring, other EGM parameters are at least as important in substrate mapping (Fig. 33.12). EGMs with an isolated or late component following an isoelectric interval (and usually but not invariably after the surface QRS) may reflect delayed activation of surviving myofibril bundles that are anatomically constrained by dense sheets of fibrosis. The importance of such ILPs was first recognized by Miller et al., who demonstrated that they were eliminated by clinically successful subendocardial resection.[93] Arenal et al. were the first to show that recording ILPs was dependent on the wavefront vector by which scar is activated, as many more patients had ILPs recorded during RV pacing compared to the conducted rhythm.[37] Similarly, ventricular extrastimuli may unmask such EGMs by causing additional interval-dependent conduction slowing within scar.[94] Sites of entrainment-defined VT isthmuses generally display such EGMs during sinus rhythm.[95] In addition to wavefront vector when mapping these potentials, the utility of targeting those ILP that decrement in response to the prematurity of extrastimuli has been established by Porta-Sanchez et al.[96] This technique, known as decrement evoked potential (or DEEP) mapping has been shown to have better specificity for VT isthmus detection than standard ILP mapping.[96]

Haqqani et al. showed that the scars of ICM patients with spontaneous VT contain a greater number and density of ILPs per unit area compared to matched control ICM patients without clinical VT.[15] These ILPs may form conduction channels in sinus rhythm that may correspond to diastolic isthmuses in VT.[97] In many cases, limited ablation of common proximal ILPs may eliminate many interconnected distal ILPs and thus block the putative channel.[97]

Multielectrode catheters facilitate high-density mapping and increased signal resolution, thus the recording of a greater number of ILPs.[98] The Bordeaux group described that 67 of 70 patients displayed late potentials when undergoing high-density endocardial and epicardial mapping with a multispline multipolar catheter.[94] They called these potentials local abnormal ventricular activities (LAVA), but they represent the same electrophysiologic phenomena as ILP, namely delayed activation of surviving myocyte bundles within dense scar. Linear multipolar catheters and multipolar grid array catheters can also facilitate rapid, high-resolution scar mapping, with the smaller orthogonal (and potentially omnipolar) bipoles of the latter delineating smaller (and thus more specific) low-voltage zones in a recent comparison[99] (Video 33.1).

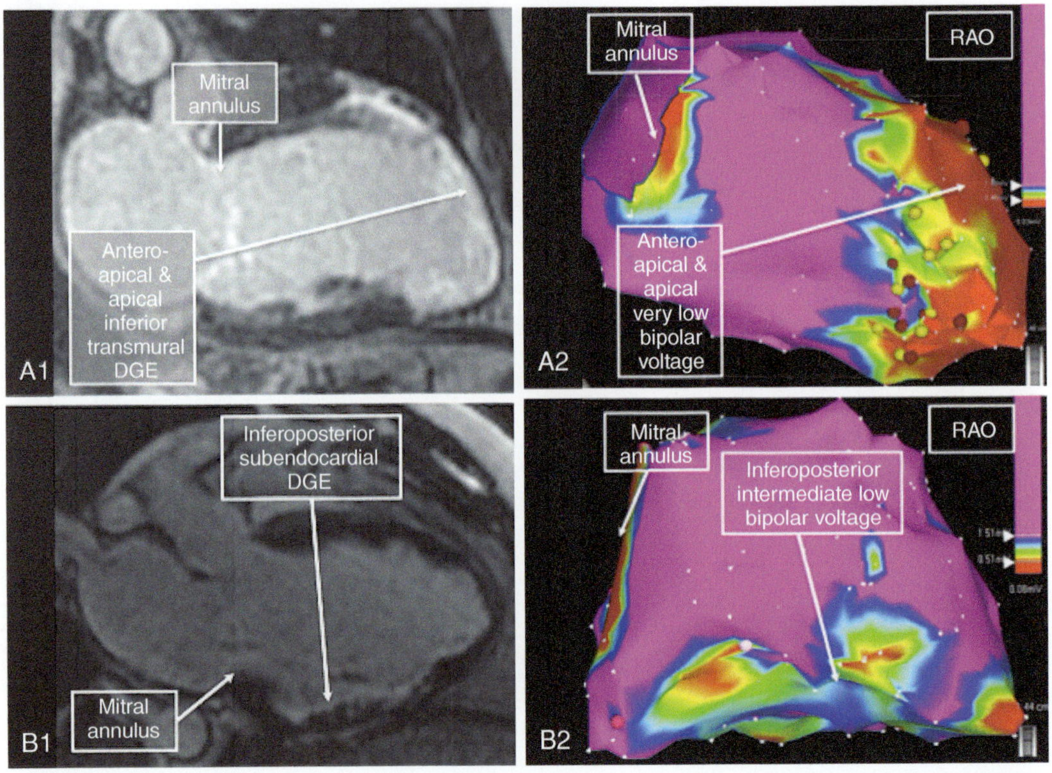

Fig. 33.13 (A1, A2) Scar imaging and mapping results from the left ventricle of a 48-year-old man with ischemic cardiomyopathy and remote anteroapical myocardial infarction. His ejection fraction was 17% on MRI and 20% by echocardiography, with an LV end-diastolic volume of 330 mL on MRI. In the two-chamber long-axis MRI view in A1, there is a large confluent area of anteroapical delayed gadolinium enhancement (DGE) with complete transmural involvement. The corresponding voltage map is shown in A2 in the right anterior oblique (RAO) projection with a regionally matched anteroapical zone of very low bipolar voltage (peak-to-peak electrogram amplitudes <0.5 mV). (B1, B2) MRI and voltage map from a 44-year-old male patient with a remote inferior MI, with ejection fraction 26% on MRI. In this case a matched inferior partial thickness infarct is defined by both modalities, with an inferior region of subendocardial DGE extending to the apex seen on the three-chamber long-axis view in B1, while B2 shows the corresponding inferior zone of intermediate bipolar voltage (0.5–1.5 mV) with patchy areas of very low voltage.

Apart from sinus rhythm EGM recording and analysis, substrate mapping relies heavily on interpreting the responses to pacing within scar. If myocardial capture of electrically excitable scar occurs, then a close analysis of the resulting pace map may give a clue to the relationship between the pacing site and the exit site of the VT from the scar. Pacing at sites of ILPs may also identify slowly conducting channels that traverse dense scar and may form VT isthmuses.[97] Long stimulus-QRS delays are frequently seen when pacing at these sites, sometimes with excellent morphology match to one or more induced VT circuits[97] (Fig. 33.14). Sites of greatest interest often display an abrupt transition from excellent to poor pace maps at closely adjacent points, highly suggestive of block in one exiting channel, with orthodromic activation along another scar exit. Additionally, VT induction during pace mapping may be predictive of critical sites in the VT circuitry.[26]

Although the postinfarct scar is conventionally considered to be predominantly subendocardial, in select patients critical reentrant circuit components may be located intramurally or on the epicardium[11,100,101] (Fig. 33.15). In anteroseptal infarct patients, the potential contribution of right ventricular septal substrate must also be recognized.[102] Importantly, due to the presence of confluent infarct scar, the interval and morphology ECG criteria used to predict epicardial exits in idiopathic and nonischemic cardiomyopathy VT are not useful in the postinfarct setting.[103] In the large referral population published by Sarkozy et al., 13% of patients underwent epicardial mapping (practically all of whom had failed prior endocardial ablation attempts) but only two-thirds of these had epicardial ablation performed and this was tempered with 14% major complication rate.[100] These and other data underscore the importance of exhaustive endocardial mapping and ablation in postinfarct VT in the first instance.[104,105] Finally, after endocardial, intramural, and epicardial substrate have been defined, it is important, particularly in patients with inferior infarct scars, to exclude the presence of endocavitary substrate in the papillary muscles.[64]

Functional Substrate Mapping

The most significant paradigm shift in substrate mapping has been the recognition that the electrophysiology of scar activation is at least as important as EGM amplitude or morphology in detecting local sites during the basal rhythm that may form critical circuit components during reentrant VT.

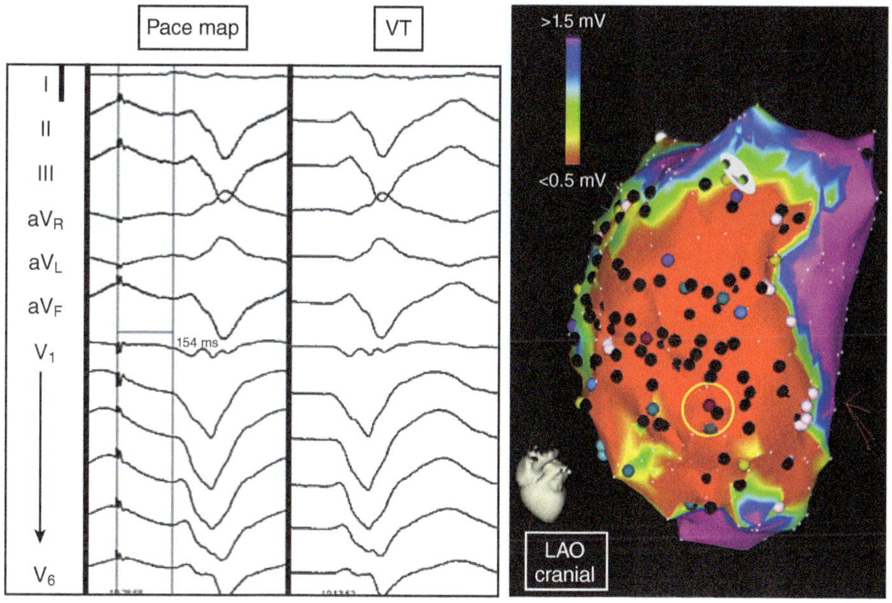

Fig. 33.14 Pacing responses during substrate mapping. A very long stimulus to QRS of 154 ms is demonstrated whilst bipolar pacing at 10 mA at 2 ms during sinus rhythm. The paced QRS morphology displays a good match to one of the induced ventricular tachycardias in this patient.

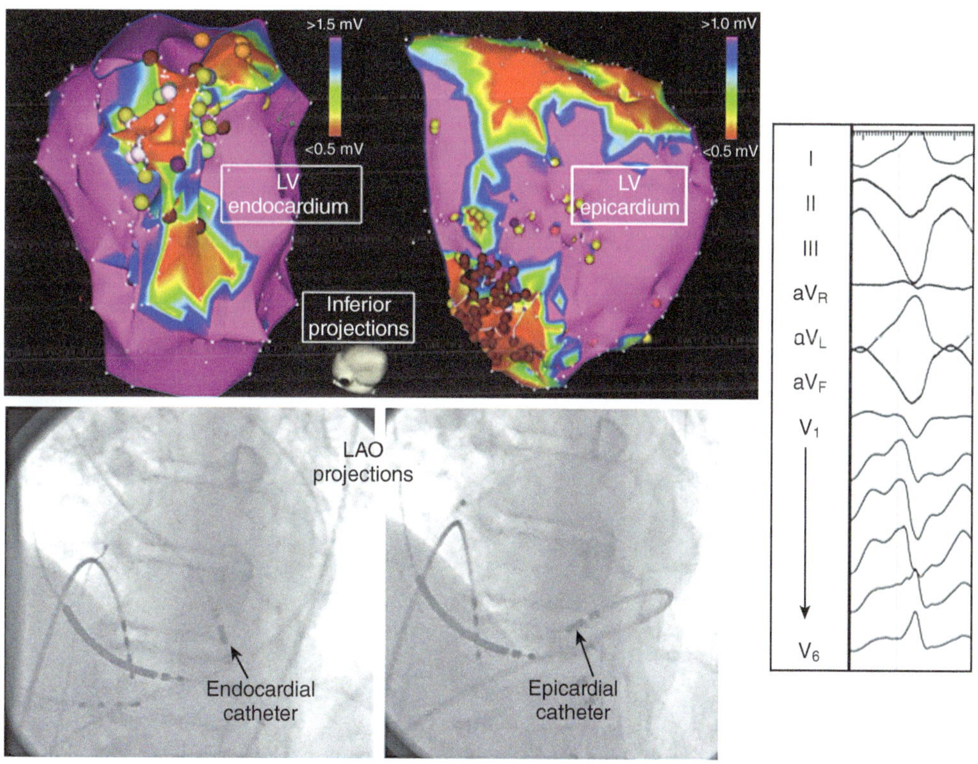

Fig. 33.15 A 69-year-old man with remote inferior myocardial infarction presented with the ventricular tachycardia (VT) displayed. Extensive endocardial mapping defined the infarct scar as shown (*top left*) but only outer loop sites were seen here on entrainment. Epicardial mapping disclosed central isthmus sites at epicardial locations opposite the best endocardial sites where ablation terminated VT and rendered it noninducible.

Tung and colleagues were the first to describe the technique of isochronal late activation mapping (ILAM) in which EGM offset annotation allows for visualization of slow conduction within the scar.[106] They found that critical VT circuit sites were only uncommonly found within the very latest activating isochrones as these sites probably represent blind ending cul de sacs. Significantly however they found that upstream regions of wavefront slowing as visualized by isochronal crowding

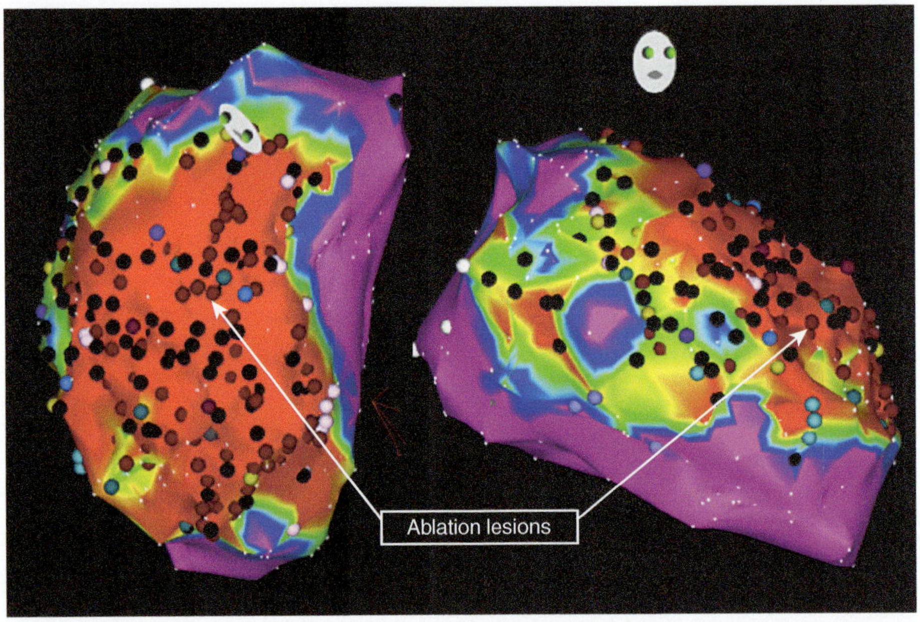

Fig. 33.16 Substrate ablation strategy demonstrating extensive scar homogenization with ablation lesions tagged as *red dots*. Ablation targets included sites of good pace map, sites of slow conduction in putative ventricular tachycardia supporting channels, and isolated late potentials.

(deceleration zones) were extremely likely to contain VT isthmus sites[106] (Fig. 33.17).

Local wavefront deceleration can also be visualized using the grid array multielectrode catheter in omnipolar mapping mode in which local conduction velocity is assessed over pairs of linear and orthogonal closely spaced small electrodes. Recent data suggest that this technique is complementary to ILAM mapping in targeting low-voltage areas of relevant to VT machinery.[107]

The useful effects of both altering wavefront activation vector as well as introducing prematurity cannot be overstated when performing functional substrate mapping and several of these techniques have been described here.

Substrate Ablation Strategies

Once detailed characterization of the substrate using these techniques is complete, a substrate-based ablation strategy can be devised. This may involve pace map–guided radial linear ablation deep into dense scar,[33] linear ablation along the scar border,[108] linear ablation connecting areas of EUS,[109] ablation of voltage or pacing-defined conduction channels,[26,110] electrical isolation of the VT machinery containing infarct core,[111] scar dechanneling,[97] or ablation of all ILPs to electrically homogenize the scar[94,105,112] (Fig. 33.16). The greatest utility of the newer functional substrate mapping approaches outlined here is to select those regions in the scar and those ILPs that most likely correlate to VT circuit sites and hence minimize unnecessary ablation.

The currently accepted endpoint of substrate-based ablation procedures is generally VT noninducibility, although multiple studies suggest that alternative endpoints such as ILP abolition on remapping may be useful.[94,105,112] Continued noninducibility of clinical VTs at later noninvasive programmed stimulation (via the ICD) appears to predict a better long-term outcome.[113] Due to its potential to eliminate all VTs that can be generated by a patient's infarct scar, complete substrate ablation (attempting to recapitulate surgical subendocardial resection) demonstrates better outcomes than ablation targeting only mappable VTs.[114]

Mapping of Polymorphic Postinfarct VT

Electrical storm due to polymorphic VT or VF is an uncommon although potentially fatal arrhythmic presentation. Unlike monomorphic VT, a mature, healed MI scar is not required to develop polymorphic VT, and this can be seen in the early postinfarct phase. While the arrhythmia itself cannot be defined by conventional activation mapping, polymorphic VT is frequently initiated by stereotypical endocardial Purkinje fiber triggering beats, which can be mapped and ablated, frequently in the scar border zone.[40,115,116] These are usually manifest as premature ventricular complexes (PVCs) that exhibit preceding Purkinje-like potentials (PLP) during endocardial mapping (Fig. 33.18). In patients with insufficient ectopy at the time of mapping, mapping of the Purkinje network and pace mapping to stored clinical PVC morphology on ICD EGMs may provide more focused ablation targets than empiric ablation of all PLPs.[117]

ABLATION LESION DELIVERY

For reasons of both efficacy and safety, open-irrigated ablation has become the gold standard for RF energy delivery and lesion formation.[66,118] The ability to cool the electrode–tissue interface with open irrigation allows for greater power delivery and

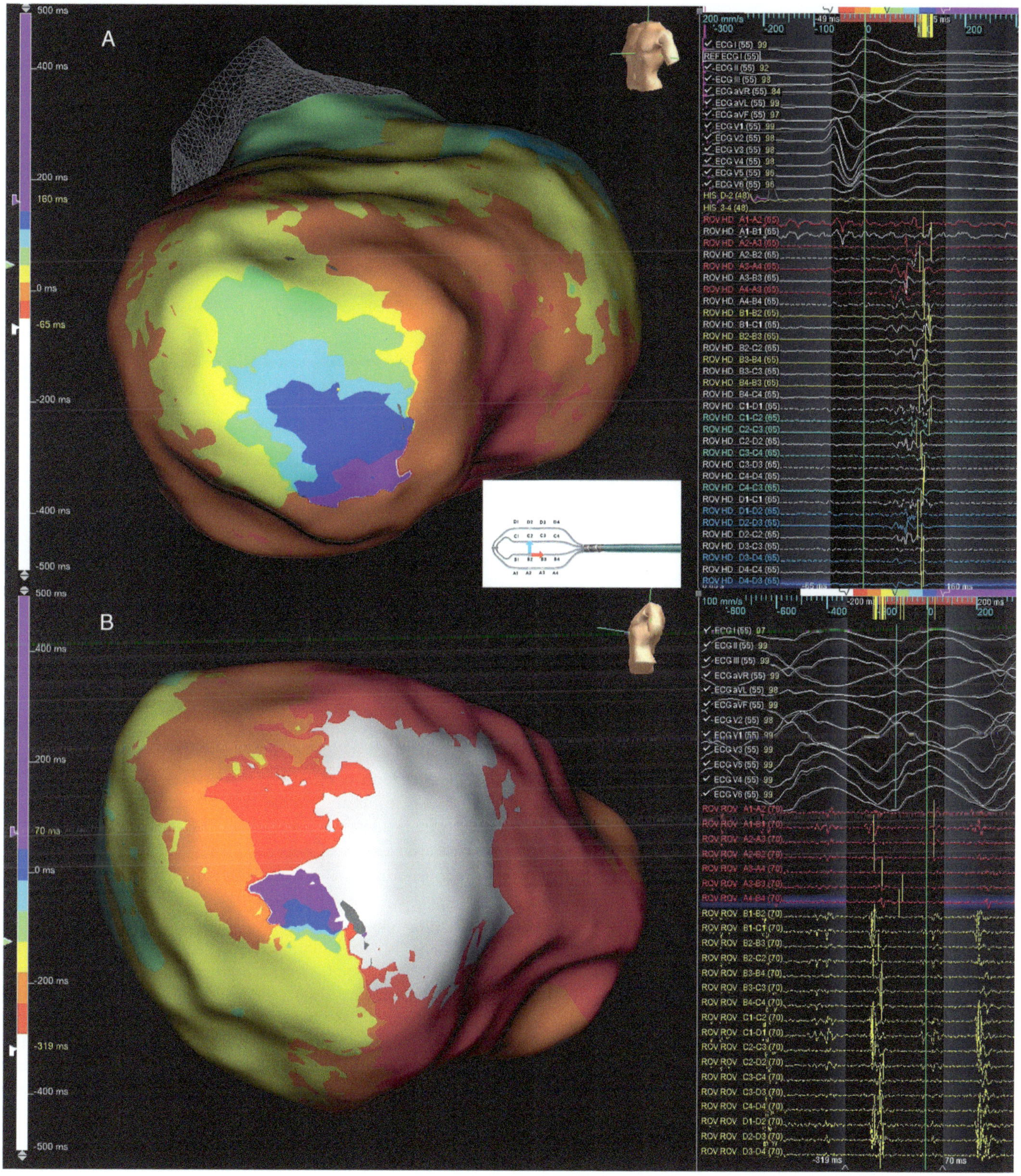

Fig. 33.17 High-density endocardial left ventricular activation maps acquired with the HD Grid (Abbott, St Paul, MN) multipolar mapping catheter (A, *inset*) in a patient with a prior anterior infarct. (A) Sinus rhythm isochronal late activation map (ILAM) with electrogram offset automatically annotated (*right*). No prematurity or altered wavefronts were necessary in order to denote significant numbers of isolated late potentials. Of the eight equally spaced isochrones, four are crowded in a small area at the apex, confirming a "deceleration" zone. (B) Activation map of the induced VT, showing an apically based, figure-of-eight dual loop reentry circuit. The late activating electrograms recorded at the apex during functional substrate mapping have become mid-diastolic potentials in VT (B, *right*).

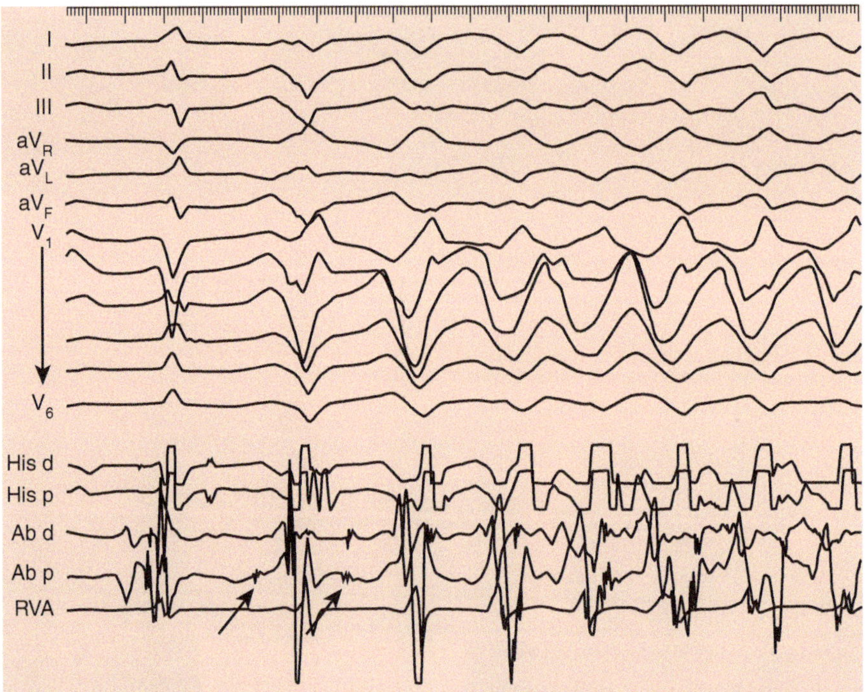

Fig. 33.18 Mapping and ablation of Purkinje triggers of polymorphic ventricular tachycardia (VT). This recording was made in a patient with frequent episodes of polymorphic VT, all preceded by right bundle branch block (RBBB) premature ventricular contractions (PVCs). In the electrophysiology lab, a run of RBBB PVCs was observed. Note the Purkinje potentials (*arrows*) recorded on the mapping catheter (labeled Ab d and Ab p), present on PVC beats and during sinus. Both the Purkinje-ventricular interval and the morphology of the PVCs change from beat to beat. Ablation of the Purkinje system trigger resulted in freedom from recurrent polymorphic VT. *d*, Distal; *p*, proximal; *RVA*, right ventricular apex.

deeper resistive heating, even within scarred myocardium.[118] Additionally, the risk of coagulum and char formation (and potential embolism) is lower when using open-irrigated electrodes.[119] The temperature cut-off is typically set around 43°C to prevent excessive heating of deep tissue with the attendant risk of steam pop and myocardial perforation (though this is less of a risk when ablating within infarcted areas of the left ventricle). Application then typically begins at a power of 30 W and is smoothly titrated to as high as 50 W if necessary in order to achieve at least a 10-Ω impedance drop. Contact force-sensing catheters allow for a more precise titrating of power throughout an application. Although concepts of force-time-power integrals to predict lesion adequacy have been validated in the atrium, no optimum values for these metrics have yet been defined for ablation in the normal or infarcted ventricle. Additionally, if deeper lesions are required for transmural ablation targets, the usual 0.9% saline irrigant can be substituted for 0.45% half-normal saline, albeit with a somewhat higher risk of steam pop formation.[120]

Several end points for individual RF energy applications are commonly used. Foremost among these is the clean termination of a tolerated VT at a site of perfect entrainment mapping during RF delivery. While this is a good sign that an effective ablation lesion has been created at a critical portion of the VT circuit, it does not imply that the circuit is permanently abolished and further ablation is often required to completely transect the diastolic isthmus and render the VT noninducible. Of course, suboptimal mapping, wide isthmuses, and deep (intramural or epicardial) arrhythmogenic tissue may also be the cause of failure to terminate VT despite producing a myocardial lesion; hence, other markers of lesion formation are required.

EGM attenuation is often used for this purpose, with the unipolar-tip EGM being most reliable given that bipolar signal attenuation may not be seen if the ring electrode contributes significantly to the bipolar EGM. The thickness of ventricular myocardium means this endpoint is often not observed despite effective lesion formation. Similarly, loss of late and isolated components of the local EGM is an encouraging sign. Loss of pace capture, or a significant rise in capture threshold, is also seen in dense scar but may be less frequently observed at the border zones where surrounding myocardium may still be captured after lesion delivery. Lesion formation can be acutely visualized using ICE, but this is a relatively insensitive technique and edema no doubt contributes significantly to the echogenic densities seen at the catheter tip, as they frequently disappear when reimaged a few minutes later. Given the limitations of all of these techniques, impedance drop (along with contact force monitoring where available) is the most frequently used marker of lesion formation in practice despite its less-than-ideal sensitivity and specificity.

Noninducibility remains the endpoint for most VT ablation procedures, particularly if VT was easily inducible at commencement. However, programmed stimulation is not entirely reliable for VT induction at the conclusion of the procedure and both perilesion edema and anesthesia may render VTs temporarily noninducible. Frankel et al. showed that noninducibility at delayed postprocedural noninvasive programmed stimulation through the ICD predicted a better VT-free medium-term outcome.[113] Alternative endpoints for substrate ablation include elimination of isolated potentials during high-density scar remapping, change in pace map morphology after linear ablation, mitral isthmus block for some inferior infarct VTs, electrical isolation of the VT machinery containing infarct core, dechanneling of previously documented conducting channels, and elimination of deceleration zones on ILAM remapping.[121]

Following catheter ablation, at least 6–12 weeks of anticoagulation are routine in order to prevent thrombus formation at endocardially denuded RF lesion sites. Recent data from the STROKE VT trial confirm that direct oral anticoagulants are superior to aspirin for this purpose, in reducing both clinical stokes and asymptomatic cerebral emboli.[52]

OUTCOMES

The efficacy of postinfarct VT ablation has been established in multiple randomized trials and prospective multicenter studies. For tolerated VTs, the historical medium-term success rates of an entrainment mapping-guided ablation procedure were variable but reasonable overall, with 67–91% of VTs successfully eliminated over 2- to 3-year follow-up.[122–124] However, these older series are generally presented with the denominator comprised of patients enrolled with reproducibly inducible mappable VT, a subgroup that represents the minority of real-world patients. The most contemporary outcome data from multicenter randomized trials using modern mapping systems and open-irrigated ablation catheters look at a larger cross-section of often extremely unwell patients with both mappable and unmappable VTs who have additional or exclusive substrate ablation performed.[7,8,47,104,114,125–127] In a recent meta-analysis of nine randomized trials of VT ablation versus medical therapy in structural heart disease patients, the vast majority of whom had postinfarct VT, Virk et al. found significant pooled reductions in VT recurrence, ICD shocks, and electrical storm with catheter ablation.[128] No mortality or heart failure benefit could be demonstrated.

While most patients can expect freedom from VTs that were specifically targeted and ablated, the development of new morphologies over time represents the single biggest reason for arrhythmia recurrence. Yokokawa et al. found that 33 of 98 patients (34%) with postinfarct VT recurred over mean 35-month follow-up following successful ablation of all clinical VTs.[129] Of the patients with recurrence, 79% had developed a new VT morphology and these were generally patients with a larger area of electroanatomically defined scar. Some data suggest similar VT-free outcomes may be achieved after repeat ablation with comparable overall survival as long as VT does not recur subsequently.[47]

Most patients with postinfarct VT have ICM and advanced structural heart disease. Not surprisingly, even if ablation achieves good arrhythmia control in these patients,[47] long-term mortality is high, up to 52% at 6 years.[130] Though the majority of these deaths are from progressive cardiac failure, some are sudden and ICD therapy is usually indicated, even after apparently successful VT ablation.

COMPLICATIONS

The nature and severity of the underlying heart disease, as well as the comorbidities frequently present in the postinfarct population (particularly peripheral vascular disease, cerebrovascular disease, and renal impairment), make scar-related VT ablation a riskier undertaking than other percutaneous procedures. Major complications occur in 5–8% of patients.[47,49] Recognized complications include death, myocardial infarction, stroke, aortic or mitral valve trauma, cardiac perforation with tamponade, heart block, coronary artery injury, cardiogenic shock, and vascular access site complications. Early mortality is seen in up to 5% of patients.[48] The incidence of complications is higher (up to 14%) if epicardial mapping and/or ablation is performed with additional risks related to pericardial bleeding, RV laceration, abdominal bleeding, phrenic nerve palsy, and coronary artery trauma.[100] Thorough procedural preparation and meticulous attention to detail during the case are mandatory to optimizing safety. Early detection of complications such as cardiac perforation with real-time ICE imaging allows for rapid intervention before end-organ damage ensues.

TROUBLESHOOTING THE DIFFICULT CASE

Catheter ablation of postinfarct scar-related VT is a complex and often challenging undertaking, and difficulties are to be expected, even in the ideal candidate (Table 33.2). The majority of the challenges surround unmappable VT morphologies where noninducibility and nontolerability frequently cause problems related to safety and efficacy. The widespread use of hemodynamic support and substrate-based ablation have helped improve both. Pleomorphic, unstable, and incessant VT can occur during the ablation procedure, often in patients who present with electrical storm, and repeated cardioversions may induce myocardial stunning.

In the era of open-irrigated ablation catheters, inadequate power delivery is rarely the cause of ablation failure in postinfarct VT and suboptimal mapping or poor contact force is more often to blame. High-resolution substrate mapping with multielectrode catheters and the use of varied and premature wavefronts during mapping, alternative access routes, and contact force sensing all have a role in overcoming these difficulties. The recognition of nonendocardial substrate and circuit components is critical to achieving success, and sequential attention may need to be directed to the epicardium, intramural tissue, RV, and papillary muscles in challenging cases.

TABLE 33.2 **Troubleshooting the Difficult Case**

Problem	Causes	Solution
Hemodynamic instability during VT	Advanced structural heart disease and ventricular dysfunction	Hemodynamic support with inotropes, IABP, LVAD, or ECMO Employ ultra-high-density multipolar mapping and terminate VT after short periods Use a predominantly substrate-based strategy in sinus rhythm
VT noninducible	Antiarrhythmic drugs GA or sedation Autonomically mediated Combination factors	Cease AAD as far in advance as possible Plan earlier ablation if possible, rather than adding more AAD after VT episodes Minimize sedation and repeat procedure awake if tolerated Aggressive programmed stimulation on isoproterenol/dopamine or epinephrine Accept noninducibility and execute substrate-based ablation strategy with alternate endpoints
Failure of ablation despite perfect entrainment map	Suboptimal entrainment map Poor catheter contact Wide isthmus Low power delivery	Review mapping data to ensure appropriate overdrive paced cycle length, concealed fusion, correct PPI and EGM-QRS interval measurement Improve contact with different catheter or approach (retrograde vs. transseptal), preformed sheath, ICE and/or contact force sensing Use GA with apnea or JET ventilation Linear lesion delivery to transect isthmus Use newer-generation open irrigated ablation catheters Use half-normal saline irrigant Use ICE to define anatomy of trabeculae/pouches etc. Use newer-generation open irrigated ablation catheters
Failure of endocardial catheter ablation	Insufficiently detailed endocardial mapping of VT circuits or substrate Insufficient ablation of surviving conduction channels within scar Critical VT circuit components are located epicardially, intramurally or endocavitary	Use multipolar or ultra-high-density mapping catheters to obtain more detailed mapping data of VT and/or substrate with varying wavefronts and prematurity Consider early RV mapping Use high-power ablation with newer-generation open irrigation catheters to obtain more complete endocardial substrate modification Early remapping of putative channels with high-density multipolar catheters Suspect early with ECG clues, diffuse early endocardial activation or lack of mid-diastolic activity Percutaneous or surgical pericardial access for epicardial mapping and ablation High-power ablation with newer-generation open irrigated catheters to create deeper lesions affecting intramural targets Use ICE to delineate papillary muscle and preoperative imaging to define papillary muscle involvement in scar

AAD, Antiarrhythmic drugs; *ECMO*, extracorporeal membrane oxygenation; *EGM*, electrogram; *GA*, general anesthesia; *IABP*, intra-aortic balloon pump; *ICE*, intracardiac echocardiography; *LVAD*, left ventricular assist device; *PPI*, postpacing interval; *RV*, right ventricle; *VT*, ventricular tachycardia.

CONCLUSIONS

Catheter ablation for postinfarct VT has become an established treatment option for patients with episodes of sustained VT and/or ICD therapies. These patients usually have advanced myocardial dysfunction and often present with electrical storm and multiple ICD shocks leading to significant morbidity and mortality. Medical options are limited in this context, and VT ablation often has a very positive mid-term clinical impact. The procedure had evolved considerably over the last few decades, and new mechanistic insights and technologies continue to drive improved safety and efficacy. Later relapse due to the emergence of new circuits accounts for the majority of VT recurrence following ablation and is reflective of both the dynamic evolution of the postinfarct ventricular substrate over time and the need for ICD therapy to mitigate against the ongoing risk of sudden death.

REFERENCES

Please refer to the e-book for a complete list of references.

34

Ablation of Ventricular Tachycardia in Nonischemic Cardiomyopathy

Frank Bogun, Konstantinos C. Siontis

KEY POINTS

- Entrainment mapping focuses on sites with concealed entrainment.
- Pace mapping and electrogram mapping focus on sites with fractionated electrograms and late potentials.
- Myocardial fibers within scar tissue are ablation targets.
- Preprocedural magnetic resonance imaging is used to assess for the presence and location of scar tissue.
- Intracardiac echo is used to assess for intracardiac structures such as papillary muscles, location of scar, or aneurysms.
- Ablation tools include 3.5-mm open-irrigated-tip catheter with bipolar ablation if necessary.
- Special ablation systems include irrigated-tip radiofrequency (RF) catheter, needle RF catheter, and bipolar or simultaneous unipolar RF ablation setup.
- RF delivery is 20–50 W for 60–120 seconds.
- Markers of success and endpoints for energy delivery are impedance drop, electrogram diminution, and pace noncapture.
- Sources of difficulty are the intramural and epicardial locations of the arrhythmogenic substrate.

DISEASE SPECTRUM

The term *nonischemic cardiomyopathy* (NICM) encompasses a spectrum of diseases, including dilated idiopathic cardiomyopathy, hereditary cardiomyopathy, cardiac sarcoidosis, and other forms of myocarditis, as well as Chagas disease, hypertrophic cardiomyopathy, amyloidosis, valvular heart disease, and arrhythmogenic right ventricular cardiomyopathy (ARVC). Most of these disease entities result in myocardial scar formation, thus creating a substrate for the subsequent development of ventricular arrhythmias. Ventricular tachycardias (VTs) are among the many clinical manifestations of disease in patients with NICM.

This chapter focuses on VT ablation in patients with idiopathic dilated cardiomyopathy, hereditary cardiomyopathy, myocarditis, cardiac sarcoidosis, ARVC, hypertrophic cardiomyopathy and Chagas disease.

ETIOLOGY AND CHARACTERIZATION OF THE ARRHYTHMOGENIC SUBSTRATE

A comprehensive evaluation using multiple diagnostic modalities is necessary to identify the etiology and to characterize the arrhythmogenic substrate in patients with NICM (Table 34.1). Commonly, no specific underlying disease process can be identified, and idiopathic dilated cardiomyopathy may be present, which often can be a sequela of myocarditis.[1] Cardiac magnetic resonance imaging (MRI) with delayed enhancement (DE-MRI) is an important modality that can offer key information regarding the etiology and the arrhythmogenic substrate in NICM.[2] Scar distribution in the cardiac MRI can indicate disease-specific patterns[3] of scarring that may be helpful in directing further workup in clarifying the underlying etiology of cardiomyopathy. It must be mentioned, however, that sarcoidosis can present diagnostic challenges, and there is no test that can definitively rule out cardiac sarcoidosis.[4] The workup for sarcoidosis requires biopsies (cardiac or noncardiac) to assess for the disease-specific histology of noncaseating granulomas.[4] A scar pattern in the DE-MRI with multifocal areas of delayed enhancement in the RV with basal septal involvement suggests, but does not prove, the presence of cardiac sarcoidosis.

It is important to keep in mind that frequent premature ventricular complexes (PVCs) may cause a reversible form of NICM. In patients who present with a cardiomyopathy of unclear etiology and who have a PVC burden >10–20%, catheter ablation of the PVC's is appropriate and may result in improvement or even reversal of cardiomyopathy.[5] Most often in these select cases, there is no delayed enhancement in the cardiac MRI, indicating that there is no other myopathic process present.

Most VTs in patients with NICM are due to reentry originating within scar tissue. DE-MRI is used as the gold standard for imaging of scar tissue (Fig. 34.1). Exact localization of the scar is of particular importance in patients with NICM. In patients with ischemic cardiomyopathy, the scar is typically located subendocardially, giving rise to VTs that can be reached by endocardial mapping. In NICM, on the other hand, intramural VT

TABLE 34.1 Arrhythmic Syndrome Diagnostic Criteria

Idiopathic dilated cardiomyopathy	Cardiomyopathy without obvious etiology despite diagnostic workup
Familial cardiomyopathy	Pathogenic mutations in cardiomyopathy genes, such as LMNA, TTN
Myocarditis	Viral infection of the myocardium resulting in acute or chronic myocarditis which may heal with or without sequelae (scar)
Sarcoid heart disease	Sarcoidosis involving the myocardium; can be part of systemic form or can be limited to the heart
Arrhythmogenic right ventricular cardiomyopathy	Predominantly right ventricular dilation and dysfunction; Task Force criteria for diagnosis
Hypertrophic cardiomyopathy	Cardiomyopathy associated with hypertrophy without obvious cause
Chagas disease	Cardiomyopathy caused by infection with the parasite *Trypanosoma cruzi*

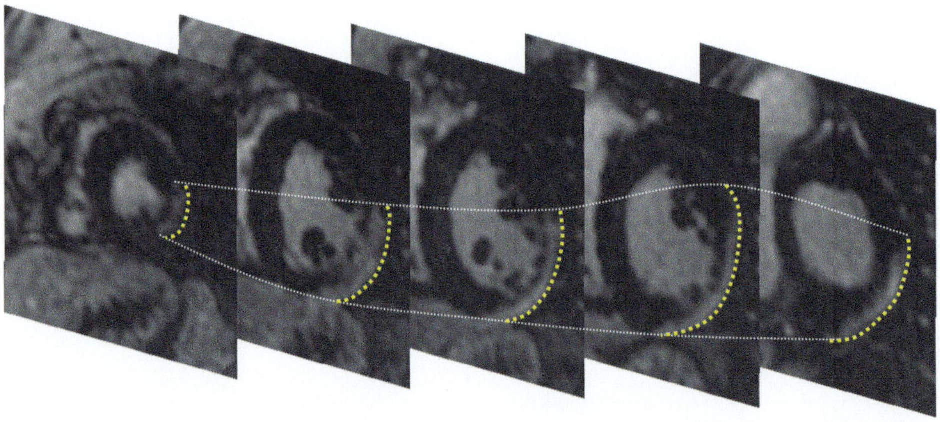

Fig. 34.1 Stack of short-axis views of a delayed-enhanced magnetic resonance image in a patient with nonischemic cardiomyopathy from base (*right*) toward apex (*left*). There is predominantly epicardial uptake of gadolinium, indicative of scar tissue (*yellow dotted lines*) in the basolateral left ventricle. (From Bogun FM, Desjardins B, Good E, et al. Delayed-enhanced magnetic resonance imaging in nonischemic cardiomyopathy: utility for identifying the ventricular arrhythmia substrate. *J Am Coll Cardiol.* 2009;53:1138–1145.)

and epicardial VTs are more frequent and may result in procedural failure if an endocardial-only approach is used.

Scar tissue can be differentiated from normal myocardium on T1-weighted MRI images, due to delayed contrast enhancement and the fact that gadolinium contrast agents shorten the longitudinal relaxation time (T1). Gadolinium contrast agents (gadolinium chelates) are unable to cross the intact cell membrane, and in the normal myocardium the tissue volume is mainly intracellular. Enhancement of the myocardium several minutes after intravenous injection of a gadolinium chelate indicates accumulation of contrast material in areas where the extracellular space is increased. In the setting of myocardial necrosis or inflammation, disruption of myocyte membranes causes an increased distribution space for gadolinium. In the setting of chronic scar formation, collagenous scar tissue has replaced the necrotic tissue, and the increase in interstitial tissue leads to an increased volume of distribution for the contrast agent, resulting in hyperenhancement.

DISEASE-SPECIFIC ARRHYTHMOGENIC SUBSTRATE

MRI, in addition to helping identify the arrhythmogenic substrate[2] and etiology, is of key importance in planning an effective ablation procedure.[6]

Idiopathic Dilated Cardiomyopathy

Reports focusing on the histologic findings in patients with dilated cardiomyopathy as well as conduction studies in these patients have demonstrated that the architecture, more than the amount of fibrosis, affects conduction velocity.[7] Discontinuous conduction resulting in unidirectional block can occur, especially in the presence of long strands of fibrosis and dense replacement fibrosis.[7,8] Based on whole-heart analyses in patients with NICM-related VT, fibrosis patterns are variable, but there is a correlation between viable myocardium and unipolar and bipolar voltage.[9] The presence of scar by DE-MRI has been correlated with the spontaneous occurrence of VT as well as the inducibility of VTs, and with outcome in patients with NICM even in the presence of preserved left ventricular (LV) function.[3,10–12] The hallmark of idiopathic dilated cardiomyopathy is the presence of mid-wall delayed enhancement. In a study by Neilan et al.,[13] intramural scarring was present in 52% of the patients. Predominant epicardial scarring was observed in 26%, and focal scarring involving insertion points was seen in 20% of the patients. There is a predominance of perivalvular scarring,[14] but the anteroseptal and inferolateral LVs have also been involved in the arrhythmogenic substrate in these patients.[15]

The presence of scarring, however, should prompt further workup including assessment for inflammation with positron-emission tomography (PET) and genetic testing, especially in the presence of a family history of cardiomyopathy.

Myocarditis

Acute myocarditis of any etiology can result in scarring and the development of cardiomyopathy. Ventricular arrhythmias are generally uncommon in acute myocarditis.[16] Among patients who have sustained arrhythmias during an acute myocarditis phase, these arrhythmias are often polymorphic VT or ventricular fibrillation.[17] In chronic myocarditis, there is intramural or epicardial scarring in addition to evidence of inflammation by endomyocardial biopsy or PET imaging.[18] In the majority of patients with ventricular arrhythmias, the scar is located intramurally, while epicardial scarring was present in about one-fourth of patients. The scar pattern is similar in patients presenting with VT late (i.e., a median of 13 months) after myocarditis.[19] It should be noted that it is not possible to distinguish between idiopathic dilated cardiomyopathy and healed myocarditis, as the scarring pattern can be similar, with predominantly intramural and epicardial distribution.[1]

Cardiac Sarcoidosis

Sarcoidosis can affect the myocardium in the form of an infiltrative cardiomyopathy with acute or chronic inflammation and subsequent scarring. The Japanese Health and Welfare Ministry criteria have been traditionally used to establish the criteria for cardiac involvement.[20] In 2014, the Heart Rhythm Society published a consensus statement including updated criteria for the diagnosis of cardiac sarcoidosis (Table 34.2).[4] A positive biopsy for the presence of noncaseating granulomas is key for making a definitive diagnosis of sarcoidosis. In the absence of a positive endomyocardial biopsy, the presence of specific criteria can be used to make a probable diagnosis of cardiac involvement provided noncaseating granulomas from an extracardiac source have been demonstrated. However, the revised 2017 Japanese guidelines allow for the diagnosis of cardiac sarcoidosis in the absence of a biopsy.[21] Hence, the diagnosis of isolated cardiac sarcoidosis is difficult and ideally requires a positive cardiac biopsy; not surprisingly, the prevalence of isolated cardiac sarcoidosis likely is underestimated[22] and requires a heightened index of suspicion. Electrogram-guided endomyocardial biopsy has the potential to increase the diagnostic yield as sarcoidosis involvement of the myocardium tends to be patchy.[23]

Granulomas start within the myocardium and reach the endocardium or epicardium via extension of the initial inflammatory lesions. In cardiac sarcoidosis, patchy, multifocal involvement, involvement of the basal septum, but also patterns involving predominantly the LV epicardium or the RV, have all been described.[24,25] Ventricular arrhythmias can occur in the acute inflammatory setting or in the chronic state when inflammatory tissue has been replaced by scar tissue. In the absence of acute inflammation, the location of scar determines the origin of most ventricular arrhythmias.[6] The presence and extent of delayed enhancement are known predictors of adverse outcomes in patients with cardiac sarcoidosis.[26] Similarly, the presence of ^{18}F-fluorodeoxyglucose (FDG) uptake in PET imaging in patients with cardiac sarcoidosis identifies patients at higher risk of VT or death.[27] Locally increased FDG uptake in the absence of a positive biopsy for sarcoidosis has been described, and the term *arrhythmogenic inflammatory cardiomyopathy* has been coined for this condition.[28] Cardiac sarcoidosis, in contradistinction to other cardiomyopathic processes, often affects the myocardium in a patchy pattern and may be missed with endomyocardial biopsies; hence, sarcoidosis is still in the differential diagnosis of an inflammatory cardiomyopathy.

TABLE 34.2 Heart Rhythm Society Diagnosis Criteria for Cardiac Sarcoidosis

1. Histologic Diagnosis
Cardiac sarcoidosis is diagnosed in the presence of noncaseating granuloma.
2. Clinical Diagnosis
Cardiac sarcoidosis is probable* if:
   a) There is extracardiac sarcoidosis
   and
   b) One or more of the following criteria:
      - Steroid ± immunosuppressant responsive cardiomyopathy or heart block
      - Unexplained ejection fraction <40%
      - Unexplained ventricular tachycardia (sustained or induced)
      - Advanced atrioventricular block
      - Patchy uptake on cardiac positron-emission tomography (in a pattern consistent with cardiac sarcoidosis)
      - Late gadolinium enhancement on magnetic resonance imaging (in a pattern consistent with cardiac sarcoidosis)
      - Positive gallium uptake (in a pattern consistent with cardiac sarcoidosis)
   and
   c) Other causes for cardiac manifestations have been excluded

*"Probable" indicates that there is sufficient evidence for making the diagnosis of cardiac sarcoidosis.
From Birnie DH, Sauer WH, Bogun F, et al. HRS expert consensus statement on the diagnosis and management of arrhythmias associated with cardiac sarcoidosis. *Heart Rhythm.* 2014;11:1305–1323.

Arrhythmogenic Cardiomyopathy

The Task Force Criteria for the diagnosis of arrhythmogenic cardiomyopathy (ARVC) were updated in 2010 (Table 34.3)[29] and will be discussed in more detail in the ARVC chapter. Of note is that limited data exist on the use of MRI in defining the arrhythmogenic substrate in patients with ARVC. Possible reasons include difficulties in imaging the thinner wall of the RV as well as differences in optimal inversion times of the RV if nulling is performed based on the LV.[30] In a study of 23 patients with ARVC who underwent both DE-MRI and endocardial voltage mapping, the DE-MRI failed to detect areas of scar in about half of the areas with low endocardial voltage, especially in the inferobasal RV.[31] Of note, the involvement of the LV in patients with ARVC has been well known and may be present in up to three-fourths of the patients. Intramyocardial LV fat as detected in multidetector computed tomography (MDCT) imaging was the most sensitive imaging finding in a recent series, but the correlation with low voltage was poor.[32] The phenotype of left-dominant arrhythmogenic cardiomyopathy caused by desmoplakin

TABLE 34.3 **Revised Task Force Criteria for the Diagnosis of ARVC/D[25]**

Right Ventricular Dysfunction and Structural Changes	
Major	Regional RV akinesis, dyskinesis, or aneurysm (echo, MRI, right ventriculography) **and** one or more criteria indicating RV dysfunction/dilatation by • ***Echocardiography:*** - PLAX RVOT ≥32 mm (corrected for body size [PLAX/BSA] ≥19 mm/m^2) - or PSAX RVOT ≥36 mm (corrected for body size [PSAX/BSA] ≥21 mm/m^2) - or fractional area change ≤33% • ***MRI:*** - Ratio of RV end-diastolic volume to BSA ≥110 mL/m^2 (male) or ≥100 mL/m^2 (female) - or RV ejection fraction ≤40%
Minor	Regional RV akinesis, dyskinesis, or aneurysm (echo, MRI, right ventriculography) **and** one or more criteria indicating RV dysfunction/dilatation by • ***Echocardiography:*** - PLAX RVOT ≥29 to <32 mm (corrected for body size [PLAX/BSA] ≥16 to <19 mm/m^2) - or PSAX RVOT ≥32 to <36 mm (corrected for body size [PSAX/BSA] ≥18 to <21 mm/m^2) - or fractional area change >33% to ≤40% • ***MRI:*** - Ratio of RV end-diastolic volume to BSA ≥100 to <110 mL/m^2 (male) or ≥90 to <100 mL/m^2 (female) - or RV ejection fraction >40% to ≤45%
Tissue Characterization	
Major	Residual myocytes <60% by morphometric analysis (or <50% if estimated), with fibrous replacement of the RV free wall myocardium in ≥1 sample, with or without fatty replacement of tissue on endomyocardial biopsy
Minor	Residual myocytes 60–75% by morphometric analysis (or 50–65% if estimated), with fibrous replacement of the RV free wall myocardium in ≥1 sample, with or without fatty replacement of tissue on endomyocardial biopsy
Repolarization Abnormalities	
Major	Inverted T waves in right precordial leads (V_1, V_2, and V_3) or beyond in individuals >14 years of age (in the absence of complete right bundle branch block QRS 120 ms)
Minor	- Inverted T waves in leads V_1 and V_2 in individuals >14 years of age (in the absence of complete right bundle branch block) or in V_4, V_5, or V_6 - Inverted T waves in leads V_1, V_2, V_3, and V_4 in individuals >14 years of age in the presence of complete right bundle branch block
Depolarization/Conduction Abnormalities	
Major	Epsilon wave (reproducible low-amplitude signals between end of QRS complex to onset of the T wave) in the right precordial leads (V_1–V_3)
Minor	- Late potentials by SAECG in ≥1/3 parameters in presence of QRS < 110 ms - Filtered QRS duration ≥114 ms - Duration of terminal QRS <40 µV ≥38 ms - Root-mean-square voltage of terminal 40 ms ≤20 µV - Terminal activation duration of QRS ≥55 ms (nadir S wave to end of QRS in V_1, V_2, or V_3)
Arrhythmias	
Major	- Sustained or nonsustained VT with left bundle branch block superior axis
Minor	- Nonsustained or sustained ventricular tachycardia of RV outflow configuration, left bundle branch block morphology with inferior axis (positive QRS in leads II, III, and aVF and negative in lead aVL), or of unknown axis - 500 ventricular extrasystoles per 24 hours (Holter)
Family History	
Major	- ARVC/D confirmed in first-degree relative (meeting Task Force criteria) - ARVC/D confirmed pathologically at autopsy or surgery in first-degree relative - Identification of a pathologic mutation during genetic testing in the patient under consideration
Minor	- ARVC/D in first-degree relative in whom Task Force criteria cannot be assessed - Premature SCD (<35 years old) caused by suspected ARVC/D in first-degree relative - ARVC/D confirmed pathologically or by current Task Force criteria in second-degree relative

ARVC/D, Arrhythmogenic right ventricular cardiomyopathy/dysplasia; *BSA*, body surface area; *PLAX*, parasternal long-axis view; *PSAX*, parasternal short-axis view; *PVC*, premature ventricular complex; *SAECG*, signal-averaged electrocardiogram; *SCD*, sudden cardiac death; *RV*, right ventricle; *RVOT*, right ventricular outflow tract; *VT*, ventricular tachycardia.

mutations, a gene implicated in the pathogenesis of ARVC, was recently described.[33]

Hypertrophic Cardiomyopathy

Hypertrophic cardiomyopathy (HCM) is the most common inherited cardiomyopathy with a prevalence approximating 1:500 in the general population.[34] The underlying genetic substrate typically includes pathogenic mutations in genes encoding sarcomeric proteins, though nonsarcomeric forms of HCM are also encountered. Even though phenotypic heterogeneity is present, the condition is universally characterized by myofiber hypertrophy and disarray resulting in pathologic wall thickening unexplained by loading conditions, causing LV outflow tract obstruction in some forms of the disease. The histologic substrate also provides the basis for early replacement fibrosis and predisposition to ventricular arrhythmias in HCM patients.[35] The presence of delayed enhancement in patients with HCM correlates with the presence of ventricular arrhythmias.[36] VT mapping and ablation procedures have been reported in a limited number of patients with HCM.[37] The value of MRI for correlation of the location of scar tissue with the origin of ventricular arrhythmias remains to be determined, however. Although no series of patients has been reported in which MRI was used systematically to map VT in patients with HCM, MRI has been helpful to indicate the arrhythmogenic substrate in data available.[37,38] Further, VF is a common mechanism of sudden death in HCM. Hocini et al. highlighted the role of Purkinje triggers in the initiation of VF in a series of HCM patients. These triggers were mapped and successfully ablated in hypertrophied segments with significant reduction in recurrent VF in all patients.[39]

Chagas Cardiomyopathy

Chagas cardiomyopathy results from myopericarditis as an immune response to infection with the parasite *Trypanosoma cruzi*, which is most prevalent in Central and South America. Neurogenic disturbances and coronary microvascular dysfunction are also implicated in the pathogenesis of the disease. Patients with Chagas heart disease are at high risk of ventricular tachyarrhythmias.[40] The arrhythmogenic substrate in Chagas cardiomyopathy typically involves the inferolateral LV. The value of scar imaging in identifying the arrhythmogenic substrate in this condition has not been systematically analyzed. Limited data with the use of DE-MR imaging suggest that more than two-thirds of patients have detectable myocardial fibrosis.[41] In one series, in the majority of cases (53%) the scar was endocardial, indistinguishable from postinfarction scarring. In only 12% of patients, the scarring was limited to the epicardium, and in 35% it was intramural,[42] with most of the scar being located in a lateral, inferolateral, and inferior wall.[43] Nevertheless, during simultaneous endocardial and epicardial electroanatomical mapping, the epicardium appears to harbor larger low-voltage areas compared to the endocardium.[44]

Familial Cardiomyopathy

Several pathogenic mutations have been reported to be associated with scar formation and a high prevalence of ventricular arrhythmias. Different mutations can result in different cardiomyopathy phenotypes including dilated cardiomyopathy and LV noncompaction cardiomyopathy. The most prevalent pathologic mutations include mutations of the *LMNA* gene and the *Titin* gene. Among 98 patients with NICM referred for VT ablation in one study, 37 (38%) had pathologic mutations for cardiomyopathy genes.[45] Patients with pathologic mutations had higher VT recurrence rates postablation. In particular, patients with LMNA mutations undergoing VT ablation procedures appear to have a poor prognosis.[46] Further, patients with TTN mutations had high recurrence rates after VT ablation[47]; it appears that the high recurrence rates were due to a high prevalence of intramural scarring in these patients. TTN mutations are often present in patients with LV noncompaction, and since intramural scarrring is prevalent in these patients, ablation procedures can be challenging and VT recurrence is not uncommon.[48]

PREABLATION WORKUP AND PROCEDURAL PLANNING

Different mapping strategies are possible as an initial approach in patients with NICM and VT. If endocardial mapping does not yield an effective ablation site, the coronary venous system can be mapped or a transcutaneous subxyphoid puncture to enter the pericardial space can be performed at a separate session (stepwise approach).[49] An alternative option to the stepwise approach is to enter the pericardial space during the first ablation procedure, before the administration of heparin or after reversal of anticoagulation, in all patients with NICM. Yet another approach is a substrate-specific approach that is guided by imaging and the location of the arrhythmogenic substrate. The location of the scar tissue often corresponds to areas critical for VT circuits in these patients.[6] The latter approach has the advantage that it only exposes patients to the increased periprocedural risk of epicardial puncture and mapping if the arrhythmogenic substrate either involves the epicardium or the intramural free wall. Furthermore, in patients with an intramural septal substrate, an upfront epicardial approach will be unnecessary and the scar depth as determined by DE-MRI can help predict the success of the ablation.[50] Unipolar mapping has been proposed as an alternative to estimate whether a deeper-seated scar is present. However, there is substantial overlap of unipolar low voltage between scar zones and regions of no scar. CMR with delayed enhancement remains the gold standard for exact demarcation of scars and, in our opinion, may be preferable over voltage mapping for defining distant scar.[51] Unipolar and bipolar voltage mapping may be beneficial if cardiac MRI is not available.

Most patients presenting for VT ablation have implantable cardioverter-defibrillators (ICDs), and historically MRI has been contraindicated (and still not performed at many institutions) in patients with implanted cardiac devices, despite mounting evidence that they can be safely performed in such patients with adequate precautions.[52,53] Even in patients with device-related imaging artifact, DE-MRIs can provide useful information regarding the substrate distribution to help guide mapping and ablation procedures of VT. In addition to DE-MRI, MDCT can also help in characterizing the arrhythmogenic substrate by identifying myocardial wall thinning. The feasibility of integrating DE-MRI and/or MDCT imaging data to the electroanatomical map has recently been demonstrated and has the potential to impact procedural management and outcomes in scar-related VT.[54]

If electrocardiographic VT documentation is available, this may help identify an area of interest.[55] ICD-stored electrograms of the VT(s) before the ablation procedure may serve as reference for induced VTs during the ablation procedure. The 12-lead ECG offers important information and may be helpful in deciding whether an arrhythmia may have an epicardial origin, particularly in the absence of a cardiac MRI.

SELECTION OF TARGET SITES FOR ABLATION

During the procedure, multipolar catheters are positioned in the high right atrium, the His bundle position, and the RV apex. It is important to have a catheter at the His position to assess for the presence of bundle branch reentry VT. The RV catheter is positioned at the RV apex, and the postpacing interval at this site is also helpful in diagnosing bundle branch reentry tachycardia, especially if the His deflection is difficult to appreciate.[56]

Programmed RV stimulation is used to induce VT. An electromagnetic mapping system is used in combination with an open irrigated-tip catheter and multielectrode catheters for mapping, navigation, and ablation. It is also helpful to use an intracardiac echo probe to identify the papillary muscles, aneurysms, or even epicardial scar to direct the mapping catheter in the correct direction.[57]

Endocardial activation and/or entrainment mapping (Fig. 34.2) is performed during VT if the VT is tolerated hemodynamically (Table 34.4). For VTs resulting in hemodynamic compromise, pace mapping and voltage mapping are performed at the same locations. VTs originating from an intramyocardial focus can be particularly challenging, since both entrainment mapping and pace mapping may only be helpful to get close to the epicardial or endocardial breakthrough sites. In case of hemodynamic compromise, percutaneous assist devices can maintain hemodynamic stability for a period of time that may be sufficient to more precisely identify breakthrough sites.[58] However, the use of hemodynamic support has not improved outcomes and may increase periprocedural complications, since large-bore arterial access is required.

Substrate mapping preceding programmed stimulation has the disadvantage of possibly rendering some VTs noninducible due to mechanical catheter contact.[59] Hence, induction of VT prior to substrate mapping may be beneficial. During substrate mapping, each point collected for the voltage map pacing is performed at sites with low voltage (bipolar voltage amplitude of <1.5 mV), late potentials (LPs), or fractionated electrograms. LPs, or local abnormal ventricular activities (LAVAs),[60] are particularly helpful in postinfarction patients to guide radiofrequency (RF) ablation (Fig. 34.3). Although their prevalence is lower in patients with NICM,[61] it appears that they are equally, if not more, helpful in NICM patients.[62] A good pace map (defined as ≥10/12 matching leads between the pace map and the targeted VT) at a site where there is an LP is useful for identifying a critical component of the reentry circuit (Fig. 34.3). A good pace map at a site without an LP is a less specific indicator of a critical site for ablation. Histologic analysis adjacent to sites where matching pace maps were identified and where ablation was performed indicates that diffuse fibrosis patterns are present in the area composing the arrhythmogenic substrate. More

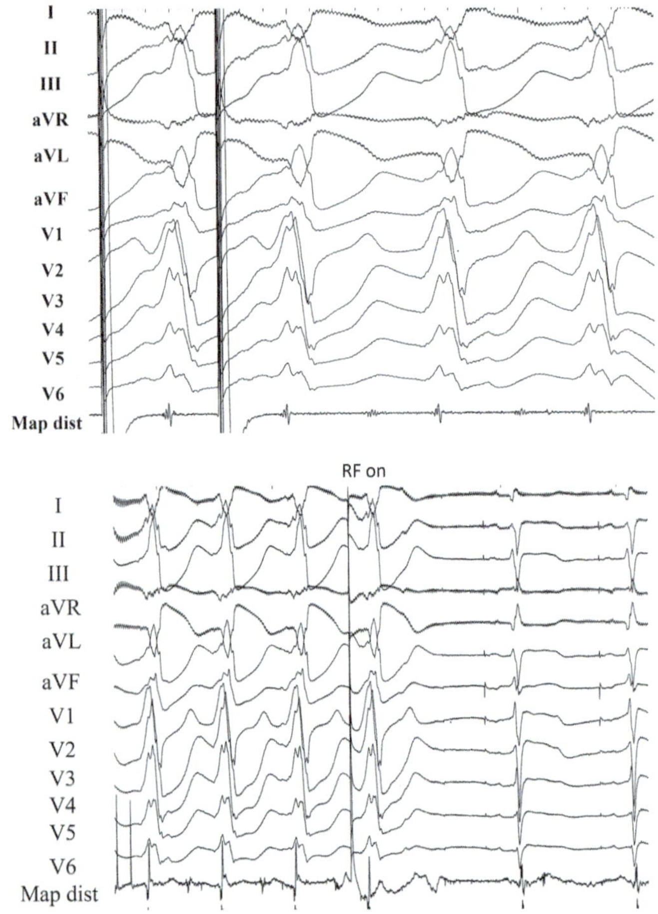

Fig. 34.2 (A) An effective ablation site in a patient with nonischemic cardiomyopathy. The catheter is located in the lateral left ventricular epicardium. There is concealed entrainment and a mid-diastolic potential during VT. The electrogram–QRS interval matches the stimulus–QRS interval (both are 230 ms). Pacing cycle length is 500 ms, and the VT cycle length is 650 ms. (B) Immediate termination of the VT shown in Fig. 34.2A when radiofrequency energy is delivered (RF on) at this location with 20 W using an open-irrigated ablation catheter.

TABLE 34.4 Target Sites for Ablation

	Target Site
During sinus rhythm	Isolated late potentials, local abnormal ventricular activity potentials
	Matching pace map (≥10/12 leads)
	Connecting low-voltage zones to areas of scar/barriers
	Deceleration zone
During ventricular tachycardia	Concealed entrainment
	Mid-diastolic potentials
	Fractionated electrograms

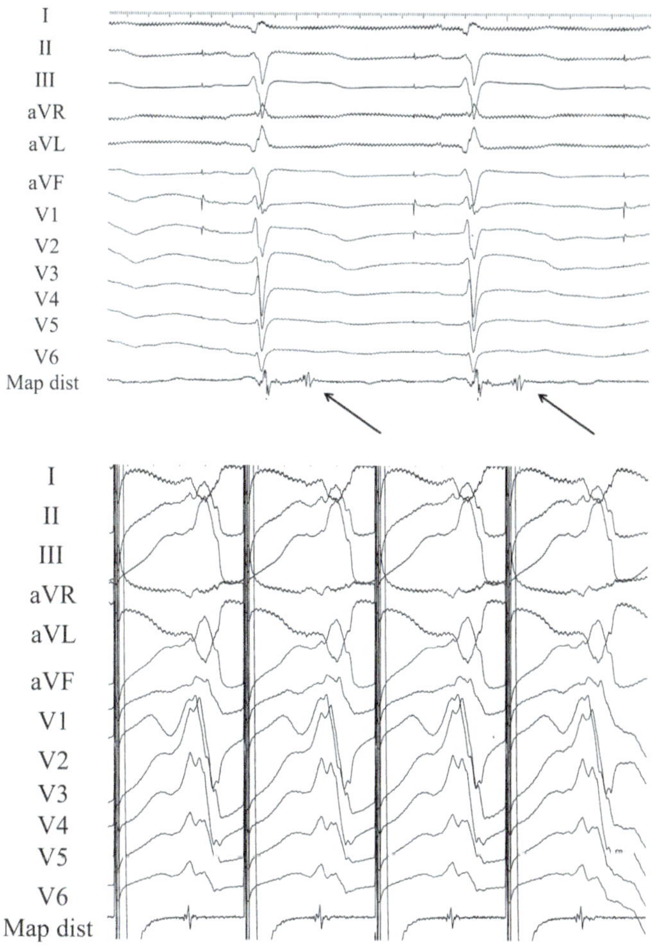

Fig. 34.3 (A) At the same site as illustrated in Fig. 34.2, isolated late potentials were present during the atrial paced rhythm (*arrows*). (B) Pacing at this location (Fig. 34.3A) during baseline rhythm showed a QRS complex that was identical to the patient's VT, with a long stimulus–QRS interval.

recently, the use of high-density substrate mapping with multipolar catheters has demonstrated the potential value of zones of conduction deceleration that are critical to arrhythmogenic circuits as ablation targets.[63]

LPs reflect fixed scar tissue (Table 34.4). They can be identified in approximately 50% of patients undergoing mapping and ablation of VT in the setting of NICM. LPs with very low amplitude may be easier to identify with a multielectrode mapping catheter with closely spaced electrodes compared to the ablation catheter. It is possible that fixed scar tissue in patients with NICM plays less of a role and that diffuse fibrosis and/or functional areas of block are more prevalent in patients in whom LPs cannot be identified. This may have important implications, since procedures with ablation over limited surface areas are less likely to eliminate VTs in these patients. Patients devoid of LPs appear to have a less favorable outcome with respect to ablation.[62] However, although none may be present on the endocardium, LPs may be found during epicardial mapping. Some patients do not have LPs or detectable scar tissue at either endocardial or epicardial locations. In these patients, the scar is often diffuse or intramural in location.

In a nonrandomized study of 93 patients with dilated NICM, two different approaches for selecting ablation targets were compared: standard ablation guided by detailed substrate, pace and activation/entrainment mapping versus "scar homogenization" targeting all abnormal electrograms in the identified scar.[64] The latter approach was associated with improved acute and long-term outcome, but results were overall inferior compared to what has been previously observed in patients with infarct-related VT.[65] Such a difference is likely attributable to the more complex arrhythmogenic substrate in NICM, particularly the common intramural distribution of the scar.

ABLATION TECHNIQUE AND ENDPOINTS

RF energy is delivered to the endocardium using open-irrigated-tip catheters. The power setting is adjusted to an impedance drop of 10–15 Ω, starting with 30–35 W, and can be increased up to 50 W. Pace capture loss at 10–20 mA, 2-ms pacing should be confirmed before the catheter is moved to a new ablation site; if an intramural focus is suspected, longer and high-power ablation lesions may be required.

Prior to an epicardial ablation, a coronary angiogram is obtained to ensure a distance of at least 1 cm from a major coronary artery. For smaller branches, a distance of 0.5 cm from the ablation catheter is usually safe. RF energy is delivered at an initial power of 20–30 W, and the power is titrated to achieve an impedance drop of 10 Ω, though energy delivery settings vary across centers and operators. The duration of the RF energy application is the same as described above for endocardial ablation. High-output pacing is performed to assess for phrenic nerve capture when ablating on the lateral LV epicardium. After the ablation, a coronary angiogram may be repeated to rule out coronary injury.

If RF energy is delivered in the coronary venous system, an irrigated-tip catheter is used with an initial power of 15 W, titrating the energy to achieve a 10-Ω impedance drop.

The endpoint of the procedure is noninducibility of VTs that were inducible in the beginning of the procedure. Piers et al. showed that in the setting of NICM elimination of all inducible VTs is superior to targeting only the VTs that have been clinically documented.[66] However, noninducibility of all VTs was only achieved in 38% of patients in that study. In a more recent study, complete noninducibility was achieved in 61% of patients and these patients had significantly more favorable long-term outcomes compared to patients with inducible VTs at the end of the procedure.[67] For cases where no VT is inducible at procedure onset, the procedural endpoint is less clear. In those patients, elimination of all late activation, defined as LPs or LAVAs, within and surrounding areas of substrate abnormality may be used as a surrogate endpoint.

DISEASE-SPECIFIC CONSIDERATIONS FOR ABLATION

Idiopathic Dilated Cardiomyopathy

The arrhythmogenic substrate can be located within the endocardium, the epicardium, or the myocardium (intramural). An imaging-guided approach has been found to be helpful (Fig. 34.4) in order to determine whether an epicardial

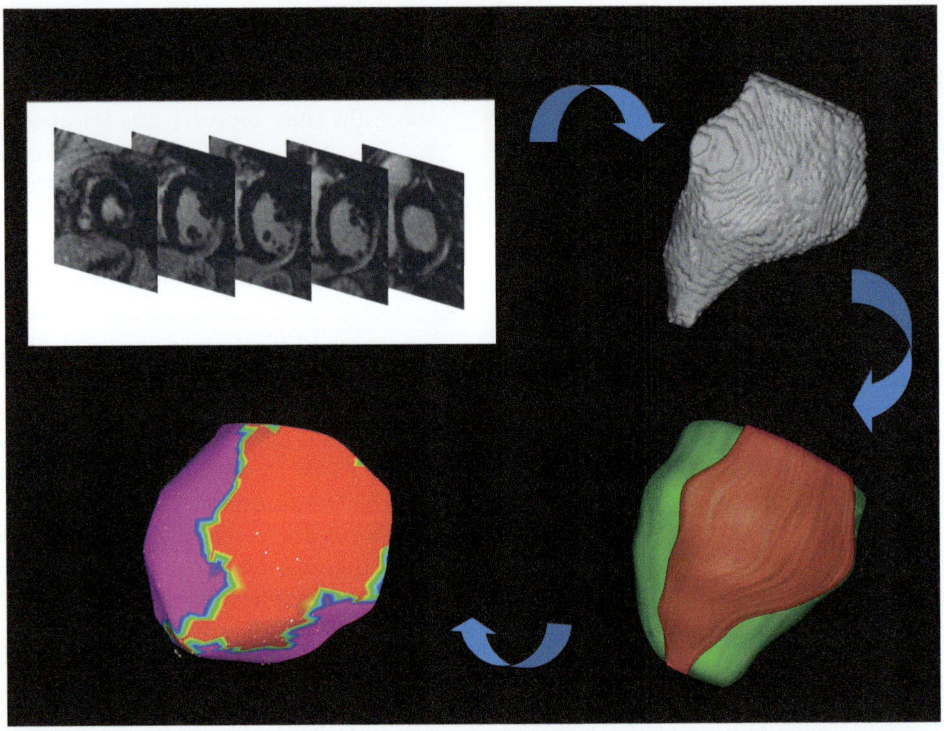

Fig. 34.4 *Top left,* Stack of short-axis views of cardiac magnetic resonance imaging from a patient with nonischemic cardiomyopathy. There is a predominant epicardial scar in the lateral left ventricle (*yellow dotted lines*). *Top right,* Three-dimensional reconstructed scar. *Bottom right,* Three-dimensional reconstruction of the epicardial surface (green) and the epicardial scar (*red*). *Bottom left,* Epicardial electroanatomical voltage map (CARTO) of the same region. Low-voltage tissue (bipolar voltage <1.5 mV) is colored in *red,* and normal voltage tissue is colored in *purple.* Three VT target sites were identified in this patient by entrainment and pace mapping they were all located in the epicardium (*yellow tags*). (From Bogun FM, Desjardins B, Good E, et al. Delayed-enhanced magnetic resonance imaging in nonischemic cardiomyopathy: utility for identifying the ventricular arrhythmia substrate. *J Am Coll Cardiol.* 2009;53:1138–1145.)

procedure may be necessary.[6,15,68] ECG criteria have been also used to determine whether a VT originates from the epicardium (Table 34.5). Intramural septal scar (Fig. 34.5A) is a particular challenge, since endocardial ablations from either side of the septum may be insufficient to reach the intramural scar. In the presence of an intramural septal scar, an epicardial ablation procedure will often be unsuccessful. There are no specific ECG criteria to suggest intramural origin of VT, but unipolar voltage mapping[51] (Fig. 34.5B) and prolonged transmural septal conduction times[69] can be helpful to identify intramural scar in the absence of a cardiac MRI. Other indicators for an intramural substrate is arrhythmia suppression,

TABLE 34.5 Electrocardiographic Criteria for Epicardial Origin of Ventricular Tachycardia

Criterion	Measure to Suggest Epicardial Origin
Pseudodelta wave[96]	≥34 ms
Intrinsicoid deflection in V_2[96]	≥85 ms
RS duration[96]	≥121 ms
Absence of q waves in inferior leads[55]	NA
Presence of q waves in lead I[55]	NA
Maximal deflection index[97]	≥0.55

when cold saline is injected into the great cardiac vein.[70] Furthermore, dual-site pace mapping has been described where paced QRS complexes from two breakout sites are averaged generating a better pace map compared to pace mapping from either side of the intramural substrate.[71] For targeting intramural septal scars, RF energy is delivered at the endocardial breakthrough sites. Deeper lesions may be achieved if the mapping catheter is positioned perpendicular to the endocardium and delivering high-power (40–50 W) RF energy for >60 seconds. Sequential unipolar ablations from either side of the septum may be necessary. Ablation delivered in a bipolar manner between the tips of two catheters may achieve even larger lesions.[72] Wire mapping of coronary septal veins can identify critical sites and guide endocardial ablation at the most proximal anatomical location.[73] Alternatively, if a septal perforator vein can be reached with an ablation catheter, cases of successful ablation of intramural ventricular arrhythmias from within that vein have been reported.[74] Coiling of perforator arteries or transcoronary venous ethanol ablation can also effectively eliminate intramural scar-related VTs.[75,76] Most recently, open-irrigated catheters with an extendable needle for intramyocardial mapping and ablation have been described for the treatment of VTs with a possibly intramural origin.[77,78] These catheters remain thus far investigational. Further, the use of half-normal saline irrigation, as well as

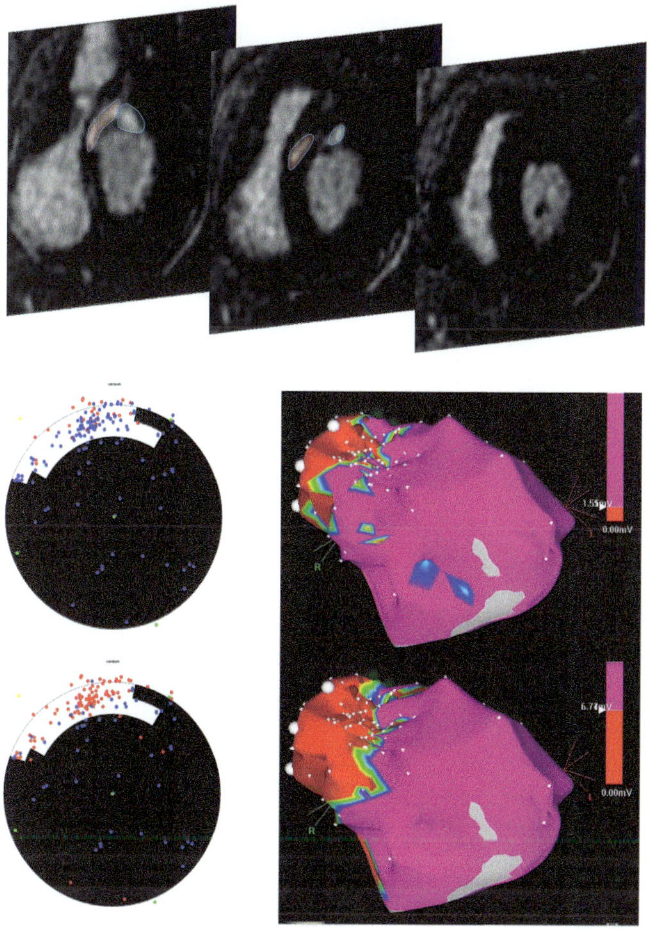

Fig. 34.5 (A) Intramural septal scar (*red area*) shown in a stacked short-axis view of a delayed enhanced cardiac magnetic resonance imaging from base (*left*) toward apex (*right*). There is an endocardial area of delayed enhancement (*green*) representing radiofrequency lesions after two failed endocardial ablation attempts. (B) *Top left*, Polar map of the area of delayed enhancement. Blue tags indicate normal voltage mapping sites with a bipolar voltage ≥1.55 mV. *Red tags* indicate low voltage (<1.55 mV). The corresponding electroanatomical map of the left ventricle is shown on the *top right panel*. The area of low voltage reflects the area where ablation lesions were delivered during prior procedures. The *bottom left panel* shows the same polar map with normal voltage mapping sites with unipolar voltage ≥6.8 mV. Sites with low unipolar voltage (<6.8 mV) are displayed in *red*. The corresponding unipolar voltage map with a cut-off value of 6.8 mV is shown to the *right*. It reflects the location of the intramural scar. (From Desjardins B, Yokokawa M, Good, E, et al. Characteristics of intramural scar in patients with nonischemic cardiomyopathy and relation to intramural ventricular arrhythmias. *Circ Arrhythm Electrophysiol.* 2013;6:891–897.)

bipolar and simultaneous unipolar RF catheter ablation, can help create larger ablation lesions that can reach deeper myocardial targets.[79,80]

A number of recent studies have reported on the outcomes of catheter ablation in idiopathic dilated NICM.[61,66,81–83] The acute success rate (complete noninducibility of any VT at the end of the procedure) ranged widely from 38% to 82%. Intermediate- to long-term VT recurrence rates ranged from 14% to 53% in these studies. In another study, the routine use of preablation substrate imaging with DE-MRI was associated with improved outcomes of VT ablation in idiopathic dilated NICM.[68] In the imaging group, RF ablation energy was delivered to areas with intramural scarring where VTs originated, hence improving outcomes, compared to a control group of patients where the precise location of intramural scarring was not known, and ablation was performed without image guidance. It remains to be shown whether other novel promising approaches of substrate characterization, mapping, and ablation that are currently under investigation may improve the acute and long-term outcomes of ablation.

More recently, a stepwise ablation approach based on imaging demonstrated that imaging is beneficial in preprocedural planning, and also predicts patients with a high risk of VT recurrence. The latter patients have a particularly high percentage of their scar volume located in deeper seated areas of the intramural myocardium[50] (Fig. 34.6).

Myocarditis

Safety and efficacy of RF ablation in patients with myocarditis has been described.[84] In the study by Dello Russo et al. involving 20 patients with chronic myocarditis, 6 (30%) required an epicardial approach to suppress VT, as endocardial ablation was ineffective. No data on MRI results were provided in this study, but imaging studies have reported epicardial involvement in almost 40% of patients with chronic myocarditis,[18] corresponding with the mapping and ablation data by Dello Russo et al.[84] In a more recent study of 23 patients with VT late after myocarditis who had endocardial and epicardial voltage mapping, most patients had epicardial low-voltage scar (14/19) while endocardial scar was uncommon (only 1 patient). DE-MRI data were consistent with this finding and demonstrated predominantly epicardial and intramural scar. The ablation strategy focused on abolition of LPs and epicardial ablation was required in 15 patients. At a median follow-up of 23 months, three-fourths of patients were free of recurrent VT.[19]

Cardiac Sarcoidosis

In patients with cardiac sarcoidosis, catheter ablation is often reserved for patients who have failed to respond to immunosuppressive therapy and antiarrhythmic medications. Most VTs in the absence of active inflammation have a reentrant mechanism and can be mapped using entrainment mapping and pace mapping depending on hemodynamic tolerance. RV involvement is common, and differentiation of cardiac sarcoidosis from arrhythmogenic RV dysplasia is important, since diagnostic criteria overlap.[85] Both noninvasive ECG and invasive electroanatomical mapping criteria can facilitate this distinction,[86,87] though genetic testing for ARVC and histologic analysis for sarcoidosis, whenever possible, provide the most definitive evidence. In patients with predominant RV involvement, the most frequent location of the reentry circuit is the paratricuspid area. In patients with epicardial scarring, an epicardial approach was necessary to eliminate VT. Similar to other forms of NICM, the location of scar tissue predicts the origin of VTs in these patients. Therefore an approach that plans the ablation procedure based on the predominant location of scarring as detected by DE-MRI is helpful in eliminating VTs in these patients.[6] In cases with intramurally located scars, the ability to eliminate VT was suboptimal.

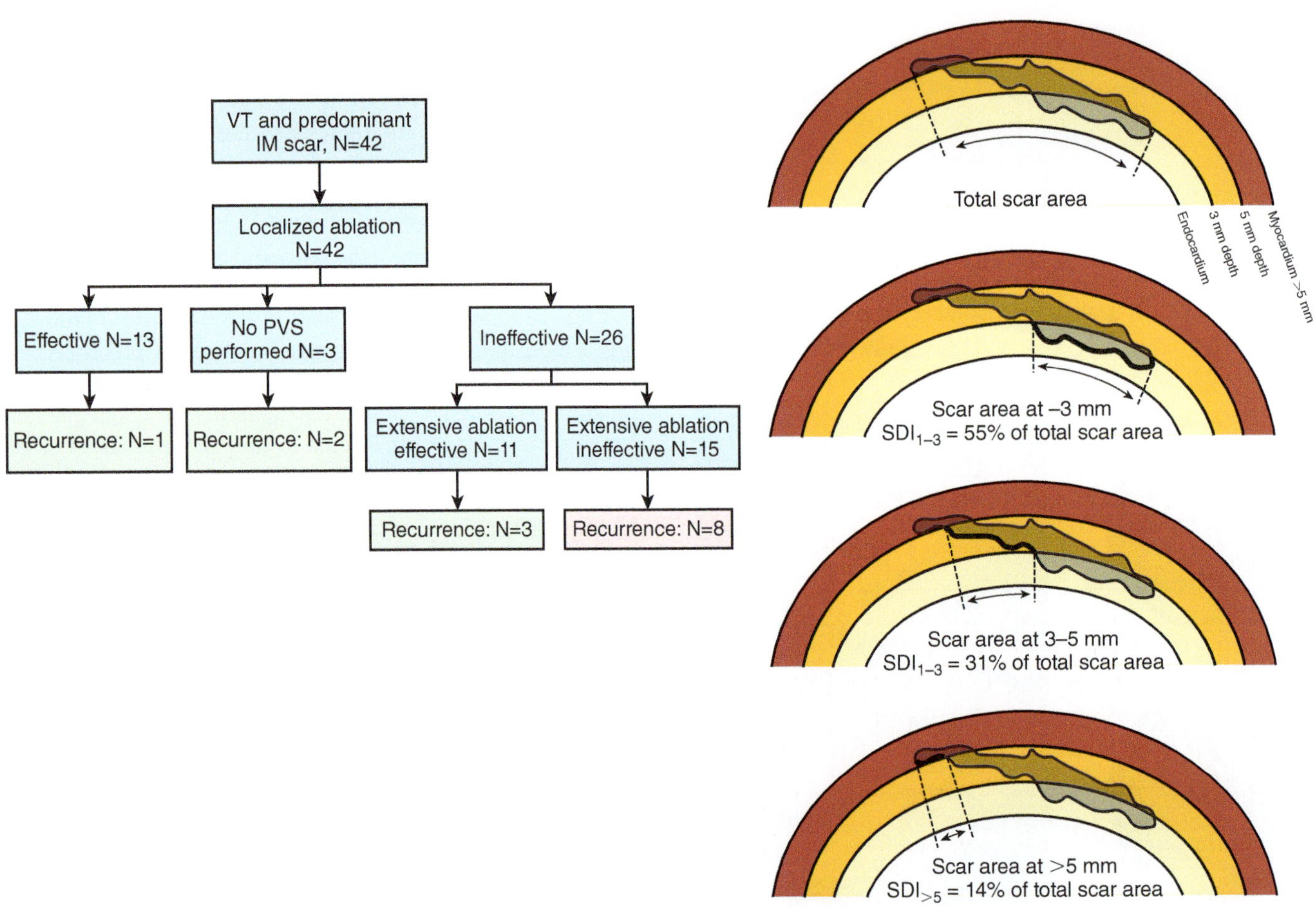

Fig. 34.6 *Left,* (A) A stepwise strategy is performed consisting of localized ablation guided by conventional mapping criteria followed by a more extensive ablation if ventricular tachycardia remained inducible. The extensive ablation was guided by the location and extent of intramural scarring on delayed enhanced cardiac magnetic resonance imaging. *Right,* (B) Demonstration of scar distribution in relation to distance of different areas of the scar from the endocardium. The scar depth index (SDI) is calculated as the percentage of the scar area seated at <3 mm, 3–5 mm, and >5 mm for SDI$_{0-3}$, SDI$_{3-5}$, and SDI$_{>5}$, respectively. Higher SDI$_{>5}$ is associated with worse acute and long-term ablation outcomes.[50] (Figure 34.6 is modified from Ghannam M, Siontis KC, Kim HM, et al. Stepwise Approach for Ventricular Tachycardia Ablation in Patients With Predominantly Intramural Scar. *JACC Clin Electrophysiol.* 2020;6:448–460.)

Several, but not all, of the patients included in this study had cardiac sarcoidosis. However, often in cardiac sarcoidosis the areas of delayed enhancement are multifocal and involve the RV and LVe; it may be difficult to predict which of the areas with delayed enhancement are arrhythmogenic based on the MRI.

Ablation outcomes in small, single-center cohorts have been generally favorable.[88] In a recent multicenter study of 158 patients with sarcoidosis-related VT, almost half of patients experienced a VT recurrence during a median follow-up of 2.5 years, but catheter ablation significantly reduced ICD shocks and need for antiarrhythmic medications.[89] Catheter ablation was also effective in eliminating VT storm in patients who presented with that arrhythmia phenotype. Active myocardial inflammation and reduced LV function preablation were the most significant predictors of adverse ablation outcome. This suggests that the timing of ablative intervention is important and ablation earlier in the disease course may be beneficial, especially in the presence of more preserved LV function and absence of inflammation. However ,many patients will require repeat ablations and concomitant treatment with immunosuppression and/or antiarrhythmic medications partly owing to the relapsing-remitting nature of myocardial inflammation in cardiac sarcoidosis.

Arrhythmogenic Right Ventricular Cardiomyopathy

The specific characteristics of ARVC relevant to VT ablation is specified in Chapter 40.

Hypertrophic Cardiomyopathy

In some series, epicardial ablation was needed in more than half of the patients with hypertrophic cardiomyopathy to eliminate targeted VTs.[37,90] Evidence of scarring is often present in the epicardium[90] but also intramurally in the interventricular septum. Extension of the scar from the septum to the epicardium may result in VT target sites being located in the epicardium (Fig. 34.7). The most common sites critical for VT were located

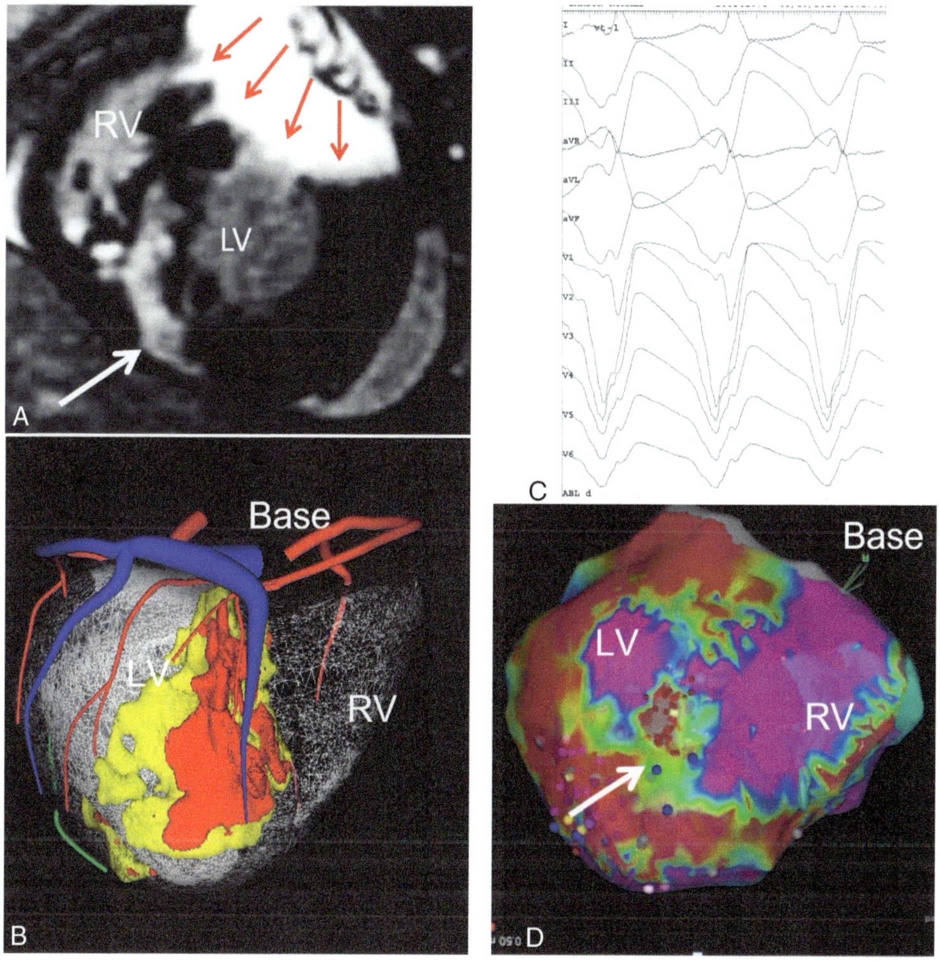

Fig. 34.7 Imaging and image reconstructions from a patient with hypertrophic cardiomyopathy who underwent ventricular tachycardia (VT) ablation. The VT was successfully ablated from the epicardium. The InHEART software was used to integrate cardiac anatomy. (A) Short-axis view of the cardiac magnetic resonance imaging (CMR) in the mid ventricular level. *Red arrows* indicate artifact from the patient's ICD. The *white arrow* indicates extension of the intramural area of late gadolinium enhancement (LGE) to the epicardium. The left and right ventricles (LV and RV) are indicated. (B) Three-D reconstruction of the CMR with the area of LGE in *yellow* (total scar) and *red* (core scar). (C) 12-lead ECG of the clinical VT of the patient. (D) Electroanatomical bipolar epicardial voltage map (CARTO) in the same orientation as the three-dimensional reconstruction of the CMR. There is low voltage in the apical and paraseptal area. A *white arrow* indicates the VT target site. VT was no longer inducible after ablation in this area.

in the LV apex (specifically in the apical form of HCM) and the RV insertion sites on the septum.[37,90]

Chagas Disease

The disease process often involves the inferolateral LV and results in aneurysm formation. In a report by Sosa et al.,[91] the majority of induced VTs had an epicardial origin. There may indeed be a predominance of epicardial circuits in Chagas disease necessitating a combined endocardial/epicardial approach. In one series, approximately 50% of VTs were eliminated from the epicardium and about 50% could be reached[92] from the endocardium, confirming the value of a combined endo/epicardial approach in patients with Chagas disease. In a more recent series of 17 patients who underwent combined endocardial and epicardial procedures, results were more favorable (83.3% acute success).[44] In a randomized trial comparing endocardial-only versus combined endocardial and epicardial ablation procedures in 30 patients with Chagasic VT, acute success was achieved in 6 patients (40%) in the endo-only group and 13 patients (86%) in the endo/epi group ($P = .021$).[93] VT recurrence at 2-year follow-up was 80% in the endo-only group and 40% in the endo/epi group ($P = .02$ by intention-to-treat). This suggests that upfront epicardial access for mapping/ablation is often beneficial in Chagasic VT.

Bundle Branch Reentry Tachycardia

Bundle branch reentry tachycardia has been described in up to one-third of patients with different forms of NICM (Fig. 34.8A),[94] although estimates from contemporary practice are lacking. Whereas it can occur in different forms of

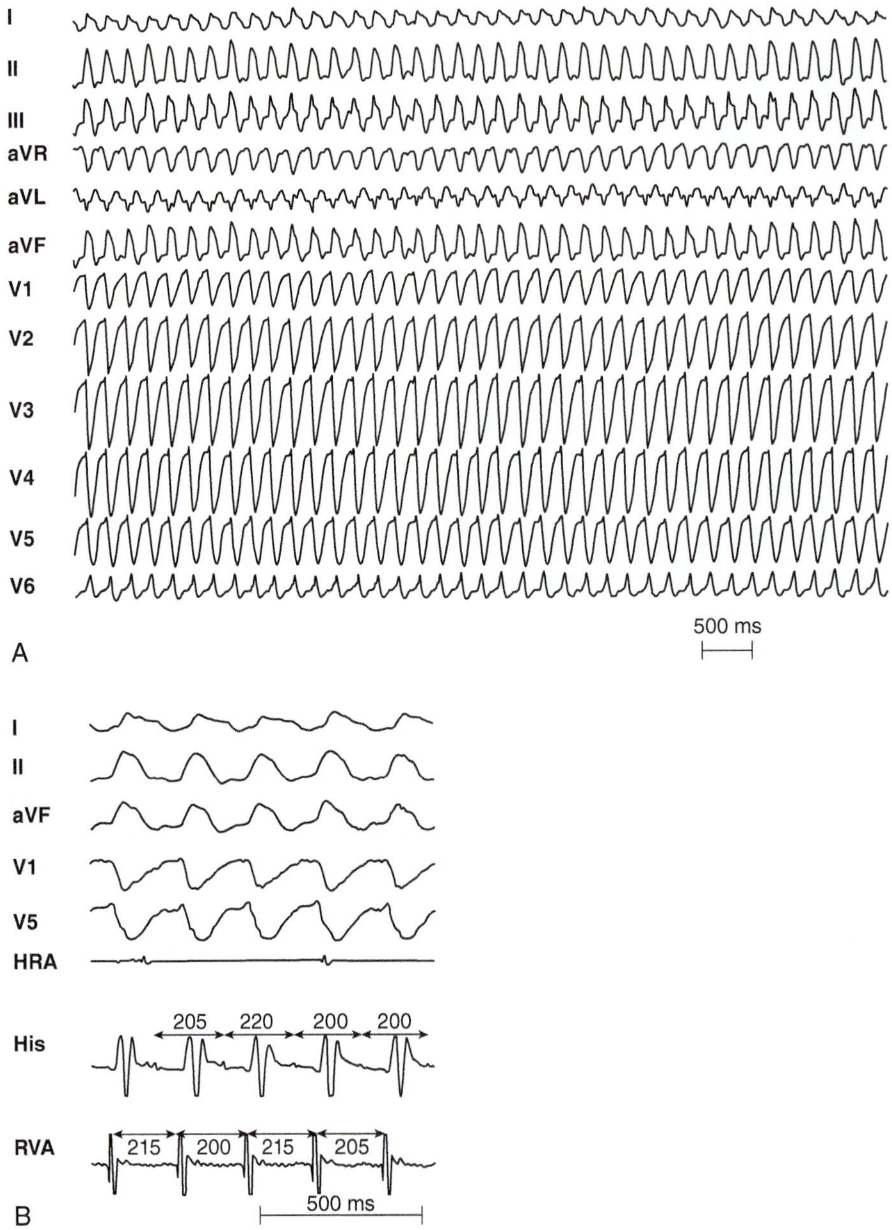

Fig. 34.8 (A) 12-lead electrocardiogram (ECG) of a clinical ventricular tachycardia (VT) in a patient with idiopathic dilated cardiomyopathy. The VT cycle length was 220 ms, with left bundle branch block inferior axis morphology. (B) Surface ECG leads I, II, aVF, V_1, and V_5, and intracardiac tracings of the high right atrium, the His position, and the right ventricular apex. The HH intervals are indicated on top of the His tracings, and the RR intervals are indicated on top of the ventricular electrograms of the right ventricular catheter. Changes in the HH interval precede changes in the RR intervals, although the changes are not identical. The VT was reproducibly inducible prior to ablation of the right bundle and was noninducible thereafter. The patient had no recurrent VT at 4-year follow-up.

cardiomyopathy, it has been found as a frequent mechanism of VT in patients with myotonic dystrophy. Its hallmark characteristic is baseline conduction abnormality with a prolonged HV interval. The left and right bundle branches are key components of the reentrant circuit. During bundle branch reentrant tachycardia, changes in the HH interval result in corresponding changes in the following VV intervals (Fig. 34.8B). Ablation of the right bundle branch usually eliminates bundle branch reentry tachycardia.

TROUBLESHOOTING THE DIFFICULT CASE

Important challenges and corresponding approaches to troubleshooting the difficult case are shown in Table 34.6. The main challenge with NICM is identifying an optimal mapping strategy in the event that the arrhythmogenic substrate cannot be identified with endocardial mapping. Epicardial mapping and ablation with a subxyphoid access (or surgical epicardial access if previous cardiac surgery was performed) can be

TABLE 34.6 Troubleshooting the Difficult Case

Problem	Causes	Solution
Unable to identify endocardial VT origin	Epicardial scar	Epicardial mapping
Unable to identify endocardial or epicardial origin	Intramural scar	Intramural ablationAblation from • Endocardial/epicardial surface for free wall scar • Left/right ventricular endocardium for septal scar
Inability to rule out BBRVT	Incorrect catheter position	• Diagnostic catheter at His position • Entrainment pacing from RV apex to assess for postpacing interval
Inability to rule out cusp VTs	Cusp is not mapped	Perform activation and pace mapping in all three aortic cusps
Inability to eliminate mid-myocardial VT	Deep-seated arrhythmogenic substrate	• High-power ablation from both sides of the myocardium sequentially • Half-normal saline • Bipolar or simultaneous unipolar ablation • Needle-tip ablation • Coronary venous or arterial ethanol ablation • Stereotectic body radiation

BBRVT, Bundle branch reentrant ventricular tachycardia; *VT*, ventricular tachycardia.

helpful depending on the underlying substrate (see the surgical ablation Chapters 37 and 41 for further details). This can be avoided to some extent by preprocedural MRI. In the presence of contraindications to MRI, such as advanced renal failure or a morbidly obese body habitus, unipolar voltage mapping is helpful in identifying an intramural or epicardial scar. In the presence of intramural scar, the breakthrough sites of the VT may need to be identified. Ablation from both aspects of the intramural scar can be considered with conventional unipolar ablation, but deeper lesions can be generated when RF ablation is performed between two ablation catheters in a bipolar manner or with the use of other techniques such as coronary venous ethanol ablation or needle-tip catheter ablation.[75–78,80] Stereotactic body radiation therapy is also being used as a noninvasive ablation option in patients with challenging substrate and prior failed conventional ablation procedures.[95] Reproducibility of acute effects across centers and data on long-term effectiveness remain under investigation.

REFERENCES

Please refer to the e-book for a complete list of references.

35

Ablation of Unstable Ventricular Tachycardia and Idiopathic Ventricular Fibrillation

Jacob S. Koruth, Iwanari Kawamura, William Whang, Vivek Y. Reddy, Srinivas R. Dukkipati

KEY POINTS

- Substrate mapping is performed to delineate the scarred myocardium in unstable ventricular tachycardia (VT).
- For ventricular fibrillation (VF), mapping is performed to identify the focal origin of triggers.
- Targets for substrate ablation include VT exit sites identified by pace mapping, sites identified by brief resetting and entrainment mapping, late and fractionated potentials, sites with local abnormal ventricular activity, and channels between dense ("electrically unexcitable") scar. Ablation to "homogenize" the scar area is an alternative effective approach.
- Targets for focal VF are premature ventricular complex (PVC) triggers preceded by Purkinje potentials or originating from the ventricular outflow tract or papillary muscle.
- Preoperative imaging such as computed tomography scan or magnetic resonance imaging may help guide the mapping strategy.
- Sources of difficulty include epicardial and intramyocardial VT circuits, and for VF ablation, PVC triggers that are difficult to induce.

INTRODUCTION

Catheter ablation of ventricular tachycardia (VT) is performed using classic methods of activation and entrainment mapping during arrhythmia to identify the critical isthmus during VT and minimize the number of ablation lesions. However, hemodynamic instability during VT often limits the extent to which these methods can be used. Approximately 33% of patients will have exclusively hemodynamically stable VTs induced at the time of electrophysiology study.[1,2] The vast majority (~66%) will have at least one hemodynamically unstable VT induced, preventing detailed entrainment or activation mapping. Even in those patients who have a mappable stable VT, it is almost invariably true that other unstable (i.e., "unmappable") VTs can also be induced. This is not surprising when one considers that the arrhythmogenic substrate is not a simple single circuit, but rather an extensive sheet of surviving myocardial fibers in a bed of scar tissue with multiple potential entry and exit points—allowing for different reentrant paths (i.e., different VTs) to be operative at any given time.[3] For other cases, the presenting arrhythmia may be ventricular fibrillation (VF), which is

Disclosures: Jacob Koruth's disclosures: Consultant–Abbott, Farapulse, Pulse Biosciences, Cardiofocus, Affera and Grant Support–Farapulse, Pulse Biosciences, Cardiofocus, Affera, Equity: Affera

Vivek Reddy's disclosures with medical companies (unrelated to this manuscript) include: Abbott (Consultant), Ablacon (Consultant, Equity), Acutus Medical (Consultant, Equity), Affera (Consultant, Equity), (Apama Medical-Boston Scientific (Consultant, Equity), APN Health (Consultant, Equity), Aquaheart (Consultant, Equity), Atacor (Consultant, Equity), AtiAN (Consultant), Autonomix (Consultant, Equity), Axon Therapies (Consultant, Equity), Backbeat (Consultant, Equity), BioSig (Consultant, Equity), Biosense-Webster (Consultant), BioTel Heart (Consultant), Biotronik (Consultant), Boston Scientific (Consultant), Cardiac Implants (Consultant, Equity), CardiaCare (Consultant, Equity), Cardiofocus (Consultant), Cardionomic (Consultant), CardioNXT / AFTx (Consultant, Equity), Circa Scientific (Consultant, Equity), CoreMap (Consultant), CoRISMA (Consultant, Equity), Corvia Medical (Consultant, Equity), Dinova-Hangzhou Nuomao Medtech (Consultant, Equity), East End Medical (Consultant, Equity), EBR (Consultant), EPD-Philips (Consultant, Equity), EP Frontiers (Consultant, Equity), Epix Therapeutics (Consultant, Equity), EpiEP (Consultant, Equity), Eximo (Consultant, Equity), Farapulse-Boston Scientific (Consultant, Equity), Fire1 (Consultant), Gore & Associates (Consultant), HRT (Consultant, Equity), Impulse Dynamics (Consultant), Intershunt (Consultant, Equity), Javelin (Consultant, Equity), Kardium (Consultant, Equity), Keystone Heart (Consultant, Equity), LuxMed (Consultant, Equity), Manual Surgical Sciences (Equity), Medlumics (Consultant, Equity), Medtronic (Consultant), Middlepeak (Consultant, Equity), Neutrace (Consultant, Equity), Newpace (Equity), Nuvera-Biosense Webster (Consultant, Equity), Philips (Consultant), Pulse Biosciences (Consultant), Restore Medical (Consultant, Equity), Sirona Medical (Consultant, Equity), Surecor (Equity), Valcare (Consultant, Equity) and Vizaramed (Equity).

Srinivas Dukkipati's disclosures include: Biosense Webster (Research grant), Manual Surgical Sciences (Equity) and Farapulse which was acquired by Boston Scientific (Equity).

intrinsically unstable. In this chapter, we discuss techniques that can be applied for catheter ablation of unstable VT and for VF.

Imaging to Characterize the Ventricular Tachycardia Substrate

Preprocedure cardiac imaging modalities facilitate risk assessment, initial target identification, and procedural planning. When using cardiac imaging to identify locations with structural characteristics that suggest sites of origin for VT, the distribution and magnitude of myocardial scar are typically the most useful information to be gained. Cardiac magnetic resonance is well suited to identify scar based on its spatial, temporal, and contrast resolution. Both severe wall thinning and greater magnitude of scar according to delayed contrast enhancement correspond with lower-voltage areas defined by electroanatomical mapping,[4,5] and critical isthmus sites for VT ablation have been shown to correlate with magnetic esonance imaging (MRI)-defined scar in ischemic cardiomyopathy[6] and nonischemic cardiomyopathy.[7] MRI may be especially helpful to identify VT substrate that is mid-myocardial or epicardial. In a study of 77 patients with scar-related VT, MRI identified septal or epicardial scar in 43% of patients with nonischemic cardiomyopathy and in 6% of ischemic cardiomyopathy patients.[8] Among the 11 patients with subepicardial scar according to the pattern of hyperenhancement, all underwent successful ablation at an epicardial site. A major advantage of MRI is the lack of ionizing radiation. However, its use remains limited in many patients with implantable defibrillators, who comprise a large proportion of patients for VT ablation. Specifying the amount of signal intensity by contrast enhancement and the amount of wall thinning that corresponds to scar depends on parameters set during processing of the study, so that assessments of scar magnitude are generally not comparable between patients.[9]

Multidetector computed tomography (MDCT) has outstanding spatial resolution, approximately 0.5–0.625 mm,[10] and can be used to delineate important landmarks such as the coronary arteries and the phrenic nerve before ablation procedures.[11] This modality has also been applied to identification of substrate for VT ablation, particularly among patients with implanted devices that preclude MRI.[12] Areas with wall thickness <5 mm detected by contrast-enhanced MDCT are correlated with voltage <1.5 mV by electroanatomical mapping, especially on the endocardial surface.[13] More severe wall thinning <2 mm is sensitive and specific for transmurality of VT substrate, such that late and fragmented potentials appear on the endocardium in patients with post–myocarditis cardiomyopathy and on the epicardium in patients with ischemic cardiomyopathy.[14] Takigawa et al. identified 41 CT channels in nine postinfarction patients by using three criteria: (1) abnormal thickness (<5 mm), (2) thickness on both edges thinner than that inside the channel, and (3) length greater than width. These CT-defined anatomical channels predicted involvement in a critical part of the VT circuit with a sensitivity of 100% and a positive predictive value of 51.2%.[15] Hybrid imaging with positron-emission tomography (PET)/CT has been used to augment scar localization,[16,17] and delayed-enhancement imaging may significantly increase the sensitivity of MDCT for detection of scar according to electroanatomical mapping.[18] The strategies that rely on preprocedure imaging were shown to be feasible in multiple centers and could simplify unstable VT ablation procedures, but randomized controlled validation is still pending.

Intracardiac echocardiography (ICE) has a unique role during VT ablation because it is used in real time, typically through an 8 or 10 F ultrasound catheter positioned in the right atrium or right ventricle (RV).[19] ICE has been used to identify the location and degree of transmurality associated with myocardial scar. One study of 17 patients with scar-related VT showed a high correlation between scar area according to wall motion abnormalities by ICE and areas identified with electroanatomical mapping.[20] Increased echo intensity by ICE imaging has also been shown to identify scar,[21] even differentiating epicardial scar on the LV lateral wall.[22]

Defining the Scar With Electroanatomical Mapping

Substrate ablation can be used for hemodynamically unstable VT. Accordingly, the definition of the ventricular scar and the arrhythmogenic areas in and around the scar with electroanatomical mapping is critical to understanding potential sites for ablation. Based on surgical mapping studies in patients with post-MI VT, there are several electrogram (EGM) characteristics during sinus rhythm that help distinguish abnormal myocardial tissue, including low voltage amplitude, prolonged EGM duration, and fractionation with late and split potentials.[23,24] Most electroanatomical maps today delineate abnormal ventricular tissue using a peak-to-peak bipolar EGM amplitude cutoff of 1.5 mV. This is largely based on the study by Marchlinski et al. that measured left ventricular (LV) and RV bipolar voltage in six patients without structural heart disease (average age 37 years, five men).[25] The distribution of bipolar EGM signals measured with a 4-mm-tip catheter showed that 95% were greater than 1.55 mV. A subsequent study in seven patients with structurally normal hearts that measured LV EGM amplitude with a 4-mm-tip catheter corroborated these findings.[26]

Bipolar voltage amplitude values <0.5 mV are typically arbitrarily defined as dense scar, and values between 0.5 and 1.5 mV as abnormal tissue, which represents the border zone (Table 35.1). This tissue often contains surviving fibrils that can be identified as split/late potentials in sinus rhythm or mid-diastolic potentials during VT. Imaging studies using contrast-enhanced CT combined with PET and MRI have evaluated and largely validated this classification based on bipolar voltage amplitude criteria.[12,16,17,27–30] However, it is important to keep in mind that the commonly used threshold for abnormal bipolar EGM amplitude is empirically derived and not necessarily reflective of histologic scar in a particular patient. Numerous factors may affect EGM features during an individual case, including angle of the electrical wavefront compared with the catheter, electrode size, interelectrode spacing, and signal filtering. Patient-specific factors such as ventricular hypertrophy may call for upward adjustment of the cutoff values used for abnormal EGMs.[31] Chronic pacing could also affect bipolar EGM amplitude, and a study in 11 post-MI patients revealed that 8% of sites had a bipolar EGM amplitude that was "reclassified" from abnormal (≤1.5 mV) to normal (>1.5 mV), or vice

TABLE 35.1 Sinus Rhythm Electrogram Characteristics for Substrate Ablation

Feature	Definition
Dense scar	Bipolar voltage amplitude <0.5 mV
Low voltage/abnormal	Bipolar voltage amplitude ≥0.5 and ≤1.5 mV
Normal tissue	Bipolar voltage amplitude >1.5 mV
Fractionated	Low amplitude (<0.5 mV), long duration (≥133 ms), an amplitude:duration ratio of ≤0.005, multiple components without an isoelectric interval
Late or isolated potential	Occurs after termination of surface QRS complexes and separated from the ventricular electrogram by an isoelectric interval of >20 ms
Local abnormal ventricular activity (LAVA)	A broad category of abnormal electrograms that includes late/isolated potentials and fractionated electrograms. Also includes abnormal electrograms in which local and far-field components are merged and coincident with QRS complex. Separation and delay of the local electrogram can often be achieved with pacing and may represent ventricular tachycardia isthmus sites.

versa, when alternating between ventricular and atrial pacing.[32] Although substrate maps generated using standard definitions of bipolar EGM amplitude generally provide robust representations of the infarct morphology, it is important to allow for flexibility in scar definitions based on the characteristics of a particular case.

In some patients, scar may be mainly midmyocardial, and the bipolar voltage maps from the endocardium and epicardium may underestimate the amount of scar or, on occasion, may display completely normal voltage. Endocardial unipolar EGM amplitude is helpful to identify the presence of intramural or epicardial substrate.[33–36] The presence of intramural or epicardial scar is suggested by the presence of an endocardial unipolar voltage <8.3 mV in the LV and <5.5 mV in the RV. Endocardial unipolar voltage maps may be used as a surrogate for bipolar voltage maps to identify scar and together with pace mapping can be used to identify VT exit sites to guide ablation.

Pace Mapping for Ventricular Tachycardia Exit Sites

By definition, a reentrant rhythm is always depolarizing some quantity of myocardial tissue. Because the small mass of myocardial tissue in the protected myocardial channels within the scar contribute negligibly to the surface QRS, the QRS complex of a VT initiates when the wavefront of activation emanates from the border of the scar. Accordingly, once the myocardial scar is defined, a brief examination of the surface QRS morphology of the target VT(s) can generally regionalize the VT exit site to a scar border.[37,38] Based on the ECG morphology of the VT, pace mapping is performed at the suspected border(s) of the scar during normal sinus rhythm to precisely localize the exit point. Unlike during VT, pacing during sinus rhythm results in omnidirectional spread of activation—which one may expect to result in a different paced-QRS morphology than the VT-QRS morphology even when pacing from the proper exit site. However, the optimal paced-QRS morphology is often only slightly different than the target VT-QRS morphology (Fig. 35.1). This is likely because when pacing at a scar border, activation proceeding into the scar is slower and contributes little to overall ventricular activation when compared with the "orthodromic" wavefront that rapidly emanates in the opposite direction into normal tissue. Not surprisingly, less optimal matches of the pace map exit sites are found when pacing along the borders of smaller scars as opposed to larger scars. Pacing deeper within the VT channel will produce a good match with latency (stimulus-QRS interval). However pacing further into the channel often results in the wavefront exiting in the opposite direction, resulting in an abrupt change of paced-QRS morphology within the VT isthmus. This abrupt change of paced-QRS morphology change can be used for defining culprit channels in nonsustained/unstable VT.[39]

Pace mapping is also affected by the rate, stimulus strength, and electrode polarity during pacing. At faster pacing rates, the "antidromic" wavefront of activation into the scar may contribute less to the QRS morphology than during slow pacing. In addition, ventricular repolarization may fuse into and modify the QRS morphology during faster pacing rates. Because it is difficult to predict the effect of these variables, pacing is ideally performed at a rate similar to the target VT rate. By presumably capturing more distant (i.e., far-field) tissue, increasing the stimulus strength can also affect the QRS morphology. We typically start pacing at low output and increase the output until several QRS complexes are captured in succession. It is interesting to note that if multiple QRS morphologies are seen at varying outputs, this is indicative of a protected region (or channel) of tissue. That is, at the lower output, only this region is captured by pacing, whereas at a higher output, the far-field tissue is also captured.

ABLATION STRATEGIES BASED ON SUBSTRATE MAPPING

Once the arrhythmogenic substrate has been defined, a number of different ablation strategies can be used. The details for substrate ablation are described in the other chapters; we briefly summarize some of these strategies.

Linear Lesions

This approach, first described by Marchlinski and colleagues,[25] involves identifying a VT exit site using standard pace mapping. Subsequently, linear lesions are placed using one of many approaches: (1) lesions extending from the "dense scar" (defined as <0.5 mV) to either anatomical boundaries or normal myocardium; (2) extending lesions along the borders of the scar

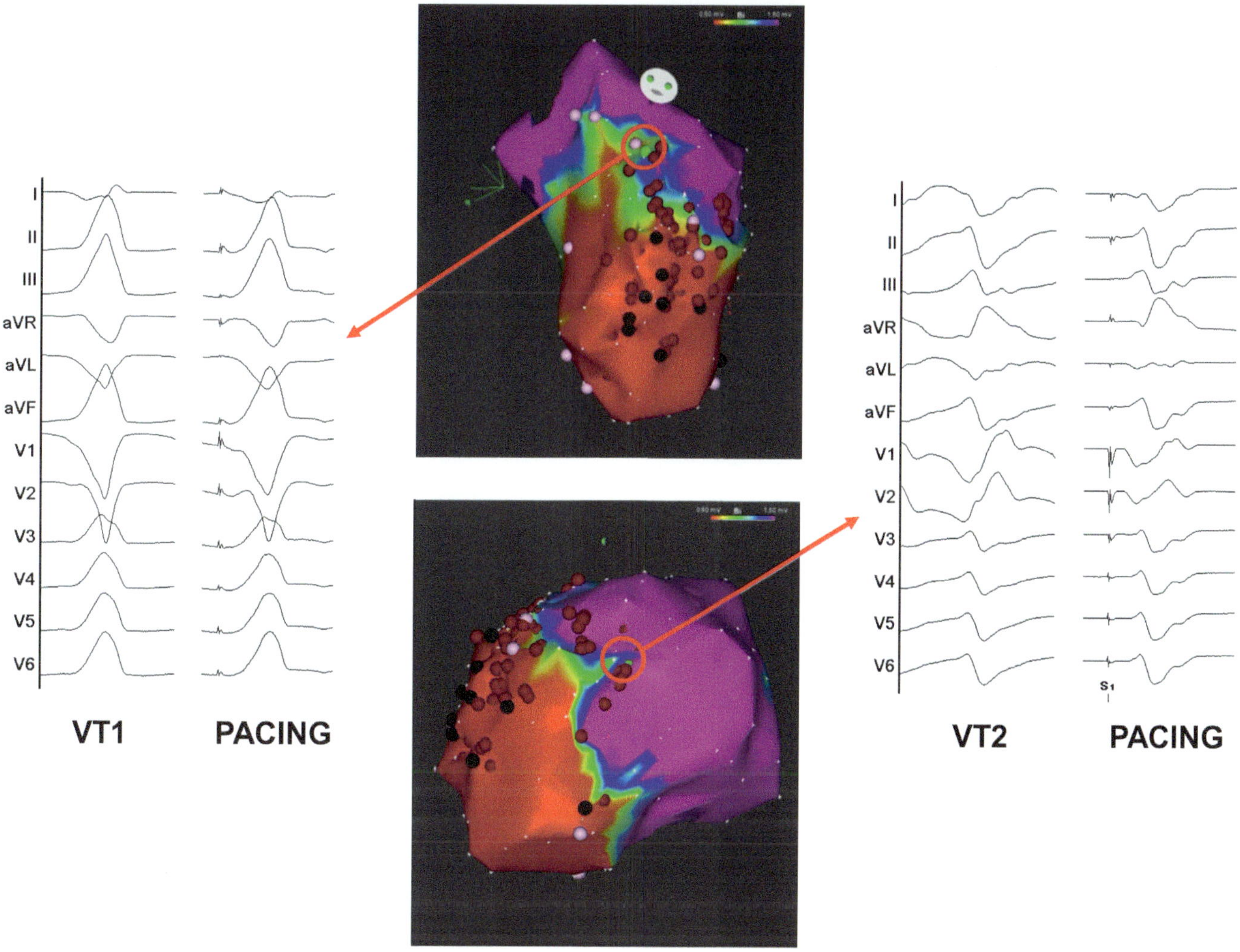

Fig. 35.1 Pace mapping along scar border to identify ventricular tachycardia (VT) exit sites. Electroanatomical mapping of the left ventricular endocardium in a patient with prior anterior myocardial infarction was performed. The bipolar voltage maps demonstrated a large anterior, septal, and apical scar (*middle upper panel*—superior left anterior oblique projection, *middle lower panel*—left lateral projection). Pace mapping was performed along the scar border to identify exit sites for two VTs (VT1, VT2). Pacing at the superior anteroseptal portion of the scar identified an excellent pace match to VT1 (*middle upper panel—red circle, green point*). Pacing from the basal lateral aspect of the scar yielded a good pace match to VT2 (*middle lower panel—red circle, green point*). These sites were subsequently ablated as they represented exit sites for the VTs. The color range in the bipolar voltage are 0.5–1.5 mV; *purple* and *red* represent normal and severely diseased tissue, respectively. *Black points*, late potentials; *pink points*, fractionated potentials; *red points*, ablation sites.

traversing/centering on these optimal pace sites (Fig. 35.2); or (3) a pair of crossing linear lesions extending from the exit site into the scar and the other along the border of the scar.

Ablation of Late Potentials/Dechanneling

EGMs with late activation and prolonged duration have been strongly correlated with VT circuits.[40,41] This criterion requires recording low-amplitude, high-frequency EGMs with multiple components of prolonged duration (fractionated potentials) or components recorded after the surface QRS that is separated by an isoelectric segment (late potential). Fractionated potentials generally refer to EGMs that have a voltage amplitude <0.5 mV, a duration of ≥133 ms, and an amplitude:duration ratio of ≥0.005, whereas late potentials refer to low-amplitude signals that are separated from the ventricular EGM by an isoelectric segment of >20 ms.[24,42–45] These late/isolated potentials are particularly interesting in that they are thought to represent candidate sites for critical portions of VT circuits and are excellent targets for ablation.[44,46,47] Conduction channels within myocardial scar may also be identified by the relatively higher voltage in these areas compared with surrounding tissue.[48,49] Decreasing the bipolar voltage definition of dense scar <0.5 mV may delineate conduction channels within the scar that may serve as VT isthmus sites. However, the specificity of conduction channels predicting VT isthmus sites is low but markedly improved when the channels contained late potentials. Fractionated and late EGMs underappreciated during sinus rhythm. Identifying these components during catheter mapping can be increased by changing the propagation wave front by mapping during RV or LV pacing as opposed to sinus rhythm.

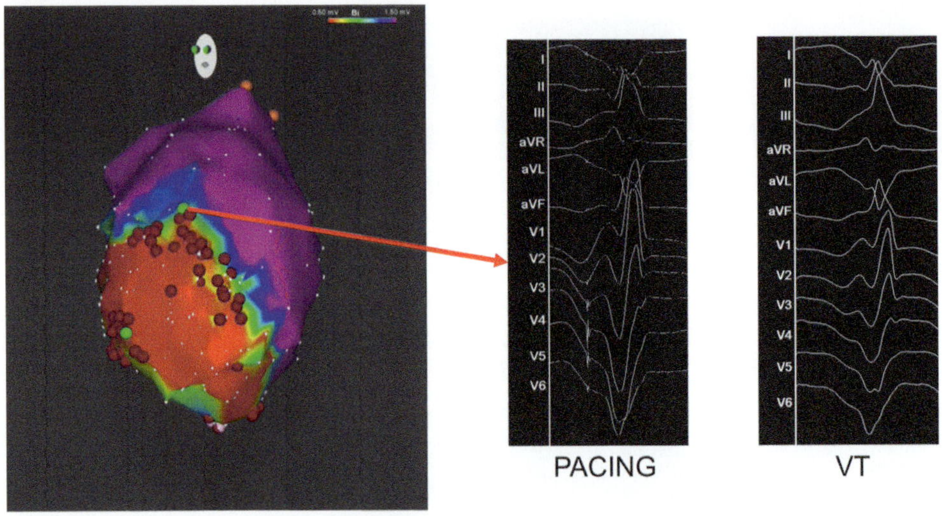

Fig. 35.2 Ablation along scar border at ventricular tachycardia (VT) exit site identified by pace mapping. A sinus rhythm bipolar voltage map of the left ventricle (LV) in a left anterior oblique projection is shown (*left*). The patient had a large scar extending from the mid-anterior wall to the apex and septum. A hemodynamically unstable VT was repeatedly induced that was pace terminated (*right*). Pace mapping was performed along the scar border to identify the VT exit site. Pacing at the anterior and superior portion of the scar identified a site (*green point*) with an excellent pace match to the VT (*middle*). Ablation (*red points*) was performed along the scar border rendering the VT noninducible. The color range in the bipolar voltage are 0.5–1.5 mV; *purple* and *red* represent normal and severely diseased tissue, respectively.

Local Abnormal Ventricular Activity Ablation

Jaïs and colleagues described a substrate-based ablation approach based on EGMs having local abnormal ventricular activity (LAVA).[50] EGMs demonstrating LAVA are defined as sharp high-frequency potentials occurring during or after the far-field EGM during sinus rhythm. At times these signals have multiple components or late/isolated potentials, but they also include EGMs where local electrical activity is merged with far-field ventricular activity or inscribed in the QRS complex. With programmed ventricular stimulation or with ventricular pacing at varying outputs, the local EGM can be delayed and separated from the far-field component consistent with delayed conduction to the region.

Homogenization

Scar homogenization is another strategy to address all potential channels that might result in reentry from the myocardial scar. Di Biase et al. described such an approach that targets any abnormal EGMs including those with more than three deflections, amplitude <1.5 mV, and duration >70 ms. The goal with ablation is elimination of abnormal EGMs or lack of capture with high-output pacing (20-mA output at 10-ms pulse width).[51]

Ablation Using Functional Substrate Mapping

Isochronal late activation map (ILAM) is an activation map that highlights areas of isochronal crowding, representing areas of slowed conduction. Each EGM is annotated at its latest activation, as this is thought to more accurately represent areas with long and fractionated signals. Irie et al. used eight isochrones for ILAM and demonstrated that only 11% of critical sites were localized to the latest isochrone, but sites critical to reentry were harbored in regions with slow conduction velocity, where three isochrones were present within a 1-cm radius.[52] Using this method to identify and ablate critical zones within the substrate, Aziz et al. reported that 70% of patients had no VT recurrence at 12 ± 10 months of follow-up. Only 18% of low-voltage area was ablated with 29-minute (21–38 minutes) radiofrequency (RF) application.[53] Reduced ablation time and procedure time may decrease acute complications and is an attractive approach for unstable VTs in the sicker population and has recently gained in popularity.

INTEGRATING THE MAPPING AND ABLATION STRATEGIES FOR ABLATION OF UNSTABLE VENTRICULAR TACHYCARDIA

The relative efficacy of the various criteria to guide identification and targeting of the "arrhythmogenic" portion of the scar is unknown and will only be fully appreciated with comparative studies. Here, we describe how we pursue VT ablation in our laboratory, with emphasis on unstable VT. For any VT ablation, we will attempt to gather preprocedure imaging to assess for the presence and location of scar, often either cardiac MRI or CT. At the onset of the ablation, we will typically attempt to induce VT with programmed stimulation to estimate the number of VTs that will require treatment, assess for VT tolerability, understand potential sites of origin by ECG, and assess inducibility as one of the possible end points of the procedure. A careful high-density ventricular map is performed to define the scar by electroanatomical mapping and tag candidate sites for ablation including late potentials and LAVA. Mapping includes epicardial access on a case-by-case basis depending on the arrhythmic substrate, the ECG morphology of any documented VTs, and the feasibility of an epicardial approach.

In cases of hemodynamically unstable VT, we use a number of strategies to identify and target putative myocardial channels within the scarred tissue including (1) resetting/entrainment mapping with hemodynamic support as needed; (2) identification of sites displaying latency and a QRS morphology similar to VT with pace mapping; (3) identification of late potentials and of areas having LAVA; (4) identification of channels within scar based on relatively higher voltage compared with surrounding tissue; and (5) pace mapping to identify densely scarred tissue with intervening channels of activation. The most direct and reliable means to identify a channel of activation is to use entrainment/resetting criteria during VT. For hemodynamically unstable VT, this can be accomplished by first performing pace mapping at the scar border to identify the putative exit site, followed by a brief induction of the unstable VT. In high-risk patients with severely depressed ejection fraction, preexisting significant congestive heart failure, or electrical storm, a percutaneous LV assist device (pLVAD) support is usually used although other approaches to support have been used. Daniele et al. demonstrated that prophylactic use of pLVAD was associated with a reduced risk of acute hemodynamic decompensation and death/heart transplant during 12 months of follow-up in high-risk patients.[54] Hemodynamically unstable VT may be rendered more stable VT with intravenous pressors and pLVAD support and thus allow for mapping during arrhythmia (Fig. 35.3).[55,56] Cohort studies of VT ablation patients have demonstrated that pLVAD support allows for greater duration of mapping during VT and results in more VT terminations during ablation.[57,58] However, the major studies to date have not shown benefits from pLVAD use with respect to VT recurrence rates.[57,59,60] Vascular complications can be an issue in patients who undergo pLVAD support.

Ideally, the ablation procedure is considered complete when all VTs inducible at the beginning of the procedure are eliminated and no additional VTs are inducible. Because the substrate modification procedure could theoretically inadvertently create new arrhythmogenic channels of activity, one is obligated to rule out this possibility. Inducibility at the end of the procedure should minimally include one RV and one LV site. In addition, if nonsustained monomorphic VT is induced, we strongly consider infusion of a sympathetic agent such as isoproterenol to determine if the VT then becomes sustained. However, complete noninducibility is not necessarily achievable in every patient—particularly those with severe ventricular dysfunction in whom a sine wave–like VT (i.e., a morphologically indeterminate VT with no isoelectric segment) is often inducible with aggressive ventricular stimulation.[26] In this situation, after all of the late potentials are eliminated, the procedure is considered complete.

ABLATION OF IDIOPATHIC VENTRICULAR FIBRILLATION

Although VF is inherently unstable as a clinical rhythm, ablation of VF by addressing triggering beats has yielded promising results. Haïssaguerre and colleagues were the first to demonstrate that in certain patients, VF can be initiated with isolated premature ventricular beats and can be treated with catheter ablation targeting these initiators.[61] After being resuscitated from recurrent (10 ± 12) episodes of primary VF, 27 patients without known structural heart disease underwent an electrophysiology study procedure.[62] This group of patients was studied because VF was initiated by isolated premature ventricular beats of identical morphology with a short coupling interval to the prior QRS complex (297 ± 41 ms) (Fig. 35.4). Endocardial mapping revealed that these triggers initiated from the RV or LV Purkinje system in 23/27 (85%) patients and from the myocardium of the RV outflow tract in 4/27 (15%) patients (Fig. 35.5). The interval from the Purkinje potential to ventricular activation varied from 10 to 150 ms during the premature beat. A Purkinje potential was also seen at these same sites during sinus rhythm but preceded the QRS by only 11 ± 5 ms. RF catheter ablation at these sites eliminated the triggering PVCs and subsequent VF in most of these patients. The mean number of RF ablation lesions required to eliminate these triggers was nine. Long-term follow-up was subsequently reported in a multicenter study of 38 patients who underwent catheter ablation of PVC triggers for idiopathic VF.[63] During a median follow-up of 63 months, seven patients (18%) had recurrent VF. Five of the seven patients underwent a repeat procedure with successful ablation of PVC triggers. Different PVCs were demonstrated in four of five patients, and a PVC that was identical to that ablated during the initial procedure was demonstrated in the remaining patient. Haïssaguerre et al. demonstrated that repetitive activity within the peripheral Purkinje system can lead to VF. This was confirmed by the reproducibility of VF induction and the consistency of distal Purkinje potentials preceding changes in ventricular activation. Importantly, they noted that only induction from the LV could induce VF but not from the RV apex.[64] Another study from same group demonstrated that in 24 patients with idiopathic VF, localized tissue alterations were present in up to 15 patients (63%), and these sites often co-located with VF drivers. These structural abnormalities covered, 5% of the ventricular surface and most frequently were located on the epicardium of the RV. Tissue abnormalities were more likely to be clustered in distinct regions. Purkinje triggers were identified in 11 patients with a higher prevalence in patients with normal ventricular myocardium compared with those with abnormal ventricular substrate (7/9 vs 4/15, $P = .033$). Of the 12 patients with idiopathic VF and structural abnormalities undergoing a substrate-based ablation, 3 (25%) also had initiating PVCs that were ablated, and 10 of these patients (83%) were free of VF recurrence during follow-up of 17 ± 11 months.[65]

Purkinje-triggered VF can also originate from the moderator band, an intracavitary structure bridging the septum to the RV free wall. It was originally thought to mainly serve a structural role, preventing RV distention and supporting the

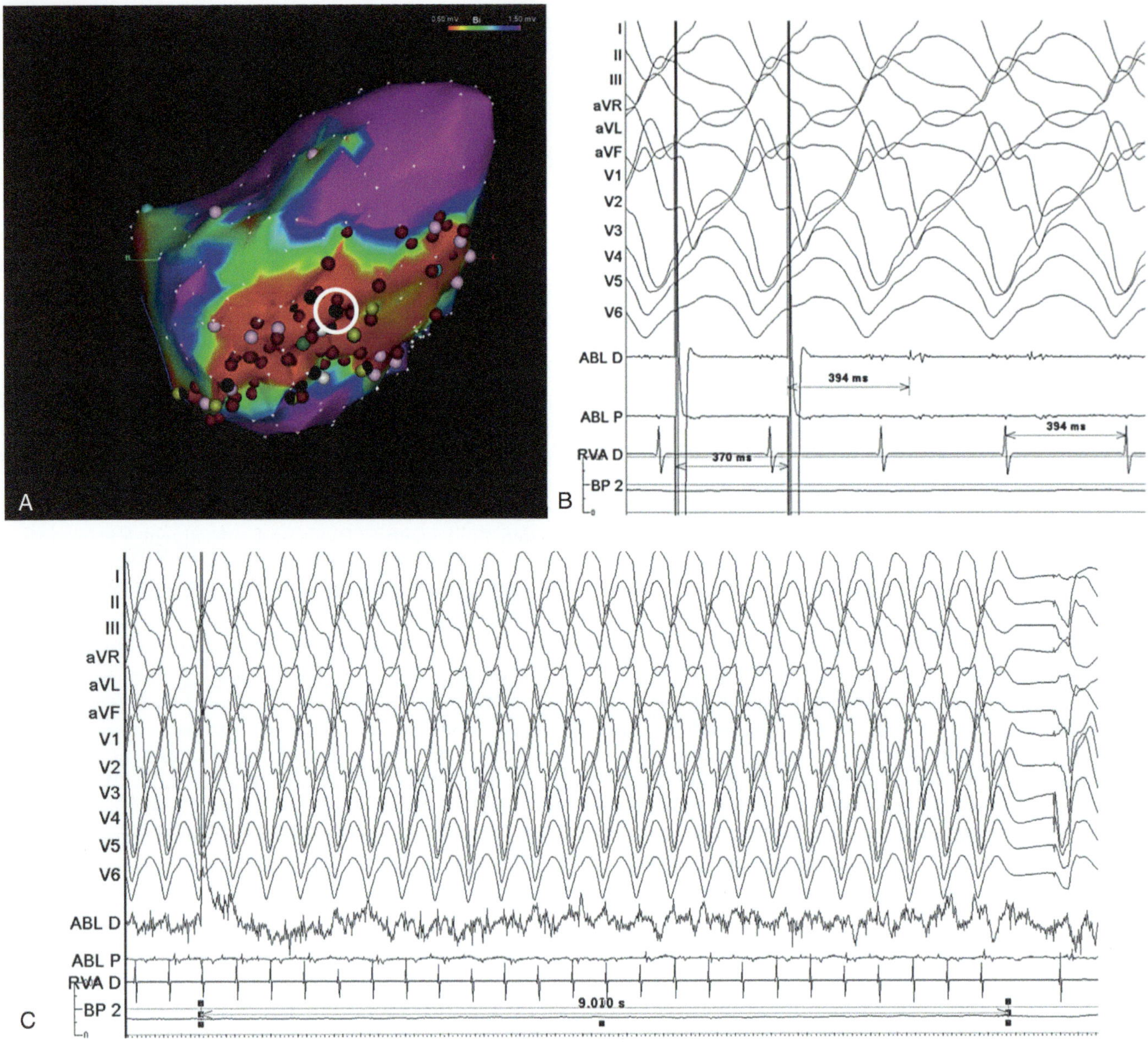

Fig. 35.3 Entrainment mapping of a hemodynamically unstable ventricular tachycardia (VT) with percutaneous left ventricular assist device (pLVAD) support. A patient with ischemic cardiomyopathy and left ventricular ejection fraction of 20% had recurrent implantable cardioverter-defibrillator shocks for VT. The patient was taken to the electrophysiology laboratory, and ventricular stimulation induced multiple monomorphic VTs, all of which were hemodynamically unstable. A pLVAD was inserted (Impella CP, Abiomed, Inc., Danvers, MA) for hemodynamic support. (A) Bipolar endocardial voltage map (inferior view) demonstrated a large inferior wall scar that had a significant amount of fractionated and late potentials. Entrainment mapping was performed during VT at a site that had a late potential (*white circle, black point*). (B) Entrainment at this site was performed during VT with the ablation catheter (ABLd). This site had diastolic potentials during VT and demonstrated entrainment with concealed fusion with a postpacing interval that was equal to the tachycardia cycle length. The blood pressure (BP 2) during VT was ~85 mm Hg and was nonpulsatile because of the pLVAD. (C) Ablation at this site terminated VT in 9 seconds. The color range in the bipolar voltage are 0.5–1.5 mV; *purple* and *red* represent normal and severely diseased tissue, respectively. *ABL D*, Ablation catheter distal electrodes; *ABL P*, ablation catheter proximal electrodes; *BP 2*, arterial blood pressure; *RVA D*, distal RV catheter electrodes. *Black points*, late potentials; *pink points*, fractionated potentials; *green points*, pace-mapping sites; *red points*, ablation sites.

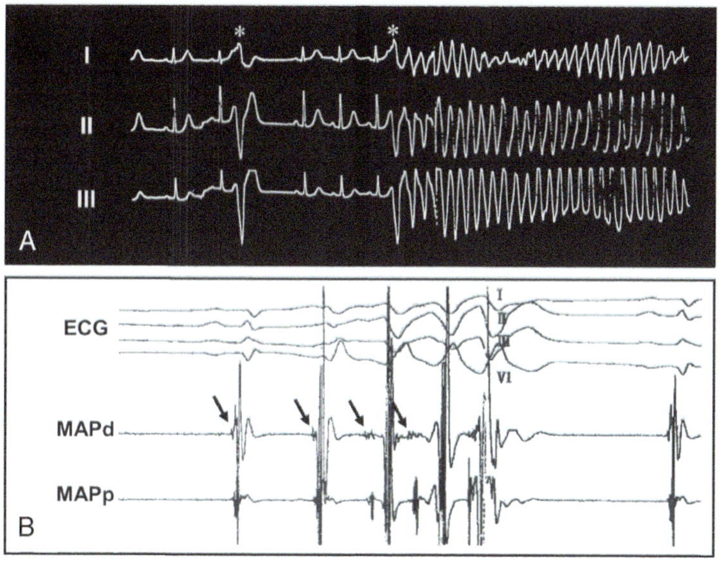

Fig. 35.4 Catheter ablation of focal ventricular fibrillation (VF). (A) In this patient with a structurally normal heart and recurrent VF, an example of monomorphic premature ventricular contractions (PVCs) (*asterisk*) initiating VF is shown. (B) In another patient with a structurally normal heart and VF, catheter mapping revealed a focal site with Purkinje potentials (*arrows*) preceding the initiating PVCs of the nonsustained polymorphic VT episode. Note that at this site, Purkinje potentials are also noted during sinus rhythm—albeit with a significantly shorter interval to the local ventricular electrogram. (Images courtesy of M. Haïssaguerre.)

papillary muscles associated with the tricuspid valve, but it also contains Purkinje fibers enabling rapid activation of the mid-free wall of the RV. The 12-lead ECG pattern of PVCs localized to the moderator band can be variable although universally have a left bundle branch block pattern and left superior frontal plane axis and are positive in leads I and aVL. Importantly, multiple exits from the moderator band have also reported.[66] Sadak et al. and others have demonstrated the efficacy of catheter ablation for moderator band arrhythmias.[67,68] A sharp Purkinje potential at the site of successful ablation can be seen preceding ventricular activation. Some patients may require repeat ablation, but long-term success rates can be excellent. To improve the stability of the ablation catheter, cryoablation instead of RF ablation has been suggested and can frequently be helpful.[68]

VF Ablation for the Patients With Channelopathies

Focal PVC triggers of VF have also been described in patients with channelopathies with otherwise structurally normal hearts and in patients with ischemic heart disease. Regarding the former, PVC triggers amenable to catheter ablation have been found in patients with either long QT syndrome or Brugada syndrome.[69] As with the other idiopathic VF patients, two types of PVC triggers have been found in both of these clinical disease states: (1) those with preceding Purkinje potentials and (2) those originating from the RV outflow tract. Nademanee and colleagues demonstrated that in nine patients with Brugada syndrome with type I ECG pattern and inducible VT/VF, abnormal EGMs were present in the RV outflow tract epicardium.[70] These EGMs demonstrated low bipolar voltage (0.94 ± 0.79 mV), prolonged duration (132 ± 48 ms), and fractionated late potentials extending beyond the QRS complex (96 ± 47 ms). Furthermore, ablation of these abnormal EGMs led to normalization of the ECG in 89% of patients and rendered all of them noninducible for VT/VF. During a follow-up of 20 ± 6 months, all patients were free of recurrent VT/VF. These findings were confirmed in larger cohorts with excellent outcomes, including that by Pappone et al.[71] Initiation of VF in the patients with early repolarization syndromes is also associated with both PVCs and depolarization abnormalities. A multicenter study led by Nademanee et al. performed detailed noninvasive and invasive mapping in 51 of 52 patients with ERS and recurrent VF episodes. They identified two phenotypes: (1) 40 patients (78%) with late depolarization abnormalities that were predominantly located in the RV epicardium and (2) 11 patients (22%) without apparent depolarization abnormalities but with PVCs associated with Purkinje sites. Overall, ablation was performed in 43 patients, and after nearly 3 years of follow-up, 91% of the patients had no VF recurrences.[72]

VF Ablation in Structural Heart Disease

Unlike the scar-related reentrant VT that is seen after an MI, it has also recently been demonstrated that certain post-MI patients with drug-refractory primary VF (i.e., VF not

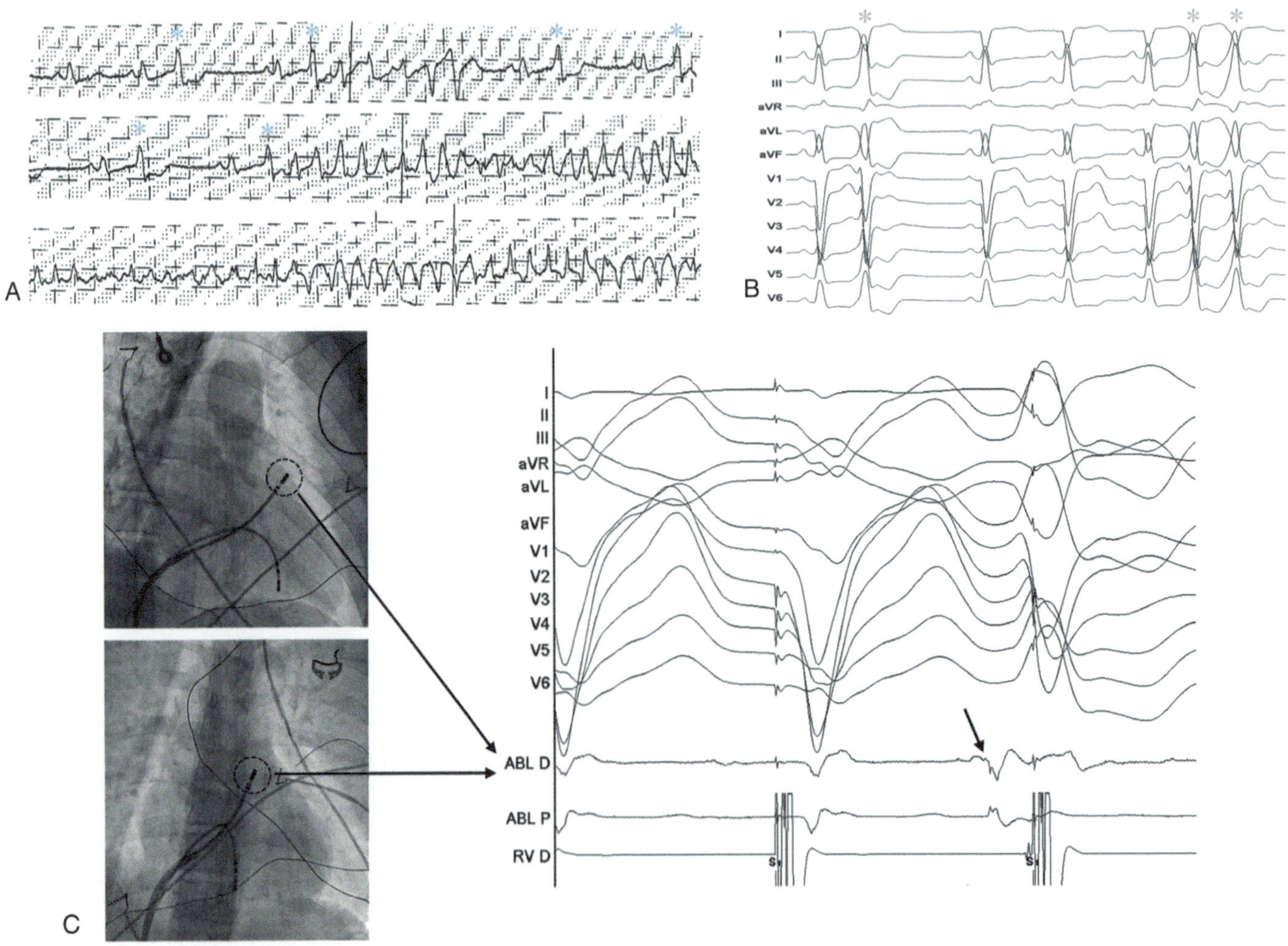

Fig. 35.5 Ventricular fibrillation (VF) initiated by right ventricular outflow tract premature ventricular contractions (PVCs). (A) In a young patient admitted for the evaluation of syncope, telemetry demonstrated unifocal PVCs (*asterisk*) initiating VF. (B) During electrophysiology study, unifocal PVCs demonstrating a left bundle branch block and inferior axis were initially seen. Subsequently, they were only inducible during ventricular pacing. (C) Fluoroscopic images in the right anterior oblique (*top left*) and left anterior oblique (*bottom left*) projections show the activation of the PVC in the anteroseptal right ventricular outflow tract (*dashed circle*). At this site, a potential (*arrow*) was seen –27 ms before the onset of the surface QRS. Ablation at this site abolished the PVCs. The patient has not had any recurrence of VF after 2 years' postablation.

preceded by monomorphic VT) also have PVC triggers of the arrhythmia.[73-77] These post-MI patients can be divided into those with a recent MI (<1 week, Figs. 35.6 and 35.7) and those with remote MIs (>1 month, Fig. 35.8). The PVC triggers were exclusively associated with Purkinje-like potentials and successfully targeted for catheter ablation. In a multicenter study, Komatsu et al. evaluated the effect of catheter ablation for post-MI refractory VF storm triggered by PVCs in 110 patients. The investigators reported that focal triggers were found to originate from the scar border zone in 88 patients (80%), and VF subsided in 92 patients (84%) during in-hospital stay after ablation. Importantly, the duration from the VF occurrence to the ablation procedure was associated with in-hospital mortality. During follow-up after discharge from hospital, only one patient developed recurrent VF storm.[78] In addition to VF, the Purkinje system may also play a role in post-MI reentrant VT that was relatively narrow (QRS complex ≤145 ms) resembling fascicular VT.[79,80] Mapping during VT demonstrated a reentrant mechanism with Purkinje potentials noted at the exit site. Even in patients with VF or VT storm related to acute coronary syndromes or acute decompensated heart failure, PVCs originating from the Purkinje network have been implicated as triggers and successfully ablated.[81-83] Purkinje-like potentials preceding PVCs triggering VF have been reported in other disease processes as well, such as myocarditis, aortic valve disease, DCM, mitral valve prolapse,[84] and amyloidosis.[82,85,86] In addition to PVCs triggers from the RVOT and Purkinje network, Herendael et al. demonstrated that VF can be triggered

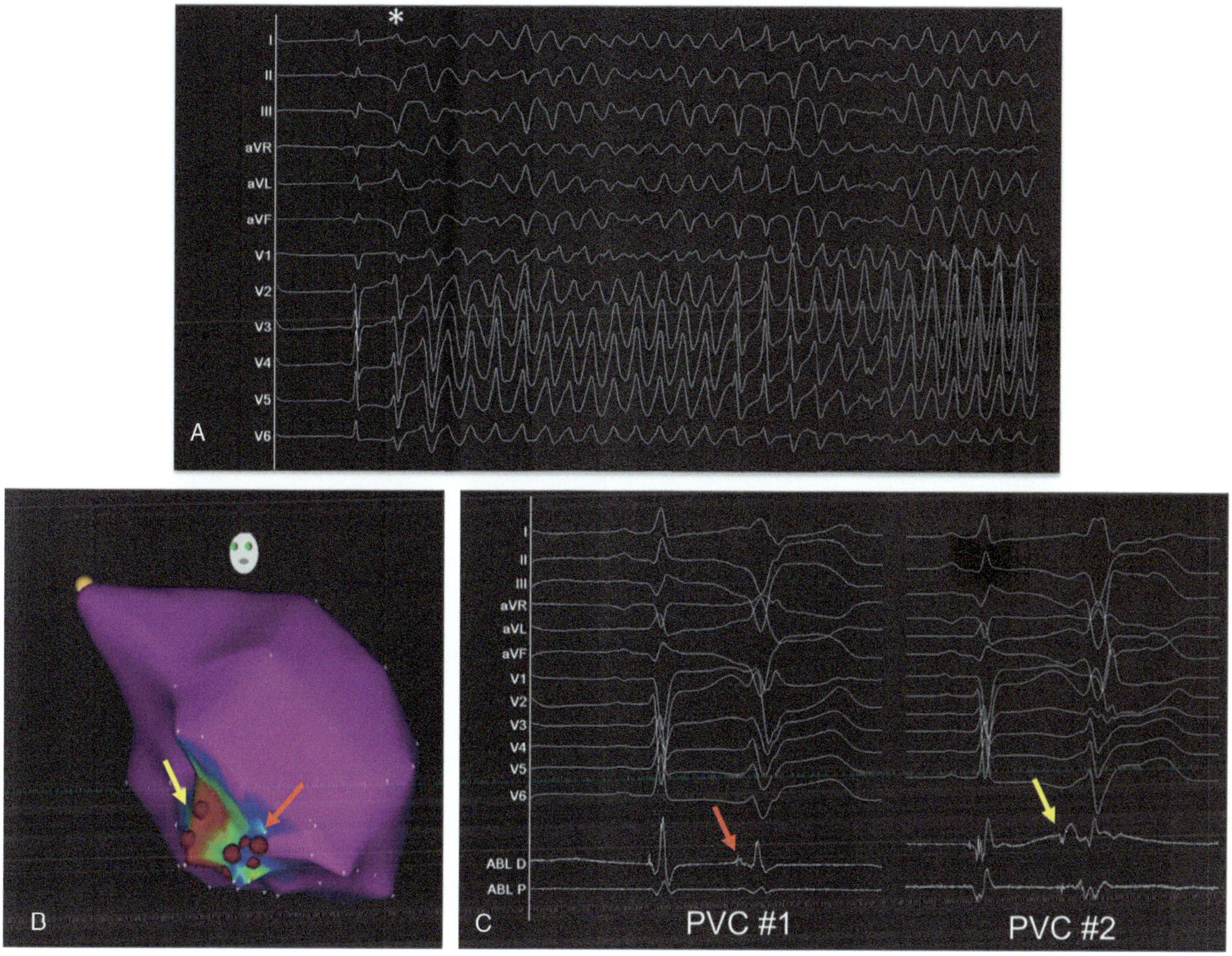

Fig. 35.6 Polymorphic ventricular tachycardia (VT)/ventricular fibrillation (VF) induced by premature ventricular contractions (PVCs) early after myocardial infarction. A 33-year-old patient developed chest pain and acute inferior myocardial infarction, which was treated with percutaneous coronary intervention and stent placement to the right coronary artery. On hospital day 2, he developed multiple episodes of polymorphic VT and VF, which were triggered by unifocal PVCs that were refractory to β-blockers, lidocaine, and amiodarone. (A) The patient was taken for electrophysiology study and spontaneously developed polymorphic VT and VF, requiring defibrillation. This was triggered by PVC #1 (*asterisk*). The patient was noted to have very frequent PVCs (#1), which also induced nonsustained polymorphic VT frequently. (B) Electroanatomical activation mapping of the left ventricular (LV) endocardium was performed, and PVC #1 was mapped to the distal LV septum (*red arrow*). (C) The earliest site of activation of PVC #1 (*left*) had a Purkinje potential (*red arrow*), which precedes the PVC by –42 ms. This Purkinje potential was also seen during the sinus rhythm complex. After ablation was performed at this early site, the morphology changed to PVC #2 (*right*). Activation mapping showed the earliest activation during this PVC to be slightly more basal location on the LV septum (see [C]–*yellow arrow*). Again at this site, Purkinje potentials were seen in sinus rhythm and preceding PVC (*yellow arrow*). This time, the Purkinje potential preceded PVC #2 by –88 ms. Ablation at this site rendered PVCs and polymorphic VT/VF noninducible. The color range is set such that *purple* represents late activation and *red* the earliest activation.

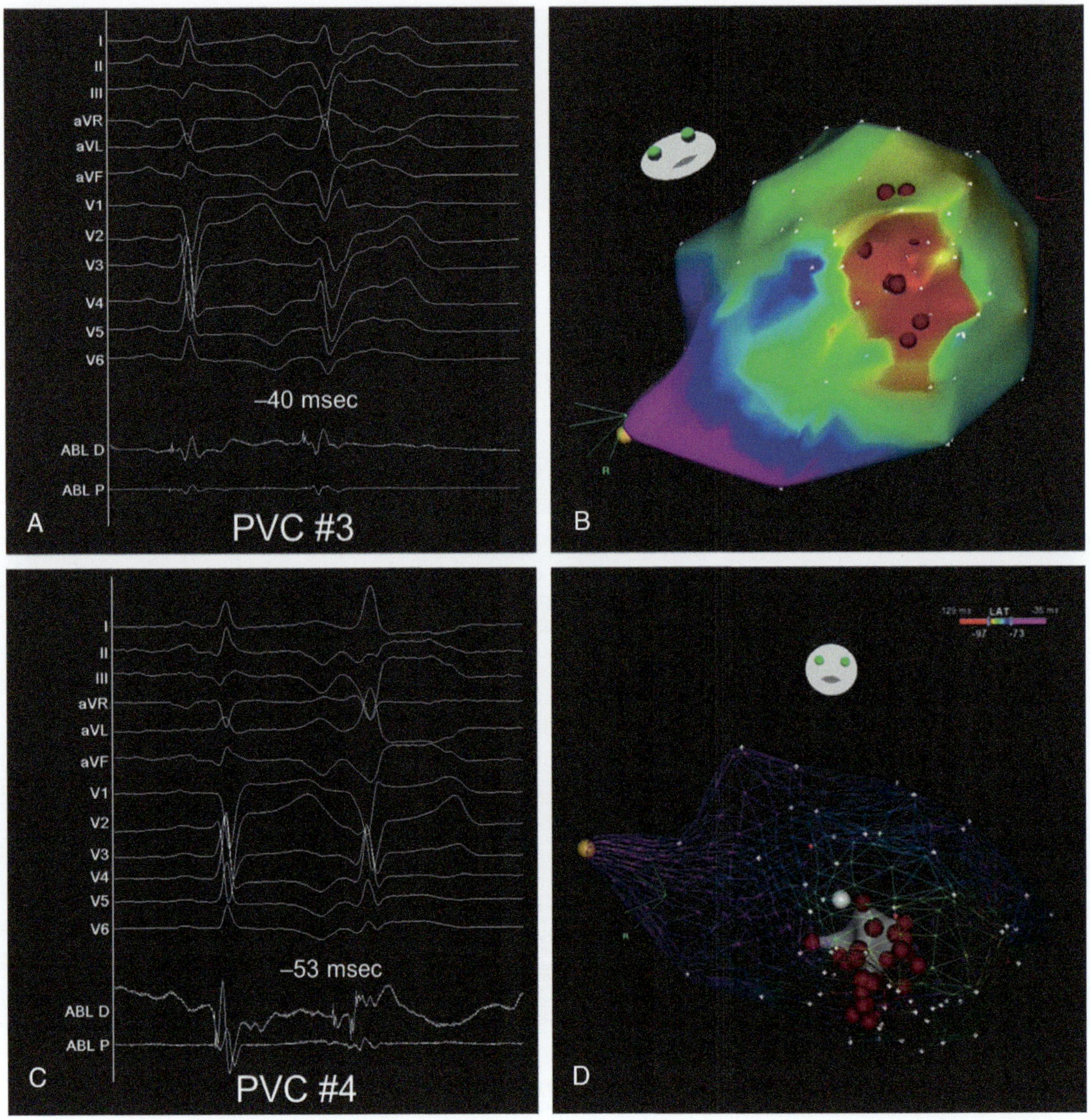

Fig. 35.7 Polymorphic ventricular tachycardia (VT)/ventricular fibrillation (VF) induced by premature ventricular contractions (PVCs) early after myocardial infarction. In the same patient as in Fig. 35.6, 2 days postablation, the patient began having unifocal PVCs and experienced sustained monomorphic VT that was of a similar morphology to the PVC. The patient was taken back to the electrophysiology laboratory. (A) The patient was noted to have very frequent PVC #3. This was of similar morphology to that seen in the first procedure (Fig. 35.6, PVC #1). Activation mapping of PVC #3 demonstrated the earliest activation to be again on the distal left ventricular (LV) septum. Again, Purkinje potentials were seen in sinus rhythm and preceding PVC #3 by –40 ms. (B) The electroanatomical activation map (shown in right anterior oblique caudal projection) of the LV endocardium showed a broad area of early activation. Ablation at this site was performed, and PVC morphology changed to PVC #4. (C) The earliest site of activation of PVC #4 had a Purkinje potential preceding the PVC by –53 ms. (D) Electroanatomical activation mapping of PVC #4 (shown in right anterior oblique projection) demonstrated that the earliest site of activation was noted be on the posteromedial papillary muscle (*gray structure*) rather than the LV endocardial wall (*mesh*). Ablation was performed on the papillary muscle and rendered all PVCs and VT/VF noninducible. This patient subsequently underwent implantable cardioverter-defibrillator implantation and has not had any further VT/VF after more than 3 years of follow-up. The color range is set such that *purple* represents late activation and *red* the earliest activation.

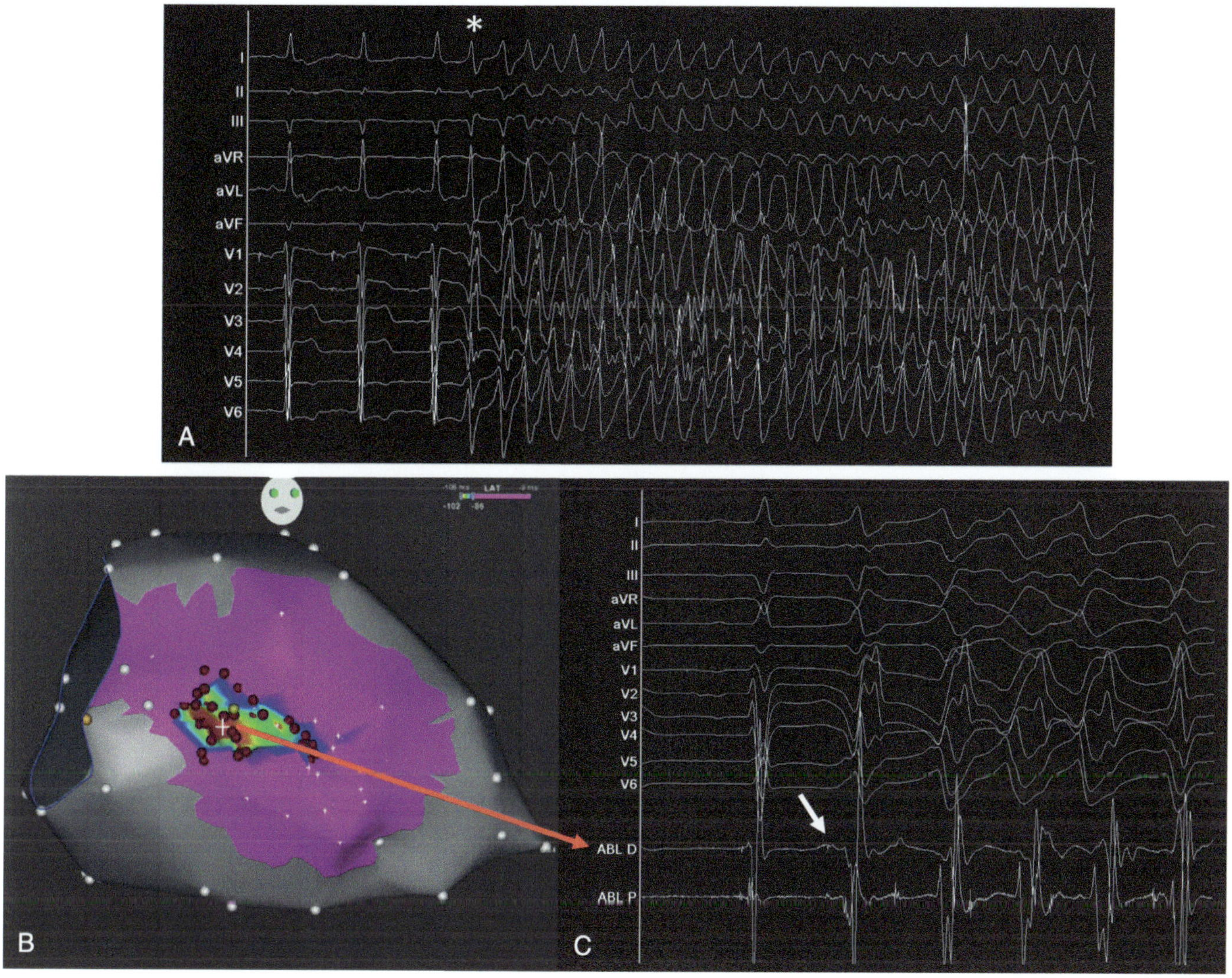

Fig. 35.8 Polymorphic ventricular tachycardia/ventricular fibrillation induced by premature ventricular contractions (PVCs) after remote myocardial infarction. A patient with remote myocardial infarction and coronary artery bypass grafting presented with cardiac arrest. He was noted to be in ventricular fibrillation (VF) and underwent defibrillation. He continued to have recurrent VF, which was triggered by a unifocal PVC. Following cardiac catheterization, the patient was taken to the electrophysiology study. (A) At the beginning of the procedure, he had spontaneous polymorphic ventricular tachycardia (VT) and then VF requiring defibrillation. This was triggered by a unifocal PVC (*asterisk*). The patient had very frequent PVCs of the same morphology. (B) Electroanatomical mapping of the left ventricular (LV) endocardium (right anterior oblique projection) demonstrated that the earliest site of activation was on the basal/mid-LV septum (*red*). (C) At this site, a Purkinje potential was seen in both sinus rhythm and preceding the PVC (*arrow*). Ablation at this site was performed, and the patient did not have any more PVCs or VT/VF. The patient was discharged and has not had any VT/VF after 1 year of follow-up. The color range is set such that *purple* represents late activation and *red* the earliest activation.

by PVCs from the LV outflow tract and papillary muscles.[87] In this series, 17 of 30 patients (57%) had PVC triggers from these locations. PVC triggers have also been reported from other myocardial locations demonstrating abnormal voltage or EGMs.[87,88]

Common to all of these patients with VF amenable to catheter ablation is the clinical demonstration of frequent PVCs initiating the arrhythmia (Table 35.2). Acute ablation success rates are near 100% when PVCs are inducible during the procedure. After discharge from the hospital, chronic success rates range from 82% to 100%. Despite the impressive clinical success rate of this therapeutic paradigm, an important practical limitation is the unknown frequency at which these patients can be identified. These patients appear to represent a highly selected cohort, thereby rendering VF ablation a rarity. Another limitation is the fact that frequent PVCs are necessary to map and VF may repeatedly occur during PVC mapping. If frequent PVCs are absent, one is limited to pace-mapping techniques to identify the target site (assuming that a 12-lead ECG of the pathologic PVCs is available)—a technique inferior to activation mapping of the pathologic PVCs.

TABLE 35.2 Catheter Ablation of Focally Triggered Ventricular Fibrillation

Study	Cardiac Pathology	No. of Patients	Distribution of FOCI	Follow-Up (Months)	Clinical Success (%)
Haïssaguerre et al.[62]	Normal	27	Purkinje = 23 RVOT = 4	24 ± 28	89
Knecht et al.[63]	Normal	38	Purkinje = 33 RVOT = 4 Myocardium = 1	63	82
Haïssaguerre et al.[69]	LQTS, Brugada	7	Purkinje = 4 RVOT = 3	17 ± 17	100
Bansch et al.[73]	CAD and MI	4	Purkinje = 4	15 ± 13	100
Marrouche et al.[74]	CAD and MI	8	Purkinje = 8	10 ± 6	88
Szumowski et al.[75]	CAD and MI	5	Purkinje = 5	16 ± 5	100
Enjoji et al.[81]	CAD and MI	2	Purkinje = 2	≥12	100
Bode et al.[82]	CAD and MI, myocarditis, valvular	7	Purkinje = 7	10	100
Hayashi et al.[83]	CAD, MI	5	Purkinje = 5	33 ± 22	100
Sinha et al.[85]	DCM	4	Purkinje = 4	12 ± 5	100
Mlcochova et al.[86]	Amyloidosis	2	Purkinje = 2	<1–8	100
Herendael et al.[87]	Normal, MI, DCM	30	Purkinje = 9 LVOT = 9 Papillary = 8 Myocardial = 4	16	83
Syed et al.[91]	Mitral valve prolapse	14	Purkinje = 11 Papillary or fascicular = 13	16	86
Santoro et al.[92]	Normal and DCM	6	Papillary = 6	58 ± 11	100
Sadek et al.[67]	Normal	7	Moderator band = 7	22 ± 12	100
Nademanee et al.[72]	ERS or JWS	51	Purkinje = 11 RV epicardium = 40	31 ± 26	91
Krummen et al.[93]	ICM and NICM	6	LV = 2 LV and RV = 4	12	83
Komatsu et al.[78]	ICM	110	Purkinje = 100	26	84
Haïssaguerre et al.[65]	Normal	24	NA	17 ± 11	83
Haïssaguerre et al.[94]	ICM, NICM, and BrS	54	NA	56 ± 30	100

CAD, Coronary artery disease; *DCM*, dilated cardiomyopathy; *LQTS*, long QT syndrome; *LVOT*, left ventricular outflow tract; *MI*, myocardial infarction; *RVOT*, right ventricular outflow tract.

CONCLUSION AND FUTURE DIRECTIONS

Hemodynamically unstable ventricular arrhythmias are amenable to catheter ablation. Currently, both scar-related VTs and certain patients with primary VF can be effectively treated with catheter ablation. For scar-related VT, instead of only trying to identify the pathway of activation during tachycardia, the scarred myocardium is identified, and strategically placed ablation lesions are used to eliminate potentially arrhythmogenic tissue. Since this substrate-based ablation strategy is performed in sinus rhythm, virtually any VT can be targeted for catheter ablation regardless of its hemodynamic effect. Irrespective of the cardiac pathology underlying the formation of the myocardial scar, a substrate-based approach to VT ablation can still be used. The demonstration that VF can be eliminated by catheter ablation in certain patients is an exciting option in the treatment of this sometimes-intractable clinical situation. Our understanding of the role of catheter ablation in primary VF and the role of the Purkinje network and the ventricular outflow tract is being refined with increased clinical experience.

Moving forward, multipolar catheters with smaller electrode size and reduced interelectrode spacing hold promise to improve the accuracy and speed with which substrate maps are acquired, although studies are required to validate voltage thresholds for abnormal tissue.[89] Noninvasive mapping techniques to identify rotor areas in VF may also offer insights for ablation beyond targeting of triggers.[90]

REFERENCES

Please refer to the e-book for a complete list of references.

36

Substrate-Based Ablation for Ventricular Tachycardia

Lohit Garg, Wendy S. Tzou

KEY POINTS

Mapping

- Arrhythmogenic substrate in ventricular tachycardia (VT) in the setting of structural heart disease is typically composed of viable but diseased myocardium within scar, which promotes reentry.
- This substrate can often be identified and effectively targeted with ablation in sinus rhythm or during pacing.
- Relevant substrate features are consistent with abnormal conduction and include (1) low-amplitude, high-frequency, bipolar signals, including local abnormal ventricular activities, most easily appreciated as late potentials in sinus rhythm; (2) sites at which pace maps demonstrate exit or central isthmus characteristics; (3) low-amplitude unipolar endocardial signals; and (4) substrate may also be directly visualized with preprocedure imaging or periprocedural intracardiac echocardiography (ICE).

Ablation Targets

- Ablation is targeted to regions identified on mapping, as above, to render substrate electrically inexcitable.
- VT noninducibilty following ablation is the most common end point.
- Also important is demonstration of entrance block (subsequent absence of conduction into the targeted region following ablation) and exit block (absence of pace capture within region that previously captured prior to ablation).

Special Equipment

- Electroanatomical mapping systems are critical for effective identification and visualization of substrate.
- ICE is extremely helpful in identifying substrate and in confirming catheter location and facilitating safety.
- Multipolar catheters can assist with higher-resolution and higher-density mapping. Irrigated-tip ablation catheters are essential for effective RF delivery.

Sources of Difficulty

- The proximity of VT substrate to other critical anatomical structures, including coronary arteries, phrenic nerve and proximal His-Purkinje system, and presence of mid-myocardial substrate each add difficulty in achieving effective VT control. However, this does not necessarily preclude the possibility of reducing VT burden with standard radiofrequency or adjunctive ablation techniques in experienced centers.

INTRODUCTION

Fibrotic tissue, and its ability to promote arrhythmogenic substrate when incorporated into living myocardium, was recognized decades ago among patients with prior myocardial infarction (MI) and ventricular tachycardia (VT). This concept was produced by the results obtained from early cardiac surgical experiences in invasive VT management, which subsequently provided the framework for contemporary catheter-based strategies for substrate modification.[1–7] Patients considered for treatment at that time were those with refractory VT following chronic, often transmural MI, which promoted both left ventricular (LV) systolic dysfunction and aneurysm formation. The initial approach included surgical resection of densely scarred aneurysms, sometimes with concomitant coronary artery bypass grafting; however, VT recurrence rates using this approach were disappointingly high, approaching 80% in some series.[8,9] Electrophysiological (EP) data collected during this era provided important information regarding (1) reentry as the mechanism in most cases and (2) localization of critical reentry elements within the subendocardium (1- to 3-mm thickness). This region harbored diseased but surviving myocytes contained within channels protected by surrounding scar or other electrically inert anatomical barriers (Figs. 36.1–36.3).[3,5,10] Guided by data as demonstrated in Fig. 36.1, subendocardial resection, among the patients who survived the surgery, led to effective arrhythmia control in >90% over a mean follow-up time of >2 years, further validating the concepts generated from the initial EP study.[5]

The involvement of scar and associated reentry in monomorphic VT among patients with nonischemic etiologies for structural heart disease (SHD) has also now become well recognized.[11–19] Therefore, the invasive treatment of VT in these patients has paralleled approaches taken for VT in the post-MI setting, focusing on modification of the arrhythmogenic substrate (Table 36.1). However, the scar distribution in nonischemic cardiomyopathy (NICM) is more heterogeneous and depends on the etiology. VT ablation in the setting of NICM more often requires epicardial access and use of adjunctive ablation techniques.

The advent of catheter ablation using radiofrequency (RF) energy as an ablation source in the 1980s, followed by rapid advancements in electroanatomical mapping tools, led to several

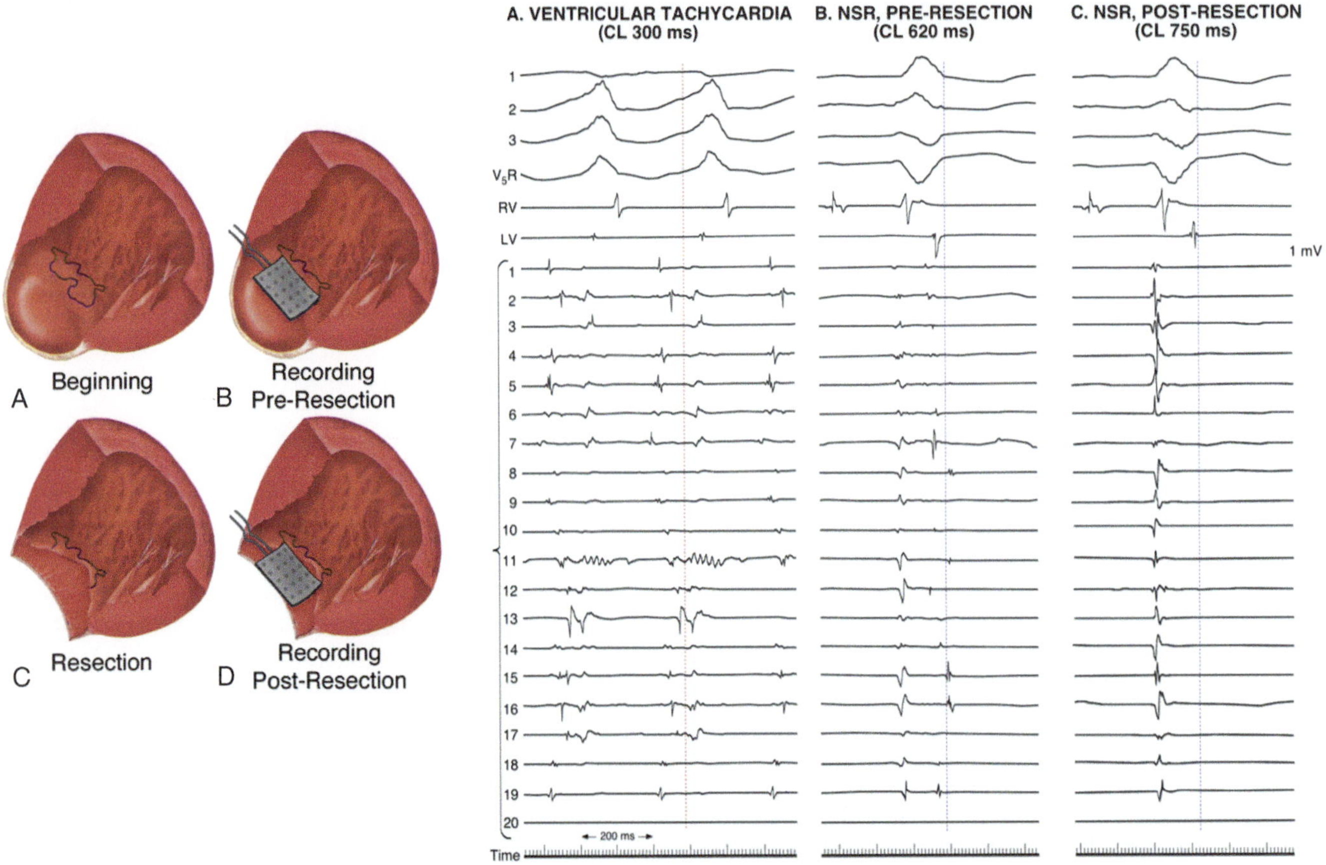

Fig. 36.1 *Left:* (A) Diagram of multipolar plaque placement in region of scar and border zone tissue prior to subendocardial resection (shown in B and C), for baseline, intraoperative electrophysiologic study. (D) Repositioning of recording plaque in same orientation for postresection electrophysiologic study. *Right:* Prior to subendocardial resection (A), ventricular tachycardia (VT) is inducible, and local recordings from the endocardium demonstrate presence of mid-diastolic potentials throughout the region of scar and border zone, and (B) similar signals are seen as late-potentials in sinus rhythm. Following resection (C), late potentials are no longer present. Acute VT noninducibility and lack of VT recurrence was achieved in most undergoing this type of procedure. (Reproduced from Miller JM, Tyson GS, Hargrove WC, Vassallo JA, Rosenthal ME, Josephson ME. Effect of subendocardial resection on sinus rhythm endocardial electrogram abnormalities. *Circulation.* 1995;91:2385–2391.)

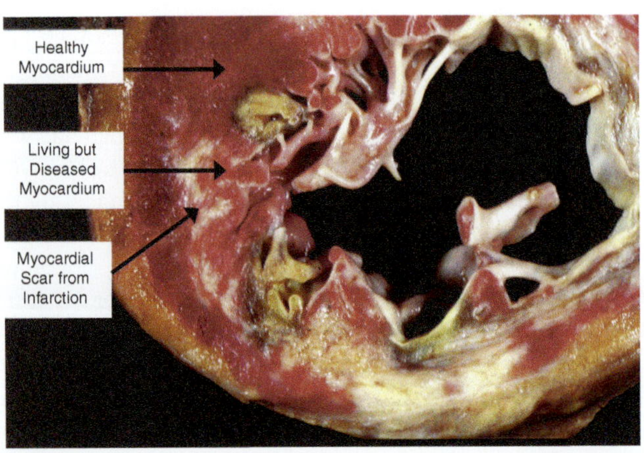

Fig. 36.2 In this cross-section of the left ventricle from a patient with prior "transmural" myocardial infection, note the heterogeneity of scar tissue intermixed with living tissue in the majority of the distribution of the infarction. (Modified from Tzou W, Marchlinski F. Electrophysiological evaluation of recurrent ventricular tachycardia. In: Saksena S, Camm AJ, et al. [eds]: *Electrophysiological Disorders of the Heart*, 2nd ed. Philadelphia: Elsevier; 2012:336.)

important milestones in our ability to effectively manage these patients. First, it became possible to "see" potentially arrhythmogenic substrate without the need for direct visualization with open-heart surgery and attendant surgical risks. Second, and perhaps most importantly, many of these characteristics could be identified and ablated during sinus rhythm, without the need for repeated and sustained VT inductions and entrainment or activation mapping.[12,20–22] As one-third of such patients have stable, hemodynamically tolerated VT that is able to be mapped for prolonged time periods or with repeated entrainment maneuvers, substrate-based ablation has become routine for most VT ablation procedures among those with SHD.[19,21–24] This approach has helped increase the number of patients that can be effectively treated and has provided important gains in preventing recurrent VT and implantable cardioverter-defibrillator (ICD) therapies. Given the relative safety and efficacy that can be achieved using substrate-based approaches, VT ablation is no longer considered a treatment of last resort for patients with SHD.[19,22,24–38]

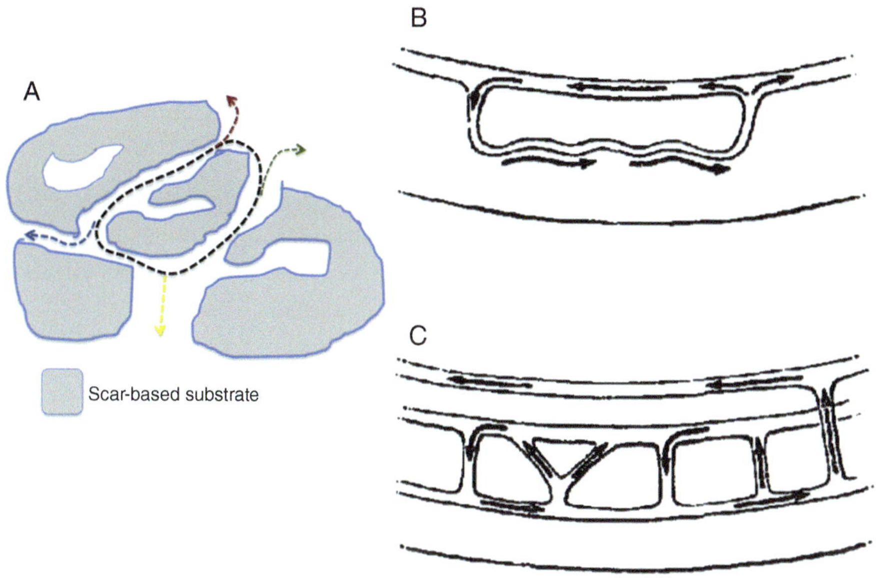

Fig. 36.3 (A) Examples of different exits (*colored, dashed arrows*) that can result from reentry involving the same substrate and central conduction circuit (*black dotted line*). Note as well that the vector of conduction through the circuit can also occur in multiple directions. The same concept is illustrated in these cartoons (B & C) of a cross-section through scarred myocardium, with multiple potential wavefronts of activation and exits (*black arrows*) using reentry circuit elements within the same substrate but on a three-dimensional scale. (B, C, Reproduced from Downar E, Kimber S, Harris L, Mickleborough LL, Sevaptsidis E, Masse S, et al. Endocardial mapping for ventricular tachycardia in the intact human heart, II. Evidence for multiuse reentry in a functional sheet of surviving myocardium. *J Am Coll Cardiol.* 1992;20:869–878.)

TABLE 36.1 **Potential Substrate Sites for Ablation**

Identified During Sinus or Paced Rhythm
Low-Amplitude Electrograms (EGMs) on Voltage Map Bipolar signals: • Endocardium: ≤1.5 mV • Epicardium: ≤1.0 mV • Dense scar: ≤0.5 mV Endocardial unipolar signals (suggesting mid-myocardial or epicardial substrate): • Right ventricle: ≤5.5 mV • Left ventricle: ≤8.3 mV

Sites Demonstrating Abnormal Local Conduction
• EGMs with multiple (>3) components of high-frequency or >80-ms duration (typically but not necessarily low voltage):
  • Present in baseline rhythm or
  • Provoked by ventricular pacing (alternate site if pacing present at baseline) or with extrastimulation mapping (a.k.a. local abnormal ventricular activities (LAVAs))
• Late potentials: distinct bipolar EGMs inscribed after end of surface QRS, separated from the initial local ventricular EGM by an isoelectric interval
• "Channels" of conduction within dense scar: EGMs recorded within dense scar
  • Elicited by decreasing color range on electroanatomical map, such that narrow channels of larger voltage surrounded by areas of extremely low voltage can be visualized
  • Often facilitated by mapping with multipolar catheters with <3.5-mm spacing between centers of adjacent electrodes
• Locations containing three isochrones of late potential or LAVA activation mapping within a 1-cm distance

Sites With Favorable Pace Map Characteristics One or more of the following: • Paced QRS matches VT QRS morphology in bundle branch block configuration, frontal plane axis, and precordial transition • Long (>40 ms) stimulus-QRS onset time • Multiple paced QRS morphologies produced with pacing at a single site
Identified While Mapping in Ventricular Tachycardia, if Tolerated • Sites with early, mid-diastolic activation (even if far-field) • Sites with characteristics of isthmus components

This chapter aims to describe various approaches for performing substrate-based VT ablation, among both ischemic cardiomyopathy and NICM for which the VT mechanism of reentry is demonstrated or presumed.

ANATOMY AND PATHOPHYSIOLOGY

The anatomical elements of a VT circuit are composed of surviving myocardial tissue within regions of electrically inert fibrotic scar tissue. Although scar is usually implicated as the source of VT in patients with SHD, the scar tissue itself is electrically inexcitable and, in and of itself, is not the actual target for ablation; this is the likely reason that surgically based resection of only dense scar had such poor efficacy in controlling VT.[8,9] The true areas of interest in such patients are the regions of surviving myocytes that are contained within or are at the border zones of these areas of fibrosis (Figs. 36.1 and 36.2). These surviving myocytes contain disrupted and reduced numbers of gap junctions, which lead to nonuniform conduction, slowing of conduction velocity, and altered refractory periods.[39,40] Differentially and abnormally conducting tissue connected in series, or channels, then provides the critical elements that allow reentry to occur and sustain. These properties include the potential to develop unidirectional block and areas of slowed conduction through which reentrant wavefronts can propagate once initiated.[40–43] An important feature of this substrate, especially in the context of understanding how modification is effective, is that these channels of conducting tissue that exist within abnormal and fibrotic substrates are numerous and are usually not fixed in conduction velocity or conduction vector. In other words, unidirectional block can be provoked within the same tissue in disparate directions depending on the site and method of initiating reentry. Using various pathways of conduction, several distinctive VTs based on QRS morphology and even cycle length can thus result from varying exits or other components of VT circuits propagating differently but within the same abnormal substrate (Fig. 36.3).[1] Identifying areas containing potential channels of conduction and rendering them electrically inert with ablation, functionally making existing scar tissue more electrically homogeneous, is the ultimate goal of contemporary substrate modification.[24,28,30–33]

The most common method used for identifying fibrotic myocardium has been to identify regions of reduced amplitude or absent bipolar electrogram (EGM) signals during sinus rhythm using a roving mapping catheter.[12] Use of an electroanatomical mapping system to record location and EGM voltage rendering a three-dimensional (3D) model is critical to all substrate modification strategies.[22] Of note, identifying areas with low-amplitude bipolar signals represents only a starting point for identification of relevant substrate. Signals within abnormal myocardium involved in reentry typically display other characteristics consistent with abnormal conduction, including high-frequency, multicomponent fractionation; prolonged duration (>80 ms) signals; or activation continuing or occurring after global ventricular activation has occurred, as manifested by the completion of the surface QRS complex (Figs. 36.1 and 36.4).[10,14,20,44] The latter, so-called late potentials (LPs), have frequently been found at critical sites within reentrant VT circuits, including 89% of isthmus sites, 57% of entrance, and 20% of exit sites.[10,20] Identification of EGMs with reduced voltage and abnormal characteristics forms the basis for substrate modification using catheter ablation.

Nonischemic Versus Ischemic VT Substrate

Most of the research discussed thus far has been based on work performed in the context of ischemic heart disease. Although these concepts have also been demonstrated to be useful and applicable to VT ablation in nonischemic heart disease, several important differences exist in ischemic versus nonischemic substrates that should be highlighted.

In contrast to the fairly predictable scar distribution encountered in patients with ischemic heart disease and VT, scar characteristics and distribution among patients with NICM can be far more heterogeneous and, relatively speaking, more 3D (Fig. 36.5). Periannular substrate is common, around the aortic or mitral valve, among patients with idiopathic dilated LV cardiomyopathy, and around the tricuspid and/or pulmonic valve among those with arrhythmogenic right ventricular cardiomyopathy (ARVC).[11,12,14,45,46] However, there is a wide variation of other presentations, especially when taking into account other nonischemic etiologies for SHD, including prior myocarditis, cardiac sarcoidosis, or other infiltrative cardiomyopathies.[47–49] Notably, NICM substrates more often involve the epicardium as well as the mid-myocardium.[14,18,46,49–53] In increasingly encountered instances, the substrate is entirely localized within the mid-myocardium or septum (Fig. 36.6).[13,53–58] Increasingly recognized is that NICM substrate for VT can be present among patients with a known history of coronary artery disease and even with a known history of prior MI (mixed cardiomyopathy), at a rate that likely exceeds a previously reported rate of 1.2%.[53,59] In fact, a seminal study among 89 patients with monomorphic VT and SHD (51% NICM), all of whom underwent endocardial and epicardial activation mapping during VT, revealed that the majority of patients had 3D VT activation equally involving both epicardial and endocardial surfaces (73% in ICM and 49% in NICM). The VT circuit components were entirely mid-myocardial, with focal breakouts observed on endocardium and epicardium in 16% ICM patients and 20% NICM patients.[53] Recognizing that VT circuits in SHD, both ischemic and nonischemic in etiology are more 3D than previously understood, is critical in planning for ablation, especially when recognizing greater challenges that are usually encountered in ablation of VT in NICM compared to ICM with more prevalence of mid-myocardial and epicardial scar.[48,49,60–63]

The presence of mid-myocardial and subepicardial scar confounds our ability to identify substrate using conventionally accepted mapping techniques. Standard bipolar voltage mapping, for instance, provides great detail with respect to the tissue with which a mapping catheter's electrodes are in direct contact, but it provides limited information regarding tissue that is deeper to the tip–tissue interface.[51,52] Limitations in identifying such substrate may be especially enhanced when using contemporary multipolar catheters with small interelectrode size and spacing, as these bipoles reflect an even narrower field of view

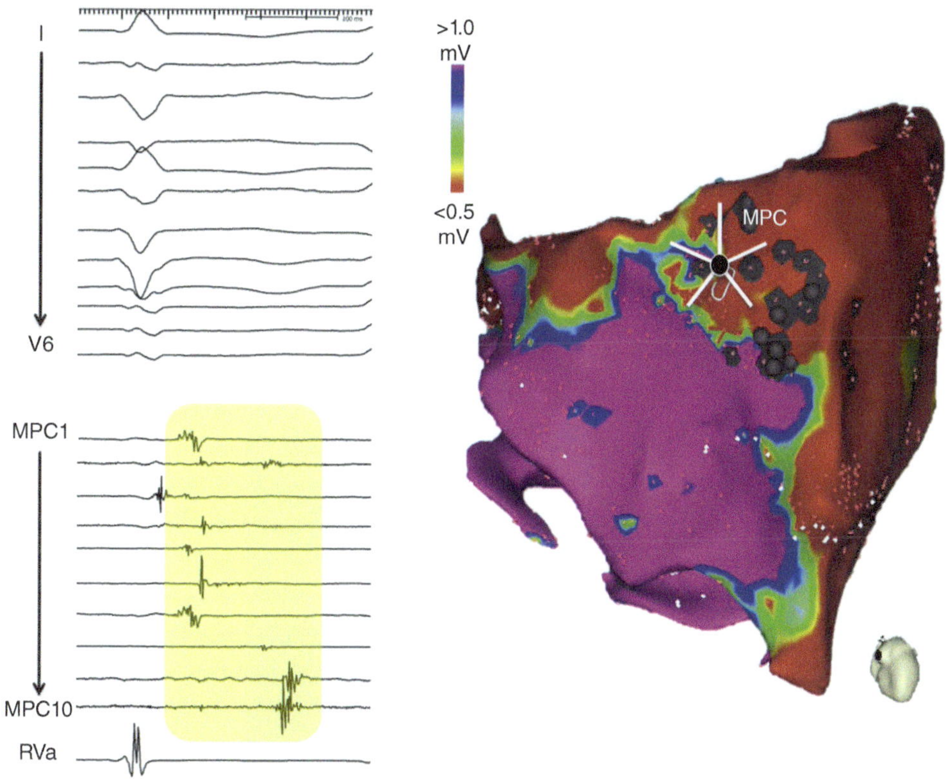

Fig. 36.4 (*Left*) Examples of diffusely present late potentials (highlighted in *yellow*), with varying degrees of conduction delay, recorded from each spline of a multipolar catheter (MPC) placed over the epicardial scar of a patient with arrhythmogenic right ventricular cardiomyopathy and ventricular tachycardia. Note the normal activation at the site of the catheter located in the right ventricular apex (RVa), which is essentially on time with the activation of the global ventricular myocardium represented by the surface QRS. (*Right*) Posterior projection of the inferior RV epicardial electroanatomical bipolar voltage map, showing the position of the MPC at which site the late potentials shown on the left were recorded.

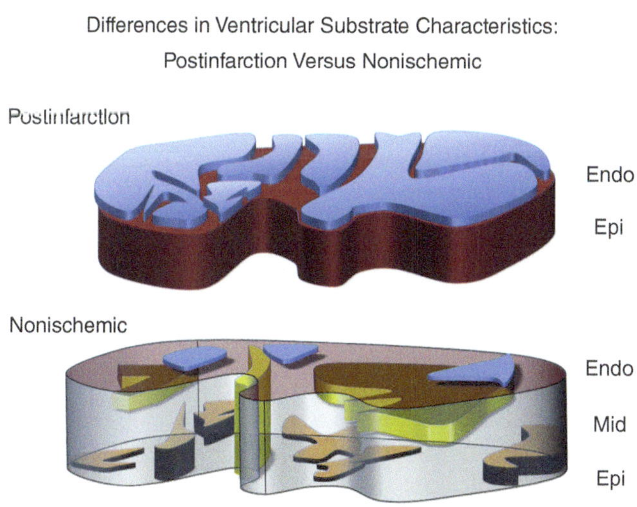

Fig. 36.5 Diagram of differences in ventricular substrate characteristics and distribution for ventricular tachycardia in the setting of ischemic versus nonischemic heart disease. (*Top*) Scar following MI (*blue shapes*) tends to be localized toward the endocardium (endo), while scar in nonischemic substrates (bottom) is more heterogenous and three-dimensional, and can involve the endo, the mid-myocardium (Mid, *yellow shapes*), and/or the epicardium (Epi, *orange shapes*).

than those with larger interelectrode spacing.[64–66] Use of unipolar mapping, during which signals are recorded between the distal electrode (cathode) and an anode placed at an electrically inert and remote location, for instance at Wilson central terminus, widens the field of view substantially.[51,52] This type of mapping compromises the ability to assess EGM detail but may allow for gross appreciation of deeper substrate abnormalities (Figs. 36.7 and 36.8).

Therefore, potentially epicardial or mid-myocardial substrate can still be identified from endocardial mapping, but with assessment of unipolar instead of bipolar EGMs. This concept was demonstrated to be valid among cohorts of VT patients with LV NICM and ARVC who underwent detailed endocardial and epicardial mapping with modest to no identifiable endocardial substrate and among whom endocardial unipolar voltage cutoffs could be validated with bipolar epicardial signal analysis.[51,52] Use of adjunctive imaging, for instance, with preprocedural cardiac magnetic resonance imaging (cMRI) or with intraprocedural intracardiac echocardiography (ICE), has also been demonstrated to be of particular value among patients with NICM and VT, based on challenges that exist in identifying substrate using only EP mapping tools.[13,67–69]

However, even once identified or recognized, additional challenges exist in effectively delivering energy and penetrating to regions of interest using standard ablation techniques, and achieving effective VT control in such patients has been repeatedly demonstrated to be challenging in observational studies and clinical trials.[19,48–50,58,60,61,70–72] Despite challenges, scar within

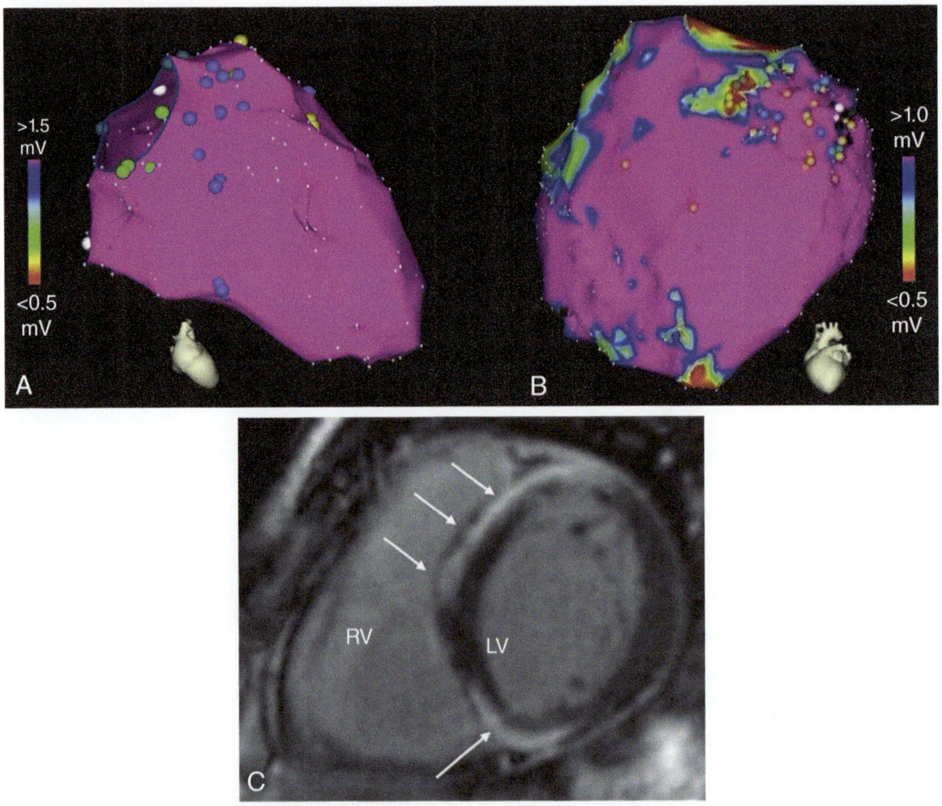

Fig. 36.6 Example of substrate localized entirely within the mid-myocardium from a patient with nonischemic cardiomyopathy and ventricular tachycardia. (A) Right anterior oblique projection of the endocardial left ventricular bipolar voltage map and (B) left anterior oblique projection of the epicardial bipolar voltage map, each demonstrating lack of apparent substrate. Areas of low voltage on the epicardium correlate with expected coronary arterial or fat distributions and are not truly indicative of abnormal substrate. (C) Cardiac magnetic resonance imaging, however, demonstrates substantial regions of delayed gadolinium enhancement, consistent with scar, within the mid-myocardium in the interventricular septum as well as the inferior left ventricle (*white arrows*).

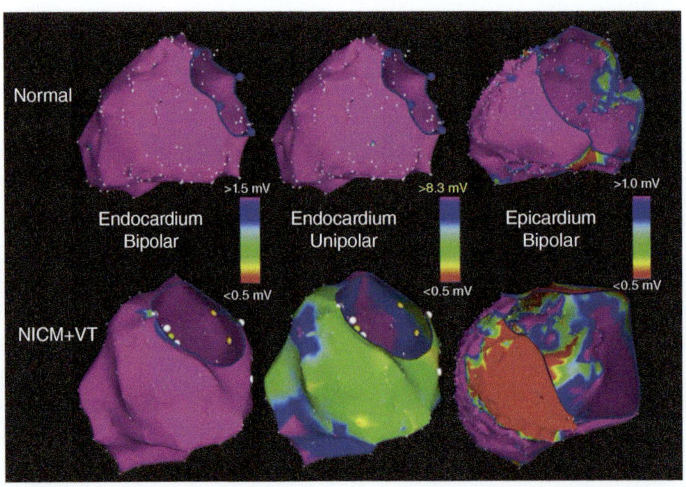

Fig. 36.7 Electroanatomical left ventricular voltage maps in posterolateral projection from a patient with structurally normal heart (*top row*) and a patient with nonischemic cardiomyopathy and ventricular tachycardia (NICM+VT, *bottom row*), with only mid-myocardial and epicardial substrate. In the normal patient, endocardial bipolar, unipolar, and epicardial voltage maps all are normal. In the NICM+VT patient, although the endocardial bipolar voltage map (*bottom left*) shows no significant abnormality, the endocardial unipolar signal assessment using a cutoff of ≤8.3 mV (bottom middle), suggests a substantial area of abnormality in the peri-mitral distribution. Epicardial abnormality is substantiated by bipolar voltage abnormality in the same distribution on epicardial mapping (*bottom right*). (Reproduced with permission from Hutchinson MD, Gerstenfeld EP, Desjardins B, et al. Endocardial unipolar voltage mapping to detect epicardial ventricular tachycardia substrate in patients with nonischemic left ventricular cardiomyopathy. *Circ Arrhythm Electrophysiol.* 2011;4:49–55.)

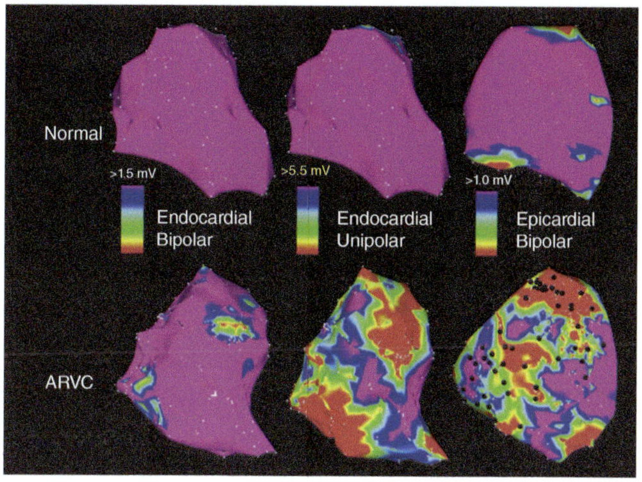

Fig. 36.8 Electroanatomical right ventricular voltage maps in right anterior oblique projection from a patient with structurally normal heart (*top row*) and a patient with arrhythmogenic right ventricular cardiomyopathy and ventricular tachycardia (ARVC, *bottom row*), with predominantly mid-myocardial and epicardial substrate. The endocardial bipolar, unipolar, and epicardial voltage maps all are normal in the patient without structural heart disease. In the ARVC patient, the endocardial bipolar voltage map (*bottom left*) shows minimal abnormality, while the endocardial unipolar voltage map, using a cutoff of ≤5.5 mV (*bottom middle*), indicates a substantial area of abnormality throughout the RV free wall, which is confirmed on the epicardial bipolar voltage map (bottom right), throughout which late potentials were identified (*black dots*). (Adapted from Polin GM, Haqqani H, Tzou W, et al. Endocardial unipolar voltage mapping to identify epicardial substrate in arrhythmogenic right ventricular cardiomyopathy/dysplasia. *Heart Rhythm.* 2011;8(1):76–83. https://doi.org/10.1016/j.hrthm.2010.09.088.)

myocardium has been demonstrated to produce a compartmentalization effect, delaying transmural conduction times and often disrupting intramural activation patterns (Fig. 36.9).[54,73] This compartmentalization effect can sometimes confer an advantage; the scar tissue that provides a barrier to transmural conduction can also sometimes be used as a reinforcing anchor for ablation lesions, assuming that the lesions can penetrate to the scar. Often, repeated ablations or use of adjunctive ablation techniques (discussed later in this chapter) is necessary to achieve success comparable to what can be achieved with less effort among patients who have had VT related to prior MI.[50,57,61–63,70,71,74–76]

MAPPING VENTRICULAR TACHYCARDIA SUBSTRATE

Several mapping approaches have been developed to identify relevant substrate for ablation and effective ventricular arrhythmia control, many of which have substantial overlap. The following sections and Tables 36.1 and 36.2 highlight the approaches that have come to form the foundation of contemporary substrate modification for VT management.

Mapping Tools

Tools that are essential for substrate-based VT mapping and ablation include an electroanatomical mapping (EAM) system and associated mapping catheter(s), which can be composed of a single bipolar electrode for point-to-point mapping (typically the ablation catheter is used in this instance) or multiple electrodes on a multipolar catheter.[12,22,65,66,77,78] The advantage of mapping with the ablation catheter is that simultaneous mapping and ablation can occur; in order to ablate in concert with mapping using multipolar catheters, either multiple access sites to the chamber being mapped must be obtained (i.e., retrograde aortic and transseptal accesses in the case of endocardial LV mapping) or catheter exchanges need to be performed.[77] However, multipolar mapping catheters confer the additional advantage of smaller electrode sizes and interelectrode spacing that allow for greater resolution, detail, and speed in mapping and potentially in better identifying channels and abnormal substrate compared to catheters with larger electrodes within areas of low voltage.[65,66,77] While such high-density mapping catheters allow for quicker and more detailed characterization of substrate in direct contact with the mapping electrodes, assessment of deeper, mid-myocardial or epicardial substrate is potentially even more compromised given the even narrower field of view.

Not required but usually helpful for both mapping and ablation is phased-array ICE. ICE provides real-time imaging to confirm catheter location and contact, assess for anatomical variations and structures such as papillary muscles that may challenge catheter movement or alter the ablation approach, assess for acute complications such as cardiac perforation and effusion or worsening systolic function, and reduce use of fluoroscopy. ICE is especially useful when epicardial or mid-myocardial substrate is present. Scar often appears as regions of increased echogenicity on ICE and can be quickly identified with initial catheter placement and image acquisition and even before any EP mapping has occurred.[68] Hyperechoic regions within the mid-myocardium or epicardium often correlate with unipolar voltage abnormalities (Fig. 36.10) and can substantiate the need for additional mapping (and ablation) on the surface opposite (i.e., the epicardium or RV side of the septum). ICE can be used in conjunction with any of the commercially available EAM systems. Currently only the CARTO system (Biosense Webster, Diamond Bar, CA) has the capability of integrating ICE images into the EAM, using the CARTO Sound catheter (Fig. 36.10D–E). This feature can be helpful in facilitating rapid 3D anatomical reconstruction of the chamber of interest, based on fusion of two-dimensional ICE images taken at different angles. It also can incorporate locations and anatomy of papillary muscles or other anatomical variables directly into the map, as well as superimpose a visual substrate reference into the map, all of which facilitate mapping and ablation. More contemporary 3D and "four-dimensional" ICE catheters have been developed, the utility of which is still to be determined in VT mapping and ablation.

VT Induction

VT induction is usually attempted at multiple junctures during a case, even for substrate-based ablation cases. At the beginning of the case, either before or after a substrate map is created, this is performed for several reasons: (1) to gain a gross understanding of the number of monomorphic VTs that may need to be

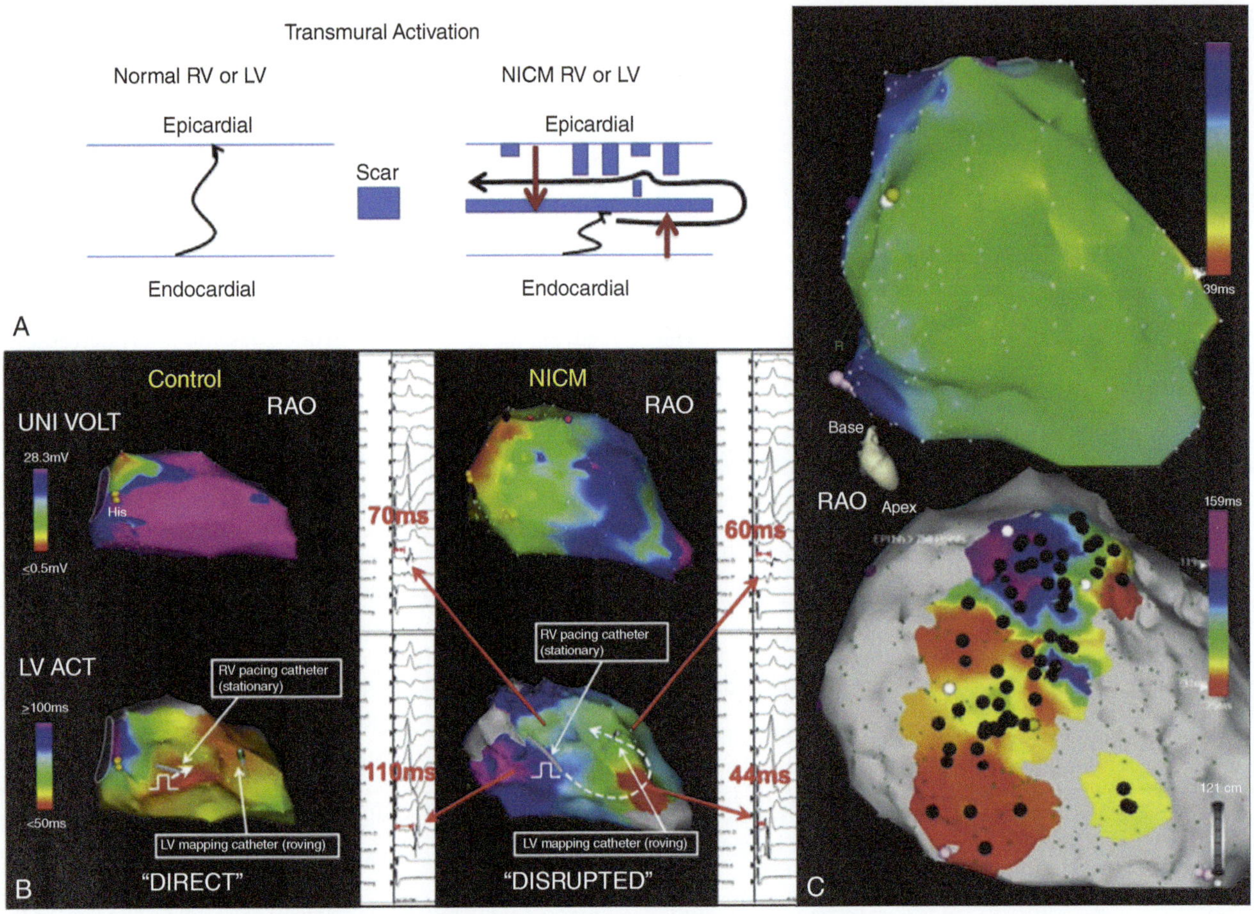

Fig. 36.9 (A) Cartoon depicting transmural electrical activation patterns (*black arrow paths*) in normal right ventricle (RV) or left ventricle (LV) (*left panel*), with earliest breakthrough activation on the epicardium generally immediately opposite the site of stimulation from the endocardium. In contrast, the presence of scar (*right panel*) can alter and delay electrical conduction, with earliest site of epicardial activation often distant or discordant from site of endocardial stimulation. In the latter example, the intramural scar provides relative compartmentalization to conduction and can be used as an anchor for ablation lesions, which need only to penetrate to the scar boundary and do not need to be transmural to effectively disrupt the potential for reentrant ventricular tachycardias to occur. (Modified from Tzou WS, Frankel DS, Hegeman T, Supple GE, Garcia FC, Santangeli P, et al. Core isolation of critical arrhythmia elements for treatment of multiple scar-based ventricular tachycardias. *Circ Arrhythm Electrophysiol.* 2015;8:353–361.) (B) Shown are right anterior oblique (RAO) projections of electroanatomical LV maps obtained from a patient without structural heart disease (*left panels*) and with nonischemic cardiomyopathy (NICM, *right panels*). The unipolar voltage map in sinus rhythm from the control patient (*top left*), demonstrates absence of mid-septal scar, and the earliest site of LV activation immediately opposite the site of RV septal pacing (*bottom left*). In the NICM patient, however, the unipolar voltage map (*top right*) demonstrates significant septal scarring (corrroborated on cardiac magnetic resonance imaging) and earliest site of LV activation (*bottom right*) more apical than the site of septal RV pacing, with marked comparative delays in transmural conduction times. (Reproduced from Betensky BP, Kapa S, Dejardins B, Garcia FC, Callans DJ, Dixit S, et al. Characterization of trans-septal activation during septal pacing: criteria for identification of intramural ventricular tachycardia substrate in nonischemic cardiomyopathy. *Circ Arrhythm Electrophysiol.* 2013;6:1123–1130.) (C) Sinus rhythm activation maps obtained from the RV endocardium (*top*) and epicardium (*bottom*) in a patient with arrhythmogenic right ventricular cardiomyopathy with extensive scarring involving the epicardial RV free wall, evidenced by extensive late potentials (*black dots*) throughout. In contrast to smooth endocardial wavefront propagation from apical anteroseptum to base within 86 ms (*top*), epicardial activation of the same patient shows progressively later activation starting from the mid-inferior RV toward the epicardial infundibulum. This occurs much later than corresponding endocardial activation and with a discordant vector suggestive of independent epicardial activation rather than multisite transmural conduction breakthrough from the endocardium. (Modified from Haqqani HM, Tschabrunn CM, Betensky BP, Lavi N, Tzou WS, Zado ES, Marchlinski FE. Layered activation of epicardial scar in arrhythmogenic right ventricular dysplasia: possible substrate for confined epicardial circuits. *Circ Arrhythm Electrophysiol.* 2012;5:796–803.)

TABLE 36.2 **End Points and Outcomes for Contemporary Substrate-Based Ablation Based on Ablation Strategy**

Ablation Strategy	Ablation End Point In Addition to VT Noninducibility	Outcomes From Index Publications
Direct Ablation at All Sites of Interest		

Local abnormal ventricular activity (LAVA) ablation	Elimination of all LAVAs, including but not limited to late potentials	• Complete LAVA elimination in 70%
		• Median follow-up 22 months
		• Complete vs. incomplete LAVA elimination:
		  • VT recurrence 32% vs. 75%
		  • Mortality 19% vs. 20%
		  • Adjusted HR for recurrent VT or death: 0.49, 95% CI 0.26–0.95, $P = .035$

Late potential abolition	Elimination of all late potentials	• Complete abolition of late potentials in 84%
		• Mean follow-up 13.4 months
		• Complete vs. incomplete late potential abolition:
		  • Acute VT noninducibility (among those inducible prior to ablation): 65.7% vs. 5.7%, $P = .005$)
		  • VT recurrence: 9.5% vs. 75%, $P < .001$

Scar homogenization	Elimination of all evidence for abnormal local conduction (late potentials and abnormal EGMs), within regions of bipolar EGM amplitude ≤ 1.5 mV	Ischemic cardiomyopathy:
		• Mean follow-up 22 months
		• Scar homogenization vs. "standard" ablation (linear lesions sets targeting putative isthmus sites):
		  • VT recurrence 19% vs. 47%, log-rank $P = .006$
		Nonischemic cardiomyopathy:
		• Mean follow-up 14 months
		• Scar homogenization vs. "standard" ablation
		  • Acute noninducibility of any VT following ablation: 69.4% vs. 42.1%, $P = .01$
		  • VT recurrence 36% vs. 61.4%, $P = .031$
		  • Adjusted hazard ratio for VT recurrence: 0.48, 95% CI 0.27–0.96, $P = .027$

Selective Ablation		

Scar dechanneling: Ablation at presumed conducting channel (CC) entrance sites within scar, characterized by
• Late potentials of shortest delay following global ventricular activation *and*
• Bipolar signal voltage ≤1.5 mV
	Elimination of all identified CCs into scar following targeted ablation at entrance sites	• Median follow-up 21 months
		• Complete scar dechanneling achieved in 84.2%
		• Additional ablation (pace mapping ± mapping) performed in 45.5%
		  • 26.1% with incomplete scar dechanneling
		• Acute VT noninducibility:
		  • 54.5% after scar dechanneling only
		  • 78.2% after scar dechanneling + additional ablation
		• Overall VT recurrence 26.7%
		• Incomplete vs. complete scar dechanneling:
		  • Recurrent VT or sudden cardiac death adjusted HR 2.54, 95% CI 1.06–6.10, $P = .037$
		• Scar dechanneling vs. scar dechanneling + additional ablation:
		  • VT recurrence 20% vs. 38%, $P = .013$
		  • Survival 95% vs. 89%, $P = .013$

Core isolation: Ablation encircling sites within scar with VT circuit isthmus features characterized by
• Bipolar signal amplitude ≤1.5 mV (≤1.0 mV when possible) *and*
• Late potentials, abnormal EGMs, or dense scar regions with channels of conduction *and*
• Pace capture with favorable pace map characteristics *or*
• Isthmus sites identified on limited activation or entrainment during VT
	• Elimination of evidence for abnormal local conduction
	• Failure to capture the ventricle with pacing from inside the ablation lesion set using a pacing output of 20 mA and pulse width of 2 ms from multiple (≥3), discrete sites that had previously demonstrated capture (exit block).
		• Mean follow-up 17.5 months
		• Core isolation achieved in 84%
		• Additional ablation (pace mapping ± mapping) performed in 27%
		• Acute VT noninducibility:
		  • 73% after core isolation alone
		  • 82% after core isolation + additional ablation
		• Overall VT recurrence 14%
		• Core isolation achieved vs. not achieved:
		  • VT recurrence HR 0.17, 95% CI 0.03–0.84, $P = .03$
		• VT-free survival based on end points:
		  • VT noninducible + core isolation: 90%
		  • VT noninducible + no core isolation: 67%
		  • VT inducible + core isolation: 83%
		  • VT inducible + no core isolation: 0%

Continued

TABLE 36.2 End Points and Outcomes for Contemporary Substrate-Based Ablation Based on Ablation Strategy—cont'd

Ablation Strategy	Ablation End Point In Addition to VT Noninducibility	Outcomes From Index Publications
Deceleration zone: Ablation targeting the areas of isochronal crowding – High-density mapping in sinus rhythm – ILAM maps generated by annotating to the latest electrogram deflection – Targeted ablation of deceleration zone defined as >3 isochrones in 1-cm radius	• Reduction of isochronal crowding in primary deceleration zone	• Mean follow-up of 12 ± 10 months • Average of 2 ± 1 DZ colocalized to putative isthmus in 95% patients • Acute VT noninducibility in 77% • 70% freedom from VT recurrence • 80% in ischemic and 63% in nonischemic cardiomyopathy • Overall survival rate 87%

HR, Hazard ratio; *CI*, confidence interval; *VT*, ventricular tachycardia. Acute VT noninducibility refers to that assessed following ablation.

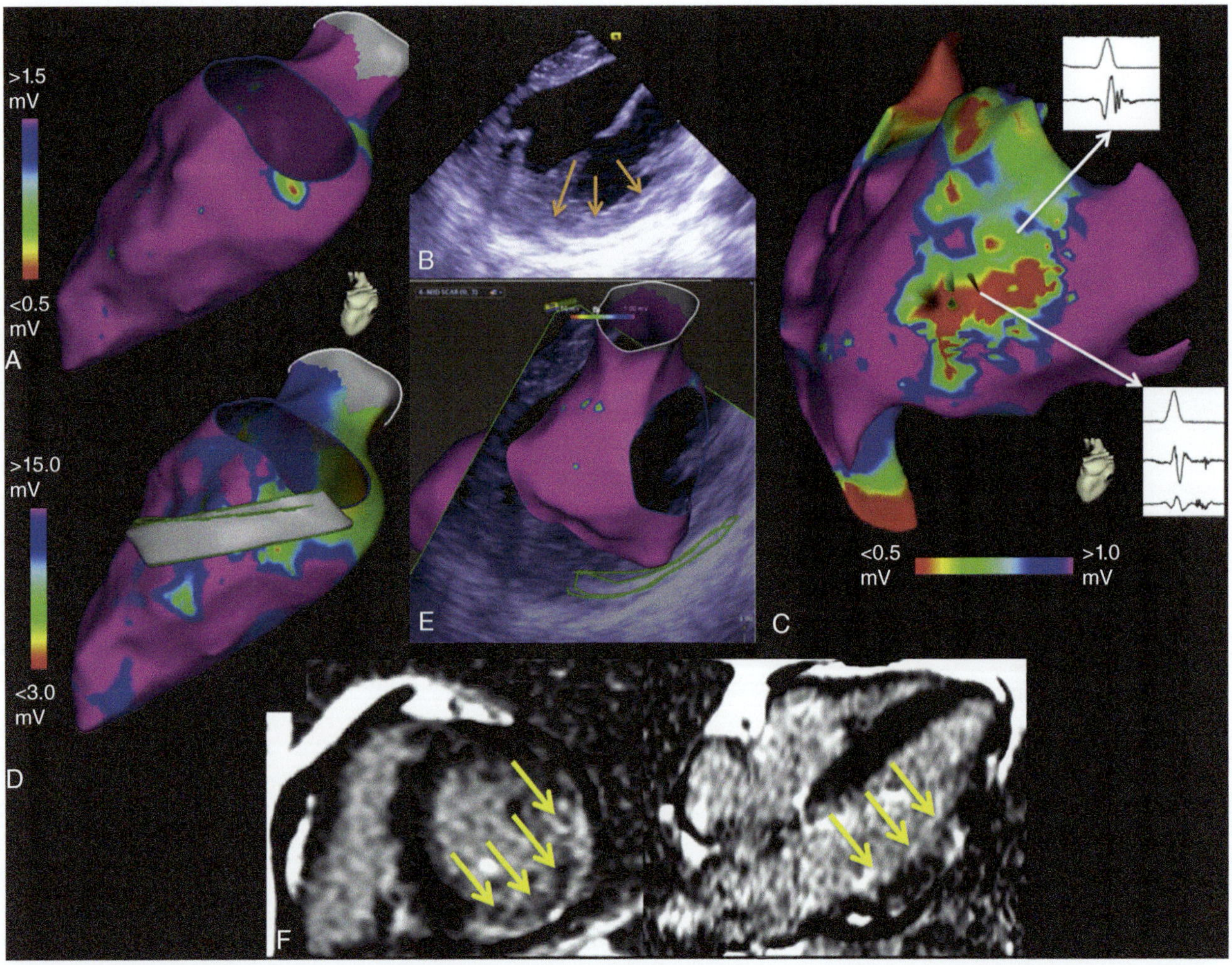

Fig. 36.10 Shown are electroanatomical maps (A, C, D), intracardiac echocardiography (ICE) with example of integration of ICE images within the electroanatomical mapping system (B, E), and cardiac magnetic resonance imaging (MRI) from a patient with nonischemic cardiomyopathy and ventricular tachycardia due to cardiac sarcoidosis. The posterolateral projection of the endocardial left ventricular (LV) bipolar voltage map (A) demonstrates no significant LV endocardial abnormality. However, real-time ICE images (B) clearly demonstrate a hyperechoic region (*orange arrows*) in the distal mid-myocardium and epicardium consistent with fibrotic substrate; in the CARTO system, two-dimensional contours of the region of interest are collected and integrated into the three-dimensional electroanatomical map (D, reconstructed three-dimensional scar location using ICE contours collected at different LV angles). Note that the scar location as seen on ICE correlates with the region of unipolar voltage abnormality in the inferolateral, perimitral annular mid-myocardium to epicardium (D). In this case, the threshold for abnormal unipolar voltage was increased, which uncovered the deeper substrate. (F) Cardiac MRI demonstrates delayed gadolinium enhancement (*yellow arrows*) in the same regions as observed on intraprocedural mapping. When epicardial access and mapping were performed (C), the bipolar voltage map also corroborates prior findings. Examples of abnormal electrograms and late potentials obtained from mapping the abnormal epicardial substrate are also shown.

targeted, which is especially relevant in the frequent instances in which 12-lead ECGs of spontaneously occurring ("clinical") VTs are unavailable; (2) to estimate potential exit sites (and potential sites to focus mapping and ablation) based on 12-lead morphology of induced VTs and acquire 12-lead templates from which subsequent pace mapping can be based; and (3) to confirm that substrate-based, reentrant VT accounts for the clinical tachycardias experienced by the patient, thus justifying proceeding with substrate modification. At subsequent intervals during ablation, VT induction is also often attempted to determine the end point for ablation (discussed in greater detail later).

Programmed electrical stimulation (PES) methods can vary, but a widely used protocol is to pace for 8 beats using constant pacing drive cycle lengths of 600 and 400 ms followed by the introduction of one to three extrastimuli until VT is induced or the ventricular effective refractory period is reached. Performing PES at multiple ventricular sites other than the right ventricular (RV) apex, such as the RV outflow tract or the LV, also can be useful in some patients in whom stimulation from the RV apex fails to induce VT. The ability to induce sustained monomorphic VT increases successively with the introduction of up to three extrastimuli. Beyond three extrastimuli, the probability of inducing monomorphic VT increases only marginally while the potential to induce polymorphic VT or VF increases more substantially.[79]

Voltage Mapping

Reference values for "normal" bipolar voltage were defined by mapping the RV and LV among six patients without SHD and with the use of the CARTO EAM system.[12] Specifically, the nadir-to-peak amplitudes of all bipolar ventricular EGM signals obtained with a mapping catheter composed of a 4-mm tip electrode and 2-mm ring electrode, separated by 1-mm interelectrode distance, were measured from the endocardial RV and LV. Among normal RVs, the mean ± standard deviation EGM amplitude was 3.7 ± 1.7 mV; although the range of normal values obtained varied from 0.4 to 11.5 mV, ≥95% of all signals were >1.44 mV. In normal LV endocardium, mean EGM amplitude was 4.8 ± 3.1 mV, with a range of 0.6–20.5 mV; ≥ 95% of all signals were >1.55 mV. For ease of use, an average normal value of >1.5 mV was then generated, and this value has persisted as the standard for identifying normal bipolar endocardial ventricular EGM amplitude or voltage.[12] Using a similar approach among eight patients with structurally normal hearts, a reference value of >1.0 mV was determined to be consistent with normal epicardial EGM amplitude, after taking care to exclude areas of major coronary arterial distribution and associated epicardial fat (within 1 cm of these regions), both of which can lead to artificially low-amplitude signals due to poor contact with the myocardium rather than reflecting true abnormality of tissue.[14]

Abnormal endocardial bipolar signal amplitude correlating with "dense scar" was derived from intraoperative VT mapping data and defined as <0.5 mV.[7,12] An essential point to emphasize is that signal analysis based on voltage alone is insufficient for identifying relevant substrate; poor catheter contact can produce low voltage that does not correlate with substrate of interest. Other features indicating abnormal conduction must also be present, including fractionation, or late or prolonged duration of activation, as described earlier.

Interrogated sites can be color-coded based on voltage amplitude and displayed on the EAM, producing a 3D reconstruction of the chamber of interest with EGM information at each site sampled by the catheter, and visually highlighting relevant substrate within which more detailed mapping and ablation should be focused. Although these values were developed and validated using the magnetic-based CARTO system (Biosense Webster, Diamond Bar, CA), other mapping systems incorporating impedance-based methods for sensing intracardiac catheter position and visualization have also been developed and are used clinically, including EnSite (Abbott, Minneapolis, MN) and Rhythmia (Boston Scientific, Minneapolis, MN). The accuracy in location, activation, and scar identification in each of these systems has been validated with in vivo, imaging, or histopathologic correlation studies.[66,78,80]

In a method similar to that which was used to determine normal bipolar endocardial signal amplitudes, reference values for normal LV and RV endocardial unipolar voltage were determined by assessing voltage characteristics among patients without SHD (six in the LV endocardial unipolar validation study and eight in the RV endocardial unipolar validation study). More than 95% of unipolar endocardial EGMs acquired from normal LVs had an amplitude >8.27 mV (mean, 19.6 ± 6.9 mV), and >95% of those acquired from normal RVs had an amplitude >5.5 mV (Fig. 36.7).[51,52] Using these reference values, endocardial LV unipolar voltage <8.3 mV accurately identified 82% of patients with confirmed epicardial scar abnormalities as defined by bipolar epicardial mapping. Among four patients in whom disparities were identified with regard to extent of endocardial unipolar and epicardial bipolar abnormalities, cardiac magnetic resonance imaging (cMRI) in two identified the presence of mid-myocardial substrate that correlated with the endocardial unipolar abnormality, thus lending support to the idea that unipolar signal analysis may be more effective in identifying mid-myocardial substrate compared to bipolar mapping.[51,67] We have additionally found that sometimes increasing the threshold for abnormal may be necessary to further bring out mid-myocardial or epicardial abnormalities on unipolar voltage assessment (Fig. 36.8). Among ARVC and RV VT patients, endocardial RV unipolar voltage reference <5.5 mV in prospective validation (Fig. 36.8) significantly correlated with epicardial bipolar voltage area both with respect to size and location ($r = 0.81$, $P = .008$).[52]

Therefore, a voltage map created in sinus (or paced rhythm) can provide starting information with minimal hemodynamic compromise regarding presence of substrate localized toward the ventricular endocardial surface (using bipolar voltage cutoffs of <1.5 mV to define scar and <0.5 mV to define dense scar), epicardial surface (bipolar signal amplitude <1.0 mV), or potentially within the mid-myocardium (LV or RV unipolar signal amplitude <8.3 mV or <5.5 mV, respectively).

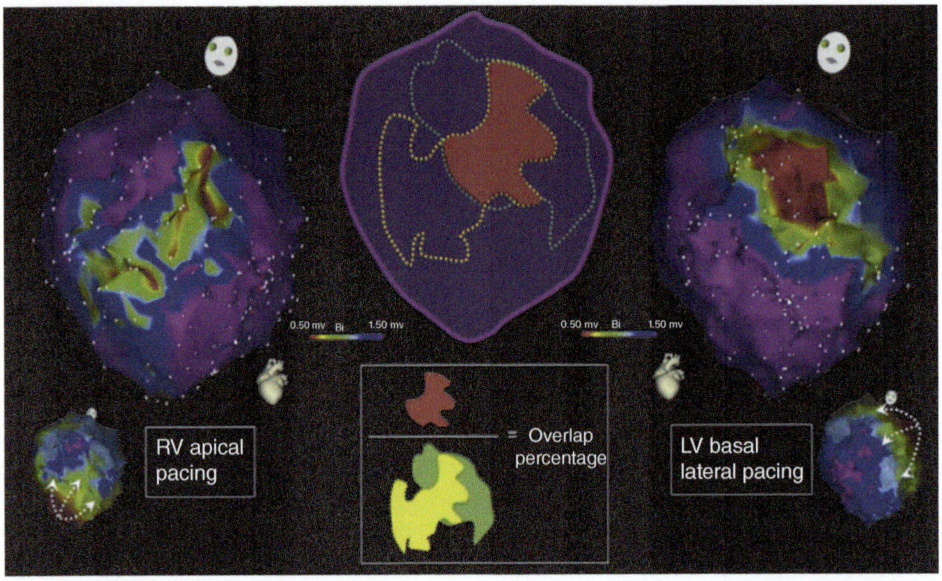

Fig. 36.11 Example of differences in distribution of substrate based on bipolar electrogram voltage and origination of wavefront of activation. (Reproduced from Tung R, Josephson ME, Bradfield J, Shivkumar K. Directional influences of ventricular activation on myocardial scar characterization: voltage mapping with multiple wavefronts during ventricular tachycardia ablation. *Circ Arrhythm Electrophysiol.* 2016;9:e004155.)

An important advance has been the recognition that the bipolar signal amplitude is also dependent on the wavefront of activation in relation to the orientation of the electrode pair, as it represents a summation of unipolar signals acquired from each electrode that comprises the bipole. Bipolar voltage produced by a wavefront that is parallel to the electrode pair (such that activation of the distal and proximal electrodes is sequential and temporally the most distinct) is typically larger than a wavefront traveling perpendicular to the electrode pair (as activation of the distal and proximal electrodes is simultaneous, thus yielding the lowest difference in unipolar signal summation).[81–83] Discordance in identifying areas of abnormal substrate, defined using usual bipolar voltage amplitude cutoffs,[12] based on wavefront of activation (e.g., sinus versus RV pacing) could be as high as 92% and is typically greatest among those patients with greater degrees of heterogeneous scar and NICM substrate (Fig. 36.11).[82] Multipolar catheters (e.g., HD GRID, Abbott, St Paul, MN, and Optrell, Biosense Webster, Diamond Bar, CA) incorporating multiple linear electrodes have been developed to help neutralize the effect of wavefront propagation on bipolar voltage amplitudes.[83]

Pace Mapping

VT exit sites, from which the rest of the ventricles are activated producing the 12-lead ECG morphology observed during VT, can usually be reasonably and quickly localized based on ECG characteristics (Table 36.1).[84,85] The process of pace mapping involves (1) using 12-lead ECG "templates" of spontaneously occurring or induced VTs to approximate exit sites within areas of abnormal substrate, as defined earlier, and (2) pacing at such sites to produce a QRS complex that either mimics the QRS complex during VT (consistent with an exit site) or has features suggestive of other central isthmus sites. Good pace map sites, meaning sites at which pacing produces a QRS complex that is similar to the VT QRS, have often been defined as those where the paced QRS matches the VT QRS complex in 10 or more leads.[86] However, a more liberal definition, which accounts for limitations in this type of mapping and is described in greater detail later, is one in which the paced QRS matches the VT QRS morphology in bundle branch block configuration, frontal plane axis, and precordial transition.[87] Even using the more liberal definition, good pace map matches are observed <30% of the time at sites demonstrated by entrainment to be central isthmus sites.[87]

Perhaps more important is the timing of the pacing stimulus, when local myocardial capture occurs relative to the onset of the evoked QRS complex which represents the activation of the global ventricular myocardium beyond the substrate. This temporal difference can provide valuable information about the captured myocardium that is relatively insulated by surrounding scar tissue, and is a marker for relative location within a potentially critical isthmus (Fig. 36.12).[44,86,87] For instance, pacing at a VT exit site should lead to more immediate activation of normal myocardium and produce a QRS complex very similar to the VT morphology with relatively short (<40 ms) stimulus-QRS time.[87,88] Pacing more proximally within a protected isthmus should produce progressively longer stimulus-QRS times. However, the more proximally within a VT isthmus that pacing is performed, especially when at early isthmus or entrance sites, the less likely it is that the paced QRS complex will match the VT QRS, and, in fact, the more likely that multiple paced morphologies reflecting multiple potential exits may be produced.[44,87,88] The reason for this phenomenon is that pacing during sinus rhythm, in the absence of functional unidirectional block that is present during VT, can lead to multidirectional wavefront propagation, which will produce a different ventricular activation and QRS morphology than when VT is ongoing and wavefront propagation within the same region is unidirectional. Furthermore, if high output is used for pacing capture, the pattern of ventricular

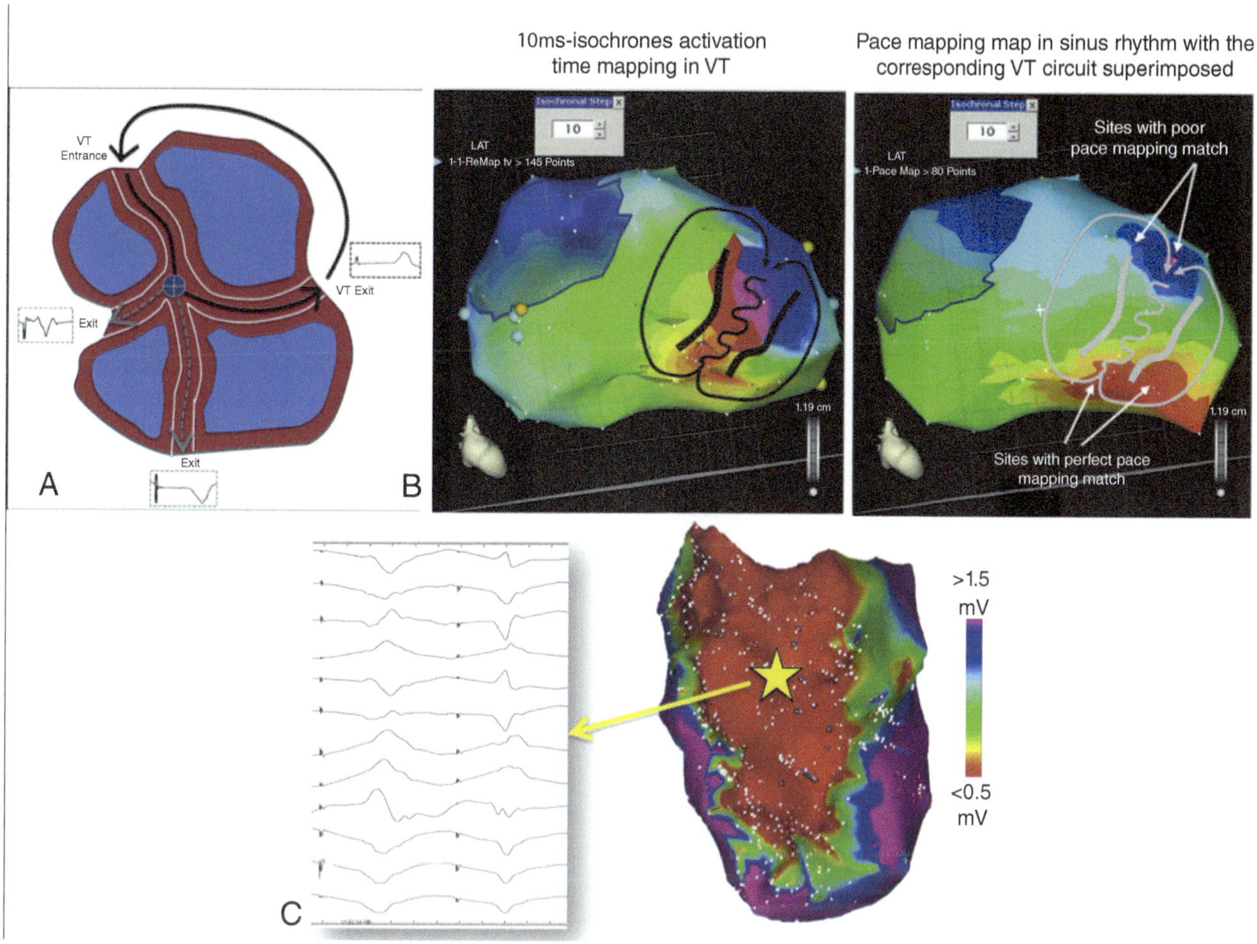

Fig. 36.12 Favorable pace map characteristics beyond QRS morphology match are demonstrated. (A) Schematic demonstrating the following concepts: (1) how pacing from a single site within scar (*blue*) can produce multiple QRS morphologies based on differential wavefront propagation and exit and (2) how stimulus-QRS times may be prolonged (>40 ms) due to underlying delayed conduction in diseased but viable tissue, as well as may vary based on relative distance of pacing and exit sites. (Reproduced from Tung R, Mathuria N, Michowitz Y, Yu R, Buch E, Bradfield J, et al. Functional pace-mapping responses for identification of targets for catheter ablation of scar-mediated ventricular tachycardia. *Circ Arrhythm Electrophysiol.* 2012;5:264–272.) (B) Displayed are right anterior oblique projections of electroanatomical maps of the LV, with activation times displayed during ventricular tachycardia (VT) and central isthmus corridor highlighted (*left*), and corresponding pace map (*right*) in a patient with prior anterior myocardial infarction. Note that the sites with best pace map matches, based only on degree of 12-lead QRS morphology match (*right*), are closest to the exit of the VT circuit; the more proximally within the VT circuit (i.e., from exit to entrance) that pacing is performed, the worse the pace map matches become. See text for further detail. (Reproduced from de Chillou C, Groben L, Magnin-Poull I, Andronache M, Abbas MM, Zhang N, et al. Localizing the critical isthmus of postinfarct ventricular tachycardia: the value of pace-mapping during sinus rhythm. *Heart Rhythm.* 2014;11:175–181.) (C) An example of multiple QRS morphologies produced pacing from the same site within dense scar, each with long stimulus-QRS time.

activation can change and produce a different QRS morphology due to a greater virtual electrode size or anodal capture, even if pacing is performed within a critical site within the VT circuit. Nevertheless, despite these limitations, pace-mapping can approximate the exit site of VT circuits and therefore can lead operators to the associated and more critical central isthmus components to which the exits are adjacent.

Local Abnormal Ventricular Activity and Late Potentials

In some cases, often in the absence of dense scar tissue, areas with diseased conduction may be obscured by higher voltage amplitudes of myocardium to which they are directly adjacent. Areas such as these, with so-called local abnormal ventricular activities (LAVAs), can sometimes be revealed by altering the wavefront of activation of the region, for instance with ventricular pacing instead of during sinus, or by uncoupling their activation from more normal tissue, for instance with ventricular extrastimuli, which serve to provoke conduction property differences and thus lead to more marked temporal differences in activation than are otherwise present with stimulation at a fixed cycle length (Fig. 36.13).[32,89–91] Several strategies have been described in which ventricular extrastimuli may be introduced to uncouple abnormal from normal myocardium, thus revealing

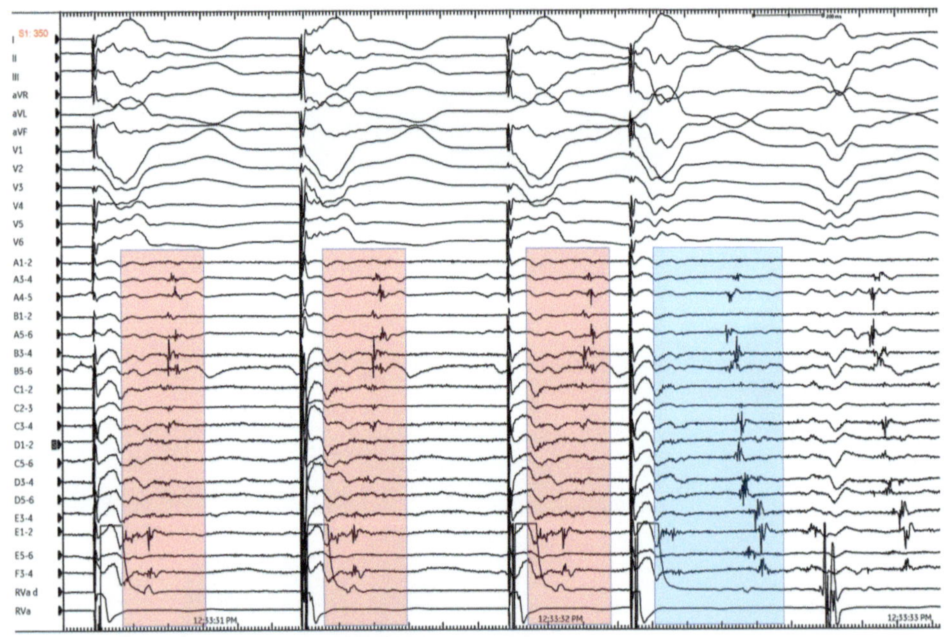

Fig. 36.13 Examples of regions with local abnormal conduction (e.g. local abnormal ventricular activities, or LAVAs), revealed with ventricular pacing at 500 ms (*Red highlight*) or with ventricular extra-stimulation (*Blue highlight*).

substrate that otherwise was obscured and assists in refining ablation targets. In 29% to 62% of cases, in fact, abnormal zones of conduction have been identified within regions of preserved bipolar voltage, emphasizing that functional assessment of substrate is also important, especially in the face of heterogeneous fibrosis.[89-91] Conversely, sometimes, in the presence of densely scarred or infarcted myocardium, small channels of surviving myocytes that participate in reentry may also be obscured, especially when using standard cutoffs for bipolar voltage defining normal and abnormal. In such cases, viable channels of conducting myocardium may be identified simply by decreasing the color range, such that tissue with larger amplitude signals can be accentuated with respect to the larger regions of extremely low voltage that may surround it. These sites can then serve as targets for pace mapping and ablation (Fig. 36.14).[92] Alternatively, multipolar catheters with smaller interelectrode distances also have shown utility in better identifying regions of relative heterogeneity with higher resolution and faster acquisition times.[65,66,77,78,93]

Similar to but more straightforward than LAVA mapping, identification of regions of late potentials recorded during normal sinus or paced rhythm can be annotated on an EAM and help highlight potentially important elements of VT circuits.[24,30,32,33,94,95] Late potentials are defined as bipolar EGM recordings that are inscribed after the end of the surface QRS complex, separated from the major initial local ventricular EGM component by an isoelectric interval. In one approach, the entire substrate-based map can be displayed as an activation map. In distinction from activation maps created during tachycardia, during which sites of earliest activation are sought, late potential maps emphasize areas of latest activation during sinus (or nontachycardia) rhythm. A fiducial, reproducibly identified component of the QRS complex is used for timing reference; with use of the typical color scale, red represents "early" and purple represents "late." Areas with the most delay in local conduction during sinus rhythm then appear as purple on the EAM. Conversely, those regions without significant conduction delay appear as red, and areas of activation with relatively intermediate slowing are color-coded with respect to the color distribution in the visible spectrum (Figs 36.15 and 36.16).[33,94,95] Another approach for highlighting areas with late potentials is to create hybrid substrate EAMs, for instance annotating late potential points as markers or tags on a standard voltage map, individually color-coded to represent relative timing following surface QRS activation.[30]

Limitations to Substrate Mapping Strategies

Although regions containing late potentials are generally recognized to be important, ablation at only sites demonstrating the most delayed conduction during sinus rhythm may not always be successful in suppressing recurrent VT and may incorporate potentially unnecessary ablation.[30,94,95] Irie and colleagues demonstrated the utility of isochronal late activation maps (ILAMs) in identifying sites of highest potential ablation yield among 33 patients with 47 scar-related VTs of mixed etiologies, then prospectively evaluating the approach in 10 additional patients.[94] In retrospective, off-line analysis, late potential maps were created with categories of activation, using the surface QRS complex as reference, distinctly divided into eight isochrones of activation following the QRS (Fig. 36.16). When correlating ILAMs with sites believed to be critical for reentry, based on mid-diastolic activity during VT with nonectopic termination

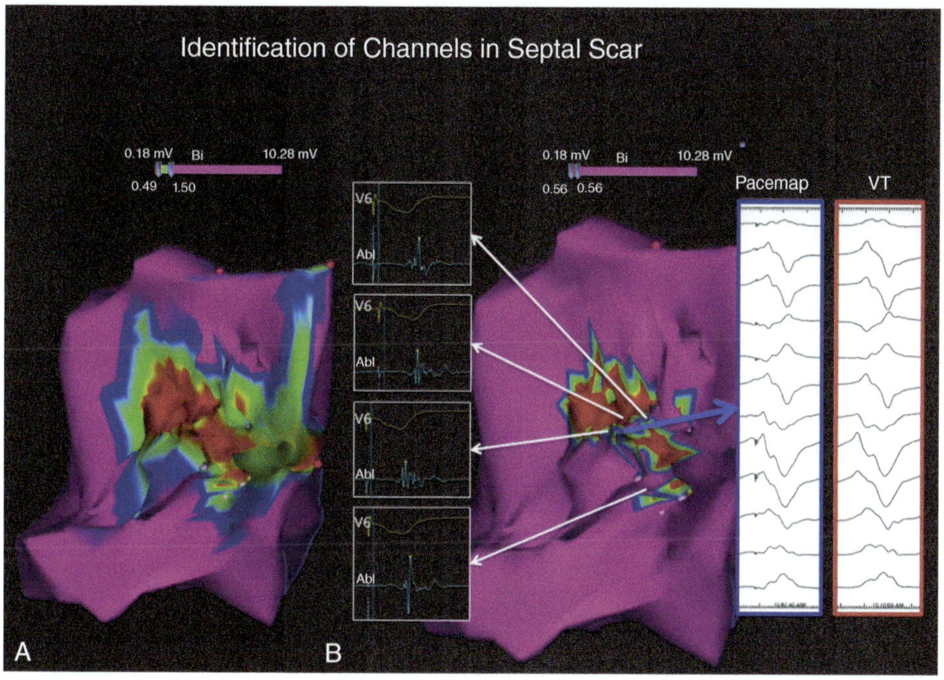

Fig. 36.14 Septal projections of endocardial electroanatomical voltage maps of the right ventricle are shown using standard bipolar voltage amplitude cutoffs (A) and decreasing the color scale threshold for abnormal in order to accentuate regions of potentially viable conduction channels within dense scar (B). (B) Evidence for residual conduction within the channels include presence of late potentials throughout (white arrows to associated bipolar electrograms recorded by the ablation catheter (Abl)) and ability to capture myocardium with pacing at these sites. Pacing from the site indicated by the blue arrow produced a 12-lead QRS complex that was a nearly identical match to the clinical ventricular tachycardia (VT).

during ablation, response to entrainment consistent with isthmus sites, or pace-mapping criteria as described earlier, only 11% of critical sites were localized to the latest activation isochrones. The majority (64%) were localized to the second and third latest isochrones; these often also were sites that demonstrated isochronal crowding, defined as regions containing >2 isochrones within a 1-cm radius, and consistent with regions of relatively delayed conduction in sinus rhythm. Aziz et al. subsequently prospectively validated this mapping technique among 127 patients (50% NICM) and demonstrated that areas of isochronal crowding of LAVAs and LPs during sinus rhythm correlated with VT termination sites in 95%.[95] While the concept behind the technique is intuitive and biologically plausible, important limitations exist in the ability of existing EAM systems to accurately automate activation mapping performed in this fashion (which is counter to how traditional activation mapping during tachycardia is performed); thus far only EnSite (Abbott, Minneapolis, MN) has this type of mapping algorithm as an automated option. Even with such an algorithm in place, however accuracy of how timing is annotated often must be manually double-checked, and, in an era where 10,000+ points are routinely acquired with high-density mapping catheters, these are salient considerations.

Despite limitations, however, the basic approaches described for mapping and ablating substrate in sinus rhythm have been effective in overall management of VT in patients with SHD, as detailed here.

CARDIAC IMAGING TO GUIDE SUBSTRATE-BASED ABLATION

As noted, multiple cardiac imaging modalities exist that may be useful in identifying VT substrate and can be integrated within EAM to potentially refine ablation and reduce procedure times.[13,22,68,69] ICE (as discussed earlier) is being increasingly used and is relatively widely available.[22,68] Preprocedural imaging with cardiac MRI (CMR) or multidetector cardiac computed tomography (MDCT), though not widely available, can provide detailed scar characteristics and identify putative VT isthmuses potentially without the need for extensive, traditional mapping.[56,69,96,97]

Multiple studies have evaluated the correlation of scar identified with CMR and EAM and successful ablation sites. CMR, in the setting of acceptable image resolution (usually including proprietary software to minimize artifact from cardiac implantable electronic devices) and registration within the EAM, has been shown to highlight targets for ablation including transmural scar areas, scar border zone, and the core scar–scar border zone junction (Fig. 36.17).[98–101] A major limitation of CMR, in addition to those mentioned earlier, is the low spatial resolution and the maximal voxel resolution of 1.4 mm^3 with 3-T MRI. Conducting channels as small as <0.2 mm have been described and could be missed with CMR. In addition, identification of scar involving the RV with CMR is challenging and has not been validated in larger studies. MDCT had a significantly higher resolution (<0.4-mm voxel size) compared to CMR. MDCT can define scar

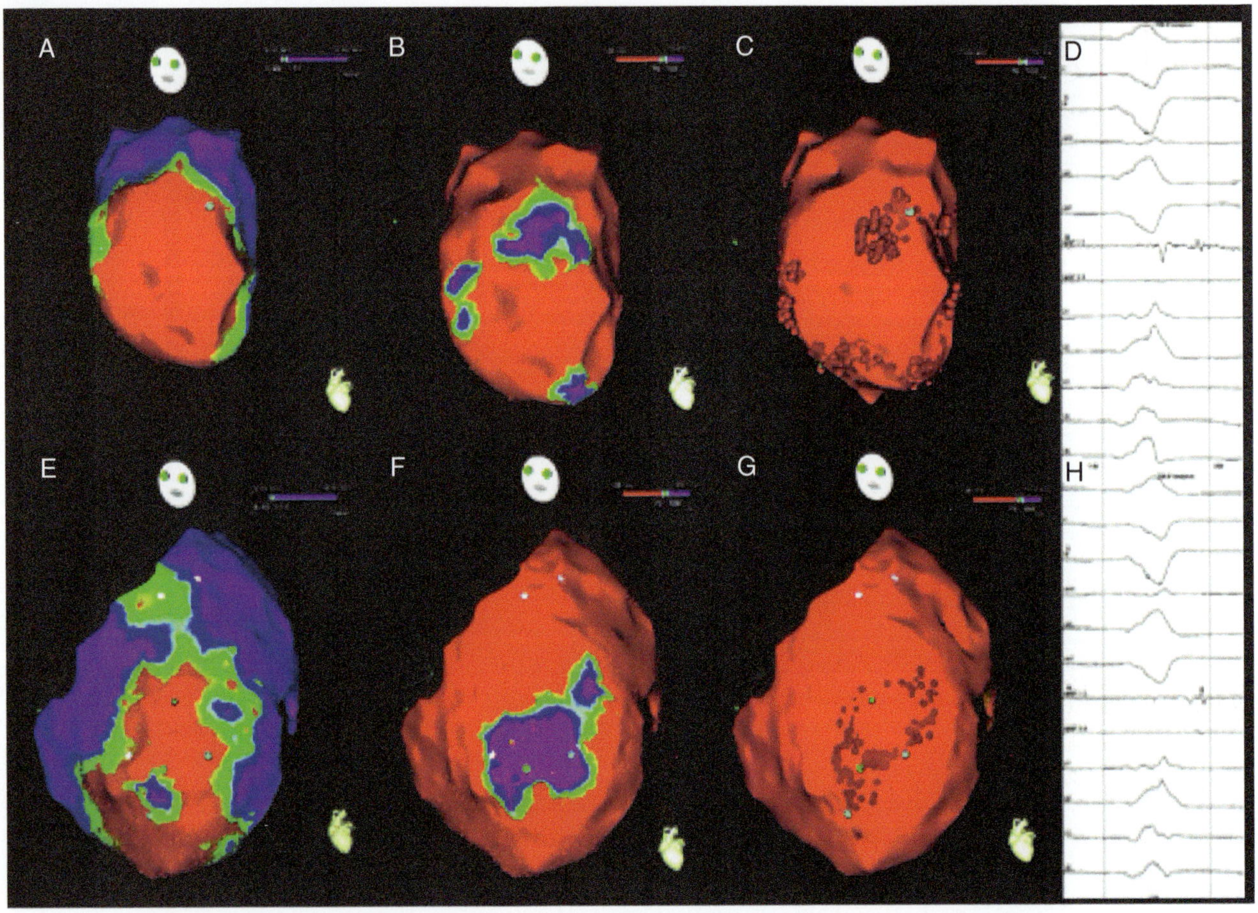

Fig. 36.15 Depicted are anteroposterior projections of electroanatomical voltage (A, E) and late potential activation (B, C, F, G) maps, obtained from the left ventricular (LV) endocardium (*top rows*) and epicardium (*bottom rows*) in a patient with prior anterior myocardial infarction and ventricular tachycardia (VT). The color scale in B, C, F, and G is adjusted such that earliest (*red*) activation is with respect to the onset of the surface QRS complex (D, H), and latest (*purple*) activation is with respect to the offset of the late potential following the QRS. Following ablation targeting late potential clusters (B, F), remapping demonstrates absence of any significant areas of delayed conduction (C, G). (Reproduced from Vergara P, Trevisi N, Ricco A, Petracca F, Baratto F, Cireddu M, et al. Late potentials abolition as an additional technique for reduction of arrhythmia recurrence in scar related ventricular tachycardia ablation. *J Cardiovasc Electrophysiol.* 2012;23:621–627.)

and correlates well with EAM in the setting of ICM VT but performs less well in identification of NICM substrate.[100,102] MDCT can identify areas of wall thinning, hypoattenuation as a result of fatty metaplasia and decreased perfusion, as well as anatomical information, including coronary arteries and epicardial fat, that could be helpful for planning an ablation.[100] There is incremental utility and promise of these modalities to assist in improving procedural speed and efficacy. However, limited availability of the tools and imaging expertise, as well as imperfect image integration and registration error (3–5 mm), even at centers with dedicated resources, can limit utility.[100,101]

SUBSTRATE-BASED ABLATION FOR ELIMINATION OF VENTRICULAR TACHYCARDIA

Contemporary VT RF ablation typically is performed with use of 3.5- to 4-mm, cooled-tip catheters. Although both open- and closed-irrigated catheters are commercially available, we typically use open-irrigated catheters with normal saline as the standard coolant at our institution. In challenging cases, open-irrigated ablation using hypotonic irrigant (usually half-normal saline) has been utsed in VT ablation in SHD, especially for repeat ablations (see discussion later).[103–105] Greater ablation lesion sizes as well as efficacy in arrhythmia control and outcomes have been demonstrated using irrigated-tip compared to standard-tip catheters.[106–109] Use of force-sensing irrigated catheters, including SmartTouch Thermocool (Biosense Webster, Diamond Bar, CA) and TactiCath (Abbott, Minneapolis, MN), has improved ability to assess adequate catheter contact during ablation and, by extension, associated improvement in lesion efficacy, although data regarding improved clinical outcomes are limited with regard to their use in VT ablation.[110–112]

With open-irrigated catheters, temperature-controlled unipolar RF ablation is typically used, with temperature limit of 40–45°C and power delivery of up to 50 W. Duration of individual lesion applications ranges from 30 seconds to several minutes and is guided by ≥1 of the following parameters used to assess acute efficacy: (1) impedance drop of ≥10 Ω from

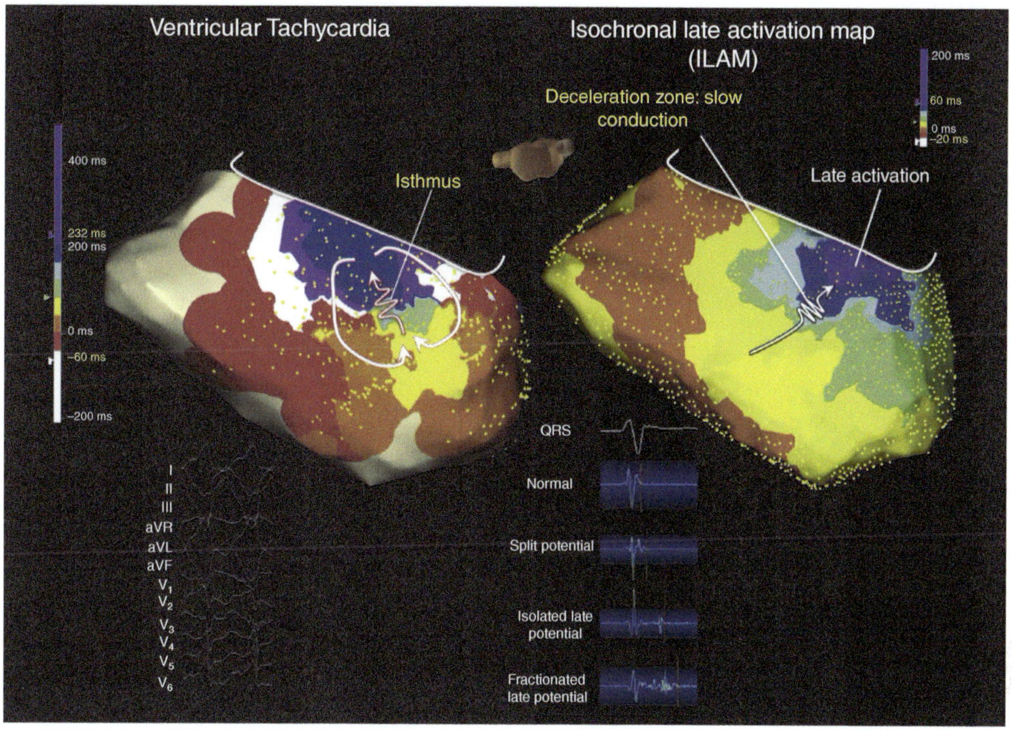

Fig. 36.16 Patient with prior inferior myocardial infarction and ventricular tachycardia (VT). (*Left*) Activation map during VT, during which an isthmus is identified, with representative circuit superimposed demonstrating pattern of figure-of-eight activation. (*Right*) In sinus rhythm, an isochronal late activation map (ILAM) is created, in which categories of late potentials are displayed based on eight equally distributed isochrones of ventricular activation. Shown on the bottom right are examples of how late-potential timing is annotated, to the offset of the local electrogram. Note that the isochrones encompassing the latest late potential activation (*blue and purple regions*) do not correlate anatomically with where the isthmus for VT was identified; in fact, the isthmus is contained within the region where only intermediately delayed late-potential regions were identified but where isochronal crowding is observed. (Bottom right panel reproduced from Irie T, Yu R, Bradfield JS, Vaseghi M, Buch EF, Ajijola OA, et al. Relationship between sinus rhythm late activation zones and critical sites for scar-related ventricular tachycardia: systematic analysis of isochronal late activation mapping. *Circ Arrhythm Electrophysiol.* 2015;8:390-399. Other figure components reproduced from Dr. Roderick Tung.)

baseline; (2) reduction in EGM amplitude or loss of late potential during ablation; (3) termination of VT not associated with ventricular ectopy with ablation, in limited cases in which ablation is performed during VT; and (4) observation of increased myocardial echogenicity on ICE at the site of ablation. These factors must also be weighed against the risk of excessive tissue heating that could lead to steam formation within myocardium, subsequent vaporization, and local myocardial rupture, a phenomenon known as "steam pop" (SP). In our experience, we have found that SPs more often occur when impedance reduction rates are rapid (1.4 Ω/s versus 0.38 Ω/s among lesions without steam pop, $P = .032$, unpublished data); these often are associated with rapid increases in tissue echogenicity observed on ICE as well (Fig. 36.18). Other clues supporting effectiveness of ablation lesions can be gleaned from response to pacing following ablation, including the following: (1) inability to capture the ablation site pacing at 10–20 mA following ablation[24,113] and (2) after a series of contiguous lesions have been applied, observing a change in paced QRS morphology compared to pacing at the same site prior to ablation, implying block along a region of prior conduction and subsequently altered exit (Fig. 36.19).[114]

Traditional Substrate-Based VT Ablation: Targeting the Putative Critical Isthmus Identified With Pace Mapping

Historically, substrate modification was first guided by pace mapping within regions of low voltage.[12,115] Recognizing that the exit site is likely to be spatially adjacent to other, more critical VT circuit components and that the critical isthmus is more likely (in >80% of cases) to be in dense scar or deeper within the border zone, a strategy of applying ablation lesions in linear distribution through sites with good pace-map matches within scar border zone and continuing the lesions into the lower-voltage scar adjacent to putative exit sites was used; length of lesion sets typically was >4 cm.[12,92,115] The concept behind doing so was to transect or disrupt other critical circuit components that were not only relevant to the "clinical" VT but also could subsequently neutralize substrate for other reentrant VTs (Fig. 36.20). The initial report using this strategy included 16 patients with ischemic cardiomyopathy (n = 9) or NICM (n = 7), among whom the median number of VT episodes in the month prior to ablation was 21 (range 6–55).[12] Following ablation, VT-free survival was achieved in the majority (75%) over a >15-month

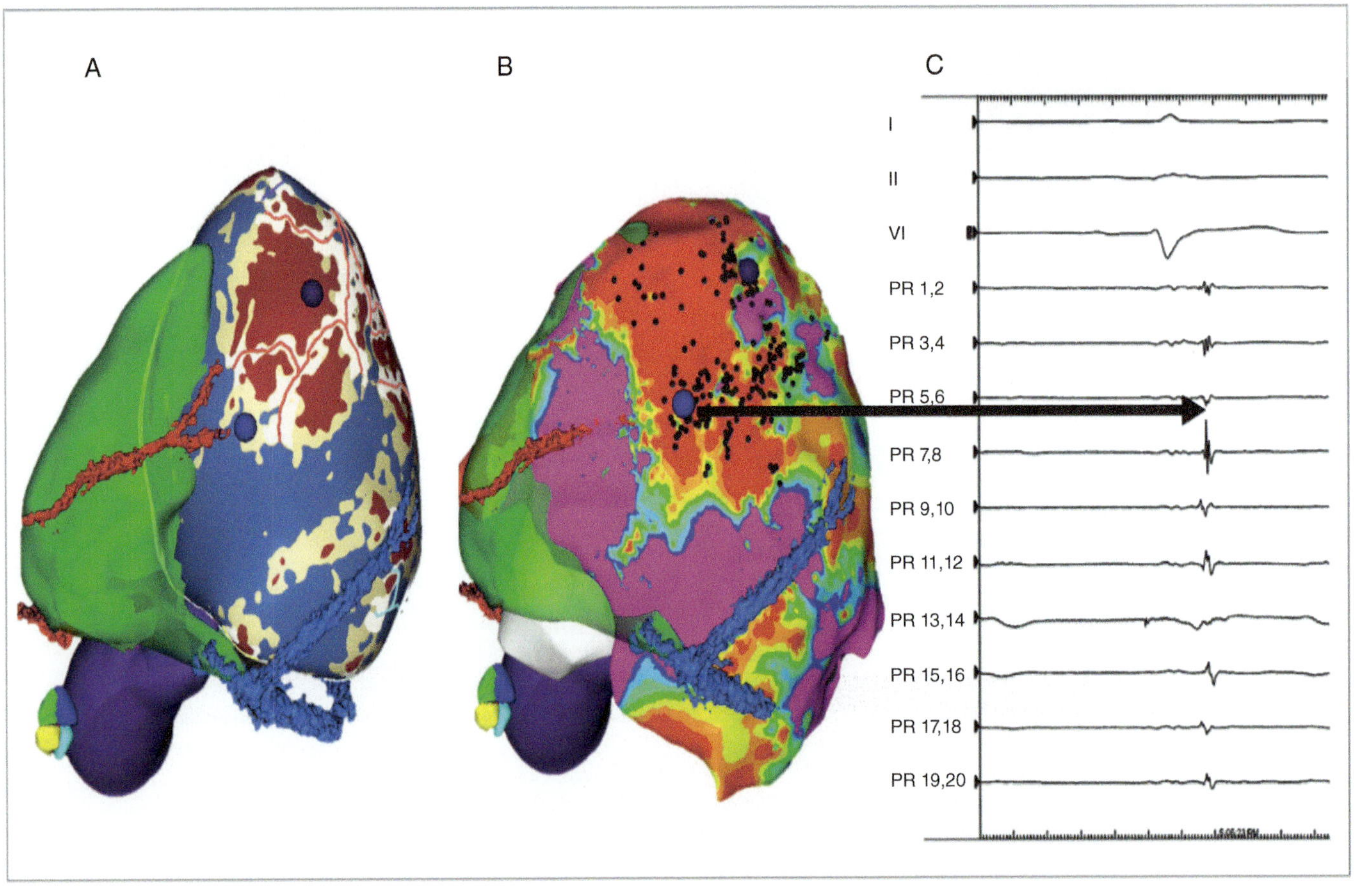

Fig. 36.17 (A) Inferior view of segmented and processed (ADAS 3D software, ADAS3D Medical) contrast-enhanced MDCT with hypoperfused (*highlighted in red*) myocardial scar regions in the apical inferolateral left ventricle and spared intervening tissues (*blue* is healthy, *yellow* is border zone, and *white* is border zone of the corridors) as candidate "channels" (*red lines surrounded by white*) for putative VT isthmus. Epicardial coronary arteries are highlighted in red and coronary venous system are highlighted in *blue*. (B) Bipolar epicardial voltage map in sinus rhythm (*red* < 0.5 mV; *purple* > 1.0 mV), highlighting a large scar area with distribution matching the ADAS 3D reconstruct. (C) Illustrates the late potentials noted within the scar region (*black* dots on B) and overall agreement with "channels" identified on MDCT. Pacing at *blue* dot on B with good pace match for clinical VT.

follow-up period. Importantly, most of those with VT recurrence had isolated recurrences, and only one patient had more frequent episodes that were amenable to pacing therapy only. Subsequent observational studies from large-volume tertiary-referral centers have reported modest success with regard to VT-free survival using this approach among patients with ischemic cardiomyopathy or NICM, ranging from 67% over a median 1-month follow-up to 71% over a follow-up of >4 years.[109,116]

This strategy of linear ablation guided by pace mapping was the first nonsurgical substrate modification strategy described to successfully ablate unmappable VT.[12] It has been the principal VT ablation approach not only in clinical practice but also in clinical trials, and it has provided the foundation from which other substrate-based ablation approaches have evolved over the last >2 decades. See Table 36.3 for a summary of the major prospective clinical trials in which substrate modification was included as the ablation approach for management of VT.[21,23,25,26,29,34–38] Details from selected studies are discussed next.

Multiple randomized clinical trials have now demonstrated that substrate-based ablation in patients with a history of VT following prior MI is superior to medical therapy in reducing recurrent VT and ICD shock burden. The multicenter Prophylactic Catheter Ablation for the Prevention of Defibrillator Therapy (SMASH-VT) Trial[25] compared ICD + catheter ablation to ICD implantation and usual medical therapy among 128 patients with MI > 1 month before enrollment and one of the following: (1) secondary-prevention ICD anticipated or implanted within 6 months of enrollment for VF, hemodynamically unstable VT, or syncope with inducible VT during invasive EP testing or (2) patients who had undergone primary prevention ICD implantation but subsequently had received appropriate ICD therapy for a single event. None of the patients enrolled were previously treated with Class I or III antiarrhythmic drugs. This was the first trial published to incorporate substrate-based ablation as first-line treatment for VT. The overall ventricular arrhythmia recurrence rates were relatively low over 2-year follow-up (12% for those undergoing ablation and 33% for those who did not), and catheter ablation was associated with a 65% risk reduction in recurrent VT events, including both antitachycardia pacing (ATP) and ICD shocks ($P = .007$), and a 73% risk

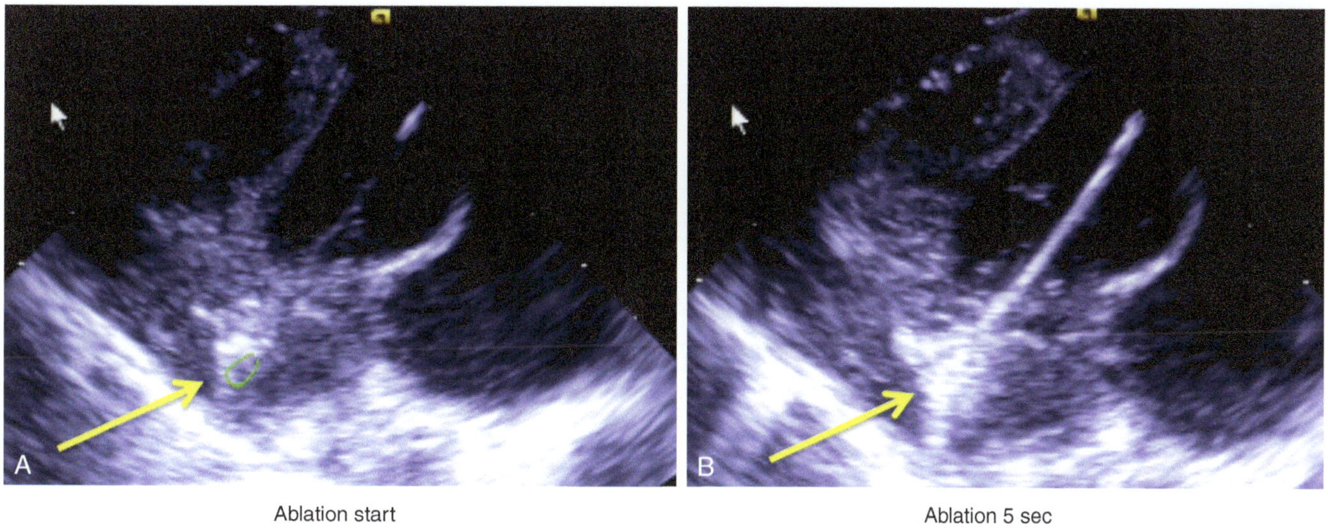

Fig. 36.18 Intracardiac echocardiography findings associated with impending steam pop during radiofrequency ablation. Note the rapid rate of increased echogenicity of the left ventricle at the ablation catheter-tip–tissue interface, as well as increased formation of bubbles within the blood pool on intracardiac echocardiography (A) from the initiation of open-irrigated radiofrequency ablation to (B) 5 seconds after application using 50 W.

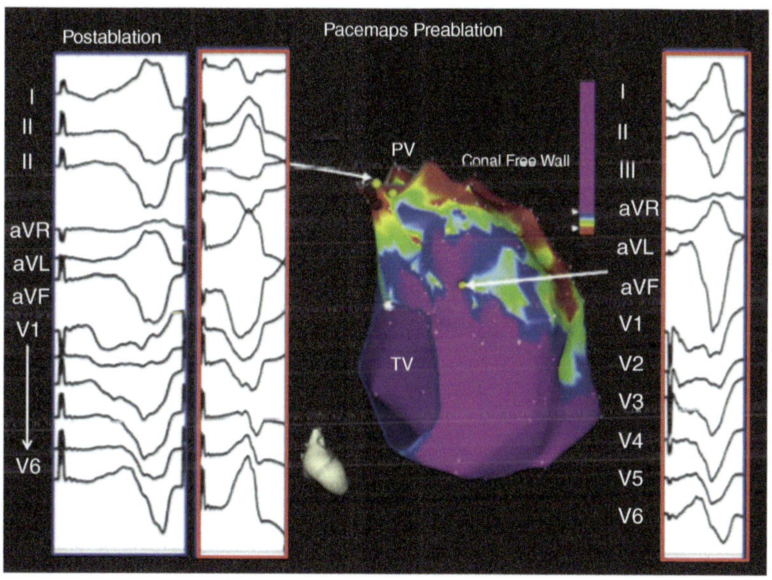

Fig. 36.19 Electroanatomical voltage map of the right ventricle reveals a large area of scar that extends from the pulmonic valve (PV) to the conal free wall. Pace maps from the conal free wall under the pulmonic valve and adjacent to the tricuspid valve prior to RFA are shown (outlined in *red*). Pacing at the same site under the pulmonic valve following ablation produces a different pace map (outlined in *blue*) from baseline, now resembling that obtained from the more inferior pacing site preablation, and with longer stimulus to QRS time, suggesting that block across the ablated region has been achieved. (Modified from Bala R, Dhruvakumar D, Latif SA, Marchlinski FE. New end point for ablation of ventricular tachycardia: change in QRS morphology with pacing at protected isthmus as index of isthmus block. *J Cardiovasc Electrophysiol*. 2010;21:320–324.)

reduction in ICD shocks alone (Fig. 36.21).[25] The study was not powered to assess a mortality difference, but there was a trend toward reduced mortality among ablation patients (9% vs. 17%, $P = .29$), which at the very least supports the relative safety of ablation even for those presenting with hemodynamically unstable VT or VF.

In a similarly designed trial based in Europe, the Catheter Ablation of Stable Ventricular Tachycardia Before Defibrillator Implantation in Patients with Coronary Heart Disease (V-TACH) randomized 107 patients with prior MI, reduced LVEF (≤50%), and VT to ICD + ablation, using the linear substrate-based ablation approach described or ICD alone.[26] Important differences between this trial and SMASH-VT were that only patients with hemodynamically tolerated VT were included and use of Class III antiarrhythmic drugs was not an exclusion criterion; in fact more than one-third of patients enrolled were treated with amiodarone at the time of randomization. Similar to results in SMASH-VT, there was a significant

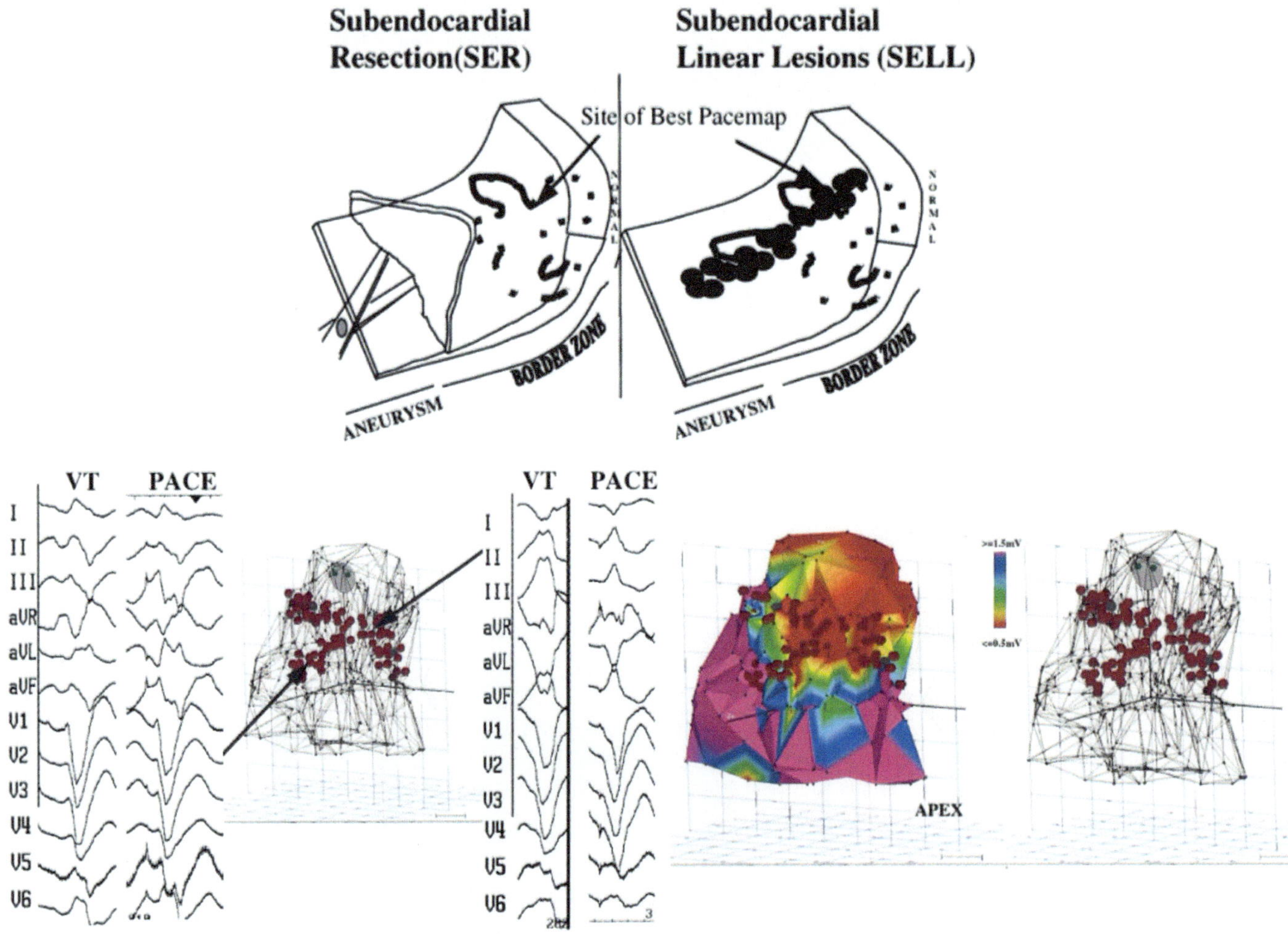

Fig. 36.20 (*Top*) Schema for suggested mechanism of linear lesion technique contrasted with surgical subendocardial resection. Subendocardial linear lesions extend from dense scar to normal endocardium, based on voltage map. Linear lesions guided by pace mapping may interrupt potential for reentry, much like subendocardial resection. (*Bottom*) Electrocardiograms of VT and pace map (PACE) identifying appropriate region for linear ablation in patient with RV cardiomyopathy. (*Left*) VT morphologies are mimicked by pace mapping at RV free wall sites, as indicated on mesh silhouette of RV. (*Right*) Color voltage map of RV in anteroposterior view, coupled with mesh figure, as in A. The 12-lead ECG during VT and pace map directed linear lesions to RV free wall. Linear lesions, identified by contiguous *dark circles*, extend from dense scar (*red*) and cross-border zone sites showing best pace maps. APEX indicates location of RV apex. (Reproduced from Marchlinski FE, Callans DJ, Gottlieb CD, Zado ES. Linear ablation lesions for control of unmappable ventricular tachycardia in patients with ischemia and nonischemic cardiomyopathy. *Circulation.* 2000;101:1288–1296.)

TABLE 36.3 Summary of Prospective Clinical Studies of Ventricular Tachycardia in Patients With Structural Heart Disease Involving Substrate-Based Catheter Ablation

Study Name (year)	N	Structural Heart Disease Type(s)	LVEF, %	Prior Amiodarone Treatment	Treatments	Mean Follow-Up, months	Freedom from Recurrent VT	Difference in ICD shocks	Survival
Catheter Ablation Following Multiple Treatments for Recurrent VT									
Cooled RF Ablation System Trial (2000)	146	ICM + NICM (18%)	31	40%	Ablation (nonrandomized)	8	44% (1-y K-M estimate)		75% (1-yr K-M estimate)
Multicenter Thermocool Ventricular Tachycardia Ablation Trial (2008)	231	ICM	25 (median)	70%	Ablation (nonrandomized)	6	53%	Median 11.5 vs. 0 (6 mo pre vs. post ablation)	82% (12 mo)

TABLE 36.3 Summary of Prospective Clinical Studies of Ventricular Tachycardia in Patients With Structural Heart Disease Involving Substrate-Based Catheter Ablation—cont'd

Study Name (year)	N	Structural Heart Disease Type(s)	LVEF, %	Prior Amiodarone Treatment	Treatments	Mean Follow-Up, months	Freedom from Recurrent VT	Difference in ICD shocks	Survival
Post-Approval Thermocool VT (2016)	249	ICM + NICM (4.6%)	30.1	68.3%	Ablation (nonrandomized)	6	62%	Median 13 vs. 0 (6 mo pre vs. post ablation)	86.6% (1 yr) 81.2% (2 yrs) 74.6% (3 yrs)
VANISH (2016)	259	ICM	31.1–31.2	65% (7% with dose ≥300 mg qd)	Ablation vs. escalated medical therapy	27.9	75.8% vs. 66.9% (VT storm), P= .08; 62.1% vs. 57.5% (Appropriate ICD shocks p 30 days), P= .19	See previous column	72.7% vs. 72.4%, P= .86
HELP-VT (2014)	227	ICM + NICM (28%)	32.7	37%	Ablation ICM vs. NICM (nonrandomized)	Median 20–27	43% vs. 23%, P= .01		91.9% vs. 87.3%, P= .307
VISTA (2015)	118	ICM	32.0–32.6	0% (16.9% on sotalol or mexiletine)	Scar homogenization vs. traditional limited ablation	12	84.5% vs. 51.7%, log rank P< .001		8.6% vs. 15%, log-rank P= .21
Gökoglan et al. (2016)	93	NICM	29–32	61%	Scar homogenization vs. traditional limited ablation	14	64% vs. 38.6%, log rank P= .031		
SURVIVE-VT	144	ICM	33–35	0	Ablation vs. antiarrhythmic drug	24	Not directly reported; Recurrent VT storm, incessant VT, slow undetected VT, or hospital admission for VT HR 0.21, 95% CI 0.08–0.57, P= .002	19.7% vs. 22.6%, P= .750	94.3% vs. 92.9%, P= .622
PARTITA (2022)	47	ICM + NICM (19%)	32.2	12%	Ablation vs. standard therapy after 1st ICD shock	24.2	69.6% vs. 50%, P= .434	8.7% vs. 41.7%, P= .039	0% vs. 33.3%, P= .004
Catheter Ablation Prior to ICD Implantation									
SMASH-VT (2007)	128	ICM	30.7–32.9	0	Ablation+ ICD vs. ICD	22.5	88% vs. 67%, P= .007	9% vs. 31%, P= .003	91% vs. 83%, P= .29
V-TACH (2010)	107	ICM	34.0 ± 9.2	35%	Ablation+ ICD vs. ICD	22.5	47% vs. 29%, P= .045	Mean 0.6 vs. 3.4 per patient per year	91.5% vs. 91.4%, P= .677
SMS (2017)	111	ICM	31.2 ± 7.1	32%	Ablation+ ICD vs. ICD	2.3 ± 1.1 years	49% vs. 52.4%, P= .84	0.7 vs. 2.1. P= .028	83% vs. 80%, p= 0.65
BERLIN-VT (2020)	159	ICM	41± 6	35%	Ablation+ ICD vs. ICD	396 ± 284 days	60.3% vs. 51.8%, P= .047	17.8% vs. 21.7%, P= .33	92.1% vs. 97.6%, P= .18
PAUSE-SCD (2022)	121	ICM + NICM (65%)	40 (30–49)	35.5%	Ablation+ ICD vs. ICD	31.3	78.3% vs. 49.2%, P= .02	10% vs. 24.6%, P= .03	91.7% vs. 93.4%, P= .62

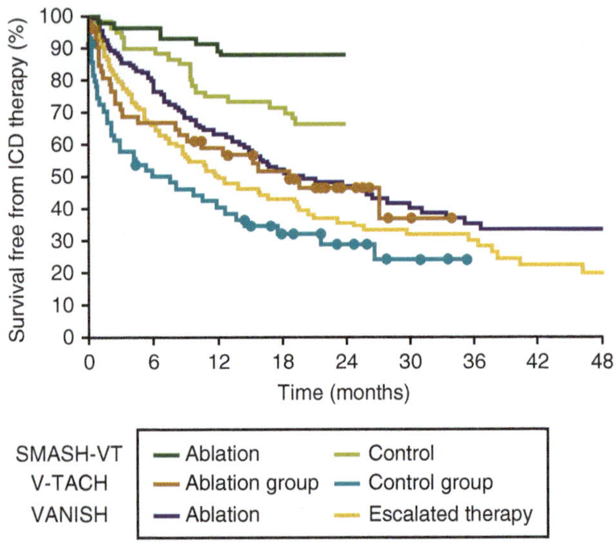

Fig. 36.21 Composite of Kaplan-Meier survival analyses of major randomized clinical trials comparing catheter ablation to usual or escalated medical therapy among patients with ventricular tachycardia (VT) following prior myocardial infarction. Survival free from any implantable cardioverter-defibrillator (ICD) therapy is displayed from the Prophylactic Catheter Ablation for the Prevention of Defibrillator Therapy (SMASH-VT trial [Reddy VY, Reynolds MR, Neuzil P, Richardson AW, Taborsky M, Jongnarangsin K, et al. Prophylactic catheter ablation for the prevention of defibrillator therapy. *N Engl J Med.* 2007;357:2657–2665]). Survival free from recurrent VT or ventricular fibrillation is displayed from the Catheter Ablation of Stable Ventricular Tachycardia Before Defibrillator Implantation in Patients with Coronary Heart Disease (VTACH) trial (Kuck KH, Schaumann A, Eckhardt L, Willems S, Ventura R, Delacrétaz E, et al. Catheter ablation of stable ventricular tachycardia before defibrillator implantation in patients with coronary heart disease (VTACH): a multicentre randomised controlled trial. *Lancet.* 2010;375:31–40). Survival free from composite end point of death occurring at any time after randomization or VT storm or appropriate ICD shock after 30-day treatment is displayed from the Ventricular Tachycardia Ablation versus Escalated Antiarrhythmic Drug Therapy in Ischemic Heart Disease Trial (VANISH, Sapp JL, Wells GA, Parkash R, Stevenson WG, Blier L, Sarrazin JF, et al. Ventricular tachycardia ablation versus escalation of antiarrhythmic drugs. *N Engl J Med.* 2016;375:111–121. doi:10.1056/NEJMoa1513614).

reduction in recurrent VT or VF among those randomized to ablation (HR 0.61, 95% CI 0.37–0.99, *P* = .045, Fig. 36.21). The absolute proportions with recurrent VT were higher in each group compared to in SMASH-VT (53% in the ablation arm and 71% in the nonablation arm over 2 years), although in the context of arguably different patient populations with respect to duration of arrhythmia history and treatment. Despite modest improvements in VT recurrence, ablation was associated with a nearly 6-fold decrease in appropriate ICD shocks per patient per year (0.6 vs. 3.4, *P* = .018).

The Substrate-Modification Study (SMS) and the Preventive Ablation of Ventricular Tachycardia in Patients With Myocardial Infarction (BERLIN-VT) Trial similarly showed decreased burden of recurrent VT or ICD therapies with prophylactic substrate-based ablation among patients with ICM and VT, randomized to either ablation + ICD or ICD alone.[34,38] However, the results appeared less favorable than those in the preceding trials. In SMS, 117 ICM patients (mean LVEF 31.2% ± 7.1%) who presented with unstable VT or VF were randomized 1:1 to ablation prior to ICD implantation or ICD implantation + medical therapy; 6 were randomized to the ablation group were excluded as they did not undergo ablation and had missing ICD data. Over an approximately 2-year follow-up, time to recurrent VT/VF (the primary end point) did not differ significantly between groups (log-rank *P* = .84), with 2-year estimated VT-free survival of 49.0% (95% CI, 33.3–62.9%) among those who underwent ablation, versus 52.4% (95% CI 36.7–65.9%) in those randomized to ICD-only. Similarly, there was no significant difference in any of the secondary end points (time to appropriate ICD therapies, cardiac rehospitalizations, serious adverse events, overall mortality, spontaneous episodes with ATP or shocks). However, in analysis incorporating time to multiple end point events, that is, burden of recurrent episodes, the patients randomized to catheter ablation had significantly reduced burden of recurrent arrhythmias in the primary end point assessment (any VT/VF) and in most analyzed recurrent VT or VF subgroups, with reductions ranging from 56% to 67% in all except those with recurrent VT/VF and ICD shock (likely given low event rates in each arm), thus confirming that ablation is effective in reducing the burden of recurrent VT in ICM.[34]

BERLIN-VT randomized 163 ICM patients (mean LVEF 41% ± 6%) to immediate (preventive group) or deferred ablation (performed only after three appropriate ICD shocks) prior to ICD implantation. Six patients (1 in the preventive and 5 in the deferred ablation group) were excluded due to withdrawal of consent, failure to meet inclusion criteria, failure to undergo any procedure, or early withdrawal; therefore, 76 patients in the preventive and 83 patients in the deferred groups were ultimately analyzed. Of note, the trial was terminated early (prior to an initially desired 208 patients) due to interim analysis indicating futility. In the preventive group, 7 patients did not undergo ablation, due to absence of inducibility or substrate (n = 4; 3 of these also did not undergo ICD implantation), refusal (n = 2), or referral to cardiac surgery (n = 1). Among the deferred ablation patients, 10 (12%) underwent ablation a median of 46 days (interquartile range 19–105 days) after ICD implantation. There was no statistically significant difference between groups in the primary composite end point (mortality and unplanned hospitalization for either symptomatic VT or VF or heart failure decompensation. However, consistent with prior trials and in a cohort with better LV systolic function than in previous trials, patients undergoing early ablation had significantly improved survival from recurrent sustained VT/VF (HR 0.62, 95% CI 0.38–1.00, *P* = .050, log-rank *P* = .047) and appropriate ICD treatment (HR 0.55, 95% CI 0.33–0.91, *P* = .020, log-rank *P* = .018).[38]

The Ventricular Tachycardia Ablation versus Escalated Antiarrhythmic Drug Therapy in Ischemic Heart Disease (VANISH) trial investigated the utility of VT ablation compared to escalated antiarrhythmic drug therapy on VT recurrence and mortality among 259 patients with ischemic cardiomyopathy and recurrent VT that was refractory to prior treatment with Class I or III AADs.[29] Patients randomized to escalated AAD had treatment administered based on amiodarone dose at baseline as follows: (1) those not on amiodarone had loading of 400 mg bid for 2 weeks then 400 mg daily for 4 weeks, followed by maintenance dosing of 200 mg daily; (2) those on amiodarone <300 mg daily had loading of 400 mg bid for 2 weeks and 400 mg daily for 1 week, then maintenance dosing of 300 mg daily; (3) those on ≥300 mg daily amiodarone were maintained at the same dose and had mexiletine 200 mg tid added to the regimen. Those randomized to ablation underwent a similar substrate-based ablation strategy as described above for the vast majority (88.6%) of cases; in the remainder, more focused ablation guided by entrainment and activation were performed. Over 4-year follow-up, primary end point events (death or VT storm or appropriate ICD shock after 30-day treatment period) were less frequent among the ablation compared to escalated AAD group (59.1% vs. 68.5%; hazard ratio for ablation patients 0.72, 95% CI 0.53–0.98, *P* = .04, Fig. 36.21); this difference was driven by trends toward decreased ICD shocks and VT storm events. Another important secondary outcome difference is that those randomized to the escalated treatment arm were 73% more likely to recur with sustained VT below the programmed ICD detection limit than those who underwent ablation (*P* = .02). Finally, for those who were already on amiodarone at the time of presentation with recurrent VT, subsequent ablation led to markedly improved rates of the primary outcome compared those randomized to escalated AAD (HR 0.55, 95% CI 0.38–0,80, *P* = .001).

Three important, multicenter, randomized trials of catheter ablation versus medical therapy were published in 2022 (Table 36.3).[35–37] The Substrate Ablation vs. Antiarrhythmic Drug Therapy for Symptomatic Ventricular Tachycardia (SURVIVE VT) Trial was conducted among nine centers in Spain, and randomized 145 ICM patients (mean LVEF 33–35%) to comprehensive substrate-based endocardial LV ablation versus AAD (61 [86%] treated with amiodarone alone or with β-blockers and 10 [14%] sotalol + β-blockers). The trial was stopped after 7 years due to slow enrollment, at which time 81% of the projected 180 patients had been enrolled. Disproportionate crossover between treatment groups occurred, with 8 patients (10.1%) randomized to ablation crossing over to AAD, and 18 (24.3%) randomized to AAD undergoing catheter ablation due to recurrent VT on AAD. Additionally, 3 patients randomized to ablation underwent repeat ablation. The primary outcome was a composite of cardiovascular death, appropriate ICD shock, unplanned heart failure hospitalization, or severe treatment-related complications over 24-month follow-up, and occurred in significantly fewer ablation (n = 71, 28.2%) versus AAD (n = 73, 46.6%) patients (HR 0.52; 95% CI 0.30–0.90; *P* = .021). Notably, the difference in the primary outcome was driven by a trend for decreased HF hospitalizations and a significantly reduced incidence of severe treatment-related adverse events/complications in the ablation versus AAD groups (9.9% vs. 28.8%; HR 0.30; 95% CI 0.13–0.71; *P* = .006). In line with previous studies, recurrence of sustained, incessant, or slow VT and hospitalization for recurrent VT was also significantly lower in the ablation versus AAD treatment arm.[35–37]

The Does Timing of VT Ablation Affect Prognosis in Patients With an Implantable Cardioverter-Defibrillator (PARTITA) and Pan-Asia United States Prevention of Sudden Cardiac Death (PAUSE-SCD) trials were notable for several important reasons.[36,37] One major common difference between these and all of the prior randomized controlled trials in VT is the inclusion of patients with NICM as well as ICM. Other distinctions are as discussed next.

PAUSE-SCD was a multicenter trial that exclusively enrolled patients in Asia (n = 180) with SHD and VT without ICDs at baseline, comprised notably of a minority with ICM (34.7%), and the majority with NICM (30.6%) and ARVC (34.7%). Patients (n = 133, mean LVEF 40%) were randomized to ICD + medical therapy or ablation + ICD. Forty-seven patients who underwent ablation but deferred ICD implantation were followed prospectively in a registry, and 12 patients withdrew consent prior to treatment, thus 121 patients (60 ablation, 61 no ablation) were assessed in intention-to-treat analysis. Catheter ablation included epicardial as well as endocardial ablation in 31 (55.4%). Over a median 31.3-month follow-up, the primary outcome (composite of VT recurrence, cardiovascular hospitalization, or death) was reached in 49.3% of the ablation group and 65.5% in the control group (HR 0.58, 95% CI 0.35–0.96, *P* = .04); the outcome was driven primarily by a significant reduction in recurrent VT in the ablation (39.4%) compared to control group (58.2%). There were also significant reductions in ICD therapies, including both ATP as well as shocks, among ablation versus control patients. Interestingly, the patients who refused ICD but underwent ablation and were followed in the registry experienced similar primary outcome events, including VT recurrence in follow-up as the randomized ablation patients did (VT recurrence 40%; primary outcome compared to randomized ablation patients (HR 1.10, 95%CI 0.61–1.98, *P* = .75).[37]

The design of PARTITA was particularly unique, as it involved two phases: phase A enrolled ICM (78%) and NICM patients (total n = 517) who met indication for primary or secondary prevention ICD implantation in a prospective registry, with the primary end point being first appropriate ICD shock for VT; phase B randomized consenting patients from phase A who experienced the primary outcome. Fifty-six (10%) of enrolled patients had ICD shock for VT (74% with an originally primary prevention indication for ICD), of whom 47 were randomized to either catheter ablation or medical therapy. At the first interim analysis at 24.2 months, significantly fewer ablation patients experienced the primary composite outcome of death or worsening HF hospitalization (HR 0.11, 95% CI 0.01–0.85, *P* = .034); the difference was still observed after excluding noncardiac deaths, which occurred disproportionately in the control arm (1 ablation patient and 6 control patients, *P* = .053). This is the first randomized control trial of VT ablation versus medical therapy to show a mortality benefit and in a population that included NICM as well as ICM patients.[36]

The weight of the clinical evidence thus indicates that this ablation approach is effective in mitigating episodes of recurrent VT and ICD shocks and improving quality of life, either when antiarrhythmic drugs have failed or as a first approach for VT management. However, despite these important relative benefits, the absolute numbers of patients with VT recurrence following ablation (as many as 46% in ICM and as high as 80% among NICM patients) have spawned additional efforts to improve upon traditional ablation end points and, by extension, longer-term VT recurrence rates.

VT Noninducibility as an Ablation End Point

The most commonly used method for determining the end point for ablation has been assessment of inducibility with PES. Inability to induce VT using the same or more aggressive stimulation with which VT was induced prior to ablation is typically considered an end point of acute success, as it often correlates with improved VT-free survival.[19,21,24,30,60] However, its predictive value is far from perfect, and there are several limitations in relying on this end point alone. First, the definition of VT noninducibility can and has been interpreted variably and, depending on which definition is used, determination of acute success can vary significantly. Using the strictest definition, lack of induction of any VT may be the most straightforward, but its positive predictive value is limited; inducing very fast VTs (cycle length [CL] <200 ms) or polymorphic VT or ventricular fibrillation (VF) with aggressive stimulation does not reliably predict recurrence of clinically significant monomorphic VT.[19,21,24] Second, defining VT noninducibility as an inability to induce clinical VT similarly has inherent limitations, as what defines "clinical" can also be interpreted variably. Many times 12-lead ECGs of spontaneous VTs are not able to be obtained, and the only available detail about clinical events may be from ICD EGMs, from which only limited information may be gleaned regarding VT CLs and, to some extent, ICD EGM morphologies.[117] Finally, even when 12-lead ECGs are available of spontaneously occurring VTs, inducing VTs of other morphologies does not necessarily mean that the latter are "nonclinical" or potentially clinically insignificant; the site and method of VT induction in the EP laboratory may produce unidirectional block and reentry through the same substrate used by the spontaneously occurring VT but which differ in wavefront propagation and exit compared to that evoked by spontaneously occurring triggers. These VTs, although they may differ in 12-lead ECG morphology, should still be considered to be potentially of clinical importance. Most commonly, failure to induce monomorphic VTs with similar 12-lead ECG morphology or within 20 ms in CL of previously observed VTs following substrate-based ablation is considered to be an acceptable acute end point.

Beyond defining VT noninducibility, there are other issues with this acute ablation end point that limit its predictive value. First, lack of inducibility before ablation confounds interpretation of noninducibility following ablation. Second, there is a known lack of reproducibility in inducing VT, especially in the setting of concomitant antiarrhythmic drug (AAD) use. Third, changes in autonomic tone and use of general anesthesia may affect VT inducibility. Fourth, ablation lesions may either expand as a result of disruption of microcirculation, with consequent myocyte loss, or regress secondary to healing and resolution of edema. Finally, patients may be too unstable to tolerate additional attempts at VT induction after ablation.[19,24,31,43,109,118–120]

Additional substrate-based ablation strategies have been developed over the last decades since the initial linear-ablation transection approach. Each is guided by specific mapping methods, as described earlier, for identifying arrhythmogenic myocardium believed to be of greatest importance. Each has aimed to improve upon determination of the standard procedural end point of VT noninducibility to achieve improved long-term outcomes. Although the mapping strategies may differ in specific approach and focus, there is substantial overlap in the general principles applied for ablation. Common goals among all are to achieve the following: (1) entrance block, or elimination of apparent conduction of excitable myocardium within targeted substrate and (2) VT noninducibility following ablation.

The following sections summarize ablation strategies that incorporate additional mapping approaches and ablation end points beyond VT noninducibility, as well as associated outcomes (Table 36.2).

LAVA and Late Potential Elimination

Once areas containing LAVAs and late potentials are identified, using mapping strategies as described above, subsequent ablation is performed throughout the sites demonstrating abnormal conduction, usually with application of relatively contiguous ablation lesions, with the goal of elimination of targeted signals from the endocardium and epicardium when feasible. Ablation continues until these targeted signals are eliminated, as confirmed by repeated mapping following ablation (Fig. 36.13).[32,33] Favorable outcomes have been achieved using these techniques in populations with both ICM and NICM with VT. In the initial description of endocardial or epicardial LAVA elimination among 70 patients (20% NICM), complete LAVA elimination (achieved among 70%) was associated with significant improvement in survival and VT recurrence (2-year event-free rates of 55% versus 20% among those in whom LAVA elimination was unable to be achieved). LAVA elimination was the only characteristic that was independently associated with event-free survival in a multivariate analysis including the VT noninducibility and underlying SHD substrate. (HR 0.49, 95% CI 0.26–0.95, $P = .035$).[32]

An impressive 90.5% freedom from VT recurrence was observed among patients (28% NICM) among whom complete abolition of late potentials was achieved, with better sensitivity (60.0% vs. 50.0%) and specificity (95.0% vs. 87.5%) in predicting recurrent VT compared to VT noninducibility.[33]

Scar Dechanneling and VT Core Isolation

Knowing that the majority of the critical VT circuit components reside within fibrotic tissue with abnormal voltage, targeting channels of conduction within these abnormal regions and achieving electrical isolation may result in better control of contemporarily documented "clinical" VTs as well as subsequent VTs that may later arise from the same substrate. Focused targeting of these putative critical elements of the circuit through identification of the possible channels and surviving myocardium within scar is the basis for the scar dechanneling and VT core isolation strategies.

In the scar dechanneling approach, Berruezo and colleagues identified regions with late potentials but focused specifically on identifying and focally targeting sites with the earliest of late

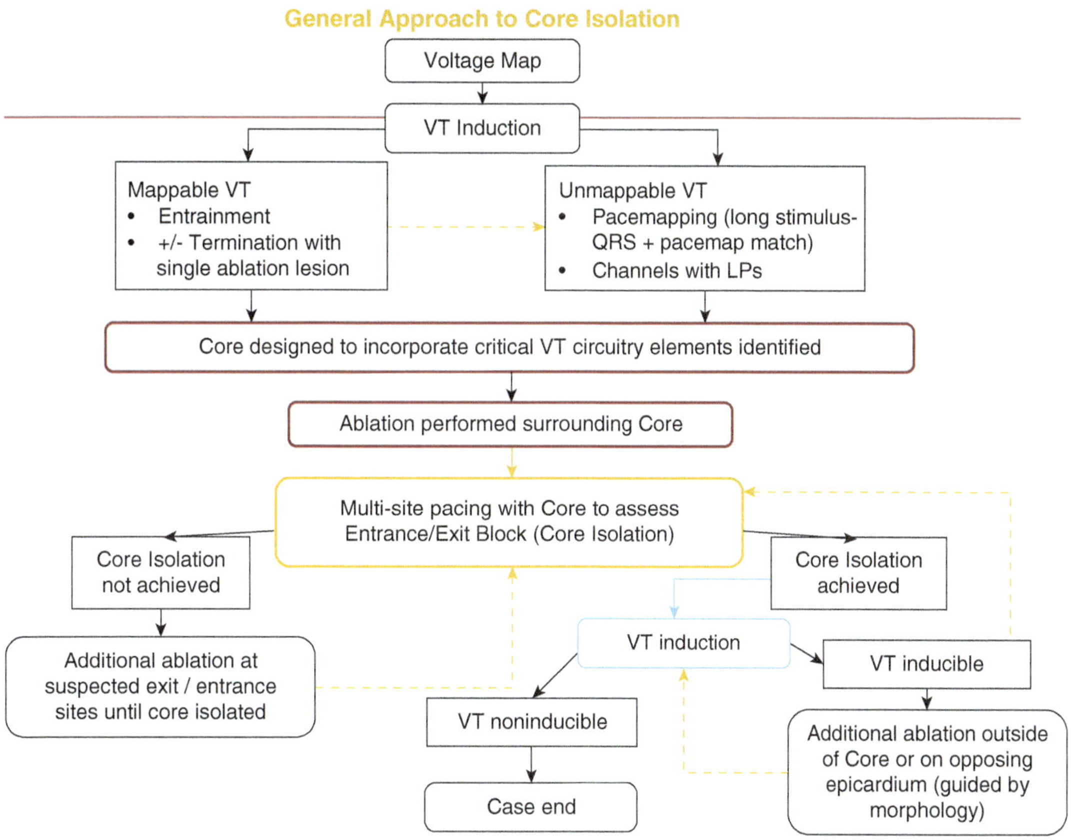

Fig. 36.22 Flowchart detailing the general approach for core isolation. *LP,* Late potential; *VT,* ventricular tachycardia. (From Tzou WS, Frankel DS, Hegeman T, Supple GE, Garcia FC, Santangeli P, et al. Core isolation of critical arrhythmia elements for treatment of multiple scar-based ventricular tachycardias. *Circ Arrhythm Electrophysiol.* 2015;8:353–361.)

potentials, speculating that these sites represent entrance sites of conduction into scar and could be focally targeted to prevent subsequent reentry within the scar.[30] After completion of a standard voltage map, specific sites were annotated with color-coded points or tags as entrance versus inner conducting channel (CC) sites, based on degree of delay in local activation. Specifically, sites with late potentials with least delay were tagged as entrance CC, and those with relatively later delay were tagged as inner CC sites. With focal ablation delivered to entrance-CC sites, commonly located at the periphery of identified scar, no evidence of delayed activation within the scarred region on remapping could be demonstrated (i.e., all late potential activity was abolished at sites in which they were demonstrated to exist prior to ablation) and without directly ablating all late potentials identified, thus providing evidence for "dechanneling" and electrical homogenization. This end point was achieved in 84.2% of 101 patients, although additional ablation using previously described approaches was also needed to achieve the most commonly accepted end point, VT noninducibility, which was achieved in 78.2%.

A related but distinct strategy for substrate modification is VT "core" isolation.[24] Using this ablation strategy, critical VT circuit components are identified using mapping strategies described earlier and summarized in Table 36.2 and Fig. 36.22, on either the endocardial or epicardial surface. When feasible, limited activation and entrainment techniques are also utilized to confirm relative importance of sites mapped during sinus rhythm. These sites of importance (Figs. 36.22 and 36.23) are annotated on the EAM. Electrical excitability of tissue within abnormal regions identified is confirmed at baseline with pacing and capture at standard output. Sites with lack of electrical excitability at baseline, as defined by extremely low voltage and inability to capture with pacing at high output, are also annotated. Once the critical circuitry elements are identified, ablation lesions are applied circumferentially around the entirety of these elements, which often but does not always correlate with the circumference of scar identified by low voltage and abnormal EGM characteristics. In the original description of this technique, among 44 patients (27% NICM, mean LVEF 31%) presenting with multiple clinical VTs and 48% with VT storm, less than half of the substrate defined as EGM amplitude <1.5 mV was targeted for isolation, indicating potential sparing of some regions of reduced voltage. In addition to entrance block within the isolated region and VT noninducibility, this technique introduced an additional procedural end point of exit block within the isolated region. Exit block, and therefore successful core isolation, was defined by failure to capture the ventricle with pacing from inside the lesion set using a pacing output of 20 mA and pulse width of 2 ms from multiple (≥3), discrete sites that had previously demonstrated capture. In the setting of incomplete core isolation or persistent VT inducibility, additional ablation was performed, either on the endocardium or epicardium, guided by subsequent mapping and VT morphology. Using this approach, we demonstrated incremental benefit

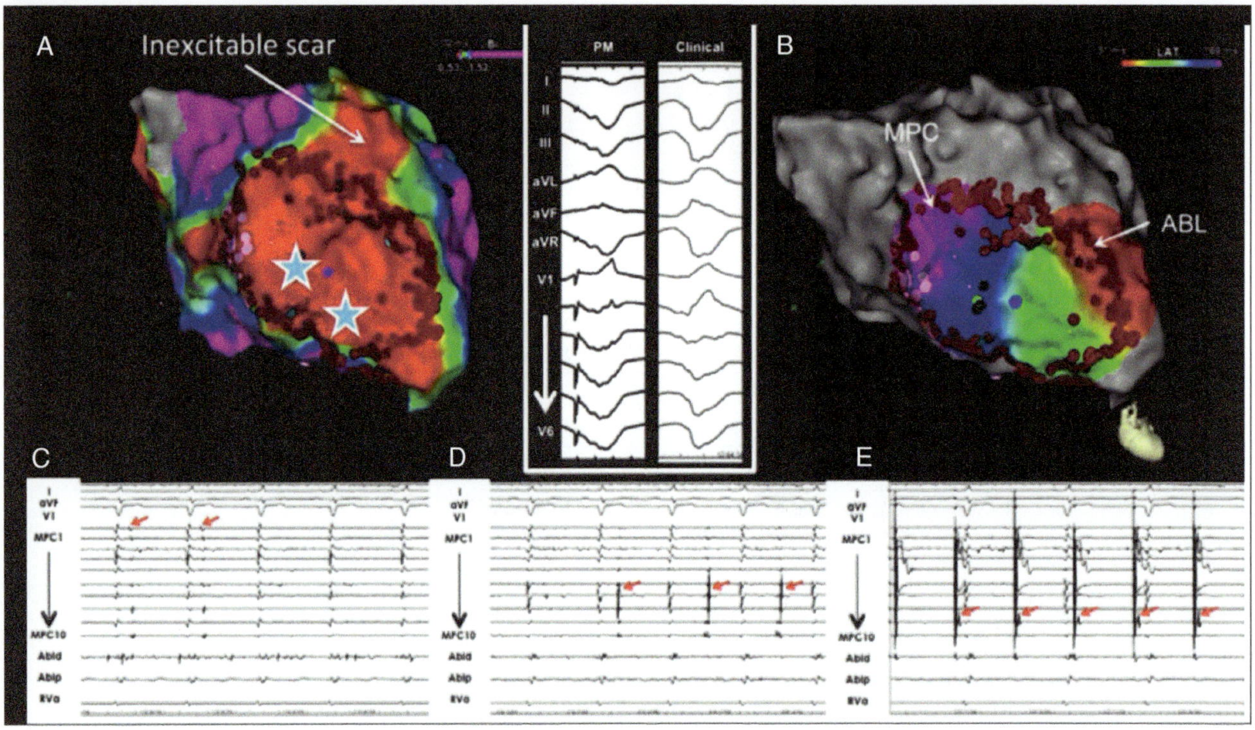

Fig. 36.23 Example of core isolation (CI) in a patient with ventricular tachycardia (VT) storm and a large anterior myocardial infarction. (A) Endocardial voltage map, anteroposterior view. The VT circuit core was defined by good pace map (PM) sites (*stars* depict examples), as defined in the text and was isolated by contiguous ablation at the junction between dense scar and border zone or regions without pacing capture at baseline. (B) Late potential (LP) activation map performed after CI identifying a single site of endocardial breakthrough within the isolated area. A multipolar catheter (MPC) was positioned within the CI area, and the ablation catheter (ABL) at the site of endocardial breakthrough. (C) Ablation at the earliest breakthrough results in CI, with entrance block demonstrated by disappearance of near-field LPs from the MPC during ablation (*arrows*). (D) After CI, dissociated potentials were recorded (*arrows*). (E) After isolation, pacing from the MPC shows local myocardial capture (*arrows*) with exit block. (Reproduced from Tzou WS, Frankel DS, Hegeman T, Supple GE, Garcia FC, Santangeli P, et al. Core isolation of critical arrhythmia elements for treatment of multiple scar-based ventricular tachycardias. *Circ Arrhythm Electrophysiol.* 2015;8:353–361.)

in VT-free survival when core isolation and VT noninducibility were both achieved (90% without VT recurrence), as well as when only core isolation was achieved (83% without recurrent VT). VT-free survival was achieved in 86% of the patients over mean follow-up of 17.5 ± 9.0 months and was significantly better than those in whom core isolation was unable to be achieved ($P = .013$).

Scar Homogenization

Perhaps the most straightforward and most extensive VT ablation strategy described is the direct ablation and elimination of all electrically excitable tissue within a scar. This approach was initially described among patients with ICM and VT without prior coronary arterial bypass graft (CABG) surgery. Comprehensive endocardial and epicardial ablation targeting substrate identified primarily using abnormal bipolar EGM amplitude was performed (Fig. 36.24), with marked improvement in VT-free survival compared to similar patients who underwent traditional VT ablation as described above (81% vs. 53%, log-rank $P = .006$).[31] A longer-term follow-up study by the same group and including more patients demonstrated improved 5-year VT-free survival of 81.4% and 66.3%, $P = .01$, among those undergoing endocardial + epicardial (n = 70) versus endocardial-only scar homogenization (n = 291), respectively. This strategy, while involving more ablation than the other strategies, is designed not only to target all possible VT circuits but to allow for multiply redundant lesions, thereby minimizing effects from conduction recovery due to nondurable lesions. However, prior CABG is usually prohibitive for percutaneous epicardial access and ablation, and technical experience as well as staff and resources to ensure safety of epicardial access likely led to the much lower observed rate of pericardiotomy-related complications in these trials compared to those reported from other experienced centers,[22,121] thus the generalizability of this technique to all patients with VT following MI is somewhat limited.

In a randomized clinical trial of 118 ICM patients with VT and in whom prior cardiac surgery was not an exclusion criterion (VISTA Trial), scar homogenization of the LV endocardium (and epicardium when needed and feasible) was compared to traditional VT ablation (Table 36.3).[28] The outcomes related to more extensive ablation and scar homogenization were encouraging, with statistically and clinically significant improvements in VT-free survival (84.5% vs. 51.7%, log-rank $P < .001$, Fig. 36.25) and without significant differences in periprocedural

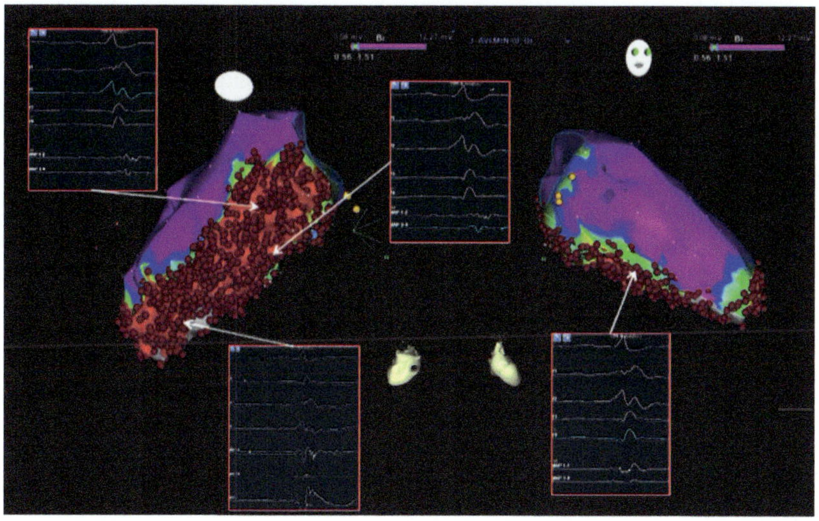

Fig. 36.24 Electroanatomical bipolar left ventricular voltage maps obtained in sinus rhythm from a patient with prior inferior myocardial infarction and drug-refractory ventricular tachycardia (VT). Representative electrograms (EGMs) obtained throughout the region of scar, based on bipolar EGM amplitude ≤0.5 mV, are shown, as is ablation lesions applied throughout the endocardial scar. (Reproduced from Di Biase L, Santangeli P, Burkhardt DJ, Bai R, Mohanty P, Carbucicchio C, et al. Endo-epicardial homogenization of the scar versus limited substrate ablation for the treatment of electrical storms in patients with ischemic cardiomyopathy. *J Am Coll Cardiol.* 2012;60:132–141.)

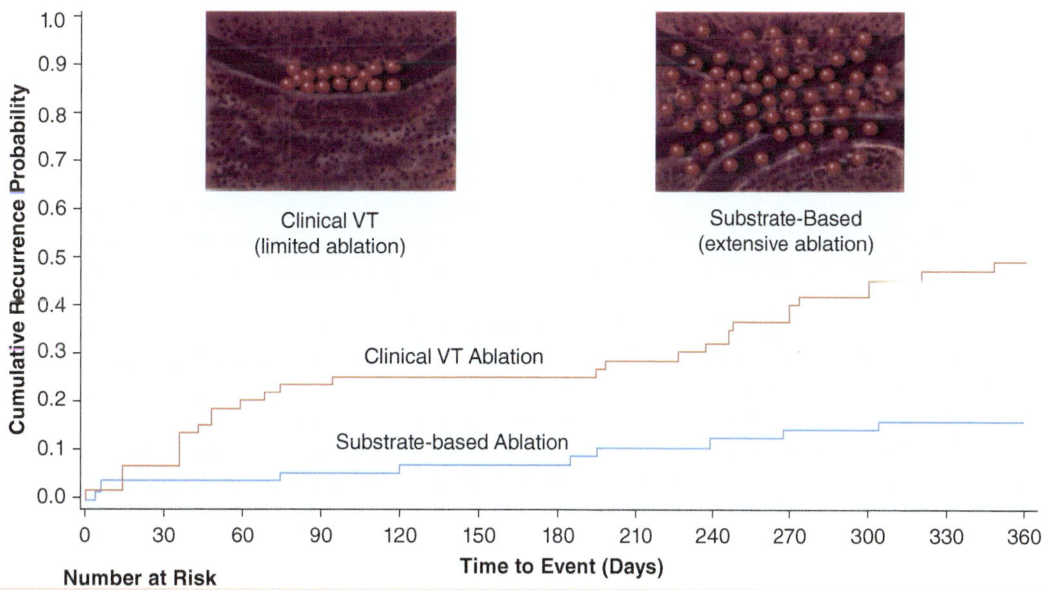

Number at Risk

Ablation Strategy													
Substrate-based	58	56	56	55	55	54	54	52	51	50	50	49	49
Clinical Stable VT	60	56	48	46	45	45	45	43	41	38	35	32	31

Fig. 36.25 Comparison in survival free from recurrent ventricular tachycardia (VT) among patients with ischemic cardiomyopathy and VT undergoing substrate-based ablation versus standard, clinical VT ablation (log-rank $P < .001$). Median time to recurrence was 7.0 months (interquartile range: 6.3–7.8 months) and 2.5 months (interquartile range: 1.2 to 8.6 months), respectively (unadjusted hazard ratio: 0.26, 95% confidence interval: 0.11–0.61]). (Modified from Di Biase L, Burkhardt JD, Lakkireddy D, Carbucicchio C, Mohanty S, Mohanty P, et al. Ablation of stable VTs versus substrate ablation in ischemic cardiomyopathy: the VISTA Randomized Multicenter Trial. *J Am Coll Cardiol.* 2015;66:2872–2882.)

complications ($P = .61$) or mortality at 12-month follow-up (8.6% in scar homogenization group vs. 15% in the traditional ablation arm, log-rank $P = .21$).

However, while this approach is straightforward and effective among patients with VT due to prior MI, using it among NICM substrates, which confer the greatest challenge in terms of VT ablation and management due to increased complexity of substrate, has not led to improved outcomes compared to other substrate-based strategies described (Table 36.3).[122]

Regardless of which specific substrate-based mapping and ablation approach is used, effective VT control can be achieved in the majority of patients (70%), as demonstrated from the cumulative experiences of 12 international tertiary-referral VT ablation centers in the International Ventricular Tachycardia Center Collaborative Group (IVTCC).[19] In fact, lack of VT recurrence in the largest and most mixed cohort of SHD patients undergoing VT ablation to date (n = 2,061, 43% NICM) was found to be associated with increased probability of VT- and transplant-free survival (Fig. 36.26), irrespective of underlying ischemic or nonischemic substrate, or severity of heart failure.[19,123] Therefore, although effective VT control can be challenging to achieve, continued progress and associated safety in substrate-based mapping and ablation techniques have made catheter ablation a more viable therapeutic option, even among the sickest of patients with SHD.

COMPLICATIONS

Procedural complications associated with substrate-based VT ablation are generally higher than reported for non-VT ablation, due to increased comorbidities that accompany SHD. Recurrent induction and attempts at mapping VT can lead to hemodynamic decompensation and substrate-based ablation might be associated with lower risk of complications especially in patients with severe cardiomyopathy. Total complications reported from large single- or multi-center studies experienced in substrate-based VT ablation have ranged from 4% to 10%,[19,21,23,28,50,116,124] and have included death in up to 3%.[19,21,23,120,124] More commonly encountered complications include vascular access complications (hematoma, arteriovenous fistula, pseudoaneurysm) in 1.6–4.7%, pericardial effusion with tamponade in 1.3–4%, usually treated with percutaneous drainage but in rare cases requiring open surgical repair in 0.1–0.7%, heart failure, cardiogenic shock or other hemodynamic instability necessitating ending the procedure in 0.3–3.2%, stroke or TIA in 0.5–0.8%, complete heart block, typically anticipated and due to targeting of basal septal substrate, in 0.8–0.9%, venous thromboembolism in 0.3–0.6%, coronary artery injury in 0.2%, incessant VT in 0.4%, and pericarditis in 0.4%.[19,21,31,50,116]

Incidence of complications varies widely depending on a number of factors, including operator experience, hospital

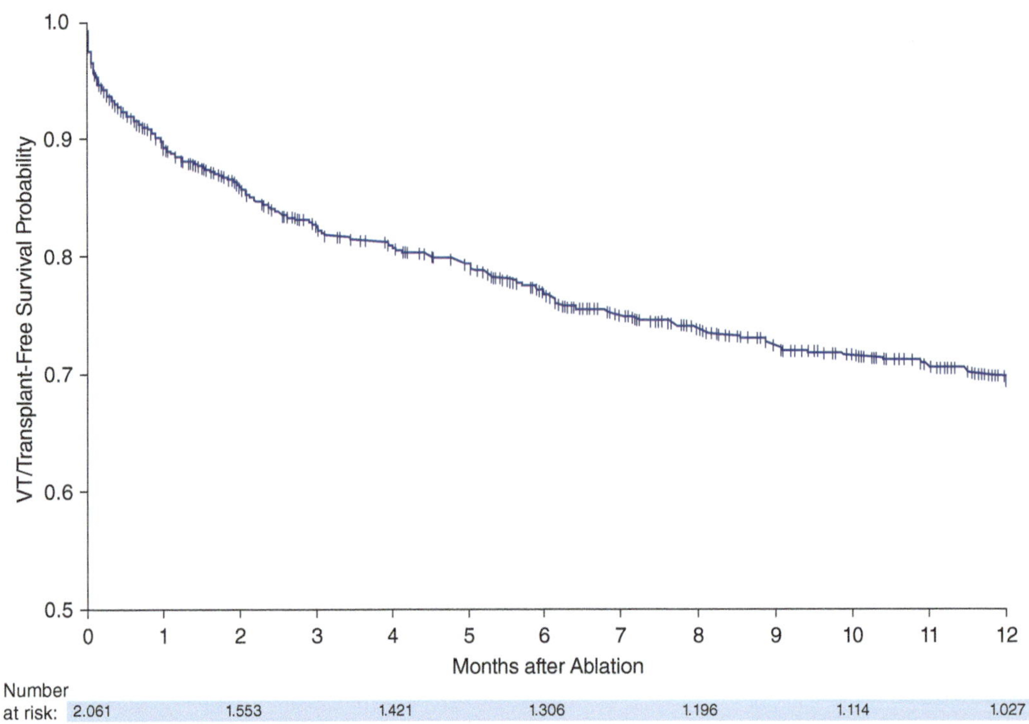

Fig. 36.26 Kaplan-Meier survival estimate of freedom from recurrent ventricular tachycardia following catheter ablation among 2,061 patients with structural heart disease, from the International Ventricular Tachycardia Center Collaborative Study. (Reproduced from Tung R, Vaseghi M, Frankel DS, Vergara P, Di Biase L, Nagashima K, et al. Freedom from recurrent ventricular tachycardia after catheter ablation is associated with improved survival in patients with structural heart disease: an international VT Ablation Center Collaborative Group Study. *Heart Rhythm.* 2015;12:1997–2007.)

ablation volume, and baseline patient comorbidities.[125] Complexity of the anticipated procedure, including need for epicardial access and ablation or repeated ablation, also can be associated with higher complication risk.[70,124]

TROUBLESHOOTING THE DIFFICULT CASE

Several challenges may arise during a substrate-based VT ablation procedure that can increase the difficulty of the case. Most of the common challenges and proposed methods with which to address the challenges have been discussed in previous sections and are summarized in Table 36.4. A common reason for failure to successfully treat VT with substrate modification is a lack of adequate mapping data in the chamber or region of interest. This can either be due to insufficient point acquisition or lack of substrate closest to the surface in which mapping is performed. The former, which most often occurs in the context of poor catheter contact and artificially produces regions of "low voltage" and the false illusion of a greater degree of substrate than is present, can also lead to unnecessary and often ineffective ablation. This problem can be alleviated in several ways. Catheter reach can be optimized by using an alternatively sized curve; this can be accomplished simply using the other curve on a bidirectional catheter (our approach is usually to use a bidirectional catheter with curves of differing radius in anticipation of this potential problem, such as F-J, D-F, etc.), or by changing the direction of the approach entirely, for instance via transseptal rather than retrograde aortic access, or vice versa. Use of a force-sensing catheter and/or ICE can also help ensure mapping (and ablation) with adequate contact with improved time efficiency as well as safety. Finally, if available, remote navigation ablation systems, such as Stereotaxis (St. Louis, MO), have demonstrated utility in improving catheter stability and shown incremental benefit, particularly in the setting of repeated ablation.[126] Conversely, sometimes mapping with a single-bipole catheter, as is the case when mapping with the ablation catheter, may not confer sufficient resolution to detect substrate of greatest interest—the most common scenario in which this may be the case is in the setting of prior MI and very dense endocardial scar, in which narrow channels of viable but diseased myocardium may be obscured and overlooked when mapping with a catheter with a larger field of view. Mapping with a multipolar catheter with electrodes that are more closely spaced,

TABLE 36.4 Troubleshooting the Difficult Case

Problem	Causes	Solution
Apparent lack of endocardial substrate (defined by low bipolar signal amplitude or signs of local abnormal conduction, e.g., fractionation, LAVAs, late potentials)	• Insufficient mapping catheter resolution • Mid-myocardial or epicardial substrate	• Change to multipolar catheter for faster and higher-density point acquisition • Assess unipolar instead of bipolar signal amplitudes among points already acquired • Use ICE to identify regions of increased echogenicity in mid-myocardium or epicardium • Obtain percutaneous epicardial access for mapping; map opposite side of septum; or map coronary venous system for suspected mid-septal substrate
Apparent lack of endocardial or epicardial substrate	• Mid-myocardial substrate	• Assess unipolar instead of bipolar signal amplitudes among points already acquired • Use ICE to identify regions of increased echogenicity in mid-myocardium • Attempt limited mapping during VT to identify most critical regions in which to focus ablation, guided by abnormalities in unipolar voltage or ICE
Ineffective radiofrequency energy delivery	Inadequate catheter contact • Inadequate ablation lesion size or depth • Inadequate mapping	• Change catheter reach, either with curve of different radius, bidirectional catheter, or direction of approach (transseptal access instead of retrograde aortic or vice versa); use force-sensing catheter and/or intracardiac echocardiography (ICE); consider use of remote navigation systems • Irrigated ablation (if nonirrigated ablation was initially utilized); • Consider use of adjunctive techniques to enhance RF lesion size (e.g., half-normal saline irrigant, bipolar ablation) • Use higher-power, irrigated-tip RF energy or lower power with longer application durations (up to several minutes) • Continue mapping: consider alternative approach for substrate identification, access to chamber of interest, or map alternative chamber adjacent to site of interest
Substrate of interest in close proximity to critical anatomical structures	• Coronary arteries on epicardium or in aortic root • Phrenic nerve on epicardium • Proximal His-Purkinje system	• Use ICE to visualize ostium of left main coronary artery in aortic root and perform coronary angiography prior to any epicardial ablation • Avoid ablating with RF energy within 5 mm of proximal major coronary artery • Consider lower-power RF energy (<30 W) or cryoablation as energy source • Ablate opposite site of interest on epicardium from endocardium using longer, higher-power RF applications ± use of adjunctive techniques • Annotate phrenic nerve course with pacing and diaphragmatic stimulation prior to epicardial ablation • Mechanically insulate or lift phrenic from epicardial surface infusing agitated saline or using peripheral angioplasty balloon within space • Avoid ablation in this region unless open conversation has occurred with patient prior to procedure regarding risk of complete heart block and need for possible device upgrade

as discussed in the mapping section, can sometimes help reveal such areas of importance. The need to serially exchange the multipolar mapping catheter for the ablation catheter once ablation proceeds can be eliminated by achieving two sites of access to the chamber of interest and can also allow for simultaneous high-resolution mapping and ablation, as described earlier.

The greatest challenge exists when substrate is predominantly mid-myocardial. In addition to performing careful analysis of unipolar EGMs or using peri- or pre-procedural imaging (ICE or MRI/MDCT, respectively) to identify such regions, limited mapping during VT may be needed to hone in on the region(s) of interest as guided by unipolar signal and ICE abnormalities, to identify the most critical sites to target with ablation with the least amount of collateral damage. Importantly, collateral damage includes ablation of sometimes substantial amounts of normal myocardium in order to reach abnormal tissue within which critically important VT circuitry may be only postulated to exist. Characteristics consistent with sites of greatest interest include regions with mid-diastolic although far-field activation with a diffusely early area of activation (>2 cm^2 within which earliest activation times are within 10 ms).[127,128]

Ablation failure can also occur due to delivery of ablation lesions of inadequate size or depth aside from the contact issue discussed above. Larger and deeper lesions can usually be achieved with irrigated versus nonirrigated catheters; so, a starting point would be ensure that ablation is performed with an irrigated-tip catheter. Assuming that these issues have been addressed, the most common setting in which larger lesions are necessary are in the mid-myocardial substrate scenario already discussed. When myocytes are exposed to a nonlethal dose of heat, the surviving cells will transiently appear to be electrically inexcitable. This hibernation period can last from minutes to weeks. The eventual result is resumption of electrical conductivity in the previously ablated regions. This lack of lesion durability is a common reason for failure and often occurs at deeper levels of myocardium targeted for ablation; it also is the likely mechanism accounting for increased VT recurrence rates following ablation among those with mid-myocardial substrate.[70,129,130] In these circumstances special, adjunctive ablation techniques such as bipolar RF delivery, use of half-normal saline irrigant with an open-irrigated catheter, needle RF ablation, and transcoronary or venous ethanol injection may be additionally helpful.[63,74,103–105,130–133] Given that many of these techniques are not standardly used in clinical practice, seeking assistance from an operator experienced in use of these techniques is recommended if considered.

Bipolar ablation involves the use of two ablation catheters to deliver RF energy as opposed to the standard unipolar ablation delivering RF current from the catheter tip to a dispersive patch. High-power bipolar ablation has been demonstrated to be effective for eliminating septal VT after previously failed ablation attempts.[132,134] The use of ethanol in coronary arteries or veins has been shown to be effective in limited circumstances, particularly for VTs involving the mid-septum or LV summit region.[74,131] Success of these approaches, however, has been limited and obviously also depends highly on the presence of fortuitous anatomy, i.e., presence of coronary arterial or venous branches through which myocyte-toxic ethanol can be delivered selectively to arrhythmogenic regions.[130,131] Use of half-normal saline (HNS) has also been demonstrated to be useful in achieving larger and deeper ablation lesions.[103–105,135] HNS has a higher impedance than normal saline; when a fluid with higher impedance surrounds an electrode through which RF is being delivered to myocardium, RF delivery to tissue is enhanced and larger lesions are observed (Fig. 36.27). This is true both for endocardial or epicardial ablation. As an extension of the latter concept, Aryana et al. showed that a higher amount of saline accumulating in the pericardium results in

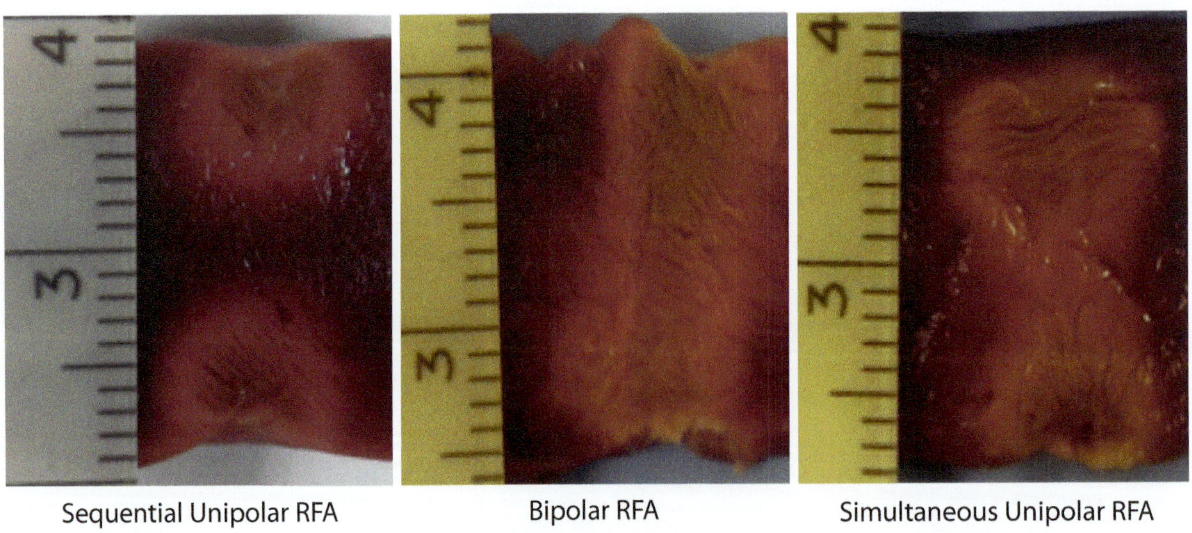

Fig. 36.27 Cross-sections of radiofrequency ablation (RFA) lesions applied to viable bovine myocardium in ex vivo preparation. Note that bipolar ablation application using the same energy (50 W), catheter-tip orientations, and RFA duration (60 s) resulted in a more densely transmural lesion than either sequential unipolar or simultaneous unipolar RFA applications. (Reproduced from Nguyen DT, Gerstenfeld EP, Tzou WS, Jurgens PT, Zheng L, Schuller JL, et al. Radiofrequency ablation using an open irrigated electrode cooled with half-normal saline. *J Am Coll Cardiol EP*. 2017. doi:10.1016/j.jacep.2017.03.006.)

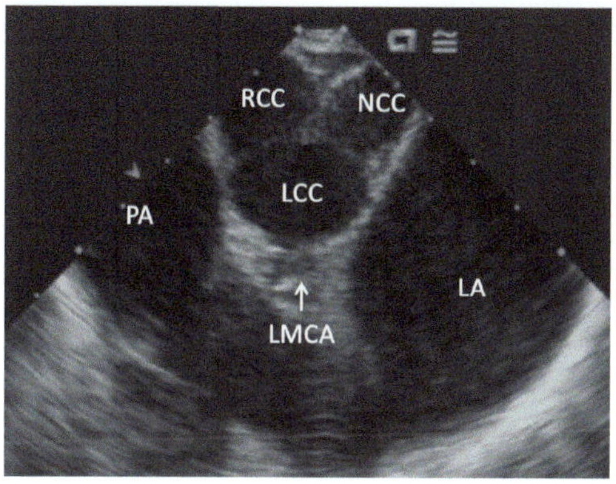

Fig. 36.28 Intracardiac echocardiography image of the aortic cusps, with os of the left main coronary artery (LMCA) visualized. *PA*, Pulmonic artery; *RCC*, right coronary cusp; *NCC*, noncoronary cusp; *LCC*, left coronary cusp; *LA*, left atrium.

smaller lesions compared to those delivered with continuous suction applied to the potential space.[136] We have observed that infusion of HNS into the pericardial space increases the efficacy of epicardial RF ablation.[103,104]

Finally, there may be anatomical barriers that prevent the effective delivery of radiofrequency or cryothermal energy. For example, proximity to the normal His-Purkinje conduction system and coronary arteries may limit the use of higher powers to critical regions targeted for ablation; these structures are most relevant to consider when targeting VT in the basal septum or on the epicardium. Fat may also protect regions of interest or limit ablation efficacy on the epicardium. ICE can be used to help identify and avoid the ostium of the left main coronary artery prior to ablation in the aortic root or pulmonic valve cusp (Fig. 36.28). Coronary angiography should be performed whenever the proximity of ablation to a coronary artery is in question; this includes the endocardium and epicardium. We generally avoid ablating with RF energy within 5 mm of a proximal major coronary artery.[22] In circumstances in which ablation in closer proximity to a coronary artery is considered to be important, use of lower-power RF energy (<30 W) or cryoablation as energy source can be considered. Also, a consideration is to ablate opposite the site of interest on the epicardium from the endocardium using longer, higher-power RF applications with or without the use of adjunctive techniques.[137]

Additionally, although phrenic nerve injury can usually be avoided, this structure should not be forgotten when performing epicardial ablation. The left phrenic nerve typically courses along the lateral aspect of the LV and can be easily identified with pacing and diaphragmatic stimulation (assuming no paralytic agents have been administered). It also is not adherent to the epicardial surface and thus can be potentially moved out of the way of an ablation site. Techniques that have been described with which this can be safely achieved include infusion of fluid (HNS may be more ideal, as discussed above) or air, avoiding iatrogenic tamponade, or inflating a peripheral angioplasty balloon within the space.[138,139]

With advances that have been made in increasing ablation efficacy in the setting of SHD, one can never neglect the potential for causing collateral damage, and caution must always be exercised in minimizing this potential.

CONCLUSION

The most common underlying mechanism for VT in the setting of SHD, either from ischemic or nonischemic causes, is scar-based reentry. Because most ventricular arrhythmias are not hemodynamically tolerated, strategies aimed at scar modification with substrate-based ablation during paced or sinus rhythm have been developed. These substrate-based approaches are enabled with electroanatomical mapping and include empiric ablation guided by pace mapping, the targeting of late potentials or local abnormal ventricular activities within scar, scar dechanneling, core isolation, and scar homogenization. Regardless of the ablation strategy used, consistent differences exist in VT-free survival outcomes based on etiology of SHD, with recurrence rates substantially higher among patients with NICM due to differences in scar distribution in the epicardium and mid-myocardium. In addition, challenges remain with regard to the safe creation of ablation lesions on endocardial, epicardial, and mid-myocardial tissue. However, despite remaining challenges in VT ablation, substrate-based ablation remains effective in controlling VT refractory to medical therapy. Newer technologies designed to overcome these challenges are in development and offer promise for improving the safety and efficacy of substrate-based VT ablation.

REFERENCES

Please refer to the e-book for a complete list of references.

37

Epicardial Approach to Catheter Ablation of Ventricular Tachycardia

Roderick Tung

KEY POINTS

- Percutaneous access to the pericardial space has improved our ability to characterize and modify arrhythmogenic epicardial scar substrates.
- Knowledge of pericardial anatomy and relevant surrounding structures is important for recognizing and reducing complications.
- Although the practice and utilization of epicardial mapping for ventricular tachycardia ablation vary, substrates with a high likelihood of epicardial scar and prior failed endocardial ablation are most likely to derive benefit from this adjunctive approach.
- Understanding fluoroscopic views for both anterior and inferior approaches for access optimizes the safety and efficacy of the percutaneous puncture.
- Surgical access can safely be performed in a sterile electrophysiology laboratory to enable catheter ablation in patients with prior cardiac surgery or adhesions via subxiphoid window for inferior wall substrates and by limited anterior thoracotomy for anterior, apical, and lateral substrates.
- Intrapericardial steroids may reduce pericarditis, although repeat access to the pericardial space is possible in the majority of patients.
- Careful attention to the anatomical course of the phrenic nerve and coronary arteries is important before radiofrequency delivery to minimize complications.
- The presence of epicardial fat can confound the diagnosis of scar in low-voltage regions and impair the penetration of radiofrequency energy delivery into the myocardium.
- The most common complication related to epicardial access is pericardial bleeding, which can result from right ventricular puncture, or trauma from mechanical sheath or catheter manipulation and ablation.
- A combined epicardial-endocardial ablation strategy provides more comprehensive two-dimensional modification of three-dimensional complex scar substrates. Observational cohort studies have demonstrated increased freedom from ventricular tachycardia recurrence with a combined strategy compared with endocardial ablation alone.

The pericardial space has been historically viewed as a region accessed only in the clinical event of a hemodynamically significant effusion to therapeutically alleviate tamponade or sample fluid for diagnosis. In 1996, Sosa et al. described a percutaneous method similar to a pericardiocentesis to access a "dry" pericardial space.[1] This innovative, yet seemingly high-risk approach opened up a new frontier in complex ablation of arrhythmias, whereby the epicardial surface of the heart could be mapped and ablated by catheters without the need for sternotomy.

The presence of epicardial reentrant circuits may be an important reason for the relatively low historical success rates (50%) of endocardial ablation for scar-mediated ventricular tachycardia (VT).[2,3] As scar is often transmural and spatially complex, epicardial ablation allows for more comprehensive modification of arrhythmogenic substrates. Since the advent of this percutaneous approach, electroanatomical mapping in the pericardial space has improved our understanding and characterization of the transmural extent and anatomical propensity of scars across a diverse range of substrates. The complications associated with this approach are related to collateral injury during access and ablation, so knowledge of the relevant anatomy is critical to maximize the safety and efficacy of the procedure.

PERICARDIAL ANATOMY

The pericardium is a continuous self-enclosed sac that consists of three layers—a serous visceral pericardium, serous parietal pericardium, and fibrous layer. Embryologically, the serous pericardium consists of a visceral layer (epicardium) and a parietal layer that is reflected onto the outer fibrous layer (epipericardium). A physiologic amount of serous fluid (20–60 mL) between the visceral and parietal layer is contained in the pericardial space to lubricate the movement of the epicardium on the parietal pericardium. The normal range of pericardial thickness is 1–3.5 mm.[4]

The pericardium serves to protect the heart from trauma, adhesions, and infection. Importantly, it suspends and anchors the heart in a fixed position in the thorax. Superiorly, the pericardium is fixed to the great arteries, surrounding the aorta and pulmonary artery several centimeters above the heart. Inferiorly, the parietal pericardium is attached and anchored to the central tendinous aponeurosis of the diaphragm. Anteriorly, pericardiosternal ligaments attach the fibrous pericardial layer to the manubrium and xiphoid process (Fig. 37.1).

The two major sinuses relevant to electrophysiologic procedures are the transverse and oblique sinuses. The transverse

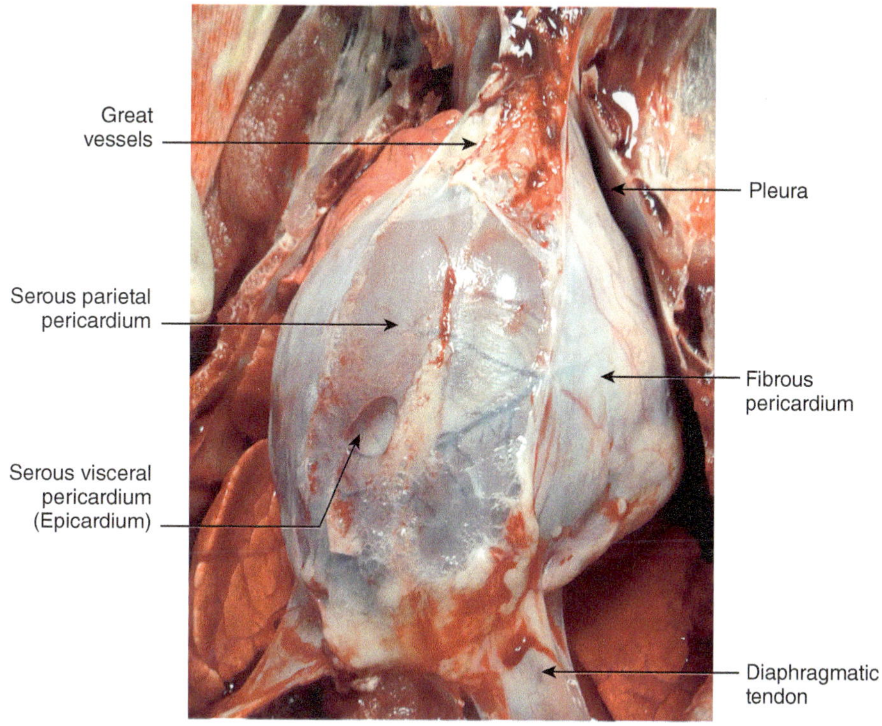

Fig. 37.1 Porcine heart in situ after percutaneous epicardial access via anterior approach. The serous visceral pericardium (epicardium) is seen through the puncture site. Removal of the sternum shows the parietal layer with the fibrous outer layer peeled off. Broad diaphragmatic attachments are seen inferiorly.

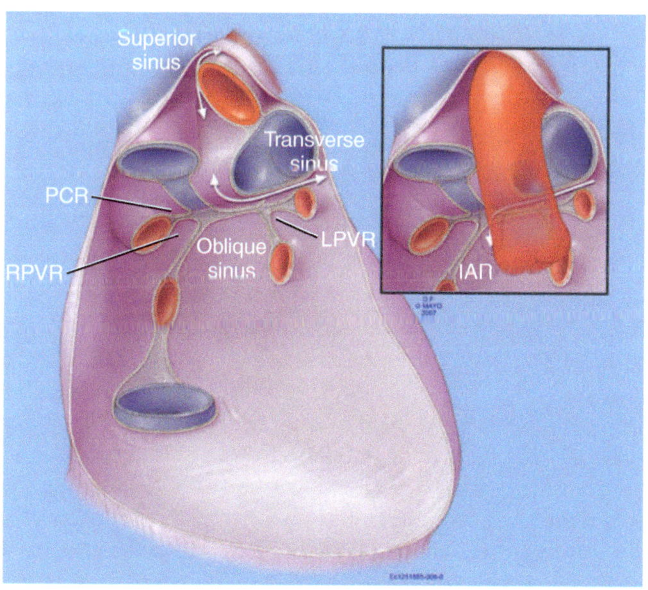

Fig. 37.2 Pericardial recesses and sinus posterior to the heart. The oblique sinus lies posterior to the left atrium. The transverse sinus lies posterior to the ascending aorta. *IAR*, Inferior atrial recess; *LPVR*, left posterior venous recess; *PCR*, posterior caval recess; *RPVR*, right posterior venous recess. (From Lachman N, Syed FF, Habib A, et al. Correlative anatomy for the electrophysiologist, Part I: the pericardial space, oblique sinus, transverse sinus. *J Cardiovasc Electrophysiol.* 2010;21:1421–1426.)

sinus lies superior to the left atrium and posterior to the ascending aorta (Fig. 37.2). The roof of the transverse sinus is marked by the right pulmonary artery as it courses through the aortic arch[5] (Fig. 37.3). It is through the transverse sinus that crossing between the left and right side of the heart can be achieved. More commonly, access from the left to the right side of the heart during percutaneous access procedures occurs anterior to the great vessels.

The oblique sinus lies directly posterior to the left atrium and anterior to the esophagus and descending aorta. It is bounded by the venous reflections of the inferior vena cava and four pulmonary veins (Fig. 37.3). As a result, manipulation in the oblique sinus is difficult because of the numerous reflections but anatomically is not required for ablation of ventricular tachycardia (VT).

Nerve fibers from the parietal layer of the pericardium transmitted by the phrenic nerve are sensitive to pain. Inflammation of this layer is responsible for the pleuritic pain of pericarditis. The phrenic nerves course along the anterior and lateral pericardial surface outside of the fibrous pericardium.

CLINICAL INDICATIONS FOR EPICARDIAL MAPPING

Access to the pericardial space for epicardial mapping is clinically indicated when a high suspicion for epicardial scar and/or VT site of origin is present. Currently, the indications for epicardial mapping and ablation are dependent on the scar substrate, prior ablation history, and electrocardiographic characteristics of the targeted VT. A European Heart Rhythm Association/Heart Rhythm Society consensus statement reported that epicardial access was performed in 17% of VT ablation cases, based on a survey among tertiary referral centers although with significant variation in practice patterns.[6] With increased cumulative experience that reinforces procedural safety and efficacy, a trend toward wider implementation is likely.

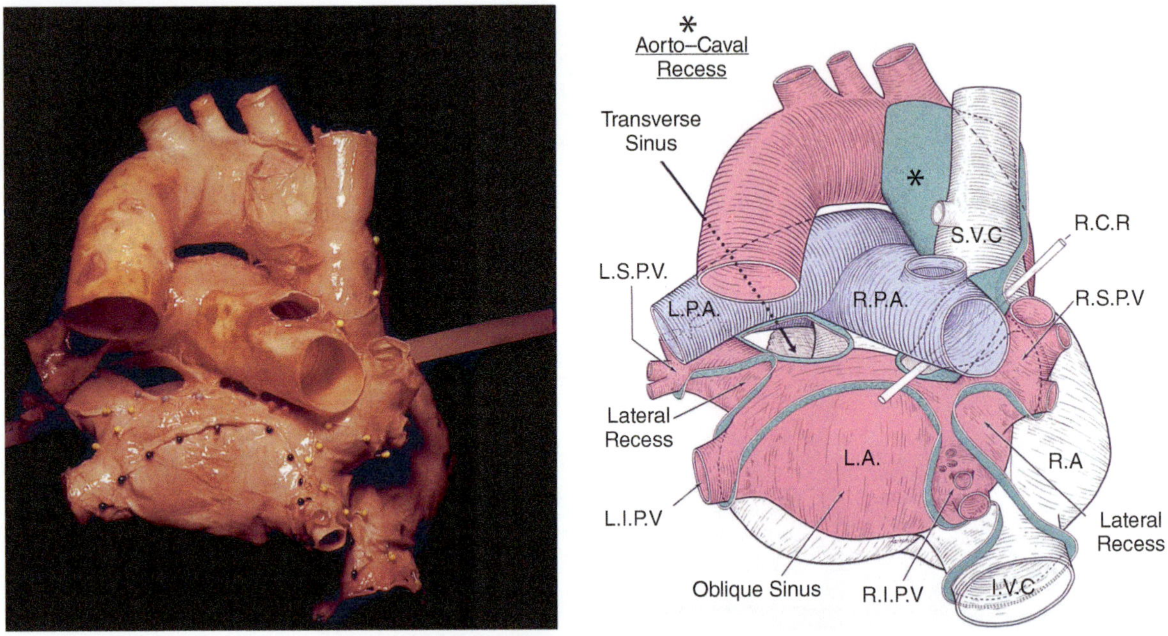

Fig. 37.3 Anatomical dissection of the posterior left atrium and great vessels intact. The oblique sinus is marked superiorly by black pins. A wooden rod is passed through the transverse sinus. *IVC*, Inferior vena cava; *LA*, left atrium; *LIPV*, left inferior pulmonary vein; *LPA*, left pulmonary artery; *LSPV*, left superior pulmonary vein; *RA*, right atrium; *RCR*, retrocaval recess; *RIPV*, right inferior pulmonary vein; *RPA*, right pulmonary artery; *RPO*, right posterior oblique; *RSPV*, right superior pulmonary vein; *SVC*, superior vena cava. (From McAlpine, UCLA Cardiac Arrhythmia Center Library, courtesy Dr. Kalyanam Shivkumar.)

The characterization of various substrates, including nonischemic cardiomyopathy (NICM),[7–8] arrhythmogenic right ventricular cardiomyopathy (ARVC),[9,10] hypertrophic cardiomyopathy (HCM),[11,12] and Chagasic cardiomyopathy[13,14] with magnetic resonance imaging (MRI) and electroanatomical mapping, has demonstrated the presence of significant epicardial scarring that is often more extensive than scar seen on the endocardial surface (Fig. 37.4A, B). In contrast, the scar of ischemic cardiomyopathy (ICM) has been reported to be wedge-shaped with primary subendocardial necrosis and variable epicardial sparing depending on the duration of coronary occlusion. This is in concert with the wavefront of necrosis theory proposed by Reimer and Jennings.[15] Earlier surgical studies that demonstrated a relative paucity of late potentials in postinfarct scars were performed predominantly on anterior infarcts with aneurysms.[16,17] In comparison with nonreperfused infarcts, reperfused infarcts have been shown to have different structural and functional scar characteristics with a patchy pattern and variable epicardial sparing.[18] In our experience, epicardial scar may be equally as extensive as endocardial scar in ICM patients without aneurysms and VT termination from the epicardium is seen in 24% to 64% of cases[19,20] (Fig. 37.5). There is no established gold standard for an epicardial circuit as criteria based on the isthmus, exit, or entire circuit offer variable definitions. Newer data from simultaneous epi-endo activation mapping show epicardial isthmus components in 61% of ICM VT circuits with epicardial breakout during QRS onset in 81% (Fig 37.6).

The implementation of epicardial mapping and ablation is highly variable and is more commonly performed at highly experienced centers.[21,22] Wider adoption of epicardial ablation is justifiable at centers with sufficiently low risk of complications. Various practice patterns range from using epicardial ablation only in the event of a previously failed endocardial ablation to using it as part of a combined comprehensive initial strategy. However, randomized prospective data are lacking. A proposed strategy for clinical decision-making to assess a patient for epicardial access is shown (Fig. 37.7).

Electrocardiographic criteria have been proposed to be suggestive of an epicardial exit site. Delayed myocardial conduction from an epicardial exit is initially slow before accessing the subendocardial conduction system, with an "outside-to-in" activation pattern. Berruezo et al. demonstrated several morphologic criteria that favored an epicardial exit site: (1) a "pseudo-delta" wave duration >34 ms, (2) QRS complex duration >200 ms, (3) delayed intrinsicoid deflection of >85 ms, and (4) RS complex duration >121 ms.[23] In NICM, a QS pattern in lead I or the inferior leads can signify the absence of "inside-to-outside" activation of the heart from the lateral and inferior walls.[24,25] However, these criteria have significant limitations where the severity of cardiomyopathy, scar burden, and conduction delay associated with antiarrhythmic drugs decrease their diagnostic specificity. In the setting of structural heart disease, these electrocardiographic criteria have been shown to lack any predictive or discriminatory value by Martinek et al.[26] in ICM and Piers et al. in NICM.[27]

Several findings on endocardial mapping can be suggestive of an epicardial site of origin. The absence of early activation sites (diastolic or presystolic) or a diffuse, broad region of activation on electroanatomical mapping suggests that the site of origin or circuit is not limited to the endocardium. In addition, poorly matched pace map sites endocardially and the inability to terminate a mappable VT with endocardial ablation are

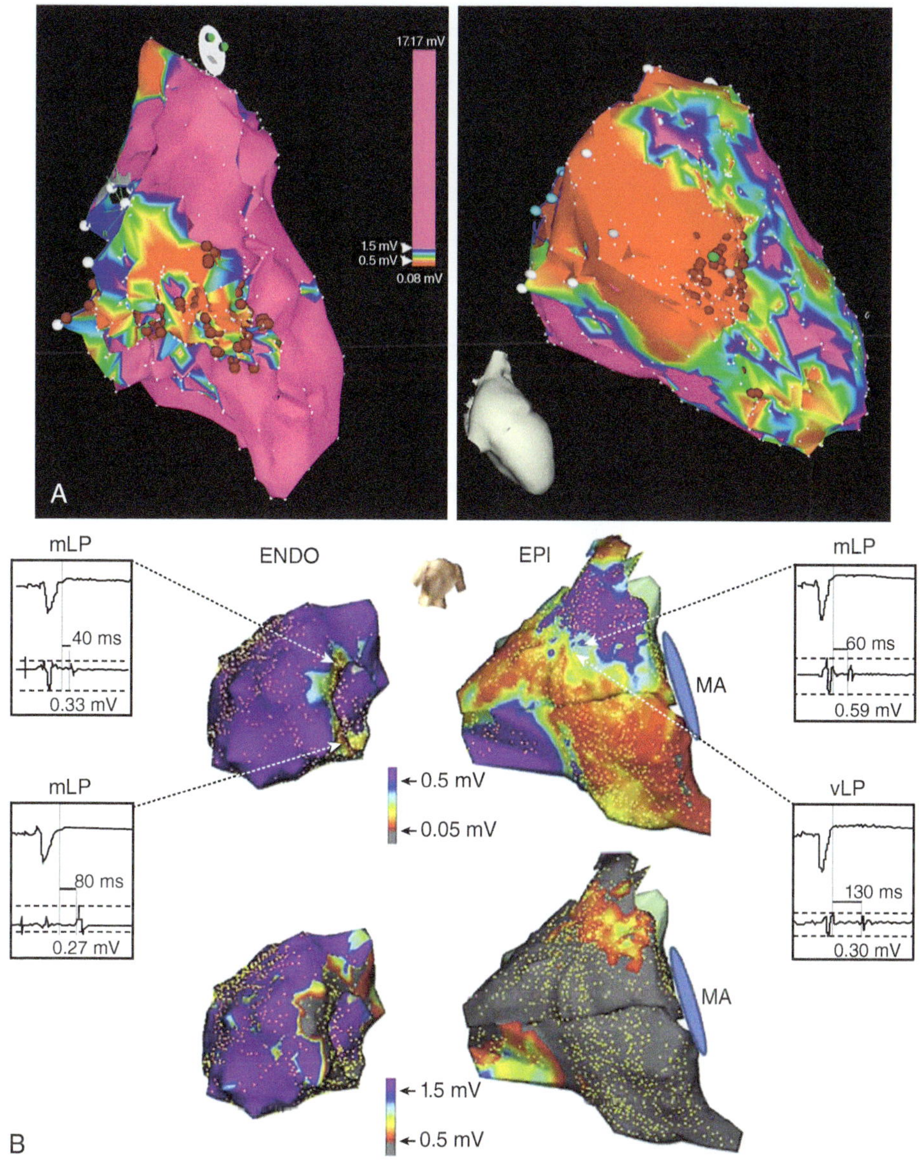

Fig. 37.4 (A) Combined epicardial and endocardial electroanatomical map of patient with arrhythmogenic right ventricular cardiomyopathy reveals more extensive epicardial scar (right anterior oblique caudal view). The *red circles* indicate ablation lesions and the termination of ventricular tachycardia was achieved at the *green circle*. (B) Electroanatomical substrate mapping of a patient with nonischemic cardiomyopathy reveals extensive epicardial scar in relation to endocardial scar. Multiple late potentials are seen within the low-voltage regions. *mLP*, Moderate late potential; *vLP*, very late potential. (From Nakahara S, Tung R, Ramirez RJ, et al. Characterization of the arrhythmogenic substrate in ischemic and nonischemic cardiomyopathy implications for catheter ablation of hemodynamically unstable ventricular tachycardia. *J Am Coll Cardiol.* 2010;55:2355–2365.)

suggestive of an intramural or epicardial VT. A unipolar display (<5.5 mV right ventricle [RV], <8.27 mV left ventricle [LV]) in patients with limited endocardial abnormalities identified by electroanatomical mapping has been proposed to identify scar at a greater depth using a "wider field of view" in patients with NICM and ARVC.[28,29]

SUBXIPHOID PERCUTANEOUS TECHNIQUE

Percutaneous puncture via subxiphoid access first described by Sosa et al.[1] uses the same approach as a pericardiocentesis. However, because of the risk of cardiac puncture in the absence of an effusion, additional modifications and cautionary steps are used. Importantly, fluoroscopy with contrast imaging and use of a curved tip needle for entering the pericardial space increase the safety and success of obtaining epicardial access.

Surgical backup is important for ablation centers attempting epicardial interventions in the event of complications, and a typed blood sample should be obtained. Before attempting access, anticoagulant, antithrombotic, and antiplatelet agents should be discontinued to minimize the risk of bleeding. In our experience, thienopyridines have been associated with the highest incidence of bleeding. To optimize safety, epicardial access is obtained before systemic heparinization, which is necessary

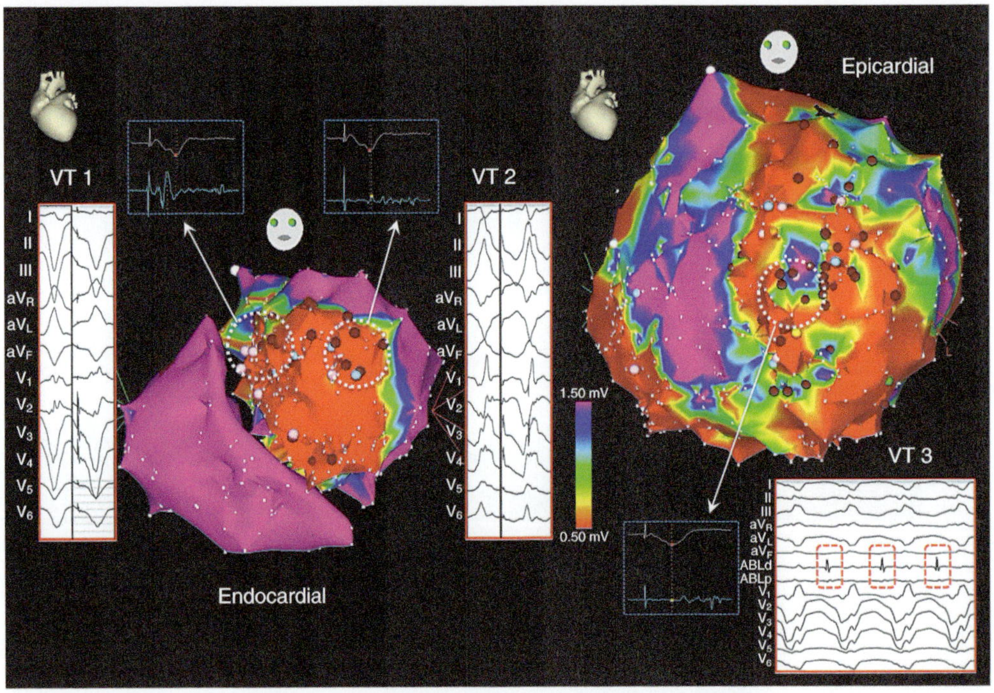

Fig. 37.5 Combined epicardial-endocardial biventricular mapping in a patient with anterior infarction. Heterogeneous epicardial scar is more extensive than dense endocardial scar. Two ventricular tachycardias were localized to the endocardium by pace mapping and the third was terminated on the epicardium at a mid-diastolic site. (From Tung R, Michowitz Y, Yu R, et al. Epicardial ablation of ventricular tachycardia: an institutional experience of safety and efficacy. *Heart Rhythm.* 2013;10:490–498.)

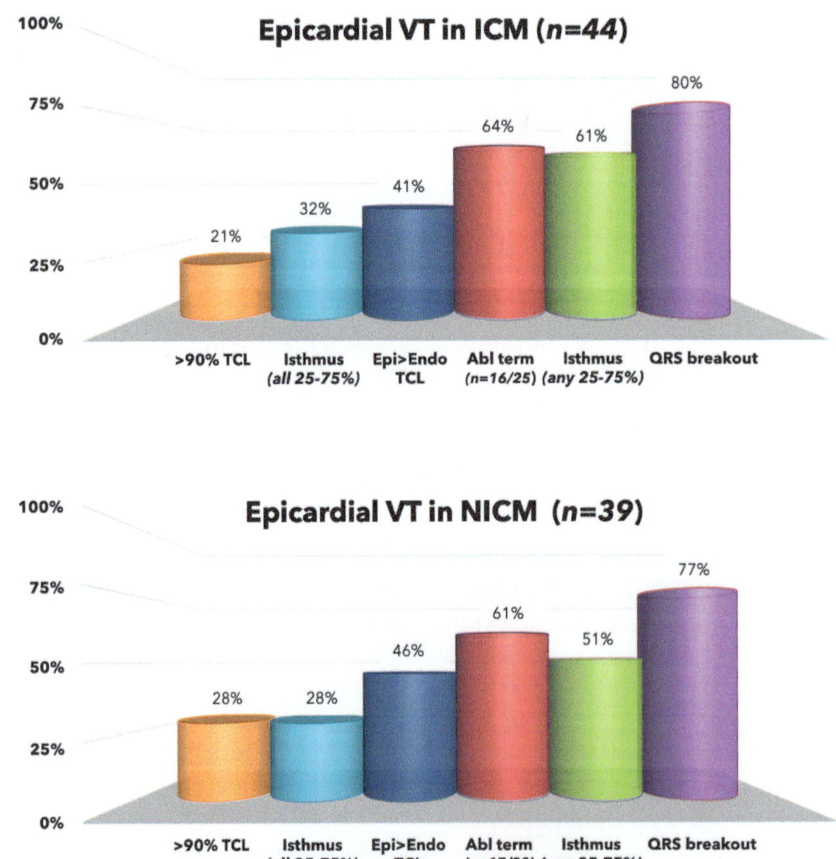

Fig 37.6 Different potential definitions of an epicardial VT circuit, based on the extent of tachycardia cycle length (TCL), isthmus components, and exit breakout region recorded on the epicardium. Termination of tachycardia is a pragmatic definition, whereas the extent of TCL identified with activation mapping is more mechanistic.

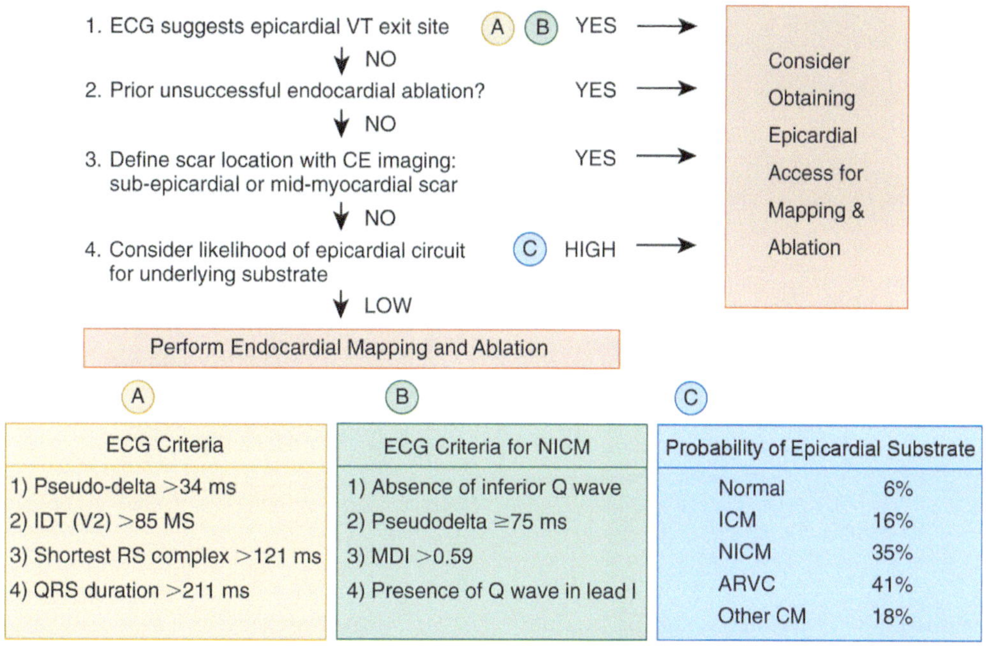

Fig. 37.7 Suggested clinical decision tree to assess the indication for epicardial mapping and ablation. (From Boyle N, Shivkumar K. Epicardial interventions in electrophysiology. *Circulation*. 2012;126(14):1752–1769.)

during endocardial mapping and ablation. In addition, we often perform epicardial mapping once access is obtained before endocardial mapping to minimize the total duration of systemic anticoagulation during the procedure.

The choice of sedation and anesthesia is an important consideration during preprocedural planning, as general anesthesia minimizes patient movement and regulates respiration. It is our opinion that epicardial access performed under general anesthesia optimizes patient safety, comfort, and overall success. However, general anesthesia may diminish the ease of VT inducibility and prolong procedural duration. This concern is more relevant when the mechanism of ventricular arrhythmia is thought to be automatic or triggered. If conscious sedation is chosen, the sedation may be deepened for the puncture and lightened after successful access is obtained.

The procedure is commenced with sterile preparation of the subxiphoid region, which is then anesthetized with topical 1% lidocaine. Antibiotics are administered at our institution to minimize any risk of bacterial pericarditis. The location of the subxiphoid process by palpation should be carefully confirmed as an anatomical miscalculation may increase the risk of the procedure. A 17-gauge curved-tipped needle, originally designed for epidural access to minimize trauma to the spinal cord, is preferred as it allows an angled guidewire course away from the myocardium when the parietal pericardium is punctured. Two lengths of Tuohy epidural needles are available at our institution: 17 gauge × 3.5 inches (90 mm, BD Medical, Franklin Lakes, NJ) and 17 gauge × 6 inches (152 mm, Hakko, Cincinnati, OH) and should be selected based on body habitus (Fig. 37.8).

At our center, the puncture site is performed one fingerbreadth left of the subxiphoid process, allowing for access through the Larrey space (trigonum sternocostale), which has been reported to be avascular.[30] A shallow entry initially directed to the left shoulder is preferred to minimize puncture of the liver with an increase toward 45 degrees after several centimeters. Manual pressure over the right upper quadrant may be applied to minimize hepatic puncture.

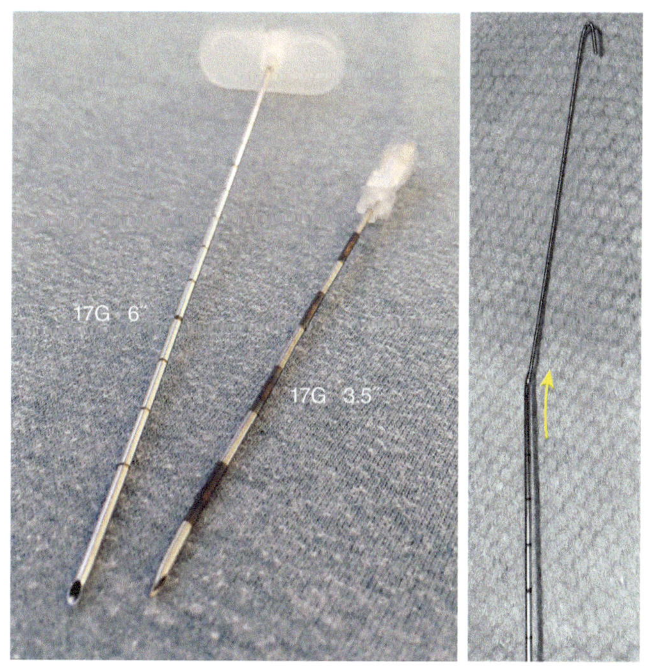

Fig. 37.8 Two lengths of commercially available epidural needles for percutaneous access. The curved tip facilitates a wire exit course out of the lumen slightly tangential to the epicardium.

Biplane fluoroscopy is useful to assess the approach of the needle for the two approaches: anterior and posterior (inferior). A helpful rule of epicardial access is to puncture at the

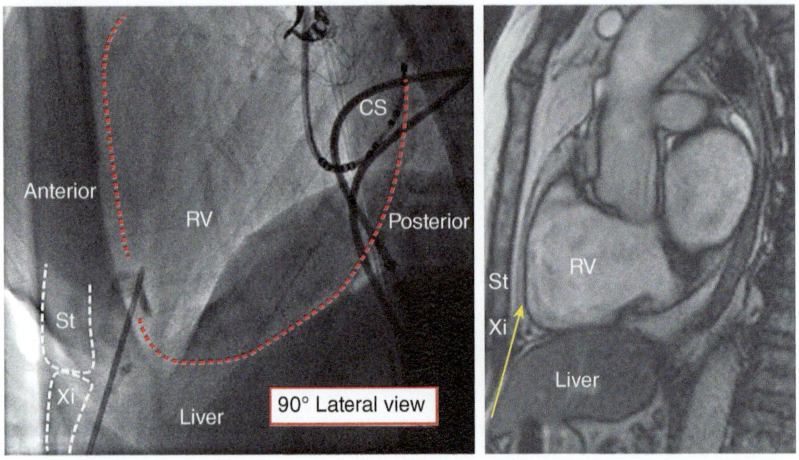

Fig. 37.9 Cross-table lateral views on magnetic resonance imaging and fluoroscopy demonstrating the anterior approach to epicardial puncture just inferior to the sternum and superior to the liver. *CS*, Coronary sinus; *Xi*, xiphoid process; *RV*, right ventricle; *ST*, sternum.

site farther away from the desired region of mapping as acute "U turns" required of the catheter course to map the region around the puncture site are technically challenging. If an anterior puncture is desired, the needle track is continued along a shallow course (<30 degrees), and a steep lateral projection is helpful at assessing the needle track just posterior to the sternum as it approaches the anterior RV (Fig. 37.9). A posterior approach requires steepening of the needle (>45 degrees) course to aim for the basal portion of the heart, which is fluoroscopically marked by the coronary sinus catheter. The right anterior oblique (RAO) projection is useful for determining a basal versus apical approach angle. The left anterior oblique (LAO) projection is helpful to identify the RV free wall, which forms the right heart border. It is our preference to approach with an angle that is more tangential to the inferior heart border visualized on LAO to minimize RV puncture. However, a puncture directed too septally increases the risk of posterior descending artery injury (Fig. 37.10). The incidence of diaphragmatic and liver puncture may be higher with a posterior approach, but the anterior approach increases the probability of puncture of the superior epigastric artery, which is the more superficial and caudal continuation of the left interior mammary artery. Frequently, the diaphragmatic attachments must be punctured before accessing the pericardial space and can be misinterpreted as the parietal pericardium.

Once the needle is advanced to the inferior heart border, cardiac pulsations, an injury current detected with alligator clips, or ventricular ectopy can all signify contact and indentation of the parietal pericardium onto the epicardium. The most sensitive period for cardiac pulsations occurs during inspiration with inferior displacement of the heart increasing the contact with the needle. A pressure sensor may be useful to improve safety for access.[31] In an awake patient, pain signals needle contact with the parietal pericardium through the fibrous layers. A minimal amount of contrast is injected to visualize "tenting" or indentation of the fibrous pericardium as large quantities of contrast injected obscure the fluoroscopic field of view (Fig. 37.11). Once the pericardium is in contact with the needle, either constant pressure or a swift calculated puncture can be executed until the puncture is felt with a "pop" or, more commonly, visualized with release of the contrast-stained pericardial outer surface. A slight withdrawal of the needle once puncture is sensed, as the pericardium releases, reduces the risk of RV perforation as the advanced needle frequently violates the anatomical plane of the RV (Videos 37.1 and 37.2). Contrast is quickly injected to confirm layering within the pericardial space, and then a guidewire is advanced along the lateral heart border in the LAO projection. New tools are being tested that may improve safety and efficacy of approach, including different needle designs and a pressure-sensing tip.[31] A "needle-in-needle" approach with initial micropuncture entry has also been shown to be feasible and may improve safety.[32,33] Insufflation of CO_2 after intentional wire exit from a coronary vein or atrial appendage may improve safety by creating a greater space for puncture from pneumopericardium.[34,35]

Before sheath cannulation, the guidewire must be confirmed to reach the left heart border in the LAO view to exclude the possibility of RV puncture with guidewire insertion into the RV outflow tract (Fig. 37.12). The optimal guidewire course for confirmation traverses several chambers and reaches the most outer portion of the fluoroscopic cardiac silhouette (Fig. 37.13). Following this, we use a smaller soft tip dilator (5 F) over the wire for further confirmation. The first aspirate of pericardial fluid is obtained via this small dilator to assess for a blood and 10–20 mL of contrast is injected.

Contrast pericardiography is helpful to confirm the pericardial puncture and to assess for adhesions, which may limit the ability to navigate the catheter and increase the probability of pericardial bleeding as these are released and dissected with the sheath and catheter during mapping and ablation (Fig. 37.14). Once this is performed, a long wire is placed across the transverse sinus or anterior to the great vessels and a long sheath is advanced under LAO projection.

We have chosen a long sheath at our center to increase the distance of the operator from the fluoroscopy tube and to minimize the risk of losing access. A steerable sheath can be used if

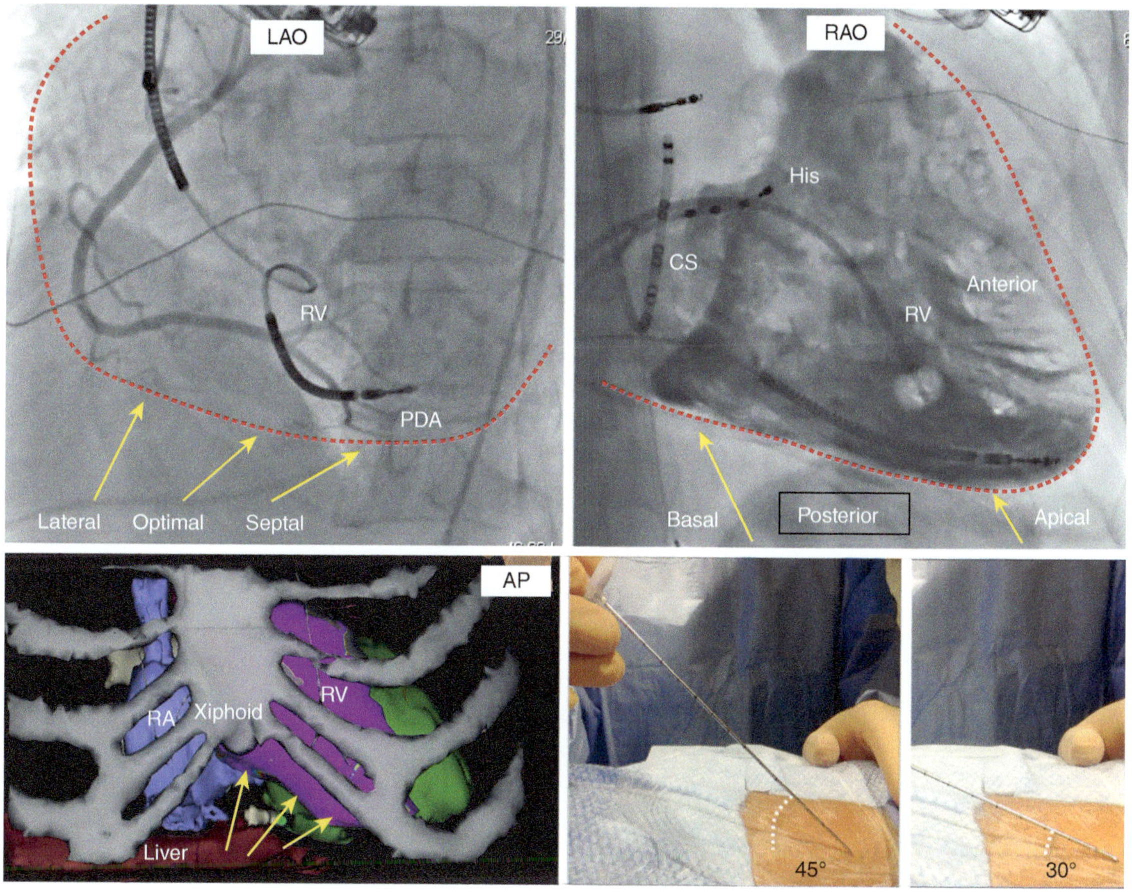

Fig. 37.10 Relevant anatomy on fluoroscopic views during percutaneous access with posterior approach. In left anterior oblique view, septal approach increases the risk of posterior descending branch puncture as shown. A lateral approach increases the risk of right ventricular puncture as the angulation is more perpendicular with the inferior surface of the heart. In right anterior oblique view, steepening the angle of entry allows the operator to adjust the depth of puncture from apical to basal. An anteroposterior view based on three-dimensional computed tomography reconstruction demonstrates the anatomical position of the right ventricle in relation to the xiphoid process.

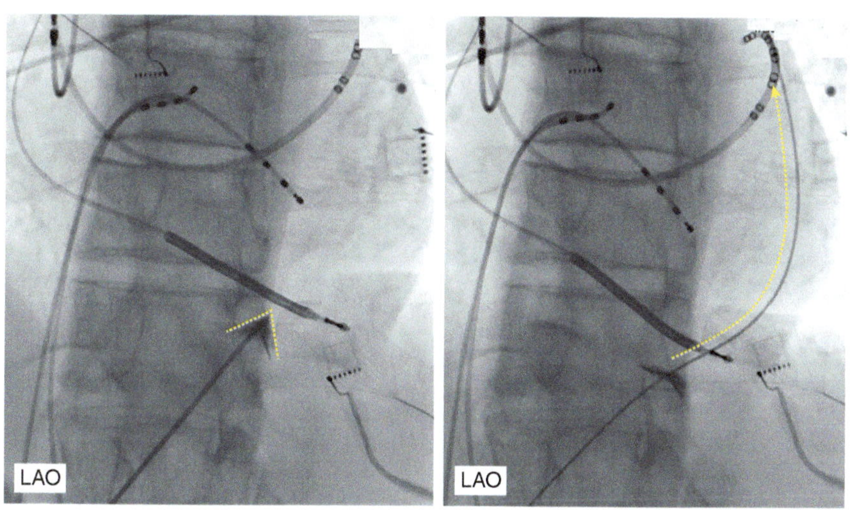

Fig. 37.11 Indentation, or tenting of the pericardium with the Tuohy needle visualized on left anterior oblique (LAO) projection. Release of the contrast-stained pericardium is seen as the guidewire is advanced superiorly toward the lateral heart border.

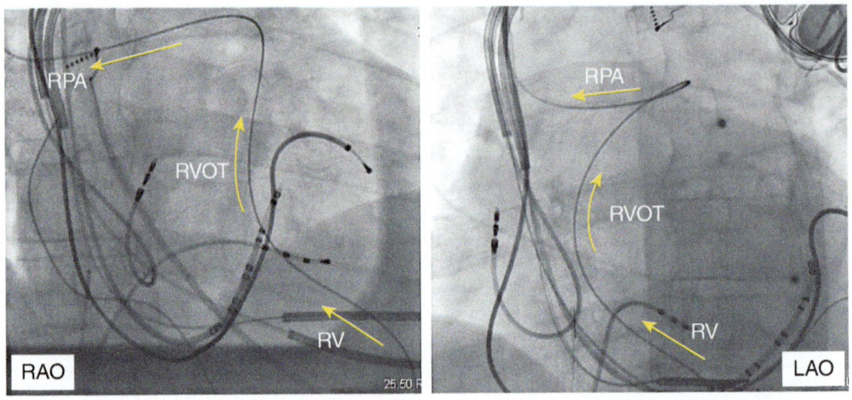

Fig. 37.12 Fluoroscopic views of the guidewire course after inadvertent right ventricular (RV) puncture. On left anterior oblique (LAO), the wire fails to cross the septum to the lateral heart border as it travels up to the right ventricular outflow tract (RVOT) out of the right pulmonary artery. *RAO*, Right anterior oblique; *RPA*, right pulmonary artery.

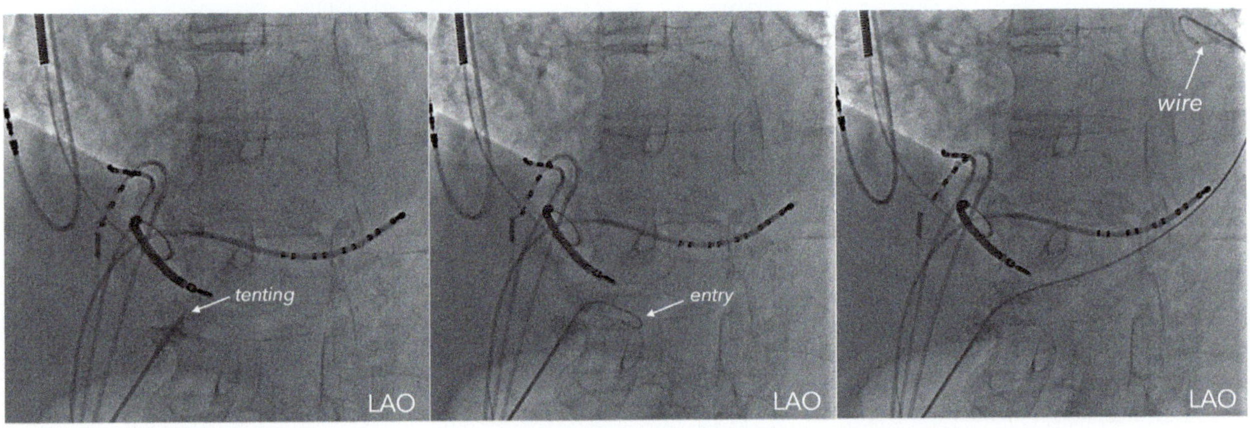

Fig. 37.13 Optimal guidewire course within pericardial space that crosses multiple chambers along the outermost cardiac border on fluoroscopy in left anterior oblique (LAO) projection. (From Boyle N, Shivkumar K. Epicardial interventions in electrophysiology. *Circulation*. 2012;126(14):1752–1769.)

small adhesions are encountered or to assist in mapping regions that are not easily accessible with a fixed sheath.[36] In addition, we use a "double-wire" technique and retain one wire to always maintain pericardial access in the case of inadvertent sheath withdrawal during mapping. It is important to minimize the amount of time that a sheath does not have a catheter protruding from it, as an exposed sheath end may lacerate coronary vessels during normal cardiac motion. We use an angiographic catheter as a "place holder" if an ablation catheter is not in the epicardial sheath for mapping or ablation.

SURGICAL ACCESS

In the case of prior cardiac surgery or clinical pericarditis, dense adhesions are likely to be encountered in the pericardial space, making a percutaneous approach less desirable. These adhesions decrease the ability for the operator to determine if the puncture is in the pericardial space, limits the ability to access all epicardial regions, and increases the risk of bleeding as adhesions are bluntly dissected without direct visualization. Sosa et al. described the feasibility of limited access to the inferior wall in patients with prior cardiac surgery.[37] Recently, Tschabrunn et al. demonstrated that percutaneous access can be obtained in patients with noncoronary artery bypass grafting surgery, although dense adhesions are often encountered and mappable regions remain limited.[38] It is our practice not to attempt percutaneous access on any patient with prior surgery because of limited access and an increased risk for complications. A recent report of subepicardial dissection requiring emergent surgery highlights the potential risk of blind dissection in the setting of severe adhesions.[39]

Soejima et al. first described epicardial access by creation of a surgical subxiphoid window to enable catheter placement into the pericardial space.[40] We have shown that a limited anterior thoracotomy can be obtained in the electrophysiologic laboratory and is useful for accessing anterior, lateral, and apical regions of the LV in contrast to subxiphoid window, which is best suited for scar located on the inferior surface of the heart[41] (Figs. 37.15 and 37.16).

The rules for hybrid ablation are similar to those for percutaneous with the following exceptions: (1) sterility is of increased importance; (2) selection of mapping and ablation tools requires special consideration; and (3) an open chest may increase defibrillation threshold because of the presence of air, necessitating preparation for internal defibrillation.[42]

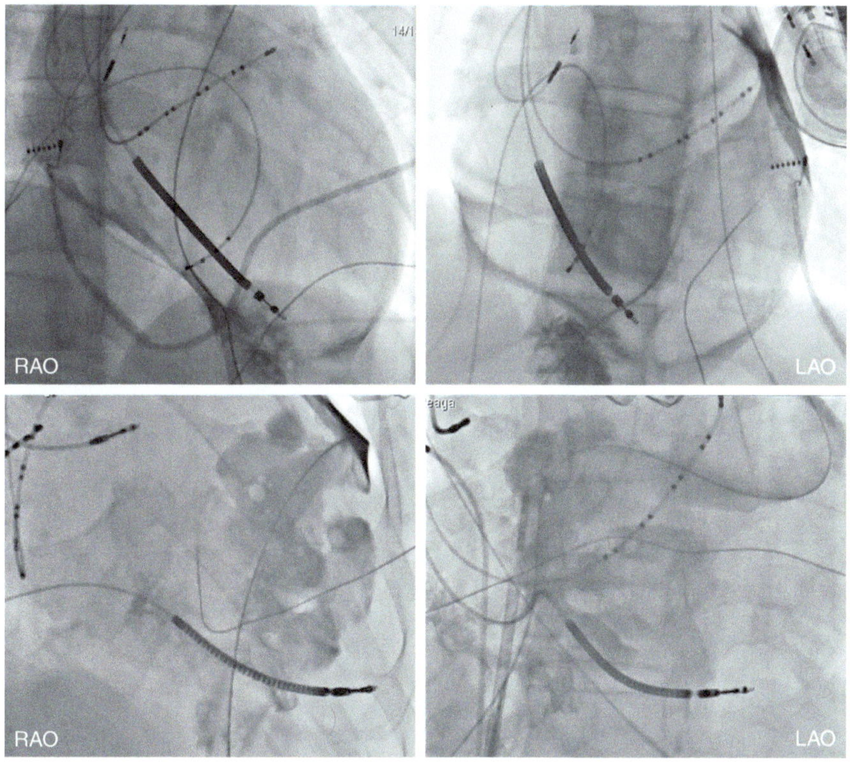

Fig. 37.14 Contrast pericardiogram in a patient without adhesions (*top*) shows even distribution of contrast from base to apex in right anterior oblique (RAO) and left and right heart borders in left anterior oblique (LAO). Loculation of contrast seen only along the course of the guidewire is shown in a patient with prior pericarditis and unsuccessful epicardial attempted access (*bottom*).

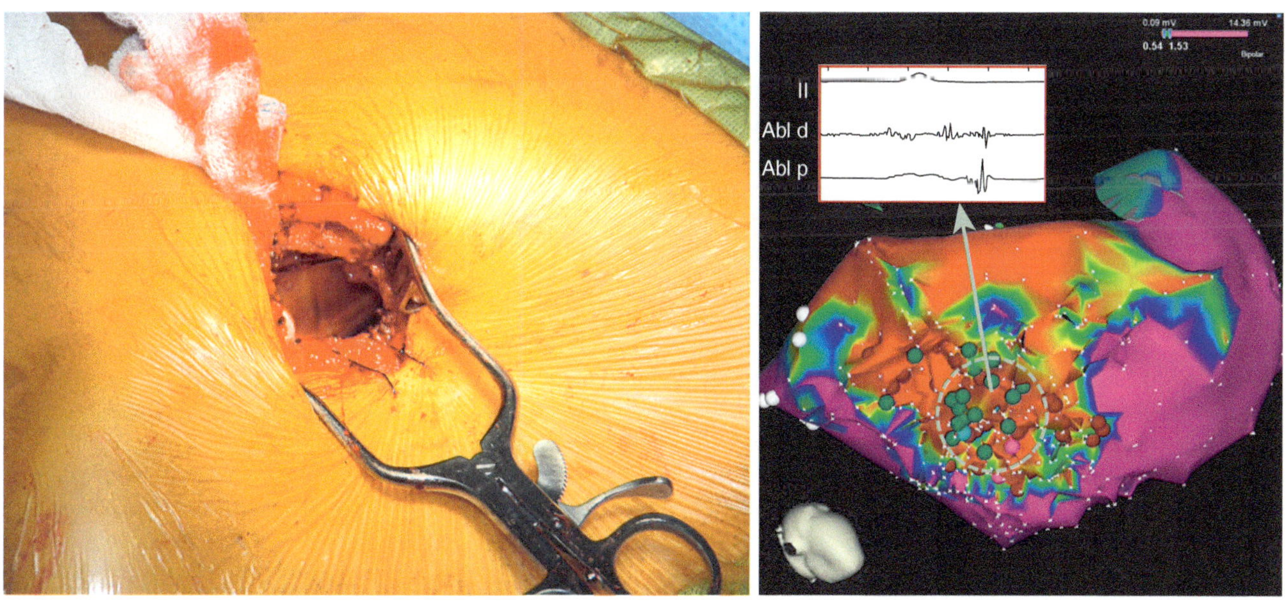

Fig. 37.15 Subxiphoid surgical window to access postinfarct inferior wall scar that contains multiple fractionated and late potentials (*green circles*). *Red circles* indicate ablation lesions.

MAPPING AND ABLATION TOOLS

After access into the pericardial space is obtained, catheter movement is typically unimpeded. The sheath can be advanced and torqued to assist in accessing regions outside of the catheter range. Epicardial mapping of VT follows the same principles of endocardial mapping, where identification of late potentials, pace mapping, and entrainment are used to localize critical isthmuses (Fig. 37.17).

Both commercially available electroanatomical mapping systems, originally validated with endocardial mapping, may be used for epicardial mapping and ablation.[43–45] There are important advantages and disadvantages for both electrofield (NavX, Abbott, St. Jude Medical, Minneapolis, MN) and magnetic-based

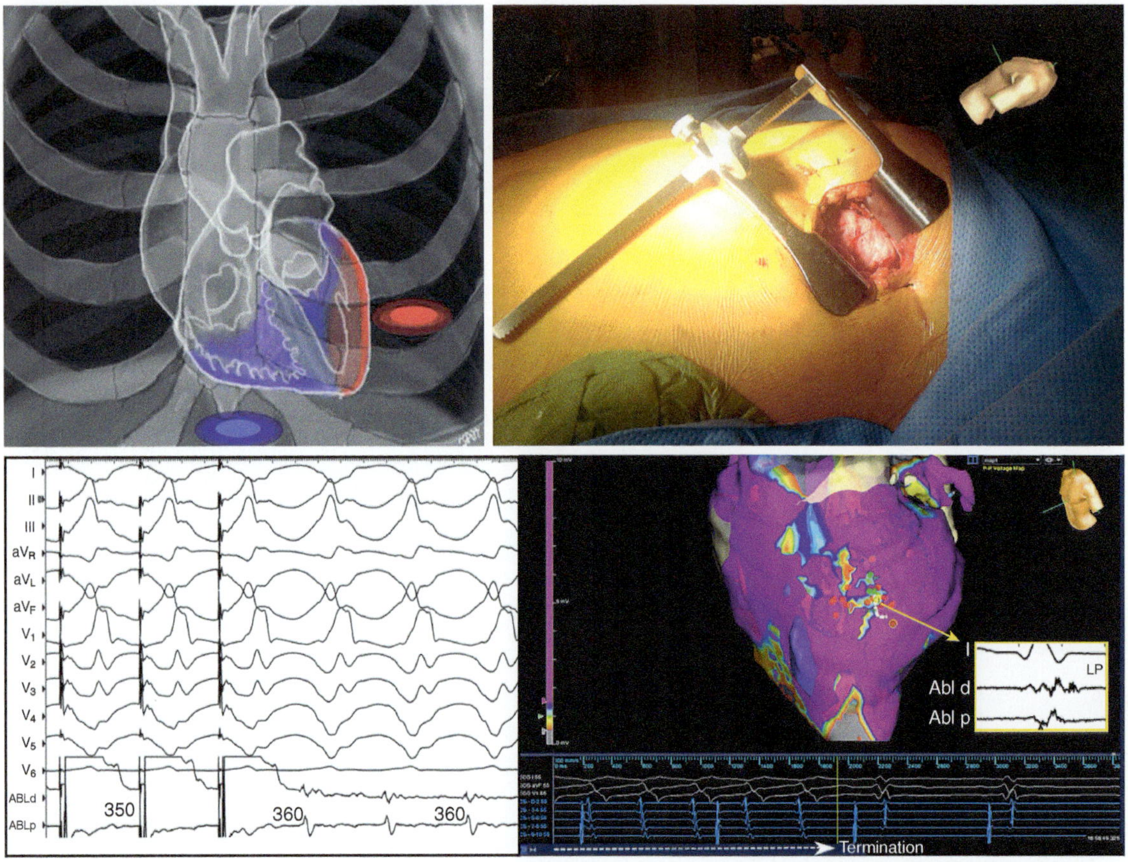

Fig. 37.16 Limited anterior thoracotomy allows access to the anterior, lateral, and apical regions of the left ventricle (*red regions* on cartoon). Entrainment and termination of ventricular tachycardia at a fractionated and late potential site within patchy epicardial postinfarct scar on the anterior wall is demonstrated.

(CARTO, Johnson & Johnson, Biosense-Webster, Diamond Bar, CA) systems. Because of the difference in impedance in the pericardial space from the blood pool, the epicardial geometry constructed with the electrofield system may appear less spherical. In addition, the relationship between simultaneously displayed endocardial maps within the epicardial shell may not be as consistent as the magnetic-based system. Registration with computed tomography (CT) or MRI can mitigate this limitation. However, compared with histopathologic scar, the correlation between both of these mapping systems is excellent[43] (Fig. 37.18). Use of a multipolar mapping catheter increases the sampling density and number of late potentials identified in a shorter period of time.

d'Avila et al. demonstrated that irrigated radiofrequency (RF) delivery resulted in larger epicardial lesions compared with nonirrigated technology (3.7 ± 1.3 mm vs. 6.7 ± 1.7 mm) because of the absence of convective cooling by blood flow.[46] In addition, ablation over regions with epicardial fat (>3 mm) with nonirrigated RF failed to create lesions, compared with 4.1 ± 2-mm lesions with irrigated RF delivery (Fig. 37.19).

However, the use of open irrigation necessitates constant drainage of the pericardial irrigant to prevent tamponade. Use of a closed-irrigation ablation systems (Chilli, Boston Scientific, Natick, MA) may offer advantages although clinical adoption is limited.[47] In a hybrid surgical open thoracotomy procedure, a closed system is particularly useful to minimize irrigant in the surgical field. Magnetic interference may also be encountered with surgical tools required for exposure (retractors) when using the magnetic-based mapping system.

Regardless of catheter choice, the practical power settings for epicardial ablation tend to be more permissive than those seen for endocardial ablation. However, the optimal power settings have not been conclusively defined. Titrated irrigated RF with a flow rate of 10–30 mL/min up to 50 W with a temperature limit of 45–50°C has been used for epicardial ablation.[19,21,22] A reduced flow rate may reduce intrapericardial fluid accumulation without compromising lesion efficacy.[48] The concern for char formation and steam pops is mitigated by less consequence in the pericardial space. In addition, the catheter orientation is always tangential to the epicardial surface, and contact force is less variable compared with a perpendicular endocardial catheter orientations, as long as there is no significant amount of accumulated irrigant in the pericardial space. Cryoablation has been evaluated in an animal model by d'Avila et al. and has been shown to create lesions comparable to cooled-tip RF (6.0 ± 1.2 mm in scar and 7.0 ± 0.7 mm in border zone tissue).[49]

CORONARY ARTERIES

Before delivering RF energy on the epicardial surface, the local anatomy within the targeted region must be assessed to minimize the risk of collateral damage. d'Avila et al. demonstrated acute and chronic coronary arterial damage with RF delivered

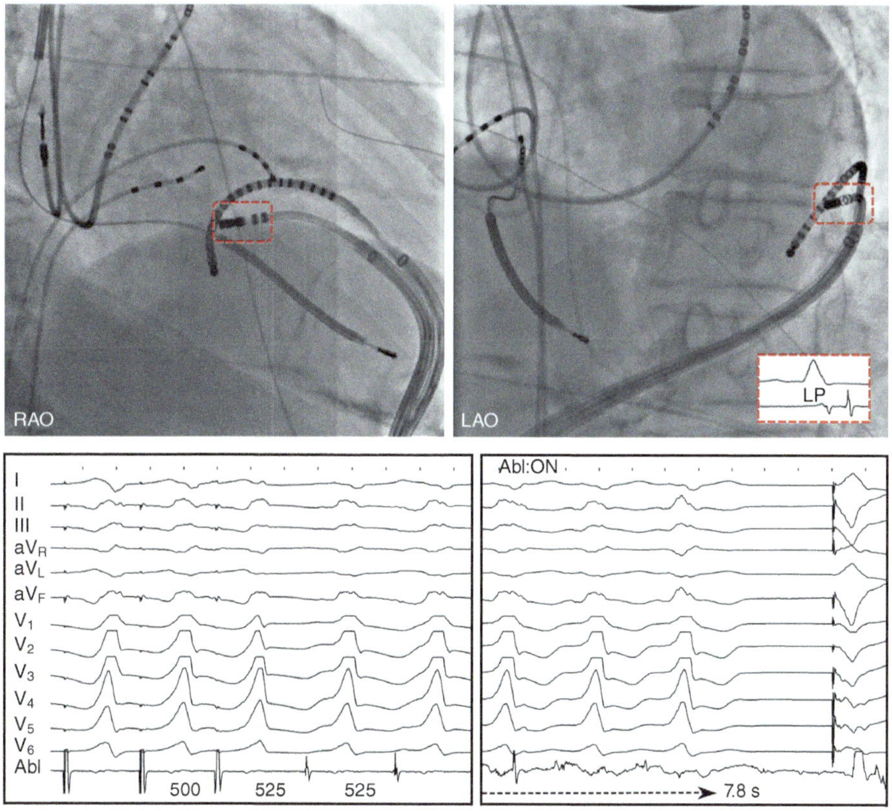

Fig. 37.17 Identification of a late potential in the midinferolateral wall in a patient with ischemic cardiomyopathy. The late potential becomes mid-diastolic during the clinical ventricular tachycardia and nearly perfect concealed entrainment is demonstrated before termination with radiofrequency on the epicardium. (Modified from Tung R, Michowitz Y, Yu R, Mathuria N, Vaseghi M, Buch E, et al. Epicardial ablation of ventricular tachycardia: an institutional experience of safety and efficacy. *Heart Rhythm.* 2013;10:490–498.)

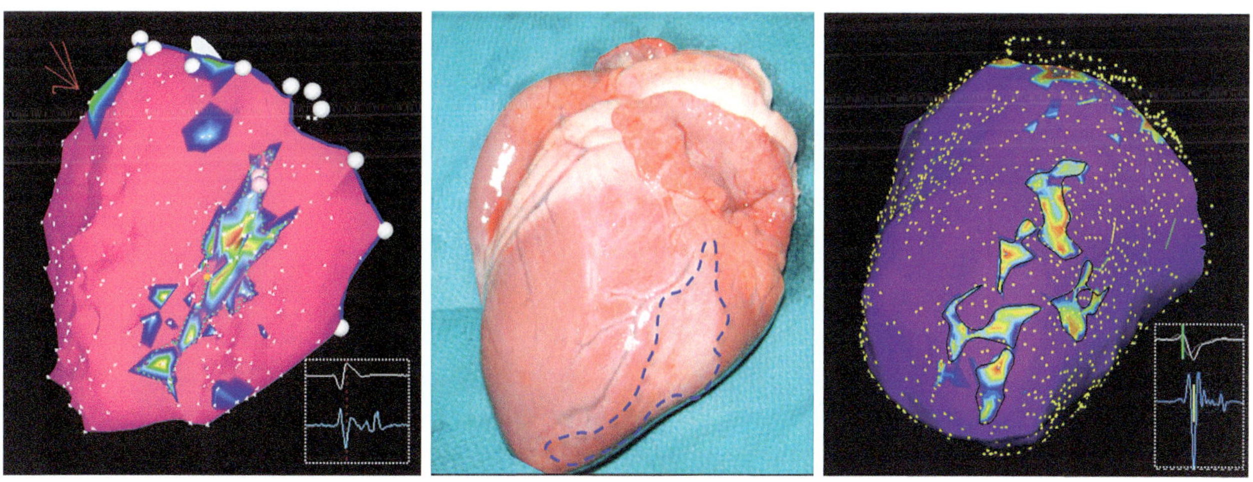

Fig. 37.18 Comparable delineation of patchy epicardial scar in porcine occlusion-reperfusion circumflex artery model using magnetic *(left)* and electrofield-based *(right)* mapping systems with late potential detection. (From Tung R, Nakahara S, Ramirez R, et al. Accuracy of combined endocardial and epicardial electroanatomical mapping of a reperfused porcine infarct model: a comparison of electrofield and magnetic systems with histopathologic correlation. *Heart Rhythm.* 2011;8:439–447.)

overlying and adjacent to the vasculature in an animal model.[50,51] Coronary vessel injury can range from spasm, to acute thrombosis, to extracellular matrix proliferation in the tunica media and late intimal hyperplasia (Fig. 37.20). Susceptibility to damage is inversely proportional to vessel size, and interposed fat and coronary veins had a protective effect on arterial injury. Of note, no coronary stenosis >70% was seen in these experiments up to 70 days after ablation.

The consensus statement recommends >5-mm distance from a coronary artery for safe ablation throughout all phases of the cardiac cycle, although many centers implement a larger safety margin of 1 cm.[6] Angiography is the most accurate method to

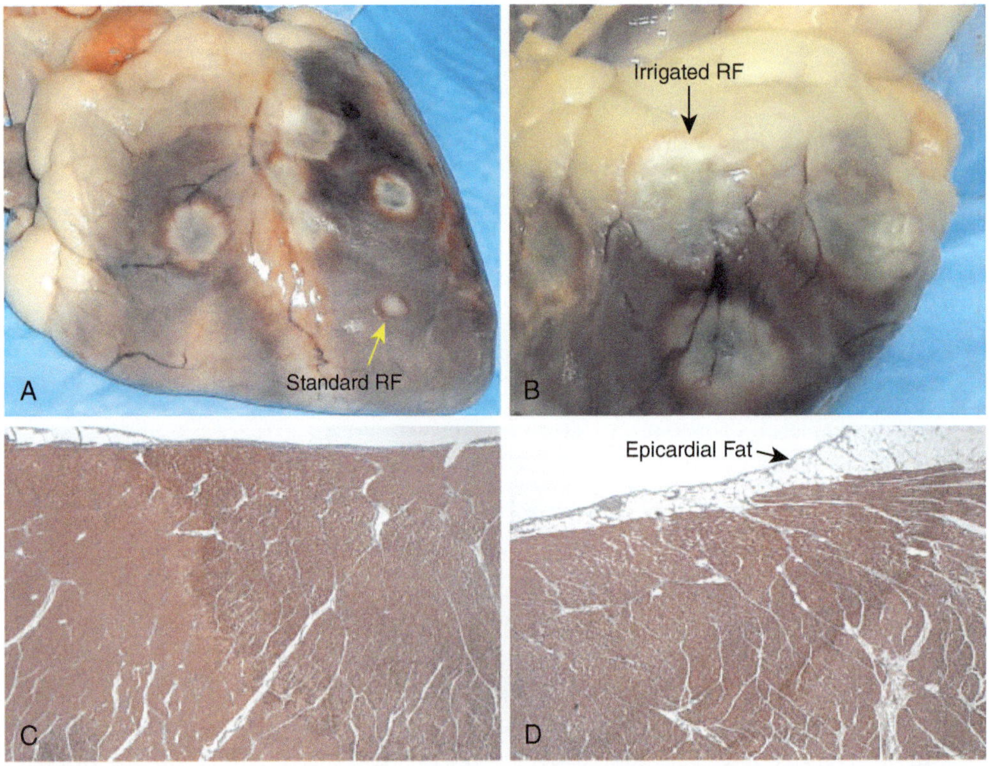

Fig. 37.19 Comparison of standard radiofrequency applications (A) with cooled-tip irrigated radiofrequency (B) in a porcine model. Irrigated technology creates greater lesions with greater diameter on the epicardium. In regions covered by epicardial fat, less attenuation of lesion depth is seen with irrigated ablation (D) compared with standard radiofrequency (C). (Modified from d'Avila A, Houghtaling C, Gutierrez P, Vragovic O, Ruskin JN, Josephson ME, Reddy VY. Catheter ablation of ventricular epicardial tissue: a comparison of standard and cooled-tip radiofrequency energy. *Circulation*. 2004;109:2363–2369.)

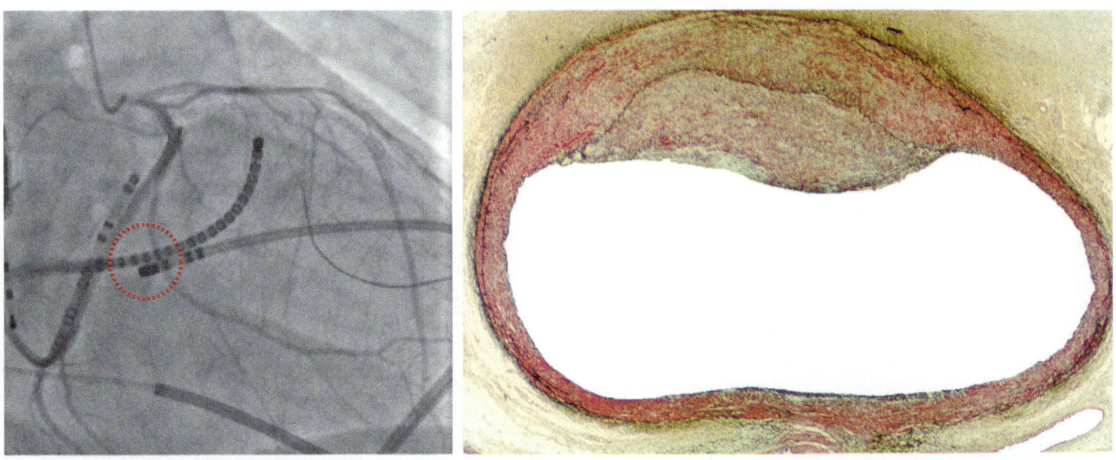

Fig. 37.20 Epicardial ablation is withheld as coronary angiography demonstrates the obtuse marginal branch in the targeted region for ablation (*left*). The chronic effects of radiofrequency ablation directly over coronary artery in a porcine model are shown where thickening and proliferation of the tunica media and intima are seen. (Modified from Tung R, Michowitz Y, Yu R, Mathuria N, Vaseghi M, Buch E, et al. Epicardial ablation of ventricular tachycardia: an institutional experience of safety and efficacy. *Heart Rhythm*. 2013;10:490-498; Viles-Gonzalez JF, de Castro Miranda R, Scanavacca M, Sosa E, d'Avila A. Acute and chronic effects of epicardial radiofrequency applications delivered on epicardial coronary arteries. *Circ Arrhythm Electrophysiol*. 2011;4:526–531.)

exclude an artery in close proximity to a target region, and at our institution, we perform an angiogram before any RF is delivered. If the myocardium supplied by the artery is sufficiently scarred, discretion is necessary to weigh the myocardium in jeopardy distal to the ablation against the clinical arrhythmic burden of the patient. However, acute coronary injury can result in ischemic ventricular fibrillation. Thyer et al. demonstrated that the injection of intracoronary cold saline during ablation resulted in lower intracoronary temperatures with lesions that spared the vessel wall in an animal model.[52]

Real-time integration of CT-derived coronary anatomy with electroanatomical mapping has been shown to be feasible after endocardial mapping.[53] However, the significance of registration errors of even 2.8 ± 1.3 mm cannot be dismissed if the target site is in close proximity to the coronary artery. Further, opacification of smaller branches of the main coronaries is not sufficient in many CT acquisitions. For these reasons, image registration does not obviate the need for coronary angiography but may be a useful adjunct once relative fluoroscopic positions are known.

PHRENIC NERVE

When ablation is performed on the lateral wall of the epicardial LV, the proximity to the left phrenic nerve should be assessed. Diaphragmatic paralysis is uncommon but can result in significant patient morbidity ranging from mild dyspnea, to orthopnea, to respiratory failure requiring mechanical ventilation. Bai et al. followed 17 patients with phrenic nerve palsy after ablation and reported resolution in all 15 patients by 8.3 ± 6.6 months.[54]

The left phrenic nerve descends behind the left brachiocephalic vein and courses over the aortic arch and pulmonary trunk. It then passes along the fibrous pericardium over the left atrial appendage (LAA) and then the lateral LV. Three anatomical courses have been described by Sanchez-Quintana et al. on gross cadaveric dissection: (1) anterior (18%, over left anterior descending); (2) lateral (59%, tip of LAA over obtuse marginal); and (3) posterior (23%, base of LAA to inferolateral wall)[55] (Fig. 37.21). The right phrenic nerve lies lateral to the right brachiocephalic vein, and the superior vena cava is not relevant to epicardial ventricular ablation.

Fan et al. demonstrated the utility of high-output pacing (>10 mA) to characterize the course of the phrenic nerve on electroanatomical mapping.[56] Attention to phrenic capture is particularly relevant in patients with NICM, who have a predilection toward basal lateral epicardial scar. Importantly, skeletal muscle relaxants and paralytics should not be administered after induction of general anesthesia as diaphragmatic capture during pacing may be impossible, giving a false indicator of being at a safe distance from the nerve.

If a targeted region is in close proximity to the phrenic nerve, separation of the epicardium from the parietal pericardium can be achieved by several methods. Buch et al. first described balloon (Meditech, Boston Scientific, Natick, MA) displacement of the phrenic nerve in humans as well as in an animal model.[57,58] Di Biase et al. compared balloon, air, saline, and a combination of air and saline in a series of eight patients and demonstrated that the combination of air and saline was most effective.[59]

EPICARDIAL FAT

Epicardial fat presents two unique challenges for mapping and ablation of VT. Because fat insulates myocardium during contact mapping, low-voltage regions are frequently detected and can be difficult to distinguish from scar. In addition when ablation is required in these regions, interposed fat impairs the efficacy of RF delivery. Reddy et al. demonstrated an anatomical propensity for epicardial fat distribution in the RV free wall and lateral wall in a CT-based study of normal subjects.[60]

For these reasons, preprocedural imaging may be useful to identify these regions for registration on electroanatomical mapping to understand the local epicardial anatomy of a targeted region[61] (Fig. 37.22). van Huls van Taxis demonstrated increased epicardial fat thickness (>7 mm) was an important cause of epicardial ablation failure where ineffective sites were significantly thicker than successful sites (16.9 ± 6.8 mm vs. 1.5 ± 2.1 mm, $P = .002$).[53]

A few studies have assessed the critical thickness of epicardial fat required to diminish underlying myocardial voltages.[45,53] A thickness of >5 mm was shown to influence bipolar electrogram voltage.[62] In a porcine study, we demonstrated that 4 mm of fat interposed between normal myocardium was sufficient to result in the registration of low voltage in the region of the left anterior descending artery.[63]

Electrogram characteristics may improve the distinction between scar versus epicardial fat in regions of low voltage registered by a mapping catheter. Reddy et al. showed the utility of electrogram duration (>50 ms), where regions exhibiting preserved electrogram width under fat demonstrated normal duration compared with localized regions of slow conduction with wider electrograms.[45] The quantification of deflections on the electrograms as a fractionation index can increase the specificity of scar detection, in addition to the presence of late potentials, which is highly specific for scar[63] (Fig. 37.23).

Ablation over epicardial fat results in decreased lesion depth because of inadequate RF penetration of conductive heating. In comparison with normal tissue, the lesion depth achieved with a 4-mm irrigated catheter over interposed fat was reduced (6.7 ± 1.7 vs. 4.1 ± 2 mm). In situations in which extensive thickness of fat is suspected over a critical site, an open surgical approach for dissection may be necessary. For epicardial LV summit arrhythmias, a percutaneous approach is of low yield because of proximity to the left coronary arterial system and significant thickness of interposed fat. One alternative for an open surgical technique in these situations is a totally endoscopic robotic approach.

INTRAPERICARDIAL STEROID AND REPEAT ACCESS

The prevention of pericarditis after instrumentation (up to 30%) serves two purposes: (1) to minimize symptomatic postprocedural irritation and (2) to optimize the ability to reaccess the space by decreasing adhesion formation. d'Avida et al. first demonstrated in a porcine model that the instillation of triamcinolone (2 mg/kg) was effective at preventing pericarditis. The relevance of this study to humans is not known.

With regard to reaccessing the pericardial space after prior instrumentation, success rates have been favorable. Roberts-Thomson reported successful repeat access in 87% (13/15) of patients, where only four received intrapericardial steroids at the initial procedure.[64] We similarly experienced successful access in 88% of patients during a repeat procedure, where 4 of 11 received prior intrapericardial steroids (250 mg methylprednisolone).[19] Schmidt et al. reported that repeat epicardial access was not possible in 25% (3 of 12) because of adhesions in a cohort of 56 patients with previous failed endocardial ablation

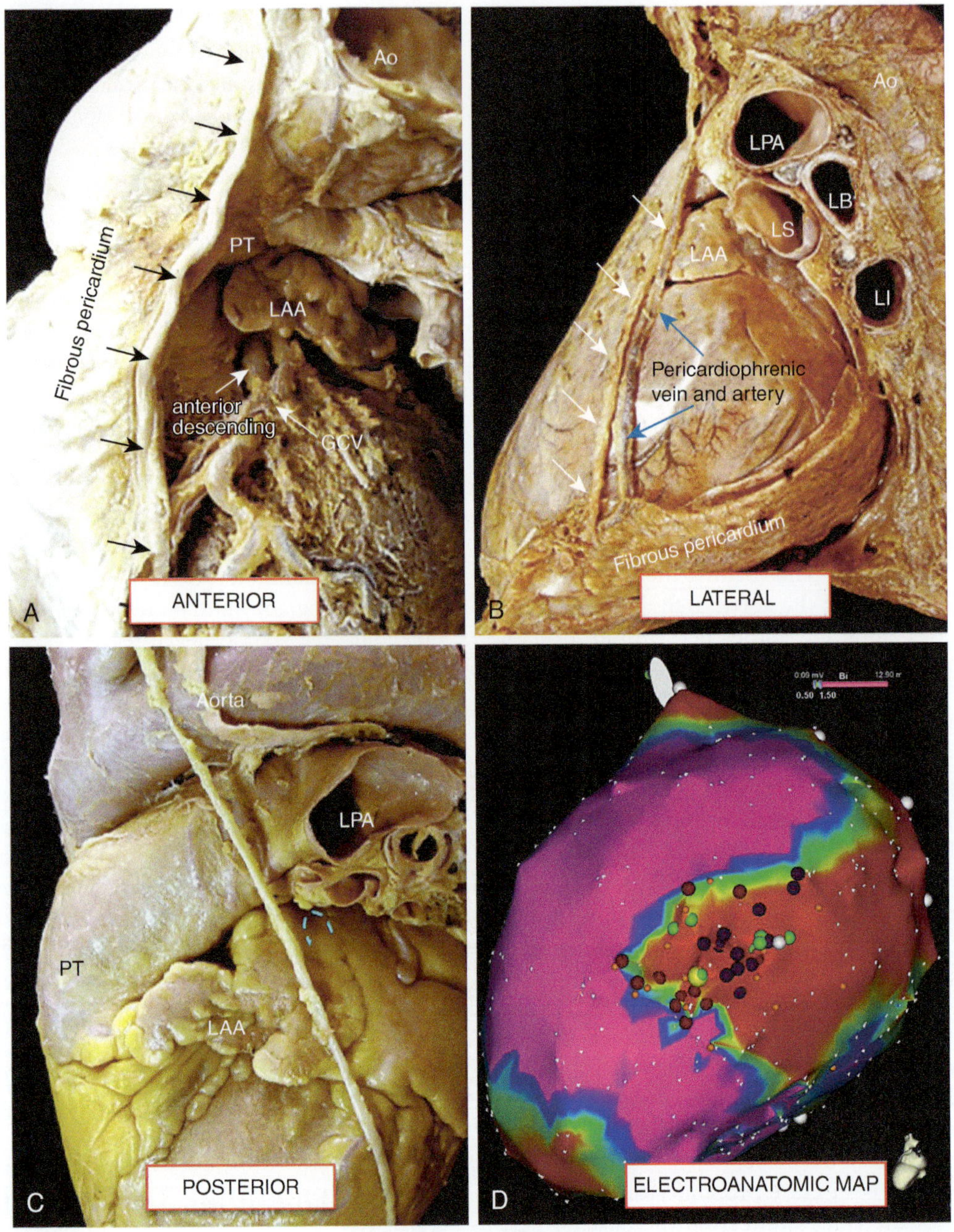

Fig. 37.21 Anatomical gross pathology dissections demonstrating three courses of the left phrenic nerve over the left ventricle: anterior, lateral, and posterior. High-output pacing before ablation along the basal lateral wall can identify regions of phrenic capture, which can be tagged on electroanatomical mapping (*dark circles.*) *Red circles* indicate ablation lesions, *green* indicates late potentials, and termination of ventricular tachycardia was achieved at the *yellow circle*, which was inferior to the course of the phrenic. *Ao*, Aorta; *LAA*, left atrial appendage; *LB*, left bronchus; *LI*, left inferior; *LPA*, left pulmonary artery; *LS*, left superior; *PT*, pulmonary trunk. (Modified from Viles-Gonzalez JF, de Castro Miranda R, Scanavacca M, Sosa E, d'Avila A. Acute and chronic effects of epicardial radiofrequency applications delivered on epicardial coronary arteries. *Circ Arrhythm Electrophysiol.* 2011;4:526–531.)

treated with systemic nonsteroidal anti-inflammatory drugs (NSAIDs).[65] In a series of 30 patients, Tschabrunn demonstrated successful repeat access in all patients, where only six received steroid administration on the initial procedure.[66] Adhesions were encountered in 23%, although blunt dissection with the sheath allowed for complete mapping in all but two patients. Although it appears from these cohorts that intrapericardial steroids are not necessary to re-access the pericardial space, there appears to be little risk.

REPORTED COMPLICATIONS

The most common complications are related to the puncture, where the course of the needle has the potential to pass through the liver, colon, diaphragm, pleural space, and RV. Pericardial bleeding is the most frequent complication that results from inadvertent puncture of the RV, which can be observed in up to 20% of cases.[21] A "dry" puncture can occur without significant bleeding, in the absence of sheath insertion. Sosa et al. reported a cumulative experience of 7%

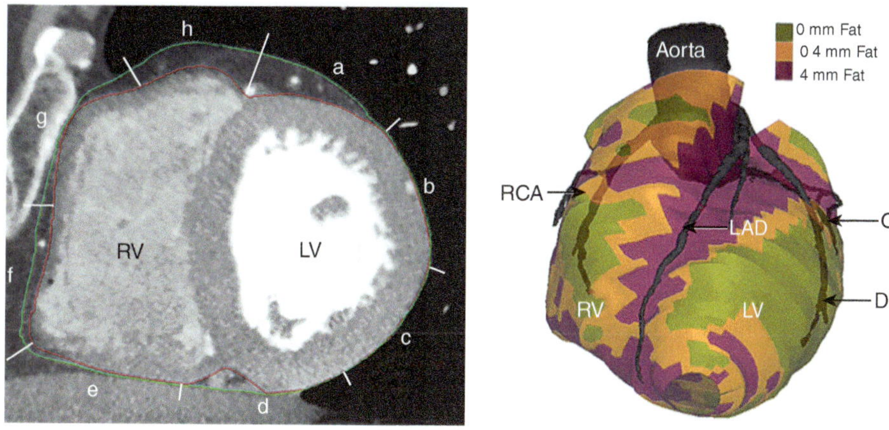

Fig. 37.22 Integration of multidetector computed tomography (MDCT) for registration of coronary anatomy and fat thickness with electroanatomical mapping. (A) MDCT short-axis slice with pericardial (*green*) and epicardial (*red*) contours divided into eight segments. MDCT-derived aorta with coronary arteries merged with the color-coded epicardial fat meshes into the final fusion image. (Modified from van Huls van Taxis CF, Wijnmaalen AP, Piers SR, van der Geest RJ, Schalij MJ, Zeppenfeld K. Real-time integration of MDCT-derived coronary anatomy and epicardial fat: impact on epicardial electroanatomic mapping and ablation for ventricular arrhythmias. *JACC Cardiovasc Imaging*. 2013;6:42–52.)

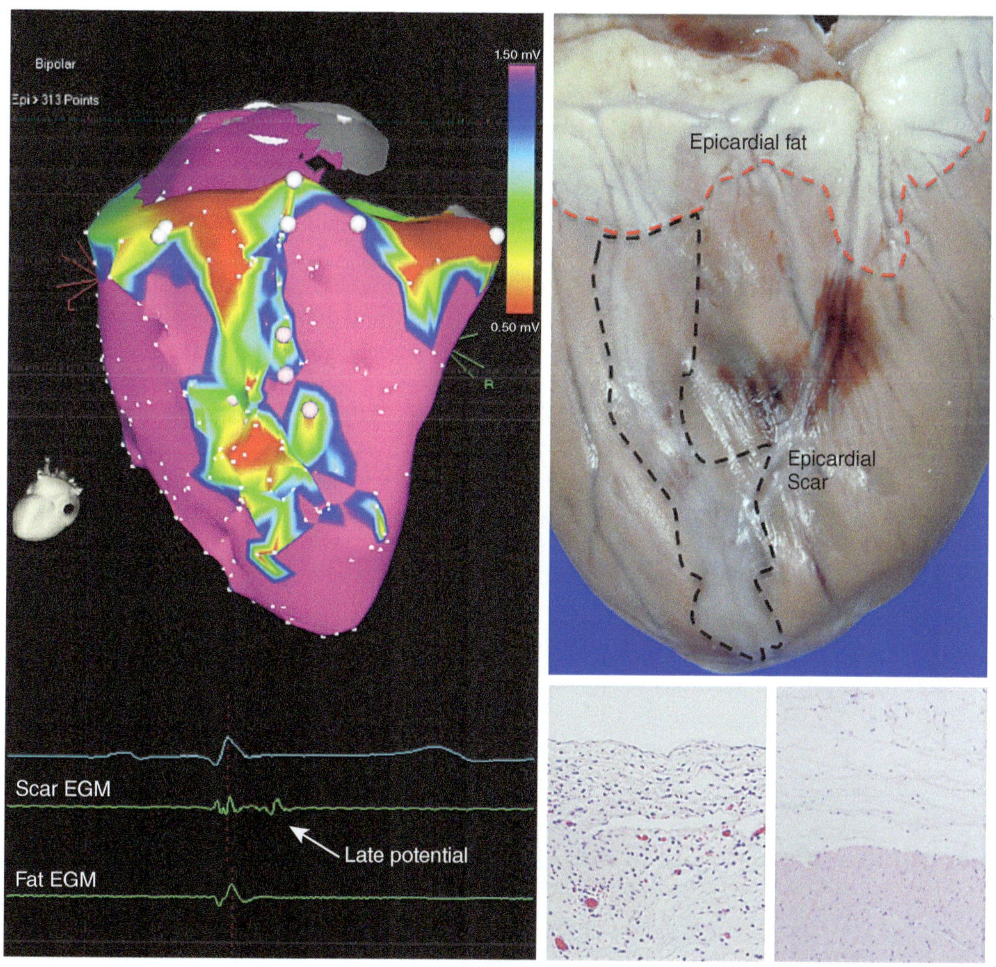

Fig. 37.23 Comparison of electrograms in regions of epicardial fat and scar in a porcine model. Fractionated electrogram and late potentials are specific for scar. (From Tung R, Nakahara S, Ramirez R, Lai C, Fishbein MC, Shivkumar K. Distinguishing epicardial fat from scar: analysis of electrograms using high-density electroanatomic mapping in a novel porcine infarct model. *Heart Rhythm*. 2010;7:389–395.)

hemopericardium (200 ± 100 mL) requiring drainage in 215 consecutive cases.[67] In two large multicenter experiences, Sacher et al. described a 5% (seven hemopericardium [>80 mL] and one coronary stenosis) incidence of acute major complications among 156 procedures, and Della Bella et al. observed major complications in 4.1% (eight tamponade and one abdominal bleed) among 222 cases.[21,22] Among 109 epicardial procedures for VT at our institution over a 7-year period, we observed a 6.7% incidence of hemopericardium (>80 mL), but no occurrence of tamponade, surgical intervention, or procedural mortality was seen.[19]

Although the vast majority of cases of pericardial bleeding can be managed effectively with a drain, the most adverse sequelae are those that require emergent surgical intervention. We have found that in cases of significant bleeding, a double drainage technique with active suction results in the most effective evacuation of the pericardial space and may stave off impending surgery.[68] Puncture or laceration of a diaphragmatic epigastric artery or liver can result in significant intraabdominal hemorrhage. Significant hypotension in the absence of a pericardial effusion should signal this potential complication. If significant hemopericardium develops after access is obtained, laceration of an epicardial vessel should be suspected. As stated previously, sheaths placed in the pericardial should be protected with a protruding catheter to minimize the potential for trauma if the relatively rigid open tip of the sheath is left exposed (Fig. 37.24). It is not uncommon to encounter bloody aspirate throughout the course of mapping and ablation that can be related to prolonged heparinization, small adhesions, mild hemorrhage from ablation lesions, or epicardial blebs. If hemopericardium develops after the sheath is removed, a double puncture or "stitching" of the RV may have occurred (i.e., inadvertent puncture of the RV after entering the pericardial space, and exit from the RV through a second puncture with the sheath reentering the pericardial space).[69]

In a case series from five centers, Koruth et al. reported unusual complications including RV pseudoaneurysm, ventricular-abdominal fistula, liver puncture with intraabdominal bleed, hepatic subcapsular hematoma, and two cases of tamponade caused by coronary sinus branch laceration[70] (Fig. 37.25). Over an 8-year period, Killu et al. reported eight atypical complications in a single-center experience during 116 attempts.[71] These complications ranged from a broken wire (0.025-in) in the pericardial space requiring snaring, two left lobe hepatic punctures, an abdominopericardial fistula, hemothorax, and phrenic nerve palsy. Recurrent chronic pericarditis and a delayed effusion 2 weeks after the procedure was also reported.

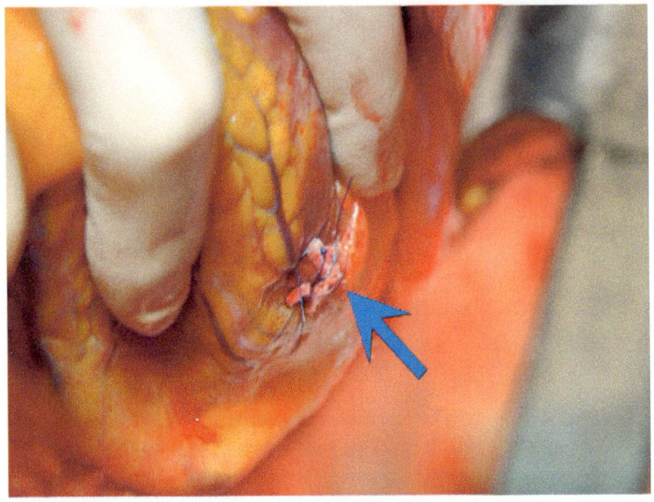

Fig. 37.24 Intraoperative picture of repaired laceration of coronary sinus branch secondary to sheath trauma that required emergent surgery for hemostasis. (From Koruth JS, Aryana A, Dukkipati SR, et al. Unusual complications of percutaneous epicardial access and epicardial mapping and ablation of cardiac arrhythmias. *Circ Arrhythm Electrophysiol.* 2011;4:882–888.)

Symptomatic pericarditis is a common postprocedural complication that occurs in up to 30% of patients after epicardial mapping and ablation. As stated previously, the effect of intrapericardial steroids on clinical pericarditis is not known. Maintaining a pericardial drain postprocedurally causes mechanical irritation that can exacerbate symptoms, and we do not routinely leave a catheter in the pericardial space if the intraprocedural bleeding is <100 mL and the fluid clears consistently with irrigation. Medical management with NSAIDs is typically sufficient although colchicine and oral steroids can be used in refractory cases.

EFFICACY

The efficacy of epicardial access and ablation has been reported in several single and multicenter cohorts and is specifically addressed in other sections in this book. These experiences are summarized in Table 37.1. Traditionally, the utility of epicardial

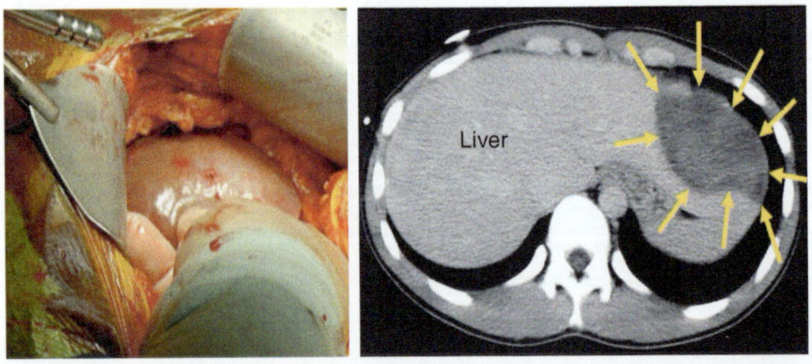

Fig. 37.25 Hepatic lobe punctures during epicardial access resulting in subcapsular hematoma. (Modified from Koruth JS, Aryana A, Dukkipati SR, Pak HN, Kim YH, Sosa EA, et al. Unusual complications of percutaneous epicardial access and epicardial mapping and ablation of cardiac arrhythmias. *Circ Arrhythm Electrophysiol.* 2011;4:882–888.)

TABLE 37.1 **Epicardial Ventricular Tachycardia Ablation Studies**

Author and Reference No.	Year	N	Substrate (n)	Epicardial Ablation (n)	Ablation Parameters	Ablation Approach	Acute Success	Follow-Up (mo)	Intermediate Success
Sosa[73]	1998	10	Chagas CM (6)	6	4-mm tip to 60°C	Pace mapping Mid-diastolic or cont. EGMs	100%	4-9	100%
Sosa[74]	2000	14	ICM (14)	7	NR	Thermal mapping Mid-diastolic or cont. EGMs	56%	14 ± 2	37%
Schweikert[75]	2003	30	Normal heart (20) ICM (7) NICM (3)	8	Closed/open tip irrigation to 50°C Mean 3 ± 1 RF applications	Activation mapping	93%	26 ± 13	58%
Sarabanda[76]	2005	56	Chagas CM (56)	56	8-mm tip to 70°C	Entrainment of pace mapping Presystolic EGMs targeted	30%	NR	NR
Cesario[8]	2006	20	ICM (12) NICM (8)	6 2	8-mm tip; 40–70 W to 55°C	Pace mapping Mid-diastolic and fract. EGMs	100%	12 ± 4	75%
Daniels[77]	2006	12	Normal	12	4-mm solid tip or irrigated; cryo	Activation/pace mapping	75%	NR	NR
Aryana[78] (magnetic navigation)	2007	24	ICM (13) NICM HCM ARVC Sarcoidosis	3	4-mm solid tip (2) or irrigated (22)	Activation/entrainment/pace mapping; late/fract. EGMs	97%	7 ± 3	83%
Garcia[9]	2009	13	ARVC (13)	13	4 mm solid tip 50 W to 55°C; closed/open irrigation 50 W to 42°C	Activation or pace mapping; focal or linear RF to LPs	92%	18 ± 13	77%
Schmidt[51]	2010	56	Normal (16) ICM (11) NICM (16) ARVC (13) Myocarditis (3)	12 10 12 10 1	irrigation RF 50 W to 43°C; median 1–12 RF applications	Activation/entrainment mapping; abnormal EGMs	69% 100% 76% 77% 66%	12 ± 5	47%
Sacher[21] (multicenter)	2010	134	ICM (51) NICM (39) ARVC (14) Other CM (13) Normal (17)	51 39 14 13 17	4- and 8-mm solid tip; closed/open irrigation from 20 to 50 W; cryo	Multiple	NR	23 ± 21	71%

Continued

TABLE 37.1 Epicardial Ventricular Tachycardia Ablation Studies—cont'd

Author and Reference No.	Year	N	Substrate (n)	Epicardial Ablation (n)	Ablation Parameters	Ablation Approach	Acute Success	Follow-Up (mo)	Intermediate Success
Nakahara[79]	2010	33	ICM (17) NICM (16)	7 10	8-mm solid tip; closed/open irrigation to 50 W	LPs and fract. EGMs	82% (ICM) 50% (NICM)	12 ± 10	82%
Nademanee[80]	2011	9	Brugada (9)	9	Open irrigation 30–50 W to 45°C, median 35 RF applications	LPs and fract. EGMs	78%	20 ± 6	78%
Bai[10] (multicenter)	2011	49	ARVC (49)	26	3.5-mm tip open irrigation	Activation or entrainment mapping; LPs and fract. EGMs	85% (endo-only ablation 52%)	39 ± 4	85%
Della Bella[22] (multicenter)	2011	218	ICM (85) NICM (67) ARVC (13) HCM (5) Normal (48)	218	Open-irrigation tip (80% of cases); 20–40 W to 45°C or Δ impedance 20 Ω Solid-tip RF (12% of cases) Cryoablation (8% of cases)	Pace/entrainment mapping	72%	17 ± 18	68%
Dello Russo[81]	2012	20	Myocarditis	6	Irrigation tip, 40 W to 43°C	Activation/entrainment/pace/ scar mapping	100%	Median 28	90%
Tung[19]	2013	95	ICD (33) NICM (45) Idiopathic (17)	71	Open/closed irrigation 4-mm catheter, 30-50 W, 45-50°C	Activation/entrainment/pace mapping; LPs, fract. EGMs	48% (NICM) 45% (ICM)	12	36% (NICM) 85% (ICM)
Sarkozy[82]	2013	56	ICM	38	Open irrigation 4-mm catheter, 50 W to 45°C	Activation/entrainment/pace mapping; LPs, fract. EGMs	59%	26	46%

ARVC, Arrhythmogenic right ventricular cardiomyopathy; *CM*, cardiomyopathy; *cont.*, continuous; *cryo*, cryoablation; *EGM*, electrogram; *endo*, endocardial; *fract.*, fractionated EGM; *HCM*, hypertrophic cardiomyopathy; *ICM*, ischemic cardiomyopathy; *LP*, late potentials; *mo*, months; *NICM*, nonischemic cardiomyopathy; *NR*, not reported; *RF*, radiofrequency.
(Modified from Boyle N, Shivkumar K. Epicardial interventions in electrophysiology. *Circulation*. 2012;126(14):1752–1769.)

mapping and ablation has been demonstrated in patient populations referred for ablation after a prior failed endocardial ablation. Therefore, significant selection bias toward enriched epicardial substrates may be present when interpreting reported cohorts. The role of epicardial ablation as a preemptive strategy, with combined epicardial-endocardial ablation, has been evaluated in ICM, ARVC, and HCM, and it appears that this more comprehensive strategy results in greater freedom from recurrent VT.[8,10,12,72]

CONCLUSION

Since the first description of percutaneous access to the pericardial space over 20 years ago, the field of VT ablation has progressed significantly into the epicardial "second dimension." Mapping and ablation within the previously inaccessible pericardial space without sternotomy have contributed to an improved mechanistic understanding of scar substrates and benefited patients with VT refractory to endocardial strategies. New tools for safely accessing the pericardial space are being developed that will broaden its use for mapping and ablation. With an appreciation for the relevant anatomy and understanding of potential complications, from common to uncommon, a reduction in adverse events is anticipated. As broader adoption of this technique has been implemented globally, future prospective studies will be needed to evaluate the role of epicardial ablation as a first-line therapeutic strategy in patients with recurrent VT.

REFERENCES

Please refer to the e-book for a complete list of references.

38

Ablation of Ventricular Tachycardia in Congenital Heart Disease

Melissa R. Robinson

KEY POINTS

- Sinus rhythm mapping is used to identify arrhythmogenic isthmuses characterized by slow conduction.
- Activation mapping is used to confirm participating isthmuses.
- Anatomic isthmuses are capable of sustaining reentry.
- Intracardiac ultrasound is used to monitor catheter stability and contact with myocardium.
- Multipolar catheters assist in high-density mapping.
- Irrigated ablation is used to achieve transmurality.
- Thick anatomic isthmuses preclude transmural block, and catheter instability is a concern.

INTRODUCTION

Ventricular tachycardia (VT) remains an important late cause of morbidity and mortality in patients with both repaired and unrepaired congenital heart disease (CHD).[1,2] As surgical repair and longitudinal care have improved for patients with CHD, increasing numbers of patients are living into adulthood. Arrhythmias may occur in conjunction with hemodynamic decline related to progressive valvular disease or ventricular dysfunction; however, they may also present as an isolated issue. The ability to successfully ablate VT has the potential to profoundly influence both quality of life and mortality in these patients.

ANATOMY

The overwhelming majority of patients with CHD and VT have underlying repaired tetralogy of Fallot (ToF). This is also the largest population of CHD patients for whom implantable cardioverters-defibrillators (ICDs) are implanted for VT, the majority for nonfatal monomorphic VT.[3] Given the relatively fast cycle lengths (median VT cycle length, 290 ms), nearly half of patients require cardioversion shocks to terminate VT, with concomitant effects on quality of life. Additionally, complications from ICDs in this population remain high.[4]

Much more rarely, VT may occur in patients with repaired ventricular septal defects (VSDs), transposition of the great arteries, Ebstein anomaly, and lesions involving the right ventricular (RV) outflow tract (RVOT). In general, however, there is typically a common factor of a ventriculotomy. Many of these patients have chronic pressure or volume overload as well, which increases myocardial fibrosis and leads to the potential for reentrant ventricular arrhythmias.

Considerable progress has been made in understanding the critical anatomical isthmuses (AIs) involved in VT in repaired ToF. Initial investigations centered on clinical, mechanoelectrical, and noninvasive factors that may predict ventricular arrhythmias in these patients.[4–6] Many factors such as QRS width, RV function, symptomatic nonsustained (NSVT), surgical technique, and older age at the time of repair will increase the likelihood of ventricular substrate capable of sustaining reentry. Despite statistical significance, these factors do not discriminate sufficiently in the individual patient.

Given the ease of measurement, the sinus rhythm QRS has been a focus of intensive study into VT risk in ToF. Although a wider QRS has been shown in many arrhythmia substrates to portend a risk of ventricular arrhythmia, the relationship may be more complex in repaired ToF. In an elegant study detailing RV activation time in relationship to QRS morphology (left [LBBB] versus right bundle branch block [RBBB]), QRS duration, as well as VT inducibility, the Leiden group described the contribution of slow conduction within the RV AIs to VT induction.[7] They found that a narrow QRS does not exclude the possibility of VT inducibility, especially in the absence of a baseline RBBB. In patients with an RBBB, a prolonged QRS may be due to an enlarged RV, block across an AI, or slow conduction, with only the latter being predictive of VT inducibility. QRS fragmentation has also recently been shown in small studies to correlate with arrhythmia risk and has been correlated with mortality.[8] However, none of these factors provide sufficient sensitivity or specificity in evaluating patients at risk for VT with repaired ToF.

The breadth of anatomical considerations in CHD and subsequent surgical repair is certainly beyond the scope of this chapter. It is also worth emphasizing that in an individual patient, the relative contributions of the initial anatomy and the surgical approach may differ. The historical era of the initial repair as well as the occasional misclassification of the initial lesion may occur, confounding the invasive electrophysiologist (e.g., double-outlet RV versus ToF). It is for this reason, among others,

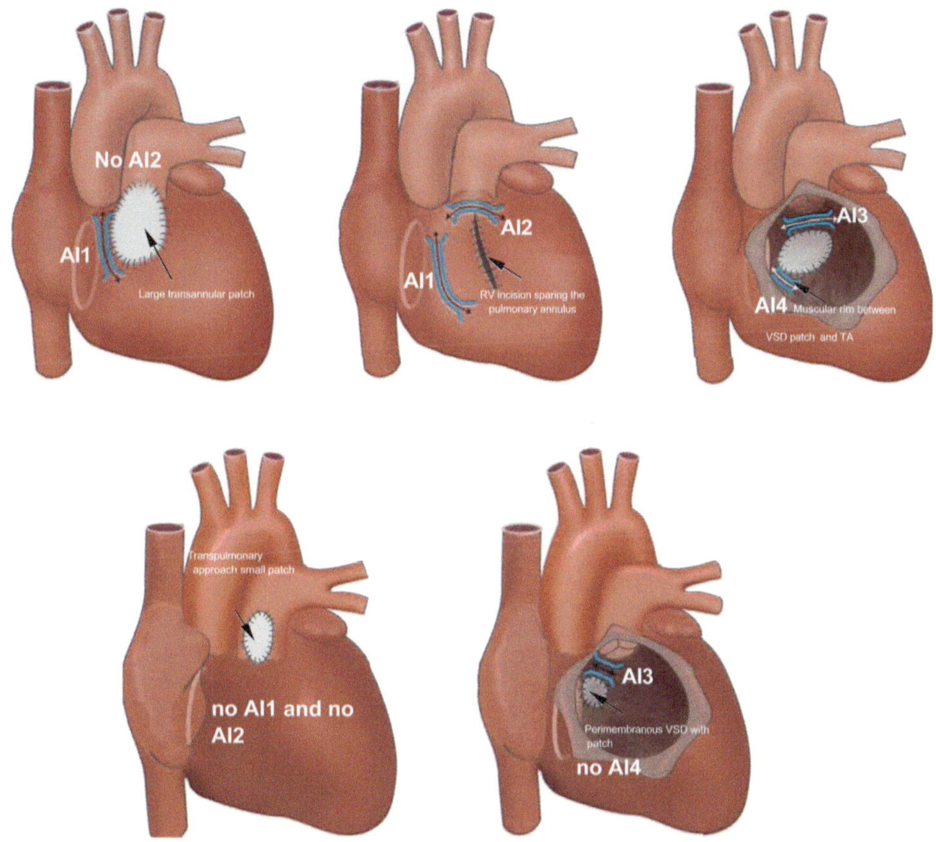

Fig. 38.1 Schematic overview of the four potential anatomical isthmuses (AIs) for ventricular tachycardia (VT) in repaired tetralogy of Fallot. AIs in repaired tetralogy of Fallot according to the surgical approach and variation of the malformation. *RV*, Right ventricle; *TA*, tricuspid annulus; *VSD*, ventricular septal defect. (From Cronin EM, Bogun FM, Maury P, et al. 2019 HRS/EHRA/APHRS/LAHRS expert consensus statement on catheter ablation of ventricular arrhythmias. *Heart Rhythm*. 2020;17:e2–e154, Fig. 38.12).

that collaboration between adult CHD specialists is highly recommended for these patients.[9] Nonetheless, a detailed discussion of the specific anatomy in ToF can be illustrative here.

Since the 1970s, primary repair in infancy has been the general approach to these patients. Unoperated patients with ToF have RVOT obstruction, sometimes quite severe, along with a VSD. The aorta overlies the VSD, and this relationship becomes important in the discussion of mapping and ablation later in this chapter. Surgical repair involves relief of the RV obstruction and patch closure of the VSD. As these are generally performed in the very young, the VSD patch material itself is quite small, but surrounding fibrosis may contribute to arrhythmogenesis in this area. There has been considerable evolution in the approach to reconstruction of the RVOT, with large transannular patches associated with long ventriculotomies giving way to transpulmonary approaches with little ventricular myocardial disruption. Some patients continue to require more involved repairs, including RV-to–pulmonary annulus (PA) conduits in the case of pulmonary atresia.

PATHOPHYSIOLOGY

Initial studies evaluating VT in ToF required invasive mapping in the operating room and narrowed the focus to the RVOT.[10] These studies were pivotal in conclusively determining the mechanism of VT as reentry and paved the way for successful surgical and, later catheter ablation.[11] In the three-dimensional (3D) electroanatomical mapping era, several early case reports hinted at important corridors facilitating reentry, but it was not until the seminal work by Zeppenfeld and colleagues that the AIs were codified in a series of 11 patients, of whom 9 had repaired ToF.[12] This was also the first study to suggest that ablation may be performed in sinus rhythm in these patients, with the putative anatomic isthmuses transected either via catheter or surgical ablation.

The critical isthmuses for reentrant monomorphic VT in ToF have now been well characterized both electrically and anatomically (Fig. 38.1). Reentry may rarely involve myocardial scar remote from these sites, such as from postcardiotomy pericarditis or coronary injury. However, it is the surgically created isthmuses from the ventriculotomy to the tricuspid valve (Isthmus 1) and from the ventriculotomy to the PA (Isthmus 2, when present), combined with the congenitally created corridors between the VSD to PA (Isthmus 3) and VSD to tricuspid valve (Isthmus 4, when present), that define the potential VT circuits in repaired ToF.

Two studies used separate anatomical specimen libraries of pediatric and adult patients with ToF to provide both gross and histologic data useful for any electrophysiologist embarking on VT ablation in this patient population[13,14] (Fig. 38.2). Notable findings were that Isthmus 1A and Isthmus 1B (extending from

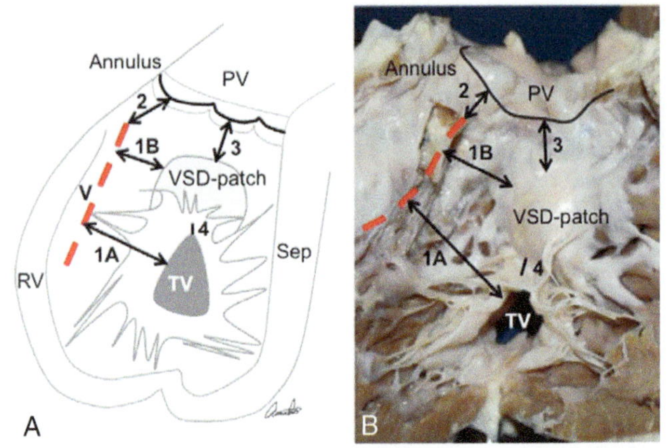

Fig. 38.2 (A), Diagram of the ventricular isthmuses in modified left anterior oblique view and (B) representative gross specimen displayed in an identical view. (1A) Ventriculotomy (V; *dotted line*)-to-tricuspid annulus. (1B) Ventriculotomy-to-ventricular septal defect (VSD) patch. (2) Ventriculotomy-to-pulmonary annulus (*solid black line*). (3) Pulmonary annulus-to-VSD patch. (4) VSD patch-to-tricuspid annulus. *PV*, Pulmonary valve; *RV*, right ventricle; *Sep*, septum; *TV*, tricuspid valve. (From Moore JP, Seki A, Shannon KM, et al: Characterization of anatomic ventricular tachycardia isthmus pathology after surgical repair of tetralogy of Fallot. *Circ Arrhythm Electrophysiol*. 2013;6(5):905–911.)

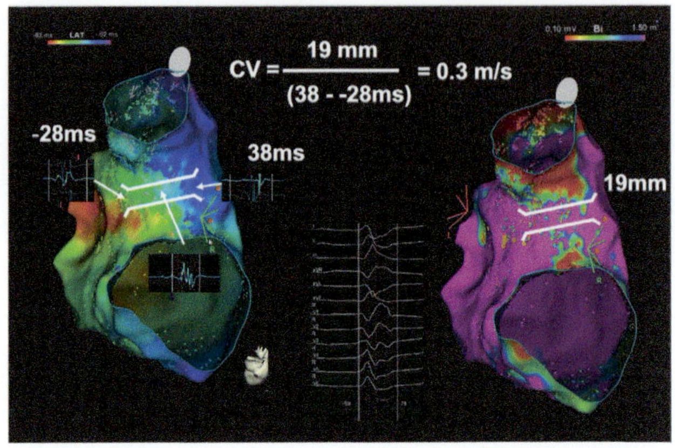

Fig. 38.3 Calculation of conduction velocity across Isthmus 3 in a patient with palpitations and tetralogy of Fallot. The isthmus length and electrogram timing at the entrance and exit of an abnormal isthmus are used to calculate conduction velocity, in this case abnormal at 0.3 m/s. This patient was found to be inducible for ventricular tachycardia at electrphysiology study prior to transcatheter pulmonary valve replacement and underwent catheter ablation.

the tricuspid valve and the VSD patch, respectively, and the ventriculotomy) were the longest and thickest of the AIs. This warrants emphasis as entrainment of reentrant VT using one of these broader isthmuses and Isthmus 3 posteriorly (between the pulmonary vein [PV] and VSD patch) often yield results consistent with an exit site. However, ablation targeting these regions exclusively are much more difficult and less successful given the length and thickness of this tissue (1–1.5 cm in Isthmus 1 versus 0.5 cm in Isthmus 3).

Another important finding from these studies was that Isthmus 3 (PA to VSD) was nearly universally present in all of the specimens, while Isthmus 4 (VSD patch to tricuspid valve) was only rarely identified (<10%). Additionally, the use of a transatrial-transpulmonary mode of correction prevents the creation of Isthmus 2. Histologic examination confirmed endocardial fibroelastosis to variable degrees at sites of prior surgery, involving all isthmuses, with a higher percent transmural fibrosis in Isthmus 3.

The presence of the AI itself is not sufficient to support reentry, of course. Reentry requires sufficiently slow conduction in order to allow time for repolarization of tissue just beyond the propagating wavefront. In another landmark study, the Leiden group characterized the AI properties in 74 consecutive repaired ToF patients referred for electrophysiology study.[15] All patients were found to have at least one AI, but the patients who were inducible for VT had longer, narrower, and more slowly conducting channels than those without inducible VT. They defined a slowly conducting AI (SCAI) as bounded by unexcitable tissue, containing abnormal voltage (<1.5 mV) and having a conduction velocity <0.5 m/s (Fig. 38.3). VT was not inducible acutely and not seen in long-term follow-up in patients with AIs having a velocity >0.5 m/s. This study lends further support to the idea of eliminating VT risk with sinus rhythm mapping in repaired ToF, potentially prophylactically.

It may be tempting to analogize reentrant VT in ToF to that seen in common acquired heart disease, such as ischemic cardiomyopathy. There are important differences, however. Slow conduction within the reentrant VT circuit in ToF is generally confined to a relatively small segment of the VT circuit. Even in the presence of significant sinus rhythm conduction delay, the majority of slow conduction occurs within the conduction system, manifest as the typical RBBB of tetralogy, not within the bulk of the ventricular myocardium.[16] It is generally relatively small areas of slow conduction, facilitated by fibrosis, that allow for reentry. This narrows down the targets of more detailed investigation and mapping considerably.

The majority of VT in CHD is related to macro reentry within the AIs discussed earlier, but focal VTs can be occasionally seen, mainly originating from the outflow tract regions in nontetralogy patients with outflow tract anomalies.[17,18] Reentry involving the His-Purkinje system has also been described and may be underrecognized as it often is in acquired heart disease–related VT as well.[18]

ARRHYTHMIA DIAGNOSIS AND DIFFERENTIAL DIAGNOSIS

Arrhythmia Diagnostic Criteria

Ventricular tachycardia in CHD	• Surface QRS morphology changes (left bundle morphology VT with underlying sinus right bundle) • Identification of anatomic isthmuses with sinus rhythm mapping • Confirmation of macroreentry mechanism with entrainment maneuvers • Rule out focal VT in rare cases

Surface Electrocardiogram

The 12-lead ECG of VT in tetralogy of Fallot will show a wide-complex, often very rapid tachycardia. Atrioventricular dissociation may be present but is often difficult to appreciate. Patients

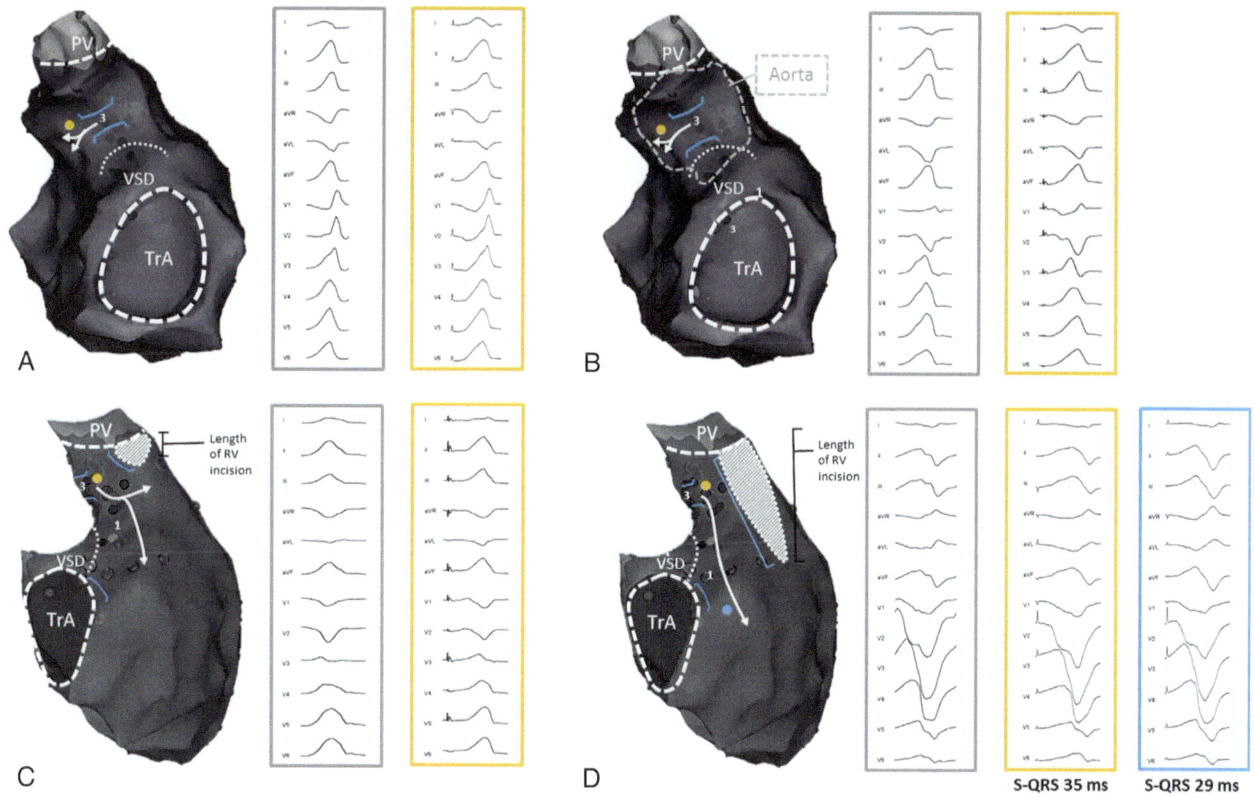

Fig. 38.4 Pace matches for right and left bundle branch block (RBBB and LBBB, respectively) ventricular tachycardias (VTs) in repaired tetralogy of Fallot. Schematic overview of right ventricular (RV) electroanatomical maps in (A, B) modified posteroanterior view and (C, D) modified right anterior oblique view. *White dashed lines* indicate electrically unexcitable borders. Anatomical isthmus (AI) 1 and AI3 are indicated between *blue brackets*. Induced VT morphologies are delineated in *gray*. *Yellow* and *blue tags* indicate pacing sites irrespective of VT morphology with corresponding paced morphology. *White arrows* indicate the presumed activation direction during VT and pacing. (A) RBBB paced match in AI3 (septal exit). (B) RBBB paced match in the coronary cusp. Note the transition break morphology in V2. (C) LBBB paced match in AI3 (free wall exit) in the presence of a small RV incision. (D) Similar LBBB paced matches in AI3 (free wall exit) and AI1 in the presence of a large RV incision. Note the increase in the S-QRS interval when pacing at the VT isthmus site (*yellow*) compared with the VT exit site (*blue*). *PV*, pulmonary valve; *TrA*, tricuspid annulus; *VSD*, ventricular septal defect. (From Brouwer C, Kapel GFL, Jongbloed RM, et al. Noninvasive identification of ventricular tachycardia-related anatomical isthmuses in repaired tetralogy of Fallot. *J Am Coll Cardiol.* 2018;4:1308–1318.)

often tolerate very rapid rates, leading observers to occasionally assume the diagnosis to be supraventricular tachycardia based on hemodynamic tolerance alone. The 12-lead morphology is generally inconsistent with aberration, with the majority of VTs being of left bundle morphology in this cohort of patients with underlying RBBB.

Although the RVOT is central to macro reentrant VT in ToF, there is no similarity in morphology to that seen in idiopathic VT from the RVOT. Global ventricular activation generally propagates from the posterior Isthmus 3, between the PA and the VSD patch, in either a clockwise direction (when observed from an anteroposterior or left anterior oblique projection) or counterclockwise direction, exiting from Isthmus 3 out laterally. Clockwise propagation produces an RBBB VT, often with a qR pattern in V1. Counterclockwise VT exits Isthmus 3, then proceeds through Isthmus 1, producing an LBBB VT pattern.[18] Precordial transition is dependent on the length of the RV incision, with longer incisions producing later precordial transitions (Fig. 38.4).

Entrainment Mapping

There are no unique investigations of entrainment mapping of VT in repaired CHD, per se. Generally, criteria used for ablation of VT in coronary artery disease are applied to reentrant circuits involving VT in CHD as well. It is worth noting that these tachycardias are often very rapid, and therefore postpacing intervals, when entraining at sites critical to the circuit, may yield return cycles that are longer than expected or cause acceleration into nonclinical rhythms. Additionally, there is the potential for figure-of-eight circuits with varying cycle lengths.[19]

MAPPING: APPROACH TO EFFICIENT MAPPING

As anatomical understanding has grown, most ablation procedures will begin with detailed substrate mapping in sinus or paced rhythm. Multipolar catheters are recommended as low-amplitude signals within regions of scar can be missed when using ablation catheters for mapping, given the large field of view. Areas of low voltage should be confirmed to have been sampled with adequate

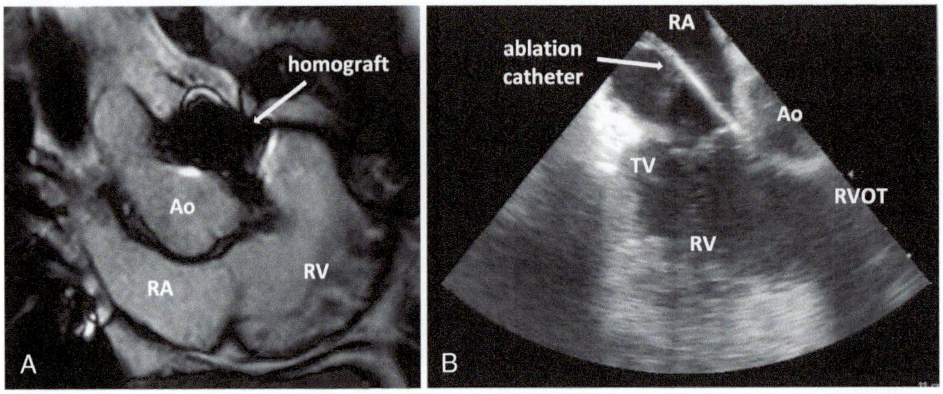

Fig. 38.5 Correlative imaging in tetralogy of Fallot useful for VT ablation. (A) Cardiac MRI showing aortic root seated in "hammock" between right atrium and postoperative outflow tract with pulmonic valve homograft. (B) Intracardiac ultrasound image with ablation catheter traversing tricuspid valve and approximating ventricular septal defect patch.

catheter contact, which can be difficult between the PA and tricuspid valve. Use of intracardiac ultrasound (ICE) is an important adjunct in this regard (Fig. 38.5). ICE can also be used to identify the tricuspid valve annulus as not to overlook conducting myocardium basal to the VSD patch (through Isthmus 4). A stabilizing or deflectable sheath may be needed to achieve adequate contact. Failure to capture with high-output unipolar pacing (10 mA at 0.2 ms) when contact is confirmed defines regions of scar.[20]

AIs are considered abnormal in the absence of continuous normal bipolar electrograms (>1.5 mV). Additionally, the conduction velocity within the isthmus can be defined by dividing the length of the AI by the difference in the local activation time at the isthmus entrance and exit. SCAIs have conduction velocities <0.5 m/s, as discussed earlier.[15]

Despite rapid tachycardia rates, many patients will tolerate activation mapping of VT (Fig. 38.6A). Normal RV function and avoidance of general anesthesia both improve hemodynamic status during VT. Mapping should focus on the previously identified AIs, especially those with calculated slow conduction (<0.5 m/s). The body of the RV is rarely participatory in the VT circuit in the absence of postsurgical myocardial scar and is often a source of catheter ectopy during mapping, which can terminate VT.

Entrainment mapping should be performed whenever feasible, with criteria used as for ischemic VT (Fig. 38.6B, C). Identification of a central isthmus site is paramount, as exit and entrance sites tend to be broad, and ablation in these regions may be associated with low rates of arrhythmia termination and prevention. Endocardial scar may require high-output pacing for entrainment, which can lead to far-field capture, confounding results. Similarly, critical sites may fall below standard scar settings in the 3D electroanatomical mapping systems. Careful signal adjudication and real-time processing may be needed to accurately identify the precise circuit.

Pace mapping for VT circuit localization may be needed when the VT is either not tolerated or not inducible. Care should be taken to target ablation in areas with excellent morphology match to the VT and a long stim-QRS interval, generally correlating with a more central isthmus site. The vulnerable central isthmus with slow conduction may be very small, but activation of the ventricle often proceeds as a wide funnel from these corridors. For example, a common VT circuit is one that propagates through Isthmus 3 (VSD to PA) and then lateral through Isthmus 1 (RV incision to TV) and then anteriorly back to the septum. Pace mapping from Isthmus 1 may yield an excellent pace map, but the stim-QRS interval will be very short and ablation here is unlikely to achieve the needed transmurality to achieve block.

Ablation Target Sites

- Participating anatomical isthmuses
- Anatomical isthmuses with slow conduction (<0.5 m/s)
- Aortic root ablation may be needed for block across Isthmus 3 (VSD to PA)

ABLATION

Ablation should target the AIs involved in the VT circuit. Irrigated ablation is recommended, and a small-curve catheter can often facilitate improved contact. The ablation catheter may need to be oriented vertically to the tissue in order to not slide on the smooth endocardial surface in the postsurgical patients, especially along Isthmus 3 (VSD to PA). High-power ablation (30–50 W) is used until loss of capture is confirmed. Cryoablation is generally not used in these cases but may be used in cases where the conduction system is in proximity to the target ablation site.

Block should be confirmed across any targeted AI (Fig. 38.7). Incomplete ablation may facilitate reentry by worsening slow conduction. Whether the aortic root should be accesses routinely in these ablations is a matter of ongoing study but is recommended by this author whenever Isthmus 3 has been targeted. It is possible to see endocardial block across Isthmus 3 in the RV and have conduction propagating via the "epicardium," which sits at the base of the aorta.

Noninducibility remains an important endpoint as well. Full programmed stimulation should be repeated both in the resting state and with adrenergic stimulation. Relatively high doses of isoproterenol may be needed (up to 10 μg/min) for VT induction.

SUCCESS

Success with catheter ablation of VT in ToF continues to improve as our understanding of the circuits and ablation targets has evolved. Success rates approach 90% when an AI can be identified and block can be achieved.[17,18] In the previously mentioned study by Kapel et al., the absence of SCAI or elimination of any SCAI

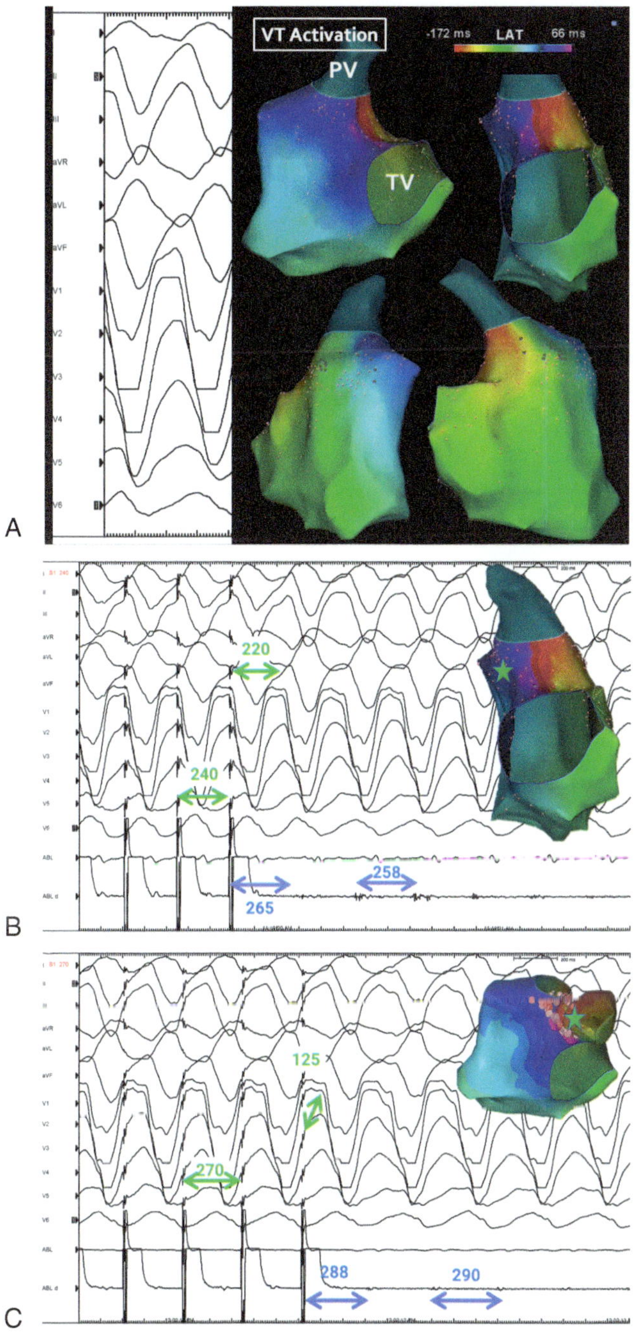

Fig. 38.6 Patient with repaired tetralogy of Fallot and recurrent ventricular tachycardia (VT). (A) Clinical VT, left bundle, left superior axis with a precordial transition in V6, cycle length 258 ms. Activation is also shown, with rapid activation across the anterior right ventricle and isochronal crowding in the posterior right ventricular outflow tract, Isthmus 3. (B) Entrainment from a site just septal to Isthmus 3, consistent with an entrance site. Note the subtle fusion seen best in the limb leads due to the wide entrance zone. Ablation along Isthmus 3 slowed the tachycardia but did not terminate it. (C) Entrainment from the aortic cusp, site opposite Isthmus 3. A mid-isthmus site is identified and ablation here was successful.

by ablation was associated with complete arrhythmia freedom in long-term follow-up.[15] Those patients not ablated or unsuccessfully ablated had a high risk of recurrence, however.

Perhaps even more so than in acquired heart disease VT ablation, complications are not frequently reported for VT ablation in this population. In repaired ToF, risks of VT ablation appear to be low, with no major complications reported in many of the larger series. However, given published studies come from highly experienced centers, interpretation of complication data is limited. Heart block can be avoided by ablation targeting an isthmus lateral to the proximal conduction system in most cases. Vascular access complications remain as with all percutaneous procedures.

RISK STRATIFICATION PRIOR TO PULMONARY VALVE REPLACEMENT

The need for pulmonary valve replacement (PVR) has long been recognized as a risk factor for ventricular arrhythmias in repaired ToF. Until recently, these patients exclusively underwent surgical replacement of the pulmonary valve, introducing the opportunity for concomitant surgical ablation of arrhythmogenic tissue. Several studies have evaluated VT risk stratification approaches pre-PVR.[21,22] These included heterogeneous groups of patients (those both with and without preoperative spontaneous VT, for example) and variable ablation protocols (some surgical and others catheter based). These studies do show, however, a high rate of inducibility both pre-PVR (up to 70%) as well as post-cryoablation alone (up to 50%), perhaps reflecting incomplete transection of the putative isthmus(es) in the operating room.

Transcatheter PVR is increasing, supplanting surgical repair in a large proportion of patients with severe pulmonary valve regurgitation after repair of ToF. This approach creates a unique challenge for electrophysiologists aiming to treat VT and prevent the development of VT in the future. Transcatheter valve designs continue to evolve with a recent iteration having a large proximal skirt that improves fixation and stability in the distal RVOT. After placement of this valve, there is prosthetic material often covering the isthmus between the native PA and the VSD patch, potentially precluding effective ablation (Fig. 38.8).[23] Given the potential for excluding critical substrate for sustaining reentrant VT, studies are being directed at prophylactic evaluation and ablation of any slowly conducting isthmuses prior to valve placement as primary prevention for VT.

SURGICAL ABLATION

Ventricular arrhythmias in CHD may herald worsening hemodynamics due to anatomical abnormalities, coronary abnormalities, worsening valvular function, or ventricular function. Presentation with VT warrants evaluation for these important hemodynamic lesions and correction when feasible. The most common lesion found is residual pulmonary regurgitation in repaired ToF with subsequent RV enlargement and disfunction. PVR can reduce recurrent VT via favorable effects on RV remodeling and hemodynamics. However, the critical AIs remain, as does the risk of recurrent VT, and should be addressed in the electrophysiology lab or the operating room if surgical PVR is planned.[24,25]

There have been several small series evaluating surgical ablation of VT guided by both preoperative or intraoperative electroanatomical mapping in CHD. Despite obvious advantages in certain patients with challenging anatomy, clinical success rates have been more modest, especially in repaired ToF, with 20–45% of patients undergoing prophylactic empiric cryoablation at the time of repair experiencing recurrent VT in high-risk cohorts.[26] These outcomes may improve as assessment for block intraoperatively

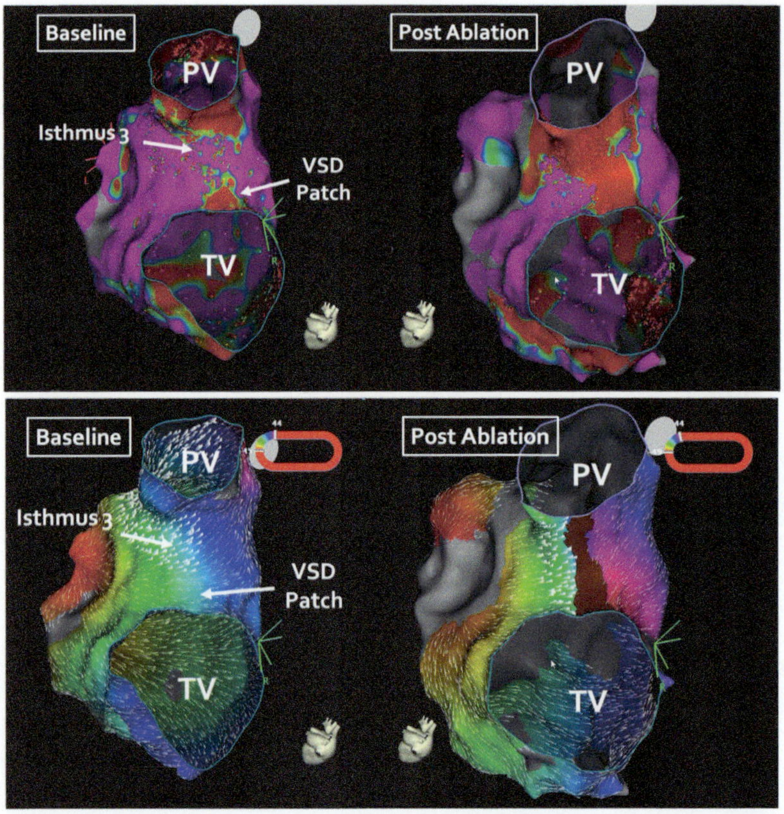

Fig. 38.7 Sinus rhythm voltage and activation at baseline and post ablation in a patient found to have slow conduction (0.33 m/s) across Isthmus 3 and inducible ventricular tachycardia prior to pulmonary valve replacement. (*Top*) Baseline voltage delineating the presence of Isthmus 3 (and absence of Isthmus 4) and voltage after ablation through this region. (*Bottom*) Propagation in sinus rhythm, with the thicker vector arrows delineating relatively slower conduction. Post ablation, conduction across Isthmus 3 is eliminated and block is achieved.

becomes standard, but currently repeat electrophysiological study is recommended postoperatively in these patients.[27]

TROUBLESHOOTING THE DIFFICULT CASE

As the approach to VT ablation in repaired ToF has been streamlined, the technical difficulty level has been reduced. However, challenging cases certainly remain, especially given the variety of anatomical considerations even within a group of patients with similar underlying pathology.

Achieving transmurality is essential for creating block across putative and definitive anatomic isthmuses for VT. Although these may be relatively thin isthmuses, interstitial fibrosis may hinder radiofrequency energy delivery via heterogeneous tissue impedance. Practically, this requires access to the contralateral side when possible. For Isthmuses 1 and 2, these require epicardial access, which is feasible only via a surgical approach. As discussed previously, in the presence of Isthmus 3 or 4, ablation of the more anterior corridors is redundant and unnecessary.

Transmural ablation of Isthmus 3 (PA to VSD patch) may require access to the aortic root.[28] The proportion of cases where trans-isthmus block cannot be achieved via the RV endocardium alone is currently unknown but may be further elucidated as more prophylactic ablations are performed pre-PVR. The aortic root, generally the right coronary cusp, sits opposite to Isthmus 3 and can provide a favorable vantage point for ablation with advantageous contact. A case requiring ablation in the aortic cusp for termination is detailed in Fig. 38.6.

The vast majority of patients with VT in ToF and valvular dysfunction will present with pulmonary insufficiency. Pulmonic stenosis as a residual valvular lesion presents a potentially more challenging substrate with significant ventricular hypertrophy. This may be a cause of ablation failure. Surgical ablation is often used in this situation, but the coronary venous system may provide another vantage point for ablation (Fig. 38.9).

Troubleshooting the Difficult Cases

Problem	Causes	Solution
Unable to induce VT	• Adrenergic dependent • Inability to elicit unidirectional block	• Use isoproterenol, sometimes high doses • Induction from sites close to AIs to facilitate block • Ablate SCAI in sinus rhythm
Poor catheter stability	• Right atrial enlargement • Smooth tissue in posterior RVOT	• Deflectable sheath • Use of intracardiac ultrasound • Consider IJ access approach • Ablate in sinus rhythm
Inability to terminate VT or create block	• Ventricular hypertrophy • Poor catheter contact • Prosthetic material • Dense scar	• Mapping in aortic root • Mapping distal coronary sinus looking for basal septal vein • Long lesions (3–4 minutes) • Half-normal saline irrigation

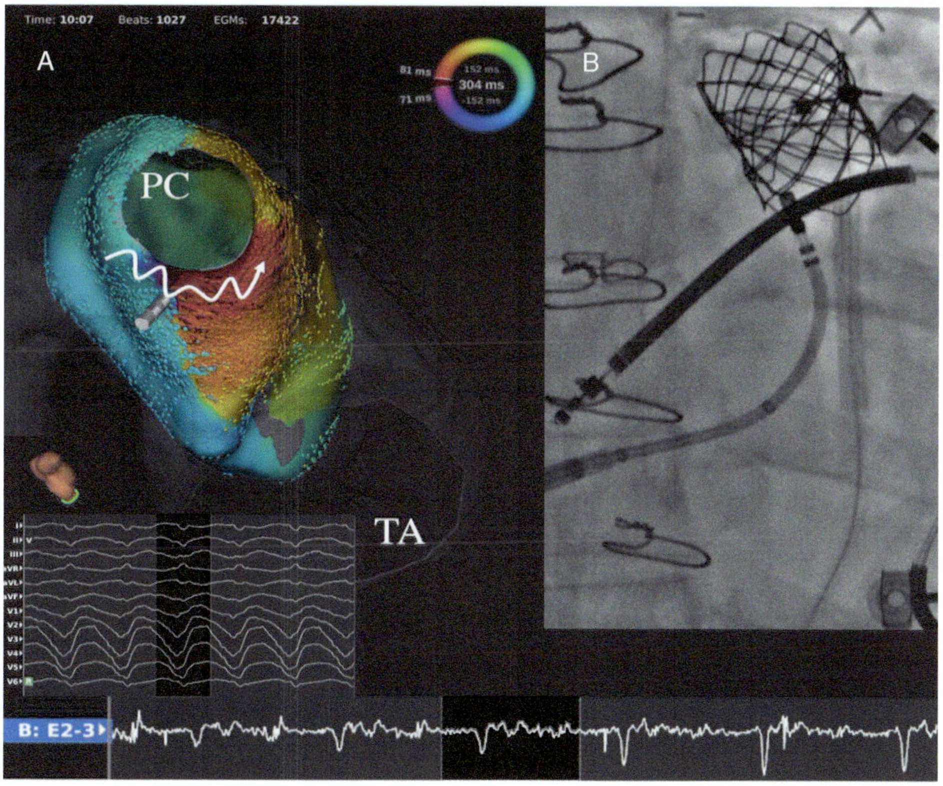

Fig. 38.8 (A) Counterclockwise circuit using Isthmus 3 traveling in myocardium partially covered by the prosthetic pulmonary valve. (B) Ablation catheter just inside the prosthetic valve. (Note: implantable cardioverter-defibrillator lead was placed in the epicardium due to vascular obstruction.) (From Combes N, Bartoletti S, Heitz F, Waldmann V. Critical isthmus of ventricular tachycardia covered by transcatheter pulmonary valve in a patient with tetralogy of Fallot. *Eur Heart J.* 2020;41:723.)

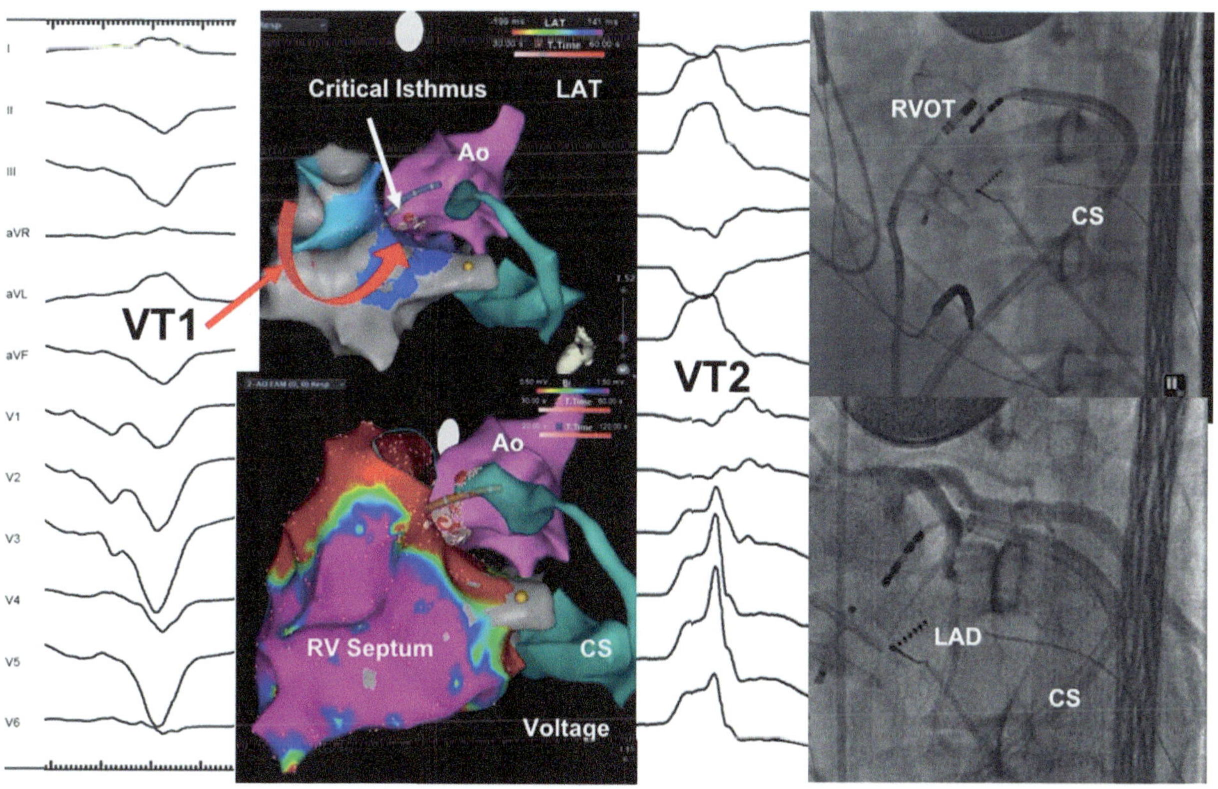

Fig. 38.9 Mapping a septal coronary vein for ventricular tachycardia (VT) in a patient with repaired tetralogy of Fallot and recurrent VT despite endocardial right ventricular, aortic root, and open surgical ablation at the time of pulmonary valve replacement for prosthetic valve pulmonic stenosis. Paired VT morphologies are shown, utilizing isthmus 3 posteriorly. Ablation within the vein terminated VT.

EBSTEIN ANOMALY

Ebstein anomaly presents a unique and rare substrate for VT. Both unoperated and postsurgical patients may present with VT, and VT is an important risk factor for sudden death in patients with Ebstein anomaly. The apical displaced tricuspid valve leads to atrialized ventricular tissue, which is subjected to myocardial stretch and fibrosis in the setting of pressure and volume overload related to tricuspid valve and RV dysfunction. In a multicenter center retrospective study, Moore and colleagues reported a series of 24 patients with Ebstein anomaly who underwent ablation for VT.[29] VT mechanisms were found to be both focal and macroreentrant, with mechanism unrelated to surgical status. However, location appeared to be less localized to the atrialized RV muscle in postoperative patients (Fig. 38.10). Ablation success was achieved in 92% of patients with no complications in the adult cohort.

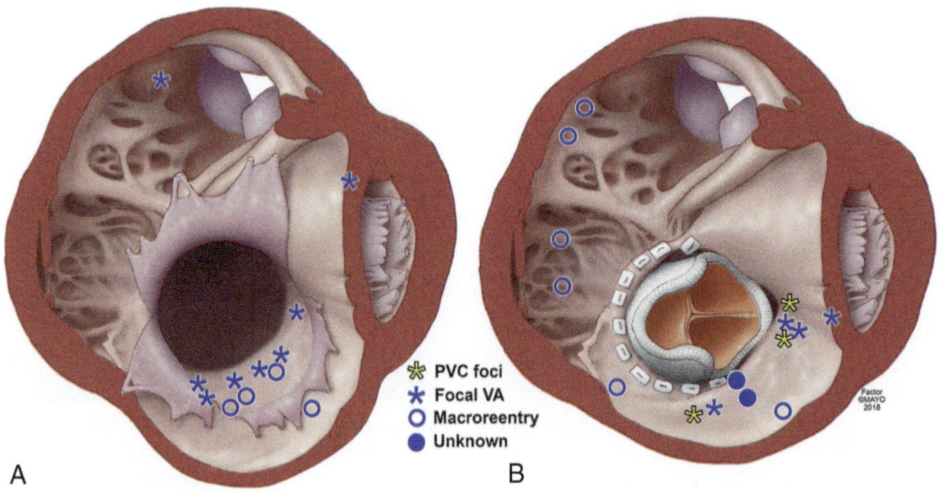

Fig. 38.10 Anatomic location of ventricular arrhythmia (VA) substrates among (A) unoperated and (B) postsurgical patients in a modified left anterior oblique view. The most common site of origin for VA in unoperated patients was the atrialized right ventricle as opposed to postsurgical patients, where VA sites of origin were more varied. *PVC*, Premature ventricular contraction. (From Moore JP, Shanoon KM, Gallotti RG, et al. Catheter ablation of ventricular arrhythmia for Ebstein's anomaly in unoperated and post-surgical patients. *J Am Coll Cardiol.* 2018;4:1300–1307.)

CONCLUSION

Ablation of VT in the setting of CHD is an important and growing need in electrophysiology. As surgical techniques and medical care have improved, many more patients are living into adulthood with CHD and may experience VT. VT ablation in repaired ToF has advanced tremendously over the last decade and a half, with AIs clearly defined and arrhythmogenic substrate able to be characterized in sinus rhythm. These advances have ushered in a new era for VT ablation in ToF, with many patients being cured of their arrhythmias.

REFERENCES

Please refer to the e-book for a complete list of references.

39

Ablation of Ventricular Tachyarrhythmias in Brugada Syndrome

Koonlawee Nademanee, Qing Lou

KEY POINTS

- Arrhythmogenic substrates of Brugada syndrome (BrS) are characterized by markedly fractionated and prolonged duration of the electrograms present over the right ventricular outflow tract/right ventricular epicardium.
- Marked epicardial and interstitial fibrosis is the pathology underlying these abnormal epicardial electrograms.
- Ablations at these substrate sites normalize the electrocardiogram pattern and prevent ventricular fibrillation recurrence.
- Catheter ablation of BrS substrates is a promising therapeutic modality for symptomatic BrS patients.

Since its discovery in the early 1990s, Brugada syndrome (BrS) has drawn worldwide attention as the leading cause of premature death in young adults who are otherwise apparently healthy individuals.[1] The syndrome was initially thought to be "a primary electrical disease" that caused ventricular fibrillation (VF) in patients with structurally normal hearts. However, several studies over the past three decades have made significant progress toward a better understanding of the syndrome's underlying pathophysiology—a complex interplay between genetics, myocardial substrate abnormalities, and channelopathy.[2,3] During the first two decades, treatment of symptomatic BrS patients was quite challenging due to limited therapeutic options: implantable cardioverter-defibrillator (ICD) and quinidine were only the two therapies for BrS patients.[2,4] However, the use of quinidine is limited by its unavailability in many parts of the world and its relatively high incidence of side effects.[5] ICD is the only proven treatment option for high-risk symptomatic patients, especially for those who have survived out-of-hospital cardiac arrest. Unfortunately, ICD implantation may not be an adequate solution for many patients (i.e., infants and young children). Given that an ICD does not prevent VF recurrence, patients with BrS with frequent VF recurrences often experience frequent ICD shocks, which adversely affect patients and pose a therapeutic conundrum for physicians; in rare instances, a heart transplant was performed to control electrical storm.[6] Fortunately, the discovery of epicardial BrS substrates in the right ventricle (RV), especially at the right ventricular outflow tract (RVOT), provides interventional electrophysiologists with an excellent target site for catheter ablation.[7,8] Indeed, ablations of Brugada epicardial substrates have been proved to be very effective and increasingly used worldwide.[8–12] This chapter discusses in detail the BrS substrates and how one can successfully eliminate them through catheter ablation and, in turn, prevent VF recurrences in BrS patients.

ARRHYTHMOGENIC SUBSTRATES

During the first two decades of BrS, repolarization was thought to be the prevailing mechanism for its electrocardiogram phenotype and electrophysiological abnormalities underlying VF.[4] The repolarization theory is based on the perfused canine RV wedge preparation that shows transmural dispersion of repolarization caused by reduction of net inward Na^+ current (NaV1.5) alongside nonuniform increases in the transient outward current (I_{to}) within the subepicardial myocardium, especially in the RVOT, causing this area to develop a notch-and-dome appearance of the epicardium action potential (AP) leading to a coved type of ST-segment elevation in the right precordial leads. If the loss of the AP dome is further accentuated, then it causes a marked shortening of the epicardial AP in certain regions, causing pronounced heterogeneity of transmembrane voltage potentials and, in turn, phase 2 reentry and triggered VF.[4]

However, during this past decade, the depolarization theory proposed by the Amsterdam group offers a different hypothesis, which contends that in BrS, the RVOT depolarizes the latest.[6] As a result, the delay in the AP of the RVOT causes the electrical gradient from the more positive RV to RVOT, leading to the ST-elevation of the right precordial leads, similar to the situation if there were a myocardial injury at the RVOT. As the RVOT depolarizes later (during repolarization of the RV), this gradient is reversed and the net current flows toward the RV, resulting a negative T wave.[13] They argue that these depolarization abnormalities are produced by severely compromised conduction including slow and/or asynchronous conduction, localized block, and absence of activation within the RVOT, creating a large potential difference with respect to the body of the RV.[13–16]

Thus, it is not surprising that our study of nine Thai BrS patients with frequent ICD discharges confirmed the presence of arrhythmogenic substrate in the RVOT characterized

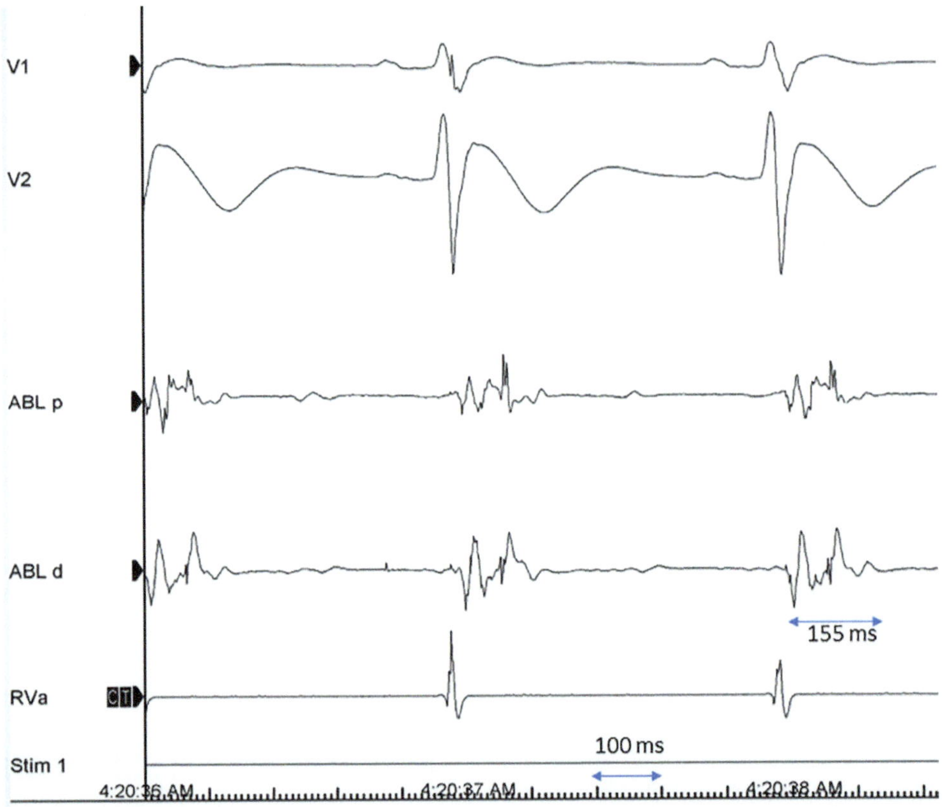

Fig. 39.1 Examples of electrograms with fractionated late potentials that represent good target sites for catheter ablation. The bipolar electrograms recorded from distal and proximal pair electrodes of the ablation catheter at the right ventricular outflow tract epicardium exhibit low-voltage electrograms with long fractionated potentials that coincide with the appearance of the coved type J-point elevation typical of Type 1 Brugada ECG pattern.

by low voltage (<1 mV), prolonged electrogram duration (>80 ms), and fractionated late potentials (Fig. 39.1). What was surprising, however, was that in all of these patients the substrates that harbored abnormal electrograms localized exclusively to the anterior RVOT epicardium and were not present in the corresponding endocardial site, clustering only in the anterior aspect of the RVOT epicardium as shown in Fig. 39.2. Ablation at these sites rendered ventricular tachycardia (VT)/VF noninducible and normalized the Brugada ECG pattern in most of the patients with no recurrent spontaneous VT/VF seen.[7]

Following the above observation, a key question then arose: What is the pathology underlying these abnormal electrograms? The answer to this question came from our multicenter collaborative study that aimed to determine the underlying pathology of BrS substrates.[14] From this study, sudden cardiac death victims with BrS family history and negative routine autopsy were found to have rich epicardial and interstitial fibrosis and reduced gap junction expressions in the RVOT,[14] coinciding with a significant increase in the collagen content in all ventricular walls over and above the normal collagen seen in age- and sex-matched controls. We also performed open thoracotomy for direct mapping and ablations in six symptomatic BrS patients with frequent ICD therapies; the indications for open thoracotomy were either to remove an infected ICD or failure to gain epicardial access percutaneously. Biopsy specimens from the substrate sites that harbored abnormal fragmented electrograms revealed epicardial and interstitial fibrosis (Fig. 39.3) despite normal cardiac imaging (computed tomography [CT] or magnetic resonance imaging {MRI]) as well a grossly normal-appearing heart on direct visualization during thoracotomy in all of these patients. Ablations were delivered on these fibrotic areas with fractionated electrograms in the RVOT/RV epicardium, Brugada ECG patterns were normalized, and ablation was effective in preventing recurrent spontaneous VF episodes as well as inducible VF by programmed electrical stimulation.

Similar findings were also observed in the explanted heart of a BrS patient who underwent heart transplantation for refractory VF and whose heart had interstitial fibrosis causing conduction delay.[6] Thus, one can confidently conclude that epicardial and interstitial fibrosis and reduced gap junction expression in the RVOT/RV are the principal pathology that underlies arrhythmogenic substrates causing the Brugada ECG pattern, abnormal fractionated low-voltage late potentials, and VF. Further, one can conclude that these myopathic changes likely result in heterogeneity of impulse conduction, conduction delay, and dispersion RV/RVOT epicardium causing reentry as the main electrophysiological mechanism.

This supposition is further strengthened by the finding that ajmaline unmasks the Brugada ECG pattern: The drug, by reducing I_{Na}, markedly delays impulse conduction in these RVOT substrate sites that have underlying fibrosis, thereby increasing the areas of the late activation and in turn increasing STE over the right precordial ECG leads. This is associated with local STE

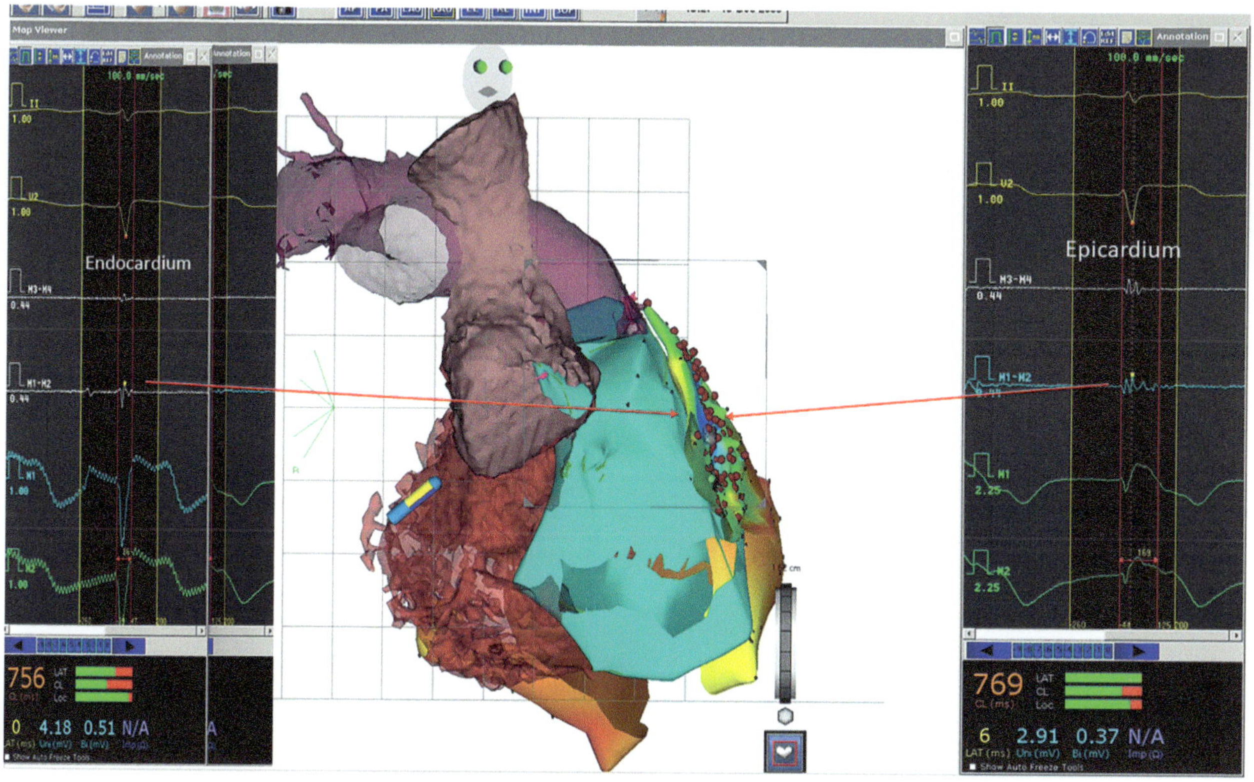

Fig. 39.2 A right lateral view of the right ventricular outflow tract (RVOT) displays the difference in ventricular electrograms between the endocardial and epicardial site of the anterior RVOT. The left and right insets display bipolar and unipolar electrograms recorded from the endocardium and epicardium from the same site of the RVOT, respectively. M1–2 and M3–4 = Bipolar electrograms recorded from the distal and proximal pairs of the catheter ablation catheter. Both M1–2 and M3–4 recordings show abnormal fractionated electrogram in the epicardium but not over the endocardial at the same site. M1 and M2 = unipolar recordings of the distal and the second electrodes of the ablation catheter. Note that the unipolar electrograms of both distal and the second electrodes over the RVOT epicardium exhibit curved type J wave elevation identical to the Brugada ECG pattern, but the unipolar electrograms on the endocardial site appear to be normal.

and local loss of amplitude of the unipolar EGMs, as detected by electrocardiographic imaging (ECGI) [Fig. 39.4]. Furthermore, as shown in the Fig. 39.5, ajmaline changes bipolar and unipolar electrograms of these fibrotic areas from relatively normal electrograms to markedly abnormal fractionated ones, coinciding with an appearance of STE in the unipolar electrograms in these areas.[15] More importantly, the unipolar electrograms after administration of the drug have a monophasic morphology resembling an action potential that is a sign of absence of local activation, similar to that recorded from a monophasic AP catheter.[13,16] This clearly shows that ajmaline unmasks the substrate by creating excitation failure, manifesting as the genesis of monophasic EGMs or as late monophasic components of unipolar EGMs in fibrotic tissue.[15] In short, ajmaline, by reducing I_{Na}, severely compromises impulse conduction in the BrS substrates and can uncover the fibrotic sites by producing fractionated EGMs, conduction block, or excitation failure that create milieu for current-to-load mismatch phenomenon that leads to VF risk and the signature Brugada ECG pattern. The drug increases about twofold the measured size of the target area for the ablation. Thus, it is imperative to use sodium channel blockers, ajmaline, procainamide, or pilsicainide to guide a successful catheter ablation of BrS substrates for better long-term outcomes.

CATHETER ABLATION OF BRUGADA SUBSTRATES

Since our initial introduction of ablation of BrS epicardial substrates, several studies have confirmed that substrate ablations of the BrS is indeed safe and effective. The procedure is recommended as a Class 2B indication for symptomatic BrS patients and has been increasingly used worldwide.[8–12,17]

Even though the anterior RVOT epicardium is a primary substrate site and that abnormal fractionated late potentials are always present in BrS patients, it is not the exclusive site of BrS substrates. Subsequent findings have revealed that about one-third of BrS patients also have a significant substrate on other part of RV, including anterior and inferior RV epicardium and, in a rare number of patients, in the left ventricular (LV) epicardium.[8,18] Thus, it is essential to be very deliberate and perform detailed mapping of the substrates in order to achieve optimal outcomes.

MAPPING

We used the Sosa technique to gain epicardial access for mapping and ablations.[19] Coronary angiography was not routinely performed. Adequate coronary anatomy is obtained through

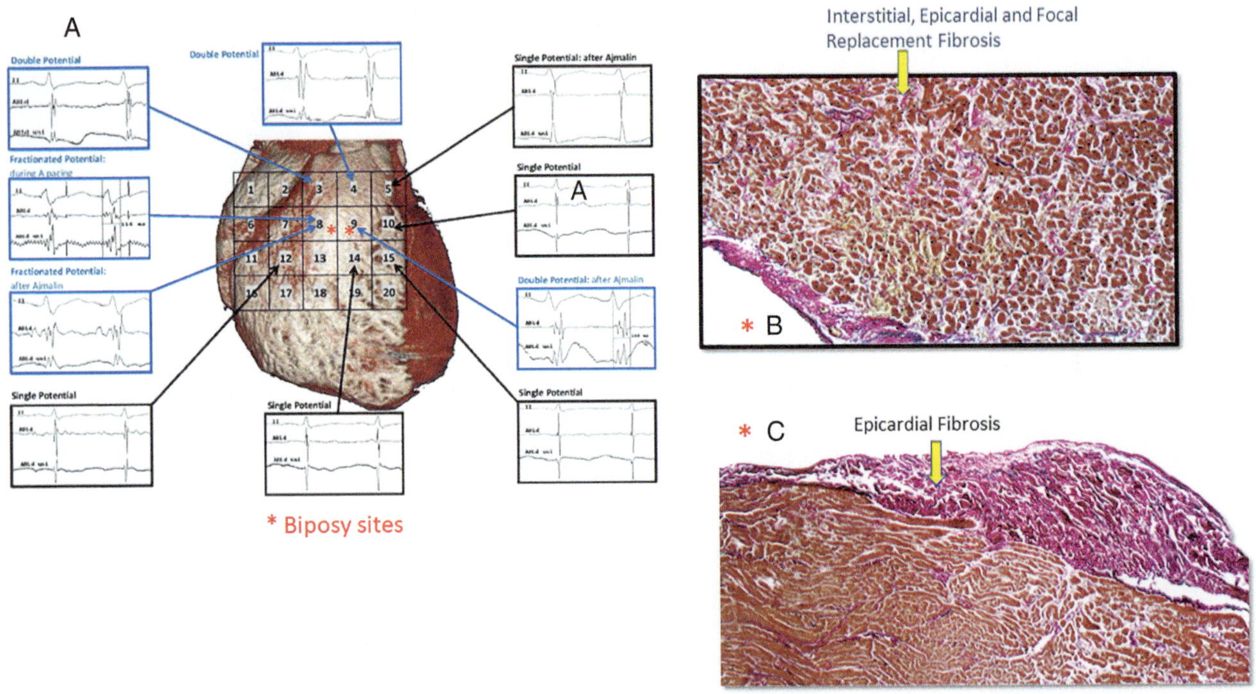

Fig. 39.3 (A) Computed tomography scan of the heart (center) of a Brugada syndrome (BrS) patient showing anatomical grid over the anterior right ventricular outflow tract. ECG lead II and a distal bipolar (0.4 mV/cm voltage scale at 30–300 Hz filter settings) and unipolar (5 mV/cm voltage scale at 0.05–300 Hz filter settings) electrogram at labeled sites given in surrounding panels. Abnormal fractionated electrograms are recorded from the biopsy sites (sites 8 and 9). Epicardial biopsy and histology studies at these sites show both thickened epicardial and interstitial fibrosis by picrosirius stain (B, C, *yellow arrows*). (From Nademanee K, Raju H, de Noronha SV, et al. Fibrosis, connexin-43, and conduction abnormalities in the Brugada syndrome. *J Am Coll Cardiol.* 2015;66(18):1976–1986.)

detailed endocardial and epicardial mapping by recognizing the location of annulus and right ventricular septum as a landmark of atrioventricular (AV) groove and interventricular septum, respectively. In our laboratory, noninvasive ECGI mapping is routinely used for quickly identifying BrS substrates and VF drivers. Endocardial and epicardial electroanatomical mapping of the RV as well as epicardial mapping of the LV can then be performed with high-density mapping catheters such as a circular mapping catheter, multielectrode catheters that have a smaller electrode interval such as Pentaray, or DecaNav (Biosense Webster) for higher resolution and high-density mapping. Image integration tools such as CARTO Merge, CartoUnivu for fluoroscopic/image integrations, and 2D-Realtime Integration with electroanatomical mapping are very helpful to create the detailed epicardial and endocardial electroanatomical map. Such maps can be displayed based on either voltage or duration of local potentials. An example of the map is shown in Fig 39.6, which was obtained from a BrS patients with multiple ICD therapies from recurrent VF episodes. ECGI mapped on Fig 39.6A clearly shows the latest activation and slow conduction are in the RVOT and RV inferior areas, which are the same sites that have low voltage and ST elevation of the unipolar electrograms, that are magnified after ajmaline administration. These areas colocalized with the ablation targeted areas that were tagged by its EGM characteristic of the abnormal low-voltage fractionated signals as shown in Fig 39.6C that are also where the VF drivers are located.

ABLATION PROTOCOL AND ENDPOINT

An irrigated-tip catheter with contact force >5g is required before RF application. The RF power is titrated from 30 to 50 W to achieve >10-Ω impedance reduction from baseline. Rapid disappearance of EGMs and a decline in recorded signal amplitude provide sufficient evidence of acute elimination of the target. A complete elimination of all substrate sites is the ideal endpoint.

EFFICACY AND SAFETY OF CATHETER ABLATION FOR BRS

Brugada substrate ablation now has been accepted as an important effective treatment modality and is being used in several centers worldwide. However, long-term outcomes are still needed. Therefore, we created a worldwide Brugada Ablation of VF Substrate Ongoing Multicenter (BRAVO) registry study of catheter ablation (ClinicalTrials.gov NCT04420078) for the treatment of symptomatic BrS patients. We enrolled 159 highly symptomatic patients (median age 42 years; 156 male patients) with BrS and spontaneous VF who underwent substrate ablation for recurrent VF episodes; 43 (27%) of them had BrS and early repolarization (ER) pattern.[20] All except five had an ICD for cardiac arrest (n = 125) or syncope (n = 34). Importantly, 140 (88%) had experienced numerous ICD shocks for spontaneous VF prior to ablation. After a single ablation procedure, 128 of 159 (81%) patients

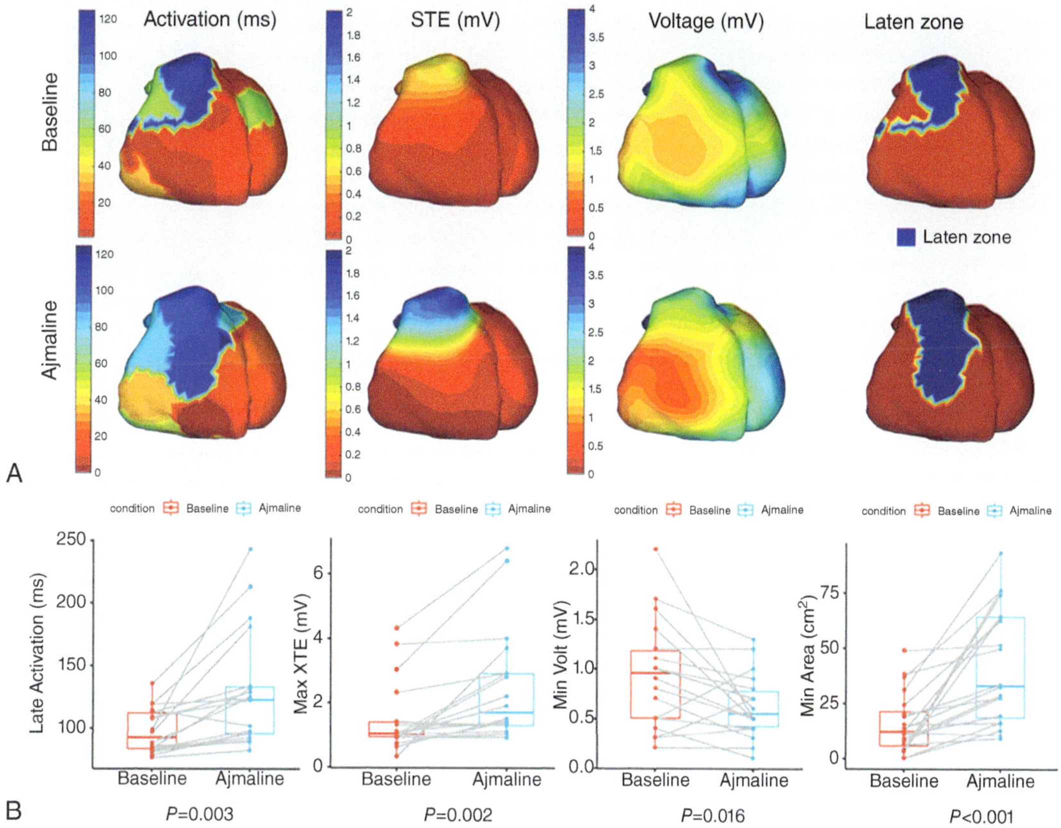

Fig. 39.4 (A) An example of electrocardiographic imaging maps from one of the study patients, displaying activation time, ST-elevation (STE), voltage, and areas of the late-activated area before and after ajmaline during sinus rhythm. (B) Results from the analyses of all patients within the late activation zone.

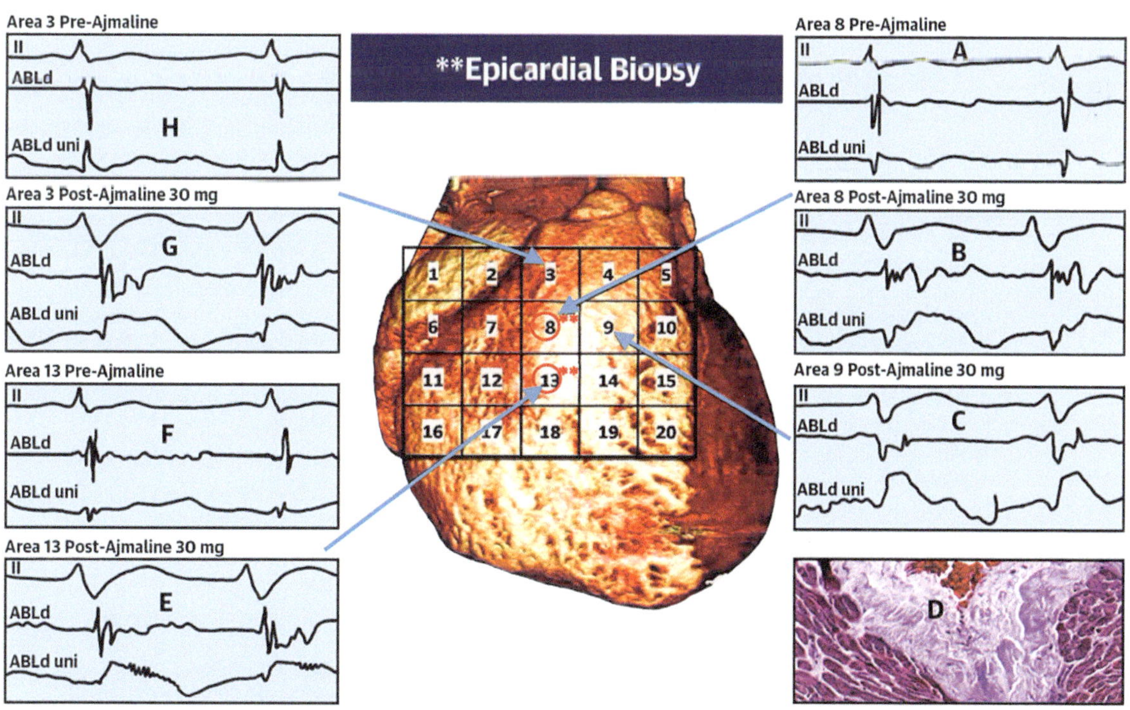

Fig. 39.5 Computed tomography scan of the heart (*center*) from one of the four BrS patients undergoing open thoracotomy mapping and ablation showing right ventricular (RV) anatomical grid. ECG lead II and a distal bipolar (0.4 mV/cm voltage scale at the filter 30–300 Hz) and unipolar electrogram (5 mV/cm voltage scale at the filter 0.05–300 Hz) are displayed in insets of the surrounding panels. Clockwise from the right: (A, B), electrograms from site 8 at baseline and after ajmaline, respectively; (C), electrograms recorded from site 9 after ajmaline; (D) histology of the biopsy specimen (Masson trichrome stain) from site 8 showing epicardial fibrosis; (E, F) and (G, H) electrograms recorded from sites 13 and 3 after ajmaline and at baseline, respectively.

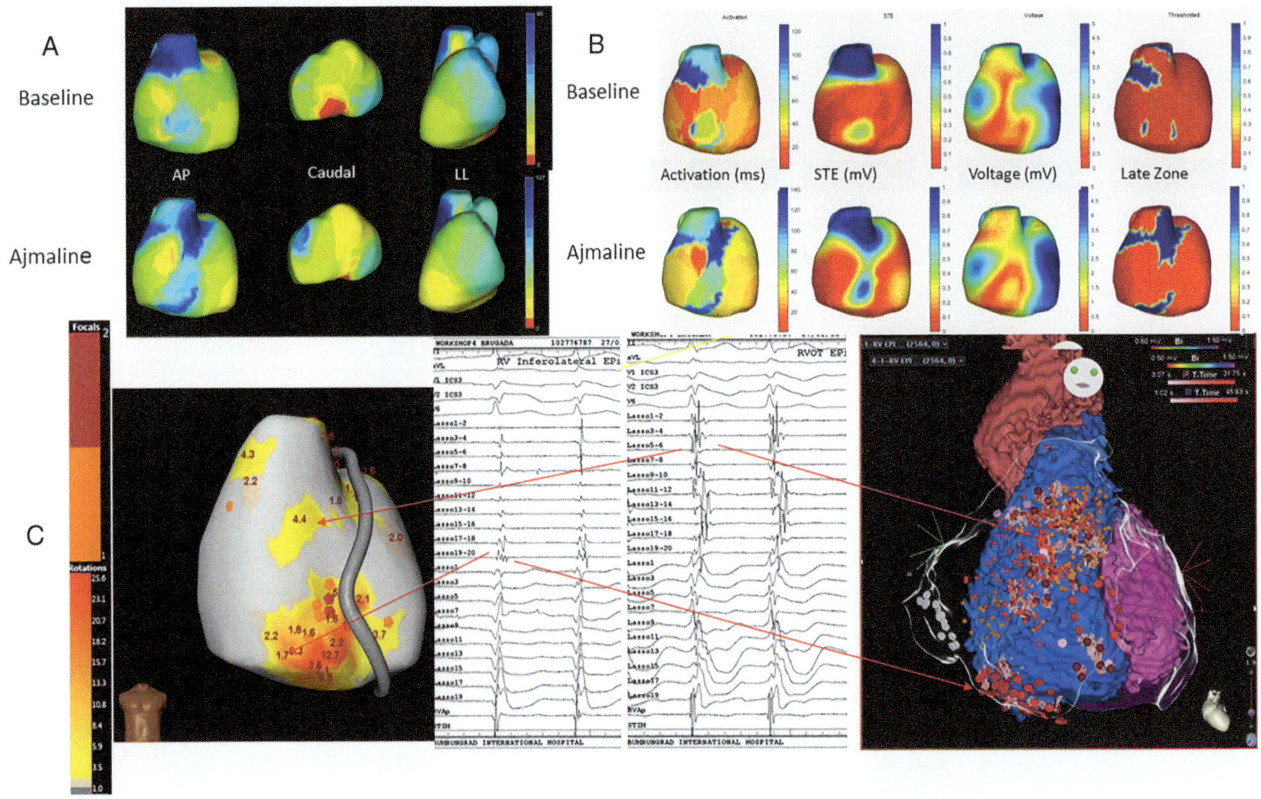

Fig. 39.6 (A) Electrocardiographic imaging (ECGI) activation map at baseline and after ajmaline administration; it shows three views of the biventricular ECGI activation map: anterior posterior (AP), bottom view (caudal), and left lateral (LL). The earliest activation is in *red,* and the latest is in *dark blue.* Note that the latest activation is at the right ventricular outflow tract (RVOT) and RV inferior areas, whereas the earliest is at the septum; there was clear slow conduction in the RVOT). (B) Biventricular maps of activation time, ST elevation (STE), voltage, and areas of the late-activated area before and after ajmaline during sinus rhythm in this patient. (C) Correlation between areas that harbor late fractionated potentials and ventricular fibrillation (VF) drivers. *Left,* Composite map of VF driver; the *shaded areas* on the composite map represent rotational activities, and the numbers on the ECGI map represent the number of rotations at each point on the heart as recorded at 5 seconds of a VF episode. The *colored hexagons* represent the number and location of epicardial focal breakthroughs. *Right inset,* Electroanatomical map is shown in the anteroposterior (AP) view. *Middle,* Tracings recorded from the RV inferior and RVOT epicardium show abnormal fractionated potential at the same sites as VF drivers and ablation sites (*red arrows*). The tracings are organized in the following fashion: top four are L1, aVL, V_1, and V_2 positioned at the third intercostal space (V1ICS3 and V2 ICS3, respectively) followed by 10 bipolar recordings from the Lasso catheter and the unipolar recordings from the Lasso poles 1, 3, 5, 7, 9, 11, 13, 15, 17, and 19. *Left middle tracing inset,* Recordings from the RV inferior epicardium, exhibiting fractionated signals from the bipolar recordings from the Lasso 17–18 and 19–20. *Other middle tracing inset,* Recordings from the RVOT epicardium, showing abnormal fractionated late electrograms in all bipolar and unipolar recordings. *Red dots* on the electroanatomical maps represent VF substrates that harbor abnormal fractionated electrograms. *Small pink dots* are the areas where RF applications were delivered. Note that this patient had extensive epicardial substrates from the RVOT, RV body, and RV inferior wall.

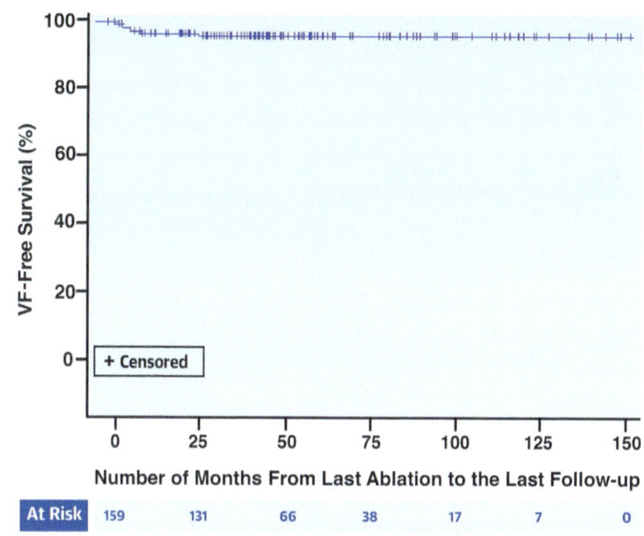

Fig. 39.7 A cumulative ventricular fibrillation–free survival Kaplan-Meier plot after the last ablation. (Reproduced from Nademanee K, Chung FP, Sacher F, et al. Long-term outcomes of Brugada substrate ablation: a report from BRAVO (Brugada ablation of VF Substrate Ongoing Multicenter Registry). *Circulation.* 2023;147. doi:10.1161/CIRCULATIONAHA.122.063367.)

remained free of VF recurrences. The number of patients free of VF recurrences increased to 153 (96%) after a repeat procedure (mean 1.2 ± 0.5 procedures, median 1), with a mean follow-up period of 48 ± 29 months from the last ablation. Fig. 39.7 shows the Kaplan-Meier VF-free survival beyond 5 years after the last ablation was 95%. Multivariable analysis showed that the only variable associated with a VF-free outcome was normalization of the Type 1 Brugada ECG, after the ablation (hazard ratio [HR] 0.078, 95% confidence interval [CI] 0.008–0.753; $P = .0274$). There were no arrhythmic or cardiac deaths. Complications included hemopericardium in 4 (2.5%) patients. The only patient who had VF recurrence after normalization of Brugada ECG pattern after ablation has combined BrS and ER syndromes (ERS).

COMBINED SYNDROME OF BRS AND ERS

A combined Brugada and early repolarization ECG pattern either in the inferior leads (II, III, and aVF) or lateral leads (V_4–V_6) or both inferior and lateral leads—the so-called J-wave syndrome—is not uncommon, especially in Southeast Asia.[18] Several studies in the past decade show that these overlapping features of BrS and ERS increased risk of recurrent VT/VF to a level higher than that posed by BrS alone.[21–24]

The combined BrS and ERS subset also presents a more difficult task than does pure BrS for catheter ablation, as VF recurrence rate after ablation is higher than that of BrS alone. This is likely because of larger substrates in the combined syndrome than those of BrS alone. In addition to the RVOT substrate sites, the combined syndrome patients commonly have substrates at the RV inferior wall and RV inferolateral areas close to the tricuspid annulus.[18]

CONCLUSION

Three decades have passed since BrS was introduced, and much has been learned about the pathophysiology of the syndrome. We have made major strides in advancing our understanding and management of the syndrome: Catheter ablation of the BrS substrates is clearly the most effective treatment modality for VF prevention in BrS. Recently, several patients who had been free of VF for several years and no longer wanted an ICD or did not want a replacement device at the end of the current ICD's battery life requested that the device be taken out. Similarly, new symptomatic Brugada patients who sought ablation treatment did not want an ICD implanted after the ablation.

However, it would be premature based on the data available to recommend catheter ablation alone without an ICD for symptomatic BrS patients, especially those who survived aborted sudden cardiac death. One also has to be mindful that BrS is part of J-wave syndrome that includes "early repolarization" syndrome, and often the two syndromes coexist. This combined BrS and early repolarization syndrome has a higher rate of VF recurrences after ablation; thus, many of those with J-wave syndrome will continue to need ICD backup. This would lead us to hypothesize that symptomatic BrS patients who have no overlapping syndrome could avoid ICD after substrate ablation if normalization of the right precordial ECG at the higher ICS lead positioning after sodium channel blocker challenge could be achieved. To address this hypothesis, we are carrying out a randomized clinical trial, Brugada Syndrome Ablation for the prevention of VF Episodes (BRAVE study, ClinicalTrials.gov NCT02704416). Once this trial is completed, it is very likely that we will have the answer as to whether we can treat symptomatic BrS patients without an ICD.

REFERENCES

Please refer to the e-book for a complete list of references.

40

Catheter Ablation of Ventricular Tachycardia in Arrhythmogenic Right Ventricular Cardiomyopathy

Alessio Gasperetti, Harikrishna Tandri

KEY POINTS

- Electroanatomical substrate in arrhythmogenic right ventricular cardiomyopathy is often epicardial.
- Ventricular tachycardia focus frequently localizes to the basal peritricuspid region in the right ventricle.
- Late potentials are frequently identified during sinus rhythm activation mapping, indicating areas of conduction slowing and unidirectional block.
- Catheter ablation, especially epicardial ablation, is associated with good long-term arrhythmia-free survival.
- Recurrences are not uncommon, and neuraxial modulation such as sympathectomy may be required in refractory patients.

INTRODUCTION

Arrhythmogenic right ventricular cardiomyopathy (ARVC) is an inherited desmosomal myopathy[1] characterized by progressive fibrofatty replacement of the myocardium, right ventricular (RV) enlargement, and malignant ventricular arrhythmias (VAs).[2–5] Several pathogenic desomosomal mutations have been reported in the last decade, and genotype–phenotype association has been systematically described, with specific desmosomal genes associated with early left ventricular (LV) involvement.[6–9]

Ventricular arrhythmias are a hallmark of arrhythmogenic RV cardiomyopathy. Frequent premature ventricular contractions (PVCs) and recurrent ventricular tachycardia (VT) may be seen in all stages of the disease and are associated with a significant risk of arrhythmic sudden cardiac death (SCD).[10] Current guidelines, therefore, recommend implantable cardioverter-defibrillator (ICD) placement in selected patients with ARVC,[11] especially those meeting Task Force criteria. Device therapy due to sustained VT and/or ventricular fibrillation (VF) is not uncommon, and in patients who fail antiarrhythmic medical therapy, catheter ablation (CA) has been shown to reduce VT burden and ICD shocks.[12,13] CA has been also proposed as an alternative to ICD implantation, especially when a device is either unavailable or undesirable,[14,15] but a definite consensus on whether CA could completely replace the need for ICDs is yet to be reached. Despite a reasonable success rate of CA, VT recurrence often occurs, and repeat procedures are not rare. In our experience, a third of the patients require more than one procedure, especially if the initial procedure was an endocardial-only approach. Nonetheless, CA is increasingly used for the management of patients with ARVC. Recent technological advances, as well as a better understanding of the pattern of cardiac scaring and an expanded role of epicardial ablation strategies, have led to improved long-term results and safer risk profiles. In this chapter, we aim to address the overall concepts of epicardial CA in ARVC, focusing on substrate characterization and ablation strategies.

SUBSTRATE FORMATION: ARRHYTHMOGENESIS AND DISEASE PHENOTYPE

The roles of inflammation and apoptosis are increasingly being recognized in ARVC and may precede phenotypic changes by several years. Myocyte apoptosis, postinflammatory fibrosis, and nonuniform fibrofatty infiltration result in a mosaic of healthy myocytes admixed in electrically inactive areas, forming a complex substrate of electrical heterogeneity.[16,17] As the disease progresses, large areas of fibrosis result in ventricular dysfunction and right heart failure. Therefore, clinical presentation varies along the course of the disease, with a wide spectrum of clinical stages, including a concealed phase (no overt structural disease), early disease phase (most commonly found and usually associated with ventricular arrhythmias and SCD), and a late disease phase (with either RV failure or biventricular failure).[18]

Frequent PVCs (monomorphic or polymorphic) in the absence of detectable structural changes on conventional imaging are often the earliest manifestations of the disease. PVCs mostly arise from the RV free wall or the floor of the RV, demonstrating a superior axis, although PVCs from the RV tract are not uncommon. Nonsustained VT can be observed especially during or shortly after exertion in the cooldown phase. As the disease progresses, fibrosis ensues, leading to formation of slow conducting channels that support sustained monomorphic VT. Risk of VF appears to be greater in the early phase of the disease, and it is not uncommon for the first presentation to be SCA. Later stages of the disease are characterized by monomorphic VTs, which are much more amenable to CA.

SYMPATHETIC MODULATION AND ARRHYTHMOGENESIS IN EARLY ARVC

The sympathetic nervous system plays an important role in arrhythmogenesis in ARVC.[19] Exercise-induced arrhythmias are often seen, and physical exertion is associated with worse phenotype expression and a higher risk of SCD.[20,21] Not surprisingly, sympathetic modulation by either β-blocker therapy, first-line antiarrhythmic therapy in ARVC, or surgical sympathetic denervation in refractory cases is associated with a reduction of VA burden and ICD shocks.[11,22] Mutations of the cardiac ryanodine receptor (RyR2) have been identified in cases of ARVC, suggesting shared mechanisms and triggers with catecholaminergic polymorphic VT (CPVT).[23] In late phases of the disease, however, the influence of sympathetic tone in triggering or maintaining VA appears to be reduced, due probably to substrate expansion and predominance of scar-dependent arrhythmias.[24]

This catecholamine-sensitive nature of VAs in ARVC is partially captured by the response of this disease to isoproterenol challenge tests. An isoproterenol test has been suggested as a potentially effective screening strategy in patients with suspected ARVC.[25] Denis et al. demonstrated that an arrhythmogenic response to infusion of high doses of isoproterenol (45 mg/min) was highly sensitive for the presence of ARVC (sensitivity 91.4%, negative predictive value 99.1%), even in early stages of the cardiomyopathy.[25] Additionally, induction of polymorphic VAs with left bundle branch block (LBBB) morphology during isoproterenol infusion, without any other identified or recognized structural heart disease, was reported as strongly suggestive of ARVC. Furthermore, Philips et al. originally reported a high degree of association between the morphology of sustained VTs induced during isoproterenol infusion (20 mg/min) and PVCs presented at baseline. Mapping and ablation of baseline PVCs eliminated the VTs with the same morphology, all originating from the RVOT and RV basal regions (border zones).[26] In this study, a high PVC burden during isoproterenol infusion was also associated with shorter VT-free survival after CA, regardless of the approach used (endocardial or endoepicardial).[27] At the same time, however, multiple limitations in the routine use of isoproterenol have been reported as well. The findings reported by Denis at al. have a relatively low specificity, partially hindering the diagnostic role of isoproterenol challenge in an all-comer population, and is a reason why its diagnostic role is not universally accepted and currently not included in the diagnostic criteria for ARVC. However, this may have prognostic significance and identify high-risk subjects who might benefit from ICD implantation.[28]

SUBSTRATE DISTRIBUTION: PATTERNS OF SCAR AND IMPLICATIONS ON ELECTROANATOMICAL MAPPING

As previously discussed, substrate expansion represents the main trigger of electrical progression of ARVC. The vast majority of VAs observed during advanced phases of the disease are in fact scar dependent and represent a good target for CA procedures.[24] The scar distribution, however, as well as the scar characteristics, are not uniform during disease evolution, and an adequate visualization of electrical substrate has strong implications in patients' management.

Technological advances in image assessment and electrical characterization of the substrate, as well as a higher sensitivity of diagnostic screening in early ARVC, have provided important insights into recognition of scar distribution (patterns) along the course of the disease. The original concept of scar distribution (the "triangle of dysplasia")[2] postulated a typical disease involvement of the RV outflow tract (RVOT) and inflow tract, the basal inferior wall, and the apex. More recent studies with CMR, later corroborated by electroanatomical mapping (EAM) techniques, showed how the apical involvement is rare in early stages of the disease, pointing instead toward the presence of a significant disease substrate in the anterior RV and in the LV posterolateral wall.[6,9,29,30] The current paradigm of substrate distribution therefore points toward early disease preferentially affecting the basal inferior area of the RV, advancing then to the basal anterior segment with time, and causing a global RV impairment in severe, advanced forms of ARVC (Fig. 40.1). The peritricuspid RV area is extensively affected, often presenting with areas of low-amplitude potentials and late potentials during sinus rhythm on EAM. Similar voltage and conduction characteristics are observed in the posterolateral basal wall of the LV. These areas may represent either a hallmark of advanced disease in case of a right-dominant form of ARVC or a precocious sign of structural alteration in those left-dominant phenotypes (i.e., those associated with a mutation in the desmoplakin gene [*DSP*]).[7,9] In the former case, a reduction of the RV function is to be expected, while most left-dominant phenotypes have been reported as with a preserved LV function.

Understanding scar distribution is crucial to CA in ARVC. Affected regions identified by systematic characterization of the EAM substrate match with regions of myocardial loss, reflecting the replacement of electrically active myocardial tissue by electrically silent fibrofatty tissue.[31,32] Low-voltage and fragmented/prolonged duration electrograms, detected within the scar and its borders, and late potentials are typically observed in RV inferobasal regions (perivalvular tricuspid areas) and in different regions of RV anterobasal, anterolateral, and infundibular walls. Isolated scar in the RVOT and apex as well as interventricular septum involvement appear to be rare in early ARVC. Additional LV epicardial inferolateral free wall involvement has also been described and appears to be more frequent than previously recognized. Importantly, while the vast majority of arrhythmias originates in the RV, an increasing amount

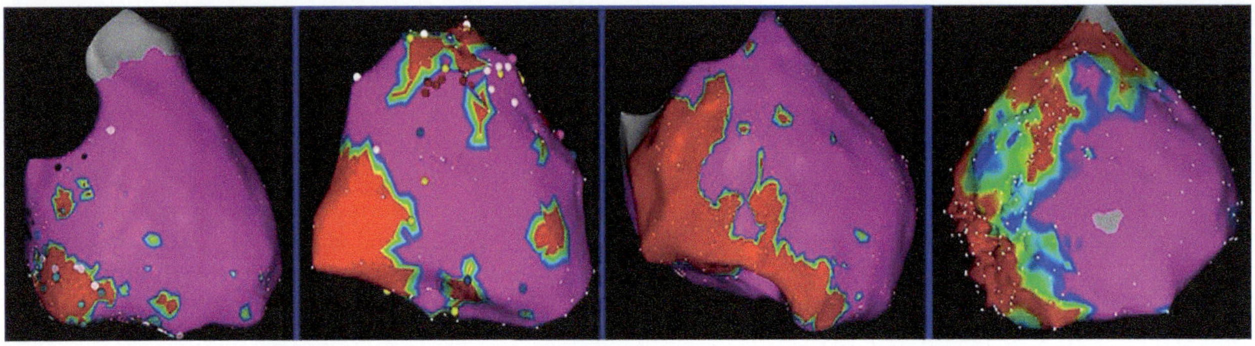

Fig. 40.1 Electroanatomical epicardial scar patterns observed in ARVC. CARTO electroanatomical voltage maps with cutoffs of 1.0 mV for low voltage and 0.5 mV for scar. *Left,* Patient with limited ARVC. Subsequent panels show scar extensions to the anterior wall, inferior wall, and the entire right ventricle.

of arrhythmias with right bundle branch morphology has been reported. The most common origin of those arrhythmias, however, has still been recognized as within the RV.[33,34]

When discussing substrate in ARVC, it is important to address not only the localization of the arrhythmic substrate (RV versus LV localization) but also the depth of its involvement. The scarring process seems to progress from the epicardium toward the endocardium gradually, with epicardial electroanatomical substrate usually predominating over endocardial.[16,18] The presence of epicardial electrical abnormality areas extending beyond the underlying endocardial electrical substrate and the identification of large epicardial scar with minimal endocardial involvement in early disease have been consistently reported.[6,12,27,35,36] This is of crucial importance while planning CA and defining ablation targets, as exclusive endocardial mapping and ablation may result in low success rates. Furthermore, by virtue of this centripetal scarring process, intramyocardial involvement is not rare and may affect procedure outcomes, as technical limitations may obviate the successful ablation of such circuits.

THE ROLE OF ENDOCARDIAL MAPPING AND ABLATION IN ARVC

Despite the growing number of epicardial interventions, the endocardial assessment remains a key step while defining the electroanatomical substrate in ARVC. Systematic voltage mapping of the endocardial surface should be primarily obtained in sinus rhythm, when feasible, and special attention must be drawn to collecting points in the peritricuspid valve region and anterior RVOT. High-density electroanatomical mapping over a larger area results in a more precise delineation of electrical scar and its surroundings. Adequate contact is critical during RV mapping, as the RV endocardial surface is heavily trabeculated, and voltage abnormalities may be exaggerated due to the inability to reach the wall, which is especially true when mapping with multielectrode catheters. Contiguous bipolar electrogram voltage abnormalities (<1.5 mV) are registered, and low-voltage areas (LVAs; <0.5 mV) represent dense scar, as validated in the literature.[17,37]

At our center, after delineating the endocardial scar, pace mapping is performed to replicate the morphology of clinical VT from the borders of the defined endocardial scar. Twelve-lead ECG documentation of VT morphology is critical, especially when mapping unstable VTs. Areas of long stimulus to QRS (S-QRS) and paced morphology similar to clinical VT are marked as possible participants in the VT circuit. VT can be briefly induced, mapped, and entrained from the scar, even if it is not tolerated, in order to get a glimpse of the participation of the endocardial surface in the VT circuit.

In the early stages of the disease, endocardial scar may be minimal or not even detectable at bipolar voltage mapping. Herein, obtaining a unipolar voltage mapping may provide valuable information regarding both presence and extension of epicardial scar, given the recognized association between unipolar endocardium LVAs (<5.5 mV) and epicardial scar.[36,38] Failure to obtain a decent pace map match through the endocardial surface also suggests the participation of subepicardial circuit. Nevertheless, it is worth mentioning that the identification of epicardial substrate does not preclude the need for endocardial ablation for procedural success as mid-myocardial circuits may be eliminated from the endocardial surface.[39] As a rare disease, most reports come from single-center studies or pooled data from tertiary centers with a high volume of epicardial procedures, and thereby, the role of endocardial ablation may be underestimated. Hence, some centers have suggested that systematic, upfront epicardial ablation may not be necessary for all patients, especially when considering the risk associated with the procedure.[13,38] Along the same lines, recent clinical studies have reported the role of a stepwise approach for CA of VT in ARVC, wherein only patients who failed a prior endocardial procedure underwent epicardial ablation.[40] In our center, when investigating patients who had their first CA performed locally, although epicardial ablation was performed in around 64% of patients, endocardial ablation alone was not associated with worse outcomes or lower VT-free survival rate.[41] Multiple indicators suggest the existence or participation of a subepicardial circuit. Prior failed endocardial ablation, VT ECG morphology, identification of islands of epicardial scar at cardiac imaging, limited electroanatomical substrate in the endocardium, lack of a good pace map while stimulating potential target areas along the endocardial surface, and failure to eliminate the VT after endocardial mapping and ablation collectively favor the value of epicardial assessment. Nevertheless, these findings should not be considered independently as none of them have been individually linked to better acute or long-term outcomes.

PERICARDIAL ACCESS

The use of percutaneous access into the pericardial space for ablative purposes was originally described by Sosa et al.[42] Since then, as a result of an improved understanding of the ARVC substrate, the technique has grown in importance as an ablation strategy and has been reported in up to two-thirds of the procedures.[13] Preprocedural contrast-enhanced multidetector computed tomography (MDCT) or CMR should be obtained for all patients to define thoracic anatomy and anticipate local anatomical constraints that might complicate or obviate access or even catheter manipulation inside the pericardial space. Of note, anticoagulation must be held before the procedure following drug-specific protocols.

In our institution, we use an anterior approach to obtain epicardial access in all patients undergoing epicardial ablation (Fig. 40.2).[43] An epidural introducer needle is inserted through a small subxiphoid puncture at a 20-degree angle; under biplane fluoroscopy guidance, the needle is carefully advanced through a shallow path toward the anterior aspect of RV silhouette. Once the needle has approached the pericardium, a small amount of contrast is injected to confirm pericardium tenting. The needle is then further advanced, and the pericardium space is accessed. Additional contrast is injected to reassure location, which is followed by the insertion of a 0.035-inch Bentson J-tipped floppy guidewire (Cook Medical, Bloomington, IN) into the pericardial space. The guidewire should freely travel inside the pericardial space, wrapping around the heart across multiple chambers. After access is established and confirmed, a long deflectable sheath is advanced over the guidewire into the pericardial space. This anterior and superficial approach allows for safer access to anterior and basal regions of both ventricles, as it avoids the interventricular groove and reduces the odds of vascular injury. In addition, the shallow path across thoracoabdominal transition reduces the risk of hepatic or bowel laceration. Periodic pericardial aspiration should be performed, and clear fluid indicates absence of myocardial injury. Pericardial drain is normally not required unless hemorrhagic fluid is observed after the end of the procedure and active bleeding is suspected. Some degree of pericarditis is uniformly reported after epicardial ablation. The extent of pericarditis is associated with several factors, including trauma to the epicardial surface, blood in the pericardium, and the extent of epicardial ablation. Since pericarditis is the most frequent untoward result of epicardial ablative therapy across several studies,[44] postprocedural anti-inflammatory medication and/or colchicine is advised. In our center, we systematically inject methylprednisolone (125 mg) into the pericardial space, as it is associated with a reduction of the extent of pericarditis after extensive ablations.[45]

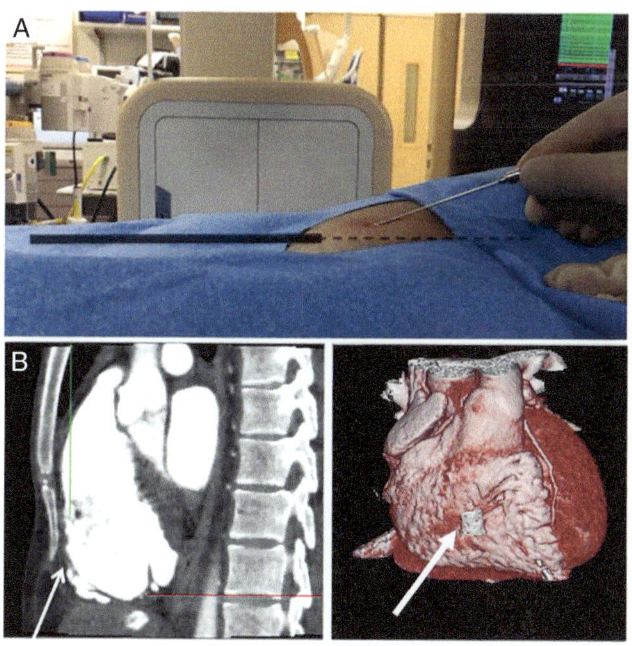

Fig. 40.2 Anterior epicardial access. (A) An epidural introducer needle is inserted through a small dermatomy, at a 20-degree angle, toward the anterior RV silhouette (*black line* = xyphoid process). (B) Thoracic computed tomography illustrating the anterior and superficial path to be followed by the needle (*white arrow*). As noted, there is a fair window between the xyphoid process and the diaphragm.

Pericardial Space: Anatomical Peculiarities

Full understanding of local anatomy is mandatory before manipulating the pericardial space (see Chapter 6). Awareness of surrounding structures and nuances of the pericardial space is fundamental to avoid complications and optimize ablation results. Access to pericardial space entails a risk of coronary injury due to trauma caused by catheter/sheath manipulation or while ablating the nearby sites. A coronary angiogram may be required to accurately define the distance between coronary arteries and the ablation site, which appears relatively safe when >1 cm.

Fat distribution along the epicardial surface must be carefully considered while mapping and ablating epicardially. Epicardial fat is primarily distributed along basal RV (perivalvar region) and extends over the proximal course of the left anterior descending artery (LAD) along the interventricular septum, the left atrial appendage, and the AV groove from the crux cordis to the basal lateral wall. Evaluation of epicardial fat thickness is also important, since it may attenuate voltage readings, with most reports supporting 4- to 5-mm thickness as a critical threshold value.[46–48] Additionally, RF application efficacy can be reduced or rendered ineffective due to epicardial fat thickness and dampening effect. Imaging methods such as computed tomography (CT) or CMR can be used for not only preprocedural evaluation (access strategy) but also the identification of regions of dense epicardial fat (mapping and ablation strategies). In that sense, image integration (CT/CMR and three-dimensional electroanatomical mapping) permits enhanced real-time appreciation of valuable anatomical features during electroanatomical mapping construction and assessment, such as scar distribution, channel delineation, epicardial fat spreading, and coronary artery locations.

EPICARDIAL ELECTROANATOMICAL MAPPING AND ABLATION STRATEGIES

Complex subepicardial and mid-myocardial circuits often participate in arrhythmogenesis in ARVC. Segmented and delayed activations within those regions provide the environment for independent VT circuits to occur, wherein the inability to create deep lesions from the endocardial surface is considered one of the central reasons leading to failed endocardial-only ablation.[42] This is particularly demonstrated by the negative relationship between the thickness of the basal wall and efficacy of the ablation lesions.[35]

Electroanatomical mapping of RV endocardium and biventricular epicardium has been increasingly used in most experienced centers. The techniques of epicardial mapping and ablation used in ARVC are not different from those used in other nonischemic cardiomyopathies. Detailed biventricular epicardium mapping allows for an extensive assessment of scar and its borders, wherein bipolar voltage >1.0 mv identifies normal myocardium.[49] The unique pattern of scar distribution in the peritricuspid region, especially in the basal inferior RV, results in reentrant circuits and, hence, superior axis VTs with late precordial transition in V_4 and V_5. Late potentials well after the QRS are frequently observed during sinus rhythm, and detailed pace mapping in this scar is often valuable in determining potential exit sites of reentrant VTs (Fig. 40.3). Multiple VT morphologies often share the same circuit (different exit sites), and channels in the basal scar are commonly involved (Fig. 40.4). Inferior axis VTs are most often related to the epicardial scar in the anterior RVOT. Careful annotation of late potentials and recording the EGMs that represent the AV groove are critical for planning ablation in ARVC. Epicardial scar often extends to the AV groove, and ablation in this region also carries a risk of injury to the right coronary artery. Further, the AV groove host a variable but often significant amount of epicardial fat, which may affect mapping quality and ablation results. Some electrogram features can help differentiate low-voltage electrograms associated with diseased myocardium from those derived from fat. Longer (>80 ms; specificity 99%) and more fractionated (≥5 deflections, sensitivity 95%; ≥8 deflections, specificity 92%) electrograms were able to discriminate myocardial scar, especially when found in combination. The presence of late potentials was highly specific for scar (99%), while bipolar low-voltage signals alone were not able to differentiate epicardial scar from fat. Unipolar voltage maps, however, appear not to be impaired by fat distribution and may be superior to identify scar swathed by fat.[50]

Although techniques of pace mapping and entrainment mapping are similar in ARVC compared to other cardiomyopathies, the importance of substrate-guided ablation cannot be overemphasized in ARVC. Isochronal late activation maps (ILAMs) during sinus rhythm and RV pacing are frequently useful in demonstrating areas of slow conduction and are often targeted for substrate-based ablation strategies (Fig. 40.5). After ablation of critical VT circuits, special attention should be devoted to systematically ablate all late potentials in the epicardial scar. Large isthmuses are often found in moderate-severe ARVC and may impair a good pace map match. In this case, linear lesions

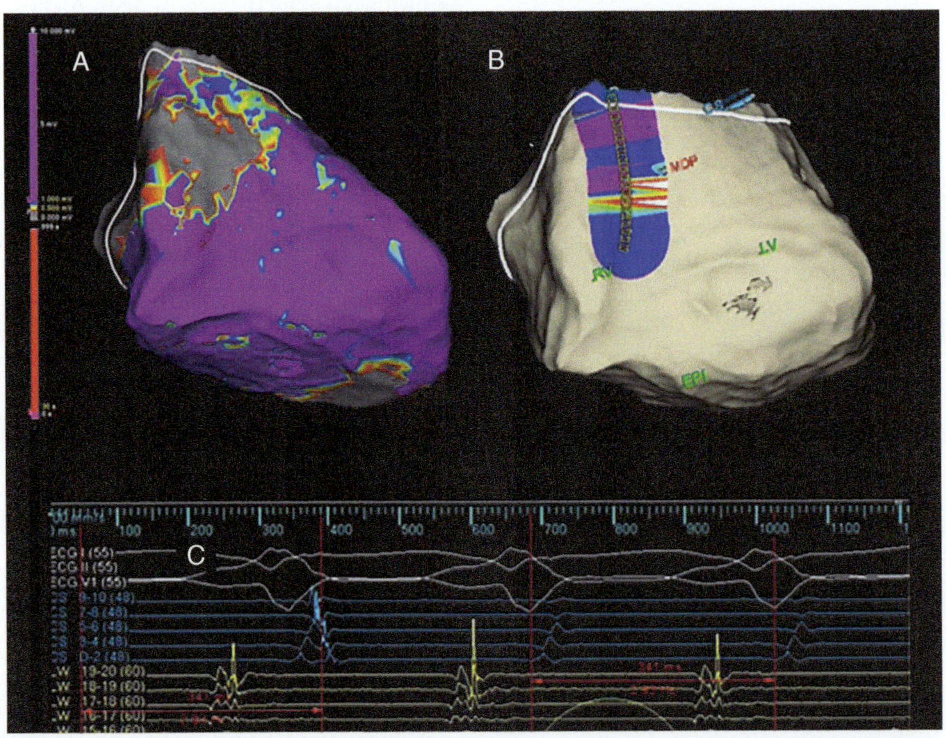

Fig. 40.3 Ensite electroanatomical epicardial voltage maps of a patient with sustained VT. Voltage cutoffs are 1.5 mV for low voltage and 0.5 mV for scar. (A) Pattern of activation through the epicardial scar during VT in a patient with ARVC. (B) Entire diastolic interval is included in the linear mapping catheter.

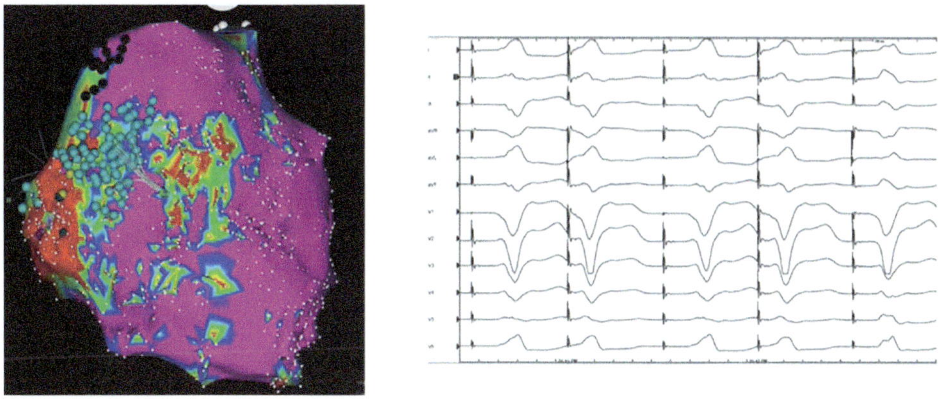

Fig. 40.4 Pace mapping within the scar demonstrates multiple exit sites that can be potential VT morphologies from the same isthmus.

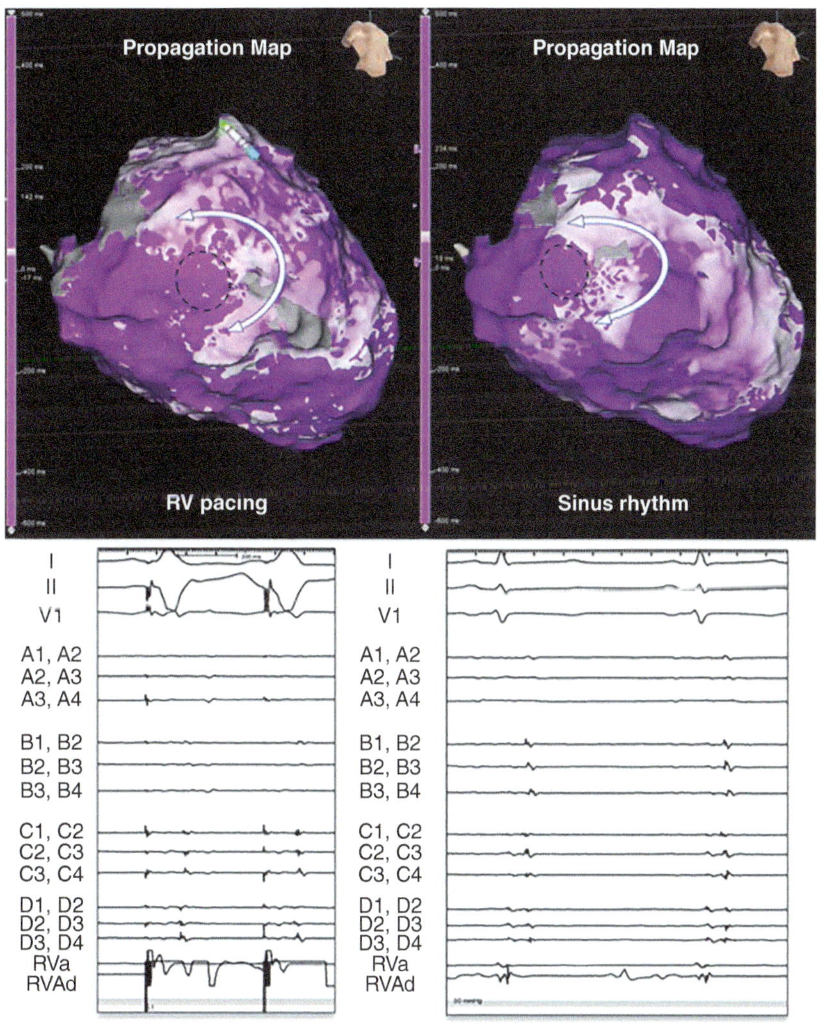

Fig. 40.5 Activation mapping during RV pacing (*left*) and sinus rhythm (*right*) showing conduction slowing around the scar border with activation around the scar. Unidirectional block within this region precedes onset of sustained ventricular tachycardia.

through isthmus or diastolic pathway, extended to valvular anatomical boundaries, scar, or preserved myocardium should be performed to achieve efficient substrate modification.

Noninducibility during programmed stimulation well after the ablation has been associated with better arrhythmic outcomes, especially when performed following isoproterenol infusion.[51–54] Mapping and systematic ablation of residual PVCs are also undertaken at some centers.[55] However, the effect of this strategy on overall outcomes remains unclear.

COMPLICATIONS

The growing importance of epicardial mapping and ablation in CA of VT has led to a consistent increase in the number of epicardial procedures performed worldwide, but the complication rates associated with the procedure remain relatively high compared to endocardial ablation alone. Pericarditis without pericardial effusion is the most frequent postoperative consequence of epicardial access, reported in up to 20–30% of patients.[44,56] Major complications occur in 4–10% of patients and often include pericardial tamponade, persistent bleeding, extensive pericardial inflammation, coronary injury, and acute myocardial infarction.[56–58] In a recent study including 100 consecutive epicardial procedures, our group reported the feasibility and safety of using an anterior approach to access the pericardium space. In this series, successful epicardial access was obtained in all patients without significant pericardial bleeding (> 80 mL), RV puncture, or need for emergent cardiac surgery. Although self-limited pericarditis was seen in all patients in this series, only two subjects required colchicine at discharge.[59] Less common complications, such as liver puncture, RV pseudoaneurysm, coronary sinus laceration, and pleuropericardial fistulas, have been also reported.[60,61] Epicardial ablation in LV free wall is associated with the risk of phrenic nerve injury, and high-voltage stimulation while mapping those regions is recommended to identify high-risk sites. In this setting, displacement of the nerve by using different strategies, such as angioplasty balloon, saline infusion, or both, has been described with variable results.[62]

OUTCOMES OF EPICARDIAL ABLATIONS IN ARVC

Several studies have consistently reported the growing importance of epicardial ablation in ARVC over the past decade. Though VT-free survival rates after ablation vary across different studies (ranging between 35% and 85%; Table 40.1), a combined endoepicardial approach has been associated with better long-term results, especially in patients who failed a prior endocardial-only ablation. Garcia et al., in a small study including 13 patients who failed endocardial VT ablation, showed that a combined endoepicardial approach rendered 77% of patients free of VT recurrence over a mean follow-up of 18 months.[35] This was then corroborated by the findings of Bai et al., who investigated the long-term results of CA in 49 ARVC patients and reported a lower VA recurrence rate associated with the combined strategy compared to endocardial-only ablation (84.6 versus 52.2%; $P < .001$).[27] Our group, in a study of 30 consecutive ARVD/C patients who underwent an epi-endo ablative strategy, reported a long-term VT-free survival of 70% (24 months) with 69% of VT critical circuits located on the epicardial surface.[12] In a recent meta-analysis including 258 patients with ARVC, a combined endoepicardial ablation was associated with lower VT recurrence rates, although it did not affect mortality compared to endocardial-only procedures.[56,63]

Although existent data suggest a potential benefit of an early epicardial approach, whether its systematic application as a first-line strategy yields additional benefit is still to be determined. Berruezo et al. investigated the role of a combined endoepicardial ablation as first-line therapy and reported low VT recurrence rates (26.8%) over a mean follow-up of 32 months. Those results, however, did not prevent the authors from suggesting that an upfront epicardial ablation may not be required for all patients, as they identified a negative correlation between the area of endocardial scar and epicardial substrate.[38] The identification of an electroanatomical scar pattern where a large endocardial substrate, given by the local bipolar LVAs, coexists with smaller areas of epicardial scar, given by endocardial unipolar-LVA, may indicate a low yield of additional epicardial mapping and ablation, especially when weighing the inherited risks associated with the procedure. Along the same lines, in a study investigating the role of an adjuvant epicardial CA, a combined approach was performed only in cases of recurrent VT or persistent VT inducibility after endocardial ablation;

TABLE 40.1 Outcomes of Catheter Ablation in Arrhythmogenic Right Ventricular Dysplasia

	Year	Patients/ Procedures (n)	Target Surface	Follow-Up Duration (months/years)	Short-Term Results	Long-Term Results and Observations
Marchlinski et al.[17]	2004	21/19	Endo (1 Epi: RBBB VT)	27 ± 22 months	No inducible VT: 73.68%	No VT recurrence: 89%
Verma et al.[66]	2005	22/-	Endo	37 months	No inducible VT: 82%	VT recurrence: 23% (1 year), 27% (2 years), and 47% (3 years)
Dalal et al.[64]	2007	24/48	Endo: No EAM: 38	32 ± 36 months	Complete success: 46% Partial success: 31% Failure: 23%	VT recurrence: 85% Cumulative VT recurrence-free survival: 75% (1.5 months), 50% (5 months), and 25% (14 months) Cumulative incidence of VT recurrence: 64% (1 year), 75% (2 years), and 91% (3 years)

TABLE 40.1 Outcomes of Catheter Ablation in Arrhythmogenic Right Ventricular Dysplasia—*cont'd*

	Year	Patients/ Procedures (n)	Target Surface	Follow-Up Duration (months/years)	Short-Term Results	Long-Term Results and Observations
Garcia et al.[35]	2009	13/—	Endo + Epi	18 ± 13 months	Noninducible monomorphic VT: 85% Eliminated all targeted VT: 92%	No VT recurrence: 77%
Bai et al.[27]	2011	49/—	Endo: Endo + Epi:	3 years	No inducibility of ablated VT or monomorphic sustained VT (endpoint): 100%	Freedom from VAs or ICD therapy: 52.2% (12/23) in G1 (Endo), 84.6% (22/26) in G2 (Epi-Endo), $P < .001$
Berruezo et al.[67]	2012	11/—	Endo + Epi: (scar dechanneling)	11 months	All clinical and induced VTs: 100%	VT recurrence: 9%
Philips et al.[12]	2012	87/175	EAM: 69% procedures Endo: 85% Endo + Epi: 9% Epi: 6%	88 ± 66 months	Clinical VT ablated: 82% Total acute success: 47% Partial acute success: 38% (inducible VTs but not clinical VT) Failure: 15%	Freedom from VT after a single procedure: 47% (1 year), 31% (2 years), 21% (5 years), and 15% (10 years) Freedom from VT after a single Endo CA: 45% (1 year), 29% (2 years), and 19% (5 years) Freedom from VT after a single Epi CA: 64%, 45%, and 45%
Santangeli et al.[13]	2015	62/121	Endo: 37% Endo + Epi (adjuvant): 63%	56 ± 44 months	No inducibility: 77% No inducibility also at NIPS: 86%	VT-free survival: 71% with a single VT episode in additional 15% (9)
Philips et al.[68]	2015	30/—	Endo + Epi	19.7 ± 11.7 months	Total acute success: 87%	VT-free survival: 83% (6 months), 70% (12 months), and 70% (24 months)
Wei et al.[69]	2017	48/70	Endo: 52 (74%) Epi: 18 (26%)	71.4 ± 45.7 months	—	VT-free survival after a single CA: 37.5% VT-free survival after last CA: 56.3% Acute procedural success was associated with longer VT-free survival
Berruezo et al.[38]	2017	41/41	Endo + Epi (1st ablation)	32.2 ± 21.8 months	Total acute success: 90%	VT-recurrence (end of follow-up): 26.8% Left-dominant AC associated with a higher risk of VT recurrence Bi/uni-LVA ratio > 0.23 was associated with limited Epi substrate
Mussigbrodt et al.[40]	2017	45/—	Endo: 23 (51%) Endo + Epi (adjuvant): 22 (49%)	31.1 ± 27.4 months	Total acute success: 84%	VT-free survival (Endo-only): 56.5% VT-free survival (Endo + Epi): 59.1% Inducibility-guided ablation strategy yielded similar long-term results regardless of the approach (Endo or Endo + Epi)
Laredo et al.[70]	2019	23/24	Endo: Epi: 17%	3.9 years (1 month–10 years)	Total acute success: 46%	VT-free survival: 75% (12 months) not predicted long-term survival

Continued

TABLE 40.1 Outcomes of Catheter Ablation in Arrhythmogenic Right Ventricular Dysplasia—*cont'd*

	Year	Patients/ Procedures (n)	Target Surface	Follow-Up Duration (months/years)	Short-Term Results	Long-Term Results and Observations
Mathew et al.[71]	2019	47/81	Endo: 52 (74%) Epi: 18 (26%)	50.8 (18.6, 99.2 months)	Total acute success: 80% Partial success: 16%	VT/VF-free survival after index CA: 36% (end of follow-up) VT/VF-free survival after multiple CA: 63% (1 year), 45% (5 years) 36% of patients underwent only endocardial CA
Mahida et al.[72]	2019	77/77	Endo: 47% Epi: 53%	3 ± 4.2 years	—	VT-free survival after the last CA: 56% (3 years) VT-free survival after the last CA (at least 1 Endo-Epi): 71% VT-free survival after the last CA (Endo-only): 47% No difference in VT-free survival was observed when comparing a single CA vs. AAD escalation
Daimee et al.[41]	2019	116/166	Endo: 36.1% Epi + Endo: 63.9%	5.2 ± 3.2 years	Total acute success: 95.8% Partial success: 4.2%	VT-free survival after first CA: 68.6% (1 year), 62.4% (2 years), and 49.8% (5 years) VT-free after last CA: 81.8% (1 year), 76.8% (2 years), and 69.6% (5 years)

AAD, antiarrhythmic drug; *CA*, catheter ablation; *EAM*, electroanatomic mapping; *Endo*, endocardial; *Epi*, epicardial; *ICD*, implantable cardioverter-defibrillator; *RBBB*, right bundle branch block; *VA*, ventricular arrhythmia; *VF*, ventricular fibrillation; *VT*, ventricular tachycardia.

endoepicardial ablation was required in 63% of patients, with an overall VT-free survival rate of 71% (mean follow-up of 56 months).[13] In our institution, while using a similar strategy, approximately two-thirds of patients underwent epicardial ablation during the first ablation procedure, and no significant difference in VT-free or ICD shock survival was observed when comparing both strategies (endocardial versus epicardial).[41]

It is worth mentioning that, besides the improved short- and long-term VT-free outcomes, VT ablation also reduces the need for antiarrhythmic drugs and ICD interventions. Though redo procedures are not rare, the value of multiple procedures is still debatable. Although early studies have failed to prove the existence of a cumulative benefit on VT-free survival rates associated with repeat procedures,[12,64] recent data seem to suggest a further reduction of VA burden after subsequent ablations.[41,65]

PERSPECTIVES

Despite the growing number of patients with ARVC undergoing epicardial CA ablation and the improving outcomes in the past decade, recurrence is not rare, and CA remains a palliative procedure in this population. The efficacy of CA in some genotype-specific forms of the disease, including biventricular disease patterns with significant LV cardiomyopathy (desmoplakin and phospholamban subtypes), has not been yet evaluated. Disease progression and the role of substrate expansion in VT recurrence are questions still unanswered. Ultra-high-density mapping of the scar along with new image integration tools may allow for targeted ablation of conducting channels (scar dechanneling) instead of extensive substrate ablation.

While scar-related reentrant VT in late ARVC is well understood, the role of CA in rapid adrenergically mediated arrhythmias in early disease remains unclear. Inability to induce the VT in the electrophysiology lab and lack of a defined substrate in the early phase limit the utility of ablative strategies. The excess of catecholamine/exercise-mediated arrhythmias, the sensitivity of the arrhythmias to isoproterenol infusion, and the favorable response to β-blockers highlight the sympathetic dysregulation encountered in ARVC. Neuraxial modulation with bilateral cardiac sympathetic denervation has shown to be beneficial in patients with structural heart disease and refractory VT, and this benefit appears to extend to ARVC patients. In our experience, bilateral cardiac sympathetic denervation significantly reduced the VT burden, the number of ICD shocks, and the need for antiarrhythmic medications in patients who failed a prior VT ablation procedure. This is especially true in young patients with rapid adrenergically mediated ventricular arrhythmias and a high burden of polymorphic PVCs. Nevertheless, further investigation is necessary to define the optimal timing of bilateral cardiac sympathetic denervation and whether different stages of the disease equally benefit from the procedure.

REFERENCES

Please refer to the e-book for a complete list of references.

41

Hybrid Approaches for Catheter Ablation of Ventricular Tachycardia

Wei-Hsin Chung, Justin Hayase, Jason S. Bradfield

KEY POINTS

- The hybrid approach is an important alternative in patients with previous cardiac surgery.
- Current approaches include subxiphoid window, limited anterior thoracotomy, video-assisted thoracoscopy, robotic-assisted, or median sternotomy.
- A thorough preprocedural plan is essential. This includes review of electrocardiography, prior mapping, and advanced imaging data with cardiac magnetic resonance imaging. Preoperative communication between electrophysiologists, surgeons, anesthesiologists, and perfusion teams is critical.
- There is no direct comparison of mapping accuracy between impedance-based and magnetic-based mapping systems and no comparison of outcomes between radiofrequency-based and cryothermal-based ablation strategies.

INTRODUCTION

Catheter ablation for ventricular tachycardia (VT) has evolved from a salvage procedure for VT recurrence to a standard treatment that can reduce hospitalizations and, potentially, mortality when performed appropriately early in the disease course.[1,2] However, the effectiveness of catheter ablation is limited by the accessibility of arrhythmogenic tissue as well as the ability to create adequate lesions and avoid collateral damage. In certain cases, surgical ablation can be performed where catheter ablation may be ineffective; however, this is limited by its invasiveness, prolonged hospital stays, and higher morbidity.[3] The concept of a hybrid surgical approach for arrhythmias emerged initially in the 1970s as a treatment for Wolff-Parkinson-White syndrome.[4] With the development of minimally invasive surgery and high-density mapping, the hybrid approach has evolved into an attractive method for treating highly complex ventricular arrhythmias. We defined *hybrid ablation* as a combination of surgical intervention for access and catheter-based mapping and ablation. In this chapter, the contemporary methods of patient selection, specific procedural considerations, outcomes, and future directions are reviewed.

PATIENT SELECTION

A hybrid approach should be considered when (1) percutaneous epicardial access is expected to be limited or not possible, (2) when a patient is undergoing a concurrent cardiac surgery, such as left ventricular assist device (LVAD) implantation, or (3) when reentry to the left ventricle (LV) via aortic valve and/or mitral valve should be avoided[5] (Fig. 41.1 and Table 41.1).

In 1996, Sosa et al. introduced a percutaneous epicardial approach for patients with Chagas cardiomyopathy associated with VT and opened a new territory of interventional electrophysiology (EP) in VT management.[6] Epicardial ablation is commonly considered in nonischemic cardiomyopathy (e.g., arrhythmogenic cardiomyopathy), which is often characterized by a perivalvular scar or primarily epicardial substrate.[7,8] This is in contrast to ischemic cardiomyopathy, which can generally be targeted with an endocardial-only approach. An important limitation of the percutaneous epicardial approach is the presence of pericardial adhesions, which not only limits access and catheter manipulation but also can lead to intrapericardial bleeding when disrupted. Although limited studies reported feasibility of percutaneous epicardial access in patients with prior cardiac surgery and pericarditis, current expert consensus is to avoid percutaneous access attempts in the postsurgical population due to limited success, limited access to the entire epicardial surface, and associated procedure risks.[9,10] Several case series have reported higher than 20% complication risk associated with percutaneous epicardial access in prior cardiac surgery patients[11,12] (Fig. 41.1D). Complications include coronary artery bypass graft disruption, pericardial bleeding, and intraabdominal bleeding.[9,12–14] Once thought to be the consequence of prior cardiac surgery, pericardial adhesions can also be encountered unexpectedly in 8% of first-time epicardial access during the procedure.[15] Other extracardiac anatomical abnormalities can affect the success of percutaneous access, such as pectus deformity and overlying bowel loops. In such circumstances, surgical ablation can provide a safer and more efficacious strategy.[16–20]

Another important application for hybrid ablation is performing this concurrently with LVAD implantation. Following LVAD surgery, percutaneous epicardial access will be extremely challenging, so this provides a window of opportunity to access the arrhythmic substrate, which may later become inaccessible. The ASSIST-ICD (Determination of Risk Factors of Ventricular

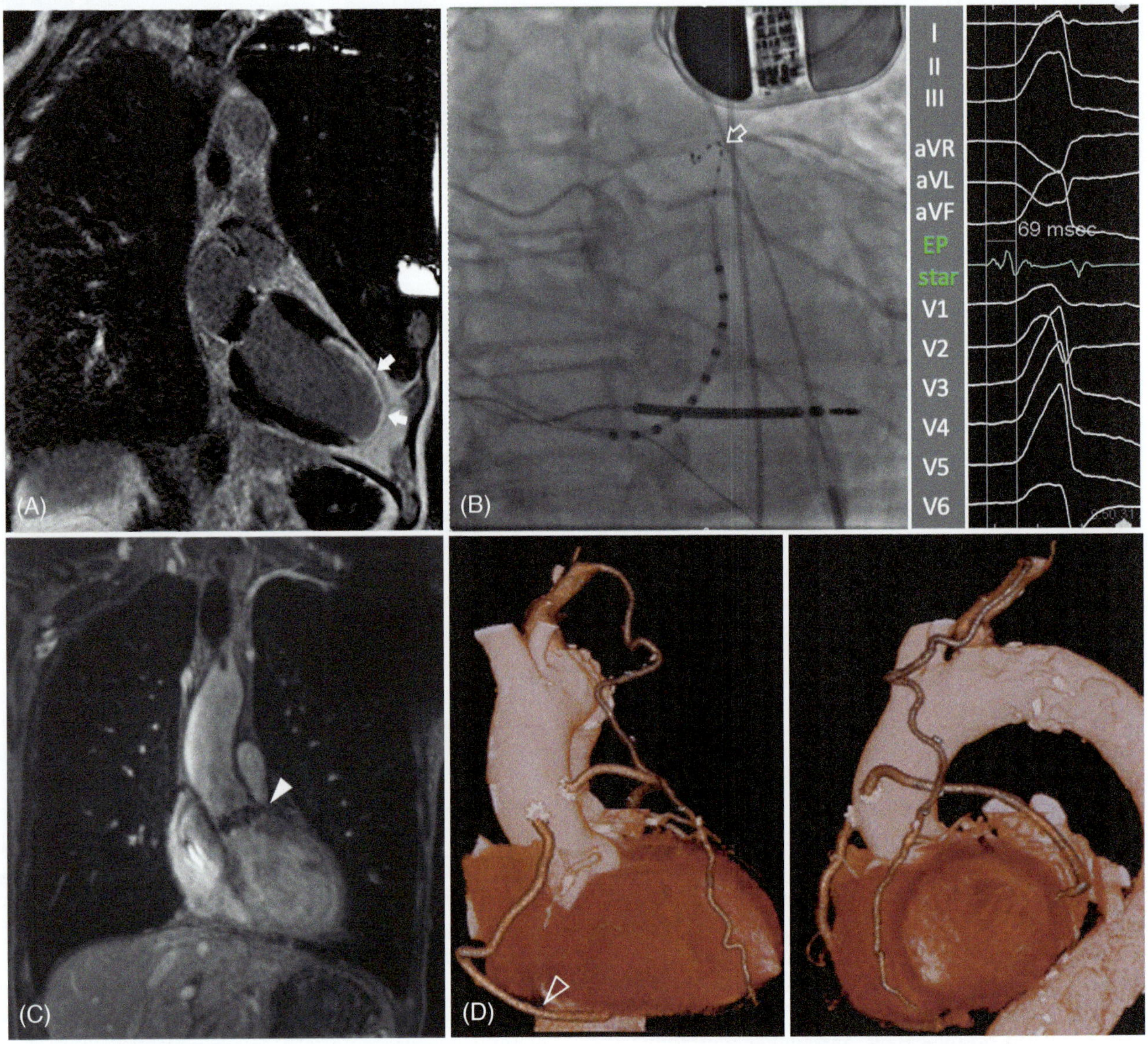

Fig. 41.1 Proposed indications for hybrid ventricular tachycardia ablation. (A) Cardiac magnetic resonance imaging (MRI) showing a large region of transmural delayed enhancement (*arrow*) of the left ventricular (LV) apex. (B) Fluoroscopic image showing an EP-star catheter (Baylis Medical, Fort Worth, TX) within the anterior interventricular vein (*clear arrow*) with early activation time of 69 ms pre-QRS in the region of the LV summit. (C) Cardiac MRI in a patient with prior surgical aortic valve repair (*solid arrowhead*). (D) Three-dimensional computed tomography reconstruction of a patient with prior coronary artery bypass surgery. Note that the graft to the distal right coronary artery (*clear arrowhead*) could be disrupted by percutaneous epicardial access.

TABLE 41.1 Indications for Hybrid Surgical Ablation Procedure and Patient Selection Considerations

Indications/Patient Selection
Epicardial substrate/difficult to reach substrate
– Prior endo/epi attempts
– Failed ablations/intramural substrate
– LV summit
Anticipated pericardial adhesion (prior cardiac surgery, prior failed percutaneous epicardial access attempts)
High-risk percutaneous access (e.g., coronary artery bypass grafts)Concomitant cardiac surgery (e.g., left ventricular assist device)

Arrhythmias After Implantation of Continuous Flow Left Ventricular Assist Device) study demonstrated the potential utility of a risk score, which may help select patient candidates for this approach.[21] The incidence of VT after LVAD implantation was around 28%–52%, which is the second most common postprocedural complication, only secondary to respiratory failure.[22,23] In patients with late ventricular arrhythmias, cardiovascular death accounts for 61.7% of mortality.[21] Further analysis also showed that the short-term mortality after electric storm is high, and 30% of patients will die within 15 days.[24] The challenges of ablation after LVAD implantation are not limited to epicardial access. Endocardial ablation in these patients is affected by difficult retrograde aortic access, suboptimal catheter manipulation in a decompressed LV cavity, physical interactions with the inflow cannula, and electromagnetic interference affecting intracardiac electrogram and three-dimensional (3D) mapping systems.[25] To circumvent these obstacles, Moss et al. performed epicardial substrate mapping and ablation intraoperatively during LVAD implantation and demonstrated the association between a higher burden of low-voltage area on electroanatomical mapping and postimplantation ventricular arrhythmias.[18] Further prospective study is required to examine the benefit of intraoperative or preoperative arrhythmia ablation in patients who are scheduled for LVAD implantation or other cardiac surgery.

Emerging indications for hybrid ablation also include LV summit arrhythmias (Fig. 41.1B) and double-valve replacement (Fig. 41.1C). Catheter ablation of ventricular arrhythmias arising from the LV summit is currently one of the most challenging procedures in clinical EP. This area is bounded by epicardial structures including the left anterior descending artery (LAD), left circumflex artery, and great cardiac vein (GCV) and covered by a thick layer of fat. Current approaches include ablation from adjacent structures including the right ventricular (RV) outflow tract, LV outflow tract, left coronary cusp, or GCV, but the failure rate remains high. There are currently a number of case reports and small case series using a hybrid approach to facilitate visualizing the region by open sternotomy.[26–28] Another emerging approach is totally endoscopic robotic epicardial surgical ablation (TERESA), which uses the DaVinci robot (Intuitive Surgical, Sunnyvale, CA) to directly visualize the LV summit and gain exposure to map and ablate via a chest port[29] (Fig. 41.2D). Further research is warranted to demonstrate the feasibility of these surgical approaches to the treatment of LV summit arrhythmias.

When mapping and ablating the LV endocardium, approaches include atrial transseptal and retrograde aortic approach. However, these approaches are not feasible in the presence of mechanical aortic and mitral valve replacement due to the high risk of catheter entrapment.[10] Other reported approaches include direct percutaneous LV puncture, interventricular puncture, and ethanol ablation.[30–32] When the morphology is not suggestive of a septal origin, an epicardial approach should be considered, but percutaneous epicardial access might achieve only a limited area of mapping that has a high risk of complications. Under such circumstances, hybrid surgical ablation can be an alternative.

PROCEDURE PLANNING

Hybrid surgical epicardial access should serve not only as a bail-out procedure but also as an upfront "tailor-made" procedure design. To plan a successful procedure, a multidisciplinary team is mandatory. The team should include cardiac EP, cardiothoracic surgery, cardiac anesthesiology, and a perfusion team. A 12-lead electrocardiogram (ECG) of the arrhythmia is essential to identify whether the site of origin of the arrhythmia is epicardial and from which region, whenever available.[33,34] Noninvasive programmed stimulation through an implantable cardioverter-defibrillator (ICD) could also be used if the tachycardia ECG is not available. Insight as to the epicardial substrate can also be obtained through careful review of previous ablation procedures, even if only endocardial. Unipolar voltage data, lack of good endocardial pace map, inability to entrain the tachycardia, and a broad outbreak in activation mapping are suggestive of an epicardial source.[35] Another crucial element in preoperative evaluation is advanced imaging to evaluate the scar such as with late gadolinium-contrast magnetic resonance imaging (Fig. 41.1A). The three-dimensional (3D) reconstruction of these images can provide valuable information in planning the surgical access approach and provide the greatest chance for a successful outcome.[36]

Attention must be paid to where the procedure will be performed. A perfusion team should be available. In some case series, the procedure is performed in the operating room with a portable 3D mapping system (NavX; Abbott, St Paul, MN).[37] Procedures can also be routinely performed in a hybrid EP laboratory, in conjunction with the cardiothoracic surgical and operation room teams.[38] It is also important to note that fluoroscopy may still be essential to deliver safe ablation since the coronary arteries are not always visible depending on the limitations of the operative window. An upfront plan for cardiopulmonary bypass may be required for patients undergoing full median sternotomy, such as for LVAD implantation but is not typically required for most stand-alone hybrid cases. ECG lead placement and defibrillator pad location are dictated by the surgical approach (Fig. 41.3A and 41.3C). It should be noted that precordial ECG leads are often displaced, even if the planned surgical window is limited, since the patient often requires a full surgical prep in the event urgent sternotomy and cardiopulmonary bypass is required. General anesthesia is used in all cases, following which a surgical epicardial window is achieved.

ACCESS SITE

Three surgical approaches can be used to achieve access: subxiphoid window, anterior/anterolateral thoracotomy, or full sternotomy (Table 41.2 and Fig. 41.2A–D). The surgical approach should be tailored to the region of interest, which can be determined by integrating clinical data from surface ECG, advanced cardiac imaging, and previous mapping.[16] This also requires detailed preoperative discussion between the electrophysiologist and cardiac surgeon.

Soejima and colleagues initially described performing the subxiphoid technique in the EP laboratory setting in six patients with recurrent VT, with failed endocardial catheter ablation and

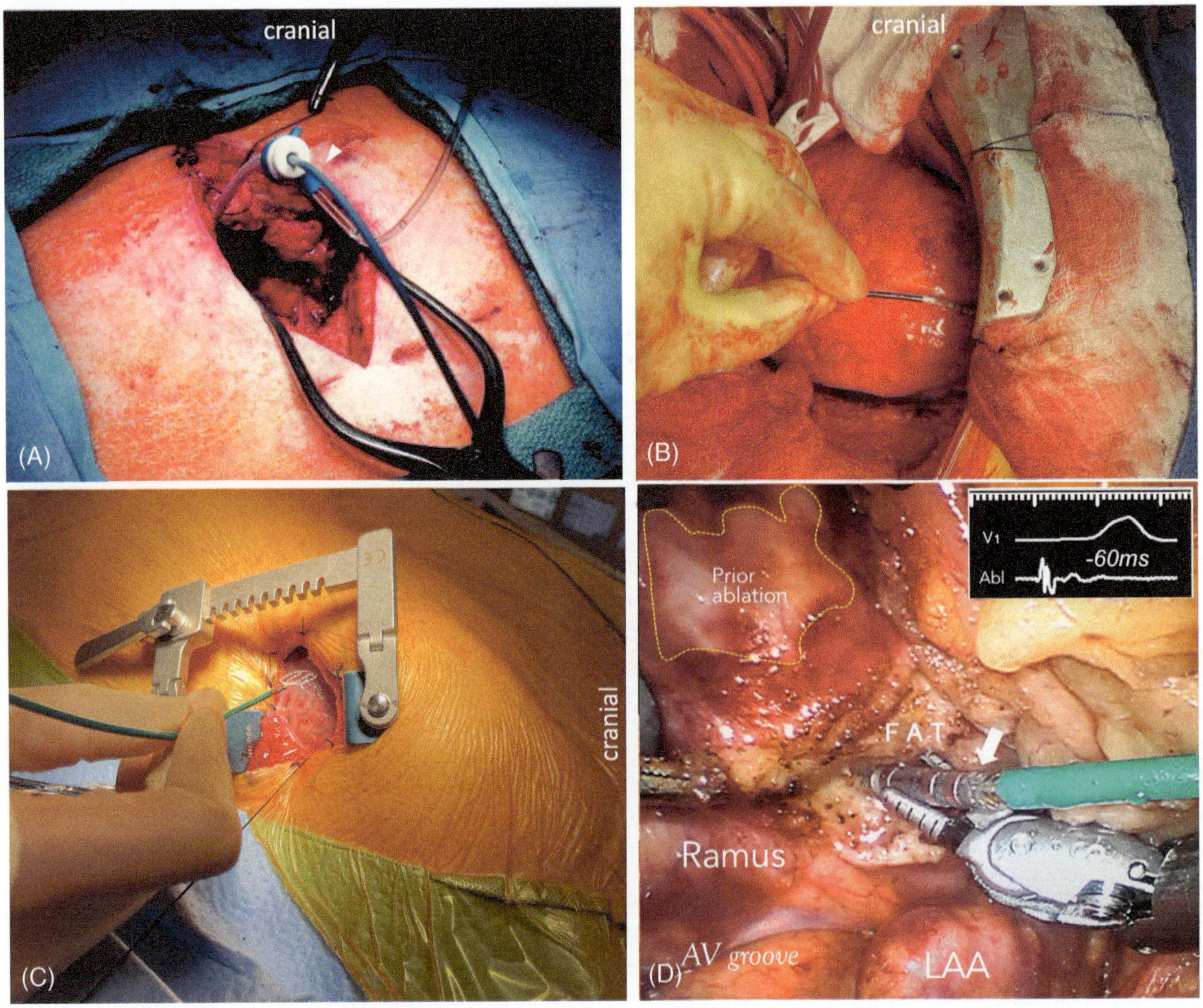

Fig. 41.2 Published approaches of surgical ventricular arrhythmia ablation. (A) Showing a 3-inch incision made at subxiphoid area under direct visualization and an 8-F sheath inserted into the pericardial space. Through the sheath, a 7-F mapping and ablation catheter (*arrowhead*, Navi Star, Biosense-Webster) was inserted into the pericardial space. (Reproduced from Soejima K, Couper G, Cooper JM, et al. Subxiphoid surgical approach for epicardial catheter-based mapping and ablation in patients with prior cardiac surgery or difficult pericardial access. *Circulation.* 2004;110(10):1197–1201). (B) Showing an open chest sternotomy, the operator mapped directly with a Livewire 2-2-2 decapolar mapping catheter on the anterolateral left ventricle (LV) (Courtesy UCLA Cardiac Arrhythmia Center). (C) Showing limited anterior thoracotomy and the operator directly mapped with an HD Grid (Abbott, Chicago, IL) (Courtesy UCLA Cardiac Arrhythmia Center). (D) Showing the robotic-assisted LV summit mapping and ablation. Note that the local activation time at the time of ablation catheter (*arrow*, Flexibility, Abbott) is 60 ms earlier than the surface electrocardiography (V_1) (Courtesy UCLA Cardiac Arrhythmia Center.)

a history of prior cardiac surgery (Fig. 41.2A).[39] Pericardiotomy was performed by opening the abdominal facias in the linea alba, veering to the left of the xiphoid, exposing the pericardium and opening horizontally. Then the pericardiotomy is extended toward the left side and blunt dissection of adhesions was performed to visualize the inferior and inferolateral ventricles. Their approach offers the advantage of creating a smaller incision, mapping epicardially, and defining the location of epicardial coronary arteries by coronary angiography, which is critical for safety.[39–41] However, visibility can be limited, and access may be challenged by a greater distance from the surgical incision to the epicardial substrate.

Limited anterior thoracotomy has several different considerations compared with subxiphoid access (Table 41.1). Single-lung ventilation may be required to aid pericardial exposure.[16] A left anterior incision is made by extending through the subcutaneous tissue and fascia and planned intercostal space (usually between third through fifth) (Fig. 41.2-C). The pericardium is then dissected off the left ventricle laterally to maximally expose the surgical field. (Video 41.1) In contrast with subxiphoid access, anterior thoracotomy facilitates anterior, anterolateral, and true apex ablation, indicating the LAD territory. In the largest series of hybrid surgical ablation, only 36% of the total estimated epicardial surface could be mapped on average due to

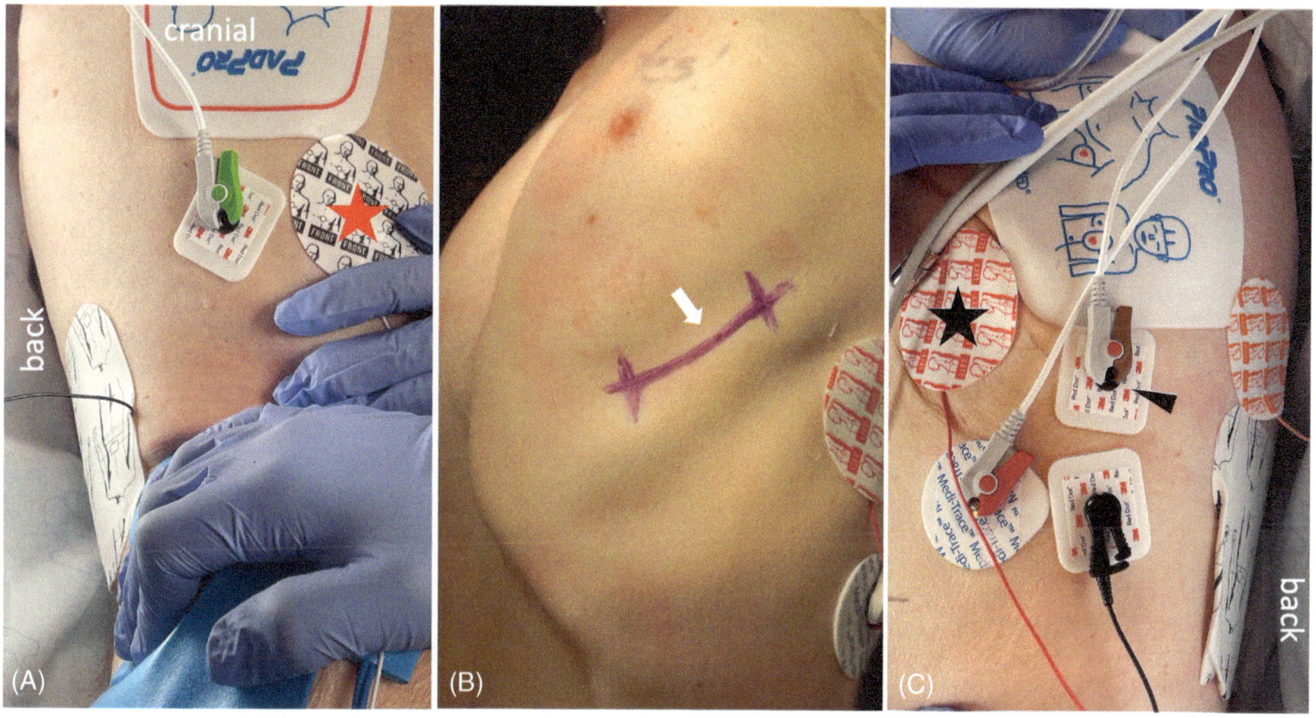

Fig. 41.3 Presurgical preparation. (A) The three-dimensional (3D) patches for the mapping system must be displaced from their usual positions to the mid-axillary line (*star*). (B) The incision is marked before sterile preparation (*arrow*) for limited anterior thoracotomy and the rearrangement of the 3D patches in Ensite system. The surgical incision can be optimized by utilizing transthoracic echocardiography to identify the left ventricular apex. (C) The precordial leads must also be either removed or placed postoriorly to expose the surgical area. Here, only V_6 was preserved (*solid arrow*).

TABLE 41.2 Hybrid Surgical Access Approach Considerations, Strengths, and Weaknesses

	ACCESS APPROACH		
	Subxiphoid	**Limited Thoracotomy**	**Open Sternotomy**
Ventilation	Normal ventilation setting	Single lung may be required	Ventilation per cardiac anesthesia
ECG leads	Usual placement of electrodes	Displaced ECG electrodes	
Accessed left ventricular segment	Inferior/inferolateral segments	Anterior/anterolateral and apical segments—tailor intercostal space to location of substrate	Maximum exposure
Adhesion during dissection	Mild adhesions may be addressed with surgical dissection	May need extensive dissection with need for oversewing	May require cardiopulmonary bypass to fully mobilize heart
Three-dimensional mapping	Impedance or magnetic system can be used	An impedance-based system may give distorted geometry if large retractors required	Either impedance or magnetic system will be influenced
Ablation catheters	Conventional EP catheters for mapping and ablation	Conventional EP catheters for mapping and ablation but may experience frequent steam pops. Surgical tools under direct vision can be used after mapping with EP catheters.	
Defibrillation	No specific concern	External cardioversion might fail	Surgical defibrillation paddles

ECG, Electrocardiographic; *EP*, electrophysiologic.

adhesions.[38] This highlights the importance of thorough preprocedural planning. Significant adhesions are more often encountered and careful dissection is required. However, ultimately, unless full sternotomy is undertaken, there are often areas that cannot be safely freed from postoperative adhesions given the limited surgical field of view. Care should be taken to protect the phrenic nerve and coronary vessels.

Several case reports have described modification of the thoracotomy approach to a video-assisted thoracoscopy.[42,43] In a case report of a patient with Brugada syndrome, the authors described using 3.5-mm ports installed in intercostal spaces II, IV, and VI with two instrument ports and one camera port.[42] The approach uses a non–rib-displacing limited thoracotomy through the third intercostal space to facilitate direct

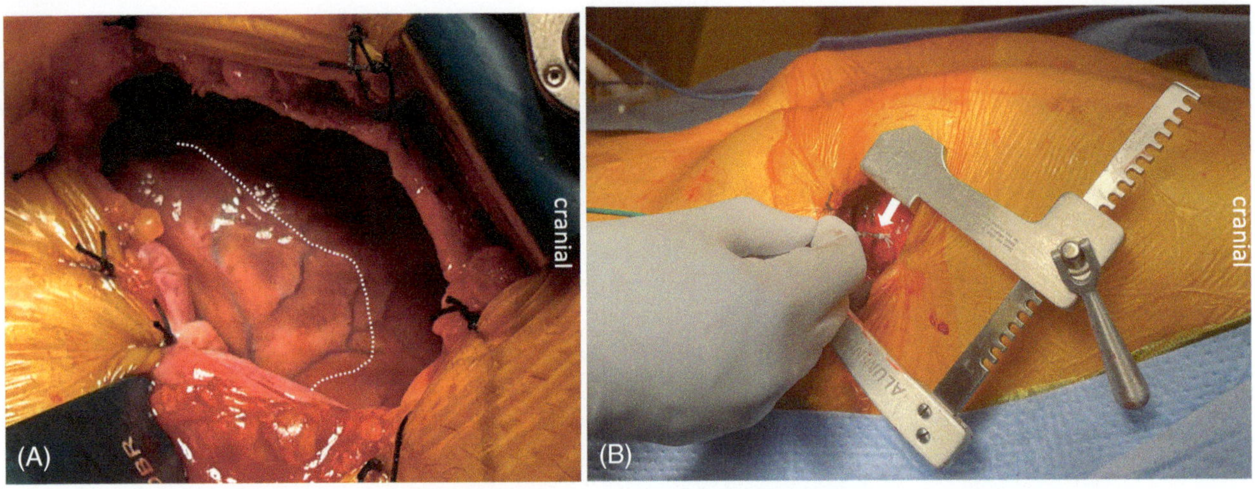

Fig. 41.4 Thoracotomy with epicardial mapping. (A) View of the directly exposed anterolateral left ventricle and infarcted zone (dotted line). (B) Direct mapping with HD Grid (Reproduced with permission of Abbott, © 2023. All rights reserved.) on the surface of epicardium. (Also see Video 41.1.)

visualization of the epicardium through a smaller incision. Mulpuru reported on endoscopic robotic-assisted (DaVinci robot) surgery as an alternative to median sternotomy and its evolution to a method for treating complex arrhythmias arising from LV summit.[44] The robotic-assisted technique has been used as a totally endoscopic LV summit ablation using a duodecapolar catheter and irrigated ablation catheter, reported by Aziz and colleagues[29] (Fig. 41.2D). A video-assisted technique with a pericardioscopic cannula (AtriCure, Mason, OH) is also reported to facilitate pericardial lysis in VT ablation by direct blunt dissection of the pericardium.[45]

Open sternotomy is considered to be a last resort. While this provides a wide field of visibility and access, this is associated with increased procedure time, risk, and comorbidity (Fig. 41.2B). This approach is usually unnecessary unless other methods have failed or a concomitant cardiac surgery is planned, such as LVAD implantation.[19,46,47] When considering mapping and ablation intraoperatively during LVAD implantation, pericardiotomy and lysis of adhesions are performed by the cardiac surgeon prior to mapping, which should be performed before cardioplegia is instituted, whenever possible. The timing of cardiopulmonary bypass is determined by the surgeon.[18] Although hybrid ablation could be considered, whether this should be performed before, during, or after LVAD implantation remains undefined.

MAPPING AND ABLATION

After the epicardium is surgically exposed, the electrophysiologist can proceed with mapping and ablation with a 3D mapping system. Both NavX (Abbott Medical, St. Paul, MN) and CARTO (Johnson & Johnson, Biosense Webster Diamond Bar, CA) systems are frequently used in hybrid procedures and, therefore, the choice should be based on operator preference. Both magnetic-based and impedance-based mapping systems can be used in hybrid procedures. However, impedance-based mapping systems may produce distorted geometry during an open chest or a thoracotomy procedure due to the change in thoracic impedance. This situation can be attenuated by filling the open chest cavity with warm sterile lactated Ringer solution.[18] A magnetic-based system, on the other hand, will be altered by surgical instruments, such as large retractors and the surgical table itself, though this effect might be attenuated by special arrangement of the patches as reported by Corona et al.[19] Briefly, the posterior patches on the back are in the usual position, and anterior patches are placed horizontally just below the umbilical line in order to limit the electromagnetic interference. Nevertheless, this approach requires knowledge for troubleshooting in setting up the mapping system, especially if the procedure is to be carried out in the operating room. Magnetic-based systems might, therefore, be more suitable for subxiphoid or thoracoscopic approaches, as these can more easily be used in a hybrid laboratory setup.

In a subxiphoid approach, precordial lead placement may not be altered, but in the thoracotomy and open chest approach, the leads must be displaced (Fig. 41.3). As a result, this affects ECG interpretation during mapping (Fig. 41.5C). If endocardial mapping is to be performed, this generally should be done after surgical access is established with confirmation of hemostasis. Following this, full heparization with an activated clotting time greater than 300 seconds should be attained if LV endocardial mapping and ablation are required.

The elevated threshold of defibrillation is another important concern during hybrid ablation. During procedures with subxiphoid, thoracotomy, and endoscopic robotic approaches, air enters into the pericardial space. This can result in failure of external defibrillation. In one case series, 2 of 10 patients experienced a failed external cardioversion and required internal defibrillation though the ICD.[16] As such, someone should be available to program the ICD to deliver a shock if external defibrillation fails.[48]

Substrate mapping, activation mapping, and pace mapping can be created by sweeping multipolar catheters (Livewire Steerable Duo-Deca or Advisor HD Grid, Abbott, or DecaNav, Biosense

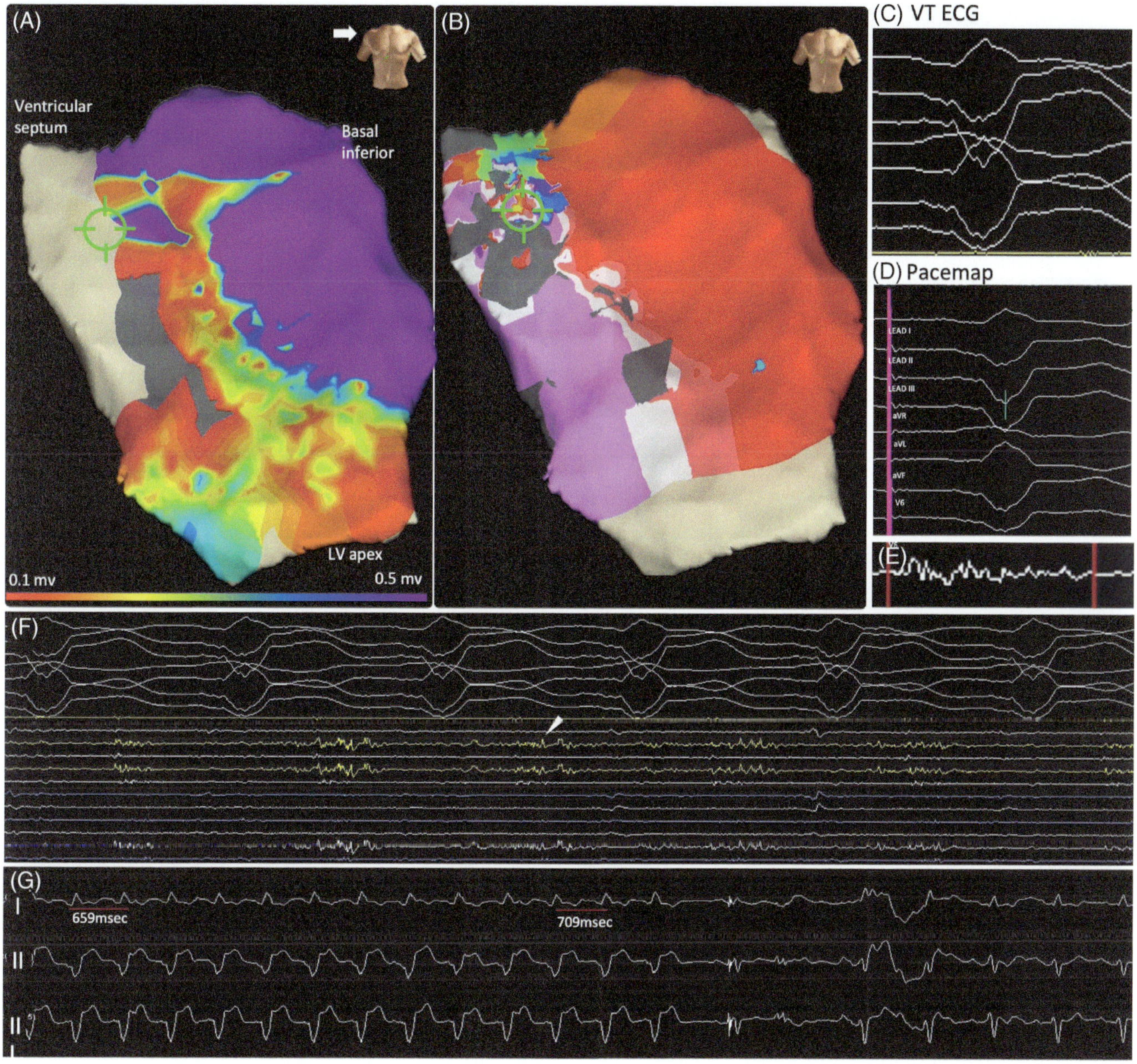

Fig. 41.5 Left ventricular (LV) epicardial three-dimensional mapping with Ensite (Reproduced with permission of Abbott, © 2023. All rights reserved.) via anterior thoracotomy in a 70-year-old man with ischemic cardiomyopathy status post four-vessel coronary artery bypass graft surgery presenting with a recurrent ventricular tachycardia (VT) after a prior endocardial radiofrequency ablation 3 months ago. (A) Limited activation map with an extensive scar over the anterior wall of the LV. Of note, the orientation (*arrow*) must be adjusted manually due to the distorted impedance after thoracotomy. (B) Isochronal map during VT with region of conduction slowing near the green target. (C) Only limited limb leads and V_6 can be observed during the procedure. (D) Excellent pace map for the clinical VT with a long stim–QRS interval was obtained from the same area where the mid-diastolic potentials were observed. (D). (E) Magnified diastolic potential. (F) Long, fractionated, mid-diastolic potential during VT. (G) Ablation with cryothermal energy resulted in prolongation of the cycle length of tachycardia from 659 ms to 709 ms and termination of VT during ablation. (Also see Video 41.2.)

Webster) along the epicardial surface as in conventional ablation (Fig. 41.4-B). VT induction and entrainment can be performed based on operator discretion. The representative case in Fig. 41.5 shows the capability of limited thoracotomy in creating a voltage map, isochronal map, and pace map, identifying mid-diastolic potential and termination of VT during ablation (Video 41.2).

An important difference between percutaneous access and surgical access is the ablation energy choice and system. Options include open-irrigated radiofrequency (RF) and cryothermal energy (Table 41.3).

A key consideration in surgical procedures is the impendence change that occurs during ablation. When ablating through a

TABLE 41.3 Hybrid Surgical Ablation Energy Sources

SURGICAL ABLATIVE ENERGY SOURCES		
Radiofrequency	**Cryothermal**	
• Conventional radiofrequency catheters (e.g., Flexability, Tacticath, SmartTouch) • Coolrail (AtriCure, Mason, Ohio)	• CryoICE (AtriCure, Mason, OH)	• CryoFlex (Medtronic, Minneapolis, MN)
• High impedance and steam pops • Able to map and pace	• Malleable probe, to fit the cardiac contour • Better catheter stability during ablation • Unable to map and pace	
Image, table 41.3		
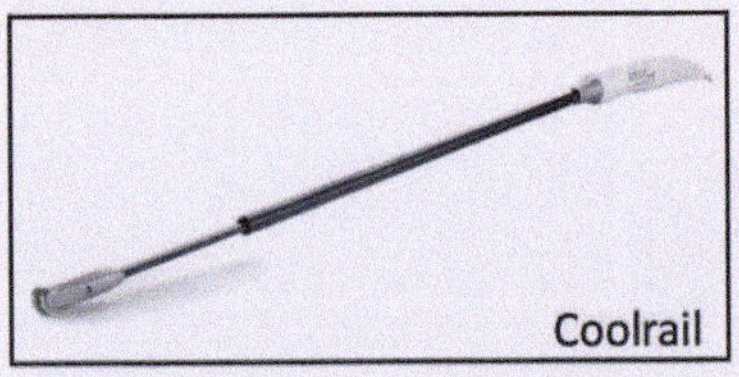	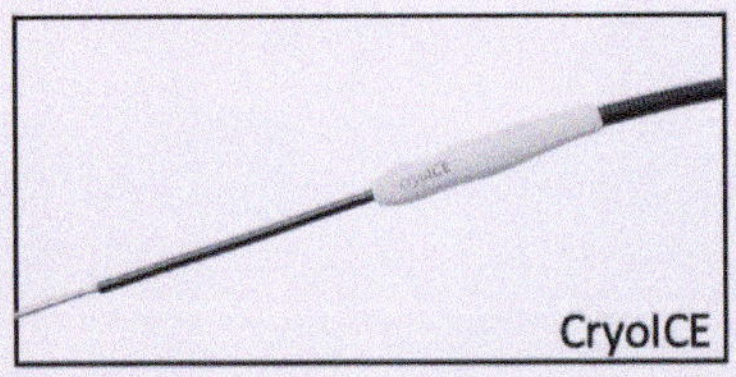	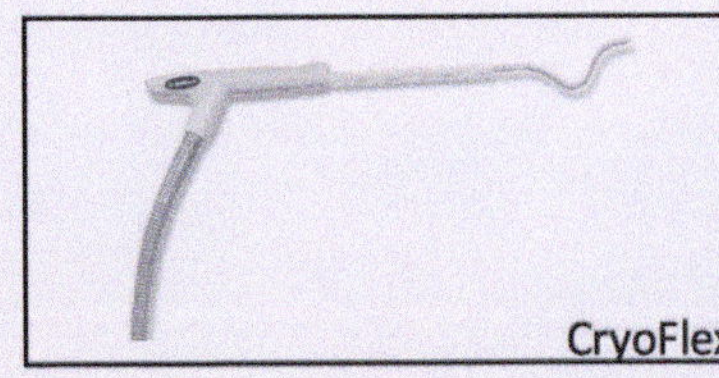

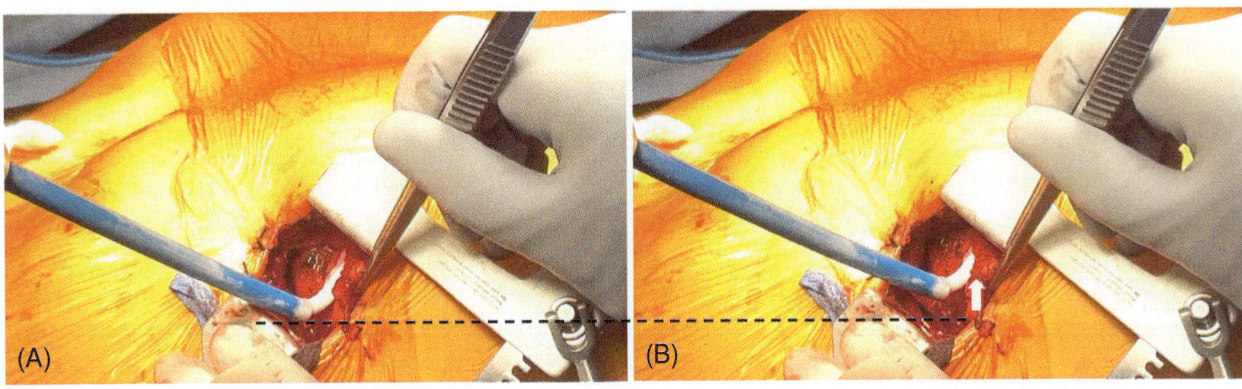

Fig. 41.6 Cryothermal energy delivery. Note the tip of CryoICE catheter with ice formation during ablation. The *arrow* indicates movement of the catheter from *dashed line* during systole (A) and diastole (B); the catheter remained stabilized on the epicardium. (Also see Video 41.3.)

standard irrigated RF catheter, like FlexAbility (Abbott Medical) and Thermocool SF (Biosense Webster), high impedance and steam pops can occur, especially during thoracotomy access or an open chest approach. This phenomenon could be caused by insufficient surrounding irrigation, since the RF ablation catheters were designed for ablation in bloodstream.[16] Manual adjustment of the RF generator impedance threshold is required to allow ablation during high impedance.

Certain ablation tools are available that were specifically designed for use within the open chest. The surgical RF ablation device, Coolrail bipolar linear ablation pen (AtriCure, West Chester, Ohio), has an internally irrigated catheter with 30-mm parallel electrodes. RF current is delivered with activation of the generator (ASU2 generator; AtriCure) in a power-controlled mode at 30 W for 40 seconds. The lesion has a larger surface area with a depth of 4–5 mm.[49,50] Rapid cooling cryothermal energy can be created by using either Argon gas (CryoFlex, Medtronic) or nitrous oxide (CryoICE, AtriCure). The surgifrost Surgical Cryoablation System consists of a flexible metal probe with an adjustable insulation sheath, which can be shaped to conform the cardiac contours. After a target temperature of −150°C and 3-minute application, the depth of the lesion could be up to 6 mm.[46] Another cryoprobe, CryoICE (AtriCure, Mason, OH), with a similar design has also been reported in ablation before LVAD implantation with a target temperature −70°C and 2.5 minutes.[20] In addition to the malleability of the cryoablation catheter, it also provides better stability during ablation with ice ball formation and tissue adhesion (Fig. 41.6) (Video 41.3). However, unlike standard RF ablation catheters, the cryoprobes are unable to map and ablate at the same time. To visualize the cryoprobe, one may use surgical ties to affix the cryoprobe to the proximal portion of a multipolar mapping catheter, leaving distal electrodes free from contacting the metal. In this way, the distal part of the catheter and the approximate location of cryoprobe can be tracked during ablation (Fig. 41.7).[37]

In conclusion, surgical tools require direct visualization of the substrate and are limited by inability to pace, map, or be visualized in 3D mapping systems. However, they can create large lesions in a shorter time. They are suitable for thoracotomy or open chest approaches and require precise

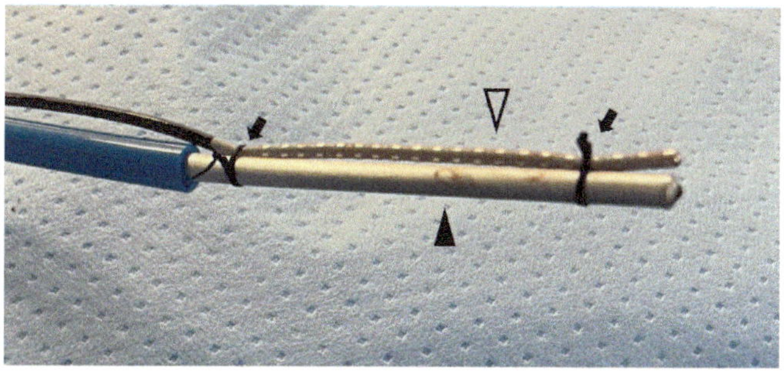

Fig. 41.7 Method for indirectly visualizing the cryoablation probe, CryoICE (AtriCure) (*solid arrowhead*), within the electroanatomical mapping system. Surgical ties (*arrow*) were used to secure the cryoprobe to the multipolar mapping catheter (*clear arrowhead*).

preoperative evaluation. Standard catheters can map, pace and be visualized on the 3D mapping system but are challenging to use in thoracotomy and an open chest approach due to impedance limitations. These standard RF catheters can be better utilized in subxiphoid surgical access with little modification needed.

SAFETY AND OUTCOME

Hemodynamic decompensation during a prolonged procedure or VT induction poses a major limitation in VT procedures despite inotrope use.[51] Patients with advanced age, marked LV dysfunction and comorbidities such as chronic obstructive pulmonary disease are at higher risk of decompensation.[52] Although a relatively safe procedure, the largest case series demonstrated a 20% short-term complication rate including generalized bleeding without focus, damage to LV during anterior thoracotomy approach requiring intraoperative repair, and damage to the epigastric artery.[38] Another important issue is postoperative pleuritic pain. The pain is related to the creation of the access, such as sternotomy, intercostal access, rib retraction, tissue injury, inflammation from the lesions, and the drain sites. Similar to other cardiac surgery patients, the pain not only affects the patient's experiences but also prolongs hospitalization.[53] The pain can be managed with systemic and regional anesthesia. Pericarditis is also common and can be managed with intrapericardial steroids or systemic colchine.[54]

The largest (N = 40) case series reported a short-term success rate, defined by noninducibility, as 50% to 80% in a group of nonischemic and ischemic cardiomyopathy patients. The success rate did not differ in subxiphoid or anterior thoracotomy approaches.[38] A case series of five patients in Europe with mixed etiology of cardiomyopathy demonstrated 80% noninducibility and one patient required a redo procedure after 21 months.[55] Kunkel and colleagues reported 100% noninducibility after the procedure and 75% VT–storm free survival in eight patients over 3.4 ± 1.7 years, with mixed cardiomyopathy.[37] Despite these encouraging results, further study is warranted to evaluate the safety and efficacy of this approach.

SUMMARY

As the complexity of ventricular arrhythmia ablation evolves, hybrid surgical access has emerged as an attractive option. The spectrum of methods includes the open chest approach, subxiphoid window, limited anterior thoracotomy, video-assisted thoracoscopy, and robotic-assisted approach. An essential part of the preoperative planning for the procedure is the communication between different subspecialties, careful patient selection, thorough imaging review, and surgical planning. Currently, there is no existing best energy source or mapping system for this highly complex patient group, and large-scale data are lacking given the rarity of this procedure. This approach can be an effective means of treating refractory ventricular arrhythmias in patients who have failed conventional treatments and who have an acceptable safety profile.

REFERENCES

Please refer to the e-book for a complete list of references.

PART 8

Miscellaneous Topics

42

Complications Associated With Catheter Ablation of Cardiac Arrhythmias

Carola Gianni, Javier E. Sanchez, J. David Burkhardt, Andrea Natale, Amin Al-Ahmad

KEY POINTS

- Clinicians involved in the care of patients undergoing catheter ablation should be familiar with complications associated with this procedure.
- Complications are often related to the anatomy and access site of the heart or vessels that are involved, targeted arrhythmia, the energy source used for ablation, the type and number of catheters used, catheter/sheath manipulation, and injury to the surrounding structures in proximity to the sites of ablation.
- Complications can occur immediately or weeks after the procedure and can range from minor to life threatening.
- Ultrasound (bedside, intracardiac) is the most valuable tool for prompt recognition of the most common ablation-related complications.
- Early recognition and treatment are key to avoid unwanted sequelae.

INTRODUCTION

Complications are a significant source of morbidity and mortality,[1–6] and clinicians involved in the care of patients undergoing catheter ablation of cardiac arrhythmias should be familiar. Complications range from minor to life-threatening and can occur anywhere from immediate moment to weeks following the procedure, and attentive patient surveillance is key to recognize and promptly treat them to avoid unwanted sequelae. We provide an overview of the most common complications associated with catheter ablation, with a focus on how to prevent, diagnose, and treat them appropriately.

VASCULAR ACCESS–RELATED COMPLICATIONS

See Table 42.1 for a list of vascular access–related complications.

Most vascular access–related complications are associated with the inadvertent puncture of structures surrounding the target vessel. The use of real-time vascular ultrasound to guide access is the single most important tool to reduce their incidence, because it allows the visualization of the needle while it is being maneuvered under the skin.[7]

Hematomas and pseudoaneurysms are usually secondary to inadequate pressure, either after sheath removal from the puncture site (artery or vein) or for inadvertent puncture of an arterial vessel/branch when obtaining venous access.[8] It is important to remember that large-bore sheaths are used for catheter ablation and many patients are on uninterrupted antithrombotic drugs and might still be heparinized at the time of sheath removal. In addition, cardiac comorbidities are common, including extensive arterial calcifications or obesity, which might hinder the ability to exert adequate pressure over the puncture site. Heparin should be fully reversed (activated clotting time [ACT] < 180 seconds), and dedicated staff should pull the sheaths and stay with the patient until hemostasis is achieved. Alternatively, vascular closure devices can be used (suture based, collagen based, external compression); when correctly deployed, they shorten the time to achieve hemostasis, but the patient should still be monitored for the occurrence of hematoma/pseudoaneurysm because suboptimal deployment is not uncommon. While most hematomas do not require intervention, neck hematomas, when voluminous, might lead to airway compression; if compression does not control bleeding, intubation and/or evacuation/surgical repair might be necessary.

When bleeding from the puncture site is prolonged, it can organize into a high-pressure sac (pseudoaneurysm), which is suspected when a nonresolving "hematoma" is present, associated with a vascular bruit. Pseudoaneurysms are diagnosed with vascular ultrasound (yin-yang sign, Fig. 42.1). Pseudoaneurysms require focused, prolonged (at least 1 hour, in our experience) compression over the neck, which can be only achieved with ultrasound-guided compression, which should be exerted until the sac is completely thrombosed (longer periods for larger sacs and wider neck).[9] When this fails (typically, obese patients or large bore sheaths) or is not feasible (requires longer times, is painful), thrombin injection into the sac is a feasible alternative, if there are no high-risk features for thrombin spillage into the main vessel (namely a large neck), leading to limb ischemia or venous thromboembolism, according to the bleeding source. When all else fails, surgical repair is indicated.

TABLE 42.1 Vascular Access–Related Complications

Hematoma* (including retroperitoneal hematoma)
Pseudoaneurysm*
Arteriovenous fistula
Hemothorax
Pneumothorax
Arterial dissection
Nerve damage
Thrombosis/thromboembolism
Infection

The most common complications are denoted with an asterisk (*).

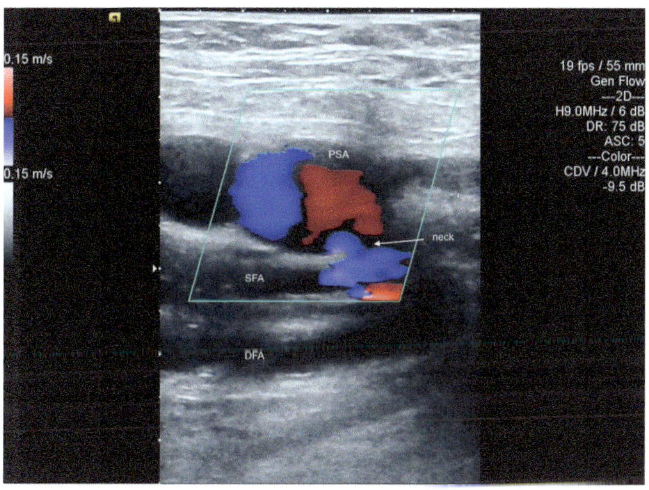

Fig. 42.1 Vascular ultrasound image (long-axis view) of a femoral pseudoaneurysm, which was effectively treated with ultrasound-guided compression. *DFA*, Deep femoral artery; *PSA*, pseudoaneurysm; *SFA*, superficial femoral artery.

Retroperitoneal hematoma occurs when a central vessel (vein or artery) is punctured above the inguinal ligament; here, pressure cannot be adequately exerted over the access site and bleeding occurs unseen, until accumulation of a significant volume of blood accumulates in the retroperitoneum. Flank pain/bruising, anemia, and tachycardia are the typical symptoms and should prompt computed tomography (CT)/magnetic resonance imaging (MRI) of the retroperitoneum. Interventional treatment (embolization/covered stenting) or surgical repair might be necessary if the bleeding does not stop, typical of patients with antithrombotic therapy and using larger-bore access sheaths.[10]

Arteriovenous fistulae occur for the inadvertent "through-and-through" access, when the sheath goes through the artery before entering the vein (on the groin, this is typical of low access sites, below the femoral bifurcation). Arteriovenous fistula is usually suspected when hearing a bruise at the level of the access site or when "arterial" (usually, brighter and with higher pressure than the pure venous counterpart) is observed when obtaining venous access in repeat procedures. Again, arteriovenous fistulae are easily diagnosed with ultrasound. Spontaneous closure is rare, and observation is indicated only for smaller sheaths, when shunts are smaller and less likely to result in limb ischemia. Interventional percutaneous treatment (covered stent/vascular plugs) or surgical repair should be considered for all other cases.

Other vascular access–related complications are less common.[11] Hemothorax and pneumothorax are complications associated with superior access (internal jugular vein and subclavian/axillary vein), with the associated inadvertent puncture of intrathoracic vessel or the lung, which are easily avoided when obtaining access with real-time ultrasound. Treatment (air/blood evacuation, repair) might be necessary when lung function is affected. Arterial dissection is seen when the needle/wire is advanced between the intima and media during arterial access; this type of dissection is self-limiting (against flow). Visualizing the wire with ultrasound inside the arterial vessel before proceeding to advance a sheath/catheter into the false lumen is the most important maneuver for the distal progression of the dissection (into the aorta). Nerve damage can result from either direct injury (inadvertent puncture) or compression by an adjacent hematoma/pseudoaneurysm. Treatment is mostly supportive, so prevention (access with ultrasound) is key. Thrombosis is observed when flow is limited within the accessed vessel: small vessel, multiple sheaths (>2) on the same side, long sheaths, lack of systemic anticoagulation, and intervascular deployment of closure devices all can lead to thrombosis (arterial or venous, according to the access site) and thromboembolism (see later). Of note, we do give heparin to all patients undergoing ablation, including right-sided procedures, with at least a bolus of 5000 IU of heparin and avoid obtaining multiple accesses on the same side. Finally, infection is rare, and usually associated with the use of vascular closure devices, which should be avoided in thin patients (collagen plug/suture exposed) and patients with active periaccess site infections.

SHEATH/CATHETER MANIPULATION–RELATED COMPLICATIONS

See Table 42.2 for a list of sheath/catheter manipulation–related complications. Pericardial bleeding result from cardiac perforation due to careless manipulation of catheters and sheaths

TABLE 42.2 Sheath/Catheter Manipulation–Related Complications

Pericardial bleeding*
Aorto–right atrial fistula
Hemothorax
Intramural myocardial dissection/hematoma
Thrombosis/thromboembolism*
Air/calcium embolism
Lead dislodgement
Cardiac valve damage
Coronary artery injury

The most common complications are denoted with an asterisk (*).

within the cardiac chambers. This includes during transseptal access, where the needle/sheaths are advanced into the pericardial space as opposed to the left atrium (LA).

When performing transseptal access, the most useful tool to avoid perforation is using intracardiac echocardiography (ICE), which, akin to vascular ultrasound, allows for the direct visualization of the needle/sheath apparatus being maneuvered in the right atrium (RA), through the septum, and into the LA. When using fluoroscopy only, multiple views are necessary to avoid a too posterior, too superior, or too inferior access, all of which can possibly lead to pericardial access and subsequent bleeding. Additionally, a too anterior access can result in access through the noncoronary cusp, leading to aortic root perforation and subsequent aorto–RA fistula if a sheath is advanced to the aorta. When this happens, the sheath should be left in place, as a bridge to surgical or percutaneous repair.[12] To avoid advancing the transseptal sheath into the pericardium/aorta, secondary confirmation of LA catheterization is necessary by means of contrast injection, oxygenated blood aspiration, and/or pressure waveform. Of note, if the sheath is advanced into the aortic root, it should not be withdrawn until the perforation is repaired (surgery, percutaneous closure device), to avoid massive bleeding into the pericardial space. None of this is necessary when the needle is directly visualized going through the septum and saline injected through it is seen freely flowing in the LA. In addition, with ICE it is possible to assess the LA dimensions (space between the septum and lateral wall) and the presence of interatrial septum anomalies (namely fibrotic or aneurysmatic), which increase the risk of lateral wall/LA appendage (LAA) perforation while pushing the needle/sheath through the septum. In these circumstances, transseptal access should be obtained in a more controlled setting; the puncture should be facilitated by applying radiofrequency (RF) electrocautery on the transseptal needle or using a dedicated RF needle/wire or using a stiffer wire with the tip positioned in one of the pulmonary veins (PVs) used to advance the sheath.

In general, during mapping and ablation, sheaths should never be advanced without a wire/catheter out of their distal end. Additionally, catheters should always be advanced under some form of real-time imaging guidance and *never* against resistance, as denoted by tactile feedback or contact force (when available). Operational awareness is important; some catheters and sheaths are stiffer than others, some areas are more delicate than others. The RVOT, the trabeculations within both atrial appendages, the LA roof near the junction with the right superior PV,[13] and the coronary sinus are very thin, and care should be observed not to exert torque or advance sheaths or catheter when any resistance is met. Similarly, advancing catheters/wires deep within the PVs or superior vena cava (SVC) can result in laceration of distal branches, resulting in slow bleeding into the pleural space and late-presenting hemothorax.

In addition to perforation and pericardial bleeding, intramural myocardial dissection/hematoma is possible if the needle/sheath or catheters are advanced against resistance throughout the endocardial wall but without reaching the epicardial space. This will create a flap and an intramural myocardial space, in which blood can accumulate leading to hemodynamic instability based on the location.[14]

Early recognition of pericardial bleeding is important to avoid tamponade and its sequelae. Anticoagulation can be reversed, fluids can be administered for preload optimization, and early pericardiocentesis can be performed without concurrent hypoperfusion. At the beginning of any cardiac ablation procedure, it is important to note the amount of baseline pericardial effusion (it might be significant!) and monitor the pericardial space throughout the procedure for any change from baseline. Again, the best tool is ICE: the pericardial space can be visualized from the RA (best with higher depth settings, i.e., > 15 mm) or RV. If this is not available, the pericardial space can be monitored on fluoroscopy by regular imaging of the heart in a left anterior oblique (LAO) projection; without significant effusion, the left cardiac silhouette is moving. However, with just fluoroscopy, it is not possible to monitor for changes in volume if a baseline effusion is present. If a de novo pericardial effusion is seen or the baseline pericardial effusion has increased its volume throughout the procedure, bleeding should be suspected—heparin is reversed, and further action is taken based on the speed of blood accumulation, which is a function of multiple factors, including chamber of perforation (high vs. low pressure), location (important translation/rotation), size of perforating sheath/catheter, concomitant drugs/diseases hindering hemostasis, and presence of adhesions. Focal perforation in low-volume chambers away from the annular plane is usually self-limiting, and conservative management without full anticoagulation reversal might be sufficient. Cardiac tamponade is also rare after cardiac surgery; adhesions prevent significant accumulation of blood within the pericardial space. However, perforation and bleeding causing loculated effusion around the LV might still lead to tamponade, usually requiring surgery for evacuation. In some cases, pericardial bleeding might be slow and can pass unobserved during the procedure. If it does not stop (typical of high-pressure chambers), patients develop hypotension over time, usually associated with pericarditis chest pain. If bleeding and effusion are suspected, prompt beside cardiac ultrasound and fluids are an important first step, with pericardiocentesis in case of tamponade physiology.

When cardiac tamponade is present (Fig. 42.2), fluids should be given, with additional pressors if hypotension is not corrected. Care should be taken to avoid high blood pressure, which can increase the speed of blood loss. Anticoagulation should be reversed; protamine is immediately used in those who received heparin (40–50 mg protamine, to achieve a goal ACT < 180 seconds). For those on uninterrupted anticoagulation and continuous active bleeding, nonspecific agents such as fresh frozen plasma (FFP) and prothrombin factor concentrates (PCCs) can be administered. Additionally, specific reversal agents can be used for warfarin (vitamin K), dabigatran (idarucizumab), or factor Xa inhibitors (andexanet alfa).[15] Platelet transfusion might be useful for patients on antiplatelet drugs or known platelet dysfunction. The patient should be typed and crossmatched for blood as well. These interventions should take place simultaneously with preparation for pericardiocentesis.

Every EP lab should have a pericardiocentesis kit available in the room, and every patient should be prepped in the subxiphoid

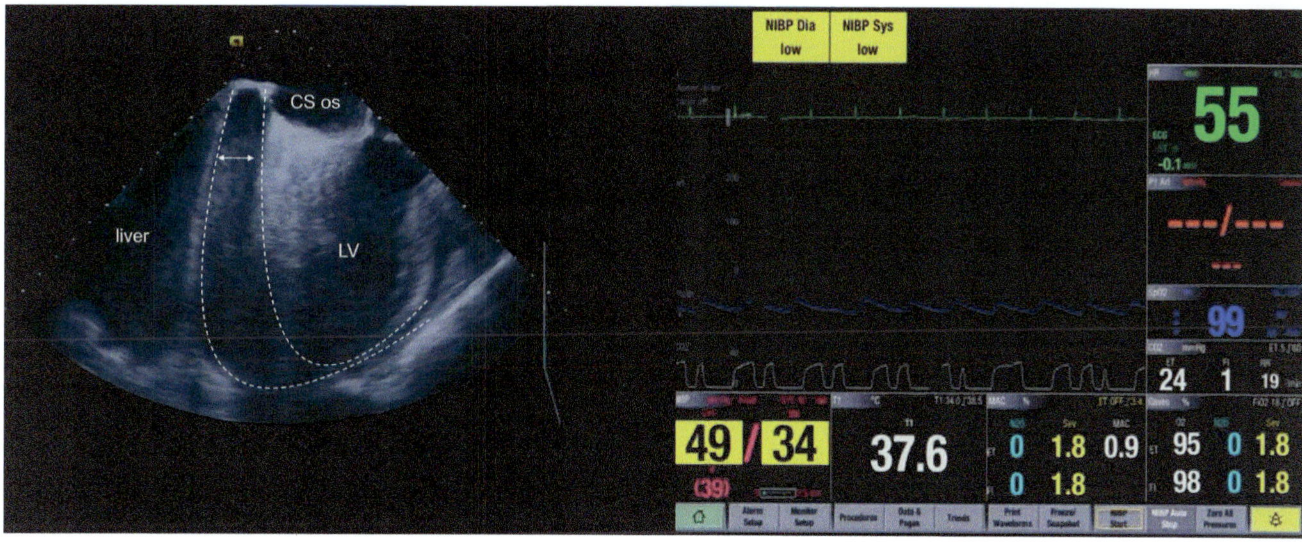

Fig. 42.2 Cardiac tamponade, with intracardiac echocardiographic image (obtained from the right atrium) showing a significant de novo effusion due to pericardial bleeding. *CS,* Coronary sinus; *LV,* left ventricle.

area at the beginning of any cardiac ablation procedure. A pericardiocentesis kit should include two types of Tuohy epidural needles (normal length and long length, for obese patients), a stiff long wire, a short 8-Fr dilator, a mid-length 8-Fr flexible/deflectable sheath, a 6-Fr pigtail catheter, and multiple 50-mL syringes. The epidural needle is preferred because its curved tip points away from the heart to avoid cardiac laceration (i.e., up for anterior pericardial access, down for inferior pericardial access).[16] The stiff wire and dilator are useful to ease the advancement of the pericardial sheath through the ligamentous subxiphoid space. A flexible/deflectable sheath is preferred so that it can be pointed in different areas of the pericardial space (closer to the bleeding source, pockets of accumulated blood). The pigtail catheter might be used in case of fast bleeding, inserted in the pericardial sheath to allow concomitant aspiration of blood by two operators from two different sites.

Subxiphoid access can be obtained with either cardiac ultrasound or fluoroscopy guidance. Either way, it is important to confirm the intrapericardial location of the wire before advancing the sheath: when using cardiac ultrasound, before advancing the wire, saline can be injected through the needle and bubbles are observed within the pericardial space; with fluoroscopy, contrast should be seen pooling in the pericardial space and the wire should travel along both the left and right heart borders in the anteroposterior/LAO projection (Fig. 42.3). If subxiphoid access to the pericardial effusion cannot be obtained (very obese patients, loculated effusion), ultrasound-guided transthoracic or transcardiac approaches might be attempted, but surgery, including emergency pericardial window, should not be delayed. Once access is obtained, the blood can be evacuated. In case of high-volume blood loss, in addition/alternative to allogenic blood transfusions, the patient can be autotransfused; an autologous blood recovery system is preferred to direct autotransfusion, which can result in a systemic inflammatory response and disseminated intravascular coagulation. Once fluid is evacuated from the pericardial space, it is important to assess the rate of bleeding (mL/min). If the rate does not decrease despite evacuation and full reversal (which might take up 30 minutes for PCC concentrates), open-chest surgical repair is most likely needed. After surgery, care should be taken to reinitiate anticoagulation as soon as possible in those patients who underwent extensive LA ablation (with or without LAA isolation), as catastrophic thromboembolism is possible, with permanent clinical sequelae or death, despite successful surgical repair. If bleeding stops, vacuum is maintained within the draining system to allow for close approximation between the parietal and visceral pericardium, thus preventing further bleeding. The drain can be removed if no further drainage is observed and there are no echocardiographic signs of blood reaccumulation. For self-limiting, low-volume effusions, the

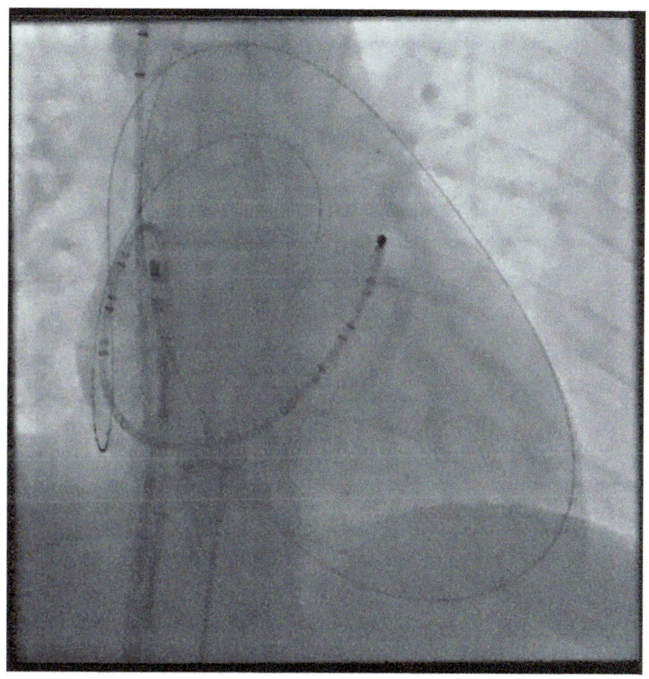

Fig. 42.3 Fluoroscopic image of the wire traveling along the left and right heart borders after subxiphoid pericardial access.

drain can be removed in the EP lab; in all other cases, the drain is kept overnight and removed after confirmation of no blood reaccumulation with bedside ultrasound.

During mapping and ablation, thrombosis can form on all dwelling long sheaths and catheters and result in pulmonary and/or systemic (left-sided procedures) thromboembolism. Thromboembolism can also be a result of the dislodgement of a preexisting clot in the LAA of patients not adequately anticoagulated in the preprocedural period. Prevention is the most important aspect, and adequate anticoagulation is key. As stated above, heparin should be given in all procedures, with a target ACT > 300–350 seconds for left-sided procedures or use of bulky catheters (multisplined, basket). To be fully therapeutic at the time of LA catheterization and/or catheter insertion, heparin should be administered early, ideally before vascular access is obtained. In addition for atrial fibrillation (AF) procedures, patients on direct anticoagulation agents should be maintained on uninterrupted or minimally interrupted (holding one dose) anticoagulation, while those on vitamin K agonists, the INR should be on target (between 2 and 3) in the periprocedural settings, from 3 weeks up to the day of the procedure.[17] LMWH/UFH bridging should never be used, as it leads to both increased bleeding and thrombotic complications compared to an uninterrupted oral anticoagulation strategy. In case of high-risk features (low EF, labile INR, nonadherence to drugs, prior LAA clot), an LAA-focused imaging study (CTA, TEE, or even ICE on the table) should be performed to exclude the presence of an LAA clot should be performed before accessing the LA.

Air embolism is a result of air introduced into the circulation through infusion lines or by suction when catheters are removed too quickly from the sheaths. Again, prevention is key—all infusion lines should be monitored for bubbles, all sheaths must be valved with closed side-ports, and catheter withdrawal should be slow and always followed by aspiration of fluid from the sheath, until blood is seen. Air can be seen on fluoroscopy and ICE (Fig. 42.4), and, when identified, any pooled air should be aspirated whenever possible, either through the sheath or by using a pigtail catheter. Pressure support (target MAP 80–90 mm Hg) is helpful, as it can promote dissolution of the air bubbles. Coronary air embolism typically involves the right coronary artery (which lies superiorly when the patient is lying supine) and presents acutely as inferior ST elevation, ventricular fibrillation (VF), and/or heart block. If pressure support does not lead to dissolution of air, coronary intervention (intracoronary air aspiration–contrast flush) might be required. Cerebral air embolism is usually detected postprocedure, with patients displaying new-onset neurologic signs. MRI or CT may reveal serpiginous hypodensities in the cerebral vasculature, indicative of air bubbles. Treatment is mostly supportive. In the setting of a retrograde (transaortic) approach, calcium embolism is a third possible embolic complication, observed when significant calcific aortic valve/aortoiliac disease is present. This can be prevented by knowing the extent of calcifications (prior ultrasound/CTA or intraprocedural vascular ultrasound/ICE) and opt for a transseptal approach or use a long sheath, avoiding catheter manipulation within the diseased vessel(s).

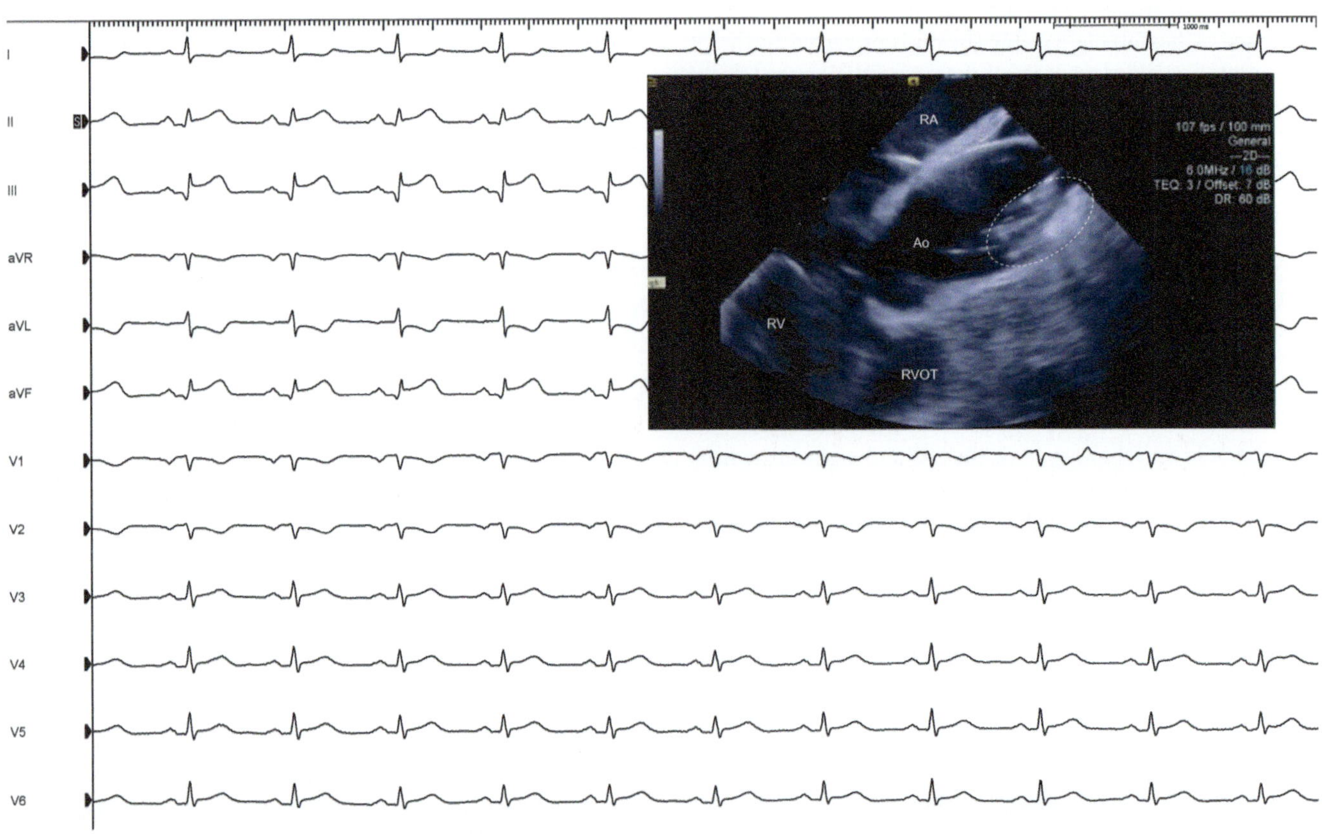

Fig. 42.4 Inferior ST elevation in the setting of air embolism, evident on the intracardiac echocardiographic image of the ascending aorta (*insert*).

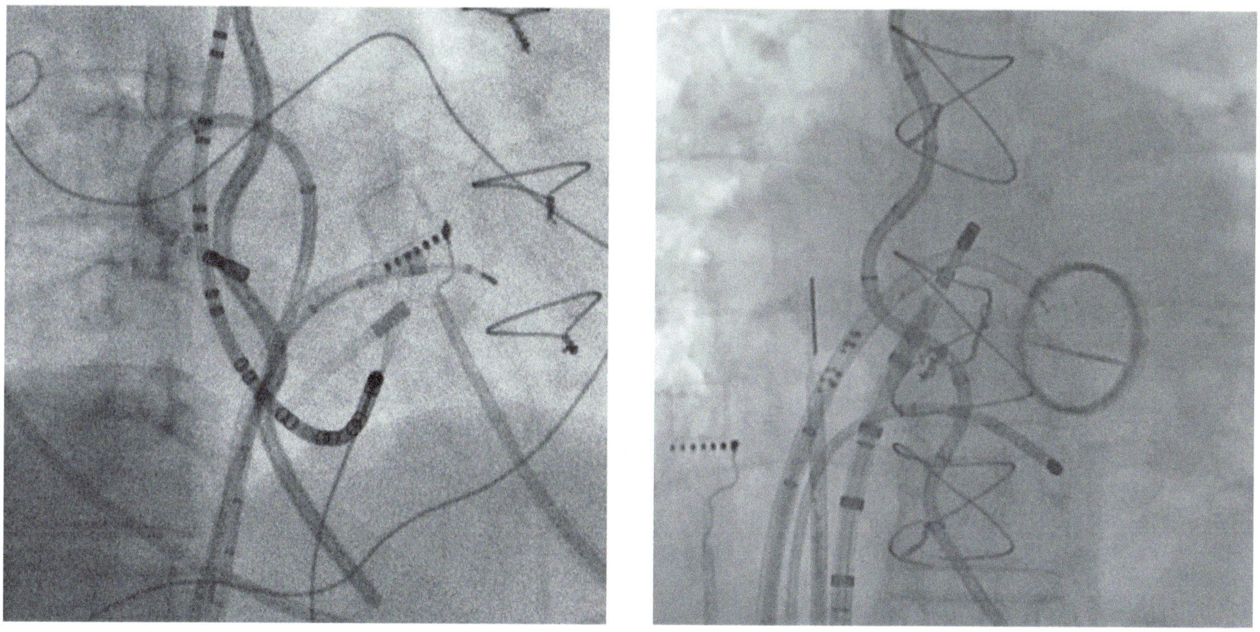

Fig. 42.5 Catheter entrapment: circular mapping catheter in a native mitral valve (*left*) and pentasplined catheter in a mechanical mitral valve (*right*).

In patients with cardiac implantable electronic devices, another possible complication occurring during catheter/sheath manipulation is lead dislodgement.[18] Most commonly, this occurs to atrial leads when performing transseptal access without making sure (with fluoroscopy or ICE) that the sheath/needle apparatus lies medial to lead. Care should also be taken when maneuvering catheters and sheath within the coronary sinus in patients with left ventricular leads, which are usually passive fixation and can be dislodged when pulling out of the vessel when the catheter/sheath is deflected. If possible, catheter ablation should be deferred up to 3 months after a device implant procedure to allow for encapsulation of the lead tip within the myocardium.[19] In the periablation setting, devices should be interrogated before and after the procedure, and in case of dislodgement, lead revision and repositioning are indicated.

Finally, cardiac valve damage can be a result of careless manipulation of mapping and ablation catheters. Mitral valve injury and avulsion can occur when a circular mapping catheter is trapped in the mitral valve apparatus from inadvertent positioning in the LV and applying counterclockwise rotation (Fig. 42.5). It is possible to free the catheter with gentle clockwise manipulation and advancement of the sheath into the LV, but surgical removal may be necessary. Prosthetic mechanical valve damage is also possible when catheters get trapped between the discs and the valvular ring, very common when using multisplined catheters (Fig. 42.5). The latter should not be used in patients with mechanical valves, and care should be taken whenever maneuvering catheters around mechanical valves.[20] Aortic valve damage usually results from attempts to cross the valve with a straight ablation catheter; to avoid perforation, the catheter should always be looped in the distal aortic arch/descending aorta before crossing the valve. This "looping" maneuver should never be performed in or around the aortic root or the coronary ostia can be engaged by the ablation catheter, resulting in traumatic coronary artery injury leading to dissection/occlusion.

ENERGY DELIVERY–RELATED COMPLICATIONS

See Table 42.3 for a list of energy delivery–related complications.

Tissue overheating with RF energy ablation is a potential cause for pericardial bleeding; it can lead to steam pops, which can be extensive and may lead to cardiac perforation.[21] Limiting the contact force, power, and time of energy delivery, as well as using irrigated-tip ablation catheters in a temperature-controlled mode (if the thermistor allows for proper temperature sensing), minimizes the risk of steam pops. It is also important to monitor the ablation catheter for sudden impedance rise and appearance of high-frequency, irregular signals on the intracardiac electrogram recordings (Fig. 42.6), signs of tissue overheating/impending steam pop and should prompt immediate

TABLE 42.3 **Energy Delivery–Related Complications**
Pericardial bleeding*
Thrombosis/thromboembolism
Pericarditis*
Atrioventricular and sinus node injury
Vagal reflexes*
Pulmonary vein and superior vena cava stenosis*
Phrenic nerve and periesophageal vagal plexus injury*
Atrioesophageal fistula
Bronchial and lung injury
Coronary artery injury
Volume overload*/acute exacerbation of heart failure

The most common complications are denoted with an asterisk (*).

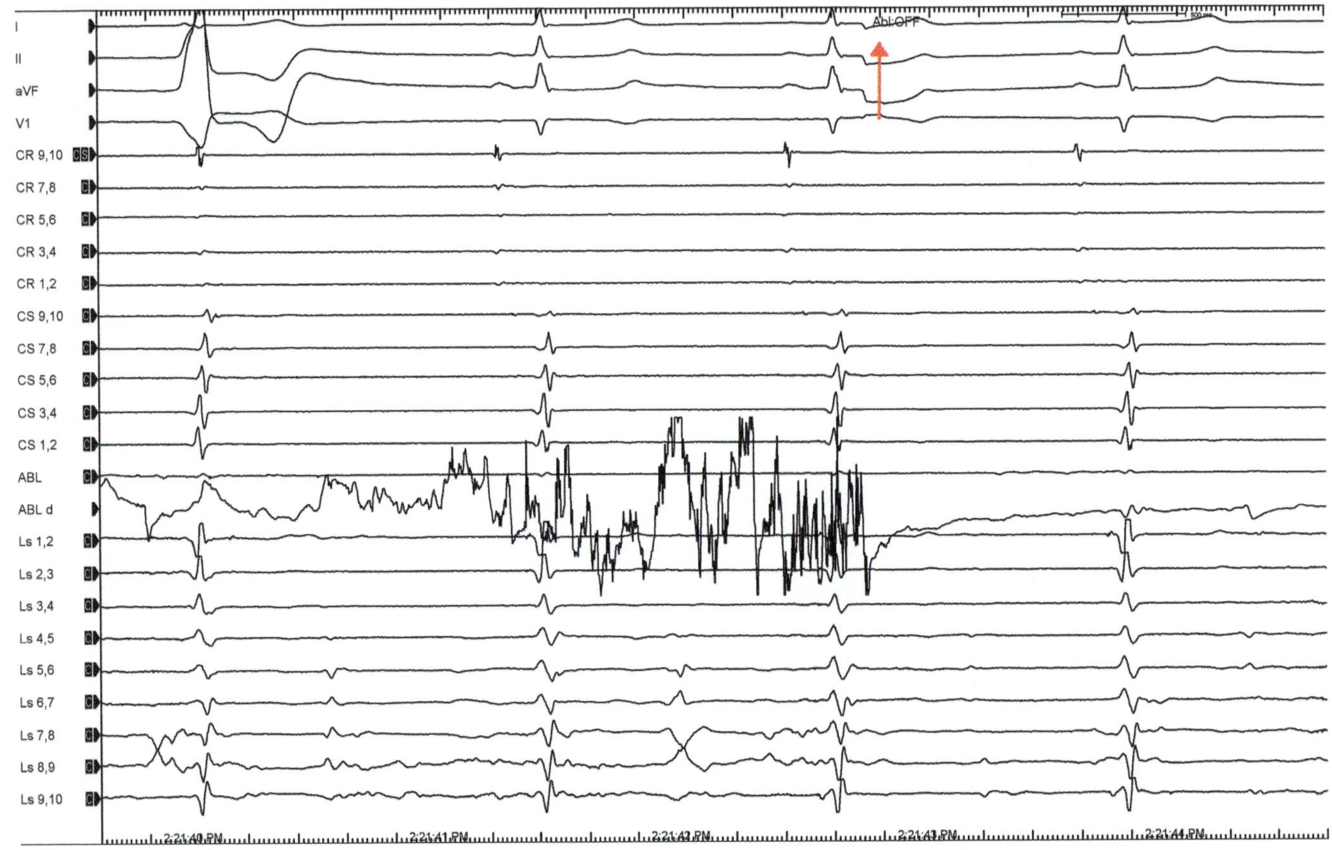

Fig. 42.6 High-frequency, irregular signals observed on the ablation electrogram recording in conjunction with steady impedance rise, both indicative of an impending steam pop; radiofrequency energy was promptly terminated (*arrow*).

termination of RF energy delivery. In the setting of RF ablation, thrombosis and thromboembolism are associated with char/thrombus formation at the tip of nonirrigated/inadequately irrigated ablation catheters; it is suspected when RF energy does not create effective lesions and impedance rise > 10–20 Ω is observed during energy delivery. The ablation catheter should be withdrawn outside of the body, the tip of the ablation catheter inspected for char formation, and char/thrombus removed before proceeding with the ablation procedure.

Unwanted injury to structures surrounding the primary ablation target is also possible. It can happen during ablation *using all commonly used energy sources (RF, cryo, pulsed field)*, although some complications are more common with specific energy sources.

Symptomatic pericarditis is a common complication of RF catheter ablation, secondary to pericardial injury and more frequently encountered with extensive ablation of thin-walled chambers or when epicardial access is obtained. Cryoablation and newly developed pulsed-field ablation (PFA) do not appear to be associated with significant pericarditis, but whether this is related to the type of energy used/mechanism of lesion formation or relatively far fewer clinical applications of these sources is yet to be determined. Onset is in the early postprocedural period, and the course is usually mild, self-limited, responding well to nonsteroidal antiinflammatory drugs or colchicine. Adjunctive steroids might be considered for refractory pain, significant ECG changes, and/or pericardial effusion. In rare cases, pericarditis can develop later (Dressler syndrome–like), with symptoms (fever, pericarditis pain, low blood pressure) presenting weeks following the ablation procedure. Diagnosis is made by ECG and beside echocardiography, which can show significant concomitant effusion, requiring pericardiocentesis. If extensive ablation or epicardial access is anticipated (epicardial ablation, phrenic nerve dislodgement), premedication with colchicine might be effective in controlling symptoms without the need of a loading dose (lower incidence of side effects). In case of epicardial access, pericardial sheaths should be removed at the end of the procedure unless there is continued bleeding. To control inflammation and pain, intermediate-acting steroids, and long-acting local anesthetics (liposomal bupivacaine) can be injected intrapericardially right before removing the sheath.[22]

Atrioventricular (AV) node injury and resulting AV block possible when targeting arrhythmias near the AV node/His bundle region, such as AVNRT, septal accessory pathways, proximal coronary sinus/septal atrial tachycardia (AT)/flutters (AFl), and septal ventricular tachycardia (VT). AV block is also possible with contralateral bundle injury when baseline bundle branch block is present at baseline. Careful mapping of the His bundle region, catheter stability, and interruption of energy delivery when signs of impending AV block (PR prolongation, fast junctional rhythm, VA block) are observed are key to avoid this complication. All energy sources can potentially cause this complication, but cryoenergy is associated with a much lower incidence of AV block. It can sometimes be used for "cryo-mapping" when mild low temperatures (up to −10°C) are

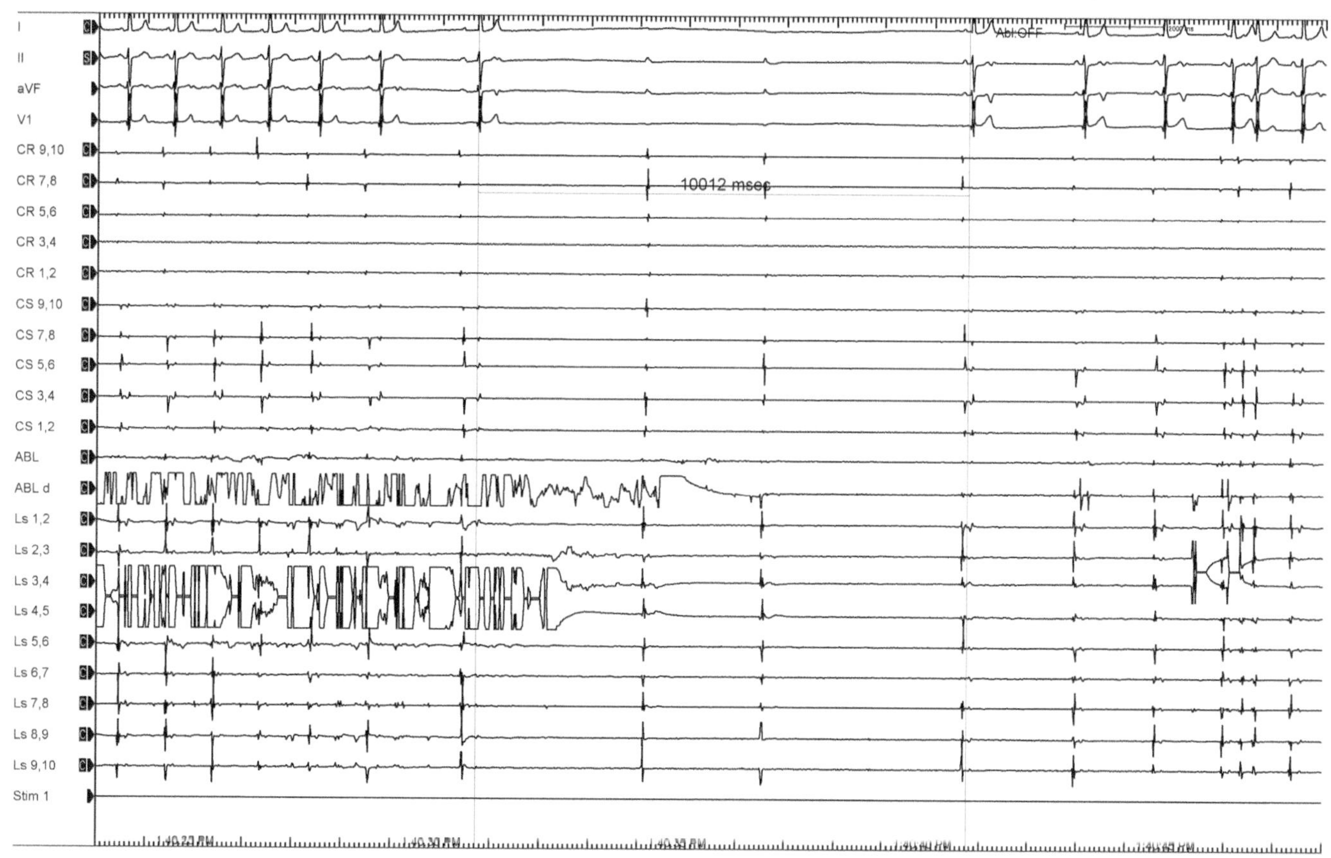

Fig. 42.7 Vagal response during ablation on the anterior aspect of the left superior pulmonary vein.

applied to create "test" lesions in high-risk areas. If AV block occurs, it is usually reversible, and ablation with lower temperatures, leading to permanent damage, can be avoided in this area. If transient AV block is observed during a procedure, overnight observation with telemetry might be needed to exclude progression to permanent AV block by means of lesion expansion or edema, especially when RF energy is used. When permanent, AV block requires implantation of a permanent pacemaker, as resumption of AV conduction after lesion maturation is rare and unpredictable. Of note, after pacemaker implantation following AV node injury (voluntary or not), patients can develop polymorphic ventricular tachycardia (VT) and subsequent sudden cardiac arrest, possibly owing to an increased sympathetic nerve activity along with prolongation of the action potential duration. The risk of such ventricular arrhythmias is reduced when pacing rates are programmed to 90 bpm for the first 3 months, with gradual reduction to the desired base rate in the following months at a rate of around 10 bpm per month (see Chapter 25).[23] Sinus node injury and sinus node dysfunction can be a result of direct injury when ablating near the superior vena cava/RA junction but also with injury of the sinus node artery during LA roof/right superior PV ablation. Damage can be reversible if energy application is immediately terminated when a sudden slowing of sinus rate is noted. A permanent pacemaker might be indicated if no sign of reversal is observed in the days following the ablation.

Vagal reflexes causing bradycardia and hypotension can occur due to inadvertent ablation of epicardial ganglionated plexi, typically during ablation around the left superior PV (Fig. 42.7). Vagal reflexes are transient, and their effects are reversed when RF energy delivery is interrupted.[24] Rarely, prolonged hypotension might occur, requiring atrial or ventricular pacing and muscarinic antagonists (atropine or glycopyrrolate) for reversal. Vagal reflexes are also almost invariably observed during PFA procedures and are thought to be a result of direct stimulation of the ganglionated plexi. Timely prophylaxis with muscarinic antagonists (ideally, prior to transseptal access) is highly effective to dampen/prevent this side effect. Similarly, with PFA it is not uncommon to stimulate bronchial nerves (cough), phrenic nerves (hiccup), sympathetic nerves (hypertension), and thoracic nerves (chest muscles contraction) during energy delivery. More profound paralysis might be needed to avoid significant chest movements, which might lead to catheter instability and nonpermanent lesions.

PV stenosis results from inflammation associated with a distal ablation, when energy (RF, cryo, laser) is delivered within the PVs (ostia and beyond).[25] To date, there is no report of PV stenosis after PFA, even with ostial energy delivery, possibly owing to the mechanism of cellular death induced by PFA (electroporation/apoptosis without resulting inflammation/fibrosis). But, as stated, more experience is needed to make any definite conclusion on the safety of PFA. Symptoms such as cough, dyspnea, hemoptysis, and recurrent pneumonia are only present in case of severe (> 70%) stenosis or multiple PV involvement. Most commonly, patients display stenosis on a follow-up imaging study, which is performed in preparation

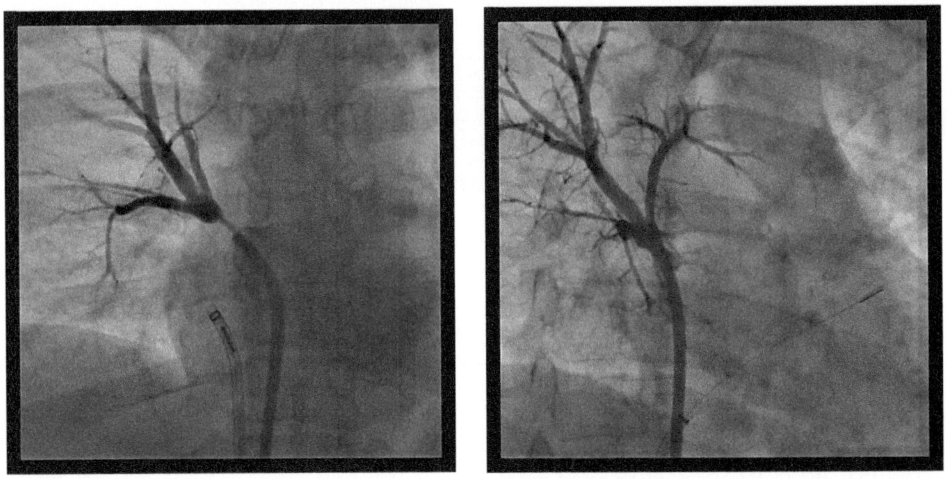

Fig. 42.8 Severe right superior pulmonary vein stenosis treated with venoplasty and stenting.

of an additional left-sided electrophysiology procedure (repeat ablation, LAA closure). The diagnosis is made by CTA/MRA or PV flow studies on echocardiography (TEE/ICE). Routine screening of asymptomatic patients might be used for newer energy sources or inexperienced operators to assess the relative incidence of PV stenosis and correct the technique if necessary. To prevent PV stenosis, energy delivery should be antral, as defined by ICE imaging or 3D mapping. A circular mapping catheter placed at the level of the PV antra is a useful marker to always perform ablation proximal to it. For symptomatic PV stenosis, moderate (50–70%) stenosis involving multiple PVs, or severe PV stenosis (Fig. 42.8), pulmonary stenting is the treatment of choice, as balloon venoplasty alone is almost inevitably associated with recurrent stenosis.[26] After stenting, surveillance with follow-up imaging is important, as recurrent stenosis is not rare. SimilarlySVC stenosis is observed with ablation within the SVC when performing SVC isolation or inappropriate sinus tachycardia ablation, with a higher incidence observed in the setting of small veins and concomitant leads/indwelling catheters. Patients usually present with SVC syndrome, and venoplasty/stenting are required.[27] To prevent SVC stenosis, energy delivery should be at the level of the RA/SVC junction, as defined by ICE or 3D mapping, and ablation performed with a segmental approach (ablation of the septal and posterior segments, including extending into the posteroseptal RA wall, is usually sufficient for isolation).

Nerve injury to the phrenic nerves and to the periesophageal vagal plexus can occur with RF, laser, and cryoenergy. PFA appears to be safe with respect to injury, but more experience is needed to conclude on the effect of PFA on pericardiac nerves; stimulation is very common, and higher doses might result in stunning, with reversible muscle weakness. Right and left phrenic nerve injury is seen when ablating within and around the SVC/right superior PV and within the LAA/left persistent SVC, respectively. As such, it is more common when energy is delivered using balloon-based technologies (cryo, laser), when energy is delivered more ostially. Left phrenic nerve injury can also be observed after epicardial ablation for VT, where the target is in the vicinity of the basal/lateral LV (substrate typical of

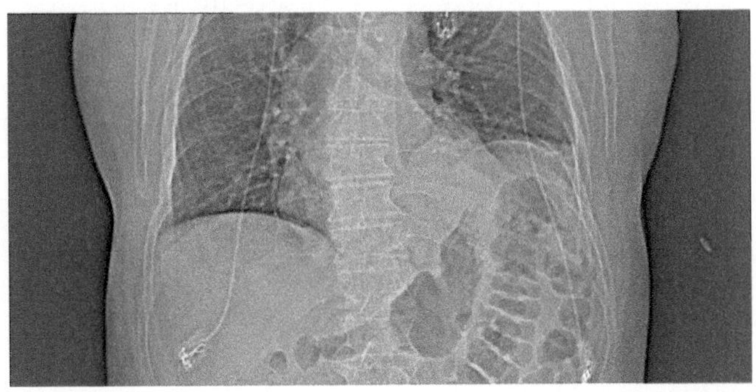

Fig. 42.9 Left phrenic nerve paralysis after distal ablation in the left atrial appendage.

nonischemic cardiomyopathy–related VT). Patients might be asymptomatic or present with dyspnea, hiccups, and cough; imaging (chest radiography, chest CT/MRI, diaphragmatic ultrasound) shows unilateral diaphragmatic elevation (Fig. 42.9) with paralysis on functional studies (fluoroscopy/ultrasound). In most cases, recovery occurs within 12 months, but damage might be permanent with associated varied limitations in physical activity. In these patients, contralateral nerve damage is catastrophic (ventilatory failure requiring permanent support), and care should be taken when performing subsequent invasive procedures around the remaining functional phrenic nerve. To prevent phrenic nerve injury, is important to delineate the course of this nerve with high-output pacing, and ablation should not be performed in sites of phrenic nerve capture whenever possible. If ablation needs to be performed in these sites (i.e., inappropriate sinus tachycardia ablation, epicardial VT ablation), an esophageal balloon can be placed in the pericardial space through a deflectable sheath (Fig. 42.10), and directed to the lateral/posterior margin of the RA so it is interposed between the phrenic nerve and the ablation catheter.[28,29] When ablating in the vicinity of the phrenic nerve, it is important to monitor their integrity during ablation. The right phrenic nerve can be paced above the site of ablation, ensuring constant capture during energy delivery; additionally, monitoring normal diaphragmatic excursion during spontaneous breathing on fluoroscopy

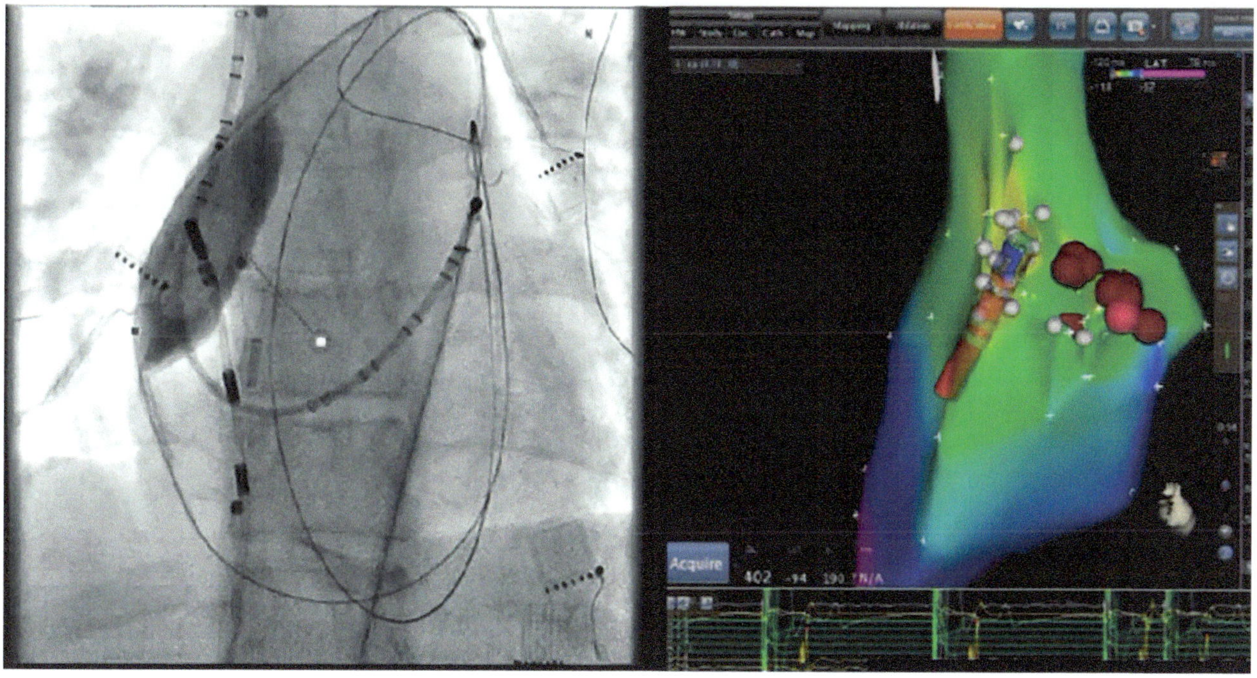

Fig. 42.10 Esophageal balloon positioned in the pericardial space, interposed between the ablation catheter and the phrenic nerve in a case of inappropriate sinus tachycardia ablation.

or ICE, or recording of the diaphragmatic compound motor action potentials can provide insight into the integrity of both nerves. Energy delivery should promptly be stopped at the first sign of phrenic nerve dysfunction (reduced excursion, weaker contraction). If this is done in a timely manner, recovery is usually observed. Periesophageal vagal plexus injury is observed with ablation of the posterior heart and can result in gastric hypomotility, with abdominal bloating and discomfort occurring hours to days after the procedure. The diagnosis is made by barium contrast imaging. As with phrenic nerve injury, spontaneous recovery is common but may require up to 12 months. Prevention involves the same strategies adopted for the prevention of esophageal injury, as outlined next.

Atrioesophageal fistula (AEF) is the most dreaded complication of AF ablation, resulting from either direct thermal injury of the anterior esophageal wall or indirect injury due to nerve/vascular damage.[30,31] AEF has been described after RF and cryoablation, but not PFA (to date). Patients typically present with symptoms 2–4 weeks following an ablation procedure involving ablation of the posterior heart, most commonly the LA posterior wall, but also coronary sinus and epicardial basal LV. Symptoms are variable and include chest pain, dysphagia, odynophagia, massive gastrointestinal bleeding, persistent fever and chills, recurrent neurologic events, and septic shock. Without prompt surgical repair, mortality is high; those who survive have a significant residual disability due to recurrent, widespread systemic embolism that occurred before repair. For early diagnosis, patient awareness is key; patients should be instructed to immediately contact the EP service if any of the aforementioned typical symptoms occur. CT of the head or chest revealing intravascular air should immediately arouse suspicion. High-resolution (1-mm slice thickness or less) CT or MRI with oral contrast can reveal the fistula, while a barium swallow is not sensitive enough. When atrioesophageal fistula is suspected, the patient should be made nil per os (strictly) and any manipulation of the esophagus, including TEE and esophagogastroduodenoscopy, should be avoided as it can precipitate massive hemorrhage (fistula disruption) and air embolism (air insufflation during endoscopy). To prevent this complication, it is important to limit RF energy delivery in areas near the esophagus. The esophageal course is variable and can change during the procedure; the only reliable way to determine its location during ablation is to perform repeated esophagography using low-osmolar water-soluble contrast or visualize its course relative to the ablation catheter on ultrasound, with the ICE catheter positioned in the LA. Luminal esophageal temperature monitoring can be a useful indicator, but it is important to know its limitations; while a rapid elevation of luminal temperature is worrisome, lack of heating does not equal safety, given variable orientation of the probe within the lumen (Fig. 42.11). The type of temperature probe used is also important, as different probes react to a change in temperature more or less rapidly, with only the one reacting more rapidly providing a reliable measurement.[32] As such, it is best to assume that the esophagus is in potential danger whenever ablation is performed at any site on the left atrial posterior wall; avoiding excess tissue contact pressure (< 10 gr), and limiting the time of RF application (moving the ablation catheter every 5–10 seconds) are important strategies to reduce the occurrence of esophageal injury. Of note, limiting the power of RF energy can be deleterious as longer delivery times are needed to obtain effective lesions; these lesions reach greater depths than the ones obtained with a high-power, short-duration strategy,[33] potentially damaging the esophagus.

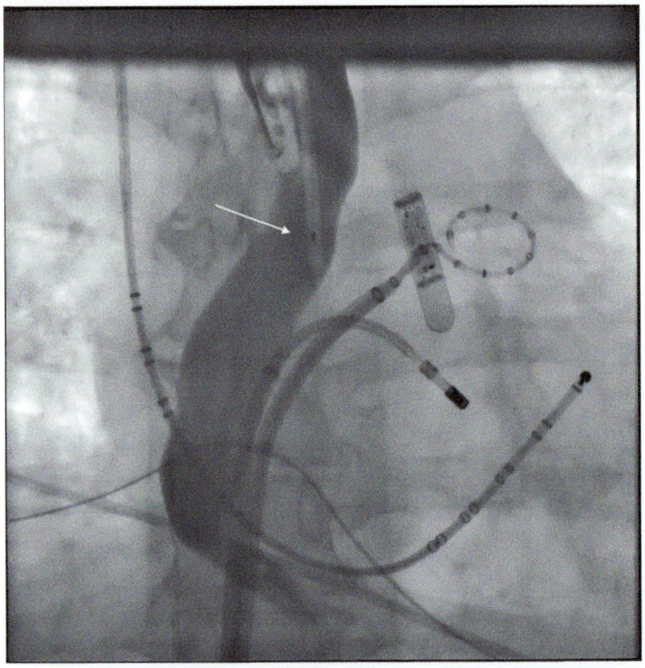

Fig. 42.11 Esophagogram to delineate the esophageal course. Note that using a temperature probe (*arrow*) is not a reliable method to assess the esophageal location and injury.

Bronchial and lung injury is a result of direct thermal injury when delivering energy (RF, laser, cryo) deep within the PVs, where they are in close relationship with the bronchial tree. Very distal ablation is rare with antral isolation techniques employed when delivering RF and laser energy, while a deep-seated cryoballoon reaching low nadir temperatures can cause thermal injury to the neighboring bronchial and lung tissues. Patients present with cough, hemoptysis, and lung consolidation; the prognosis is usually benign, with symptoms resolving once inflammation has resolved, but cases of atriobronchial fistula have been reported, a fatal complication.[34] Prevention is key, with proximal seal, avoidance of low nadir temperature, and adjusting the cryoablation time according to the time-to-isolation of the treated PV.

Coronary artery injury is a specific complication occurring in the setting of ablation of arrhythmias originating around the aortic coronary cusps, coronary venous system, or on the epicardial surface of the ventricles.[35] When RF/cryoenergy is applied close to the coronary arteries, these can be susceptible to heat–freeze damage, which may result in spasm, stenosis, and occlusion with associated thrombus formation. In theory, PFA can affect the coronary circulation, by producing spasm (direct stimulation of afferent nerves) or endothelial damage (reversible or irreversible electroporation, a function of transmurality of energy delivery) and care should be taken when delivering higher doses in critical areas. During ablation in the coronary cusps, real-time visualization of the right coronary and left coronary ostia with ICE is the gold standard to avoid ablation within the coronary arteries. The ablation catheter can be visualized in real-time on ICE and the distance between the tip and the coronary ostia can be assessed. Additionally, electrograms might also point to an intracoronary location if, when mapping in the right or left coronary cusp, atrial electrograms are seen instead of ventricular ones, which would be expected in a coronary cusp location (Fig. 42.12). Ablation within the coronary venous system is not associated with an increased risk of coronary artery injury when using irrigated-tip ablation catheters, possibly owing to the relatively high flow of the combined effect of irrigation/blood circulation leading to effective heat dissipation. During epicardial ablation of non–scar-related ventricular arrhythmias, where the ablation target lies within normal tissue, repeat selective angiography might be necessary to delineate the epicardial coronary circulation in real-time to avoid ablation in the proximity of the main coronary arteries.

When an externally irrigated ablation catheter is used, attention should be paid to the volume infused to prevent volume overload, which is common after complex atrial and ventricular arrhythmia procedures.[36] Monitoring of the fluid status (weight gain, lung ultrasound) is important, and a short course of diuretics (intravenous or oral) might be appropriate to avoid congestion or acute exacerbation of heart failure. The latter is also observed during or after scar-related VT ablation in patients with chronic systolic heart failure associated with ischemic and nonischemic cardiomyopathy. Frequent VT induction

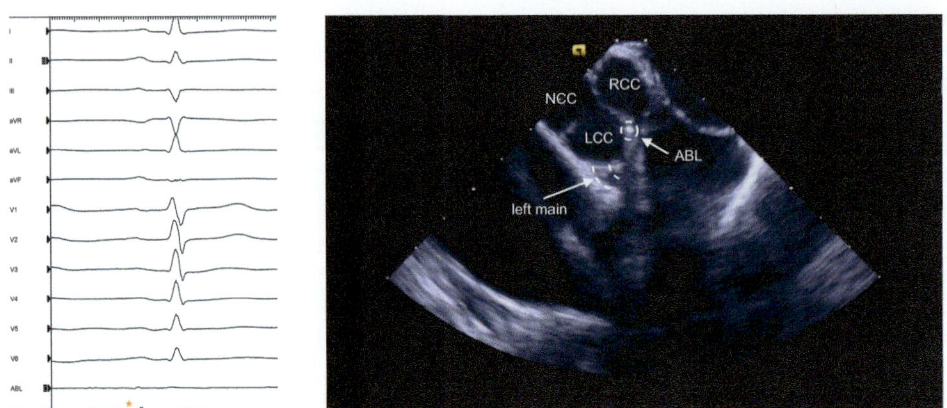

Fig. 42.12 Electrograms of the ablation catheter when inside the left main coronary artery, displaying an atrial electrogram (*star*) instead of the expected ventricular electrogram. On the right, intracardiac echocardiography image showing the location of the ablation catheter (ABL) in relation to the left main coronary artery.

and prolonged mapping during the VT may be attempted, and multiple shocks may be required to terminate unstable VTs, leading to a state of cardiogenic shock. Deployment of hemodynamic support systems may be helpful, but a better strategy is to perform a substrate-based ablation strategy (see Chapter 36) with limited ablation of abnormal electrograms or full scar homogenization, for which VT induction and mapping are not required to achieve longer-term success.[37]

EPICARDIAL CATHETER ABLATION–RELATED COMPLICATIONS

See Table 42.4 for a list of complications occurring in the setting of epicardial catheter ablation procedures (see Chapter 37). Epicardial access and ablation can result in a variety of uncommon serious complications, which every operator performing these procedures should be aware of.[38] Most critical complications occur during percutaneous subxiphoid pericardial access, but ablation-related complications should also be mentioned.

To minimize bleeding, systemic anticoagulation with heparin should not be administered or its effects must be reversed if already administered before attempting pericardial access. Inadvertent puncture of surrounding structures is always possible when the needle blindly passes from the skin to the pericardial space. Arterial vessels of the rectus muscle, diaphragm, and anterior chest wall may be punctured, leading to catastrophic bleeding into the abdominal or mediastinal space. In addition, it is possible to puncture the left lobe of an enlarged liver in patients with congestive heart failure or hepatopathies (especially with inferior epicardial access approaches), or the lung in patients with emphysema (anterior epicardial access approach). Mediastinal, intraperitoneal, and intrapleural bleeding might be unrecognized until a large amount of blood has accumulated. Unexplained hypotension associated with localizing pain (abdominal, chest) should prompt a search for intraabdominal or intrathoracic bleeding with bedside ultrasound or CT imaging. Early diagnosis and prompt management (arterial embolization, surgical repair with hematoma evacuation) are key to avoid grave sequelae, including death.

Inadvertent puncture of the RV is relatively common and are usually benign if only the needle or guidewire has entered the chamber. RV perforations may be easily recognized with a contrast injection and, if ICE is used, the wire can be seen floating within the RV/pulmonary artery. If the needle is within the RV, it should be slightly retracted until contrast is seen surrounding the heart within the pericardial space, and access can proceed as usual. In case the sheath had been introduced into the RV, a second attempt to obtain proper pericardial access while leaving the first sheath in place should be performed. At the end of the procedure, percutaneous closure of the RV perforation with transcatheter closure devices can be attempted before removing the sheath.[39] If this is not possible or it fails, prompt drainage of the subsequent pericardial bleed is necessary after removing the sheath, and surgical repair should be anticipated in case of continuous bleeding. Although rare, "through-and-through"/double RV perforation is also possible; in such cases, the needle enters and exits the RV at the time of access. This might not be recognized, and the procedure can be uneventful until the catheter and sheath are removed and copious bleeding at the end of the procedure ensues, an inevitable surgical emergency.[40] Inadvertent puncture of epicardial coronary vessels is also common with epicardial access; it is not uncommon to aspirate 10–30 mL of bloody drainage after a "dry" puncture. However, if a large amount of blood is aspirated or bleeding is not self-limited, percutaneous intervention (embolization/covered stenting) and surgical repair might be necessary.

During sheath and catheter manipulation, air may be inadvertently introduced into the pericardial space.[13] Intrapericardial air can cause elevation of the defibrillation threshold[40] of transthoracic defibrillators (external patches, single coil leads), resulting in VT/VF refractory to shock.[41] Care should be taken to avoid entry of significant amounts of air, and when air is recognized on fluoroscopy, it should be promptly evacuated from the pericardial space. During mapping and ablation using externally irrigated ablation catheters, it is important to closely monitor volume of irrigation fluid that is instilled within the closed pericardial space, which might lead to cardiac tamponade if the fluid is not continuously aspirated.

Finally, ablation in the epicardial space is associated with injury of the coronary vessels and phrenic nerves, and epicardial access and ablation always cause symptomatic pericarditis; for specifics about these complications, see earlier sections.

TABLE 42.4 Epicardial Catheter Ablation–Related Complications
Puncture of the liver, lung, arterial vessels of the rectus muscle, diaphragm, and anterior chest
Right ventricular perforation
Puncture of epicardial coronary vessels
Elevated defibrillation thresholds secondary to intrapericardial air
Cardiac tamponade secondary to catheter irrigation
Phrenic nerve injury

ACKNOWLEDGMENTS

The authors would like to thank Takumi Yamada and G. Neal Kay, authors of the previous edition of this chapter, for providing insight toward the creation of this new version.

REFERENCES

Please refer to the e-book for a complete list of references.

43

Atrial Transseptal Catheterization

Shumpei Mori, Kalyanam Shivkumar

KEY POINTS

- A detailed understanding of the individual anatomy of the atrial septum and its relationship with surrounding structures is fundamental for safe atrial transseptal catheterization.
- Although a biplane fluoroscopy-guided approach with Brockenbrough needle had been the historical standard for atrial transseptal catheterization, it has been largely replaced by an intracardiac echocardiography-guided approach.
- Other specialized tools, such as radiofrequency-assisted transseptal needles, have further improved the efficacy and safety of the atrial transeptal catheterization.

INTRODUCTION

Access to the left heart via the atrial transseptal catheterization was first described in 1959 as an alternative technique to the conventional transaortic approach.[1] Despite subsequent technical refinements,[2–4] atrial transseptal catheterization was initially adopted only by few highly specialized institutions, because of the higher risk of potentially life-threatening complications. The development and widespread implementation of radiofrequency (RF) catheter ablation for the treatment of cardiac arrhythmias in the 1990s renewed interest in this procedure.[5] Along with wide application of the RF catheter ablation for atrial fibrillation (AF),[6] currently, atrial transeptal catheterization has been considered a fundamental skill for any interventional electrophysiologists.[7] Although the general technique of this procedure has not changed substantially over the years, important technological advances have made the procedure significantly easier and safer.[8–14] This chapter reviews the anatomy, indications, techniques, and outcomes related to the atrial transseptal catheterization.

ANATOMIC CONSIDERATIONS FOR TRANSSEPTAL CATHETERIZATION

A detailed understanding of the anatomy of the atrial septum and its surrounding structures[15] in each case is fundamental to safely perform atrial transseptal catheterization.

The anatomical true septum is defined as the partition that can be penetrated without exiting to the extracardiac space. Within the area that right atrium (RA) faces the left atrium (LA), the true atrial septum is confined at the floor of the fossa ovalis and its anterior limbus (Fig. 43.1).[16] The floor of the fossa ovalis is the primary septum, and its anterior limbus is referred to as the anteroinferior muscular buttress derived from the vestibular spine.[17] The superior free margin of the primary septum is seen as the flap valve in the LA, that is attaching to the anterosuperior interatrial fold (Fig. 43.2). Compared to the thin primary septum, the anteroinferior muscular buttress is the thick muscular atrial septum located between the fossa ovalis and coronary sinus orifice (Fig. 43.2). The location of this buttress corresponds to the medial attachment of the Eustachian valve. The tendon of Todaro runs within this buttress.[17] The buttress, at its cranial end, is connected with the central fibrous body beneath the noncoronary aortic sinus to fix the atrial septum to the fibrous skeleton of the heart (Fig. 43.3).[18] Even though they are referred to as the secondary septum, the anterosuperior, superior, posterior, and inferior limbus of the fossa ovalis is the interatrial groove/fold, which is not the true septum (Figs. 43.4 and 43.5).[16] The anterosuperior interatrial groove/fold is related to the aortic root and ascending aorta. The superior interatrial groove/fold is adjacent to the superior vena cava. The posterior interatrial groove/fold is close to the right pulmonary veins and right phrenic nerve. The inferior interatrial groove/fold is related to the inferior vena cava (Figs. 43.4 and 43.5). The inferior interatrial groove is in continuity with the inferior pyramidal space.[19] The inferior pyramidal space is the epicardial space wedging from the inferior crux of the heart toward the central fibrous body, carrying the coronary sinus, atrioventricular nodal artery, and atrioventricular node (Fig. 43.2). Therefore, any invasive procedures outside the fossa ovalis and anteroinferior muscular buttress should not be deemed as the true atrial transseptal catheterization. They are the approach to perforate the free wall of the RA toward the subepicardial fibroadipose tissue or into the pericardial space, which is associated with cardiac perforation[20] and/or inadvertent damage to the adjacent structures,[21,22] with potential consequence of catastrophic complications.

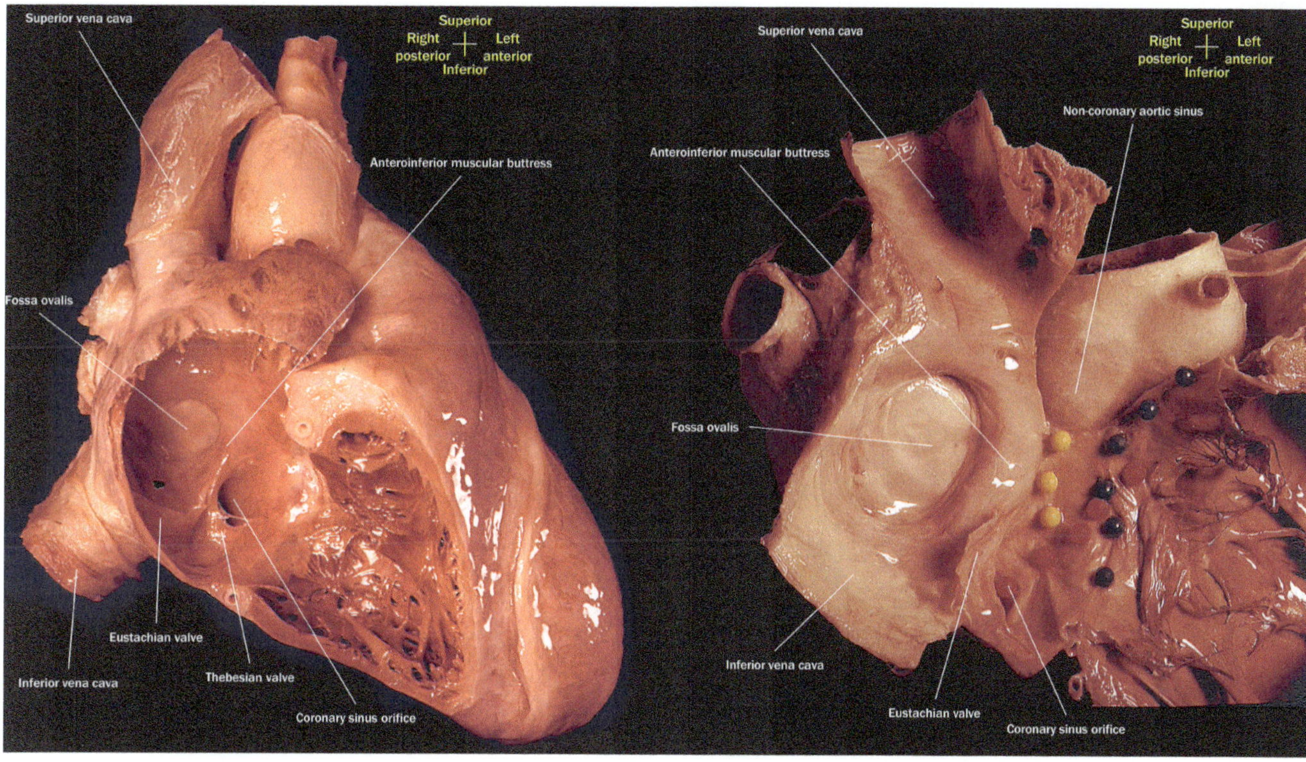

Fig. 43.1 The fossa ovalis viewed from the right anterior oblique direction. The thickness of the limbus of the fossa ovalis is less prominent in the heart on the *left*. (Illustration courtesy of UCLA Cardiac Arrhythmia Center, Wallace A. McAlpine MD Collection.)

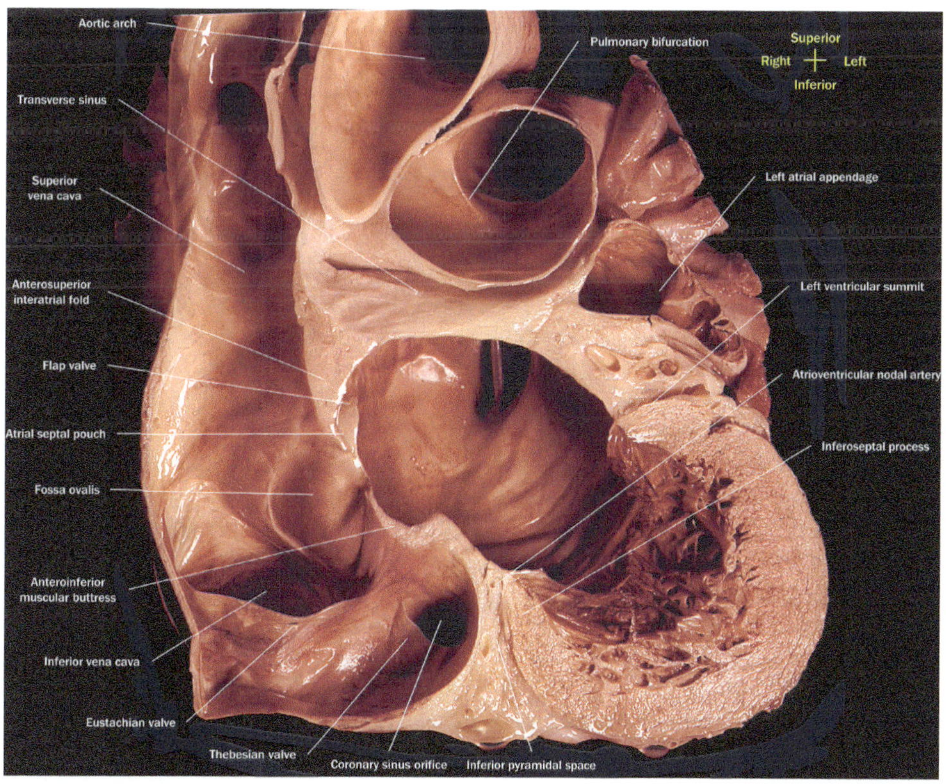

Fig. 43.2 The fossa ovalis viewed from the frontal direction. The frontal plane cut is made at the level of anterior limbus of the fossa ovalis. The anterior limbus between the fossa ovalis and the coronary sinus corresponds to the anteroinferior muscular buttress. It is the muscular true atrial septum, which contains the tendon of Todaro and connects to the central fibrous body beneath the noncoronary aortic sinus. The relationship between the flap valve of the primary septum and the anterosuperior interatrial fold, the so-called secondary septum, is well appreciated. The atrial septal pouch is created between the free flap valve and the interatrial fold. This part, when evaluated in two-dimensional imaging, can be confused as double atrial septum. (Illustration courtesy of UCLA Cardiac Arrhythmia Center, Wallace A. McAlpine MD Collection.)

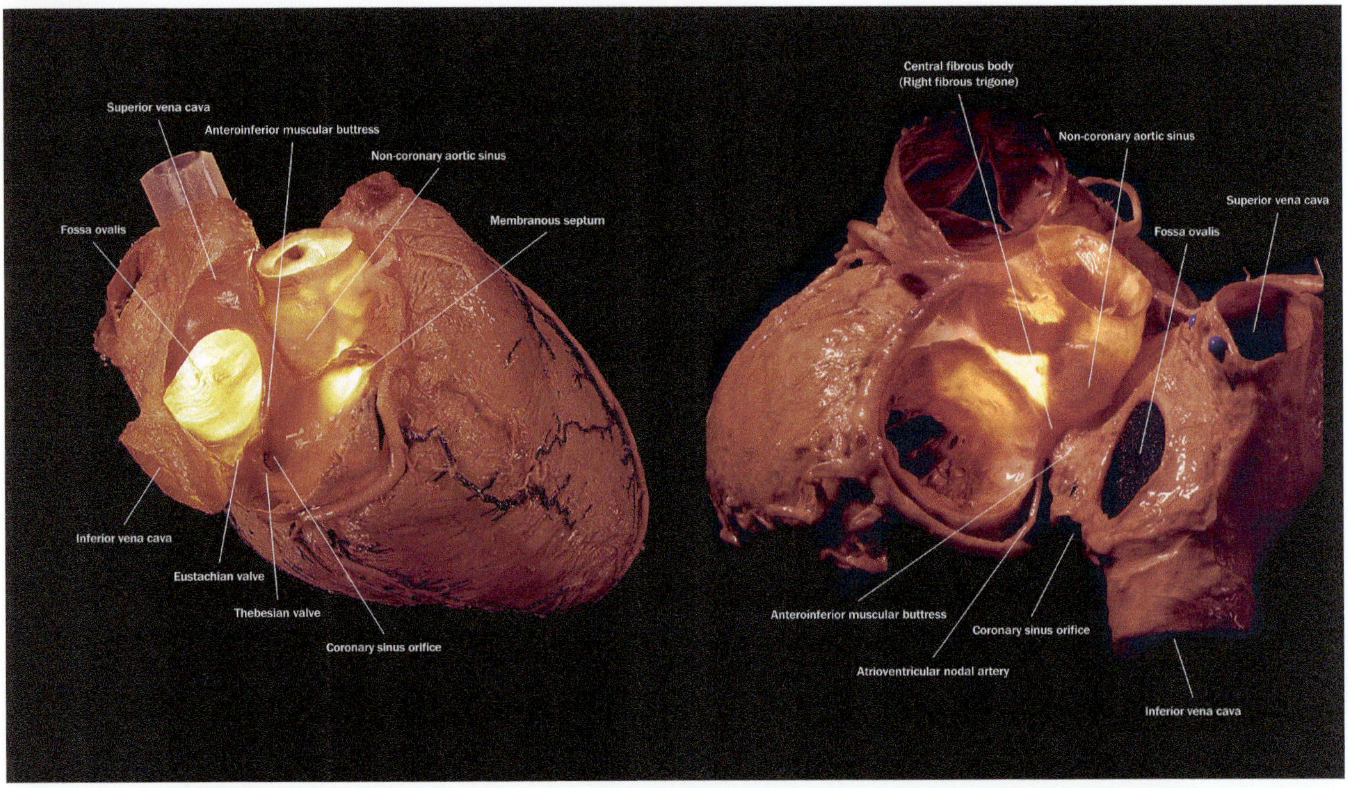

Fig. 43.3 The fossa ovalis viewed from both right atrial (*left*) and left atrial side (*right*). The size of the fossa ovalis is relatively large in both hearts. *Right,* Unusual dissection—the removal of the left atrium through removal of the primary septum and division of the interatrial fold and anteroinferior muscular buttress. Usually from the left atrium, without transillumination, fossa ovalis cannot be visually detected. Only the flap valve of the primary septum is observed as the crescent-shaped slit-like pocket near the anterosuperior margin of the fossa ovalis, right posterior to the noncoronary aortic sinus. In the right panel, the connection of the anteroinferior muscular buttress to the central fibrous body is well appreciated. The triangular space between the mitral annulus and the anteroinferior muscular buttress carries the atrioventricular nodal artery originating from the left circumflex artery, initially filled with the subepicardial adipose tissue of the inferior pyramidal space. (Illustration courtesy of UCLA Cardiac Arrhythmia Center, Wallace A. McAlpine MD Collection.)

When viewed from within the RA, the fossa ovalis appears as a crater-like translucent depression (Figs. 43.1–43.3). Only the primary septum at the floor of the fossa ovalis, which is a fibromembranous structure with a thickness ranging from 0.5 to 1.5 mm, is the suitable anatomical location for the atrial transeptal catheterization. Although there are wide individual variations, in general, the normal fossa ovalis is a longitudinally oblong structure, and the average size of the fossa ovalis is approximately 20 × 15 mm.[23–25] Considering its thickness (Fig. 43.5), the anterior limbus (anteroinferior muscular buttress) should not be routinely targeted for atrial transseptal catheterization even though it is the true septum.

Notably, the thickness of the interatrial groove/fold (secondary septum) surrounding the fossa ovalis is not always a distinct and prominent structure (Figs. 43.1 and 43.2).[15] Thus, when withdrawing the transseptal sheath and needle from the superior vena cava toward the fossa ovalis, operators cannot always expect the conventional visual motion showing the "final jump," corresponding to the passage of the tip of the dilator from the superior interatrial groove into the fossa ovalis. Similarly, the first jump cannot always be expected as the gap at the junction between the superior vena cava and the RA appendage; this gap is less distinct (Figs. 43.1 and 43.2).

Initially, the site of penetration tends to be located in the superior half of the fossa ovalis due to the superior shift of the puncture system.[23] Technical advancement involving intracardiac echocardiography (ICE)[9] and RF-assisted transseptal needles[13] makes it feasible to select the site of penetration. Currently, the site of penetration can be adjusted according to the main target structures, such as the pulmonary vein, LA appendage, and mitral valve.[26]

When the heart is viewed from an attitudinal perspective, the RA is located right, anterior, and inferior relative to the LA. As a result, the plane of the atrial septum is not described by the anteroposterior sagittal plane and generally is not located vertically. Instead, the plane of the atrial septum is tilted toward right anteroinferior direction (Fig. 43.4). When viewed from superior direction, the plane of the atrial septum directs toward left anterior direction (Fig. 43.6).

Fluoroscopically, therefore, the right anterior oblique direction can show less foreshortened image of the primary septum at the floor of the fossa ovalis (Fig. 43.7 and Video 43.1). This is the best view direction to confirm the tip of the dilator in the fossa ovalis and separate the fossa ovalis from the noncoronary aortic sinus (Fig. 43.7). The atrial septum is still tilted inferiorly

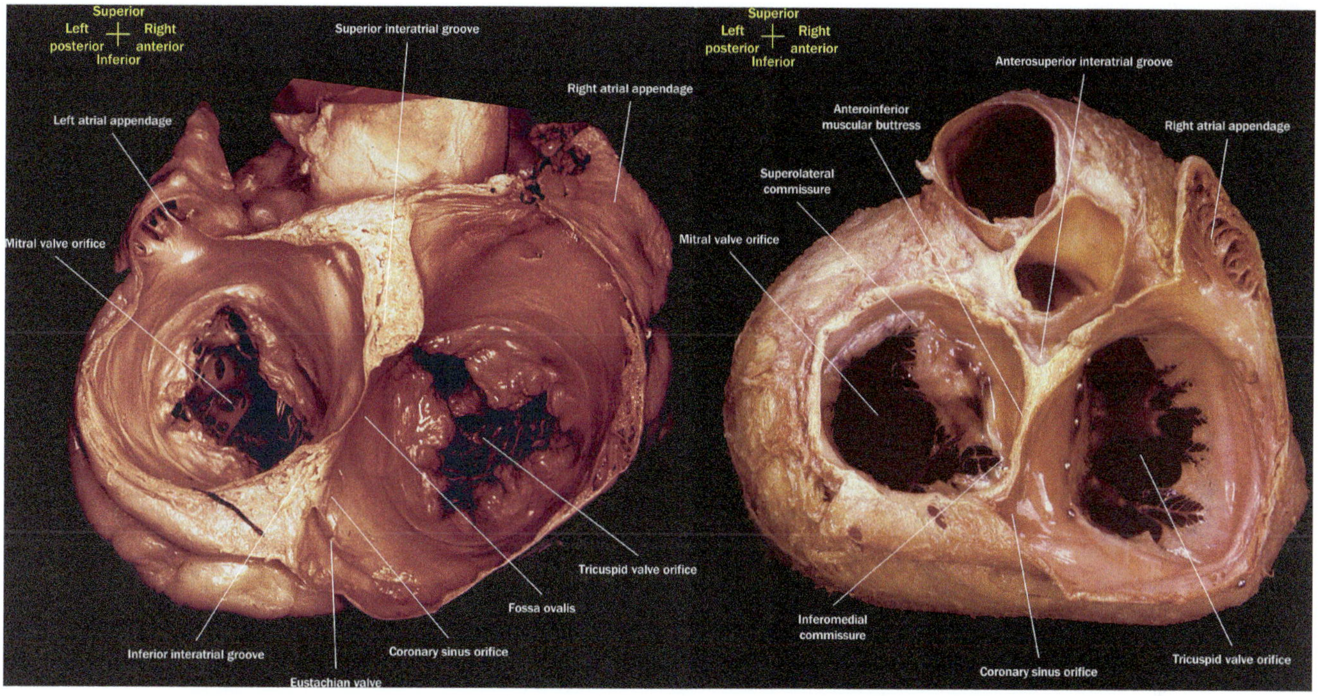

Fig. 43.4 The vertical cut of the fossa ovalis *(left)* and anteroinferior muscular buttress *(right)* viewed from the right posterosuperior direction. The *right panel* is more apical cut anterior to the fossa ovalis, compared to the *left panel* bisecting the fossa ovalis. The difference in the thickness between the primary septum and anteroinferior muscular buttress is appreciated. *Left,* Thick superior and inferior interatrial folds, that contains the subepicardial adipose tissue of the interatrial groove, compatible with the lipomatous hypertrophy. Thus, these folds are not the septum, even if they are referred to as the secondary septum. En face views of both atrioventricular valves are obtained. They show the topographic relationship between the superolateral and inferomedial commissures of the mitral valve, as well as superolateral location of the orifices of the left and right atrial appendages. (Illustration courtesy of UCLA Cardiac Arrhythmia Center, Wallace A. McAlpine MD Collection.)

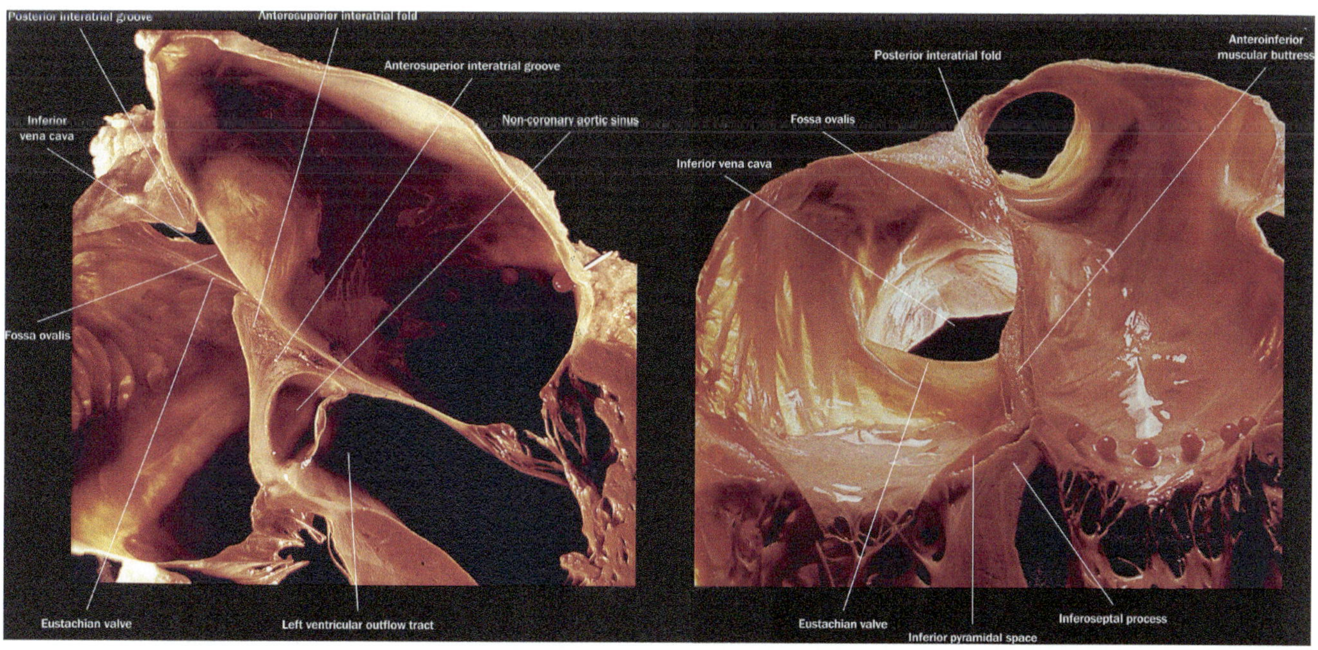

Fig. 43.5 The horizontal cut of the fossa ovalis viewed from the superior direction. The *left panel* showing the bottom of the noncoronary aortic sinus is a more superior cut plane than the *right panel* showing the four-chamber view. Similar to the superior vena cava, the inferior vena cava is the septal side structure located beneath the fossa ovalis. In addition to the primary septum at the floor of the fossa ovalis, the anteroinferior muscular buttress is also the true muscular atrial septum located between the fossa ovalis and the coronary sinus orifice toward the central fibrous body. Thus, it is beneath the level of the noncoronary aortic sinus (*right*). The floor of the triangle of Koch faces the basal inferoseptum of the left ventricle, also referred to as the inferoseptal process, intervened by the subepicardial adipose tissue of the inferior pyramidal space (*right*). (Illustration courtesy of UCLA Cardiac Arrhythmia Center, Wallace A. McAlpine MD Collection.)

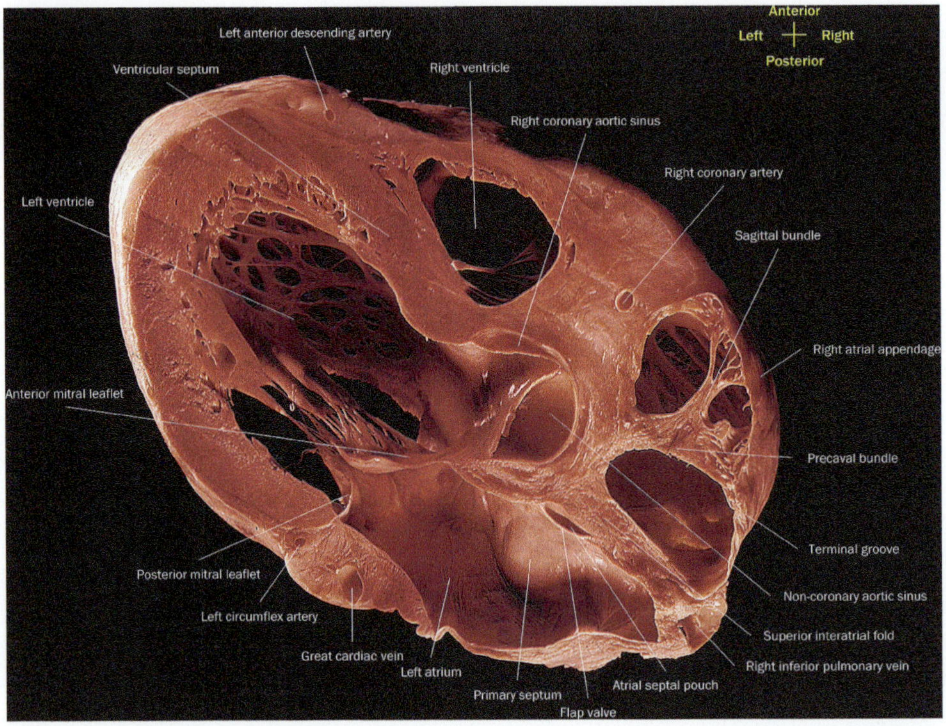

Fig. 43.6 The horizontal cut at the level of the junction between the superior vena cava and the right atrial appendage, viewed from the superior direction. This is the section superior to the fossa ovalis, showing the flap valve of the primary septum and atrial septal pouch. This section is more superior than the *left panel* in Fig. 43.5. This also demonstrates that the tricuspid annulus is located inferior relative to the mitral annulus. (Illustration courtesy of UCLA Cardiac Arrhythmia Center, Wallace A. McAlpine MD Collection.)

to the observer, because the LA leans on the RA (Fig. 43.7). The perfect en face view of the fossa ovalis can be obtained from the right anterior oblique and caudal direction. The tangential view of the primary septum at the floor of the fossa ovalis is obtained from the left anterior oblique direction (Fig. 43.7). It shows the primary septum as the linear structure tilting toward the right anterior direction (Figs. 43.7 and 43.8). Once the tip location is confirmed in the fossa ovalis away from the aortic root using the right anterior oblique projection, this is the best view to be used for puncture and to proceed the system into the LA.

In the current clinical practice of catheter ablation, it is common to have three-dimensional datasets obtained from either cardiac computed tomography or cardiac magnetic resonance imaging before the procedure. Even if fine three-dimensional reconstruction (Figs. 43.7, 43.8) is not readily available, clinicians can readily assess the clinical anatomy relevant to the atrial transseptal catheterization by applying slab-maximum or minimum intensity projection images from the right and left anterior oblique directions, in addition to regular axial image (Fig. 43.9). Extent of the tilting and rotation direction of the atrial septum shows wide individual variation (Fig. 43.10), which can be affected by age, body weight, size of the both atria, rotational position of the heart, position of the diaphragm, and elongation and dilatation of the ascending aorta.[25,27] Less-tilting atrial septum renders the conventional approach using Brockenbrough needle difficult due to potential superior shift of the needle tip.[23] As optimal right and left anterior oblique directions are variable, reflecting the large variation in the rotational position of the atrial septum within the living-heart,[27] right and left anterior oblique angulations need to be customized for each patient.

INDICATIONS AND CONTRAINDICATIONS FOR ATRIAL TRANSSEPTAL CATHETERIZATION

A transseptal approach is recommended for any interventional approaches targeting the structures in the left heart. It works as the alternative to the conventional retrograde transaortic approach, with different merits and limitations. For instance, the atrial transseptal catheterization can avoid arterial access, thus minimizing the time needed for complete postprocedural vascular recovery. When retrograde transaortic approach to the left ventricle (LV) is contraindicated, such as the presence of severe aortic valve disease, a mechanical aortic prosthesis, significant aortic atherosclerosis, and/or an aortic aneurysm, the transseptal approach is not the only but the first alternative access to the LV. During catheter mapping of left-sided accessory pathways, antegrade transseptal approach showed no difference in total procedure time or fluoroscopy time compared with retrograde transaortic approach. However, the retrograde approach was associated with a higher incidence of periprocedural complications or crossover to the other technique.[28] Atrial insertion of the accessory pathway is easy to access from the antegrade approach, whereas ventricular insertion can be readily accessed from the retrograde approach. Although the retrograde approach is often preferred to antegrade approach for

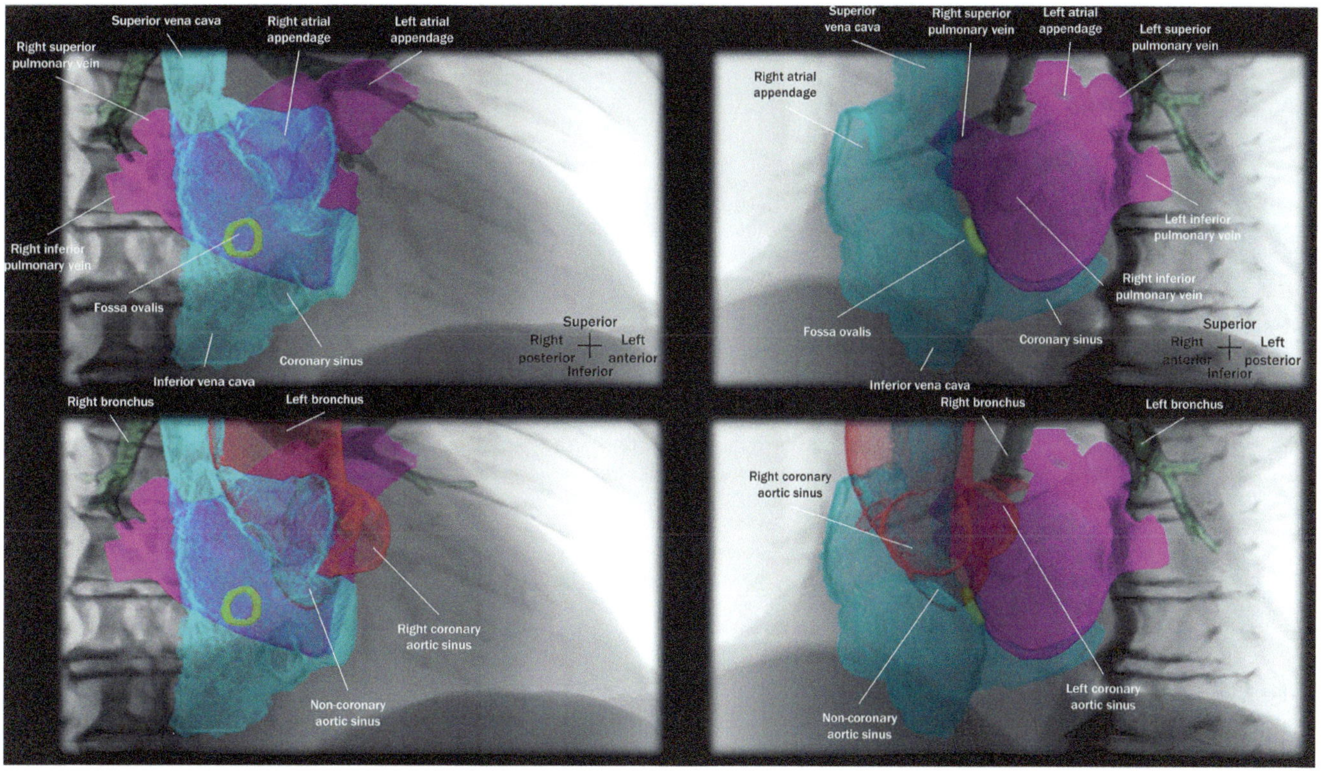

Fig. 43.7 The virtual fluoroscopic image with shell-like reconstructions of the right atrium, left atrium, bronchi, and proximal aorta viewed from the right anterior oblique direction (*left panels*) and left anterior oblique direction (*right panels*). The proximal aorta shown in the *lower panels* is removed in the *upper panels*. The *yellow structure* demarcates the fossa ovalis in this case. Thus, the right anterior oblique projection is important to obtain an en face view of the fossa ovalis, separating it from the noncoronary aortic sinus and posterior wall of the sinus venarum. The right anterior oblique view shows the most foreshortened image of the coronary sinus. On the other hand, proceeding with the system should be done by referring to the left anterior oblique projection, as it should show an en face image of the puncture system and the extent of the left atrium. Understanding these structural anatomical relationships is fundamental to performing safe left atrial transseptal catheterization. (Refer to Video 43.1.)

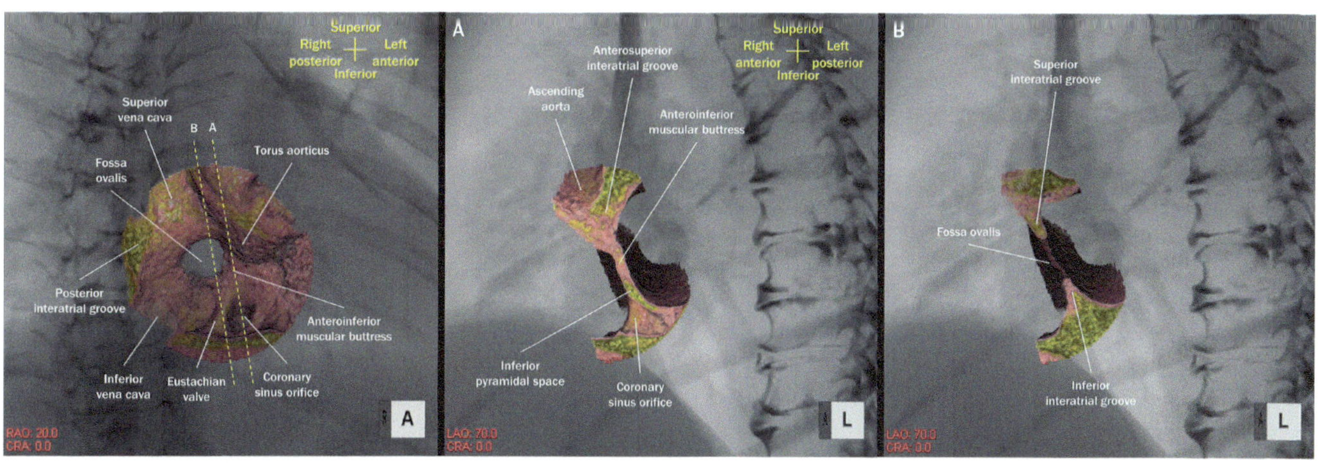

Fig. 43.8 Virtual dissection around the fossa ovalis with virtual fluoroscopic image viewed from the right anterior oblique direction (*left panel*) and left anterior oblique direction (*middle and right panels*). (A, B) *Yellow dashed line* in the *left panel* corresponds to the cutting plane shown in the *middle and right panels*, respectively. An almost en face view of the fossa ovalis is obtained from the right anterior oblique direction, and the tangential view of the fossa ovalis is obtained from the left anterior oblique direction. The angulation should be adjusted individually according to each rotational position of the atrial septum evaluated from the preprocedural imaging. The anteroinferior muscular buttress is seen superior to the coronary sinus behind the central fibrous body at the bottom of the noncoronary aortic sinus (*middle*). The fossa ovalis is sandwiched between the superior and inferior interatrial folds (*right*).

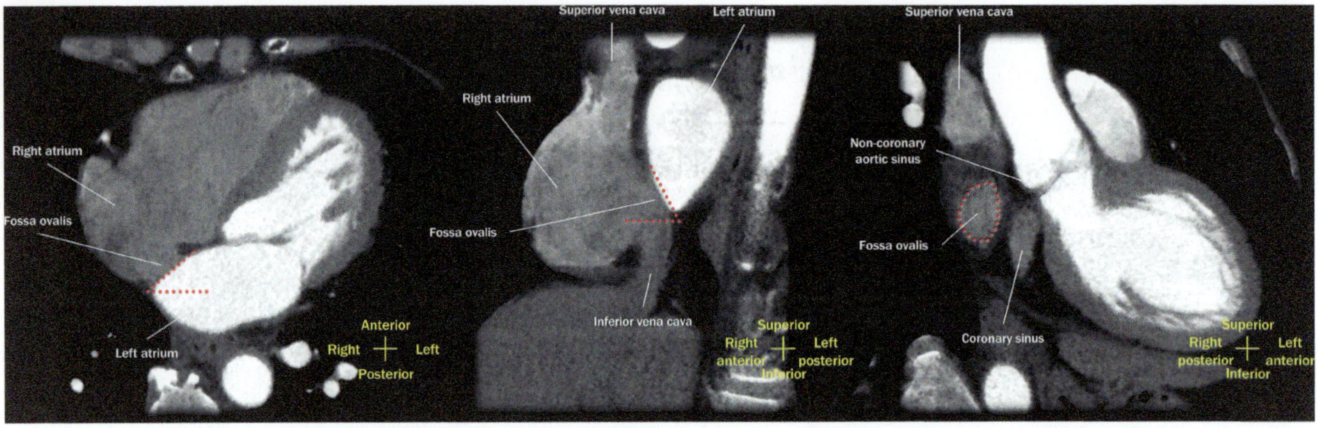

Fig. 43.9 Three quick views that should be evaluated to prepare for the atrial transseptal catheterization using the preprocedural imaging. If preprocedural cardiac computed tomography or cardiac magnetic resonance imaging is available, there is no reason not to assess individual anatomy by these quick reconstructions. A 3- to 5-mm slab minimum (or sometimes maximum) intensity projection images are created using horizontal section (*left*), left anterior oblique section corresponding to the bicaval view (*middle*), and the right anterior oblique and caudal section (*right*). Size and relative location of the fossa ovalis with surrounding structural anatomy can be readily assessable, which may affect the individualized transseptal puncture strategy.

mapping and ablation of ventricular tachycardia, certain structures (e.g., superolateral papillary muscles) may be more easily sampled with an antegrade approach.[29] The presence of LA thrombus or mobile mass constitutes a relative contraindication to the transseptal catheterization. In addition, transseptal catheterization should be avoided for patients in whom persistent right-to-left shunting would be unfavorable (e.g., concomitant LV assist device).

INTRAPROCEDURAL PATIENT MANAGEMENT: SEDATION AND ANTICOAGULATION

Proper procedural sedation is important to avoid unpredictable patient movements during the transseptal catheterization. Also, adequately controlled respiration is necessary to prevent significant shifts of the transseptal sheath and needle positioning. During inspiration, a catheter positioned in the RA might shift superiorly by an average of 9 mm,[30] which could result in inadvertent puncture outside the fossa ovalis.

The practice of uninterrupted warfarin or non–vitamin K antagonists during AF ablation is commonly used. Significant reduction in periprocedural thromboembolism with an uninterrupted anticoagulant strategy was shown compared with low-molecular-weight heparin bridging.[31] Although the incidence of major bleeding complications did not differ between the two anticoagulation strategies, minor bleeding was significantly less common in patients with uninterrupted warfarin therapy.

Before the widespread implementation of intraprocedural imaging with ICE, systemic anticoagulation was typically withheld until the achievement of LA access to minimize the risk of major bleeding (e.g., inadvertent puncture of the aorta or cardiac perforation). However, delaying the initiation of systemic anticoagulation until after transseptal puncture may increase the risk of sheath-associated thrombus formation (Fig. 43.11 and Video 43.2). The administration of heparin before LA access is recommended, particularly when ICE is available to optimize the puncture site.[32] In addition, lower levels of anticoagulation (activated clotting times of 250–300 seconds) are associated with an increased incidence of both sheath-associated and in situ thrombosis in patients undergoing AF ablation; using a higher target activated clotting time (ACT; 300–350 seconds) may decrease this occurrence.[33]

TECHNIQUES AND TOOLS FOR TRANSSEPTAL CATHETERIZATION

General Considerations

The basic tools for atrial transseptal catheterization are the transseptal sheath and needle (Fig. 43.12). Standard nonsteerable transseptal sheaths (e.g., LAMP series or SL series, St. Jude Medical, St. Paul, MN) are available in two sizes (8 F and 8.5 F) and different lengths ranging from 63 to 81 cm with built-in 67- to 85-cm dilators. The system can accommodate a 71- to 89-cm Brockenbrough needle or a standard 0.032-inch guidewire. Steerable sheaths (e.g., Agilis, St. Jude Medical, St. Paul, MN) are usually available in only one size (8.5 F) and two lengths (61 cm or 71 cm) and can also accommodate a 71- to 89-cm transseptal needle or a 0.032-inch guidewire.

The design of the transseptal needles is standardized and consists of a proximal hub containing a flange with a pointed end and a distal end. A pointed end works as the arrow to indicate the plane of the needle curvature (Fig. 43.13). The great majority of transseptal punctures are performed with the standard needle curvature (BRK, St. Jude Medical), although different curvatures might be needed for large (BRK-1) or very small (BRK-2) atria. The choice of transseptal sheath and needle can be tailored to the operator's preference and/or individual patient anatomy; however, for AF ablation procedures, the use of steerable sheaths has been shown to improve freedom from recurrent of arrhythmia and decrease fluoroscopy time.[34] The use of a larger-diameter curve for the steerable sheath is quite useful in

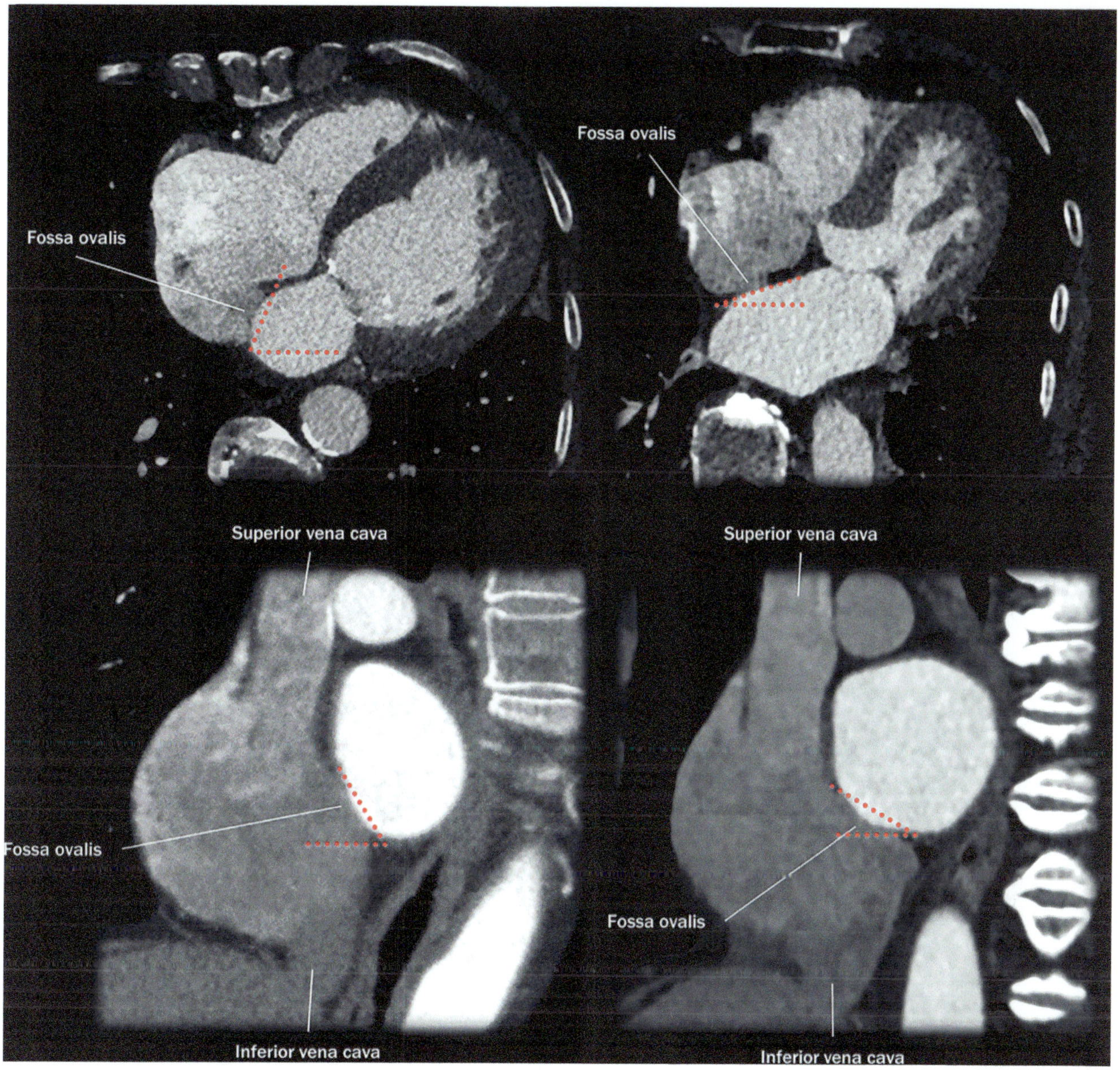

Fig. 43.10 Individual variation of the structural anatomy of the fossa ovalis. The rotational position evaluated with the horizontal section (*top*) and tilting evaluated with the left anterior oblique section (*bottom*) of the primary septum at the floor of the fossa ovalis are markedly variable. Preprocedural understanding of these variations should affect the individualized strategy during the atrial transseptal catheterization.

patients with dilated atria or when ablation beyond around the mitral valve or within the LV is required.

Fluoroscopy-Guided Transseptal Catheterization

The fluoroscopy-guided technique is still commonly used for atrial transseptal catheterization.[20] A correct understanding of the fluoroscopic anatomy based on conventional landmarks is crucial (Figs. 43.7 and 43.8). To locate the approximate region of the fossa ovalis, it is important to obtain the en face view of the atrial septum to avoid foreshortening of the fossa ovalis. The biplane angulation should be adjusted based on individual rotational position of the atrial septum, which can be estimated from the preprocedural images (Figs. 43.9 and 43.10) or the diagnostic catheters positioned in standard locations, such as the coronary sinus, bundle of His, and noncoronary aortic sinus.[35,36] The most important angulation is the optimal right anterior oblique projection, as it can separate the fossa ovalis from the aortic root and posterior atrial wall. Generally, the coronary sinus catheter is most foreshortened from this projection (Fig. 43.7). The left anterior oblique projection is adjusted to be perpendicular to the right anterior oblique projection. The fossa ovalis is generally located right posterior to the noncoronary aortic sinus (Figs. 43.1, 43.3, 43.7, and 43.9). The location of the noncoronary aortic sinus is recognized as the torus aorticus or right aortic mound when viewed from within the RA (Figs. 43.8 and 43.14). However, the location of the fossa ovalis relative to the noncoronary aortic sinus is variable according to the depth of aortic wedging into the heart.[25] If the aortic root,

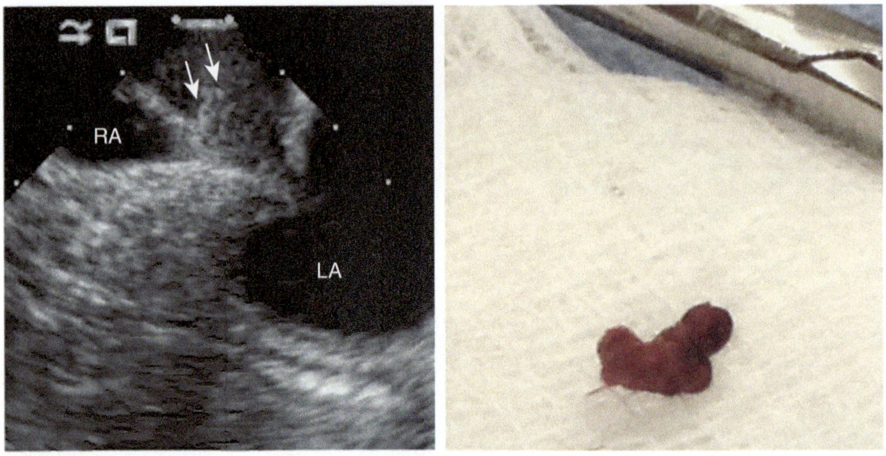

Fig. 43.11 *Left,* Intracardiac echocardiography (ICE) image showing a large thrombus (*arrows*) adherent to the junction of the transseptal sheath and dilator during fossa tenting. This thrombus occurred despite therapeutic systemic anticoagulation (international normalized ratio, 3.0; activated clotting time, 360 seconds). ICE allows the operator to identify such thrombi before passing the sheath into the systemic circulation. *Right,* A 3 × 2-mm thrombus aspirated from the transseptal sheath in the left panel. (Refer to Video 43.2.)

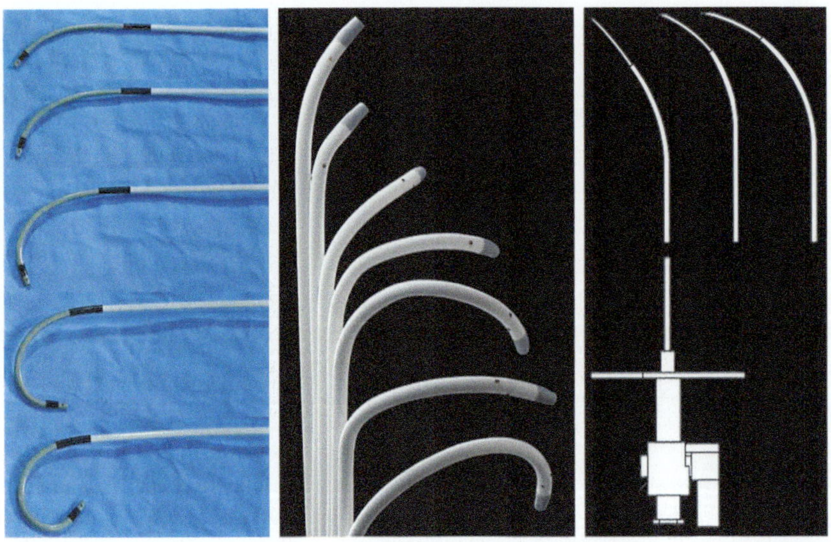

Fig. 43.12 A variety of transseptal sheath shapes and lengths are available, and their selection is based on operator experience and the specific procedure performed. These sheaths all have small side holes for infusion, as well as radiopaque markers for fluoroscopic visualization. Because of their rigidity and navigability, we find deflectable sheaths *(left)* to be useful for a variety of applications. The degree of curvature of the transseptal needle *(right)* can be tailored to individual patient anatomy.

due to its elongation or dilatation, is deeply wedged into the heart, the location of the fossa ovalis is shifted superiorly relative to the aortic root.[25] When the transseptal approach is obtained via the standard route from the femoral vein, the fossa ovalis is located superior and slightly left anterior to the orifice of the inferior vena cava (Figs. 43.1, 43.3, 43.7, and 43.8). A long guidewire is typically inserted from the femoral vein into the superior vena cava. The transseptal sheath-dilator assembly is then advanced over the guidewire until the dilator tip reaches the level of the tracheal carina. The guidewire is then withdrawn, the transseptal dilator is flushed with heparinized saline, and the transseptal needle (flushed with heparinized saline and connected to a small syringe with contrast) is inserted into the sheath-dilator system. The transseptal needle should be advanced under fluoroscopy and positioned when the tip is just inside the distal end of the dilator. The proper orientation of the pointer hub (and needle tip) largely depends on the individual patient's anatomy,[36,37] the rotational direction of the atrial septum (Fig. 43.10). Thus preprocedural assessment of the rotational direction of the fossa ovalis in the axial image is important (Figs. 43.9, 43.10, and 43.13). A position around 4 o'clock is typically adequate to maintain the needle perpendicular to the plane of the fossa ovalis (Fig. 43.13).[35,36] The direction of the hub should be paralleled with the direction of the flush port of the sheath, which also indicates the direction of the curve of the sheath (Fig. 43.13). At this stage, the transseptal sheath/dilator/needle system are slowly withdrawn. When crossing the superior vena cava–RA appendage junction, the tip dives inferiorly

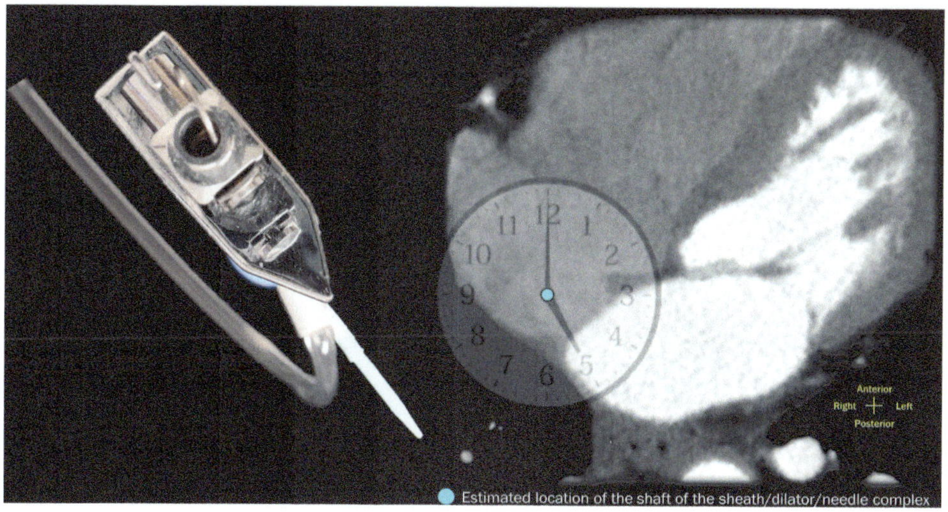

Fig. 43.13 The anatomical basic concept of clock-based indication of the optimal direction of the hub of the Brockenbrough needle, flash port of the sheath, and tip of the sheath/dilater. The optimal direction is affected by the location of the shaft of the sheath/dilater/needle complex, size of the fossa ovalis, and rotational position of the fossa ovalis evaluated in the horizontal section viewed from the inferior direction.

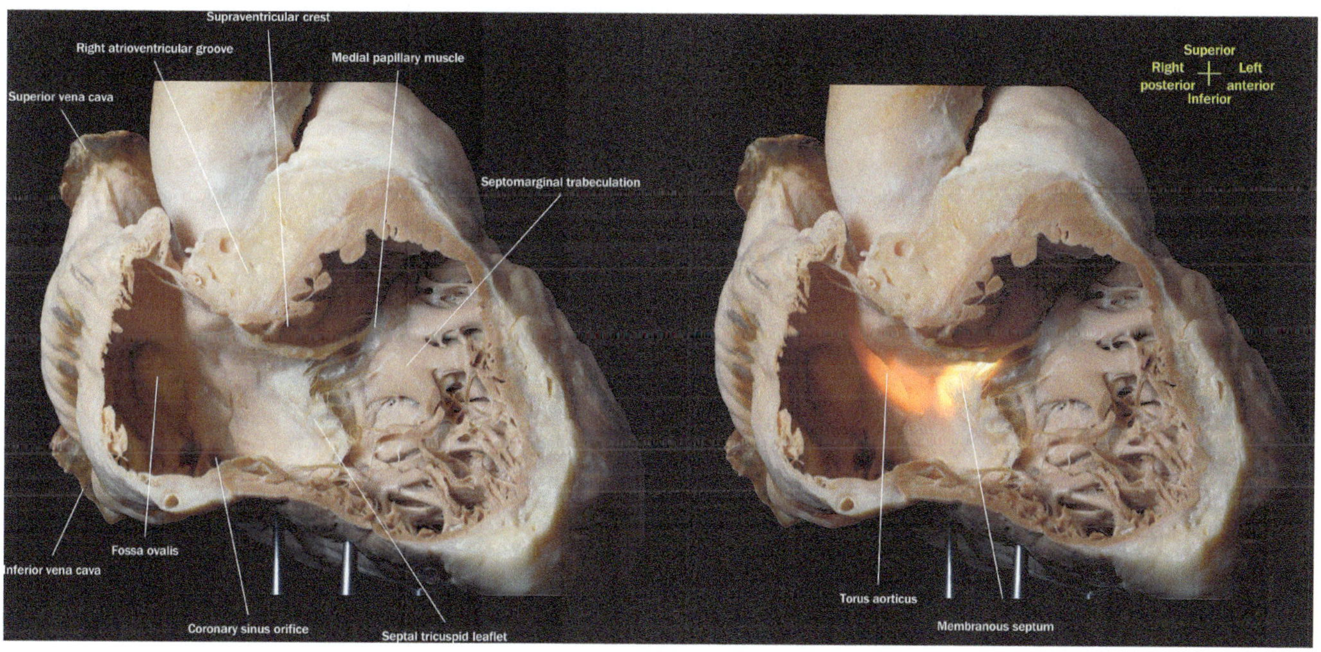

Fig. 43.14 The opened right heart viewed from the shallow right anterior oblique direction. Transillumination with the light source placed in the aortic root (*right*) indicates the location of the noncoronary aortic sinus bulging toward the right atrium located left anterior to the fossa ovalis and superior to the coronary sinus orifice. This bulge is referred to as the torus aorticus or right aortic mound, which is not the atrial septum. It is fundamental to avoid the transseptal puncture into this region, which can induce catastrophic complication. The membranous septum is also transilluminated and is divided into atrioventricular and interventricular portions by the septal tricuspid leaflet.

and posteriorly (i.e., rightward in the left anterior oblique projection). This drop is, however, not always detectable as appreciated by projection images viewed from the left anterior oblique direction (Figs. 43.9 and 43.10). At this point, before further withdrawing the system, the orientation of the dilator tip should be confirmed in the bilateral projections. In the right anterior oblique direction, the orientation of the dilator tip should be right superoposterior to the coronary sinus catheter, placed at the center of the estimated location on the noncoronary aortic sinus and the posterior cardiac silhouette. Once appropriately oriented in the right anterior oblique projection, the system is further withdrawn in the left anterior oblique projection. A second drop is typically readily recognizable compared to the first drop. It is seen when passing from the superior limbus into the fossa ovalis (Fig. 43.15). Once the fossa ovalis is engaged, the direction of the dilator tip is reconfirmed in the right anterior oblique projection. The dilator tip located at the fossa ovalis should show synchronous pulsatile motion with the catheter

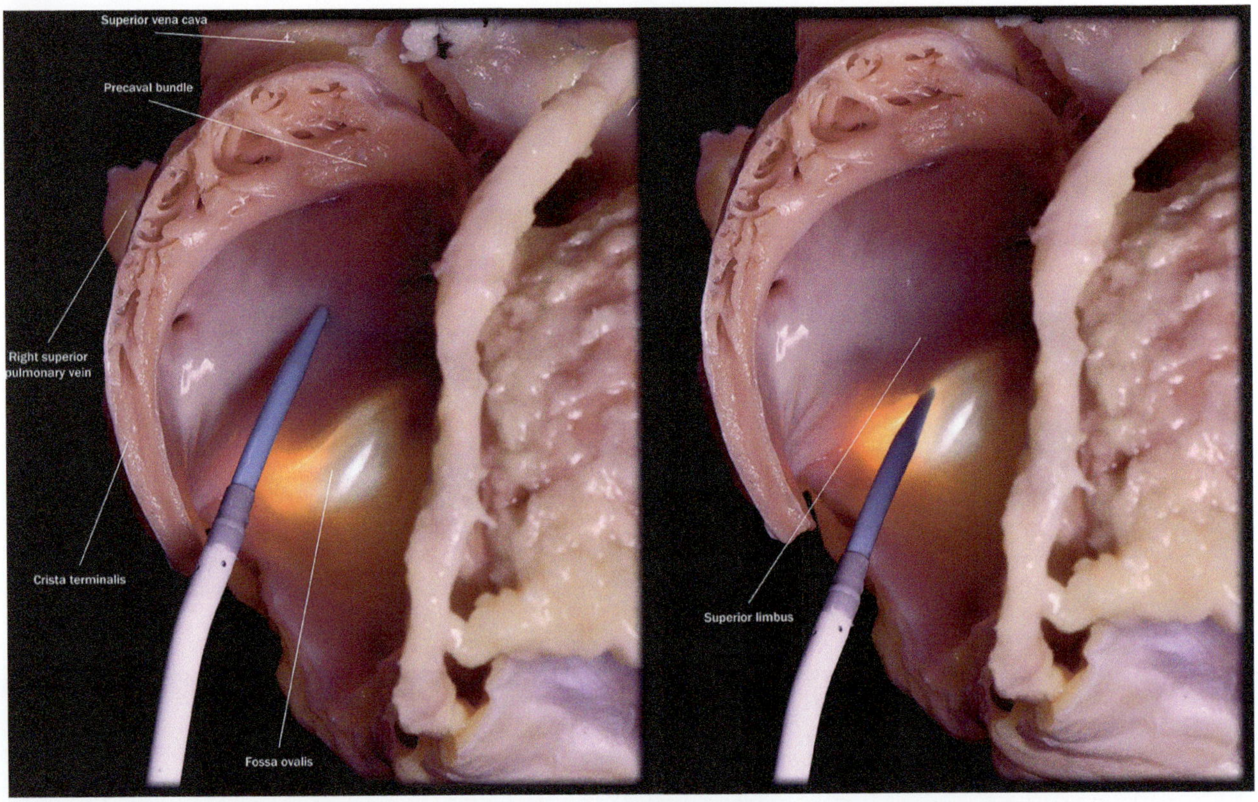

Fig. 43.15 Engagement of the system into the fossa ovalis viewed from the right anterior oblique direction. When the transseptal sheath/dilator/needle system are slowly withdrawn, the tip passes the superior limbus (*left*) and dives into the fossa ovalis (*right*), which is readily recognizable.

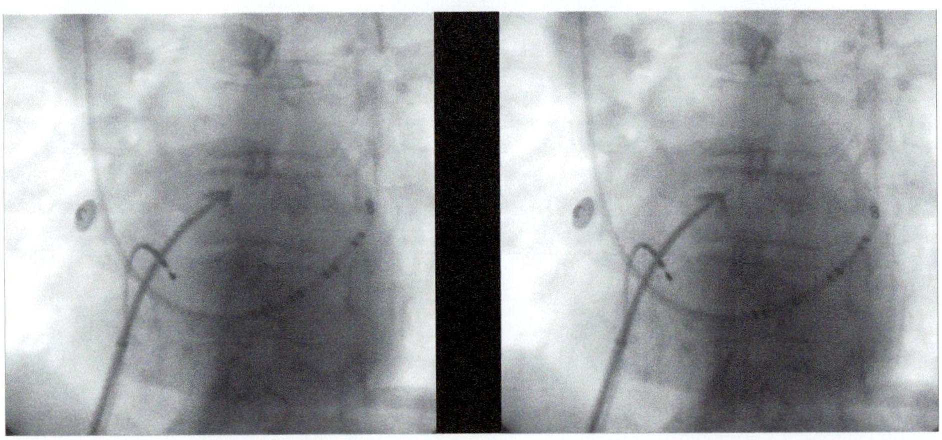

Fig. 43.16 Left anterior oblique views during the transseptal puncture. The small amount of contrast injection via the needle shows tenting of the primary septum at the floor of the oval fossa (*left*). The needle successfully penetrates the primary septum (*right*). The multipolar electrodes are placed at His region and coronary sinus.

placed in the coronary sinus. Once the proper orientation of the dilator tip is achieved and double-checked from the bilateral projection, small quantities of dye may be injected through the transseptal needle (Fig. 43.16) to confirm the tenting of the primary septum at the floor of the fossa ovalis. If no tenting is observed or if contrast injection results in diffuse staining of the septum, the needle is likely outside the fossa ovalis. When appropriate positioning cannot be confirmed, it is advisable to repeat the whole maneuver to engage the true fossa ovalis. This requires withdrawing the needle from the body, flushing of the entire system to remove clots, reintroducing the guidewire into the sheath-dilator system, readvancing the system to the level of the tracheal carina, and repeating the process of engaging the fossa ovalis. Sometimes, when pushing the needle against the fossa ovalis, the whole system moves up superiorly toward superior limbus instead of tenting the fossa ovalis,[23] especially in the case with less tilted atrial septum or dilated RA (Fig. 43.10). Thus, preprocedural assessment of the fossa ovalis from the left anterior oblique direction is important (Figs. 43.9 and 43.10). This superior shift typically indicates that the curve on the

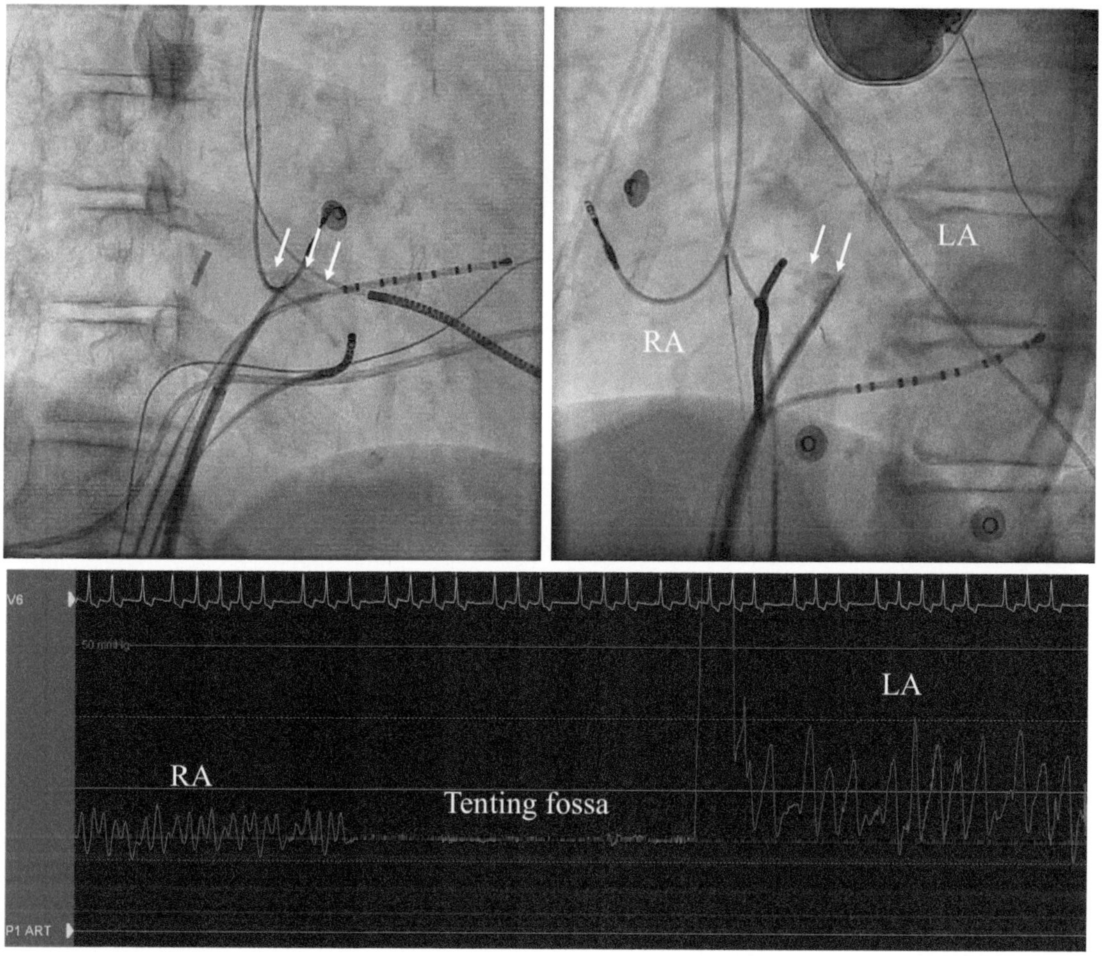

Fig. 43.17 Fluoroscopic images in the right anterior oblique (*top left*) and left anterior oblique (*top right*) projections during transseptal catheterization under fluoroscopic guidance. Contrast medium is injected through the Brockenbrough needle to demonstrate tenting of the interatrial septum (*arrows*). A decapolar catheter is placed at the septal tricuspid annulus to record a His-bundle electrogram; this gives a fluoroscopic landmark for the posterior and inferior aspect of the aortic root. Note permanent pacing leads in the right atrium (RA) and right ventricle. Alternatively, continuous pressure transduction can be performed through the transseptal needle. *Bottom*, Characteristic right atrial pressure tracing; dampening of the waveform is noted when tenting of the fossa ovalis occludes the needle lumen. After crossing, the left atrial (LA) waveform is obtained. (Refer to Video 43.3.)

transseptal needle is relatively insufficient. Although this superior shift or slip of the needle is common,[23] manual recurving of the needle will be necessary to avoid this, by bending the mid-distal shaft of the needle to better reach the septum. Once the needle is appropriately tenting the fossa ovalis, the needle is advanced against the fossa ovalis and gently pushed forward until it enters the LA using the left anterior oblique direction (Fig. 43.16). An additional contrast injection confirms the correct positioning within the LA by seeing that the contrast dilutes within the LA and enters the LV. Correct positioning of the needle in the LA may also be obtained by confirming an appropriate pressure tracing (Fig. 43.17 and Video 43.3). If the injected contrast passes upward or a systemic arterial pressure tracing is recorded from the transseptal needle, puncture of the aortic root is likely. It is imperative that inadvertent aortic puncture is recognized to avoid introducing the transseptal dilator and/or sheath into the aorta. If this happens, however one cannot remove the wire or the dilater or sheath from the aorta, but consider surgery or transcatheter occluder of the potential fistula.[38] Once the transseptal needle is within the LA, counterclockwise torque may be applied to the whole system to prevent inadvertent puncture of the posterior wall of the LA. It is useful to then gently advance the entire system into the LA with the needle exposed until the dilator passes through the fossa ovalis. Once the dilator is positioned within the LA, the needle is withdrawn just inside the tip of the dilator to prevent inadvertent puncture of the LA wall. The needle should remain within and near the tip of the dilator to provide support for the subsequent crossing of the transseptal sheath. Failure to maintain adequate support from the dilator/needle combination will result in failure to cross with the transseptal sheath and possibly the loss of LA access. By holding the dilater, then the sheath should be advanced into the LA by checking the left anterior oblique projection toward the lateral LA wall. The left bronchus can be used as the marker to indicate the location of the proximal left superior pulmonary vein, thereby implying the approximate

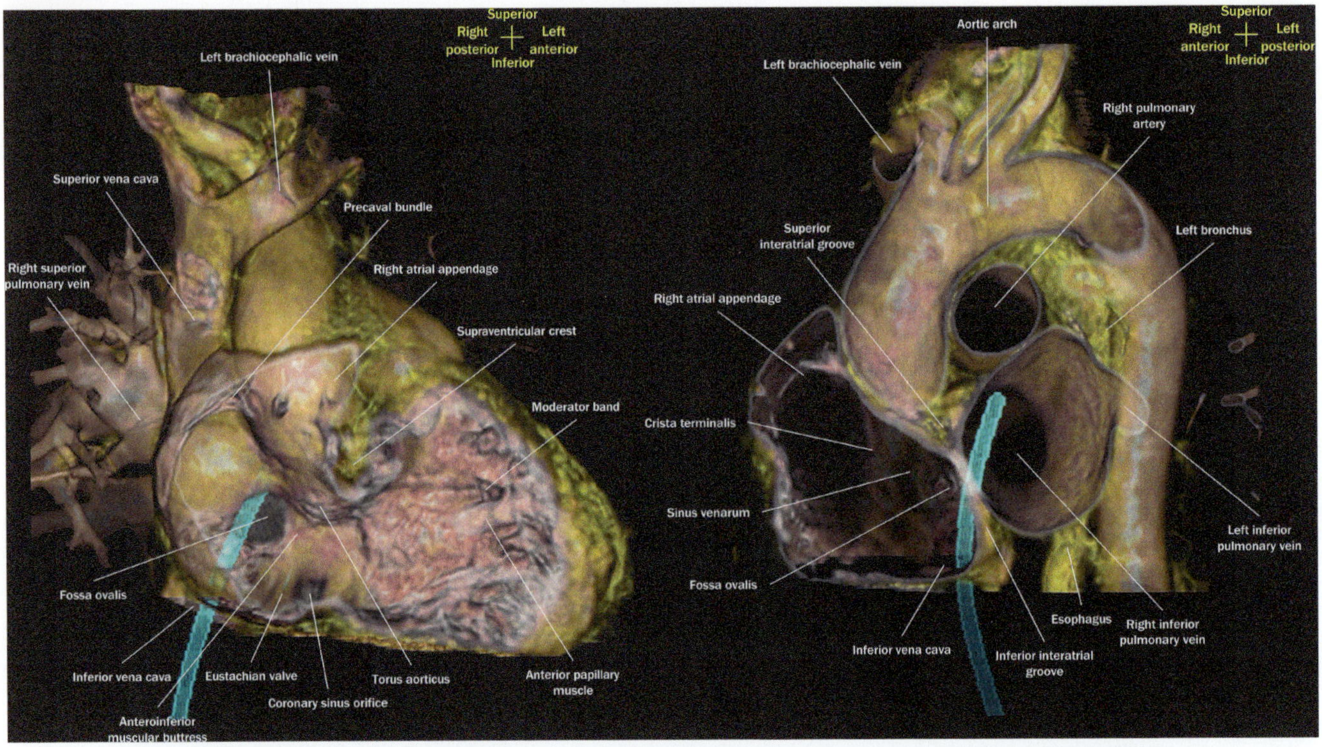

Fig. 43.18 Virtual dissection images with virtual transseptal sheath viewed from the right anterior oblique direction (left) and left anterior oblique direction (right). Three-dimensional living heart anatomy is appreciated. The oval fossa in this case is relatively closer to the noncoronary aortic sinus, and thus it is located left anterosuperior relative to the orifice of the inferior vena cava. The primary septum at the floor of the oval fossa is less tilting, which commonly renders superior puncture within the fossa ovalis due to superior shift of the system during the fluoroscopy-guided approach. (Refer to Videos 43.4 and 43.5.)

location of the level of the LA roof (Fig. 43.7). The dilator and needle are then gently withdrawn together under continuous aspiration to prevent entrainment of air within the transseptal sheath and subsequent air embolism. Figs. 43.18 and 43.19 shows the three-dimensional location of the virtual sheath within the LA (Videos 43.4 and 43.5).

Intracardiac Echocardiography-Guided Transseptal Catheterization

There are two commercially available transducers for ICE: mechanical (i.e., radial) and phased-array systems. The radial transducer is mounted on a 9-F, nonsteerable catheter and emits an imaging beam at a 15-degree forward angle, perpendicular to the long axis of the catheter. The transducer rotates at 1800 rpm and produces a 360-degree imaging plane. The fixed, 9-MHz transducer frequency provides excellent near-field resolution; however, far-field structures are poorly visualized, necessitating imaging proximate to the structure of interest (Fig. 43.20 and Video 43.6).

The phased-array transducer contains 64 elements with frequencies ranging from 5 to 10 MHz (AcuNav, Siemens Medical, Mountain View, CA; View Flex Xtra, St. Jude Medical, St. Paul, MN). This platform provides greater flexibility in imaging both adjacent and remote structures (imaging depth of up to 15 cm) (Fig. 43.20 and Video 43.6). The transducer is mounted on an 8- or 10-F catheter that can be deflected in four directions (anterior, posterior, right, and left) in addition to 360-degree axial rotation. Its steerability and low profile allow the transducer to be navigated throughout any cardiac chamber of interest. The phased-array transducer is also capable of full spectral and color Doppler measurements, greatly enhancing the physiologic data achievable.

The relevant views to facilitate transseptal puncture are obtained with the imaging transducer positioned in the mid-RA. To provide consistency between patients in imaging technique, we initially position the transducer facing the tricuspid annulus, to obtain the "home view." From the "home view," gentle clockwise rotation to the catheter brings into sequential view the inferomedial and superolateral papillary muscles, the mitral valve and LA appendage, the left pulmonary veins, the posterior wall of the LA, the right pulmonary veins, the sinus venarum and crista terminalis, and the RA appendage (Fig. 43.21 and Video 43.7).[39] The structures in the LA are all visualized through the fossa ovalis. Optimal plane should be any planes between the one showing the LA appendage and the one showing posterior wall, but selecting the plane that shows the widest LA free wall should be safe. Once the optimal plane has been determined, the transseptal puncture can be obtained with the same methodology used for fluoroscopy-guided access, with the additional advantage that ICE allows for direct real-time visualization of the relationships between the fossa ovalis, the needle-dilator-sheath system, and the LA wall (Fig. 43.22). Experienced operators can use ICE as the only modality to guide the transseptal puncture to eliminate the radiation exposure.

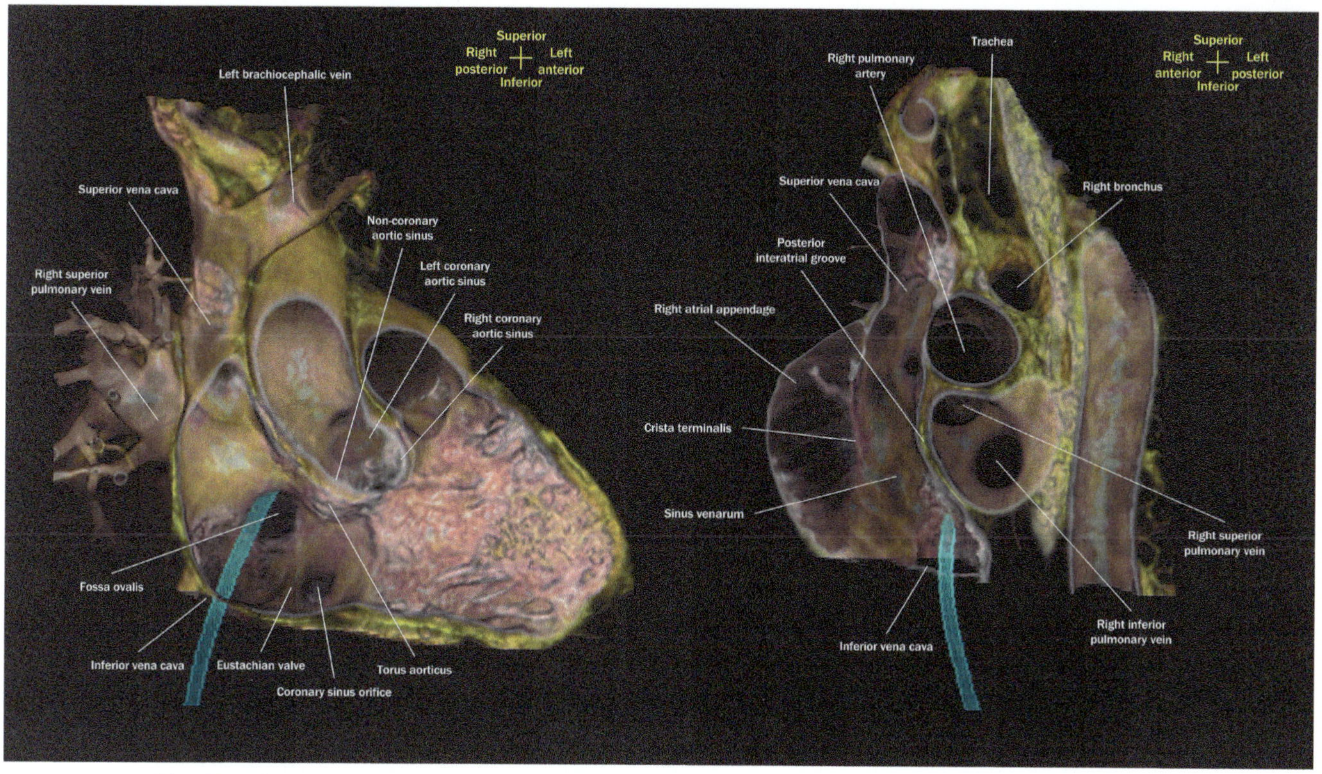

Fig. 43.19 Further progressive virtual dissection is made on the Fig. 43.18 to show the structural anatomy behind. The aortic root can be seen (left) behind the right arial appendage, and the superior vena cava and sinus venarum can be seen (*right*) behind the ascending aorta. Importantly, the right panel shows the plane posterior to the fossa ovalis. Thus, the partition between the both atria is not the primary septum, but the posterior interatrial fold, also referred to as the Sondergaard groove or Waterston groove. Understanding the neighborhood structural anatomy around the fossa ovalis is fundamental. (Refer to Videos 43.4 and 43.5.)

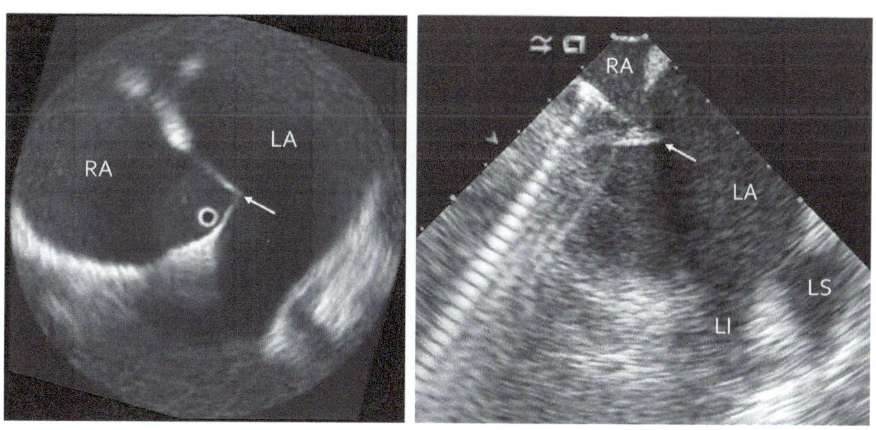

Fig. 43.20 Tenting of the fossa ovalis with the transseptal needle (*arrows*) as visualized by mechanical (*left*) and phased-array (*right*) intracardiac echocardiography (ICE). Note the superior far-field imaging achieved with phased-array ICE. *LA*, Left atrium; *LI*, left inferior pulmonary vein; *LS*, left superior pulmonary vein; *RA*, right atrium. (Refer to Video 43.6.)

One of the main advantages of ICE-assisted transseptal puncture is the possibility to determine the optimal site of the septum through which to obtain access (Fig. 43.23 and Video 43.8) for the specific procedure performed.[26] Individualizing the puncture site is very difficult using a fluoroscopy-only approach. Distance between the atrial septum and the free wall of the LA atrium can be easily appreciated to avoid cardiac perforation. The general concept to optimize the location of septal crossing is that bulky devices require adequate working distance within the LA to appropriately align the device to the target structure. Thus, in general, a posterior crossing is optimal when targeting structures near the atrioventricular junction, including the LA appendage[40] and the mitral valve.[41,42] On the other hand, anterior crossing is favorable to access the structure distant from the atrioventricular junction, including the pulmonary veins and posterior wall of the LA. For the pulmonary vein isolation

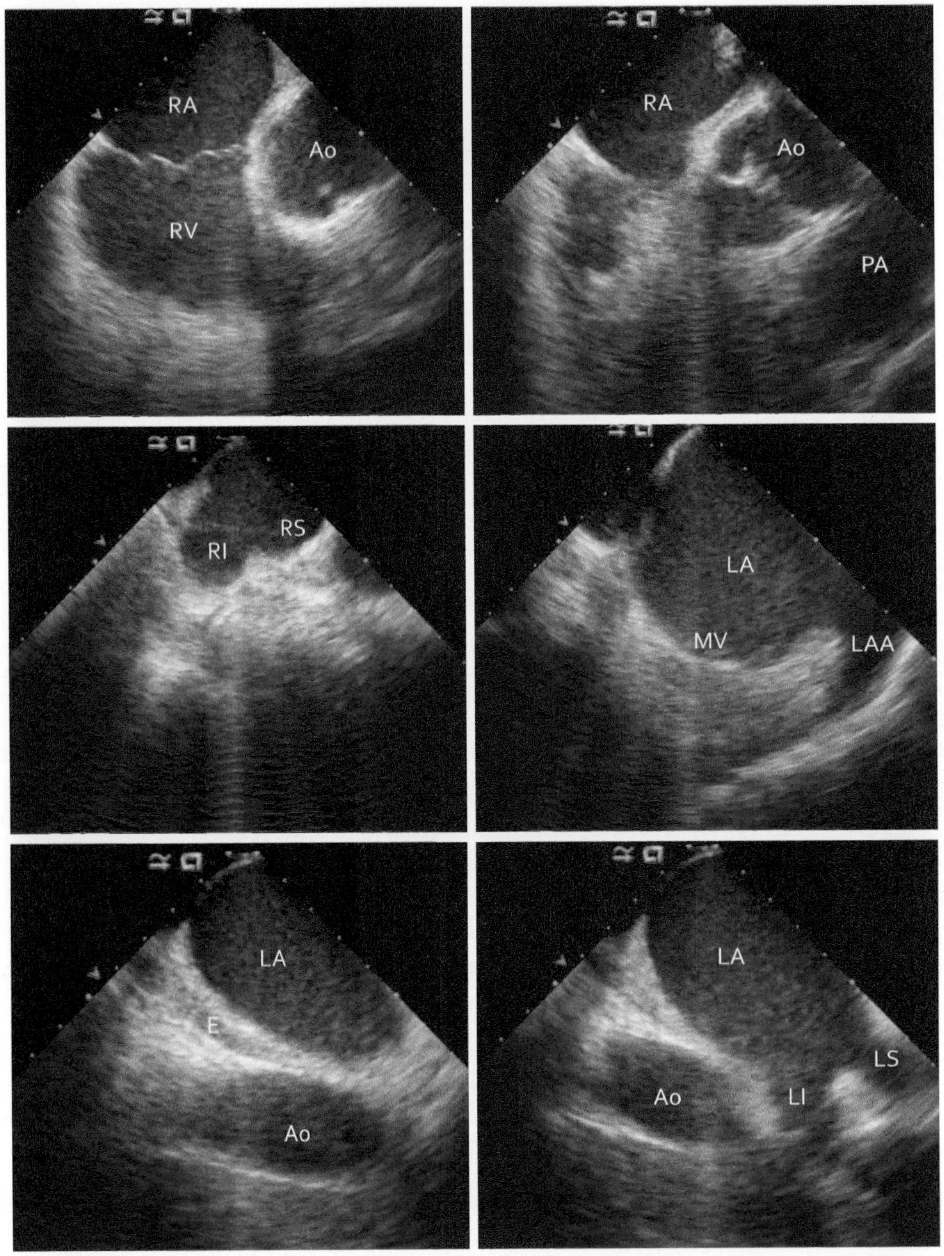

Fig. 43.21 Phased-array intracardiac echocardiography images obtained by placing the imaging transducer in the mid right atrium. The "home view" is shown in the top left. Sequential imaging planes (clockwise, *top left* to *middle left*) are obtained by rotating the catheter in a clockwise fashion; all of the relevant anatomy to guide transseptal puncture is visualized. *Ao*, Aorta; *E*, esophagus; *LA*, left atrium; *LAA*, left atrial appendage; *LI*, left inferior pulmonary vein; *LS*, left superior pulmonary vein; *MV*, mitral valve; *PA*, pulmonary artery; *RA*, right atrium; *RI*, right inferior pulmonary vein; *RS*, right superior pulmonary vein; *RV*, right ventricle. (Refer to Video 43.7.)

using RF ablation catheter, however, optimal location of puncture seems not consistent, affected by each operator's preference. Either anterior or posterior puncture will be favorable for left pulmonary vein and warfarin ridge (LA ridge). However, posterior puncture brings working distance very short for the right pulmonary veins as the posterior limbus is identical to the antrum of the right pulmonary veins. Thus, for the right pulmonary veins, anterior crossing should be favorable. In similar fashion, as the pulmonary venous component and LA appendage form the superior structure, an inferior approach can secure the working distance. On the contrary, the mitral valve is a relatively inferior structure compared to the pulmonary venous component and LA appendage, and superior puncture is feasible especially for the medial scallops and inferomedial commissures. The important thing is that the optimal site of puncture should not be determined only by the target structures. Considering the huge variation in individual structural anatomy, including the distance to the target structure, size of the fossa ovalis, size of each atrium, and rotational position of the heart, preprocedural appreciation of individual three-dimensional

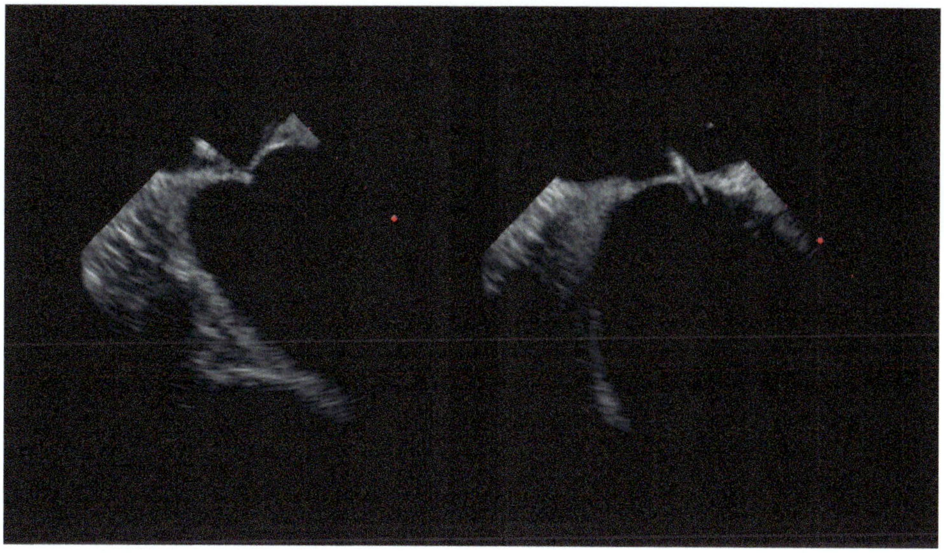

Fig. 43.22 Phased-array intracardiac echocardiography showing the tenting of the primary septum at the floor of the oval fossa (*left*) and the sheath after successful puncture (*right*).

anatomy is fundamental to determine the optimal puncture site in each case (Figs. 43.9 and 43.10).

Other Techniques and Imaging Modalities

Some operators perform AF ablation with two dedicated sheaths in the LA. There are three commonly used techniques to obtain double transseptal puncture: (1) dedicated punctures for each sheath; (2) a single puncture through which two sheaths are placed with a double-wire technique; and (3) a single puncture after which the ablation catheter is advanced into the LA alongside the original sheath through the original puncture site. Using separate puncture sites minimizes interaction between the two transseptal sheaths, thereby facilitating AF ablation. However, the choice is largely based on operator preference.

Transesophageal echocardiography (TEE) has also been used to guide transseptal catheterization, especially in the setting of structural heart disease intervention with an incremental benefit compared with a fluoroscopy-based approach.[8,12,43] The major limitations of TEE-guided approach include the requirement for general anesthesia, need for an additional operator to manipulate the probe, and the risk of esophageal trauma from probe passage (particularly relevant given the extent of systemic anticoagulation during LA access).

Fluoroless Transseptal Catheterization

A completely fluoroless technique has been recently described.[44,45] This approach typically involves a combined use of ICE and the three-dimensional mapping system in lieu of the standard fluoroscopic projections. In brief, the RA anatomy is reconstructed with a mapping catheter or with ICE, and the location of the fossa ovalis is marked. The transseptal sheaths and coronary sinus catheter are positioned without the aid of fluoroscopy under direct ICE guidance. For the transseptal access, either the standard Brockenbrough needle or the RF-assisted needle (NRG RF Transseptal Needle, Baylis Medical, Montreal, Canada) can be used; the latter can also be directly visualized on the mapping system owing to its exposed electrode on the needle tip. The challenges with this approach include the inability to directly visualize the location of the temperature probe for esophageal temperature monitoring and the need for optimal acoustic windows to fully rely on ICE imaging. The advantages consist of the lack of fluoroscopic exposure for the patient, the operator, and the laboratory staff, as well as the benefit of not wearing lead aprons.

APPROACH TO THE DIFFICULT TRANSSEPTAL CATHETERIZATION

Although atrial transseptal catheterization is an essential aspect of many electrophysiology studies, difficulties may present at various stages of the procedure (Table 43.1). Along with the improvements in tools, the potential risk of complication may decrease. On the other hand, technical improvement has rendered transseptal puncture more often performed for difficult cases, including patients with congenital heart disease, atrial septal closure device, and repeated catheterizations. In addition to detailed preprocedural anatomical evaluation, integration of available tools into an organized approach for troubleshooting is required to overcome challenging cases.[46]

Anatomic Variants of the Atrial Septum

Morphologic variations in the structure of the atrial septum are common and present unique challenges for transseptal catheterization. The distortion of the intracardiac anatomy may alter the reliability of the standard fluoroscopic technique in these cases. The most common abnormality of the atrial septum is the patent foramen ovale, an embryologic remnant that is encountered in 20–30% of patients.[24,47] Generally, the site of communication is located at the anterosuperior part of the fossa ovalis, which is close to the proximal aorta. ICE or TEE imaging can readily identify this occurrence (Fig. 43.24 and Video 43.9). Fluoroscopic clues of inadvertent crossing through the patent

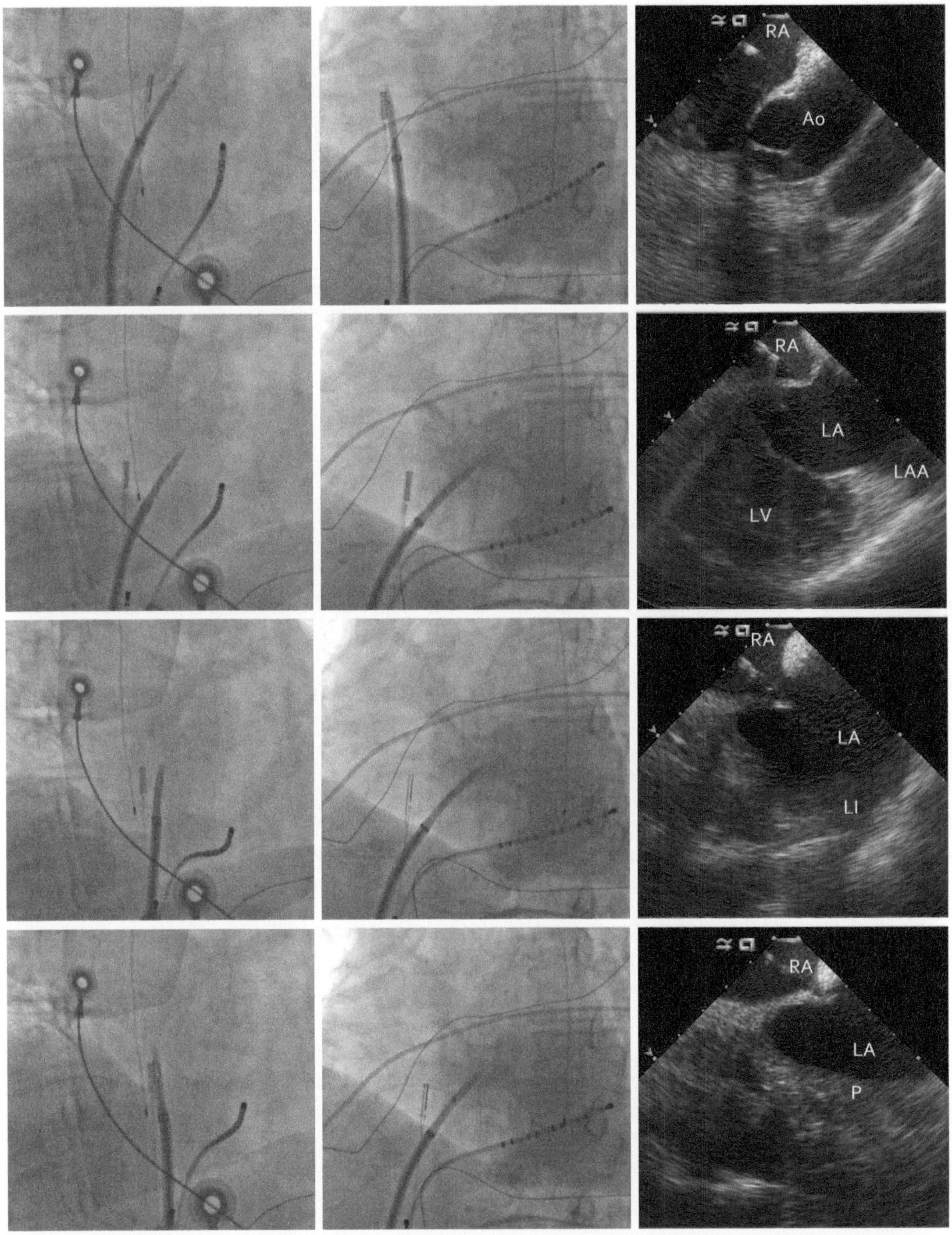

Fig. 43.23 Phased-array intracardiac echocardiography (ICE) (*right*), right anterior oblique (*left*), and left anterior oblique (LAO; *middle*) fluoroscopic images taken during transseptal catheterization. Each of the four rows of images is taken simultaneously with the transseptal apparatus positioned at different locations. In the first row, the transseptal needle is directed toward the aortic root at the level of the sinutubular junction; note the anterior and superior fluoroscopic appearance obtained from this location (relative to the coronary sinus [CS] catheter). In the second row, the transseptal needle has been withdrawn and rotated in a clockwise manner; the needle is now directed toward the left atrial appendage (LAA) and mitral valve. This angle of crossing is often favorable to facilitate: (1) left ventricular access for ventricular tachycardia ablation; (2) mapping the mitral annulus during accessory pathway ablation; or (3) placement of an LAA closure device. In the third row, the transseptal needle has been rotated farther in a clockwise manner; now the needle is directed toward the left-sided pulmonary veins. Note the relatively parallel alignment of the transseptal sheath and the CS catheter. This is the optimal angle of crossing for pulmonary vein isolation. In row 4, the transseptal apparatus has been rotated farther clockwise posteriorly. The needle is now directed toward the posterior left atrium wall (P); inadvertent puncture of the atrial wall can occur with this approach. ICE is particularly helpful at illustrating the distance available for crossing in each orientation. Note the similarity in transseptal sheath position in the LAO projection for positions 2–4. *Ao,* Aorta; *LA,* left atrium; *LI,* left inferior pulmonary vein; *LV,* left ventricle; *RA,* right atrium. (Refer to Video 43.8.)

TABLE 43.1 Troubleshooting the Difficult Case

Problem	Possible Risk	Solution
Patent foramen ovale (PFO)	Inadvertent access through PFO, difficult catheter manipulation	Use fluoroscopy or imaging to avoid fossa cannulation and to puncture the fossa in a conventional location
Atrial septal aneurysm	Inadvertent puncture of the posterior left atrial wall	Use of intracardiac echocardiography; guidewire-based transseptal apparatus
Thickened interatrial septum (e.g., postsurgical, prior transseptal catheterization)	Inability to obtain left atrial access, inadvertent cardiac perforation	Intracardiac echocardiography to target the thinnest part of the septum; radiofrequency-assisted transseptal needle
Presence of an atrial septal closure device	Inability to obtain left atrial access, device dislodgement	Intracardiac echocardiography to visualize the native septum suitable for puncture or to guide access when direct puncture of the device is necessary

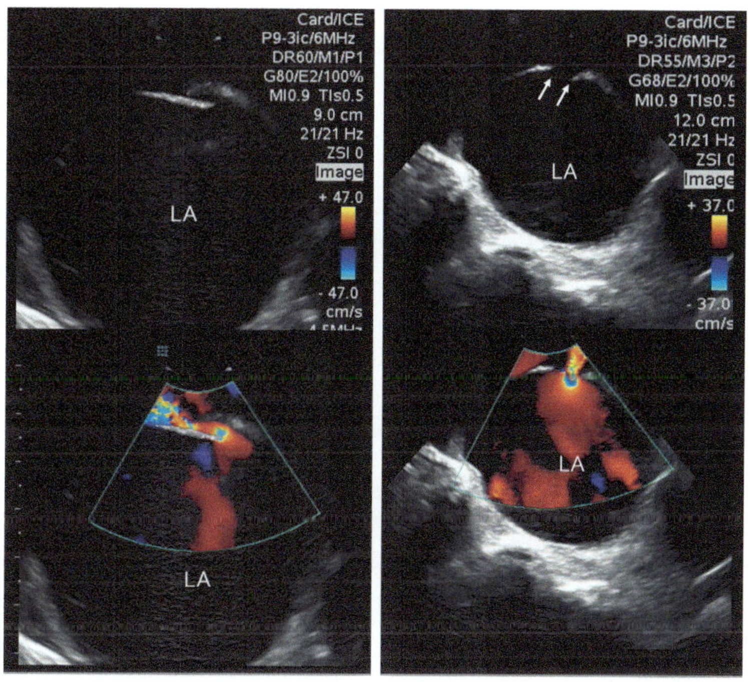

Fig. 43.24 Phased array intracardiac echocardiography images from patients with a patent foramen ovale (PFO; *left*) and an ostium secundum atrial septal defect (ASD; *right*). Corresponding color Doppler images are shown (bottom). The relatively superior and anterior location of the PFO makes catheter manipulation challenging when used for transseptal access. In contrast, the relatively posterior location and large size of the secundum ASD are favorable for direct left atrial (LA) access. (Refer to Video 43.9.)

foramen ovale include septal crossing without needle deployment. A transseptal access via the patent foramen ovale greatly impedes catheter navigability during AF ablation.[48]

The presence of an atrial septal aneurysm, defined as a greater than 10-mm excursion of the septum during the respiratory cycle, is particularly prevalent in patients with a patent foramen ovale.[49] The common fluoroscopic manifestation is excessive tenting into the LA without needle deployment. Although intraprocedural identification of an atrial septal aneurysm can be difficult using fluoroscopy alone, any preprocedural imaging, including transthoracic echocardiography (TTE), cardiac computed tomography, and cardiac magnetic resonance imaging, can easily detect this anatomy. Thus, careful evaluation of the preprocedural imaging of each case is fundamental, and not only for detecting this anatomy. In many cases, the degree of septal tenting can be dramatic, extending to the lateral LA wall.[50] In such cases, a relatively small distance is available for sheath crossing and the risk of cardiac perforation is increased. ICE can be useful to fine-tune the direction of needle crossing, thereby maximizing the space available for crossing (Fig. 43.25 and Video 43.10).

Less common congenital atrial septal malformations such as the double atrial septum (Fig. 43.26 and Video 43.11),[51] cor triatriatum, and atrial septal pouch[52] pose specific challenges (Fig. 43.6). It is important to know that double atrial septum seen in two-dimensional imaging can be nothing but the manifestation of the flap valve,[24] as detection of the three-dimensional feature of the slit-like flap valve is sometimes challenging by only two-dimensional imaging. Because of alterations in blood flow within the pouch, this anatomy may predispose to thrombus formation, which may contraindicate the transseptal puncture.

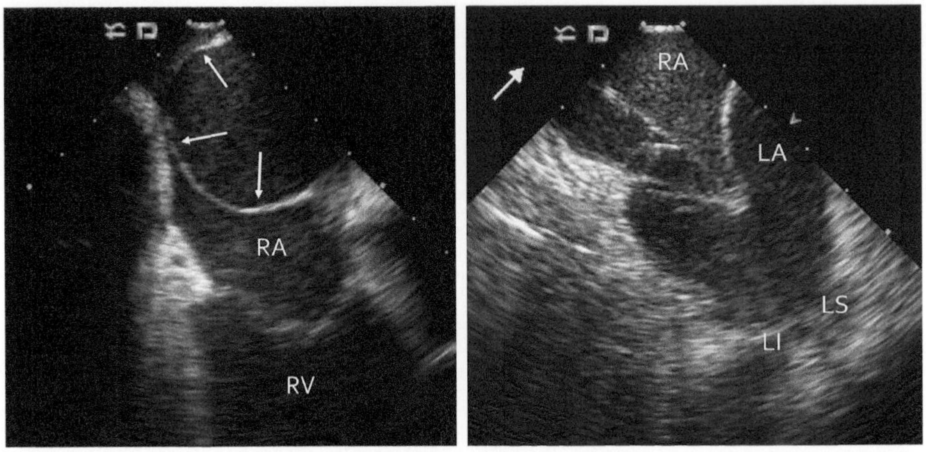

Fig. 43.25 Phased-array intracardiac echocardiography (ICE) images taken from two patients with an interatrial septal aneurysm. The type of billowing fossa (*arrows*; *left*) often impedes catheter manipulation in the right atrium (RA). When the transseptal needle is advanced into the fossa ovalis (*right*), the hypermobile and redundant septal wall often tents far into the left atrium (LA). Using ICE to fine-tune the transseptal needle position to maximize the distance available for sheath crossing may avoid inadvertent perforation of the LA wall. *LI*, Left inferior pulmonary vein; *LS*, left superior pulmonary vein; *RV*, right ventricle. (Refer to Video 43.10.)

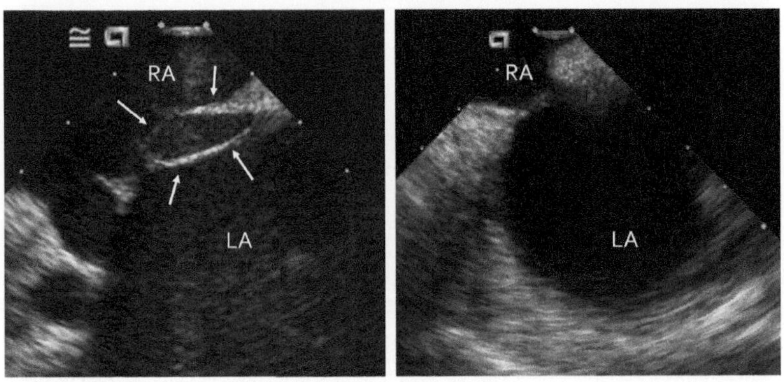

Fig. 43.26 Phased-array intracardiac echocardiography (ICE) images taken from two patients with abnormalities of the interatrial septum. *Left*, Double interatrial septum; the two layers of the septum are marked with opposing *arrows*. In this case, ICE was useful to guide transseptal access through the inferior aspect of the fossa where the septum was fully fused. *Right*, Lipomatous hypertrophy of the septum. *LA*, Left atrium; *RA*, right atrium. (Refer to Video 43.11.)

Lipomatous hypertrophy of the atrial septum is found in up to 2.2% of patients, and its presence is associated with advancing age, obesity, and atrial arrhythmias.[53] The fatty infiltration characteristically forms thick interatrial groove but spares the fossa ovalis. Thus, it produces the classic "dumbbell"-shaped atrial septum (Figs. 43.26 and 43.27). The residual fossa may be quite small, thus limiting the surface area available for sheath crossing (Fig. 43.27).

Thickening of the atrial septum poses the biggest challenge. A thick atrial septum is common after repetitive transseptal catheterization or prior cardiac surgical procedures.[54] These cases require the operator to exert significantly more forward pressure to cross the septum, with the resultant potential for inadvertent puncture of the LA free wall once the needle crosses the atrial septum. In these cases, a detailed survey with the ICE may identify heterogeneity in the degree of thickness, thereby permitting catheterization in a more favorable location (Fig. 43.28 and Video 43.12). Septal crossing of the sheath may also be facilitated in these cases by using the RF-assisted transseptal needles[13] or minimizing the diameter of the transseptal sheath rather than using a sheath with a larger outer diameter such as steerable sheaths.

Transseptal Catheterization in the Presence of an Interatrial Septum Closure Device

Traditionally, the presence of an atrial septum closure devices was considered a contraindication to transseptal puncture, because of a perceived risk of trauma to the device, potential device dislodgement, and postprocedural shunt. Feasibility and safety of transseptal puncture in the presence of an atrial septum closure device have been reported, either via a portion of the native septum not covered by the device or through the device itself.[55,56] No procedure-related complications were encountered, and no residual shunt was observed in any patient. The potential target zone is anywhere at the intact segment of the primary septum (Fig. 43.29 and Video 43.13) or anywhere at the interatrial groove or anteroinferior muscular buttress, both of which are thicker than the primary septum and have a risk of cardiac perforation or damage to the surrounding structures. Thus, when

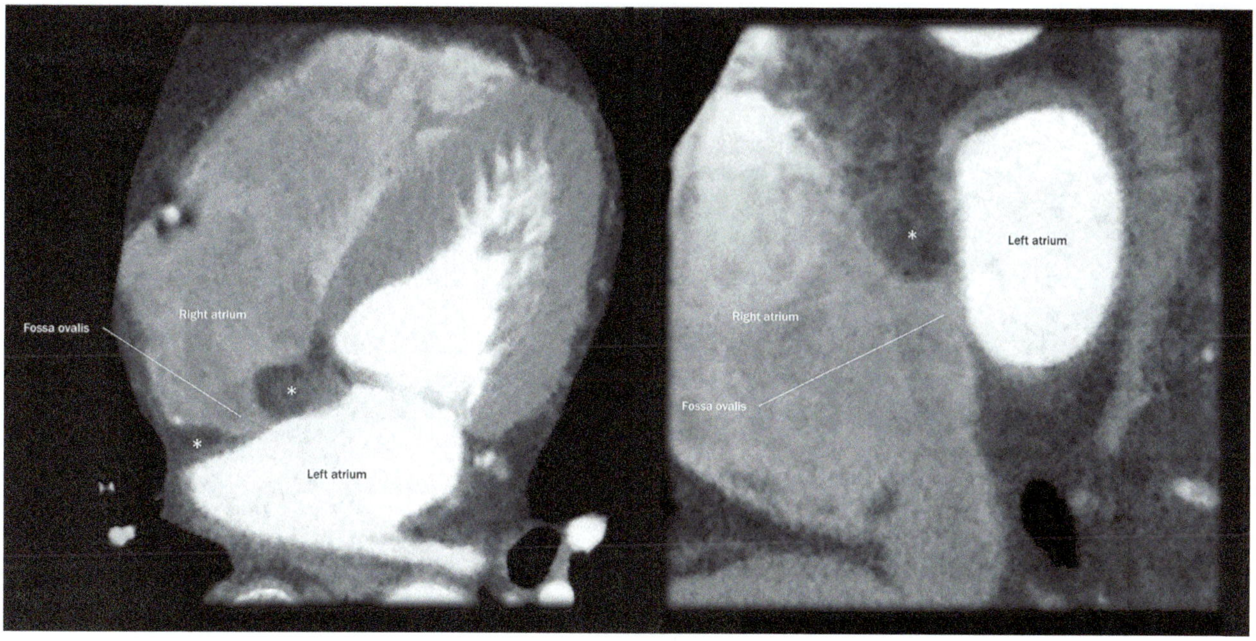

Fig. 43.27 Cardiac computed tomographic images showing the lipomatous hypertrophy (*asterisks*) surrounding the fossa ovalis. *Left and right,* Horizontal and vertical sections of the fossa ovalis, respectively.

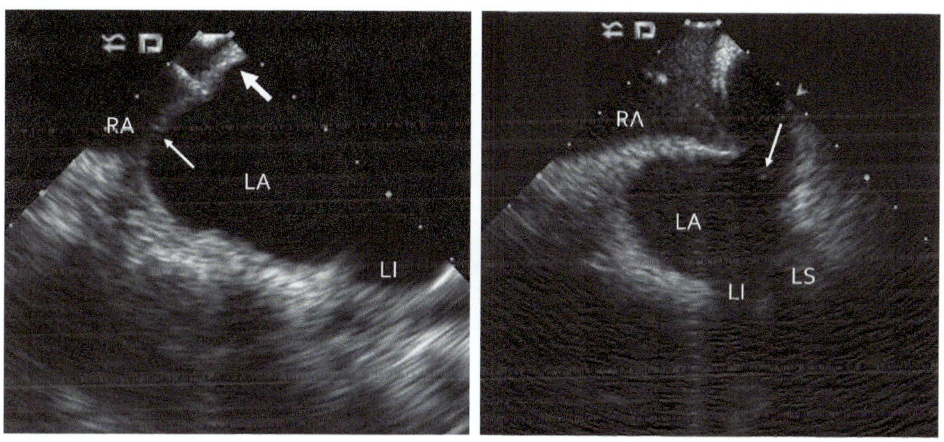

Fig. 43.28 Phased-array intracardiac echocardiography (ICE) images taken from two patients during transseptal access, highlighting the value of ICE in optimizing the location of septal crossing. *Left,* Significant heterogeneity in fossa thickness is seen; the superior aspect of the fossa is 5 mm (*large arrow*) and the inferior aspect is 2 mm (*small arrow*). Crossing a thicker aspect of the septum requires more force and may increase the risk of procedure complications. *Right,* Taken during an atrial fibrillation ablation procedure. Although the orientation of crossing is typically quite favorable, this patient has an abnormal atrial morphology and relatively mobile atrial septum. This results in only 5 mm of distance between the transseptal needle (*arrow*) and the posterior wall of the left atrium (LA). An inferior approach was challenging in this case because of the relative thickness of the fossa. *LA,* Left atrium; *LI,* left inferior pulmonary vein; *LS,* left superior pulmonary vein; *RA,* right atrium. (Refer to Video 43.12.)

planning the peridevice approach, detailed preprocedural three-dimensional planning is the key to secure its safety (Fig. 43.30).

Superior Approach to Transseptal Catheterization

A superior transseptal approach has been described for the placement of endocardial LV pacing leads,[57] as well as in patients with interruption of the inferior vena cava in the setting of left isomerism undergoing AF ablation procedures.[58,59] In a case series of three patients with interruption of the inferior vena cava, transseptal puncture was performed via the right internal jugular vein using either a large curved 8-F sheath (Mullins or SL-3, St. Jude Medical, St. Paul, MN) or a Brockenbrough needle manually bent to achieve a 150-degree angle. A RF-assisted technique from a superior approach has been described.[60,61] A novel pigtail wire is commercially available to allow superior transseptal access, minimizing the need for wire exchange (Fig. 43.31).

Transseptal Catheterization in Patients With Congenital Heart Disease

Patients with surgically repaired congenital heart disease are encountered with increasing frequency in clinical practice.

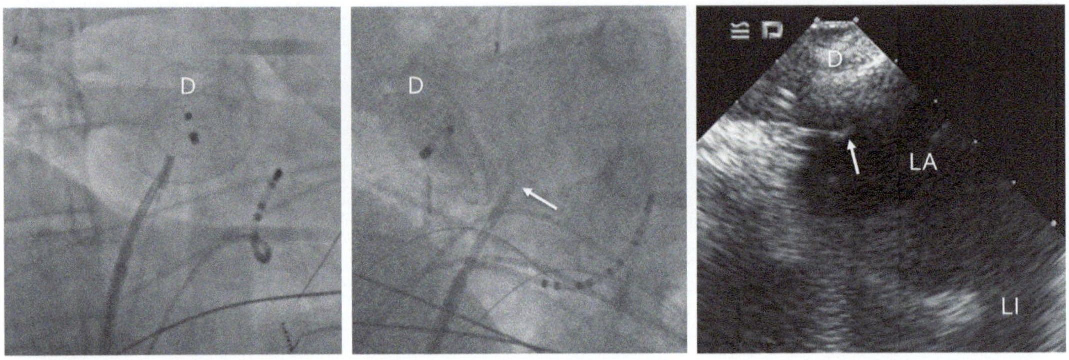

Fig. 43.29 Fluoroscopic (right anterior oblique, *left*; left anterior oblique [LAO], *middle*) and phased-array intracardiac echocardiography (ICE; *right*) images taken during transseptal catheterization of a patient with a percutaneous septal occlusion device (D). Septal crossing can be performed either around or through the device. In this case, ICE identified an intact segment of the fossa present below the device. The position of the sheath during fossa tenting (*arrow*) is seen in the LAO and ICE images. *LA*, Left atrium; *LI*, left inferior pulmonary vein. (Refer to Video 43.13.)

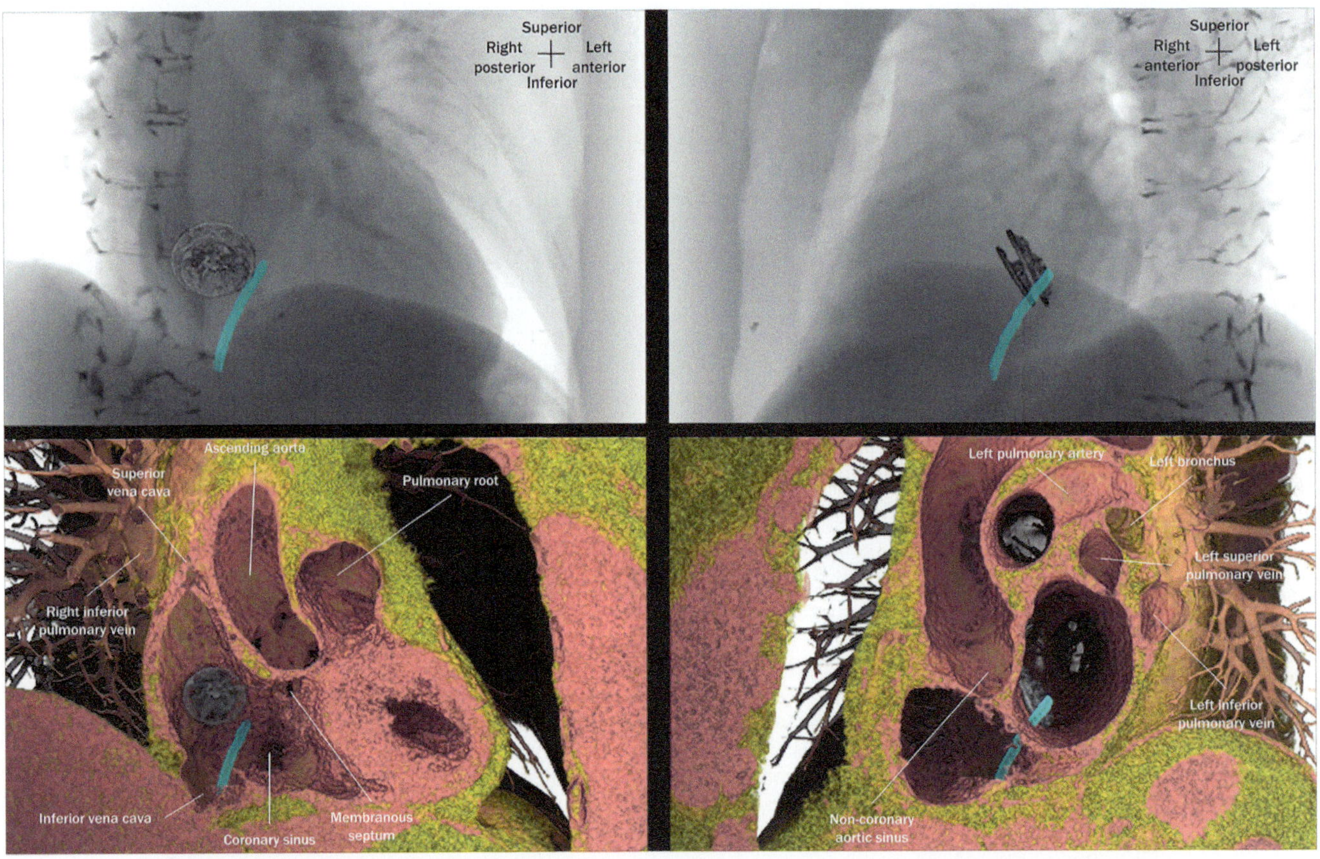

Fig. 43.30 Preprocedural planning of the transseptal puncture in a patient with percutaneous septal occlusion device. Virtual fluoroscopic images (*top*) and virtual dissection images (*bottom*) are reconstructed using the preprocedural cardiac computed tomography and viewed from the right anterior oblique direction (*left*) and left anterior oblique direction (*right*). The virtual transeptal puncture system is also reconstructed in sky blue. In this case, as the entire native primary septum at the oval fossa is covered by the device, the transseptal puncture at the anteroinferior muscular buttress (anterior limbus) is simulated.

Many of these patients have complex arrhythmias related to their postsurgical substrate. Planning based on comprehensive preprocedural evaluation of the three-dimensional anatomy is critical to achieve successful transseptal catheterization. The most common congenital abnormalities that provide challenging atrial access are D-transposition of the great arteries repaired with an atrial switch procedure and patients with Fontan circulation. In both of these clinical scenarios, patients commonly present with atrial flutter circuits. Often, operators need to puncture the surgical graft to access the target atrium (Fig. 43.32).[62] Regardless of whether these grafts are composed of native atrial tissue or synthetic materials, their relative thickness can impede crossing with conventional tools.[63] These procedures are facilitated by a combination of detailed preprocedural

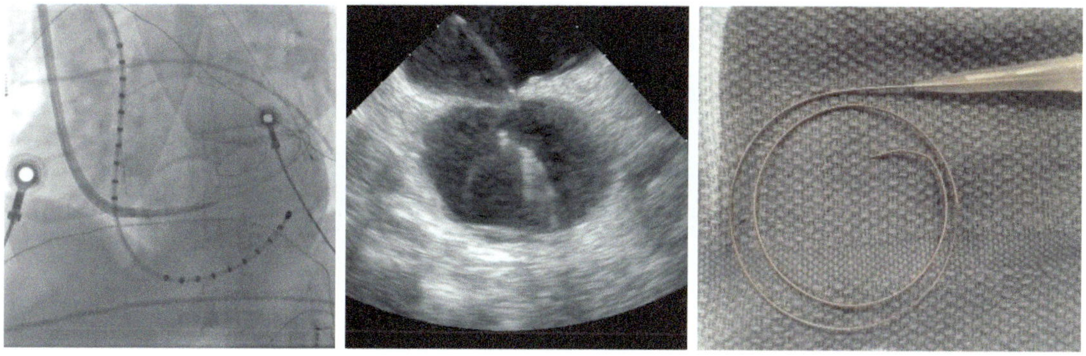

Fig. 43.31 Transseptal catheterization using a superior approach. *Left,* Left anterior oblique fluoroscopic image demonstrates transseptal access using a superior approach. A deflectable sheath (Agilis small curl, St. Jude Medical) is positioned in the right atrium via the right internal jugular vein and deflected superiorly to engage the fossa ovalis. Direct visualization is achieved with intracardiac echocardiography (*middle*). *Right,* Access is performed with a dedicated radiofrequency wire and an exchange pigtail wire (ProTrack, Baylis Medical). The pigtail wire is advanced in the left atrium to favor advancement of the dilator and sheath in the left atrium.

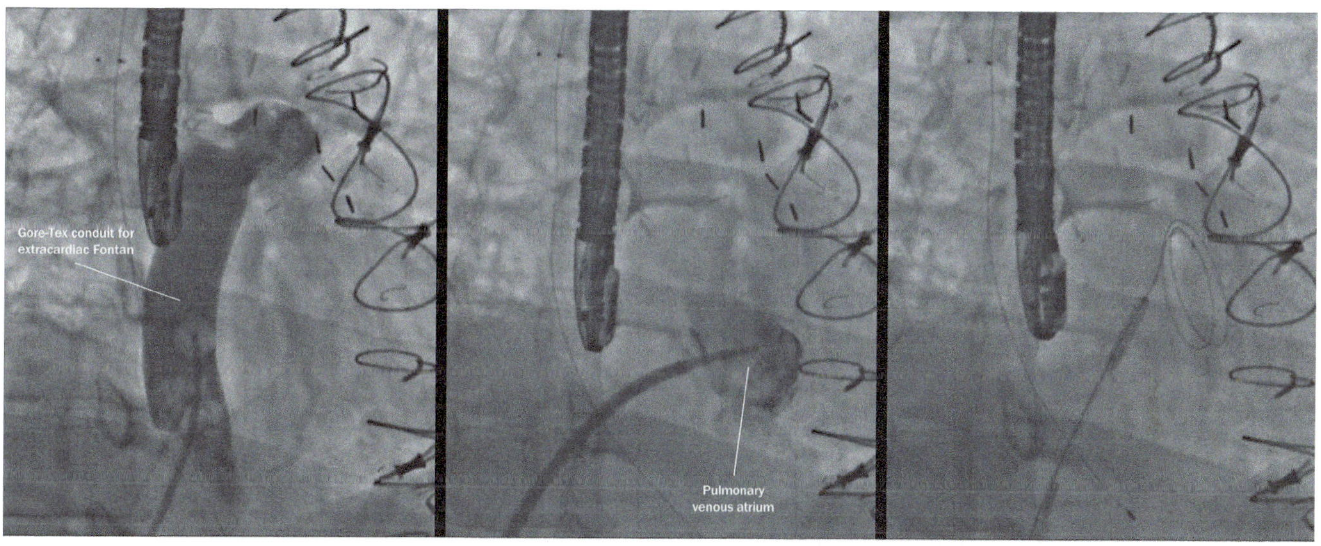

Fig. 43.32 Fluoroscopic images viewed from the right anterior oblique direction showing conduit angiogram (*left*) in a patient with extracardiac Fontan palliation, dilator of transseptal sheath crossing conduit into pulmonary venous atrium (*middle*), and Toray valvuloplasty wire coiled in the atrium with angioplasty balloon inflated across conduit crossing (*right*).

planning, intraprocedural contrast angiography,[64] and real-time ultrasound imaging.

PROCEDURAL COMPLICATIONS AND TOOLS TO LOWER THEIR RISKS

For experienced operators, the anticipated rate of complications during transseptal catheterization should be less than 1%,[20] especially when real-time echocardiographic imaging is used. The most common complication is cardiac perforation, which can occur within both atria. Injury of the aortic root, including aortoatrial fistula and aortic dissection, caused by the anterior puncture outside the fossa ovalis is less common but potentially critical.[21,38] Preprocedural evaluation of the structural anatomy in each case and the use of real-time imaging and/or fluoroscopic landmarks are critical to avoid these complications. Contrast opacification of the fossa ovalis and or intracardiac catheter landmarks can help define the appropriate plane of crossing when ultrasound is not available. The use of continuous pressure transduction through the transseptal needle can identify inadvertent aortic puncture, thereby avoiding subsequent dilation and sheath crossing. Other complications include pulmonary or systemic embolism with either air or thrombus. Diligent sheath and wire management should greatly mitigate or eliminate the possibility of inadvertent air embolism. After removal of needle and dilator, or when exchanging electrode catheters, slow aspiration of sheath contents until all air is withdrawn from sheath and/or side port/hub chamber followed by flushing of the sheath with heparinized saline should effectively preclude the introduction of air into the LA.

Novel technologies have been developed to facilitate transseptal catheterization in patients with difficult anatomic barriers.

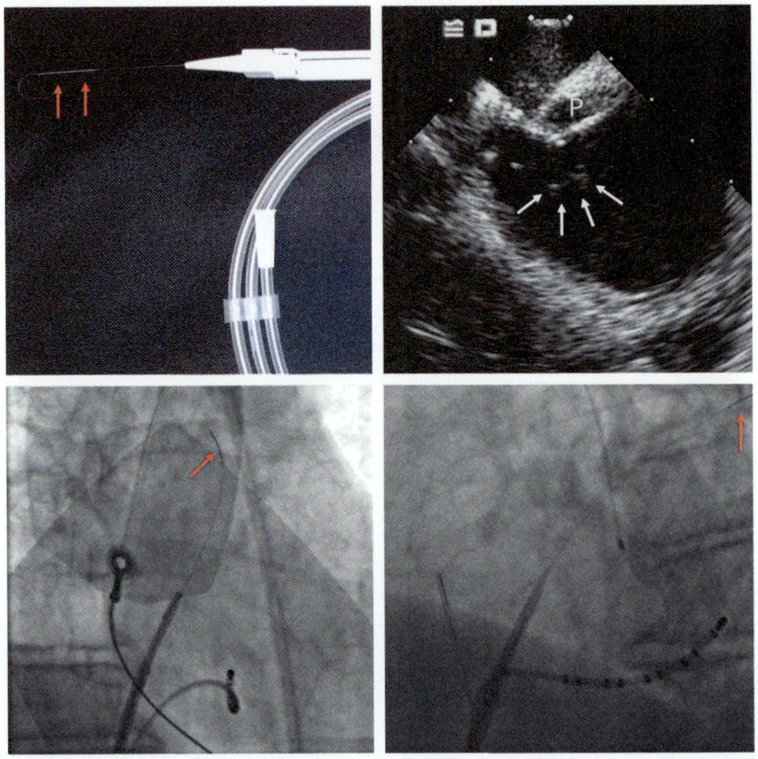

Fig. 43.33 Transseptal access using the SafeSept transseptal guidewire (Pressure Products, San Pedro, CA). This 0.014-inch × 135-cm "J"-shaped nitinol guidewire is equipped with a radiopaque coil on the shaft that allows for visualization under fluoroscopy (*red arrows*). The wire assumes a J shape after it pierces the fossa (*top right, white arrows*), thus allowing for advancement within the left atrium with minimal risk for perforation. After crossing, the J wire is advanced into the left pulmonary veins and provides support for sheath crossing. (Refer to Video 43.14.)

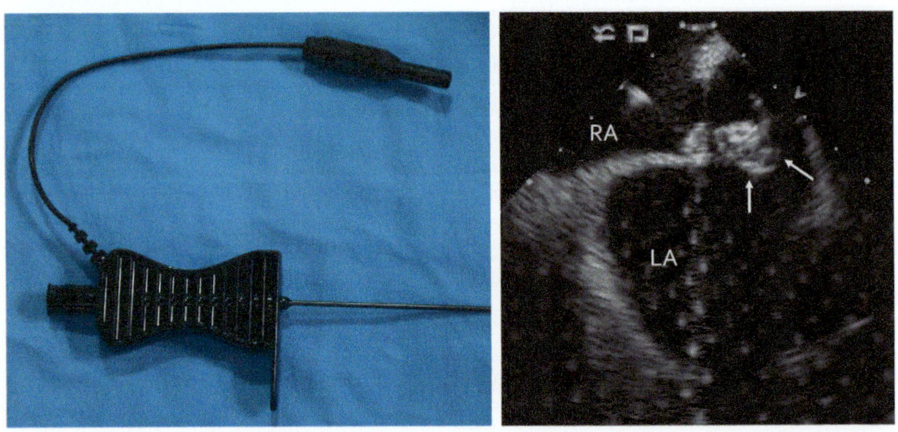

Fig. 43.34 Transseptal access using the NRG radiofrequency transseptal needle (Baylis Medical, Montreal, Canada). The needle hub is shown (*left*). The side port is connected to the radiofrequency (RF) generator, and the distal port can be used for pressure transduction. A phased-array intracardiac echocardiography image is shown (*right*). Note both the characteristic echo artifact and microbubble formation (*arrows*) during RF application. *LA*, Left atrium; *RA*, right atrium. (Refer to Video 43.15.)

The SafeSept transseptal guidewire (Pressure Products, San Pedro, CA) is a 0.014-inch × 135-cm "J"-shaped nickel titanium (nitinol) guidewire with a sharp tip that has been specifically designed to perforate the fossa ovalis with minimal applied pressure. Introduced through a standard Brockenbrough transseptal needle while tenting the fossa, the wire assumes a J shape after it pierces the fossa, thus allowing for advancement within the LA with minimal risk of perforation (Fig. 43.33 and Video 43.14).[65]

The RF-assisted transseptal needle (NRG RF Transseptal Needle, Baylis Medical, Montreal, Canada) is available in 56- to 91-cm lengths, so the system can be used with a full spectrum of transseptal sheaths. The RF energy is delivered through a dedicated generator, with a power setting of 10 W for 2 seconds (unipolar mode) (Fig. 43.34 and Video 43.15). This secures a lower failure rate and pericardial effusion rate.[13,66]

A RF-assisted puncture can also be performed by applying RF energy from a surgical electrocautery system to the proximal hub of a standard Brockenbrough needle,[10] with the generator programmed to 20 W in the cut mode.

A pigtail RF wire (Supracross, Baylis Medical, Montreal, Canada) has a 180-cm length and 0.035-inch diameter, and it is insulated to the tip allowing delivery of RF energy to cross the atrial septum from a superior approach. The distal portion of the wire forms a 2.5-cm-diameter pigtail shape, which facilitates tracking of the dilator/sheath transseptal apparatus (Fig. 43.30).

CONCLUSION

Atrial transseptal catheterization represents a fundamental skill for any interventional electrophysiologist. Although its basic technique has not substantially changed over the past 50 years, important technical advancements, including an integration of the real-time ICE, have refined the safety and efficacy of the procedure. Other specialized tools, such as RF-assisted transseptal needles, have further improved the safety of this common procedure. Through these improvements, currently atrial transseptal catheterization can be applied safely even for those with challenging anatomy. Regardless of these technical improvements, however, a detailed evaluation of the anatomy of the atrial septum and its relationship with surrounding structures in each case are always fundamental.

ACKNOWLEDGMENTS

We thank individuals who have donated their bodies and tissues for the advancement of education and research. Special thanks to One Legacy Foundation and the NIH SPARC Program, which formed the basis for obtaining donor hearts for research and for funding this effort. We are also grateful to Prof. Warwick J. Peacock, Dr. Grace Chang, and Mr. Edwin Ng with the UCLA Surgical Sciences Laboratory and all the staff members of the UCLA Donated Body Program, Translational Research Imaging Center (Department of Radiology) at UCLA, and Translational Pathology Core Laboratory at UCLA for their supports in dissection, image acquisition, and histologic preparation. We would like to thank the family of Dr. Wallace A. McAlpine; his daughters, Ms. Laurel Flowers, Ms. Kim Renteria Clark, and Ms. Leigh McAlpine Whitten, and his son, Mr. Fraser McAlpine, for helping us locate the works of Dr. McAlpine. We thank Mr. Michael Papalucas, who expertly digitized the original slides made by Dr. McAlpine. Finally, we would like to thank Dr. Pasquale Santangeli and Dr. Mathew D. Hutchinson, authors of the previous edition of this chapter, for providing excellent insights and figures/videos as part of the sources for this new version.

REFERENCES

Please refer to the e-book for a complete list of references.

44

Ablation of Cardiac Arrhythmias in Pediatric Population

Maully Shah, Christopher Janson, Chandra Srinivasan, Dustin Nash, Shashank Behere

KEY POINTS

- Children have the same variety of arrhythmia mechanisms as adults but with a different distribution and often in different clinical settings.
- Despite physical similarities of older children to adults, children are not just little adults when it comes to the choice to proceed with and techniques for performing ablation; however, virtually all the techniques used in adults, including epicardial approaches, can be performed in pediatric patients.
- Ablation in infants and very small children carries a variety of special risks and should be undertaken only after failure of medical therapy and in the most experienced hands.
- The presence of structural congenital heart disease significantly complicates any ablation procedure, demanding that the operator be familiar with both the structural and electrophysiologic (EP) issues at hand, particularly if atrioventricular discordance is present.
- Atrial flutter and fibrillation are rare arrhythmias in the pediatric population in the absence of congenital heart disease but may be amenable to catheter-based therapies.
- Atrial ectopic tachycardia, junctional ectopic tachycardia, and the permanent form of junctional reciprocating tachycardia can all manifest as incessant tachyarrhythmias with a dilated cardiomyopathy in children. Ablation therapy may be particularly helpful in such cases if it can be performed safely.
- Coronary artery injury from radiofrequency (RF) ablation can occur when the ablation site is in close proximity to a coronary artery and is probably unrecognized in most cases where it occurs. Consequently, coronary angiography should be considered before the use of RF ablation of some posteroseptal substrates, particularly in smaller children.
- Minimization of fluoroscopy exposure with the use of nonfluoroscopic and lower-dose fluoroscopic techniques is feasible and seems prudent during all catheter-based EP procedures in children.
- For ablation in children, safety should always take precedence over efficacy. Consequently, when cryotherapy can be effective, it is often the technology of first choice.
- The Pediatric and Congenital Electrophysiology Society/Heart Rhythm Society (PACES/HRS) Expert Consensus Statement on the use of Catheter Ablation in Children[1,2] are useful guides for procedural indications and general recommendations in these patient populations but do not replace the need for clinical judgment and patient-specific decision-making.

INTRODUCTION

The explosion in understanding and management of most arrhythmias in adults over the past 50 years is both reflected and amplified in the field of pediatrics. The application of procedures or devices commonly used in the management of arrhythmias in adults remains somewhat delayed in children because of technical issues related to size or lack of regulatory approval. Other issues, such as a smaller number of patients and a higher diversity of clinical characteristics and age, have limited the ability to perform controlled therapeutic trials, even multicenter ones. Despite these limitations, a combination of continued technical developments in the miniaturization of devices, multicenter retrospective reviews and registries, occasional controlled clinical trials, and the use of pharmacologic agents approved by the U.S. Food and Drug Administration for adults has resulted in almost equivalence in the armamentarium of adult and pediatric electrophysiologists.[3–7]

This chapter concentrates primarily on two categories of rhythm disorders: arrhythmias that are mechanistically similar or identical to those in adults (>18 years) but whose presentation and management is complicated by the presence of young age or congenital heart disease (CHD); and arrhythmias that are either unique to pediatric patients or are observed only rarely in adults (Table 44.1). Most of the material in this chapter relates to children without CHD unless specified in the text. Atrial and ventricular tachyarrhythmias in the patient with CHD are addressed in Chapters 14 and 38, respectively.

TABLE 44.1 Comparison of Arrhythmias/ Conditions in Children and Adults

Arrhythmias/Conditions Not Typically Observed in Adults
Ectopic atrial tachycardia
Junctional ectopic tachycardia
Permanent junctional reciprocating tachycardia
Double atrioventricular nodes
Alternative Presentations of Arrhythmias/Conditions Commonly Observed in Adults
Atrioventricular nodal reentrant tachycardia
Preexcitation syndromes in infants
Preexcitation syndromes with congenital heart disease
Ventricular tachycardia with tetralogy of Fallot
Atrial reentry with congenital heart disease
Arrhythmias/Conditions with Similar Management in Adults and Children
Preexcitation syndromes after infancy
Congenital long QT syndrome
Right ventricular outflow tract ventricular tachycardia
Arrhythmogenic right ventricular dysplasia
Benign accelerated idioventricular rhythm

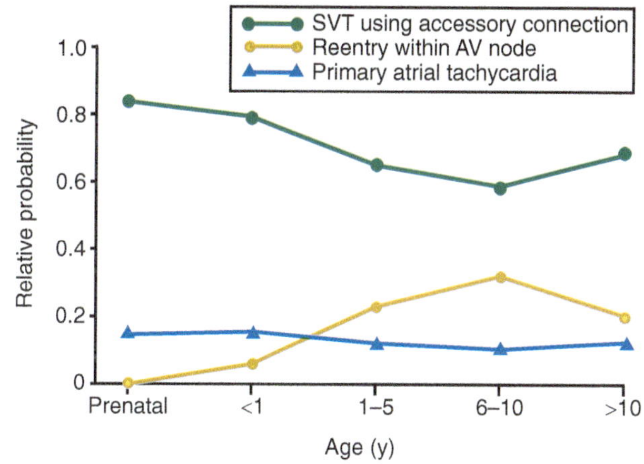

Fig. 44.1 Distribution of supraventricular tachycardia mechanisms as a function of age in pediatric patients. The percentage of patients with primary atrial tachycardias remains relatively constant, while there is a shift from accessory pathway mediated tachycardias to atrioventricular nodal reentry from infancy to adolescence. (From Ko JK, Deal BJ, Strasburger JF, Benson DW Jr. Supraventricular tachycardia mechanisms and their age distribution in pediatric patients. *Am J Cardiol.* 1992;69:1028–1032.)

ARE CHILDREN JUST LITTLE ADULTS?

The notion that children are simply small adults may apply to older teens. However, for many procedures, what seems like only a difference of scale can have dramatic implications, which begin with the diagnosis, extend from the initial recommendation for an ablation to the technical performance of the procedure,[8] and end with the long-term risks of producing radiofrequency (RF) lesions in developing myocardium[9,10] and near coronary arteries.[11 14] Safety recommendations that define institutional, procedural, and personnel recommendations for performing catheter ablation in children based on age and patient size will be reviewed in detail in the relevant sections of this chapter.

On average, children are obviously smaller than adults, resulting in smaller cardiac chambers, thinner and perhaps more fragile tissues, smaller coronary arteries, and smaller distances between structures, such as the posterior septum and the atrioventricular (AV) node, or the AV ring and the coronary arteries. Not so obviously, children may be dissimilar from adults in ways other than size. Arrhythmia mechanisms overlap but are proportionately very different.[15–18] Incessant arrhythmias are much more common,[19] probably based on lack of symptom recognition in infants and small children, better early tolerance, and late morbidity and mortality if left untreated, which ensures that most patients will not reach adulthood with their arrhythmias. Accessory pathway (AP) locations are skewed toward the right side,[3,4,20] at least partially related to the simultaneous presence of structural CHD.[21–23] In addition, developing myocardium appears to have the potential for spontaneous cure of an arrhythmia[18,24] but also the potential for both RF and cryothermal lesion growth with time.[9,10]

Arrhythmia Mechanisms

The arrhythmias seen in pediatric patients are typically the more treatable varieties. Ventricular tachycardia (VT) is relatively rare in children, accounting for less than 5% of all tachycardias and only 20% of wide-complex tachycardias.[25,26] Supraventricular tachycardia (SVT),[27,28] which accounts for the vast majority of arrhythmias in children, is most likely to result from a concealed or manifest accessory AV pathway (Fig. 44.1),[18] portending well for possible catheter ablation therapy. In the absence of a history of surgery for structural CHD, APs probably underlie about 75% of all SVTs in children[18] and account for about 95% of SVTs in neonates,[34,35] compared with 30% to 40% of SVTs in adults.[19,20] Atrioventricular nodal reentrant tachycardia (AVNRT) and primary atrial tachycardias (ATs; both reentrant and automatic)[21] each appear to account for about half of the remaining SVTs (see Fig. 44.1).[11] Atrial fibrillation (AF) is seen uncommonly in pediatric patients in the absence of structural or CHD ("lone" AF) and only rarely is problematic enough to justify catheter ablation with pulmonary vein (PV) isolation. However, there are circumstances under which either ablation of an isolated ectopic PV focus or full wide area PV isolation is a reasonable approach.[29,30]

The Decision to Ablate: Safety Versus Efficacy

One overriding theme in the management of arrhythmias in children compared with adults is an emphasis on safety over efficacy. Although there are few cases at any age in which safety is not an important concern, the relatively benign course of many arrhythmic conditions in childhood, the potential disruption that therapies such as permanent pacing cause for a child, and the fact that parents are usually the decision-making surrogate for the child often lead to a different decision tree for children than for adults. Further, for some situations and technologies (e.g., the potential for coronary artery damage with RF energy application at the AV groove), the size of the patient and of the heart may be important. The 2014 and 2016 Pediatric and Congenital

Electrophysiology Society/Heart Rhythm Society (PACES/HRS) Expert Consensus Statement on the use of Catheter Ablation in Children[1,2] provides guidance for patient selection for catheter ablation, but scientific guidelines and recommendations do not replace the need for clinical judgment and patient-specific decision-making. Furthermore, recommendations may need modifications based on contemporary data and new technological developments that improve the safety and success of catheter ablation.

Ablation in patients with Wolff-Parkinson-White (WPW) syndrome is an excellent example of how decision-making may be highly age-dependent.[31] In this chapter, the term *WPW* will be used to describe the condition of preexcitation on the surface electrocardiogram (ECG), with or without coexisting tachycardia. Because of a variety of concerns, even the most symptomatic infant with WPW and paroxysmal SVT is only rarely a candidate for ablation.[1,31–33] Myocardial injury[9,10] and potentially severe coronary injury[11–14,32] are more likely with RF ablation in this age group. Although the introduction of cryoablation has changed this situation somewhat, there remain a number of reasons to be cautious in managing infants with ablation procedures.[33,34] Perhaps most important is that about 40% of APs in infants spontaneously stop functioning during the first year of life,[35,36] and an additional third of patients are unlikely to have symptoms between infancy and early childhood.[37] In children larger than 15 kg who have symptomatic arrhythmias, the balance between risks and benefits clearly shifts toward ablation therapy, but usually only if the ablation can be performed safely.[1,31] In contrast to the situation in infants, even asymptomatic WPW patients between the ages of 10 and 18 years may be managed more aggressively than adults.[38] Unlike asymptomatic adults who are unlikely to ever have symptoms,[39,40] the older child with a high-risk pathway is exactly the type of patient who may present with sudden arrhythmic death as their initial symptom, leading to the recommendation that such patients should undergo risk stratification, with those who are at high risk being offered catheter ablation as a therapeutic option.[38,40] Further, the guidelines for sports participation in patients with WPW recommend considering risk stratification before approval.[41] Other age-dependent differences in management decisions are addressed in the discussions of individual arrhythmias.

Use of Cryoablation in Children

Catheter-based cryoablation was approved for use in the United States in 2003 for ablation of AVNRT. Since then, there have been a variety of reports in children, primarily focused on its use in AVNRT and expansion to other arrhythmia substrates.[1,42–48] Cryoablation has several potential advantages over RF ablation, including (1) reversible cryomapping before the production of a permanent lesion,[51] (2) adherence of the catheter tip to the endocardium upon freezing, (3) a well-defined edge of the cryolesion, (4) minimal effects on adjacent coronary arteries,[49,50] and (5) a lower incidence of thrombus.[51] The first four of these issues are particularly relevant to small children because of the close proximity of a variety of critical cardiac structures to the ablation target and the reported potential for RF lesion growth in immature myocardium.[9] In fact, the most common major complication during RF ablation in pediatric patients is AV block,[3,4,52–54] and there also appears to be a higher potential for coronary artery injury in this patient group,[11–14] even during slow-pathway (SP) modification[12] (see full discussion later under AVNRT).

Despite frequent use of the technology for septal tachycardia substrates, there are no reports of permanent AV block with cryoablation,[1,55–58] even in children as small as 20 kg,[57] in the presence of a His potential (Fig. 44.2) and in various forms of CHD associated with displaced or less predictable AV conduction systems.[59]

The primary disadvantage of cryoablation is that inherent in its high level of safety is a smaller lesion size than for RF ablation. Another disadvantage is the unidirectional nature of the catheter, which impedes endocardial mapping. With a few exceptions,[58] even aggressive application of cryoenergy has not yielded similar long-term success rates to RF for ablation of nonseptal APs.[60–66]

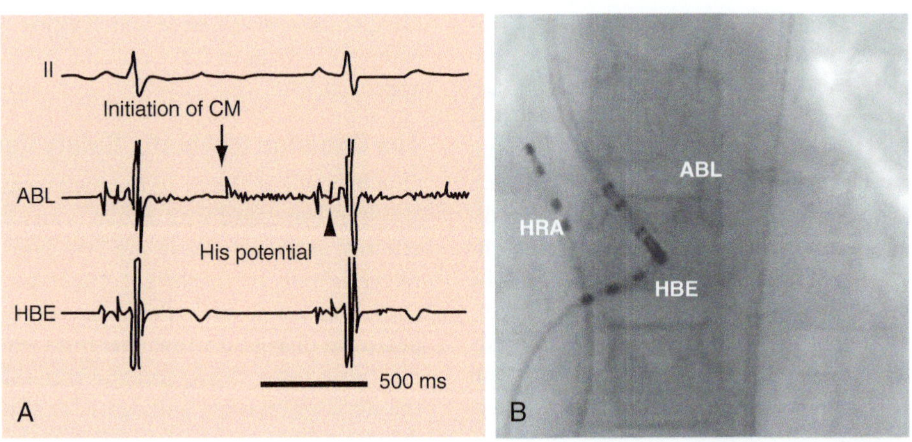

Fig. 44.2 Successful cryoablation at location with His potential in a patient with junctional ectopic tachycardia. (A) Identical His potentials are clearly seen from the ablation catheter (retrograde approach through the aortic valve) and from the His catheter (in a usual position) just before initiation of cryomapping (CM). (B) Fluoroscopic images in the anteroposterior view shows cryoablation catheter overlapping the image of the His position catheter. *ABL,* Ablation; *HBE,* His-bundle electrogram; *HRA,* high right atrium.

Atrioventricular Nodal Reentrant Tachycardia

The incidence of AVNRT gradually increases during childhood from being rare during infancy to 10–15% in young school-aged children and almost 50% in older teenagers.[1,18] Overall, AVNRT accounts for approximately 30% of all pediatric ablations[1,3,4,67] and approximately 10% of congenital heart ablations.[68,69]

Age-Dependent Changes in the AV Node

The increased incidence of AVNRT with advancing age is postulated to be the result of maturational changes of the AV node. Key histologic alterations observed are a gradual increase in fibrofatty tissue distorting the initial tightly packed architecture of the transitional cell zone and its relationship with the compact AV node.[70] With the gradual expansion of the AV muscular septum, there is an increase in the calculated surface area of the triangle of Koch (KT), a change in the shape of the AV node and its relative position within KT.[70] This phenomenon also shifts the positions of the rightward and leftward posterior extensions of the compact AVN, from relatively close to each other in the very young to wide apart in adolescents and young adults.[70] The overall incidence of dual node physiology is 25% of children without documented SVT but electrophysiology studies have shown that the occurrence is disproportionate in adolescents vs. younger children (44% vs. 15%),[71] once again suggesting that developmental histologic and morphologic changes in the AV node and AV septal junction area may favor dual node physiology in older children.

Pathophysiology of AVNRT in Children

The seminal work by Jackman et al. reporting the successful RF ablation of AVNRT targeting antegrade SP signals ("Asp") launched the era of AVNRT ablation and proved the existence of targetable separate atrial insertion zones for SP conduction.[72] Morphologic studies confirm the existence of rightward and leftward inferior extensions of the compact AV node and provide an embryological basis for their existence,[71,72–74] while newer studies incorporating connexin genotypic data challenge the traditional perspective that rightward and leftward inferior inputs are discrete entities.[75] Similar to AVNRT in adults, these extensions provide anatomical substrates for SP catheter ablation in children.

Compared to adult patients, there are several key differences in the electrophysiology characteristics of AVNRT in children (1) eliciting longitudinal dissociation curves in AV node conduction by programmed stimulation based on the classic definition for dual AV node physiology—a 50-ms increase in the atrium-to-His bundle (AH) interval for a 10-ms decrement in the atrium-to-atrium (AA) interval, is possible in only approximately 60% of children with AVNRT (Fig. 44.3).[76–80] In fact, AVNRT could theoretically take place with minimal or no change in the AH interval at the transition point between the fast pathway (FP) and SP, a condition in which the change in AH would be of no value in identifying dual pathways. Therefore, less stringent criteria may be necessary to define dual AV nodal physiology in children.[76,78–82] (2) Younger children have faster

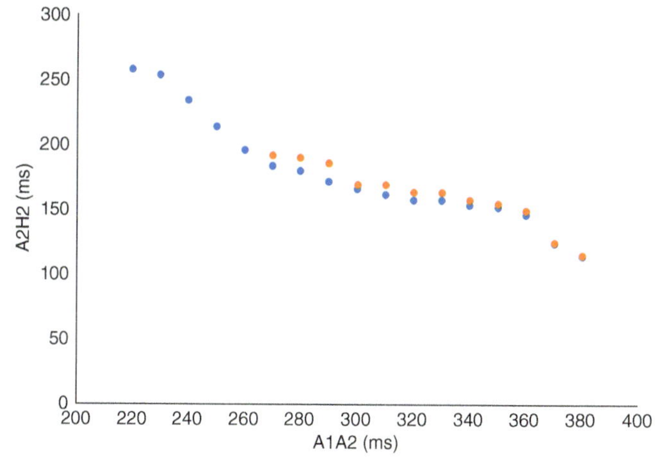

Fig. 44.3 A smooth atrioventricular (AV) node function curve without evidence of dual AV node pathways was present (*blue dot*) prior to ablation in a 7-year-old with atrioventricular nodal reentrant tachycardia. Ablation in the slow-pathway zone resulted in loss of the "tail" of the curve (*orange dot*). A_1A_2, Interval between atrial deflection of the last drive cycle and the extrastimulus; A_2H_2, AH interval at the His-bundle catheter after the extrastimulus.

conduction in the SP compared to older children and adults,[116,117] and the magnitude of the AH jump at the FP effective refractory period (ERP) appears less pronounced in younger children and increases with age in adolescence.[77–80] (3) Evidence of sustained SP conduction (SSPC), also known as the *crossover* phenomenon, where the PR interval ≥ RR interval during decremental atrial pacing seems more predictive of inducible AVNRT in children than the presence of an AH jump[81,83] (Fig. 44.4). (4) The 2:1 AV conduction during AVNRT, which can be mistaken for AT on the surface ECG (Fig. 44.5A), is observed frequently in young patients and must be distinguished from AT with 2:1 AV conduction by specific maneuvers. This can be seen in typical and atypical AVNRT (Fig. 44.5B, C). The block is functional regardless of whether a His-bundle potential is observed on nonconducted beats.[84]

Atypical AVNRT

In adult series, approximately 10% of AVNRT deviates from the parameters of using rightward inferior SP as the antegrade limb, and the FP as the retrograde limb, either due to the presence of retrograde SP activation, and/or the presence of a distinct antegrade SP, falling into the category of atypical AVNRT. The site of earliest retrograde atrial activation is at the coronary sinus os (CSO) or within the proximal 1–2 cm of the CSO (Fig. 44.5B). In patients with fast-slow AVNRT, multiple AH jumps may be observed during programmed atrial extrastimulation (AES), which is consistent with presence of multiple SPs. Data on atypical AVNRT are relatively scarce in pediatric and adult series.[85] Although the majority of atypical AVNRT can be successfully ablated with targeting of the "usual" rightward inferior SP, it is not curative in all cases of atypical AVNRT, suggesting the existence of SP inputs in other anatomical locations including the mid or superior septum, left side of the septum, or distal CS.[86] The exact incidence of atypical AVNRT is not well described,

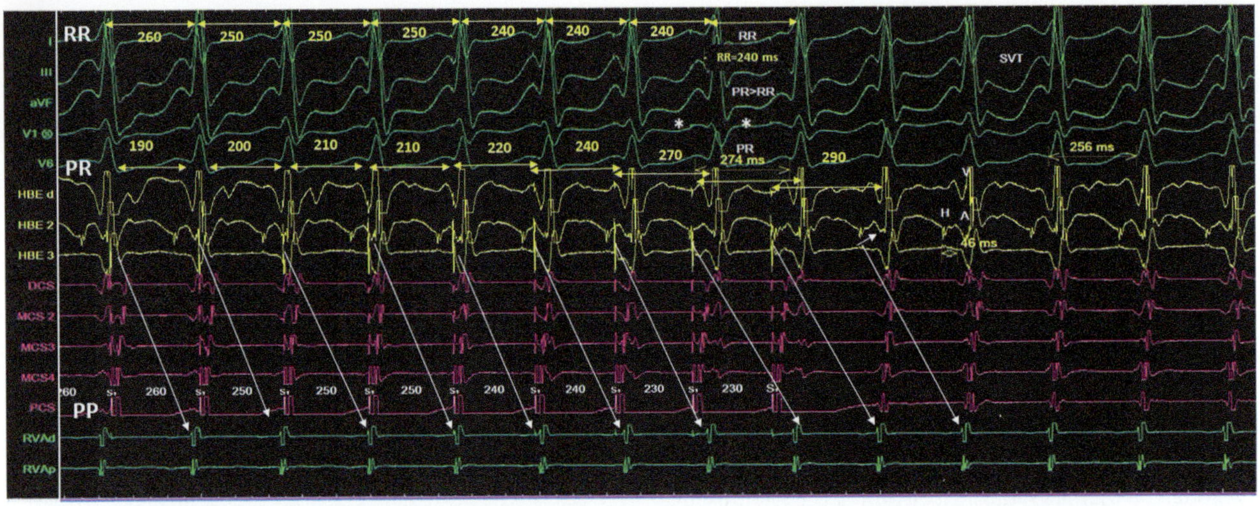

Fig. 44.4 ECG measurements during incremental atrial pacing from proximal coronary sinus (CS) catheter in a 9-year-old patient with atrioventricular nodal reentrant tachycardia without evidence of dual AV node physiology. ECG leads (I, III, aVF, V_1, V_6) and five channels from a decapolar catheter in the CS: DCS, MCS 2, MCS 3, MCS 4, PCS, hexapolar catheter in the His bundle (HBE), and quadrupolar catheter in the RV apex (RVA) are displayed. PR, RR, and RR intervals measured with a paper speed of 100 mm/s. PR intervals (*) represent PR intervals > RR interval (PR/RR = 1.17), indicating sustained slow-pathway conduction (SSPC) with induction of AVNRT.

A

B

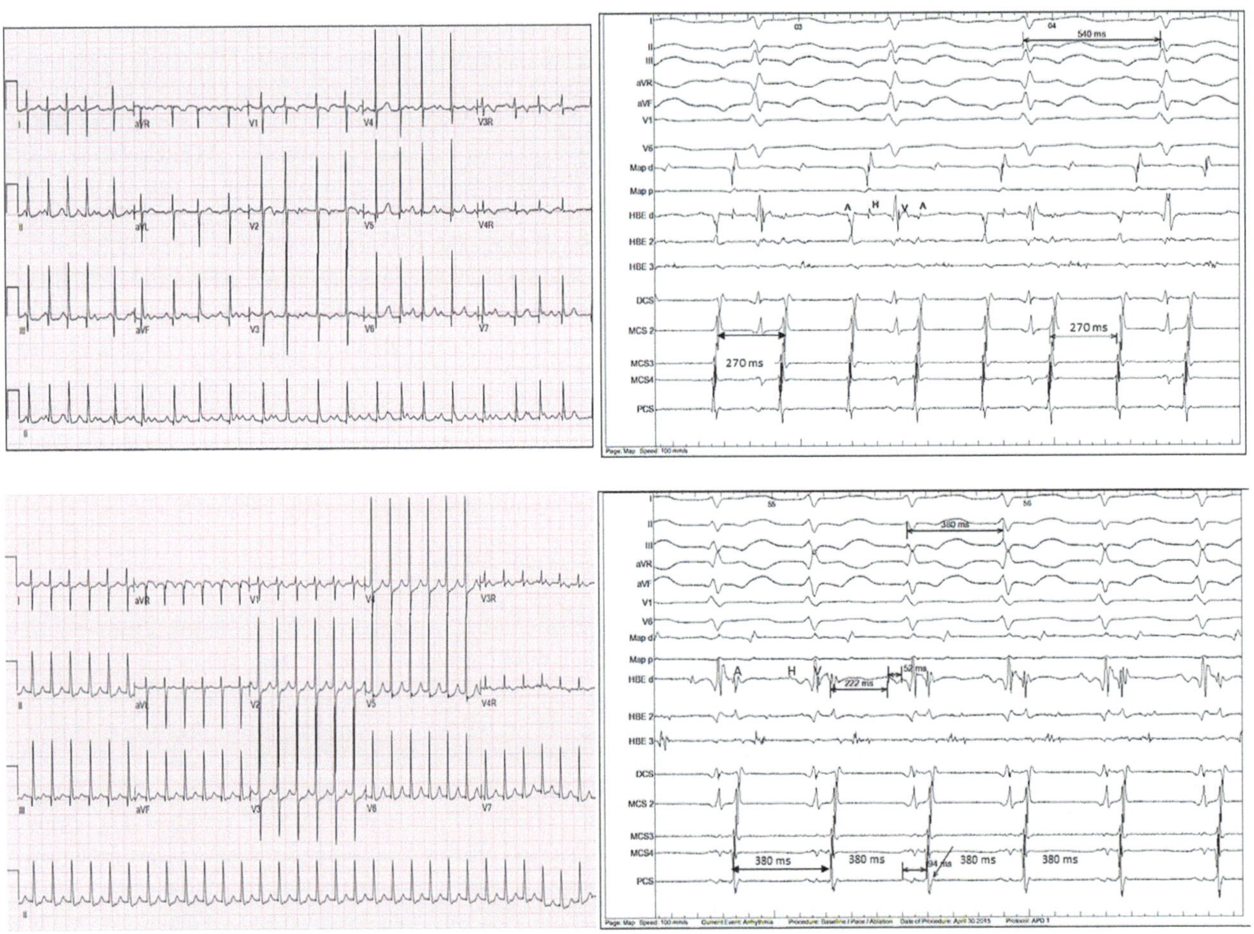

Fig. 44.5 (A) ECG shows an irregular rhythm (RR interval 280–560 ms) in a 12-year-old complaining of palpitations that was initially diagnosed as atrial tachycardia with variable AV conduction in the emergency department. Intracardiac signals in the same patient show induction of fast-slow atrioventricular nodal reentrant tachycardia (AVNRT) with 2:1 AV block. A His-bundle potential is absent on blocked beats; AV block occurred in the supra-Hisian region. Earliest retrograde atrial activation is seen in PCS during atypical AVNRT. (B) ECG and intracardiac electrograms in the same patient after fast-slow AVNRT transitioned to 1:1 AV conduction when atrial cycle length was longer (380 ms). Earliest retrograde atrial activation is once again seen in PCS. Five standard ECG leads, five channels from a decapolar catheter in the coronary sinus (distal to proximal), three-channel recording from the His bundle (HBE), and two-channel recording from the map catheter in the right atrium are displayed.

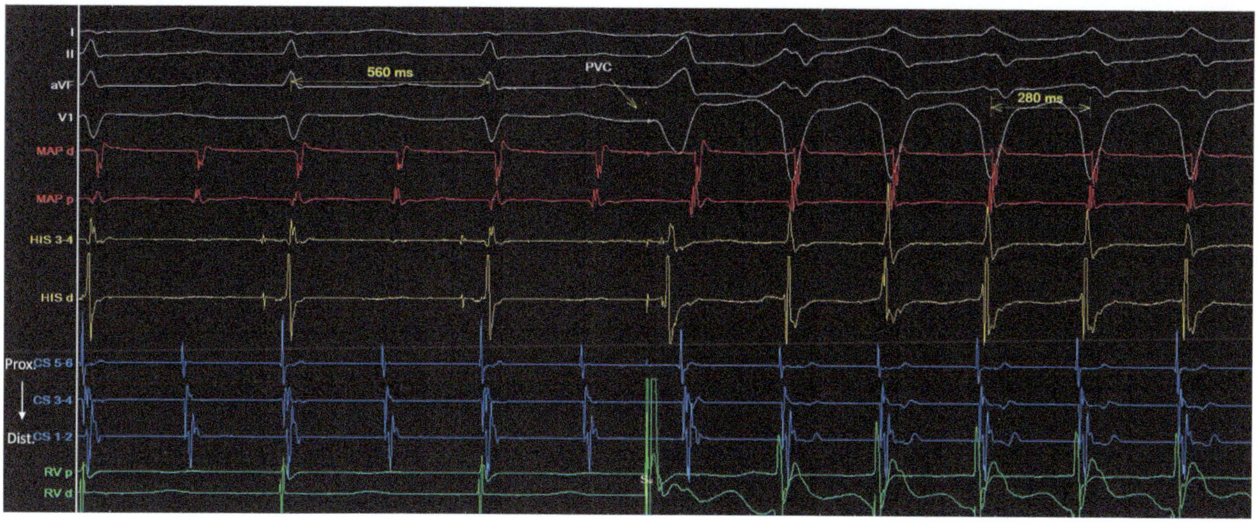

Fig. 44.5, Cont'd (C) Typical AVNRT with 2:1 block in a different patient. A His-bundle potential is absent on blocked beats. A ventricular extrastimulus (PVC) introduced during 2:1 AV block results in 1:1 conduction indicating the AV block is functional and the level of block is in the lower common pathway. During 1:1 AV nodal conduction, there is aberrancy with left bundle block.

but we suspect it is underdiagnosed and is likely responsible for some portion of recurrences. In one large pediatric study, the incidence of atypical AVNRT was 8% and was significantly associated with recurrent AVNRT.[87]

Dual AV Node Nonreentrant Tachycardia

The phenomenon of dual fast and slow AV conduction of single atrial beats, also termed "AV nodal double fire," is sometimes seen in adolescents. Rarely, tachycardia is manifested, which is characterized by a sinus beat that leads to consecutive double antegrade conduction via the FPs and SPs, resulting in two ventricular depolarizations (Fig. 44.6). The interval between the two QRS complexes is usually fixed but may be complicated by bundle branch block or intraventricular conduction disturbances. This unusual arrhythmia may be mistaken for AF or VT on the surface ECG. Dual AV node nonreentrant tachycardia (DAVNNT) can also initiate or convert into AVNRT. SP modification is usually the recommended therapy.

Unique Considerations for Pediatric/CHD AVNRT Ablation

The following are some of the unique considerations in children and patients with CHD once a decision has been made to perform SP modification.

Triangle of Koch

The dimensions of Koch triangle (KT) vary directly and significantly with weight, height, age, and body surface area, with the latter being the strongest predictor.[88] In children ≤15 kg, or BSA ≤0.6 m^2, the length of KT may be ≤5–7 mm, approximating the diameter of the lesion generated by a standard 4-mm electrode catheter tip used to deliver RF energy (Fig. 44.7). Intuitively, one would expect that a smaller KT would limit safe delivery of RF ablation energy and risk injury to the AV node.

We use 3D electroanatomical mapping to depict "personalized" KT dimensions prior to SP ablation.[89] The boundary of the KT is defined by the lowest His-bundle recording site, the septal tricuspid valve (TV) annulus, and the posterior margin of the CSO as a surrogate of tendon of Todaro. The AV node lies superior and anterior to the CSO. It is also useful to obtain geometry of the CSO including the roof and the floor. One caveat is that when the CS is cannulated from the femoral vein the catheter tends to rise toward the roof of the CS, and when cannulated from a superior vessel such as the internal jugular vein, it lies in the floor of the CS. Therefore, when the CS cannulation is from the femoral vein, it should be assumed that the proximal electrodes of the catheter are closer to the AV node, and ablation at any point higher may be associated with a higher risk of AV node injury. To gain better knowledge of the individual CSO and CS anatomy, a direct angiogram of the CS may be of additional value.

Mapping the Slow Pathway

Catheter ablation of AVNRT in children and in patients with CHD has seen a continual refinement of safety and efficacy in the current era.[90–95] Similar to adults, AVNRT is usually ablated by targeting the SP input to the circuit. In most patients with structurally normal hearts, the anatomy of the inferior KT is predictable, allowing for anatomical targeting of the area of ablation, at least for the rightward inferior SP input, which plays a critical role in the majority of AVNRT. Classic SP potential can also be identified and targeted (Fig. 44.8A) within this anatomical region. Another useful method is to insert resetting atrial extrastimuli to confirm the anatomical location of the antegrade slow limb of AVNRT (Fig. 44.8B), since a single atrial extrastimulus delivered close to the atrial component of the AVNRT circuit should be able to reset the tachycardia.[94] This method allows us to identify the site

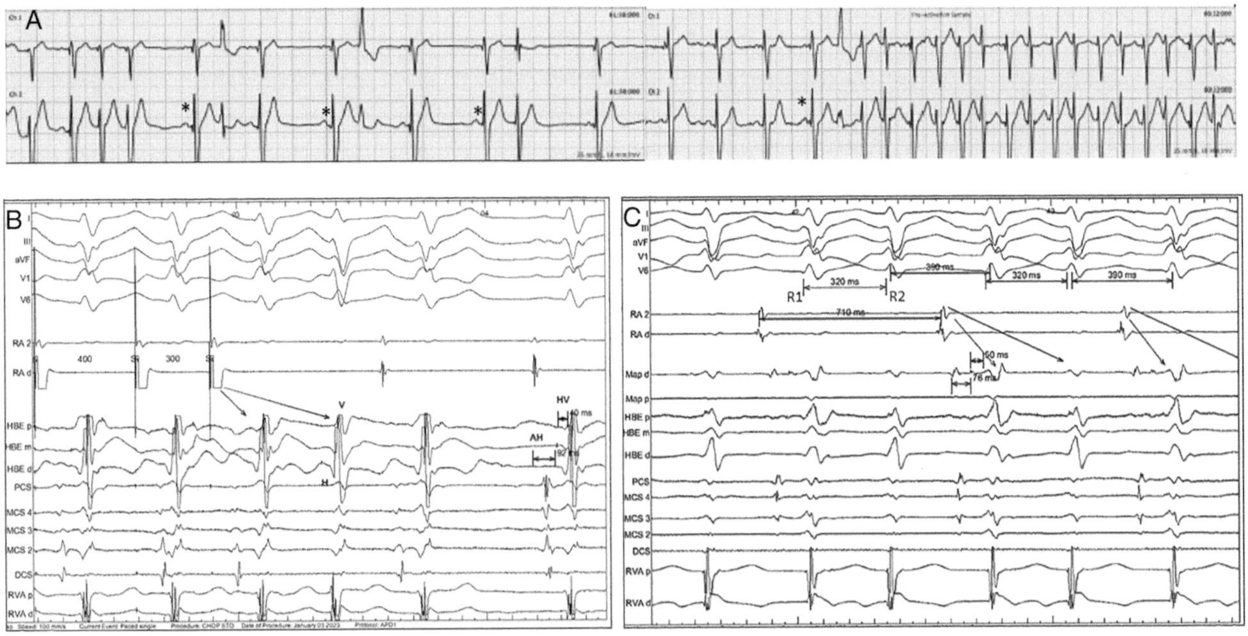

Fig. 44.6 (A) Ambulatory monitoring in a 16-year-old boy with palpitations shows salvos of irregular tachycardia interrupted by frequent "ectopic beats." Electrophysiology study confirmed ventricular "double fire" following a single sinus node activity. One P wave (*) is followed by two QRS complexes (BBB in second QRS on several beats) due to consecutive antegrade conduction via fast and slow pathways from the AV node. (B) Programmed atrial extrastimulus (400/300 ms) initiates a "two-for-one" response without an AH jump. (C) Dual AV node nonreentrant tachycardia with fixed cycle length between the two QRS complexes (R1-R2: 320 ms).

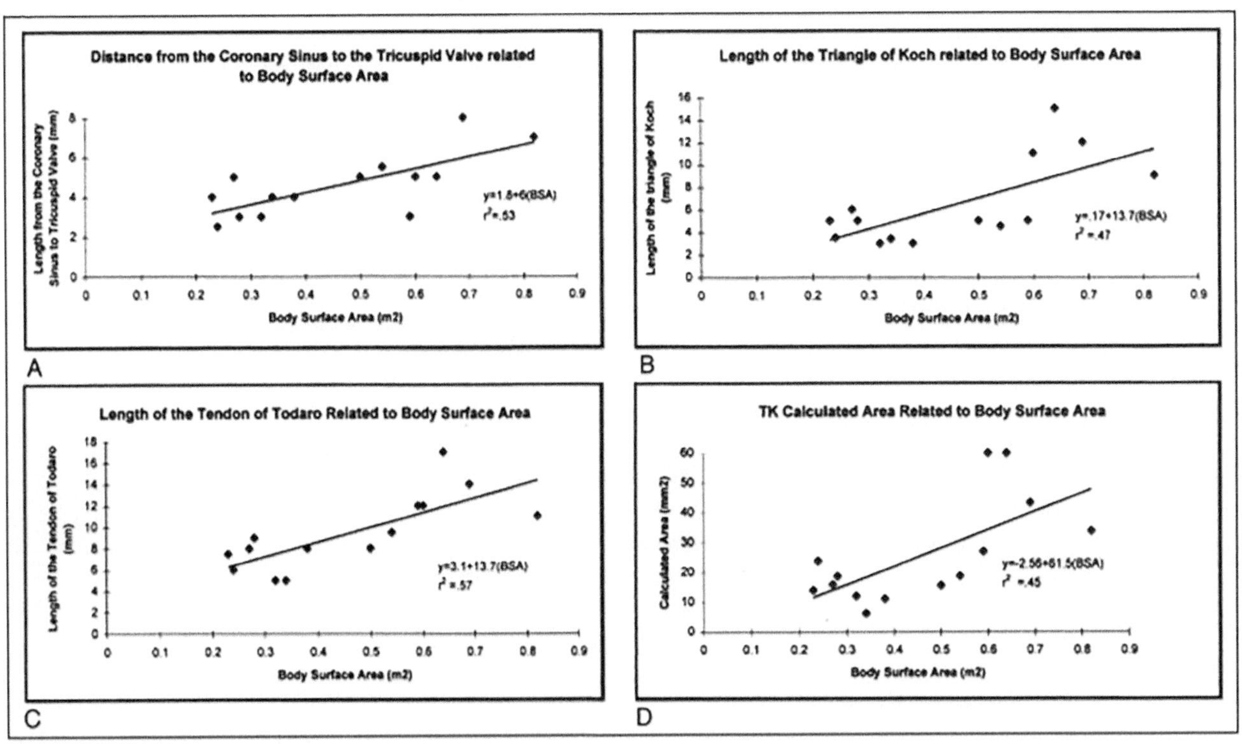

Fig. 44.7 The relation of the dimensions of the Koch triangle to subject weight. The distance from the coronary sinus to the tricuspid valve (A), the length of the Koch triangle (the distance from the coronary sinus to the central fibrous body) (B), the length of the tendon of Todaro (C), and the calculated area of Koch triangle (D) are plotted against subject weight. The corresponding simple regression line and equation are included on each plot. (From Goldberg CS, Caplan MJ, Heidelberger KP, Dick MM. The dimensions of the triangle of Koch in children. *Am J Cardiol.* 1999;83(1):117–120.)

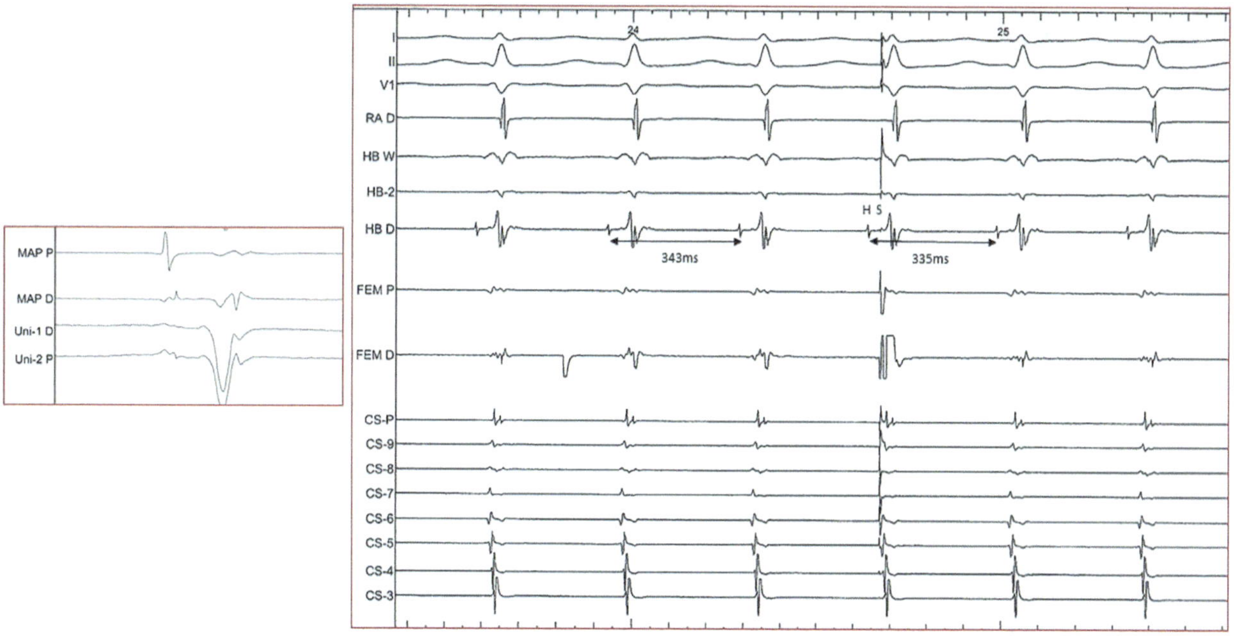

Fig. 44.8 (A) Map catheter in the inferior triangle of Koch with "dome and spike" appearance of slow pathway potential, Asp during sinus rhythm (B). Three standard ECG leads (I, III, V_1), eight-channel recording from the CS, three-channel recording from the His bundle, and single-channel recording from the high right atrium are displayed. Example of resetting response during slow-fast atrioventricular nodal reentrant tachycardia. Premature atrial stimulus delivered close to the rightward inferior slow-pathway extension, 45 ms after the His Bundle potential advances the next His Bundle potential by 8 ms.

most likely to interrupt the SP input. It is especially helpful in refining the target when AVNRT remains inducible after initial attempts at ablating the rightward inferior SP or in cases referred after failed ablation of the rightward inferior SP where other anatomical sites of SP input must be explored.[94] Low-voltage bridge (LVB) mapping combines the anatomical map with voltage data assessing for low-amplitude signal (antegrade SP signal) and allows a visual representation of the SP inputs.[95–100] Not all patients present a characteristic low-voltage target. Propagation mapping, when used in conjunction with voltage mapping, has been proposed to further improve the localization of the SP. A propagation map from the prior voltage map is evaluated, marking a "wave collision" at the site of wavefront convergence in KT (Fig. 44.9A–D and Video 44.1),[98,99] The LVB strategy to guide ablation has been described in children with good short-term and medium-term outcomes, with lower fluoroscopy and procedural times,[97–102] but sole reliance on this type of mapping strategy without electrophysiology correlation may lead to misinterpretation as 3D maps are highly dependent on point density, selection of voltage thresholds, and subjective interpretation. In particular, the successful ablation site using this technique is often on or slightly superior (toward the AV node) in location compared with the propagation wave collision point.[99] Thus, it may be safer to use cryoablation when using this mapping technique for SP ablation. However, the technique may be limited when dealing with atypical AVNRT or SP targets other than the rightward inferior SP. It should be noted that the "old school" approach of a combined anatomical and electrogram (EGM)-guided RF ablation continues to be practiced in the current era in many pediatric centers with excellent outcomes regarding safety and long-term success.[91,101–103]

Unique Considerations for Pediatric/CHD AVNRT Ablation

While the approach to mapping and ablation of AVNRT target SPs is quite similar in both adults and children with structurally normal hearts, the ablation of AVNRT in patients with CHD warrants special mention due to its unique aspects.[68,69,93,105] In general, AVNRT ablation in complex CHD has lower success rates (82%), higher recurrence rates (20%), higher complication rates (14%), and higher procedural and fluoroscopic times.[93] Atypical AVNRT is seen in up to 36% of AVNRT in CHD.[93] There are numerous challenges to the usual assumptions made in AVNRT ablation in a normal heart. The compact AV node itself may be displaced, sometimes predictably so (e.g., inferior displacement in AV canal defects; Fig. 44.10), but sometimes in a manner that is harder to predict (e.g., heterotaxy syndromes).[69] In some cases, there may even be twin AV nodes (described later in this chapter).[105] The inferior KT may be distorted from its normal arrangement, naturally due to the underlying lesion (e.g., tricuspid atresia) or unnaturally secondary to surgical intervention in the area (e.g., tricuspid annuloplasty rendering some portion of electrically active tissue inaccessible). A detailed understanding of the patient's underlying anatomy and subsequent interventional and surgical history is critical. Additional imaging that may be incorporated into the 3D electroanatomical map (CT, MRI) may provide better understanding. Real-time visualization of the region of interest with intracardiac echo can be valuable. Steerable sheaths and remote magnetic navigation (where available) are important

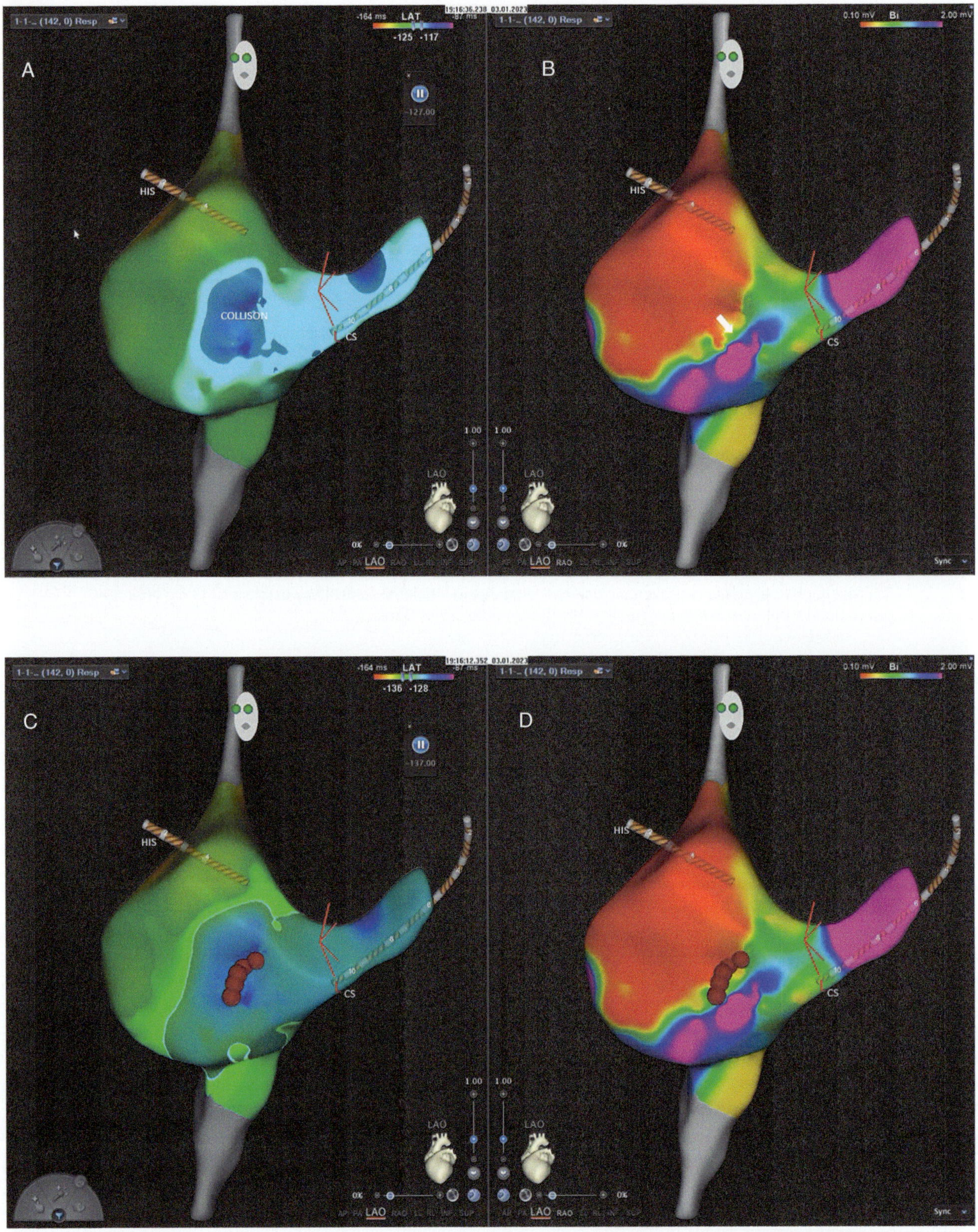

Fig. 44.9 An example of an LAO view of the atrial septum obtained in a patient with typical atrioventricular nodal reentrant tachycardia displaying a propagation map (Video 44.1, A) and a voltage map (B) acquired using the CARTO 3 system (Biosense Webster Inc., Diamond Bar, CA). The His-bundle markers ("His") and the CS are designated. The wavefront collision is seen in KT and marked by the "COLLISION" label. In the voltage map on the *right*, the *red area* on the atrial surface represents a voltage <0.1 mV correlating with the TV annulus, with the color gradient changing to *purple* with voltages >2.0 mV toward the CS. *Intermediate colors* represent voltage data between the low-voltage and the high-voltage values. The low-voltage bridge is depicted by the *arrow* (B). RF lesions (*red dots*) applied in sinus rhythm are superimposed on the previous propagation (C) and voltage maps to depict site of successful slow pathway ablation guided by a low-voltage bridge (D).

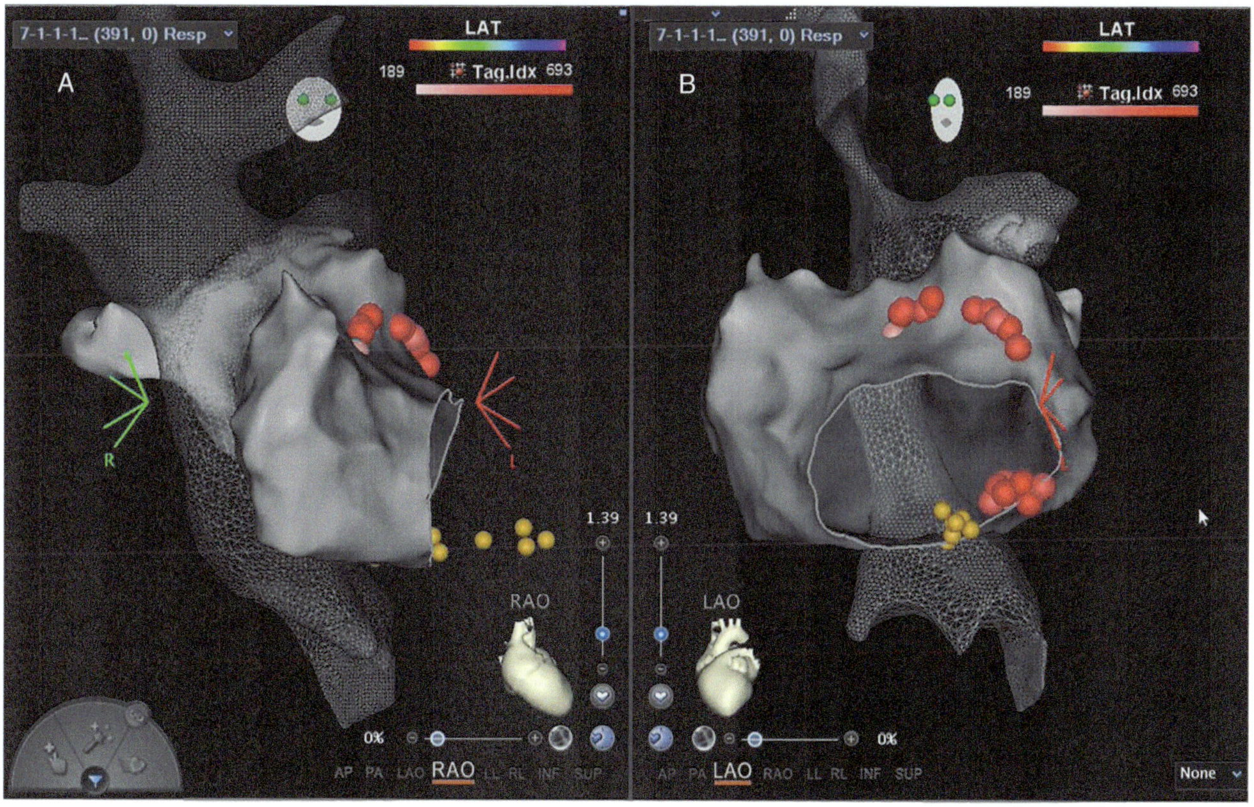

Fig. 44.10 CARTO 3D anatomical map with 3D CTA overlay of patient with right unbalanced complete common AV canal defect, status post Fontan palliation who underwent EP study for atypical atrioventricular nodal reentrant tachycardia with multiple slow pathways. *Gold tags* represent the inferiorly displaced His bundle. RF lesion tags (*red*) placed along multiple slow-pathway inputs forming retrograde limbs of tachycardia.

considerations from a technical standpoint to achieve adequate tissue contact. The position of the compact AV node must be estimated by combining anatomical information with identified His-bundle potentials to provide an electroanatomical outline. In our practice, once AVNRT is confirmed as the mechanism of tachycardia, we will map out SP potentials (in sinus rhythm), performing resetting maneuvers to get as close to the culprit antegrade SP as possible (Fig. 44.8). If the SP is the retrograde limb, we map the retrograde activation.

Choice of Ablation Energy and Relation to Outcomes

Traditionally the choice between cryoenergy and RF has involved balancing safety and efficacy. In adult series, metanalyses have yielded a similar acute success rate, but a higher late recurrence rate with cryoablation, even when accounting for cryocatheter tip size.[102] RF ablation is more commonly associate with AV block, as high as 0.75% in some analyses.[92,104] In the pediatric context, large single-center series demonstrate excellent acute success rates (98% to 99%) and low medium-term recurrence rates with RF ablation of AVNRT with a risk of AV block approaching zero.[91,103,104] Cryoablation also has a similarly high acute success rate with no significant risk of AV block.[91,103] With cryoablation, failure of focal ablation and need for lengthier and high-density linear ablation are associated with higher recurrence rates, though this may represent a limitation of the technique when the substrate may be distinct from the typical rightward inferior extension.[106–108] Interestingly, younger age of ablation appears to correlate with a lower recurrence rate, although longer follow-up assessment will be important.[109,110] Based on the success and safety of cryoablation in the treatment of pediatric AVNRT, the U.S. Food and Drug Administration recently approved cardiac cryoablation focal catheters (Freezor and Freezor Xtra, Medtronic Inc. Minneapolis, MN), the first and only ablation catheters approved for pediatric use in the current era.

Energy Delivery and Slow Pathway Ablation Endpoints

Special attention is given to the stability of intracardiac EP catheters, and His-bundle recording is mandatory during energy delivery. Standard RF settings used for adult AVNRT ablations are used for pediatric AVNRT ablation, but SP ablation can be performed successfully with a low incidence of recurrence using low energy and temperature.[111] Also, repeated short-duration (15–20 seconds) RF applications are sometimes applied instead of a continuous 60-second lesion at the site of accelerated junctional rhythm (AJR). When AJR develops, VA conduction is carefully monitored to ensure there is no injury to the FP. In some cases, overdrive atrial pacing is performed at CL 10% to 15% faster than the rate of AJR to monitor for stable antegrade AV node conduction. AJR during RF and lack of inducibility of AVNRT following RFA even with isoproterenol infusion are considered markers of RFA success, as opposed to presence or absence of SP conduction and single echo beats. In patients with continuous AV node conduction curves prior to ablation, nonindicibility of AVNRT with either elimination of sustained SP conduction or shortening of the FPERP after ablation is an acceptable end point.[81–83] The latter supports the hypothesis of removal of electrotonic inhibition on the FP after successful SP modification or complete ablation.

The cryoablation technique involves identifying the SP target in the usual fashion as with RF during sinus rhythm. AJR is usually not seen with cryoablation and therefore cannot guide lesion delivery. Cryoablation is performed during sinus rhythm in patients with clear-cut dual AV node physiology. It may need to be performed during SVT in patients with continuous antegrade dual AVN conduction curves or in patients with atypical AVNRT when mapping earliest retrograde atrial activation is necessary. Note that the successful site for cryoablation of the SP is usually found in the mid-septal region of KT, which is superior to the usual successful site for RF ablation. The risk of catheter dislodgement at time of SVT termination is low due to cryoadhesion. Cryoablation lesions are placed reaching −75°C to −80°C. When ablating in sinus rhythm, atrial extrastimulus testing to evaluate for SP conduction is performed 45–60 seconds after initiation of cryoablation. If there is no termination of SP conduction, the lesion is stopped, and further mapping is pursued for a new location. If the SP is eliminated (or modified), a single 4-minute lesion is applied at that location before moving to a new site. If the disappearance of SP conduction is noted, the patient undergoes a "freeze–thaw–freeze" lesion set consisting of a 4-minute lesion, a 30-second warmup, and a second 4-minute lesion. Further "insurance" lesions are placed at the discretion of the operator. The PR interval is monitored throughout the period when cryoenergy is delivered and the lesion is interrupted promptly if any lengthening is observed. The majority of pediatric centers use a 6-mm-tip cryocatheter, but if success cannot be achieved, operators will use an 8-mm-tip cryocatheter[107] or crossover to RF. The procedural endp oint of cryoablation has traditionally been complete elimination of SP conduction because when the same end point as RFA was used—a maximum of single AV nodal echo beat, the recurrence rate for cryoablation was more than double as that seen with RFA.[104] Collins et al. suggested reduction in SSPC and decrease in maximal AH interval with A1A2 pacing or atrial overdrive pacing as markers for successful SP cryoablation in children.[90] Prolongation of the FPERP period during cryoablation with shortening of FPERP after termination of lesion has also been cited as a marker for SP modification.[112] Recent data show that similar to successful RFA of SP, presence of residual SP conduction with single echo beat after multiple cryolesions is not associated with recurrence when there is noninducible SVT.[113]

Risk of AV Block

The possibility of ablation-induced complete heart block deserves special attention in the pediatric patient for two reasons. First, the risk of heart block is theoretically higher in smaller patients, simply because of a number of geometric differences.[88] Despite these potential problems, the reported incidence of ablation-induced complete heart block does not appear to be significantly higher in infants and children than in adults.[91,105] However, should AV block occur, the consequences of permanent pacing in a young child are far more grave than in an adult, involving technical factors of pacemaker implantation with epicardial lead placement, multiple pacemaker and lead revisions over a lifespan, decades of a ventricular paced rhythm with potential hemodynamic impairment, and alternations in quality of life. These issues should affect both the decision to ablate and the energy choice when ablating near the normal AV conduction system. To date, there are still no reported cases in the literature of permanent AV block with the use of cryoablation; however, a theoretical risk still exists. Regardless of the technique(s) used to map the SP, great care must be taken to avoid ablating progressively higher in the KT when initial lesions fail to terminate inducible AVNRT. As a rule, we avoid RFA any higher than the superior margin of the CSO, as this is associated with an increased risk of AV block.

Coronary Artery Injury—General Considerations for Atrioventricular Nodal Reentrant Tachycardia and Accessory Pathway Ablation

Acute and late coronary artery injury has been reported after RF ablation for AP-mediated tachycardias in children, adults, and animals.[11–13,32,114] These cases have involved both left- and right-sided coronary arteries, as well as a posterior descending branch of the right coronary artery during ablation of a right posteroseptal AP.[11,12] Blaufox et al. reported a case of coronary damage involving the posterior left ventricular branch coming off a right dominant coronary system, during SP modification in a 30-month-old 15.5-kg child with AVNRT. ST elevation in the inferior leads was noted minutes after RF application, managed conservatively and documented to have resolved at 2-month follow-up angiography.[12] We also observed a 16-year-old 80-kg female who developed inferior ST elevation within moments of an RF application at the inferior CSO. ST changes resolved within 15 minutes; angiography confirmed occlusion of a left posterior branch arising from the right dominant coronary system, which was successfully ballooned within 20 minutes of onset. The patient subsequently has had a reassuring clinical course with normal ECG, normal stress test, and no residual SVT (Fig. 44.11).

These cases illustrate that coronary artery injury may occur with SP ablation for AVNRT and has the potential to be missed. Infants and young children may be at particular risk. The inflammatory component of tissue injury caused by RF energy has been shown to invade layers of the right coronary artery, leading to acute narrowing, when RF energy is applied to the atrial side of the lateral tricuspid annulus in pigs.[14,32] Further maturation of this injury can result in significant late coronary stenosis.[14] The reported incidences of coronary injury after RF ablation were 0.03% in children and 0.06% in adults.[4] However, in a study in which coronary angiography was performed before and after RF ablation for AP-mediated tachycardias, there was a 1.3% reported incidence of coronary artery injury.[115–117] Therefore, unless evidence for coronary artery injury is actively sought, it will go undiagnosed and underreported. Understanding these factors is critical to preventing injury.

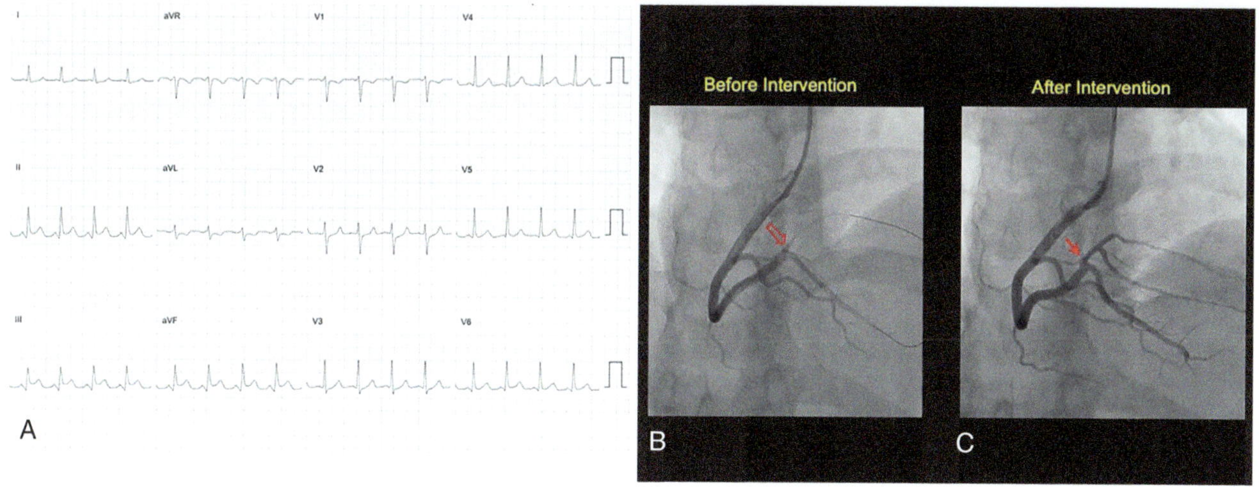

Fig. 44.11 ECG (A) shows ST-elevation inferior leads within moments of an RF application at the inferior CSO. Selective right coronary arteriogram (B) confirmed occlusion of a left posterior branch arising from the right dominant coronary system, which was successfully treated with angioplasty (C).

Summary and Recommendations

Specific precautions when ablating AVNRT in children are shown in Table 44.2. It is recommended that cryotherapy be considered as first choice for ablation in children <15 kg. Selective coronary arteriography should be considered when performing RFA in the posteroseptal region, especially in children <15 kg. In the presence of CHD, a detailed understanding of the individual anatomy and conduction system variations is key to performing a safe and successful ablation.

Accessory Pathways in the Pediatric Population

AV reentrant tachycardia (AVRT) involving an AP is the most common form of tachyarrhythmia seen in children and accounts for the largest percentage of catheter ablation procedures performed at pediatric centers.[3,4,18,23,24,118,119] AVRT may manifest as early as fetal life, but the frequency peaks during the first year of life and early adolescence. Most patients present with orthodromic reciprocating tachycardia (ORT). Antidromic reentrant tachycardia is a rare occurrence in children with WPW. Preexcited AF with rapid anterograde conduction over the AP is the most concerning presentation at any age (Fig. 44.12).[23,120–123] Although the reported risk of SCD in WPW is numerically low, data strongly suggest that the incidence of life-threatening events in asymptomatic children with WPW may be much higher than in adults.[122–124] With emerging studies contradicting data from an older era that loss of AP conduction with noninvasive testing can identify WPW patients at a low risk of a cardiac event, the threshold for catheter ablation in patients with WPW is lower in current clinical practice.[91,125,126] AP ablation in contemporary pediatric studies demonstrates high rates of acute success (92% to 97%) and low rates of complications (Table 44.3).[3,4,118,119] Recurrence rates are less well-defined but range from 7% to 12% in the present era.

TABLE 44.2 Precautions for Ablation of Atrioventricular Nodal Reentry Tachycardia in Children
• Cryoablation is the safest energy modality for children weighing <15 kg. • When the CS is cannulated via the femoral vein, it is oriented to the roof of the CS (i.e., near the superior margin of the CSO and closer to the AV node). Ablation at any point higher may be associated with a higher risk of AV block. • Before RFA especially in children weighing <15 kg, selective coronary angiography of the coronary artery supplying the posterior septum should be considered. If a coronary artery branch is <2–3 mm from an RFA site, delivery of RF energy should be used with caution and postablation coronary angiography should be considered.

Mapping and Ablation of Accessory Pathways

In general, mapping of APs in children follows similar principles as that in adults, but some differences are worth noting. In younger children, one of the technical difficulties is inserting multiple intracardiac diagnostic EP catheters due to the small caliber of venous structures. A few alternative solutions include replacing the high right atrium catheter with a transesophageal bipolar or multipolar electrode that is connected to the EP recording system (Fig. 44.13). A single multipolar catheter can be used to record the right ventricular EGM from distal poles and the His-bundle EGM from proximal poles. Children have robust anterograde and retrograde AV nodal conduction which can create challenges in concealed AP mapping due to fusion and inability to isolate AP conduction.[110] This is commonly observed in the setting of septal APs but has also been described in children with concealed left-sided AP. In this latter scenario, when mapping in SVT is not an option, pacing from the LV can unmask eccentric VA conduction and facilitate mapping.[127] An additional method to isolate AP conduction from fusion with AV node conduction is intravenous

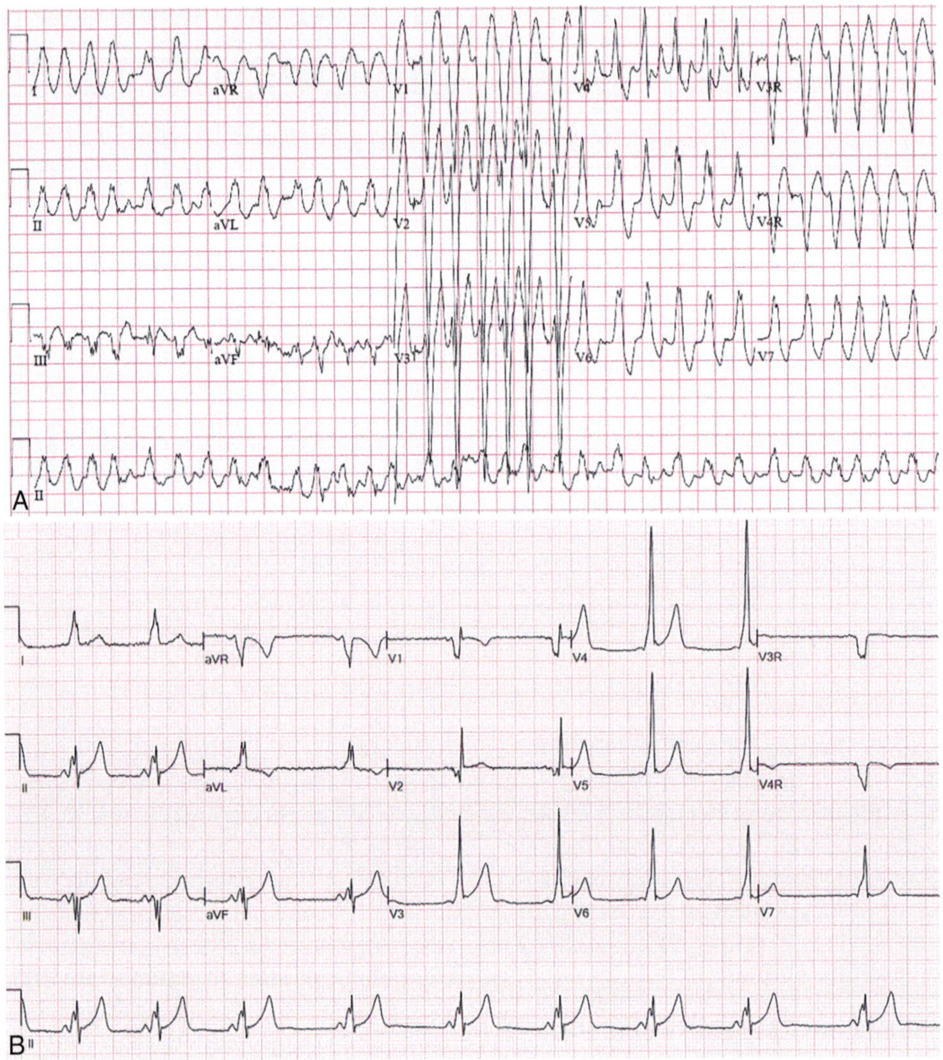

Fig. 44.12 (A) ECG shows a wide-complex irregular rhythm in a 15-year-old with palpitations and syncope suggesting preexcited atrial fibrillation. (B) Post DC cardioversion, the ECG shows WPW with QRS morphology similar to the preexcited atrial fibrillation. A right midseptal AP was successfully ablated.

TABLE 44.3 Summary of Outcomes of Pediatric Ablation Registries

Study	Era	Number of Cases	Acute success	Recurrence	Complications
NICOR; Walsh et al., 2021[118]	1999–2018	Total N = 7069 (n = 4187 AP)	92% (all AP)	2% repeat AP ablation	0.1% AV block for APs
EUROPA; Krause at al., 2020[119]	2012–2017	Total N = 683 (n = 380 AP)	94% (all AP)	7% AP (follow-up: 1 year)	0.7% major complications 0% AV block requiring pacemaker
MAP-IT; Dubin et al., 2019[81]	2014–2016	Total N = 948* (n = 669 AP)	96% (all AP) 97% cAP 95% WPW	7% cAP 7% WPW (follow-up: 10 ± 5 months)	2.5% 0.1% AV block requiring pacemaker
PAPCA; van Hare et al., 2004[3]	1999–2003	Total n = 2761	94% (all AP) 96% cAP 93% WPW	15% cAP 11% WPW (follow-up: 1 year)	4% overall cohort 3% AV block for septal APs
PCAR; Kugler et al., 1997[4]	1991–1996	Total n = 3653	90% (all AP)	23% AP (follow-up: 3 years)	3.2% overall cohort 0.7% AV block

*Atrioventricular nodal reentrant tachycardia or atrioventricular reentrant tachycardia; no congenital heart disease.

AP, Accessory pathway; *AV*, atrioventricular; *cAP*, concealed accessory pathway; *WPW*, Wolff-Parkinson-White syndrome.

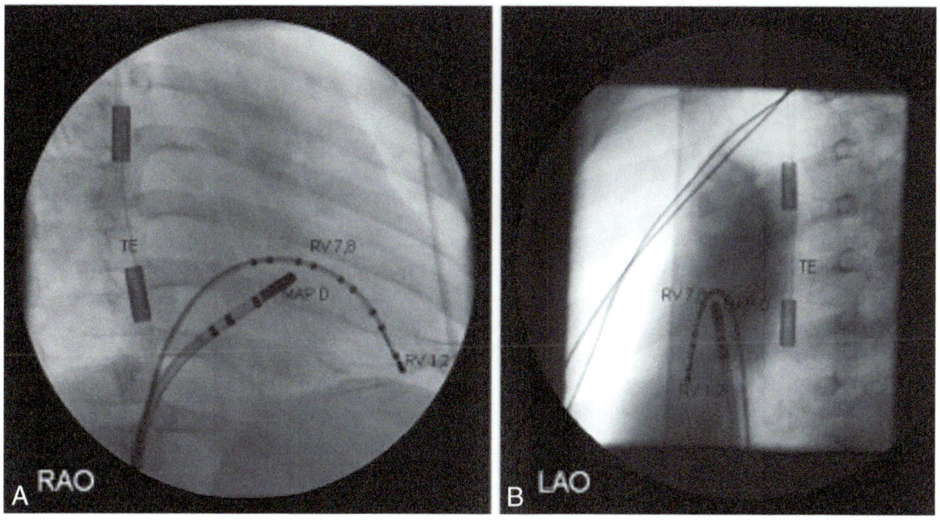

Fig. 44.13 Example of catheter ablation with two intracardiac catheters. AP (A) and lateral (PA) fluoroscopic views in a 9-month-old (7-kg) child with junctional ectopic tachycardia. To reduce number of intracardiac and intravascular catheters in a small child, a bipolar transesophageal (TE) catheter was used to pace and record EGMs from the left atrium, and a 4-F decapolar catheter was placed from the left femoral vein in the RV to record His-bundle EGMs (RV 7,8) and to pace and record EGMs from RV (RV 1,2). The cryoablation catheter (7 F) is placed from the right femoral vein. A 4-F decapolar CS catheter (not shown) is usually placed from the right internal jugular vein.

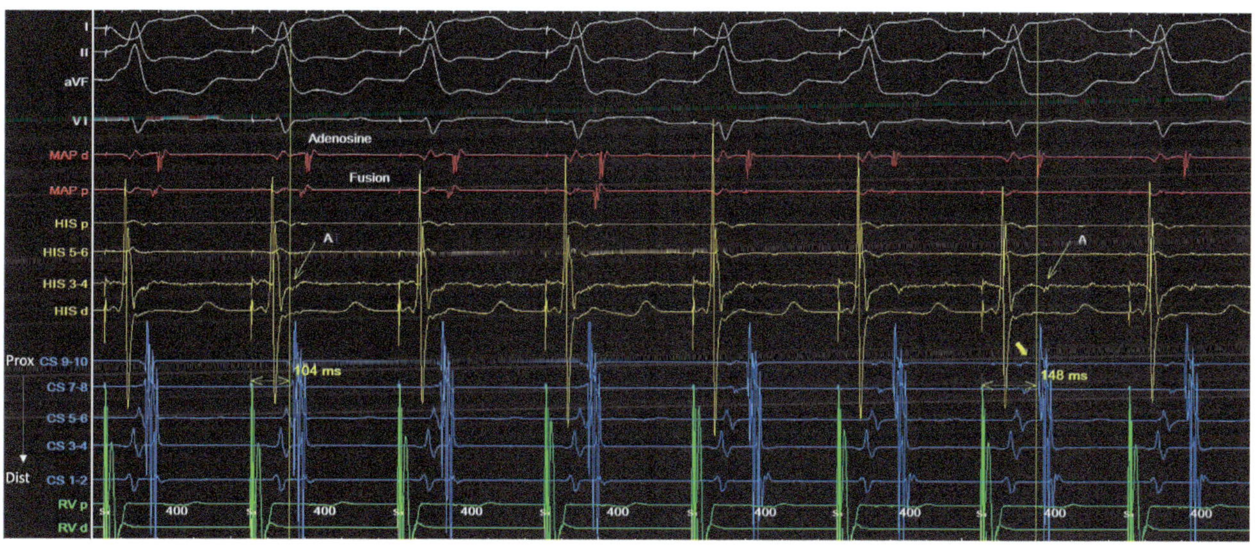

Fig. 44.14 Intravenous adenosine administered during ventricular pacing in a patient with a right posteroseptal AP. During the first four beats, retrograde atrial activation is fused between the AV node and AP. Following AV block with adenosine, the proximal CS (9-10) shows earliest atrial activation (*solid arrow*).

adenosine administration (Fig. 44.14). Adenosine prolongs conduction in the AV node, causes AV block transiently, and shortens AP refractoriness.[128] We typically administer intravenous adenosine prior to AP ablation in sinus rhythm to look for dormant preexcitation as well with ventricular pacing to eliminate AP fusion with AV node conduction. Administration of intravenous adenosine is then repeated at intervals during the postablation "waiting period" to identify early AP recurrence.[129] When there is a reversible injury to the AP as in the perilesional zone of RFA, the AP is partially depolarized, making it unexcitable, and refractory to impulse conduction. Adenosine by causing membrane hyperpolarization makes the pathway reexcitable and thereby unmasks dormant AP conduction.[128–130] Administering adenosine only postcatheter ablation is insufficient proof of ablation success as a fraction of AP with decremental and nondecremental conduction are adenosine sensitive in children.[131]

Another challenge is identification of AP potentials in children. There is considerable literature in adults on the importance of targeting AP potentials, but in our experience a discrete AP potential (separate from atrial and ventricular EGMs) is less commonly identified at the site of ablation success in children; rather, it is more likely buried within a fractionated continuous signal.[132] Whether this difference relates to heart

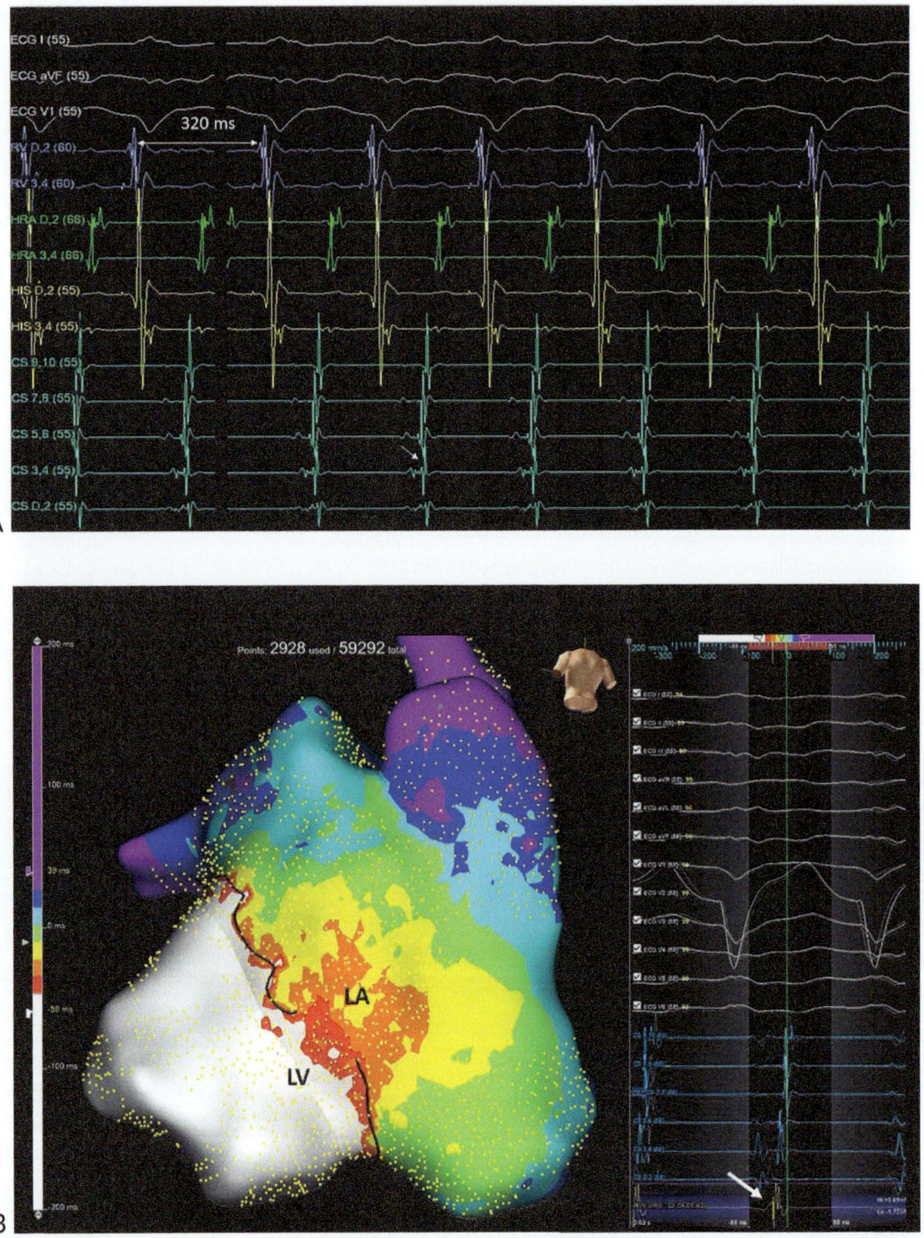

Fig. 44.15 (A) Wide- complex SVT (CL 320 ms) with LBBB morphology with eccentric retrograde atrial activation and earliest activation in CS 3,4 (*arrow*). V-A-H-V response to ventricular overdrive pacing with PPI-TCL <115 ms and SVT termination with His synchronous PVCs confirmed orthodromic SVT with concealed left-sided AP. (B) Localization of left free wall AP was performed using Advisor HD Grid Sensor Enabled mapping catheter (Abbott Inc.). Isochronal activation maps obtained by open window mapping show retrograde conduction over a left free wall AP during SVT (Video 44.2). *Black lines* denote block of conduction across the mitral valve annulus. Activation breakout into the left atrium occurred at site of AP insertion (*white circle*). Ablation at the white circle eliminated AP conduction within 3 seconds. At the site of successful ablation, the ablation catheter demonstrated fused ventricular and atrial signals that were qualitatively similar to the signal recorded by the HD Grid catheter (*arrow*). *LA*, Left atrium; *LV*, left ventricle.

size, age-related tissue conduction velocity, other age-related differences in AP physiology or our failure to appreciate the AP potential in a small heart despite differential pacing techniques is not clear. Multiple APs are seen in 3% to 13% of children undergoing ablation.[132–135] When multiple APs are close to each other, it may be difficult to distinguish between an oblique pathway, discrete pathways, or a single pathway with multiple insertions.[135] In the current era, nearly all pediatric centers use 3D electroanatomical mapping (EAM) with either zero or minimal fluoroscopy for catheter ablation in North America, which has been demonstrated to increase the success rate of pediatric AP ablation, compared to fluoroscopy alone.[136] Multipolar mapping catheters have been used to perform high-density mapping along the annulus, and the open-window mapping (OWM) technique can identify a site of breakout activation across the annulus, representative of AP insertion (Fig. 44.15A, B and

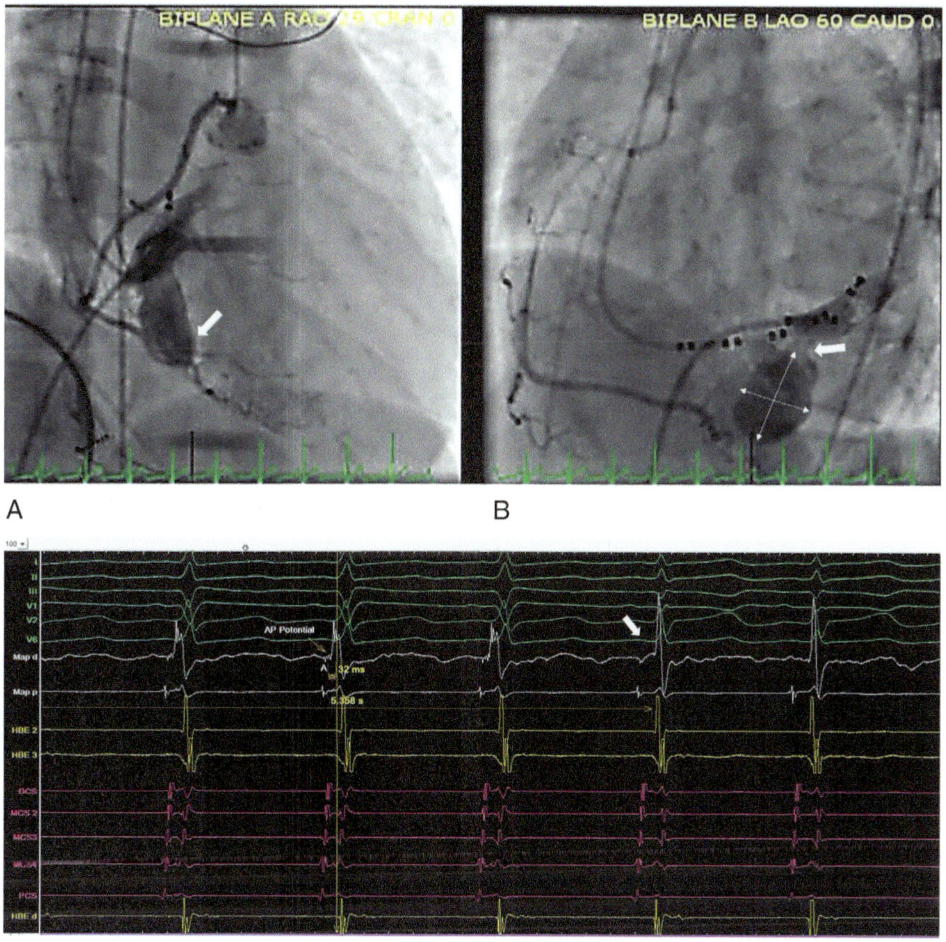

A B C

Fig. 44.16 A 15 year-old patient with WPW and SVT with two prior failed ablations. During the third procedure, a simultaneous injection of contrast in the coronary sinus with selective right coronary angiogram in the RAO (A) and LAO (B) views showed a large diverticulum measuring 14 mm × 10 mm. The posterolateral branch of RCA was close to the base of the diverticulum. The AP was successfully ablated in the neck of the diverticulum (*arrow*) using an irrigated-tip catheter with a power of 35 W. The CS was cannulated with a decapolar 2-5-2 catheter from the right internal jugular vein. (C) Intracardiac electrograms in preexcited sinus rhythm during RF ablation in the neck of the diverticulum (Fig. 44.14B). Six standard ECG leads, five-channel recording from a decapolar catheter in the coronary sinus (distal to proximal), and three-channel recording from the His bundle (HBE) are displayed. There is an AP potential on both the distal and proximal electrodes of the Map catheter at the site of successful ablation with ventricular activation preceding the surface ECG delta wave by 32 ms. RFA successfully eliminated AP in 5.3 seconds (*solid arrow*).

Videos 44.2, 44.3, and 44.4). Specifically, the OWM technique uses a high-density mapping (Advisor HD Grid Sensor Enabled catheter, Abbott Inc.) and includes both atrial and ventricular signals in the same window of interest, with computer annotation of the local signal demonstrating the steepest slope (i.e., maximal dV/dt).[137] When there is failure to identify AP using available mapping techniques, one must consider the possibility of APs in unusual locations such as aortomitral continuity, coronary cusps, left anteroseptal area under the aortic cusp, atrial appendage (AA), and epicardial area related to the CS myocardial extension over the middle and posterior cardiac veins.[138–142] Posteroseptal epicardial APs may occur in association with a CS diverticulum, which can be identified by direct coronary sinus angiography (Fig. 44.16A–C).[142,143]

Several pediatric centers favor cryoablation over RFA for all AP ablation procedures. Some pediatric centers perform cryoablation for right-sided APs and others predominantly use RFA while reserving cryoablation for APs in proximity to the conduction system.[46,47,144–146] Poor electrode–tissue contact seems to be the main source of ablation failure of AP. A catheter inversion technique to achieve deflection of the tip to a parallel orientation to the septum under the hinge of the TV is useful for para-Hisian APs.[144] If ablation is performed during AVRT, RV pacing is performed at similar cycle length (or 10 ms faster) to prevent catheter dislodgement from ablation site should AVRT terminate with ablation. This is not an issue with cryoablation due to cryoadhesion. The use of long sheaths has helped mitigate this problem to some degree, but the sheath needs to be

TABLE 44.4 **Tips for Pediatric Accessory Pathway Ablation by Anatomical Location**

AP Site	Approach	Tips and Tools	Risks//Precautions	Recent Pediatric Data
Anteroseptal	• Inferior: RFV • Superior: RIJV • Retrograde in aortic cusp (NCC)	• Cryoablation • "Breath holds" or ↓ tidal volume during ventilation to ↓ diaphragmatic excursion • ABL curved underneath the TV septal leaflet and back towards the TVA for direct AP contact • Consider long sheath for catheter stability (e.g., Swartz SR1, Abbott Inc. MN). • Map AP in SVT to isolate AP conduction. • Target ventricular insertion to minimize injury to compact AV node (larger VEGM on ABL)	• AV block • Susceptible to mechanical trauma (AP bump)	• Acute success: 83–89%[3,4,47,57,67,91,146] Recurrence: 18%[146]
Midseptal	• Inferior: RFV	• Cryoablation • Map AP in SVT to isolate AP conduction • Target ventricular insertion to minimize injury to compact AV node (larger VEGM on ABL)	• AV block	• Acute success: 73–83%[3,4,67,91,146] Recurrence: 19%[146]
Posteroseptal	• Inferior: RFV • Map RPS and LPS • Consider Map in CSO/CS branches	• Consider CS angiogram for coronary venous anatomy and to evaluate for diverticulum • Consider CAG for proximity to CA • Low-power RF (irrigated or nonirrigated) in CS • Consider cryoablation within CS	• Perforation • Coagulum formation • Coronary artery injury	• Acute success: 94%[3,4,67,91.140]
Right free wall	• Inferior: RFV • Superior: RIJV for right anterior, anterolateral AP	• "Breath holds" or ↓ tidal volume during ventilation to ↓ diaphragmatic excursion • Consider fixed and steerable long sheaths for catheter stability (e.g., Swartz SR1, SR 2, SR3, Agilis NxT Steerable Introducer Sheath, Abbott Inc., Destino steerable sheaths, Oscor, Germany)	• Coronary artery injury	• Acute success: 89–96%[3,4,20,67,174–176] • Recurrence 5%[91]
Left free wall	• Transseptal • Retrograde CS	• Microelectrode fixed multipolar catheter that can be advanced to GCV, AIV (e.g., EPstar 6F decaploar with lumen and 2-F octapolar, Baylis Medical, Inc) • For aneurysmal or fibrotic atrial septum • NRG RF Transseptal Needle, or VersaCross RF transseptal wire, (Baylis Medical Inc.)	• Perforation • Thromboembolism	• Acute success: 96–99%[3,46,7,91] • Recurrence 7%[91]
"Off the AV annulus" AP	• For EPI AP, consider: percutaneous API ablation[149,315] • Surgical ablation (e.g., AA-AP)	• Map ipsilateral atrial appendage for right and left atrial appendage-ventricular APs • Map aortic cusps for anteroseptal APs • Map MCV, GCV, VoM, AIV for APs involving CS-ventricular connections • Low-power irrigated RF in CS branches • Angiogram to visualize CS diverticulum • CAG for proximity of ablation site to CA	• Perforation of tip of AA • CA occlusion/injury	—

AA, Atrial appendage; *AIV*, anterior interventricuar vein; *AP*, accessory pathways; *AV*, atrioventricular; *CA*, coronary artery; *CAG*, coronary arteriogram; *CS*, coronary sinus; *CSO*, coronary sinus ostium; *f/up*, follow-up; *FV*, femoral vein; *GCV*, great cardiac vein; *MCV*, middle cardiac vein; *N*, number; *RIJ*, right jugular vein; *VEGM*, ventricular electrogram; *VoM*, vein of Marshall; *WPW*, Wolff-Parkinson-White syndrome.

manipulated to allow the ablation catheter tip to be positioned in parallel with the AV valve. There is significant experience and research on the use of contact force (CF) irrigated-tip RF ablation catheters in adults, but its safety and efficacy for AP ablation in children have been reported in only a small series of patients.[147,148] It is also not known if a transmural lesion is required for successful AP ablation in children given that all current CF ablation catheters have an irrigated tip. A concrete protocol for use of CF in pediatrics still does not exist and there remains minimal evidence on the benefit of CF in ablation of pediatric APs. Rarely, the AP may have to be approached via an epicardial route.[149] Practical tips for pediatric AP ablation and contemporary outcomes by anatomical locale are listed in Table 44.4.

Accessory Pathways in Infants

There are three special considerations in infants that make management of symptoms secondary to an AP different from that in an older child or adult. First, the risk of a sustained reentrant primary AT, such as AF, is very close to zero in the small,

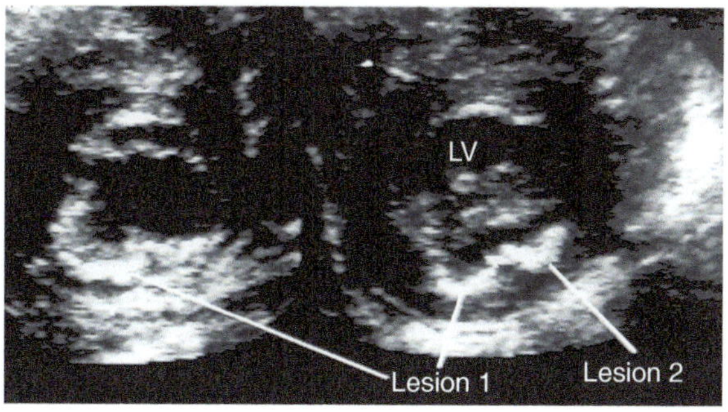

Fig. 44.17 Short-axis echocardiogram of an infant who died suddenly 2 weeks after an ablation procedure for two left-sided accessory pathways. Immediately after resuscitation, two large echo-dense regions were seen in the left ventricle (LV) despite radiofrequency applications being placed from an atrial approach. These echo-dense lesions correlated with the findings on postmortem examinations. (From Erickson CC, Walsh EP, Triedman JK, Saul JP. Efficacy and safety of radiofrequency ablation in infants and young children <18 months of age. *Am J Cardiol.* 1994;74:944–947.)

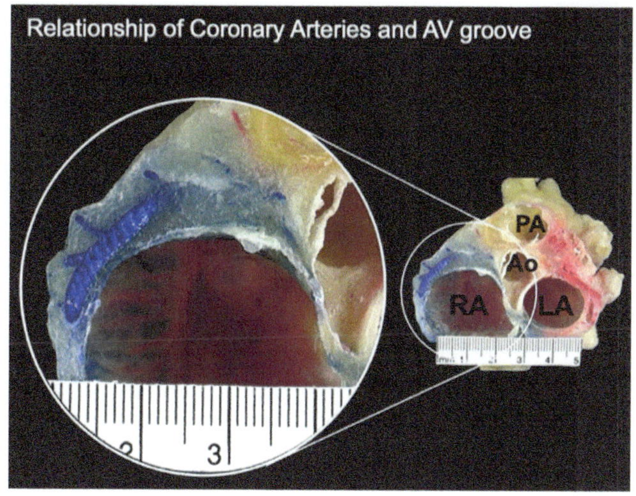

Fig. 44.18 Paraffin-preserved cross section on an infant heart at the level of the AV grooves showing the relationship of the right (*blue*) and left (*pink*) circumflex coronary arteries to the tricuspid and mitral valve annulus, respectively. Note the coronary arteries are <2 mm from the endocardial surface of the AV grooves. *Ao*, aorta; *LA*, left atrium; *PA*, pulmonary artery; *RA*, Right atrium.

structurally normal heart, making the risk of sudden death in infants with WPW very low.[18,24,150] Second, as noted earlier, AP function may spontaneously disappear by 1 year of age.[24,36] Finally, the known risks of any catheterization, combined with the specific risks of catheter ablation in this age group,[34,151–154] suggest that pharmacologic control should be aggressively pursued before ablation is attempted.

In humans, myocardial cell division probably occurs through approximately 6 months of age.[155] Although this finding could potentially protect the myocardium from long-term complications secondary to early injury, ventriculotomy scars produced in newborn puppies,[156] RF ablation lesions in immature lambs,[9] and cryoablation lesions in infant swine[50] appear to increase in size during subsequent development. In addition, in contrast to mature ablation scars from adult animals, late lesions from the neonatal lambs were often histologically invasive and poorly demarcated from the surrounding tissue.[9] The potential clinical importance of these results is underscored by a reported sudden death 2 weeks after an AP ablation in a 5-week-old, 3.2-kg infant.[157] An echocardiogram from the infant at the time of a brief resuscitation, as well as autopsy findings, revealed relatively large lesions extending into the left ventricle from the intended mitral groove ablation site (Fig. 44.17). Another heightened risk in infants is coronary artery damage because of the potentially close proximity of the coronaries to the ablation catheter and the reduced capacity for protective cooling during RF application in any small coronary artery (Fig. 44.18). Although most reports of coronary damage in the literature have been limited to the posterior septum or a nondominant right coronary artery,[13,14] complete occlusion of the left circumflex artery was reported in a 5-week-old, 5.0-kg infant undergoing RF ablation of a left lateral AP.[11]

Despite these disturbing cases, nonpharmacologic therapy will be necessary in a small subset of infants with AP-mediated tachycardia.[154,158] As discussed previously, cryotherapy may offer other advantages for small children. (1) It allows for reversible loss of tissue function.[159–161] (2) It is less harmful to coronary arteries, even when they are in very close contact,[50,162] because of the differing effects of cold and heat on connective tissue and the vascular inflammatory response. Coronary artery flow also protects the vessel through local warming during cryotherapy, similar to the way in which blood flow protects through local cooling during RF energy application. (3) Cryolesions are smaller than RF lesions, contributing to the ability to safely create cryolesions even adjacent to the His bundle.[163,164]

If technical or other considerations require the use of RF energy, considerable caution should be used. RF lesion size is related to catheter tip size, RF power, tip temperature, and lesion duration. Therefore, the following technical modifications should be adopted (Table 44.5). The development of real-time intracardiac echocardiography (ICE) is useful in monitoring catheter location and lesion size and may also help reduce some procedural risks, but the size (8 F to 9 F) of the ICE probe may limit its use in very small children.[165]

The 2016 Consensus Statement[1] provided multiple recommendations related to ablation in infants and small children. Most importantly, based on a variety of data, the document recommends an approximate cutoff of 15 kg to differentiate

TABLE 44.5 Precautions for Ablation of Accessory Atrioventricular Connections in Infants

Cryoablation is the preferred technique.

When radiofrequency (RF) ablation is necessary:

- Deliver energy as far on the atrial side as possible.
- Use a 5-F RF ablation catheter*
- Perform a test application with low-temperature RF delivery (50°C) before high-temperature delivery.
- Limit maximal target temperature to 60°C.
- Use short-duration RF delivery of 7–10 × time to effect with 30- to 40-second maximal delivery.

*Note: There is only one commercially available 5-F ablation catheter (Marinr, Medtronic Inc.).

TABLE 44.6 **Associations of Wolff-Parkinson-White Syndrome and Congenital Heart Disease***

Lesion	No. of Patients	No. of Patients With WPW	Prevalence (%)
Ebstein	234	21	8.97[a]
L-TGA	588	8	1.36[a]
HCM	300	3	1.00[a]
Pulmonary valve disease	424	2	0.47
Tricuspid atresia	458	2	0.44
VSD-membranous	2659	10	0.38
DORV	955	3	0.31
HLHS	666	2	0.30
MVP	1096	3	0.27
Dextrocardia	427	1	0.23
Trisomy 21	916	2	0.22
TOF-pulmonary atresia	556	1	0.18
TOF	2520	3	0.12
AV canal defect	2058	2	0.09
D-TGA (all)	2156	2	0.09
Coarctation	2862	1	0.04[a]
D-TGA/IVS	704	0	0.00
Mitral atresia	417	0	0.00
Total	20,303	66	0.33

AV, Atrioventricular; *DORV,* double-outlet right ventricle; *HCM,* hypertrophic cardiomyopathy; *D-TGA,* transposition of the great arteries with D-looped ventricles; *HLHS,* hypoplastic left heart syndrome; *IVS,* intact ventricular septum; *L-TGA,* "corrected" transposition of the great arteries; *MVP,* mitral valve prolapse; *TOF,* tetralogy of Fallot; *VSD,* ventricular septal defect.

[a]$P < .01$ compared with general population estimate of 0.30%.

indications for ablation, recognizing that an exact size or age should not be specified for individual patients. Further, it specifies that catheter ablation in the very smallest children (3–7 kg and <6 months of age) should be reserved for life-threatening arrhythmias, or refractory ones after multiple failed attempts at medical management, which may include various combination therapies. Some of the general recommendations are that ablation should be performed by an experienced pediatric electrophysiologist who undertakes the various strategies to reduce risk described earlier.

Accessory Pathways in Patients With Congenital Heart Disease

Although it is not strictly a pediatric issue, the combination of structural heart disease and arrhythmia is clearly encountered more often by pediatric electrophysiologists than by others. In unselected patients with CHD, preexcitation syndromes are statistically increased in patients with Ebstein malformation, L-transposition of the great arteries, or hypertrophic myopathy (Table 44.6).[22,166–168] Of course, preexcitation also occurs in other patients with CHD but with an incidence not statistically higher than in the general population.

Anatomy

The association of WPW with Ebstein anomaly and with the left-sided TV in L-transposition probably has its basis in the embryology of TV formation.[169,170] The mitral valve and the anterior leaflet of the tricuspid valve are fully delaminated early in development; however, the posterior and septal leaflets of the TV are not even fully formed by 3 months' gestation. Ebstein anomaly appears to occur when there is arrested development of tricuspid valve formation sometime between delamination of the anterior and of the posterior leaflets (Fig. 44.19). The high prevalence of preexcitation combined with anatomical findings of accessory connections in a number of selected cases of Ebstein anomaly[169–171] suggests that the arrested valve development results in remnants of muscular or specialized tissue connections that cross the AV groove. In fact, multiple pathways are common in these patients, often with a combination of a posteroseptal pathway and one or more additional free-wall pathways.[168]

Pathophysiology

The electrophysiology of the APs in patients with CHD is not particularly unique. Bidirectional, anterograde-only, and retrograde-only APs have been reported. Further, these patients have the same range of tachyarrhythmias found in patients with structurally normal hearts: orthodromic and antidromic AV reciprocating tachycardias and other SVTs (e.g., AVNRT, atrial flutter [AFL]/AT) with bystander participation of an anterogradely conducting AP. However, the physiologic and clinical implications of the tachycardia may be markedly different in patients with CHD.

Abnormal hemodynamics, increased incidence of isolated atrial and ventricular ectopy, sometimes poor tolerance of antiarrhythmic therapy, and the need for surgical repair that accompanies CHD all contribute to an increased need for aggressive arrhythmia management in this patient population. However, abnormal anatomy and atypical or displaced conduction systems may also enhance the difficulty and risks of catheter ablation (Fig. 44.20). Although RF catheter ablation is difficult in these patients, results have been good enough to recommend the procedure in all patients who require subsequent surgical repair to avoid postoperative arrhythmias as a complication and in most symptomatic patients older than 1 year of age who have significant structural lesions.

A review of the reported cases of RF ablation in patients with CHD revealed that most of the patients had Ebstein malformation of a right-sided tricuspid valve.[22,169–172] However, a significant proportion had more complex anatomy, with AV valve discordance (right atrium to left ventricle, left atrium to right ventricle—S,L,L or I,D,D) and often heterotaxy.[173,174] Multiple pathways are extremely common in this group, occurring in 30% to 80% of patients, compared with 5% to 10% of patients without CHD.[168,171,172] Like the patients with Ebstein malformation, those with AV discordance had all of their APs associated with the tricuspid valve regardless of atrial situs, AV

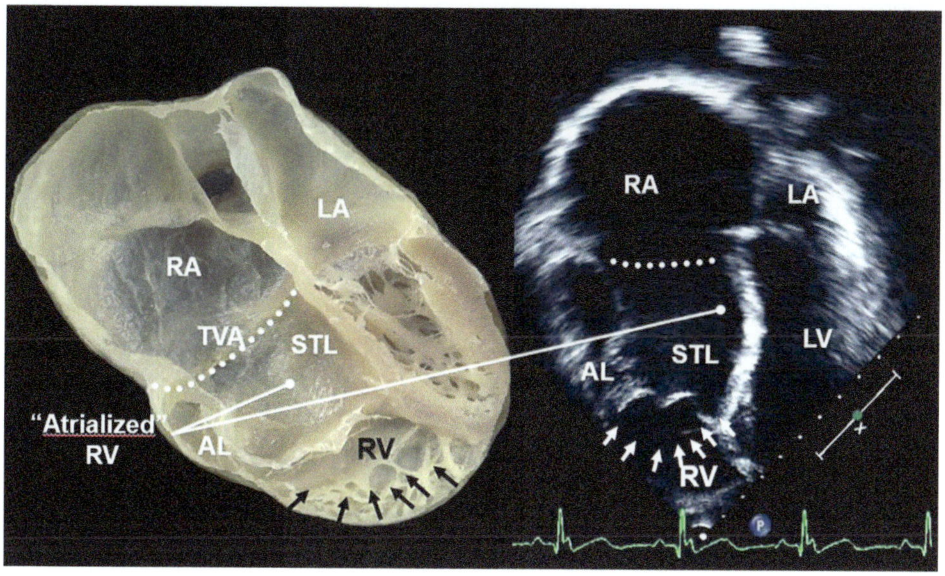

Fig. 44.19 Paraffin-preserved specimen of Ebstein anomaly with a corresponding apical four-chamber echocardiographic view. There is apical displacement of the hinge points of the septal and posterior leaflets of the tricuspid valve into the right ventricle. The portion of the right ventricle between the annulus fibrosus and the plane of leaflet coaptation is the atrialized RV, which is functionally integrated into the right atrium. The annulus fibrosis remains at its usual level (*dotted line*). The "true" RV (*black arrows*) is below the hinge-points of the affected leaflets. Note the thin wall of the atrialized RV. *AL*, anterior leaflet of the tricuspid valve; *LA*, left atrium *RA*, Right atrium; *RV*, right ventricle; *STL*, septal leaflet of the tricuspid valve; *TVA*, "true" tricuspid valve annulus.

relationship, or valve function.[170,175] This finding is in contrast to the more random location of APs reported for patients without CHD. Hypertrophic cardiomyopathy is the exception: APs are more likely to be on the normal left-sided mitral valve.[176,177]

Mapping and Ablation in Patients With Ebstein Anomaly

Ebstein anomaly poses several unique challenges to AP mapping and ablation.[176] A major difficulty lies in identification of appropriate ablation targets along the true tricuspid annulus, where atrialized RV myocardium generates low-amplitude and/or fractionated ventricular signals. Differentiation of atrial and ventricular signals can be difficult, leading to a lack of specificity in predicting a successful ablation site. In fact, very early ventricular activations, which might be termed "pseudo" AP potentials, can often be seen near the AV groove (Fig. 44.21). APs with fractionated ventricular EGMs corresponded anatomically to sites of atrialized RV and were associated with higher atrial-to-ventricular signal ratios than controls.[178] As the multiple components within these fractioned EGMs can complicate differentiation of atrial and ventricular signals during activation mapping, the investigators recommend the delivery of extrastimuli at the AP refractory period to separate atrial and ventricular components.[178] Techniques for visualizing the plane of the true AV ring include right atrial and ventricular angiography, right coronary angiography, or introduction of a multielectrode microcatheter into the right coronary artery, although this latter technology is currently not available available.[179,180] Another challenge in this population is the frequent occurrence of broad APs, with a study reporting 26% prevalence of such APs, defined by the site of early activation and ablation success measuring >1 cm in width. Challenges of mapping include right atrial and TV annular enlargement, which can interfere with catheter stability; long sheaths and deflectable sheaths can facilitate catheter stability and contact (Table 44.7).[176,180,181] The above challenges are magnified in older patients who have large hearts with poorly defined AV grooves.

Another unique anatomical challenge in Ebstein's is the existence of a prominent ridge along the inferior right AV groove, observed in 45% of examined specimens in a recent report. The presence of the ridge correlated to the clinical history of an AP, and the authors speculate that the ridge may be a part of the developmental process that leads to AV electrical connections. The authors hypothesize that such a ridge may interfere with catheter stability and energy delivery.[182–184] Visualization of such a ridge intraprocedurally may be accomplished via right atrial angiogram in RAO projection or via ICE.[184] The ridge may also form the substrate for a broad wavefront of activation, which may complicate mapping.[182,184] It should be noted that coronary damage has been reported on multiple occasions in patients with Ebstein anomaly, probably because of the thin RV wall and often diminutive right coronary artery.[13] Consequently, despite the tendency to use higher-power ablation systems with active or passive cooling for difficult cases, such technologies should be used only if an adequate distance between the catheter tip and the artery has been documented. The definition of adequate here depends on the size of the nearby coronary artery: the larger the size, the safer the ablation. Further, strong consideration should be given to the use of cryotherapy, at least as a

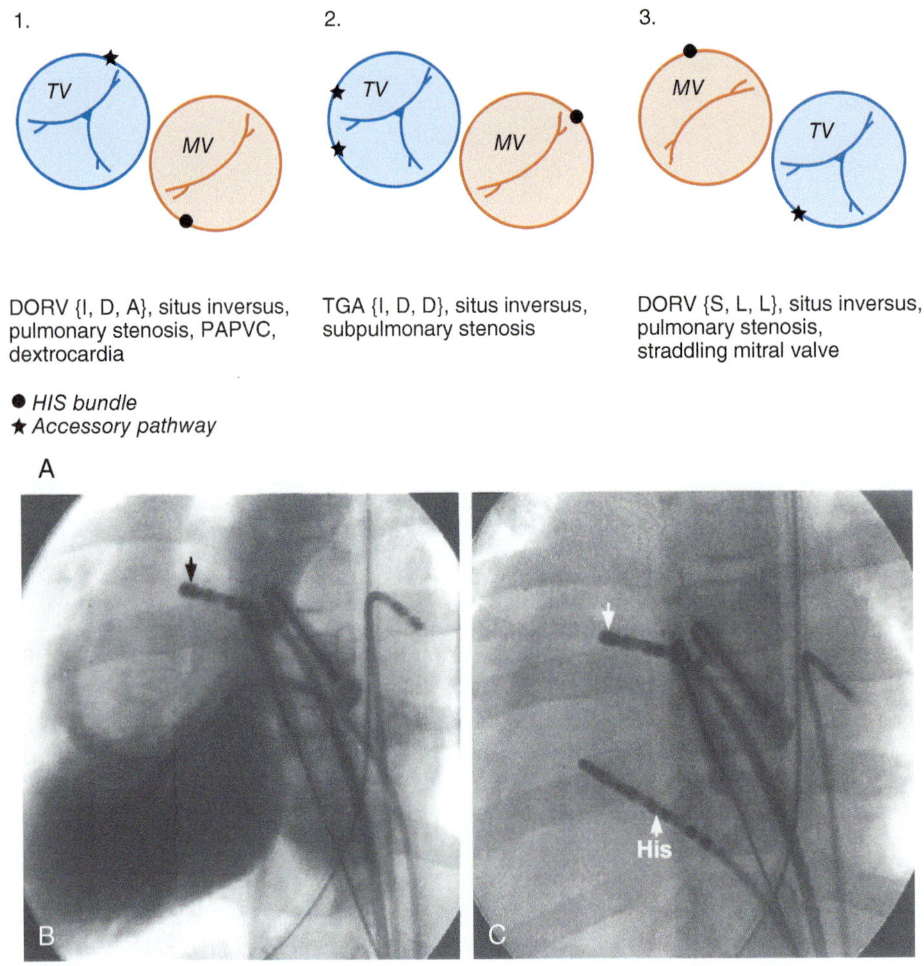

Fig. 44.20 (A) Cartoon demonstrating the locations of the mitral valve (MV), tricuspid valve (TV), His bundle, and accessory pathways in three patients with preexcitation syndromes and atrioventricular discordance. Patient 1 corresponds with B and C. The angiogram in the anteroposterior projection (C) illustrates the importance of defining the anatomy of the atrioventricular (AV) valves. The decapolar catheter (*bottom white arrow* in C) was advanced from the left-sided inferior vena cava across the MV and positioned with the second pair of electrodes at the His bundle. The mapping catheter (*black arrow* in B, *upper white arrow* in C) was advanced from the inferior vena cava across the atrial septum to the right-sided (anatomical) left atrium and positioned at the location of the accessory pathway, which in this case was at the superior and anterior portion of the left-sided TV. The unmarked catheter is an atrial pacing catheter in the left-sided right atrium. *DORV*, Double-outlet right ventricle; *PAPVC*, partial anomalous pulmonary venous connection; *TG(A)*, transposition of the great arteries. (From Saul JP, Walsh EP, Triedman JK. Mechanisms and therapy of complex arrhythmias in pediatric patients. *J Cardiovasc Electrophysiol.* 1995;6:1129–1148.)

mapping tool. Safety is enhanced, and the adhesion of the catheter may be particularly useful in larger patients.

In general, 80% to 90% of patients can be rendered arrhythmia free by the procedure, with relatively infrequent major complications such as permanent AV block.[22,180,183] Recurrence rates have been reported to be as high as 40%, particularly if multiple pathways are present, although there is a trend toward lower recurrences in the recent era.[172,183] Practical tips for mapping and ablation of APs in Ebstein anomaly are presented in Table 44.7.

Atrioventricular Discordance

Ablation procedures in patients with heterotaxy and/or AV discordance require special considerations.[185] First, detailed echocardiography and angiography are instrumental in defining the complex anatomy of the atria, the AV ring, and the coronary sinus, so that the cameras and catheters can be positioned appropriately (see Fig. 44.22). Second, careful attention must be given to locating the normal conduction system. In virtually all patients with AV discordance, the AP has been associated with the tricuspid valve, whereas the His bundle has been associated more closely with the mitral valve. As predicted by Ho et al.,[186] the normal conduction axis is often located at an anterior position along the AV groove. Once the "normal" and abnormal conduction fibers are located, electrophysiologic study and RF ablation of the APs can proceed with less risk of damage to the normal conduction system.

Mapping and ablation require detailed knowledge of the anatomy[185] and often innovative approaches. For instance, in cases of atrial inversion (right atrium on the left, or vice versa)

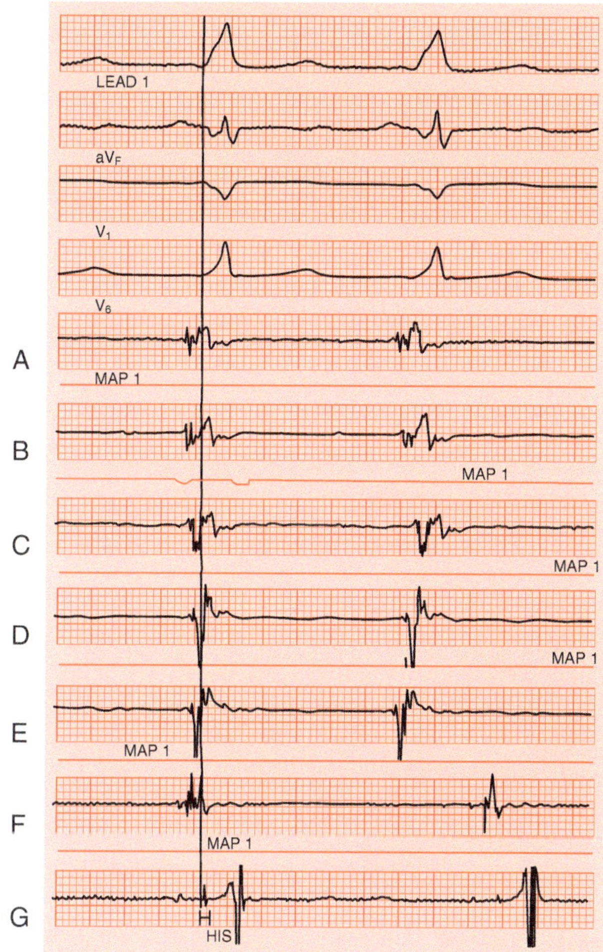

Fig. 44.21 Electrograms near the accessory pathway in a patient with Ebstein malformation. Electrograms *A* through *F* were recorded with the distal pair of an ablating catheter very near the point of successful ablation shown in *F*. Note early ventricular activation in *A* through *D*, despite lack of success. Electrograms in *D* and *E* were not significantly different, but *E* had transient success. *F*, Point of permanent success, probably has the earliest activation; however, the differences are much clearer in retrospect. The *dark vertical line* marks the point of earliest surface QRS activation for all electrograms. *G* shows the position of the atrial and HIS electrograms. Pathway location was posterior septal. (From Saul JP. Ablation of atrioventricular accessory pathways in children with and without congenital heart disease. In Huang SK, ed. *Radiofrequency Catheter Ablation of Cardiac Arrhythmias: Basic Concepts and Clinical Applications.* Mt. Kisko, NY: Futura; 1994:365–396.)

with AV discordance (I,D,D), an atrial approach to the right-sided tricuspid valve may require a reverse transseptal procedure from the left-sided inferior vena cava and right atrium to the right-sided left atrium. If present, the coronary sinus in such cases will also be reversed. AVNRT may also be present in these patients, requiring identification of the SP of an AV node that is typically along the anterior mitral annulus. Clearly, the need for a detailed understanding of the anatomy in these cases cannot be overemphasized.

Twin Atrioventricular Nodes

In hearts with normal or inverted atrial situs, but discordant AV connections (S,L,L or I,D,D), the anterosuperior ventricle is a

TABLE 44.7 Tips for Mapping and Ablation of APs in Ebstein Anomaly

Anatomical Challenge	Useful Strategies
Identification of the true AV annulus	• Right coronary angiogram • Right atrial angiogram
Difficulty in differentiation of atrial and ventricular signals	• Extrastimulus testing at pathway ERP to separate AEGM and VEGM • Differential pacing sites to reverse the activation wavefront
Catheter stability due to atrial dilation	• Long or deflectable vascular sheath
Prominent ridge	• RA angiogram and/or ICE to visualize ridge • Deflectable vascular sheath
Potential for coronary injury	• Coronary angiography • Consider cryoablation
Potential for perforation due to RV myocardial thinning	• Consideration cryoablation

AEGM, atrial electrogram; *AV*, Atrioventricular; *VEGM*, ventricular electrogram; *ERP*, effective refractory period; *ICE*, intracardiac echocardiography; *RV*, right ventricle; *R*, right atrium.

morphologic left ventricle that carries with it the mitral valve.[185] As Anderson and others,[185,186] have described, the AV node in corrected transposition is typically situated superior and anterior in the atrial wall, near the anterolateral quadrant of the mitral valve (Fig. 44.22). The penetrating bundle then runs in the fibrous continuity between the right-sided mitral valve and the anterior cusp of the posterior great artery, eventually linking to the left bundle branch on the right side of the ventricular septum. The right bundle branch then penetrates the ventricular septum to emerge in the inferior left-sided right ventricle. A second AV node that is often present more inferiorly, in the normal area of the triangle of Koch, can also link to the ventricular conduction fibers posteriorly, usually inferior to a ventricular septal defect. If the posterior and anterior ventricular bundle branches link together, a conduction sling (Fig. 44.22), sometimes referred to as a *Monckeberg sling*, is formed.[187–189] These anatomical findings provide the substrate for a host of different modes of ventricular excitation or preexcitation and AV reciprocating tachycardias. However, before the publication of a 1994 report,[187] there had been no electrophysiologic documentation of this phenomenon.

Epstein et al. reported on seven of these patients, all of whom had AV discordance (2-S,L,L and 1-I,D,D) and characteristics consistent with the diagnosis of two separate AV nodes (twin or double).[190] Five of the seven patients also had a malaligned AV canal defect. The electrophysiologic findings included (1) the existence of two discrete, nonpreexcited QRS morphologies, each with an associated His-bundle EGM and a normal His-to-ventricle (HV) interval; (2) decremental as well as adenosine-sensitive anterograde and retrograde conduction; and (3) inducible AV reciprocating tachycardia with anterograde conduction over one AV node and retrograde conduction over the other. Ventricular premature beats placed into tachycardia

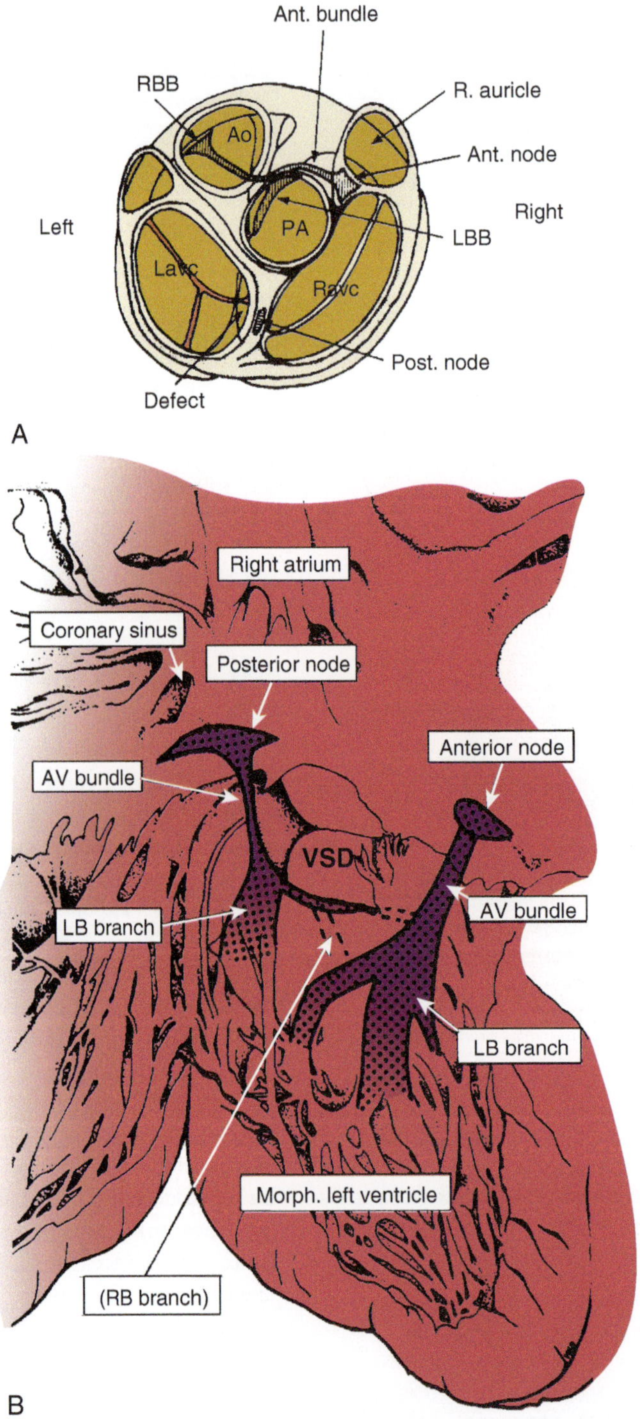

Fig. 44.22 (A) Diagram of the base of the heart and the atrioventricular (AV) conduction system in L-transposition of the great arteries (corrected) as seen from above. Note the bicommissural mitral valve on the *right* and the tricommissural tricuspid valve on the *left*. The AV node may lie posteriorly (Post. Node) in the septum in a somewhat normal location, anteriorly on the right-sided mitral valve (Ant. Bundle), or in both places. *LBB,* Left bundle branch; *RBB,* right bundle branch. (From Anderson RH, Arnold R, Wilkinson JL. The conducting system in congenitally corrected transposition. *Lancet.* 1973;1:1286-1288.) (B) Diagram of the conduction system from a patient with corrected transposition in a crisscross heart, with AV valve anatomy similar to that shown in (A). Note the dual conduction system with both the posterior and anterior AV nodes penetrating into the ventricles, and near connection of the conduction systems within the ventricle. (From Symons JC, Shinebourne E(A) Joseph MC, et al. Criss-cross heart with congenitally corrected transposition: report of a case with d-transposed aorta and ventricular preexcitation. *Eur J Cardiol.* 1977;5:493.)

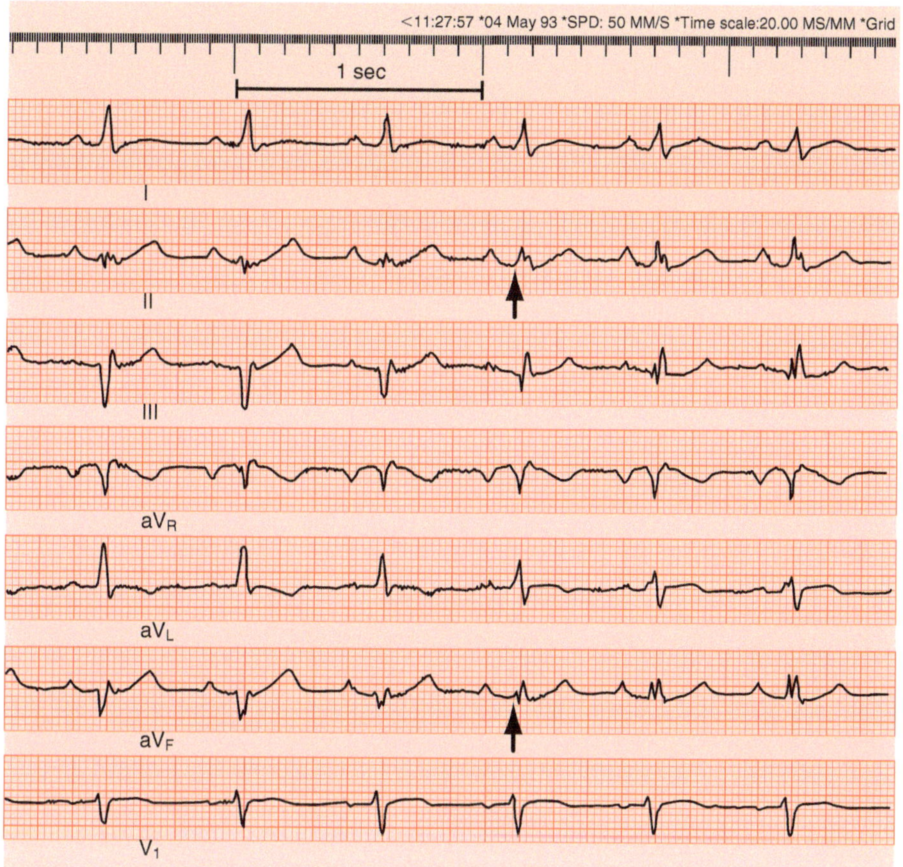

Fig. 44.23 Six-lead electrocardiograms in a patient with L-looped ventricles and common atrioventricular (AV) canal. Note spontaneously changing QRS morphology without obvious changes in the PR interval (*arrows*). The first morphology has a superior axis consistent with nonpreexcited rhythm from a posterior location as in common AV canal. The other morphology was presumed to be from a second anterior AV node as per the electrophysiologic study findings (see text). (From Saul JP. Ablation of atrioventricular accessory pathways in children with and without congenital heart disease. In Huang SK, ed. *Radiofrequency Catheter Ablation of Cardiac Arrhythmias: Basic Concepts and Clinical Applications.* Mt. Kisko, NY: Futura; 1994:365–396.)

while the His was refractory could preexcite the atrium, indicating that the tachycardia involved two AV connections. In all cases, applications of RF energy at the site of the bidirectional pathway resulted in transient junctional acceleration with an identical QRS morphology to that generated by anterograde conduction over the targeted AV node and modified or eliminated both anterograde and retrograde conduction at that site. Although there is a possibility that one or the other of these pathways was a Mahaim-type AV fiber, their locations, and the presence of near-normal HV intervals, retrograde conduction, orthodromic tachycardia, and junctional-type acceleration during RF ablation all favor a second AV node. The precise etiology may make little difference for the medical management of such patients but is important if damage to the better of the two conduction systems is to be avoided during ablation procedures performed before surgery in these patients with complex anatomy.

One patient with AV discordance and complete common AV canal was particularly illustrative of the features described. Two QRS morphologies were seen during normal rhythm, each with a normal PR interval (Fig. 44.23). One of the QRS morphologies (#1) was more typical of an endocardial cushion defect with a superior axis. At electrophysiology study, QRS morphology #1 could be produced by posterior atrial pacing and had an HV interval of about 50 ms with the His potential found posteriorly in the ventricle (Fig. 44.24). The other QRS morphology (#2) could be produced by anterior atrial pacing and had an associated HV interval (from the posterior His) of only 20 ms, but the QRS appearance did not strongly suggest preexcitation (see Fig. 44.24). The anterograde effective refractory period (ERP) of this anterior pathway was approximately 200 ms. Earliest ventricular activation was near the septal remnant regardless of QRS morphology. A regular tachycardia involving (1) QRS morphology #1 (see Fig. 44.25); (2) a 1:1 A/V relation; (3) a minimum ventriculoatrial (VA) interval of 70 ms; and (4) earliest retrograde atrial activation at the left anterior AV groove near the midline (tricuspid side of common valve) could be reproducibly induced with ventricular pacing. Ventricular premature beats placed into tachycardia while the His was refractory could preexcite the atrium, indicating that the tachycardia involved two AV connections. Retrograde VA conduction was all via the anterior pathway, was decremental, and had an ERP of 230 ms. Application of RF energy near the point of earliest retrograde conduction (anterior and to the left) resulted in transient

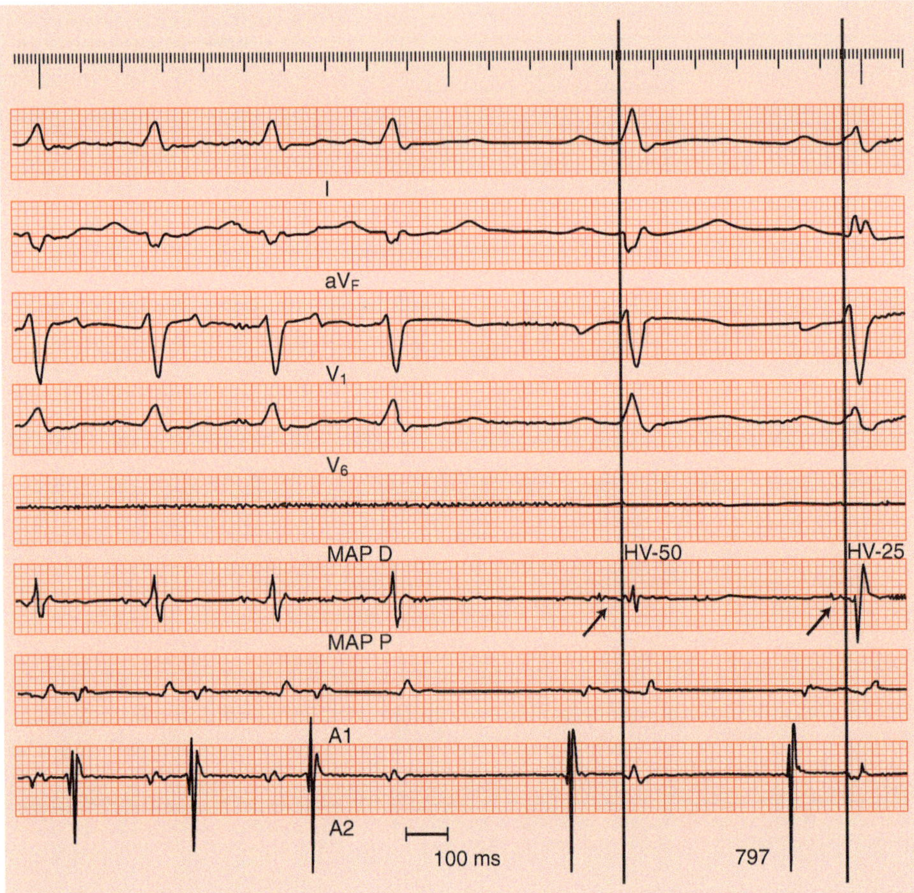

Fig. 44.24 Intracardiac recordings in same patient as Fig. 44.22 with L-loop ventricles and common atrioventricular (AV) canal. Note HV interval of 50 ms during the tachycardia and the first sinus beat after spontaneous termination. QRS morphologies for the tachycardia and this beat were identical. Also note shorter His-to-ventricle interval of 25 ms during the last beat, which is the anterior AV node QRS morphology. (From Saul JP. Ablation of atrioventricular accessory pathways in children with and without congenital heart disease. In Huang SK, ed. *Radiofrequency Catheter Ablation of Cardiac Arrhythmias: Basic Concepts and Clinical Applications.* Mt. Kisko, NY: Futura; 1994:365–396.)

junctional acceleration of QRS rhythm #2, followed by a sudden change to a regular slower rhythm of QRS #1 (Fig. 44.25). After RF application, VA conduction was eliminated, and tachycardia was noninducible. These findings illustrate the following important features (1) there were two anterograde conduction pathways, one posteroseptal and one anteroseptal; (2) both pathways were on the left (tricuspid) side of the common AV ring; (3) both pathways had slow conduction properties; (4) retrograde conduction occurred over only the anterior pathway; and (5) tachycardia was orthodromic, anterograde posterior, and retrograde anterior. The presence of the specialized conduction sling connecting the twin AVNs may be more difficult to characterize, and one report has suggested that the absence of a resetting phenomenon is electrophysiological evidence of the sling operating as a part of the SVT circuit involving twin AV nodes.[191]

Patient Size and Structural Disease

One observation that is difficult to prove statistically but seems clear from our own experience is that the smaller chamber size in smaller patients is a technical asset in catheter ablation.[192] Although larger patient size may be useful when the retrograde approach to left-sided accessory connections is used, smaller patient size appears to be helpful for catheter stabilization during an atrial approach, particularly in patients with structural heart disease and potentially very large hearts. Consequently, earlier intervention during childhood is preferable to waiting for near-adult size.

Recurrence Risk in CHD

The incidence of recurrence of tachycardia or preexcitation in patients who were initially successfully ablated has been reported to be 8% to 40%.[22,193–195] An increased risk of recurrence has been reported with right-sided pathways and with multiple pathways.[22,193–195] Both of these conditions occur with increased frequency in this patient population, and, in combination with the complex anatomy, this probably accounts for the high recurrence rate.

Summary and Recommendations

Catheter ablation is recommended for persistent SVT related to accessory AV connections or twin AV nodes in CHD patients, as an alternative to medical therapy when medical therapy is

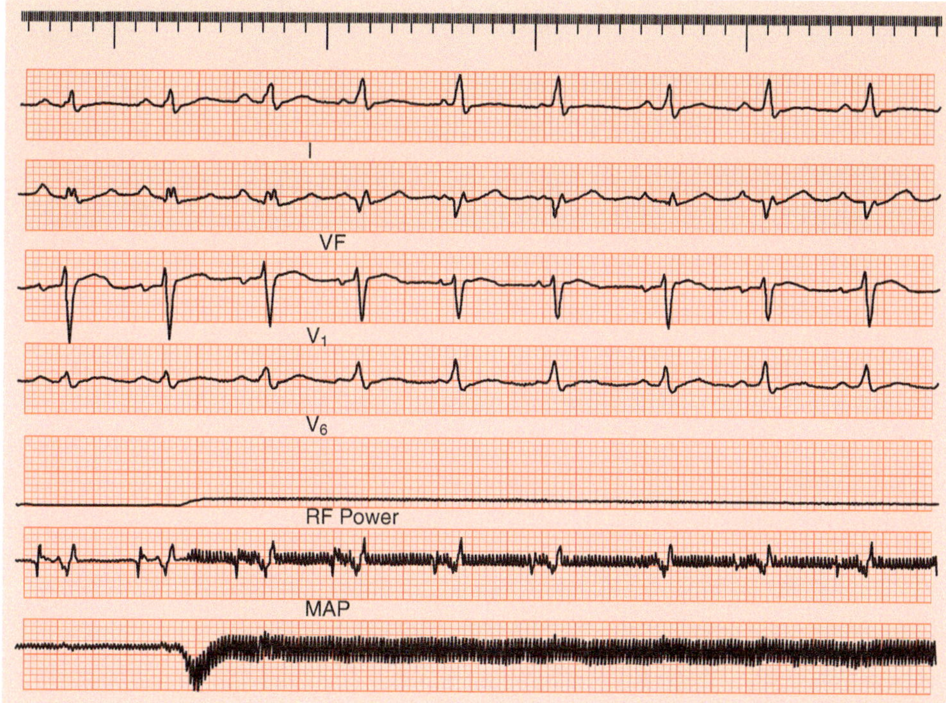

Fig. 44.25 Response to radiofrequency (RF) ablation at the location of the anterior atrioventricular (AV) node in the same patient as in Figs. 44.22 and 44.23. Within 1 second after application of RF energy, the PR interval shortened, presumably because of junctional acceleration. Approximately 1 second later, the junctional acceleration stopped, and the PR interval lengthened with a change in QRS morphology consistent with loss of the morphology associated with the anterior AV node that had a shorter His-to-ventricle interval. *MAP*, Monophasic action potential. (From Saul JP. Ablation of atrioventricular accessory pathways in children with and without congenital heart disease. In Huang SK, ed. *Radiofrequency Catheter Ablation of Cardiac Arrhythmias: Basic Concepts and Clinical Applications.* Mt. Kisko, NY: Futura; 1994:365–396.)

either not effective or associated with hemodynamic or intolerable side effects in any patient. Ablation of any tachycardia substrate before planned surgical intervention for CHD should also be considered as SVT may complicate the post operative course and surgical procedures may preclude future access to AP substrates (e.g., atrioventricular valve replacement).

Some procedural recommendations for catheter ablation in patients with CHD include: (1) an attempt should always be made to carefully identify the location of the normal AV conducting system, particularly in patients with AV discordance; (2) the anatomical TV is the most likely location for accessory connections; (3) smaller patient size may be an asset; (4) an atrial approach should probably be attempted first for connections around the tricuspid annulus (right- or left-sided); (5) the true AV groove should be well identified, using either atrial and ventricular EGM balance, a coronary angiogram, or, if available, a coronary mapping wire in larger patients; (6) consider twin AV nodes as the substrate for reentrant tachycardia in patients with AV discordance and malaligned AV canal defects who have two distinct QRS morphologies that both have normal PR intervals; and (7) consider cryoablation for APs in close proximity to the AV node.

Atrial Flutter or Fibrillation in the Absence of Other Heart Disease

In the pediatric patient, atrial reentry tachycardias are relatively rare in the absence of either structural or functional heart disease. The term *lone atrial flutter or fibrillation* has been applied here, referring to the isolated nature of the arrhythmia findings. However, both of these tachyarrhythmias are occasionally observed in pediatric patients. There are two age ranges for presentation. Perhaps the most common is during the third trimester of fetal life, when AFL accounts for up to one-third of fetal tachycardias,[196] often lasting through delivery and leading to ventricular dysfunction. Neonatal AFL almost universally resolves without recurrence if it can be managed successfully during fetal and early neonatal life.[197] Consequently, ablation therapy for such infants should not be necessary and has never been reported.

A second presentation peak occurs during adolescence, when both AFL and AF may occur generally in the absence of any identifiable gross structural, hormonal, or chemical cause.[198,199] In some cases of "lone" AFL, endomyocardial biopsy has revealed myocarditis.[198] Though rare, refractory organized atrial reentrant arrhythmias have been described in the setting of diffuse atrial scarring with electrical silence, and mechanical paralysis in the absence of atrial dilation or any systemic or neurodegenerative disorders.[200] These occur in the context of partial or progressive atrial standstill. Such a presentation could be seen rarely manifesting in pediatric age group leading to refractory intra-atrial reentrant arrhythmias in the absence of CHD (Fig. 44.26). An intracardiac EPS and 3D electroanatomical voltage mapping will often be revealing in such cases.

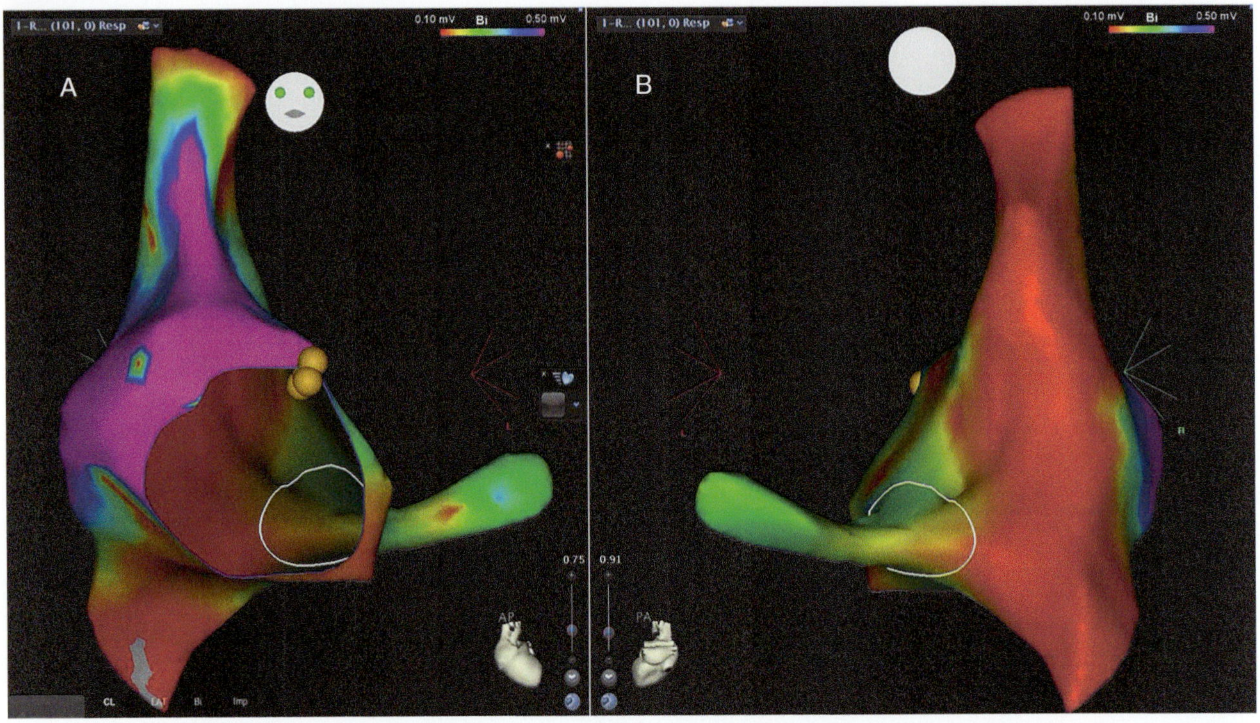

Fig. 44.26 Three-dimensional voltage maps on anteroposterior (A) and posteroanterior (B) projections of right atrium and coronary sinus in a 7-year-old boy with *SCN1B* variant affecting $Na_v1.5$ sodium current demonstrating extensive "scarring" (voltage color scale range: 0.1–0.5 mV, "purple" indicates voltage >0.5 mV). This patient developed drug refractory intra-atrial reentrant tachycardia in the setting of structurally normal heart.

AF and AFL could also be the manifestation of a yet undiagnosed or ill-defined cardiac channelopathy.[198,201]

There have been few studies on outcomes of lone AF in the young. In one multicenter series of 18 patients ≤21 years of age presenting with AF, 39% were noted to have inducible AVNRT or AVRT involving a concealed AP, all of whom were successfully ablated with no recurrences over a mean follow-up of 1.7 years, suggesting that AF was triggered by one of these mechanisms.[199] In the largest multicenter study of 241 healthy children ≤21 years with AF, 39% had AF recurrence, an incidence that was similar with and without treatment.[202] Although initial management should be conservative, multiple recurrences in this age group despite medical therapy may lead to a need for ablation therapy similar to the scenario in adults. The use of catheter ablation has been reported for both AF and AFL in young patients. Success rates were >90% for the AFL subgroup in a relatively large series of patients in the Pediatric Ablation Registry.[4] Acute success has also been reported in a few small series of normal adolescent patients with paroxysmal AF by targeting foci in the pulmonary veins (PVs), crista terminalis, or left atrium.[203–205]

Specific technical details for ablation of either AFL or AF in teenagers are not particularly different from those in adults and are not repeated here; however, there are some differences in decision-making and approach that may be important. Most importantly, the decision of when to ablate can be quite different, particularly for AF. After conversion from a first episode of AF or AFL, either no therapy or a drug to block the AV node response is adequate. After recurrence, the threshold for ablation of AFL can be similar to that in adults and a majority of cases involve the cavotricuspid isthmus as the critical site for reentry.[198]

The use of ablation therapy for the rare cases of AF in pediatric patients is also appealing, but the high emphasis on safety over efficacy mandates that a decision to perform wide area circumferential isolation of all PVs and/or left atrial linear ablation in this age group be considered only after failure of multiple antiarrhythmic agents and ruling out triggering substrates such as ectopic AT (EAT), AVRT or AVNRT. In the largest multicenter pediatric AF study to date, only ablation of a non-AF substrate (AP, SP, or other focal arrhythmia mechanism) was associated with longer freedom from AF recurrence. Empiric PVI did not prolong freedom from AF recurrence.[202] Thus, the technique chosen should be the most conservative in terms of safety because complications such as PV stenosis and stroke can be devastating to a child. Finally, an operator experienced with ablation for AF should be included in the procedure. This is a population where coming back for a second procedure should take precedence over a higher-risk first procedure.

Focal Atrial Tachycardia in the Child

Focal AT (FAT) is characterized by atrial activation starting rhythmically at a small area (focus) from which it spreads centrifugally.[206] Mechanistically, FAT may be due to one of three basic arrhythmia mechanisms: reentry, automaticity, and triggered activity. FATs are differentiated into those due to abnormal automaticity and those not due to abnormal automaticity (so-called nonautomatic FATs or NAFAT).[207]

TABLE 44.8 Sites of Ectopic Atrial Tachycardia in Children

Anatomical Sites	Reported Incidence from Published Studies[208–210,216]
Right atrial appendage	3–25%
Tricuspid annulus	15–20%
Crista terminalis	4–28%
Free wall of right atrium	8–11%
Left atrial appendage	5–34%
Pulmonary veins	14–44%
Mitral annulus	9–17%
Free wall of left atrium	3%
Interatrial septum/perinodal area	14%

EAT is often a term that is applied to focal AT of abnormal automaticity. EAT is an uncommon rhythm disorder that accounts for 5% to 20% of SVTs in children[208–210] but less than 2% of SVTs in adult series. It involves abnormally rapid impulse generation from a single atrial focus outside the sinus node (Table 44.8). Because the tachycardia is frequently incessant, the presentation is accompanied by a functional left ventricular myopathy in 50% to 75% of cases.[209–212] EAT may resolve spontaneously in some patients, particularly in those presenting at <6 months of age (>70% spontaneous resolution).[213,214] In many cases, conventional antiarrhythmic drug therapy is not effective.[213–215] The fact that ventricular function usually returns to normal if the arrhythmia can be controlled has led to an aggressive search for other therapies, most notably catheter ablation.[1,215–217]

EAT is a nearly incessant tachycardia with wide fluctuations in atrial rate, which often parallel the autonomic state and respond to isoproterenol in a similar way to sinus rhythm (Fig. 44.27).[207] Typically, the ectopic focus rate changes gradually with a "warm-up" at initiation, and a "cool down," sometimes associated with exit block, at termination. Programmed atrial stimulation is usually of little value in the initiation of EAT, and neither atrial stimulation nor direct current (DC) cardioversion is useful for terminating it. Finally, the reset response of the EAT focus to single premature atrial stimuli can be almost identical to that of the normal sinus node.[207]

Most cases of EAT are not associated with specific pathologic abnormalities of either cardiac or skeletal muscle. However, single focus and multifocal EAT may be found in association with RAS/MAPK pathway disorders (RASopathies).[218] Pathologic findings have been either normal or limited to nonspecific fibrosis, cellular hypertrophy, and patchy fatty infiltrates, all of which may be secondary to the tachycardia-induced myopathy.[219] In some cases, histopathology examination has shown the presence of ectopic nodal structures at the site of successful catheter ablation of EAT. Other etiologies involve expression of HCN4 and connexins at atrial sites remote from the sinus node responsible for EAT.[220,221] Clues to the etiology of EAT may come from the use of RF catheter therapy. First, it has been observed that EAT almost always involves a small area of tissue or a single cell, because it is eliminated within a few seconds after application of RF energy.[216] Second, just before successful elimination of the foci, the ectopic rate often accelerates, consistent with enhanced automaticity observed in response to RF energy in other tissue (Fig. 44.28).[222] Finally, the foci seem to cluster in a few specific areas of the right and left AAs, and near or within the pulmonary venous ostia (Fig. 44.29). These findings all suggest that EAT involves subtle electrical changes in otherwise normal tissue from trabeculated atria or connections between the primitive atria and the systemic veins.

NAFAT is an uncommon tachycardia mechanism in pediatric patients with structurally normal hearts presenting as paroxysmal SVT.[223,224] Most patients in this series with structurally normal hearts had a single focus, located in the right atrium, amenable to catheter ablation.[224] Tachycardia is reproducibly initiated with atrial extrastimuli, more commonly in reentry as opposed to triggered activity.[223,224]

Therapy

Virtually every class of antiarrhythmic agent has been used as pharmacologic therapy for EAT. Although no single class or agent appears to be universally effective, the best results have been observed with Class IC and Class III agents,[7,213,214,225] with amiodarone perhaps the most effective.[226] Recent studies have shown ivabradine, which blocks the I_f current and slows spontaneous phase 4 depolarization, to be effective in incessant FAT.[227,228]

In contrast to pharmacologic therapy, catheter ablation for EAT arising from a single focus has been acutely successful in 90% to 100% of cases without significant complications.[216,229] Because of the high success rates of catheter ablation and the morbidity of drug therapy, the question of drug therapy has generally been reduced to one of whether it should be attempted at all in patients with severe ventricular dysfunction—and, if so, for how long—while waiting for spontaneous reversion to sinus rhythm. Consistent with this assessment, both EAT and NAFAT as with other forms of SVT, are considered a Class I indication for catheter ablation for patients >15 kg with ventricular dysfunction.[1]

Mapping and Ablation

Most incessant EATs can be successfully mapped using a bipolar signal from the distal electrode pair of a single map/ablation catheter referenced to a single fixed intraatrial signal. Comparison with the beginning of the surface P wave, when it can be identified, is very useful to identify timing in relation to some known measure of early atrial activation. Map signals that precede the surface P wave by >20 ms are most likely to indicate a successful location.[216] Although virtually all early ablation series were done with such basic mapping techniques, there are many situations in which more sophisticated mapping is useful or even necessary. High-density mapping can be performed with a variety of technologies and levels of sophistication.

A simple decapolar catheter, which provides four or more nearby timing points to the distal bipole, yields a great deal of directional information. Early distal timing with sequentially later timing of the proximal pairs suggests that the tip is indeed

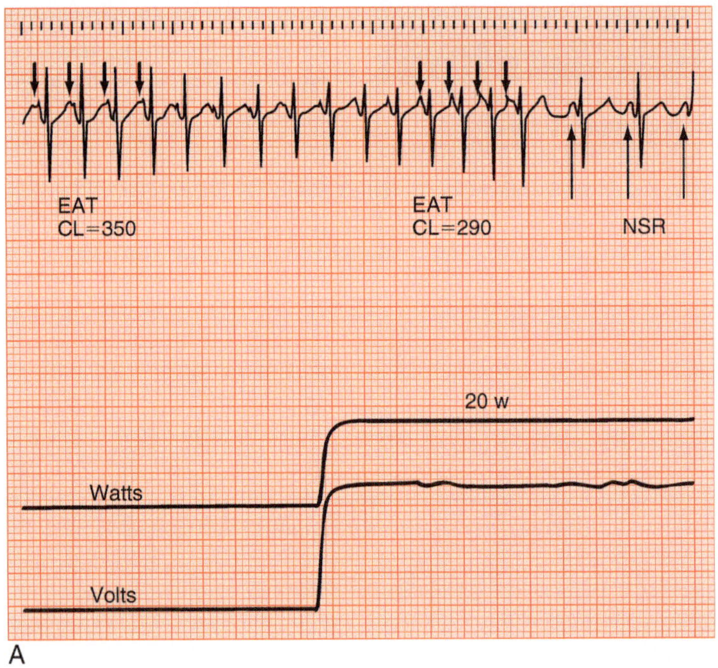

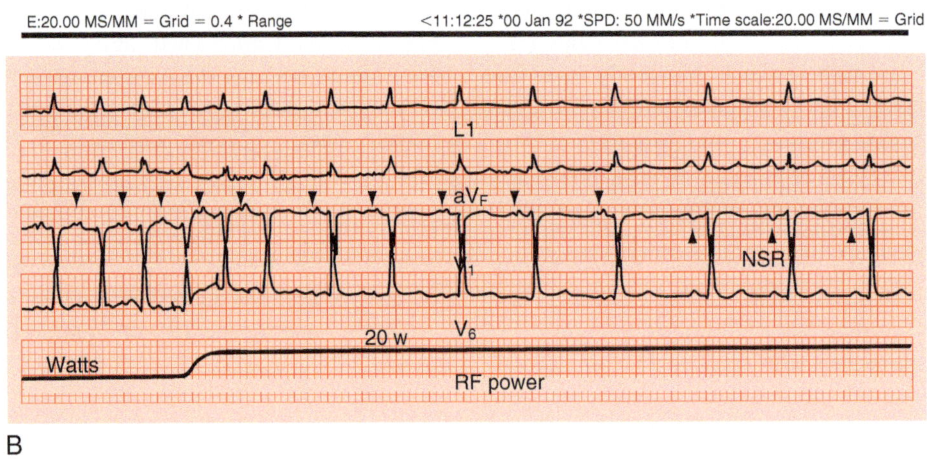

Fig. 44.27 Ectopic atrial tachycardia (EAT) ablation. (A) Note how ectopic P waves (*arrows*) terminate after a brief period of acceleration. (B) EAT slows briefly, then terminates. In both cases, the changes occur soon after radiofrequency (RF) application. In other cases, the ectopic focus may stop immediately at the onset of application of RF energy.

near the ectopic focus. However, even very early timing of the distal bipole when proximal timing is equivalent indicates that activation is approaching the catheter from a different location. This situation often arises when an anterior right upper PV focus is being mapped from within the high posterior right atrium. Timing may be early all along the catheter in the right atrium, but it will be earlier and sequential when the tip is in the right upper PV. In such a case, ablation will be successful only when it is applied on the left atrial/PV side of the atrial wall.

This example also highlights the value of 3D multipoint mapping. There are a few considerations when choosing the best 3D technology for EAT mapping, including the following. (1) Some foci are intermittently active, particularly under sedation or anesthesia, making sequential activation mapping frustrating or impossible. (2) The location of right PV and near-septal foci may not be discernible from either the surface ECG or preliminary mapping, necessitating mapping in both the left and the right atria. (3) Some patients have multiple foci. (4) Some pediatric patients are too small for certain mapping technologies, particularly if remote areas of the left atrium must be accessed. Given these considerations, we have found that for clearly incessant EATs sequential mapping technologies that allow simultaneous display and comparison of both the atria work well and provide the most flexibility. The CARTO (Biosense Webster Inc.) and EnSite (Abbott Inc.) mapping systems both have all these characteristics. However, for intermittent or potentially multiple foci, sequential mapping technologies may be frustrating, particularly if the focus activity is sensitive to catheter tip pressure. High-definition or ultra-high-definition contact maps created by multielectrode mapping catheters with small and closely spaced electrodes have started to become the widely adopted approach particularly in incessant and easily

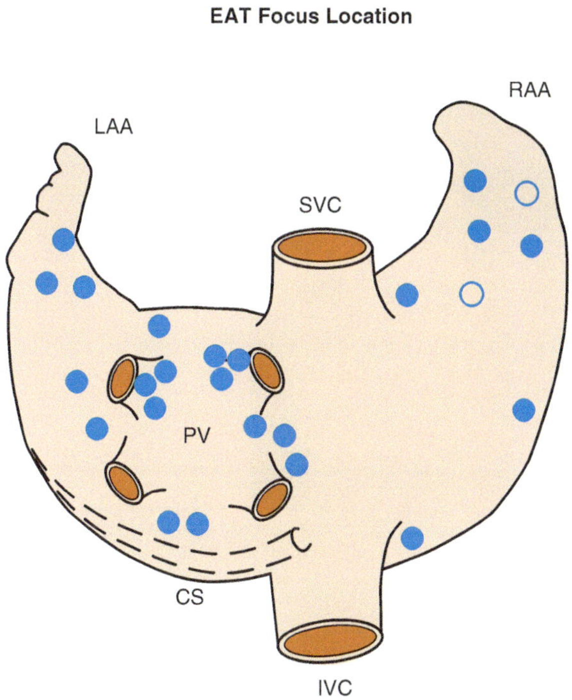

Fig. 44.28 Location of ectopic atrial tachycardia foci in whom detailed mapping was possible. *Closed circles* indicate sites of successful ablation, and *open circles* indicate foci that could not be eliminated. *IVC*, Inferior vena cava; *LA(A)*, left atrial appendage; *PV*, pulmonary vein; *RAA*, right atrial appendage; *SVC*, superior vena cava. (From Walsh EP. Ablation of ectopic atrial tachycardia in children. In: Huang SK, ed. *Radiofrequency Catheter Ablation of Cardiac Arrhythmias: Basic Concepts and Clinical Applications.* Mt. Kisko, NY: Futura; 1994:421–443.)

inducible sustained ATs. In pediatric population, this is more commonly achieved using either the PentaRay catheter coupled with CARTO 3 mapping system (Biosense Webster Inc., Diamond Bar, California) or the Advisor HD grid (Abbott, Inc.), coupled with the EnSite Precision cardiac mapping system and, less commonly, the IntellaMap Orion basket (which is contraindicated for age <8 years and needs special regulatory approval and parental consent) mapping catheter coupled with Rhythmia HDx(Boston Scientific, Marlborough, MA) mapping system.[230]

For nonsustained EAT, a technology that allows for simultaneous single-beat noncontact mapping, such as the Endocardial Solutions Inc. (ESI) balloon, was a promising concept. However, the ESI system is no longer available for clinical use and is of historical significance. Consequently, no existing system deals with all four of the considerations noted earlier. Regardless of the technology used, if foci are intermittently active and either multilead P-wave morphologies or multipolar intra-atrial activations have been recorded during EAT, pace mapping may also be a useful adjunct to identify the focus site.[231]

In general, failure to eliminate EAT through catheter ablation is less dependent on the ablation technology than on obtaining a good map with early activation and the number of foci present. Because the normal atria are rarely more than 3 to 4 mm thick, most ablation technologies can easily create transmural lesions using standard settings. Therefore, techniques for creating larger lesions, such as active and passive tip cooling and high-powered generators, should rarely, if ever, be necessary. In fact, because most pediatric EAT foci are in the left atrium and often near the ostium of a PV, less destructive ablation technologies (using

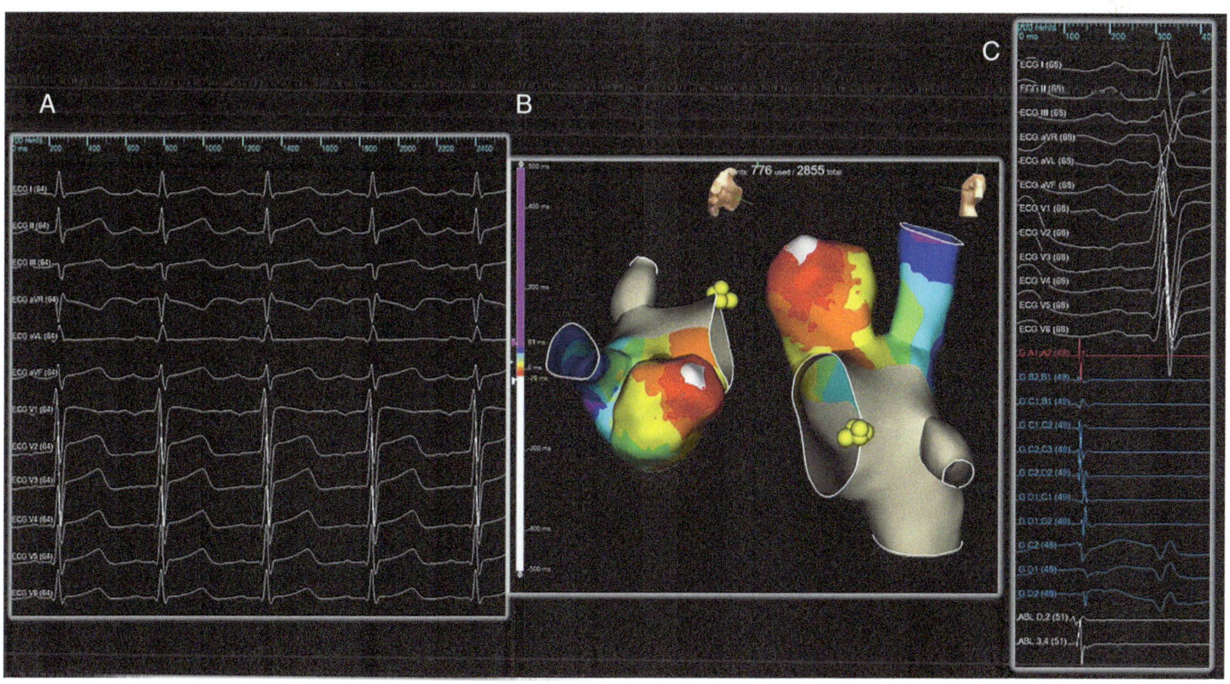

Fig. 44.29 A 15-year-old with right atrial tachycardia since birth that has been managed with antiarrhythmic medications presents for catheter ablation (A). The P-wave axis on ECG mimics a sinus P wave, but PR is slightly prolonged and there is a negative P wave in lead V_1 during atrial tachycardia. Mapping performed with Advisor HD Grid using Ensite X Cardiac Mapping System and VoXel Mode (Abbott Inc.). Atrial tachycardia was localized to the tip of the right atrial appendage (B). Successful ablation site had a bipolar signal that preceded P wave by 40 ms and QS complex in unipolar signal preceded by a small R (C). *Yellow dots,* His bundle.

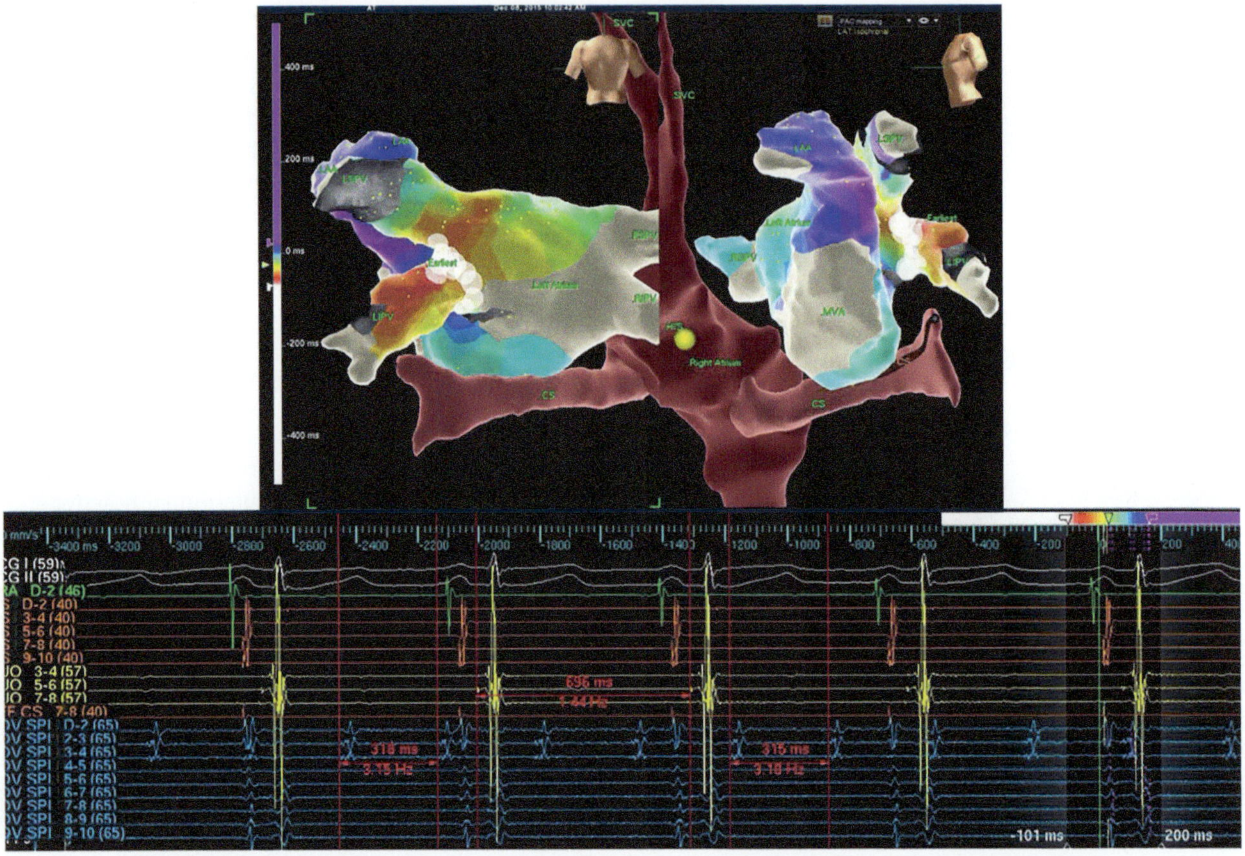

Fig. 44.30 A 11-year-old boy presenting with incessant ectopic atrial tachycardia from left inferior pulmonary vein. Three-dimensional geometry of left atrium and right atrium with coronary sinus in posteroanterior (*top left*) and left lateral (*top right*) projections with activation map of atrial tachycardia. Circumferential isolation of left inferior pulmonary vein (*white lesions*) performed. Electrograms (*bottom half*) demonstrates exit block to tachycardia within left pulmonary vein ostia (*blue channels*, 318 ms). Surface and other intracardiac electrograms (right atrium, *green*; coronary sinus, *orange*; His bundle, *yellow*) demonstrate sinus rhythm at 696 ms.

lower temperature, power, and duration) or cryotherapy may be most appropriate in the child.

The AAs remain a challenging site for focal AT ablation. From a diagnostic standpoint, right AA tachycardia can mimic sinus tachycardia as P-wave morphology appears similar to sinus. A relatively long PR interval and negative P waves in leads V_1–V_2 during tachycardia allows ECG differentiation from sinus rhythm. AA varies significantly in shape, size, and orientation to adjacent cardiac structures. Compared with the proximal AA, distal AA, complicated with a multilobulated morphology, thin wall, and relatively low blood flow, often restricts catheter mobility and delivery of effective energy to the desired point. Part of the tachycardia may have an epicardial origin. In addition, AA is a highly mobile structure that limits catheter maneuverability and consistent contact during ablation, even with a steerable sheath. The risk of complications, such as perforation from catheter manipulation or rupture from ablation steam pop, may thus increase with inadvertent manipulation and multiple procedures. Endocardial RF ablation at the tip of the AA can be performed safety and successfully but with extreme caution (Fig. 44.30A–C). We perform an AA angiogram for anatomical visualization before ablation, use high-density mapping (Videos 44.5 and 44.6), and use an irrigated-tip catheter to deliver RF energy with a temperature limited to 40–42°C. RF energy is started at 15 W and gradually increased up to a power of 25–30 W at the tip and to 30–35 W at the AA base with careful impedance monitoring (Video 44.6). Ablation at the base of the appendage appears to be safer than the tip, but reaching the accurate target may be difficult due to pectinate muscle ridges or the ablation energy may not penetrate the wall. Risk of injury to the phrenic nerve during left AA focal AT ablation should also be considered. In such situations of high-risk or procedure failure, alternative methods include surgical resection via sternotomy, a totally thoracoscopic approach for appendectomy of the left AA or isolation of the AA orifice with the cryoballoon.[232–234] Endocardial mapping of AA should be performed to locate the AT focus before surgical appendectomy to ensure complete removal of arrhythmia substrate without residual foci in the stump or base of the excised AA.

Alternative approaches to focal ablation could be adopted for certain sites. Isolation of a single "culprit" PV was performed in an 11-year-old patient presenting with incessant focal PV tachycardia from a left inferior PV (Fig. 44.27). It is often useful to include 3D imaging such as cardiac CT scan as part of preprocedural planning, which helps in assessment of pulmonary venous anatomy and ostial dimensions. Isolation of distal left superior vena cava (SVC) at the level of roof of left atrium

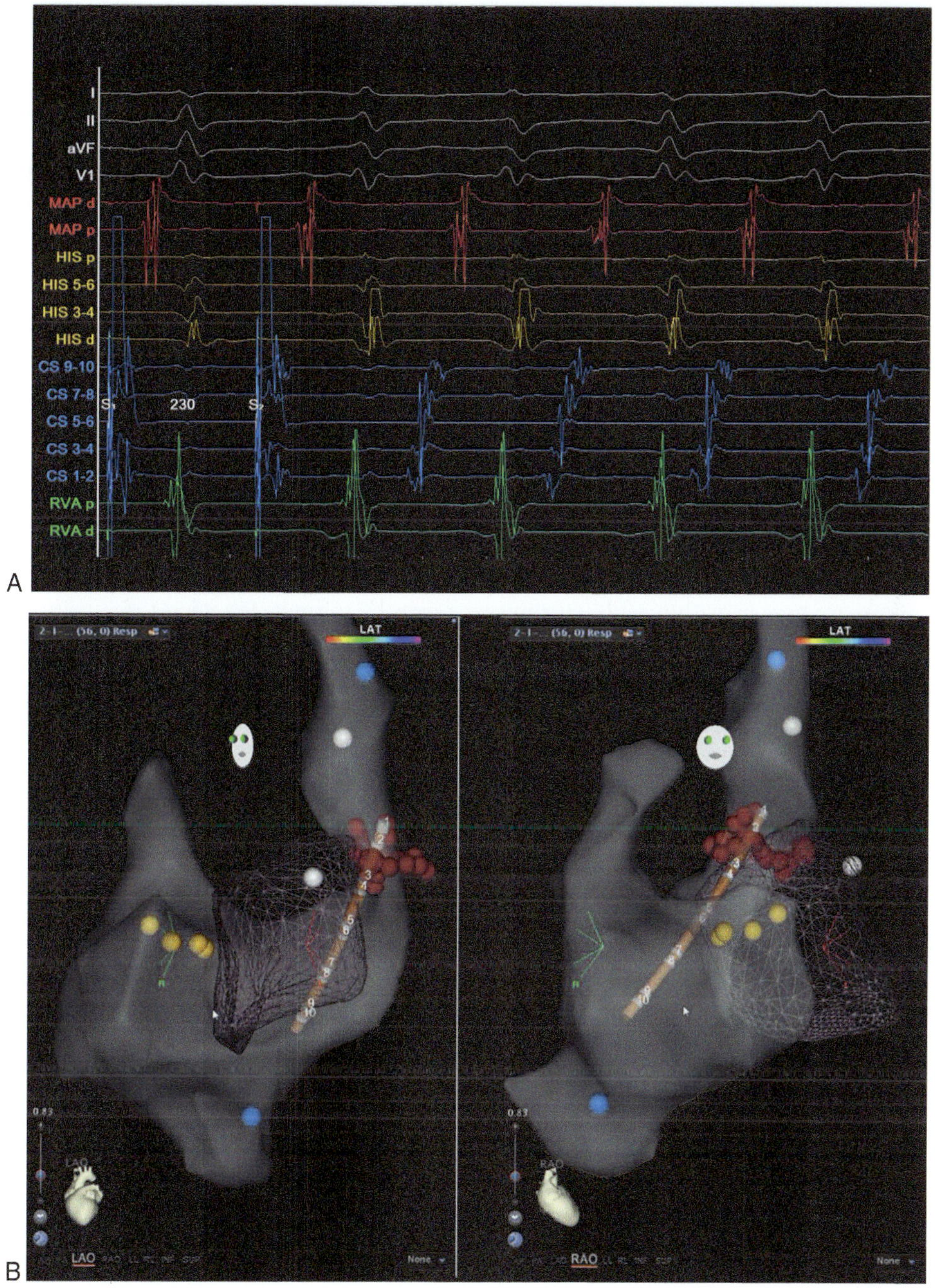

Fig. 44.31 (A) An 8-year-old boy with normal intracardiac anatomy, absent right superior vena cava (SVC), persistent left SVC draining to coronary sinus, presenting with paroxysmal symptoms of palpitations, found to have reproducibly inducible 1:1 short VA narrow QRS complex supraventricular tachycardia (SVT) with "eccentric" (earliest atrial activation near distal left SVC at the level of roof of left atrium), consistent with focal microreentrant atrial tachycardia. There was no evidence of conduction via extranodal atrioventricular accessory connection. SVT rendered noninducible after isolation of distal left SVC with irrigated radiofrequency catheter ablation. (A) Induction of SVT by single atrial extrastimulus from mid-coronary sinus (surface electrocardiograms and intracardiac electrograms shown: high right atrial recording (*red*, Map channels), coronary sinus electrograms (*blue*, CS channels), right ventricular apex (*green*, RVA channels), His-bundle catheter displaced (*yellow*, HIS channels); (B) three-dimensional geometry of right atrium, left SVC draining into coronary sinus (*gray*), partial left atrium (*wire mesh*). Decapolar catheter shadow positioned inside coronary sinus and distal SVC. Irrigated radiofrequency catheter applications in circular ring fashion (*red lesions*) isolating distal left SVC below the electrodes 1 and 2.

resulted in noninducibility of focal microreentrant AT from this region in an 8-year-old with normal intracardiac anatomy, absent right SVC, and persistent left SVC draining to coronary sinus (Fig. 44.31A, B).

Ablation of Atrial Tachycardia in Infants and Small Children

Catheter ablation may be become necessary in infants and small children in case of incessant medically resistant AT, particularly those who have developed or at risk of tachycardia-mediated cardiomyopathy. Few technical differences between the use of catheter ablation in these small patients versus other groups are worth emphasizing. One must be mindful of the number and size of vascular sheaths that are being used. Catheter ablation may be performed with fewer than the typical set of reference mapping and diagnostic catheters. The number of vascular sheaths could be conserved by using a transesophageal diagnostic electrode catheter positioned behind the left atrium recording atrial EGMs to serve as the reference catheter for mapping AT (Fig. 44.13). Finally, safe catheter ablation in this age group requires not only knowledge of pediatric electrophysiology but also personnel in the catheterization laboratory who are mindful of the needs of the critically ill infant.

Complications

Beyond the usual complications of any ablation procedure, there are few unique complications to EAT ablation. Both of these topics are covered elsewhere in this textbook. Although some EAT foci in children are near or within a PV, eliciting concerns about stenosis, clinically significant stenosis, has not been reported for a pediatric case. The potential for damage to the sinus node or to the right phrenic nerve for foci that occur along the crista terminalis should be considered, and the phrenic nerve should be well mapped-out before delivering ablation energy along the right atrial free wall. This is particularly important in patients who have had prior heart surgery because the phrenic nerve and pericardium are often fixed in place on the atrial surface. Cryoablation during simultaneous upstream phrenic nerve pacing can be a safe and effective approach in such cases.[235] Ablation in the AA should be performed with caution due to risk of perforation or thrombus formation as discussed, previously.

Ventricular Tachycardia in the Absence of Heart Disease

VT is uncommon in pediatric patients without structural and/or electrical heart disease. The reported incidence of nonsustained or sustained VT is estimated to be between 0.1 and 0.8 per 10,000 children.[1,2,236-237] The majority (>50%) of patients with idiopathic left or right VT have a very good long-term prognosis, with a large proportion of patients not requiring medical or invasive treatment with spontaneous cessation of arrhythmias during follow-up and with the option of curative ablation for symptomatic cases.[1,2,236-238] The clinical presentation and its clinical course vary greatly, ranging from to an incidental finding during monitoring without symptoms to palpitations, syncope, heart failure from incessant tachycardia-induced cardiomyopathy, and, rarely, VF, and sudden death.

Focal Ventricular Tachycardia

Idiopathic focal VT (IVT) is commonly detected during the early teenage years. Presentation can range from asymptomatic to symptoms of congestive heart failure due to tachycardia-induced cardiomyopathy. Proposed mechanisms include abnormal automaticity or triggered activity.[1,2,236] The most common location in children is the right ventricular outflow tract (RVOT) followed by the left ventricular outflow tract (LVOT).[1,2,238-239] Less commonly but similar to the adult population, the foci may be localized to the mitral and tricuspid valve annulus, papillary muscles, or the RV moderator band (Fig. 44.32A–E and Video 44.7).[240-242] Note that in infants and very young children, the QRS duration may be relatively narrow during VT and 1:1 ventricular atrial association may be occasionally present due to robust AV node conduction.

Outflow Tract Tachycardia

RVOT tachycardia (RVOT-VT) accounts for 60% to 80% of VT in children with a structurally normal heart. The focus is typically located in the posteroseptal region or the RV free wall below the pulmonary valve.[235-238] Less commonly, the focus is above the pulmonary valve or near the His bundle (Fig. 44.33A–E).[240,241] LVOT tachycardia (LVOT-VT) may arise from the coronary cusps, aortic root, aortic-mitral valve continuity, superior base of the left ventricular septum, anterior interventricular vein, and, rarely, LV summit (Fig. 44.34).[242-247]

All children with VT need a thorough evaluation including physical examination, family history inquiry, ECG, ambulatory monitoring, exercise stress testing if age appropriate, echocardiography, and cardiac magnetic resonance imaging (MRI). Other potentially malignant forms of VT may mimic idiopathic outflow tract VT including arrhythmogenic RV cardiomyopathy (ARVC), catecholamine sensitive polymorphic VT (CPVT), and Brugada syndrome. Idiopathic focal outflow VT be sustained or nonsustained and may be sensitive to adenosine, Valsalva maneuvers, calcium channel blockers, and β-blockers. ECG localization criteria of focal VT has been described in adult patients[248,249]; the same criteria are used in children but may be less sensitive and specific in infants and younger children due to differences in size, physical growth, and developing cardiac structures. For patients who fail medical treatment and undergo catheter ablation, the reported acute success is 90% to 95% with a recurrence rate of approximately 10%.[2,250-252] However, these results are limited to small series of patients. Indications for catheter ablation in children with idiopathic VT are published in the 2014 PACES/HRS expert consensus statement on the evaluation and management of ventricular arrhythmias in the child with a structurally normal heart.[2]

Mapping and Catheter Ablation of Idiopathic VT in Children

In general, catheters are positioned in the His-bundle region, RV apex RVOT, and CS. When vascular size or access is a limitation, we often use a fixed multipolar catheter (e.g., HIS-RV or HV Express catheter, Access Point Technologies EP Inc.) to simultaneously record and pace from the His bundle and RV apex. A multielectrode catheter that can be advanced as far as possible into the great cardiac vein or anterior interventricular vein is used (e.g., EPstar 6F decapolar with lumen and 2F EPstar octapolar, Baylis Medical, Inc). When possible ICE is used, especially when ablating near the aortic and pulmonary valves, in the coronary cusps, papillary muscle, and RV moderator band (Figs. 44.32 and 44.34).

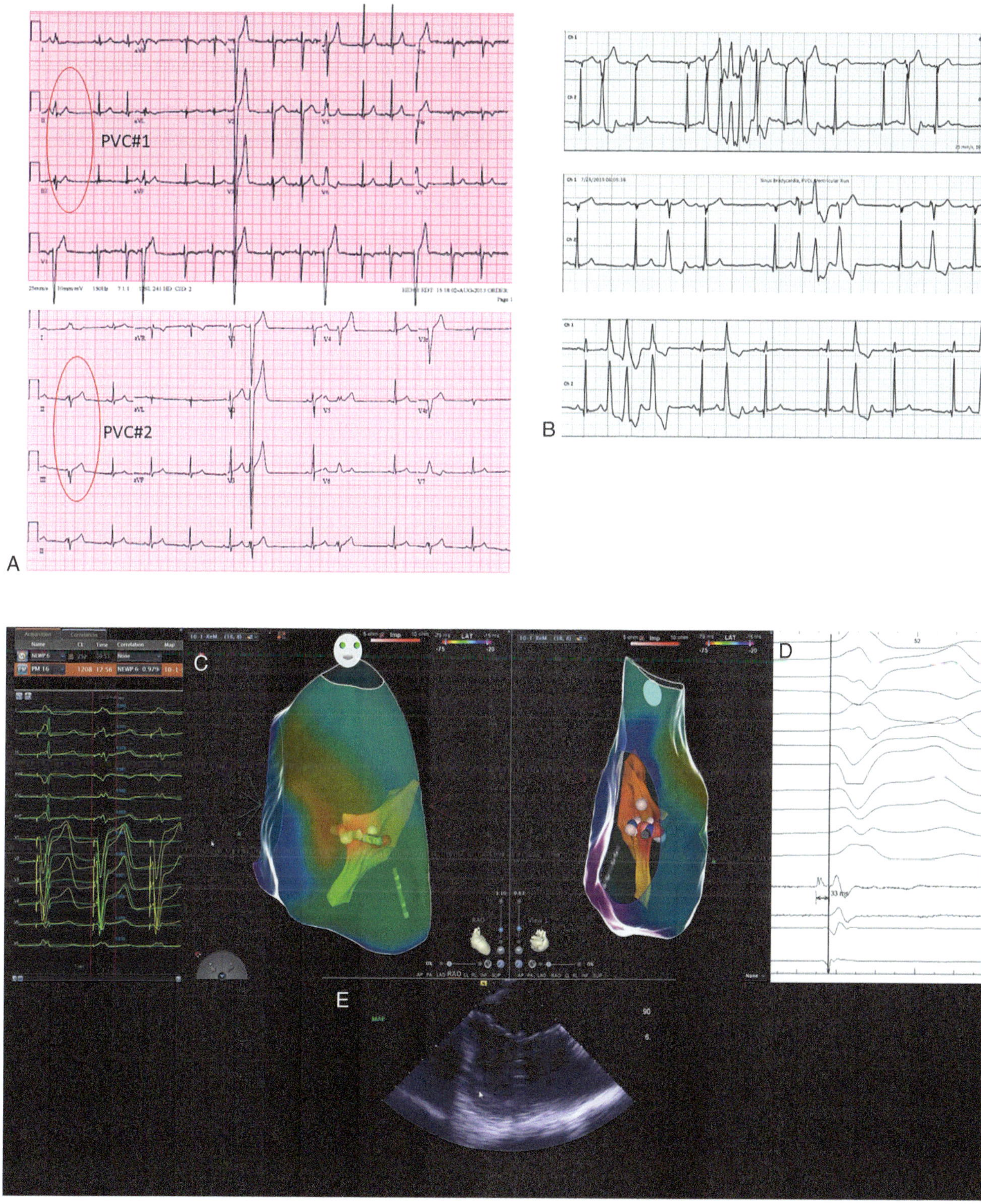

Fig. 44.32 Example of relatively narrow QRS premature ventricular contractions with LBBB morphology, superior QRS axis, and late transition in lead V_5 on ECG with "inferior lead discordance" (A) and nonsustained "polymorphic VT" on ambulatory monitoring (B) in a 14-year-old with palpitations. PVCs were mapped to the right ventricular moderator band (MB) with multiple exit sites resulting in "polymorphic" complexes. Pace mapping from middle of the moderator band using PASO (CARTO 3, Biosense Webster Inc.) automated template matching for PVCs yielded a 97% match for PVC#1 and 96% for PVC#2. Ventricular electrogram at site of successful ablation from the middle of the moderator band preceded the surface ECG QRS by 33 ms (D). A series of RF lesions using an irrigated-tip CF ablation catheter (Thermocool SmartTouch, Biosense Webster Inc.) abolished PVCs. (E) Video 44.7.

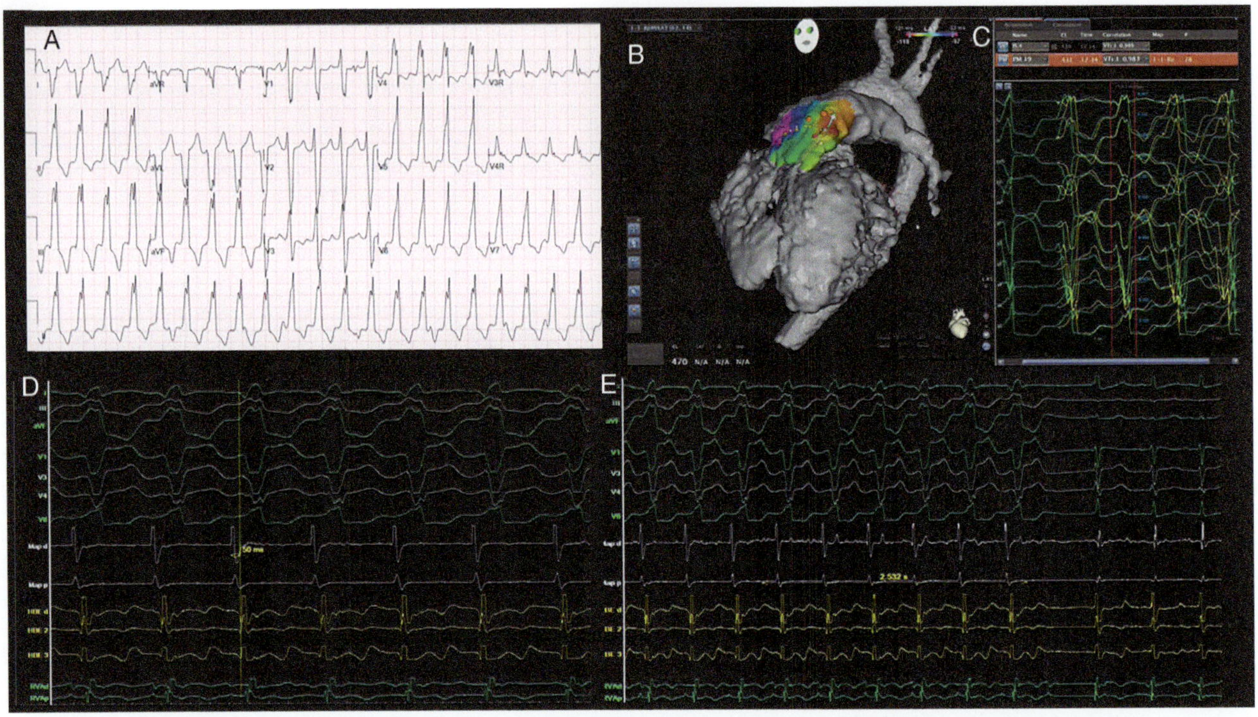

Fig. 44.33 Ablation of right ventricular outflow tract (RVOT) tachycardia in a 12-year-old patient with incessant VT (130 bpm) and tachycardia-induced cardiomyopathy (LVEF 20%). (A) ECG shows LBBB with inferior QRS axis in the frontal plane, R-wave notching in inferior leads, and R/S transition ≥lead V_3. (B) Electroanatomical activation map in the same patient with 3D image reconstruction of RV, LV, and RVOT using MRI generated by CARTO 3 (Biosense Webster, Diamond Bar, CA). The VT focus originated just underneath the left posterior leaflet of the pulmonary valve. (C) Using the quantitative morphology matching software (PaSo software, CARTO 3, Biosense Webster), pace mapping at the site of earliest origin of VT resulted in a PaSo coefficient value of 0.983. (D) The earliest activation at the distal tip of the ablation catheter preceded the QRS complex by 50 ms. (E) RF ablation (25 W, 31°C) with an irrigated 3.5-mm tip catheter (Thermocool Smarttouch SF Catheter, Biosense Webster Inc.) at site of earliest activation terminated VT in 2.5 seconds with no recurrence at 2-year follow-up. LVEF normalized to 60% in 6 months after RFA.

Preprocedural imaging with cardiac CT or CMR is routinely performed for merging with the 3D electroanatomical map that is obtained during the EP procedure. In addition, ventricular angiography, coronary sinus venography, and selective coronary arteriography (Fig. 44.34) is performed on a case-by-case basis to assess anatomical site of ablation and distance from neighboring structures.

Induction of focal VT may be challenging if the patient is not in the arrhythmia spontaneously. Induction of focal VT may require both rapid atrial and ventricular pacing especially if the mechanism is triggered automaticity. Sometimes, induction is linked to a critical heart rate, which may depend on autonomic tone, and pharmacologic agents may help or hurt induction. Once induced, activation mapping is performed by either point-by-point mapping with a standard ablation catheter or initially by a high-density multielectrode mapping catheter (e.g., PentaRay, Biosense Webster, Diamond Bar, CA; Advisor HD Grid, Abbott Inc, North Chicago, IL; Orion, Boston Scientific Inc. Marlborough, MA) in the chamber of interest to identify the site of earliest activation. The site of earliest activation is then fine-tuned by obtaining the earliest signal on the bipolar EGM recorded by the catheter's distal tip and preceding the surface QRS in conjunction with a QS unipolar EGM. Discrete potentials associated with myocardial extensions may be found in the semilunar valve cusps and it is important to recognize the far-field (subvalvular activation) and near-field potentials and reversal during VT (Fig. 44.34B). Pace mapping is particularly useful in identifying the site of focal VT origin. Computer-generated pace maps for automated comparison of paced morphology to VT template is available on modern mapping systems (e.g., CARTO PASO module, Biosense Webster, Inc.) (Fig. 44.33C). For outflow tract VT, if mapping in the RVOT and LVOT fails to identify the site of origin, mapping is extended above the semilunar valves and special attention is paid to the EGMs recorded from the coronary sinus as mapping may need to be extended to great cardiac vein and anterior interventricular vein. In the current era, most pediatric centers use 3D electroanatomical mapping for VT ablation procedures, and nuances of each commercially available mapping system have been previously described.[253]

The mapping and ablation techniques are very similar to those implemented in the adult population. However, special care must be taken when flexing and torquing the catheter in the ventricle and outflow tracts of young patients. Particularly, the catheter tip should not be advanced if the tip is perpendicular to the RVOT because of the risk of perforation. For left-sided VTs, patients should be adequately anticoagulated throughout the procedure. When using the retrograde aortic approach for

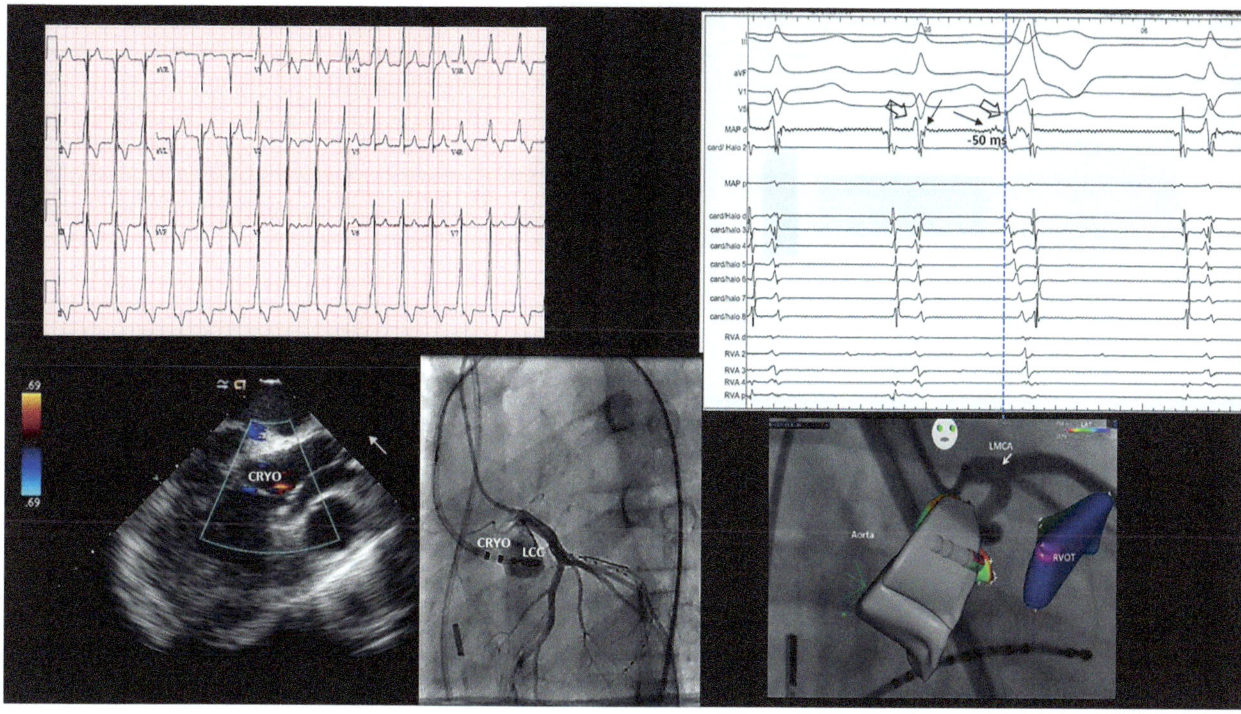

Fig. 44.34 A 14-year-old with structurally normal heart presenting with incessant ventricular tachycardia and cardiomyopathy with LVEF of 25%. Multimodality imaging used to ablate VT in a critical area (left coronary cusp). (A) ECG shows VT with RBBB and inferior QRS axis. (B) VT was mapped to the left coronary cusp. A sharp potential, after the ventricular electrogram in the endocardial recording from the cryoablation catheter (CRYO) at the site of successful ablation in the left coronary cusp was also recorded on the same site 50 ms before the onset of the QRS complex (*arrow*) during a spontaneous ventricular premature beat. The near field ventricular signal is also 20 ms early (*open arrow*). (C) Intracardiac ultrasound was used to monitor the tip of the ablation catheter and also assess for aortic valve regurgitation during ablation. (D) Selective left main coronary artery (LMCA) angiography was performed just prior to cryoablation with catheter at the site of ablation. The multipolar microcatheter is in the anterior interventricular vein with the distal electrode pair 10 ms early that the surface QRS of the PVC. (E) Frozen RAO frame of LMCA cine-angiogram integrated with a 3D electroanatomic map using the CARTO 3 System and CartoUnivu module (in an 8-year-old patient to avoid two femoral arterial catheters in a young child). *RVOT*, Right ventricular outflow tract. Cryoablation immediately interrupted all spontaneous ventricular ectopy. LVEF% normalized within 3 months after ablation.

LVOT VT, extreme caution must be used when attempting to cross the aortic valve and the catheter tip should not be pushed against closed valve leaflets or inadvertently slide into the coronary arteries.[254] The catheter tip should be curled into a "J" loop or "pigtail" curve in the aorta itself and then gently prolapsed across the aortic valve into the LV under fluoroscopic and/or ICE guidance. A long sheath may be needed in some instances to guide the ablation catheter across the aortic valve and into the LV. Manipulating the ablation catheter to cross the aortic valve can cause traumatic disruption of the intima in the aortic root, resulting in antegrade aortic dissection.[255]

We use RF energy to ablate most focal VT, but cryoablation can also be used and may be beneficial in some locations. Irrigated-tip RFA is rarely required in the RVOT as most of the foci are superficial and larger lesions may risk perforating the thin RV free wall of a young patient. For left-sided idiopathic focal VT, non–irrigated- or irrigated-tip RF is used. The latter may be beneficial in ablating LV papillary muscle VT, intramural VT, and areas of low blood flow or when there is a greater concern for thromboembolism. We have used cryoablation when ablating aortic cusp VT (Fig. 44.34). The major consideration has been its inherent stability due to cryoadhesion when ablating in a mobile aortic root and to prevent collateral injury. In all cases, before performing catheter ablation, an aortic root or selective coronary arteriogram is performed when the ablation catheter is positioned at the site of intended ablation (via a separate arterial access) to ensure a safe distance (>5–10 mm) from the coronary ostium. In the pediatric EP laboratory, this is of even greater importance as most pediatric electrophysiologists are not trained in coronary interventions and free-standing children's hospitals may not have immediate access to a coronary interventional cardiologist to manage coronary complications. When using a cryoablation catheter in the aortic cusp location, it should be manipulated with caution due to its unidirectional curve and stiff shaft. Our preference is to use the 6-mm-tip small-curve cryocatheter (Freezor, Medtronic Inc.) for aortic cusp VT in children. Cryoablation may also be safer (but may be less effective) when ablation is performed in coronary veins that are in close proximity to neighboring coronary arteries, such as the LV summit region. In addition to its safety and cryoadhesion features, cryoablation has a lesser tendency than RF energy to induce automaticity. This may be particularly useful for ablating VT arising from the RV moderator band, RV anterior papillary muscle, and LV papillary muscles that are surrounded by a dense network of Purkinje fibers that tends to induce hemodynamically unstable ventricular arrhythmias in response to RF energy.[256]

Fascicular Ventricular Tachycardia

Fascicular VT, idiopathic left VT, verapamil-sensitive VT, or Belhassen tachycardia arises from the mid to apical left ventricular septum.[257,258] It is the second most common cause of VT, accounting for 15% of IVT in children.[2,259] On ECG, right bundle branch block with a left anterior hemiblock is seen. Detailed EP studies have suggested the mechanism of this tachycardia is due to a reentry circuit usually involving the left posterior fascicle and adjacent abnormal Purkinje tissue with slow, decremental calcium-dependent conduction. The entrance site of the slow conduction zone is thought to be near the base of the LV septum, whereas the exit site is more apical. During tachycardia, the retrograde limb consists of Purkinje tissue from the left posterior fascicle. The anterograde limb is composed of abnormal Purkinje tissue adjacent to the left posterior fascicle that boasts slow, decremental conduction that is verapamil sensitive and insulated from the surrounding myocardium.[258] Less common sites of reentry include the left anterior fascicle or the left upper septal fascicle. Intravenous verapamil terminates the VT in 90% of patients however oral verapamil is less efficacious with a 20% recurrence of VT.[2,259] The prognosis is typically benign with some reports of spontaneous resolution. Treatment with verapamil until the patient reaches the appropriate size for catheter ablation may be considered. The success rate of catheter ablation is approximately 77% to 90% with a recurrence rate of approximately 20%.[2,259]

Catheter ablation is performed as originally demonstrated by targeting the LPF, guided by earliest Purkinje potentials and late diastolic potentials during VT.[258–261] This technique requires induction of VT, as success is determined by termination of VT during the ablation lesion and the lack of inducibility following ablation. Inducibility of VT may be challenging in the pediatric population, as most cases are performed under general anesthesia. In addition, the critical substrate is vulnerable to mechanical injury and simple placement of a LV catheter may induce the VT noninducible. To overcome these challenges, previously described substrate-based approaches during sinus rhythm include either ablation of the slow conduction zone adjacent LPF, creating an anatomical linear ablation to transect the middle or distal portion of LPF, or ablation of the most distal LPF fibers at the Purkinje–myocardial interface.[262–264] Fishberger et al. reported a high degree of acute success and no complications or recurrences in a small series of children ablated during sinus rhythm with just partial fascicular block using a substrate-based approach.[265] Regardless of technique used, when placing a catheter in the LV, the operator should be careful to avoid aortic valve damage, catheter entrapment in the sub–mitral valve apparatus, left bundle branch block, and cardiac tamponade.

Premature Ventricular Contractions

Premature ventricular contractions (PVCs) are frequent in healthy neonates, infants, and children. Nearly 20% of the neonates have uncomplicated ventricular ectopy consisting of uniform PVCs or couplets.[2] This decreases to 10% in toddlers and school-age children and increases to 20% to 30% of the normal adolescents.[2] Most patients are asymptomatic and do not need intervention, but surveillance is recommended for ectopy burden >10% on 24-hour ambulatory monitoring.[2] Adults with high PVC burden can develop LV dilation, dysfunction, and strain, consistent with a cardiomyopathy, which is reversible with catheter ablation of the PVCs.[266] Evidence in children with similar ectopy burden is limited, and there seems to be considerable variability in susceptibility to PVC-related cardiomyopathy even in children with a high PVC burden.[267–269] Catheter ablation may be indicated for patients with ventricular dysfunction in association with PVCs to restore cardiac synchrony and normal cardiac function.[2]

ARRHYTHMIAS UNIQUE TO THE PEDIATRIC PATIENT

A variety of issues may account for differences between adults and children in the incidence or prevalence of an arrhythmia (see Table 44.2). For the arrhythmia labeled *congenital* junctional ectopic tachycardia (JET), the issue is definitional, because its congenital nature has been presumed based on presentation with incessant junctional tachycardia before 6 months of age and familial tendencies. Patients with other incessant tachycardias, including EAT (discussed in section on Focal Atrial Tachycardia) and the permanent form of junctional reciprocating tachycardia (PJRT), may present as children because they are unlikely to reach maturity with their arrhythmia because of a tendency to develop ventricular dysfunction and congestive heart failure secondary to the tachycardia. Finally, the cardiac substrate for arrhythmia is clearly age dependent, in terms of both myocardial cellular development and the presence of structural CHD.

Junctional Ectopic Tachycardia

In the pediatric population, unlike in adults, JET (also termed focal or automatic junctional tachycardia) is seen in two relatively distinct settings: postoperative and congenital (Fig. 44.35) (also see Chapter 23).[270–272] The electrophysiologic characteristics of both varieties are similar to those of EAT,[270] suggesting they are also caused by abnormal automaticity, in this case arising from either low in the AV node or high in the His-Purkinje system. However, direct intracellular recordings have not been obtained.

The postoperative and congenital forms of JET differ primarily in their duration and response to therapy.[270–272] Postoperative JET is (1) strongly associated with ventricular septal defect repair, either alone or at the time of repair of more complex anomalies (Table 44.9)[272]; (2) usually transient, lasting between 1 and 4 days; and (3) responds well to cooling and intravenous magnesium as well as other antiarrhythmic agents.[273–275] These observations strongly suggest that the tachycardia is a response to trauma and inflammation induced at the time of the repair. In contrast, congenital JET is (1) typically not associated with structural CHD[271]; (2) incessant (see Fig. 44.35D); (3) has a positive family history in as many as 50% of cases[271,275]; (4) anecdotally does not respond to cooling; (5) is associated with the maternal lupus anti-SSA and

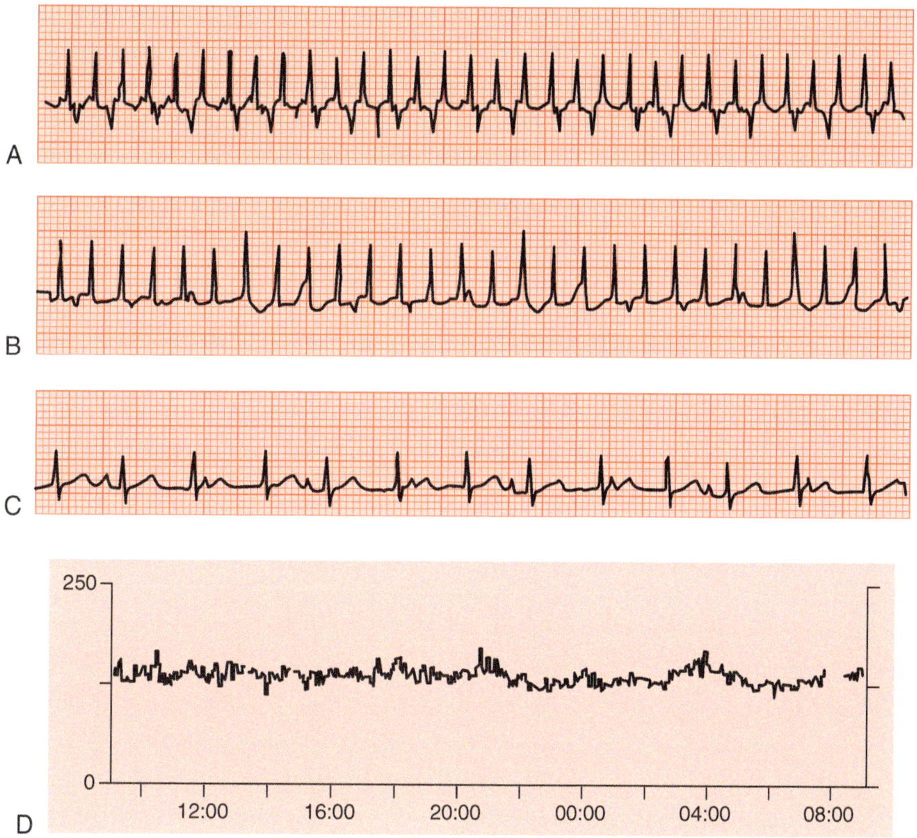

Fig. 44.35 Junctional ectopic tachycardia in a 6-week-old infant at presentation (A), 24 hours after intravenous amiodarone was begun (B), and when controlled on oral amiodarone (C). Note the ventricular rate of over 300 bpm with ventricle-to atrium (VA) Wenckebach before amiodarone (A). After 24 hours of intravenous amiodarone, the ventricular rate decreased to approximately 260 bpm and there was occasional VA block (B). After control on amiodarone, the ventricular rate was normal at about 120–130 bpm (C). Over 24 hours (D), there was "normal" rate variability, but there was still junctional rhythm with occasional sinus capture throughout, as shown in (C). (From Saul JP, Walsh EP, Triedman JK. Mechanisms and therapy of complex arrhythmias in pediatric patients. *J Cardiovasc Electrophysiol.* 1995;6:1129–1148.)

TABLE 44.9 Association of Postoperative Junctional Ectopic Tachycardia and Congenital Heart Disease

Lesion	No. of Patients	No. of Patients With JET	Prevalence (%)	*P* Value
TOF	378	28	7.4	.00005
VSD	285	9	3.2	.004
TGA/VSD	57	9	15.8	.23
Fontan	266	6	2.3	.997
Truncus	33	4	1.2	.824
CCAVC	177	4	2.3	.999
PAB	111	2	1.8	.999
HLHS	94	1	1.1	.999
MVR	50	1	2.0	.999
TGA/IVS	261	—	—	.02
Coarct/Arch	375	—	—	.0001
ASD	273	—	—	.001
PDA	201	—	—	.009
Systemic-PA shunt	192	—	—	.015
Total	2,753	64	2.3	—

ASD, Atrial septal defect; *CCAVC*, complete common atrioventricular canal; *coarct*, coarctation; *HLHS*, hypoplastic left heart syndrome; *IVS*, intact ventricular septum; *JET*, junctional ectopic tachycardia; *MVR*, mitral valve replacement; *PA*, pulmonary artery; *PAB*, pulmonary artery band; *PDA*, patent ductus arteriosus; *TGA*, transposition of the great arteries; *TOF*, tetralogy of Fallot; *VSD*, ventricular septal defect.

anti-SSB antibodies in some cases[276]; and (6) may spontaneously resolve but over a period of months to years.[62,277] Both JET types may result in severe hemodynamic compromise and appear to be exacerbated by both endogenous and exogenous adrenergic stimulation, and both arrhythmias seem to respond well to amiodarone (see Fig. 44.35C).[271,272]

The etiology of the congenital type, other than being "familial," is unclear. An extensive histologic evaluation was performed by Bharati et al.[278] in two patients who presented at or before 6 months of age. In one case, there were acute inflammatory changes at the summit of the ventricular septum and more chronic changes throughout the heart, including fibroelastosis, suggesting myocarditis. In the other, there were a variety of abnormal anatomical findings in the area of the AV node, including leftward displacement of the node and an abnormal central fibrous body. Multiple Purkinje-like tumor cells were found by Rossi et al.[279] in a third patient who did not present until 13 months of age, differentiating him slightly from the congenital group. Together these findings remain somewhat unsatisfying, because they fail to provide a unifying etiology consistent with the familial tendencies, and most patients do not present with findings of myocarditis. Dubin et al.[277] described a patient with both congenital AV block and JET, suggesting a link between the two diagnoses. The mother had Sjögren syndrome and was strongly positive for anti-SSA and anti-SSB antibodies. Recently, whole exome sequencing identified the *TNNI3K* gene as a cause of familial conduction system disease and congenital junctional ectopic tachycardia, suggesting that there may be a genetic basis for JET.[276]

Therapy

The propensity for JET to eventually resolve spontaneously and the potential risk of AV block from catheter ablation of the JET focus in the AV junction suggest that JET may initially be best treated medically by minimizing adrenergic stimulation and beginning either intravenous or oral amiodarone, particularly in infants.[280–287] Ivabradine is a promising agent in the treatment of both congenital and postoperative JET usual as adjunctive therapy but also as monotherapy, suggesting with its low side effect profile that it is worth trying in new patients and patients not adequately managed with other agents or experiencing side effects.[286–288] Now, there are also a number of case reports,[280–285] a recent case series mostly in noninfants[289] and a single multicenter series,[286] that demonstrate that with both RF and cryoablation, it is possible to eliminate the JET in about 85% of patients while preserving AV conduction. Importantly, despite similar success rates in the multicenter series, AV block did occur in 3 of 17 patients (18%) undergoing RF ablation.[289,290] If JET is either resistant to medical therapy, persistent after a prolonged period of control, or producing intractable hemodynamic compromise or ventricular dysfunction, ablation has a Class I indication in any size patient, but the initial use of cryoablation was also included as Class I specifically in patients ≤15 kg.[1]

Mapping and Ablation

The multicenter series of patients undergoing ablation[286] did provide evidence that cryoablation is equally successful to and much safer than RF ablation for JET; however, it did not provide specifics on exactly how the ablations were performed. The specific details in the small number of reported cases of successful JET ablation[280–285] provide a few overarching recommendations to use when approaching these patients. In most younger patients with incessant JET, the region of interest has ended up in the anterior septum near the bundle of His. In older patients, successful ablation has been reported in the posteroseptal region,[289] with the site sometimes identified by the use of retrograde atrial activation as a guide. This region corresponds to the site used for SP modification and should be associated with a low incidence of permanent AV block. However, the data presented may be most consistent with frequent paroxysms of AVNRT triggered by junctional escape beats, and other reports have not found mapping of earliest retrograde activation to be useful.[289] Before ablation, the catheter should be moved very slightly posterior to that site, attempting to minimize the His activation from the distal ablation tip, similar to the methodology used in the past for FP ablation. Most prior reports of successful elimination of JET without subsequent AV block have used this technique with brief, lower-power applications of RF energy. However, there is clearly a risk of AV block in children with this technique. Saul[290] demonstrated earliest His activation during tachycardia with retrograde mapping just under the aortic valve in a 10-year-old child with intermittent incessant tachycardia (Fig. 44.2). The proximity to the AV conduction system makes it ideal for both cryomapping and cryoablation, with successful elimination of the JET and preservation of the AV node, despite a catheter signal and location suggesting very close proximity to the His bundle. Finding a site for ablation may be challenging when there no retrograde conduction. Shah et al.[280] performed successful cryoablation (Fig. 44.13) without permanent AV block at a site with a His potential and then torquing the catheter to get a small atrial and large ventricular EGM (small A/V ratio). An intravenous infusion of a short-acting β-blocker (esmolol) was used to slow the JET rate, enabling overdrive atrial pacing during ablation, which allowed for assessment of AV node function. Periodic interruption of atrial pacing was used during cryothermal application to check for persistence or termination of JET.[280] In the current era, cryoablation should be the energy of choice for JET ablation regardless of age or size of the patient to preserve intact AV nodal conduction.

Permanent Form of Junctional Reciprocating Tachycardia

Like EAT and JET, PJRT is an often-incessant tachycardia that is typically recognized in infancy or childhood, either by detection of a rapid heart rate on a routine examination or because of the accompanying myopathy observed in many patients. First described by Coumel et al.,[291] the tachycardia is characterized by a narrow QRS rhythm with variable rates, a retrograde P-wave axis, and an RP interval that is longer than the PR interval. PJRT represents approximately 4% of the SVTs seen in infants[19] and in the past accounted for 10% of pediatric patients referred for catheter ablation.[20] Because of its incessant nature, there were relatively more cases seen in the early days of RF ablation, whereas now only new cases of this rare condition are seen.

As is now clear from the results of EP studies, surgical and catheter ablation results, and anatomical data,[292–294] PJRT is caused by an orthodromic reciprocating tachycardia involving a slowly conducting concealed AP, making the name a misnomer. It is the slow and decremental retrograde conduction in the AP that leads to both the ECG characteristics and the incessant nature of the rhythm.

Therapy

Similar to other tachycardias caused by APs, PJRT may resolve spontaneously in some patients.[24] However, in many patients, PJRT is notoriously difficult to control medically. Catheter ablation has now proven to be a highly effective technique for eliminating these fibers with minimal risk of AV block.[295,296] Also, the precise AP localization provided by current mapping techniques and the demonstrated points of successful ablation have elucidated the fact that these APs are not always posteroseptal but can occur in almost any location along the AV groove (Fig. 44.36).

Mapping and Ablation

As with any other AP, the methodology for ablation of PJRT pathways depends on their location. Because many of the pathways are posteroseptal, ablation within the mouth or veins of the coronary sinus is often necessary. Mapping should virtually always be performed during tachycardia. Electrogram characteristics, EP techniques, and mapping techniques are somewhat different for PJRT pathways than for typical nondecremental APs (Fig. 44.37). It is often impossible to confirm an AP as the retrograde conduction pathway using the standard technique of atrial preexcitation by a ventricular premature beat while the His is refractory, because the retrograde conduction decrements after premature ventricular stimulation. However, atrial "post excitation" may be seen due to decremental conduction. Further, the VA interval is usually long, with a long isoelectric segment between the ventricular and atrial signals, and an AP potential may be present in as many as 75% of cases.[297] Finally, the pathways must usually be mapped and ablated in tachycardia because it is often not possible to achieve reliable exclusive AP conduction during ventricular pacing. This is the result of either competitive retrograde AV node conduction or retrograde block at any cycle length longer than that of the tachycardia.

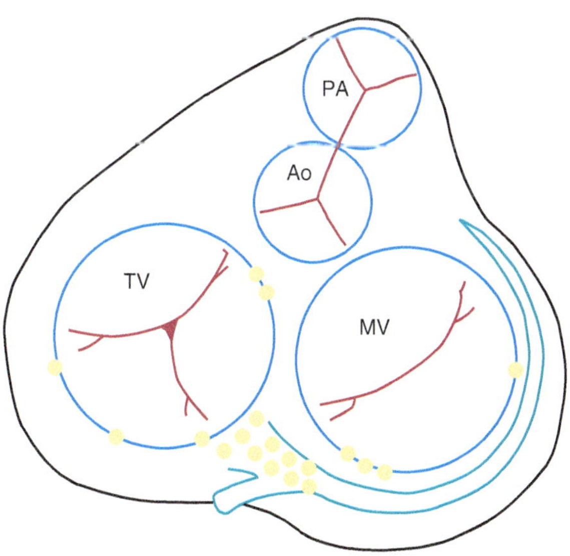

Fig. 44.36 Schematic diagram of accessory pathway locations in patients with permanent form of junctional reciprocating tachycardia (PJRT) as identified by radiofrequency ablation. *Circles* represent accessory pathways causing the tachycardia. Eleven pathways were in the typical location either within or just outside the mouth of the coronary sinus, four were elsewhere along the tricuspid annulus, and four along the mitral annulus. *Ao*, Aorta; *MV*, mitral valve; *PA*, pulmonary artery; *TV*, tricuspid valve. (From Ticho BS, Walsh EP, Saul JP. Ablation of permanent junctional reciprocating tachycardia. In: Huang SK, ed. *Radiofrequency Catheter Ablation of Cardiac Arrhythmias: Basic Concepts and Clinical Applications.* Mt. Kisko, NY: Futura;1994:397–409.)

Complications and Recommendations

Despite the proximity to the AV node, AV block has not been reported in the larger series of patients who have undergone RF ablation.[294–297] However, it is now clear from both animal[162] and patient data that if RF energy is used to ablate posteroseptal pathways inside the coronary sinus, there is a significant risk of coronary damage, particularly if ablation is performed near a terminating branch of the right coronary or left circumflex artery.[12] This issue and the possibility that subclinical coronary damage occurs much more often than has been previously recognized were discussed earlier in the section on AVNRT and are probably most applicable in the setting of posteroseptal PJRT pathways.[290] We recommend the following for pediatric patients undergoing posteroseptal ablation of an AP: (1) coronary angiography should be considered before application of RF energy along the posterior AV groove, particularly near the septum, or within the coronary sinus; (2) if a small coronary artery is within 2 to 3 mm of an ablation site, cryotherapy is the preferred initial ablation choice; (3) if cryotherapy is either unavailable or ineffective, RF energy application should be minimized by reducing either catheter size, the temperature set point, or maximum power and/or duration; and (4) high-energy RF application with active or passive cooled-tip technology should be avoided or used with extreme caution.

Despite these safety concerns, the high efficacy and relative safety of ablation for PJRT, combined with the fact that pharmacologic therapy is often ineffective, have led to PJRT being included with most other SVT categories in the 2016 Consensus Statement,[1] where ablation is considered as a class I recommendation for patients >15 kg or any patient with ventricular dysfunction.

Other General Considerations in the Peditric Patient

Complications

A distinct risk of vascular injury, secondary to thrombus or embolus formation, exists with any catheterization in smaller children but is particularly present with any interventional or prolonged diagnostic catheterization.[298] Therefore it is not surprising that vascular complications, including microembolism

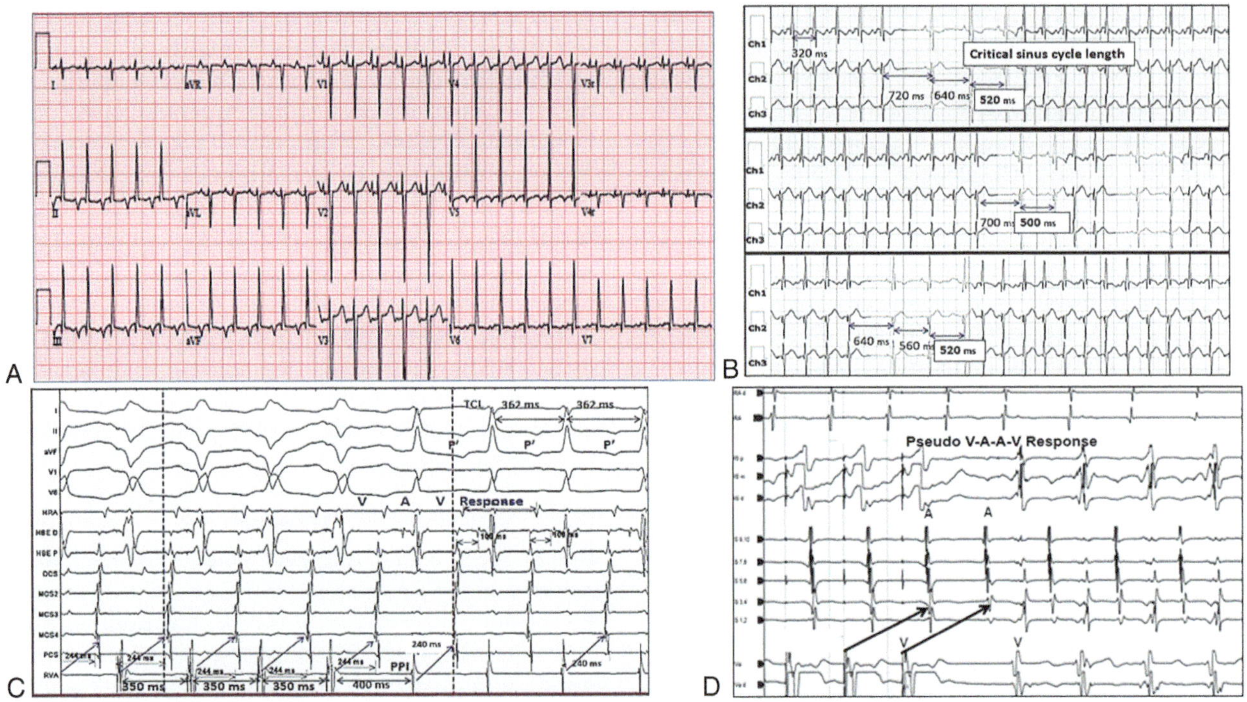

Fig. 44.37 Example of permanent junctional reciprocating tachycardia in a 3-year-old child with tachycardia induced cardiomyopathy. (A) 15-lead ECG shows long RP tachycardia with RP′ ≥50% of tachycardia cycle length and negative P waves in II, III, aVF, and V_5–V_6 leads. (B) Ambulatory monitoring in the same child shows spontaneous termination of PJRT, which is reinitiated at a critical cycle length (approximately 500 ms) without a premature atrial contraction or prolongation of the PR interval. (C) During EP study, VA interval during entrainment ventricular pacing approximates the VA interval during tachycardia, thus favoring atrioventricular reentrant tachycardia over atrioventricular nodal reentrant tachycardia and the atrial activation pattern during ventricular pacing is identical to that during tachycardia. The postpacing interval approximates the TCL, which also favors AVRT via a septal bypass tract (PPI-TCL = 38 ms). Cessation of ventricular pacing produces a V-A-V response. (D) In another patient with PJRT, cessation of ventricular pacing produces a pseudo V-A-A-V response due to decremental conduction of AP (*arrows*).

to the foot and arterial occlusion[299] have been reported with catheter ablation. Of note, however, the incidence of these problems appears to be quite low, even in the smallest patients, probably because of meticulous heparinization, a tendency not to use the retrograde arterial approach in most pediatric centers, and the current availability of smaller (4 F) diagnostic and ablation catheters. Production of new[300] or increased valvar regurgitation has been reported in pediatric patients after use of the retrograde arterial approach, providing an additional reason to avoid this approach in smaller patients. The risk of acute coronary damage has been addressed extensively, but it should also be noted that only limited data in humans are available, and no data on late coronary function have been reported in animals, children, or adults.

Sedation and Anesthesia

The pain and discomfort of an RF ablation procedure do not appear to be very much higher than for a typical diagnostic catheterization, even accounting for the pain some patients feel during the actual RF application. Therefore, general anesthesia is by no means necessary. Some advantages include avoiding uncontrolled patient movement that may dislodge the catheter may inadvertently occur at a critical point in the procedure, particularly if the RF application produces pain. It may also make the procedure much more tolerable, and children are then more willing to return for follow-up procedures, if needed. The effects of anesthesia strategy on arrhythmia inducibility and procedural outcomes were evaluated by Janson et al.[301] in a multicenter retrospective study of 6621 children using data from the National Cardiovascular Data Registry's Improving Pediatric and Adult Congenital Treatment Registry. They reported no differences between general anesthesia and monitored anesthesia care in SVT or EAT inducibility, acute ablation success, or major adverse events, but general anesthesia was associated with higher rates of non-inducibility in PVC/VT cases. It is generally recommended that patients 12 years of age and younger and patients with moderate or complex CHD have the procedure performed in collaboration with an anesthesiologist who has expertise with pediatric and/or CHD patients, as appropriate.[1]

Fluoroscopic Exposure

Fluoroscopy as a risk factor for malignancy is an issue at every age but may be of more theoretical concern in children and young adults for a variety of reasons. The most obvious of course is that the malignant potential of radiation exposure generally manifests itself after many years, so the risk in any population or individual will be related to the number of life-years expected after the procedure, a number that increases with decreasing age of the exposure. A second factor is that radiation exposure in children who are still growing and have more cell divisions is generally considered to have more malignant potential than adults. Third, some of the longest and most complicated cases occur in adolescents and young adults with complex CHD, a group already subject to excess radiation exposure because of multiple prior catheterizations for nonarrhythmia indications.

For all these reasons, a variety of pediatric investigators have focused on techniques to reduce radiation exposure during catheter ablation procedures.[302–306] As with all diagnostic radiation, a variety of basic technical modifications can be performed to strive for exposure, which is as low as reasonably achievable (ALARA).[307] These techniques include lower frame rate, field reduction, reduced output, last image hold, and of course minimizing the use of fluoroscopy to when absolutely necessary. One study focusing on ALARA techniques alone was able to produce significantly lower radiation exposure than historical controls.[307] However, the alternative approach has been to use nonfluoroscopic techniques, which depend on impedance- or magnetic-based 3D mapping localization to define the relevant chamber anatomy and the location of ablation applications. Numerous studies have now demonstrated the feasibility of these techniques to significantly and dramatically reduce fluoroscopy for ablation of any arrhythmia, and to even eliminate fluoroscopy exposure entirely for simpler procedures like AV node modification and AP ablation.[303–309] Although theoretically any radiation exposure elevates the risk of late neoplasm, the ancillary use of these nonfluoroscopic techniques to reduce radiation exposure has lowered fluoroscopy times to levels below those of most diagnostic catheterizations.

The use of 3D nonfluoroscopic, electroanatomical mapping system was considered: Class I for assisting mapping and ablation of postoperative tachyarrhythmias in patients with moderate or complex CHD and Class IIa as a primary tool or adjunct to fluoroscopy during ablation procedures in all pediatric patients to reduce radiation exposure in accordance with the ALARA principle and provide electroanatomical mapping for more complex procedures.[1]

Ablation on Mechanical Circulatory Support Devices

The need for mechanical circulatory support (MCS) for the management of physiologically malignant arrhythmias is not unique to pediatric patients. In addition to the use of ECMO for acute management in patients with hemodynamic compromise, a variety of reports have described ablation procedures performed successfully on ECMO.[310–311] The relevant technical issues include transporting the patient on ECMO from the intensive care unit to the catheterization laboratory, avoiding the ECMO cannulae with the electrophysiologic and ablation catheters and possibly adjusting flow temporarily to avoid overcooling of an RF catheter or heating of a cryocatheter when the target site is in the flow path of an ECMO catheter.

Catheter ablation in children on other forms are of MCS are rare but the use of the Impella device (Abiomed Inc., Danvers, MA) has been reported for systemic right ventricular support during catheter ablation of intra-atrial reentrant tachycardia in a patient with D-TGA status post Mustard procedure.[312] In our own experience, we have performed catheter ablations for incessant tachycardia (EAT, AVRT) induced cardiomyopathy in two children with Impella devices (Impella 5 via transaxillary artery in one and Impella 2.5 via femoral artery in the other using the EnSite Velocity in one and EnSite X with VoXel Mode, in the other [Abbott Inc.]). We did not note any mapping interference when using the EnSite Velocity but there was interference with ablation catheter tip navigation when EnSite VoXel magnet-based mapping was used, especially when the ablation catheter (Tacticath Contact Force, Sensor Enabled, Abbott Inc.) was in the same plane as the Impella device even though 3D mapping was in the right side of the heart. Electromagnetic interference has previously been reported when the Impella device is used with magnet-based mapping systems and can be reduced by impedance-based mapping or transiently switching the Impella device off (if tolerated) while creating the electroanatomical map.[313] This illustrates that 3D system selection may be important for procedure planning.[313]

Left ventricular assist devices (LVADs) also generate electromagnetic interference that causes high-frequency noise artifacts on 12-lead ECG and may interfere with mapping especially when surface ECG waveforms are used as a reference for intracardiac signals.[314] We performed ablations on two patients with LVADs (HeartMate II, HeartMate 3 from Abbott, Inc.). Both patients had EAT-induced cardiomyopathy with a right atrial focus. We did not encounter EMI that interfered with electroanatomical mapping of the right atrium but as expected there was high-frequency noise artifacts on the surface ECG. This was remedied by applying a low-pass filter, which significantly improved the waveform tracing and quality of the ECG.[314]

Epicardial Ablation Techniques

Epicardial techniques have taken a more and more consistent role in ablation of VT in adult patients[315] and are covered elsewhere in this textbook. In addition, the technique has had limited use for a variety of arrhythmias in pediatric patients.[149,316,317] Upadhyay et al.[149] reported 10 procedures from two centers in nine children with EAT (n = 1), WPW (n = 3), and ventricular tachycardia (n = 5), with a 70% success rate and no significant complications. Patient ages ranged from 8 to 19 years, and none had previous operations for CHDs. The primary conclusion is that the technique can be performed safely and effectively in pediatric patients and can be considered in selected cases when endocardial ablation has been unsuccessful.

SUMMARY

Children are usually smaller than adults, but in general, ablation techniques used in adults should not simply be miniaturized to fit the size of the pediatric patient. Multiple factors, including the distribution of arrhythmia mechanisms, ongoing myocardial development, and potentially increased risk of vascular injury and AV node damage, as well as the effects of smaller cardiac size, should all influence the ablation technique. An overriding theme in the child should be that safety takes precedence over efficacy. There are numerous similarities between adult and pediatric patients. Specifically, regardless of age, it seems clear that a variety of techniques and approaches are necessary to successfully ablate substrates in all locations of the heart. At present, because of a paucity of technology approved for use in children, there is a high rate of off-label technology utilization in this population. While new devices and technology typically undergoes thorough preclinical testing, human clinical trials, postapproval studies and postmarketing surveillance in adults, pediatric electrophysiologists often need to improvise novel ways of using these technologies that have not been rigorously tested for safety and effectiveness in children and in patients with CHD. Recently, the FDA has recognized the particular challenges of device development in the pediatric arena and has instituted several regulatory programs to help address these issues.[318]

ACKNOWLEDGMENT

The authors are grateful to Tammy Sweeten, electrophysiology lab specialist at The Children's Hospital of Philadelphia, for her assistance with figures in this chapter.

We thank Dr. J.P. Saul for Figures 44.1, 44.2, 44.17, 44.20 to 44.25, 44.27, 44.28, 44.35, and 44.36, which were previously published in "Special Considerations for Ablation in Pediatric Patients." In Huang SK, 4th ed. *Catheter Ablation of Cardiac Arrhythmias*. Elsevier: 2019:664–687.

REFERENCES

Please refer to the e-book for complete references.

INDEX

Note: Page numbers followed by "*f*" indicate figures and "*t*" indicate tables.

B

H

I

J

K

L

M

Q

R

W

X